Koss' Diagnostic Cytology
AND ITS HISTOPATHOLOGIC BASES

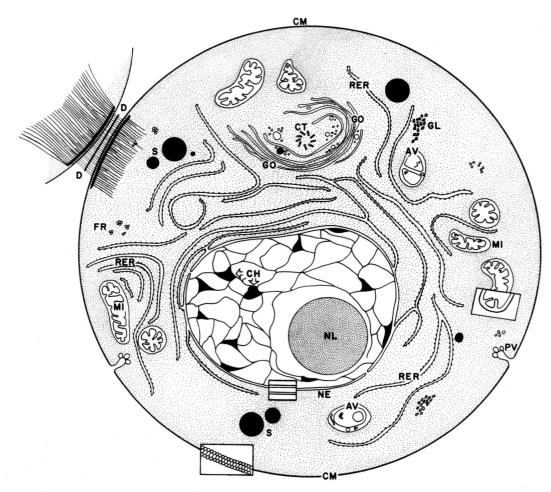

Schematic representation of a cell. Portions of cell membrane, nuclear envelope, and mitochondrion are enlarged to show unit membrane structure.

AV = autographic vacuole
CH = chromocenters
CM = cell membrane
CT = centriole in cross section
D = desmosome
FR = free ribosomes, as polyribosomes
GL = glycogen
GO = Golgi complex

MI = mitochondria
NE = nuclear envelope (membrane) with pores
NL = nucleolus
PV = pinocytotic vesicles
RER = "rough" endoplasmic reticulum with ribosomes attached to it
S = granules (secretion and storage)

Koss' Diagnostic Cytology

AND ITS HISTOPATHOLOGIC BASES

FIFTH EDITION

VOLUME ONE

EDITOR

▬ LEOPOLD G. KOSS, MD, Dr.h.c., Hon. FRCPathol (UK)

Professor and Chairman Emeritus
Department of Pathology
Montefiore Medical Center
The University Hospital for the Albert Einstein College of Medicine
Bronx, New York

COEDITOR

▬ MYRON R. MELAMED, MD

Professor and Chairman
Department of Pathology
New York Medical College
Westchester Medical Center
Valhalla, New York

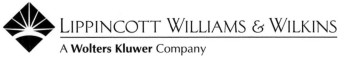

LIPPINCOTT WILLIAMS & WILKINS

A **Wolters Kluwer** Company

Philadelphia • Baltimore • New York • London
Buenos Aires • Hong Kong • Sydney • Tokyo

Acquisitions Editor: Jonathan Pine
Managing Editor: Joyce Murphy
Developmental Editor: Grace Caputo, Dovetail Content Solutions
Marketing Manager: Adam Glazer
Project Manager: David Murphy
Manufacturing Manager: Ben Rivera
Production Services: Maryland Composition
Design Coordinator: Holly Reid McLaughlin
Cover Design: Christine Jenny
Printer: Quebecor World Kingsport

Library of Congress Cataloging-in-Publication Data

Koss' diagnostic cytology and its histopathologic bases / editor, Leopold G. Koss,
coeditor, Myron R. Melamed.—5th ed.
    p. ; cm.
  Rev. ed. of: Diagnostic cytology and its histopathologic bases / Leopold G. Koss. 4th
ed. c1992.
  Includes bibliographical references and index.
  ISBN 0-7817-1928-3
  1. Cytodiagnosis. 2.   Histology, Pathological.   I. Koss, Leopold G. II. Melamed, Myron
R., 1922–   III. Koss, Leopold G. Diagnostic cytology and its histopathologic bases.
IV. Title: Diagnostic cytology and its histopathologic bases. [DNLM: 1.   Cytodiagnosis. 2.
Neoplasms—pathology. 3.   Pathology, Clinical. QY 95 K856 2005]
RB43.K67 2005
616.07'582—dc22

                                                        2005005149

To my teachers in science and to my teachers in humanities, and most of all to the memory of my parents and sister, Stephanie, who perished during the Holocaust.

L.G.K.

In loving memory of Barbara, my wife.

M.R.M.

Contributors

Alberto G. Ayala, MD
Deputy Chief of Pathology
The Methodist Hospital
Houston, Texas

Carol E. Bales, BA, CT(ASCP),
CT(IAC), CFIAC
Independent Quality Assurance
Consultant
Staff Cytotechnologist
Providence St. Joseph Medical
Center
Burbank, California

Peter H. Bartels, MD, PhD
Professor Emeritus
Optical Sciences Center
University of Arizona
Tucson, Arizona

Linda A. Cannizzaro, PhD
Professor of Pathology
The Albert Einstein School of
Medicine
Director of Cytogenetics
Montefiore Medical Center
Bronx, New York

Nancy P. Caraway, MD
Associate Professor of Pathology
The University of Texas
MD Anderson Cancer Center
Houston, Texas

Bogdan Czerniak, MD, PhD
Professor of Pathology
University of Texas
MD Anderson Cancer Center
Houston, Texas

Ronald A. DeLellis, MD
Professor of Pathology and Laboratory
Medicine
Brown Medical School
Pathologist-in-Chief
Rhode Island Hospital and the Miriam
Hospital
Providence, Rhode Island

Abdelmonem Elhosseiny, MD
Professor of Pathology
University of Vermont College of
Medicine
Attending Pathologist
Fletcher Allen Health Care
Burlington, Vermont

Rana S. Hoda, MD, FIAC
Associate Professor of Pathology
Director of Cytopathology
Medical University of South Carolina
Attending Pathologist
Hospital of Medical University of
South Carolina
Charleston, South Carolina

Ruth L. Katz, MD
Professor of Pathology
The University of Texas
Chief, Research Cytopathology
MD Anderson Cancer Center
Houston, Texas

Andrzej Kram, MD, PhD
Visiting Fellow
University of Texas
MD Anderson Cancer Center
Houston, Texas

Britt-Marie Ljung, MD
Professor of Pathology
University of California at San
Francisco
San Francisco, California

Carlos A. Rodriguez, MD, MIAC
Adjunct Professor of Pathology
Tucuman National University Medical
School
Chief, Department of Pathology
Hospital Instituto de Maternidad y
Ginecologia
Tucuman, Argentina

Miguel A. Sanchez, MD
Associate Professor of Pathology
Mount Sinai School of Medicine
New York, New York
Chief, Department of Pathology and
Laboratory Medicine
Englewood Hospital
Englewood, New Jersey

Rosalyn E. Stahl, MD
Assistant Clinical Professor of
Pathology
Mount Sinai School of Medicine
New York, New York
Associate Chief, Department of
Pathology and Laboratory Medicine
Englewood Hospital
Englewood, New Jersey

Deborah Thompson, MS
Senior System Analyst
Optical Sciences Center
University of Arizona
Tucson, Arizona

Tomasz Tuziak, MD, PhD
Visiting Fellow
University of Texas
MD Anderson Cancer Center
Houston, Texas

Muhammad B. Zaman, MD
Clinical Professor of Pathology
New York Medical College
Chief, Cytopathology
CBL Path
Marmaroneck, New York

Preface

Thirteen years have elapsed since the publication of the fourth edition of this book. In the interim, a large number of books and atlases on the subject of cytopathology have been published. Some of these books are lavishly illustrated with color photographs and a few have benefited from an excellent layout. Therefore, a legitimate question may be asked—whether a new edition of an ''older'' book (so characterized by a young cytopathologist testifying in a court case) is justified.

The colossal effort involved in updating this book was undertaken not to produce an atlas or a synoptic book that may appeal to readers favoring easy fare, but to create a textbook that covers, in depth, the broad field of human pathology through the prism of cells and corresponding tissue lesions. This book reflects half a century of practical and research experience of the principal author, now assisted by a trusted friend and colleague, Dr. Myron R. Melamed.

In rewriting this book, particular attention has been devoted to the interpretation of the increasingly important aspirated cell samples, colloquially known as fine needle aspiration biopsies or FNAs. A book on this topic, by Koss, Woyke, and Olszewski, published in 1992 by Igaku-Shoin, is out of print and no longer available. In the previous editions of *Diagnostic Cytology*, the topic was treated as a single, very large chapter, originally written by the late Dr. Josef Zajicek and his associates from the Karolinska Hospital in Stockholm; it was updated in the fourth edition by this writer. As this fifth edition was being planned, it became paramount to expand the single chapter into a series of chapters, each addressing in depth the topics at hand. We were fortunate to secure the help of several distinguished colleagues whose names are listed as authors of their chapters. The chapters written by the principal author and editor of this book (LGK) carry no author's name. All the contributions were carefully reviewed and revised by the senior editor; thus, the blame for any insufficiencies falls on his shoulders. Inevitably, some duplications of information occurred and were not eliminated. It was interesting to see how different observers look at the same, or similar, issues from a different vantage point. Innovations in the practice of cytopathology and, when available, data on molecular biology and cytogenetics have been incorporated into the discussion of organs and organ systems. Therefore, it is hoped that the book will continue to fulfill its role as a source of knowledge and references of value to the cytopathologists, the cytopathologist-in-training, the practicing pathologists, the cytotechnologists, and even some basic science investigators who may be interested in the clinical approach to a discussion of human cells and tissues. With the exception of some irreplaceable black-and-white photographs or drawings, the book is illustrated in color.

Another aspect of cytopathology that has emerged in the 1990s, to the dismay of many, has been the legal responsibility that cytopathologists have to assume if a diagnostic verdict is alleged to have led to significant damage or sometimes even death of a patient. Although there are many who are attempting to soften the blow to their egos and pockets of their insurance company by contriving complex defense maneuvers, the bottom line remains, as it has always been, that the patients come first and are entitled to competent services by laboratories. This has been one of the guiding principles in this new edition, wherein considerable attention has been devoted to avoidance of errors.

This book took over five years to complete. It is hoped that the readers will find it informative and useful. With the aging process taking its toll, it is unlikely that future editions of this book, if any, will be written or edited by the same authors.

Leopold G. Koss, M.D.
New York, 2005

Preface to First Edition, 1961

The concept of diagnostic cytology as presented in this work has been greatly influenced by the efforts of Dr. George N. Papanicolaou. His contributions to our knowledge of the cytologic presentation of cancer have changed the status of cytology from a largely theoretical field of knowledge to a widely accepted laboratory procedure.

In the present work the widely used expression "exfoliative cytology" has been replaced by "diagnostic cytology." The method is not based on examination of exfoliated cells alone; material may be also obtained from organs that do not yield any spontaneously exfoliating cells. Cytology has ceased to be an adjunct to other methods of diagnosis; rather, it has become a primary source of information in many fields of medicine, such as gynecology, urology, and thoracic surgery, to name only a few. It is our feeling that the pathologist competent in examination of cytologic preparations should not suggest the possibility of a diagnosis but must learn to establish a diagnosis, in much the same way as on examination of histologic evidence. A laboratory of diagnostic cytology should be operated on the same principles as a laboratory of surgical pathology.

The purpose of the authors in the present volume is to outline and explain the principles of diagnostic cytology for the use of practicing pathologists and others who may be interested in this challenging field. The authors hope that this book will fill a gap in the library of manuals on methods of laboratory diagnosis.

This book consists of two parts: the first has been devoted to a brief résumé of basic cytology and cytopathology, the second part to special diagnostic cytology of organs. Each organ or system has been treated as follows:

1. Normal histology and cytology
2. Benign cytopathologic aberrations
3. Cytopathology of cancer

In some instances additional subdivisions were required. The pathology and the cytology of the female genital tract have been discusses in a some-what more detailed manner because of great current interest.

Throughout an attempt has been made to interpret the cellular alterations in terms of patters of disease. A description of histologic changes therefore precedes or accompanies, whenever possible, the discussion of the cytologic patterns.

The practice of diagnostic cytology is very time-consuming, and much of the task of screening smears is usually delegated to lay screeners or cytotechnologists. The role of trained cytotechnologists cannot be emphasized sufficiently, and their skill is a tremendous asset to the pathologist, to the laboratory, and last, but not least, to the patient. Since it is hoped that this book will also help in teaching and training of cytotechnologists, certain basic concepts of anatomy, histology,

cytology, and tissue pathology have been included. To those among the readers who will find these passages cumbersome, the authors express their apologies. However, it was felt that the book would be of greater practical value if the entire field of human pathology on the cellular level were presented in as complete a manner as possible.

Among the numerous applications of cytologic technics, one stands out very clearly. It is the place of cytology in the detection and the diagnosis of early, clinically silent cancer of various organs, such as cervix uteri, endometrium, bronchus, bladder, stomach, etc. Cytology has been primarily responsible for our increasing but still fragmentary knowledge of this group of diseases. Therefore, special emphasis in this book has been placed on the histologic and cytologic presentation of early cancer.

Statistical data pertaining to the value of cytology as applied to various organs have been omitted except for statements emphasizing specific points. The authors are satisfied that in their hands the method has proved to be highly reliable and accurate, and there are also other laboratories where the same standards prevail. The concept of a "false negative" cytologic diagnosis is as absurd as the concept of a "false negative" biopsy. Cytology is no substitute for a tissue biopsy but may be made equally reliable, especially in situations where a biopsy is not contemplated or not possible. As in other forms of laboratory diagnosis, it is practically impossible to avoid all errors in cytologic findings by comparison with histologic sections and thorough follow-up of patients are among the surest methods to improve and polish one's knowledge and to avoid the pitfalls of cellular morphology.

It is apparent that it would be beyond the scope of any volume to attempt to illustrate all the variations of normal and abnormal cells; therefore, the authors consider illustrations merely as an aid in the interpretation of the written word. The photographs, prepared by one of us (GRD), are chiefly in black and white and are based largely on material from Cytology and Pathology Laboratories at Memorial Hospital. Except when noted, the cytologic material was stained by Papanicolaou's technic, and the histologic material with hematoxylin and eosin. Use of more color photography would have raised the price of the book to prohibitive levels. The beautiful color pictures in Papanicolaou's Atlas* may be profitably consulted in conjunction with the present text.

Since this book has no precedent, undoubtedly there will be some errors of judgment and omission. The authors will be grateful for criticism and corrections from the readers.

Leopold G. Koss, M.D.
Grace R. Durfee, B.S.

---

* Papanicolaou GN. *Atlas of Exfoliative Cytology.* Cambridge, Massachusetts: The Commonwealth Fund by Harvard University Press, 1954 (Supplement I, 1956, Supplement II, 1960).

Acknowledgments

Several people were either essential or very helpful during the preparation of this book. Without the help of my secretary, Ms. Cordelia Silvestri, this book could never have been completed. Besides her extraordinary secretarial talents, she kept me and all the other authors on a short leash, kept records (and copies) of all the manuscript pages, and of archives as they built up. I thank Dr. Myron (Mike) R. Melamed, who consented to be a coeditor of this book. We have been friends and colleagues for half a century, having met while serving in the U.S. Army during the Korean War. Besides writing or revising several chapters, Mike always found time to discuss various aspects of this book with me and the publishers. The many other contributors, authors and coauthors, listed in the opening pages of this book and again as authors of various chapters, were willing to complete and deliver their work on time and suffered in silence at the indignities heaped upon them by the senior editor in reference to their text and photographs.

At Montefiore Medical Center, besides Ms. Silvestri, Mr. Barry Mordin patiently executed many of the tables and digitized many illustrations and diagrams. My colleagues Drs. Antonio Cajigas, Magalis Vuolo, and Maja Oktay assisted in finding missing references and offered helpful comments. Dr. Victoria Saksenberg, a cytopathology fellow (2003–2004), reviewed several manuscripts and translated them from American to Queen's English. Several cytotechnologists, particularly Gina Spiewack, were always willing to look for unusual cells needed as illustrations. A very special and heartfelt thanks to my dear friend and colleague of many years, Dr. Klaus Schreiber, who was always helpful in selecting illustrative material to be incorporated into the book. He was also willing to patiently listen to conceptual or practical problems and helped to find solutions. I thank Dr. Diane Hamele-Bena, now at Columbia-Presbyterian Medical Center, who prepared the beautiful drawings for Chapter 28. Special thanks to two old friends of mine, Professors Claude Gompel of Brussels, Belgium, who contributed several drawings, and Stanislaw Woyke of Warsaw and Szcecin, Poland who, generously allowed the use of several photographs. The support of Dr. Michael Prystowsky, the Chairman of Pathology at Montefiore/Einstein, during the long gestational period of this book was very much appreciated.

To all of these people, my deepest thanks and gratitude.

Leopold G. Koss, M.D.

To the Readers

The magnification factors of the color photographs taken with objectives 10×, 20 or 25×, or 40× are not included in the legends. Only unusual magnifications, such as very low power, very high dry power (objectives 60–80×), and oil immersion are listed. Two families of stains were pre-dominantly used: Papanicolaou stain for fixed smears and one of the hematologic stains (May-Grünwald-Giemsa or Diff-Quik) for aspiration smears. Tissue sections were gen-erally stained with hematoxylin and eosin. Exceptions are noted.

Table of Contents

General Cytology

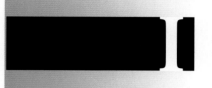

Diagnostic Cytology: Its Origins and Principles

1

EARLY EVENTS: THE BIRTH OF MICROSCOPY AND CLINICAL CYTOLOGY

Diagnostic cytology is the culmination of several centuries of observations and research. Although it is beyond the scope of this overview to give a detailed account of the past events, the readers may find a brief summary of these developments of interest.

Although some cells can be seen with the naked eye, for example, birds' or reptiles' eggs, it was the invention of the microscope that led to the recognition that all living matter is composed of cells. The term **microscope** was proposed in 1624 by an Italian group of scientists, united at the Academia dei Licei in Florence. The group, among others, included the great astronomer, Galileo, who apparently was also a user of one of the first instruments of this kind (Purtle, 1974). The first microscopes of practical value were constructed in Italy and in Holland in the 17th century. The best instrument, constructed by the Dutchman, **Anthony van Leeuwenhoek (1632–1723)** allowed a magnification of ×275. Leeuwenhoek reported on the miraculous world of microscopy in a series of letters to the Royal Society in London. His observations ranged from bacteria to spermatozoa. Interested readers will find illustrations of Leeuwenhoek's work and further comments on him and his contemporaries in the excellent book entitled *History of Clinical Cytology* by Grunze and Spriggs (1983). For nearly 2 centuries thereafter, these instruments were costly, very difficult to use and, therefore, accessible only to a very small, wealthy elite of interested scientists, most of whom were amateurs dabbling with microscopy as a diversion. Many of these microscopes were works of art (Fig. 1-1). Using one of these microscopes with a focusing adjustment, the Secretary of the Royal College in London, **Robert Hooke**, observed, in 1665, that corks and sponges were composed of little boxes that he called **cells** (from Latin, *cellula* = chamber) but the significance of this observation did not become apparent for almost 200 years. The great 17th century Italian anatomist, Malpighi, was also familiar with the microscope and is justly considered the creator of histology. The event that, in my judgment, proved to be decisive in better understanding of

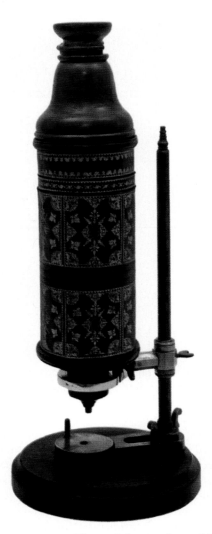
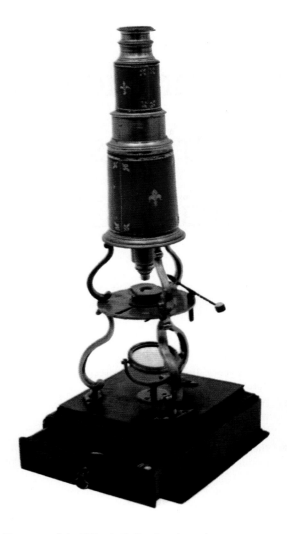

Figure 1-1 **Two beautiful 17th century microscopes.** (Courtesy of the Billing's Collection, Armed Forces Institute of Pathology, Washington, DC.)

cell and tissue structure in health and disease was the invention of achromatic lenses that allowed an undistorted view of microscopic images. In the 1820s, the construction of compound microscopes provided with such optics occurred nearly simultaneously in London (by Lister, the father of Lord Lister, the proponent of surgical antisepsis) and in Paris (by the family of opticians and microscope makers, named Chevalier). These microscopes, with many subsequent improvements, were easy to use, could be mass-produced at a reasonable price, and thus became available to a great many interested professional investigators, leading to a better understanding of cell structure and, indirectly, to an insight into the mechanisms of cell function and, hence, of life processes. Although, even in the age of molecular biology, much remains to be discovered about the interplay of molecules leading to cell differentiation and function, some progress has been made (see Chaps. 3 and 7) and more can be expected in the years to come.

Nearly all the microscopic observations during the first half of the 19th century were conducted on cells because the techniques of tissue processing for microscopic examination were very primitive. Early on, the investigators observed

that animal cells from different organs varied in size and shape and that some were provided with specialized structures, such as cilia. Perhaps the most remarkable record of these observations was an atlas of microscopic images by a French microscopist, **André François Donné,** published in Paris in 1845. The atlas was the first book illustrated with actual photomicrographs of remarkable quality (Fig. 1-2), obtained by the newly described method of Daguerre. The observations by many early observers led to the classification of normal cells and, subsequently, tissues as the backbone of normal cytology and histology. In the middle of the 19th century, the pioneering German pathologist, **Rudolf Virchow,** postulated that each cell is derived from another cell (*omnis cellula a cellula*). This assumption, which repeatedly has been proved to be correct, implies that at some time in a very distant past, probably many million years ago, the first cell, the mother of all cells, came to exist. How this happened is not known and is the subject of ongoing investigations.

By the middle of the 19th century, several books on the use of the microscope in medicine became available. In the book, *The Microscope in its Applications to Practical Medi-*

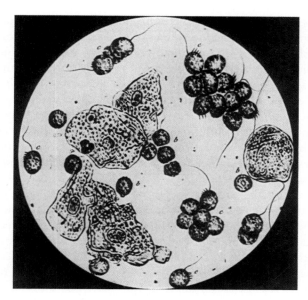

Figure 1-2 Reproduction of Figure 33 from *Donné's Atlas,* published in 1845. The daguerreotype represents "vaginal secreta" and shows squamous cells, leukocytes, identified as "purulent globules" (*b*), and *Trichomonas vaginalis* (*c*). Note the remarkable pictorial quality of the unstained material.

cine, that appeared in two editions (1854 and 1858), **Lionel Beale** of London described the cells as follows: "A cell consists of a perfectly closed sac containing certain contents. The most important structure within the cell wall, in most instances, is the nucleus, upon which the multiplication of the cell . . . (and other functions) . . . depend. It must be borne in mind, however, that in some cells, such as the human blood corpuscles (erythrocytes, comment by LGK) a nucleus is not to be demonstrated. Within the nucleus there usually exists . . . a clear bright spot. This is the nucleolus." Beale further classified cells into several categories according to their shapes (*scaly or squamous cells, tesselated cells* [epithelial cells lining serous membranes, LGK], polygonal cells, columnar cells, spherical cells, spindle-shaped cells, fusiform cells, etc.)*,* thus describing the entire spectrum of cell configuration. He further described cells derived from various organs (including the central nervous system) and reported that some cells were ciliated, notably those of the trachea, bronchus, fallopian tubes and portions of the endocervical canal. Beale also reported that "some cells have a remarkable power of multiplication . . . distinguished for the distinctness and number of its nuclei" (cancer cells). Beale described the use of the microscope to identify cancer of various organs that he could distinguish from a benign change of a similar clinical appearance. It is evident, therefore, that by the middle of the 19th century, approximately 150 years ago, there was considerable knowledge of the microscopic configuration of human cells and their role in the diagnosis of human disease.

Perhaps the most important series of observations pertinent to this narrative was the recognition that cells obtained from clinically evident cancerous growths differed from normal cells. The initial observations on cancer cells is attributed to a young German physiologist, **Johannes Müller,**

who, in 1838, published an illustrated monograph entitled *On the Nature and Structural Characteristics of Cancer and Those Morbid Growth That Can Be Confounded With It.* In this monograph, Müller discussed at some length the differences in configuration of cells and their nuclei in cancer when compared with normal cells. Müller's original observations on the differences between normal and cancerous cells were confirmed by several investigators. For example, in 1860, Beale identified and described cancer cells in sputum. It may come as a surprise to some of the readers that as early as 1845 and 1851, a German microscopist, working in Switzerland and writing in French, **Hermann Lebert,** used cell samples aspirated from patients by means of a cannula for the diagnosis of cancer. In 1847, **M. Kün** of Strasbourg, about whom little is known, described a needle with a cutting edge useful in securing material from subcutaneous tumors, examined as smears (Grunze and Spriggs, 1983; Webb, 2001).

Virchow, often considered the father of contemporary pathology, and who was Müller's pupil, was a superb observer at the autopsy table and a good microscopist. He recognized and described the gross and microscopic features of a large number of entities, such as infarcts, inflammatory lesions, leukemia, and various forms of cancer. However, his views on the origin of human cancer were erroneous because he believed that all cancers were derived from connective tissue and not by transformation of normal tissues (Virchow, 1863). For this reason, he had difficulties in accepting the observations of two of his students and contemporaries, **Thiersch** in 1865 and **Waldayer** in 1867, who independently advocated the origin of carcinomas of the skin, breast, and uterus from transformed normal epithelium. Because Virchow wielded a tremendous influence in Germany, not only as a scientist but also as a politician (he was a Professor of Pathology in Berlin as well as a Deputy to the German Parliament, a socialist of sorts, who fought with the famous Chancellor, Bismarck), views that were in conflict with his own were often rejected, thus delaying the development of independent scientific thought. It took about 40 years until the confirmation of Thiersch's and Waldayer's concepts of the origin of carcinomas was documented by **Schauenstein** for the uterine cervix in 1908 (see Chap. 11). It took many more years until the concept of a preinvasive stage of invasive cancer, originally designated as *carcinoma in situ* by **Schottlander and Kermauner** in 1912, was generally accepted and put to a good clinical use in cancer detection and prevention.

These are but a few of the early contributions that have bearing on diagnostic cytology as it is known today. In addition to the contributors mentioned by name, there were many other heroes and antiheroes who made remarkable contributions to the science of human cytology during the second half of the 19th century, and this brief narrative doesn't do justice to them. The interested reader should consult a beautifully illustrated book on the history of clinical cytology by Grunze and Spriggs (1983).

Still, in spite of these remarkable developments, the widespread application of cytology to the diagnosis of human disease did not take place until the 1950s. Although sporadic publications during the second half of the 19th century and the first half of the 20th century kept the idea of cytologic diagnosis alive, it was overshadowed by developments in histopathology.

THE ERA OF HISTOPATHOLOGY

The Beginning

Although cells teased from tissues were the main target of microscopic investigations during the first half of the 19th century, consistent efforts have been made to develop methods of tissue processing. Thus, in the 1858 edition of Beale's book, several pages are dedicated to the methods of hardening soft tissue samples by boiling and to the methods of preparation of transparent, thin sections suitable for microscopic examination with hand-held cutting instruments. Subsequently, various methods of tissue fixation were tried, such as chromium salts, alcohol, and ultimately, formalin and the manual cutting instruments were replaced by mechanical microtomes around 1880. Simultaneously, many methods of tissue staining were developed. There is excellent evidence that, by 1885, tissue embedding in wax or paraffin, cutting of sections with a microtome, and staining with hematoxylin and eosin were the standard methods in laboratories of pathology, as narrated in the history of surgical pathology at the Memorial Hospital for Cancer, now known as the Memorial Sloan-Kettering Cancer Center (Koss and Lieberman, 1997).

Two events enhanced the significance and value of tissue pathology. One was the introduction of the concept of a **tissue biopsy,** initially proposed for diagnosis of cancer of the uterine cervix and endometrium by **Ruge and Veit** in 1877, who documented that the microscope is superior to clinical judgment in the diagnosis of these diseases. However, the term **biopsy** is attributable to a French dermatopathologist, **Ernest Besnier,** who coined it in 1879 (Nezelof, 2000). The second event was the introduction of **frozen sections,** popularized by Cullen in 1895, which allowed a rapid processing of tissues and became an essential tool in guiding surgeons during surgery (see also Wright, 1985). With these two tools at hand, the study of cells was practically abandoned for nearly a century. Next to autopsy pathology, the mainstay of classification of disease processes during the 18th and 19th centuries, histopathology became the dominant diagnostic mode of human pathology, a position that it holds until today. Histopathology is based on **analysis of tissue patterns, which is a much simpler and easier task than the interpretation of smears that often requires tedious synthesis of the evidence dispersed on a slide.** Further, histopathology is superior to cytologic samples in determining the relationship of various tissues to each other, for example, in identifying invasion of a cancer into the underlying stroma.

Current Status

The introduction of histopathology on a large scale led to the rapid spread of this knowledge throughout Europe and the Americas. The ever-increasing number of trained people working in leading institutions of medical learning was capable of interpretation of tissue patterns supplementing clinical judgment with a secure microscopic diagnosis. Further, the tissue techniques allowed the preparation of multiple identical samples from the same block of tissue, thus facilitating exchanges between and among pathologists and laying down the **foundation of accurate classification of disease processes, staging and grading of cancers and systematic follow-up of patients, with similar disorders, leading to statistical behavioral studies of diseases of a similar type.** Such studies became of critical importance in evaluating treatment regimens, initially by surgery or radiotherapy and, even more so, after the introduction of powerful antibiotics and anti-cancer drugs that were active against diseases previously considered hopeless. Nearly all clinical treatment protocols are based on histologic assessment of target lesions. Histologic techniques were also essential in **immunopathology** that allowed the testing of multiple antibodies on samples of the same tissue. Such studies are difficult to accomplish with smears, which are virtually always unique.

THE RETURN OF CYTOLOGY

Papanicolaou and the Cytology of the Female Genital Tract

The beginnings of the cytology of the female genital tract can be traced to the middle of the 19th century. The microscopic appearance of cells from the vagina was illustrated by several early observers, including Donné and Beale, whose work was discussed above (see Fig. 1-2). In 1847, a Frenchman, **F.A. Pouchet,** published a book dedicated to the microscopic study of vaginal secretions during the menstrual cycle. In the closing years of the 19th century, sporadic descriptions and illustrations of cancer cells derived from cancer of the uterine cervix were published (see Chap. 11).

However, there is no doubt whatsoever that the current resurgence of diagnostic cytology is the result of the achievements of **Dr. George N. Papanicolaou** (1883–1962), an American of Greek descent (Fig. 1-3). Dr. Pap, as he was generally known to his coworkers, friends, and his wife Mary, was an anatomist working at the Cornell University with a primary interest in endocrinology of the reproductive tract. Because of his interest in the menstrual cycle, he developed a small glass pipette that allowed him to obtain cell samples from the vagina of rodents. In smears, he could determine that, during the menstrual cycle, squamous cells derived from the vaginal epithelium of these animals followed a pattern of maturation and atrophy corresponding to maturation of ova. He made major contributions to the understanding of the hormonal mechanisms of ovulation and menstruation and is considered to be one of the pioneering contributors to reproductive endocrinology.

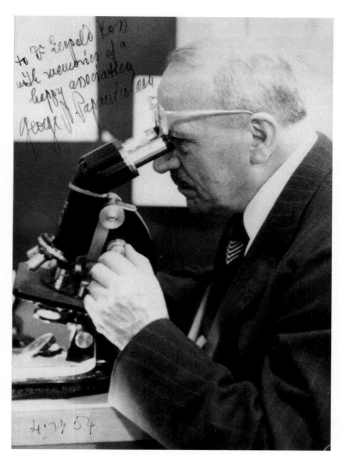

Figure 1-3 George N. Papanicolaou, 1954, in a photograph inscribed to the author.

However, his fame is based on an **incidental observation of cancer cells in vaginal smears of women** whose menstrual cycle he was studying. Papanicolaou had no training in pathology and it is, therefore, not likely that he himself identified the cells as cancerous. It is not known who helped Papanicolaou in the identification of cancer cells. It is probable that it was James Ewing who was at that time Chairman of Pathology at Cornell and who was thoroughly familiar with cancer cells as a consequence of his exposure to aspiration biopsies performed by the surgeon, Hayes Martin, at the Memorial Hospital for Cancer (see below). Papanicolaou's initial contribution to the subject of "New Cancer Diagnosis," presented during an obscure meeting on the subject of the Betterment of the Human Race in Battle Creek, MI, in May, 1928, failed to elicit any response. Only in 1939, prodded by Joseph Hinsey, the new Chairman of the Department of Anatomy at Cornell, had Papanicolaou started a systematic cooperation with a gynecologist, **Herbert Traut,** the Head of Gynecologic Oncology at Cornell, who provided him with vaginal smears on his patients. It soon became apparent that abnormal cells could be found in several of these otherwise asymptomatic patients who were subsequently shown to harbor histologically confirmed carcinomas of **the cervix and the endometrium.** Papanicolaou and Traut's article, published in 1941 and a book pub-

lished in 1943, heralded a new era of application of cytologic techniques to a new target: the discovery of **occult** cancer of the uterus. Papanicolaou's name became enshrined in medical history by the term **Pap smear,** now attached to the cytologic procedure for cervical cancer detection. The stain, also invented by Papanicolaou and bearing his name, was nearly universally adopted in processing cervicovaginal smears.

Papanicolaou's name was submitted twice to the Nobel Committee in Stockholm as a candidate for the Nobel Award in Medicine. Unfortunately, he was not selected. As a member of the jury told me (LGK) many years later, the negative decision was based on the fact that Papanicolaou had never acknowledged previous contributions of a Romanian pathologist, **Aureli Babés** (Fig. 1-4), who, working with the gynecologist C. Daniel, reported in January 1927 that cervical smears, obtained by means of a bacteriologic loop, fixed with methanol and stained with Giemsa, were an accurate and reliable method of diagnosing cancer of the uterine cervix. On April 11, 1928, Babés published an extensive, beautifully illustrated article on this subject in the French publication, *Presse Médicale*, which apparently had remained unknown to Papanicolaou. One of the highlights

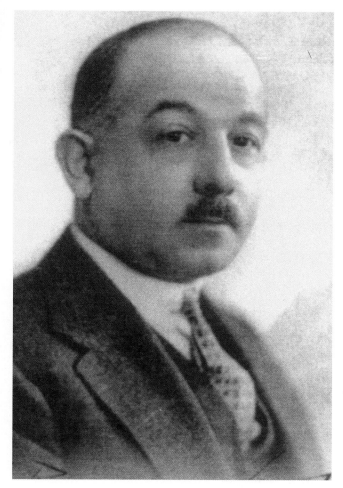

Figure 1-4 Aureli Babés. (Courtesy of Dr. Bernard Naylor, Ann Arbor, MI.)

of Babés' article was the observation that a **cytologic sample may serve to recognize cancer of the uterine cervix before invasion.** Babés' observations were confirmed only once, by an Italian gynecologist, Odorico Viana in 1928, whereas Papanicolaou's work stimulated a large number of publications and received wide publicity. Both Babés' and Viana's articles were translated into English by Larry Douglass (1967 and 1970).

The reason for Papanicolaou's success and Babés' failure to attract international attention clearly lies in the differences in geographic location (New York City vs. Bucharest) and in timing. If Papanicolaou's 1928 article were his only publication on the subject of cytologic diagnosis of cancer, he would have probably remained obscure. He had the great fortune to publish again in the 1940s and his ideas were slowly accepted after the end of World War II, with extensive help from Dr. Charles Cameron, the first Medical and Scientific Director of the American Cancer Society, which popularized the Pap test. A summary of these events was presented at a meeting of the American Cancer Society (Koss, 1993).

The Pap Smear: The Beginning

The value of the **vaginal smear** as a tool in the recognition of occult cancers of the uterine cervix and the endometrium was rapidly confirmed in a number of articles published in the 1940s (Meigs et al, 1943 and 1945; Ayre, 1944; Jones et al, 1945; Fremont-Smith et al, 1947). It soon became apparent that the vaginal smear was more efficient in the discovery of cervical rather than endometrial cancer and the focus of subsequent investigations shifted to the uterine cervix. In 1948, **Lombard et al** from Boston introduced the concept of the vaginal smear as a screening test for cancer of the uterine cervix.

Because the vaginal smear was very tedious to screen and evaluate, the proposal by a Canadian gynecologist, **J. Ernest Ayre,** to supplement or replace it with a cell sample obtained directly from the uterine cervix under visual control was rapidly and widely accepted. In 1947, Ayre ingeniously proposed that a common wooden tongue depressor could be cut with scissors to fit the contour of the cervix, thus adding a very inexpensive tool that significantly improved the yield of cells in the cervical sample. **Ayre's scraper or spatula,** now made of plastic, has remained an important instrument in cervical cancer detection.

In 1948, the American Cancer Society organized a national conference in Boston to reach a consensus on screening for cervical cancer. The method was enthusiastically endorsed by the gynecologists but met with skepticism on the part of the participating pathologists. Nonetheless, the first recommendations of the American Cancer Society pertaining to screening for cervical cancer were issued shortly thereafter. In 1950, **Nieburgs and Pund** published the first results of screening of 10,000 women for occult cancer of the cervix, reporting that unsuspected cancers were detected in a substantial number of screened women. This seminal article, followed by a number of other publications, established the Pap test as a standard health service procedure. Further

support for the significance of the test was a series of observations that the smear technique was helpful in discovering precancerous lesions (initially collectively designated as **carcinoma in situ**), which could be easily treated, thus preventing the development of invasive cancer.

Unfortunately, no double-blind studies of the efficacy of the cervicovaginal smear have ever been conducted, and it became the general assumption that the test had a very high specificity and sensitivity. The legal consequences of this omission became apparent 40 years later.

The Pap Smear From the 1950 to the 1980s

Although the American pathologists, with a few notable exceptions (Reagan, 1951), were reluctant to acknowledge the value of the cervicovaginal smear, toward the end of the 1960s, an ever-increasing number of hospital laboratories were forced to process Pap smears at the request of the gynecologists. In those years, the number of pathologists trained in the interpretation of cytologic material was very small, and it remained so for many years. The responsibility for screening and, usually the interpretation of the smears, was assumed by cytotechnologists who, although few in number, were better trained to perform this function than their medical supervisors. With the support of the National Cancer Institute, several schools for training of cytotechnologists were established in the United States in the 1960s. These trained professionals played a key role in the practice of cytopathology. This time period has also seen the opening of several large commercial laboratories dedicated to the processing of cervicovaginal smears. New books, journals, and postgraduate courses offered by a number of professional organizations gave the pathologists an opportunity to improve their skills in this difficult field of diagnosis.

Several very successful programs of cervix cancer detection were established in the United States and Canada, and it became quite apparent that the mortality from cancer of the uterine cervix could be lowered in the screened populations. As a consequence, by the end of the 1980s, **a 70% reduction in the mortality** from this disease was recorded in several geographic areas where mass screening was introduced. **However, in none of the populations screened was cancer of the cervix completely irradicated.**

The Pap Smear From the 1980s to Today

In the 1970s and early 1980s, several articles commenting on the failure of the cervicovaginal smear in preventing the developments of invasive cancer of the uterine cervix appeared in the American literature and in Sweden (Rylander, 1976; Fetherstone, 1983; Koss, 1989; summary in Koss and Gompel, 1999). The reports did not fully analyze the reasons for failure and were generally ignored. In 1987, however, an article in the *Wall Street Journal* by an investigative journalist, **Walt Bogdanich,** on failure of laboratories to identify cancer of the cervix in young women, some who were mothers of small children, elicited a great deal of attention. It prompted the Congress of the United States in 1988 to promulgate a law, known as the Amendment to the Clinical Laboratory Improvement Act **(CLIA 88),** governing the practice of gynecologic cytology in the United States. The implications of the law in reference to practice of cytopathology are discussed elsewhere in this book (see Chap. 44). Suffice it to say, cytopathology, particularly in reference to cervicovaginal smears, has become the object of intense scrutiny and legal proceedings against pathologists and laboratories for alleged failure to interpret the smears correctly, casting a deep shadow on this otherwise very successful laboratory test.

As a consequence of these events, several manufacturers have proposed changes in collection and processing of the cervicovaginal smears. The collection methods of cervical material in **liquid media,** followed by automated processing with resulting **"monolayer"** preparations, have been approved by the Food and Drug Administration (USA). Other manufacturers introduced apparatuses for automated screening of conventional smears. New **sampling instruments** were also developed and widely marketed, notably endocervical brushes. All these initiatives were designed to reduce the risk of errors in the screening and interpretation of cervicovaginal smears. These issues are discussed in Chapters 8, 11, 12, and 44.

DEVELOPMENTS IN NONGYNECOLOGIC CYTOLOGY

Historical Overview

At the time of early developments in general cytology in the 19th century, summarized above, numerous articles were published describing the application of cytologic techniques to various secreta and fluids, such as sputum, urine, effusions, and even vomit for diagnostic purposes. These contributions have been described in detail in Grunze and Spriggs' book. The recognition of lung cancer cells in sputum by **Beale** in 1858 was mentioned above.

As lung cancer became a serious public health dilemma in the 1930s and 1940s, **in Great Britain, Dudgeon and Wrigley** developed, in 1935, a method of "wet" processing of smears of fresh sputum for the diagnosis of lung cancer. The method was used by **Wandall** in Denmark in 1944 on a large numbers of patients, with excellent diagnostic results. Woolner and McDonald (1949) at the Mayo Clinic and Herbut and Clerf (1946) in Philadelphia also studied the applications of cytology to lung cancer diagnosis. In the late 1940s and early 1950s, Papanicolaou, with several coworkers, published a number of articles on the application of cytologic techniques to the diagnosis of cancer of various organs, illustrated in his Atlas. In the United Kingdom, urine cytology was applied by **Crabbe** (1952) to screening of industrial workers for cancer of the bladder and gastric lavage techniques by **Schade** (1956) to screening for occult gastric cancer, a method extensively used in Japan for population screening. Esophageal balloon technique was applied on a large scale in China for detecting precursor lesions of esophageal carcinoma. Screening for oral cancer has been shown to be successful in discovering occult carcinomas

in situ. **Thus, conventional cytologic techniques, when judiciously applied, supplement surgical pathology in many situations when a tissue biopsy is either not contemplated, indicated, or not feasible.** It needs to be stressed that cytopathology has made major contributions to the recognition of early stages of human cancer in many organs and, thus, contributed in a remarkable way to a better understanding of events in human carcinogenesis and to preventive health care. These, and many other applications of cytologic techniques to the diagnosis of early and advanced cancer and of infectious disorders of various organs, are discussed in this text.

THE ASPIRATION BIOPSY (FNA)

The Beginning

Ever since syringes or equivalent instruments were introduced into the medical armamentarium, probably in the 15th century of our era, they were used to aspirate collections of fluids. With the introduction of achromatic microscopes and their industrial production in the 1830s, the instrument became accessible to many observers who used it to examine the aspirated material. It has been mentioned above that a French physician, **Kün,** and a German-Swiss pathologist, **Lebert,** described, in 1847 and 1851, the use of a cannula to secure cell samples from palpable tumors and used the microscope to identify cancer. Sporadic use of aspirated samples has been described in the literature of the second half of the 19th century and in the first years of the 20th century. An important contribution was published in 1905 by two British military surgeons, **Greig and Gray,** working in Uganda who aspirated the swollen lymph nodes, by means of a needle and a syringe, of patients with sleeping sickness to identify the mobile trypanosoma (see Webb, 2001 for an excellent recent account of early investigators).

In the 20th century, to my knowledge, the first aspiration biopsy diagnosis of a solid tumor of the skin (apparently a lymphoma) was published by **Hirschfeld** (1912), who was the first person to use a **small-caliber needle.** He subsequently extended his experience to other tumors, but was prevented by World War I from publishing his results until 1919. Several other early observers reported on the aspiration of lymph nodes and other accessible sites (Webb, 2001).

The most notable development in diagnostic aspiration biopsy was a paradoxical event. **James Ewing,** the Director of the Memorial Hospital for Cancer in New York City and also a Professor of Pathology at Cornell University Medical School, was a dominant figure in American oncologic pathology between 1910 and 1940. Although Ewing has made great contributions to the classification and identification of human cancer, he was adamantly opposed to tissue biopsies because they allegedly contributed to the spread of cancer (Koss and Lieberman, 1997). Because of the ban on tissue biopsies, a young surgeon and radiotherapist at the Memorial Hospital, **Hayes Martin,** who refused to treat patients without a preoperative diagnosis, began to aspirate palpable tumors of various organs by means of a large-caliber needle and a Record syringe. The material was prepared in the form of air-dried smears, stained with hematoxylin and eosin by Ewing's technician, **Edward Ellis.** Tissue fragments (named *clots*) were embedded in paraffin and processed as cell blocks. Palpable lesions of lymph nodes, breast, and thyroid were the initial targets of aspiration. The material was interpreted by Ewing's associate and subsequent successor (and my Chief–LGK), **Dr. Fred W. Stewart.** In response to a specific query, the reasons for this development were explained many years later in a letter dated June 30, 1980, written by Dr. Fred W. Stewart to this writer.

> Martin and Ewing were at sword's point on the need for biopsy proof prior to aggressive surgery or radiation (in neck nodes since Hayes Martin dealt exclusively in head and neck stuff) and the needle was a sort of compromise. Ewing thought biopsy hazardous—a method of disease spread. The material was seen mostly by me (FWS). Ewing, at the time, was quite inactive. Eddie Ellis merely fixed and stained the slides. He probably looked at them—he was used to looking at stuff with Ewing and really knew more about diagnoses than a lot of pathologists of the period. The needle really spread from neck nodes to the various other regions, especially to the breast, of course.

The method proved to be very successful and accurate with very few errors or clinical complications. Martin and Ellis published their initial results in 1930 and 1934. In 1933, Dr. Fred W. Stewart published a classic article, "The Diagnosis of Tumors by Aspiration," in which he discussed, at length, the pros and cons of this method of diagnosis, its achievements, and pitfalls, based on experience with several hundred samples. As Stewart himself stated in a letter (to LGK), he was "damned by many for having advocated this insecure and potentially harmful method of diagnosis, without a shred of proof." For a detailed description of these events, see Koss and Lieberman (1997). In fact, the method of aspiration pioneered by Martin has remained a standard diagnostic procedure at Memorial Sloan-Kettering Cancer Center until today (2004), the only institution in the world where the procedure has remained in constant use for more than 75 years. There is no evidence that the Memorial style aspiration smear was practiced on a large scale anywhere else in the world. The method was described and illustrated by John Godwin (1956) and again in the first edition of this book (1961) by John Berg, but has met with total indifference in the United States.

In Europe, on the other hand, the interest in the method persisted. Thus, in the 1940s, two internists, **Paul Lopes-Cardozo** in Holland and **Nils Söderström** in Sweden, experimented on a large scale with this system of diagnosis, using **small-caliber needles and hematologic techniques** to process the smears. **Lopes-Cardozo and Söderström** subsequently published books on the subject of thin-needle aspiration. Although both books were published in English, they had virtually no impact on the American diagnostic scene, but were widely read in Europe.

Current Status

Working at the Radiumhemmet, the Stockholm Cancer Center, the radiotherapist-oncologist, **Sixten Franzén,** and his student and colleague, **Josef Zajicek,** applied the thin-needle technique first to the prostate and, subsequently, to a broad variety of targets, ranging from lesions of salivary glands to the skeleton. Franzén et al (1960) described a syringe (initially developed for the diagnosis of prostatic carcinoma) that allowed performance of the aspiration with one hand, whereas the other hand steadied the target lesion (see Chap. 28). As nonpathologists, these observers used air-dried smears, stained with hematologic stains. In the 1970s, special aspiration biopsy clinics were established in Stockholm and elsewhere in Sweden to which patients with palpable lesions were referred for diagnosis. The technique soon became an acceptable substitute for tissue biopsies. An extensive bibliography, generated by the Swedish group, supported the value and accuracy of the procedure (Zajicek, 1974, 1979; Esposti et al, 1968; Löwhagen and Willems, 1981).

It can be debated why the aspiration biopsy flourished in Sweden, whereas initially it was unequivocally rejected in the United States (see Fox, 1979). This writer believes that the Swedish success was caused, in part, by inadequate services in biopsy pathology because, by tradition, in the academic Departments of Pathology (that are the mainstay of Swedish pathology), research took precedence over services to patients, a situation quite different from that in the United States (see exchange of correspondence between Koss, 1980, and Söderström, 1980). A further reason for the Swedish success was the government-sponsored health system, based on salaries, which offered no monetary rewards to surgeons and other clinicians for the performance of biopsies. Therefore, the creation of aspiration diagnostic centers offering credible and rapid diagnoses was greeted with enthusiasm. This is yet another major point of difference with the situation in the United States, where surgeons (and sometimes other specialists) feel financially threatened if the biopsies are performed by people encroaching on their "turf."

Although the Swedish authors published in English and also contributed to this book (editions 2, 3, and 4), the impact of thin-needle aspiration techniques on the American scene initially has been trivial and confined to a few institutions and individuals. The radical change in attitude and the acceptance of the cytologic aspirates in the United States may be due to several factors. Broad acceptance of exfoliative cytologic techniques (Pap smears) for detection and diagnosis of cervix cancer, subsequently extended to many other organs, clearly played a major role in these developments. The introduction of new imaging techniques, such as imaging with contrast media, computed tomography, and ultrasound, not only contributed to improved visualization of organs but also to **roentgenologists' ability to perform a number of diagnostic procedures by aspiration of visualized lesions,** hitherto in the domain of surgeons (Ferucci, 1981; Zornoza, 1981; Kamholz et al, 1982). After timid beginnings in the early 1970s, documenting that the use of a thin needle was an essentially harmless and diagnostically beneficial procedure, a new era of diagnosis began which initially forced the pathologists to accept the cytologic sample as clinically valid and important. In those days, most pathologists had to struggle to interpret such samples. Thus, once again, the pathologists were forced into an area of morphologic diagnosis for which they were not prepared by training or experience.

The current enthusiasm for this method in the United States is surely related to the Swedish experience that insisted that the **interpreter of the smears (i.e., the cytopathologist) should also be the person obtaining cell samples of palpable lesions directly from patients.** In fact, many of the leaders in this field were trained in Sweden, particularly by the late Dr. **Torsten Löwhagen.** This was the exact opposite of the situation in the 1960s, when Swedish observers repeatedly visited the Memorial Hospital for Cancer in New York City to learn the secrets of the aspiration biopsy. Nowadays, by performing the procedure and by interpreting its results, the pathologists assume an important role in patient care. Without much doubt, **aspiration cytology has become an elixir of youth for American pathology,** making those who practice it into clinicians dealing with patients, not unlike the pioneers of pathology in the 19th century.

At the time of this writing (2004), biopsy by aspiration, also known as **thin- or fine-needle aspiration biopsy (FNA),** has become an important diagnostic technique, sometimes replacing but often complementing tissue pathology in many clinical situations. The targets of the aspiration biopsy now **encompassed virtually all organs of the human body,** as discussed in Chapter 28 and subsequent chapters. Within recent years, numerous books, many lavishly illustrated, have been published on various aspects of aspiration cytology. With a few exceptions, these books do not address the key issue of the aspiration biopsy: it is a **form of surgical pathology, practiced on cytologic samples** (Koss, 1988). Only those who have expertise in tissue pathology are fully qualified to interpret the aspirated samples without endangering the patient. These aspects of aspiration cytology are discussed in Chapter 28.

CYTOLOGIC SAMPLING TECHNIQUES

Diagnostic cytology is based on **four basic sampling techniques:**

- Collection of exfoliated cells
- Collection of cells removed by brushing or similar abrasive techniques
- Aspiration biopsy (FNA) or removal of cells from palpable or deeply seated lesions by means of a needle, with or without a syringe. Aspiration biopsy (FNA) procedures are described in Chapter 19 for lung and pleura and Chapter 28 and subsequent chapters for all other organs.
- Intraoperative cytology (see below)

Exfoliative Cytology

Exfoliative cytology is based on spontaneous shedding of cells derived from the lining of an organ into a body cavity, whence they can be removed by nonabrasive means. Shedding of cells is a phenomenon based on constant renewal of an organ's epithelial lining. Within the sample, the age of these cells cannot be determined: some cells may have been shed recently, others may have been shed days or even weeks before. A typical example is the **vaginal smear** prepared from cells removed from the posterior fornix of the vagina. The cells that accumulate in the vaginal fornix are derived from several sources: the squamous epithelium that lines the vagina and the vaginal portio of the uterine cervix, the epithelial lining of the endocervical canal, and other sources such as the endometrium, tube, the peritoneum, and even more distant sites (Fig. 1-5). These cells accumulate in the mucoid material and other secretions from the uterus and the vagina. The vaginal smears often contain leukocytes and macrophages that may accumulate in response to an inflammatory process, and a variety of microorganisms such as bacteria, fungi, viruses, and parasites that may inhabit the lower genital tract.

Another example of exfoliative cytology is the **sputum.** The sputum is a collection of mucoid material that contains cells derived from the buccal cavity, the pharynx, larynx,

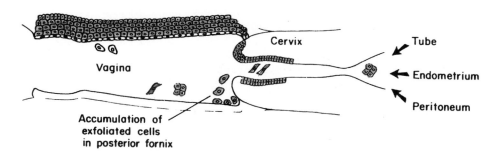

Figure 1-5 Exfoliative cytology. A schematic representation of the cross section of the vagina, uterine cervix, and the lower segment of the endometrial cavity. Cells desquamating from the epithelial lining of the various organs indicated in the drawing accumulate in the posterior vaginal fornix. Thus, material aspirated from the vaginal fornix will contain cells derived from the vagina, cervix, endometrium, and sometimes fallopian tube, ovary, and peritoneum. Common components of vaginal smears include inflammatory cells, bacteria, fungi, and parasites such as *Trichomonas vaginalis* (see Fig. 1-2). Red indicates squamous epithelium, blue represents endocervical epithelium, and green is endometrium.

and trachea, the bronchial tree and the pulmonary alveoli, as well as inflammatory cells, microorganisms, foreign material, etc. The same principle applies to **voided urine** and to a variety of **body fluids (effusions).** The principal targets of exfoliative cytology are listed in Table 1-1.

It is evident from these examples that a cytologic sample based on the principle of exfoliated cytology will be characterized by a great variety of cell types, derived from several sources. An important feature of exfoliative cytology is the poor preservation of some types of cells. Depending on type and origin, some cells, such as squamous cells, may remain relatively well preserved and resist deterioration, whereas other cells, such as glandular cells or leukocytes, may deteriorate and their morphologic features may be distorted, unless fixed rapidly. In addition, spontaneous cleansing processes that naturally occur in body cavities may take their toll. Most cleansing functions are vested in families of cells known as *macrophages* or *histiocytes* and *leukocytes*. These cells may either phagocytize the deteriorating cells or destroy them with specific enzymes (see Chap. 5). A summary of principal features of exfoliative cytology is shown in Table 1-2. The exfoliated material is usually examined in smears, filters, and cell blocks or by one of the newer techniques of preservation in liquid media and machine processing (see below).

Abrasive Cytology

In the late 1940s and 1950s, several new methods of securing cytologic material from various body sites were developed. The purpose of these procedures was to enrich the sample with cells obtained directly from the surface of the target organ. The **cervical scraper or spatula,** introduced by Ayre in 1947, allowed a direct sampling of cells from the squamous epithelium of the uterine cervix and the adjacent endocervical canal (Fig. 1-6). A **gastric balloon** with an abrasive surface, developed by Panico et al (1950), led to the development of devices known as **esophageal balloons,** extensively used in China for the detection of occult carcinoma of the esophagus in high-risk areas (see Chap. 24). A number of **brushing instruments,** suitable for sampling

---

TABLE 1-2
PRINCIPAL FEATURES OF EXFOLIATIVE CYTOLOGY

- The technique is applicable to organs with easy clinical access whence the samples can be obtained.
- The samples often contain a great variety of cells of various types from many different sources.
- The cellular constituents are sometimes poorly preserved.
- The samples may contain inflammatory cells, macrophages, microorganisms, and material of extraneous origin.
- The signal advantage of exfoliative cytology is the facility with which multiple samples can be obtained.

TABLE 1-1
PRINCIPAL TARGETS OF EXFOLIATIVE CYTOLOGY

Target Organ	Techniques*	Principal Lesions To Be Identified	Incidental Benefits
Female genital tract	Smear of material from the vaginal pool obtained by pipette or a dull instrument. Fixation in alcohol or by spray fixative.	Precancerous lesions and cancer of the vagina, uterine cervix, endometrium, rarely fallopian tubes, ovaries	Identification of infectious agents, such as bacteria, viruses, fungi, or parasites (Chapters 8–18)
Respiratory tract	Sputum: either fresh or collected in fixative (smears and cell blocks)	Precancerous states mainly carcinoma in situ and lung cancers	Identification of infectious agents, such as bacteria, viruses, fungi, or parasites (Chapters 19 and 20)
Urinary tract	Voided urine; fresh or collected in fixative (smears and cytocentrifuge preparations)	Precancerous states, mainly flat carcinoma in situ and high grade cancers	Identification of viral infections and effect of drugs (Chapters 22 and 23)
Effusions (pleural, peritoneal, or pericardial)	Collection of fluid: fresh or in fixative (smears and cell blocks)	Metastatic cancer and primary mesotheliomas	(Chapters 25 and 26)
Other fluids (cerebrospinal fluid, synovial fluid, etc.)	Collection in fixative Cytocentrifuge preparations	Differential diagnosis between inflammatory processes and metastatic cancer	Identification of infectious agents (viruses, fungi) (Chapter 27)

*For further details of sample collection see this and other appropriate chapters. For further technical details, see Chapter 44.

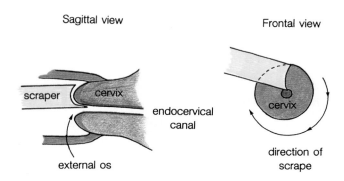

Sagittal view

Frontal view

Figure 1-6 **Method of obtaining an abrasive sample (scraping) from the uterine cervix by means of Ayre's scraper.** Red indicates squamous epithelium and blue indicates endocervical mucosa.

various organs, were also developed (see below). Several such instruments were developed for the sampling of the uterine cervix (see Fig. 8-45).

Endoscopic Instruments

The developments in optics led to the introduction of rigid endoscopic instruments for the inspection of hollow organs in the 1930s and 1940s. Bronchoscopy, esophagoscopy, and sigmoidoscopy were some of the widely used procedures. In the 1960s, **new methods of endoscopy** were developed based upon transmission of light along flexible glass fibers. This development led to the construction of flexible, **fiberoptic instruments** permitting visual inspection of viscera of small caliber or complex configuration, such as the secondary bronchi or the distal parts of the colon, previously not accessible to rigid instruments. The fiberoptic instruments are provided with small brushes, biopsy forceps, or needles that permitted a very precise removal of cytologic samples or small biopsies.

The introduction of fiberoptic instruments **revolutionized the cytologic sampling of organs of the respiratory and gastrointestinal tracts** and, to a lesser extent, the urinary tract. The brushes could be used under direct visual control for sampling of specific lesions or areas that were either suspect or showed only slight abnormalities (Fig 1-7). The

method became of major importance in the search for early cancer of the bronchi (including carcinoma in situ) and of superficial cancer of the esophagus and stomach (see Chaps. 20 and 24). Transbronchial aspiration biopsies of submucosal lesions could also be performed. The introduction of fiberoptic sigmoidoscopes and colonoscopes contributed to a better assessment of abnormalities that were either detected by roentgenologic examination or were unsuspected. Colonic brush cytology proved to be useful in searching for recurrences of treated carcinoma or in the search for early carcinoma in patients with ulcerative colitis (see Chap. 24).

The cytologic samples obtained by brushings, with or without fiberoptic guidance, differ markedly from exfoliated samples. The cells are removed directly from the tissue of origin and, thus, do not show the changes caused by degeneration or necrosis. Inflammatory cells, if present, are derived from the lesion itself and are not the result of a secondary inflammatory event. The sample is usually scanty and careful technical preparation is required to preserve the cellular material. The methods of smear preparation are described in Chapters 8 and 44.

Since fiberoptic instruments can also be used for tissue biopsies of lesions that can be visualized, one must justifiably ask why cytologic techniques are even used. Experience has shown, however, that brush specimens result in sampling of a wider area than biopsies. This is occasionally of clinical value, particularly in the absence of a specific lesion. Brushing and aspiration techniques also allow the sampling of submucosal lesions. A summary of the principal features of abrasive cytology is shown in Table 1-3.

Washing or Lavage Techniques

Washing techniques were initially developed as a direct offshoot of rigid endoscopic instruments. On the assumption that cells could be removed from their setting and collected in lavage fluid from lesions not accessible or not visible to the endoscopist, small amounts of normal saline or a similar solution were instilled into the target organ under visual control, aspirated, and collected in a small container. A pioneering effort by Herbut and Clerf in Philadelphia (1946)

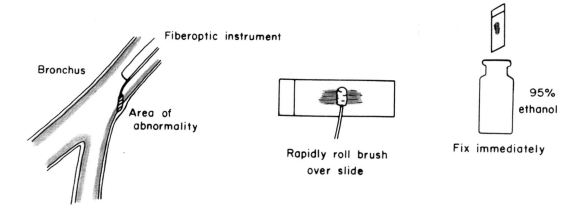

Figure 1-7 **Bronchial brushing under fiberoptic control.** Method of securing a brush sample from bronchus. Blue indicates bronchial epithelium.

TABLE 1-3

PRINCIPAL FEATURES OF ABRASIVE CYTOLOGY

- The method allows direct sampling of specific targets, such as the surface of the uterine cervix or a bronchus.
- With the use of fiberoptic instruments direct samples of accessible internal organs may be secured.
- The cells obtained by abrasive techniques are derived directly from the tissue and thus are better preserved than exfoliated cells and require different criteria for interpretation.
- Subepithelial lesions may be sampled by brushing or aspiration techniques.
- Care must be exercised to obtain technically optimal preparations.

defined the technique of bronchial washings for the diagnosis of lung cancer. The esophagus, colon, bladder, and occasionally other organs were also sampled in a similar fashion (see corresponding chapters).

With the development of flexible fiberoptic instruments, brushings largely replaced the washing techniques. However, several new lavage techniques were developed. The three principal techniques are the **peritoneal lavage** (described in Chap. 16), **bronchoalveolar lavage** (described in Chap. 19), and **lavage or barbotage of the urinary bladder** (described in Chaps. 22 and 23).

Because relatively large amounts of fluid are collected during these procedures, the samples cannot be processed by a direct smear technique. The cells have to be concentrated by centrifugation, filtering, or cell block techniques described in Chapter 44.

The principal targets of abrasive cytology, washings, and lavage are shown in Table 1-4.

Body Fluids

The cytologic study of body fluids is one of the oldest applications of cytologic techniques, first investigated in the latter half of the 19th century. The purpose is to determine the cause of fluid accumulation in body cavities, such as the pleura, pericardium (effusions), and the abdominal cavity (ascitic fluid). Primary or metastatic cancer and many infectious processes can be so identified (see Chaps. 25 and 26).

Other applications of this technique pertain to cerebrospinal fluid and other miscellaneous fluids, described in Chapter 27. The cell content of the fluid samples must be concentrated by centrifugation, sedimentation, or filtration as described in Chapter 44. The material is processed as smears, filter preparations, or cell block techniques.

Aspiration Cytology (FNA)

The technical principles of aspiration cytology are discussed in Chapter 28. The technique of aspiration of the

lung and mediastinum is discussed in Chapters 19 and 20. Organ-specific features are described in appropriate chapters. The principal features of the technique are summarized in Table 1-5.

Intraoperative Cytology

Intraoperative consultations by frozen sections are a very important aspect of practice in surgical pathology that is often guiding the surgeon's hand. Supplementing or replacing frozen sections by cytologic **touch, scrape, or crush preparations** has been in use in neuropathology for many years (Eisenhardt and Cushing, 1930; McMenemey, 1960; Roessler et al, 2002) (see Chap. 42) and more recently has been receiving increased attention in other areas of pathology as well (summary in Silverberg, 1995).

Methods

The smears are prepared by forcefully pressing a clean glass slide to the cut surface of the tissue. Good smears may also be obtained by scraping the cut surface of the biopsy with a small clean scalpel and preparing a smear(s) from the removed material. Crushing small fragments of tissue between two slides and pulling them apart is particularly useful in assessing lesions of the central nervous system where obtaining large tissue samples for frozen sections may be technically difficult, but may also be applied to other organs.

As with aspiration biopsy samples, the smears may be air-dried and stained with a rapid hematologic stain or fixed and stained with either Papanicolaou or hematoxylin and eosin, depending on the preference and experience of the pathologist. These techniques are described in greater detail in Chapters 28 and 44.

Applications

Intraoperative cytology is applicable to all organs and tissues. As examples, biopsies of the breast (Esteban et al, 1987), parathyroid (Sasano et al, 1988), uterine cervix (Anaastasiadis et al, 2002), and many other tissue targets (Oneson et al, 1989) may be studied. Recently, several communications evaluated the results of cytologic evaluation of **sentinel lymph nodes** in breast cancer (Viale et al, 1999; Llatjos et al, 2002; Creager et al, 2002a) and malignant melanoma (Creager et al, 2002b).

Advantages and Disadvantages

When compared with a frozen section, the smears are much **easier, faster, and cheaper** to prepare. Thus, the principal value of intraoperative cytology is a **rapid diagnosis.** Intraoperative cytology is of special value if the tissue **sample is very small and brittle** (as biopsies of the central nervous system) but sometimes of other organs, such as the pancreas, that are not suitable for freezing and cutting (Kontozoglou and Cramer, 1991; Scucchi et al, 1997; Blumenfeld et al, 1998).

The **interpretation** of smears is **identical to** that of material obtained by **aspiration biopsy, discussed in appropriate chapters.** As is true with other cytologic preparations,

TABLE 1-4

PRINCIPAL TARGETS OF ABRASIVE CYTOLOGY WASHINGS AND LAVAGE TECHNIQUES

Target Organ	Technique*	Principal Lesions to Be Identified	Incidental Benefits
Female Genital Tract			
Uterine cervix, vagina, vulva, endometrium	Scrape or brush; smear with immediate fixation in alcohol or spray fixative	Precancerous states and early, cancer and their differential diagnosis	Cancerous processes in other organs or the female genital tract may be identified (ovary, tube); identification of infectious processes (Chapters 12, 14, and 16)
Peritoneal fluid collection and washings	Fluid sample: collect in fixative	Residual or recurrent cancer of ovary, tube, endometrium, or cervix	(Chapter 16)
Respiratory Tract			
	Bronchial brushing; bronchial washings and lavage; bronchoalveolar lavage	Identification of precancerous states, lung cancer, and infections	Recognition of infectious agents; chemical and immunologic analysis of fluids in chronic fibrosing lung disease (Chapters 19 and 20)
Buccal Cavity and Adjacent Organs			
	Direct scrape smear; fixation as above	Identification of precancerous states and cancer	(Chapter 21)
Urinary Tract			
	Bladder washings or barbotage; processed fresh or fixed	Identification of carcinoma in situ and related lesions	Monitoring of effect of treatment; DNA analysis by flow cytometry or image analysis (Chapter 23)
Gastrointestinal Tract			
Esophagus	Brush or balloon smears; fixation as above	Identification of precancerous states (mainly carcinoma in situ and dysplasia), early cancer, or recurrent cancer after treatment	
Stomach	Brush, rarely balloon; smears, fixation as above		(Chapter 24)
Colon	Brush; smears, fixation as above	Monitoring of ulcerative colitis	
Bile ducts and pancreas	Aspiration of pancreatic juice (essentially obsolete); brushing	Diagnosis of cancer of the biliary tree and pancreas	

*Techniques of collection of cell samples in liquid media and processing by specially constructed machines or apparatuses are described in Chapter 44.

the interpretation of intraoperative smears requires training and experience. However, even in experienced hands, a correct diagnosis may be difficult or impossible if the target tissue contains only very small foci of cancer, which can only be identified by special techniques such as immunocytochemistry, as is the case in some sentinel lymph nodes.

By nearly unanimous consensus of the authors of numerous articles on this topic, **false-positive cancer diagnoses are very rare in experienced hands** (specificity approaches 100%), but **failures to recognize a malignant tumor are not uncommon.** The **sensitivity** and overall accuracy of the method are approximately 80% to 85%.

Clearly, in many cases of cancer, the intraoperative cytology will obviate the need for frozen sections and will replace frozen sections in special situations.

Application of Cytologic Techniques at the Autopsy Table

It is gratifying that several observers proposed the use of **cytologic techniques at the autopsy table,** as first described by Suen et al in 1976. The technique, based on touch preparations or needle aspiration of visible lesions, offers the option of a **rapid preliminary diagnosis** that may be of value to the clinicians and pathologists. Further, this approach is an **excellent teaching tool** of value in training house officers in cytology. Ample evidence has been provided that this simple and economical technique should be extensively used (Walker and Going, 1994; Survarna and Start, 1995; Cina and Smialek, 1997; Dada and Ansari, 1997).

TELECYTOLOGY

New developments in microscopy, image analysis, and image transmission by microwaves, telephone, or the Internet have generated the possibility of exchange of microscopic material among laboratories and the option of consultations with a distant colleague. The concept was applied to histopathology (summary in Weinstein et al, 1996, 1997)

and expanded to cytology (Raab et al, 1996; Briscoe et al, 2000; Allen et al, 2001; Alli et al, 2001).

As a **consultation system,** the method is particularly appealing for solo practitioners in remote areas who can benefit from another opinion offered by a large medical center in difficult cases. On an experimental basis, the system was applied to cervicovaginal smears (Raab et al, 1996), breast aspirates (Briscoe et al, 2000), and a variety of other types of specimens (Allen et al, 2001).

The accuracy of the system in reference to cervicovaginal smears was tested by Alli et al (2001) comparing the diagnoses established by several pathologists on glass slides and digital images. The diagnostic agreement in this study was low to moderate, although the levels of disagreement were relatively slight. Discrepancies were also reported in reference to other types of material (Allen et al, 2001).

Although theoretically very appealing and possibly useful in select situations such as the diagnosis of breast cancer in a patient in the Antarctica, cut off from access to medical facilities for 6 months a year, there are significant problems with telecytology. A smear contains thousands of images that should be reviewed before reaching a diagnostic verdict. Transmitting and receiving this large number of images is time consuming at both ends. Finding a suitable consultant who would be willing and able to spend hours reviewing microscopic images on a television screen would not be practical as a daily duty. Reservations about the use of preselected fields of view in diagnostic telecytology were also expressed by Mairinger and Geschwendter (1997).

On the other hand, **telecytology as a teaching tool** has already achieved much success and will continue to be a desirable addition to any teaching system.

THE ROLE OF CLINICIANS IN SECURING CYTOLOGIC SAMPLES

The quality of the cytologic diagnosis depends in equal measure on the excellence of the clinical procedure used to secure the sample, the laboratory procedures used to process the sample, and the skills and experience of the interpreter. The **clinical procedures** used to secure cytologic samples from various body sites and organ systems are discussed in appropriate chapters. The success and failure of the method often calls for close collaboration between the clinician and the cytopathologist. **Experience and training cannot be described in these pages except for outlining of a few basic principles:**

- **Familiarity with diagnostic options** available for the specific organ or organ system;
- **Securing in advance all instruments and materials** needed for the procedure;
- **If necessary or in doubt, a discussion between and among colleagues** to determine the optimal procedure, which may be of benefit to the patient.

The choice of methods depends on the type of information needed. Cancer detection procedures, for example, those used for detecting precursor lesions of carcinoma of the uterine cervix, have a different goal than diagnostic procedures required to establish the identity of a known lesion.

The issue of turf, that is, who is best qualified to perform the procedure, is often dictated by clinical circumstances. A skilled **endoscopist or interventional radiologist** cannot be replaced and must be thoroughly familiar with the optimal technique of securing diagnostic material. In many ways, the diagnostic cytologic sample is **similar to a biopsy** where the territories are well defined, that is, the clinician obtaining the sample for the pathologist to interpret. However, in diagnostic cytology, there are **gray areas,** such as the needle aspiration of palpable lesions (FNA), where special skills must be applied for the optimal benefit to the patient. In such situations, optimal training and experience should prevail (see Chap. 28).

In general, material for cytologic examination is obtained either as **direct smears,** prepared by the examining physician, gynecologist, surgeon, trained cytopathologist, or paramedical personnel from instruments used to secure the samples at the time of the clinical examination, or as **fluid specimens,** that are forwarded to the laboratory for further processing. Regardless of the method used, **it is essential for the clinician to provide accurate clinical and laboratory data** that are often extremely important in the interpretation of the material.

Of the two procedures, the preparation of smears is by far the more difficult.

Preparation of Smears

Smears can be prepared from material **obtained directly from target organs** by means of simple instruments (e.g., the uterine cervix) or **from brushes** used to sample hollow organs (e.g., the bronchi or organs of the gastrointestinal tract). For most diagnostic purposes, **well-prepared, well-fixed, and stained smears are easier to interpret than air-dried smears, which have different microscopic characteristics, unless the observer is trained in the interpretation of this type of material.** Still, many practitioners of **aspiration biopsies (FNAs),** particularly those who follow the Swedish school, favor **air-dried smears fixed in methanol and stained with hematologic stains** (see Chap. 28). In this book, every effort has been made to present the cytologic observations based on the two methods side-by-side.

It is important to place as much as possible of the material obtained on the slide and to prepare a **thin, uniform smear.** Thick smears with overlapping cell layers are difficult or impossible to interpret. Considerable skill and practice are required to prepare excellent smears by a single, swift motion without loss of material or air drying.

Preparation of **smears from small brushes used by endoscopists to investigate hollow organs may be particularly difficult.** A circular motion of the brush on the surface of the slide, while rotating the brush, may result in an adequate smear. Too much pressure on the brush may result

in **crushing of material.** If the person obtaining diagnostic material is not familiar with the technical requirements of smear preparation, competent help must be secured in advance. If none is available, the brushes can be **put into liquid fixative and forwarded to the laboratory for smear preparation.**

Except in situations in which the preparation of air-dried material is desirable (see above and Chap. 28), **immediate fixation of material facilitates correct interpretations.** Two types of fixatives are commonly used: **fluid fixatives and spray fixatives.** Both are described in detail in appropriate chapters and summarized in Chapter 44.

In addition to the customary commonly available fixatives, such as 95% alcohol, new commercial fixatives have become available. One such fixative is CytoRich Red (TriPath Corp., Burlington, NC) that has found many uses in the preparation of various types of smears. This fixative preserves cells of diagnostic value while lysing erythrocytes (see Chaps. 13 and 44 for further discussion of this fixative). In general fixation of smears, 15 minutes is more than adequate to provide optimal results. **Errors of patient identification or occurrence of "floaters," or free-floating cells, may cause serious diagnostic mishaps. If automated processing** of a cytologic sample is desired, the commercial companies provide vials with fixatives accommodating collection devices or cell samples. For further discussion of these options, see Chapters 8 and 44.

Spray fixatives provide another option. Their makeup and mode of use are described in detail in Chapter 44. When correctly used, spray fixatives protect the smears from drying by forming an invisible film on the surface of the slides. If spray fixatives are selected (and they usually are easier to handle than liquid fixatives), they should be applied **immediately** after the process of smear preparation has been completed. The use of spray fixative requires some manual dexterity, described in detail in the appendix to Chapter 8.

Collection of Fluid Specimens

Fluid specimens may be obtained from a variety of body sites, such as the respiratory tract, gastrointestinal tract, urinary tract, or effusions, and the clinical procedures used in their collection are described below. As is discussed in detail in Chapter 44, **unless the laboratory has the facilities for immediate processing of fluid specimens, it is advisable either to collect such specimens in bottles with fixative prepared in advance or to add the fixative shortly after collection. The common fixative of nearly universal applicability to fluids is 50% ethanol or a fixative containing 2% carbowax in 50% ethanol** (see Chap. 44). It is sometimes advisable to collect bloody fluids with the addition of **anticoagulants, such as heparin. Ether-containing fixatives should never be added to fluids.**

The volume of the fluid rarely need be larger than 100 ml. Screw cap bottles of 250-ml content, containing 50 ml of fixative, are suitable for most specimens. Generally, the volume of the fixative should be the same or slightly in excess of the volume of the fluid to be studied. **The fluids**

may be processed either as smears or cell blocks. The methods of preparation are described in Chapter 44.

BASIC PRINCIPLES OF THE INTERPRETATION AND REPORTING OF CYTOLOGIC SAMPLES

Diagnostic cytology is the **art and science** of the interpretation of cells from the human body that either exfoliate (desquamate) freely from the epithelial surfaces or are removed from tissue sources by various procedures, summarized above. The **cytologic diagnosis,** which is often more difficult than histologic diagnosis, **must be based on a synthesis of the entire evidence available,** rather than on changes in individual cells. If the cytologic material is adequate and the evidence is complete, a definitive diagnosis should be given.

Clinical data are as indispensable in cytologic diagnosis as they are in histologic diagnosis. Definitive cytologic diagnosis must be supported by all the clinical evidence available. Of the greatest possible importance in maintaining satisfactory results in diagnostic cytology is the **uniformity of the technical methods employed in each laboratory.** The cytologic diagnoses are frequently based on minute alterations of cytoplasmic and nuclear structure. These alterations may not be very significant, per se, unless one can be sure that variations due to the technique employed can be safely eliminated. However, as in any laboratory procedure, **situations may arise in which the evidence is too scanty for an opinion, and this fact must be reported appropriately.** The imposition of rigid reporting systems, such as the **Bethesda system** for reporting cervicovaginal material, summarized in Chapter 11, and found to be of value in securing epidemiologic or research data, may sometimes deprive the pathologist of diagnostic flexibility. These issues are discussed at length in reference to all organs and organ systems.

Before attempting the cytologic diagnosis of pathologic states, it is very important to acquire a **thorough knowledge of normal cells** originating from a given source. "Normal" includes variations in morphology caused by physiologic changes that depend on the organ of origin. Moreover, the cells may show a variety of morphologic changes that, in the absence of cancer, may result in substantial cellular abnormalities. Among these, one should mention primarily **inflammatory processes of various types; proliferative, metaplastic, degenerative, and benign neoplastic processes;** and, finally, **iatrogenic alterations** that occasionally may create a truly malicious confederacy of cellular changes set on misleading the examiner.

The understanding of the basic principles of cell structure and function, although perhaps not absolutely essential in the interpretation of light microscopic images, nevertheless adds a major dimension to the understanding of morphologic cell changes in health and disease. Furthermore, basic sciences have already been of value in the diagnosis of human disease. For these reasons, in the initial chapters of this book, there is a reasonably concise summary of some of the basic knowledge of cells and tissues.

QUALITY CONTROL

Much has been said lately about **quality control** in cytology. On the assumption that this branch of human pathology is practiced with the skill and technical expertise similar to that observed elsewhere in medicine today, **the best quality control is generated by the follow-up of patients.** Constant referral to tissue evidence and the clinical course of the disease and, if death intervenes, to the postmortem findings, are the only ways to secure one's knowledge. It is a pity that currently there is a pervasive tendency to regard a postmortem examination as a tedious and generally wasteful exercise. There is abundant evidence that, in spite of enormous technical progress, the **autopsy** still provides evidence of clinically unsuspected disease in a significant **percentage of patients. Diagnostic cytology must be conceived of and practiced as a branch of pathology and of medicine. Any other approach to this discipline is not beneficial to the patients.**

BIBLIOGRAPHY

Allen EA, Ollayos CW, Tellado MV, et al. Characteristics of a telecytology consultation service. Hum Pathol 32:1323–1326, 2001.

Alli PM, Ollayos CW, Thompson LD, et al. Telecytology: Intraobserver and interobserver reproducibility in the diagnosis of cervical-vaginal smears. Hum Pathol 32:1318–1322, 2001.

Anastasiadis PG, Romanidis KN, Polichronidis A, et al. The contribution of rapid intraoperative cytology to the improvement of ovarian cancer staging. Gynecol Oncol 86:244–249, 2002.

Ayre JE. Selective cytology smear for diagnosis of cancer. Am J Obstet Gynecol 53:609–617, 1947.

Ayre JE. A simple office test for uterine cancer diagnosis. Can Med Assoc J 51:17–22, 1944.

Babès A. Diagnostique du cancer utérin par les frottis. Presse Méd 36:451–454, 1928.

Beale LS. The Microscope and Its Application to Practical Medicine, 2nd ed. London, John Churchill, 1858.

Berg JW. The aspiration biopsy smear. In Koss LG. Diagnostic Cytology and Its Histopathologic Bases, 1st ed. Philadelphia, JB Lippincott, 1961.

Blumenfeld W, Hashmi N, Sagerman P. Comparison of aspiration, touch and scrape preparations simultaneously obtained from surgically excised specimens. Effect of different methods of smear preparation on interpretive cytologic features. Acta Cytol 42:1414–1418, 1998.

Bogdanich W. The Pap test misses much cervical cancer through laboratory errors. Wall Street J, p 1, Nov. 2, 1987.

Briscoe D, Adair CF, Thompson LD, et al. Telecytologic diagnosis of breast find needle aspiration biopsies. Acta Cytol 44:175–180, 2000.

Cina SJ, Smialek JE. Prospects for utilization and usefulness of postmortem cytology. Am J Forensic Med Pathol 18:331–334, 1997.

Crabbe JGS. Exfoliative cytologic control in occupational cancer of the bladder. Br Med J 2:1072–1074, 1952.

Creager AJ, Geisinger KR, Shiver SA, et al. Intraoperative evaluation of sentinel lymph nodes for metastatic breast carcinoma by imprint cytology. Mod Pathol 15:1140–1147, 2002a.

Creager AJ, Shiver SA, Shen P, et al. Intraoperative evaluation of sentinel lymph nodes for metastatic melanoma by imprint cytology. Cancer 94:3016–3022, 2002b.

Cullen TH. A rapid method of making permanent specimens from frozen sections by the use of formalin. Bull Johns Hopkins Hosp 6:67, 1895.

Dada MA, Ansari NA. Post-mortem cytology: A reappraisal of a little used technique. Cytopathology 8:417–420, 1997.

Donné AF. Cours de Microscopie Complémentaires des Etudes Medicales. Atlas execute d'après Nature au Microscope-Daguerreotype. Paris, Balliere, 1845.

Douglass LE. Odorico Viana and his contribution to diagnostic cytology. Acta Cytol 14:544–549, 1970.

Douglass LE. Further comment on the contribution of Aurel Babes to cytology and pathology. Acta Cytol 11:217–224, 1967.

Dudgeon LS, Wrigley CH. On demonstration of particles of malignant growth in the sputum by means of the wet film method. J Laryngol Otol 50:752–763, 1935.

Eisenhardt L, Cushing H. Diagnosis of intracranial tumors by supravital techniques. Am J Pathol 6:541–552, 1930.

Esposti PL, Franzen S, Zajicek J. The aspiration biopsy smear. *In* Koss LG (ed). Diagnostic Cytology and its Histopathologic Bases, ed 2. Philadelphia, JB Lippincott, 1968, pp 565–596.

Esteban JM, Zaloudek C, Silverberg SG. Intraoperative diagnosis of breast lesions. Comparison of cytologic with frozen section technics. Am J Clin Pathol 88:681–688, 1987.

Ferucci JT, Wittenberg J. Interventional Radiology of the Abdomen. Baltimore, Williams & Wilkins, 1981.

Fetherstone WC. False-negative cytology in invasive cancer of the cervix. Clin Obstet Gynecol 23:929–937, 1983.

Fox CH. Innovation in medical diagnosis. Lancet 1:1387–1388, 1979.

Frable WJ. Needle aspiration biopsy. Past, present, and future. Hum Pathol 20: 504–517, 1989.

Franzén S, Giertz G, Zajicek J. Cytologic diagnosis of prostatic tumours by transrectal aspiration biopsy. A preliminary report. Br J Urol 32:193–196, 1960.

Fremont-Smith M, Graham RM, Meigs JV. Vaginal smears as an aid in the diagnosis of early carcinoma of the cervix. N Engl J Med 237:302–304, 1947.

Godwin JT. Aspiration biopsy: Technique and application. Ann NY Acad Sci 63:1348–1373, 1956.

Greig EDW, Gray ACH. Note on the lymphatic glands in sleeping sickness. Lancet 1:1570, 1904.

Grunze H, Spriggs A. History of Clinical Cytology: A Selection of Documents, 2nd ed. Darmstadt, E Giebeler Verlag, 1983.

Herbut PA, Clerf LH. Bronchogenic carcinoma; diagnosis by cytologic study of bronchoscopically removed secretions. JAMA 130:1006–1012, 1946.

Hirschfeld H. Bericht ueber einige histologischmikroskopische und experimentelle Arbeiten bei den boesartigen Geschwuelsten. Z Krebsforsch 16:33–39, 1919.

Hirschfeld H. Ueber isolierte aleukaemische Lymphadenose der Haut. Z Krebsforsch 11:397–407, 1912.

Hooke R. Micrographia. London, Jo. Martin and Ja. Allestry, 1665.

Jones CA, Neustaedter T, MacKenzie LL. The value of vaginal smears in the diagnosis of early malignancy; preliminary report. Am J Obstet Gynecol 49: 159–168, 1945.

Kamholz SL, Pinsker KL, Johnson J, Schreiber K. Fine needle aspiration biopsy of intrathoracic lesions. NY State J Med 82:736–739, 1982.

Kline TS. Aspiration Biopsy Cytology, ed 2. New York, Churchill Livingstone, 1988.

Kontozoglou TE, Cramer HM. The advantages of intraoperative cytology: Analysis of 215 smears and review of the literature. Acta Cytol 35:154–164, 1991.

Koss LG. Cervical (Pap) smear: New directions. Cancer 71:1406–1412, 1993.

Koss LG. Diagnostic Cytology and Its Histopathologic Bases, 4th ed. Philadelphia, JB Lippincott, 1992.

Koss LG. The Papanicolaou test for cervical cancer detection: A triumph and a tragedy. JAMA 261:737–743, 1989.

Koss LG. Aspiration biopsy: A tool in surgical pathology. Am J Surg Pathol 12(Suppl 1):43–53, 1988.

Koss LG. On the history of cytology (editorial). Acta Cytol 24:475–477, 1980.

Koss LG. Thin needle aspiration biopsy (editorial). Acta Cytol 24:1–3, 1980.

Koss LG, Gompel C. Introduction to Gynecologic Cytopathology with Histologic and Clinical Correlations. Baltimore, Williams & Wilkins, 1999.

Koss LG, Lieberman PH. Surgical pathology at Memorial Sloan-Kettering Cancer Center. *In* Rosai J (ed). Guiding the Surgeon's Hand. The History of American Surgical Pathology. Washington DC, The American Registry of Pathology, Armed Forces Institute of Pathology 1997.

Koss LG, Woyke S, Olszewski W. Aspiration Biopsy: Cytologic Interpretation and Histologic Bases, 2nd ed. New York, Igaku-Shoin, 1992.

Kün M. New instrument for the diagnosis of tumors. Mon J Med Sci 7:853–854, 1847.

Lebert H. Trait Pratique des Maladies Cancereuses et des Affections Curables Confundues avec le Cancer. Paris, JB Balliere, 1851.

Lebert H. Physiologie Pathologique Recherches Cliniques, Expérimentales et Microscopiques. Paris, JB Baillière, 1845.

Linsk JA, Franzén S. Clinical Aspiration Cytology, 2nd ed. Philadelphia, JB Lippincott, 1989.

Ljung B-M, Drejet A, Chiampi N, et al. Diagnostic accuracy of fine-needle aspiration biopsy is determined by physician training in sampling technique. Cancer Cytopathol 93:263–268, 2001.

Llatjos M, Castella E, Fraile M, et al. Intraoperative assessment of sentinel lymph nodes in patients with breast carcinoma: Accuracy of rapid imprint cytology compared with definitive histologic workup. Cancer 96:150–156, 2002.

Lombard HL, Middleton M, Warren S, Gates O. Use of vaginal smear as a screening test. N Engl J Med 239:317–321, 1948.

Lopes-Cardozo P. Clinical Cytology using the May-Grünwald-Giemsa Stained Smear. Leyden, L Staflen, 1954.

Löwhagen T, Willems J-S. Aspiration biopsy cytology in diseases of the thyroid. *In* Koss LG, Coleman DV (eds). Advances in Clinical Cytology. London, Butterworth, 1981, pp 201–231.

Mairinger T, Geschwendter A. Telecytology using preselected fields of view: The future of cytodiagnosis or a dead end? Am J Clin Pathol 107:620–621, 1997.

Martin HE, Ellis EB. Aspiration biopsy. Surg Gynecol Obstet 59:578–589, 1934.

Martin HE, Ellis EB. Biopsy by needle puncture and aspiration. Ann Surg 92: 169–181, 1930.

McMenemey WH. An appraisal of smear-diagnosis in neurosurgery. Am J Clin Pathol 33:471–479, 1960.

Meigs JV, Graham RM, Fremont-Smith M, et al. The value of vaginal smear in the diagnosis of uterine cancer: Report of 1015 cases. Surg Gynecol Obstet 81:337–345, 1945.

Müller J. On the Nature and Structural Characteristics of Cancer and Those Morbid Growth Which May Be Confounded With It (Translated from the 1838 German edition by C. West). London, Sherwood, Gilbert & Piper, 1840.

Nezelof C. Biopsy: A recent term. Newsletter of the History of Pathology Society, August 2000.

Nieburgs HE, Pund ER. Detection of cancer of the cervix uteri: Evaluation of comparative cytologic diagnosis: A study of 10,000 cases. JAMA 142: 221–225, 1950.

Oneson RH, Minke JA, Silverberg SG. Intraoperative pathologic consultation: An audit of 1,000 recent consecutive cases. Am J Surg Pathol 13:237–243, 1989.

Paget J. Lectures on Tumours. London, Longman, 1853.

Panico FG, Papanicolaou GN, Cooper WA. Abrasive balloon for exfoliation of gastric cells. JAMA 143:1308–1311, 1950.

Papanicolaou GN. Atlas of Exfoliative Cytology. Cambridge, MA, Harvard University Press, 1953; Suppl 1, 1956; Suppl 2, 1960.

Papanicolaou GN. New cancer diagnosis. *In* Proceedings 3rd Race Betterment Conference. Battle Creek, Michigan, Race Betterment Foundation, 1928, p 528.

Papanicolaou GN, Traut HF. Diagnosis of Uterine Cancer by the Vaginal Smear. New York, Commonwealth Fund, 1943.

Papanicolaou GN, Traut HF. The diagnostic value of vaginal smears in carcinoma of the uterus. Am J Obstet Gynecol 42:193–206, 1941.

Pouchet FA. Théorie Positive de l'Ovulation Spontanée et de la Fécondation des Mammifères et de l'Espèce Humaine Basée sur l'Observation de toute la Série. Atlas. Paris, Baillière, 1847.

Purtle H. History of microscopy. *In* The Billings Microscope Collection, ed 2. Washington DC, The Armed Forces Institute of Pathology 1974.

Raab SS, Zaleski MS, Thomas PA, et al. Telecytology: Diagnostic accuracy in cervical-vaginal smears. Am J Clin Pathol 105:599–603, 1996.

Rather LJ. The Genesis of Cancer: A Study in the History of Ideas. Baltimore, Johns Hopkins University Press, 1978.

Reagan JW. The cytological recognition of carcinoma in situ. Cancer 4:255–260, 1951.

Roessler K, Dietrich W, Kitz K. High diagnostic accuracy of cytologic smears of central nervous system tumors: A 15-year experience based on 4,172 patients. Acta Cytol 46:667–674, 2002.

Rubin IC. Pathological diagnosis of incipient carcinoma of uterus. Am J Obstet 62:668–676, 1910.

Ruge C, Veit J. Anatomische Bedeutung der Erosionen an dem Scheidentheil. Centralbl f. Gynaekologie, 1:17–19, 1877.

Rylander E. Cervical cancer in women belonging to a cytologically screened population. Acta Obstet Gynecol Scand 55:361–366, 1976.

Sasano H, Geelhoed GW, Silverberg SG. Intraoperative cytologic evaluation of lipid in the diagnosis of parathyroid adenoma. Am J Surg Pathol 12: 282–286, 1988.

Schade ROK. Cytological diagnosis of gastric carcinoma. Gastroenterologia 85: 190–194, 1956.

Scucchi LF, Di Stefano D, Cosentino L, Vecchione A. Value of cytology as an adjunctive intraoperative diagnostic method. An audit of 2,250 consecutive cases. Acta Cytol 41:1489–1496, 1997.

Silverberg SG. Intraoperative cytology: Promise, practice, and problems. Diagn Cytopathol 13:386–387, 1995.

Söderström N. Thin needle aspiration biopsy. Letter to the editor. Acta Cytol 24:468, 1980.

Söderström N. Fine-Needle Aspiration Biopsy: Used as a Direct Adjunct in Clinical Diagnostic Work. Stockholm, Almqvist & Wiksell, 1966.

Stewart FW. The diagnosis of tumors by aspiration. Am J Pathol 9:801–812, 1933.

Suen KC, Yermakov V, Raudales O. The use of imprint technic for rapid diagnosis in postmortem examinations: A diagnostically rewarding procedure. Am J Clin Pathol 65:291–300, 1976.

Survarna SK, Start RD. Cytodiagnosis and the necropsy. J Clin Pathol 48: 443–446, 1995.

Thiersch C. Der Epithelialkrebs namentlich der Haut. Leipzig, W Engelmann, 1865.

Van Leeuwenhoek A. Letters to the Royal Society. Philos Trans R Soc Lond 9:121, 1674; 12:1040, 1679; 22:552, 1702.

Viale G, Bosari S, Mazzarol G, et al. Intraoperative examination of axillary sentinel lymph nodes in breast carcinoma patients. Cancer 85:2433–2438, 1999.

Virchow R. Die Krankhaften Geschwuelste. Berlin, August Hirschwald, 1863.

Virchow R. Die Cellularpathologie in ihrer Begruendung auf physiologische und pathologiscge Gewebelehre. Berlin, August Hirschwald, 1858.

Walker E, Going JJ. Cytopathology in the post-mortem room. J Clin Pathol 47: 714–717, 1994.

Wandall HH. A study on neoplastic cells in sputum as a contribution to the diagnosis of primary lung cancer. Acta Chir Scand 91(Suppl 93):1–43, 1944.

Webb AJ. Early microscopy: History of fine needle aspiration (FNA) with particular reference to goitres. Cytopathology 12:1–6, 2001.

Webb AJ. Through a glass darkly (the development of needle aspiration biopsy). Bristol Med Chir J 89:59–68, 1974.

Weinstein RS. Static image telepathology in perspective. Hum Pathol 27: 99–101, 1996.

Weinstein RS, Bhattachryya AK, Graham AR, et al. Telepathology: A ten-year progress report. Hum Pathol 28:1–7, 1997.

Woolner LB, McDonald JR. Diagnosis of carcinoma of lung: Value of cytologic study of sputum and bronchial secretions. JAMA 139:497–502, 1949.

Wright JR Jr. The development of frozen section technique, the evolution of surgical biopsy, and the origins of surgical pathology. Bull Hist Med 59: 295–326, 1985.

Zajicek J. The aspiration biopsy smear. *In* Koss LG (ed). Diagnostic Cytology and its Histopathologic Bases, 3rd ed. Philadelphia, JB Lippincott, 1979, pp 1001–1104.

Zajicek J. Aspiration Biopsy Cytology. Part 1. Cytology of Supradiaphragmatic Organs. Basel, S Karger, 1974.

Zajicek J. Aspiration Biopsy Cytology. Part 2. Cytology of Infradiaphragmatic Organs. Basel, S Karger, 1979.

Zornoza J. Percutaneous Needle Biopsy. Baltimore, Williams & Wilkins, 1981.

The Basic Structure of the Mammalian Cell

2

A cell is a self-contained fundamental unit of life. All cells are tridimensional, space-occupying structures, although when spread on a glass slide and viewed through the light microscope, they appear to be flat. Each mammalian cell has **three essential components: cell membrane, cytoplasm, and nucleus** (Fig. 2-1 and see Frontispiece and Fig. 3-1). The cell membrane encloses the transparent cytoplasm. Within the cytoplasm, enclosed in its own membrane or envelope, there is a smaller, approximately spherical dense structure—the nucleus. **The nucleus is the principal repository of deoxyribonucleic acid (DNA),** the molecule governing the genetic and functional aspects of cell activity (see Chap. 3). Although some mammalian cells, such as erythrocytes or squamous cells, may lose their nucleus in the final stages of their life cycle, even these final events are programmed by their DNA. **All nucleated cells are classified as eukaryotic cells (from Greek, *karion* = kernel, nucleus) in contrast with primitive cells, such as bacteria, wherein the DNA is present in the cytoplasm but is not enclosed by a membrane as a distinct nuclear structure (prokaryotic cells).** Many of the fundamental discoveries pertaining to the molecular biology of cells were made in prokaryotic cells, documenting that all basic biochemical manifestations of life have a common origin. Families of cells differ from each other by their structural features (morphology) and by their activities, all programmed by DNA. The recognition of these cell types and their alterations in health and disease is the principal task of diagnostic cytology. ***All cells share the fundamental structural components*** that will be described in these pages.

MICROSCOPIC TECHNIQUES USED IN EXAMINATION OF CELLS

Cells can be examined by a variety of techniques, ranging from the commonly used light and electron microscopy to newer techniques of confocal and digital microscopy. Additional information on cell structure, derivation, and function can be obtained by immunocytochemistry and by in situ hybridization of cell components. The techniques required for special procedures will be described in the appropriate chapters. This brief summary will serve as an introduction to the description of the fundamental structure of the cell.

Light Microscopy

Bright-Field Light Microscopy
Bright-field light microscopes are optical instruments that allow the examination of cells at magnifications varying from 1× to 2,000×, using an appropriate combination of lenses. The highest resolution of the commonly used light microscopes, that is, the ability of the instruments to visualize the smallest objects, is limited by the wavelength of the visible spectrum of light, which is about 0.5 μm. The principles of bright-field light microscopy have been described in numerous books and manuals and need not be repeated here. It is assumed that the readers have a working knowledge of these instruments. Suffice it to say that the **quality of the optics used, skill in the adjustment of the illumination, and the depth of the microscope's focus are essen-**

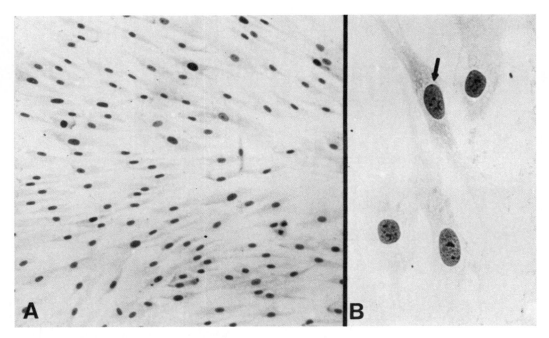

Figure 2-1   Benign human fibroblasts from a female patient in tissue culture. *A.* Low-power view shows the relationship of the cells, which do not overlap each other. *B.* High-power view shows delicate cytoplasm, generally oval or round nuclei with small multiple nucleoli. Sex chromatin indicated by arrow (*A:* ×250; *B:* ×1,000) (Alcohol fixation, Papanicolaou stain. Culture by Dr. Fritz Herz, Montefiore Hospital. From Koss LG. Morphology of cancer cells. *In* Handbuch der allgemeinen Pathologie, vol. 6, Tumors, part I. Berlin, Springer, 1974, pp 1–139.)

tial in evaluating the cellular preparations. In practice of clinical cytology, bright-field microscopy satisfies nearly all requirements for the diagnostic assessment of cells. The same technique is used in assessing the results of special stains and of immunocytochemistry.

Preparation of Cells for Bright-Field Light
Microscopic Examination

The cells are usually prepared for a light microscopic examination in the form of **direct smears** on commercially available glass slides of predetermined thickness and optical quality. Samples of cells suspended in fluid may be placed on glass slides by means of a special centrifuge, known as a **cytocentrifuge,** or a similar apparatus. A cell suspension may also be **filtered across a porous membrane.** The cells deposited on the surface of such membranes may either be examined directly or may be placed on glass slides by a process of **reverse filtration.** Cell samples may also be studied in histologic-type sections, after embedding of the sediment in paraffin (a technique known as the **cell block).** For details of these techniques, see Chapter 44.

Fixation.   Fixation of cell preparations is a common procedure having for its purpose the best possible **preservation of cell components** after removal from the tissue of origin. A variety of fixatives may serve this purpose, all described in Chapter 44. However, diagnostic techniques may also be based on **air-dried cell preparations, either unfixed or postfixed in methanol,** which introduce a number of use-

ful artifacts. Such techniques are used in hematology and in aspiration biopsy samples.

Staining.   Optimal results in bright-field microscopy are obtained on stained preparations that provide visible contrast and discrimination among the cell components. A variety of stains, described in Chapter 44, can be used to best demonstrate various cell components. Common stain combinations use hematoxylin and its variants as the nuclear stain and eosin or its many variants as the cytoplasmic stain. Examples of stains of this type include the **hematoxylin-eosin stain** and the **Papanicolaou stain,** which allow for a good visualization of the principal components of the cell, by contrasting the nucleus and the cytoplasm. Other stains in common use include methylene blue, toluidine blue, and **Giemsa colorant** that provide less contrast among cell components but have the advantage of rapidity of use. An example of cells fixed in alcohol and stained by the Papanicolaou method is shown in Figure 2-4.

Phase-Contrast Microscopy

Phase-contrast microscopy utilizes **the difference in light diffraction** among the various cell components and special optics that allow the visualization of components of **unstained cells.** The **Nomarski technique** is a variant of phase contrast microscopy that is particularly useful in the **study of cell surfaces.** Either technique may be applied to the study of **living cells** in suspension or culture and, when coupled with time-lapse cinematography or a television system, may provide a continuous record of cell movements and behavior. These techniques are particularly useful in experimental systems, as they may document the differences in cell behavior under various circumstances, for example, after treatment of cultured cells with a drug or during a genetic manipulation. The systems also allow the study of events, such as **movement of chromosomes during cell division,** or mitosis. An example of the application of the Nomarski technique to a cell culture is shown in Figure 2-2 .

Fluorescent Microscopy

Cells or cell components stained with fluorescent compounds or **probes** can be visualized with the help of microscopes provided with special lenses and a **source of fluorescent light,** such as a mercury bulb or a laser, tuned to an appropriate wavelength, exciting fluorescence of the probe. In highly specialized commercial systems, the amount of fluorescence can be measured in individual cells or families of cells, and may serve to quantify various cell components. A somewhat similar system is used in **flow cytometry** (see

Chap. 47). Fluorescence microscopy is particularly valuable in the procedures known as **in situ hybridization,** with the purpose of documenting the presence of chromosomes, chromosomal aberrations, or individual genes (see Fig. 2-31 and Figs. 4-26, 4-27, and 4-29). Fluorescent microscopy is also useful in identifying certain **components of cell cytoplasms or cell membranes,** using specific antibodies. Application of fluorescent microscopy and other techniques to the study of **living cells** was summarized in a series of articles on biologic imaging in the journal, *Science*, 2003.

Confocal Microscopy

Using a system of complex optics and a laser, the technique, combined with phase and fluorescent microscopy in complex and costly instruments, allows the **visualization of cells and tissues in slices,** separated from each other by approximately 1 μm. The images of the slices can be combined on a computer to give a three-dimensional picture of the cell or tissue and their components. This technique is applicable to individual cells or cell clusters that can be examined layer-by-layer.

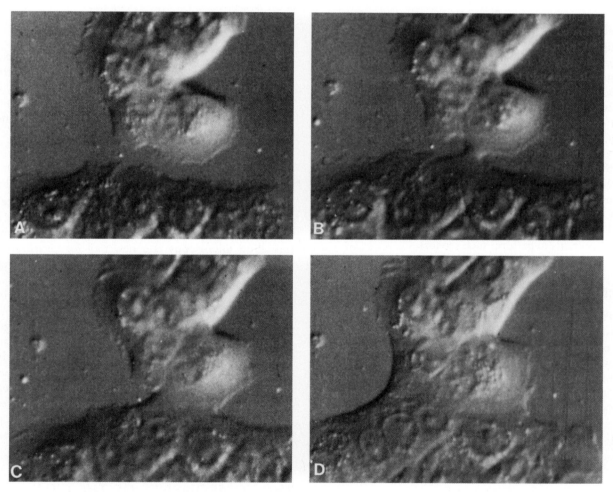

Figure 2-2   Time-lapse cinematography, using Nomarski interference contrast optics, shows events in the merging of two colonies of cultured human cancer cells, line C41. (In this technique the cell nuclei are seen in the form of craters wherein are located the nucleoli shown as small elevations.) *A.* Beginning of sequence: two adjacent colonies. *B.* Sixteen minutes later: a cytoplasmic bridge between the two colonies has been established. *C.* Twenty-six minutes later: the area of merger has increased in size. *D.* Ninety-five minutes later: the merger has progressed to the point at which several cells in both colonies are fused. (Courtesy of Dr. Robert Wolley, Montefiore Hospital.)

Digital Microscopy

With the wide availability of sophisticated computers, it has become possible to **transform cell images into digits, that is, numerical values.** The images are recorded by television or digital cameras, transformed into numerical values and stored in the computers' memory, on videotape, or on a videodisc. The original images can be reconstituted when needed. Such images, often of outstanding quality, can be manipulated with the help of special software. Images from several different sources can be assembled into plates suitable for publications or special displays. The colors of the displays can be adjusted for optimal quality of images. Many new plates in this book have been prepared with this technique. Digital microscopy can also be applied to electron microscopic images (Shotton, 1995).

Digital microscopy has been extensively applied in **analytical and quantitative studies of cells and cell components.** These techniques allow discrimination among families of cells of similar appearance but different biologic or clinical significance. They can also be applied to a variety of **measurements of cell components, such as DNA,** as discussed in Chapter 46. Variants of these techniques have been used in commercial instruments for automated or semiautomated analysis of cell populations.

Digital microscopy is suitable for direct transmission of images via cable or satellites to remote locations **(telepathology or telecytology)** for **teaching or diagnostic purposes,** as discussed in Chapters 1 and 46. Demonstration projects of this technology have documented that such images are of good quality when examined at the receiving stations. The images can be studied under variable magnification factors, thus allowing for diagnostic opinions. Transmissions of images by Internet have been extensively used for teaching. It is conceivable that, in the future, central telepathology consultation centers will be established to advise pathologists on difficult cases. At present, the systems are limited by cost, the speed of transmission, and by the availability of knowledgeable consultants to perform such services.

Electron Microscopy

Transmission Electron Microscopy

Transmission electron microscopic technique utilizes certain **optical properties of a fixed beam of electrons** to illuminate the object. The images are captured on photographic plates. Extremely thin sections of tissues or cells (50 to 100 nm) and staining with heavy metals are required. Special fixation and embedding techniques must be used. The method allows a unique insight into the fine structure of the cell. Most of the images in this chapter were obtained by this technique.

Scanning Electron Microscopy

In the commonly used mode, the scanning electron microscopy technique utilizes a **rapidly moving beam of electrons to scan the surface of cells** or other objects. The cells are dehydrated, fixed, and coated with a thin metallic layer, usually of gold and palladium. The metal forms an exact

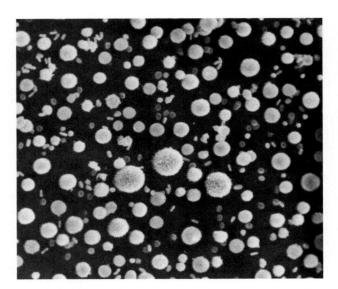

Figure 2-3 **Scanning electron microscope view of cells in pleural effusion.** The small doughnut-like cells are erythrocytes, the large chestnut-like cells are cancer cells. Intermediate-sized cells are macrophages, mesothelial cells, and leukocytes. The surfaces of the large cancer cells are covered by microvilli. (×300.) (Courtesy of Dr. W. Domagala, Montefiore Hospital.)

replica of the cell surface. The beam of electrons glides over the metallic surface, and the reflected electrons form an image that may be registered on a photographic plate (Fig. 2-3) or on a fluorescent screen. Scanning electron microscopy is also applicable to the **freeze-fracture technique,** described below.

Other Techniques

Several other special techniques, such as **interference microscopy** and **x-ray diffraction microscopy,** have been used for a variety of investigative purposes. **Scanning-tunneling microscopy** is a new tool for visualization of surfaces of molecules such as DNA. This technique has no applications to diagnostic cytology.

Magnetic resonance, a technique widely used in imaging of the human body **(MRI),** is applicable to the study of tissues in vitro and to histologic sections as **magnetic resonance microscopy** (Huesgen et al, 1993; Sbarbati and Osculati, 1996; Johnson et al, 1997). The technique is based on magnetic gradients that produce a shift in hydrogen ions' alignment in water content of the living tissues, creating images that can be captured by computer and recorded on a photographic plate. Because of its low resolution, the practical value of this technique remains to be determined.

THE COMPONENTS OF THE CELL

The components of the cell will be described under three main headings: **the cell membrane, the cytoplasm, and the nucleus** (see Frontispiece). Whenever possible, the description will comprise light and electron microscopic observations. The purely morphologic description has limited bearing on the intimate biochemical interrelationship of the cell components. The reader is referred to Chapter 3 and the appended references for further information.

The Cell Membrane

The cell membrane is the outer boundary of the cell, **facilitating and limiting the exchange of substances between the cell and its environment.** In light microscopy, the membrane of well-fixed mammalian cells cannot be seen. The cell's periphery appears as a thin condensation (Fig. 2-4).

In transmission electron microscopy, the cell membrane appears as a well-defined line measuring approximately 75 Å in width (Fig. 2-5). **The membrane is composed of three layers,** each about 25 Å thick (see Frontispiece and Fig. 2-18). The inner and the outer dense (electronopaque) layers are separated by a somewhat wider lucent central layer. Similarly constructed membrane systems are observed in a variety of intracytoplasmic components within the cell, such as the mitochondria and the endoplasmic reticulum (see below). The term **unit membrane** is often used in reference to cell membranes in general.

Davson and Danielli (1952) proposed that the plasma membrane is composed of a double lipid layer coated by polypeptide chains of protein molecules. This concept was acceptable so long as it readily explained certain physicochemical characteristics (semipermeability) of cell membranes. However, it has become evident that the cell membrane, far from being a passive envelope of cell contents, plays a critical role in virtually every aspect of cell function. Thus, **the cell membrane regulates the internal environment of the cell, participates actively in recognition of the external environment and in transport of substances to and from the cell, determines the immunologic**

makeup of the cells, and accounts for the interrelationship of cells.

The initial insight into the makeup and function of the cell membrane was based on the study of erythrocytes. Their membrane is made up of a **double layer (bilayer) of lipids,** formed by molecules provided with chains of fatty acids. The lipid molecules have one water-soluble (or hydrophilic) end and a water-insoluble (or hydrophobic) end. In the cell membrane, the electrically charged hydrophilic ends of the lipid molecules form the inner and the outer surfaces of the cell membrane, whereas the uncharged, hydrophobic chains of fatty acids are directed toward the center of the cell membrane, away from the two surfaces. Cholesterol molecules add structural rigidity to the cell membrane. Protein molecules of various sizes, functions, and configurations are located within the lipid bilayer **(integral proteins)** but also extend beyond the cell membrane, either to the outside or to the inside of the cell or both. Such **transmembrane proteins** provide communication between the cell environment and cell interior. The number, makeup, position, and mobility of the protein molecules account for specific, individual properties of cells and tissues by forming specific receptor molecules. Cell membranes are further characterized by molecules of carbohydrates that attach either to the lipids (glycolipids) or to the proteins (glycoproteins) and which are the repository of the immunologic characteristics of the cell.

On the inner (cytoplasmic) aspect of the cell membrane, other protein molecules have been identified **(peripheral proteins).** Their function appears to be structural in **maintaining the integrity of the cell membrane and in providing communication between the cell membrane and the interior of the cell** (Fig. 2-6).

This complex asymmetric structure of the cell membrane cannot be demonstrated by conventional electron micros-

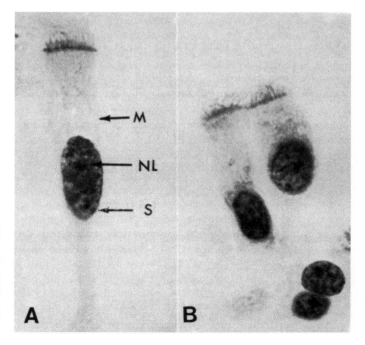

Figure 2-4 Human bronchial cells, oil immersion. *A.* The focus was on the region of the cell membrane (M) and the nucleus. Within the latter there is a single nucleolus (NL) and several chromocenters. A sex chromatin body (S) adherent to the nuclear membrane may be observed. In this photograph the cilia appear to be anchored in a thick portion of the cytoplasm or a terminal plate. *B.* The focus was on cilia and their points of attachment within the cell. These are dense granules or basal corpuscles. The basal corpuscles form the so-called terminal plate.

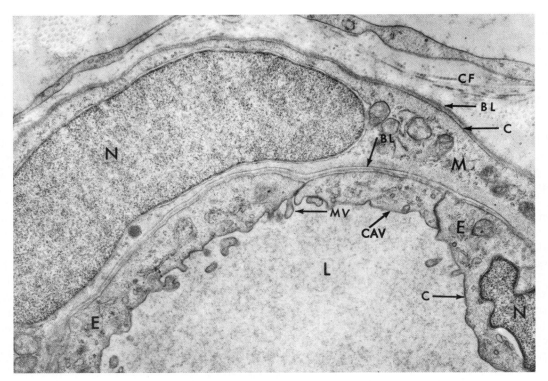

Figure 2-5   Electron micrograph of a segment of an arteriole. L = lumen, E = endothelial cells, M = smooth muscle cell, N = nucleus. Caveolae (CAV) and microvilli (MV) are evident in the endothelial cell. C = cell membrane; CF = collagen fibers with characteristic periodicity. Basement laminae (membranes) (BL) separate the endothelial cells from the muscle cells and the muscle cells from the connective tissue. (×16,000.)

copy. Therefore, to study the problem, special techniques have been applied, such as freeze-fracture. The **freeze-fracture technique** consists of three steps: very rapid freezing of cells and tissues, fracturing the tissue with an instrument, and preparation of a metal replica of the fractured surface that can be examined in the scanning electron microscope. It has been determined that the fracture lines are not distributed in a haphazard fashion but, rather, run along certain predetermined planes.

Freeze-fracture of cell membranes disclosed **two surfaces** that, by agreement, have been named the **P face** and **E face** (Fig. 2-7). The P face represents the inner aspect of the cell membrane and contains numerous protruding protein particles. The E face represents the outer part of the cell membrane, which is relatively smooth, except for pits corresponding to the protein particles attached to the P face. A few protein particles usually remain attached to the E face. The density and distribution of the protein particles varies from cell type to cell type and may be substantially modified by immunologic and chemical methods, indicating that the position of these particles within the cell membrane is not fixed. Thus, **the cell membrane is now thought to be a fluid-mosaic membrane,** as first proposed by Singer and Nicholson (1972). It may be conceived as a viscous structure that can adapt itself to changing needs and conditions by being permissive to movements of large molecules, such as protein particles. Fixation of cells solidifies the membrane. The freeze-fracture images represent only snapshots of the position of the protein particles at the time of fixation.

The freeze-fracture technique may also be used to study the structure of cell junctions (see Fig. 2-16) and the interior of other cell membranes, such as the nuclear envelope (see Fig. 2-27).

The **basic structure of intracellular membranes,** such as those composing the endoplasmic reticulum or mitochondria, appears to be **essentially similar to that of the cell membrane,** but differs in lipid/protein ratios and associated proteins and enzymes, reflecting the diversity of functions.

Cytoplasmic Interactions

Extensive work has been performed in recent years to establish links between the cell membrane and the cytoplasm. It is quite evident that this must be a very intimate association, as cell function depends on signals and nutrients received through the cell membrane. Also, the export of substances manufactured by the cell (or products of cell metabolism) must be regulated by interaction between the cytoplasm and the cell membrane.

Molecular biologic investigations of recent years have identified numerous protein molecules that contribute to the function of the cell membrane as a flexible link between the environment and the interior of the cell. Each one of these molecules interacts with other molecules and theseinteractions are growing increasingly complex. So far, only

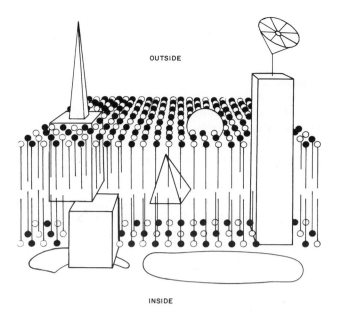

Figure 2-6 Schematic representation of the current concepts of cell membrane. The membrane is made up of two layers of lipids (*pins*), with points directed toward the center (uncharged hydrophobic ends) and pinheads (electrically charged hydrophilic ends) toward the two surfaces. The *black pinheads* indicate molecules of cholesterol, which add rigidity to the cell membrane. Integral protein molecules, represented by geometric figures of various shapes, are located within the bilipid layer, but also protrude from both surfaces. Symbolic representation of an emitting and receiving (dish) antennae show the cell's communications with its environment. On the inner aspect of the cell membrane, peripheral proteins (spectrin, actin) have been identified. These probably lend structural support to the membrane and provide communication between the cell membrane and the cytoplasm.

small fragments of this knowledge have emerged. At the time of this writing (2004), no clear, cohesive picture has been formulated to explain how the cell membrane functions. Suffice it to say that there is good evidence that the cell membrane plays an important role in virtually every aspect of cell function in health and disease. Luna and Hitt (1992) discussed the **interaction between the cell skeleton and cell membrane as one example** of these interactions. Among the components of the cell skeleton that interact with the cell membrane are the intermediate filaments and tubules, described further on in this chapter.

The cell membrane is also the site of molecules that define the immunologic features of the cell. For example,

the clusters of differentiation (CD) and blood group antigens discussed elsewhere in this book, are located on the cell membranes.

Coated Pits, Vesicles, and Caveolae: Mechanisms of Import and Export

Import, export, and transport of a variety of molecules within the cytoplasm takes place through pits and vesicles formed by invagination of cellular membranes. The largest of such vesicles observed on cell surfaces are known as **pinocytotic vesicles.** The pits and vesicles are coated by molecules of a complex protein, **clathrin,** which appears to be present in all cells. Clathrin is composed of three heavy and three light protein chains that form the scaffolds of the coats. Clathrin requires the cooperation of other proteins known as *adaptors* to fulfill its many functions, which include **capturing, sorting, and transporting molecules.** The molecular mechanisms of endocytosis have been extensively studied (Gillooly and Stemark, 2001). It may be assumed that each pit or vesicle is provided with specific receptors to a molecule or molecules of importance to the cell, and that it will recognize and selectively capture this molecule or molecules from thousands of molecules circulating within the fluid bathing the cell. Once the selected substance is captured, the vesicle closes and sinks into the cytoplasm to deliver its cargo to its appropriate destination. However, nature is extremely economical, and there is excellent evidence that the fragment of cell membrane that is used to form a vesicle is recirculated and returned to the surface in a different location to serve again. A similar mechanism is observed in removal or **phagocytosis** of hostile substances (or organisms, such as bacteria) that are recognized by the receptors on the cell surface. Removal of accumulated extracellular debris is another phagocytic function usually performed by specialized cells **(macrophages)** in a similar manner (see Fig. 5-13). A number of genetic disorders are now thought to be associated with **defective mechanisms of intracellular membrane transport** (Olkkonen and Ikonen, 2000).

A reverse mechanism occurs in **export of molecules,** which are packaged into vesicles formed within the cell (mainly in the Golgi apparatus) (see below) and travel to the surface. The vesicles attach to the inner aspect of the cell membrane by means of specific receptors. After the merger, the cell membrane splits open, and the content of the vesicles is discharged into the circulating fluid bathing the cell.

Besides clathrin-coated pits, the cell membrane also forms specific small invaginations (50 to 100 nm in diameter) that are known as **caveolae.** In cross-section, the caveolae appear as small, spherical vesicles in the adjacent cytoplasm (see Fig. 2-5). They are particularly prevalent in endothelial cells, smooth muscle cells, and type I pneumocytes (Schlegel et al, 1998; Couvet et al, 1997). The caveolae are composed of **caveolins,** a family of integrated membrane proteins, which interact with a number of signaling molecules and thus regulate the cell's responses to its environment (Okamoto et al, 1998). Thus, caveolins have been **implicated in cells' response to injury** and may play a role in human breast cancer (Engelman, 1998).

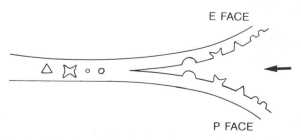

Figure 2-7 Principle of freeze-fracture. The sharp wedge (*arrow*) separates the frozen membrane into two faces (P and E; see text) without disturbing the position of intermembrane protein particles or structures (see Figs. 2-16 and 2-27).

Specialized Structures of Cell Surfaces

Transmission electron microscopy has been helpful in elucidating some of the structural details of specialized structures of cell surfaces and the manner in which cells are attached to each other.

The Glycocalix

Specialized techniques of electron microscopy serve to demonstrate an ill-defined, **fuzzy layer of material on the free surfaces of cells**. This layer is referred to as **glycocalix** and appears to be composed primarily of glycoproteins containing residues of sialic acid. Although the thickness and, presumably, chemical makeup of glycocalix vary from one type of cell to another, its occurrence is a rather generalized phenomenon, the exact function of which is not well understood.

Cilia and Flagella: Motile Cell Processes

The cilia and flagella may be readily identified by light microscopy. Both are mobile extensions of the cell membrane and are capable of rapid movements. A **flagellum** is usually a single, elongated mobile part of the cell, as observed in spermatozoa. **Cilia** are shorter and multiple, usually functioning (batting) in a synchronous manner, for example, in cells lining the bronchial epithelium (see Fig. 2-4), or other epithelia, such as that of the fallopian tube and the endocervix. Cells bearing cilia are usually **polarized**; that is, they have a **specific spatial orientation** in keeping with their function: the cilia are usually oriented toward the lumen of an organ or tissue. The cilia are anchored in a thick, flat portion of the cell cytoplasm immediately adjacent to the surface, referred to as a **terminal plate** (see Fig. 2-4A). Careful observation reveals that the terminal plate is composed of a series of dense granules, or basal corpuscles, each belonging to a single cilium (see Figs. 2-4B and 2-8). **Cilia are rare in cancer cells.**

There is a remarkable **uniformity of ultrastructure of the motile cell processes** throughout the animal and the plant kingdoms. Each cilium or flagellum contains **11 microtubules,** of which **two are single and located within the center, and nine are double (doublets) and located at the periphery** (Figs. 2-9 and 2-10). The structure of the cilia and flagella is very similar to that of the centrioles (see below). Species differences do exist in the manner in which the cilia and the flagella are anchored within the cytoplasm (see Fig. 2-8).

Within recent years, considerable insight has been gained into the function of the cilia and flagella. These cell processes are composed of an intricate system of protein fibrils that glide against each other in executing the movements, which require a substantial input of energy, provided by mitochondria. For details of the current concepts of movements, see Satir (1965) and Sale and Satir (1977).

Microvilli and Brush Border

Microvilli are **short, slender, regular projections on free surfaces of cells** that can be visualized in electron micros-

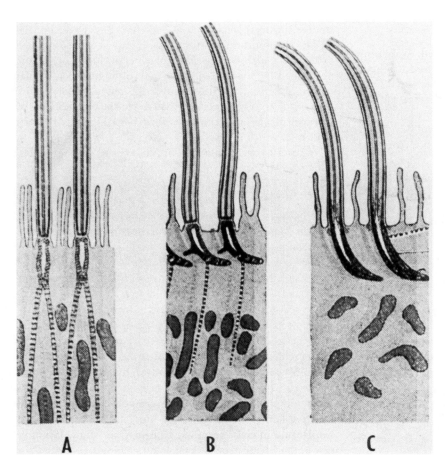

Figure 2-8 Diagrammatic representation of the structure of the ciliary apparatus (*A*) of a mollusk (*Elliptio*), (*B*) an amphibian (*Rana*), and (*C*) a mammal (mouse). Note the differences in attachment to the cytoplasm. (Fawcett DW. Laryngoscope 64:557–567, 1954.)

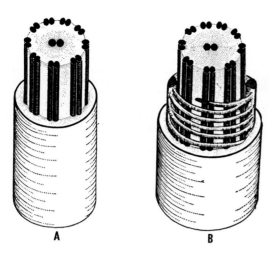

Figure 2-9 Diagrammatic representation of a cilium (**A**) and of the principal piece of mammalian sperm flagellum (**B**). Note the similarity of the basic structure, with two single microtubules in the center and nine double microtubules at the periphery. This structure of cilia is encountered throughout the plant and the animal kingdoms. (Fawcett DW. Laryngoscope 64:557–567, 1954.)

copy or light microscopy. The term **brush border** or **striated border** is applied to specialized cell surfaces provided with microvilli. The brush border is observed on the free surface of the intestinal mucosa (Fig. 2-11A and see Fig. 2-15). The regular, finger-like intestinal microvilli, delimited by the plasma membrane, measure approximately 1 μm in length and serve the function of increasing the useful surface of the cell. A similarly organized brush border is observed in the proximal segment of the renal tubules. Microvilli may be observed by light microscopy on the surface of various **normal human cells**, as **short, delicate, hair-like striations, best observed in air-dried and stained cells, spread on glass slides.** Scanning electron microscopy shows microvilli, as finger-like, slender structures, projecting from the surface of the cell. **Long and irregular microvilli that occur on the surfaces of cancer cells are much easier to**

see in light microscopy and are occasionally of diagnostic help. These observations are discussed in detail in Chapter 7 and are illustrated in Figures 7-7 to 7-14.

Cell Contacts

The relationship of cells to one another within the same tissue or within adjoining tissues is of paramount importance for the structural integrity and function of all organs (see Fig. 2-11). These relationships are regulated by cell membranes, which form a variety of cell contacts and cell attachments. It is not known as yet whether the cell attachments are formed on predetermined specialized areas of cell surfaces, or incidental to haphazard cell contacts.

From the morphologic point of view, a number of structural cell contacts have been identified. These are the **desmosomes,** the **junctional complexes,** and the **gap junctions** (Fig. 2-12).

The Desmosomes and Hemidesmosomes

The structure of cell attachments, especially within the epithelia, has been of interest to biologists and pathologists alike for over a century. Early on, it has been noted in light microscopy that, within the squamous stratified epithelia, the cells are attached to each other by means of cytoplasmic extensions, named **intercellular bridges.** In phase microscopy, fine fibrils, named *tonofibrils,* may be seen converging on the areas connecting the unfixed, unstained cells. For many years, it has been known that, in the centers of the intercellular bridges, there existed small dense structures, variously referred to as *granules* (Ravier) or *nodes* (Bizzozero) and currently referred to as **desmosomes.** Electron microscopic studies have demonstrated that the desmosomes represent **points of adhesion of two adjacent cells** (see Figs. 2-11 to 2-13). The cytoplasm of adjacent cells remains firmly attached at the points of desmosomal adherence but, owing to artifacts of

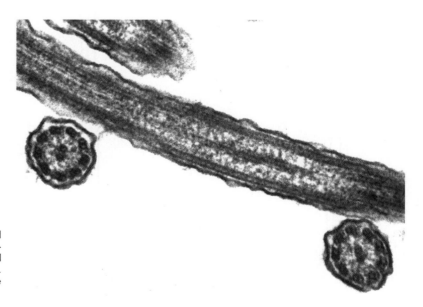

Figure 2-10 Electron micrograph of cross- and longitudinal sections of cilia from human endocervical cells. The nine peripheral double microtubules and the two central single microtubules are well shown. (×80,000.) (Courtesy of Dr. H. Dembitzer, Montefiore Hospital.)

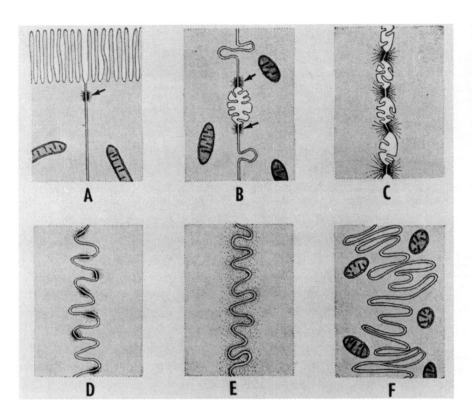

Figure 2-11 Diagrammatic representation of several types of specialization found on the surfaces of contact between adjacent cells. *A.* On the interface between columnar epithelial cells of the intestine, desmosomes (*arrow*) are frequently seen near the free surface showing striated border. *B.* On the contact surfaces of liver cells, desmosomes occur (*arrows*) on either side of the bile capillary. Near these are stud-like processes that project into concavities on the surface of the adjacent cell. *C.* In the stratified squamous epithelium of the rodent vagina, the cell surfaces are adherent at the desmosomes and retracted between, giving rise to the so-called intercellular bridges of light microscopy. A continuous system of intercellular spaces exists between bridges. Projecting into these spaces are a few short microvilli. *D.* In the stratum spinosum of the tongue, adjoining cells have closely fitting corrugated surfaces. Numerous desmosomes are distributed over the irregular surface. *E.* The partially cornified cells of the superficial layers of stratified squamous epithelium apparently lack desmosomes, but the ridges and grooves of the cell surfaces persist. *F.* An extraordinarily elaborate intercrescence of cell surfaces is found in the distal convoluted segment of the frog nephron. (Fawcett DW. Structural specializations of the cell surface. *In* Palsy SL (ed). Frontiers in Cytology. New Haven, Yale University Press, 1958.)

fixation, it shrinks elsewhere. The elongated desmosome-bound portions of the cytoplasm constitute the intercellular bridges seen in light microscopy. Recent studies show that molecules of C-cadherin are an essential component of desmosomes (He et al, 2003).

The **fine structure of a desmosome,** or *macule adherens* (from Latin = adhesive area; plural, *maculae* adherentes), is fairly uniform in most tissues examined to date: within each cell, at the region of localized contact of two cells, there is a dense plaque adjacent to the cell membrane, made up of converging cytoplasmic actin microfilaments (tonofibrils). The two cell membranes do not appear modified. Within the intercellular substance, there is a dense central lamina. Very slender filaments run between the central lamina and the adjacent cell membranes (see Fig. 2-13).

The desmosomal apparatus is operational in all epithelia and many other tissues, but the details of the structure may vary from one tissue type to another. For instance, the squamous epithelium of the genital tract may be structurally somewhat different from the squamous epithelium of other

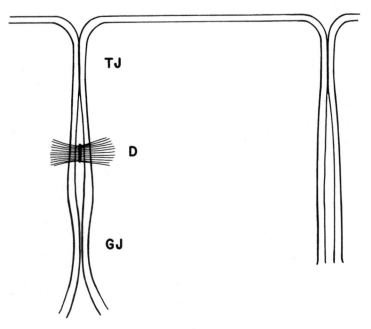

Figure 2-12 Diagrammatic representation of the three principal types of cell junctions. The tight junction (TJ) is formed by fusion of the two outer layers of adjacent cells. It is impermeable to most molecules. The gap junction (GJ) serves the purposes of cell-to-cell communication. The desmosomes (D) are button-like, extremely tough cell junctions that are particularly well developed in protective epithelia, such as the squamous epithelium.

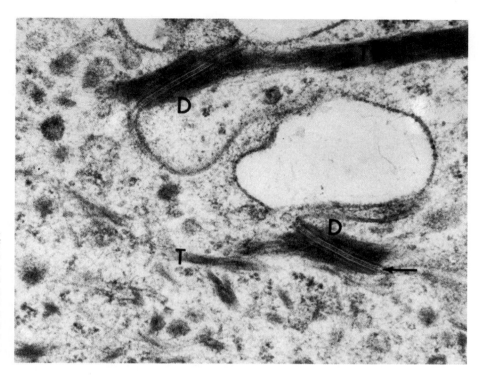

Figure 2-13 Desmosomes and actin-filaments (tonofibrils). Epidermis of human vulva. Electron micrograph of a portion of two adjoining epithelial cells showing actin filaments attached to two desmosomes (D). The filaments do not transverse cell boundaries. Note within the intercellular space a central dense lamina (*arrow*), a part of the desmosome structure. Bundles of filaments (T) may be observed within the cytoplasm. (×54,400.)

organs. Burgos and Wislocki (1956) demonstrated the existence of intercellular canaliculi in the rodent vagina during estrus. Such canaliculi conceivably serve as channels for metabolites, etc. and, perhaps, are instrumental in bringing about the marked cyclic changes in the vaginal epithelium in these animals (see Fig. 2-11).

Recent investigations of cytoskeleton (see below) disclosed that desmosomes are biochemically complex structures containing many different **filamentous proteins,** some of which are **desmosome specific.** Among the latter, specific adhesion proteins (**adherins**) have been identified in cytoplasmic plaques. Other protein components of desmosomes are **desmoplakins** and **desmogleins.** The desmosomes also contain intermediate filaments of various molecular weights. It has been documented that the makeup of desmosomes varies in different cell and tissue types (Franke et al, 1982, 1994). With the development of specific monoclonal antibodies to these proteins, the presence of desmosomal proteins may now be used as a means of tissue identification and diagnosis of diseases (Franke et al, 1989, 1994; Schmidt et al, 1994).

Hemidesmosomes (half-desmosomes) are observed at the attachment points of epithelial basal cells to the basement lamina. The half-desmosome is morphologically somewhat similar to the desmosome: there is a thickening of a limited area of the cytoplasm of a basal cell adjacent to the cell membrane, upon which converge cytoplasmic fibrils. However, the apposed basement membrane shows merely a slight thickening, which contains slender filaments. An intermediate thickening, or membrane, is usually present within the fibrils of the hemidesmosome (Fig. 2-14). Jones et al (1994) documented that the hemidesmosomes serve as **connectors between the extracellular matrix and the intermediate filaments in the cytoplasm of the cell.** The mechanisms of cell adhesion molecules to the extracellular matrix were reviewed by Hutter et al (2000).

The Junctional Complexes

Farquhar and Palade (1963) described a particular type of attachment of epithelial cells, known as the junctional complex, located along the lateral surfaces of the cells adjacent to the lumen (Fig. 2-15). The junctional complex is composed of **three parts.** The **tight junction** (*zonula occludens*), closest to the lumen, represents an area of fusion of the outer leaflets of the plasma membranes of two adjacent cells. The molecular mechanisms of formation of this junction were discussed by Knox and Brown (2002). This cell junction contains the adhesion molecule, E-cadherin (Franke et al, 1994). The **intermediate junction** (*zonula adherens*) is characterized by the presence of an intercellular space, separating areas of cytoplasmic density occurring in each of the participating cells. The third part of the junctional complex is a **desmosome** (*macula adherens*). On the surface of certain epithelia, for example, in the small intestine, the tight junctions form an occlusive network that is essentially not permeable to molecules, even of a very small size, and, presumably, synchronizes the function of these epithelia. Thus, nutrients cannot penetrate the seal between the cells, but are absorbed by the cell surfaces facing the lumen. A similar arrangement is encountered on the surfaces of many other epithelia in contact with a fluid medium, such as the renal tubules, bile canaliculi, and ependymal cells. Freeze-fracture of tight junctions shows a continuous network of ridges and grooves at the site of membrane fusion (Fig. 2-16A).

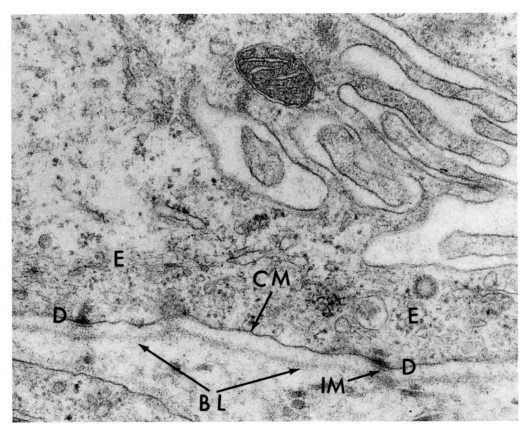

Figure 2-14   **Half-desmosomes.** Electron micrograph of the basal portion of the epithelial cell (E) of rat bladder and the basement lamina (BL). The half-desmosomes (D) are fan-shaped areas of increased density owing to numerous converging fine fibrils. An intermediate membrane (IM) is present between the cell membrane (CM) and the basement lamina. Dense material, possibly fibrillar, located between the cell membrane and the basement lamina completes the half-desmosome. (×54,600.)

The Gap Junctions (Nexus Junctions)

First observed in the cardiac muscle and, subsequently in a variety of other tissues, the gap or nexus junctions were identified as **specialized areas of cell contact.** In transmission electron microscopy, gap junctions appear as well-demarcated areas of merger between two adjacent cells, somewhat less than 200 Å in thickness. The junction is composed of seven layers, three of which are electron-translucent and are sandwiched in between electron-dense layers (see Fig. 2-12). The central electron-lucent zone (or gap) is composed of small hexagonal subunits, forming the **channels of communication between adjacent cells** (Revel and Karnovsky, 1967). Freeze cleaving confirmed that the gap junction is a highly specialized area of cell contact, displaying membrane-associated particles in a hexagonal array (see Fig. 2-16B). There are at least two different types of gap junctions, with a somewhat different arrangement of particles.

The gap junction channels are composed of a diverse family of proteins, named **connexins** (Donaldson et al, 1997). **The gap junctions have multiple functions: they provide cell-to-cell communications of essential metabolites and ions and may serve as electrical synapses** (Leitch, 1992). It has been shown that defects in connexins may be associated with human diseases (Paul, 1995; Spray, 1996). Thus, the gap junctions and the associated proteins are essential to function and integrity of tissues.

The Cytoplasm and Organelles

The cytoplasm is the component of the cell, located between the nucleus and the cell membrane. Depending on the type and origin of the cell, the cytoplasm may present a variegated light microscopic appearance. Its **shape, size, and staining properties vary greatly** and will be described in detail for the various tissues and organs. In living cells, there is an intense movement of particles within the cytoplasm.

In conventional **light microscopy,** various products of cell metabolism may be seen in the cytoplasm, often appearing as **granules** or **vacuoles.** The latter are round or oval structures, generally with an unstained or a faintly stained center. Their contents may be identified by special techniques.

Electron microscopic investigation of cells, coupled with sophisticated biochemical methods, has shed considerable light on the basic structure of the cytoplasm and of the major organized cytoplasmic components or organelles.

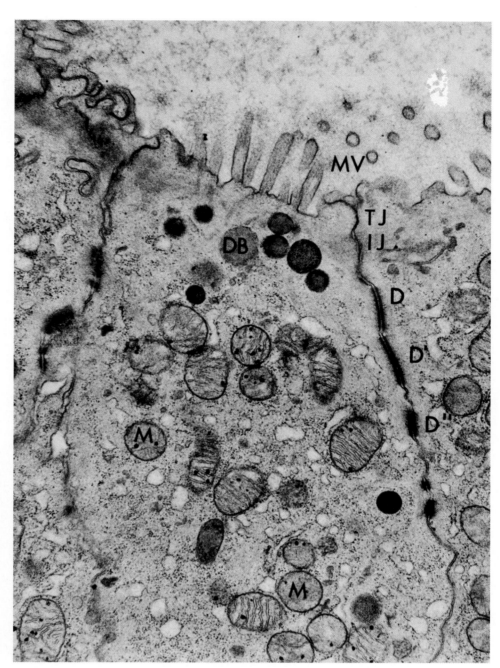

Figure 2-15 Junctional complex. Electron micrograph of intestinal-type epithelium observed in a rare nasal tumor of man. The component of the junctional complex may be observed: tight junction (TJ), intermediate junction (IJ), and the desmosome (D). Other desmosomes (D', D") may be observed below. Note also the microvilli (MV), seen in longitudinal and cross section, and mitochondria (M), some with intramitochondrial dense granules. Also note dense bodies (DB), which may represent secretory granules (×22,800.) (Courtesy of Dr. Robert Erlandson, Sloan-Kettering Institute for Cancer Research, New York.)

Ultrastructure of the Cytoplasm

The cytoplasm is composed of **organized cell components, or organelles,** the **cytoskeleton,** and a **cytoplasmic matrix.** The organized components of the cytoplasm comprise the membranous systems, ribosomes, mitochondria, lysosomes, centrioles, microbodies, and miscellaneous structures.

The Membranous System

The membranous system **is composed of the endoplasmic reticulum and the Golgi complex.**

The Endoplasmic Reticulum

The endoplasmic reticulum is a closed **system of unit membranes** forming tubular canals and flattened sacs or cisternae that subdivide the cytoplasm into a series of compartments. The membranes of the endoplasmic reticulum may be "rough," that is, covered with **numerous attached granules composed of ribonucleic acid (RNA) and proteins (RNP granules or ribosomes;** see below), or **"smooth,"** free of any particles. The amount and structural forms of endoplasmic reticulum vary from one cell type to another. In general, **rough endoplasmic reticulum** is abundant in cells with **marked synthesis of proteins** for export—for instance, in the pancreas or the salivary glands, see Figure 2-17. In light microscopy, the RNA-rich cytoplasmic areas (once named *ergastoplasm*) stain bluish with hematoxylin. This feature is commonly observed in metabolically active cells. **Smooth cytoplasmic reticulum is abundant in cells that synthesize various steroid hormones.**

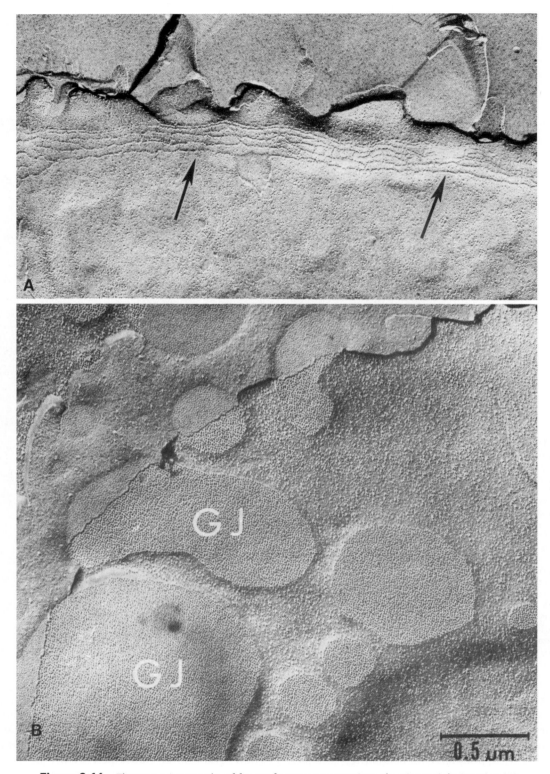

Figure 2-16   Electron micrographs of freeze-fracture preparations showing a tight junction (*A*) and a gap junction (*B*). *A.* The tight junction (zonula occludens) appears in freeze-fracture images as a continuous meshwork of ridges and grooves representing the sites of membrane fusion (*arrows*). Epidermis of the transparent catfish (*Kryptoterus*). *B.* The appearance of gap junctions is quite different from the tight junction in that they are made up of plaques (GJ) of closely packaged particles. The particles measure about 9 nm in diameter and are believed to be the sites at which hydrophilic channels bring about electrical coupling between cells. Myocardium of a tunicate (*Ciona*). (Unpublished data of RB Hanna and GD Pappas, Albert Einstein College of Medicine, New York. Courtesy of Dr. Pappas.)

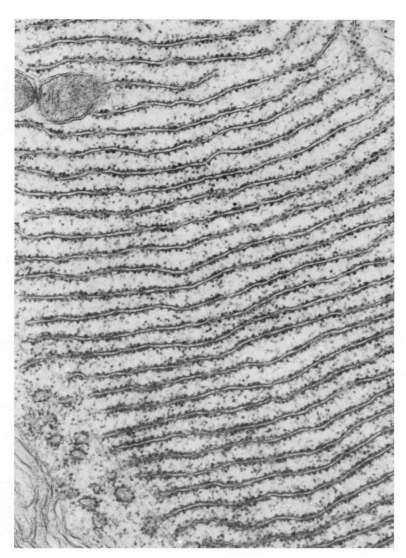

Figure 2-17 "Rough" endoplasmic reticulum. Electron micrograph of an epithelial cell of a human submaxillary gland. Note the ribosomes (RNP particles) attached to the membranes of the endoplasmic reticulum. Free ribosomes are also present in the space between the membranes. (×43,000.) (Courtesy of Dr. Bernard Tandler, Sloan-Kettering Institute for Cancer Research, New York.)

The Golgi Complex

First described by Golgi in 1898, this organelle consists of a **series of parallel, doughnut-shaped flat spaces or cisternae and spherical or egg-shaped vesicles demarcated by smooth membranes** (Fig. 2-18). In epithelial cells with secretory function, the Golgi complex is usually located between the nucleus and the luminal surface of the cells. Present evidence suggests that the Golgi complex **synthesizes and packages** cell products for the cells' own use and for export (Fig. 2-19). For example, the Golgi complex synthesizes structural proteins, such as the components of the asymmetric unit membrane observed in the urothelium (Hicks, 1966; Koss, 1969; see Chapter 22). The synthesis of the protein products occurs within the cisternae of the Golgi complex. The **products for export** are packaged in the form of **vesicles lined by a single smooth membrane** derived from pinched off ends of the cisternae and is released into the cytoplasm (Fig. 2-20). A review of the mechanisms of protein sorting by the Golgi apparatus was provided by Allan and Balch (1999).

The Ribosomes

The ribosomes are submicroscopic particles measuring between 150 and 300 Å in diameter, depending on the technique used, and are composed of **RNA and proteins** in approximately equal proportions. They are ubiquitous and have been identified in practically all cells of animal and plant origin. In the cytoplasm, the ribosomes may be either floating free or they may be attached to the outer surface of the endoplasmic reticulum (see Fig. 2-17). It appears likely that the two types of ribosomes exercise different functions: the **free ribosomes** are primarily engaged in the production of proteins for the cell's own use, whereas **attached ribosomes** are responsible for protein production for export. A marked concentration of ribosomes (and hence proteins) confers upon the cytoplasm a basophilic staining (see above).

Each ribosome is composed of two, approximately round subunits of unequal size and has been compared to a **Russian doll.** Ribosomes may be joined together by strands of messenger RNA (mRNA) to form **aggregates or polyribosomes** that thus resemble a string of beads. The string may be either

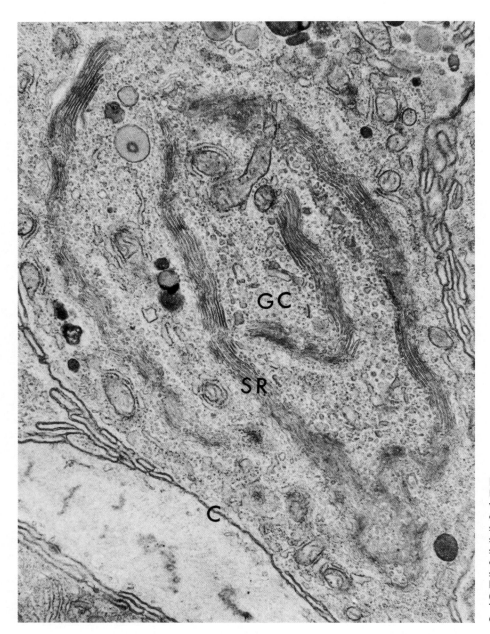

Figure 2-18 **Inactive Golgi complex.** Electron micrograph of human labial salivary gland. In this type of cell, the Golgi complex (GC) is composed mainly of a series of parallel membranes made up of smooth reticulum (SR). Note the absence of ribosomes (see Fig. 2-17). C = cell (plasma) membrane; its three-layer structure, with a translucent middle layer is well seen in this photograph. (×17,300.) (Courtesy of Dr. Bernard Tandler, Sloan-Kettering Institute for Cancer Research, New York.)

open or closed. Ribosomes are attached to the membranes of the endoplasmic reticulum by the larger subunit.

The **ribosomal RNA (rRNA)** is manufactured in the nucleolus and transferred into the cytoplasm where it becomes associated with the protein component. At the conclusion of the process of protein synthesis, the ribosomal subunits are separated and return to the cytoplasmic pool. The details of the **mechanism of protein synthesis** are discussed in Chapter 3. Ribosome-like structures may also be observed within the nucleus, presumably representing various types of RNA.

The Mitochondria

Although the mitochondria were first observed in light microscopy in the latter part of the 19th century, their structure and function have become better known only within the last 50 years. These organelles are present in all eukaryotic cells.

Mitochondria are **small, usually elongated structures,** usually less than 0.5 μm in width and less than 7 μm in length. Even within the same cell, the mitochondria may **vary substantially in size and configuration,** assuming spherical, cigar-, club-, or tennis racquet–like shapes. However, the basic **structure** of a mitochondrion, initially described by Palade in 1953, is uniform. Each mitochondrion is **composed of two membranes, located one within the other.** The outer shell of the mitochondrion is a continuous, closed-unit membrane. Running parallel to the outer membrane is a morphologically similar **inner membrane** that forms numerous crests or invaginations **(cristae mitochondriales),** subdividing the interior of the organelle into a series of communicating compartments (Fig. 2-21 and see Frontispiece and Fig. 2-15). Frequently, the cristae are approximately at a right angle to the long axis of the mitochondrion, but they may also be oblique or, for that matter, longitudinal. There is no

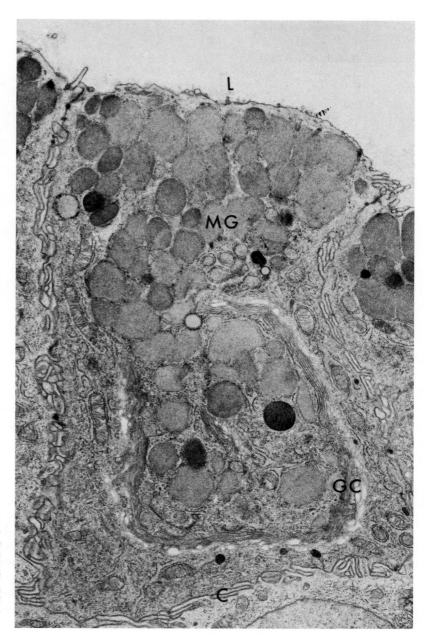

Figure 2-19   Active Golgi complex. Electron micrograph of a human labial salivary gland. Note the enormous accumulation of mucous granules (MG) within the Golgi complex (GC) and above it, toward the lumen (L) of the acinus. The basic structure of the Golgi complex is maintained. C = cell (plasma) membrane (see Fig. 2-18). (×8,700.) (Courtesy of Dr. Bernard Tandler, Sloan-Kettering Institute for Cancer Research, New York.)

known relationship between the orientation of the cristae and the function of the organelle. A homogeneous material or **mitochondrial matrix,** containing a mixture of molecules and enzymes, fills the interior of the organelle.

The size and configuration of the mitochondria may vary according to the nutritional status of an organ. For instance, the mitochondria of the liver may become very large in some deficiency states, only to return to normal with resumption of a normal diet. Mitochondrial enlargement may also be caused by poor fixation of material. The latter is the probable background of a cell change known as *cloudy swelling* to light microscopists.

Accumulation of fat, hemosiderin, and proteins may be observed in the immediate vicinity of the mitochondria. This probably occurs because of the role of the mitochondria in **energy-producing oxidative processes.** Indeed, the key role of the mitochondria within the cell is that

of carriers of energy-producing complex enzyme systems. Several oxidative systems have been identified within the mitochondria: Krebs cycle enzymes, fatty acid cycle enzymes, and the enzymes of the respiratory chain, including the cytochromes. Most importantly, the formation of energy-producing adenosine triphosphate (ATP) from phosphorus and adenosine diphosphate (ADP) takes place within the mitochondria. The ATP is exported into the cytoplasm where it serves as an essential source of energy for the cell.

It has been documented that the **mitochondria possess their own DNA** that is independent of nuclear DNA and is responsible for independent protein synthesis and for the **mitochondrial division cycle.** This supports the concept that the mitochondria are quasi-independent organelles, living in symbiosis with the host cell, which they supply with energy. It is a matter for an interesting

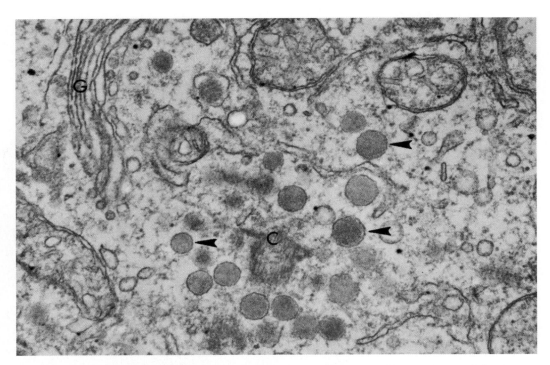

Figure 2-20   Ultrastructural features of a calcitonin-producing medullary carcinoma of the thyroid. Numerous electron-opaque secretory granules bound by a single membrane may be noted (arrowheads). The peripheral cisternae of the Golgi complex (G) show accumulation of electron-opaque substance; hence, the assembly of the secretory granules is probably a function of the Golgi apparatus. (×54,400.) (Koss LG. Morphology of cancer cells. *In* Handbuch der allgemeinen Pathologie, vol. 6, Tumors, part I. Berlin, Springer, 1974, pp 1–139.)

speculation that mitochondria may represent **primitive bacteria** that, at the onset of biologic events, became **incorporated into the primordial cell,** and this association became permanent for mutual benefit. Thus, **two genetic systems exist within a cell,** one vested in the mitochondria and the other in the nucleus. The two systems are interdependent, although the exact mechanisms of this association are not understood.

The **mitochondrial DNA** has been extensively studied, and its structure has been determined. It is a small molecule of **double-stranded DNA containing only 37 genes** (13 structural genes encoding proteins, 22 transfer RNA genes, and 2 genes encoding ribosomal RNAs). **All mitochondria of the zygote are contributed by the ovum; hence, all of mitochondrial DNA is of maternal origin.** Because muscle function depends heavily on energy systems vested in mitochondria, it is not surprising that **various muscular disorders have been observed in association with abnormalities of mitochondrial DNA** (Moraes et al, 1989; Fadic and

Johns, 1996; and DiMauro and Schon, 2003). Such disorders are transmitted exclusively by females to their offspring. There is also recent evidence that **mitochondria participate in the phenomenon of programmed cell death or apoptosis.** The issue is discussed at length in Chapter 6.

In **cells characterized by an abundance of mitochondria** (**oncocytes,** sometimes named **Hürthle cells,** and tumors composed of oncocytes **oncocytomas**), which may occur in the salivary glands, thyroid, kidney, breast, and sometimes in other organs, the mitochondrial DNA may be modified (Welter et al, 1989). For description of oncocytes and oncocytomas, see appropriate chapters.

The Lysosomes (Lytic Bodies) and the Autophagic Vacuoles

The lysosomes, or cell **disposal units,** are the organelles participating in the **removal of phagocytized foreign material.** Occasionally, the lysosomes also digest **obsolete frag-

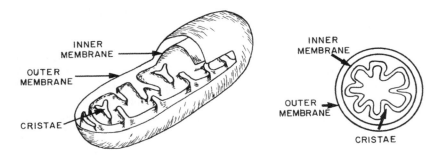

Figure 2-21   Schematic representation of a mitochondrion shown in longitudinal section (*left*) and cross-section (*right*). For details, see text.

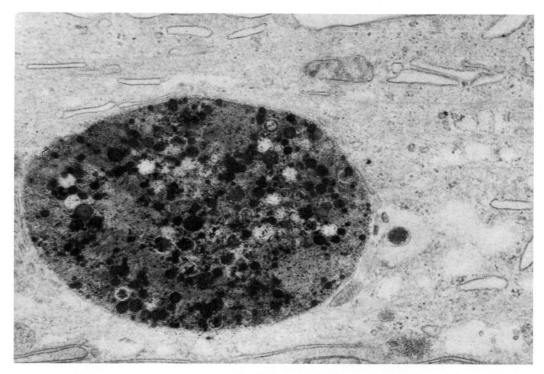

Figure 2-22   **Electron micrograph of epithelial cell, rat urinary bladder.** Large oval body containing droplets of dense lipid-like material and clear vesicles. The body is probably a disposal unit and, as such, related to autophagic vacuoles and lysosomes. (×38,000.)

ments of cytoplasm and organelles, such as mitochondria, for which the cell has no further use. The term **autophagic vacuoles** or *residual bodies* has been suggested for such structures. In electron microscopic preparations, the lysosomes may be identified as spherical or oval structures of heterogeneous density and variable diameter (Fig. 2-22). The lysosomes contain several **hydrolytic enzymes,** acid phosphatase being the first one identified, that serve to digest the phagocytized material. It is of interest to note that granules commonly observed in neutrophilic leukocytes belong to the family of lysosomes inasmuch as they contain "packaged" digestive enzymes that assist in the dissolution of phagocytized bacteria.

The origin of at least some lysosomes has been traced to certain regions of smooth endoplasmic reticulum (Novikoff et al, 1973) that is intimately associated with the inner (active) face of the Golgi complex.

It appears that, in some cells at least, the outer membrane of the lysosome may merge with the cell membrane. This is followed by extrusion of the contents of the lysosome into the extracellular space. This process is the reverse of pinocytosis, or phagocytosis (see above).

The lysosomes appear to play an important role in certain **storage diseases,** for example, in **Tay Sachs disease.** This is one of several known inborn or hereditary defects of metabolism wherein the deficiency of an enzyme (hexosaminidase A) results in accumulation of a fatty substance, ganglioside, in lysosome-like vesicles in cells of the central nervous system. In several other uncommon diseases (such as metachromatic leukodystrophy) and certain granulomatous dis-

orders (**malakoplakia,** see Chap. 22), abnormalities of lysosomes play a major role.

The Peroxisomes or Microbodies

The peroxisomal family of organelles is characterized by storage of enzymes involved in **metabolism of hydrogen peroxide.** The most commonly encountered enzyme is catalase. Morphologically, peroxisomes are vesicular structures that, in nonhuman cells, are often provided with a dense **central core** or **nucleoid** (Fig. 2-23). Occasionally, the core has a crystalloid structure. Microbodies were extensively studied in liver cells and cells of the renal proximal convoluted tubules of rats. It has been shown that, under certain circumstances, peroxisomes are capable of becoming very large and, apparently, of dividing (Lavin and Koss, 1973). Whether these organelles have an independent DNA system, such as that of the mitochondria, is not known.

The Centrioles

The centrioles are cytoplasmic organelles that play a key role during cell division. Each interphase animal cell contains a pair of centrioles, short tubular structures, usually located in the vicinity of the concave face of the Golgi complex. As the cell is about to enter mitosis, another pair of centrioles appears, and each pair travels to the opposite poles of the cell and becomes the **anchoring point of the mitotic spindle.** The formation of the mitotic spindle from microtubules is described below.

The origin of the second pair of centrioles has not been fully clarified; apparently it is synthesized de novo from pre-

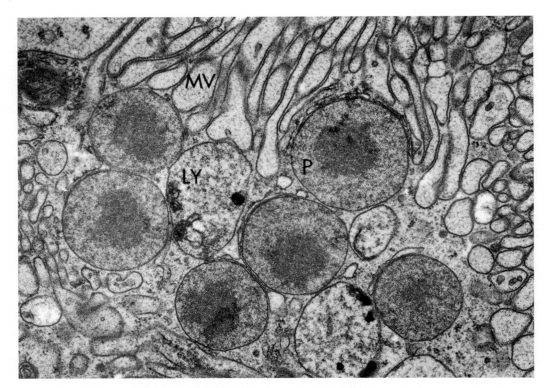

Figure 2-23 **Peroxisomes (P) or microbodies in proximal tubules of rat kidney.** Note the central dense core or nucleoid. Ly = lysosomes; MV = microvilli. (× 19,800.) (Lavin P, Koss LG. Effect of a single dose of cyclophosphamide on various organs in the rat. IV. The kidney. Am J Pathol 62:169, 1971.)

cursor molecules in the cytoplasm (Johnson and Rosenbaum, 1992). This event is induced and directed in an unknown fashion by the original pair of centrioles. Each pair of centrioles is surrounded by a **clear zone, the centrosome,** which, in turn, is surrounded by a slightly denser area or the **astrosphere.** Within each pair, the centrioles are placed at right angles to each other. Thus, in a fortuitous electron micrograph, one centriole will appear in a longitudinal section and the other in cross section. In the cross section, each **centriole appears as a cylindrical structure with a clear center and nine triplets or groups of three microtubules** (Fig. 2-24). Thus, **the basic structure of the centriole, first described by de Harven and Bernhard in 1956, closely approximates that of cilia and flagella** (see Figs. 2-9 and 2-10). It has been suggested that the centrioles are at the origin of cilia. If this were the case, it would indicate that the centrioles might multiply manyfold. It has been observed that formation of the sperm flagellum takes place from one of the centrioles, while the other remains inactive.

The Cytoskeleton

The skeleton of the cells and, hence, the structures maintaining their physical shape, facilitating their motion, and providing structural support to all cell functions, is provided by a **family of fibrillar proteins.** Several techniques were developed that allow the isolation of these proteins and the production of specific **monoclonal or polyclonal antibodies** that can be used to identify these proteins and to localize them within cells. By techniques of molecular biology, the

precise composition of such proteins has been determined and the genes responsible for their formation identified and sequenced (see Chap. 3). This work is not only of theoretical value but has also led to strides in immunocytochemistry, particularly relative to intermediate filaments (see below and Chap. 45).

The cytoskeleton is fundamentally composed of **three types of fibrillar proteins,** initially classified by their diameter in electron microscopic photographs: the **actin filaments** (microfilaments, tonofilaments), **intermediate filaments,** and **microtubules.** They will be described in sequence.

Actin Filaments (Microfilaments, Tonofilaments)

The ubiquitous actin filaments, measuring **5 to 7 nm in diameter,** are observed in all cells of all vertebrate species. In electron microscopy, they can be recognized as **bundles of longitudinal cytoplasmic filaments** crisscrossing the cytoplasm and often converging on specific targets such as desmosomes (see Fig. 2-13). The actin filaments are found within virtually all structural cell components and **interact with many other proteins that regulate their length.** The fundamental structure of these elongated fibrillar proteins is helical, with two different ends: this latter feature allows the filaments to attach to two different molecules and function as an intermediary polarized link. The actin filaments are **easily polymerized** (i.e., they form structures composed of several actin units). This is probably the mechanism that allows actin filaments to form tight meshworks in conjunction with other proteins. Among the latter, it is important to men-

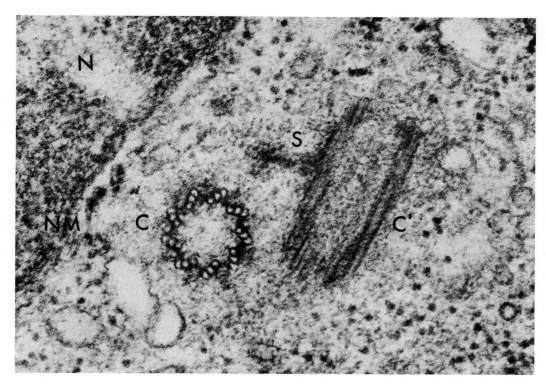

Figure 2-24 **Centrioles.** Electron micrograph of thymus of DBA mouse. Two centrioles are seen in this electron micrograph: one (C) in cross section, showing nice triplets of tubules, and the other (C') in oblique section and apparently at a right angle to (C). Centriole satellite (S) is attached to C'. This may represent the point of anchorage of the tubules of the mitotic spindle. N = nucleus; NM = nuclear membrane. (×94,000.) (Courtesy of Dr. Etienne de Harven, Sloan-Kettering Institute for Caner Research, New York.)

tion the **links of actin filaments to a contractile protein, myosin,** accounting for motion and contractility of cells and of cell appendages such as cilia and flagella. Other linkages occur with **transmembrane proteins,** such as spectrin, ensuring the communications between the cell membrane and cell interior. Thus, actin microfilaments perform several essential functions within cells as linkage filaments coordinating the activity of divergent cell components.

Intermediate Filaments

The group of cytoplasmic filaments was initially identified in electron microscopy because of their **diameter (7 to 11 nm);** hence, intermediate filaments (IFs) are larger than actin microfilaments and smaller than microtubules (see the following section). This group of filaments assumed an important role in immunocytochemistry and histochemistry as **markers of cell derivation and differentiation** by means of **specific antibodies** that serve to identify the presence and the distribution of IFs in cells and tissues (see Chap. 45). The genes governing the synthesis of IFs have been identified by molecular biology techniques and applied to studies of cell differentiation across species, documenting that these genes belong to the fundamental cellular genes in primitive multicellular organisms, such as worms, mollusks, and perhaps even plants (Nagle, 1988 and 1994). It is of interest, though, that the **precise function of the IF proteins is obscure,** as they do not appear to participate in any life cycle events.

Several subspecies of IF proteins have been identified, differing from each other by relative molecular mass (M_r) and anatomic distribution (Table 2-1). Their significance in immunocytochemistry is discussed in Chapter 45. Perhaps the best known of the IFs are the **keratins,** which have been extensively studied in the epidermis of the skin (Sun et al, 1984; Franke et al, 1989). As shown in Figure 2-25, there are several subfamilies of keratin filaments (proteins) forming pairs, each composed of one basic and one acidic protein (see Fig. 2-25A). Each type of squamous epithelium (skin, cornea, other epithelia) may be represented by a special pair of proteins of high relative molecular mass. With the change of epithelial type from a single layer to multilayer epithelium, different keratin genes, producing proteins of increasing molecular mass are activated (see Fig. 2-25B). This mechanism may be important in understanding the change known as *squamous metaplasia* (see Chap. 6).

Of note is the identification of **lamins,** structural proteins of the nucleus, and its components. These proteins contribute to the **formation of the nuclear membrane and the nuclear pore complexes.** They may play a role in the organization of interphase chromosomes (see below).

Microtubules

Microtubules, measuring between **22 and 25 nm in diameter,** have long been recognized and identified by light microscopy as the **constituents of the mitotic spindle.** The determination of their existence in the interphase cells re-

TABLE 2-1
CHARACTERISTICS AND DISTRIBUTION OF INTERMEDIATE FILAMENTS (IF) IN TISSUES

Type	M_r (daltons)	Tissue Distribution
Keratins		
Form: acid types 9–19	40,000–68,000	Epithelia (specific types associated with specific
Pairs: neutral – basic types 1–8		epithelial types and their maturation)
Desmin	53,000	Muscle fibers of all types
Vimentin	57,000	Cells of mesenchymal origin and some epithelial
		cells, such as mesothelium, thyroid, endometrium
Glial fibrillary proteins (GPF)	55,000	Glial cells, Schwann cells
Neurofilaments	68,000; 160,000; 200,000	Dendrites and axons; body of neuronal cells
Lamins	60,00–80,000	Form nuclear skeleton and various nuclear
		structures; similar to cytoplasmic IF

For further discussion of intermediate filaments, see Chapter 45.
Modified with permission from Nagle RB. Intermediate filaments: A review of the basic biology. Am J Surg Pathol, *12* (Suppl. 1): 4–16, 1988.

quired electron microscopy. The understanding of their chemical makeup, function, and molecular biology is an ongoing process. Microtubules are **hollow, tube-like structures,** which appear to be universally present in all cells, and are synthesized from precursor molecules of **tubulin.** As described earlier (see Figs. 2-9 and 2-10), **microtubules are an integral component of cilia, flagella, and centrioles** (see Fig. 2-24). Microtubules, like actin filaments (see above), are polarized, that is, they have one "minus" and one "plus" end; hence, they can be attached to two different molecules and form a bridge between them.

The principal role for microtubules and associated pro-

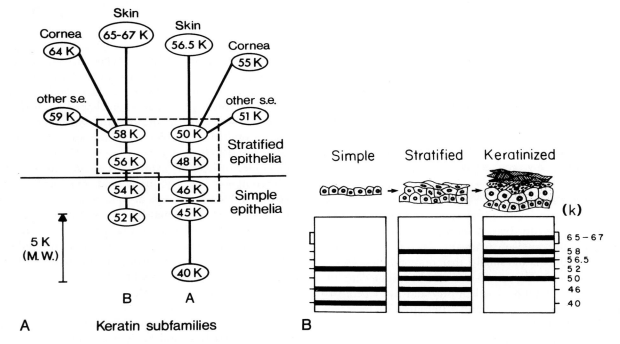

Figure 2-25 *A.* A unifying model of keratin expression. Keratins of subfamilies A (acidic) and B (basic) are arranged vertically, according to their relative molecular mass (molecular weights). The drawing indicates that keratin proteins of A and B type form pairs, with proteins of increasing relative molecular mass (M_r) making their appearance as epithelia mature from simple to stratified. K = kilodaltons; s.e. = stratified epithelia. *B.* A schematic drawing showing the embryonic development as well as the postulated evolutionary history of human epidermis. The bottom part of the drawing shows a simplified diagram of electrophoretic analysis of keratins of increasing M_r, expressed in kilodaltons (numbers on right) corresponding to the evolution of epithelia from simple to stratified to keratinized. K = kilodaltons; s.e. = stratified epithelium. (Sun TT, et al. Classification, expression, and possible mechanisms of evolution of mammalian epithelial keratins: A unifying model. *In* Levin AJ, et al (eds). Cancer Cells, vol. 1. Cold Spring Harbor, New York, Cold Spring Harbor Laboratory, 1984, pp 169–176.)

teins is their **participation in cellular events requiring motion.** Cilia and flagella are a good example of this function in which microtubules perform a sliding movement in association with a protein, dynein, and an energy-producing system, adenosine triphosphate (ATP).

The **mitotic spindle** is synthesized by the cells undergoing mitosis from molecules of tubulin. The **spindle formation may be inhibited** by some drugs, such as colchicine and vinblastine, **or enhanced** by Taxol, a potent anti-cancer drug, derived from the bark of a tree, the western yew (*Taxus brevifolia*). These drugs are commonly used in experimental work involving cell division. During cell division, **the centrioles serve as an organizing center for the mitotic spindle** (see above). From the centrioles, located at the opposite poles of the cell, the microtubules attach to the condensed double chromosomes arranged at the metaphase plate (see Chap. 4) and participate in the migration of the single chromosomes into the two daughter cells. Once the mitosis is completed, the spindle microtubules are depolarized and redistributed in the cytoplasm. Undoubtedly, microtubules perform yet other functions within the cell: they may be associated with movements of coated pits and pinocytotic vesicles to and from cell membranes and are associated with cell motion.

Storage of Products of Cell Metabolism Within the Cytoplasm

The identification of the many varied materials produced and stored within the cells was successfully accomplished before the era of electron microscopy. The identification of **lipids, glycogen, mucin, and pigments,** such as bile, hemosiderin, melanin, and lipofuscin, goes back to the 19th century. Electron microscopy has shed considerable light on their ultrastructure, the mechanisms of accumulation, and their relationship to various cytoplasmic organelles. Thus, lipids often accumulate in close rapport with mitochondria (see above). The role of the Golgi complex in the production of mucus and other cell products, and in formation of storage vesicles, was discussed above. The production of various **polypeptide hormones** in the pancreatic islet cells and other cells with endocrine function, accumulating in the form of endocrine cytoplasmic vesicles, has been documented (see Fig. 2-20). The histochemical or immunocytochemical **identification of the nature of various cell products** stored in the cytoplasm may play a **crucial role in diagnosis** of some cell and tissue disorders. As an example, the presence of mucin may be of value in the differential diagnosis of an adenocarcinoma, whereas the presence of melanin may establish the diagnosis of a malignant melanoma. The identification of specific hormones by immunocytochemistry is often of assistance in classifying tumors with endocrine function (see Chap. 45).

The Cytoplasmic Matrix

The space within the cytoplasm, not occupied by the membranous system, the cell skeleton, or by the organelles, is referred to as the *cytoplasmic matrix*. The matrix is composed of **proteins and free ribosomes.** There is still little knowledge about the makeup of the proteins constituting the bulk of the cytoplasmic matrix. It is quite certain that the matrix contains all of the **amino acids necessary for protein synthesis,** various **forms of RNA, and enzymes** (see Chap. 3). Under the impact of various chemicals or heat, the matrix may be irreversibly **coagulated; this is the principle of cell fixation.** In electron micrographs, the matrix appears as a homogeneous substance, occasionally containing fine granules, fibrils, or filaments.

The Nucleus and Its Membrane

The Nuclear Membrane

The nucleus is enclosed within the nuclear membrane, or **nuclear envelope,** composed of **two electron-dense membranes,** each measuring approximately 75 Å in thickness and separated from each other by a clear zone measuring from 200 to 400 Å in width. On the **inner (nuclear)** side of the nuclear membrane, there is a **layer of filaments (fibrous lamina),** about 300 Å in thickness, which presumably enhances the resilience of the membrane and may play a role in the anchorage of chromosomes. The **outer membrane** of the nuclear membrane resembles rough endoplasmic reticulum because numerous ribosomes are attached to it; thus, it may be considered as a part of the cell's inner membrane system. The nuclear membrane is characterized by the presence of **nuclear pores** (Fig. 2-26). A pore is an area where there is a **fusion of the two dense layers of the nuclear envelope.** A complex array of protein molecules with a central channel, about 9 nm in diameter **(nuclear pore complex),** constitutes the nuclear pore. The nuclear pores serve as **exchange channels between the nucleus and the cytoplasm.** Freeze-fracture of the nuclear membrane discloses that the **distribution of the nuclear pores is random** and does not follow any geometric pattern (Fig. 2-27). Still, the nuclear pores form a close relationship with individual chromosomes and their **number may be chromosome dependent.** For example, it has been shown that the number of nuclear pores is increased in aneuploid cancer cells with elevated DNA content and, hence, elevated number of chromosomes (Czerniak et al, 1984). This is in keeping with the new data on the organization of the normal interphase nucleus (see below). The nuclear membrane **disappears during the late prophase** of the mitosis and is **reformed during the late telophase** (for stages of mitosis, see Chap. 4). The probable mechanism of formation of the nuclear membrane is discussed below.

The intact nuclear envelope shows a **remarkable resistance to trauma** or corrosive chemicals such as acids or alkali. When a cell is exposed to such agents, the cytoplasm usually disintegrates fairly rapidly, but the nuclear envelope usually remains intact, protecting the contents of the nucleus. **This remarkable property of the nuclear envelope is utilized in many techniques of nuclear isolation,** for example, in measuring DNA content by flow cytometry (see Chap. 47).

The Nucleus

The nucleus is the principal repository site of DNA and, therefore, is the **center of events governing metabolic and**

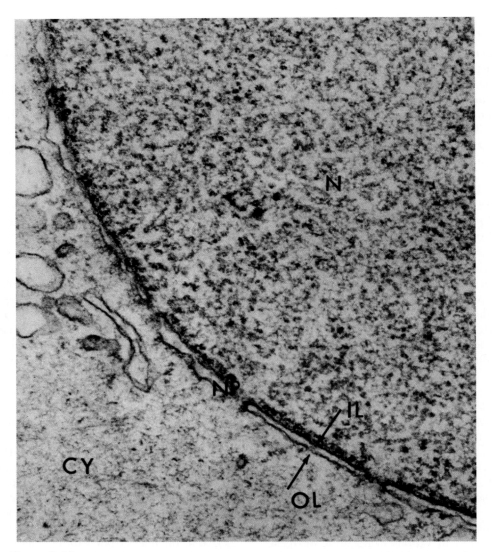

Figure 2-26   **Area of nucleus.** Electron micrograph of an epithelial cell, rat bladder; N = nucleus. Note the nuclear envelope, consisting of two membranes, the inner (IL) and the outer (OL), separated by a translucent space. The inner (nuclear) aspect of the nuclear membrane appears thick because of the presence of a fibrous lamina. Nuclear pores (NP) are well in evidence. Nuclear contents appear granular; CY = cytoplasm. (×64,000.)

reproductive processes of the cell. The basic concepts pertaining to the mechanism of DNA structure and function are described in Chapter 3. The events in cell division (cell cycle and mitosis) are described in Chapter 4.

Resting or Interphase Nucleus

In light microscopy of appropriately stained preparations, the **"resting" or interphase nuclei** of normal cells are seen as a **large, usually spherical structure** located within the cytoplasm. In stained preparations, the nucleus is surrounded by a **distinct, thin peripheral ring, representing the nuclear membrane.** The **location** of the nucleus depends on cell shape: in cells of approximately spherical, oval, or spindly configuration, the nucleus usually occupies a central position; in cells of columnar shape, which are usually polarized, the nucleus is frequently located in the vicinity of the distant cell pole, away from the lumen of the organ. The **shape** of the normal nucleus may vary: it is usually

spherical but may be oval, elongated, or even indented, and, hence, kidney-shaped, depending on cell type. In **polymorphonuclear leukocytes and megakaryocytes,** the nuclei form two or more lobes. Located **within the nucleus** is an important organelle, the **nucleolus,** which may be single or multiple (see below).

The dominant **chemical component** of the interphase nucleus is a **mixture of DNA and associated histones and nonhistone proteins (known in the aggregate as nuclear chromatin)** that readily reacts with dyes such as hematoxylin, that confer upon the nucleus a bluish stain of variable intensity (see Frontispiece and Fig. 2-1).

The **double-stranded DNA** within the nucleus can also be stained with a highly specific stain, the **Feulgen stain** (Fig. 2-28), which is extensively used in quantitative analysis of DNA. The total DNA can also be visualized and quantitated with the use of **specific fluorescent reagents (probes),** such as **propidium iodide or DAPI,** extensively

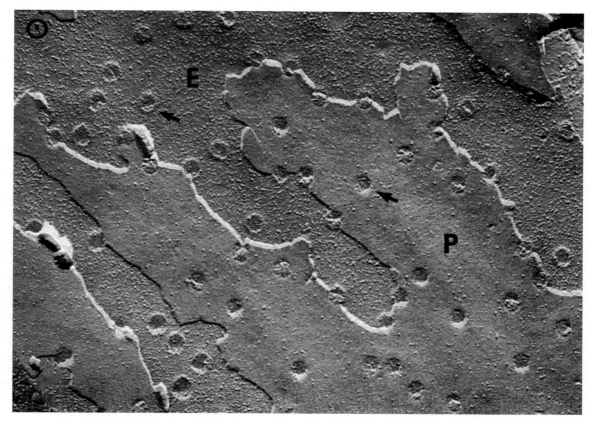

Figure 2-27   Freeze-fracture replica of the nuclear membrane of a urothelial cell, showing random distribution of the nuclear pores (*arrows*) on face E and face P. Note the fine granules of intermembrane proteins in the background. (Approx. ×50,000.) (Courtesy of Dr. Bogdan Czerniak.)

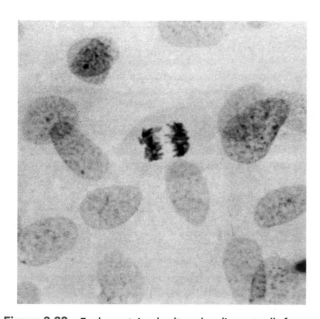

Figure 2-28   Feulgen-stained cultured malignant cells from an experimental carcinoma of the bladder (line BC 7, probably fibroblastic). The stain is specific for double-stranded DNA; hence, only the nuclei are stained. Note the increase in the intensity of staining of the condensed chromosomal DNA in the mitotic figures. (×1,000.) (Culture by Dr. Fritz Herz, Montefiore Hospital. Koss LG. Morphology of cancer cells. *In* Handbuch allgemeinen Pathologie, vol. 6, Tumors, part I. Berlin, Springer, 1974, pp 1–139.)

used in molecular biology and quantitative and analytical cytology (see Chap. 47).

The **size of the nucleus** depends substantially, but not absolutely, on its **DNA content. During the cell cycle,** described in Chapter 4, the **DNA content of the nucleus doubles during the synthesis phase (S-phase) and remains double until the cell divides. The diameter of nuclei with a double amount of DNA is about 40% larger** than that of nuclei in the resting phase of the cell cycle. Thus, the assessment of the nuclear size, an important feature in recognition of cancer cells, must always be compared with a population of normal cells. For further discussion of this issue, see Chapter 7.

In well-fixed and stained cells, within the homogeneous background of the nucleus (sometimes referred to as nuclear "sap"), one can observe a fine network of thin, thread-like linear condensations, known as the **linin network.** Located at various points in the network are small, dark **granules of odd shapes, the chromocenters.** The chromocenters are composed of an **inactive form of DNA,** composed of sequences that do not participate in the biologic activities; therefore, they are designated as **constitutive heterochromatin.** Constitutive heterochromatin may also be identified in chromosomal preparations around the centromeres (see Chap. 4). This form of chromatin should be distinguished from **another form of condensed chromatin that may occur in only some cells and that is called facultative**

heterochromatin. An example of the latter is the **sex chromatin body** (also known as the **Barr's body** after the person who described it), which is a condensed portion of one of the two X chromosomes and, therefore, is seen only in females or male individuals with genetic abnormalities, such as excess of X chromosome (Klinefelter's syndrome) (see Chaps. 4 and 9 for further discussion of this condition). The **sex chromatin body is seen as a triangular dark structure, attached by its base to the inner side of the nuclear membrane, with the tip of the triangle pointed toward the center of the nucleus.** The identification of the sex chromatin body is of value in the recognition of some genetic disorders and occasionally cancer cells (see Chaps. 7, 26, and 29).

Interphase Nucleus in Electron Microscopy

Except for the nuclear membrane, described above, the ultrastructure of the interphase nucleus does not cast much light on its organization. The area of the nucleus is filled with finely granular material, or **nuclear "sap" (nucleoplasm),** wherein one can observe scattered ribosomes. The filamentous proteins, lamins, may sometimes be observed as a network of fine filaments attached to the nuclear membrane. The **chromatin** may be seen as **overlapping electron-dense or dark areas at the periphery of the nucleus,** undoubtedly representing **fragments of chromosomes** attached to the nuclear membrane (see below—structure of interphase nucleus). The correlation of the electron microscopic images with specific chromosomes has been poor, even with the use of immunoelectron microscopy, wherein specific genes or proteins can be identified by antibodies usually labeled with colloidal gold.

The Nucleus in Cycling Cells

In a cell population that is proliferating and, therefore, is characterized by mitotic activity, the appearance of the nonmitotic nucleus may change. Besides the **enlargement,** caused by the increase in DNA during the **S-phase of the cell cycle** (see above), the granularity of the nucleus may increase substantially during the **prophase of the mitosis because of early condensation of parts of chromosomes** in the form of chromatin granules. Although such events are more common in cancer cells (see Chap. 7), they may also occur in normal cells undergoing cell division.

The Nucleolus

In a normal interphase resting nuclei, the nucleoli are seen as **round or oval structures of variable sizes,** averaging about 1 μm in diameter, occupying a small area within the nucleus. The location of the nucleoli is variable but, in light microscopy, they are usually located close to the approximate center of the nucleus, rarely at the periphery. The **number of nucleoli per nucleus** varies from one to four but usually only one nucleolus is observed. The reason for the variable number of nucleoli is their **origin in the nucleolar organizer loci, located on each of the two homologues of chromosomes 13, 14, 15, 21, and 22.** Thus, theoretically, 10 nucleoli per cell should be seen. However,

the small nucleoli merge shortly after the birth of the cell, thus reducing the total number of these organelles.

Thanks to the work of Caspersson and his colleagues in Sweden (1942, 1950), much is known about the **natural sequence of events in the life of a nucleolus.** The nucleoli are born within the nucleolar organizer loci in the designated portion of the chromosomes by accumulation of proteins and **ribonucleic acid (RNA),** which "explodes" the center of the chromosomal fragment (Figs. 2-29 and 2-30). The **chromosomal DNA of the nucleolus organizing locus forms a rim surrounding the RNA-rich central space and is easily recognized as the nucleolus-associated chromatin.** After merger of small nucleoli, the larger nucleolus, or nucleoli, occupies a central role in the life of a cell as the center of production of RNA (see Chap. 3). The nucleolus disappears at the onset of cell division, only to be reborn again in the daughter cells after mitosis.

The **size of the nucleoli** in interphase cells **varies according to the function of the cell.** In metabolically active cells, such as cells processing or secreting various products, the nucleoli are larger than in quiescent cells with limited metabolic activities. For example, in mucus-secreting intestinal epithelial cells, the nucleoli are larger than in squamous cells, which perform an essentially passive protective function. Under some circumstances, such as an **injury requiring rapid repair** when the cells are forced to produce a large amount of protein, the **accumulation of large amounts of RNA causes the nucleoli to become multiple and very large** and measure up to 4 or 5 μm in diameter. Large nucleoli of irregular configuration are common in cancer cells (see Chap. 7).

An important feature of the nucleoli in light microscopy is their **staining affinities.** The **center** of the nucleolus accepts **acidophilic dyes,** such as eosin, and therefore stains red. The periphery, that is, **the nucleolus-associated chromatin,** retains the staining features of DNA and, therefore, stains **blue with basophilic dyes.** In Feulgen stains, the nucleolus-associated chromatin accepts the dye, but the center of the nucleolus remains unstained.

The Nucleolus in Electron Microscopy

The ultrastructure of the nucleolus has been extensively studied because of its role as the center of production of RNA (see Chap. 3). The nucleolus is composed of electron-dense and electron-lucent areas. Occasionally, at the periphery of the nucleolus, a distinct dense zone corresponding to the nucleolus-organizing region of a chromosome may be distinguished. The core of the nucleolus corresponds to the granular and fibrillar products of ribosomal RNA in various stages of synthesis.

Organization of the Interphase Nucleus

Although the light microscopic structure and ultrastructure of the nucleus have been well known for many years, as summarized above, until the 1980s, no tools were available to probe the organization of the interphase nucleus. It was commonly thought that during interphase, the nuclear chromatin represented uncoiled chromosomal DNA, forming a structure of incredible complexity. Although individ-

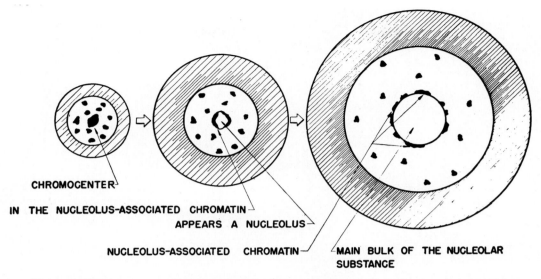

CHROMOCENTER

IN THE NUCLEOLUS-ASSOCIATED CHROMATIN

APPEARS A NUCLEOLUS

NUCLEOLUS-ASSOCIATED CHROMATIN

MAIN BULK OF THE NUCLEOLAR SUBSTANCE

Figure 2-29 Diagram of development of nucleolus from nucleolus-associated chromatin. (Caspersson TO. Cell Growth and Cell Function–A Cytochemical Study. New York, WW Norton, 1950.)

ual genes could be identified and localized on individual chromosomes by molecular biologic techniques (see Chap. 3), the overall organization of the interphase nucleus remained a mystery. On the other hand, considerable knowledge was accumulated in reference to the nucleus during mitosis, giving rise to the study of cytogenetics (see Chap. 4). Thus, it became known that the normal human cell contains **46 chromosomes, arranged in 22 pairs of nonsex chromosomes or autosomes and two sex chromosomes, either 2 X (in females) or XY (in males).** Thus, each chromosome had its double and both are known as **homologues.**

The introduction of **fluorescent probes,** first to specific segments of individual chromosomes and then to whole chromosomes, has now allowed us to study the **position and configuration of chromosomes in interphase cells.** The techniques are known as **fluorescent in situ hybridization (FISH),** and **chromosomal "painting"** techniques. A number of initial studies, conducted mainly on human cells in culture, suggested that, contrary to previous assumptions, individual chromosomes could be identified in interphase cells.

However, only a recent study of terminally differentiated human bronchial cells (Koss, 1998) could document that **all chromosomes retain their identity during the interphase** (Fig. 2-31). Further, it was shown that the **two homologues of the same chromosome were located in different portions of the nucleus and were in close apposition to the nuclear membrane.** By measuring angles formed by two homologues, it could be documented that the **position of individual chromosomes in interphase cells is constant** and is probably maintained in normal cells throughout the entire cell cycle. It was also documented that, in the bronchial cells, the **configuration of the two homologues was somewhat different,** suggesting that they may participate differently in cell function, as has been previously documented for X chromosome (Lyon's hypothesis, see Chap. 4). These studies strongly suggest that the **fundamental organization of the nuclear DNA is orderly throughout the life of the cell** and explains the orderly transmission of the genetic material from one generation of cells to another. The peripheral position of the chromosomes on the nuclear membrane also strongly suggested that **each homologue might be responsible for the formation of its own proprietary segment of the nuclear membrane** during the telophase. It was also suggested that the **nuclear pores,** which are the portals of exit (or entry) of the nuclear products (such as RNA) into the cytoplasm, might be formed at the points of junction of adjacent segments of the nuclear

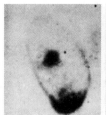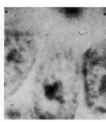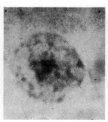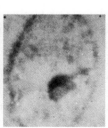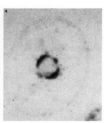

Figure 2-30 Actual photographs of development of nucleolus inside the nucleolus-associated chromatin in a neurocyte (Feulgen stain). (Caspersson TO. Cell Growth and Cell Function–A Cytochemical Study. New York, WW Norton, 1950.)

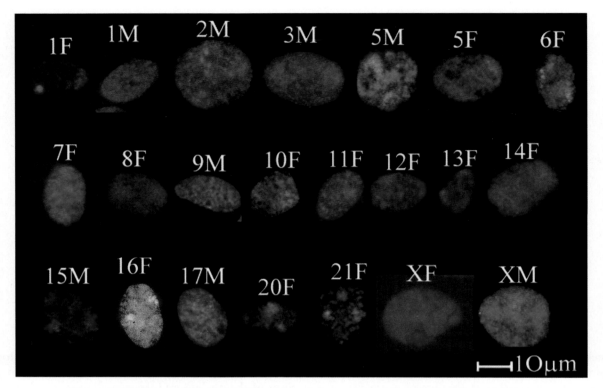

Figure 2-31   **The position and configuration of chromosomes in terminally differentiated bronchial cells (oval nuclei) or goblet cells (spherical nuclei) stained with FISH.** The two homologues of each chromosome are clearly located in different territories of the nucleus. The location of the autosomes on or adjacent to the nuclear membrane is evident. Identification numbers of chromosomes and the sex of the donor (F or M) are indicated. Only one signal was generated for the X chromosome in a male (XM). The differences in configuration and size of territories of the two autosomes (one "compact" and one "open") are best seen in chromosomes 1F, 1M, 5M, 5F, 7F, 8F, 9M, 10F, 12F, 15M, 20F, and XF. Similar differences were noted for other chromosomes but are not well shown.

membrane. The consequences of these observations may have a significant impact on our understanding of nuclear structure and function.

The Basement Membrane

The basement membrane is a complex structure that occurs at the **interface of epithelia and the underlying connective tissue.** There are several component parts to the basement membrane. Best seen in the electron micrograph is a thin, condensed, usually uninterrupted electron-opaque layer, known as **basal lamina** (see Figs. 2-5 and 2-14). Basal lamina is separated from the epithelial cell membranes by a narrow, electron-lucent layer known as **lamina lucida.** Crossing the lamina lucida are the cell junctions, known as **hemidesmosomes,** described above, that anchor epithelial cells to the basal lamina (see above and Fig. 2-14). On the side of the connective tissue, the basal lamina is in close contact with **collagen fibrils.** Basal lamina is also observed in nonepithelial tissues, for example, surrounding **smooth-muscle cells.** Within recent years, the basement membranes have been the subject of intensive studies, for several reasons. The basement membranes are a product of interaction between the epithelial cells and the connective tissue; hence,

they form a barrier that has been shown to be important in a variety of diseases. Cell surface receptor molecules, known as **integrins,** are an important factor in regulating the relationship of the cells to the extracellular matrix (Giancotti and Ruoslanti, 1999). Some examples of diseases affecting the basement membrane are disorders of the renal glomeruli, certain skin disorders, and invasive cancer. **Cancer cells,** even in invasive or metastatic cancers, **are capable of reproducing the basal lamina,** although it may be functionally deficient.

The principal functions of the basement membrane appear to be the support and anchorage of cells, such as epithelial cells, and, most likely, a regulatory role in the activity of some other cells, such as the smooth muscle. **Basal lamina also serves as a template in epithelial regeneration.** Major **chemical components** of the basement membrane include several complex proteins, such as laminins, collagen types IV and V, fibronectin, proteoglycans, and other adhesion molecules. The interrelationship of these components with each other, and the cells that produce it, is complex and not fully understood at this time. The relationship of cancer suppressor genes with various adhesion molecules and, hence, the basement membrane, in the genesis of benign tumors and formation of metastases in malignant tumors, is discussed in Chapters 3 and 7.

BIBLIOGRAPHY

Afzelius BA, Mossberg B. Immotile cilia. Thorax 35:401–404, 1980.

Allan BB, Balch WE. Protein sorting by directed maturation of Golgi compartments. Science 285:63–66, 1999.

Allfrey VG. Nuclear ribosomes, messenger-RNA and protein synthesis. Exp Cell Res (Suppl) 9:183–212, 1963.

Amos LA, Klug A. Arrangements of subunits in flagellar doublet microtubules. J Cell Sci 14:523–549, 1974.

Anderson S, Bankier AT, Barrell BG, et al. Sequence and organization of the human mitochondrial genome. Nature 290:457–465, 1981.

Baines AI. A spectrum of spectrins. Nature 312:310–311, 1984.

Baserga R, Huang C-H, Rossini M, et al. The role of nuclei and nucleoli in the control of cell proliferation. Cancer Res 36:4297–4300, 1976.

Baserga R, Nicolini C. Chromatin structure and function in proliferating cells. Biochim Biophys Acta 458:109–134, 1976.

Beard ME, Novikoff AB. Distribution of peroxisomes (microbodies) in the nephron of the rat. A cytochemical study. J Cell Biol 42:501–518, 1969.

Beebe TP Jr, Wilson TE, Ogletree DF, et al. Direct observation of native DNA structures with the scanning tunneling microscope. Science 370:370–372, 1989.

Bennet V, Cohen CM, Lux SE, Palek J (eds). Membrane Skeletons and Cytoskeletal-Membrane Associations. UCLA Symposia on Molecular and Cellular Biology, New Series, vol 38, 1986.

Berlin RD, Oliver JM, Ukena TE, Yin HH. The cell surface. N Engl J Med 292:515–520, 1975.

Bernier-Valentin F, Rousset B. Interaction of tubulin with cellular membranes. J Submicrosc Cytol 16:97–98, 1984.

Bershadsky AD, Vasiliev JM. Cytoskeleton. New York and London, Plenum Press, 1988.

Biological Imaging: Series of papers. Science 300:82–102, 2003.

Boesze-Battaglia K, Schimmel R. Cell membrane lipid composition and distribution: Implications for cell function and lessons learned from photoreceptors and platelets. J Exper Biol 200:2927–2936, 1997.

Borisy GBG, Cleveland DW, Murphy DB (eds). Molecular Biology of the Cytoskeleton. Cold Spring Harbor Laboratory, Cold Spring Harbor, New York, 1984.

Brachet J, Mirsky AE (eds). The Cell, 6 vols. New York, Academic Press, 1959–1961.

Brasseur R, Pillot T, Lins L, et al. Peptides in membranes: Tipping the balance of membrane stability. Trends in Biochem Sciences 22:167–171, 1997.

Bretscher MS. Endocytosis: Relation to capping and cell locomotion. Science 224:681–686, 1984.

Bretscher MS. Membrane structure: Some general principles. Science 181:622–629, 1973.

Brodsky FM. Living with clathrin: Its role in intracellular membrane traffic. Science 242:1396–1402, 1988.

Brodsky FM. Clathrin structure characterized with monoclonal antibodies. I. Analysis of multiple antigenic sites. J Cell Biol 101:2047–2054, 1985.

Brown WM. Polymorphism in mitochondrial DNA of humans as revealed by restriction endonuclease analysis. Proc Natl Acad Sci USA 77:3605–3609, 1980.

Burgos MH, Wislocki GB. Cyclical changes in guinea pig's uterus, cervix, vagina and sexual skin, investigated by histological and histochemical means. Endocrinology 59:93–118, 1956.

Cann RL, Stoneking M, Wilson AC. Mitochondrial DNA and human evolution. Nature 325:31–36, 1987.

Caplan MJ. Membrane polarity in epithelial cells: Protein sorting and establishment of polarized domains. Am J Physiol 272:425–429, 1997.

Carmo-Fonseca M, David-Ferreira JF. Interaction of intermediate filaments with cell structure. Electr Microsc Rev 3:115–141, 1990.

Caro LG, Palade GE. Protein synthesis, storage, and discharge in the pancreatic exocrine cells. J Cell Biol 20:473–495, 1964.

Case JT, Wallace DC. Maternal inheritance of mitochondrial DNA polymorphisms in cultured human fibroblasts. Somatic Cell Genet 7:103–108, 1981.

Caspersson T, Santesson L. Studies on the protein metabolism of the cells of epithelial tumors. Acta Radiol (Suppl 46):1–105, 1942.

Caspersson TO. Cell Growth and Cell Function. A Cytochemical Study. New York, WW Norton & Co., 1950.

Churchill J, Churchill A. Lysosomes. London, Ciba Foundation Symposium, 1963.

Ciba Foundation Symposium 108: Basement Membranes and Cell Movement. London, Pitman, 1984.

Cooper D, Schermer A, Sun TT. Biology of disease. Classification of human epithelia and their neoplasms using monoclonal antibodies to keratins: Strategies, applications, and limitations. Lab Invest 52:243–256, 1986.

Couchman JR, Hook M, Rees DA, et al. Adhesion, growth and matrix production by fibroblasts on laminin substrates. J Cell Biol 96:177–183, 1983.

Couvet J, Shengwen L, Okamoto T, et al. Molecular and cellular biology of caveolae. Paradoxes and plasticities. Trend Cardiovasc Med 7:103–110, 1997.

Cowin P, Garrod DR. Antibodies to epithelial desmosomes show wide tissues and species cross-reactivity. Nature 261:148, 1983.

Cricenti A, Selci S, Felici AC, et al. Molecular structure of DNA by scanning tunneling microscopy. Science 245:1126–1127, 1989.

Czerniak B, Koss LG, Sherman A. Nuclear pores and DNA ploidy in human bladder carcinomas. Cancer Res 44:3752–3756, 1984.

Dainiak N. Surface-membrane–associated regulation of cell assembly, differentiation, and growth. Blood 78:264–276, 1991.

Dalton AJ, Felix MD. Cytologic and cytochemical characteristics of the Golgi substance of epithelial cells of the epididymis in situ, in homogenates and after isolation. Am J Anat 94:171–187, 1954.

Davies E. Intercellular and intracellular signals and their transduction via the plasma membrane-cytoskeleton interface. Semin Cell Biol 4:139–147, 1993.

Davson H, Danielli JF. The Permeability of Natural Membranes, 2nd ed. London, Cambridge University Press, 1952.

De Pierre JW, Karnovsky ML. Plasma membranes of mammalian cells. A review of methods for their characterization and isolation. J Cell Biol 56:275–303, 1973.

deDuve C. The lysosome. Sci Am 208:64–72, 1963.

deDuve C, Baudhuin P. Peroxisomes (microbodies and related particles). Physiol Rev 46:323–357, 1966.

deDuve C, Wattiaux R. Functions of lysosomes. Ann Rev Physiol 28:435–492, 1966.

deHarven E, Bernhard W. Etude au microscope electronique de l'ultrastructure du centriole chez les vertebres. Z Zellforsch 45:378–398, 1956.

Dell'Angelica EC, Klumperman J, Stoorvogel W, Bonifacino JS. Association of the AP-3 adaptor complex with clathrin. Science 280:431–434, 1998.

Dembitzer HM, Herz F, Schermer A, et al. Desmosome development in an in vitro model. J Cell Biol 85:695–702, 1980.

DeRosier DJ, Tilney LG. The form and function of actin: A product of its unique design. *In* Shay JW (ed). Cell and Muscle Motility. The Cytoskeleton. New York, Plenum Press, 5:139–169, 1984.

DiMauro S, Schon EA. Mitochondrial respiratory-chain diseases. N Engl J Med 348:2656–2668, 2003.

Dingle JT, Fell HB (eds). Lysosomes in Biology and Pathology. Amsterdam, North Holland, 1969.

Domagala W, Koss LG. Configuration of surfaces of human cancer cells in effusions. A scanning electron microscope study of microvilli. Virch Archiv B (ZellPathol) 26:27–42, 1977.

Donaldson P, Eckert R, Green C, Kistler J. Gap junction channels: New roles in disease. Histol Histopathol 12:219–231, 1997.

Dustin P. Microtubules. New York, Springer-Verlag, 1970.

Easton JM, Goldberg B, Green H. Immune cytolysis: Electron microscopic localization of cellular antigens with ferritin-antibody conjugates. J Exp Med 115:275–288, 1962.

Engel J, Odermatt E, Engel A, et al. Shapes, domain organizations and flexibility of laminin and fibronectin, two multifunctional proteins of the extracellular matrix. J Mol Biol 150:97–120, 1981.

Engelman JA, Lee RJ, Karnezis A, et al. Reciprocal regulation of Neu thyrosine kinase activity and caveolin-1 protein expression in vitro and in vivo. Implications for human breast cancer. J Biol Chem 273:20448–20455, 1998.

Essner E, Novikoff AB. Cytologic studies on two functional hepatomas, interrelations of endoplasmic reticulum, Golgi apparatus, and lysosomes. J Cell Biol 15:289–312, 1962.

Estabrook RW, Holowinsky A. Studies on content and organization of respiratory enzymes of mitochondria. J Biophys Biochem Cytol 9:19–28, 1961.

Euteneuer U, McIntosh JR. Polarity of some motility-related microtubules. Proc Natl Acad Sci USA 78:372–376, 1981.

Fadic R, Johns DR. Clinical spectrum of mitochondrial diseases. Semin Neurol 16:11–20, 1996.

Farquhar MG, Palade GE. Junctional complexes in various epithelia. J Cell Biol 17:375–412, 1963.

Fawcett D. Cilia and flagella. *In* Brachet J, Mirsky AE (eds). The Cell, vol 2. New York, Academic Press, 1961, pp 217–297.

Fawcett DW. The Cell, 2nd ed. Philadelphia, WB Saunders, 1981.

Fawcett DW. The mammalian spermatozoon: A review. Dev Biol 44:394–436, 1975.

Fawcett DW. The membranes of the cytoplasm. Lab Invest 10:1162–1188, 1961.

Featherstone C. Coming to grips with Golgi. Science 282:2172–2174, 1998.

Flagg-Newton J, Simpson I, Loewenstein WR. Permeability of the cell-to-cell membrane channels in mammalian cell junction. Science 205:404–407, 1979.

Franke WW. Nuclear lamins and cytoplasmic intermediate filament proteins: A growing multigene family. Cell 48:3–4, 1987.

Franke WW, Appelhans O, Schmid E, et al. Identification and characterization of epithelial cells and mammalian tissue by immunofluorescence microscopy using antibodies to prekeratin. Differentiation 15:7–25, 1979.

Franke WW, Jahn L, Knapp AC. Cytokeratins and Desmosomal Proteins in Certain Epithelioid and Nonepithelial Cells. *In* Osborn M, Weber K (eds). Current Communications in Molecular Biology: Cytoskeletal Proteins in Tumor Diagnosis. Cold Spring Harbor, New York, Cold Spring Harbor Laboratory, 1989, pp 151–172.

Franke WW, Koch PJ, et al. The desmosome and the syndesmoses: Cell junctions in normal development and malignancy. Princess Takamatsu Symposia 24:14–27, 1994.

Franke WW, Moll R, Schiller DL, et al. Desmoplakins of epithelial and myocardial desmosomes are immunologically and biochemically related. Differentiation 23:115, 1982a.

Franke WW, Schiller DL, Moll R, et al. Diversity of cytokeratins: Differentiation specific expression of cytokeratin polypeptides in epithelial cells and tissues. J Mol Biol 153:933–959, 1981.

Franklin RJ, Caron M, Stiles GL. Mechanism of membrane-receptor regulation. N Engl J Med 310:1570–1578, 1984.

Freddo TF. Mitochondria attached to desmosomes in the ciliary epithelia of human, monkey and rabbit eyes. Cell Tissue Res 251:671–675, 1988.

Friend DS, Gilula NB. Variations in tight and gap junctions in mammalian tissues. J Cell Biol 53:758–776, 1972.

Fuchs E, Cleveland DW. A structural scaffolding of intermediate filaments in health and disease. Science 279:514–519, 1998.

Fuchs E, Weber K. Intermediate filaments: Structure, dynamics, function, and disease. Ann Rev Biochem 63:345–382, 1994.

Gabbiani G, Kapanci Y, Barazzone P, Franke WW. Immunochemical identification of intermediate-sized filaments in human neoplastic cells: A diagnostic aid for the surgical pathologist. Am J Pathol 104:206, 1981.

Geiger B. Membrane-cytoskeleton interaction. Biochem Biophys Acta 737:335–341, 1983.

Giancotti FG, Ruoslahti E. Integrin signaling. Science 285:1028–1032, 1999.

Giles RE, Blanc H, Cann HM, Wallace DC. Maternal inheritance of human mitochondrial DNA. Proc Natl Acad Sci USA 77:6715–6719, 1980.

Gillooly DJ, Stenmark H. A lipid oils the endocytosis machine. Science 291:993–994, 2001.

Goerlich D, Mattaj IW. Nucleocytoplasmic transport. Science 271:1513–1518, 1996.

Goldman AE, Green KJ, Jones JC, et al. Intermediate filaments: Their interactions with various cell organelles and their associated proteins. J Submicrosc Cytol 16:73–74, 1984.

Goodenough UW, Heuser JE. Structural comparison of purified dynein proteins with in situ dynein arms. J Mol Biol 180:1083–1118, 1984.

Gray MW, Burger G, Lang BF. Mitochondrial evolution. Science 283:1476–1481, 1999.

Green DE, MacLennan DH. Structure and function of the mitochondrial cristae membrane. Bioscience 19:213–222, 1969.

Hagenau F. The ergastoplasm: Its history, ultrastructure, and biochemistry. Int Rev Cytol 7:425–483, 1958.

Hall A. Rho GTPases and the actin cytoskeleton. Science 279:509–514, 1998.

Hansma PK, Elings VB, Marti O, Bracker CE. Scanning tunneling microscopy and atomic force microscopy: Application to biology and technology. Science 242:209–216, 1988.

Hartl FU, Neupert W. Protein sorting to mitochondria: Evolutionary conservations of folding and assembly. Science 247:930–938, 1990.

He W, Cowin P, Stokes DL. Untangling desmosomal knots with electron tomography. Science 302:109–113, 2003.

Henderson D, Geisler N, Weber K. A periodic ultrastructure in intermediate filaments. J Mol Biol 155:173–176, 1982.

Hicks RM. The function of the Golgi complex in transitional epithelium. Synthesis of the thick cell membrane. J Cell Biol 30:623–643, 1966.

Hirokawa N, Keller TCS III, Chasan R, Mooseker M. Mechanism of brush border contractility studied by the quick-freeze deep-etch method. J Cell Biol 96:1325–1336, 1983.

Hockenbery D, Nunez G, Milliman C, et al. Bcl is an inner mitochondrial membrane protein that blocks programmed cell death. Nature 348:4180–4186, 1990.

Hodges GM, Muir MD. A scanning electron-microscope study of the surface features of mammalian cells in vitro. J Cell Sci 11:233–247, 1972.

Holder JW, Elmore E, Barrett JC. Gap junction function and cancer. Cancer Res 53:3475–3485, 1993.

Holt IJ, Harding AE, Morgan-Hughes JA. Deletions of muscle mitochondrial DNA in patients with mitochondrial myopathies. Nature 331:717–719, 1988.

Huesgen CT, Burger PC, Crain BJ, Johnson GA. In vitro MR microscopy of the hippocampus in Alzheimer's disease. Neurology 43:145–152, 1993.

Hutter H, Vogel BE, Plenefisch JD, et al. Conservation and novelty in the evolution of cell adhesion and extracellular matrix genes. Science 287:989–994, 2000.

Hynes RO, Schwarzbauer JE, Tamkun JW. Fibronectin: A versatile gene for a versatile protein. In Basement Membrane and Cell Movement. Ciba Foundation Symposium 108: Basement Membrane and Cell Movement. London, Pitman, 1984, pp 75–92.

Izzaurralde E, Adam S. Transport of macromolecules between the nucleus and the cytoplasm. RNA 4:351–364, 1998.

Johnson GA, Benveniste H, Engelhardt RT, et al. Magnetic resonance microscopy in basic studies of brain structure and function. Ann NY Acad Sci 30:139–147; 147–148, 1997.

Johnson KA, Rosenbaum JL. Replication of basal bodies and centrioles. Curr Opin Cell Biol 4:80–85, 1992.

Jones JC, Asmuth J, Baker SE, et al. Hemidesmosomes: Extracellular matrix/intermediate filament connectors. Exp Cell Res 213:1–14, 1994.

Katz SI. The epidermal basement membrane: Structure, ontogeny and role in disease. In Ciba Foundation Symposium 108: Basement Membrane and Cell Movement. London, Pitman, 1984, pp 243–259.

Kelly DE, Shienvold FL. The desmosome: Fine structural studies with freeze-fracture replication and tannic acid staining of sectioned epidermis. Cell Tissue Res 172:309–323, 1976.

Kelly RB. Pathways of protein secretion in eukaryotes. Science 230:25–32, 1985.

Knox AL, Brown NH. Rap1 GTPase regulation of adherens junction positioning and cell adhesion. Science 295:1285–1288, 2002.

Korn ED, Carlier MF, Pantaloni D. Actin polymerization and ATP hydrolysis. Science 238:638–644, 1987.

Kornberg RD. Chromatin structure: A repeating unit of histones and DNA. Science 184:868–871, 1974.

Koss LG. Characteristics of chromosomes in polarized normal human bronchial cells provide a blueprint for nuclear organization. Cytogenet Cell Genet 82:230–237, 1998.

Koss LG. Electron microscopy in cytology. Acta Cytol 29:195–196, 1985.

Koss LG. The asymmetric unit membrane of the epithelium of the urinary bladder of the rat. An electron microscopic study of a mechanism of epithelium maturation and function. Lab Invest 21:154–168, 1969.

Kumar NM, Gilula NB. Molecular biology and genetics of gap junction channels. Semin Cell Biol 3:3–16, 1992.

Kurtz SM. The fine structure of the lamina densa. Lab Invest 10:1189–1208, 1961.

Kuznetsov G, Nigam SK. Folding of secretory and membrane proteins. New Engl J Med 339:1688–1695, 1998.

Lang F, Busch GL, Ritter M, et al. Functional significance of cell volume regulatory mechanisms. Physiol Rev 78:247–306, 1998.

Lavin P, Koss LG. Effect of a single dose of cyclophosphamide on various organs in the rat. IV. The kidney. Am J Pathol 62:169–180, 1973.

Lazarides E. Intermediate filaments as mechanical integrators of cellular space. Nature 283:249–256, 1980.

Lee G, Arscott PG, Bloomfield VA, Evans DF. Scanning tunneling microscopy of nucleic acids. Science 244:475–477, 1989.

Lefkowitz RJ, Caron MG, Stiles GL. Mechanisms of membrane-receptor regulation. Biochemical, physiological and clinical insights derived from studies of the adrenergic receptors. N Engl J Med 310:1570–1578, 1984.

Leitch B. Ultrastructure of electrical synapses: Review. Electron Microsc Rev 5:311–339, 1992.

Levin ER. Endothelins. N Engl J Med 333:356–363, 1995.

Liotta LA, Rao NC, Barsky SH, Bryant G. The laminin receptor and basement membrane dissolution: Role in tumour metastasis. In Basement Membranes and Cell Movement (Ciba Foundation Symposium 108), 1984, pp 146–162.

Love R, Soriano RZ. Correlation of nucleolini with fine nucleolar constituents of cultured normal and neoplastic cells. Cancer Res 31:1030–1037, 1971.

Luna EJ, Hitt AL. Cytoskeleton-plasma membrane interaction. Science 258:955–964, 1992.

Madri JA, Prat BM, Yurchenco PD, Furthmayr H. The ultrastructural organization and architecture of basement membranes. In Ciba Foundation Symposium 108: Basement Membrane and Cell Movement. London, Pitman, 1984, pp 6–24.

Malhotra SK. The Plasma Membrane. New York, John Wiley, 1983.

Marsh M, McMahon HT. The structural era of endocytosis. Science 285:215–220, 1999.

Marx JL. A potpourri of membrane receptors. Science 230:649–651, 1985.

Maul GG (ed). Nuclear Envelope and the Nuclear Matrix. New York, Alan R. Liss, 1982.

McCarthy JB, Furcht LT. Laminin and fibronectin promote the directed migration of B16 mouse melanoma cells in vitro. J Cell Biol 98:1474–1480, 1984.

McManus ML, Churchwell KB, Strange K. Regulation of cell volume in health and disease. N Engl J Med 333:1260–1266, 1995.

McNutt NS, Weinstein RS. Membrane ultrastructure at mammalian intercellular junctions. In Butler JAV, Noble D (eds). Prog Biophys Mol Biol 26:45–101, 1974.

Mermall V, Post PL, Mooseker MS. Unconventional myosins in cell movement, membrane traffic, and signal transduction. Science 279:527–533, 1998.

Mills JW, Mandel LJ. Cytoskeletal regulation of membrane transport events. FASEB 8:1161–1165, 1994.

Mitchison T, Kirschner M. Microtubule dynamics and cellular morphogenesis. In Borisy CG, Cleveland DW, Murphy DB (eds). Molecular Biology of the Cytoskeleton. Cold Spring Harbor Laboratory, Cold Spring Harbor, New York, 1984, pp 27–44.

Moore MS, Mahaffey DT, Brodsky FM, Anderson RGW. Assembly of clathrin-coated pits onto purified plasma membranes. Science 236:558–563, 1987.

Moraes CT, DiMaura S, Zeviani M, et al. Mitochondrial DNA deletions in progressive external opthalmoplegia and Kearns-Sayre syndrome. N Engl J Med 320:1293–1299, 1989.

Moreau MF, Chretien MF, Dubin J, et al. Transposed ciliary microtubules in Kartagener's syndrome. A case report with electron microscopy of bronchial and nasal brushings. Acta Cytol 29:248–253, 1985.

Moses M. Breakdown and reformation of the nuclear envelope at cell division. In Proceedings of the 4th Int. Conf. on Electron Microscopy. Berlin, Springer-Verlag, 1960, pp 230–233.

Mueller H, Franke WW. Biochemical and immunological characterization of desmoplakins I and II, the major polypeptides of the desmosomal plaque. J Mol Biol 163:647-671, 1983.

Mukherjee S, Ghosh RN, Maxfield FR. Endocytosis. Physiol Rev 77:759–803, 1997.

Nagle RB. A review of intermediate filament biology and their use in pathologic diagnosis. Mol Biol Rep 19:3–21, 1994.

Nagle RB. Intermediate filaments: A review of the basic biology. Am J Surg Pathol 12(Suppl 1):4–16, 1988.

Novikoff AB, Holtzman E. Cells and Organelles, 2nd ed. New York, Holt, Rinehart and Winston, 1976.

Novikoff AB, Novikoff PM, Davis C, Quintana N. Studies on microperoxisomes. V. Are microperoxisomes ubiquitous in mammalian cells? J Histochem Cytochem 21:737–755, 1973.

Okamoto T, Schlegel A, Scherer PE, et al. Caveolins, a family of proteins for organizing 'preassembled signal complexes' at the plasma membrane. J Biol Chem. 273:5419–5422, 1998.

Olkkonen VM, Ikonen E. Genetic defects of intracellular-membrane transport. N Engl J Med 343:1095–1102, 2000.

Osborn M, Weber K (eds). Current Communications in Molecular Biology: Cytoskeletal Proteins in Tumor Diagnosis. New York, Cold Spring Harbor Laboratory, 1989.

Osborn M, Altmannsberger M, Debus E, Weber K. Differentiation of the major human tumor groups using conventional and monoclonal antibodies specific for individual intermediate filament proteins. Ann NY Acad Sci 455: 649–668, 1985.

Osborn M, Geisler N, Shaw G, Weber K. Intermediate filaments. Cold Spring Harbor Symp Quant Biol 46:413–430, 1982.

Osborn M, Weber K. Biology of disease. Tumor diagnosis by intermediate filament typing: A novel tool for surgical pathology. Lab Invest 48:372–394, 1983.

Palade GE. Symposium: Structure and biochemistry of mitochondria: Electron microscope study of mitochondrial structure. J Histochem Cytochem 1: 188–211, 1953.

Palade GE, Porter KR. Studies on endoplasmic reticulum: I. Its identification in cells in situ. J Exper Med 100:641–656, 1954.

Pappas GD, Waxman SG. Synaptic fine structure-morphological correlates of chemical and electronic transmission. *In* Pappas GD, Purpura DP (eds). Structure and Function of Synapses. New York, Raven Press, 1972, pp 1–43.

Parry DA, Steinert PM. Intermediate filament structure. Curr Opin Cell Biol 4: 94–98, 1992.

Paul DL. New functions of gap junctions. Curr Opin Cell Biol 7:665–672, 1995.

Payne GS, Schekman R. Clathrin: A role in the intracellular retention of a Golgi membrane protein. Science 245:1358–1365, 1989.

Payne GS, Schekman R. A test of clathrin function in protein secretion and cell growth. Science 230:1009–1014, 1985.

Pierce GB Jr, Midgley AR, Ram SJ. The histogenesis of basement membranes. J Exp Med 117:339–348, 1963.

Pollard TD, Cooper JA. Actin and actin-binding proteins. A critical evaluation of mechanisms and functions. Annu Rev Biochem 55:987–1035, 1983.

Pollister AW. Nucleoproteins of nucleus. Exp Cell Res (Suppl) 2:59–74, 1952.

Porter KA (ed). The cytoplasmic matrix and the integration of cellular function. J Cell Biol 99, 1, part 2. New York, Rockefeller Univ. Press, 1984.

Porter KA, Tucker JB. The ground substance of the living cell. Sci Amer March, 57–67, 1981.

Porter KR. An Introduction to the Fine Structure of Cells and Tissues, 2nd ed. Philadelphia, Lea & Febiger, 1964.

Quax W, Khan PM, Quax-Jeuken Y, Blomendal H. The human desmin and vimentin genes are located on different chromosomes. Gene 38:189–196, 1985.

Raff EC. Genetics of microtubule system. J Cell Biol 99:1–10, 1984.

Raff RA, Mahler HR. The nonsymbiotic origin of mitochondria: The question of the origin of the eukaryotic cell and its organelles is reexamined. Science 177:575–582, 1972.

Ramaekers F, Huysmans A, Moesker O, et al. Monoclonal antibody to keratin filaments, specific for glandular epithelia and their tumors. Lab Invest 49: 353–361, 1983.

Raviola E, Goodenough DA, Raviola G. Structure of rapidly frozen gap junctions. J Cell Biol 87:273–279, 1980.

Reddy JK, Krishnakantha TP, Rao MS. Microbody (peroxisome) proliferation in mouse kidney induced by methyl clofenapate. Virchows Arch (B) 17: 295–306, 1975.

Remedios CGD, Bardden JA (eds). Actin: Structure and function in muscle and non-muscle cells. Sydney, Academic Press, 1983.

Revel JP, Karnovsky MJ. Hexagonal arrays of subunits of intercellular junctions of the mouse heart and liver. J Cell Biol 33:C7–C12, 1967.

Rhodin JAG. An Atlas of Ultrastructure. Philadelphia, WB Saunders, 1963.

Roberts K, Hyams IS (eds). Microtubules. New York, Academic Press, 1979.

Rodrigues-Boulan E, Nelson WJ. Morphogenesis of the polarized epithelial cell phenotype. Science 245:718–725, 1989.

Rothman JE, Wieland FT. Protein sorting by transport vehicles. Science 272: 227–234, 1996.

Rouiller C. Physiological and pathological changes in mitochondrial morphology. Int Rev Cytol 9:227–292, 1960.

Rungger-Brandle E, Gabbiani G. The role of cytoskeletal and cytocontractile elements in pathologic processes. Am J Pathol 110:361–392, 1983.

Ruoslahti E, Pierschbacher MD. New perspectives in cell adhesion: RGD and integrins. Science 238:491–497, 1987.

Sabatini DD, Kreibich G, Morimoto T, Adesnik M. Mechanisms for the incorporation of proteins in membranes and organelles. J Cell Biol 92:1–22, 1982.

Sale WS, Satir P. The direction of active sliding of microtubules in Tetrahymena cilia. Proc Natl Acad Sci USA 74:2045–2049, 1977.

Sanborn E, Koen PF, McNable JD, Moore G. Cytoplasmic microtubules in mammalian cells. J Ultrastruct Res 11:123–138, 1964.

Satir P. Structure and function in cilia and flagella. Protoplasmatologia III E, pp 1–52, 1965.

Satir P. On the evolutionary stability of the 9 + 2 pattern. J Cell Biol 12: 181–184, 1962.

Sbarbati A, Osculati F. Tissual imaging by nuclear magnetic resonance. Histol Histo Pathol 11:229–235, 1996.

Schatz G, Dobberstein B. Common principles of protein translocation across membranes. Science 271:1519–1526, 1996.

Schekman R, Orci L. Coat protein and vesicle budding. Science 271:1526–1533, 1996.

Schlegel A, Volonte D, Engelman JA, et al. Crowded little caves: Structure and function of caveolae. Cell Signal 10:457–463, 1998.

Schlessinger D. Ribosomes: Development of some current ideas. Bacteriol Rev 33:445–453, 1969.

Schliwa M. The Cytoskeleton. Vienna, New York, Springer-Verlag, 1985.

Schmelz M, Duden R, Cowin P, Franke WW. A constitutive transmembrane glycoprotein of Mr 165,000 (desmoglein) in epidermal and nonepidermal desmosomes. I. Biochemical identification of the polypeptide. Eur J Cell Biol 42:177–183, 1986.

Schmidt A, Heid HW, Schafer S, et al. Desmosomes and cytoskeletal architecture in epithelial differentiation: Cell type-specific plaque components and intermediate filament anchorage. Europ J Cell Biol 65:229–245, 1994.

Shaw G, Weber K. The distribution of the neurofilament triplet proteins within individual neurones. Exp Cell Res 136:119–125, 1981.

Shotton DM. Robert Feulgen Prize Lecture 1995. Electronic light microscopy: present capabilities and future prospects. Histochem Cell Biol 104:97–137, 1995.

Singer SJ, Nicholson GL. The fluid mosaic model of the structure of cell membranes. Science 175:720–731, 1972.

Singh S, Koke JR, Gupta PD, Malhotra SK. Multiple roles of intermediate filaments. Cytobios 77:41–57, 1994.

Sjöstrand FS. Fine structure of cytoplasm. The organization of membranous layers. Rev Mod Phys 31:301–318, 1959.

Sleigh MA. Cilia and Flagella. London, Academic Press, 1974.

Spray DC. Molecular physiology of gap junction channels. Clin Exp Pharmacol Physiol 23:1038–1040, 1996.

Staehelin LA. The structure and function of intercellular junctions. Int Rev Cytol 39:191–283, 1974.

Steven AC, Hainfeld JT, Trus BL, et al. Conformity and diversity in the structures of intermediate filaments. Ann NY Acad Sci 455:371–380, 1985.

Stevens A, Lowe J. Histology. London, Gower Medical Publishing, 1992.

Stewart M. Intermediate filament structure and assembly. Curr Opin Cell Biol 5:3–11, 1993.

Stoekenius W. The molecular structure of lipid-water systems and cell membrane model studies with electron microscope. *In* Harris RJC (ed). Interpretation of Ultrastructure. New York, Academic Press, 1963, pp 349–367.

Stubblefield E, Brinkley BR. Architecture and function of the mammalian centriole. *In* Warren KB (ed). Formation and Fate of Cell Organelles. New York, Academic Press, 1967, pp 175–218.

Sun TT, Eichner R, Schermer A, et al. Classification, expression, and possible mechanisms of evolution of mammalian epithelial keratins: A unifying model. *In* Levine AJ, Van de Wonde GF, Topp WC, Watson JD (eds). The Transformed Phenotype: Cancer Cells, vol 1. Cold Spring Harbor Laboratory, Cold Spring Harbor, New York, 1984, pp. 169–176.

Sun TT, Scheffer CG, Tseng A, et al. Monoclonal antibody studies of mammalian epithelial keratin. A review. Ann NY Acad Sci 455:307–329, 1984.

Sun TT, Shih CH, Green H. Keratin cytoskeletons in epithelial cells: Growth, structural and antigenic properties. Cell Immunol 83:1, 1979.

Sun TT, Shih CH, Green H. Keratin cytoskeletons in epithelial cells of internal organs. Proc Natl Acad Sci USA 76:2813–2817, 1979.

Thomas L. Organelles as organisms. *In* The Lives of a Cell. Notes of a Biology Watcher. New York, Viking, 1974.

Timpl R, Martin GR. Components of basement membranes. *In* Furthmayr H (ed). Immunochemistry of the Extracellular Matrix. Boca Raton, CRC Press, 1982, pp 119–150.

Timpl R, Fujiwara S, Dziadek M, et al. Laminin, proteoglycan, nidogen and collagen IV. Structural models and molecular interactions. *In* Basement Membranes and Cell Movement (Ciba Foundation Symposium 108), 1984, pp 25–43.

Toner PG, Carr KE. Cell Structure. An Introduction to Biological Electron Microscopy. Edinburgh, Churchill Livingstone, 1971.

Tucker JB. Spatial organization of microtubule-organizing centres and microtubules. J Cell Biol 99:55s–62s, 1984.

Tucker JB, Mathews SA, Hendry KAK, et al. Spindle microtubule differentiation and deployment during micronuclear mitosis in paramecium. J Cell Biol 101:1966–1976, 1985.

Underwood JCE (ed). Pathology of the Nucleus. Berlin, Springer-Verlag, 1990.

Unwin N, Henderson R. The structure of proteins in biological membranes. Sci Am 250:78–94, 1984.

Vallee RB, Bloom GS, Theurkauf WE. Microtubule-associated proteins: Subunits of the cytomatrix. J Cell Biol 99:38s–44s, 1984.

Verner K, Schatz G. Protein translocation across membranes. Science 241: 1307–1318, 1988.

Wallace DC. Mitochondrial disease in man and mouse. Science 283: 1482–1488, 1999.

Wallace DC. Mitochondrial DNA mutations and neuromuscular disease. Trend Genet 5:9–13, 1989.

Warfield RKN, Bouck GB. Microtubule-macrotubule transitions: Intermediates after exposure to the mitotic inhibitor vinblastine. Science 86:1219–1221, 1974.

Weber K, Osborn M. Cytoskeleton: Definition, structure and gene regulation. Path Res Pract 75:128–145, 1982.

Weeds A. Actin-binding proteins-regulators of cell architecture and motility. Nature 96:811–816, 1982.

Welter C, Kovacs G, Seitz G, Blin N. Alteration of mitochondrial DNA in human oncocytomas. Genes Chromosomes Cancer 1:79–82, 1989.

Wheatley DN. The Centriole: A Central Enigma of Cell Biology. New York, Elsevier, 1982.

Wickner WT, Lodish HF. Multiple mechanisms of protein insertion into and across membranes. Science 30:400–407, 1985.

Willis EJ. Crystalline structures in the mitochondria of normal human liver parenchymal cells. J Cell Biol 24:511–514, 1965.

Wilson L (ed). The Cytoskeleton, Cytoskeletal Proteins, Isolation and Characterization. New York, Academic Press, 1982.

Yaffe MP. The machinery of mitochondrial inheritance and behavior. Science 283:1493–1497, 1999.

Yamamoto T. On the thickness of the unit membrane. J Cell Biol 17:413–422, 1963.

Yunis JJ, Yasmineh WG. Heterochromatin satellite DNA and cell function. Science 174:1200–1209, 1971.

How Cells Function: Fundamental Concepts of Molecular Biology*

3

Molecular biology is a branch of the biologic sciences that attempts to explain life and its manifestations as a series of chemical and physical reactions. The critical event that led to the development of this new science was the discovery of the fundamental **structure of deoxyribonucleic acid (DNA)** by Watson and Crick in 1953. Few prior developments in biology have contributed so much and so rapidly to our understanding of the many fundamental aspects of cell function and genetics. Although, so far, the impact of molecular biology on diagnostic cytology has been relatively modest, this may change in the future. Therefore, some of the fundamental principles of this new science are briefly summarized. The main purpose of this review is to describe the events in DNA replication, transcription, and translation of genetic messages; to clarify the new terminology that has entered into the scientific vocabulary since 1953; and to explain the techniques that are currently used to probe the functions of the cell. It is hoped that this review will enable the reader to follow future developments in this still-expanding field of knowledge. Of necessity, this summary touches upon only selected aspects of molecular biology, representing a personal choice of topics that, in the judgment of the writer, are likely to contribute to diagnostic cytology. For reasons of economy of space, with a very few exceptions, the names of the many investigators who con-

---

* For a glossary of terms used in this chapter, see appendix at end of chapter.

tributed to this knowledge are not used in this text. Readers are referred to other sources listed in the bibliography for a more detailed record of individual contributors and additional information on specific technical aspects of this challenging field.

Molecular biology is easily understood because it is logical and based on the simple principles of organic chemistry. Hence, basic knowledge of organic chemistry is necessary to understand the narrative. Every attempt has been made to tell the story in a simple language.

THE CELL AS A FACTORY

Although the main morphologic components of the cell have been identified by light and electron microscopy (see Chap. 2), until 5 decades ago, the understanding of the mechanisms governing cell function has remained elusive and a matter for conjecture. Molecular biology has now shed light on some of these mechanisms, although, at the time of this writing (2004), much remains to be discovered. The living cell is best conceived as a **self-contained miniature factory that must fulfill a number of essential requirements necessary to manufacture products, either for its own use or for export** (Fig. 3-1). A cell is a three-dimensional structure contained within the **cell membrane**, which is a highly sophisticated, flexible structure (see Chap.

2). The membrane not only protects the cell from possible hostile elements or environmentally unfavorable conditions, but it is also capable of **selective intake of materials that are important and necessary to the survival of the cell;** this latter property is vested in specialized molecular sites: **the membrane receptors** (see Chap. 2). The cell exports finished products by using intricate mechanisms in which the cell membrane is an active participant. The membrane is also provided with a series of devices, such as **cell junctions, which allow the cell to live in harmony and to communicate with its neighbors.**

The cell is constructed in a sturdy fashion, thanks to the **cell skeleton** composed of microfilaments, intermediate filaments, and microtubules (see Chap. 2). The cell is capable of producing the components of its own skeleton and of regulating their functions. The **energy needs** of the cell are provided by the metabolism of foodstuffs, mainly sugars and fats, interacting with the energy-producing systems, adenosine 5′-triphosphate (ATP), vested primarily in the mitochondria. **The machinery that allows the cell to manufacture or synthesize products for its own use or for export,** mainly a broad variety of proteins, **is vested in the system of cytoplasmic membranes, the smooth and rough endoplasmic reticulum, and in the ribosomes** (see Chap. 2). **Disposal** of useless or toxic products is vested in the system of **lysosomes** and related organelles. As a signal advantage of most cells over a manmade factory, the cell is

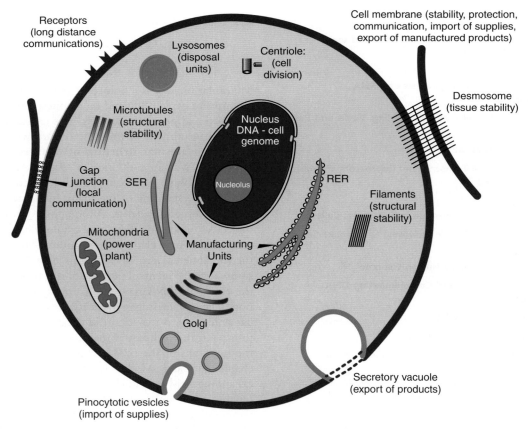

Figure 3-1 A schematic view of a cell as a factory. The functions of the various structural components of the cell are indicated. SER = smooth endoplasmic reticulum; RER = rough endoplasmic reticulum.

provided with a **system of reproduction** in its own image, in the form of **cell division or mitosis** (see Chap. 4). Thus, aged and inadequately functioning cells may be replaced by daughter cells, which ensure the continuity of the cell lineage, hence of the tissue, and ultimately of the species. The equilibrium among cells is also maintained by a **mechanism of elimination of unwanted or unnecessary cells** by a process known as **apoptosis, or programmed cell death.** Apoptosis plays an important role during embryonal development, wherein unnecessary cells are eliminated in favor of cells that are needed for construction of tissues or organs with a definite function. Apoptosis also occurs in adult organisms and may play an important role in cancer. The mechanisms of apoptosis are complex and consist of a cascade of events, involving the mitochondria and the nuclear DNA, discussed at length in Chapter 6.

It is quite evident from this brief summary that a highly sophisticated system of organization, which will coordinate its many different functions, must exist within each cell. Furthermore, within multicellular organisms, these functions vary remarkably from cell to cell and from tissue to tissue; hence, they must be governed by a flexible mechanism of control. The **dominant role in the organization of the cell function is vested in the DNA,** located in the cell's nucleus. The mechanisms of biochemical activities directed by DNA and the interaction of molecules encoded therein is the subject of this summary.

DEOXYRIBONUCLEIC ACID (DNA)

Background

The recognition of the microscopic and ultrastructural features of cells and their fundamental components, such as the nucleus, the cytoplasm with its organelles, and the cell membrane, all described in Chapter 2, shed little light on the manner in which cells function. The key questions were: How does a cell reproduce itself in its own image? How are the genetic characteristics of cells inherited, transmitted, and modified? How does a cell function as a harmonious entity within the framework of a multicellular organism?

The facts available to the investigators during the 100 years after the initial observations on cell structure were few and difficult to reconcile. The developments in organic chemistry during the 19th century documented that the **cells are made up of the same elements as other organic matter, namely, carbon, hydrogen, oxygen, nitrogen, phosphorous, calcium, sulfur,** and very small amounts of some other inorganic elements. Perhaps the most critical discovery was the synthesis of urea by Wöhler in 1828. Soon, a number of other organic compounds, such as various proteins, fats and sugars, were identified in cells. Of special significance for molecular biology was the observation that **all proteins are composed of the same 20 essential amino acids.** A further important observation was that most **enzymes,** hence substances responsible for the execution of many chemical reactions, **were also proteins.** The cell ceased to be a chemical mystery, but it remained a functional puzzle.

The observations by the Czech monk, Gregor Mendel (or Mendl), who first set down the laws governing **dominant and recessive genetic inheritance** by simple observations on garden peas, opened yet another pathway to molecular biology. Was there any possible link between biochemistry and genetics? The phenomenon of mitosis, or cell division, and the presence of chromosomes were first observed about 1850, apparently by one of the founding fathers of contemporary pathology, Rudolf Virchow. Several other 19th-century observers described chromosomes in some detail and speculated on their possible role in genetic inheritance, but, again, there was no obvious way to reconcile the chromosomes with the genetic and biochemical data.

In 1869, a Swiss biochemist, Miescher, isolated a substance from the nuclei of cells from the **thymus** of calves, named **thymonucleic acid,** and since renamed **deoxyribonucleic acid or DNA.** The relationship between DNA and the principles of genetic inheritance, as defined by Mendel, was not apparent for almost a century. A hint linking the chromosomes with the "thymonucleic" acid was provided by Feulgen and Rossenbach, who, in 1924, devised a DNA-specific staining reaction, which is known today as the **Feulgen stain.** It could be shown that chromosomes stained intensely with this stain (see Fig. 2-28). Interestingly, in the 1930s, the Swedish pioneer of cytochemistry, Torbjörn Caspersson, suggested that thymonucleic acid could be the substance responsible for genetic events in the cell.

It was not, however, until 1944 that Avery, MacCarty, and MacLeod, working at the Rockefeller Institute in New York City, described a series of experiments documenting that **DNA was the molecule responsible for morphologic changes in the bacterium,** *Diplococcus pneumoniae,* thus providing firm underpinning to the principle that the genetic function was vested in this compound. The universal truth of this discovery was not apparent for several more years, particularly because bacterial DNA does not form chromosomes. The understanding of the mechanisms of the function of DNA had to await the discovery of the fundamental structure of this molecule by Watson and Crick in 1953. For a recent review of these events, see Pennisi (2003).

Structure

DNA was once described as a "fat, cigar-smoking molecule that orders other molecules around." In fact, the molecule of **DNA is central to all events occurring within the cell.** In bacteria and other relatively simple organisms not provided with a nucleus **(prokaryotes),** the DNA is present in the cytoplasm. In higher organisms **(eukaryotes),** most of the DNA is located within the nucleus of the cell. In a nondividing cell, the DNA was thought to be diffusely distributed within the nucleus. Recent investigations, however, strongly suggest that even in the nondividing cells, the chromosomes retain their identity and occupy specific territories within the nucleus (Koss, 1998). For further details of the nuclear structure, see Chapter 2. During cell division, the DNA is condensed into visible chromosomes (see Chap. 4). Small amounts of DNA are also present in other cell organelles, mainly in the mitochondria; hence, the suggestion that mitochondria represent previously independent bacterial organisms that found it advantageous to live in symbiosis with cells (see Chap. 2). To understand how DNA performs the many essential functions, it is important to describe its structure. **DNA forms the well-known double helix,** which can be best compared to an ascending spiral staircase or a twisted ladder (Fig. 3-2). The staircase has a supporting external structure, or **backbone,** composed of molecules of a pentose sugar, **deoxyribose,** bound to one another by a molecule of **phosphate.** This external support structure of the staircase is organized in a highly specific fashion: the organic rings of the sugar molecules are alternately attached to the phosphate by their 5′ and 3′ carbon molecules* (Fig. 3-3). This construction is fundamental to the understanding of the **synthesis of nucleic acids, which always proceeds from the 5′ to the 3′ end, by addition of sugar molecules in the 3′ position.** The **steps of the staircase** (or rungs of the ladder) are **formed by matching molecules of purine and pyrimidine bases,** each attached to a molecule of the sugar, deoxyribose, in the backbone of the molecule (Fig. 3-4; see Fig. 3-2). The purines are **adenine (A)** and **guanine (G);** the pyrimidines are **thymine (T)** and **cytosine (C).** It has been known since the 1940s, thanks to the contributions of the chemist, Chargaff, that in all DNA molecules, regardless of species of origin, the proportions of adenine and thymine on the one hand, and of guanine and cytosine on the other hand, were constant. This information, combined with data from x-ray crystallography of purified molecules of DNA, allowed Watson and Crick to construct their model of the DNA molecule. In it, the purine, adenine, and the pyrimidine, thymine (the **A-T bond),** and cytosine and guanine (the **C-G bond)** are always bound to each other. The triple C-G bond is stronger than the double A-T bond (see Figs. 3-2 and 3-4). This **relationship of purines and pyrimidines is immutable,**

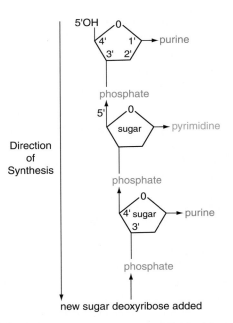

Figure 3-3   **Schematic representation of the backbone of DNA** and the direction of synthesis from 5′ to 3′, indicating positions of carbons in the molecules of sugar.

except for the **replacement of thymine by uracil (U) in RNA** (see below), and is the basis of all subsequent technical developments in the identification of matching fragments of nucleic acids (see below). The term **base pairs (bp)** is frequently used to define one matching pair of nucleotides and to define the length of a segment of double-stranded DNA. Thus, a DNA molecule may be composed of many thousands of base pairs. It is of critical importance to realize that the sequence of the purine-pyrimidine base pairs varies significantly, in keeping with the encoding of the genetic message, as will be set forth below.

Packaging

DNA is an enormous molecule. If fully unwrapped, it measures about 2 meters in length (but only 2 nm in diameter) in each single human nucleus. Each of the 46 individual human chromosomes contains from 40 to 500 million base pairs and their DNA is, therefore, of variable length, but still averages about 3 cm. It is evident, therefore, that to fit this gigantic molecule into a nucleus measuring from 7 to 10 μm in diameter, it must be folded many times. The **DNA is wrapped around nucleosomes,** which are cylindrical structures, composed of proteins known as *histones* (see Fig. 4-5). This reduces the length of the molecule significantly. Further reduction of the molecule is still required, and it is assumed that DNA forms multiple coils and folds to form a compact structure that fits into the space reserved for the nucleus. An apt comparison is with a wet towel that is twisted to rid it of water and then folded and refolded to form a compact ball. The interested reader is referred to a delightful book by Calladine and Drew (1997) that explains in a simple fashion what is known today about packaging of DNA. Be it as it may, individual chromosomes are

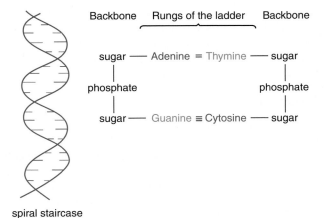

spiral staircase

Figure 3-2   **Fundamental structure of DNA shown as a twisted ladder** (*left*). The principal components of the backbone of the ladder and of its rungs are shown on the *right*. It may be noted that the triple bond between purine (guanine) and the pyrimidine (cystosine) is stronger than the double bond between adenine and thymine.

---

* *The 5′ and 3′ designate carbons in the sugar molecules that distinguish them from carbons 5 and 3, occurring in pyrimidine and purine base.*

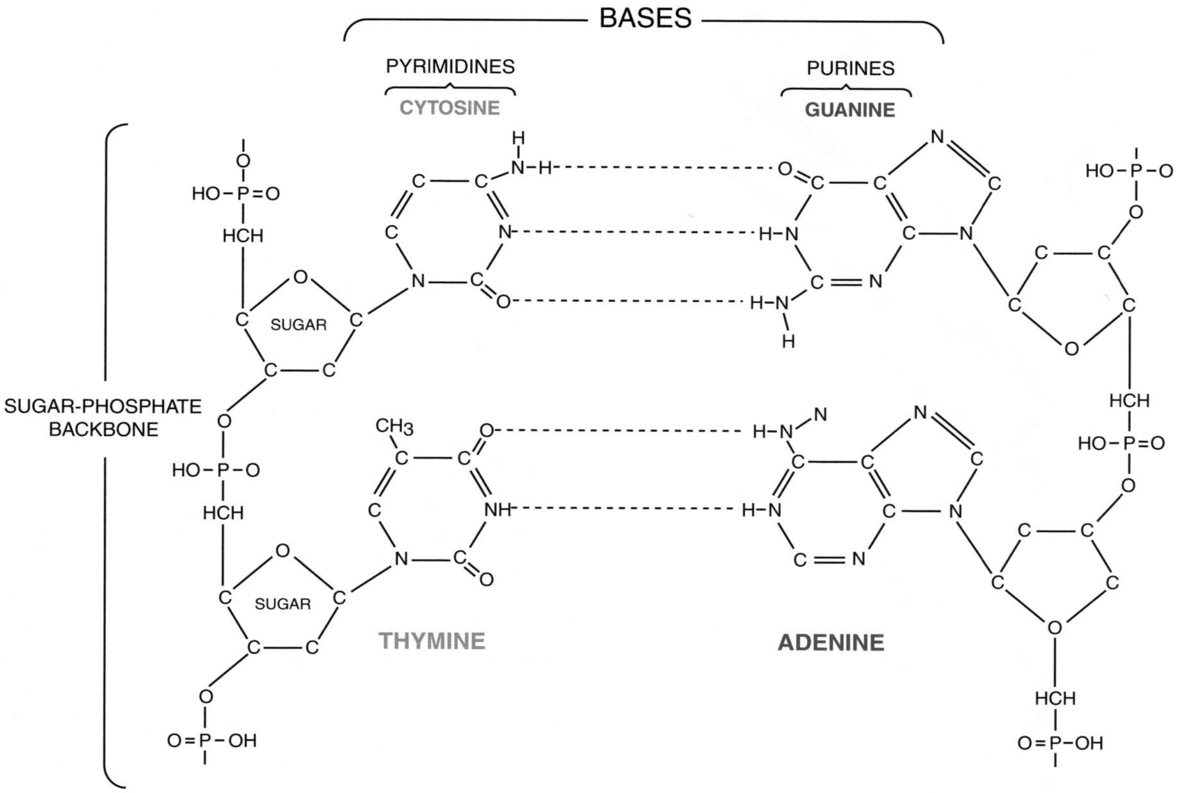

Figure 3-4   Two steps in the DNA ladder. The ladder is shown opened out (uncoiled).

Replication

The elegance and simplicity of the structure of the double helix resolved the secret of inheritance of genetic material. Because the double helix is constructed of two reciprocal, matching molecules, it was evident to Watson and Crick that **DNA replication can proceed in its own image:** the double helix can be compared to a zipper, composed of two corresponding half-zippers. Each half of the zipper, or one strand of DNA, serves as a template for the formation of a mirror image, complementary strand of DNA (Fig. 3-5). Hence, the first event in DNA replication must be the separation of the two strands forming the double helix. The precise mechanism of strand separation is still not fully understood, although the enzyme primase plays an important role. A further complication in the full understanding of the mechanisms of DNA replication is that the DNA molecule is wrapped around nucleosomes (see above). How the nucleosomal DNA is unwrapped and replicated, or for that matter transcribed (see below), is not fully understood as yet.

The synthesis of the new strand, governed by enzymes known as **DNA polymerases,** follows the fundamental principle of A-T and G-C pairing bonds and the principle of the 5'-to-3' direction of synthesis, as described above. Because the two DNA strands are reciprocal, the synthesis on one strand is continuous and proceeds without interruption in the 5'-to-3' direction. The synthesis on the other strand also follows the 5'-to-3' rule but must proceed in the opposite direction; hence, it is discontinuous (Fig. 3-6). The segments of DNA created in the discontinuous manner are spliced together by an enzyme, ligase. When both strands of DNA (half-zippers) are duplicated, two identical molecules (full-zippers) of DNA are created. This fundamental basis of DNA replication permits the daughter cells to inherit all the characteristics of the mother cell that are vested in the DNA. Replication of DNA takes place during a well-defined period in a cell's life, the **synthesis phase or S-phase of the cell cycle, before the onset of cell division (mitosis)** (see Chap. 4). By the time the cell enters the mitotic division, the DNA, in the form of chromosomes; is already duplicated. Each chromosome is composed of two identical mirror-image DNA segments (chromatids), bound together by a centromere (see Fig. 4-2). It is evident that the mechanism of DNA replication is activated before mitosis, when the chromosomal DNA is not visible under the light microscope, because the chromosomes are markedly elongated.

The exact sequence of events leading to the entry of the cell into the mitotic cycle is still under investigation and may be influenced by extracellular signals (see review by Cook, 1999). Whatever the mechanism, a family of proteins, **cyclins,** causes the resting cell to enter and progress through the phases of the cell division. For a review of cyclins, see the article by Darzynkiewicz et al (1996) and Chapter 4.

It is also known that the **replication of the chromo-**

composed of multiple coils of DNA, as shown in Figure 4-5 and discussed at some length in Chapter 4.

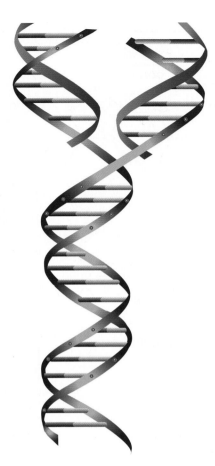

Figure 3-5 **The DNA molecule and its manner of replication.** Each base pair and its respective sugar–phosphate helix comes apart and induces synthesis of its complementary chain.

DNA Replication (trigger : primase)

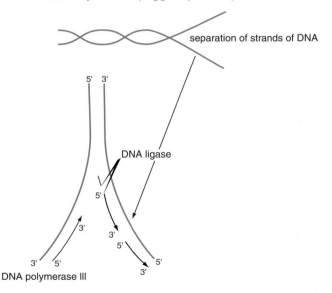

Figure 3-6 **Events in DNA replication.** Following the 5′ to 3′ direction of synthesis, one strand replicates in a continuous manner, whereas the complementary second strand replicates in shorter segments that must be bound (spliced) together by the enzyme, ligase.

somes is not synchronous and that some of them replicate early and others replicate late. It has been proposed that those genes common to all cells that ensure the fundamental cell functions and "housekeeping" chores, replicate during the first, early part of the S-phase, whereas the tissue-specific genes replicate late. During other phases of the cell cycle, the mechanism of DNA replication is either inactive or markedly reduced.

If one considers that during the lifetime of the human organism, DNA replication occurs billions of times and that even single **errors of replication** affecting critical segments of DNA may result in serious genetic damage that may lead to clinical disorders (see below), it is evident that efficient mechanisms of replication control must exist that will eliminate or neutralize such mistakes. Work on bacteria suggests that there are at least three controlling steps in DNA replication: selection of the appropriate nucleotide by DNA polymerases; recognition of the faulty structure by another enzyme; and finally, the repair of the damage. In eukaryotic cells, the molecule **p53,** which has been named **"the guardian of the genome,"** appears to play a critical role **in preventing replication errors** prior to mitosis. As discussed in Chapter 6, cells that fail to achieve DNA repair will be eliminated by the complex mechanism of **apoptosis.** Regardless of the technical details, it is quite evident that these control mechanisms of DNA replication in multicellular organisms are very effective.

Transcription

Once the fundamental structure of DNA became known, attention turned to the manner in which this molecule governed the events in the cell. There were two fundamental questions to be answered: How were the messages inscribed in the DNA molecule (i.e., how was the genetic code constructed?) and how were they executed? It became quite evident that the gigantic molecule of DNA could not be directly involved in cell function, particularly in the formation of the enzymes and other essential molecules. Furthermore, it had been known that protein synthesis takes place in the cytoplasm and not in the nucleus; hence, it became clear that an intermediate molecule or molecules had to exist to transmit the messages from the nucleus to the cytoplasm (see Fig. 3-8A). The best candidate for this function was **RNA.** RNAs, or the **ribose nucleic acids,** were analyzed at about the same time that the basic chemical makeup of DNA became known, in the 1940s. They were known to **differ from DNA in three respects: the sugar** in the molecule was **ribose,** instead of deoxyribose (hence the name); the molecule, instead of being double-stranded, was **single-stranded** (although there are some exceptions to this rule, notably in some viruses composed of RNA); and the **thymine** was replaced by a very similar base, **uracil** (Fig. 3-7). Several forms of RNA of different molecular weight (relative molecular mass) were known to exist in the cytoplasm and the nucleus. However, they appeared to be stable and, accordingly, not likely to fulfill the role of a messenger molecule that had to vary in length (and thus in molecular mass)

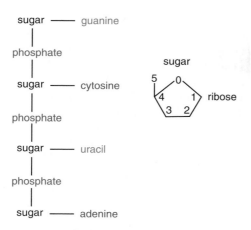

Figure 3-7   Fundamental structure of an RNA molecule and its sugar, ribose.

to reflect the complexity of the messages encoded in the DNA. The molecule that was finally identified as a **messenger RNA, or mRNA,** was difficult to discover because it constitutes only a small proportion of the total RNA (2% to 5%) and because of its relatively short life span. The DNA code is **transcribed** into mRNA with the help of specific enzymes, **transcriptases** (Fig. 3-8A). The transcription, which occurs in the nucleus on a single strand of DNA, follows the principles of nucleotide binding, as described for DNA replication, except that in RNA, thymine is replaced by a similar molecule, uracil (Fig. 3-8B). As will be set forth in the following section, each molecule of mRNA corresponds to one specific sequence of DNA nucleotides, encoding the formation of a **single protein molecule, hence a gene.** Because the size of the genes varies substantially, the mRNAs also vary in length, thus in molecular mass, corresponding to the length of the polypeptide chain to be produced in the cytoplasm. The identification of and, subsequently, the in vitro synthesis of mRNA proved to be critical in the further analysis of the genetic code and in subsequent work on analysis of the genetic activity of identi-

fiable fragments of DNA. For a recent review of this topic, see articles by Cook (1999) and Klug (2001).

Reannealing

In experimental in vitro systems, **the bonds between the two chains of DNA can be broken** by treatment with alkali, acids, or heat. Still, the affinity of the two molecules is such that once the cause of the strand separation is removed, the two chains will again come together, an event known as **reannealing.** These properties of the double-stranded DNA became of major importance in gene analysis and molecular engineering.

MOLECULAR TRAFFIC BETWEEN THE NUCLEUS AND THE CYTOPLASM

Although it has been known for many years that the nucleus is provided with gaps in its membrane, known as the **nuclear pores** (see Chap. 2 and Fig. 2-26), the precise function of the nuclear pores was unknown. Within recent years, some light has been shed on the makeup of the nuclear pores and on the mechanisms of transport between the nucleus and the cytoplasm. The nuclear pores are composed of complex molecules of protein that interact with DNA (Blobel, 1985; Gerace et al, 1978; Davies and Blobel, 1986). Further, specific molecules have been identified that assist in the export of mRNA and tRNA from the nucleus into the cytoplasm and import of proteins from the cytoplasm into the nucleus across the nuclear pores. Proteins, known as **importins** and **exportins** have now been identified as essential to the traffic between the nucleus and the cytoplasm. The interested readers are referred to a summary article by Pennisi (1998) and the bibliography listed.

The Genetic Code

The unraveling of the structure of DNA and its mechanism of replication was but a first step in understanding the mech-

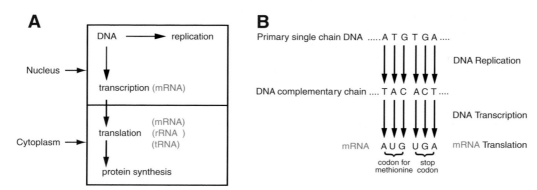

Figure 3-8   *A.* A diagrammatic representation of the principal nuclear and cytoplasmic events in protein formation. *B.* DNA replication, transcription, and translation for the amino acid methionine and for the stop codons, indicating the beginning and the end of protein synthesis. Note the replacement of thymine (T) by uracil (U) in mRNA. It is evident that the process could be reversed; by unraveling the composition of a protein and its amino acids, it is possible to deduce the mRNA condons, thereby the DNA code for this protein.

anism of cell function. The subsequent step required deciphering the message contained in the structure. Since neither the sugar molecule nor the phosphate molecule had any specificity, **the message had to be contained in the sequence of the nucleotide bases (i.e., A,G,T, and C),** as was suggested by Watson and Crick shortly after the fundamental discovery of the structure of the DNA. It was subsequently shown that the **DNA code is limited to the formation of proteins from the 20 essential amino acids.** The specific sequences of nucleotides that code for amino acids could be defined only after the pure form of the intermediate RNA molecules could be synthesized.

By a series of ingenious and deceptively simple experiments, it was shown that **different clusters of three nucleotides coded for each of the 20 amino acids,** the primary components of all proteins. A sequence of three nucleotides, encoding a single amino acid, is known as a **codon** (Fig 3-9B). **A series of codons, corresponding to a single, defined polypeptide chain or protein, constitutes a gene.** As discussed in the foregoing, the code inscribed in the DNA molecule is transcribed into mRNA, which carries the message into the cytoplasm of the cell wherein protein formation takes place (see Fig. 3-8A). The code, therefore, was initially defined, not as a sequence of nucleotides in the DNA, but as it was transcribed into RNA. Because there are four nucleotides in the RNA molecule (A,G,C, and U, substituting for T), and three are required to code for an amino acid, there are 4 X 4 X 4 or 64 possible combinations. These combinations could be established by using synthetic

RNA. Thus, the identity of the triplets of nucleotides, each constituting a codon, could be precisely established (see Fig. 3-9). It may be noted that only **one amino acid, methionine, is coded by a unique sequence,** AUG (adenine, uracil, guanine). It was subsequently proven that the **codon for methionine initiated the synthesis of a sequence of amino acids constituting a protein.** In other words, every protein synthesis starts with a molecule of methionine, although this amino acid can be removed later from the final product. All other amino acids are encoded by two or more different codons. There are also three nucleotide sequences that are interpreted as termination or **"stop"** codons. The stop codons signal the end of the synthesis of a protein chain.

Once the RNA code was established, it became very simple to identify corresponding nucleotide sequences on the DNA by simply substituting U(racil) by T(hymine). This reciprocity between DNA and RNA base sequences was also subsequently utilized in further molecular biologic investigations (see Fig. 3-8B).

MECHANISMS OF PROTEIN SYNTHESIS OR mRNA TRANSLATION

The unraveling of the genetic code and the unique role of proteins still did not clarify the precise mechanisms of the synthesis of proteins, often composed of thousands of amino acids. It is now known that protein formation,

GENETIC CODE

1st position (5')	2nd position				3rd position (3')
	U	**C**	**A**	**G**	
U	Phe	Ser	Tyr	Cys	U
	Phe	Ser	Tyr	Cys	C
	Leu	Ser	*Stop*	*Stop*	A
	Leu	Ser	*Stop*	Trp	G
C	Leu				U
	Leu	Pro	etc.		C
	Leu				A
	Leu				G
A			etc.		U
					C
					A
	Met				G
G			etc.		U
					C
					A
				Gly	G

EXAMPLES OF CODONS

CUC leucine	UUU phenylalanine	CCC proline	GGG glycine	AUG methionine

Figure 3-9 Examples of codons for several amino acids using the first, second, and third position of the mRNA nucleotides, uracil (U), cytosine (C), adenine (A), and guanine (G). It may be noted that 19 amino acids have multiple codes (for example, tyrosine [Tyr] is coded by UAU and UAC). There is but one code for methionine (Met), namely AUG, indicating the beginning of a protein. There are several stop codons, indicating the end of protein synthesis (see Fig. 3-8B).

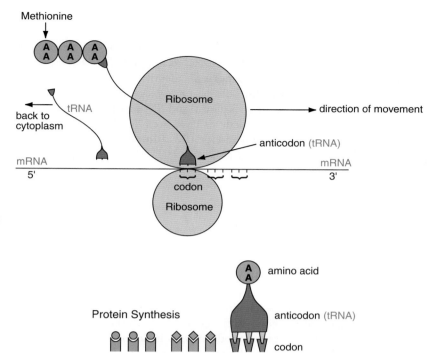

Figure 3-10 **Schematic representation of protein formation.** mRNA glides along a groove separating the two components of the ribosome in the 5′ to 3′ direction. Each codon is matched by an "anticodon," carried by transfer RNA (tRNA), that one-by-one brings the amino acids encoded in mRNA to form a chain of amino acids or a protein. The protein synthesis begins with methionine and stops with a stop codon. Once the tRNA has delivered its amino acid, it is returned to the cytoplasm to start the cycle again. AA = amino acid.

or **translation of the message encoded in mRNA,** takes place in the cytoplasm of the cell and requires two more types of RNA. One of these is **ribosomal RNA (rRNA),** which accounts for most of the RNA in the cell and is the principal component of **ribosomes.** These granule-like organelles are each made up of one small and one larger spherical structure separated by a groove, thus somewhat resembling a Russian doll (see Fig. 2-17). The third type of RNA is the **transfer RNAs (tRNA),** which function as carriers of the 20 specific amino acids that are floating freely in the cytoplasm of the cell. For a recent review of this topic, see the article by Cech (2000).

The synthesis of proteins occurs in the following manner: mRNA, carrying the message for the structure of a single protein, enters the cytoplasm, where it is captured by the ribosomes. The synthesis is initiated by the codon for methionine. The mRNA slides along the ribosomal groove, and the **sequential codons are translated one by one into specific amino acids that are brought to it by tRNA.** Each molecule of tRNA with its specific **anticodon sequences that correspond to the codons,** carries one amino acid

(Fig. 3-10). In translation, the same principles apply to the matching (pairing) of nucleotides and the direction of synthesis, from the 5′ to the 3′ end, as those discussed for DNA replication and transcription into mRNA. The amino acids attach to each other by their carboxy (COOH)—and amino (NH)—terminals and form a protein chain. The synthesis stops when a stop codon is reached and the protein is released into the cytoplasm where it can be modified before use or export (Fig. 3-11). The specific sequence of events in translation is currently under intense scientific scrutiny. It is generally assumed that inaccurate translation results in formation of a so-called nonsense protein that is apparently recognized as such and is either not further utilized or is destroyed.

UNIQUENESS OF PROTEINS AS CELL BUILDING BLOCKS AND BASIS OF PROTEOMICS

The deciphering of the genetic code led to one inescapable conclusion: The **code operates only for amino acids, hence proteins, and not for any other structural or chemical cell components, such as fats or sugars.** Therefore, proteins, including a broad array of enzymes, are the core of all other cell activities and direct the synthesis or metabolism of all other cell constituents. By a feedback mechanism, the synthesis and replication of the fundamental molecules of DNA or RNA are also dependent on the 20 amino acids that form the necessary enzymes. Proteins execute all events in the cell and, thus, may be considered the plenipotentiaries of the genetic messages encoded in DNA and transmitted by RNA. One must reflect on the extraordinary simplicity

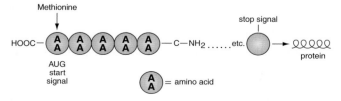

Figure 3-11 **The basic structure of a protein.** All amino acids have one acid carboxymolecule ending COOH and one amino ending C-NH2. The end product is usually coiled and folded in a manner that ensures its specificity. AA = amino acid.

of this arrangement and the hierarchical organization that governs all events in life.

The recognition of the unique role of proteins in **health** and **disease** has led to the recently developed techniques of **proteomics.** The purpose of proteomics is the identification of proteins that may be specific for a disease process, leading to development of specific drugs (Liotta and Petricoin, 2000; Banks et al, 2000). Micromethods have been developed that allow **protein extraction and identification** from small fragments of tissue (Liotta et al, 2001).

DEFINITION OF GENES

Once the mechanism of protein formation had been unraveled, it became important to know more about the form in which the message is carried in the DNA. Briefly, from a number of studies, initially with the fruit fly, *Drosophila*, then with the mold, *Neurospora*, it could be demonstrated that each protein, including each enzyme, had its own genetic determinant, called a *gene*. With the discovery of the structure of DNA and the genetic code, a **gene is defined as a segment of DNA, carrying the message corresponding to one protein or, by implication, one enzyme.** The significance of the precise reproduction of the genetic message became apparent in 1949, when Linus Pauling and his colleagues suggested that sickle cell anemia, characterized by a deformity of the shape of red blood cells, was a "molecular disease." The molecular nature of the disease was established some years later by Ingram, who documented that sickling was due to the **replacement of a single amino acid** (hence, by implication, one codon in several hundred) in two of the four protein chains in hemoglobin. This replacement **changes the configuration of the hemoglobin molecule** in oxygen-poor environments, with resulting deformity of the normal spherical shape of red blood cells into curved and elongated structures that resemble "sickles." More importantly still, sickle cell anemia behaves exactly according to the principles of heredity established by Mendel. If only one parent carries the gene, the offspring has a "sickle cell trait." If both parents carry the gene, the offspring develops sickle cell anemia.

To carry the implications of these observations still further, if the genes are segments of nuclear DNA, then they should also be detectable on the metaphase chromosomes. With the development of specific genetic probes and the techniques of in situ hybridization, to be described below, the presence of normal and abnormal genes on chromosomes could be documented.

REGULATION OF GENE TRANSCRIPTION: REPRESSORS, PROMOTERS, AND ENHANCERS

Once the principles of the structure, replication, and transcription of DNA were established, it became important to learn more about the precise mechanisms of regulation of these events. If one considers that the length of the DNA

chain in an *Escherichia coli* bacterium is about four million base pairs and that of higher animals in excess of 80 million base pairs, these molecules must contain thousands of genes. How these genes are transcribed and expressed became the next puzzle to be solved. Since it appeared that the fundamental mechanisms could be the same, or similar, in all living cells regardless of species, these studies were initially carried out on bacteria, which offered the advantage of very rapid growth under controlled conditions that could be modified according to the experimental needs.

The French investigators, Jacob and Monod, demonstrated that the functions of genes controlling the utilization of the sugar, lactose, by the bacterium *E. coli*, depended on a feedback mechanism. The activation or deactivation of this mechanism depended on the presence of lactose in the medium. It was shown that the transcription of the gene encoding an enzyme (β-galactosidase) that is necessary for the utilization of lactose, is regulated by an interplay between two DNA sequences, the **repressor** and the **operator.** The activation or deactivation of the repressor function is vested in the operator. The repressor function, which prevents the activation of the family of enzymes known as **transcriptases,** is abolished at the operator site by the presence of lactose. In the absence of lactose, the repressor gene is active and blocks the transcription at the operator site. Once the operator gene is derepressed by the lactose, the β-galactosidase gene is transcribed into the specific mRNA by the enzyme, RNA polymerase. The activity of the RNA polymerase is triggered by two sequences of bases located on the DNA molecule, one about 35 and the other about 10 bases **ahead of the site of transcription,** or **upstream.** These DNA sequences are known as **promoters** and they are recognized by RNA polymerase as a signal that the transcription may begin **downstream,** that is, at the first nucleotide of the DNA sequence (gene) to be transcribed (Fig. 3-12). The promoter is provided with specific, very short nucleotide sequences, or **"boxes,"** which regulate still further the transcription of DNA into mRNA (the discussion of boxes will be expanded below). The terms *upstream* and *downstream* have become incorporated into the language of molecular biology to indicate nucleotide sequences located on the DNA either before or after a specified gene or sequence of genes.

In the cytoplasm of the bacterium, the mRNA, which contains the sequences necessary for the transcription of the β-galactosidase, together with two other adjacent genes (providing additional enzymes necessary for utilization of lactose by the bacterium) is transcribed into the three enzymes. The name **operon** was given to a sequence of the three genes that are transcribed into a single mRNA molecule. Subsequently, similar regulatory mechanisms were observed for other genes on prokaryotic cells, confirming the general significance of these observations.

The search for similar mechanisms in eukaryotic cells began soon thereafter. An important difference in mRNA between prokaryotic and eukaryotic cells must be stressed: The mRNA of prokaryotes contains information for several proteins (an operon), whereas the mRNA of eukaryotic cells

Figure 3-12 Regulation of the *lac* (lactose) gene expression in *Escherichia coli*. The transcription of the genes identified as *operon*, encoding the enzymes for utilization of the sugar lactose, may be blocked at a site named *operator* by a protein, the *repressor*, which is deactivated in the presence of lactose. The transcription of DNA into mRNA is initiated at a site known as the *promoter* region. The *boxes* indicate specific nucleotide sequences necessary in activation of RNA polymerase, the enzyme essential in transcription (see Fig. 2-14).

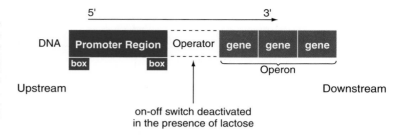

encodes only one protein, an advantage in the manipulation of this molecule.

Promoter sequences were also recognized in DNA of nucleated, eukaryotic cells. In such cells, two sequences of bases are known to occur: one of them is the so-called **CAT box** (a sequence of bases 5'-CCAAT-3', occurring about 80 to 70 bases upstream, and the other, a **TATA box** (a sequence of 5'-TATAAA-3'), occurring about 30 to 25 bases upstream. The RNA polymerase activity begins at base 1, and it continues until the gene is transcribed. The end of the transcription is signaled by another box composed of **AATAA** sequence of bases (Fig. 3-13). At the beginning of the transcription, at its initial or 5' site, the mRNA acquires a "cap" of methylguanidine residues, which presumably protects the newly formed molecule from being attacked by RNA-destroying enzymes (RNAses). At the conclusion of the transcription, the mRNA is provided with a sequence of adenine bases (AAAAA), also known as the **poly-A tail.** As always, the RNA is transcribed from the 5' end to the 3' end.

Subsequently, other DNA sequences important in the transcription of eukaryotic genes, named *enhancers*, were also discovered. It is of interest that the enhancer sequences may be located at a distance of several hundred or even several thousand nucleotides from the promoter site. It has been proposed that the enhancer sequences act through DNA loops that may bring together the enhancer site and the gene, thereby facilitating its transcription. Subsequently, the discovery of specific promoter and enhancer sequences of DNA played a major role in molecular engineering (see below).

Exons and Introns

Once the principles of the genetic code were unraveled, it was thought that the transcription of DNA into mRNA was a simple one-on-one process, resulting in a direct copy of the DNA sequence into an RNA message. It was noted first in 1977 that the message contained in DNA genes was, in fact, substantially modified: **the mRNA was often considerably shorter than the anticipated length,** with segments that were removed before RNA left the nucleus. The **removed segments of RNA were called introns,** and their removal required "splicing" or bringing together the **remaining portions of RNA, called exons** (Fig. 3-14).

The presence of introns complicated enormously the sequencing of mammalian genes, because it became evident that large portions of the DNA molecule, although transcribed, carried no obvious message for translation in the cytoplasm. In fact, there is still much speculation but little factual knowledge about the reasons for the existence of introns. It is generally thought that they exercise some sort of a regulatory function in RNA transcription.

Additional studies documented that **only a small proportion (about 5%) of human DNA encodes for protein genes.** The remaining bulk of the molecule represents **noncoding DNA.** Whether this is an appropriate term for the DNA, with completely unknown function and significance, remains to be seen. It is of interest, though, that in the noncoding DNA, there are repetitive nucleotide sequences (also known as **short tandem repeats, inverted repeats,** and **interspersed repeats**) that vary from individual to individual and thereby allow **genetic fingerprinting** (see below).

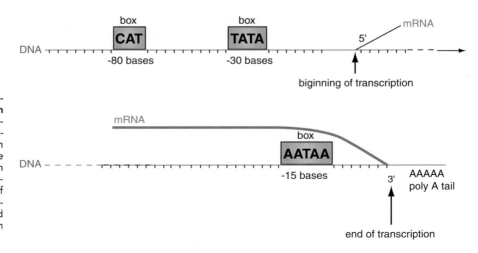

Figure 3-13 A schematic representation of mammalian gene transcription showing the position of specific nucleotide sequences (*boxes*) regulating the beginning and the end of the transcription process (see text). A sequence of adenine bases (poly-A tail) is added to mRNA upon completion of the transcription of a mammalian gene. The mRNA is composed of inactive sequences (introns) and active sequences (exons). The introns are excised and the exons combined (spliced) to form the final mRNA message.

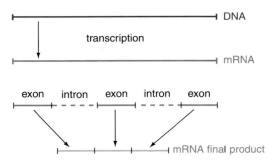

Figure 3-14 Schematic representation of transcription of mammalian genes. The splicing of the exons is shown in the *bottom* part of the diagram.

REGULATION OF GENE EXPRESSION IN EUKARYOTIC CELLS

Although some of the mechanisms of gene encoding, transcription, and translation have been elucidated, the understanding of the fundamental principles of gene expression in complex multicellular organisms is still very limited. Some progress has been reported in the studies of embryonal differentiation in a small worm, *caenorhabditis elegans*, which has only 19,000 genes that have been sequenced (Ruvkun and Hobert, 1998). Whether these studies are applicable to humans remains to be seen. It is important to realize that a **zygote, composed of the DNA complements of an ovum and a spermatozoon, contains all the genes necessary to produce a very complex multicellular organism.** It is quite evident that, during the developmental process, genes will be successively activated and deactivated until a mature, highly differentiated organism has reached its full development. It is known now that **unneeded cells are eliminated by the process of apoptosis** (see Chap. 6). Still, how these events are coordinated is largely unknown at this time. Here and there, a gene or a protein is discovered that interacts with other genes and proteins and activates or deactivates them. Recently, **double-stranded RNA molecules,** known as *interference RNA* **(iRNA),** have been shown to play an important role in gene deactivation (Ashrafi et al, 2003; Lee et al, 2003). These relationships are increasingly complex and constantly changing, suggesting that the **blueprint for gene expression in eukaryotic cells in complex multicellular organisms has not been discovered as yet** and most likely will remain elusive for some time. It could be documented, though, that given appropriate circumstances, **all genes can be found in every cell.** This has been dramatically documented by **cloning of sheep and other animals using nuclei derived from mature epithelial cells.** Long-suppressed genes can also be activated in instances when growth processes are deregulated, for example, in cancer. It is of interest that certain genetic sequences that are likely to be involved in gene activation appear to be highly preserved (conserved) in all multicellular organisms, including insects, strongly supporting the concept of unity of all life.

If these issues of activation of genes during fetal development may be considered esoteric, there is unfortunately

equally limited understanding of gene expression in mature cells. It is known that the transcription of mRNA can occur only off one strand of the DNA molecule. Hence, the separation of the two strands of DNA is an important prerequisite of gene transcription. Clearly, during the normal activity of a mature cell, all active genes necessary for the cell's survival and function must be activated and deactivated at one time or another. It is generally assumed that the separation and reannealing of the DNA strands and gene expression and repression are due to various proteins binding to each other and to specific regions of the DNA, but the precise knowledge of these events currently eludes us.

RESTRICTION ENZYMES (ENDONUCLEASES) AND SEQUENCING OF DNA

Although considerable progress was made in understanding the mechanisms of gene transcription after the discovery of the principles of the genetic code and the repressor-operator system in bacteria, the exact makeup of genes (i.e., the sequence of codons) in eukaryotic cells remained a mystery, largely because of the enormous size of the DNA molecules. Although chemical methods for analysis and sequencing of DNA were known, they shed little light on the arrangement of bases, hence on the genetic code of genes. The discovery of **restriction enzymes (endonucleases)** in the 1970s significantly modified this situation. Restriction enzymes that were capable of breaking down foreign DNA were discovered in bacteria.

It soon became evident that these enzymes were highly specific because they **recognized specific sequences of nucleotides or clusters of nucleotides** and, thus, could be used to cut DNA at specific points. The enzymes were **named after the bacterium of origin.** For example, the bacterium *E. coli* gave rise to the enzyme *Eco*Rl, *Bacillus amyloliquefaciens* to enzyme *Bam*HI, *Haemophilus influenzae* to enzyme *Hind*III, and so on. These enzymes recognize a sequence of four, six, or eight bases in the corresponding complementary chains of DNA (Fig. 3-15). Because the frequency of sequential four bases is greater than that of six or eight bases, the enzymes recognizing a sequence of four bases will cut the DNA into smaller pieces than the enzymes recognizing a larger number of sequential nucleotides. Moreover, because the two chains of DNA are complementary, they may or may not be cut in precisely the same location. As a consequence, the ends of the DNA fragment of the two chains may be of unequal length, leading to the so-called **sticky ends,** in which one chain of the DNA will be longer than the other. This feature of DNA fragments obtained by means of restriction enzymes is most helpful in recombinant DNA studies (see below).

The restriction enzymes were the tools needed to **cut very large molecules of DNA into fragments of manageable sizes** that could be further studied. Perhaps the most important initial observation was that **DNA fragments could be separated from each other by creating an elec-**

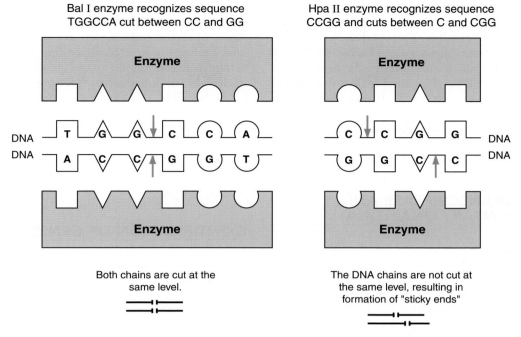

Bal I enzyme recognizes sequence
TGGCCA cut between CC and GG

Hpa II enzyme recognizes sequence
CCGG and cuts between C and CGG

Both chains are cut at the
same level.

The DNA chains are not cut at
the same level, resulting in
formation of "sticky ends"

Figure 3-15   Restriction enzymes (endonucleases). Two examples of these enzymes, one cutting DNA at the same location in both chains (*left, arrows*) and the other at different points in the DNA chains (*right, arrows*) leaving "sticky ends" (*right*).

tric field (electrophoresis) in loosely structured gels of the sugar, agarose. The DNA fragments are separated from each other by size, with smaller fragments moving farther in the gel than larger fragments, and by configuration, with circular fragments moving farther than the open fragments of similar length. The fragments can be visualized by staining with DNA-specific dyes, such as ethidium bromide, or by radioactive labels that give autoradiographic signals on photographic plates (Fig. 3-16). Thus, a restriction map of a DNA molecule can be produced. Each fragment can also be removed intact from the gel for chemical analysis or sequencing of bases or transferred onto nitrocellulose paper for hybridization studies with appropriate probes (see below). Several methods of analysis of the DNA fragments, known as *base sequencing* were developed, leading

to precise knowledge of the sequence of bases. The technical description of sequencing methods is beyond the scope of this summary, and the reader is referred to other sources for additional information. Currently, automated instruments are used for this purpose.

SEQUENCING OF THE ENTIRE HUMAN GENOME

In 2001, simultaneous publications from the International **Human Genome Project** (Lander et al, 2001) and a commercial company, Celera (Ventner et al, 2001), nearly **three billion nucleotide codes,** organized in about **30,000 genes,** became known. The promise of this tedious and time-

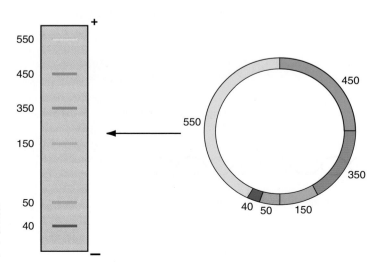

Figure 3-16   Restriction map of a circular molecule of DNA *(right)* on agarose gel *(left).* The figure indicates that size of DNA fragments in thousands of bases (kilobases; kb). DNA fragments of various length labeled with radioactive compound may be sorted out by electrophoresis on agarose gels.

consuming work is the identification of genes and gene products (proteins) specific for disease processes (Collins, 1999; Collins and Guttmacher, 2001; McKusick, 2001; Subramanian et al, 2001; Guttmacher and Collins, 2002; Collins et al, 2003). Because the number of individual proteins is probably in the millions, it is quite evident that each of the ± 30,000 human genes is capable of producing multiple proteins. A number of techniques such as **proteomics** (discussed above) and **microarray techniques** (briefly discussed below and in Chap. 4) address these issues under the global name of **transitional research.**

REVERSE TRANSCRIPTASE AND COMPLEMENTARY DNA (cDNA)

As described above, the transcription of the message from DNA to RNA is governed by a family of enzymes, known as *transcriptases.* An important advance in molecular biology was the discovery of the enzyme **reverse transcriptase** by Baltimore and by Temin and Mizutani in 1970, based on observation of replication mechanisms of RNA viruses **(retroviruses)** in mammalian cells. The genetic code of these viruses is inscribed in their RNA and **they cannot replicate without the help of the host cells.** The viruses were shown to carry a nucleotide sequence encoding an enzyme, **reverse transcriptase,** which allows them to **manufacture a single chain of complementary DNA (cDNA) from the nucleotides available in the host cell.** The single-stranded cDNA, which contains the message corresponding to the viral RNA genome, is copied into a double-stranded DNA by an enzyme, DNA polymerase. This double-stranded DNA molecule is incorporated into the native DNA of the host cell. **The host cell is now programmed to produce new viral RNA.** The viral RNA, upon acquiring a new capsule at the expense of the host membrane, becomes the reconstituted virus, which leaves the host cell to start the reproductive cycle in another cell (Fig. 3-17).

Reverse transcriptase became an extremely important enzyme in **gene identification and replication in vitro.** By means of reverse transcriptase, any fragment of RNA can now be fitted with a corresponding strand of synthetic cDNA, based on the customary principle of matching of nucleotides, described earlier. This fragment of cDNA can be duplicated by DNA polymerase into a double-stranded fragment that can be incorporated into a **plasmid** or other vector for replication in bacteria (see below). Conversely, any fragment of DNA, after separation of the strands, can be matched with synthetic RNA, which can be utilized to produce a single- or double-stranded cDNA by means of reverse transcriptase.

IDENTIFICATION OF GENES

The understanding of the relationship between DNA, mRNA, and proteins has greatly facilitated the task of identifying DNA sequences that code for various cell products. By starting with phages and viruses, and then moving on to eukaryotic cells, the science of identification and sequencing of genes with a known final product became relatively simple. The starting point can now be a sequence of amino acids in a protein product, such as a hormone. An isolated or synthetic mRNA in the presence of reverse transcriptase and a mixture of nucleotides can be used to construct a segment of the cDNA corresponding to the protein product encoded by the mRNA (Fig. 3-18). Considerable progress in techniques of gene identification has been applied to the Human Genome Project (see above).

The sequencing of nucleotides in a DNA fragment allows a computer-based comparison with other known sequenced genes. Such comparisons enable the identification of genes across various species of eukaryotic cells to determine partial or complete preservation of genes in various stages of evolution. With the use of this technique, it could be shown that certain genes may be common to humans and many other

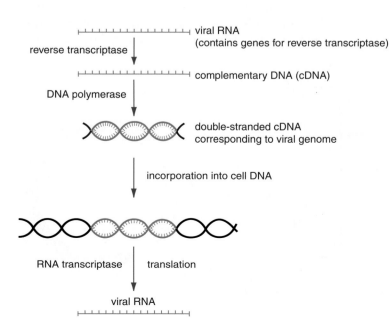

Figure 3-17 **Function of reverse transcriptase in a replication of RNA viruses (retroviruses).** The enzyme, expressed in the virus, utilizes nucleotides of the host cell to manufacture a chain of DNA corresponding to the viral RNA (complementary or cDNA). The cDNA is replicated to form a double-stranded DNA, which is incorporated into the host DNA, thereby ensuring the replication of viral RNA.

Study of Human Genes

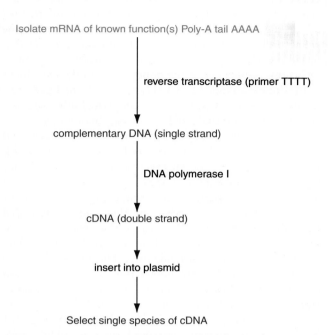

Isolate mRNA of known function(s) Poly-A tail AAAA

↓

reverse transcriptase (primer TTTT)

↓

complementary DNA (single strand)

↓

DNA polymerase I

↓

cDNA (double strand)

↓

insert into plasmid

↓

Select single species of cDNA

Figure 3-18   Sequence of events in the identification of genes. The beginning point is the isolation of a protein with a known function, for example, a hormone. This, in turn, leads to the identification of the appropriate mRNA to form a suitable cDNA and, finally, replication of the double-stranded cDNA in a DNA replication system, such as a plasmid.

species, including insects, suggesting a common ancestry to all multi-cellular organisms.

Computer analysis of sequences of nucleotides also permits the search for genes or DNA sequences, not interrupted by the boxes, indicating the beginning and the end of mRNA transcription. Such uninterrupted sequences of DNA are called **open-reading frames.** Each reading frame encodes an appropriate mRNA and a protein product. Open-reading frames represent a convenient way of presenting genetic components of smaller DNA molecules, such as viruses (see Chap. 11).

DNA CLONING IN VITRO

The concept of reproducing genes, or fragments of genes, in vitro was based on a number of discoveries and technical improvements that have occurred since the late 1970s, most of them briefly summarized in the preceding pages. The ability to separate fragments of DNA by restriction enzymes, their identification, and their sequencing represented the first step in this chain of events. It has been known for many years that bacteria possess not only genetic DNA but also **"parasitic" DNA, known as phages and plasmids.** The DNA of these parasitic species replicates within the bacteria, exploiting the machinery of DNA replication belonging to the host cell. The sequencing of phages and plasmids, and their dissection by restriction enzymes, led to a marriage of these methods and to molecular engineering.

It was mentioned previously that some restriction enzymes cut DNA chains in an uneven manner, leaving "sticky" ends. This observation became of capital importance in DNA replication in vitro or for DNA cloning. Thus, it became possible to **insert into a plasmid or phage a piece of DNA from another species,** utilizing the "sticky ends" as points of fusion. The replication in bacteria of the engineered parasitic DNA would ensure that the **DNA insert would also be replicated.** Plasmid DNA particularly proved to be extremely useful because it can be cut with the same enzymes as the DNA of other species, again with formation of sticky ends. A further useful feature of the plasmids was their role in conferring on bacteria resistance to specific antibiotics. It was of particular value that the **plasmid known as pBR322 carried two drug-resistance genes, one to ampicillin and one to tetracycline.** Thus, by inserting a fragment of foreign DNA into the plasmid at the site of one of the resistance genes, this gene is destroyed. By inserting the plasmid into a bacterium, one could expect the plasmid to multiply. However, the growth of the bacteria, hence that of the plasmids and of the foreign DNA, could be controlled by the antibiotics represented by the intact gene (Fig. 3-19). This option proved to be

1. Cut specific DNA gene with enzymes creating sticky ends

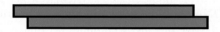

2. Cut pBR 322 plasmid with enzymes creating sticky ends site A

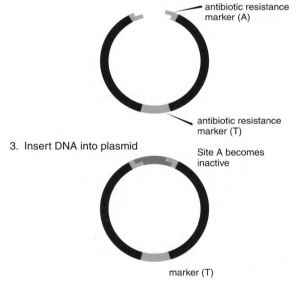

antibiotic resistance marker (A)

antibiotic resistance marker (T)

3. Insert DNA into plasmid

Site A becomes inactive

marker (T)

4. Insert modified plasmids into bacterium

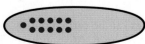

5. Extract DNA

Figure 3-19   Principles of DNA cloning using the plasmid pBR322, which has two antibiotic-resistant sites to the drugs ampicillin (A) and tetracycline (T). If only one of these two sites is used for insertion of DNA fragments (in this example, site A), the growth of the carrier bacterium can still be controlled by tetracycline. The figure does not show the restriction enzymes used in cutting the DNA.

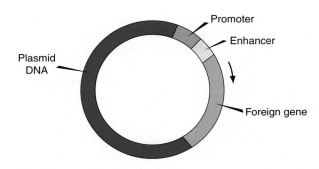

Figure 3-20   Model of a DNA construct in which promoter and enhancer sequences from another source were incorporated into the plasmid. Any nucleotide sequence, either derived from an actual DNA or synthesized in vitro, can be inserted. In this manner, almost any gene or portion of a gene can be replicated and studied.

important in ensuring that cloned DNA would not somehow escape and infect or contaminate other cells and perhaps even multinucleated organisms. This issue was of major concern at the onset of this research.

Many different plasmids are now in use. They can be selected for specific purposes and their nucleotide sequences can be matched with the sequences of the DNA fragments to be inserted. The use of this technique and its variants, notably the use of the so-called **cosmids,** combining some sequences of phages with plasmids, created a system in which **any fragment of DNA could be grown in bacteria in a test tube.** With the passage of time, techniques became available for constructing artificial sticky ends of DNA segments, thereby enlarging still further the options of this technology. To ensure replication, such fragments can also be provided with promoter or enhancer sequences taken from another, irrelevant fragment of DNA—for example, of viral origin. Constructs composed of various fragments of DNA or cDNA can be made and inserted into plasmids or vectors (Fig. 3-20). If one considers that **fragments of DNA may represent specific genes,** responsible for the synthesis of important proteins, the mechanism was in place for in vitro **production of useful products** such as hormones. Other applications of this technology include specific sequences of DNA, which may now be isolated or synthesized and reproduced in vitro, to serve as **probes for testing for the presence of unknown genes** or infectious agents, such as viruses.

METHODS OF GENE ANALYSIS AND IDENTIFICATION

Southern Blotting

The analysis of genes can be carried out by a blotting technique devised in 1975 by E. M. Southern. The technique is based on the principle of DNA replication, described above, specifically the immutable and constant association of purine and pyrimidine bases (G-C and A-T), and the constant direction of replication or transcription from the 5' to 3' end. The assumption of the technique is that two fragments of DNA will unite (anneal, hybridize), if they have complementary nucleotide sequences.

To perform the examination, **fragments of DNA,** obtained by means of one or more restriction enzymes, **are separated by electrophoresis** in the loosely structured gel of the sugar, agarose. The fragments, which travel in the gel according to size (the smaller the fragment, the farther it will move), are then treated with an alkaline solution or by heating, which breaks the bonds between the two chains of the double-stranded DNA. The gels, with the DNA fragments, are then treated with an appropriate buffer solution, and the **DNA is transferred** by capillary action to a matching sheet of nitrocellulose paper (or another suitable solid support material). The fragments of DNA on the nitrocellulose paper, representing an exact replica of the fragments separated in agarose gel, can be processed in several different ways. They can be **removed for sequencing** or gene amplification technique (see below), **or** they can be **annealed (matched) with "probes"** to determine whether the unknown DNA contains normal or abnormal genes or fragments of genes of known identity. The probes can be a DNA fragment of known composition, purified mRNA, or cDNA that is **labeled,** by a process known as **nick translation,** with a radioactive compound such as phosphorus (P^{32}). The bands can also be visualized by labeling the DNA probe with a fluorescent compound, such as ethidium bromide. Most DNA probes used today are fairly short specific sequences of DNA, rarely numbering more than several hundred nucleotides. After washing in a suitable solution to remove surplus probe and to ensure appropriate conditions of correct matching of the probe with the target DNA, the nitrocellulose paper is placed on top of a photographic plate, which must be developed in a darkroom for several days until the radioactivity of the label produces a signal on the photographic emulsion. After developing, the plate will reveal the **position of the fragments of DNA matching the probe** (Fig. 3-21). The fragment can be assessed in several ways: its size can be determined by comparison with a control probe of known size (usually expressed in thousands of nucleotide bases; kb). The expression of a gene can be studied according to the **size of the radioactive band** when compared with controls: a broader band will usually signify a higher activity of the gene, a narrower band indicates a reduced activity. Gene abnormalities can be detected by slight differences in the position of a gene on the blot. These comparisons are usually carried out by presenting the findings side by side as a **series of lanes,** each lane corresponding to one analysis (Fig. 3-22).

Southern blotting can be carried out under **stringent** and **nonstringent conditions,** defined by the experimental setting, such as salinity, temperature, and the size of the DNA probe. Under **stringent conditions,** the annealing of the nucleotides (hybridization) will take place only if the test molecule and the probe have **precisely matching nucleotide sequences.** Under **nonstringent conditions,** the annealing of the fragments may occur when the **nucleotide sequences are approximate,** and precise matching of fragments is not necessary. To give an example from an area of importance in diagnostic cytology, the presence of **human papillomaviruses (HPV),** in general, may be determined by hybridization of cellular DNA with a cocktail of probes

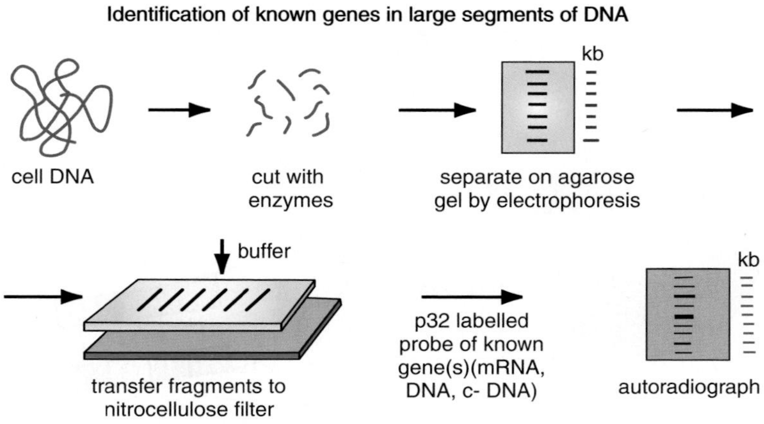

Identification of known genes in large segments of DNA

cell DNA → cut with enzymes → separate on agarose gel by electrophoresis →

buffer

transfer fragments to nitrocellulose filter → p32 labelled probe of known gene(s)(mRNA, DNA, c- DNA) → autoradiograph

kb

Figure 3-21 **Principles of Southern blotting** (developed by E.M. Southern, 1975). Kb indicates kilobases, the size of DNA fragments in a blot.

under nonstringent conditions. Under these circumstances, all HPVs have a sufficient number of similar nucleotide sequences to attach to the unknown DNA. If, however, the search is for a specific viral type, the hybridization must be performed under stringent conditions (see Chap. 11).

Dot (Spot) Hybridization

Dot hybridization is a variant of the Southern technique in which the target DNA is not treated with endonucleases but **placed in minute amounts (spotted) onto a filter membrane** and denatured by heat or treatment with alkali. The probe is labeled as described above, hybridized to the filter, and an autoradiograph is obtained. The procedure, requiring only minute amounts of target DNA, may serve as a screening test against several labeled probes. This technique and its variants have been adopted to the **DNA and RNA microarrays** that allow the recognition of known genetic sequences in unknown DNA or RNA.

In Situ Hybridization With DNA Probes

The technique of in situ hybridization is based on principles similar to Southern blotting. Instead of hybridizing fragments of DNA on a piece of nitrocellulose paper, **the target of in situ hybridization is naturally occurring DNA, which may be present in the nucleus of a cell or on a chromosome.** The purpose of in situ hybridization is to identify the presence of a gene or another DNA sequence (such as a DNA virus) and to identify its location within the target. The procedure shares some of the basic principles with Southern blotting: The target DNA, such as nuclei in a tissue section, a smear, or a chromosomal preparation, must be denatured to separate the two strands. This is usually done by heating or by treatment with hydrochloric acid or alkali. The nick-translation **labeled DNA probe** is then applied under stringent or nonstringent conditions (Fig. 3-23). The label may be a **radioactive compound** (such as radioactive phosphorus, sulfur, or tritiated thymidine) that requires the use of a photographic emulsion to document

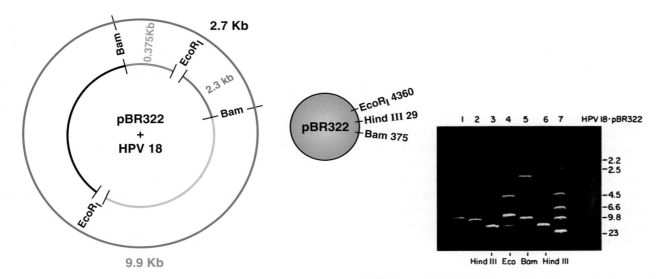

Figure 3-22 **Southern blot of a human papillomavirus type 18**, carried in the plasmid pBR322. *Left.* Sites of activity of several restriction enzymes (*EcoR*1, *Hind*III, *Bam*HI) and the size of DNA fragments in kiobases (Kb). *Right.* Southern blot in which the DNA fragments were separated according to size (indicated on the right). The "lanes" are numbered on top to compare the sizes of fragments in several experiments.

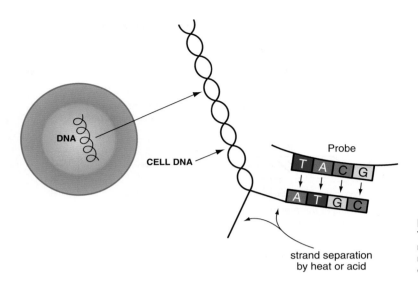

Figure 3-23 Principle of in situ hybridization (ISH). The strands of the nuclear DNA are separated and matched with a probe that may be DNA or mRNA. The reannealing will occur when the nucleotide sequences of the native DNA and of the probe match.

a positive reaction, after a lengthy period of incubation. The probe may also be labeled with a **biotin-avidin complex** that allows the demonstration of the results by a peroxidase-antiperoxidase reaction visible under a light microscope. The latter procedure is much faster but less sensitive than the radioactive label. The results of in situ hybridization of a cervical biopsy with DNA from HPV types 11 and 16 are shown in Chapter 11. **Hybridization of entire chromosomes or their segments,** to determine the location of a particular gene, is based on essentially the same principles. The technique of **fluorescent in situ hybridization (FISH)** is particularly valuable in this regard. Using probes labeled with fluorescent compounds, the **location of chromosomes** in the interphase human nucleus (see Fig. 2-31 and Chap. 4), the **number of chromosomes in a nucleus, the presence of specific genes or gene products** could be identified. By the use of specific probes, the abnormalities of chromosomes in several forms of human cancer could be defined and documented (see Chap. 4).

In Situ Hybridization With mRNA

mRNA may also be used in a hybridization system in situ. The **mRNA probes** may be developed from known DNA sequences of genes or segments of genes, or they may be synthesized according to a sequence of amino acids in a protein molecule. Such mRNA probes will **hybridize with corresponding sequences of DNA or cDNA.** By using the ingenious techniques of molecular engineering, it is also possible to construct **"antisense" probes** that will hybridize with mRNA and thus **reveal the presence of actively transcribing genes in situ.** Such probes have been used by Stoler and Broker to detect mRNA of HPV in tissue sections from the uterine cervix (see Chap. 11).

Restriction Fragment Length Polymorphism

Restriction fragment length polymorphism (RFLP) is another form of gene analysis by Southern blotting, which is carried out by comparing the effects of selected restriction

endonucleases on unknown DNA. **The addition or subtraction of a single nucleotide in the DNA sequence may alter significantly the recognition sites for the endonucleases.** Therefore, a comparison of the size and position of the DNA fragments on the blot may reveal similarities or differences between the DNAs from two individuals. It has been documented that each person has **unique DNA sequences that are akin to genetic fingerprints,** based mainly on the structure of noncoding DNA (see above). The RFLP technique has found application in human genetics, in the study of cancer, and in forensic investigations. A somewhat similar technique is based on the individual variations in **short tandem repeats** in noncoding DNA and is known as **variable number tandem repeats,** which is used for purposes similar to those for the RLFP technique.

Northern Blotting

Northern blotting (so named to differentiate it from Southern blotting, but not named after a person) is based on **techniques of isolation of RNA** from rapidly frozen cells or tissues. Among the RNAs, a small proportion (about 2%) represents mRNA that can be identified and separated by virtue of its poly-A tail (see above). The RNA of interest is separated by size, using **agarose gel electrophoresis** (with a denaturing solution, such as formamide, added), and transferred to a stable medium, such as nitrocellulose paper, by techniques similar to those used in Southern blotting. The subsequent hybridization procedure is carried out with appropriate probes, which may consist of DNA or cDNA. **The identification of the appropriate mRNA molecule indicates that a gene (or a DNA sequence) is not only present but has also been actively transcribed,** information that cannot be obtained by Southern blot analysis. The issue is of importance in the presence of several similar or related genes, as it allows the identification of a gene that is active under defined circumstances.

Western Blotting

Western blotting is a technique similar to Southern and northern blotting, except that the matching involves proteins rather than DNA or RNA, and the **probe is an antibody to a given protein.** The technique has been particularly useful in determining whether an antibody produced in an experimental system matches the amino acid sequence of an antigen and as an important step in **quantitation of gene products** by means of an antigen-antibody reaction. The technique may also be used to determine whether a protein produced in vitro matches a naturally occurring protein. The technique is important in verifying the purity of synthetic genes and gene products. As an example, a hormone produced in vitro may be matched with a hormone extracted from an appropriate tissue. See above comments on proteomics.

Polymerase Chain Reaction

In 1985, Saiki and associates described a new ingenious method of **DNA amplification**—now known as **polymerase chain reaction or PCR.**

The principle of the technique is the observation that if the synthesis by **DNA polymerase** of a segment of double-stranded DNA is initiated at both ends of the two complementary chains, the replication will continue until the entire molecule is reproduced. In order to initiate this synthesis, three conditions have to be met:

1. The **two chains of the target DNA molecule** must be separated **by heating.**
2. The **complementary two fragments of DNA or primers,** corresponding to known sequences of nucleotides at the two ends of the target molecule, also known as **flanking sequences,** must be synthesized. Thus, the exact sequence of nucleotides of the target molecule has to be known in advance.
3. DNA polymerase capable of functioning at high temperatures **(heat-stable polymerase)** must be identified.

The most commonly used, **Taq polymerase,** was derived from a bacterium, *Themes aquaticus,* living in a hot geyser in Yellowstone National Park. The concept was proposed by an employee of a then-fledgling biotechnology company, the Cetus Corporation. The employee, Kary B. Mullis, received a Nobel Prize for his contribution (Rabinow, 1995).

The principle of the method is as follows: a target segment of double-stranded DNA is heated to separate the complementary strands. Two short sequences of **synthetic DNA,** known as **primers,** each corresponding to a specific flanking nucleotide sequence of the target DNA **are mixed with the target DNA.** The primers mark the beginning and the end of the synthesis. The primers bind **(anneal)** to the flanking sequence of the target DNA, based on the fundamental principles of DNA replication. In the presence of a "soup" containing a mixture of the four essential nucleotides (A,C,G,T), the **heat-stable polymerase** copies the sequence of nucleotides in each strand of the target DNA (a function known as **primer extension**), creating two double-stranded DNA sequences. The mixture is then cooled to facilitate **reannealing** of the complementary DNA strands.

In the second cycle, the two copies of the newly created double-stranded DNA are again separated **(denatured)** by heat, thus creating four copies. Using the same primers and the same procedure, the four copies will become eight. The procedure may be repeated over several cycles of amplification. Each cycle consists of primer extension, denaturation, and reannealing, conducted under various conditions of time and temperature. After 20 cycles, the number of copies of the original target DNA fragment will grow to over 1 million (exactly 1,048,576 copies). The results are tested by Southern blotting techniques for the presence of the now-amplified segment of DNA, which may be a gene or a part thereof. The technique may reveal the presence of a single copy of a small gene, such as an infectious virus, that would not be detectable by any other technique (Fig. 3-24).

The PCR technique and its variants has found many applications in various aspects of basic and forensic and even agricultural sciences. The technique can be applied to individual **cells in situ** and to the identification of DNA viruses and of bacteria. The ability to amplify minuscule amounts of DNA will continue to find an ever-increasing applicability in various fields, particularly with introduction of new thermostabile polymerases, improved machines, known as **thermal cyclers,** and full automation of the process.

Denaturing Gradient Gel Electrophoresis

A clever way of discovering mutations in genes is the technique of **denaturing gradient gel electrophoresis (DGGE).** The concept of this technique is based on **differences in melting point (separation) of DNA double-stranded chains** in acrylamide gels mixed with a denaturing solution of urea and formamide. A gradient of the denaturing solution is created in an acrylamide gel, and the **gene product** obtained by polymerase chain reaction (PCR) is **electrophoresed** in the gel for about 8 hours. The gel is stained with ethidium bromide, which binds to DNA, and the bands are visualized under ultraviolet light. **DGGE separates DNA fragments based on nucleotide sequence rather than size.** Differences as small as a single nucleotide change will result in bands in a different position on the gel.

Monoclonal and Polyclonal Antibodies

The subject of monoclonal and polyclonal antibodies and their role in immunochemistry in tissues and cells is considered in detail in Chapter 45. Because the techniques were developed as a consequence of progress in molecular biology and because they are particularly useful in diagnostic histopathology and cytopathology, they will be briefly described here.

In 1975, Kohler and Milstein observed that splenic **B lymphocytes of mice, programmed to produce a specific antibody by injection of an antigen, could be fused with cultured plasma cells.** Plasma cells are, in essence, living factories for the production of immunoglobulins. As a con-

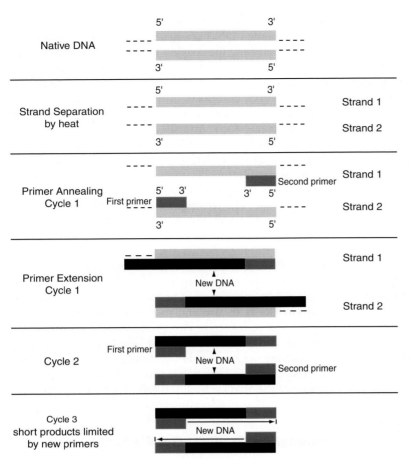

Figure 3-24 Polymerase chain reaction, a method of amplification of specific segments of DNA. Diagrammatic presentation of the first three cycles of polymerase chain reaction in the presence of a heat-resistant DNA polymerase in a suspension of nucleotides A, T, G, and C. The initiating sequences of DNA or primers are constructed in vitro, according to the desired known flanking sequences of nucleotides, identifying a gene or a part thereof. The mixture is cooled after each cycle. The result, after three cycles, is a short segment of DNA, limited by primers, that can be reproduced in several million copies after 30–40 cycles. The segment can be tested for the presence of a normal gene of a modification thereof.

sequence of the fusion, they produced the specific immunoglobulin or antibody expressed in the B lymphocytes. It is now possible to generate antibodies of varying degrees of specificity to almost any protein. As an example, highly specific antibodies to various species of intermediate filaments can be produced and used to localize and identify the presence of such filaments by immunohistologic and immunocytologic techniques. Another example is the production of antibodies to cell surface antigens (CDs) and various oncogene products that are important in classification of lymphomas and leukemias. Specific cell products, such as hormones, may also be identified by this technique.

APPLICABILITY OF MOLECULAR BIOLOGY TECHNIQUES TO DIAGNOSTIC CYTOLOGY

Several of the developments discussed in the preceding pages proved to be of direct or indirect value in diagnostic cytology. Molecular biologic techniques can be applied to the **identification of many infectious agents,** such as bacteria, fungi, and viruses. Of special significance in diagnostic cytology has been the characterization of **HPV** that may play a role in the genesis of cancer of the uterine cervix, vagina, vulva, and the esophagus, discussed

in appropriate chapters. The techniques of **in situ hybridization** have been applied in a number of diagnostic situations, for example, in the determination of the presence of various types of HPV in precancerous lesions and cancer of the various organs wherein this virus may be carcinogenic. The molecular techniques have also shed some light on the events in human cancer, which are discussed in Chapter 7. In this regard, in situ hybridization techniques with probes to chromosomes or chromosomal segments have been shown to be of value in documenting chromosomal and genetic abnormalities useful in the diagnosis and prognosis of cancer cells in various situations, discussed in appropriate chapters. **Southern blotting techniques** have been applied, among others, to the study of apoptosis, an important phenomenon in diagnostic cytology (see Chap. 5). There are also several diagnostic applications of Southern blotting, for example, to the diagnosis of malignant lymphoma and nasopharyngeal carcinoma in aspirated samples of lymph nodes (Lubinski et al, 1988; Feinmesser et al, 1992). **In situ amplification techniques,** applicable to cytologic preparations, were discussed by O'Leary et al (1997). The presence of various oncogenes and tumor suppressor genes can be documented and quantitated by **immunocytologic techniques,** and some of these approaches have been shown to be of prognostic significance (for example, in breast cancer, see Chap. 29). **Proteomic evaluation,** previously applied to tissues

(Liotta et al, 2001; Paweletz et al, 2001) can also be applied to archival cytologic material (Fetsch et al, 2002).

Other techniques that may be applicable to cytologic samples are **microarrays** and **comparative genomic hybridization.** As briefly mentioned above, the **DNA microarray technology** is the consequence of the human genome project and is based on principles of in situ hybridization. **DNA of unknown samples** is hybridized **against a large array of known genes,** placed on a slide or a plate. The matching genes may be identified by a color reaction and the collection and analysis of observations requires a computer analysis (recent reviews include Golub et al, 1999; Khan et al, 2001; Welsh et al, 2001). King and Sinha (2001) described at length the promise and pitfalls of this technology. Macoska (2002) discussed the utility of DNA microarrays as a tool in prognosis of human cancer (see also Chap. 4).

Comparative genomic hybridization compares the unknown DNA against a metaphase karyotype of known cells. Excess or loss of chromosomes or their segments is analyzed in a computerized microscope (Kallioniemi et al, 1992; Maoir et al, 1993; Houldsworth and Chaganti, 1994; Wells et al, 1999; Baloglu et al, 2001) (see also Chap. 4).

Immunocytochemistry is discussed in Chapter 45.

THOUGHTS FOR THE FUTURE

The question of whether molecular biology will soon provide answers to the question, "How cells function?" is difficult to answer at this time. It is evident that the fundamental questions pertaining to the role of DNA, RNA, and proteins in cell function and heredity have been answered to some degree within the last 50 years. There remain, however, many questions of mechanisms of the interplay and the relationship among an ever-growing number of genes and proteins that somehow manage to keep the healthy cell working as a harmonious whole. A special puzzle of interest to the readers of this book is the sequence of events in cancer, discussed in Chapter 7. For many reasons, the issue is complicated because many of the genes implicated in cancer also participate in the life events of normal cells, such as DNA replication and cell cycle regulation. Some years ago, I compared the present status of molecular biology research to a swarm of woodpeckers, each attempting to identify a worm (by analogy, a protein). It would be difficult, if not impossible, to attempt to understand how the tree grows by a synthesis of the knowledge gained by the entire swarm of woodpeckers (Koss, 1989).

The great chemist, Erwin Chargaff, who contributed significantly to Watson and Crick's discovery of DNA structure, had this to say in an article in *Science* published in 1971:

"In the study of biology, the several disciplines exist next to each other, but they do not come together. We have no real idea of the inside of a living cell, for we lack what could be called a science of compressed spaces; we lack a scientific knowledge of a whole; and while a sum can be subdivided, this is not true of a whole. I know full well, science progresses from the simple to the complex. I, too, have been taught that one must begin at the bottom; but shall we ever emerge at the top?"

APPENDIX

GLOSSARY OF TERMS COMMONLY USED IN MOLECULAR BIOLOGY

AAAA . . . :   sequence of adenine molecules terminating the chain of mRNA (poly-A tail)

allele: an alternative form of a gene

alternative splicing: a regulatory mechanism by which variations in the incorporation of a gene's exons, or coding regions, into mRNA lead to the production of more than one related protein, or isoform

amplification: enhancement of a gene(s), usually using a specific enzyme

annealing: fusion of two matching molecules (chains) of DNA or DNA with mRNA

anticodon: a sequence of nucleotides in transfer RNA (tRNA), corresponding to a codon sequence for one specific amino acid, inscribed on mRNA; a mechanism used in translation of mRNA messages into proteins

antioncogene(s):   genes believed to counteract the effect of oncogenes (see Rb gene and p53)

antisense: a strand of DNA that has the same nucleotide sequence as mRNA; a strand of mRNA that has the same nucleotide sequence as DNA

AUG (adenine, uracil, guanine):   a base sequence (codon) on mRNA signaling the amino acid methionine, which initiates the synthesis of a protein

Baml: widely used restriction enzyme (endonuclease), derived from *Bacillus amyloliquefaciens* (see restriction endonuclease)

base pairs: matching pairs of nucleotides, such as adenine (adenine–thymine or guanine–cytosine) in the two matching strands of the DNA molecule

bases: colloquial designation of pyridine and pyrimidine bases (nucleotides) that enter into the makeup of nucleic acids (see base pairs)

box: a sequence of nucleotides of known constant composition serving as a signal for the beginning of a transcriptional event or the end of it

capsid: protein coat of viral particles

chromosome walking: a technique that allows a rapid search for gene identification and location on a chromosome

codon: a sequence of three nucleotides encoding one amino acid; the code is usually expressed in RNA nucleotide sequences (see AUG)

construct: a DNA or RNA vector, such as a plasmid or a virus, engineered to express a nucleotide sequence. The constructs are often provided with promoters and enhancers borrowed from other cells or viruses

cDNA (complementary DNA): a molecule of DNA complementary to RNA, usually generated by means of the enzyme reverse transcriptase

cut (DNA): synchronous breaking (cutting) of both chains of a double-stranded molecule of DNA, usually accomplished with the help of one of the enzymes known as *restriction enzymes* or *endonucleases*. The cut may result in smooth ends or uneven (sticky) ends of the DNA chain. If a single strand of DNA is affected, the term "nick" is used (see nick translation)

denaturing gradient gel electrophoresis (DGGE): a method of discovering genetic changes based on differences in DNA melting (separation of double-stranded DNA into single chains) caused by substitution of one or more bases

dot blot: analysis of several small samples of DNA of unknown makeup to identify the presence of a known DNA or mRNA sequence, such as the presence of a virus

downstream: an event happening before the main biologic event. For example, a signal encoded in the DNA that has to be recognized by the appropriate enzyme before transcription into mRNA can take place. The concept is based on the constant direction of all transcriptional events in nucleic acids from the 5′ end of the sugar molecule to the 3′. A **downstream event, therefore,** must happen in the direction of the 3′ end of the molecule. The exact opposite is true of an "upstream" event

EcoRI: a widely used restriction enzyme (endonuclease), derived from *Escherichia coli* (see restriction endonuclease)

enhancers: DNA sequences known to promote transcription

episome (episomal): a circular gene or gene fragment, not integrated into host DNA

exon: the sequence of nucleotides in a gene corresponding to a final product (e.g., a protein [Cfr. intron]) a region of a gene that codes for a protein

five prime (5′): pertains to carbon location in the molecule of sugar (ribose, deoxyribose) in the chain of nucleic acids. The synthesis of nucleic acids (and their products) always proceeds in the direction of 5′ to 3′, the 3′ indicating the location of carbon in the sugar molecule to which the next molecule of phosphate attaches itself

frame-shift mutation: the addition or deletion of a number of DNA bases that is not a multiple of three, thus causing a shift in the reading frame of the gene. This shift leads to a change in the reading frame of all parts of the gene that are downstream from the mutation, often leading to a premature stop codon and, ultimately, to a truncated protein

gene: a segment of DNA (or corresponding RNA) encoding one protein; each gene is composed of exons and introns

gene library: a collection of genes, usually corresponding to one species, such as human

genetic engineering: methods of gene replacement, substitution or propagation in vitro, serving to produce molecules of biologic value, such as hormones, to treat genetic diseases, or to modify plant or animal species

genome: a collection of genes representing the entire endowment of an organism, also reflected in a single normal cell (other than a gamete). Not all of the genes inscribed in the DNA will be active at any given time

genomics: the study of the functions and interactions of all the genes in the genome, including their interactions with environmental factors

heteroduplex: double-stranded DNA wherein the two strands are of different origin, such as two individuals of the same species, or two related, but not identical, DNA viruses. Such strands often show differences in nucleotide sequences that will prevent their perfect match. The matching or absence thereof can be visualized under the electron microscope under stringent and nonstringent conditions. The method is used to document similarities and differences between and among DNA sequences, for example, in typing of DNA viruses, such as the HPV

heterozygous: having two different alleles at a specific autosomal (or X chromosome in a female) gene locus

homozygous: having two identical alleles at a specific autosomal (or X chromosome in a female) gene locus

initiation codon: the sequence of nucleotides indicating the beginning of protein synthesis, usually AUG coding for methionine

intron: (intervening sequence): a part of the gene inscribed in DNA that is transcribed into mRNA, but is excised before the final molecule of mRNA is produced by splicing of exons

jumping genes: transposable segments of DNA accounting for adaptation of some species to environmental conditions

lac (operon): a sequence of genes in *E. coli*, regulating the metabolism of the sugar lactose

ligase: an enzyme binding together fragments of DNA

linker: a segment of DNA (usually synthetic), that contains a nucleotide sequence corresponding to a restriction enzyme; used in gene splicing (binding) and in genetic engineering

melting (DNA): separation of the two chains of double-stranded DNA molecule by heat, acid, alkali, or a denaturing solution (urea and formamide)

missense mutation: substitution of a single DNA base that results in a codon that specifies an alternative amino acid

motif: a DNA-sequence pattern within a gene that, because of its similarity to sequences in other known genes, suggests a possible function of the gene, its protein product, or both

mRNA: messenger RNA, a link between the DNA and the production of proteins. mRNA is transcribed off DNA and translated into a protein molecule

mutation: a spontaneous or artificial change in sequence of nucleotides, resulting in a modified protein product

myc (c-myc): an oncogene located in the nucleus of cells

nick: a cut of one of the two chains of DNA. This technique is useful in incorporation of one type of DNA into another

nick translation: a technique for labeling DNA with radioactive or optical probes, such as biotin, useful in in situ hybridization and similar analytical procedures

nonsense: a genetic message that does not correspond to a viable or useful product (e.g., a protein) that is often destroyed

nonsense mutation: substitution of a single DNA base that results in a stop codon, thus leading to the truncation of a protein

northern blotting (analysis): analysis of unknown RNA performed by electrophoretic isolation of RNA sequences and subsequent match with a molecule (gene) of RNA or DNA of known composition

oncogene(s): growth-promoting genes, initially identified in rodent cells and found to be essential in malignant transformation of these cells by RNA viruses. Many similar genes have since been identified in virtually all multicellular organisms, including humans (see protooncogenes and *myc* and *ras*, as examples of oncogenes)

operator: a region of DNA that regulates the use of a metabolite (e.g., a sugar), working in tandem with a repressor gene

operon: a metabolic function of the cell, usually associated with repressor and operator genes

p2l: protein product of ras oncogene; another p21 is a protein associated with p53

palindrome: a self-complementary nucleotide sequence, often recognized by restriction enzymes

phage: a bacterial virus, the target of some of the initial studies on DNA, still very useful in molecular engineering

p53: a gene known as "guardian of the genome," essential in prevention of DNA transcription errors and often mutated in various forms of human cancer

plasmid: a self-replicating fragment of circular, double-stranded DNA, living in bacteria and sometimes conferring upon the host organism the ability to resist antibiotics. Extensively used in various forms of molecular manipulation and engineering

point mutation: the substitution of a single DNA base in the normal DNA sequence

polyadenylation: sequence of adenyl molecules (see AAAA . . .)

polymerase: enzymes that mediate the assembly of DNA or RNA fragments into a cohesive larger unit

polymerase chain reaction (PCR): a technique of DNA amplification, based on the use of initiation sequences of a gene (a primer) and a thermostable DNA polymerase. The technique can be used to reproduce innumerable copies of a single DNA segment or a gene

promoter: a sequence of DNA nucleotides signaling the attachment of RNA polymerase as an initiation point of mRNA transcription; such sequences are extensively used in molecular engineering

protooncogene: widely disseminated growth-regulating genes; when overexpressed or modified (mutated), these genes become oncogenes

ras: an oncogene commonly found in many malignant human tumors

Rb gene (retinoblastoma gene): a regulatory gene first identified in patients with the rare malignant tumor of the retina. Its congenital absence leads to the development of the tumor; hence, this is the prime example of an antioncogene

regulatory gene: genes regulating the function of other genes, such as a repressor gene

restriction endonuclease: enzymes of bacterial origin that cut nucleic acids at the site of a predetermined nucleotide sequence (see examples under Bam1 and EcoRl)

restriction enzyme: colloquial for restriction endonuclease restriction fragment length

restriction fragment length polymorphism (RFLP): a technique of comparison of DNA fragments obtained by restriction enzymes, very useful in identification of individuals and extensively used in comparative genetics and forensic work

reverse transcriptase: an enzyme capable of translating a message inscribed in RNA into the corresponding DNA, known as complementary DNA (cDNA)

RNA splicing: attachment of exons to each other, after excision of introns, to form a final molecule of mRNA. The term is also used in other forms of gene manipulation

rRNA: ribosomal RNA, mainly produced in the nucleolus and a component part of ribosomes, cytoplasmic organelles, essential in the formation of proteins

single-nucleotide polymorphism (SNP): a common variant in the genome sequence; the human genome contains about 10 million SNPs

Southern blotting: a method of DNA analysis first described by Southern (1975), in which unknown DNA is cut into fragments. The fragments are isolated by electrophoresis, transferred to a suitable paper, and matched for the presence of known genes with labeled probes that are usually DNA, but can also be RNA

start codon: see initiation codon

sticky ends: double-stranded DNA in which one chain is longer than the other, often the result of cutting with a restriction enzyme. This technique is very useful in combining two disparate molecules of DNA

stop codon: a codon that leads to the termination of a protein rather than to the addition of an amino acid. The three stop codons are TGA, TAA, and TAG

suppressor gene: a gene that prevents another gene's expression

template: a term used to define a nucleotide sequence in DNA, to be transcribed into RNA

tRNA: transfer RNA, essential in synthesis of proteins (see anticodon)

transcription: formation of RNA from a DNA

transduction: transfer of genetic material from one cell to another by means of a vector, such as a virus

transfection: transfer (infection) of DNA or RNA from one cell to another by means of a vector

translation: the mechanism of protein formation from messages inscribed in RNA

vector: an agent, such as a plasmid or a virus, capable of multiplication in bacteria or other living cells, that can be used to transfer genetic information encoded in DNA or RNA

western blotting: matching of protein molecules, one of known composition and the other unknown. The method is extensively used in testing the specificity of immunologic reagents (such as antibodies) with an antigen of known makeup

BIBLIOGRAPHY*

Fundamental Contributions

Avery OT, MacLeod CM, MacCarthy M. Studies on the chemical nature of the substance inducing transformation of pneumococcal types. J Exp Med 79: 137–158, 1944.

Chargaff E. Preface to a grammar of biology. Science 172:637–642, 1971.

Chargaff E. Structure and function of nucleic acids as cell constituents. Fed Proc 10:654-659, 1951.

Crick FHC, Barnett L, Brenner S, Watts RJ. General nature of genetic code for proteins. Proc Natl Acad Sci USA 47:1227–1232, 1961.

Crick FHC, Watson JD. The complementary structure of deoxyribonucleic acid. Proc R Soc [Am] 223:80–96, 1954.

Jacob F, Monod J. Genetic regulatory mechanisms in the synthesis of proteins. J Mol Biol 3:318–356, 1961.

Koss LG. From koilocytosis to molecular biology: The impact of cytology on the concepts of early human cancer. Mod Pathol 2:526–535, 1989.

Mullis K, Fallona F, Scharf S, et al. Specific enzymatic amplification of DNA in vitro: The polymerase chain reaction. Cold Spring Harbor Symposia in Quantitative Biology, 51:263–273, 1986.

Pauling LH, Itano A, Singer SJ, Wells IC. Sickle cell anemia: A molecular disease. Science 110:543–548, 1949.

Watson JD, Crick FHC. Genetic implications of the structure of deoxyribonucleic acid. Nature 171:964–967, 1953.

Watson JD, Crick FHC. Molecular structure of nucleic acids: A structure for deoxyribose nucleic acid. Nature 171:737–738, 1953.

General Reviews

Alberts B, Bray D, Lewis J, Raff M, et al. Molecular Biology of the Cell, 2nd ed. New York and London, Garland Publishers, 1989.

Blow JJ (ed). Eukaryotic DNA replication. Oxford, New York, Tokyo, IRL Press at Oxford University Press, 1996.

Calladine CR, Drew HR. Understanding DNA. The molecule and how it works, 2nd ed. San Diego and New York, Academic Press, 1997.

Chambers DA (ed). DNA. The Double Helix. Perspective and Prospective at Forty Years. Ann NY Acad Sci, vol 758, 1995.

Fenoglio-Preiser CM, Willman CL. Molecular biology and the pathologist. Arch Pathol Lab Med 111:601–619, 1987.

Pennisi E. A hothouse of molecular biology. Science 300:278–282, 2003.

Pennisi E. DNA's cast of thousands. Science 300:282–285, 2003.

Sklar J. DNA hybridization in diagnostic pathology. Hum Pathol 16:654–658, 1985.

Watson JD, Tooze J, Kurtz DT. Recombinant DNA. A Short Course. New York, Scientific American Books, WH Freeman, 1992.

Wallace SS, Van Houten B, Kow YW (eds). DNA damage. Effects on DNA structure and protein recognition. Ann NY Acad Sci, vol 726, 1994.

For works pertaining to molecular genetic changes in cancer, see Chapter 7

DNA Structure, Replication, and Transcription

Cook PR. The organization of replication and transcription. Science 284: 1790–1795, 1999.

Eickbush T. Exon shuffling in retrospect. Science 283:1465–1467, 1999.

Gilbert W. Genes-in-pieces revisited. Science 228:823–824, 1985.

Gilbert W. DNA sequencing and gene structure. Science 214:1305–1312, 1981.

Goldman MA, Holmquist GP, Gray MC, et al. Replication timing of genes and middle repetitive sequences. Science 224:686–692, 1984.

Klug A. A marvelous machine for making messages. Science 292:1844–1846, 2001.

Kornberg R, Klug A. The nucleosome. Sci Am (Feb) 52–66, 1981.

Koss LG. Characteristics of chromosomes in polarized normal human bronchial cells provide a blueprint for nuclear organization. Cytogenet Cell Genet 82: 230–237, 1998.

Lewin R. On the origin of introns. Science 217:921–922, 1982.

Loeb LA, Kunkel TA. Fidelity of DNA synthesis. Ann Rev Biochem 52:429–457, 1982.

Mitchell PJ, Tijan R. Transcriptional regulation in mammalian cells by sequence-specific DNA binding protein. Science 245:371–378, 1989.

Ptashne M. How gene activators work. Sci Am 260:40–47, 1989.

Radman M, Wagner R. The high fidelity of DNA duplication. Sci Am 259:40–46, 1988.

Richter JD, Theurkauf WE. The message is in the translation. Science 293: 60–63, 2001.

Schleiff R. DNA binding by proteins. Science 241:1182–1187, 1988.

Southern EM. Detection of specific sequences among DNA fragments separated by gel electrophoresis. J Mol Biol 98:503–517, 1975.

Struhl K. A paradigm for precision. Science 293:1054–1055, 2001.

Nuclear Import and Export (Nuclear Pores)

Blobel G. Gene gaiting: A hypothesis. Proc Nat Acad Sci USA 82:8527–8529, 1985.

Davies LI, Blobel G. Identification and characterization of a nuclear pore complex protein. Cell 45:699–709, 1986.

Gerace L, Blobel G. The nuclear envelope lamina is reversibly depolymerised during mitosis. Cell 19:277–287, 1980.

Gerace L, Blum A, Blobel G. Immunocytochemical localization of the major polypeptides of the nuclear pore complex-lamina fraction. J Cell Biol 79: 546–566, 1978.

Izaurralde E, Adam S. Transport of macromolecules between the nucleus and the cytoplasm. RNA 4:351–364, 1998.

Kutay U, Lipowsky G, Izaurralde E, et al. Identification of a tRNA-specific nuclear export receptor. Mol Cell 1:359–369, 1998.

Melchior F, Gerace L. Two-way trafficking with Ran. Trend Cell Biol 8:175–179, 1998.

Pemberton LF, Blobel G, Rosenblum JS. Transport routes through the nuclear pore complex. Curr Opin Cell Biol 10:392–399, 1998.

Pennisi E. The nucleus's revolving door. Science 279:1129–1131, 1998.

Siomi MC, Eder PS, Kataoka N, et al. Transportin-mediated nuclear import of heterogeneous nuclear RNP proteins. J Cell Biol 138:1181–1192, 1997.

Stade K, Ford CS, Guthrie C, Weis K. Exportin 1 (Crm1p) is an essential nuclear export factor. Cell 90:1041–1050, 1997.

Ullman K, Powers M, Forbes D. Nuclear export receptors: from importin to exportin. Cell 90:967–970, 1997.

Events in Cell Cycle

Darzynkiewicz Z, Gong J, Juan G, et al. Cytometry of cyclin proteins. Cytometry 25:1–13, 1996.

Hartwell LH, Weinert TA. Checkpoints: Controls that ensure the order of cell cycle events. Science 246:629–634, 1989.

Laskey RA, Fairman MP, Blow JJ. S phase of the cell cycle. Science 246:609–614, 1989.

McIntosh, JR, Koonce MP. Mitosis. Science 246:622–628, 1989.

Murray AW, Kirschner MW. Dominoes and clocks: The union of two views of the cell cycle. Science 246:614-621, 1989.

RNA

Ashrafi K, Chang FY, Watts JL, et al. Genome-wide RNAi analysis of Caenorhabditis elegans fat regulatory genes. Nature 421:268–272, 2003.

Joyce GF. RNA evolution and origins of life. Nature 338:217–224, 1989.

Lee SS, Lee RY, Fraser AG, et al. A systematic RNAi screen identifies a critical role for mitochondria in C. elegans longevity. Nat Genet 33:40–48, 2003.

Meegan JM, Marcus PI. Double-stranded ribonuclease coinduced with interferon. Science 244:1089–1091, 1989.

Ross J. The turnover of messenger RNA. Sci Am (Apr):48–55, 1989.

Schulman LDH, Abelson J. Recent excitement in understanding transfer RNA identity. Science 240:1591–1592, 1988.

Sharp PA. Splicing of messenger RNA precursors. Science 235:766–771, 1987.

Waldrop MM. Did life really start out in an RNA world? Science 246:1248–1249, 1989.

Regulation of Gene Expression

Marx JL. Homeobox linked to gene control. Science 242:1008–1009, 1988.
Ruvkun G, Hobert O. The taxonomy of developmental control in *Caenorhabditis elegans*. Science 282:2033–2041, 1998.
Selden RF, Skoskiewicz MJ, Russel PS, Goodman HM. Regulation of insulin-gene expression. Implication for gene therapy. N Engl J Med 317:1067–1076, 1987.

Proteins and Proteomics

Banks RE, Dunn MJ, Hochstrasser DF, et al. Proteomics: New perspectives, new biomedical opportunities. Lancet 356:1749–1756, 2000.
Cech TR. The ribosome is a ribozyme. Science 289:878–879, 2000.
Chung K-N, Walter P, Aponte GW, Moore H-PH. Molecular sorting in the secretory pathway. Science 243:192–197, 1989.
DeGrado WF, Wasserman ZR, Lear JD. Protein design, a minimalist approach. Science 243:622–628, 1989.
Filie A, Simone N, Simone C, et al. Proteomic evaluation of archival FNA patient samples of papillary thyroid carcinoma and follicular variant of papillary thyroid carcinoma yields distinct protein fingerprints with potential diagnostic applications. Mod Pathol 14:53, 2001.
Kraut J. How do enzymes work? Science 242:533–540, 1988.
Liotta LA, Kohn EC, Petricoin EF. Clinical proteomics. Personalized molecular medicine. JAMA 286:2211–2214, 2001.
Liotta L, Petricoin E. Molecular profiling of human cancer. Nat Rev Genet 1:48–56, 2000.
McKnight SL, Kingsbury R. Transcriptional control signals of a eukaryotic protein-coding gene. Science 217:316–324, 1982.
Panizo A, Roberts D, Al-Barazi H, et al. Utilization of cytology smears and manual microdissection for proteomic analysis. Mod Pathol 14:59, 2001.

Restriction Enzymes

Berman HM. How EcoRI recognizes and cuts DNA. Science 234:1482–1483, 1986.
Meselson M, Yuan R. DNA restriction enzyme from *E. coli*. Nature 217:1110–1114, 1968.
Roberts RJ. Restriction and modification enzymes and their recognition sequences. Nucleic Acids Res 11:35–67, 1983.

Enhancers and Promoters

Beckwith JR, Zipser D (eds). The Lactose Operon. Cold Spring Harbor New York, Cold Spring Harbor Laboratory, 1970.
Losick R, Chamberlin MJ (eds). RNA Polymerase. Cold Spring Harbor New York, Cold Spring Harbor Laboratory, 1976.
Mathis DJ, Chambon P. The SV40 early region TATA box is required for accurate in vitro initiation of transcription. Nature 290:310–315, 1981.
Schleif R. DNA looping. Science 240:127–128, 1988.
Youderian P, Bouvier S, Susskind M. Sequence determinants of promoter activity. Cell 30:843–853, 1982.

Restriction Fragment Length Polymorphism (RFLP)

Botstein D, White RL, Skolnick M, Davis RW. Construction of a genetic linkage map in man using restriction fragment length polymorphism. Am J Hum Genet 32:314–331, 1980.
Kan YW, Dozy AM. Polymorphism of DNA sequence adjacent to human beta globin structural gene: Relationship to sickle mutation. Proc Natl Acad Sci USA 75:5631–5635, 1978.
Vogelstein B, Fearon ER, Hamilton S, Feiberg AP. Use of restriction fragment length polymorphisms to determine clonal origin of human tumors. Science 227:642–645, 1985.

Reverse Transcriptase

Baltimore D. Viral RNA-dependent DNA polymerase. Nature 226:1209-1211, 1970.
Panganiban A, Fiore D. Ordered interstrand and intrastrand DNA transfer during reverse transcription. Science 241:1064–1069, 1988.
Temin HM, Mizutani S. Viral RNA-dependent DNA polymerase. Nature 226:1211–1213, 1970.

Genetic Disorders and Sequencing of Human Genome

Antonarakis SE. Diagnosis of genetic disorders at the DNA level. N Engl J Med 320:153–163, 1989.
Caskay CT. Disease diagnosis by recombinant DNA methods. Science 236:1223–1229, 1987.
Collins FS. Shattuck lecture: Medical and societal consequences of the human genome project. N Engl J Med 341:28–37, 1999.
Collins FS, Guttmacher AE. Genetics moves into the medical mainstream. JAMA 286:2322–2324, 2001.
Collins FS, Morgan M, Patrinos A. The human genome project: Lessons from large-scale biology. Science 300:286–290, 2003.
Gingcras TR, Roberts RJ. Steps toward computer analysis of nucleotide sequences. Science 209:1322–1328, 1980.
Guttmacher AE, Collins FS. Genomic medicine—a primer. N Engl J Med 347:1512–1520, 2002.
Lander ES, Linton LM, Birren B, et al. Initial sequencing and analysis of the human genome. Nature 409:860–921, 2001.
McKusick VA. The anatomy of the human genome. A neo-vesalian basis for medicine in the 21st century. JAMA 286:2289–2295, 2001.
McKusick VA. Mapping and sequencing the human genome. N Engl J Med 320:910–915, 1989.
McKusick VA. The morbid anatomy of the human genome: A review of gene mapping in clinical medicine. Medicine 65:1–33, 1986; 66:1–63, 1987; 67:1–19, 1988.
Subramanian G, Adams MD, Venter JC, Broder S. Implications of the human genome for understanding human biology and medicine. JAMA 286:2296–2307, 2001.
Venter JC, Adams MD, Myers EW, et al. The sequence of the human genome. Science 291:1304–1351, 2001.

Genetic Engineering

The new harvest: Genetically engineered species. Science 244:1275–1317, 1989.
Abelson J, Butz E (eds). Recombinant DNA. Science 209:1317–1435, 1980.

Polymerase Chain Reaction

Landegren U, Kaiser R, Caskey CT, Hood L. DNA diagnostics—molecular techniques and automation. Science 242:229–237, 1988.
Rabinow P. Making PCR. A story of biotechnology. Chicago, Univ. of Chicago Press, 1995
Rogers MF, Ou C-Y, Rayfield M, et al. Use of polymerase chain reaction for early detection of the proviral sequences of human immunodeficiency virus in infants born to seropositive mothers. N Engl J Med 320:1649–1654, 1989.
Saiki RK, Gelfand DH, Stoffel S, et al. Primer-directed enzymatic amplification of DNA with a thermostable DNA polymerase. Science 239:487–491, 1988.
Young LS, Bevan IS, Johnson MA, et al. The polymerase chain reaction: A new epidemiological tool for investigating cervical human papillomavirus infection. Br Med J 298:14–18, 1989.

RNA In Situ Hybridization

Angerer RC, Cox KH, Angerer LM. In situ hybridization to cellular RNAs. Genet Eng 7:43, 1985.
Stoler MH, Broker TR. In situ hybridization detection of human papillomavirus DNAs and messenger RNAs in genital condylomas and cervical carcinoma. Hum Pathol 17:1250–1258, 1986.
Strickland S, Huarte J, Belin D, et al. Antisense RNA directed against the 3' noncoding region prevents dormant mRNA activation in mouse oocytes. Science 241:680–684, 1987.

Application of Molecular Biologic Techniques to Diagnostic Cytology (partial listing, see also Chapters 4, 6, and specific chapters)

Baloglu H, Cannizzaro LA, Jones J, Koss LG. Atypical endometrial hyperplasia shares genomic abnormalities with endometrioid carcinoma by comparative genomic hybridization. Hum Pathol 32:615–622, 2001.
Feinmesser R, Miyazaki I, Cheung R, et al. Diagnosis of nasopharyngeal carcinoma by DNA amplification of tissue obtained by fine-needle aspiration. N Engl J Med 326:17–21, 1992 (see also correspondence, ibid, pp 1291–1292).
Fetsch PA, Simone NL, Bryant-Greenwood PK, et al. Proteomic evaluation of archival cytologic material using SELD affinity mass spectrometry: Potential for diagnostic applications. Am J Clin Pathol 118:870–876, 2002.

Golub TR, Slonim DK, Tamayo P, et al. Molecular classification of cancer. Science 286:531–537, 1999.

Houldsworth J, Chaganti RSK. Comparative genomic hybridization: An overview. Am J Pathol 145:1253–1260, 1994.

Kallioniemi A, Kallioniemi O-P, Sudar D, et al. Comparative genomic hybridization for molecular cytogenetic analysis of solid tumors. Science 258:818–821, 1992.

Khan J, Wei JS, Ringner M, et al. Classification and diagnostic prediction of cancers using gene expression profiling and artificial neural networks. Nat Med 7:673–679, 2001.

King HC, Sinha AA. Gene expression profile analysis by DNA microarrays. Promise and pitfalls. JAMA 286:2280–2288, 2001.

Liotta L, Kohn EC, Petricoin EF. Clinical proteomics: Personalized molecular medicine. JAMA 286:2211–2214, 2001.

Lubinski J, Chosia M, Huebner K. Molecular genetic analysis in the diagnosis of lymphoma in fine needle aspiration biopsies. I. Lymphomas vs. benign proliferative disorders; II. Lymphomas vs. nonlymphoid malignant tumors. Anal Quant Cytol Histol 10:391–398; 399–404, 1988.

Macoska JA. The progressing clinical utility of DNA microarrays. CA Cancer J Clin 52:50–59, 2002.

Maoir SD, Speicher MR, Joes S, et al. Detection of complete and partial chromosome gain and losses by comparative genomic in situ hybridization. Hum Genet 90:590–610, 1993.

O'Leary JJ, Landers RJ, Chetty R. In situ amplification in cytological preparations. Cytopathol 8:148–160, 1997.

Paweletz CP, Trock B, Pennanen M, et al. Proteomic patterns of nipple aspirate fluids obtained by SELDI-TOF. Potential for new biomarkers to aid in the diagnosis of breast cancer. Dis Markers 17:301–307, 2001.

Wells D, Sherlock JK, Handyside AH, Delhanty JDA. Detailed chromosomal and molecular genetic analysis of single cells by whole genome amplification and comparative genomic hybridisation. Nucleic Acids Res 27:1214–1218, 1999.

Welsh JB, Zarrinkar PP, Sapinoso LM, et al. Analysis of gene expression profiles in normal and neoplastic ovarian tissue samples identifies candidate molecular markers of epithelial ovarian cancer. Proc Natl Acad Sci USA 98:1176–1181, 2001.

Monoclonal Antibodies

Huse WD, Sastry L, Iverson SA, et al. Generation of a large combinatorial library of the immunoglobulin repertoire in phage lambda. Science 246:1275–1281, 1989.

Kohler G, Milstein C. Continuous culture of fused cells secreting antibody of predefined specificity. Nature 256:495–497, 1975.

Koss LG. Cytochemistry [editorial]. Acta Cytol 28:353–355, 1984.

Variable Number of Tandem Repeats

Nakamura Y, Leppert M, O'Connell P, et al. Variable number of tandem repeats (VNTR) markers for human gene mapping. Science 235:1616–1622, 1987.

Principles of Cytogenetics*

Linda A. Cannizzaro

The events governing the developmental evolution of cells as they progress from the fertilized ovum to mature tissues are not fully understood as yet. It is known, however, that this process involves extensive **proliferation and differentiation of embryonal stem cells** and their **selective destruction** by programmed cell death or **apoptosis** (see Chap. 6). These processes are governed by messages inscribed in the nuclear deoxyribose nucleic acid (DNA) (see Chap. 3). The key feature in cell proliferation is **cell division.**

There are two forms of cell division, one occurring during the formation of **gametes** (e.g., the spermatozoa and ova), known as **meiosis,** and the other affecting all other cells (**somatic cells**) known as **mitosis.** The **purpose of meiosis** is to **reduce the number of chromosomes by one half** (in humans from 46 to 23) in the gametes, so that the union of a spermatozoon and an ovum (fertilization of the ovum) will result in an organism that carries the full complement of chromosomes (in humans, 46) in its somatic cells. The **purpose of mitosis** is the reproduction of somatic cells, each carrying the full complement of chromosomes. Both forms of cell division are discussed in this chapter.

---

* For a brief glossary of essential cytogenetic terms, see the end of chapter.

The events encompassing the life of a cell from its birth until the end of the mitotic division are known as **the cell cycle,** during which the **genomic identity** of the cell, vested in the **DNA,** must be preserved. Molecular genetic technology has considerably advanced our knowledge of the processes involved in the progression of the cell cycle. The normal cell cycle has developed complex mechanisms for the detection and repair of damaged DNA. Upsetting the intricate balance of these cellular processes has dramatic and usually tragic consequences. **Dysregulation of meiosis** oftentimes is manifested as a **genetic disorder,** while **dysregulation of mitosis** may result in a **malignant disorder.**

Since the demonstration of the specificity of chromosomal changes in many disease states and their utilization in diagnosis, the cytogenetic aspects of human diseases have become of direct concern to the practicing physician. This chapter summarizes the salient features of cell division, as well as some of the inherited and malignant conditions that directly result from faulty or anomalous events during meiosis and mitosis. Recent introduction of several powerful molecular cytogenetic methods has facilitated the identification of chromosomal alterations previously irresolvable by high-resolution cytogenetic analysis. These technologies, including the recent mapping of the human genome (Caron et al, 2001; International Human Genome Sequencing Consortium, 2001; Venter et al, 2001; Peltonen and McKusick, 2001) have enormously impacted our knowledge of human genetic disease and the contributions made by these innovations will be made evident in the forthcoming narrative.

THE CELL CYCLE

The cell cycle is composed of several phases, which have, for their purpose, the preservation of the genomic heritage of the cell to be transmitted to the two daughter cells.

The phases of the cell cycle are as follows:

- G_0 (resting phase)
- G_1 (gap^1)
- S (synthesis)
- G_2 (gap^2)
- M (mitosis)

The events in the phases of cell cycle are described below.

Events Preparatory to Cell Division

Genetic information in the form of DNA is stored within the interphase nucleus in thread-like, tangled structures called **chromatin.** During the process of cell division, the DNA condenses and divides into several distinct pairs of linear segments or **chromosomes.** Each time the cell divides, the hereditary information carried in the chromosomes is passed on to the two newly formed cells. The DNA in the nucleus contains the instructions for regulating the amount and types of proteins made by the cell. These instructions are copied, or transcribed, into messenger RNA

(mRNA), which is transported from the nucleus to the ribosomes located in the cytoplasm, where proteins are assembled (see Chap. 3).

Most somatic cells spend the greater part of their lives in G_0, or the resting phase of the cell cycle, because such cell populations are not actively dividing.

Before a cell can divide, it must double its mass and duplicate all of its contents. This ensures the ability of the daughter cells to begin their own cycle of growth followed by division. Most of the work involved in preparing for division goes on invisibly during the **growth phase of the cell cycle, known as the** *interphase,* which comprises the G_1, S, and G_2 phases of the cell cycle (Fig. 4-1). The interphase nucleus is the seat of crucial biochemical activities including the synthesis of proteins and the duplication of its chromosomal DNA in preparation for subsequent cell division.

Cell Division

The **process of cell division** (see Fig. 4-1) can be readily visualized in the microscope and consists of two sequential

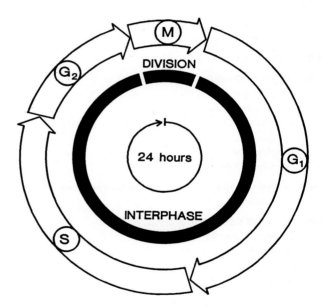

Figure 4-1 **Schematic presentation of the phases of the mitotic cycle.** After the *M phase*, which consists of nuclear division (mitosis) and cytoplasmic division (cytokinesis), the daughter cells enter the interphase of a new cycle. Interphase begins with the G_1 *phase* in which the cells resume a high rate of biosynthesis after a relatively dormant state during mitosis. The *S phase* starts when DNA synthesis begins and ends when the DNA content of the nucleus has been replicated (doubled); each chromosome now consists of two sister chromatids. The cell then enters the G_2 *phase*, which ends with the start of mitosis (M). The latter begins with mitosis and ends with cytokinesis. During the early part of the M phase, the replicated chromosomes condense from their elongated interphase state and can be seen in the microscope. The nuclear membrane breaks down, and each chromosome undergoes organized movements that result in the separation of its pair of sister chromatids as the nuclear contents are divided. Two nuclear membranes then form, and the cytoplasm divides to generate two daughter cells, each with a single nucleus. This process of cytokinesis ends the M phase and marks the beginning of the interphase of the next cell cycle. Although a 24-hour cycle is shown in this figure, cell cycle times vary considerably in cells, with most of the variability being in the duration of the G_1 phase. (Courtesy of Dr. Avery Sandberg, Scottsdale, AZ.)

events: **nuclear division (mitosis)** followed by **cytoplasmic division (cytokinesis).** The cell-division phase is designated as the *M phase* (**M = mitosis**). The period between the end of the M phase and the start of DNA synthesis is the *G₁ phase* (**G = gap**). In G₁, RNAs and proteins, including the essential components needed for DNA replication, are synthesized without replication of DNA. Once all the ingredients are synthesized in G₁, DNA replication takes place in the ensuing synthesis phase **(S-phase)** of the cell cycle.

The period between the completion of DNA synthesis and the M phase is known as the *G₂ phase,* in which additional cellular components are synthesized in preparation for the cell's entry into mitosis. The interphase thus consists of successive G₁, S, and G₂ phases that normally constitute 90% or more of the total cell cycle time (see Fig. 4-1).

However, following the completion of mitotic division, most normal somatic cells leave the division cycle and enter a **postmitotic resting phase (G₀),** rather than the new **G₁ phase.** The unknown **trigger mechanism for cell division** is activated during the G₀ phase; as a result, the cell enters G₁ phase and is committed to divide (Brachet, 1985; Levitan, 1987; Therman, 1993; Nicklas, 1997; Hixon and Gualberto, 2000). In fact, experiments have shown that the point of no return, known as the *restriction point* (**R point),** occurs late in G₁. After cells have passed this point, they will complete the rest of the cycle at their normal rate, regardless of external conditions. The time spent by cells in G₂ and S phases is relatively constant (Brachet, 1985; Gardner, 2000). One interesting exception is the epidermis of the **skin,** in which **some cells remain in the G₂ phase** and thus are able to undergo rapid division in wound healing.

Studies of the cell cycle in yeast have shown that the **cell proceeds from one phase of the cell cycle to the next by passing through a series of molecular checkpoints** (Li and Murray, 1983). These checkpoints determine whether the cell is ready to enter into the next phase of the cell cycle. These biochemical checkpoints involve the synthesis of new proteins and degradation of already existing proteins. Both the S phase and the M phase are activated by related **protein kinases,** which function at specific stages of the cell cycle. Each kinase consists of at least two subunits, one of which is **cyclin,** so named because of its role in the cell cycle. There are several cyclins involved in regulating entry into different parts of the cell cycle, and they are degraded after serving their purpose or as the cell progresses in the cycle and through mitosis (Rudner and Murray, 1996; Amon, 1999; Cerrutti et al, 2000; Gardner, 2000).

The cells of the human body divide at very different rates. Some cells, such as mature neurons, heart and skeletal muscle, and mature red blood cells, do not divide at all or perhaps only under most exceptional circumstances. Other cells, such as the epithelial cells that line the inside and outside surfaces of the body (e.g., the intestine, lung, and skin), divide continuously and relatively rapidly throughout the life of the individual. The behavior of most cells falls somewhere between these two extremes. Most somatic cells rarely divide, and the duration of their cell cycle may be 100 days or more.

The **average time for the mitotic cycle** in most cell types is about 16 hours in human and other mammalian cells, distributed as follows: S phase, approximately 6 to 8 hours; G₁ phase, 6 to 12 hours; G₂ phase, 4 hours; and M phase, 1 to 2 hours (see Fig. 4-1). The M, and especially G₁, phases may show considerable variation in duration. Most of the available evidence suggests that these periods are **longer in cancer cells** than in benign cells, or at least in benign cell populations that normally have a rapid turnover. Many tissues require more than 16 hours to complete the mitosis (Miles, 1979).

Even though it takes a minimum of 7 to 8 hours for a cell to duplicate its entire chromosomal DNA, individual chromosomes or segments of chromosomes are replicated asynchronously, some of them sooner and faster than others. Thus, some chromosomes, or their segments, will have completed DNA synthesis before others begin. This asynchrony does not follow a simple pattern. The synthesis does not necessarily begin at one point and spread uniformly along the chromosome, but may start at several places on a single chromosome, while others wait their turn for DNA replication. A reproducible phenomenon is the **late replication of one of the two X chromosomes** in normal female cells or in cells with more than one X chromosome. Apparently, this X chromosome finishes its DNA replication later than any other chromosome in the cell. The number of late-replicating X chromosomes is usually one less than the total number of X chromosomes in the cell (Moore, 1966; Sandberg, 1983a, 1983b).

The chromosomes are not visible under the light **microscope except during the M phase of the cell cycle.** The physical condition of the chromosomes during interphase (e.g., G₁, S, and G₂) is not known, but their invisibility is probably caused, at least in part, to their enormous elongation. The older notion that the chromosomes lose their linear structure and become dissolved in the nucleoplasm is unlikely, and it introduces unnecessary complexities into the analysis of nuclear and chromosomal dynamics (van Holde, 1989; Miles, 1964, 1979).

Recent studies of chromosomes, utilizing fluorescent probes for chromosomal "painting," suggest that the chromosomes **retain their distinct identity during the interphase** and that their position in the nucleus may be relatively constant throughout the life of the cell (Nagele et al, 1995; Koss, 1998).

CHROMOSOME STRUCTURE

Soon after a chromosome becomes visible in the early part (prophase) of mitotic division, it is already doubled into a pair of **identical chromatids** (Fig. 4-2A). This pair remains joined together at one point, the **centromere** (also called the *primary constriction*). The centromere divides the chromosome into a **short (from French, p = petit)** and **a long (q, the next letter after p) arm**

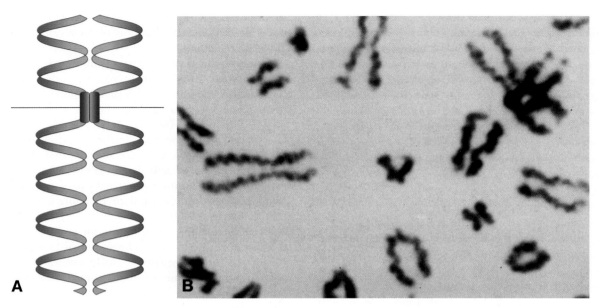

Figure 4-2   *A.* Schematic presentation of the organization of a human chromosome showing short (p), long (q) arms and the centrometre. *B.* Metaphase of human chromosomes exhibiting major coils in the chromatids. (Courtesy of Dr. Charles Miles.)

region. The centromere connects the chromosome to the spindle fibers during mitotic division. Associated with the centromere are proteinaceous structures, known as **kinetechores,** to which the microtubules of the spindle mechanism are attached (see below). Normal chromosome ends are capped by **telomeres.** These short repeat DNA **sequences are essential for maintaining the structural integrity of the chromosome** by preventing the ends from fusing with other chromosomes. If the telomere sequences are lost or broken off, an end-to-end fusion of two chromosomes can occur.

In suitable preparations, it is clear that each chromatid is in the form of a single helical coil, sometimes referred to as the **major coil** (see Fig. 4-2B). In some plant species, the strand making up the major coil is composed of smaller or **minor coils** (i.e., the chromatid is a **coiled coil**). It is to be noted that the minor coil is too large to be the Watson-Crick double helix of DNA, which may be found as fine strands at the next level of resolution. The chromosomal structure at metaphase would consist of two chromatids, each of which is coiled-coiled coil, the smallest coil being the DNA double helix. This is a useful model to keep in mind, but it may represent an oversimplification. Electron micrographs of whole human chromosomes at metaphase exhibit what has been called a *folded fiber structure,* in which the fibers appear sharply but randomly bent or angulated into meshwork (Fig. 4-3). These fibers, assuming there is a protein coat, are about the right dimensions for DNA molecules. The evidence appears to be consistent with the view that each chromatid represents a tangle of single-strand DNA, forming the Watson-Crick double helix (Fig. 4-4) (Dupraw, 1966; Miles, 1964; Bahr, 1977; Therman, 1993). There are several theories pertaining to the relationship of the primary DNA molecule to the organization of the chromosome and chromosomal banding. An example of this proposal by Comings is shown in Figure 4-5.

STAGES OF MITOSIS

Living things grow and maintain themselves in large measure because their cells are capable of multiplying by successive division. The steps observed in nuclear division are called **mitosis** or, more precisely, **mitotic division.** Although the stages of nuclear division are not sharply demarcated, they are conveniently referred to as:

- prophase
- prometaphase
- metaphase
- anaphase
- telophase (Fig. 4-6; see Fig. 4-1)

Mitosis is a complex process, which includes a breakdown of the nuclear envelope, chromatin condensation, and chromosome segregation. A brief description of these stages will first be given to provide a framework for a more detailed discussion.

Prophase proceeds from the first visible signs of cell division until the breakdown of the nuclear envelope. During the **prophase,** the **chromosomes have condensed** and appear as long rod-like structures. **Prometaphase** starts with the disruption of the nuclear envelope. **Metaphase** is the period during which the **chromosomes become aligned on the central metaphase plate. Anaphase** begins with the abrupt **separation of the chromatids into daughter chromosomes** as they proceed toward opposite poles of the cell. Finally, the nuclear membrane becomes reconstituted during **telophase.**

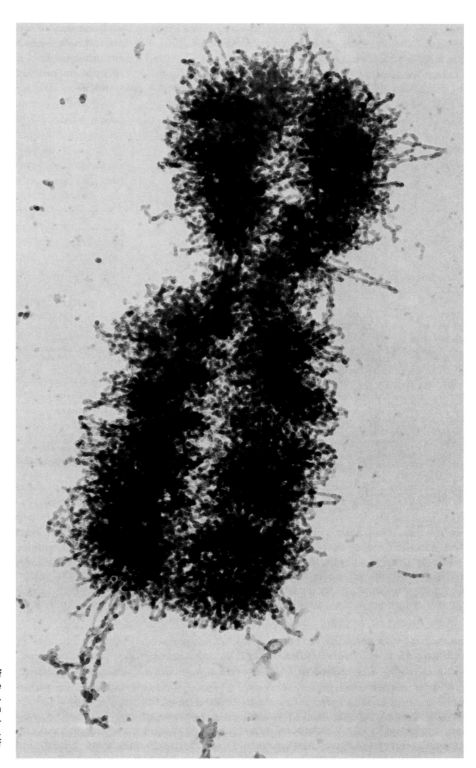

Figure 4-3   *A.* **Electron micrograph of a whole mount of a human chromosome showing the A-folded fiber structure.** The diameter of the fiber is about 20nm (200 Å). Reduced from the original magnification of ×28,000. (Courtesy of Dr. Gunter Bahr, Armed Forces Institute of Pathology, Washington, D.C.)

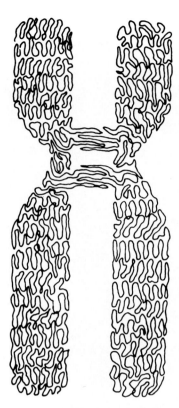

Figure 4-4 Idealized schematic drawing of a human submetra-centric chromosome at metaphase. Portions of the 2 spindle fibers are shown attached to the as yet unseparated centrometre. Each chromatid exhibits a major coil but no finer structure can be seen with the light microscope.

Prophase

The transition from the G₂ phase to the M phase of the cell cycle is not a sharply defined event. The chromatin, which is diffuse in interphase, slowly **condenses into well-defined chromosomes,** the exact number of which is a characteristic of the particular species; each chromosome has duplicated during the preceding S phase and consists of **two sister chromatids** joined at a specific point along their length by the **centromere.** While the chromosomes are condensing, **the nucleolus** begins to disassemble and **gradually disappears.**

Within the nucleus itself, the first sign of prophase is an accentuation of the **chromocenters** and a net-like pattern (Fig. 4-7B; see Fig. 4-6A). Several condensations of chromatin appear at the periphery of the nucleus, whence thin strands of chromatin extend into the center of the nucleus (see Fig. 4-7B). In females, the inactive X chromosome (Barr body) is larger than other chromocenters and is readily visible as a triangular condensation of chromatin (see Fig. 4-7). These strands and chromocenters are the condensing chromosomes. By this time, the chromosomes are probably doubled into the two chromatids or daughter chromosomes-to-be, but the double structure is sometimes difficult to visualize (Fig. 4-8A; see Fig. 4-6B). It is more evident in chromosomes that have been exposed to colchicine (a drug that inhibits mitosis) and which have been treated

with **hypotonic salt solutions.** With the breakdown of the nuclear membrane, the chromosomes are quite distinct and are arranged into a circular position, known as a **hollow spindle** or **prometaphase rosette** (see below) (see Figs. 4-6C and 4-8B,C).

At the beginning of prophase, the **cytoplasmic microtubules,** which are part of the cytoskeleton (see Chap. 2), disassemble, forming a large pool of tubulin molecules. These molecules are then reused in the construction of the main component of the mitotic apparatus, the **mitotic spindle.** This is a bipolar fibrous structure, largely composed of microtubules, that assembles initially outside the nucleus. The focus for the spindle formation is marked in most animal cells by the **centrioles** (see Chap. 2). The cell's original pair of centrioles replicates by a process that begins immediately before the S phase to give rise to **two pairs of centrioles,** which separate and travel to the opposite poles of the cell (see Fig. 4-6D). Each centriole pair now becomes part of a **mitotic center** that forms the focus for a radial array of microtubules, the **aster** (from Latin, *aster* = star). Initially, the two asters lie side by side, close to the nuclear envelope. By late prophase, the bundles of polar microtubules that interact between the two asters (seen as polar fibers in the light microscope) preferentially elongate and appear to push the two asters apart along the outer part of the nucleus. In this way, a **bipolar mitotic spindle** is formed.

Prometaphase

Prometaphase starts abruptly with the **disruption of the nuclear envelope,** which breaks up into membrane fragments that are indistinguishable from bits of endoplasmic reticulum (see Fig. 4-6C). These fragments remain visible around the spindle during mitosis. Specialized structures called **kinetochores** develop on either face of the centromeres and become attached to a special set of microtubules, called **kinetochore fibers** or **kinetochore microtubules.** These fibers radiate in opposite directions from the sides of each chromosome and interact with the fibers of the bipolar spindle. The chromosomes are thrown into agitated motion by the interactions of their kinetochore fibers with other components of the spindle.

Metaphase

In phase cinematography of living cells, the chromosomes may be seen to undergo slow to and fro writhing movements until they finally become aligned on an **equatorial plane.** This plane bisects the mitotic spindle. As a result of their prometaphase oscillations, arrangement of all the chromosomes is such that their centromeres lie in one plane. The kinetochore fibers seem to be responsible for aligning the chromosomes halfway between the spindle poles and for orienting them with their long axes at right angles to the spindle axis. Each chromosome is held in tension at the metaphase plate by the paired kinetochores, with their associated fibers pointing to opposite poles of the spindle (see Figs. 4-6D and 4-8D).

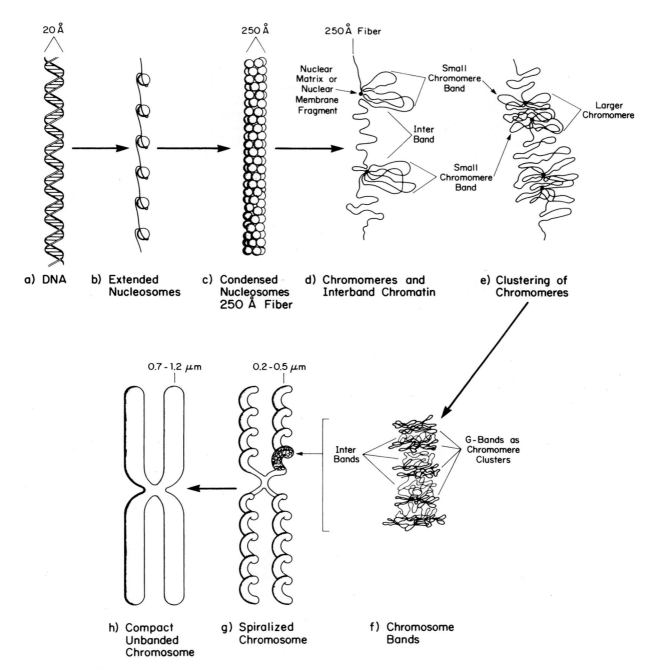

20 Å

250 Å   250 Å Fiber

Nuclear
Matrix or
Nuclear
Membrane
Fragment

Small
Chromomere
Band

Larger
Chromomere

Inter
Band

Small
Chromomere
Band

a) DNA   b) Extended
Nucleosomes   c) Condensed
Nucleosomes
250 Å Fiber   d) Chromomeres and
Interband Chromatin   e) Clustering of
Chromomeres

0.7 - 1.2 μm   0.2 - 0.5 μm

Inter
Bands

G-Bands as
Chromomere
Clusters

h) Compact
Unbanded
Chromosome   g) Spiralized
Chromosome   f) Chromosome
Bands

Figure 4-5   Single-stranded model of chromosomal structure. This suggests that a single DNAB protein (DNP) fiber, beginning at one telomere, folds upon itself to build up the width of the chromatid and eventually progresses to the opposite telomere without lengthy longitudinal fibers, with no central core and no half- or quarter-chromatids. The centromere region in this metacentric chromosome is depicted as the result of fusion of two telocentric chromosomes, with retention of the individual centromere regions. The fibers at the point of chromatid association briefly interdigitate. (Courtesy of Dr. D. Comings.)

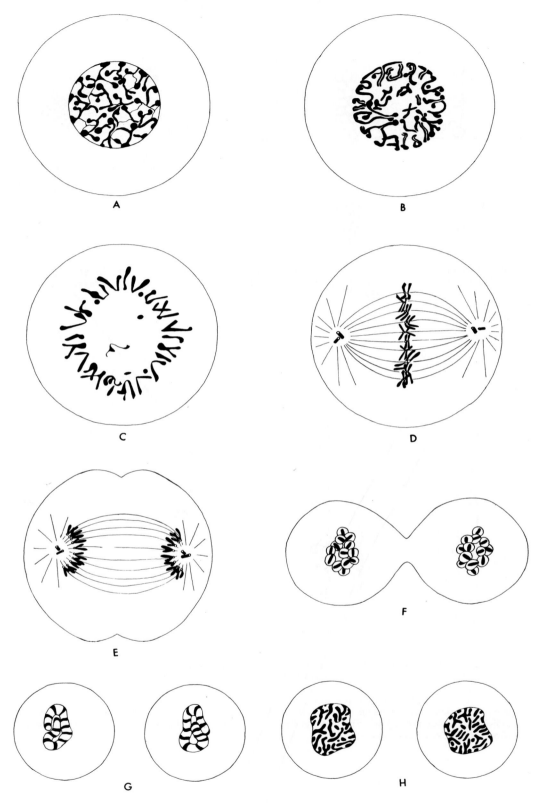

Figure 4-6   Diagrammatic presentation of human mitotic division. *A.* Mitosis begins with accentuation of the network pattern in the nucleoplasm and of the peripheral chromatin masses (chromocenters), which are presumably parts of the chromosomes. *B.* Further condensation of the chromosomes, some of which are now distinctly double (i.e., divided into chromatids). There is a breakdown of the nuclear membrane. *C.* At or shortly after the breakdown of the nuclear membrane (the conventional end of prophase), the chromosomes are arranged on the periphery of an equatorial plate, forming a so-called hollow spindle (it is not clear, however, that the spindle has as yet formed). *D.* The spindle at metaphase, with the equatorial plate viewed on end. The relative size of the centrioles, shown here as small rods, is exaggerated. *E.* Late anaphase: The chromosomes have divided, and the daughter

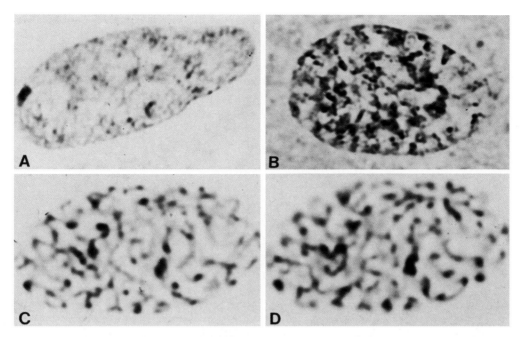

Figure 4-7 **Interphase appearance and stages of prophase condensation.** *A.* Interphase nucleus with sex chromatin body. Note the network of fine chromatin threads. *B.* An early stage of prophase showing accentuation of the chromatin network and of the peripheral chromocenters. (*C,D*) A somewhat later stage of prophase. The same nucleus photographed at two focal levels. (*A,B,* ×3,900; *C,D,* ×4,350). (From Miles CP. Chromatin elements, nuclear morphology and midbody in human mitosis. Acta Cytol 8:356–363, 1964.)

Anaphase

The metaphase may last for several hours. As if triggered by a special signal, anaphase begins abruptly as the **paired kinetochores on each chromosome separate,** allowing each chromatid to be pulled slowly toward a spindle pole (see Fig. 4-6E). All chromatids are moved toward the pole they face at the same speed. During these movements, **kinetochore fibers shorten** as the chromosomes approach the poles. At about the same time, the **spindle fibers elongate** and the two poles of the polar spindle move farther apart. Soon after separation, the chromosomes appear at both poles as dark-staining masses (see Fig. 4-8E). The anaphase stage typically lasts only a few minutes.

In the meantime, the cell has become elongated, and a constriction furrow begins to appear at the level of the metaphase equator (see Figs. 4-9A and Fig. 4-6F). This process of cytoplasmic division is called **cytokinesis.** Although cytokinesis usually follows chromosomal division, the two processes are not necessarily dependent on one another. **Chromosomal division may occur without cytokinesis** (thereby producing a cell with double the normal complement of chromosomes). Less commonly, in some lower species, anucleated cytoplasm may undergo successive divisions.

The constriction furrow extends between the two daughter cells until only a narrow strand of cytoplasm is left. At this point, a distinct granule, the **midbody,** may sometimes be seen at the narrowest part of the cytoplasmic strand (see Fig. 4-9B). The midbody is formed, at least in part, by the spindle fibers compressed into a tight bundle. The precise significance and fate of the midbody are not known.

Telophase

Some details of telophase are worthy of attention. In late anaphase, after or during cytokinesis, the compact mass of chromosomes begins to swell. In optimal material, each chromosome appears to form a distinct small vesicle, possibly by inducing the formation of a proprietary segment of the nuclear membrane, as suggested by Koss (1998) (Fig. 4-10; see Fig. 4-6F). In abnormal divisions, the process may sometimes end at this stage, with the cell thus containing numerous micronuclei (Fig. 4-11). Normally, the vesicles seem to fuse rapidly together to form a convoluted tubule (see Figs. 4-12 and 4-6G). Probably the vesicle and tubule membranes break down

groups form compact masses at the two poles. A furrow has appeared in the cytoplasm, marking the onset of cytokinesis. *F.* Early telophase: Each chromosome appears to form a small vesicle. *G.* The vesicles fuse to form a convoluted tubule with chromosomes at right angles to the long axis. Where the tubule walls contact one another, they apparently break down, leaving a continuous nuclear membrane around the chromosomes. *H.* In the final recognizable stage of telophase, the nucleus tends to resemble prophase, with chromosomes still partly condensed. The convoluted appearance is still evident. (Courtesy of Dr. C.P. Miles.)

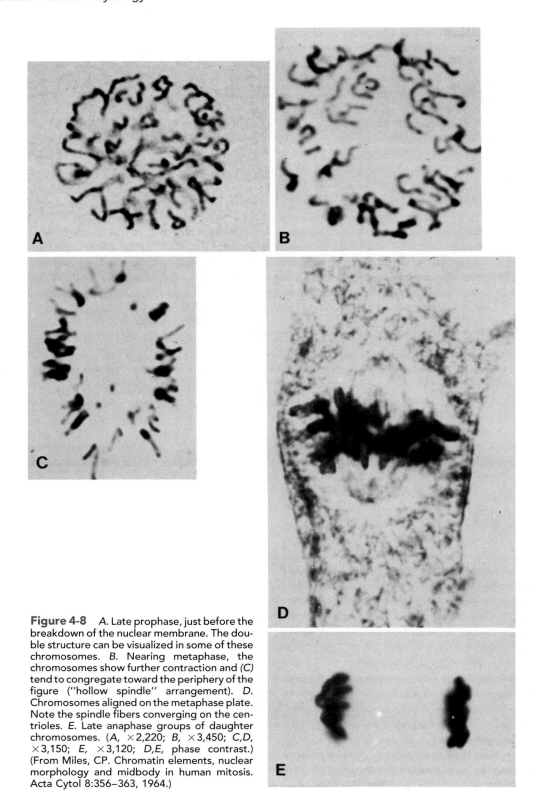

Figure 4-8 *A.* Late prophase, just before the breakdown of the nuclear membrane. The double structure can be visualized in some of these chromosomes. *B.* Nearing metaphase, the chromosomes show further contraction and *(C)* tend to congregate toward the periphery of the figure ("hollow spindle" arrangement). *D.* Chromosomes aligned on the metaphase plate. Note the spindle fibers converging on the centrioles. *E.* Late anaphase groups of daughter chromosomes. (*A,* ×2,220; *B,* ×3,450; *C,D,* ×3,150; *E,* ×3,120; *D,E,* phase contrast.) (From Miles, CP. Chromatin elements, nuclear morphology and midbody in human mitosis. Acta Cytol 8:356–363, 1964.)

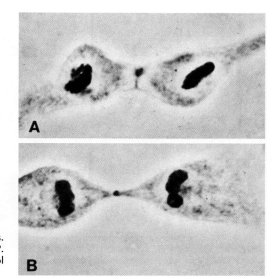

Figure 4-9   *A.* Division of the cytoplasm (cytokinesis). *B.* Later stage of cytokinesis. The midbody is the small central granule (phase contrast ×1,560). (From Miles, CP. Chromatin elements, nuclear morphology and midbody in human mitosis. Acta Cytol 8:356–363, 1964.)

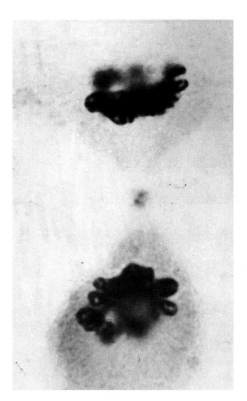

Figure 4-10   Beginning of telophase reconstruction. Each chromosome appears to form a small vesicle. The dark double structure at the center of the spindle conceivably represents a divided midbody (phase contrast ×2,250). (From Miles, CP. Chromatin elements, nuclear morphology and midbody in human mitosis. Acta Cytol 8:356–363, 1964.)

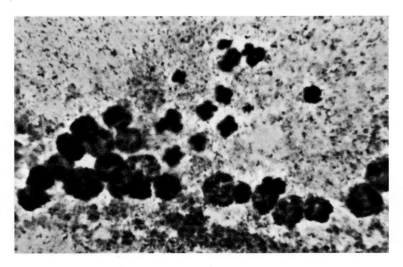

Figure 4-11   **Abnormal mitosis with micronuclei**, presumably formed through failure of chromosomal vesicles to coalesce (colchicine-treated culture; aceto-orcein stain ×1,610). (From Miles, CP. Chromatin elements, nuclear morphology and midbody in human mitosis. Acta Cytol 8:356–363, 1964.)

at points of contact so that, ultimately, a continuous nuclear membrane is formed around both groups of daughter chromatids.

The elongating chromosomes now appear at right angles to the tubule walls, thus to some extent, mimicking prophase appearances (see Figs. 4-13, 4-6H, and 4-12B). The outline of the nucleus gradually becomes less convoluted, and nucleolar material appears at the inner edges of the nucleus. The reticular appearance of the telophase nucleus (Fig. 4-14) gradually fades into the less-distinct interphase pattern.

As the separated daughter chromatids arrive at the poles, the kinetochore fibers disappear. The polar fibers elongate still farther, the condensed chromatin expands once more, the nucleoli begin to reappear, and the mitosis comes to an end.

Cytokinesis

As described above, the cytoplasm divides by a process known as *cleavage*, which usually starts sometime during late anaphase or telophase. The membrane around the middle of

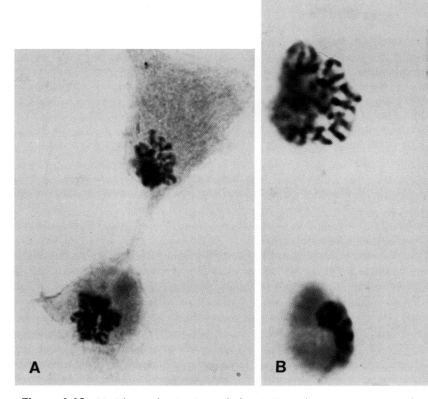

Figure 4-12   **Vesicles coalescing into tubules.** *A.* Note chromosomes arranged at right angles to the long axis of the tubule (aceto-orcein stain ×1,120; *B*, 1,610). (From Miles, CP. Chromatin elements, nuclear morphology and midbody in human mitosis. Acta Cytol 8:356–363, 1964.)

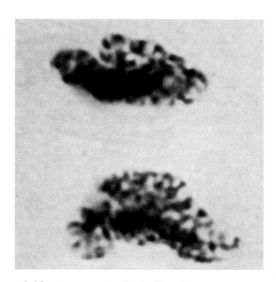

Figure 4-13 Late stages of telophase beginning to mimic prophase appearance. One daughter nucleus still shows tubule structure (aceto-orcein stain, ×3,150). (From Miles, CP. Chromatin elements, nuclear morphology and midbody in human mitosis. Acta Cytol 8:356–363, 1964.)

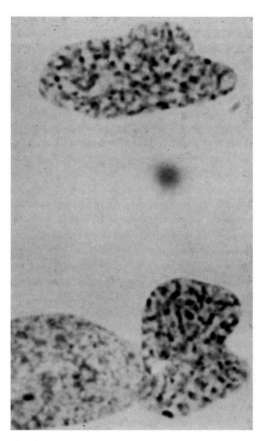

Figure 4-14 Telophase. The daughter nuclei still appear somewhat convoluted, but no suggestion of tubule remains. (Part of an interphase nucleus impinges on one daughter nucleus.) Some of the spoke-like chromosomal elements appear distinctly double, as does the larger bipartite chromocenter in one nucleus (the sex chromatin body?) (aceto-orcein stain ×2,520). (From Miles, CP. Chromatin elements, nuclear morphology and midbody in human mitosis. Acta Cytol 8:356–363, 1964.)

the cell, perpendicular to the spindle axis and between the daughter nuclei, is drawn inward to form a **cleavage furrow,** which gradually deepens until it encounters the remains of the mitotic spindle between the two nuclei (see Figs. 4-6F and 4-9). This narrow bridge, which contains a dark granule, the **midbody,** may persist for some time before it finally breaks at each, leaving two completed, separated daughter cells (Miles, 1979; Alberts, 1983; Brachet, 1985; Levitan, 1988; Edlin, 1990; Therman, 1993).

THE NORMAL HUMAN CHROMOSOME COMPLEMENT

Before 1956, the number of human chromosomes was believed to be 48, and the XX-XY mechanism of sex determination was assumed to work in the same way as it does in the fruit fly, *Drosophila*. Both of these notions about human chromosomes were eventually proved wrong. The year 1956 is often given as the beginning of modern human cytogenetics; indeed, the discovery by Tjio and Levan in 1956 that the **human chromosome number is 46** (Fig. 4-15), and not 48, was the starting point for subsequent spectacular developments in human cytogenetics. Contemporary techniques (use of colchecine/colcemid, culture methodologies, hypotonic treatment) confirmed that normal human cells have 46 chromosomes, **two sex chromosomes** (X,X or X,Y) **and 44 autosomes.** These can be seen and classified in the metaphase stage of cell division.

In 1970, Caspersson and his colleagues applied fluorescence microscopy, which they had originally used to study plant chromosomes, to the analysis of the human karyotype. They discovered that the chromosomes consist of differentially fluorescent cross bands of various lengths. Careful study of these bands made possible the identification of all human chromosomes. This discovery was followed by a host of different **banding techniques.** The most commonly employed technique is **trypsin or G-banding** (see Fig. 4-15). Chromosome preparations are pretreated with trypsin before staining them with Giemsa stain (hence, Giemsa or G-banding). By means of such banding, **each chromosome (homologue) can be identified** by the resulting alternating light and dark band patterns specific to that particular chromosome. Another banding procedure, which gives only slightly different results, involves staining with a fluorescent dye, **quinacrine dihydrochloride,** which thus yields quinacrine or **Q-bands.** These bands fluoresce under ultraviolet light with varying degrees of brightness, similar to the light and dark bands produced by G-banding. The banding of elongated prophase or prometaphase chromosomes makes it possible to define chromosome segments and breakpoints even more accurately (Bergsma, 1972; Yunis, 1974; Hsu, 1979; Emery and Rimoin, 1983; Mange and Mange, 1990). The **C-banding technique** is used to highlight the constitutive chromatin region of the chromosomes, usually the centromeres and the long arm of chromosome Y. The chromosomal preparations are exposed to barium hydroxide–saturated solution and stained with Giemsa.

With the exception of the sex chromosomes X and Y,

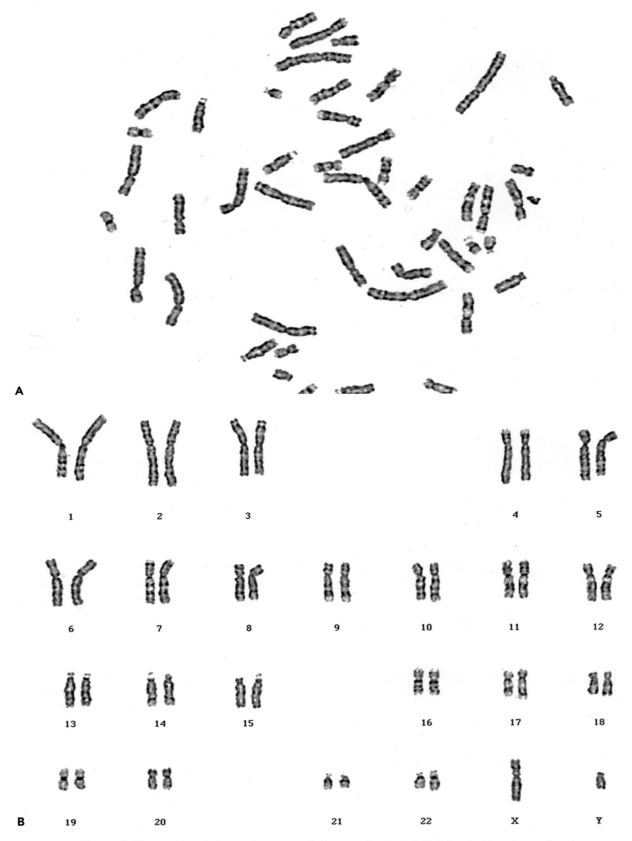

Figure 4-15   *A.* G-banded metaphase spread of a normal male cell. *B.* G-banded karyotype of a normal male cell showing the band characteristics of each pair of homologues, as well as of the sex chromosomes (X and Y).

the chromosomes occur in pairs, each pair composed of two identical chromosomes or **homologues** (from Greek, *homo* = same). Each pair of chromosomes has been numbered from 1 to 22 in order of length. The pairs are further divided into seven subgroups designated 1–3, 4–5, 6–12, 13–15, 16–18, 19–20, 21–22, or by letter A, B, C, D, E, F, and G, respectively (Fig. 4-16; see Fig. 4-15). The centromere, or primary constriction, is in a constant position on any given chromosome. In the terminology commonly employed for human chromosomes, the chromosome is *metacentric* **if the centromere is located at the center of the chromosome,** thus making both arms equal in length; **a chromosome is** *submetacentric* **if one arm is longer than the other; a chromosome is** *acrocentric* **(***acro* = **end) or** *subtelocentric* **if the centromere is located very close to the end of the short arm.**

The pairs of chromosomes at metaphase can be accurately classified into the **seven groups** by using the characteristics of length and centromere position. The two groups of acrocentric chromosomes, D (13–15) and G (21–22), for example, are easily identifiable, especially in colchicine-treated preparations. Colchicine prevents (among other effects) the centromere from dividing but does not interfere with chromatid separation. Thus, the acrocentrics remain joined at one end and come to resemble a wishbone or an old-fashioned clothespin. However, distinguishing chromosomes within groups was difficult and, sometimes impossible, until banding techniques were discovered.

Additions or deletions of portions of the chromosomes are designated by chromosome numbers and band numbers followed by p or q and + or − signs. In this manner, a precise identification of chromosomal segments, which are missing, added, or translocated can be achieved. Specialized nomenclature has been established to denote changes in chromosome number and structure (ISCN, 1995).

The ability to identify every chromosome by number has led to a slight change in the rule correlating number with chromosomal length. It has been found that the chromosome that accounts for Down's syndrome (see below) is, in fact, the shortest and not the next-to-shortest chromosome. However, to preserve the synonym **trisomy 21** for Down's syndrome, the shortest chromosome is designated as 21 and the next-shortest chromosome is designated as 22.

Certain other chromosomal features, although not of great importance in identifying particular homologues, may ultimately be of significance in the study of pathology. **The long and short acrocentrics** (13–15 and 21–22 groups) often exhibit a small structure on the short arms, called a **satellite.** Satellites, when well visualized, consist of short, thin filaments surmounted by a tiny mass of chromatin. Satellites are close to the limits of resolution, and they can rarely be observed on all the acrocentrics within one cell. Failure to demonstrate them is probably due to technical difficulties. It is known, though, that some individuals show very **conspicuous satellites,** although, once again, not on all of the acrocentrics; there has been no convincing evidence that these larger satellites are related to any disease state.

Individual or familial differences may also be observed in the **size and centromere position** of chromosomes in normal persons. Size differences were first clearly shown for the **Y chromosome** (Sandberg, 1985a, 1985b).

In addition to cytogenetic techniques for identifying individual chromosomes and their bands, sub-bands, and structures (Fig. 4-17), techniques have been developed recently for **identifying chromosomes based on unique DNA sequences within each chromosome.** This approach allows the recognition of specific chromosomes, or their parts, in interphase nuclei, thus dispensing with the more laborious process of metaphase preparation, or in situations when metaphases cannot be obtained. **Fluorescent in situ hybridization (FISH)** with molecular "paint" probes to specific chromosomes and their components has become an established laboratory technique (see Fig. 2-31). It allows the analysis of cells and tissues for the presence of chromosomal abnormalities. However, detailed karyotype analysis still requires optimal metaphases for their construction (Cannizzaro and Shi, 1997; Montgomery et al, 1997).

Heterochromatin

Another feature of chromosomes that shows familial differences, probably unrelated to disease, is the **secondary constriction.** (The **primary constriction** is at the centromere where the spindle fibers attach during mitosis; see earlier.) Readily visible in the microscope are secondary constrictions in the long arms near the centromere on chromosomes 1, 9, and 16. In normal cells, these constrictions are seen only occasionally and seldom in more than one homologue in a given cell. These constrictions are usually observed near centromeric sites on most chromosomes. At these sites, most chromosomes have small blocks of chromatin that replicate their DNA after the other chromosomal segments have completed DNA synthesis **(e.g., late-labeling DNA).** Such sites can also be selectively stained with the C-banding technique, centromeric heterochromatic stain (Fig. 4-18). In many species, such dark-staining, late-labeling segments are referred to as **heterochromatin.** In some species, these segments do not decondense in the interphase nucleus but rather remain as dark-staining masses of chromatin called **chromocenters.** In general, such **heterochromatin segments are genetically inert** (do not contain functioning genes and do not synthesize RNA). They are believed to have something to do with maintaining the structure of the chromosome; the material, therefore, is called **constitutive heterochromatin.** The latter is differentiated from **facultative heterochromatin,** which is condensed in some cells and not in others and, in contrast to constitutive heterochromatin, reflects some of the stable differences in genetic activity adopted by different cell types (e.g., embryonic cells seemingly contain very little, and some highly specialized cells contain a great deal of heterochromatin). Facultative heterochromatin is not known to contain the large number of highly repeated DNA sequences (satellite DNAs), which is characteristic of constitutive heterochromatin (Bahr, 1977; Lima-de-Faria, 1983; Therman, 1993). Although chromocenters (except for the sex chromatin body; see below) may vary in their appearance in the nuclei of human cells and, in some, they are difficult to visualize, only

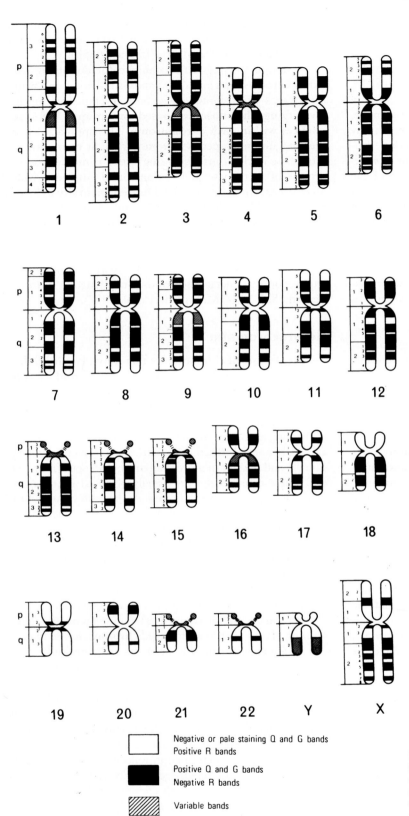

Figure 4-16 Ideogram illustrating Q- and G-bands in human chromosome complement. R-bands are the reverse of G-bands. The short arms of the chromosomes are designated as p and the long arms as q. (From Bergsma, D. [ed]. Paris Conference, 1971, Standardization of human cytogenetics. Birth Defects 8:7, 1972.)

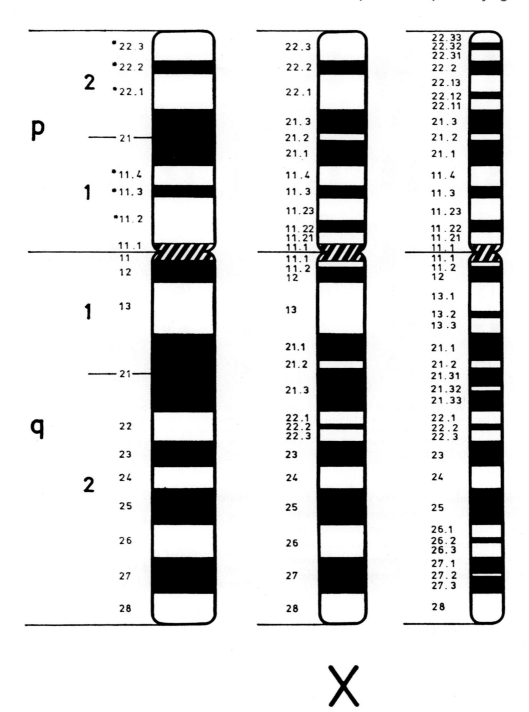

Figure 4-17 **Schematic presentation of the bands in the normal X chromosomes at different levels of staining resolution.** The X chromosome of the *left* has 17 bands besides the centromeric one, the one in the *middle* has 26 bands, and the one on the *right* has 38 bands. The use of special methodology allows the resolution of some bands into sub-bands (e.g., band Xq*23* into Xq*23.1* B *3*). (From ISCN. An international system for human cytogenetic nomenclature, Mitelman F (ed). Basel, Switzerland, S. Karger, 1995.)

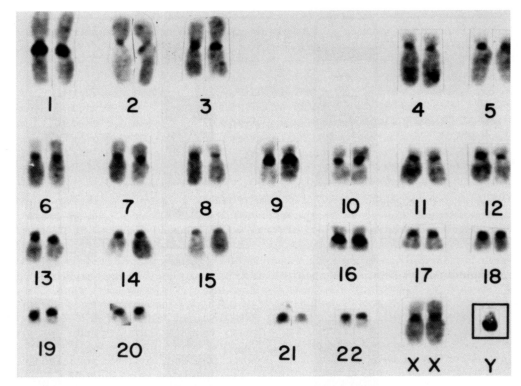

Figure 4-18   C-banded karyotype of a normal female cell, with constitutive heterochromatin of the various chromosomes staining dark. Note in particular the relatively large C-bands in chromosomes 1, 9, and 16, with each showing polymorphism of these bands. The *inset* shows a Y chromosome from a male cell demonstrating the dark staining of its long arms with this procedure. (Courtesy of Dr. Avery Sandberg.)

polymorphonuclear leukocytes are an exception. In the nuclear lobes of these cells, the constitutive heterochromatin of chromosome 1 and, perhaps other chromosomes, is observed as a **peripheral chromocenter.** With a somewhat similar technique, the C-band **heterochromatin of chromosome 9 can be identified in interphase nuclei of lymphocytes.**

GERM CELL FORMATION, MEIOSIS, AND SEX DETERMINATION

Germ Cell Formation

As has been stated, most human cells contain 46 chromosomes. The germ cells, sperm and ovum, constitute an important exception. Since the individual develops from the union of sperm and ovum, to preserve the proper somatic number of 46, these cells can have only 23 chromosomes each. Thus, the developing germ cell must lose half its chromosomes. The product of the union of the spermatozoon and the ovum, or the **zygote,** will then receive 23 chromosomes from the mother and 23 from the father. A type of cell division known as **meiosis** fulfills these requirements (Fig. 4-19).

It is clear that normal development will require that the zygote receive a set of similar chromosomes (e.g., one No. 1, one No. 2, and so on) from each parent. A set of 23 maternal or paternal chromosomes is a **haploid set,** and the final two sets of homologues form a **diploid set.**

Meiosis

The fundamental mechanism of meiosis serves to ensure that each germ cell acquires a precise set of 23 homologues, including **either an X or a Y chromosome.** Meiosis essentially consists of **two separate divisions, referred to as the first and the second meiotic divisions** (see Fig. 4-19).

First Meiotic Division

The prophase sequence of this division has been divided into several stages named **leptonema, zygonema, pachynema, diplonema,** and **diakinesis.** The chromosomes in **leptonema** (from Greek, *lepto* = thin and *nema* = thread) condense out as long convoluted threads. In **zygonema** (from Latin, *zygo* = pair), homologous chromosomes come together and pair, point for point, along their lengths. This process is called *synapsis of the homologues,* and the closely aligned synapsed pair is called a **bivalent.**

At the beginning of **pachynema** (from Greek, *pachy* = thick), pairing is complete, and the chromosomes become shorter and thicker. By this stage, each homologue may appear doubled into its two chromatids; hence, four units are seen, and the **bivalent** has become a **tetrad.** In diplonema (from Latin, *diplo* = double), the homologues begin to move away from one another, but they usually continue to remain joined at one or more points along their lengths. The involved segments near such points will resemble an X, or a cross, hence the name *chiasma* (plural, chiasmata) for such points.

In **diakinesis,** the tetrad continues to loosen, until at the

PROPHASE I

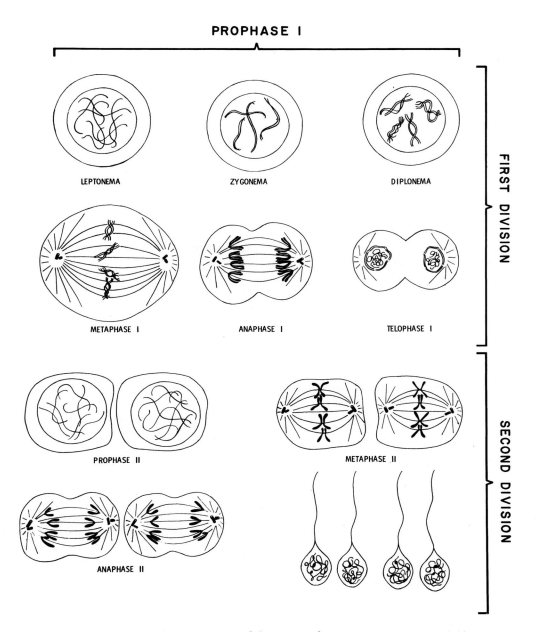

Figure 4-19   **Diagrammatic presentation of the stages of meiosis** (spermatogenesis). (Courtesy of Dr. C.P. Miles.)

first meiotic metaphase, the homologues separate completely and pass to opposite poles.

Crossover

The appearance of chiasmata is associated with **the reciprocal exchange of segments of homologous chromatids** that had tightly synapsed together in the earlier stage. Perhaps this process can be more readily grasped if we visualize the paternal homologue as a single column of soldiers that becomes aligned with a similar column, the homologue of maternal origin. If a few of the soldiers simply exchange places with an equal number from the opposite group, the composition of each column becomes completely different, but the general appearance of the column remains unchanged. In genetic terms, a crossover has occurred, and each column now represents a new combination of soldiers (Fig. 4-20).

Chromosomal segments cannot be exchanged quite so readily as soldiers in a column, since breaks in the chromosomes are probably necessary, and each break apparently prevents the occurrence of a similar break in the near vicinity. Consequently, the synapsed chromosomes seldom exchange more than one or two segments. Thus, the final germ cell does not necessarily receive unaltered paternal or maternal homologues. **Many of its chromosomes will consist of rejoined segments from both parents.** Although the behavior of the X chromosome in female meiosis is similar to that of the autosomes, the behavior of the X and Y in male meiosis is an exception to the rule. **The X and Y chromosomes in the developing spermatocyte do not synapse together** and, consequently, do not exchange segments by crossing over. Instead, the human X and Y chromosomes pair at the distal

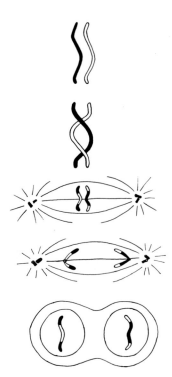

Figure 4-20 Schematic presentation of crossover of genetic material during first meiotic division. (Courtesy of Dr. C.P. Miles.)

ends of their short arms during male meiosis. There is formation of a synaptonemal complex between X and Y chromosomes in this region. Recent molecular studies have shown that there is DNA homology between X and Y chromosomes at their distal short arms, where there is a single obligatory crossing over between X and Y during meiosis. As a result, loci mapping in this region do not show strict sex linkage; accordingly, this homologous segment of the X and Y chromosomes is referred to as the **pseudoautosomal region** (Sandberg, 1983a).

Second Meiotic Division
The second meiotic division is much more akin to a somatic or mitotic division, with separation of the chromatids. All of the resulting daughter cells are haploid, that is, contain 23 chromosomes. As a result of crossing over in meiosis I, the genetic content of each haploid cell is a mixture of paternal and maternal genes.

Meiosis not only serves the fundamental need of reducing the chromosomal number of the germ cells but also constitutes a kind of lottery that vastly increases the possibilities for genetic variation. Not only does each germ cell draw at random one or the other homologue, but these homologues may themselves have already been altered through reciprocal exchange of segments. Meiosis is the principal reason for the enormous diversity, even among members of the same family (Roberts and Pembrey, 1985).

Sex Determination
The **sex chromosomes,** the male Y and the female X, differ from the **nonsex chromosomes or autosomes.**

Whereas the female has two X chromosomes, the male has only one X and one Y. During the process of meiosis, each germ cell ends up with a precise haploid set of autosomes. **In sperm, each haploid set will also include either an X or a Y** chromosome. Thus, by chance, roughly 50% of sperm will bear an X and 50% a Y. Since the mother has only one kind of sex chromosome, **all of the ova contain a single X.** If an ovum is fertilized by an X-bearing sperm, a female zygote will result (46,XX); if by a Y-bearing sperm, the offspring will be male (46,XY). Thus, it is the paternal chromosome that determines the sex of the child (Ohno et al, 1962; Miles, 1979; Levitan, 1988; Mange and Mange, 1990).

Chromosomal Nondisjunction

Mitosis and meiosis are not perfect mechanisms. Occasionally, homologous chromosomes or chromatids will fail to disjoin from one another (Fig. 4-21). This results in the two chromosomes migrating to the same pole rather than to different poles. This process is known as *nondisjunction.* **Numerical abnormalities** in the form of either additional or fewer chromosomes in the daughter cells **are a result of such chromosomal misdivisions.**

THE SEX CHROMATIN BODY AND ABNORMALITIES OF SEX CHROMOSOMES

In 1952, Barr and Bertram noticed that, in some neuronal nuclei of a cat's brain, a tiny dark granule migrated from the nucleolus to the nuclear membrane in the course of reaction to injury. These investigators noted that the dark granule appeared in some animals but not in others and, by checking their records, found that the tiny granule was found only in female and not in male cats. It was soon established that this difference extended to other tissues and to other mammals, including humans. The granule is now known as the **sex chromatin body** or as a **Barr body** and **represents a condensed X chromosome** (see Fig. 4-7A).

The significance of this finding for the study of abnormal sexual development was not lost on investigators who began to examine various types of patients with abnormalities of the sex chromatin body. One relatively common type is **Klinefelter's syndrome,** a condition in males that includes a slender body build, infertility, small testes, and, occasionally, gynecomastia. In cells of about 90% of such patients, a sex chromatin body was observed. It was thought initially that patients with Klinefelter's syndrome were genetic females. Subsequent cytogenetic analysis disclosed that most of these patients had a supernumerary sex chromosome, with a 47,XXY karyotype (Fig. 4-22).

The opposite situation was observed in patients with **Turner's syndrome or gonadal dysgenesis.** These patients are **females at birth** but have a poor development of secondary sex characteristics and fail to menstruate at puberty. Other stigmata of Turner's syndrome include a **webbed neck, a wide angle of the forearms, pigmented**

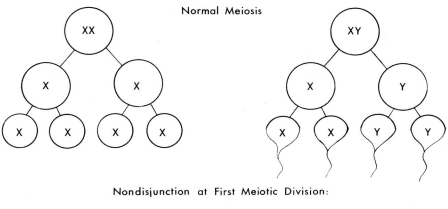

Normal Meiosis

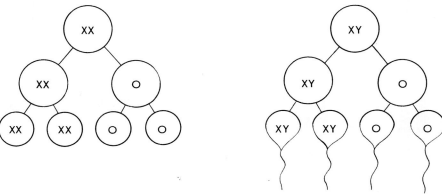

Nondisjunction at First Meiotic Division:

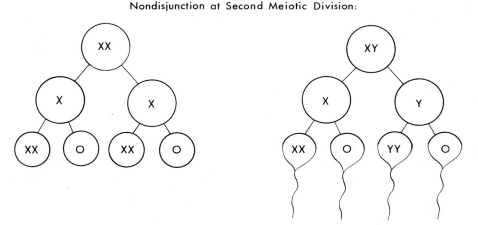

Nondisjunction at Second Meiotic Division:

Figure 4-21 The hypothetical mechanism that produces abnormal germ cells (ova and sperm). The diagrams are simplified by considering only sex chromosomes and by ignoring the production of polar bodies in oogenesis. (From Miles, CP. Human chromosome anomalies: Recent advances in human genetics. Stanford Med Bull 19:1–18, 1961.)

nevi, and coarctation of the aorta. In the cells of the presumed females with this syndrome, the sex chromatin body could not be found and the patients were thought to be genetic males. Cytogenetic analysis disclosed that the majority of **these patients lack one X chromosome** and that the **karyotype is 45,X** (see Chap. 8). In the remaining patients with this disorder, still **other chromosomal abnormalities may be observed.** Thus, some patient's cells may contain a normal X plus an X in which a part of the short or long arm has been deleted. In other cases, the abnormal X may contain, in lieu of the short arm, an additional long arm. **Such chromosomes**

with two identical homologous arms are called isochromosomes. Moreover, both in Turner's syndrome and in other cases of gonadal congenital abnormalities, the **chromosome complement may differ from cell to cell,** one cell line being (for example) normal 46,XX and another cell line with a 45,X complement, resulting in **mosaicism.** There are many more complex examples of mosaicism on record. The clinical appearance or phenotype of such patients varies markedly, but the complexities are too numerous to be discussed here. For further comments on Turner's syndrome and its recognition in cervico-vaginal smears, see Chapter 9.

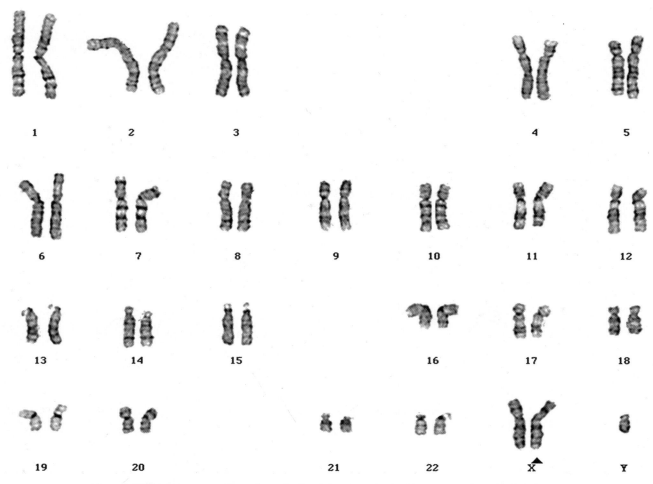

Figure 4-22 **Karyotype of a male with Klinefelter's syndrome or 47, XXY.** The arrowhead points to an additional X chromosome.

These and similar discoveries stimulated intensive analyses of patients with sexual maldevelopment. Moreover, with the knowledge that patients with Klinefelter's syndrome were occasionally somewhat mentally defective, surveys were conducted on patients in mental institutions and prisons. These surveys revealed, not only more cases of XXY, but also cases of XXXY and XXXXY. Such **male individuals with three and four X chromosomes tend to show a more severe mental deficiency** and may have skeletal and other abnormalities.

Women with three (Fig. 4-23), four, five, and even

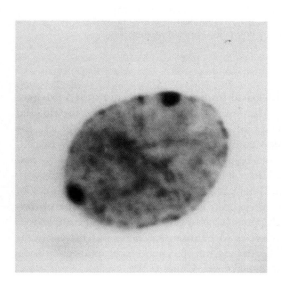

Figure 4-23 Nucleus from a female with a 46, XXX karyotype showing two sex chromatin or inactivated X chromosomes instead of the usual one present in normal (46,XX) females.

more X chromosomes have been described (Fig. 4-24). Those with three X chromosomes have been referred to as *superfemales* or allusion to a comparable situation in the fruit fly, *Drosophila*. However, the term, *super* refers strictly to the chromosomes, since in humans such **women are virtually normal.** Even with four X chromosomes, there may be only slight menstrual irregularities. There is some tendency to mental deficiency, however, and patients with five X chromosomes are usually severely retarded (Miles, 1961; Ohno et al, 1962; Moore, 1966; Sandberg, 1983a, 1983b, 1985a, 1985b; Schinzel, 1984; Mange and Mange, 1990).

With Q-staining, **the Y chromosome** is very **brightly fluorescent** and forms the so-called **Y-body** in interphase nuclei. Y-bodies can be demonstrated in a wide variety of cell types, including buccal mucosa, lymphocytes, and amnion cells. The most common anomaly of the Y chromosome is the XYY syndrome.

Origin of the Sex Chromatin Body

The finding of individuals with three or more X chromosomes has shed definitive light on the origin of the sex chromatin body. The cells of individuals with three X chromosomes have, at most, two sex chromatin bodies; individuals with four X chromosomes have at most three; and with five Xs, there are at most four sex chromatin bodies per cell. Thus, the maximum number of **sex chromatin bodies per cell is always one less than the number of X chromosomes.** This conforms to a theory proposing that the sex chromatin body consists of most, or all, of a single X chromosome. Since we know that, after the very early stage of sex determination in the fetus, only one X is necessary for normal development, it is plausible that the other or others become and remain condensed (fixed differentiation) in the somatic cells. The process of **random inactivation** of one of the X chromosomes, first postulated by Lyon, is called **lyonization,** and the af-

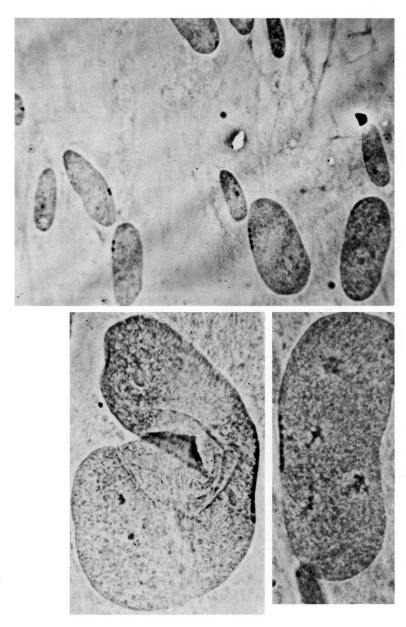

Figure 4-24   Female cells in tissue culture showing 2, 4, 8, and 16 sex chromatin bodies (tetraploid, octaploid, 16-, and 32-ploid cells). The sex chromatin bodies are concentrated in a single segment of the cell membrane. (From Miles CP. Prolonged culture of diploid human cells. Cancer Res 24:1070–1081, 1964.)

fected chromosome is presumed to be inert, not participating in the manufacture of RNA.

The chromatin that makes up the sex chromatin body is referred to as **facultative heterochromatin** as opposed to **constitutive heterochromatin** (see above), which occurs in large or small blocks near the centromeres of all chromosomes and which, so far as is known, is a permanent feature of the chromosome in all stages of development, including mitosis and meiosis. Facultative heterochromatin, on the other hand, appears in one or the other X chromosome, at random, in females at about the blastula stage.

Extra Sex Chromatin Bodies in Polyploid Cells

It may be worth pointing out that one may occasionally observe extra sex chromatin bodies in basically normal tissues. This is caused **by doubling of the entire chromosomal complement (tetraploidy).** Each X chromosome will be doubled, but the differentiation of the two Xs was previously fixed; hence, despite four X chromosomes, there will be only two, not three, sex chromatin bodies. Extreme degrees of **chromosomal duplication or polyploidy** may

occur by virtue of this doubling mechanism. It is also of note that extra sex chromatin bodies may be a useful guide in identifying cancer cells with abnormal chromosomal content. Thus, as discussed in Chapters 7, 12, and 29, finding an extra Barr body in a suspect cell supports the possibility that the cell is malignant.

ABNORMALITIES OF AUTOSOMES

Down's Syndrome (Trisomy 21)

Abnormalities involving sex chromosomes are neither the most common nor the most serious of chromosomal abnormalities. Of those that involve autosomes, the most important, at least in terms of incidence, is **Down's syndrome.** Down's syndrome is characterized **by severe mental retardation,** characteristic facial and other physical abnormalities, and is almost always related to an extra small acrocentric (G-group) chromosome 21, resulting in a karyotype with 47 chromosomes (Fig. 4-25).

In a small percentage of cases of Down's syndrome, the extra chromosome may become attached to another long acrocentric (D-group) chromosome. Less commonly, it may

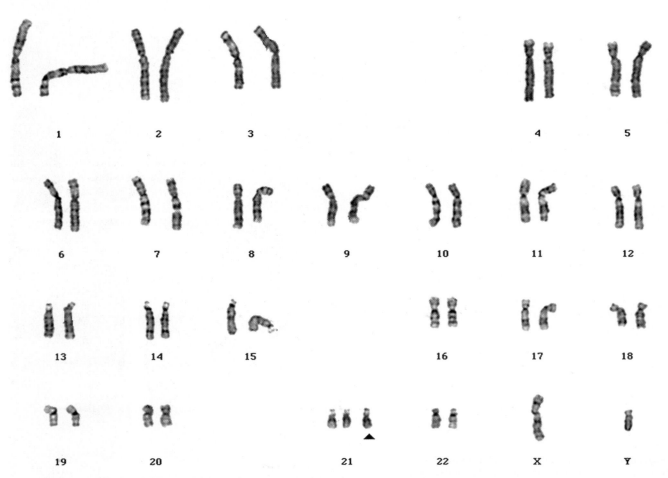

Figure 4-25 **Karyotype of a male with Down's syndrome or 47,XY, + 21.** The extra chromosome 21 is indicated by the arrowhead.

become attached to another G-group chromosome. **The attachment of one chromosome or a portion of one chromosome to another chromosome is referred to as a translocation,** and such cases are referred to as *translocation Down's syndrome.* The distinction is important since simple trisomy 21 occurs sporadically, although with an increased incidence in children of older mothers.

Translocation **Down's syndrome,** on the other hand, **often occurs in families** since the abnormal chromosome may be passed on from a parent to the offspring. Cases of Down's syndrome have also been described in which the karyotype appears normal. In some of these, however, there is suggestive evidence that a small portion of a G-group chromosome has been translocated; the segment is simply too small to be detected cytogenetically but can be detected with molecular techniques. A number of cases have been described that involve deletions or **total absence (monosomy) of a G-group chromosome.** These result in severe mental retardation and other abnormalities but are not so distinctive as Down's syndrome. Children with Down's syndrome have **an increased risk of leukemia, especially acute leukemia.**

Other Trisomy Syndromes

Patients with abnormalities involving other autosomes are less common, and the resultant abnormalities are more variable. An additional E group chromosome 18 results in **trisomy 18 or Edwards syndrome.** Such patients demonstrate abnormalities of the central nervous system and other quasi-specific features, such as low-set ears, small jaw, and flexion deformities of the limbs. These infants seldom survive beyond 1 year.

An additional D-group chromosome 13, is known as **trisomy 13 or Patau syndrome.** Patients demonstrate more severe congenital defects than trisomy 18 patients. Such infants are born with an underdeveloped brain and eyes, cleft palate, extra digits, and cardiac abnormalities. They seldom survive beyond a few weeks of life.

In both trisomy 13 and 18, the extra chromosomes may be translocated and fixed onto another homologue in the karyotype. With the newer banding techniques, trisomies have been reported involving chromosomes 8 and 9 or portions of chromosomes 7, 8, 9, and 10 **(partial trisomies)** and others. All of these involve severe mental retardation with a variety of other congenital abnormalities.

Chromosomal Deletion Syndromes

Total absence (monosomy) of **autosomes,** larger than those in the G group, is probably incompatible with fetal development to term. Loss of part of the short arm of **chromosome 5** results in the so-called **cat-cry (cri-du-chat) syndrome.** Apart from the unusual cry in infants, this syndrome does not have any of the characteristic clinical features typical for the trisomy syndromes 21, 13, and 18. These children, who are mentally deficient, may survive for some years. **Deletion of the short arm of chromosome 4** is less common and leads to more severe anomalies. Congenital abnormalities associated with deletions of various autosomes have been described. If

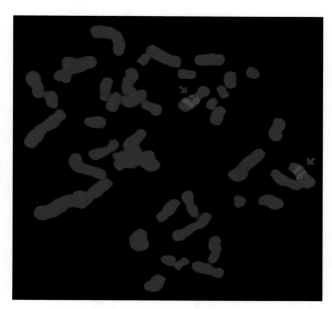

Figure 4-26 Metaphase spread of fluorescent in situ hybridization analysis of patient suspected of having Williams syndrome or deletion 7q11. The green signal on each chromosome is hybridization to a chromosome 7–specific sequence. The red signal on both chromosomes is the signal from the ELN gene probe. In this case, the patient did not contain the ELN gene deletion and did not have Williams syndrome.

portions of both the long and short arm of the same chromosome are deleted, **the ends may heal together and form a ring (ring chromosome)** with developmental abnormalities similar to those with simple deletions.

Microdeletion Syndromes

Detection of some deletions is beyond the resolution of standard cytogenetic analysis. The genes responsible for a specific syndrome such as **Williams syndrome** where the elastin (ELN) gene is deleted, are not resolvable at the cytogenetic level, even by high-resolution chromosome analyses. In such cases, **fluorescent in situ hybridization (FISH) analysis is performed with a probe, which contains the gene itself or a nearby gene to detect the missing gene** (Fig. 4-26). A number of microdeletions of specific chromosome regions have been described in association with several specific syndromes (Table 4-1). These syndromes can now

TABLE 4-1	
MICRODELETION SYNDROMES	
Prader-Willi	15q11–13
Angelman	15q11
Langer-Giedion	8q24
Miller-Dieker	17p13.3
DiGeorge/VCF	22q11
Rubenstein-Taybi	16p13
Williams	7q11
Retinoblastoma	13q14
Aniridia/Wilms	11p13

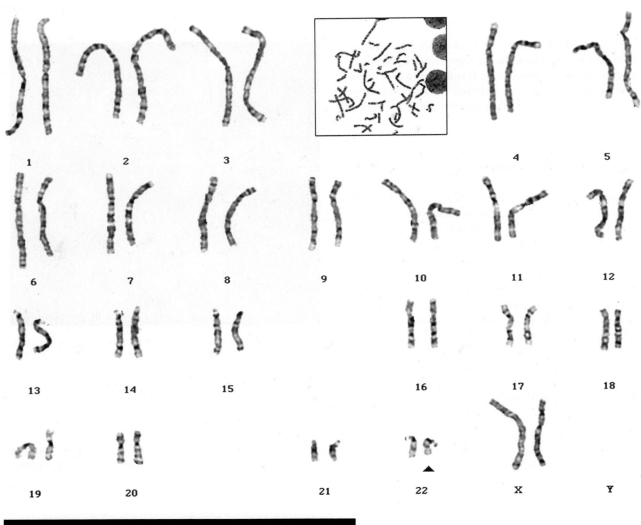

1   2   3   4   5

6   7   8   9   10   11   12

13   14   15   16   17   18

19   20   21   22   X   Y

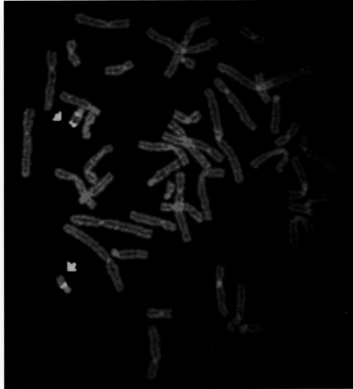

Figure 4-27   *Top.* High-resolution karyotype of female suspected of having Velo-cardio-facial (VCF) syndrome and carrying a deletion in the long arm of chromosome 22. The arrowhead points to the chromosome suspected of containing the deletion. *Bottom.* Metaphase spread after fluorescent in situ hybridization analysis with probe specific for the VCF region. Normal chromosome 22 contains two signals, and the deletion containing chromosome 22 shows just one fluorescent signal.

be diagnosed by FISH analysis with commercially available DNA probes, standardized and FDA approved for such purposes (Fig. 4-27).

Structural Chromosome Alterations

There are two major types of structural alterations, which can occur in chromosomes as a result of a breakage event: (1) that which involves **rearrangement within one chromosome** and (2) that which results from breakage and reunion events in **two or more chromosomes** (Miles, 1961; Daniel, 1988; Borgaonkar, 1989; Edlin, 1990). Unlike nondisjunction events, which result in loss or gain of select chromosomes, breakage can occur anywhere within a chromosome resulting in an unlimited number of rearrangements. Such events usually result in an unbalanced genetic complement, with some events more lethal than others. Breakage can either occur spontaneously or it can be induced by a mutagenic agent.

Breakage within a single chromosome can result in **duplications, deletions, inversions, isochromosomes, and ring formation.** In each case, the **breakpoint region** is the location of a break in a chromatid or a chromosome and is defined by the exact band involved. A **duplication** is a result of unequal crossing over or unequal sister chromatid exchange, which leads to duplication of a specific chromosome segment, oftentimes in association with deletion of another segment. A **deletion** is the loss of a chromosome segment where a break has occurred either within the chromosome arm (interstitial deletion) or at the end of the chromosome arm (terminal deletion).

An **inversion** results from two breaks occurring within the same chromosome. The segment between the breakpoint regions rotates 180°, and the broken ends fuse together. For example, a chromosome with the sequence AB-CDEF, if broken between B and C and between D and E, becomes ABDCEF after the inversion. Inversions may originate from either chromatid or chromosomal breaks. There are two types of inversions, **paracentric** where breaks occur on the same arm on one side of the centromere, in contrast with a **pericentric** inversion in which the breaks occur on both sides of the centromere. In a paracentric inversion, the intra-arm exchange may lead to no apparent altered morphology. In a pericentric inversion, if the breaks are equidistant from the centromere, no apparent change in morphology may occur; but when they are not of equal distance, an abnormal chromosome will result.

An **isochromosome** is a symmetric chromosome composed of duplicated long or short arms formed after misdivision of the centromere in a transverse plane. A **ring** chromosome is formed when breakage occurs simultaneously at two different points on the same chromosome. The resulting "sticky" ends then become rejoined together to form the ring. As a result of the formation of either an isochromosome or a ring, there usually is a significant loss of genetic material along with an associated abnormal clinical phenotype.

Rearrangements that involve more than one chromosome result in the occurrence of dicentrics, insertions, and translocations. A **dicentric** is a chromosome, which has **two centromeres** and is formed by breakage and reunion of two chromosomes. An **insertion** results from transfer of one chromosome's segment into another chromosome. This event involves two breaks in each of the involved chromosomes, and a segment of one chromosome is inserted into the site of breakage in the other.

A **translocation** occurs as a result of breakage followed by **transfer of chromosome material between the involved chromosomes.** There are two types of translocations: **reciprocal,** where there is an **even exchange of material between two different chromosomes,** and **Robertsonian,** when two acrocentrics fuse in the centromere region to **form a single chromosome.** Translocations and other chromosome alterations have a significant effect on the ability of the cell to undergo error-free cell division. Rearranged chromosome material, in the form of a translocation or inversion, will increase the likelihood of acquiring an unbalanced gamete. During the cell division process of translocation chromosomes, loops are formed by homologous segments resulting in partial monosomy or trisomy for the involved regions. In addition, studies of patients with **mental retardation** show an increased frequency **of reciprocal chromosome translocations.** These findings show that there is an increased potential for loss or gain of genetic material, which would ultimately show a phenotypically detrimental effect, usually in the form of mental/growth retardation of the offspring. Similar observations have not been reported for Robertsonian translocations.

CHROMOSOMES AND HUMAN CANCER

Cancer is a genetic disease of cells caused by DNA damage, often occurring after exposure to an environmental trauma. Such damage is expressed as perturbations in the expression of genes, which control a variety of cellular processes. Cytogenetic analyses demonstrated that some tumor types might have well-defined chromosome changes. Consistency of such changes in association with clinical data may provide diagnostic and prognostic information regarding the tumors' developmental stage and the potential for progression. Detection of a specific chromosome alteration prior to, during, and subsequent to chemotherapy or radiation treatment, is a quantitative measurement, which has been successfully used to determine the efficacy of a specific therapeutic regimen in some malignant diseases. The breakpoint regions involved in consistent cancer-related chromosome alterations have provided important clues as to where the **cancer-associated genes** are located, and the **nature of their protein products.** Drugs, specifically directed at these products, have now been developed.

The most accurate genetic information pertains to leukemias, lymphomas, related hematologic disorders, and some tumors of childhood. For most solid human cancers, including nearly all carcinomas, the information on the sequence of genetic events leading from precancerous lesions to invasive cancer is still fragmentary. The proposed sequence of genetic events in progression of colonic polyps to carcinomas is discussed in Chapter 7. There is hope that the determination of the human genetic code, discussed in Chapter 3 and the opening pages of this chapter, may lead to further progress, but it is likely that the road will be long and tedious.

Chromosomal Changes

Primary Chromosomal Changes

First recognized by Nowell and Hungerford (1960), the most consistent primary chromosomal change in human neoplasia is the **Philadelphia chromosome (Ph +),** which is diagnostic of chronic myelogenous leukemia (CML) (Fig. 4-28). This is a translocation in which a segment of the long arm of chromosome 22 is attached to the long arm of chromosome 9 (Nowell and Hungerford, 1960; Rowley, 1973; Groffen et al, 1984). This rearrangement or **translocation** is an excellent example of a chromosome alteration that characterizes a specific disease and which has been explored at the molecular level and has led to a remarkable development of an anticancer drug (see below). With advances in chromosomal banding techniques, it became possible to identify not only the exact chromosomes involved in the karyotypic changes but also subchromosomal segments.

When leukemia or a solid tumor is consistently characterized by one karyotypic anomaly, be it numerical or morphologic, this is considered **a primary or specific cytogenetic event characterizing this disease.** Unfortunately, in common solid tumors, particularly carcinomas, it is very rare to observe a single cytogenetic event. Hence, a series of such tumors must be studied to ascertain whether a change recurs with sufficient frequency to qualify as the primary event. This technique has been used in formulating the possible sequence of events in colonic cancer (Vogelstein and Kinzer, 1998; also see Chapter 7). For most human carcinomas, such a recurrent change has not been convincingly established. It is possible that the primary event in these tumors is submicroscopic, requiring molecular approaches to determine its nature.

Is the primary cytogenetic change causally related to neoplasia? In Ph-positive CML and in some lymphomas, the answer appears to be in the affirmative. In some types of leukemia, there is suggestive evidence that the primary chromosomal abnormalities are the first event leading to the onset of disease. In these conditions, known genes are modified in their structure or activity, with resulting formation of

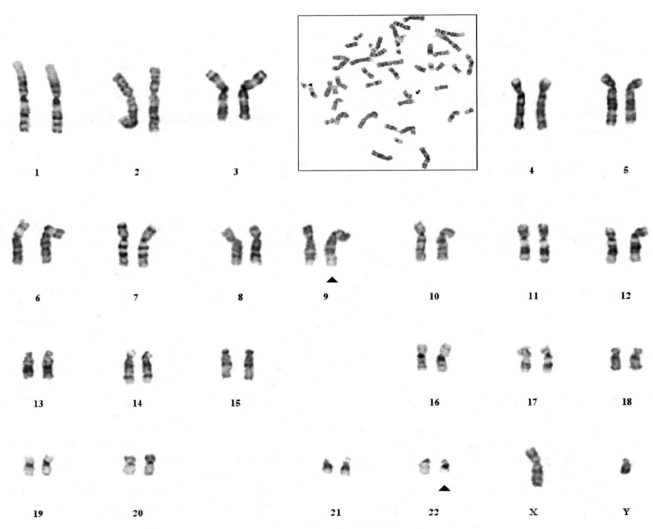

Figure 4-28 Karyotype of a male diagnosed with Philadelphia chromosome positive (PH +) chronic myelogenous leukemia (CML) showing the classic t(9;22)(q34;q11.2) chromosome rearrangement (*arrowheads*). Note the shortened chromosome 22, first observed by Nowell and Hungerford in 1960.

abnormal gene products (Knudson, 1986). The reorientation of genes from differing chromosome regions most often results in an **abnormal fusion product.** For example, the abnormality of the **bcr-abl** oncogene may be **the first** manifestation of chronic myelogenous leukemia (see below) whereas, in Burkitt's lymphoma, **a translocation of segments between chromosomes 8 and 14 results in activation of the** *myc* **oncogene** (Sheer, 1997) (see also below).

Still, the possibility exists that the primary karyotypic change reflects prior events at the molecular level, necessary for the specific chromosomal change to occur (Cannizzaro, 1991; Cahill, 1999). In most leukemias and lymphomas in which the primary chromosomal change has been established, the underlying molecular events have not yet been demonstrated because the abnormalities usually involve large segments of DNA that contain numerous genes. The identification of single genes is not possible until appropriate molecular probes become available. This problem is even greater in conditions in which entire chromosomes are involved, for example, an extra chromosome 8 in leukemia, an extra chromosome 7 in bladder cancer, or a missing chromosome 7 in secondary leukemia. Thus, the deciphering of the molecular basis of most leukemias, lymphomas, or solid tumors is still far off, even if the primary karyotypic change is known. At the same time, it must be stressed that the primary chromosomal change can serve as an important guide to the gene(s) involved. For this reason, it is crucial to rigorously establish the primary changes in as many tumors as possible.

The presence of primary chromosomal changes in **benign tumors** does not indicate that a malignant transformation will occur. This is true whether the primary changes consist of translocations (**e.g., t[3;12] in lipomas or t[12;14] in uterine leiomyomas**), deletions (**e.g., 22q- in meningioma**), or **loss or gain of entire chromosomes (e.g., +8 in benign salivary gland tumors).** This suggests that the **primary chromosomal changes in benign tumors probably involve genes that are concerned with cellular proliferation but not with malignant transformation.** This may also apply to the secondary chromosomal changes, which may be quite complex in these tumors. Much remains to be established, particularly at the molecular level, in the genetics of benign tumors. Such information should go a long way toward increasing our understanding of the consequence of chromosomal abnormalities in various conditions.

Primary chromosomal changes have been determined in some carcinomas (e.g., 3p in **small-cell lung cancer** and in **renal adenocarcinoma**) (Kovacs et al, 1987; Sandberg, 1990; Heim and Mitelman, 1995). For most carcinomas, however, the primary chromosomal changes have not been established as yet. Because these tumors are characterized by numerous and complex chromosomal changes it is possible that the primary event is masked. The other strong possibility is that these tumors are associated with gene changes at the molecular level that are not discernible with currently used techniques (Mark, 1977; Sandberg, 1985; Mark and Dahlenfors, 1986; Sandberg, 1987; Heim and Mitelman, 1995; LeBeau and Rowley, 1995; Sheer, 1997; Vogelstein and Kinzler, 1998; Meltzer and Trent, 1998).

Secondary Chromosomal Changes

With the passage of time and the evolution of a malignant tumor, whether leukemia or solid cancer, secondary chromosomal abnormalities are often observed. In solid tumors, such changes are often complex and numerous. Except for known secondary changes occurring in some leukemias, such as i(17)q in chronic myelogenous leukemia (CML); +8 in acute leukemia (AL); −Y or −X in acute myelogenous leukemia (AML) with t(8;21), the **secondary chromosomal changes apparently follow a random pattern and invariably appear to be associated with the progression of disease** (Sandberg, 1986; Sandberg, 1990; Harrison et al, 1999). In other words, a leukemia or a solid tumor is at its lowest level of aggressive behavior when it is associated only with the primary karyotypic change. More aggressive behavior is associated with the acquisition of additional chromosomal abnormalities.

What is particularly challenging is the **wide range of secondary changes** that may be present in a tumor. In **extreme cases, the chromosome count can range from hypodiploidy to hypertetraploidy, and the karyotypes are different for each cell throughout this range.**

A rough idea of these abnormalities may be gained by measuring the DNA content of the tumor cell by image analysis or flow cytometry (see Chaps. 46 and 47). It is likely that the secondary chromosomal changes play a crucial role in the biology of a tumor, that is, invasiveness, metastatic spread, and drug responsiveness. The therapy-resistant cells may ultimately emerge as the dominant cell line in the tumor or leukemia. Thus, in designing successful therapy for various malignant conditions, the presence of additional complex chromosomal changes and their biologic consequences remains an important and difficult obstacle. Cytogeneticists and molecular biologists will ultimately have to come to grips with the nature, significance, and mechanisms responsible for these secondary changes. For example, in carcinomas of the breast, lung, colon, and prostate, the nature and significance of the secondary changes must be elucidated if progress is to be made in the control and cure of these cancers. For comments on specific cytogenetic abnormalities in various solid tumors, see specific chapters. There is some hope that the use of **microarray technology** will facilitate this investigation (Marx, 2000; also see below).

Leukemias

Because culturing lymphoblasts in vitro is easy, consistent chromosome changes have been found in association with specific types and developmental stages of leukemias and lymphomas. The appearance of a specific chromosome alteration, whether it is a **translocation, deletion, inversion, or amplification,** provides clues as to which genes are responsible for the pathogenesis and progression of the disease. This information has facilitated the production of **DNA probes** able to detect disease-specific alterations in both interphase and metaphase stages. Such probes are now being used routinely to provide an accurate diagnosis of a defined malignant condition and to establish which therapeutic regimens are the most effective.

Cytogenetics has made a greater impact on the diagnostic and clinical aspects of leukemias than on any other groups of diseases. Thus, it has been shown that acute leukemias, which in the past were thought to be a homogeneous group by criteria established by a French-American-British (FAB) consensus agreement that relied heavily on cellular morphology and immunology and, in fact, consisted of a **number of subgroups,** each characterized by a specific cytogenetic change (Tables 4-2 and 4-3).

As aforementioned, chronic myelogenous leukemia (CML) was the first disease to be characterized by a specific chromosomal change, the Philadelphia (Ph) chromosome. The Ph chromosome is diagnostic of the disease, although it may also be seen in some acute lymphocytic leukemia (ALL) and acute nonlymphocytic leukemia (ANLL) cases. The translocation breakpoint of the 9;22 rearrangement, which generates the Ph chromosome differs in CML and ALL, and involves different sequences at the molecular level for each of these diseases (Cannizzaro et al, 1985).

The appearance of secondary chromosomal changes in Ph-positive CML usually consist of additional Ph chromosomes; an i(17q), +8, or +19, heralds the onset of the blastic phase of this disease before clinical evidence is apparent. It is quite likely that additional variants of leukemias will be defined cytogenetically. Each year, a few new subentities are reported and additional classification of leukemias based on molecular analysis is probable.

Prognosis, Treatment, and Follow-Up

The cytogenetic findings in acute leukemias are an independent prognostic factor. Primary chromosomal changes appear to decide the behavior and prognosis. Additional quantitative and qualitative chromosomal changes are also of prognostic significance. The additional secondary karyotypic changes modify the prognosis, usually for the worse. Generally, the presence of cytogenetically normal cells improves the prognosis of acute leukemia and related disorders, such as myelodysplasia; the absence of normal cells worsens it. Also, the increasing complexity of the karyotypic picture **(major karyotypic abnormalities [MAKA] versus minor karyotypic abnormalities [MIKA])** increases the chances of a poor prognosis.

Cytogenetic analysis of bone marrow cells is an essential part of follow-up in acute leukemias. Thus, the presence of only a rare cell, with a primary chromosomal change demonstrated at the time of the original diagnosis, indicates

---

TABLE 4-2
RECURRING CHROMOSOME ABNORMALITIES IN MYELOID MALIGNANCIES

Disease	Chromosome Abnormality	Involved Genes*
CML	t(9;22)(q34;q11)	ABL-BCR
CML, blast phase	t(9;22) with +8, +Ph, +19, or i(17q)	ABL-BCR
AML-M2	t(8;21)(q22;q11)	ETO-AML1
APL-M3	t(15;17)(q22;q12)	PML-RARA
AMMoL-M4Eo	inv(16)(p13q22)	MYH11-CBFB
	t(16;16)(p13;q22)	
AMMoL-M4/AmoL-M5	t(9;11)(p22;q23)	AF9-MLL
	other t(11q23)	MLL
	del(11)(q23)	
AML	+8	
	+21	
	−7 or del(7q)	
	−5 or del(5q)	
	−Y	
	t(6;9)(p23;q34)	DEK-CAN
	t(3;3)(q21;q26) or	
	inv(3)(q21q26)	EVI1
	del(20q)	
	t(12p) or del(12p)	
Therapy-related AML	−7 or del(7q) and/or	
	−5 or del(5q)	
	t(11q23)	MLL
	der(1)t(1;7)(q10;p10)	

* Genes are listed in order of citation in karyotypes: e.g., for CML, ABL is at 9q34 and BCR is at 22q11.
AML-M2, acute myeloblastic leukemia with maturation; AMMoL, acute myelomonocytic leukemia; AMMoL-M4Eo, acute myelomonocytic leukemia with abnormal eosinophils; AmoL, acute monoblastic leukemia: AML, acute myeloid leukemia; APL-M3, M3V, hypergranular (M3) and microgranular (M3V) acute promyelocytic leukemia; CML, chronic myelogenous leukemia.
LeBeau MM, Rowley JD. Cytogenetics. In: Hematology, 5th ed. Beutler E, Lichtman MA, Coller B, Kipps TJ, eds. McGraw Hill, NY, 1995, pp 98–106.

TABLE 4-3

RECURRING CHROMOSOME ABNORMALITIES IN MALIGNANT LYMPHOID DISEASES

Disease	Chromosome Abnormality	Involved Genes*
Acute lymphoblastic leukemia		
Pre-B	t(1;19)(q23;p13)	PBX1-TCF3(E2A)
B(Sig+)	t(8;14)(q24;q32)	MYC-IGH
	t(2;8)(p12;q24)	IGK-MYC
B or B-myeloid	t(8;22)(q24;q11)	MYC-IGL
	t(9;22)(q34;q11)	ABL-BCR
	t(4;11)(q21;q23)	AF4-MLL
	hyperdiploidy (50–60 chromosomes)	
	del(9p),t(9p)	
T	del(12p),t(12p)	
	t(11;14)(p15;q11)	RBTN1-TCRA
	t(11;14)(p13;q11)	RBTN2-TCRA
	t(8;14)(q24;q11)	MYC-TCRA
	inv(14)(q11q31)	TCRA-IGH
Non-Hodgkins lymphoma		
B	t(8;14)(q24;q32)	MYC-IGH
	t(2;8)(p12;q24)	IGK-MYC
	t(8;22)(q24;q11)	MYC-IGL
	t(14;18)(q32;q21)	IGH-BCL2
	t(11;14)(q13;q32)	CCND1-IGH
T or B (Ki−1+)	t(2;5)(p23;q35)	
Chronic lymphocytic leukemia		
B	t(11;14)(q13;q32)	CCND1-IGH
	t(14;19)(q32;q13)	IGH-BCL3
	t(2;14)(p13;q32)	IGH
	t(14q)	
	+12	
	del(13)(q14)	
T	t(8;14)(q24;q11)	MYC-TCRA
	inv(14)(q11q32)	TCRA/D-IGH
	inv(14)(q11q32)	TCRA/D-TCL1
Multiple myeloma		
B	t(11;14)(q13;q32)	CCND1-IGH
	t(14q)	
Adult T-cell leukemia	t(14;14)(q11;q32)	TCRA-IGH
	inv(14)(q11q32)	TCRA/D-IGH
	+3	

* Genes are listed in order of citation in karyotype; e.g., for pre-B ALL, PBX1 is at 1q23 and TCF3 is at 19p13.
LeBeau MM, Rowley JD. Cytogenetics. In: Hematology, 5th ed. Beutler E, Lichtman MA, Coller B, Kipps TJ, eds.
McGraw Hill, NY, 1995, pp 98–106.

that a remission is not complete or that imminent relapse is likely to occur.

Molecular cytogenetics has now contributed to the therapy of chronic myelogenous leukemia. As has been discussed above, the principal abnormality, resulting in a Ph chromosome, is a translocation of segments of chromosomes 9 and 22. The product of this translocation is a protein known as **bcr-abl-tyrosine kinase.** Recently, an inhibitor of this kinase (Gleevec) has been developed and put to clinical use in treatment of chronic myelogenous leukemia with remarkable results (Druker et al, 2001a, 2001b; Mauro and Druker, 2001). Some patients responded to the drug with return to normal blood count

and disappearance of the leukemic process. The long-term effects of this drug are still unknown at the time of this writing (2004). Interestingly, the drug also appears to be effective in **gastrointestinal stromal tumors** (Joensuu et al, 2001) although these tumors do not express bcr-abl-tyrosine kinase (see Chap. 24).

It is now clear that the chromosomal changes in leukemia can be of critical value in the treatment of these diseases. With the accumulation of appropriate data suitable for analysis in other conditions, such as solid tumors, it is possible that the cytogenetic findings will provide another prognostic parameter in addition to the customary assessment of tumor grade and stage.

Bone Marrow Transplantation

Cytogenetic studies in bone marrow transplantation (BMT) can determine whether the cells in the bone marrow are of donor or host origin. This can be accomplished when the leukemic cells are characterized by a specific anomaly or when the sex of the donor and host differ. The finding of even an occasional abnormal cell following BMT strongly suggests that leukemic cells are still present in the host's marrow. **FISH analysis with DNA probes specific for an altered chromosome region or for a sex chromosome,** has proved valuable in rapid and accurate determination of the presence or absence of donor cells in BMT patients (Garcia-Isodoro et al, 1997; Tanaka et al, 1997; Korbling, 2002).

Lymphomas

The definition of karyotypic abnormalities in Burkitt's lymphoma (BL) in cytogenetic terms is a translocation between segments of chromosomes 8 and 14, that is, [t(8;14)(q23; q32)] is one of the milestones in cancer cytogenetics. The demonstration that some BL cases have variant translocations [e.g., t(2;8)(p12;q24) or t(8;22)(q24;q11)] is an example of the cytogenetic characterization of subtypes of this tumor (Zech et al, 1976). The **identification of the molecular events** associated with the cytogenetic changes in BL pertaining to various **immunoglobulin genes** and the **oncogene c-*myc*** constitutes one of the exciting developments in human neoplasia.

Subsequent to the description of chromosomal changes in BL, several specific changes were established for other types of lymphoma (see Table 4-3), of T-cell or B-cell origin. These changes were then correlated with corresponding molecular events, such as the changes in the various T-cell receptors and **bcl** genes. The chromosomal changes described in lymphomas have been correlated with their histology and immunophenotype, as well as with prognosis. Although progress in the cytogenetic aspects of lymphomas has not been as decisive as in leukemias (particularly of the acute variety), the introduction of a universally acceptable classification system of lymphomas by WHO contributed to a meaningful correlation with cytogenetic findings (see Chap. 31).

Solid Tumors

Hematopoietic neoplasms account for fewer than 10% of human cancers; the remaining cancers are solid tumors. Unfortunately, because of the difficulty in culturing in vitro, the cytogenetic analysis of solid tumors has not kept pace with cytogenetics of leukemias and lymphomas. Further, the presence of multiple clonal abnormalities in many solid tumors, observed in later developmental stages, makes it difficult to ascertain which chromosome alterations are responsible for the tumor's pathogenesis. Improvements in short-term culture techniques and chromosome banding methods, in conjunction with earlier diagnosis of tumors, have helped to overcome some of these difficulties.

Consistent chromosome alterations, which possibly represent primary changes of specific genome regions, have now been identified in some carcinomas, such as **breast,** **lung, kidney, prostate, and colon** (Table 4-4) (First International Workshop on Chromosomes in Solid Tumors, 1986; Second International Workshop on Chromosomes in Solid Tumors, 1987; Sandberg, 1990; Heim and Mitelman, 1995; Sheer, 1997; Meltzer and Trent, 1998). Such regions have been found to contain either **a tumor-suppressor gene or an oncogene,** which are believed to be involved in either the pathogenesis or progression of the tumor to malignant transformation. It has been shown in various tumors that the number of chromosome alterations reflects the number of mutations occurring at the molecular level. As the number of chromosome alterations increases, so does the malignant potential of the tumor, ultimately evolving into a disease less likely to have a good prognosis.

Advances in methodology have made possible the detailed examination of the karyotypes of several tumor types, such as some sarcomas, testicular and kidney cancers, and neuroblastoma (Sandberg, 1985, 1990). These advances have led to the description of a number of specific chromosomal changes in solid tumors, which have opened the door to more detailed molecular definition of the genes involved in the tumors' behavior and progression. As in leukemias, the combination of cytogenetic and molecular analysis is likely to lead to a definition of subtypes within existing tumor groups. These may influence the diagnosis, classification, development of therapeutic approaches, and prognostic aspects of these tumors. An example of the impact of genetics on solid tumors is the discovery of breast cancer genes 1 and 2 (BRCA1 and BRCA2) that, if mutated, put a woman at risk for the development of breast or ovarian cancer (Vogelstein and Kingler, 1998; also see Chaps. 16 and 29). Still further advances may be expected with molecular classification of disease processes or **genomics** (Golub et al, 1999; Dohner et al, 2000; Guttmacher and Collins, 2002).

Normal Karyotypes in Cancer

The presence of **normal diploid karyotypes** in preparations from leukemic cells or solid tumors has generally been assumed to be due to the presence of normal cells, although it cannot be ruled out with certainty that such cells are not cancerous or leukemic and may, in fact, have a submicroscopic genetic change not discernible with cytogenetic techniques. The normal cells in such preparations as bone marrow in leukemia may be of normoblastic, fibroblastic, or uninvolved leukocytic origin. In solid tumors, a similar situation may be encountered and, in all probability, the diploid cells are of fibroblastic (or other stromal cell) and/or leukocytic origin.

There is no doubt, however, that many cancer cells have a diploid DNA content, measured by flow cytometry and image analysis of cancer of the breast and other organs (summary in Koss et al, 1989; see also Chaps. 46 and 47).

At the molecular level, it is possible that a diploid cell is altered in some way. Such submicroscopic alterations can be detected by molecular techniques and are usually defined as **loss of heterozygosity (LOH).** LOH involves the removal or inactivation of a tumor suppressor gene and it can be brought about by various mechanisms (Knudson, 1986; Lewin,

TABLE 4-4
RECURRING CHROMOSOME ABNORMALITIES IN HUMAN SOLID TUMORS

Tumor Type	Primary Karyotype Abnormalities
Bladder	+7; del(10)(q22–q24); del(21)(q22)
Brain, rhabdoid tumor	−22
Breast (adenocarcinoma)	−17; i(1q); der(16)t(1;16)(q10;p10)
Colon (carcinoma)	+7; +20
Ewing's sarcoma	t(11;22)(q24;q12)
Giant cell tumors	+8
Glioma	+7; −10; −22; −X; +X; −Y
Kidney (renal cell)	del(3)(p14–p21); del(3)(p11–p14)
Liposarcoma	translocations of 12q13–q14
Liposarcoma (myxoid)	t(12;16)(q13;p11)
Lung (adenocarcinoma)	del(3)(p14p23); +7
Lung (small cell)	del(3)(p14p23); +7
Lung (squamous cell)	+7
Meningioma	−22; +22; −Y; del(22)(q11–q13)
Neuroblastoma	del(1)(q32–p36)
Ovarian carcinoma	+12; +7; +8; −X
Prostate	del(10)(q24); +7; −Y
Retinoblastoma	i(6p); del(13)(q14.1q14.1)
Rhabdomyosarcoma	t(2;13)(q37;q14);t(1;13)(p36;q14)
Synovial sarcoma	t(X;18)(p11;q11)
Testicular carcinoma	i(12p)
Thyroid (adenocarcinoma)	inv(10)(q11q21)
Uterus (adenocarcinoma)	+10
Wilms' tumor	del(11)(p13p13); del(11)(p15p15)

Meltzer PS, Trent JM: Chromosome rearrangements in human solid tumors. In: The genetic basis of human cancer, Vogelstein B, Kinzler KW, eds. McGraw Hill, NY, 1998.

1997). To document LOH, the tumor DNA is cut into segments of varying length by an endonuclease (see Chap. 3). The resulting DNA fragments are separated by gel electrophoresis, and the segment with a selected gene is marked by binding a labeled cDNA. Because of individual variability, the two DNA fragments containing the genes that are derived from maternal and paternal chromosomes will be of different lengths and will appear as two bands on the gel. If one gene is mutant and, therefore, fails to bind the cDNA, there will be only one band (hence, loss of heterogeneity; LOH).

ADVANCES IN GENETIC DIAGNOSTIC TECHNIQUES

The use of higher-resolution molecular cytogenetic techniques, such as **fluorescent in situ hybridization (FISH)** and **multicolor hybridization analysis (M-FISH/SKY),** have contributed enormously to the advancement of knowledge about the regions of the genome that are involved in the development and progression of genetic and malignant diseases. These techniques utilize **DNA probes and libraries to identify and position DNA sequences along the length of a chromosome** and require actively dividing cells. On the other hand, techniques such as **comparative genomic hybridization (CGH)** and **DNA hybridization arrays** require only DNA or RNA of the target cells or tissues and do not depend on cell division. Each of these techniques is discussed in further detail below.

Fluorescent In Situ Hybridization

Fluorescent in situ hybridization (FISH) is a molecular cytogenetic technique, which permits **direct visualization of a DNA sequence on a specific chromosome site.** DNA sequences ranging in size from <1 kb to several hundred megabases can be rapidly and accurately positioned at a specific chromosome site. The DNA probe is first labeled with an immunofluorescent compound such as biotin-11-dUTP or digoxigenin-11-dUTP, and is then **hybridized overnight either to metaphase chromosome or interphase preparations.** The resultant fluorescent signal where homologous sequences have joined together is detected under ultraviolet light with filters capable of resolving wavelengths specific to the fluorescent compound (Fox et al, 1995).

This technology has facilitated **the construction of a**

physical map of genome regions, which play a critical role in genetic or malignant disorders. As mentioned above, DNA probes are now commercially available and are designed to detect microdeletions such as the absence of the elastin (ELN) gene at chromosome region 7q11, associated with the appearance of **Williams syndrome.** Deletion of the ELN gene is not detectable by either standard- or high-resolution cytogenetic analysis, but is easily detected with fluorescent in situ hybridization. Commercial probes can detect the sequences that would be lost if the microdeletion event occurred, in addition to containing a probe, which would identify the chromosome itself, in this case a chromosome 7–specific sequence (see Fig. 4-26).

In addition to sequence-specific probes, probes have been constructed that are able to identify **whole chromosomes or chromosome arms.** Such **"painting" probes** are generated, either by flow sorting of select chromosomes or by microdissecting chromosome bands directly from a metaphase preparation. Painting probes have been used to identify and define **structural and numerical alterations of chromosomes in the metaphase and in the interphase stage** (see Fig. 2-31) (Ried et al, 1998; Koss, 1998; Ludecke et al, 1989).

Spectral Karyotyping and Multicolor FISH

Spectral karyotyping (SKY) and multicolor FISH (M-FISH) are adaptations of the FISH technology and are being used to identify unusual structural and numerical chromosome alterations, particularly in neoplastic diseases. This technology uses a combination of specialized filters along with at least five different immunofluorescent compounds that are combined in different proportions to produce a range of different colors, so that a specific color precisely and consistently identifies each chromosome. Multicolor/spectral karyotyping makes it possible to identify the origin of chromosome material, which produces a marker chromosome arising from a rearrangement of sequences from two or more differing chromosomes (Ried et al, 1997; Veldman et al, 1997; Chudoba et al, 1999; Hilgenfeld et al, 1999; Ning et al, 1999).

Chromosome Microdissection

This is another relatively new technique, which helps to define chromosome segments or marker chromosomes that are not identifiable by conventional cytogenetic techniques. A chromosome region of unknown identity is dissected out of a metaphase either manually, using a microdissecting needle, or with a laser. DNA is isolated from the micro dissected fragments, labeled with a fluorescent tag, and a **micro-FISH** probe is constructed. The resulting DNA probe will **hybridize to corresponding sequences on normal chromosomal metaphases** to identify the origin of the unknown segment. This technique has been successfully used to **identify the origin of marker chromosomes** in both genetic and malignant diseases (Ludecke et al, 1989; Cannizzaro, 1996; Cannizzaro, 1997). It has also proved useful in generating DNA probes directly from commonly altered genome regions in an effort to determine how and which genes are repositioned as a result of the alteration.

One of the most important uses of the FISH technology is the determination of a **gene's orientation in relation to another gene or group of genes** after either a translocation or an inversion (Shi and Cannizzaro, 1996; Cheng et al, 2001). A **gene placed in a new position as a result of a chromosome alteration will most likely produce an altered form of the gene product.** For example, as described, a translocation between the long arms of chromosomes 9 and 22, results in producing the **Ph chromosome,** and is diagnostic of chronic myelogenous leukemia (CML) (see Fig. 4-28). This 9;22 translocation results in fusing DNA sequences, **bcr** (breakpoint cluster region) from chromosome 22, and the protooncogene, **abl,** from chromosome 9, and produces an altered gene product **(bcr:abl).** Sequences from the two involved chromosomes are labeled with two different immunofluorescent compounds, one producing a green signal, and the other producing a red signal. Fusion of bcr:abl sequences from the two chromosomes can then be detected as a yellow signal produced by the overlapping red and green signals from each of the

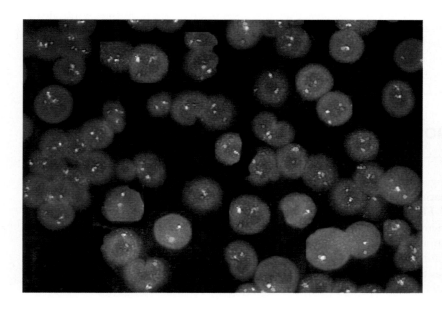

Figure 4-29 The Philadelphia chromosome results from a translocation t(9;22)(q34;q11.2) which fuses the c-abl proto-oncogene on chromosome 9 to the bcr (breakpoint cluster region) on chromosome 22. A probe detects the bcr/abl gene fusion (Philadelphia chromosome) in interphase cells. The bcr sequences are directly labeled with SpectrumGreen fluorophore and the abl sequences are directly labeled with SpectrumOrange fluorophore. Separated green and red signals indicate unrearranged chromosomes 22 and 9 respectively, while yellow signal indicates fusion of bcr/abl sequences. The majority of interphase cells show fusion signals and confirms diagnosis of patient with PH+ CML.

involved chromosomes (Fig. 4-29). This **translocation event is detectable in the interphase,** permitting a diagnosis even in those cases where the patient's cells are not dividing and, hence, do not form metaphases or have been subjected to chemotherapy or radiation therapy. Similar translocation or fusion products can now be detected and identified for several different malignant events because of consistency of the altered DNA sequences.

Comparative Genomic Hybridization

In recent years, the technique of comparative genomic hybridization (CGH) has been introduced. This technique can generate a genetic profile of a tumor cells' DNA in interphase. The signal advantage of this technique is that it **requires only a small amount of tumor DNA** (2 μg per experiment). The labeled tumor DNA is **hybridized with normal metaphases,** competing with a differently labeled tumor DNA of known makeup. The resulting hybridized metaphases **are analyzed by a computer program that determines gains or losses of individual chromosomes.** CGH studies of a variety of tumors have yielded a significant amount of new information regarding regions of the ge-

nome, which contain potential tumor suppressor genes or candidate tumor promoter genes. In many of these tumors, this technology has detected alterations in genome regions that had not been detected previously either by cytogenetic or molecular analysis (DuManoir et al, 1993; Ried et al, 1997).

Regions of the genome that are either under- or overrepresented in sequence copy number are easily identified as fluorescent red or green regions in comparison with the normal genome (Fig. 4-30). In certain tumors, such as lung, breast, ovary, and prostate, a significant amount of new information has been obtained to identify regions of the genome, which may contain potential oncogene or tumor suppressor loci (Kallioniemi et al, 1992; Houldsworth and Chaganti, 1994; Zitzelsberger et al, 1997).

As an example of this technique, Figure 4-31 shows the results of CGH applied to DNA samples of endometrial glands in atypical hyperplasia and endometrioid carcinoma (Baloglu et al, 2001). Gains in chromosome 1 and gains and losses in chromosomes 8 and 10 were the most frequent genetic abnormalities that were common to both processes, suggesting their similarity or identity (for further comments, see Chap. 14).

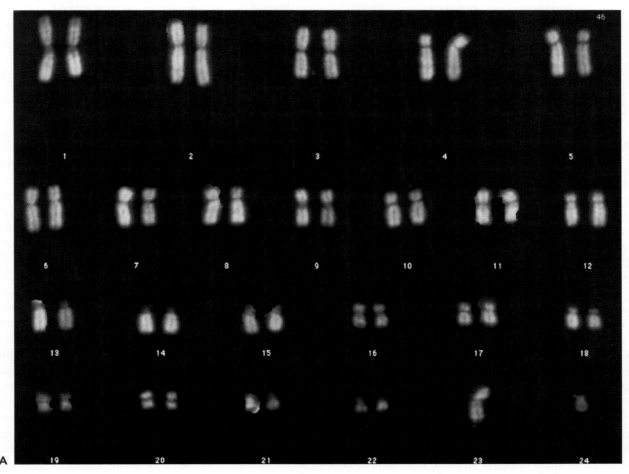

Figure 4-30 A. Karyotype produced from comparative genomic hybridization (CGH) analysis of an adenocarcinoma from a lung biopsy. Fluorescent **red signals** along several chromosome regions indicate areas of the genome, which are **underrepresented.** Fluorescent **green signals** along several chromosomes, especially chromosomes 1, 7, and 8 indicate areas of the genome, which are **overrepresented** in this tumor.

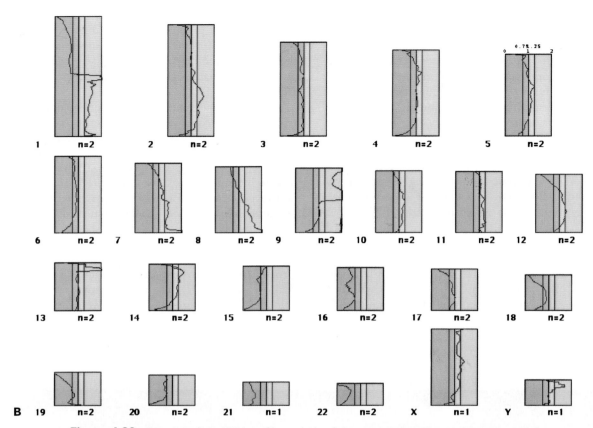

Figure 4-30 (*continued*) *B.* CGH profile analysis of the same tumor showing the ratios of the tumor DNA to the reference DNA. The critical values of DNA are represented by three vertical lines in the center of each map. The tracings either below or above the outer lines represent chromosomal gains (right) or losses (left), corresponding to the karyotype shown in *A*.

DNA Microarray

The emergence of a new technology known as **microarray analysis** has caused a surge in new information about which genes are involved in different forms of cancer. Previous to the initiation of the microarray system, each cancer was studied on a gene-by-gene basis, primarily using **Northern blot analysis or reverse transcriptase-PCR (RT-PCR)** analyses to determine the level of expression of a specific gene in a cancer. The microarray technology consists of a **slide or chip dotted with DNA from thousands of genes,** which can serve as probes for detecting which genes may be active in cancer cells from different types and stages of tumors. The **mRNA** is obtained from fresh tumor tissue and serves as a template to create the **corresponding cDNA.** The cDNA from cancer cells is given a red fluorescent label, while those from normal cells get a green label. Equal amounts of the two cDNAs are applied to the array; a red signal indicates higher expression of the gene in cancer cells, a green signal indicates higher expression of the gene in normal cells, while a yellow signal indicates an equal expression of that gene in both normal and cancer cells (Fig. 4-32). As a result, it is now possible to determine the level of expression of an enormous number of genes corresponding to a particular type and stage of cancer (Schena et al, 1995;

DeRisi et al, 1996; Shalon et al, 1996; Brown and Botstein, 1999; Freeman et al, 2000; Rosenwald et al, 2002; summary in Macosca, 2002).

The microarray analyses have been performed on some leukemias and some solid tumors. Preliminary studies of a series of patients with either AML or ALL show two distinct patterns of gene expression (Golub et al, 1999). Similar results were obtained in a subsequent study of patients with diffuse large-cell lymphoma, a common type of non-Hodgkin's lymphoma. In a study of 40 patients, the microarray gene expression profiles indicated the patients could be divided into two groups, with one group expressing genes turned on in B cells in the spleen and lymph nodes during an immune response, while the other group did not express these genes, but expressed a set of genes, which are stimulated to divide an antigen. The expression profiles also correlated well with prognosis of the two groups of patients, with the first group faring better than the second (Freeman et al, 2000). A recent study of breast cancer occurring in patients with either BCG1 or BCG2 mutations suggested some differences between these two groups of tumors do occur but their significance is unknown (Hedenfalk et al, 2001).

Microarray analyses are becoming an important tool to sort out the differences in different types and stages of can-

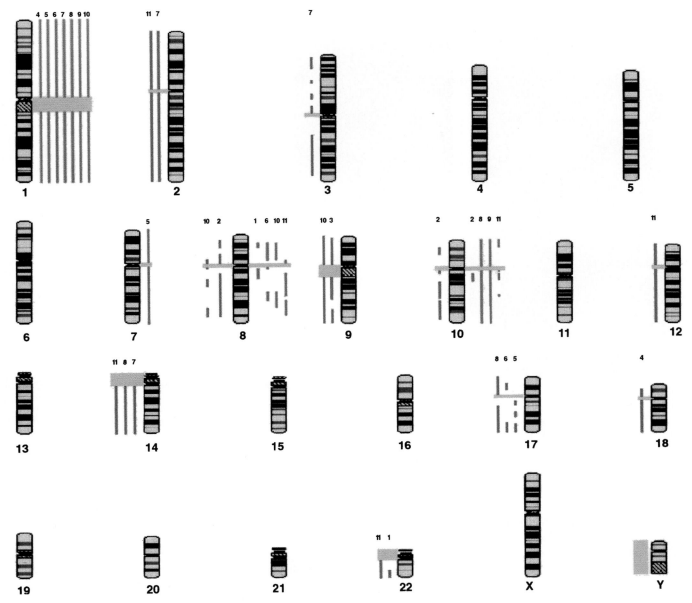

Figure 4-31   Synthetic profiles of comparative genomic hybridization (CGH) of atypical hyperplasias and endometrioid carcinomas, showing gains (green) and losses (red) in individual chromosomes. Yellow masks denote noninformative areas excluded from analysis. The case designation is by numbers on top of bars. Cases 1 to 5 are atypical endometrial hyperplasias with minimal (case 1), moderate (cases 2 and 3), and marked (cases 4 and 5) nuclear abnormalities. The remainder is cases of well-differentiated (low-grade) endometrioid carcinoma (cases 6, 7, 8, and 9), poorly differentiated (high-grade) endometrioid carcinoma (case 10), and the squamous component of a poorly differentiated carcinoma (case 11).

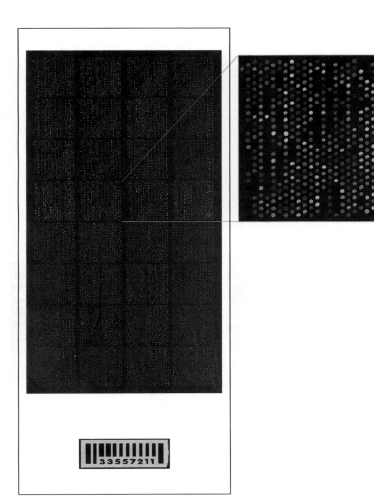

Figure 4-32 cDNA microarray analysis of squamous cell carcinoma of the head and neck region (HNSCC). RNA from HNSCC was compared to RNA from normal, adjacent epithelium. The array contains 27,323 cDNA clones. Red spots = overexpression in HNSCC; green spots = underexpression in HNSCC; yellow spots = equal expression in HNSCC and normal tissue; black = no expression in either sample. The interpretation of microarray results is difficult and time-consuming. (Courtesy of Drs. Thomas J. Belbin, Michael B. Prystowsky, and Geoffrey Childs, Albert Einstein College of Medicine and Montefiore Medical Center, Bronx, NY.)

cer; however, the **interpretation of findings is extremely difficult.** It is hoped that ultimately this information will help in the development of new drugs designed to influence specific target cells and, thus, will enhance the effectiveness of a therapeutic regimen.

APPENDIX

GLOSSARY OF CYTOGENETIC TERMS

p: short arm of a chromosome (from French, *petit*)

q: long arm of a chromosome (letter following p)

+: (plus sign): added chromosome (+8) or chromosomal segment (8q+)

−: (minus sign): lost (deleted) chromosome (−7) or chromosomal segment (5q−)

t: translocation (exchange) between chromosomes and chromosomal segments
Example: t(9;11)(q31;q21.1) = translocation involving breaks at band q31 on chromosome 9 and band q21.1 on chromosome 11

del: deletion, followed by chromosome number, arm (short = p, long = q) and, if known, band number.
Example: del(13q14) = deletion from chromosome 13 of band 14 located on the long arm of the chromosome (location of retinoblastoma gene)

i: isochromosome, followed by chromosome number and arm.
Example: i(5p), duplication of short arm of chromosome 5 (change observed in bladder cancer)

inv: inversion, upside-down position of a segment of a chromosome

BIBLIOGRAPHY

Alberts B, Bray D, Lewis J, et al. Molecular Biology of the Cell. New York, Garland Publishing, 1983.

Amon A. The spindle checkpoint. Curr Opin Genet Dev 9:69–75, 1999.

Bahr GF. Chromosomes and chromatin structure. *In* Yunis JJ (ed). Molecular Structure of Human Chromosomes. New York, Academic Press, 1977, pp 144–149.

Baloglu H, Cannizzaro LA, Jones J, Koss LG. Atypical endometrial hyperplasia shares genomic abnormalities with endometrioid carcinoma by comparative genomic hybridization. Hum Pathol 32:615–622, 2001.

Bergsma D (ed). Paris Conference (1971), Standardization in human cytogenetics. Birth Defects 8:7, 1972.

Borgaonkar DS. Chromosomal Variation in Man. A Catalog of Chromosomal Variants and Anomalies, 5th ed. New York, Alan R. Liss, 1989.

Brachet J. Molecular Cytology, vol 1. The Cell Cycle. Orlando, FL, Academic Press, 1985.

Brown PO, Botstein D. Exploring the new world of the genome with DNA microarrays. Nat Genet 21:33–37, 1999.

Cahill DP, Kinzler KW, Vogelstein B, Lengauer C. Genetic instability and darwinian selection in tumors. Trend Genet 15:M57–M60, 1999.

Cannizzaro LA. Special techniques in cytogenetics. In SR Wolman, S Sell (eds). Cytogenetic Markers of Human Cancer. Totowa, NJ, Humana Press, 1997, pp 461–477.

Cannizzaro LA. Chromosome microdissection: A brief overview. Cytogenet Cell Genet 74:157–160, 1996.

Cannizzaro LA. Gene mapping in cancer. Cancer Genet Cytogenet 55:139–147, 1991.

Cannizzaro LA, Nowell PC, Belasco JB, et al. The breakpoint in 22q11 in a case of Ph-positive acute lymphocytic leukemia interrupts the immunoglobulin light chain gene cluster. Cancer Genet Cytogenet 18:173–177, 1985.

Cannizzaro LA, Shi G. Fluorescent in situ hybridization (FISH) for DNA probes in the interphase and metaphase stages of the cell cycle. In Pollard JW, Walker JM (eds). Methods in Molecular Biology, Basic Cell Culture Protocols, vol 75. Totowa, NJ, Humana Press Inc, 1997.

Caron H, van Schaik B, van der Mee M, et al. The human transcriptome map: Clustering of highly expressed genes in chromosomal domains. Science 291:1289–1292, 2001.

Caspersson T, Zech L, Johansson C, Modest EJ. Identification of human chromosomes by DNA-binding fluorescent agents. Chromosoma 30:215–227, 1970.

Cerrutti L, Simonis V. Controlling the end of the cell cycle. Curr Op Genet Dev 10:65–69, 2000.

Cheng L, Ramesh KH, Wei D, et al. t(11;19) (q23;p.3.3) rearrangement in a patient with therapy related acute myeloid leukemia. Cancer Genet Cytogenet 129:17–22, 2001.

Chudoba I, Plesch A, Lorch T, et al. High-resolution multicolor-banding: A new technique for refined FISH analysis of human chromosomes. Cytogenet Cell Genet 84:156–160, 1999.

Daniel A (ed). The Cytogenetics of Mammalian Autosomal Rearrangements. New York, Alan R. Liss, 1988.

DeRisi J, Penland L, Brown PO, et al. Use of a cDNA microarray to analyse gene expression patterns in human cancer. Nat Genet 14:457–460, 1996.

Dohner H, Stilgenbauer S, Benner A, et al. Genomic aberrations and survival in chronic lymphocytic leukemia. N Engl J Med 343:1910–1916, 2000.

Druker BJ, Sawyers CL, Kantarjian H, et al. Activity of specific inhibitor of the BCR-ABL tyrosine kinase in the blast crisis of chronic myeloid leukemia and acute lymphoblastic leukemia with the Philadelphia chromosome. N Engl J Med 344:1038–1042, 2001.

Druker BJ, Talpaz M, Resta DJ, et al. Efficacy and safety of a specific inhibitor of the BCR-ABL tyrosine kinase in chronic myeloid leukemia. N Engl J Med 344:1031–1037, 2001.

Du Manoir S, Speicher MR, Joos S, et al. Detection of complete and partial chromosome gains and losses by comparative genomic in situ hybridization. Hum Genet 90:590–610, 1993.

DuPraw EJ. Evidence for a "folded-fibre" organization in human chromosomes. Nature 209:577–581, 1966.

Edlin G. Human Genetics. A Modern Synthesis. Boston, Jones and Bartlett Publishers, 1990.

Emery AEH, Rimoin DL (eds). Principles and Practice of Medical Genetics, vols 1 and 2. Edinburgh, Churchill Livingstone, 1983.

First International Workshop on Chromosomes in Solid Tumors. Cancer Genet Cytogenet 19:1–197, 1986.

Fox JL, Hsu PH, Legator MS, et al. Fluorescence in situ hybridization: Powerful molecular tool for cancer prognosis. Clin Chem 41:1554–1559, 1995.

Freeman WM, Robertson DJ, Vrana KE. Fundamentals of DNA hybridization arrays for gene expression analysis. Biotechniques 29:1042–1055, 2000.

Garcia-Isidoro M, Tabernero MD, Garcia JL, et al. Detection of the Mbcr/abl translocation in chronic myeloid leukemia by fluorescence in situ hybridization: Comparison with conventional cytogenetics and implications for minimal residual disease detection. Hum Pathol 28:154–159, 1997.

Gardner RD. The spindle checkpoint: Two transitions, two pathways. Trend Cell Biol 10:154–158, 2000.

Golub TR, Slonim DK, Tamayo P, et al. Molecular classification of cancer: Class discovery and class prediction by gene expression monitoring. Science 286:531–537, 1999.

Groffen J, Stephenson JR, Heistercamp N, et al. Philadelphia chromosomal breakpoints are clustered within a limited region, bcr, on chromosome 22. Cell 36:93–99, 1984.

Guttmacher AE, Collins FS. Genomic medicine—A primer. N Engl J Med 347:1512–1520, 2002.

Harrison CJ, Radford-Weiss I, Ross F, et al. Fluorescence in situ hybridization analysis of masked (8;21) (q22;q22) translocations. Cancer Genet Cytogenet 112:15–20, 1999.

Hedenfalk I, Duggan D, Chen Y, et al. Gene-expression profiles in hereditary breast cancer. N Engl J Med 344:539–548, 2001.

Heim S, Mitelman F. Cancer Cytogenetics, 2nd ed. New York, John Wiley & Sons, 1995.

Hilgenfeld E, Padilla-Nash H, Schrock E, Ried T. Analysis of B-cell neoplasias by spectral karyotyping (SKY). Curr Top Microbiol Immunol 246:169–174, 1999.

Hixon ML, Gualberto H. The Control of Mitosis. Front Biosci 5:50–57, 2000.

Houldsworth J, Chaganti RSK. Comparative genomic hybridization: An overview. Am J Pathol 145:1253–1260, 1994.

Hsu TC. Human and Mammalian Cytogenetics. An Historical Perspective. New York, Springer-Verlag, 1979.

International Human Genome Sequencing Consortium: Initial sequencing and analysis of the human genome. Nature 409:860–921, 2001.

ISCN. An international system for human cytogenetic nomenclature, Mitelman F (ed). Basel, Switzerland, S. Karger, 1995.

Joensuu H, Roberts PJ, Sarlomo-Rikala M, et al. Effect of tyrosine kinase inhibitor STI571 in a patient with a metastatic gastrointestinal stromal tumor. N Engl J Med 344:1052–1056, 2001.

Kallioniemi A, Kallioniemi O-P, Sudar D, et al. Comparative genomic hybridization for molecular cytogenetic analysis of solid tumors. Science 258:818–821, 1992.

Knudson AG Jr. Genetics of human cancer. Ann Rev Genet 20:231–251, 1986.

Korbling M, Katz RL, Khanna A, et al. Hepatocytes and epithelial cells of donor origin in recipients of peripheral-blood stem cells. N Engl J Med 346:738–746, 2002.

Koss LG. Characteristics of chromosomes in polarized normal human bronchial cells provide a blueprint for nuclear organization. Cytogenet Cell Genet 82:230–237, 1998.

Koss LG, Czerniak B, Herz F, Wersto RP. Flow cytometric measurements of DNA and other cell components in human tumors: A critical appraisal. Hum Pathol 20:528–548, 1989.

Kovacs G, Szäucs S, De Riese W, Baumgartel H. Specific chromosome aberration in human renal cell carcinoma. Int J Cancer 40:171–178, 1987.

LeBeau MM, Rowley JD. Cytogenetics. In Beutler E, Lichtman MA, Coller B, Kipps TJ (eds). Hematology, 5th ed. New York, McGraw Hill, 1995, pp 98–106.

Levitan M. Textbook of Human Genetics, 3rd ed. New York, Oxford University Press, 1988.

Lewin B. Genes VI. New York, Oxford University Press, 1997.

Li R, Murray AW. Feedback control of mitosis in budding yeast. Cell 66:519–531, 1991.

Lima-de-Faria A. Molecular Evolution and Organization of the Chromosome. Amsterdam, Elsevier, 1983.

Ludecke H-J, Senger G, Claussen U, Horsthemke B. Cloning defined regions of the human genome by microdissection of banded chromosomes and enzymatic amplification. Nature 338:348–350, 1989.

Macoska JA. The progressing clinical utility of DNA microarrays. CA Cancer J Clin 52:50–59, 2002.

Mange AP, Mange EJ. Genetics: Human Aspects, 2nd ed. Sunderland, Mass, Sinauer Associates, 1990.

Mark J. Chromosomal abnormalities and their specificity in human neoplasia: An assessment of recent observations by banding techniques. Adv Cancer Res 24:165–222, 1977.

Mark J, Dahlenfors R. Cytogenetical observations in 100 human benign pleomorphic adenomas: Specificity of the chromosomal aberrations and their relationship to sites of localized oncogenes. Anticancer Res 6:299–308, 1986.

Marx J. DNA arrays reveal cancer in its many forms. Science 289:1670–1672, 2000.

Mauro MJ, Druker BJ. Chronic myelogenous leukemia. Curr Opin Oncol 13:3–7, 2001.

Meltzer PS, Trent JM. Chromosome rearrangements in human solid tumors. In Vogelstein B, Kinzler KW (eds). The genetic basis of human cancer. New York, McGraw Hill, 1998.

Miles CP. The chromosomes and the mitotic cycle. In Koss LG. Diagnostic Cytology and Its Histopathologic Bases, 3rd ed. Philadelphia, JB Lippincott, 1979.

Miles CP. Chromatin elements, nuclear morphology and midbody in human mitosis. Acta Cytol 8:356–363, 1964.

Miles CP. Prolonged culture of diploid human cells. Cancer Res 24:1070–1081, 1964.

Miles CP. Human chromosome anomalies: Recent advances in human cytogenetics. Stanford Med Bull 19:1–18, 1961.

Montgomery KD, Keitges EA, Meynes J. Molecular cytogenetics: Definitions, clinical aspects, and protocols. In Barch MJ, Knudsen T, Purbeck J (eds). AGT Cytogenetics Laboratory Manual, 3rd ed. Philadelphia, Lippincott-Raven, 1997

Moore KL (ed). The Sex Chromatin. Philadelphia, WB Saunders, 1966.

Nagele R, Freeman T, McMorrow L, Lee H. Precise spatial positioning of chromosomes during prometaphase: Evidence for chromosomal order. Science 270:1831–1835, 1995.

Nicklas RB. How cells get the right chromosomes. Science 275:632–637, 1997.

Ning Y, Laundon CH, Schrock E, et al. Prenatal diagnosis of a mosaic extra structurally abnormal chromosome by spectral karyotyping. Prenat Diagn 19:480–482, 1999.

Nowell PC, Hungerford DA. A minute chromosome in human chronic granulocytic leukemia. Science 132:1497, 1960.

Ohno S, Klinger HP, Atkin NB. Human oogenesis. Cytogenet 1:42–51, 1962.

Peltonen L, McKusick VA. Dissecting human disease in the postgenomic era. Science 291:1224–1229, 2001.

Ried T, Liyanage M, du Manoir S, et al. Tumor cytogenetics revisited: Comparative genomic hybridization and spectral karyotyping. J Mol Med 75:801–814, 1997.

Ried T, Schrock E, Ning Y, Wienber J. Chromosome painting: A useful art. Hum Mol Genet 7:1619–1626, 1998.

Roberts JAF, Pembrey ME. An Introduction to Medical Genetics, 8th ed. Oxford, England, Oxford University Press, 1985.

Rosenwald A, Wright G, Chan WC, et al. The use of molecular profiling to predict survival after chemotherapy for diffuse large-B-cell lymphoma. N Engl J Med 346:1937–1947, 2002.

Rowley JD. A new consistent chromosomal abnormality in chronic myelogenous leukemia identified by quinacrine fluorescence and Giemsa staining. Nature 243:290–293, 1973.

Rudner AD, Murray AW. The spindle assembly checkpoint. Curr Op Cell Biol 8:773–780, 1996.

Sandberg AA. The Chromosomes in Human Cancer and Leukemia, 2nd ed. New York, Elsevier Science Publishing, 1990.

Sandberg AA. The usefulness of chromosome analysis in clinical oncology. Oncology 1:21–33, 1987.

Sandberg AA. Cytogenetics of the leukemias and lymphomas. *In* Luderer AA, Weetall HH (eds). The Human Oncogenic Viruses: Molecular Analysis and Diagnosis of Malignancy. Clifton, NJ, Humana Press, 1986, pp 1–41.

Sandberg AA (ed). The Y Chromosome. Part A. Basic Characteristics of the Y Chromosome. New York, Alan R. Liss, 1985a.

Sandberg AA (ed). The Y Chromosome. Part B. Clinical Aspects of Y Chromosome Abnormalities. New York, Alan R. Liss, 1985b.

Sandberg AA. Application of cytogenetics in neoplastic diseases. CRC Crit Rev Clin Lab Sci 22:219–274, 1985.

Sandberg AA (ed). Cytogenetics of the Mammalian X Chromosome. Part A. Basic Mechanisms of X Chromosome Behavior. New York, Alan R. Liss, 1983a.

Sandberg AA (ed). Cytogenetics of the Mammalian X Chromosome. Part B. X Chromosome Anomalies and Their Clinical Manifestations. New York, Alan R. Liss, 1983b.

Schena M, Shalon D, Davis RW, Brown PO. Quantitative monitoring of gene expression patterns with a complementary DNA microarray. Science 270:467–470, 1995.

Schinzel A. Catalogue of Unbalanced Chromosome Aberrations in Man. Berlin, Walter de Gruyter, 1984.

Second International Workshop on Chromosomes in Solid Tumors. Cancer Genet Cytogenet 28:1–54, 1987.

Shalon D, Smith SJ, Brown PO. A DNA microarray system for analyzing complex DNA samples using two-color fluorescent probe hybridization. Genome Res 6:639–645, 1996.

Sheer D. Chromosomes and cancer. *In* Cellular and Molecular Biology of Cancer, 3rd ed. Oxford, England, Oxford University Press, 1997.

Shi G, Cannizzaro LA. Mapping of 29 YAC clones and identification of 3 YACs spanning the translocation t(3;8) (p14.2;q24.1) breakpoint at 8q24.1 in hereditary renal cell carcinoma. Cytogenet Cell Genet 75:180–185, 1996.

Tanaka K, Arif M, Eguchi M, et al. Application of fluorescence in situ hybridization to detect residual leukemic cells with 9;22 and 15;17 translocations. Leukemia 11:436–440, 1997.

Therman E, Susman M. Human Chromosomes: Structure, Behavior, Effects, 3rd ed. New York, Springer-Verlag, 1993.

van Holde KE. Chromatin. New York, Springer-Verlag, 1989.

Veldman T, Vignon C, Schrock E, et al. Hidden chromosome abnormalities in hematological malignancies detected by multicolor spectral karyotyping. Nat Genet 15:406–410, 1997.

Venter JC, Adams MD, Myers PW, et al. The sequence of the human genome. Science 291:1304–1351, 2001.

Vogelstein B, Kinzler KW (eds). The Genetic Basis of Human Cancer. New York, McGraw Hill, 1998.

Yunis JJ (ed). Human Chromosome Methodology, 2nd ed. New York, Academic Press, 1974.

Zech L, Haglund V, Nilson N, Klein G. Characteristic chromosomal abnormalities in biopsies and lymphoid cell lines from patients with Burkitt and non-Burkitt lymphomas. Int J Cancer 17:47–56, 1976.

Zitzelsberger H, Lehmann L, Werner M, et al. Comparative genomic hybridization for the analysis of chromosomal imbalances in solid tumors and heamatological malignancies. Histochem Cell Biol 108:403–417, 1997.

Recognizing and Classifying Cells

Light microscopic examination of stained cells in smears is the method of choice of diagnostic cytology. It allows classification of most normal cells as to type and tissue of origin. It also allows the recognition of cell changes caused by disease processes, discussed in general terms in Chapters 6 and 7 and, more specifically, in subsequent chapters.

GENERAL GUIDELINES

The study of cells in smears should take place at several levels:

■ A rapid review of the smear with a 10× objective provides information on the makeup of the sample and its cell content. This preliminary review will tell the observer whether the smear is appropriately fixed and stained and will provide initial information on its composition. Smears containing only blood or no cells at all are usually considered inadequate, with some very rare exceptions.

■ If the smear contains cells other then blood cells, it should be examined with care. A careful review of the material or **screening of smears** with a 10× objective is usually required to identify abnormal cells that may be few in number. Screening is **mandatory** in cancer detection samples from "well" patients. A microscope stage should be utilized. The methods of screening are described in Chapter 44.

■ The screening of the smear should lead to the **preliminary assessment of the sample** and answer the following questions: (1) Does the cell population correspond to the organ of origin? (2) If the answer is positive, the next question pertains to the status of the cell population: (a) is it normal? (b) does it show nonspecific abnormalities of little consequence to the patient? or (c) Does it show abnormalities pertaining to a recognizable disease state that can be identified?

To answer these questions, fundamental principles of cell classification must be presented.

CELL CLASSIFICATION

An Overview of the Problem

In general, **the derivation, type of cells, and sometimes their function, are reflected in the cytoplasm,** whereas the **nucleus offers information on the status of the DNA,** which is of particular value in the diagnosis of cancer. Some cells that lack distinct cytoplasmic or nuclear features may be very difficult to classify. Nuclear and nucleolar changes in cancer are described in detail in Chapter 7.

Knowledge of the rudiments of histology is necessary for cell classification. For all practical purposes, the **cells encountered in cytologic samples are of epithelial and nonepithelial origin.** The most common cell types will be discussed here. Other cell types will be described as needed in appropriate chapters.

With the development of **monoclonal or polyclonal antibodies** to specific cell components, still further insights into cell derivation and function can be achieved by **immunocytochemistry.** An immunochemical analysis of the **components of the cell skeleton,** such as the intermediate filaments, of **cell products,** such as various hormones, and of immunologic features vested in the cell membrane, allows additional analysis and classification of cells (see Chap. 45).

An additional point must be made in reference to the **comparison of tissue sections and cells** of the same origin.

In **tissue sections, the cells** are often cut "on edge" and are **seen in profiles. In cytologic preparations, the cells are whole** and are generally flattened on a glass slide, usually affording a much better analysis of the cell components. A schematic comparison of histology and cytology is shown in Figure 5-1. A description of the principal tissue and cell types observed in diagnostic cytology is provided below.

Epithelial Cells

An epithelium **(plural: epithelia)** is a **tissue lining the surfaces of organs or forming glands and gland-like structures.** Similar epithelia may occur in various organs and organ systems. There are four principal groups of epithelia: (1) **squamous epithelia,** synonymous with protective function; (2) **glandular epithelia with secretory functions;** (3) **ciliated epithelia;** and (4) **the mesothelia.**

Squamous Epithelium

Histology

The squamous epithelium is a multilayered epithelium that lines the surfaces of organs that are in direct contact with the external environment. Two **subtypes** of this epithelium can be recognized: the **keratinizing type,** occurring in the **skin** and the **outer surface of the vulva** and the **nonkeratinizing type,** occurring in the **buccal cavity, cornea, pharynx, esophagus, vagina and the inner surface of the vulva,** and the **vaginal portio of the cervix.** The differences between the two subtypes of squamous epithelium reside in their mechanisms of maturation and formation of the superficial layers, discussed below.

Squamous epithelium is organized in **multiple layers.**

Starting at the bottom of the epithelium, resting on the lamina propria, to the top of the epithelium, facing the surface, four principal layers can be distinguished, although the separation of the layers is arbitrary. The bottom, **basal layer,** is composed of small cells. Immediately above are the **parabasal layers,** composed of two or three layers of somewhat larger cells, which blend with the next **intermediate layers,** composed of several layers of larger cells. The fourth **superficial layers** of the squamous epithelium are composed of a variable number of layers of the largest cells.

The epidermis of the skin is the prototype of squamous epithelium (Fig. 5-2). The features conferring special **strength** on this epithelium are **keratin filaments of high relative molecular mass,** and numerous **desmosomes,** cell junctions that are very difficult to disrupt (Fig. 5-3; see also Fig. 2-13).

The growth of the squamous epithelium is in the direction of the surface, that is, the **cells move from the basal layer, to parabasal layers, to intermediate layers, to superficial layers.** The most superficial cells are cast off. Under conditions of health, the small **cells of the basal layer** are the only cells in this type of epithelium that are **capable of mitosis.** It should be noted that the **cells of the basal layer have several different functions:** some anchor the epithelium to the basement lamina, some provide new basal cells to ensure the survival of the epithelium, and some produce cells that are destined to mature and thus form the bulk of the epithelium. **There are no morphologic differences among the basal cells with different functions.**

As the cells transit from the basal to the more superficial layers, they are programmed to **gradually increase the size**

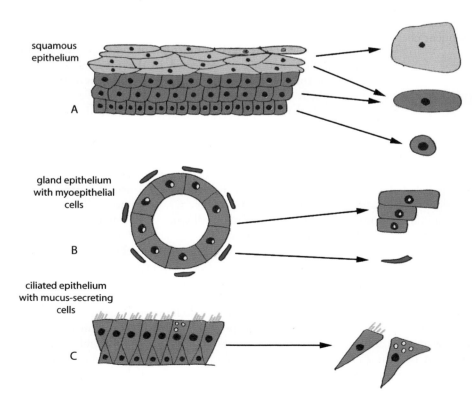

squamous
epithelium

A

gland epithelium
with myoepithelial
cells

B

ciliated epithelium
with mucus-secreting
cells

C

Figure 5-1 Comparison of histology and cytology of three common types of epithelia. *A.* Squamous epithelium. The cells are provided with a rigid skeleton of intermediate filaments; hence, they are resistant to injury. The cells vary in size and configuration, depending on the layer of origin. Cells from the superficial layer are large, with abundant cytoplasm and small nuclei. Cells from the intermediate and parabasal layers are smaller and have an open, spherical nuclei (vesicular nuclei). Cells from the basal layer are still smaller, but the nuclear structure is identical with that of parabasal cells. *B.* Glandular epithelium. These epithelia are usually quite fragile and are often injured, hence, poorly preserved. The cells may vary in size from cuboidal to columnar. Small contractile myoepithelial cells often accompany glandular cells. *C.* Ciliated epithelium with mucus-secreting cells. The ciliated cells are readily recognized because of the flat, cilia-bearing surface and a thing, tail-like opposite end. The mucus-producing cells (goblet cells) are of a similar configuration but have no cilia, and their cytoplasm is distended with mucus-containing vacuoles.

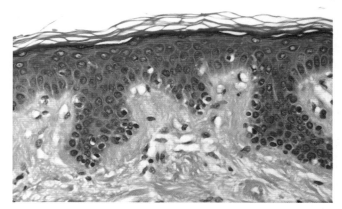

Figure 5-2   Histologic section of normal human skin as an example of squamous epithelium with protective function. Note the small cuboidal cells of the basal layer adjacent to connective tissue of the dermis (*bottom*). The surface is formed by several "basket-weave" layers of anucleated squames. The bulk of the epithelium is composed of intermediate cells. Scattered cells with clear cytoplasm are the Langerhans' cells, representing the immune system.

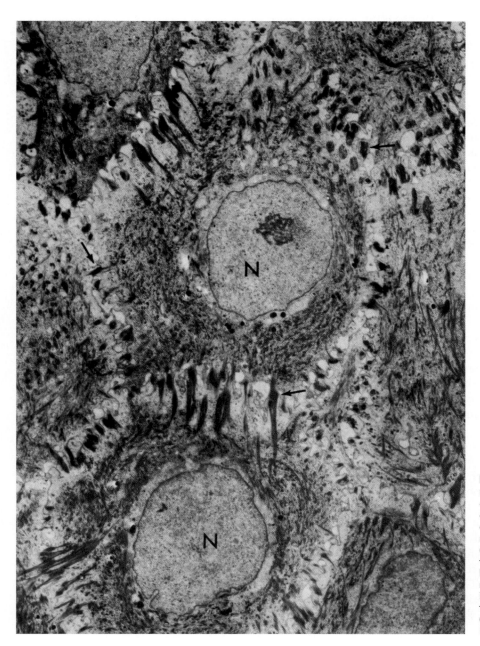

Figure 5-3   Electron micrograph of middle layer of human epidermis. The nuclei (N) are surrounded by a perinuclear clear zone free of filaments. The remaining cytoplasm shows an abundance of intermediate filaments forming aggregates (bundles) seen in longitudinal, oblique, or transverse section. Many of the filament bundles terminate on the numerous desmosomes, some identified by arrows. The integrity of the desmosomes accounts for the cohesion of this type of epithelium. (×18,000.) (Courtesy of the late Dr. Philip Prose, New York University, New York.)

of their cytoplasm. The increase in the size of the cytoplasm is accompanied by an increase in the intermediate keratin filaments of high relative molecular weight (see Fig. 2-27). As the cells progress through the stages of maturation, they are bound to each other by desmosomes, until they reach the superficial layer, where the desmosomes disintegrate to allow shedding of the most superficial cells. The process of **cytoplasmic maturation is accompanied by nuclear changes.** The nuclei of the basal, parabasal, and intermediate layers of squamous cells appears as spherical, **open (vesicular)** structures, measuring approximately 8 μm in diameter. As the cells transit from the intermediate to superficial layers, their nuclei **shrink and become condensed (nuclear pyknosis).**

The differences between the two subtypes of the squamous epithelium are evident in the superficial layers: in the **nonkeratinizing squamous epithelium,** the superficial cells are cast off, **while still retaining their nuclei** (see Chaps. 8 and 19). In the **keratinizing squamous epithelium,** such as the epidermis of the skin, the superficial cells continue to accumulate keratin filaments, which obliterate the nucleus until the cell becomes an anucleated, keratin-filled shell **(anucleated squames).** The anucleated squames of the epidermis form a superficial **horny layer,** which provides the best protection against injury (see Fig. 5-2).

Under abnormal circumstances, formation of a horny layer may also occur in nonkeratinizing squamous epithelia, resulting in white patches visible with the naked eye, and, therefore, known as **leukoplakia** (from Latin, *leukos* = white and *plax* = plaque). This condition may occur in the uterine cervix or the buccal cavity and is described in the appropriate chapters.

Squamous epithelia are also provided with cells with **immune function,** the **Langerhans' cells,** characterized by clear, transparent cytoplasm (see Fig. 5-2). These cells appear to mediate a broad variety of immunologic responses of the squamous epithelia to environmental and internal stimuli (summary in Robert and Kupper, 1999).

Cytology

Cells derived from squamous epithelia are usually quite resilient to manipulation and often retain their shape because of high keratin content. In general, these cells tend to be **flat, polygonal, and sharply demarcated,** and they **vary in size according to the layer of origin.** The smallest cells, measuring about 10 μm in diameter, are the **basal cells,** which are very rarely seen in normal states. **Parabasal cells,** derived from the parabasal layers, are somewhat larger, measuring from 10 to 15 μm in diameter. **Intermediate cells,** derived from the intermediate layers, are still larger, measuring from 15 to 40 μm in diameter. The **superficial cells** are the largest, measuring from 40 to 60 μm in diameter. The cells derived from the **basal, parabasal, and intermediate layers** show spherical nuclei, resembling open vesicles, with delicate chromatin, hence the term **vesicular nuclei,** measuring about 8 μm in diameter. The **superficial squamous cells** derived from non-keratinizing squamous epithelium, show small, **condensed, and dark nuclei** that are often encircled by a narrow clear cytoplasmic zone of

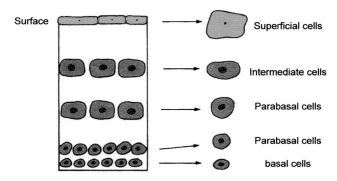

Figure 5-4 Diagrammatic representation of a squamous epithelium (other than epidermis of the skin), comparing the morphologic designation of cell types and their derivation from various epithelial layers.

contraction. Such nuclei are referred to as **pyknotic nuclei** (from Greek, *pyknos* = dense) (Figs. 5-4 and 5-5). **Anucleated squames,** derived from keratinizing squamous epithelium, appear as polygonal, transparent structures without visible nuclei. The **staining characteristics of the cytoplasm** in cytologic preparations presumably depends on the species of keratin filaments. The cytoplasm of the superficial cells is usually eosinophilic. The cytoplasm of cells from the lower cell layers is usually basophilic. These staining properties may be modified by exposure to air-drying, which often results in a tinctorial change from basophilic to eosinophilic.

Other Protective Epithelia

Variants of squamous epithelium, often highly specialized, may be observed in a variety of organ systems, for example, in the lower urinary tract and the larynx. The special features of these epithelia and the cells derived therefrom are described in the appropriate chapters.

Epithelia With Secretory Function

Histology

These epithelia are found mainly in organs with secretory functions and **exchanges with the external environment,**

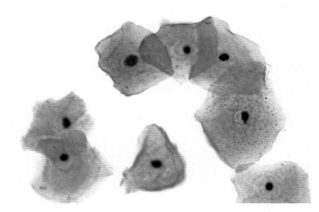

Figure 5-5 Mature squamous cells characterized by production of a large, resilient cytoplasmic surface. The condensed (pyknotic) nucleus is comparatively small. This cell type is eminently suited for the exercise of protective function. (Human buccal epithelium.)

such as food intake, **principally in the digestive tract and associated glands.** Similarly structured epithelia also occur in other locations, such as the male and female genital tracts. Secretory epithelia that **line the surfaces of organs,** such as the intestine and the endocervix, form **invaginations or crypts,** or may be organized in **glands** connected with the surface by **ducts.** Single cells of secretory type may also occur as a component of other epithelial types, for example, as **goblet cells** in the ciliated epithelium of the respiratory tract (see Fig. 5-1).

Secretory epithelia are usually made up of a **single layer of cuboidal or columnar cells with a clear or opaque cytoplasm and vesicular nuclei** (see Figs. 5-1 and 5-6). The nuclei are often located at the periphery of the cells, away from the lumen of the organ. The cytoplasm contains the products of cell secretion, such as mucus. The replacements for such epithelial cells are provided by small, intercalated **basal cells (reserve cells),** which, under circumstances not clearly defined, replace obsolete glandular cells. The third component of secretory epithelia **observed only in glands and ducts,** such as salivary glands and ducts, is a peripheral layer of elongated cells with contractile properties, known as the **myoepithelial cells** (see Fig. 5-1). The function of the myoepithelial cells is to propel the product of cell secretions into excretory ducts and beyond.

Ultrastructural features of secretory epithelia were discussed in Chapter 2. The cells are provided with a large **Golgi apparatus** wherein the synthesis of the products of secretion takes place. The superficial cells form **tight junctions** that protect the internal environment of such epithelia.

Cytology

When well preserved, the secretory cells are **cuboidal or columnar** in shape, averaging from 10 to 20 μm in length and 10 μm in width. Their **cytoplasm is transparent** because of accumulation of products of secretion, usually mucus (Fig. 5-7). The products of secretion are packaged in small cytoplasmic vacuoles. It is important to note that secretory cells are often **polarized,** that is, they display one flat surface facing the lumen of the organ. Through that

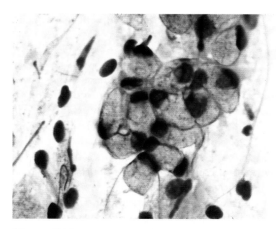

Figure 5-7 Mucus-secreting endocervical cells. The cytoplasm of these cells is filled with mucus, which remains unstained. The nuclei are pushed to the periphery. Compare with electron micrographs of somewhat similar cells (see Figs. 1-15 and 1-19). This is a good example of a glandular cell with the cytoplasmic features geared to excretory function.

surface, the cells products are discharged. The **nuclei** of the secretory cells are **open (vesicular),** averaging about 8 μm in diameter. The nuclei are either clear (transparent) or show moderate granularity, and are often provided with **small nucleoli.** The cytoplasm of cells derived from secretory epithelia is fragile and difficult to preserve. Thus, when these cells are removed from their site of origin, they often have poorly demarcated borders and their shape may be distorted. The cytoplasm of most secretory cells accepts pale basophilic stains.

The myoepithelial cells are seen **only in aspirated samples** and are recognized by their small, comma-shaped, dark nuclei, surrounded by a very narrow rim of cytoplasm (see Chap. 29).

Ciliated Epithelia

Histology

The ciliated epithelia are characterized by **columnar, rarely cuboidal cells with one ciliated surface** that is facing the lumen of the organ. Such cells occur mainly in the **respiratory tract,** where they line the bronchi (see Fig. 1-4 and Chap. 19) but may be also found in the **endocervix,** the **fallopian tube,** and the **endometrium** during the secretory phase. As an incidental finding, ciliated cells may be **occasionally observed in almost any secretory epithelium.** Very often, the ciliated cells are accompanied by secretory cells that produce mucus or related substances, for example, **goblet cells** in the respiratory tract (see Fig. 5-1). The ciliated epithelia are often **stratified,** that is, composed of several layers of cells but, as a rule, the cilia develop only on the superficial cells facing the lumen. Such epithelia also contain small, intercalated **basal cells or reserve cells,** which are the source of regeneration of the epithelial cells.

The **cilia** are mobile structures, normally moving in unison in a single direction. In the respiratory tract, the ciliated bronchial cells are covered with a layer of mucus, which is propelled by the cilia in a manner similar to a moving side-

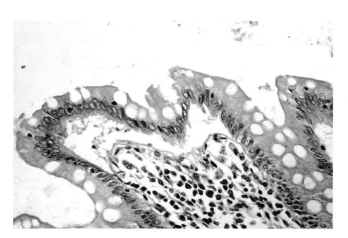

Figure 5-6 Columnar epithelium of normal human colon. Note the opaque columnar cells and very many clear goblet cells. (H & E.)

walk. Particles of dust or other inhaled foreign material are trapped in the mucus (see Chap. 19).

Cytology

The recognition of ciliated cells is easy. These cells are usually of **columnar,** less often of **cuboidal configuration,** and have **one flat surface** on which the cilia are readily visible under the microscope (see Figs. 1-4 and 5-1). The cilia are anchored in **basal corpuscles** that form a distinct dense layer **(terminal plate)** near the flat cell surface. If the cilia are destroyed, the presence of a flat cell surface provided with a terminal plate may be sufficient to recognize ciliated cells. Usually, the **cilia have a distinct eosinophilic appearance that differs from the usually basophilic cytoplasm.** The length and width of these cells vary. The ciliated cells of the respiratory tract measure about 20 to 25 μm in length and about 10 μm in diameter. Other ciliated cells may be smaller.

In the respiratory tract, the columnar cells usually show one flat, cilia-bearing surface and a comma-shaped, narrow cytoplasmic tail, representing the point of cell attachment to the epithelium (see Fig. 5-1 and Chap. 19). The clear or somewhat granular vesicular **nuclei,** measuring about 8 μm in diameter, are usually located closer to the narrow, whip-like end of the cells. In other organs, the ciliated cells may be of cuboidal configuration and have more centrally located nuclei of a similar type.

It is of importance to note here that ciliated cells **are very rarely observed in cancer.**

Mesothelia

Histology

Organs contained within body cavities, such as the lung, the heart, and the intestine, are all enclosed within protective sacs lined by specialized epithelia of mesodermal origin. These sacs, known as the **pericardium** for the heart, **pleural cavity** for the lungs, and **peritoneal cavity** for the intestine, are lined by an epithelium composed of a single layer of flat cells, known as **mesothelial cells.** The sacs are closed and, therefore, the epithelial layer is uninterrupted, lining all surfaces of the cavity (Fig. 5-8A). Under normal circumstances, the **sacs are filled with only a thin layer of fluid** that facilitates the gliding of the two surfaces of mesothelial

cells against each other (see Fig. 5-8B). It is the **function of the mesothelial cells to regulate the amount and composition of this fluid.** Therefore, the mesothelial cells are **osmotic pumps** provided with pinocytotic vesicles and microvilli on both flat surfaces.

Under abnormal circumstances, when the amount of fluid in the body cavity is increased (a condition known as **effusion**), the two opposing layers of the mesothelium separate, and the mesothelial cells may form a **multilayered epithelium** composed of larger, cuboidal cells (see Chap. 25).

Cytology

Upon removal from one of the body cavities, the cuboidal mesothelial cells may form sheets or clusters, in which the adjacent, flattened surfaces of the cells are separated from each other by clear gaps **("windows")** filled by microvilli (Fig. 5-8C). When these cells appear singly, they are usually spherical and measure about 20 μm in diameter. The **perinuclear portion of the cytoplasm of mesothelial cells is usually denser than the periphery** because of an accumulation of cytoplasmic organelles and filaments in the perinuclear location (see Chap. 25). The clear or faintly granular nuclei of mesothelial cells are usually spherical, measuring about 8 μm in diameter. Occasionally, tiny nucleoli can be observed.

Nonepithelial Cells

Endothelial Cells

Endothelial cells lining the intima of blood vessels have many similarities with mesothelial cells but are very rarely observed in diagnostic cytology, except in aspirated samples and in circulating blood (see Chaps. 28 and 43). These cells are best recognized in capillary vessels or as a layer of elongated cells surrounding sheets of epithelial cells. They may be immunostained with **clotting Factor VIII.**

Tissues With Highly Specialized Functions

There are numerous specialized types of tissues in the body. These are found, for example, in the **central nervous system;** in the **endocrine glands,** such as thyroid or the adrenal cortex; in highly specialized organs, such as the **kidney, liver, pancreas;** and in the **reproductive organs.** Their description can be found in appropriate chapters.

Supporting Systems

A complex multicellular organism cannot function without an appropriate **supporting apparatus** that includes structural support and a well-regulated **system of transport, communications, and defense.** Many of the supportive functions are vested in tissues such as the muscles, nerves, bone marrow and cells derived therefrom, which are described as needed in various chapters. However, the system of defense (immunity) is of interest in the context of this book. The fundamental significance of the **immune system** has received renewed emphasis within recent times when the **acquired immunodeficiency syndrome (AIDS)** be-

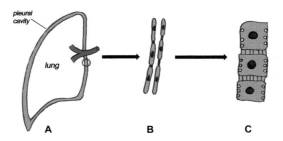

Figure 5-8 Diagrammatic representation of mesothelial sacs, using the pleural cavity as example. The cavity is actually a potential space between the two layers of pleura that enclose the lung (*A*). The *circled area* is shown in detail in a histologic cross section (*B*) and as a sheet of mesothelial cells in a cytologic preparation (*C*).

came widespread (see below). AIDS patients are unable to cope with a relatively low-grade malignant tumor (Kaposi's sarcoma), which becomes a highly aggressive neoplasm, and have low resistance to multiple infectious agents with resulting death. An understanding of the basic features of cells of the immune system in human cytology is sufficiently important to provide a brief summary of the salient facts.

The Immune Cell System

The basic concepts of the mechanism of resistance to diseases (immunity) were outlined by Metchnikoff at the turn of the 20th century. The recent years brought with them major progress in our understanding of the role that certain cellular elements play in immunity. A major review of the current understanding of the makeup and function of the immune system can be found in articles by Delves and Roitt (2000).

Immunology may be defined as the study of an organism's response to injury, particularly if the latter is due to foreign and harmful agents, for example, bacteria or viruses. **Immunity** is a natural or acquired state of resistance to diseases or disease agents, and it comprises all mechanisms that play a role in the identification, neutralization, and elimination of such agents. Although, in most instances, immunity has for its purpose the preservation of the host organism, certain immune processes may be injurious, not only to the disease agents but also to the host. Furthermore, the host may become immune to certain components of **self,** with resulting **autoimmune disorders** or diseases. **Loss of immunity** may be congenital **(primary)** or **secondary,** caused by pathologic events, such as HIV-1 infection in AIDS. For a review of primary immunodeficiencies, see Rosen et al, 1995.

Immunity has two broad components: cellular and humoral. Although both have the same purpose, namely, the protection of the host, their modes of action are different, even though they are dependent on each other. The **cell-mediated immunity,** vested primarily in T lymphocytes, is directed mainly against primary viral infections and against foreign tissues (such as transplants). **Humoral immunity,** vested primarily in B lymphocytes, acts primarily against bacterial infections. **Macrophages (histiocytes),** cells with phagocytic function, are the third family of cells involved in the function of the immune system. The activities of the **T and B lymphocytes** and of the macrophages are closely integrated by an intricate system of chemical **signals, known as lymphokines or cytokines.** The failure of one of the links in this complex interrelationship may result in severe clinical disorders, such as AIDS. A brief and highly simplified account of the basic cellular components of the immune system and their interaction is provided below.

The Lymphocytes

Until about 1970, the lymphocytes were thought to represent a single family of cells, recognized as small, spherical cells (about 8 μm in diameter), with an opaque, round nucleus, and a narrow rim of basophilic cytoplasm. Within the past 30 years, enormous progress has been made in subclassification of lymphocytes and in understanding their life cycle and function. There are two principal classes of lymphocytes: the B lymphocytes and the T lymphocytes.

B Lymphocytes

The family of B lymphocytes was first identified by immunocytochemistry. With labeled monoclonal **antibodies to immunoglobulins,** it could be verified, first by fluorescence technique and, subsequently, by the peroxidase-antiperoxidase technique that some, but not all, lymphocytes secreted immunoglobulins (Fig. 5-9). The immunoglobulin-secreting cells were first observed in chickens provided with a large perianal lymphoid organ, known as the **bursa of Fabricius** (Parson's nose). The bursa was shown to be the organ of origin of these cells; hence, they were named **B lymphocytes or B cells.** The B lymphocytes can also be characterized by several **clusters of differentiation** based on features of the cell membrane (see below).

The end stage of maturation of B cells is the **plasma cell,** known to be programmed to secrete one single type of immunoglobulin. The puzzle to be solved pertained to the mechanisms that enabled B cells to recognize, from the vast diversity of antigens, that one which would lead to the

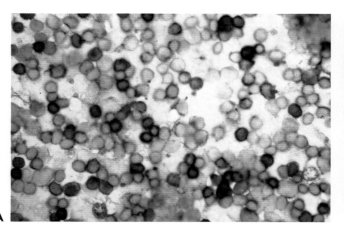
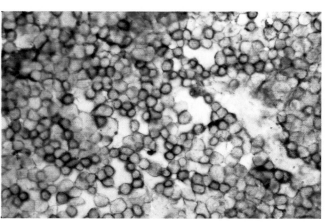

Figure 5-9   **Cytospin preparation of a lymphocyte suspension from a normal human tonsil,** using an anti-lambda (A) and anti-kappa (B) antibody and peroxidase-antiperoxidase stain. Cells expressing lambda- or kappa-light chains (dark periphery) are B lymphocytes.

formation of a specific immunoglobulin directed against this antigen.

Immunoglobulins are composed of four protein chains: two **heavy chains** and two **light chains,** the latter designated as **kappa (κ)** and **lambda (λ)** (see Chap. 45). Each one of the four chains has a **constant component,** common to all immunoglobulins, and a **variable region** that reflects the specificity of the molecule. The variable region of the light chains is the "recognition region," capable of identifying one of a broad variety of antigens.

In humans, the B cells originate in the bone marrow **from stem cells,** common to all hematopoietic cells. The cells develop by a series of fairly well-defined stages, prior to their release into general circulation, from which they populate primarily the **lymphoid organs** (e.g., the lymph nodes and the spleen). The most important development in the understanding of B cells was the mechanism of their immunologic diversity. Tonegawa (1983) proposed that, during the development of the B cells, a series of **gene rearrangements** occurs, resulting in many thousands of diverse B cells, each with the specific capability of recognizing a different antibody. The genes, known as **D** (diversity), **J** (joining), and **V** (variable region) for the heavy chains and **V** and **J** for the light chains, are located on several chromosomes: chromosome 14 (encoding the heavy chains), chromosome 2 (encoding the **κ** -light chains), and chromosome 22 (encoding the **λ**-light chains). It could be documented that there are several D and J genes and several hundred V genes, for both the heavy and the light chains. It is clear that this diversity of genes allows an almost astronomical number of variations in the programming of a B cell, each containing one VDJ gene combination for the heavy chain and a VJ combination for the light chain. **Each B cell is programmed to produce one antibody, which is expressed on the surface of the cell** (review in Stavnezer, 2000).

The principal groups of antibodies belong to several groups of immunoglobulins, each with a different immunologic advantage. The **IgM** antibodies stimulate phagocytosis and bacterial killing; **IgG** antibodies stimulate phagocytosis; **IgA** antibodies protect mucous membranes against invaders; **IgE** antibodies play a role in the elimination of parasites by activating eosinophils leading to release of histamine.

This diversity of B cells enables them to recognize most antigens that they may encounter; if the "fit" of the antibody is not perfect, a further somatic mutation may occur in the B cells, searching for a perfect fit. Once a correct antigen-antibody match is found, the B cell (with the help of specialized T cells) may reproduce itself in its own image and create a clone of cells directed against the specific antigen. Mission accomplished, the B cells will die, with the exception of a few **"memory cells"** that may persist and be called into action again if the same invader (antigen) threatens the system.

The various stages of B lymphocyte maturation in the bone marrow have also been recognized, because each is fairly accurately characterized by morphologic and immunologic changes. The recognition of the maturation stages of the B cell is the basis for contemporary classification of

malignant proliferation of lymphocytes, such as leukemias or malignant lymphomas (see below and Chap. 31).

Plasma Cells

Plasma cells are the end stage of the development of B cells and are **major providers of specific immunoglobulins.** Normal plasma cells are somewhat larger than lymphocytes and are morphologically readily recognized because of their eccentric nucleus with a spoke-like arrangement of chromatin (Fig. 5-10). The cytoplasm contains an accumulation of immunoglobulins that may form eosinophilic granules or **Russel's bodies.** As is consistent with their secretory status, the plasma cells contain abundant rough endoplasmic reticulum, as seen in electron microscopy (see Chap. 2).

Malignant tumors composed of plasma cells are known as *myelomas* or *plasmacytomas.*

T Lymphocytes

The group of lymphocytes, known as T lymphocytes, was first recognized as a relatively small subset of lymphocytes (about 10% to 30%) that failed to react with antibodies to immunoglobulins characterizing B cells (see above). Subsequently, it was documented that this group of lymphocytes was derived from the **thymus;** hence, their designation as **T lymphocytes or T cells.** The next characteristic identified in T cells was their ability to form rosettes with sheep erythrocytes (Fig. 5-11), which documented that they also possess surface receptors, albeit different from those of B cells.

The T cells were also shown to be capable of **mitotic activity and proliferation in vitro,** when stimulated by plant-derived substances known as *lectins.* The lectins commonly used for this purpose are phytohemagglutinin, pokeweed agglutinin, and concanavalin A. **Stimulated resting T lym-**

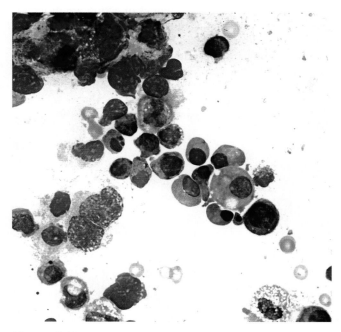

Figure 5-10   Plasma cells in ascetic fluid (case of multiple myeloma). Note the characteristic eccentric position of the nuclei. May Grunwald Giesma stain, OM ×160.

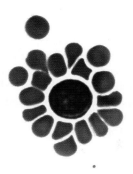

Figure 5-11 Human T lymphocyte surrounded by a rosette of sheep erythrocytes. (Oil immersion.)

phocytes convert to lymphoblasts, large cells with large nuclei, often containing one or more visible nucleoli.

Subsequent work showed that there are several **subtypes of T cells.** The gene rearrangements, described for B cells, also occur in T cells. The subtypes of T cells can be identified by antibodies to their membrane receptors (epitopes), known as **clusters of differentiation (CD)** (see below). The two most important subtypes are the **helper-inducer group,** also known as the **CD4 or T4 lymphocytes,** and the **suppressor-cytotoxic group,** also known as the **CD8 or T8 lymphocytes** (see Table 5-1). The cytotoxic cells are capable of destruction of foreign tissue and virus-infected cells. A third important group of T lymphocytes is the **"natural killer cells" (NK cells).**

The T lymphocytes are also capable of recognizing molecules belonging to the bearer (the so-called **human leukocyte antigen or major histocompatibility complex [HLA]**) and, thereby, are essential in prevention of immunologic response to "self." For a major review of the HLA system, see Klein and Sato, 2000.

The principal role for the T lymphocytes in the immune system is **coordination of the activities of the entire immune system** by means of substances known as **lymphokines, cytokines,** or **interleukins.** These substances can **stimulate the growth of the bone marrow cells (hemopoietic colony-stimulating factor), stimulate macrophages, and control the maturation of B lymphocytes.** Severe damage to a subset of T lymphocytes may produce a major defect in the immune response of patients. As mentioned above, the **destruction of the T4 (helper-inducer group) by the human immunodeficiency virus type I (HIV-1) leads to AIDS.** Robert and Kupper (1999) summarized the current state of knowledge of T cells.

Recognition of various types and subtypes of lymphocytes has led to the contemporary classification of **malignant lymphomas,** discussed in Chapter 31.

The Cluster of Differentiation (CD) System

Research into the diversity of lymphocytes has led to the discovery of numerous **antibodies to various stages of lymphocyte development** and function. These antibodies correspond to **clusters of differentiation (CD), epitopes (re-**

ceptors) found on the membranes of these cells. The CDs are numbered and have various degrees of specificity. There are more than 1,000 different antibodies to well over 100 CDs. Some of the antibodies were mentioned above: the CD 4 antibody recognizing the "helper" T cells and CD 8 recognizing the "suppressor" T cells. It is beyond the scope of this chapter and this book to list all of the CDs available today. A few of the most commonly used CDs in cytologic preparations are listed in Table 5-1. It is particularly important to recognize that different laboratories may use differently numbered CDs for the same purpose, which, in most cases, reduces itself to two questions: **(1) Is the cell population of lymphocytic origin? and (2) If the answer to the first question is positive, what is the precise characterization of the disorder?** The significance of this approach is of value in diagnostic cytology of poorly differentiated tumors and in classification of malignant lymphomas and leukemias. The reader is referred to appended references and to Chapters 31 and 45 that describes the value of these antibodies in practice of diagnostic cytology.

The Macrophages (Histiocytes)

In 1924, Aschoff described the **reticuloendothelial system** as a variety of cell types occurring in many organs that participate in body defenses by **phagocytosis.** The cells of the **reticuloendothelial system comprise immobile and mobile cells.** The immobile cells, such as the endothelial cells or Kupffer cells in the liver, respond to the local needs

TABLE 5-1	
CLUSTERS OF DIFFERENTIATION	
Selected Cluster of Differentiation	**Distribution**
CD2	T cells, NK subset
CD3	Thymocytes and mature T cells
CD4	Helper/inducer T cells, monocytes
CD5	T cells, B-cell subset, brain
CD7	Earliest T-lineage marker, most T cells, NK cells, ALL, 10% AML
CD8	Suppressor/cytotoxic T cells, NK subsets
CD10	Early B and T precursors, pre-B ALL, granulocytes, kidney epithelium (CALLA)
CD15	Granulocytes, Reed-Sternberg cells
CD20	B cells
CD30	Activated B and T cells, Reed-Sternberg cells carcinoma
CD45	Leukocyte common antigen, multiple isoforms
CD56	NK, T subset
CD138	Plasma cells (not mature B cells)

NK, natural killer cells; B CLL, B-cell chronic lymphocytic leukemia; AML, acute myeloblastic leukemia; ALL, acute lymphocytic leukemia; CALLA, common acute lymphoblastic leukemia antigen. (Courtesy of Dr. Howard Ratech, Montefiore Medical Center.)

of the organ wherein they are located. **The mobile cells are the macrophages or histiocytes.**

The **macrophages,** which are characterized by their **capacity to engulf (phagocytize)** foreign particles, such as bacteria, fungi, protozoa, and foreign material, may achieve very large sizes and, therefore, are highly visible in light microscopy. The term *macrophage* (i.e., a cell capable of engulfing large particles) was originally suggested for this group of cells by Metchnikoff, to **differentiate them from polymorphonuclear leukocytes capable of engulfing only very small particles (microphages).** The term *histiocyte* was originally coined to suggest cells with properties similar to those of macrophages, yet found predominantly in tissues. The two terms are used interchangeably, although the current trend is to favor the term *macrophage.* Both terms will be used simultaneously in this work to acknowledge wide usage of the terms *histiocyte* and *histiocytosis* in pathology. The inability of macrophages to perform the phagocytic function results in a number of life-threatening disorders (Lekstrom-Himes and Gallin, 2000).

Current evidence suggests that **macrophages are derived from monocytes of bone marrow origin** (see Chap. 19). The actual differentiation and maturation of macrophages takes place in the target tissue. The activation of precursor cells into macrophages is mediated by T lymphocytes by means of specific soluble factors or lymphokines. The changes occurring during activation may be conveniently observed in tissue cultures in vitro. The round, small precursor cells become markedly enlarged when spread on glass and acquire a number of dense cytoplasmic granules, which

have been identified as lysosomes by electron microscopy (Fig. 5-12).

Once differentiated, the **macrophages in the tissue may remain mobile** or may lose their mobility and become **fixed.** This occurs particularly in certain chronic inflammatory processes, such as tuberculosis. In the latter situation, the macrophages **assume an epithelial configuration** in clusters or sheets **(epithelioid cells),** usually accompanied by **multinucleated giant cells.**

In diagnostic cytology, macrophages play an important role and their recognition is sometimes essential. **Macrophages may be mononucleated or multinucleated. Mature mononucleated macrophages** in light microscopy are cells of variable sizes. The nucleus is round or kidney-shaped. The cytoplasm is filled with small vacuoles but often contains granules or fragments of phagocytized material. In actively phagocytizing cells, the nucleus is often peripheral (Fig. 5-13A). In scanning electron microscopy, the macrophages have been shown to have surfaces provided with flanges and ridges that are fairly characteristic of these cells (see Chap. 25).

The **multinucleated macrophages (polykaryons)** result from fusion of mononucleated macrophages and may reach huge sizes (Mariano and Spector, 1974). In some of these cells, the nuclei are arranged at the periphery in an orderly fashion **(Langhans' or Touton's cells).** In other multinucleated macrophages, the nuclei are dispersed throughout the cytoplasm (Fig. 5-13B).

Macrophages are activated by lymphokines from specifically sensitized T lymphocytes. Activated macrophages are

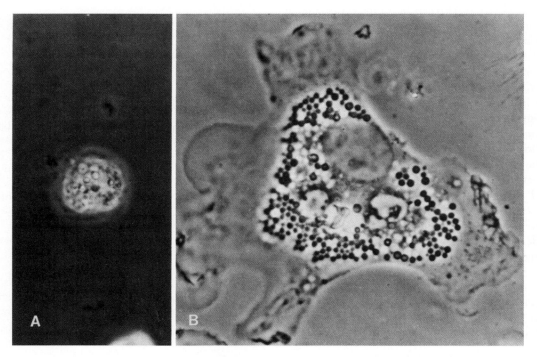

Figure 5-12 **Unstimulated and stimulated rat peritoneal macrophages in tissue culture** (phase contrast microscopy). *A.* Unstimulated macrophage. The cell is small, rounded, and shows no cytoplasmic activity of note. The nucleus is central. *B.* Stimulated macrophage. Note the large size of the cell containing numerous lysosomes that appear as dark cytoplasmic granules. The nucleus is eccentric. (×4,400.) (Adams DD, et al. The activation of mononuclear phagocytes in vitro: Immunologically mediated enhancement. J Reticuloendothel Soc 14:550, 1973.)

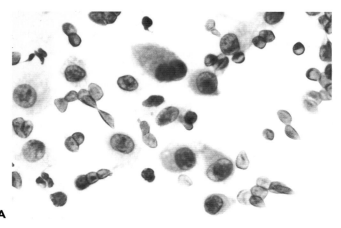

A

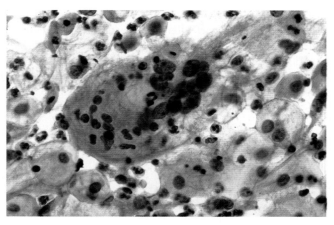

B

Figure 5-13   **Macrophages.** *A.* Mononucleated macrophages (ascitic fluid). Note the peripheral position of the nuclei within the finely vacuolated cytoplasm. *B.* Large multinucleated macrophage (vaginal smear), surrounded by squamous and inflammatory cells. There is evidence of phagocytosis of cells and cell fragments in the cytoplasm.

also capable of secreting numerous products that, in turn, may regulate functions of lymphocytes and help in disposing of phagocytized particles.

Macrophage deficiencies have been observed in AIDS wherein these cells may be infected by HIV-1. In some situations, **close contacts between macrophages and cancer cells** have been observed (Fig. 5-14). The significance of these observations is not clear.

Phagocytic Properties of Cells Other Than Macrophages

Wakefield and Hicks (1974) have shown that, under certain experimental circumstances, cells of bladder epithelium are capable of phagocytosis of erythrocytes. It is also known

that cells of endometrial stroma may acquire phagocytic properties at the time of menstrual bleeding. Sporadic examples of phagocytosis by benign and malignant cells have been observed. Little is known about the biologic circumstances that lead to these events.

Cancers Derived From the Immune Cell System

The observations summarized above have led to further characterization of the origin of many malignant diseases derived from cells that constitute the immune cell system. Most **chronic lymphocytic leukemias, non-Hodgkin's lymphomas, Burkitt's lymphomas, and all Waldenström's macroglobulinemias are of B-cell origin,** whereas the neoplastic cells of some **non-Hodgkin's lymphomas,** the rare **Sézary syndrome,** and 1% to 2% of patients with **chronic lymphocytic leukemia** are of **T-cell origin. Multiple myeloma is derived from plasma cells.** The cells of leukemic reticuloendotheliosis and histiocytic medullary reticulosis are thought to arise from macrophage precursors. For further comments on classification of lymphomas, see Chapter 31.

The Blood Cells

Only a brief mention of blood cells will be made here. **Erythrocytes** and **leukocytes** may be found with reasonable frequency in cytologic material and knowledge of their morphologic features is essential. Since hematology is not a part of this book, the reader is referred to other sources for a more detailed discussion.

Well-preserved **erythrocytes** in cytologic material indicate fresh bleeding, resulting from breakage of blood vessels. This injury may be due either to a physiologic process, such as menstrual bleeding, a disease process, a mechanical trauma, or iatrogenic procedure.

As a rule, the **neutrophilic polymorphonuclear leukocytes** are associated with **acute inflammatory processes.** In small numbers, they may be physiologically present in cytologic material of various origins.

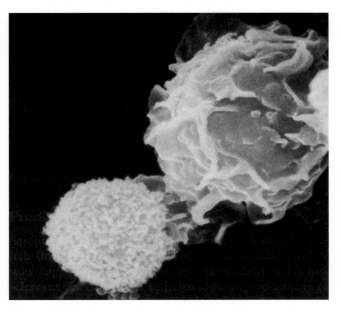

Figure 5-14   Scanning electron micrograph of an extensive contact between a macrophage, shown as a large cell characterized by surface ruffles, and a small lymphocyte with surface covered by microvilli. (Pleural effusion. Approx. ×4,000.) (Courtesy of Dr. W. Domagala, Montefiore Hospital, New York.)

Eosinophilic polymorphonuclear leukocytes (eosinophils) are associated with **allergic processes,** such as asthma or hay fever or response to a **parasitic infection.** In other situations, the role of **basophilic polymorphonuclear leukocytes (basophils)** remains obscure. **Megakaryocytes** may be observed in cytologic material, as described in Chapters 8, 19, 25, 30, and 47.

BIBLIOGRAPHY

Acuto O, Reinherz EL. The human T-cell receptor: Structure and function. N Engl J Med 312:1100–1111, 1985.

Adams DO, Hamilton TA. The cell biology of macrophage activation. Annu Rev Immunol 2:283–318, 1984.

Adams DO, Biesecker JL, Koss LG. The activation of mononuclear phagocytes in vitro: Immunologically mediated enhancement. J Reticuloendothel Soc 14:550–570, 1973.

Aschoff L. Das reticulo-endotheliale System. Ergebn Inn Med Kinderheilkd 26:1–118, 1924.

Blackman M, Kappler J, Marrack P. The role of the T-cell receptor in positive and negative selection of developing T cells. Science 248:1335–1341, 1990.

Brunstetter M-A, Hardie JA, Schiff R, et al. The origin of pulmonary alveolar macrophages. Arch Intern Mod 127:1064–1068, 1971.

Cohn ZA. The structure and function of monocytes and macrophages. Adv Immunol 9:163–214, 1968.

Cooper MD. B lymphocytes: Normal development and function. N Engl J Med 317:1452–1456, 1987.

Delves PJ, Roitt IM. The immune system. N Engl J Med 343:37–49, 108–117, 2000.

Dinarello CA, Mier, JW. Lymphokines. N Engl J Med 317:940–945, 1987.

French DL, Laskov R, Scharff MD. The role of somatic hypermutation in the generation of antibody diversity. Science 244:1152–1157, 1989.

Golde DW, Territo M, Finley TN, Cline MJ. Defective lung macrophages in pulmonary alveolar proteinosis. Ann Intern Med 85:304–309, 1976.

Guillet J-E, Lai M-Z, Briner TJ, et al. Immunological self, nonself discrimination. Science 235:865–870, 1987.

Ham AE, Cormack DH. Ham's Histology, 9th ed. Philadelphia, JB Lippincott, 1987.

Harmsen AG, Muggenburg BA, Snipes MB, Bice DE. The role of macrophages: In particle translocation from lungs to lymph nodes. Science 230:1277–1280, 1985.

Huber R. Structural basis for antigen-antibody recognition. Science 233:702–703, 1986.

Jerne NK. The generative grammar of the immune system. Science 229:1057–1059, 1985.

Johnston RB Jr. Monocytes and macrophages. N Engl J Med 319:747–752, 1988.

Jondal M, Hohn G, Wigzell H. Surface markers on human T- and B-lymphocytes. A large population of lymphocytes forming non-immune rosettes with sheep red blood cells. J Exp Med 136:207–215, 1972.

Kishimoto T, Goyert S, Kikutani H, et al. CD antigens 1996. Blood 89:3502, 1997

Klein J, Sato A. The HLA system. First of two parts. N Engl J Med 343:702–710, 782–786, 2000.

Knapp W, Borken B, Gilks WR, et al. Leukocyte typing IV. White cell differentiation antigens. Oxford, England, Oxford University Press, 1989 and 1992

Kronenberg M, Siu G, Hood LE, Shastri N. The molecular genetics of the T-cell antigen receptor and T-cell antigen recognition. Annu Rev Immunol 4:529–591, 1986.

Lay WH, Mendes N-F, Bianco C, Nussenzweig V. Binding of sheep red blood cells to a large population of human lymphocytes. Nature 230:531, 1971.

Leeson CR, Sydney T. Textbook of Histology, 5th ed. Philadelphia, WB Saunders, 1985.

Lekstrom-Himes JA, Gallin JI. Immunodeficiency diseases caused by defects in phagocytes. N Engl J Med 343:1703–1714, 2000.

Lewin KJ, Harell GS, Lee AS, Crowley LG. Malacoplakia. An electron-microscopic study: Demonstration of bacilliform organisms in malacoplakic macrophages. Gastroenterology 66:28–45, 1974.

Marchalonis JJ. Lymphocyte surface immunoglublins. Science 190:20–29, 1975.

Mariano M, Spector WG. Formation and properties of macrophage polykaryons; (Inflammatory giant cells). J Pathol 113:1–19, 1974.

Marrack P, Kappler J. The T cell receptor. Science 238:1073–1079, 1987.

Metchnikoff E. Immunity in Infective Diseases. London, Cambridge University Press, 1905.

Milstein C. From antibody structure to immunological diversification of immune response. Science 231:1261–1268, 1986.

Nathan CF, Karnovsky ML, David JR. Alterations of macrophage functions by mediators from lymphocytes. J Exp Med 133:1356–1376, 1971.

Nelson DS. Immunobiology of the Macrophage. New York, Academic Press, 1976.

Nossal GJV. Immunologic tolerance: Collaboration between antigen and lymphokines. Science 245:147–153, 1989.

Nossal GJV. The basic components of the immune system. N Engl J Med 310:1320–1325, 1989.

Novikoff PM, Yam A, Novikoff AB. Lysosomal compartment of macrophages: Extending the definition of GERL. Cell Biol 78:5699–5703, 1981.

Oettinger MA, Schatz DG, Gorka C, Baltimore D. RAG-1 and RAG-2, adjacent genes that synergistically activate V (D) J recombination. Science 248:1517–1523, 1990.

Robert C, Kupper TS. Inflammatory skin diseases, T cells, and immune surveillance. N Engl J Med 341:1817–1828, 1999.

Rosen FS, Cooper MD, Wedgwood RJP. The primary immunodeficiencies. N Engl J Med 333:431–440, 1995.

Royer HD, Reinherz EL. T Lymphocytes: Ontogeny, function, and relevance to clinical disorders. N Engl J Med 317:1136–1142, 1987.

Sinha AA, Lopez MT, McDevitt HO. Autoimmune diseases: The failure of self-tolerance. Science 248:1380–1387, 1990.

Smith KA. Interleukin-2: Inception, impact, and implications. Science 240:1169–1176, 1988.

Sprent J, Gao EK, Webb SR. T cell reactivity to MHC molecules: Immunity versus tolerance. Science 248:1357–1363, 1990.

Stavnezer J. A touch of antibody class. Science 288:984–985, 2000.

Stevens A, Lowe J. Histology. London, Grover, 1992.

Strominger JL. Developmental biology of T cell receptors. Science 244:943–950, 1989.

Tonegawa S. Somatic generation of antibody diversity. Nature 302:575–581, 1983.

Unanue ER, Allen PM. The basis for the immunoregulatory role of macrophages and other accessory cells. Science 236:551–557, 1987.

Vernon-Robert B. The Macrophage. London, Cambridge University Press, 1972.

von Boehmer H, Kisielow P. Self-nonself discrimination by T-cells. Science 248:1369–1372, 1990.

Wakefield JSJ, Hicks RM. Erythrophagocytosis by the epithelial cells of the bladder. J Cell Sci 15:555–573, 1974.

Walker KR, Fullmer CD. Observations of eosinophilic extracytoplasmic processes in pulmonary macrophages. Progress report. Acta Cytol 15:363–364, 1971.

Warnke RA, Weiss LM, Chan JKC, et al. Tumors of the lymph nodes and the spleen. Washington DC, Armed Forces Institute of Pathology, 1995.

Wehle K, Pfitzer P. Nonspecific esterase activity of human alveolar macrophages in routine cytology. Acta Cytol 32:153–158, 1988.

Weiss SJ. Tissue destruction by neutrophils. N Engl J Med 320:365–376, 1989.

Yeager HJ, Zimmet SM, Schwartz SL. Pinocytosis by human alveolar macrophages: Comparison of smokers and non-smokers. J Clin Invest 54:247–251, 1974.

Morphologic Response of Cells to Injury

6

The purpose of diagnostic cytology is to **recognize processes that cause cell changes that are identifiable under the light microscope,** supplemented, when necessary, by cytochemistry, immunocytochemistry, electron microscopy, or molecular biologic techniques (see Chaps. 2, 3, and 45). In this chapter the causes and effects of various forms of injury to the cells are discussed. Benign and malignant neoplasms (tumors) will be discussed in Chapter 7.

CAUSES OF CELL INJURY

Injury to the cells may be caused by numerous agents and disease states. A brief listing of the most significant sources of recognizable cell abnormalities observed in diagnostic cytology is as follows:

I. **Physical and Chemical Agents**
  A. Heat
  B. Cold
  C. Radiation
  D. Drugs and other chemical agents
II. **Infectious Agents**
  A. Bacteria
  B. Viruses
  C. Fungi
  D. Parasites
III. **Internal Agents**
  A. Inborn, sometimes hereditary genetic defects of cell function
    1. Storage diseases (e.g., Tay-Sachs and Gaucher's diseases)
    2. Metabolic disorders (e.g., phenylketonuria)
    3. Faulty structure of essential molecules (e.g., sickle cell anemia)
    4. Miscellaneous disorders
  B. Diseases of the immune system
    1. Inborn immune deficiencies
    2. Acquired immune deficiencies
    3. Autoimmune disorders
IV. **Disturbances of Cell Growth**
  A. Benign (self-limiting)
    1. Hyperplasia
    2. Metaplasia
  B. Tumors or neoplasms **(see Chap. 7)**
    1. Benign
    2. Malignant

CELLULAR RESPONSE TO INJURY AT THE LIGHT MICROSCOPIC LEVEL

Cells have limited ability to express their response to injury. They may respond:

- **by dying** (necrosis or apoptosis)
- **by undergoing a morphologic transformation** that may be transient or permanent
- **by mitotic activity** that again may be either transient or sustained, normal or abnormal, and may result in normal or abnormal daughter cells and subsequent generations of cells.

Although the mechanisms of cellular responses to injurious agents are still poorly understood because they are the result of complex molecular changes, it appears reasonable to assume that **a cell will attempt to maintain its morphologic and functional integrity, either by mobilizing its own resources against injury, or by seeking assistance from other cells specializing in defensive action.** The latter type of response is triggered by cell **necrosis,** a form of cell death, which results in an **inflammatory process,** with participation of leukocytes and macrophages. The significant morphologic responses of cells to various forms of injury are summarized below.

CELL DEATH

In cells, as in all other forms of life, death is an inevitable event. Death may follow a specific programmed pathway, or it may occur as an incidental event. Programmed cell death was first described and named **apoptosis** (from Greek, *apo* = from and *ptosis* = falling or sinking) by Kerr et al in 1972 (see also Searle et al, 1982 and Kerr et al, 1994). Apoptosis was first recognized as a purely morphologic phenomenon affecting cells, to be differentiated from **necrosis,** a form of cell death that occurred incidentally caused by an event or events not compatible with cell survival. The sequence of events in the two processes is compared in Figure 6-1. Within the recent years, apoptosis has received an enormous amount of attention from molecular biologists because of its importance in developmental biology and in a number of diseases, such as stroke and cancer.

Apoptosis

Morphology

The most significant studies of apoptosis in man have been conducted on cells in culture or on lymphocytes. There is comparatively little information on apoptosis in epithelial cells. Apoptotic cells are characterized by nuclear and cytoplasmic changes. The nuclear changes are a **condensation of the nuclear chromatin, first as crescentic caps** at the periphery of the nucleus, **followed by further fragmentation** and break-up of the nucleus (Fig. 6-1 top). The fragmentation of the chromatin into small granules of approximately equal sizes is known as **karyorrhexis** (from Greek, *karyon* = nucleus, *rhexis* = breakage), which has now been

recognized as a manifestation of apoptosis (Fig. 6-2). The cytoplasm of many apoptotic cells may show shrinkage and membrane blisters. It appears, however, that the cytoplasm may remain relatively intact in squamous cells. As the next stage of cell disintegration, fragments of nuclear material with fragments of adjacent cytoplasm (that may contain various organelles) are packaged into membrane-enclosed vesicles (**apoptotic bodies**). These packages of cellular debris are phagocytized by macrophages, **without causing an inflammatory reaction** in the surrounding tissues. One important consequence of apoptosis is that the cell DNA is chopped up into fragments of variable sizes composed of **multiples of 185 base pairs.** When sorted out by electrophoresis, they form a **"DNA ladder"** of fragments of diminishing sizes. Because the breaks occur at specific points of nucleotide sequences, they can be recognized by **specific probes identifying the break points in the DNA chain.** The probes, either labeled with a fluorescent compound or peroxidase, allow the recognition of cells undergoing apoptosis, either by fluorescent microscopy, flow cytometry, or by microscopic observation (Li and Darzynkiewicz, 1999; Bedner et al, 1999). A so-called **TUNNEL** reaction is a method of documenting apoptosis in cytologic or histologic samples (Gavrieli et al, 1992; Li and Darzynkiewicz, 1999; Sasano et al, 1998).

Sequence of Biologic Events

In paraphrasing a statement by Thornberry and Lazebnik (1998), apoptosis is reminiscent of a well-planned and executed military operation in which the target cell is isolated from its neighbors, its cytoplasm and nucleus are effectively destroyed, and the remains (apoptotic bodies) are destined for burial at sea, leaving no traces behind. Much of the original information on the sequence of events in apoptosis was obtained by studying the embryonal development events in the small worm (nematode), *Caenorhabditis elegans.* These studies have documented that apoptosis occurs naturally during the developmental stages of the worm to eliminate unwanted cells. It is caused by a **cascade of events,** culminating in the activation of proteolytic enzymes that effectively destroy the targeted cell. A somewhat similar, but not identical, sequence of events was proposed for mammalian cells.

Apoptosis in mammalian cells is triggered by numerous injurious factors, some known, such as viruses, certain drugs, radioactivity, and some still unknown (summary in Thompson, 1995; Hetts, 1998; review in Nature, 2000). For example, the loss of T4 cells by the human immunodeficiency virus in acquired immunodeficiency syndrome (AIDS) is caused by apoptosis. However, the pathway to apoptosis is extremely complicated because normal cells contain **genes that prevent it and genes that promote it.** This equilibrium has to be disrupted for the cells to enter the cycle of death.

In brief, it is assumed today that "death signals," received by the cytoplasm of the cell and mediated by a complex sequence of molecules, lead to activation of proteolytic enzymes, known as **caspases** that destroy the cytoplasmic proteins, including intermediate filaments, and attack the nu-

APOPTOSIS

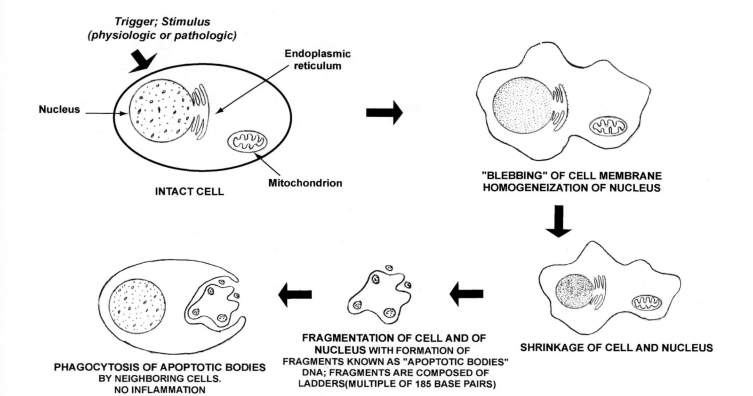

**Trigger; Stimulus
(physiologic or pathologic)**

Nucleus

Endoplasmic
reticulum

Mitochondrion

INTACT CELL

**"BLEBBING" OF CELL MEMBRANE
HOMOGENEIZATION OF NUCLEUS**

SHRINKAGE OF CELL AND NUCLEUS

**FRAGMENTATION OF CELL AND OF
NUCLEUS** WITH FORMATION OF
FRAGMENTS KNOWN AS "APOPTOTIC BODIES"
DNA; FRAGMENTS ARE COMPOSED OF
LADDERS(MULTIPLE OF 185 BASE PAIRS)

PHAGOCYTOSIS OF APOPTOTIC BODIES
BY NEIGHBORING CELLS.
NO INFLAMMATION

NECROSIS

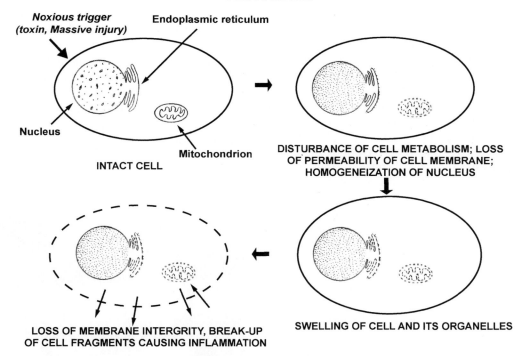

**Noxious trigger
(toxin, Massive injury)**

Endoplasmic reticulum

Nucleus

Mitochondrion

INTACT CELL

**DISTURBANCE OF CELL METABOLISM; LOSS
OF PERMEABILITY OF CELL MEMBRANE;
HOMOGENEIZATION OF NUCLEUS**

SWELLING OF CELL AND ITS ORGANELLES

**LOSS OF MEMBRANE INTERGRITY, BREAK-UP
OF CELL FRAGMENTS CAUSING INFLAMMATION**

Figure 6-1   Diagrammatic representation of apoptosis (*top*) and necrosis (*bottom*). For explanatory comments, see text. (Drawings by Professor Claude Gompel modified from diagrams by Dr. T. Brunner, Department of Pathology, University of Bern, Switzerland.)

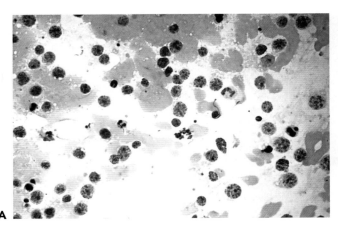 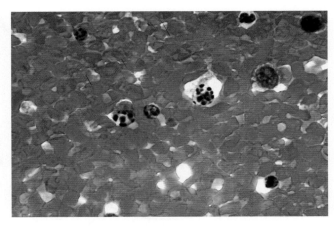

A

B

Figure 6-2   Apoptosis. *A.* Apoptosis (karyorrhexis) of malignant lymphoma cells in an aspirate of lymph node. *B.* Apoptosis of cells of malignant lymphoma in bloody pleural effusion. (*B,* High magnification.)

clear lamins, causing the collapse of the nuclear DNA structure. However, the intermediate steps of this sequence of events are enormously complicated. An injury to the molecule p53 (guardian of the genome; see Chap. 3) appears to be an important event (Bennett et al, 1998). Recent studies have documented that genes located on the **mitochondrial membrane** play a critical role in apoptosis (Brenner and Kroemer, 2000; Finkel, 2001). These genes belong to two families: **Bcl,** a protooncogene, which **protects the cells from apoptosis,** and **Bax, which favors apoptosis** (Zhang et al, 2000). If the proapoptotic molecule prevails, there is damage to the mitochondrial membrane with release of cytochrome C into the cytoplasm. Cytochrome C acts to transform a ubiquitous protein molecule known as *zymogen* into caspases.

Numerous articles on the subject of apoptosis have appeared in recent years, each addressing a small fragment of the complex puzzle. The key recent articles are cited or listed in the bibliography. The significance of apoptosis goes much beyond a simple morphologic and molecular biologic summary. It is generally thought that the mechanisms of apoptosis, besides playing a key role during embryonal development, may play a **key role in cancer and in important degenerative processes** such as Alzheimer's disease. In **cancer, suppression of apoptosis** may be one of the causes of cell proliferation, so characteristic of this group of disorders. This may explain the role of **oncogenes, such as Bcl or Myc,** as protecting the cells from apoptosis. It is considered that changes or mutations in molecules controlling DNA damage in replication (such as p53) or molecules governing events in the cell cycle (such as Rb) play a role in these events. It has been proposed that, in degenerative disorders of the brain, such as Alzheimer's disease, apoptosis may destroy essential centers of memory and control of body functions.

Necrosis

Cells may also die as a consequence of nonapoptotic events, globally referred to as **necrosis.** Some of the known causes

of necrosis are exposure to excessive heat, cold, or cytotoxic chemical agents. There is considerably less information on this type of cell death than on apoptosis, and the main difference is the **absence of typical morphologic changes and no evidence of activation of the cascade of events characterizing apoptosis** (see Fig. 6-1 bottom).

Morphology

Cells undergoing nonapoptotic forms of necrosis may show extensive **cytoplasmic vacuolization** (Fig. 6-3). The nuclear changes include homogeneous, dense chromatin known as **nuclear homogenization or pyknosis** (from Greek, *pyknos* = thick), nuclear enlargement, and breakdown of nuclear DNA, which however, **does not form the DNA ladder,** characteristic of apoptosis. Necrosis may result in destruction of the cell membranes, resulting in disintegration of the cell and **formation of cell debris** leading to an inflammatory process. The nuclear material may form fragments or streaks, often recognizable because they stain blue with the common nuclear dye, hematoxylin. Similar events may occur by physical injury to fragile cells if they are inappropriately handled during the technical preparation of

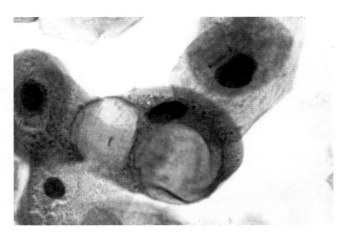

Figure 6-3   Radiation effect on squamous cells. Huge cytoplasmic vacuoles signify cell death. (High magnification.)

smears or other diagnostic material. In some cancers, the presence of nuclear necrosis is widespread and may be of diagnostic value (see oat cell carcinoma in Chap. 20).

It is often quite impossible to determine morphologically whether a cell died as a consequence of apoptosis or necrosis. There is little doubt that there may be many pathways leading to cell death. What is significant, however, is **the role played by necrotic cells as a trigger of inflammatory events,** whereas cells dying of apoptosis, as a rule, do not cause any inflammatory reaction.

Sequence of Biologic Events
Cell necrosis may be caused by many of the types of cell injury listed in the opening page of this chapter. Thus, there is a significant overlap between the two modes of cell death. It is not known today why the differences in the mode of dying occurs if the trigger of cell death is the same. It is generally believed that cell necrosis may begin in a manner similar to apoptosis, that is, by activation of a cell membrane molecule or a "death signal," which is followed by mitochondrial swelling, but this differs from the events in apoptosis because it **does not lead to caspase activation** (Green and Reed, 1998). Obviously, much is still unknown about cell necrosis, its mechanisms, and consequences.

OTHER EXPRESSIONS OF CELL RESPONSE TO INJURY

"Reactive" Nuclear Changes

It is not uncommon to observe, in material from various sources and under a variety of circumstances, but mainly in the presence of inflammatory processes, minor nuclear abnormalities such as **slight-to-moderate nuclear enlargement, slight irregularities of the nuclear contour, increase in granularity of the chromatin, and occasionally the presence of somewhat enlarged nucleoli** (Fig. 6-4). Such abnormalities are often classified as **"reactive nuclear changes."** Virtually nothing is known about the mecha-

nisms of such changes and their clinical significance is often puzzling. In many situations, such nuclear abnormalities occur in tissues adjacent to cancer. In cervical smears, the terms *atypia of squamous cells of unknown significance* (**ASCUS**) or *atypia of glandular (endocervical) cells of unknown significance* (**AGUS**) have been introduced to describe such phenomena. The term AGUS is no longer used. It is known that, in some patients with such changes a malignant lesion will be observed in the uterine cervix with the passage of time (see Chap. 11). Similar abnormalities may be observed in the so-called **repair reaction** and in **metaplasia,** discussed below. Thus, the term **reactive nuclear changes** is rather meaningless and reflects our ignorance of events leading to such nuclear abnormalities.

Multinucleation: Formation of Syncytia

It is not known why reaction to injury results in formation of multinucleated cells. These may occur as a consequence of a bacterial or viral infection, during a regenerative process, as in injured muscle, or for reasons that remain obscure. Multinucleation may be observed in cells of various derivations, such as macrophages, cells derived from organs of mesenchymal origin, or in epithelia.

The mechanism of formation of multinucleated cells by epithelioid cells was discussed in Chapter 5. Under unknown circumstances, apparently **normal epithelial cells** may form **multinucleated giant cells or syncytia** (from Latin, *syn* = together and *cyto* = cell) by cell fusion or **endomitosis,** that is, nuclear division not followed by division of the cytoplasm.

Regardless of mechanism of formation, such cells may be observed in the bronchial epithelium (see Chap. 19) and, occasionally, in other glandular epithelia (Fig. 6-5). In multinucleated cells caused by cell fusion, the cell membranes separating the cells from each other disappear. **Multinucleation** can be produced **in vitro** by the action of certain viruses, such as the Sendai virus, and **in vivo** in humans by herpesvirus and other viral infections. Thus, it is conceivable that the formation of true syncytia in epithelial cells is the reflection of a viral infection, although the causative agent may not be evident. To our knowledge, there is **no known diagnostic or prognostic significance** of the presence of

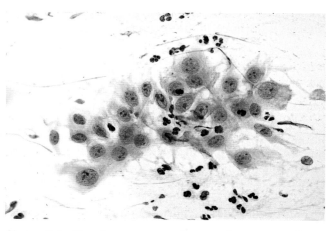

Figure 6-4 **Reactive squamous cells.** Note the presence of large nuclei and of prominent nucleoli in what is commonly referred to as a "repair reaction."

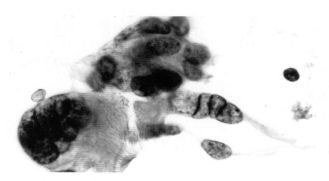

Figure 6-5 **Multinucleation of benign ciliated bronchial cells.** Note the presence of three nuclei in one of the cells and innumerable nuclei in a large cell on the left. (High magnification.)

multinucleated epithelial cells. Such cell changes **must not be confused with cell groupings or clusters, wherein cell membranes may not be visible under the light microscope, but are easily demonstrated by electron microscopy.** The term *syncytia* has been proposed by some observers to define clusters of small cancer cells in cervical smears in some cases of carcinoma in situ of the uterine cervix (see Chap. 12). The use of this term under these circumstances is erroneous.

Other Forms of Cell Injury

Nuclear abnormalities, seen in healthy or diseased tissue, are **nuclear creases** or **grooves,** folds observed in the nuclei of many cell types, and in many organs. Frequent and conspicuous nuclear grooves may be observed in some benign and malignant tumors but are not tumor-specific. The significance or mechanism of this nuclear feature is unknown (see Chaps. 7, 8, 21, and 41).

Nuclear cytoplasmic inclusions, observed as a **sharply defined clear zone in the nucleus,** are more common in certain malignant tumors but may also occur in cells derived from normal organs (see Fig. 7-19A). It can be documented by electron microscopy that the abnormality is caused by **infolding of the cytoplasm into the nucleus** (Fig. 6-6B). The reason for the mechanism of these events is unknown.

Other manifestations of cell damage may include the **loss of specialized cell appendages, such as cilia.** The loss of cilia may occur in otherwise well-preserved cells or it may be accompanied by a peculiar form of cell necrosis, often associated with viral infection (**ciliocytophthoria**) (see Chap. 19). **Loss of cell contacts** is another form of cell injury that may be caused, for example, by antibodies directed against desmosomes observed in skin disorders, such

as pemphigus (see Chaps. 19, 21, and 34). It should be noted that, in cancer, the relationship of cells to each other is often quite abnormal as discussed at some length in Chapter 7.

Cytoplasmic Vacuolization

This phenomenon may reflect a partial or temporary disturbance in the permeability of the cell membrane, resulting in formation of multiple, clear, spherical cytoplasmic inclusions **(vacuoles) of variable sizes** (see Fig. 6-3). Most vacuoles contain water and water-soluble substances. The viability of such cells is unknown, although extensive vacuolization may be a manifestation of cell death, for example, caused by radiotherapy. Small cytoplasmic vacuole formation may also occur as a consequence of **cell invasion by certain microorganisms,** such as *Chlamydia trachomatis* and other infectious agents (see Chap. 10). Storage of **fat** may also result in the formation of cytoplasmic vacuoles.

Cytoplasmic Storage

Under special circumstances, the cell may also store other products of cell metabolism that can be recognized under the light or electron microscope. Thus, **glycogen, bile, melanin pigment** (normally present in the epidermis of the skin and in the retina), and **iron,** derived from disintegrating hemoglobin molecules **(hemosiderin or hematoidin)** may accumulate in abnormal locations (see Fig. 7-24B). Another pigment, **lipofuscin,** thought to represent products of cell wear and tear, may also be seen, usually in perinuclear locations. Because hemosiderin, melanin, and lipofuscin form brown cytoplasmic deposits that may look similar under the light microscope, the use of special stains may be required for their identification (see Chap. 45). The identification of these pigments may be of critical significance in the differential diagnosis of a melanin-producing, highly malignant tumor, the malignant melanoma. Under some circumstances, **salts of calcium** may form irregularly shaped amorphous or concentrically structured deposits within the cytoplasm. Such deposits are usually recognized by their intense blue staining with hematoxylin. Also, a variety of **crystals,** either derived from amino acids or from inorganic compounds, may accumulate in cells. The implications of these findings is discussed in the appropriate chapters.

Storage Diseases

In a variety of inherited storage diseases, caused by deficiencies of specific lysosomal enzymes, such as Gaucher's disease, Niemann-Pick disease, von Gierke's disease, Tay-Sachs disease, Hand-Schüller-Christian disease, and other very rare disorders, the **products of abnormal cell metabolism** may accumulate, mainly in macrophages, but also in the cytoplasm of other cell types. As a general rule, such cells become markedly enlarged. Several of these disorders can be identified under the light microscope because of the specific appearance of the large cells. Some of these disorders may be recognized in aspirated cell samples and are discussed in Chapter 38. Most commonly, however, such cells are seen

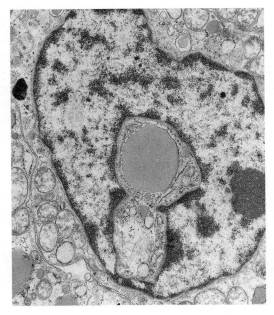

Figure 6-6 Electron micrograph of an intranuclear cytoplasmic inclusion in a cell from renal carcinoma. Note cytoplasmic organelles within the nucleus. (High magnification.) (Courtesy of Dr. Myron Melamed, Valhalla, NY.)

STAGES OF PHAGOCYTOSIS

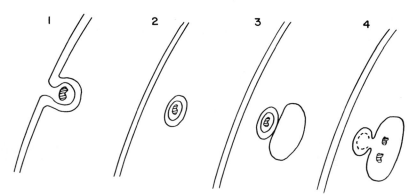

Figure 6-7 **Diagrammatic representation of the stages of phagocytosis.** (1) The foreign particle is trapped in a vesicle formed by invagination of the cell membrane. (2) It sinks into the depth of the cytoplasm, and (3) merges with a cytophagic vacuole (lysosome). (4) The enzymes contained in the cytophagic vacuole digest the foreign material. The mechanism is similar to that of pinocytosis.

in bone marrow samples. The description of the specific cell changes may be found in hematology manuals.

Phagocytosis

Phagocytosis, or ingestion of foreign particles by cells, has already been discussed in Chapter 2. Although phagocytosis, strictly speaking, cannot be considered a form of cell reaction to injury, it is often enhanced in disease processes such as inflammation and cancer. The sequence of events in phagocytosis is shown in Figure 6-7. The cells principally involved in phagocytosis are the **macrophages,** which accumulate visible particles of foreign material in their cytoplasm (Fig. 6-8). Occasionally, however, **epithelial and mesothelial cells,** and particularly **cancer cells,** are also capable of the **phagocytic function** and may display the presence of foreign particles, cell fragments, or even whole cells in their cytoplasm. A special form of phagocytosis is **erythrophagocytosis,** in which whole red blood cells are engulfed by macrophages, but also sometimes by cells of other types (see Chap. 25). The precise mechanisms of these phenomena are now being studied (Caron and Hall, 1998). A special situation is represented by an uncommon disorder, **malacoplakia,** observed mainly in the urinary bladder but also in

other organs. In it, the cytoplasmic lysosomes of macrophages lack certain enzymes necessary for the destruction of phagocytized coliform bacteria. As a consequence, the lysosomes become enlarged and readily visible as the so-called **Michaelis-Guttmann** bodies. Such bodies may undergo calcification (see Chap. 22).

LONG-TERM EFFECTS OF CELL INJURY. REPAIR AND REGENERATION

Localized cell damage and death, resulting from physical or infectious causes, leads to a **replacement or regeneration** of the injured tissue, sometimes referred to as **repair.** The **source of replacement** is the neighboring cells of the same type. Thus, an epithelium will be replaced by epithelial cells and the regeneration of the connective tissue will be provided by fibroblasts. Theoretically, the growth of cells leading to regeneration should cease when the restoration of the injured tissue is complete. In practice, this is not always so: the newly formed tissue is sometimes less than perfect and its growth may continue beyond the confines of the original tissue, sometimes resulting in a hyperplasia, and even a so-called **pseudotumor.** Alternatively, a portion of the injured tissue may be replaced by collagen-forming connective tissue, with resulting formation of a **scar.** In experimental systems, regeneration has been exhaustively studied in the liver after partial hepatectomy and in the epithelium of the urinary bladder, after destruction with the cytotoxic drug, cyclophosphamide (see Chap. 22).

In general, the **first event in the regeneration process of the injured epithelium,** usually occurring within approximately 24 hours after the onset of injury, is an intense **mitotic activity** in the normal cells surrounding the injured tissue. Cell division is apparently triggered by biochemical signals, from the injured cells. The **mitotic activity in tissue repair is not always normal: abnormal mitotic figures may be observed.** The mitotic activity results in the formation of young epithelial cells that migrate into the defect to form **a single layer of epithelial cells bridging the gap** caused by the injury. With the passage of time, the epithelium becomes multilayered. The **newly formed young epithelial cells are often atypical** and are characterized by the

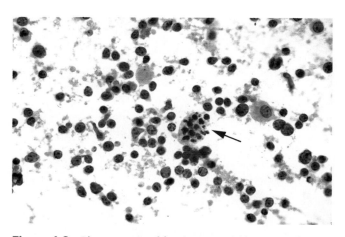

Figure 6-8 **Phagocytosis of foreign material by macrophages.** A so-called tingible body macrophage (arrow) in an aspiration smear from a normal lymph node.

presence of a basophilic cytoplasm, reflecting the intense production of ribonucleic acid (RNA) and proteins in the rapidly proliferating cells. However, the most conspicuous finding in such cells is **nuclear abnormalities** in the form of large nuclei of uneven sizes, often provided with multiple, **large, and irregular nucleoli reflecting the cell's requirement for RNA** (see Fig. 6-4). Such cells may mimic nuclear and nucleolar abnormalities of cancer and are one of the **major potential pitfalls in diagnostic cytology.** The term *repair* has been proposed to define certain benign abnormalities observed **in endocervical cells** in cervical smears although, in many such cases, there is no evidence of prior epithelial injury. Similar changes may also be observed in other organs (see Chaps. 10, 19, and 21).

The reaction to injury may also involve **connective tissue,** with resulting intense proliferation of fibroblasts. The **proliferating fibroblasts are usually large and have a basophilic cytoplasm,** not unlike proliferating fibroblasts in culture. **Large nuclei and conspicuously enlarged nucleoli** are a landmark of such reactive changes. The presence of **abnormal mitotic figures** may be noted, resulting in patterns reminiscent of malignant tumors of connective tissue or sarcomas (Fig. 6-9). Such self-limiting abnormalities may occur in muscle, fascia, or subcutaneous tissue, and they are referred to as **infiltrative or pseudosarcomatous fasciitis.**

The **molecular biology** of tissue regeneration and repair has been shown to be extremely complex. It can be assumed, in general, that under normal conditions of regeneration, there are two sets of biochemical factors working in tandem: factors inducing mitosis and, thereby, stimulating cell proliferation and factors arresting the cell proliferation, once the repair has been completed. Studies of regeneration of hepatocytes (Michalopoulos and DeFrances, 1997), wound healing (Martin, 1997), and amphibian limb regeneration (Brockes, 1997) have shown the enormous complexity of the system. Numerous genes, perhaps activated by the initial necrosis of the target tissue, enter into the equation, resulting in production of new cells and tissues. There is little known about the molecular signals that arrest the proliferative process upon completion of the repair. Some years ago,

poorly characterized chemical factors, named *chalones,* were thought to be the "stop" signal, but essentially no information emerged within the recent years. The interested reader is referred to the bibliography for further information on this subject.

The results of regeneration of repair are frequently far from perfect, particularly for epithelia, and may result in a number of abnormalities that will be described in the following sections.

BENIGN EPITHELIAL ABNORMALITIES CONSIDERED TO REPRESENT A REACTION TO CHRONIC INJURY

Basal Cell Hyperplasia

In this lesion, which may affect almost any epithelium, **the number of layers of small basal cells is increased,** so that up to one-half or even more of the epithelial thickness is occupied by small cells (Fig. 6-10). It is generally assumed, although it remains unproved, that basal cell hyperplasia is the result of a chronic injury. The **true significance of this abnormality and its mechanism of formation remain unknown.** It is sometimes assumed that this lesion is a precursor lesion of cancer, but the evidence for this is lacking. Because the events take place in the deeper layers of the epithelium, the cells resulting from the multiplication of the basal layer are not represented in samples obtained from the epithelial surface, unless there is an epithelial defect with loss of superficial cell layers. The lesion is of greater practical importance when the **small basal cells are removed by an instrument** or are found in an aspiration biopsy. Because of a large nuclear surface and, hence, an increased nucleocytoplasmic ratio (see Chap. 19), and the occasional presence of nucleoli, such cells may be sometimes mistaken for a malignant lesion composed of small cells.

Metaplasia

By definition, metaplasia is **the replacement of one type of epithelium by another** that is not normally present in

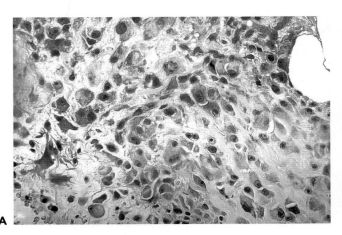

A

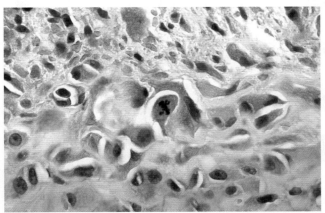

B

Figure 6-9 A benign reactive process known as infiltrative fasciitis. *A.* Note large fibroblasts with prominent nuclei and nucleoli. *B.* A quadripolar mitosis is evident in the center of the field.

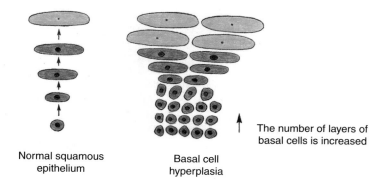

Figure 6-10 Schematic illustration of basal cell hyperplasia in squamous epithelium. The process may also involve other types of epithelia.

a given location. **In most instances, during the metaplastic process, a columnar or glandular epithelium is replaced by squamous epithelium or by cells with unusual characteristics, such as the mitochondria-rich oncocytes.** Metaplasia may occur as a result of an injury or chronic irritation caused by an inflammatory process or a mechanical trauma, for example, the pressure of a stone on an epithelium. With few exceptions, however, **the mechanisms of metaplastic replacement are generally not understood,** although lack of vitamin A may induce keratinization of epithelia in vivo or in vitro.

An example of metaplasia is the **replacement of the columnar mucus-producing epithelium** of the endocervix or of the ciliated bronchial epithelium **by squamous epithelium,** colloquially referred to as **squamous metaplasia** (Fig. 6-11). The epithelial replacement may be partial or total, complete or incomplete, and the resulting squamous epithelium may be mature or immature. The latter may be composed of squamous cells, showing **abnormalities of cell shape and, occasionally, nuclear enlargement,** when compared with normal. Some metaplastic cells may show **very large nuclei,** possibly the result of increased DNA, although there is currently no understanding of this observation. The **newly formed metaplastic epithelium very often retains some features of its predecessor.** For example, metaplastic squamous epithelial cells replacing mucus-producing endocervical epithelium may contain mucus.

In some organs and organ systems, for example in the bronchus, it is thought by some that squamous metaplasia of the bronchial epithelium may represent a steppingstone in the development of lung cancer. It is quite true that certain intraepithelial malignant lesions may resemble metaplasia, but the relationship of the two remains enigmatic. For further discussion of this important subject, see Chapter 20.

In human cytologic material derived from some organs, such as the endocervix or the bronchi, the presence of squamous metaplasia may be recognized under certain circumstances that will be described in the appropriate chapters.

The transformation of epithelial cells into cells known as **oncocytes (Hürthle cells)** may be observed in organs such as the salivary glands, thyroid, breast, and kidney. The oncocytes are rich in **mitochondria** that fill the cytoplasm. Such cells are characterized by unusual respiratory pathways and have been shown to have **abnormalities of mitochondrial DNA** (see Chap. 2). Virtually nothing is known about the mechanisms of their occurrence. The diagnostic significance of these cells will be discussed in the appropriate chapters.

Hyperplasia

The term *hyperplasia*, indicating **excessive growth,** may be applied to tissues or to individual cells. In light microscopy, the term is most often applied to an increase in the number of cell layers in a normally maturing epithelium (Fig. 6-12) or to an increase in the number of glandular structures, as in the endometrium. For whole organs, the term **hypertrophy** is used to indicate an increase in volume. For individual cells, the term must be used with great caution because it may indicate a benign process (as in cardiac muscle), but also a precancerous event or even cancer, when used in reference to epithelial cells. Unfortunately, in practice, these simple definitions are not always easy to follow. Quite often, the hyperplastic process is associated with abnormalities of component cells and the term **atypical hyperplasia** has been applied to such lesions. Atypical hyperplasia may pose significant diagnostic problems because the subsequent course of events cannot be predicted. Some of these lesions may regress or they may remain unchanged for many years. Other such lesions may progress to cancer if untreated (see Chaps. 11, 12, and 13).

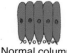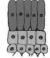

Figure 6-11 **Schematic summary of events in squamous metaplasia of the glandular-type epithelium.** Such events are common in the uterine cervix and the bronchus and occasionally occur in other glandular epithelia.

Normal columnar epithelium

Partial metaplasia: several layers of squamous cells appear beneath the columnar cells

Complete metaplasia: the columnar epithelium has been replaced by squamous epithelium

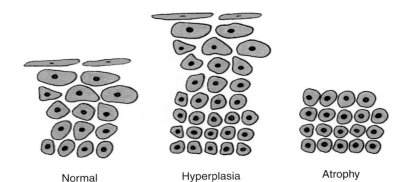

Normal　　　　Hyperplasia　　　　Atrophy

Figure 6-12 Schematic presentation of events in epithelial hyperplasia and atrophy in squamous epithelium.

The recognition of hyperplasia in cytologic material is impossible unless the cells show notable abnormalities, as they may occur in the atypical variant.

Atrophy

Atrophy is the opposite of hyperplasia; it indicates a **reduction in the volume of an organ** or, in the microscopic sense, a reduction in the **number of cells within an organ or a tissue,** or a reduction in the size or volume of individual cells. In the practice of microscopy, the atrophy of certain tissues may be recognized. For example, the number of cell layers in a squamous epithelium may be reduced (see Fig. 6-13) or there may be a reduction in the size of the component cells of an organ. Sometimes, epithelial atrophy may be identified in cytologic material, for example, in smears from the female genital tract (see Chap. 8).

SPECIFIC NONNEOPLASTIC DISEASE PROCESSES AFFECTING CELLS

Inflamatory Disorders

Inflammation is a common form of **tissue reaction to injury.** The reaction is usually caused by **bacterial, viral,** or **fungal agents,** but it may also occur as a **response to tissue necrosis, foreign bodies, and injury by therapy.** The inflammatory processes always involve a **participation of the immune system,** which is represented at the site of reaction by polymorphonuclear leukocytes of various types, lymphocytes, plasma cells, and macrophages in various proportions, depending on the causes of the inflammatory reaction and its natural course. The recognition of the type of inflammation may help in assessing the type of injury to the participating cells. It is convenient to classify inflammatory reactions as acute, subacute, chronic, and granulomatous.

Acute Inflammation

The acute inflammatory-type response to injury is characterized by **necrosis** and breakdown of cells and tissues. Because of damage to capillaries and sometimes to larger blood vessels, **blood and blood products (fibrin)** are invariably present. The dominant inflammatory cells participating in this process are **neutrophilic polymorphonuclear leuko-**cytes, usually accompanied by small populations of lymphocytes. The combination of necrotic material, cell debris, red blood cells, fibrin, and leukocytes, known collectively as **purulent exudate (pus),** give a characteristic cytologic picture that is readily identified. Although the term "acute" for this inflammatory process suggests an event of short duration (and most of them are), some reactions of this type may persist for prolonged periods, sometimes lasting several years. The **outcome** of the acute inflammatory reaction is either **healing,** associated with **tissue regeneration** and repair of the damage, or a transition to a chronic inflammatory process.

Subacute Inflammation

Subacute inflammation is an infrequent variant of the acute inflammatory process, characterized by minimal necrosis of the affected tissues and the presence of **eosinophilic polymorphonuclear leukocytes** (eosinophils) and lymphocytes. Such reactions may also be observed in the presence of parasites, which appear to be able to mobilize eosinophils. There are no documented specific cell changes associated with this type of inflammatory reaction.

Chronic Inflammation

The chronic type of inflammation is, by far, the most interesting in diagnostic cytology because it **may cause perceptible cell changes.** As the name indicates, the reaction is usually of long duration. The dominant inflammatory cells are **lymphocytes, plasma cells, and macrophages,** which may be mononucleated or have multiple nuclei. Besides evidence of phagocytosis, the macrophages may show nuclear abnormalities in the form of nuclear enlargement and hyperchromasia. Rarely, **plasma cells** may be the dominant cell population, **especially in the nasopharynx and the oropharynx;** when this occurs, the possibility of a malignant tumor composed of plasma cells (multiple myeloma) must be ruled out. Epithelial cells and fibroblasts may show various manifestations of regeneration and repair, as discussed in the preceding pages.

Granulomatous Inflammation

Granulomatous inflammation is a form of chronic inflammation characterized by the formation of nodular collections (granules) of modified macrophages resembling epithelial cells, hence known as **epithelioid cells.** The epi-

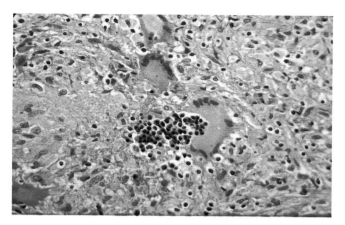

Figure 6-13   Tuberculosis of lymph nodes. Note several multi-nucleated giant cells (Langhans' cells) in the center of a spherical lesion composed of small epithelioid cells, forming a granuloma.

thelioid cells are often accompanied by **multinucleated giant cells,** which have been shown to result from fusion of epithelioid cells (Mariano and Spector, see Chap. 4). The multinucleated cells observed in tuberculosis and related disorders are known as **Langhans' giant cells** (Fig. 6-13). Similar cells may occur as a reaction to foreign material and are then known as **foreign-body giant cells.** The causes of granulomatous inflammation have been recognized: infections with *Mycobacterium tuberculosis* and related acid-fast organisms and some species of fungi are most commonly observed. In AIDS, microorganisms that are not necessarily pathogenic in normal humans, may also cause this type of inflammatory reaction. For other examples of granulomatous inflammatory process, see Chapters 10, 19, and 29.

RECOGNITION OF SPECIFIC INFECTIOUS AGENTS IN CYTOLOGIC MATERIAL

Inflammatory processes pertaining to various organs and organ systems will be discussed in appropriate chapters. Hence, this is but a brief overview of this field.

Bacteria

Very few bacterial agents cause specific cell changes, beyond the inflammatory reactions described above. Occasionally, however, specific microscopic images may be observed. Thus, the presence of the so-called **clue cells** in cervicovaginal smears is suggestive of an infection with *Gardnerella vaginalis* (see Chap. 10). ***Chlamydia trachomatis*** causes cell changes in the form of cytoplasmic inclusions. The cell changes in granulomatous inflammation, described above, occasionally may be observed in various cytologic preparations and in aspiration biopsy material.

Fungi

Fungal agents are easily identified by species in several diagnostic media. They are most commonly found, however, in pulmonary material, spinal fluid, and aspiration biopsies (see appropriate chapters for a description of these organisms).

Parasites

Parasitic agents are not commonly seen in the Western world, but are exceedingly common in the developing coun-

TABLE 6-1

CYTOPATHIC CHANGES CAUSED BY COMMON HUMAN VIRUSES

Virus	Cytoplasm	Nucleus	Inclusions
Herpesvirus (simplex of type 1 and type 2)	Enlarged in multinucleated cells	Early changes: ground-glass (opaque) nuclei, frequent multinucleation with nuclear Late stage: molding intranuclear inclusions	Eosinophilic intranuclear (in late stage)
Cytomegalovirus	May contain small satellite inclusions	Large inclusions with clear zones of "halos"	Mainly basophilic, sometimes eosinophilic large intranuclear inclusions with halos and smaller "satellite" inclusions in nucleus and cytoplasm
Human papillomavirus	Large, sharply demarcated perinuclear clear zones due to cytoplasmic necrosis (koilocytes)	Enlarged, sometimes pyknotic Virus documented by immunologic techniques, electron microscopy, or DNA hybridization in situ	None
Human polyomavirus	Normal or enlarged	Enlarged; chromatin replaced by a large inclusion (decoy cells)	Large, basophilic, homogeneous; no halo or satellite inclusion

tries. Several examples of parasites are given in the text (see appropriate chapters). The most important of these is the obligate intracellular parasite of uncertain classification, **Pneumocystis carinii**, which is the cause of a pneumonia that occurs with high frequency in AIDS patients (see Chap. 19). Cytologic samples are commonly used for the identification of this agent.

Viruses

Viral agents may cause recognizable cell changes. A summary of the cytologic findings in infections with the most common viruses is provided in Table 6-1. Additional information is provided in chapters dealing with specific organs.

Therapeutic Agents

Radiotherapy, cryotherapy, and a number of drugs, most of them belonging to the group of cytotoxic chemotherapeutic agents, may cause significant cell abnormalities. Because of the diversity of these effects, which are organ related, the changes will be described in the appropriate chapters.

BIBLIOGRAPHY

Adams DO, Hamilton TA. The cell biology of macrophage activation. Annu Rev Immunol 2:283–318, 1984.

Apoptosis. Nature 407:769–816, 2000.

Arends MJ, Morris RG, Wyllie AH. Apoptosis. The role of the endonuclease. Am J Pathol 136:116–122, 1990.

Bedner E, Li X, Gorczyca W, et al. Analysis of apoptosis by laser scanning cytometry. Cytometry 35:181–195, 1999.

Bennett M, Macdonald K, Chan S-W, et al. Cell surface trafficking of Fas: A rapid mechanism of p53-mediated apoptosis. Science 282:290–293, 1998.

Bonikos DS, Koss LG. Acute effects of cyclophosphamide on rat urinary bladder muscle. An electron microscopical study. Arch Pathol 97:242–245, 1974.

Brenner C, Kroemer G. Mitochondria-the death signal integrators. Science 289:1150–1153, 2000.

Brockes JP. Amphibian limb regeneration: Rebuilding a complex structure. Science 276:81–87, 1997.

Caron E, Hall A. Identification of two distinct mechanisms of phagocytosis controlled by different Rho GTPases. Science 282:1717–1720, 1998.

Cohn ZA, Parks E. The regulation of pinocytosis in mouse macrophages. II. Factors inducing vesicle formation. J Exp Med 125:213–230, 1967.

Cohn ZA, Parks E. The regulation of pinocytosis in mouse macrophages. III. The induction of vesicle formation by nucleosides and nucleotides. J Exp Med 125:457–466, 1967.

Cohn ZA, Parks E. The regulation of pinocytosis in mouse macrophages. IV. The immunological induction of pinocytotic vesicles, secondary lysosomes and hydrolytic enzymes. J Exp Med 125:1091–1104, 1967.

DiBerardino MA, Holckner NJ, Etkin LD. Activation of dormant genes in specialized cells. Science 224:946–952, 1984.

Fawcett DW. Surface specialization of absorbing cells. J Histochem Cytochem 13:75–91, 1965.

Finkel E. The mitochondrion: Is it central to apoptosis? Science 292:624–626, 2001.

Frankfurt DS. Epidermal chalone. Effect on cell cycle and on development of hyperplasia. Exp Cell Res 64:140–144, 1971.

Gavrieli Y, Sherman Y, Ben-Sasson SA. Identification of programmed cell death in situ via specific labeling of nuclear DNA fragmentation. J Cell Biol 119:493–501, 1992.

Green DR. A Myc-induced apoptosis pathway surface. Science 278:1246–1247, 1997.

Green DR, Reed JC. Mitochondria and apoptosis. Science 281:1309–1312, 1998.

Hetts SW. To die or not to die. An overview of apoptosis and its role in disease. JAMA 279:300–307, 1998.

Holter H. Pinocytosis. Int Rev Cytol 8:481–504, 1959.

Iverson OH. What is new in endogenous growth stimulators and inhibitors (chalones)? Pathol Res Pract 180:77–80, 1985.

Karrer HE. Electron microscopic study of the phagocytosis process in lung. J Biophys Biochem 7:357–365, 1960.

Kerr JFR. Shrinkage necrosis: A distinct mode of cellular death. J Pathol 105:13–20, 1971.

Kerr JFR, Winterford CM, Harmon BV. Apoptosis. Its significance in cancer and cancer therapy. Cancer 73:2013–2026, 1994.

Kerr JFR, Wyllie AH, Currie AR. Apoptosis: A basic biological phenomenon with wide-ranging implications in tissue kinetics. Br J Cancer 26:239–257, 1972.

Li X, Darzynkiewicz Z. The Schrodinger's cat quandary in cell biology: Integration of live cell functional assays with measurements of fixed cells in analysis of apoptosis. Exper Cell Res 249:404–412, 1999.

Majno G, Joris I. Apoptosis, oncosis, and necrosis. An overview of cell death. Am J Pathol 146:3–16, 1995.

Martin BF. Cell replacement and differentiation in transitional epithelium: A histological and autoradiographic study of the guinea-pig bladder and ureter. J Anat 112:433–455, 1972.

Martin P. Wound healing-aiming for perfect skin regeneration. Science 276:75–81, 1997.

Marx JL. Cell growth control comes under scrutiny. Science 239:1093–1094, 1988.

Marzo I, Brenner C, Zamzami N, et al. Bax and adenine nucleotide cooperate in mitochondrial control of apoptosis. Science 281:2027–2031, 1998.

Michalopoulos GK, DeFrances M. Liver regeneration. Science 276:60–66, 1997.

Mignotte B, Vayssiere JL. Mitochondria and apoptosis. Eur J Biochem 252:1–15, 1998.

Omerod MG. The study of apoptotic cells by flow cytometry. Leukemia 12:1013–1025, 1998.

Policard A, Bessis M. Micropinocytosis and rhopheocytosis. Nature 194:110–111, 1962.

Rowan S, Fisher DE. Mechanisms of apoptotic cell death. Leukemia 11:457–465, 1997.

Rustad RC. Pinocytosis. Sci Am 204:121–130, 1961.

Sasano H, Yamaki H, Nagura H. Detection of apoptotic cells in cytology specimens: An application of TdT-mediated dUTP-biotin nick end labeling to cell smears. Diagn Cytopathol 18:398–402, 1998.

Sbarra AJ, Karnovsky ML. The biochemical basis of phagocytosis. 1. Metabolic changes during the ingestion of particles by polymorphonuclear leukocytes. J Biol Chem 234:1355–1362, 1959.

Schwartzman RA, Cidlowski JA. Apoptosis: The biochemistry and molecular biology of programmed cell death. Endocr Rev 14:133–151, 1993.

Searle J, Kerr JFR, Bishop CJ. Necrosis and apoptosis: Distinct modes of cell death with fundamentally different significance. Pathol Annual 17:229–259, 1982.

Sen S, D'Incalci M. Apoptosis. Biochemical events and relevance to cancer chemotherapy. FEBS Letters 307:122–126, 1992.

Snyderman R, Goetzl EJ. Molecular and cellular mechanisms of leukocyte chemotaxis. Science 213:830–837, 1981.

Soengas MS, Alarcon RM, Yoshida H, et al. Apaf-1 and caspase-9 in p53 dependent apoptosis and tumor inhibition. Science 284:156–159, 1999.

Steller H. Mechanisms and genes of cellular suicide. Science 267:1445–1449, 1995.

Tang DG, Porter AT. Apoptosis: A current molecular analysis. Pathol Onc Res 2:117–131, 1996.

Thompson CB. Apoptosis in the pathogenesis and treatment of disease. Science 267:1456–1462, 1995.

Thornberry NA, Lezebnik Y. Caspases: Enemies within. Science 281:1312–1316, 1998.

Trauth BC, Klas C, Peters AMJ, et al. Monoclonal antibody-mediated tumor regression by induction of apoptosis. Science 245:301–305, 1989.

Walker PR, Sikorska M. New aspects of the mechanism of DNA fragmentation in apoptosis. Biochem Cell Biol 75:287–299, 1997.

Wyllie AH. Apoptosis. ISI Atlas Sci Immunol 1:192–196, 1988.

Wyllie AH. The biology of cell death in tumours. Anticancer Res 5:131–136, 1985.

Wyllie AH, Kerr JFR, Currie AR. Cell death: The significance of apoptosis. Int Rev Cytol 68:251–356, 1980.

Zhang L, Yu J, Park BH, et al. Role of BAX in the apoptotic response to anticancer agents. Science 290:989–992, 2000.

Fundamental Concepts of Neoplasia: Benign Tumors and Cancer

7

The term **neoplasia** (from Greek, *neo* = new and *plasis* = a moulding) indicates the formation of new tissue or a **tumor** (from Latin for swelling) that may be benign or malignant. The primary task of diagnostic cytology is the microscopic diagnosis and differential diagnosis of malignant tumors or cancers and their precursor lesions. This chapter presents an overview of these groups of diseases that will attempt to correlate current developments in basic research with a description of morphologic changes observed in tissues and cells.

BRIEF HISTORICAL OVERVIEW

Cancer has been recognized by ancient Greeks and Romans as **visible and palpable swellings or tumors,** affecting various parts of the human body. In fact, the very name of cancer (from Greek, *karkinos,* and Latin, *cancer* = crab) reflects the invasive properties of the tumors that spread into the adjacent tissues and grossly mimic the configuration of a crab and its legs. Ancient Greeks were even aware that the prognosis of a *karkinoma* (**carcinoma**) of the breast was poor but also cited alleged examples of healing the disease by amputation. Over many centuries, numerous attempts were made based on clinical and autopsy observations to separate "tumors" caused by benign disorders, such as inflammation, from those that inexorably progressed and killed the patient, or true cancers. These distinctions could not be objectively substantiated until the introduction of the microscope as a tool of research. As was narrated in Chapter 1, the first recognition of microscopic differences between malignant and benign cells is attributed to Johannes Müller (1836). Müller's work stimulated numerous investigators, including his student Rudolf Virchow, considered to be the founder of contemporary pathology, and led to the recognition of various forms of human cancer in the 19th century. The observations on microscopic makeup of cancer subsequently led to the recognition of precursor lesions or precancerous states. The reader interested in the history of evolution of early human thoughts pertaining to cancer is referred to the books by M.B. Shimkin (1976), L.J. Rather (1978), and to the first chapter of this book.

In the first half of the 20th century, many attempts were made to shed light on the causes and sequence of events in cancer. Only a very few of these contributions can be mentioned here. As early as 1906, Boveri suggested that cancers are caused by chromosomal abnormalities. Differences in glucose metabolism between benign and cancerous cells were documented by Otto Warburg (1926), who believed that cancer was caused by insufficient oxygenation of cells or anoxia. Early measurements of cell components documented differences in nuclear and nucleolar sizes between benign and malignant lesions of the same organs (Haumeder, 1933; Schairer, 1935). The investigations of the sequence of events in experimental cancer supported the concept of two stages of development—**initiation** and **promotion.** The principal contributors of this theory were Friedwald and Rous (1944) and Berenblum and his associates (summary in 1974) who documented that cancer of the skin in animals (usually rabbits) may be produced more efficiently if the target organ, treated with a carcinogenic agent (such as tar) was treated with a second, noncarcinogenic agent, acting as a promoter. Knudson (1971, 1976) proposed the **"two hit" theory of cancer,** in reference to retinoblastoma, a tumor of the eye. The theory assumed that two events may be necessary for this cancer to occur—a genetic error that may be either congenital or acquired, followed by another carcinogenic event that again could be either genetic or acquired. With the discovery that the **retinoblastoma gene** (Rb gene; see below) is damaged or absent in some patients with retinoblastoma, the theory has proved to be correct. Subsequent developments in molecular studies of cancer led to the discovery of numerous **tumor-promoting genes (oncogenes)** and **tumor suppressor genes,** discussed later. It has been documented within recent years that the transformation of normal cells into cancerous cells is a **multistep genetic process** that is extremely complex. It is virtually certain today that carcinogenesis in various organs may follow different and, perhaps, multiple pathways. So far, there are only a very few genetic abnormalities that may represent common denominators of several cancers, such as the **mutations of the p53 gene,** discussed later, but the events preceding these mutations are in most cases still hypothetical and obscure.

None of these observations has shed much light on the morphologic and behavioral differences between cancer cells and benign cells, which are the principal topics of this book. Nonetheless, there is no further doubt that **all tumors, whether benign or malignant, are genetic diseases of cells.**

BENIGN TUMORS

Definition

Benign tumors are **focal and limited proliferations of morphologically normal or nearly normal cells, except for their abnormal arrangement and quantity.** Benign tumors may occur in any tissue or organ and are characterized by:

- **Limited growth**
- **A connective tissue capsule**
- **The inability to either invade adjacent tissue or metastasize**

Classification

The most common benign tumors of epithelial origin are **papillomas,** usually derived from the squamous epithelium or its variants, such as the urothelium lining the lower urinary tract, and **adenomas** or **polyps,** derived from glandular epithelia (Fig. 7-1). Papillomas and polyps are visible to the eye of the examiner as pale or reddish protrusions from the surface of the epithelium of the affected organ. Microscopically, these tumors are characterized by a proliferation of epithelial cells, surrounding a core composed of connective tissue and capillary vessels. In some benign tumors of epithelial origin, such as **fibroadenomas of the breast,** the relationship of the epithelial structures and connective tissue is complex (see Chap. 29). Benign tumors **may also originate from any type of supportive tissue** (e.g., fat, muscle, bone) and usually **carry the name of the tissue of origin,** such as **lipoma, myoma, or osteoma** (Table 7-1).

Causes

The causes of benign tumors have not been fully elucidated but, in some of these tumors, **chromosomal abnormalities** have been observed (see Chap. 4 and Mitelman, 1991). The molecular significance of these abnormalities is not clear at this time. More importantly, Vogelstein and his group at Johns Hopkins observed that a **tumor suppressor gene named APC** (from **a**denomatous **p**olyposis **c**oli) is frequently mutated in benign polyps of patients with familial polyposis of colon, a disease characterized by innumerable colonic polyps and often leading to colon cancer. This gene

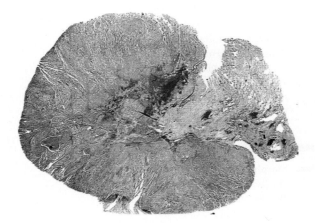

Figure 7-1   **Low-power view of rectal polyp.** Note the central stalk of connective tissue and the benign glandular epithelium forming a mushroom around the stalk but also covering the stalk.

TABLE 7-1

CLASSIFICATION AND NOMENCLATURE OF HUMAN TUMORS*

Tissue Origin	Benign	Malignant (Cancer)
Stratified protective epithelium	Papilloma	Squamous or epidermoid carcinoma; urothelial carcinoma
Columnar epithelium, including that of glands	Adenoma or polyp	Adenocarcinoma, mucoepidermoid carcinoma
		Occasionally epidermoid carcinoma
Mesothelia	Benign mesothelioma	Malignant mesothelioma
Supportive tissues of mesodermal origin	...omas according to the type of tissue involved (i.e., fat-lipoma, bone-osteoma)	Sarcoma (with designation of tissue type; i.e., liposarcoma, osteogenic sarcoma)
Lymphoid tissues	Hyperplasia	Malignant lymphomas
Blood cells		Leukemia
Tumors composed of several varieties of tissue	Benign teratomas	Malignant teratomas

* This simplified classification, although allowing a general orientation in tumor types, should not be taken too rigidly. A variety of malignant tumors may show a mixture of different types. Furthermore, combinations of sarcomas and carcinomas may occur. Special designations have been attached to a variety of benign and malignant neoplasms of some organs or systems. As the need arises, such diseases will be described in the text.

appears to **interfere with adhesion molecules maintaining the normal integrity of colonic epithelium.** The mutation of the APC gene may be a stepping stone to the development of colonic cancer (summary in Kinzer and Vogelstein, 1996). Although at this time no definitive information is available in reference to other benign tumors, it appears likely that they also occur as a consequence of mutations affecting genes essential in maintaining the normal relationship of cells.

Another known cause of benign tumors is certain **viruses.** Thus, **papillomaviruses** may cause benign tumors in various species of animals. Certain types of the human papillomaviruses (HPVs) are the cause of benign skin and genital warts and papillomas of the larynx; other types, designated as "oncogenic," are implicated in the genesis of cancer of the uterine cervix and other organs (see Chap. 11). It has been shown that some of the protein products, of the oncogenic types (which may also be involved in the formation of benign tumors), interact with protein products of genes controlling replication of DNA (p53) and the cell cycle (Rb) (see Chap. 11). No such information is available in reference to HPVs associated with benign tumors and the mechanisms of formation of warts remain an enigma at this time.

Cytologic Features

In general, **the cells of benign epithelial tumors differ little from normal,** although they may display evidence of proliferative activity in the form of mitotic figures. In general, the epithelial cells tend to **adhere well to each other** and form flat clusters of cells with clear cytoplasm and small nuclei, wherein cell borders are clearly recognized, resulting in the so-called **honeycomb effect** (Fig. 7-2).

Benign tumors of mesenchymal origin, such as tumors of fat **(lipomas),** smooth muscle **(leiomyomas),** or connective tissue **(fibromas),** can be sampled only by needle aspiration biopsies. In smears, the **cell population resembles the normal cells of tissue of origin** (i.e., fat cells, smooth muscle cells, or fibroblasts). As a warning, some malignant tumors of the same derivation may be composed of cells that differ little from their benign counterpart (see Chap. 24).

However, some benign tumors, such as **tumors of endo-**

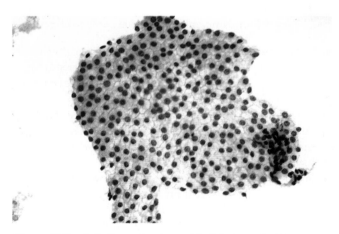

Figure 7-2 Cells from a benign epithelial tumor. In this example from prostatic hyperplasia, there is a flat sheet of cells of nearly identical sizes. The cell borders among cells are recognizable as thin lines, giving the "honeycomb" effect.

crine or nerve origin, **may show significant abnormalities in the form of large, hyperchromatic, sometimes multiple nuclei** that explain why the DNA pattern of such tumors may be abnormal (Agarwal et al, 1991). In the presence of such abnormal cells, the cytologic diagnosis of benign tumors may be very difficult. Benign tumors caused by human papillomaviruses, such as skin warts and condylomas of the genital tract or bladder, may show significant cell abnormalities that may mimic cancer to perfection.

Benign tumors of many organs show specific microscopic features that may allow their precise recognition, as will be discussed in detail in appropriate chapters. On the other hand, in some organs, such as the endometrium, the distinction between benign proliferative processes, known as atypical hyperplasia, and low-grade cancer may depend on the preference of the observer (see Chap. 14).

Behavior

Some benign tumors may **regress spontaneously,** such as skin warts. However, most benign tumors do not regress but achieve a certain size and then either stop growing or continue to grow at a very slow rate. Still, the size alone may interfere with normal organ function and may require removal. Other reasons for therapy may be necrosis or hemorrhage within the benign tumor that may cause acute discomfort to the patient. Also, a **benign tumor may occasionally give rise to a malignant tumor** although, on the whole, this is a **rare event.** The mechanisms and causes of such transformations are unknown, except for the colon, where it was shown, in high-risk populations, that a series of successive genetic abnormalities may lead from benign colonic polyps to cancer of the colon (see below).

MALIGNANT TUMORS (CANCERS)

Definition

Fully developed primary malignant tumors are characterized by several fundamental features that apply to all cancers:

- **Autonomous proliferation** of morphologically abnormal cells results in abnormal, often characteristic tissue patterns and leads to the formation of a visible or palpable swelling or tumor.
- **Invasive growth** involves growth of cancerous tissue beyond the boundaries of tissue of origin. The invasion may extend into adjacent tissues of the same organ and beyond.
- **Formation of metastases** involves growth of colonies of cancer cells in distant organs, which again can proliferate in an autonomous fashion. For metastases to occur, the cancer cells must have the ability to enter either the lymphatic or blood vessels. Spread of cancer through lymphatics is known as **lymphatic spread** and leads to metastases to lymph nodes. Spread of cancer

through blood vessels is known as **hematogenous spread** and may result in metastases to any organ in the body, whether adjacent to the tumor or distant (see Chap. 43).

The terms **recurrent cancer** and **recurrence** indicate a relapse of a treated tumor.

Classification

Cancers originating from epithelial structures or glands are known as **carcinomas,** whereas cancers derived from tissues of middle embryonal layer origin (such as connective tissue, muscle, bone) are classified as **sarcomas.** The names of yet other cancers of highly specialized organs or tissues may reflect their origin, for example, **thymus = thymoma** and **mesothelium = mesothelioma.** Cancers of blood cells are known as **leukemias,** and cancers of the lymphatic system as **lymphomas** (see Table 7-1).

Carcinomas and sarcomas may be further classified according to the type of tissue of origin, which is often reflected in the component cells. Carcinomas derived from **squamous epithelium,** or showing features of this epithelial type, are classified as **squamous or epidermoid carcinomas.** In this text, the term "squamous carcinoma" will be applied to tumors with conspicuous keratin formation, whereas tumors with limited or no obvious keratin formation will be referred to as "epidermoid carcinomas." Carcinomas derived from **gland-forming epithelium** or forming glands are classified as **adenocarcinomas.** There are also carcinomas that may combine the features of these two types of cancer and are, therefore, known as **adenosquamous** or **mucoepidermoid carcinomas.** Carcinomas of highly specialized organs may reflect the tissue of origin, for example, **hepatoma,** a tumor of liver cells.

Sarcomas are also classified according to the tissue of origin, such as **bone (osteosarcoma), muscle (myosarcoma),** and connective tissue or **fibroblasts (fibrosarcoma).** Again, tumors derived from highly specialized tissues may carry the name of the tissue of origin, for example, **glial cells** of the central nervous system (**glioma**) or pigment-forming cells, melanoblasts (**melanomas**).

Yet other tumors may show **combinations of several tissue types (hamartomas and teratomas),** or reflect certain common properties, such as production of hormones (**endocrine tumors**). In certain age groups, tumors that show similar morphologic characteristics (although not cells of origin) have been grouped together as **small-cell malignant tumors of childhood.** The feature of all these tumors will be discussed in appropriate chapters.

Immunochemistry may be of significant help in classifying tumors of uncertain origin or type (see below and Chap. 45).

Risk Factors and Geographic Distribution

Only about 5% of all malignant tumors occur in children and young adults. Most cancers are observed in people past the age of 50. In fact, it can be stated that **advancing age is a risk factor for cancer.** The reasons for this are speculative and most likely are based on reduced ability of the older organism to control genetic abnormalities that are likely to occur throughout the life of an individual but are better controlled in the younger age groups. A possible candidate is capping of chromosomes by **telomeres** that protect the ends of chromosomes from injury and that are reduced with age (de Lange, 2001). Another important risk factor is **immunosuppression,** particularly in patients with AIDS (Frisch et al, 2001).

Epidemiologic data from various continents and countries suggest that **certain cancer types may preferentially occur in certain populations.** For example, gastric cancer is very common in the Japanese, whereas cancer of the nasopharynx and esophagus is common in the Chinese. On the other hand, prostatic cancer is much less frequent in Japan than in the United States, where the disease is particularly common among African-Americans. Such examples could be multiplied. Epidemiologic studies have attempted to identify the causes of such events with modest success. It is known, for example, that among the Japanese living in Hawaii and the mainland United States, the rate of gastric carcinoma drops rapidly, and the change is attributed to a different diet. Several other environmental risk factors have been identified, but there are still huge gaps in our understanding of these events. The search for factors that may account for the geographic disparities is still in progress.

Causes

The first observations on the causes of human cancer had to do with **environmental factors.** Thus, an epidemic of lung cancer was observed in the 1880s in Bohemia (today the Czech Republic) in miners extracting tar that was subsequently shown to be radioactive (see Chap. 20). In the 1890s, after the onset of industrial production of organic chemicals, some chemicals were shown to cause bladder tumors (see Chap. 23). Asbestos has been linked with malignant tumors of the serous membranes (mesotheliomas; see Chap. 26), cigarette smoking with lung cancer, and exposure to ultraviolet radiation with skin cancers and melanomas. Many of these relationships have been studied by **cancer epidemiology,** a science that attempts to document in an objective, statistically valid fashion the relationship of various factors to cancer.

Another association of cancer is with infectious agents, such as **viruses** and **bacteria** (Parsonnet, 1999). Several **RNA viruses,** today known as retroviruses, have been shown to cause malignant tumors and leukemias in mice and other rodents, among them mammary carcinoma (Bittner, 1947; Porter and Thompson, 1948) and erythroleukemia in mice (de Harven, 1962). The ability of certain **DNA viruses,** such as the simian virus 40 (SV 40), to modify the features and the behavior of cells in culture has also been documented (Dulbecco, 1964). Such modified cells, when injected into the experimental animal, produce tumors capable of metastases.

In humans, a number of **DNA viruses** have been impli-

cated in various malignant processes. As previously mentioned, **human papillomaviruses (HPVs)** of certain types have been linked with cancer of the uterine cervix (see Chap. 11) and the esophagus (see Chap. 24). Another DNA virus, the **Epstein-Barr virus (EB virus)** was implicated in Burkitt's lymphoma and nasopharyngeal carcinoma. **Virus of hepatitis B** has been implicated in malignant tumors of the liver (hepatomas), whereas a newly discovered **herpes virus type 8** has been found in association with vascular tumors, known as Kaposi's sarcoma, and certain types of malignant lymphomas in patients with AIDS.

Bacteria, notably *Helicobacter pylori,* have now been implicated in the origin of **gastric carcinoma** and, perhaps, the uncommon **gastrointestinal stromal tumors (GISTs)** (see Chap. 24).

However, **the vast majority of human cancers occur in the absence of any known risk factors.** With the onset of molecular biology, the study of members of families with known high risk for certain cancers (**cancer syndromes;** see below) has led to the observations that they carried certain genetic abnormalities that were either recessive or dominant. These abnormalities have led to the studies of molecular underpinning of the events leading to cancer, discussed below.

Grading and Staging

Grading of cancers is a subjective method of analysis of cancers that attempts to describe the histologic (and sometimes cytologic) **level of deviation from normal tissue or cells of origin. Grading is expressed in Roman numbers or equivalent phrases.** If the histologic pattern of a cancer resembles closely the makeup of the normal tissue, and is composed of cells that closely resemble normal, it may be graded as **well differentiated,** or **grade I.** On the other extreme are cancers that barely resemble the tissue of origin, if at all, and are composed of cells that differ significantly from normal; such cancers can be classified as **poorly differentiated,** or **grade III.** Most cancers fall somewhere between the two extremes and are therefore classified as **moderately well differentiated,** or **grade II.** There are also systems of **grading based** exclusively on the **configuration of nuclei of cancer cells,** particularly in breast cancer (see Chap. 29). Several objective methods of measurements of cancer cells and their nuclei have been introduced to replace subjective grading (review in Koss, 1982). Grading may have some bearing on behavior of cancer, inasmuch as poorly differentiated tumors may be more aggressive than well differentiated. Grading is most valuable as a modifier of cancer staging.

Staging of cancers is based on an internationally accepted code **to assess the spread of cancer at the time of diagnosis. The TNM system** includes tumor size and extent of invasion (**T**), the involvement of the regional lymph nodes by metastases (**N**), and the presence or absence of distant metastases (**M**). The **T** group is usually subclassified and ranges from Tis (tumor in situ) or To, indicating a cancer confined to the tissue or organ of origin, to T1, T2,

T3 and T4, indicating tumor size and, in some instances, the depth of invasion.

Clinical staging is based on the results of inspection and palpation, now usually supplemented by radiologic techniques, such as magnetic resonance imaging (MRI) or ultrasound. **Pathologic staging** is based on examination of tissues surgically removed from the patient. The pathologic stage of a tumor may be higher than the clinical stage because, on microscopic examination, spread of cancer may be discovered in tissues that were clinically not suspect of harboring disease. **The TNM system (sometimes combined with grading) is particularly useful in assessing the prognosis.** To tumors have a much better outcome than T3 or T4 tumors. Tumors without metastases have a better prognosis than tumors with metastases. The TNM system is very useful in comparing the results of treatment of various malignant diseases in different institutions.

Behavior

In principle, all invasive cancers, if untreated, should lead to the death of the patient. However, even in untreated patients, **the behavior of cancers may be extremely variable;** some types of malignant tumors progress very slowly and take many years to spread beyond the site of origin, whereas other cancers progress and metastasize very rapidly, such as some cancers composed of small, primitive cells. In experimental systems, arrest and regression of malignant tumors was accomplished by a variety of manipulations (e.g., Silagy and Bruce, 1970) or by replacement of damaged genes and chromosomes. There is no doubt that occasionally, but very rarely, a **spontaneous regression** of human cancer can occur. Gene replacement therapy, however, has not been successful to date in human cancer.

Although **statistical data** are available today in reference to **prognosis** of most tumor types, experience shows that the **rules do not always apply to individual patients.** Except for the recognition of some cancer types with notoriously rapid progression, the classification of tumors by histologic (or cytologic) types may have limited bearing on behavior that is sometimes dependent on the organ of origin. For example, patients with squamous carcinomas of the cervix have a generally better prognosis and live longer than patients with cancers of identical type of the esophagus. As a group, adenocarcinomas of the breast are likely to be more aggressive and produce metastases sooner and more frequently than adenocarcinomas of the endometrium. In most common cancers, the behavior is better correlated with tumor stage than histologic type or grade, although grading may be a modifier of staging. The behavior of tumors of the same stage but different grades may vary. Tumors of higher grade often behave in a more aggressive fashion.

PRECURSOR LESIONS OF HUMAN CANCER

Although the concepts of precursor lesions of cancers were proposed in the early years of the 20th century (see Chap. 1),

the existence and significance of these processes was firmly established during the last half of the 20th century. It is now known, with certainty, that **tumors of epithelial tissue origin or carcinomas are preceded by abnormalities confined to the epithelium** (Fig. 7-3). All these precursor lesions were initially classified as **carcinoma in situ,** and are now subdivided into several categories with names such as **dysplasia** or **intraepithelial neoplasia. Some of these lesions may be graded** by numbers (grade I, II, or III); by

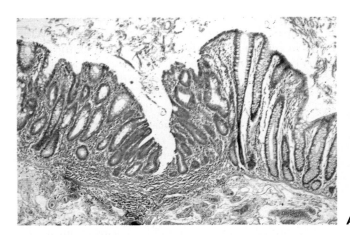

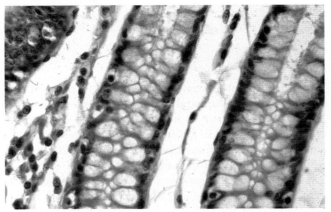

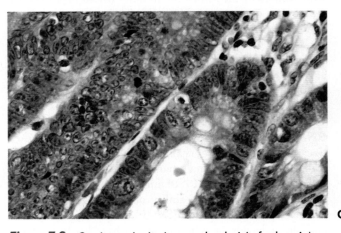

Figure 7-3 Carcinoma in situ (severe dysplasia) of colon. *A.* Low power view of normal (*right*) and **abnormal** (*left*) colonic epithelium. *B,C.* The differences between the makeup of benign glands (*B*) lined by mucus-producing cells with small nuclei, and the malignant epithelium (*C*) composed of cells with no secretory function, very large nuclei, and evidence of mitotic activity are shown.

adjectives, such as "mild," "moderate," or "severe"; or, within recent years, as **"low-grade"** or **"high-grade"** lesions. The **grading** has been used to indicate the makeup of these lesions—that is, the **degree of morphologic abnormality**—when compared with normal tissue of origin. Lesions resembling closely the epithelium of origin, albeit composed of abnormal cells, are classified as "low grade." Lesions showing less or little resemblance to the epithelium of origin, usually composed of small abnormal cells, are classified as "high grade." The grading has some bearing on the behavior of the precursor lesions, although in practice it has a rather **limited value and reproducibility,** as will be set forth in appropriate chapters.

The **general characteristics of precursor lesions of carcinomas** are as follows:

- **The lesions are confined to the epithelium of origin.**
- **They are composed of** cells showing abnormalities that are similar but not necessarily identical to fully developed cancers.
- **Their discovery is usually the result of a systematic search,** usually by cytologic techniques (e.g., in the uterine cervix, lung, oral cavity, urinary bladder, or esophagus) or incidental biopsies (e.g., colon). Although some precursor lesions may produce clinical abnormalities visible to the eye, such as redness, they do not form visible tumors. The discovery of precursor lesions is one of the main tasks of diagnostic cytology.
- **The behavior of precancerous lesions is unpredictable.** Some of these lesions are capable of progression to invasive cancer but the likelihood of **progression varies significantly from organ to organ.** For example, in the urinary bladder at least 70% to 80% of untreated precursor lesions (flat carcinomas in situ and related lesions) will progress to invasive cancer, whereas, in the uterine cervix, the likelihood of progression does not exceed 20% (see Chaps. 11 and 23). The data for other organs are not secure because the system of discovery of precancerous lesions is not efficient. It must be noted that molecular genetic studies of precancerous lesions of the urinary bladder disclosed the presence of abnormalities that may also be observed in fully developed cancer. Similar observations were made in the sequence of events leading to cancer of the colon.

Progression of Intraepithelial Lesions to Invasive Cancer

Epidemiologic studies have shown that, as a general rule, precursor lesions occur in persons several years younger than persons with invasive cancer of the same type. Hence, it is assumed that **several years are required for an intraepithelial lesion to progress to invasive cancer.** For invasion to take place, the cells of the precursor lesion must break through the barrier separating the epithelium from the underlying connective tissue and, hence, **must breach the basement membrane.** One of two possible events must be assumed:

- The cells composing the precancerous lesions acquire new characteristics that allow them to breach the basement membrane.
- The basement membrane becomes altered and becomes a porous barrier to the cells.

Although the molecular mechanisms of such events are unknown at this time, there is evidence that some of the genes involved in carcinogenesis affect the adhesion molecules on cell membranes (see below). This relationship, when unraveled, may explain the mechanisms of invasion. Another, as yet unexplored, possibility is that the **basement membrane is breached by ingrowing or outgrowing capillary vessels,** thus paving the way for cancer cells to escape their confinement.

CURRENT TRENDS IN MOLECULAR BIOLOGY OF HUMAN CANCERS

Overview of the Problem

Cancer is a disease of cells that escape the control mechanisms of orderly cell growth and acquire the ability to proliferate, invade normal tissues, and metastasize. It is generally assumed that cancer is a **clonal disorder derived** from a single transformed cell (see below). The fundamental research issue was to determine whether cancer was the result of stimulation of cell growth, damage to the mechanisms regulating normal cell replication, or both. Marx (1986) referred to this dilemma as the Yin and Yang of cell growth control, referring to the old Chinese concept of contradictory forces in nature.

There were several significant problems with the study of molecular events in cancer. One of them was the **heterogeneity of cancer cells**—the observation that few, if any, cancer cells were identical. This phenomenon of cancer cell diversity was extensively studied by Fidler et al (1982, 1985), who documented that, in experimental tumors in mice, some cancer cells were capable of forming metastases and others were not. It has also been known for several years that the number and type of chromosomal abnormalities increased with the progression of cancer, reflecting the genomic instability in the cancer cells (recent review in Kiberts and Marx, 2002). Nowell (1976), who studied this phenomenon in leukemia, called it **clonal evolution.** In cytogenetic studies of fully developed solid cancers, the number of chromosomes in individual cancer cells is often variable and other aberrations of chromosomes may also occur (see Chap. 4). It is not an exaggeration to state that advanced human cancer represents a **state of genetic chaos.** The diversity of cancer cells, even within the same tumor, made it very difficult to assess whether observed molecular genetic abnormalities had universal significance or were merely an incidental single event (recent reviews in Tomlison et al, 2000, and Hahn and Weinberg, 2002).

The type of material that was available to the basic science investigators also posed similar problems. Fragments of cancerous tissues available for such purposes were usually derived from advanced tumors that were likely to show a great deal of heterogeneity and genetic disarray. In vitro culture of human cancers is technically difficult, and the cell lines derived therefrom usually represented a single clone of cells that is not necessarily representative of the primary tumor.

Further complications arose when DNA or RNA were extracted from such tissue samples for molecular analysis. Besides tumor cells, such tissues always contained an admixture of benign cells from blood vessels, connective tissue stroma, inflammatory cells, and remnants of the normal organ of origin. The question as to what constituted tumor-specific findings, rather than findings attributable to normal cells, was often difficult to resolve. Many of these difficulties persist.

Some solutions to these dilemmas came from several unrelated sources. One of them was the discovery of **growth-promoting DNA sequences,** known as **oncogenes,** and their precursor molecules, the **protooncogenes,** in an experimental system of transformed rodent cells. The protooncogenes and oncogenes could be isolated and sequenced. The search could now begin for matching sequences in the DNA extracted from normal human tissues and cancer. The protooncogenes and oncogenes and their role in cancer are described below.

Another breakthrough occurred with the study of the patterns of occurrence of **retinoblastoma,** an uncommon malignant tumor of the retina in children. Knudson (1971) anticipated that a fundamental genetic abnormality accounted for the familial pattern of this disease. This abnormality was subsequently identified as a deficiency or absence of a gene located on chromosome 13, which was named the **retinoblastoma (Rb) gene** (see below for further discussion). Similar studies of **families with "cancer syndromes"** were also conducted. Such families, described by a number of investigators (Gardner, 1962; Li and Fraumeni, 1969; summaries in Lynch and Lynch, 1993; Fearon, 1997; Varley et al, 1997; Frank 2001) were characterized by a high frequency of occurrence of cancers in various organs. The most important cancer syndromes are listed in Table 7-2. By a variety of techniques known as **linkage analysis,** the genetic abnormalities could be identified and the genes localized—first to chromosomes, then to segments of chromosomes, and, finally, to the specific location on the affected chromosome. The isolation and sequencing of such genes were an essential step in studying their function and interaction with other genes.

Of special value in this research were **families with congenital polyposis of the colon,** a disease process in which the patients develop innumerable benign colonic polyps and, unless treated, invasive cancer of the colon sooner or later. A group at The Johns Hopkins medical institutions in Baltimore, MD, led by Vogelstein, Fearon, and others, undertook a systematic study of genetic changes occurring

---

TABLE 7-2

MOLECULAR GENETICS OF SOME CANCER SYNDROMES PERTINENT TO DIAGNOSTIC CYTOLOGY

Syndrome	Tumor Suppressor Gene	Chromosomal Location	Clinical Significance— Target Organs	Cytologic Targets
Familial polyposis coli	APC	5 q	colon cancer	metastatic cancer (liver, effusions, etc.)
Hereditary retinoblastoma	RB 1	13 q	eye: retinoblastoma bone: osteosarcoma	primary or metastatic
Breast cancer (less commonly ovarian and tubal cancer)	BRCA 1 BRCA 2	17 q 13 p	breast, ovary breast, pancreas	primary or metastatic primary or metastatic
Li-Fraumeni	p53	17 p	diverse malignant tumors	primary or metastatic
Multiple endocrine neoplasia (MEN 1)	MEN 1	11 q	tumors of endocrine organs [thyroid, parathyroid, adrenal, pancreas (islands of Langerhans), pituitary]	primary or metastatic
Multiple endocrine neoplasia (MEN 2)	RET*	10 q	thyroid: medullary carcinoma, adrenal: pheochromocytoma	primary or metastatic
Renal ca (part of von Hippel-Lindau syndrome)	VHL	3 p	kidney: carcinoma	primary or metastatic
Wilms' tumor	WT 1	11 p	kidney: Wilms' tumor	primary or metastatic
Peutz-Jeghers syndrome	STK 11+	19 p	associated with minimal deviation endocervical adenocarcinoma	endocervical adenocarcinoma
Hereditary melanoma	P16 CDK4	9 q 12 q	skin: malignant melanoma	metastatic tumors

* oncogene
+ inactivation of protein kinases

q = long arm of chromosome
p = short arm of chromosome

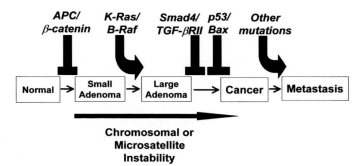

Figure 7-4 Sequence of molecular events in the development of carcinoma of colon. (Courtesy of Dr. Bert Vogelstein, Johns Hopkins Medical Institutions, Baltimore, MD.)

in benign colonic polyps, polyps with atypical features, early cancer, and invasive colonic cancer. These studies led to a **model of carcinogenesis** in the colon that postulated a sequence of genetic abnormalities leading from normal epithelium to polyps to cancer (Fig. 7-4). Although this model is not likely to be applicable to all cancers of the colon, let alone other organs, it stimulated a great deal of research on carcinogenesis. Perhaps the most important developments, resulting directly or indirectly from the studies of familial cancer, were the discovery of the role played by regulatory genes **(tumor suppressor genes) in the events of cell cycle** and the **relationship of genes involved in cancer genesis with adhesion molecules** that regulate the relationship of cells to each other and to the underlying stroma. These observations are discussed below.

Another development that proved to be of significance in this research was the **Human Genome Project,** which provided a great deal of information on the distribution of genes on human chromosomes. Although the map of the human genome has been completed and the significance and role played by most of the genes remain unknown, commercial probes to many of these genes have become available that allow the study of genetic abnormalities in various human cancers. The emerging information is, unfortunately, enormously complex and so far has shed little light on the initial events, or sequence of events, in solid human cancer. Still, the genome project led to the discovery of the human breast cancer genes BRCA1 and BRCA2, to be discussed below.

Protooncogenes and Oncogenes

The first significant observation shedding light on the molecular mechanisms of cancer was the discovery of **oncogenes** in the 1980s (summary in Bishop, 1987). The oncogenes were first identified in experimental systems in which cultured, benign rodent cells were infected with **oncogenic RNA viruses (retroviruses)** and were transformed into cells with malignant features. The viral RNA, by means of the enzyme reverse transcriptase is capable of producing cDNA that is incorporated into the native DNA (genome) of the cell, which becomes the source of viral replication. It has been observed that **regulatory genes of host DNA, named protooncogenes,** which may be incidentally appropriated by the viral genome, **are essential in the transformation of the infected cells into cells with malignant features.** The "stolen" **host cell genes,** when either **overexpressed or modified** (mutated), **become a growth-promoting factor that has been named an oncogene** (Fig. 7-5). The first oncogenes discovered were named *ras* (**r**etrovirus-**a**ssociated **s**arcoma or **ra**t **s**arcoma). Several variants of the *ras* oncogenes were subsequently discovered and described with various prefixes, such as **Ki-*ras*, Ha-*ras*,** and **N-*ras*,** reflecting the initials of the investigators.

Shortly after the discovery of the first protooncogenes and oncogenes and their sequencing, their presence could be documented by Southern blotting and similar techniques in DNA from normal human tissues, in human tumors, and in cell lines derived therefrom. On the assumption that the study of oncogenes will provide the clue to the secrets

Retroviruses (RNA)

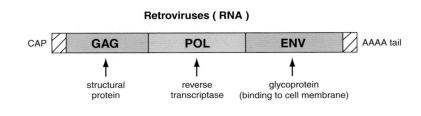

Oncogenic Retrovirus (Rous')

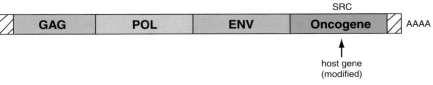

Figure 7-5 Schematic representation of the origin of an oncogene (sarcoma or src gene) in an experimental system in which malignant transformation of cultured cells is achieved by means of a retrovirus.

of abnormal cell proliferation in cancer, the search for other oncogenes and growth-promoting factors began in earnest and led to the discovery of a large number of such genes that have now been sequenced and traced to their chromosomal sites.

Two fundamental modes of oncogene function have been identified—**overexpression (amplification)** of a normal protooncogene product, and a **point mutation,** a single nucleotide change in an exon of the gene, leading to a modified protein product. It is known that some oncogenes can be activated because their original chromosomal site has been disturbed by breakage and **translocation of chromosomal segments,** as observed in lymphomas and leukemias (see below). They may also be overexpressed in chromosomal fragments, such as C-*myc* oncogene, observed in the **double-minute chromosomes** of neuroblastoma (see Chap. 4).

The protooncogenes and the oncogenes exercise their activity **through their protein products,** many of which have been identified. For example, the genes of the *ras* family encode a group of proteins of 21,000 daltons, known as p21. Contrary to the initial hopes that all oncogenes would have a simple, well-defined function in the transformation of benign into malignant cells, it is now evident that the oncogenes are a diverse family of genes, with different locations within the cell and different functions. Several oncogenes have been traced to the nucleus (e.g., *myc, myb, fos, jun*), presumably interacting directly with DNA. Other proteins encoded by oncogenes have an affinity for cell membranes (e.g., *ras, src, neu*) or the cytoplasm (e.g., *mos*). These latter two groups of oncogenes appear to interact, on the one hand, with cytoplasmic and cell membrane receptors and, on the other hand, with enzymes, such as tyrosine kinase, that play a role in DNA replication. It is possible that the oncogenes located on cell membranes are instrumental in capturing circulating growth factors that stimulate proliferation of cells.

In **solid human tumors,** the activation or overexpression of various oncogenes has been shown to be a **common event,** unlikely to establish a simple cause-effect relationship between oncogene activation and the occurrence of human cancer. The presence of oncogene products could be demonstrated either by molecular biology techniques or by immunocytochemistry in many different human cancers. As an example, the presence of the *ras* oncogene product, p21, has been documented by us and others in gastric, colonic, and mammary cancer cells, and in several other human tumors (Czerniak et al, 1989, 1990, 1992). In cytochemical studies, it was noted that oncogene products are **variably expressed by cancer cells,** some of which stain strongly and some that do not stain at all, suggesting heterogeneity of oncogene expression. It is possible that the expression of the oncogene products is, to some extent, cell cycle dependent (Czerniak et al, 1987). With image analysis and flow cytometric techniques (see Chaps. 46 and 47), the amount of the reaction product can be measured (Fig. 7-6). Press et al (1993) stressed that immunocytologic microscopic techniques with specific antibodies are probably more reliable in assessing the expression of an oncogene in tissues than

is the Southern or northern blotting technique. The blotting techniques require the destruction of the tissue samples and, therefore, fail to provide information on the makeup of the destroyed tissue and on the proportion of normal cells in the sample.

However, there is no agreement on the diagnostic or prognostic value of such measurements in human solid tumors, with a few exceptions. For example, the elevated expression of the product of the **oncogene HER2** (also known as **c-erbB2),** a transmembrane receptor protein, indicates poor prognosis and rapid progression of breast cancers in about 25% of affected women (Slamon et al, 1989). In fact, an **antibody to the protein product of this gene** has been developed commercially for human use and is of benefit in prolonging life in some women with advanced metastatic breast cancer (see Chap. 29). This is one of the first indications that knowledge of the oncogenes or tumor-promoting factors may be of benefit to patients. Although oncogenes play an important role in human cancer, their precise role is complex (summary in Krontiris, 1995). Weinstein (2002) suggested that individual cancers are "addicted" to their specific oncogenes and suggested that oncogene suppression may lead to cure.

As on example, the drug Gleevac (Novarrtis) has been shown to be effective against chronic myclogenous leukemia by blocking the oncogenic protein **bcr = abl,** the product of chromosome translocation.

Tumor Suppressor Genes and Gatekeeper Genes

The oncogene story became even more complicated with the identification of genes known collectively as tumor suppressor genes or gatekeeper genes. As previously mentioned, this research has been stimulated by studies of **families with cancer syndromes** (recent summary in Fearon, 1997; see Table 7-2). The first such gene discovered was the **retinoblastoma (Rb) gene,** located on the short arm of chromosome 13. Retinoblastoma is an uncommon, highly malignant eye tumor of childhood that occurs in two forms: (1) a familial form, in which usually both eyes are affected, and (2) a sporadic form, in which one eye is affected. Following treatment of retinoblastoma, other cancers, such as osteogenic sarcoma, may develop in the affected children. Thus, the defect of the Rb gene may have multiple manifestations.

It was postulated by Knudson in 1971 that retinoblastomas are the consequence of two mutational events **(two-hit theory of cancer).** The familial form of retinoblastoma implied a hereditary defect of some sort, supplemented by a single additional sporadic mutation, leading to cancer. In the sporadic form, two mutational events were anticipated against a normal genetic background. In retinoblastoma, the gene on chromosome 13 was frequently deficient or absent, thus fulfilling the first requirement of Knudson's hypothesis. This gene has now been sequenced and its anti-tumor activity has been confirmed in vitro by Huang et al in 1988. It has been learned in recent years that the protein **product of the Rb gene regulates the expression** of one of the proteins regulating the cell cycle, known as **D cyclins,** which govern the transition of cells from G_0 to G_1 stage of

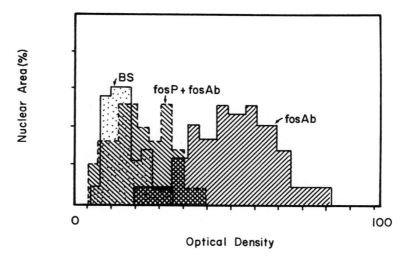

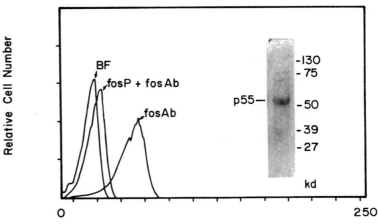

Figure 7-6 Measurement of *fos* p55 by computer-assisted image analysis (*top*) and flow cytometry (*bottom*). BS = background staining; *fos*P + *fos*Ab = antibody to *fos* product p55 blocked by p55; *fos*Ab = expression of unopposed antibody to p55; BF = background fluorescence. (*Bottom right*) Western blot of MCF7-KO protein extract incubated with antibody to c-*fos* p55. (Czerniak B, et al. Quantitation of oncogene products by computer-assisted image analysis and flow cytometry. J Histochem Cytochem 38:463, 1990.)

mitosis. It is postulated that **the absence of, or damage to, the Rb gene deregulates the cell cycle, leading to cancer.**

Another important regulatory gene is **p53**, a protein product of the gene located on the short arm of the chromosome 17 (Levine et al, 1991). p53 is a DNA binding protein that **regulates the transcription of DNA, its repair** by a cascade of other proteins, and is, therefore, considered to be a "**guardian of the genome**" (Lane, 1992). If a transcriptional error occurs, the replication is stopped until the error is repaired. The mechanism of arrest is mediated by a cell cycle inhibitor, protein $p21^{WAF1/CIP1}$, which is different from the p21 protein of the *ras* gene. If the repair is not executed, the cell may enter into the cycle of programmed cell death or **apoptosis,** discussed in detail in Chapter 6.

The natural p53 product is short-lived and difficult to demonstrate; however, a gene mutation leads to a modified protein that has a much longer life span and can be demonstrated by a variety of techniques, including immunocytochemistry. **Loss of heterozygosity of p53** (inactivation or mutation of one of the two identical genes within the cell) is a very **common event** in many human cancers of various organs, mainly in advanced stages (see later text). However, in some cancers, such as high-grade cancer of the endome-

trium, the mutation of p53 is presumed to occur as an early event (see Chap. 13). The presence of mutations of the Rb gene and of the p53 protein has been shown to confer a poor prognosis on some cancers, such as cancers of the bladder (Esrig et al, 1993; Sarkis et al, 1993), some malignant lymphomas (Ichikawa et al, 1997), and chondrosarcomas (Oshiro et al, 1998).

Other tumor suppressor genes include the recently identified **breast cancer genes, BRCA1 and BRCA2** (see Table 7-2). The mutations of these genes have been observed in a larger proportion of Jewesses of Eastern European (Ashkenazi) origin than in other comparable groups of women (recent summary in Hofmann and Schlag, 2000). Although some of these women are at an increased risk for breast, and, to a lesser extent, ovarian and tubal cancer, and deserve close follow-up, the extent of risk for any individual patient cannot be assessed. In some of these women, preventive measures, such as a prophylactic mastectomy and oophorectomy have been proposed (Schraq et al, 1997). Clearly, many such dilemmas will occur as new risk factors for cancer are discovered. Silencing of tumor suppressor genes may be caused by **methylation** that does not involve DNA mutations (recent summary in Herman and Baylin, 2003).

Another set of genes involved in malignant transformation of normal cells into cancer cells is the **susceptibility genes,** considered by Kinzer and Vogelstein (1998) as "**caretakers of the genome.**" These genes, when mutated or inactivated, contribute indirectly to the neoplastic process, probably by regulating the relationship of the transformed cells to connective tissue stroma. Such genes have been observed in a colon cancer syndrome known as the **hereditary nonpolyposis colorectal cancer** (summary in Kinzer and Vogelstein, 1996). These observations bring into focus another critical issue in reference to cancer, namely **the relationship of cancer cells to adhesion molecules** that normally maintain order within the tissue and are critical in understanding the mechanism of cancer invasion and metastases. Several such molecules, such as **cadherins** (Takichi, 1991), **integrins** (Albelda, 1993), **lamins** (Liotta et al, 1984), and **CD44** (Tarin, 1993), have been studied and have been shown to be of significance in cancer invasion and metastases.

It is the consensus of most investigators that cancer is a **multistep process** that includes **sequential and progressive accumulation of oncogenes and inactivation of growth-regulating genes.**

Microsatellite Instability

Another **mechanism of cancer formation** is instability of microsatellites, which are repetitive DNA sequences scattered throughout the genome. It has been noted that about 15% of colon cancers with a relatively normal chromosomal component display abnormalities of microsatellites (Gryfe et al, 2000; de la Chapelle, 2003). It is of note that the **two pathways of colon cancer,** i.e., chromosomal instability and microsatellite instability, result in different tumors with different behavior pattern and prognosis. The tumors with **chromosomal instability** are aneuploid, occur mainly in descending colon, and have a poor prognosis when compared with tumors with **microsatellite instability,** which tend to be diploid and occurring mainly in ascending colon (de la Chapelle, 2003).

Gene Rearrangement in Malignant Lymphomas and Leukemias: Effects of Translocations

Chromosomal abnormalities in leukemias have been studied since the onset of contemporary genetics. The **Philadelphia chromosome** (Ph), a shortened chromosome 22, described by Nowell and Hungerford in 1960 in chronic myelogenous leukemia, was the first documented chromosomal abnormality characteristic of any human cancer (see Chap. 4). With the availability of the techniques of chromosomal banding and molecular biology, the genetic changes in this group of diseases could be studied further. Many of these fundamental observations are of diagnostic and prognostic value. In many disease processes within this group of cancers, an **exchange of chromosomal segments** or **translocation** is observed (see Chap. 4 for a discussion of cytogenetic changes in human cancer). Thus, it has been shown that the Ph chromosome is the result of a translocation of portions of the long arm of chromosome 22 to the long arm of chromosome 9 [abbreviated as t(q9;q22)]. In certain forms of malignant lymphoma (notably in lymphomas of Burkitt's type), there is a reciprocal translocation between segments of chromosomes 14 and 18 (Fig. 7-7).

The results of a translocation can be:

- Activation of a gene
- Silencing of a gene
- Formation of a novel protein by fusion of coding sequences of participating chromosomes

It is the last property that has served as a template for development of a new drug (Gleevec, Novartis) that is effective **against the product of chromosomal translocation in chronic myelogenous leukemia.** The new agent also appears to be active against a group of gastrointestinal tumors known as GIST (see Chap. 24).

Many genes affected by translocations have been localized, identified, and sequenced (Mitelman and Mertens, 1997). It is now known that the genes involved are often related to the principal sites encoding immunoglobulin genes. Adjacent genes often encode for certain oncogenes. For example, the 14:18 chromosomal translocation in B-cell lymphomas affects a gene known as **bcl-2** and, in Burkitt's lymphoma, the c-**myc** gene. Both the bcl-2 and c-myc genes have been shown to be **inhibitors of programmed cell death or apoptosis** and it is assumed that their mutation prevents apoptosis of genetically deficient cells and, thus, contributes to an unregulated proliferation of abnormal cells or cancer (Sanchez-Garcia, 1997).

Tumor Clonality: Loss of Heterozygosity

Another molecular feature that is common in cancer is loss of heterozygosity. The observation is based on the premise

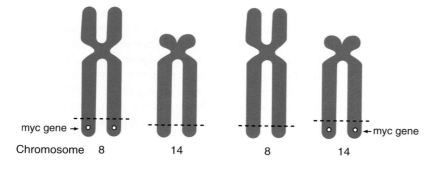

myc gene →

Chromosome   8   14   8   14

← myc gene

Figure 7-7   Reciprocal translocation between fragments of chromosomes 8 and 14 in Burkitt's lymphoma. The translation activates the myc gene and an adjacent immunoglobulin gene.

that the **two chromosomal homologues** in each cell **are not identical,** as one is of paternal and the other of maternal origin. It is assumed that **all cancer cells are derived from a single progenitor cell that carries the characteristics of only one parent and not both. One of the two genes may be inactivated or mutated.** This phenomenon, known as **loss of heterozygosity (LOH),** could be first documented by studying the clonality of **X chromosome expression** in human cancer using **markers to inactive chromosomal DNA.** The most informative of these markers is X-linked human androgen receptor or **Humara** that can be effectively used in the detection of clonality of various disorders, whether malignant or benign (Willman et al, 1994). LOH can also be determined by Southern blotting searching for differences in expression of specific genes between the normal and malignant cells of the same person, using DNA amplified by polymerase chain reaction.

Angiogenesis

Another critically important factor in growth of cancer is supply of nutrients necessary to sustain the growth of cancer cells. A network of capillary vessels sustains the growth of cancer (Folkman and Klagsbrun, 1987). The molecules responsible for growth of capillaries have been identified and drugs directed against these factors are under development (Folkman, 1995). In the broad assessment of factors leading to cancer by Hahn and Weinberg (2002), **angiogenesis** is considered to be one of the five fundamental factors in the genesis of human cancer, the other four being resistance to growth inhibition, evasion of apoptosis, immortalization, and independence from mitotic stimulation.

In animal models, suppression of angiogenesis leads to regression of end-stage cancers (Bergers et al, 1999).

Immortality of Cancer Cells

In 1965, Hayflick pointed out that **normal cells have a limited life span and die after 50 generations.** These constraints are not applicable to **cancer cells,** which **are theoretically immortal,** as pointed out by Cairns (1975). Contrary to normal cells, given favorable conditions necessary for survival, cancer cells can live forever, and, in fact, they do so in tissue cultures. The reasons for the ability of cancer cells to proliferate without constraints are complex and not fully understood. One of the likely reasons is that cancer cells are deficient in control mechanisms protecting normal cells from faulty reproduction of DNA. In favor of this concept is the presence of the genetic defects, such as a **mutated p53,** in some cancer cells. This heritable defect in DNA control mechanisms may explain why the initial genetic changes lead to a cascade of events that result in ever increasing molecular (and chromosomal) disorders, discussed previously.

It is also possible that the chromosomes in cancer cells have a better mechanism of survival that prevents them from entering senescence, customary in normal cells. The guilty party may be the group of enzymes known as **telomerases,** enzymes governing the formation of telomeres, or the terminal endings of chromosomes (Blackburn, 1990). In normal cells, the length of the telomeres shrinks with age, presumably preventing the chromosomes from normal replication and leading to cell death after the 50 generations observed by Hayflick. **Telomerases may be overexpressed in cancer** and provide additional telomeres, thus preventing the senescence of chromosomes and leading to the immortality of cancer cells (Haber, 1995). **Measuring the elevated expression of telomerase** in cells has been used in the diagnosis of cancer (see Chap. 26).

The observations on the role of telomeres and telomerase in normal and cancerous cells are somewhat paradoxical; longevity of cells (and, by implications, multicellular organisms) and cancers have a common denominator. It is a matter for pure speculation at this time whether the efforts at extending the span of normal human life will inevitably lead to cancer. The same reasoning may, perhaps, be applied to the efforts at **reversal of the malignant process by replacing damaged genes with intact genes.** Such procedures have been repeatedly and successfully performed in vitro on tissue cultures but, so far, there is no reported evidence known to us of a successful application of such a procedure to multicellular organisms in vivo. It remains to be seen what long-term consequences this sort of a genetic manipulation of complex organisms may produce.

Animal Models

Many of the relationships among genes in cancer cells have been studied in experimental models in mice and rats wherein, by special manipulations on ova, certain genes can be removed or inserted. **Knockout mice** (summary in Majzoub and Muglia, 1996) and **transgenic animals** (summary in Shuldiner, 1996) are models of gene suppression or enhancement. It is still questionable whether such animal models have direct or even indirect bearing on human cancer where rescue mechanisms surely exist that prevent single gene abnormalities from transforming normal cells into cancer cells. Nonetheless, some of the animal models shed light on mechanisms of some human cancer (see Chap. 23).

MOLECULAR BIOLOGY AND DIAGNOSTIC CYTOLOGY

The techniques of molecular biology, described in Chapter 3, have had, thus far, a relatively small impact on diagnostic cytology, and have not as yet, and perhaps never will, replace the light microscope as the principal diagnostic tool. Nonetheless, it is evident that some of these techniques already play an important role in the diagnosis, prognosis, and even treatment of human cancer and that this role may increase with the passage of time.

Some of these developments pertain to:

■ Identification and quantitation of various gene products

by in-situ hybridization and immunocytochemistry, DNA, RNA, tissue arrays and proteomics
- Analysis of DNA replication and cell proliferation
- Determination of cell death (apoptosis and necrosis, see Chap. 6)
- Documentation of chromosomal abnormalities by fluorescent in situ hybridization (FISH) and other techniques (see Chap. 4)
- Application of molecular biologic techniques to the identification of cancer cells (as an example, see Williams et al, 1998, Keesee et al, 1998)
- Identification and characterization of viral agents that may play an important role in the genesis of human cancer
- Identification of infectious agents that may directly or indirectly influence the natural history of cancer

Some of the early work documented that it was possible to perform **cytogenetic studies** on aspirated samples (Kristoffersson et al, 1985). Subsequently, **gene rearrangement in aspirated cell samples** of malignant lymphoma was documented (Lubinski et al, 1988). Cleaving the patient's DNA with an appropriate endonuclease and an analysis of the DNA product by Southern blotting disclosed patterns characteristic of the disease. Such techniques have been applied to aspirated **samples of lymph nodes.** If necessary, scanty DNA samples can be subjected to polymerase chain reaction (PCR; see Chap. 3) to amplify the genes of interest. This technique has been used by Feimesser et al (1992) to document the presence of **Epstein Barr virus (EBV)** in cells aspirated from neck lymph nodes in patients with presumed **nasopharyngeal carcinoma.** Because EBV is commonly associated with this tumor, its presence was confirmatory of the diagnosis.

The fluorescent in situ hybridization technique (FISH) has been repeatedly used in aspirated samples to document **numerical abnormalities of various chromosomes** in cancer cells (early example in Veltman et al, 1997; review in Wolman, 1997; see Chaps. 23 and 26 for further comments). The presence of **chromosomal translocations** by probes to hybrid transcripts was documented by Åkerman et al (1996) in Ewing's sarcoma and in mantle cell lymphoma by Hughes et al (1998). **Reverse transcriptase polymerase chain reaction (RT-PCR)** to identify rare cancer cells in the bone marrow and circulating blood is described in Chapter 43. Nilsson et al (1998) used this technique to study translocations in synovial sarcoma.

Studies of **apoptosis** using the TUNEL reaction (see Chap. 6) have been repeatedly performed. As this chapter is being revised (2004), these techniques, including **DNA, RNA arrays, and proteomics,** are in their infancy. Still, the early experience has shown that aspirated cell samples are suitable for molecular genetic analysis and offer one major advantage—the sampling can be repeated, if needed, without surgical removal of the lesion and without harm to the patient. Li et al (1995) documented that DNA extracted from archival cell samples is suitable for polymerase chain reaction.

Application of these techniques in reference to tumors of various organs is discussed in appropriate chapters. Examples include **molecular characterization of neuroblastoma** (Fröstad et al, 1999), determination of **telomerase activity** in fluids (Mu et al, 1999), detection of **chromosomal aberrations in squamous cancer by FISH** (Veltman et al, 1997), characterization of **Ewing's sarcoma** by reverse transcriptase polymerase chain reaction on archival cytologic samples (Schlott et al, 1997), and detection of loss of heterozygote in breast aspirates (Chuaqui et al, 1996).

MORPHOLOGIC CHARACTERISTICS OF CANCER CELLS

Identification of cancer cells by a light microscopic examination is an accepted means of cancer diagnosis, **with certain limitations.** The limitations may occur under two sets of circumstances. On the one hand, self-limiting, hence, benign, **proliferative or reparative processes may occasionally mimic cancer** (see Chap. 6 and Fig. 6-10); on the other hand, **cancer cells may not differ sufficiently from normal cells of the same origin for secure microscopic identification.** Both of these sources of error are avoidable, to a certain extent, by experience and by knowledge of the clinical history. However, there are few experienced observers who will not have recorded their occasional diagnostic failure and mistakes.

Although it is very tempting to consider identification of cancer cells as a science, the truth is that it is still largely an art, which is based on visual experiences that are recorded by the human memory in a manner that defies our current understanding. **Cancer cells, like normal cells, are composed of a nucleus and a cytoplasm.** The nucleus contains DNA and is therefore responsible for the replication of the genetic material and other events governed by DNA (see Chap. 3). As shown by electron microscopy, the cytoplasm of cancer cells contains all of the organelles necessary for energy production and other cell functions. **Thus, cancer cells are endowed with all the necessary components to sustain life and, to some extent, preserve the genetic characteristics of the tissue of origin.**

The **principal morphologic differences between benign cells and cancer cells** are shown schematically in Figure 7-8 and are summarized in Table 7-3. The differences are based on **cell size** and **configuration, interrelationship of cells, cell membrane, characteristics of the nucleus,** and **mitotic activity.** These will be discussed in sequence.

The Cytoplasm

Cell Size

The size of cancer cells usually differs from normal cells of the same origin. However, **physiologic variability in cell sizes also occurs in benign tissues.** This is particularly evident in epithelial tissues, such as squamous epithelium, wherein component cells may undergo substantial size

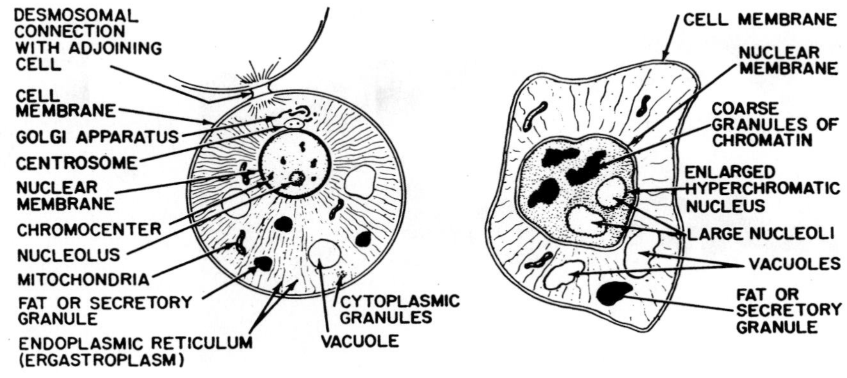

Figure 7-8 Schematic representation of the principal differences between a hypothetical benign cell (*left*) and a malignant cell (*right*). The differences, detailed in Table 7-3, pertain to cell configuration; nuclear size, shade, and texture; nucleolar size and shape; and the cell-to-cell relationship. The last is symbolized by the desmosome present on the benign cell and absent on the malignant cell to emphasize the reduced adhesiveness among cancer cells.

changes during normal maturation (see Fig. 5-4). **Cancer cells vary in size beyond the limits usually associated with physiologic variation.** Extreme size changes may be occasionally recorded; very large, sometimes multinucleated giant cells and very small cancer cells may occur. More importantly, a population of cancer cells is rarely made up of cells of equal size. **The cancer cells usually vary in size among themselves (anisocytosis)** (Fig. 7-9). These differences may be enhanced in air-dried smears stained with hematologic stains (Fig. 7-9D). However, **cell size alone is not a sufficient criterion for the diagnosis of cancer in the absence of nuclear abnormalities.**

Very little is known about the biologic events regulating cell size. It is perhaps of interest that deficiency in vitamin B_{12}, which affects the synthesis of DNA by a complex mechanism, may result in cell gigantism (see Chap. 10). It may

TABLE 7-3

PRINCIPAL MORPHOLOGIC DIFFERENCES BETWEEN NORMAL CELLS AND CANCER CELLS

	Benign Cells	Cancer Cells
Cell size	Variable within physiologic limits	Variable beyond physiologic limits
Cell shape	Variable within physiologic limits and depends on tissue type	Abnormal shapes frequent
Nuclear size	Variable within limits of cell cycle	Significant variability (anisonucleosis)
Nucleocytoplasmic ratio	Variable within physiologic limits	Commonly altered in favor of nucleus
Nuclear shape	Generally spherical, oval, or kidney-shaped	Aberrations of shape and configuration
Chromatin texture (nondividing nucleus)	Finely granular texture, "transparent"	Coarsely granular texture, "opaque"
Hyperchromasia	Rare	Common
Multinucleation	Not characteristic	Not characteristic
Nucleoli	Small, regular in shape, limited in number	Enlarged, of irregular configuration, increased in number
Nucleolini	Small and of constant size	Enlarged and of variable sizes
Adhesiveness	Excellent (except in lymph nodes, spleen, bone marrow)	Poor
Cell junctions	According to tissue type	No conclusive evidence of abnormalities
Growth pattern in culture	Contact inhibition	No contact inhibition
Number of cell generations in culture	± 50	Unlimited
Effects of lectins	Not agglutinable*	Agglutinable
Ultrastructure of cell surface in scanning electron microscope	Ridges, ruffles and blebs (microvilli in specific sites only)*	Microvilli of variable configuration on the entire surface†
Mitotic rate	As needed for replacement*	Elevated
Mitoses	Bipolar*	Aberrant forms
Placement of mitoses in epithelium	Basal layer only*	Not confined to basal layer
Cell cycle duration	16–22 hr	Normal or longer

* For exceptions, see text.
† In effusions and other fluids. Configuration still unknown in many situations.

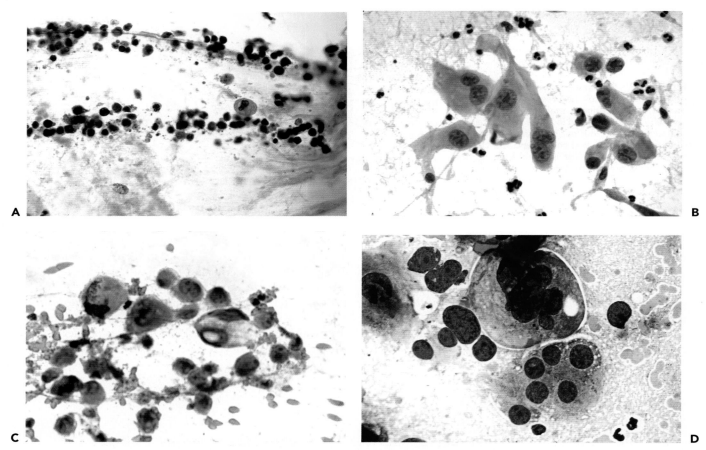

Figure 7-9 Variable sizes and configuration of cancer cells and their nuclei. *A.* Small cell (oat cell) carcinoma of lung, bronchial brush smear. *B.* Large cells. Adenocarcinoma of lung, needle aspiration biopsy (FNA). *C.* Gastric carcinoma, metastatic to vertebra, aspirated sample. Note the variability of cell and nuclear sizes and shapes. *D.* Mesodermal mixed tumor, ascitic fluid. Note bizarre, multinucleated giant cancer cells, next to smaller cells; the features are enhanced in this air-dried Diff-Quik–stained smear.

be inferred, therefore, that the abnormal sizes of cancer cells are the result of DNA abnormalities of a yet unknown nature.

Cell Configuration

Unusual, abnormal cell shapes may be observed in cancer cells, especially in advanced cancer (Fig. 7-9C), although cancer cell configuration may mimic, sometimes in a grotesque fashion, normal cells of the same origin. The configuration of cancer cells does not necessarily depend on the physical relationship of cancer cells to each other or to the supporting connective tissue, as had been claimed. For example, bizarre configuration may be observed in human cancer cells growing freely in effusions (see Chap. 26).

It must be added, however, that **bizarre configuration of cells may also be observed in benign processes,** particularly those associated with rapid proliferation of cells of either connective tissue or epithelial origin. Therefore, once again, **nuclear and clinical features** must be considered before rendering the diagnosis of cancer. There has been no substantial research on the factors governing cell shapes in cancer. It is likely that the configuration of cancer cells

is encoded in the nuclear DNA, and translated by RNA governing the formation of structural proteins.

Cell Adhesiveness

One of the principal traits of cancer cells is their poor adhesiveness to each other. Thus, in smears prepared from an aspirated sample of a malignant tumor, the abundant cancer cells may appear singly or in loosely structured aggregates, whereas this phenomenon cannot be fully appreciated in the corresponding histologic preparation (Fig. 7-10). Also, a smear from the corresponding benign tissue will yield cells mainly arranged in tightly fitting, orderly clusters, wherein the cell borders can be often identified (see Fig. 7-2).

There are some **differences in the adhesiveness of cells of various tumor types.** Generally speaking, cancer **cells of epithelial origin tend to form clusters and aggregates,** even when allowed to proliferate freely (Fig. 7-10B). Poor adhesiveness is more evident in anaplastic, poorly differentiated tumors than in well differentiated tumors. On the other hand, the cells of most nonepithelial tumors, particularly **malignant lymphomas and sarcomas,** rarely, if ever, form clusters and **tend to remain single** (Fig. 7-11).

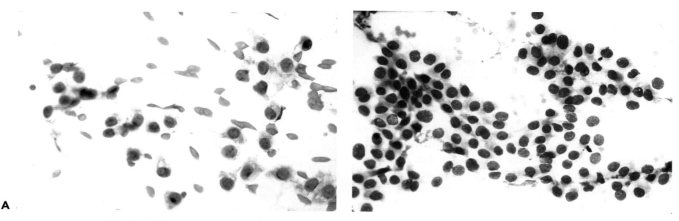

Figure 7-10   **Poor adhesiveness of cancer cells.** *A.* Aspirate of mammary carcinoma. The cancer cells are dispersed. *B.* Aspirate of pulmonary adenocarcinoma. The cell cluster is loosely structured. (*A:* Pap stain; *B:* May-Grünwald-Giemsa stain.)

The original observations pertaining to **decreased adhesiveness of cancer cells** were made by Coman (1944) who measured with a micromanipulator the force required to separate cells of squamous carcinoma and found it to be significantly lower when compared with normal squamous epithelium. Using a different technique, McCutcheon et al (1948) made similar observations on cells of adenocarcinomas of various origins. The causes of poor adhesiveness of cancer cells are not well understood. Coman (1961) pointed out that calcium played a major role because its removal diminished the adhesiveness. The possible **deficiencies in cell-to-cell attachments and junctions** were studied, using a variety of techniques. Normal tissues have an elaborate apparatus of cell attachments (e.g., junctional complexes, gap junctions, desmosomes, and hemidesmosomes) holding the cells together (see Chap. 2). All of these organelles have also been observed in cancer, both human and experimental. For example, Lavin and Koss (1971) showed that cultured cancer cells are capable of forming morphologically normal desmosomes. In searching for qualitative and quantitative differences in cell junctions between normal urothelium and urothelial cancer, Weinstein et al (1976) could find none

and stated that in cancer "there is neither concrete nor compelling circumstantial evidence which supports the popular notion that junctional defects contribute to those properties which are the hallmarks of malignant growth, namely, invasiveness and the ability to metastasize." This view was confirmed in a subsequent review by Weinstein and Paul (1981).

Molecular biologic investigations, summarized earlier, strongly suggest that **alterations of adhesion molecules may be the cause of poor adhesiveness of cancer cells.** As has been stated, there is evidence that oncogenes and modified tumor suppressor genes interact with the adhesion molecules. This research is still in early stages. It has been repeatedly shown that an overexpression of adhesion signaling molecules (focal adhesion kinase) is associated with malignant transformation (Oktay et al, 2003).

From a practical point of view, **poor adhesiveness of cancer cells gives a distinct advantage to some techniques of cell sampling.** Aspiration of a cancer, whether human or experimental, by means of a needle and syringe, will usually yield abundant cells, compared with normal tissue of similar origin. The only exceptions to this rule are normal

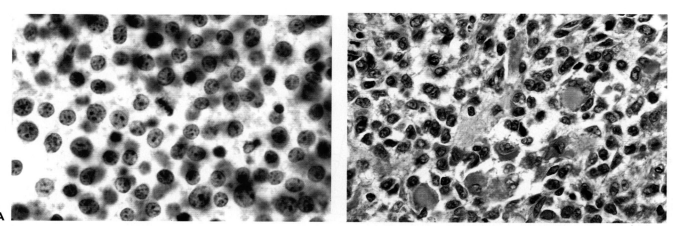

Figure 7-11   **Dispersed cancer cells.** *A.* Malignant lymphoma. Note mitosis and prominent nucleoli. *B.* Rhabdomyosarcoma. Note bizarre cell shapes and cells with eosinophilic cytoplasm, characteristic of this tumor.

lymphoid organs, the spleen, and the bone marrow, which yield abundant cells also in the absence of cancer. Scraping of cancers located on the surface of organs may yield abundant free cancer cells. Cancers may spontaneously shed (exfoliate) cells into adjacent body cavities.

Cell Membranes

The interrelationship of cancer cells may also depend on cell membranes. The first objective evidence that the membrane of cancer cells may differ from that of normal cells was based on the observation of **patterns of cell growth in tissue culture.** When **normal (diploid or euploid) cells are grown on hard surfaces,** such as glass or plastic, **they show contact inhibition,** or stop growing when their borders contact each other. After the initiation of a tissue culture from a fragment of tissue or a cluster of cultured cells, the cells multiply actively and migrate away from the inoculum. This migration takes place because of an undulating movement of cell membranes. The cell migration stops once the cell membranes come in contact with each other in the state of confluent monolayer. Simultaneously, the undulations of the cell membranes cease, the mitotic rate drops precipitously, and the synthesis of DNA, RNA decrease sharply. Although contact inhibition can be manipulated by various experimental means, it generally characterizes benign cells in culture.

In contrast, **cancer cells grown on glass or plastic surfaces do not show contact inhibition.** Their growth does not stop when a confluent monolayer is formed and the cells form multilayered accumulations (piling up) (Fig. 7-12). Ambrose (1968) pointed out that malignant cells are also capable of changing the direction of their movements more frequently than normal cells. Contact inhibition may be lifted when benign cells are transformed in vitro into malignant cells by viral or chemical agents.

The precise mechanisms of the differences in the behavior of normal and cancer cells in vitro remain to be elucidated. However, it is virtually certain that these behavior patterns are governed by adhesion molecules and growth

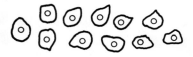
BENIGN CELLS

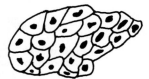
MALIGNANT CELLS

Figure 7-13 Schematic representation of effect of lectins on benign (*top*) and malignant cells (see text).

factors, as has been shown by Segall et al (1996) in reference to cultured cells of rat mammary carcinoma.

Besides behavior in culture, there are other observations that point out fundamental differences in membrane structure between benign and malignant cells. For example, there are significant differences in the effects of various substances of plant origin, known as **lectins,** such as wheat germ agglutinin (WGA) and concanavalin A (ConA), on the membranes of various benign and virus-transformed cells in culture. The general effect of lectins can be summarized as follows: (1) **dispersed benign cells are not agglutinated by lectins** and remain in suspension, and (2) **malignant cells of similar origin are agglutinated by lectins** and form clumps (Fig. 7-13). The agglutinability of benign cells may be briefly enhanced by the action of proteolytic enzymes. Also, the benign cells are agglutinable during the mitotic cycle, except the prophase. Some embryonal cells, although normal, are also agglutinable by lectins. It appears logical that the differences are based on the presence of agglutina-

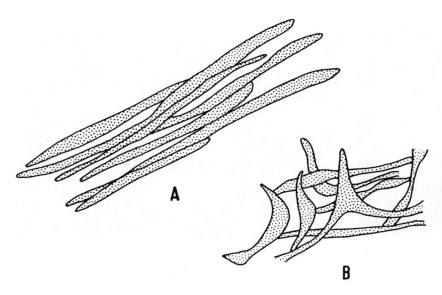

Figure 7-12 A. Growth pattern of BHK-21 benign fibroblasts growing on a glass or smooth cellulose acetate surface. B. Growth pattern of PPY polyoma-transformed (malignant) cells on glass (rough or smooth) or cellulose acetate (rough or smooth). Note overlapping of cell processes. (Ambrose EJ. The surface properties of mammalian cells in culture. In The Proliferation and Spread of Neoplastic Cells. Baltimore, Williams & Wilkins, 1968, pp 23–37.)

tion sites (receptors) on the cell surface. These sites are exposed on the surface of malignant cells and are hidden on the surface of benign cells (Ben-Basset et al, 1971; Inbar et al, 1972). It must be noted that certain **lectins,** such as phytohemagglutinin and concanavalin A, **stimulate proliferation of T lymphocytes,** with resulting formation of large, immature cells (blasts) that are capable of mitotic division. This function may also reflect the presence of appropriate receptors on the surface of the cells.

Although the biochemical and biophysical differences between membranes of benign and malignant cells require further elucidation, certain fundamental structural differences have been discovered by **electron microscopy.**

Scanning and transmission electron microscopic studies of benign and malignant human cells in some tissues and in cancer cells suspended in effusions or in urine, disclosed major differences in cell surface configuration. In general, **the surfaces of benign cells, such as squamous cells, lymphocytes, macrophages, or mesothelial cells, display** either ridges, blebs, or uniform microvilli. The surfaces of most (but not all) malignant cells of epithelial origin (carcinomas) are covered with microvilli of variable sizes and configuration (Fig. 7-14A,B). One notable exception is the **oat cell carcinoma** of lung origin, wherein the surfaces of cancer cells are smooth. The microvilli on the surfaces of benign cells differ from microvilli observed on surfaces of cancer cells. **In benign epithelial cells of glandular origin, the microvilli are polarized** (i.e., confined to one aspect of the normal cell, usually that facing the lumen of a gland or organ) and are of uniform and monotonous configuration. **The microvilli of epithelial cancer cells cover the entire cell surface,** vary in size and length, sometimes forming clumps of very long microvilli. In some tumors, notably **carcinomatous mesothelioma,** tufts of long microvilli characterize the malignant cells. The microvilli on the surface of some cancer cells may be seen under the light microscope and are helpful in recognizing cancer cells (see Chaps. 26 and 27). The mechanisms of formation of

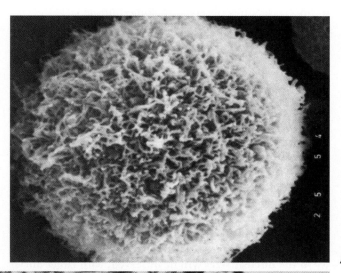

A

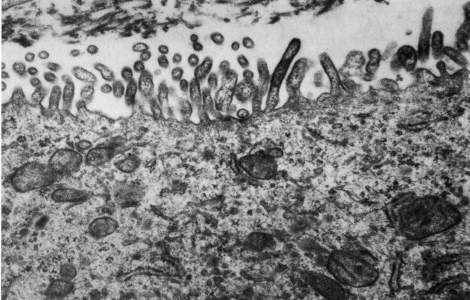

Figure 7-14 *A.* Scanning electron micrograph of a breast cancer cell in effusion. The surface is covered by innumerable microvilli of variable length and configuration. *B.* Transmission electron micrograph of the surface of a cancer cell of ovarian origin, in effusion. Note the innumerable microvilli of various lengths, thicknesses, and configurations. (*A:* ×4,600; *B:* ×25,000.) (*A:* Domagala W, Koss LG. Configuration of surfaces of human cancer cells in effusions. Virchows Arch 26:27–42, 1977. *B:* Courtesy of Dr. W. Domagala.)

B

microvilli have not been investigated so far. For the same reason, the relationship of microvilli on the surfaces of cancer cells to their agglutinability with lectins is not clear. Possibly, the two phenomena are connected in a manner that remains to be elucidated.

The Nucleus

Nuclear abnormalities are the dominant morphologic feature of cancer cells that allow their recognition in microscopic preparations. The key changes observed are:

- Nuclear enlargement, particularly in reference to the area of the cytoplasm [altered nucleocytoplasmic (N/C) ratio] in favor of the nucleus
- Irregularity of the nuclear configuration and contour
- Altered nuclear texture; hyperchromasia and coarse granulation of chromatin
- Abnormalities of sex chromatin in females
- Changes in nuclear membrane
- Nucleolar abnormalities
- Abnormalities of cell cycle and mitoses
- Special features observed in some tumors

These abnormalities will be discussed in sequence.

Size

The size and, hence, **the area of the nucleus** in smear and other cytologic preparations **depends on DNA content. The relationship is not linear.** For example, the **doubling of the amount of DNA** that occurs during the S-phase of the normal cell cycle **results in doubling of the nuclear volume, however, the nuclear diameter increases by only 40%,** a calculation based on principles of geometry. Because the nucleus in smears is flattened on the surface of the glass slide, the **nuclear diameter,** corresponding approximately to the largest cross section of the nucleus, is the dominant feature observed under the microscope.

In a normal cycling population of cells, some variability in the nuclear sizes will be observed, with larger nuclei representing cells in S, G2 phases of the cell cycle. However, under normal circumstances, the proportion of cycling normal cells is small, rarely surpassing 1% to 2%. **In most, but not all, populations of malignant cells, nuclear enlargement is a common feature, often encompassing a large proportion of cancer cells.** Because the cytoplasm of such cells is often of approximately normal size, the area of the nucleus is disproportionately enlarged, resulting in an **increase of the nucleocytoplasmic (N/C) ratio.** Because the increase in the nuclear size usually reflects an increase in the amount of DNA, in malignant tumors with approximately normal DNA content, the nuclear enlargement may not be evident but other nuclear abnormalities, discussed below, may be observed.

The amount of DNA in nuclei can be measured by techniques of image cytometry or flow cytometry (see Chaps. 46 and 47). These techniques show that in many, but not all, cancer cells there is an increase in the amount of DNA. However, **because of heterogeneity of cancer cells in many cancers, the amount of DNA varies from one can-cer cell to another,** although it can be increased in many cells; some cells may have the normal (diploid) or even subnormal amounts of DNA. **Consequently, the size of cancer cell nuclei within the same cancer often varies, a phenomenon named anisonucleoisis (nonequal nuclei),** and this feature is also common in cancer (see Fig. 7-9B–D).

Because heterogeneity or the variability of size of cancer cell nuclei would make a characterization of any given cancer nearly impossible, the concept of **DNA ploidy** was established, **based on the DNA content in the dominant population of cancer cells in a given cancer and disregarding the deviant DNA values.** The concept is based on comparison of normal amount of DNA (**diploid or euploid cells**) with the DNA content in the dominant population of cancer cells. In some cancers, the DNA ploidy of cancer cells may be equal to normal (**diploid tumors**). When the DNA content deviates from normal, the tumors are **aneuploid.** Aneuploid tumors may have a DNA content below normal (**hypodiploid aneuploid tumors**), or above normal (**hyperdiploid aneuploid tumors**). Several groups may be recognized among aneuploid tumors, for example, when the dominant DNA content is one and a half times higher than normal, the tumors are classified as **triploid;** when it is twice the normal, the tumors are classified as **tetraploid.** Various other deviations from normal may occur that are neither triploid nor tetraploid (Fig. 7-15). The DNA ploidy of a tumor or a given cell population is often expressed as **DNA index, expressing the ratio between the ploidy of the tumor cell population compared with the normal index of one.** Thus, the DNA index of a tetraploid tumor, which has twice the amount of DNA, is 2.0 and that of a triploid tumor 1.5 (see Chap. 47).

If the **increase in the diameter of the nucleus** represents an increase in the amount of nuclear DNA, it also indicates an **increase in the number of chromosomes.** The number of chromosomes in cells is determined in spreads of metaphases. The total number of chromosomes is often increased in cancer cells. Not all chromosomes are affected, some chromosomes may retain their normal number and configuration, whereas others may show numerical and morphologic abnormalities (see Chap. 4). There is a fairly good concordance between the DNA content and the number of chromosomes per cell. However, once again to reflect the heterogeneity of cancer cells, the term **stem line**, rather than ploidy, is used in the classification of human tumors based on cytogenetic findings. Again, the stem line designates the dominant cell population with an approximately constant number of chromosomes. The stem line may be **diploid** or **euploid** (corresponding to 46 chromosomes), or **aneuploid, corresponding to abnormalities in the number of chromosomes.** Thus, one can recognize triploid tumors, corresponding to 69 chromosomes, tetraploid tumors (92 chromosomes), or tumors with variable deviations from normal, in keeping with the terminology of DNA ploidy. It is evident from this information that **the size of the cancer cell nucleus in smears depends, to a large extent, on the number of chromosomes or tumor stem line.** This was documented many years ago in a study conducted by Miles and Koss (1966). The aggregate length of all chromo-

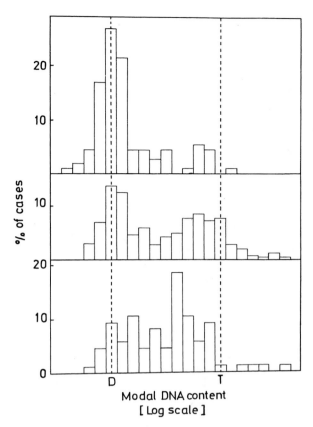

Figure 7-15 **Dominant DNA ploidy values, as determined by Feuglen spectrophotometry,** of 111 carcinomas of the corpus uteri (*top*), 392 squamous cell carcinomas of the cervix uteri (*middle*), and 85 carcinomas of the large bowel (*bottom*). D and T signify diploid and tetraploid DNA levels, respectively. It may be noted that for all three cancer sites the dominant modal DNA content is predominantly aneuploid although some cancers are diploid, and a few are tetraploid. (Atkin NB. Cytogenetic studies on human tumors and premalignant lesions: The emergence of aneuploid cell lines and their relationship to the process of malignant transformation in man. *In* Genetic Concepts and Neoplasia. Baltimore, Williams & Wilkins, 1970, pp 30–56.)

somes was measured in cells of several cultured cell lines and compared with the sizes of the nuclei (Fig. 7-16). A diploid embryonal rhabdomyosarcoma with 46 chromosomes (Fig. 7-16A,B) had small, bland nuclei. Cultured cells from several epidermoid carcinomas, with stem lines between 59 and 70 chromosomes, show larger nuclei (Fig. 7-16D–F). A malignant melanoma, with a stem line of 123 chromosomes (Fig. 7-16G), shows the largest nuclei. In Figure 7-16 panels C through G, abnormalities of nuclear chromatin are also observed (see below).

Another approach to document numerical or functional abnormalities of chromosomes in individual cancer cells is the technique of **in situ hybridization,** based on biotinylated (and hence visible in light microscopy) or fluorescent specific probes to entire chromosomes, or to chromosomal segments, such as centromeres, or to individual genes. The principles of the technique were discussed in Chapter 4. The technique examines **interphase nuclei** and, thus, may be applied to any population of cells. The basic assumption of the technique is that, in normal cells, there are two homo-

logues of each chromosome. The presence of more than two signals indicates a chromosomal abnormality that, for all intents and purposes, is diagnostic of cancer, unless the patient has a congenital abnormality in chromosomal numbers, such as trisomy of chromosome 21. The technique has been used as a diagnostic tool to document the presence of chromosomal abnormalities in cells from different body sites, such as effusions, bladder washings, and material from aspiration biopsies (Cajulis et al, 1993, 1997). With the development of new probes, the technique can be applied to the search for aberrant genes, translocations, etc. (summaries in Glassman, 1998; Luke and Shepelsky, 1998). Examples of this technique are shown in Chapters 4 and 23.

As previously discussed and in Chapter 4, **besides numerical abnormalities, the chromosomes in cancer cells may show a variety of other changes, such as translocations and marker chromosomes.**

It is evident from the earlier discussion that **nuclear size alone may be helpful in the diagnosis of malignant tumors with elevated DNA or chromosomal content but will fail in the recognition of tumors with normal or nearnormal DNA content (diploid or near-diploid tumors).** If the changes in nuclear size are subtle, the microscopist should always **compare the nuclear size of the unknown cell with a microscopic object of known size,** such as an erythrocyte (7 μm in diameter) or the nucleus of a recognizable benign cell. Subtle differences in size are of limited diagnostic help and the search for other nuclear features is necessary.

Irregularities of the Nuclear Configuration and Contour

The configuration of the nuclei in normal cells usually follows the shape of the cytoplasm. Most nuclei, in benign spherical or polygonal epithelial cells, are spherical. In cells of columnar shape, the nuclei are usually oval. Nuclei of elongated epithelial cells, fibroblasts, or smooth muscle cells are often elongated and sometimes spindle-shaped. Nuclear configuration of highly specialized cells probably reflects highly specialized functions. Thus, the nuclei of macrophages may be kidney-shaped and those of polymorphonuclear leukocytes and megakaryocytes show lobulations. It is not known, at this time, why this is so or what factors influence the shape of the nucleus. Hypothetically, it would be logical to assume that nuclear configuration and shape are optimal for most efficient nucleocytoplasmic exchanges and, hence, cell function in any given cell type. **Still, the nuclei of all benign cells have a smooth nuclear contour.**

The configuration of the nuclei of cancer cells also generally follows the configuration of the cells. Thus, most spherical or polygonal cancer cells have approximately spherical or oval nuclei. Elongated or "spindly" cancer cells have elongated nuclei. However, these nuclei often show **abnormalities of the nuclear contour,** best observed in spherical or oval nuclei. These abnormalities may be subtle, in the form of **small protrusions or notches,** in the nuclear membrane that may be difficult to observe and may require a careful inspection of the target cells (Fig. 7-17). Less often, the nuclei may show **fingerlike protrusions** that were at-

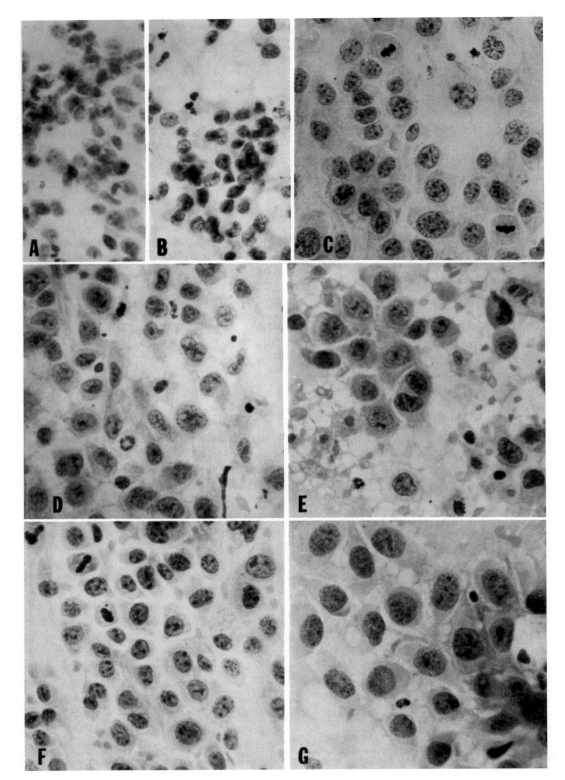

Figure 7-16 Impression smears of tumors with varying chromosomal numbers. *A,B.* Same tumor, an embryonal rhabdomyosarcoma with 46 chromosomes and a normal karyotype. *C.* A soft part sarcoma, 47 chromosomes. *D–F.* Epidermoid carcinomas with stemlines of 59, 66–67, and 70 chromosomes, respectively. *G.* Represents a malignant melanoma with stemline of 123 chromosomes. Note that the diploid tumor (*A,B*) exhibit small, relatively bland nuclei. All of the aneuploid tumors, even the one (*C*) with one extra chromosome, exhibit large hyperchromatic pleomorphic nuclei. (All oil immersion.) (Miles CP, Koss LG. Diagnostic traits of interphase human cancer cells with known chromosome patters. Acta Cytol 10:21–25, 1996.)

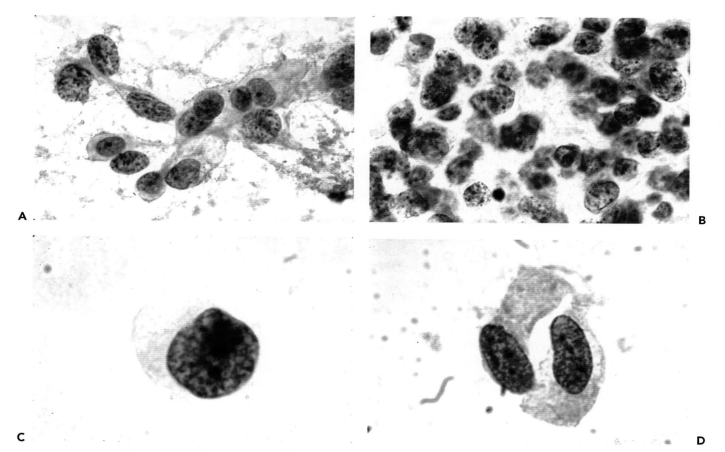

Figure 7-17   Abnormalities of the nucleus in cancer cells. *A.* Aspirate of pancreatic carcinoma. *B.* Aspirate of neuroblastoma. *C,D.* Urothelial carcinoma. Coarse granulation of chromatin and subtle abnormalities of nuclear contour (notches and protrusions) may be observed in all photographs. (Pap stain; *A*: high magnification; *B–D*: oil immersion.)

tributed in the very few pertinent studies to the presence of long marker chromosomes (Atkin and Baker, 1964; Atkin, 1969; Kovacs, 1982). It must be noted that **dense nuclear protrusions** ("nipples"), possibly an artifact, also occur in certain benign cells, such as endocervical cells (see Chap. 8).

In elongated cancer cells and most nonepithelial cells with elongated nuclei, the abnormalities of the nuclear contour are more difficult to recognize, although sometimes spinelike protrusions may be observed at one pole. In bizarre cancer cells that are sometimes multinucleated, bizarre configuration of nuclei may be observed (see Fig. 7-9D).

The abnormalities of the nuclear configuration and contour, particularly when associated with nuclear enlargement and an increase in the nucleocytoplasmic ratio, raise a high level of suspicion for the diagnosis of cancer and are usually associated with other stigmata of cancer cells.

Several observers attempted to correlate the configuration of nuclei of human tumors in histologic sections with behavior and prognosis (Miller et al, 1988; Borland et al, 1993). The observations reported may reflect a fixation artifact and, more remotely, the chromosomal makeup of the tumors studied.

Nuclear Texture: Hyperchromasia and Coarse Granulation of Chromatin

Dark staining of interphase nuclei of cancer cells with appropriated dyes, such as hematoxylin or acetic orcein, is known as **hyperchromasia. Hyperchromasia is usually associated with changes in configuration of nuclear chromatin, which shows coarse granulation** and may be associated with a **thickening of the nuclear membrane** (Fig. 7-17). By contrast, normal fixed and stained nuclei have a transparent nucleoplasm, with a fine network of filaments of **constitutive chromatin,** which forms small dense granules known as **chromocenters.** In females, the **sex chromatin body** (Barr body), representing **facultative chromatin,** may be observed as a dense, semicircular structure attached to the nuclear membrane (see Chaps. 2 and 4).

Tolles et al (1961) documented objectively the presence of hyperchromasia in cancer cells from the uterine cervix by measuring the extinction coefficients. Several studies based on computerized image analysis also documented that the changes in nuclear texture are an objective parameter separating cancer cells from normal cells of the same origin (see Chap. 46). The reasons for coarse granulation of chromatin are essentially unknown and have not received any attention from molecular biologists. A few speculative thoughts can be offered. There is evidence that **the condensed DNA of some cancer cells has a lower melting point than DNA of normal cells.** In other words, the two chains of DNA in cancer cells are easier to separate than the two chains of normal DNA (Darzynkiewicz et al, 1987). The issue has been studied further by Darzynkiewicz and his associates (1987) who suggested that the condensation of chromatin is associated with structural nuclear proteins. Atkin (1969) spoke of "**telophase pattern**" of chromatin in cancer cells, suggesting similarities in the distribution of coarsely granular DNA in cancer cells with chromatin distribution in normal telophase. Another analogy may be offered with condensation of chromosomes in prophase of mitosis. However, neither analogy corresponds to the reality because only a small fraction of cancer cells displaying hyperchromasia are undergoing mitosis. The only reasonable conclusion that is permissible, at this time, is that the **DNA in cancer cells has undergone significant structural changes of unknown nature** that accounts for hyperchromasia and coarse granulation of chromatin. Stein et al (2000) proposed that the abnormalities of nuclear structure in cancer reflect altered gene expression. However, the mechanisms and function of these changes are enigmatic. Gisselsson et al (2000, 2001) attributed the nuclear abnormalities to **chromosomal breakage and fusion** of fragments **(breakage fusion bridges).** The concept is interesting and warrants further exploration but fails to explain the coarse granularity of chromatin so common in the nuclei of cancer cells.

It must also be stressed that **hyperchromasia and coarse granularity of chromatin may be absent in cancer cells**. Numerous examples of invasive cancer of various organs have been observed wherein **nuclei of cancer cells are enlarged but completely bland and transparent**. In some of these cells, **enlarged nucleoli** can be observed. These abnormalities are most often observed in clusters of cells with generally abnormal configuration and are usually accompanied elsewhere by more conventional cancer cell abnormalities. Thus, the finding of **cell clusters with large bland nuclei is, a priori, abnormal** and should lead to further search for evidence of cancer.

It must also be stressed that **nuclear enlargement and hyperchromasia may occur in normal organs,** such as the embryonal adrenal cortex and endocrine organs, for example, the acini of the thyroid gland (see Chap. 30). Thus, the provenance of the material is of capital significance in assessing the value of the microscopic observations.

Abnormalities of Sex Chromatin in Females

Sex chromatin body (Barr body) represents the inactive X chromosome in female cells (see Chap. 4). The formula pertaining to the number of Barr bodies visible on the nuclear membrane, is X minus 1, X representing the total number of X chromosomes in a cell. Thus, a patient with 3 X chromosomes will have two Barr bodies. Because the naturally occurring excess of X chromosomes is exceedingly rare, **the presence of two or more sex chromatin bodies in a nucleus is clear evidence of genetic abnormality that**

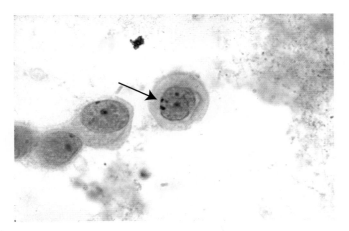

Figure 7-18 Breast cancer cell with two sex chromatin bodies (arrow). For further examples, see Chapters 26 and 29. (Orcein stain; oil immersion.)

may be observed in cancer cells (Fig. 7-18). The finding is particularly helpful in situations where other nuclear stigmata of cancer are not clearly evident and may have prognostic significance in mammary carcinoma (see Chap. 29). We found it to be of particular value in identifying cells of mammary carcinoma in effusions and in recognizing cancerous changes in cervicovaginal smears (see Chaps. 11 and 26).

Abnormalities of Nuclear Membrane

It has been previously mentioned that in many cancer cells displaying coarse granularity of chromatin, **the nuclear membrane appears thickened**. On close scrutiny, the thickness of the nuclear membrane is variable and irregular. It is not known whether this optical feature of a cancer cell nucleus, which is sometimes of diagnostic value, represents an **actual physical change in the structure of the nuclear membrane or merely a deposition of chromatin granules (or modified chromosomes) along the nuclear envelope**. Electron micrographs of cancer cells strongly suggest that deposition of chromatin (and hence chromosomes) on the nuclear membrane is the more likely explanation of this phenomenon.

Another feature of cancer cells is the **increase in the number of nuclear pores** (Czerniak et al, 1984). Although this observation has no practical value because the freeze-fracture techniques required are too cumbersome for a clinical laboratory, the observations have some bearing on understanding the metabolic processes in cancer. The Czerniak study, which was based on cells of urothelial tumors, disclosed a **relationship between DNA ploidy and the density of the nuclear pores;** the pore density was higher in tumors with increased amounts of DNA (and hence the number of chromosomes). On the other hand, the density of the pores in reference to the nuclear volume remained approximately constant. Because the nuclear pores represent a link between the nucleus and the cytoplasm, the observation suggests that the increased exchanges between the nucleus and the cytoplasm take place in cancer cells. As has been discussed in Chapter 2, the observation supports the hypothesis that the formation of nuclear pores is closely related to organization of chromosomes in the nucleus. Further studies of this observation are clearly indicated (Koss, 1998).

Multinucleation in Cancer Cells

Cancer cells with two or more nuclei are fairly common. In some cells, such as the **Reed-Sternberg cells** in Hodgkin's disease, the finding of the specific arrangement and configuration of the nuclei is of great diagnostic significance (see Chap. 31). However, in other tumors, the phenomenon is fairly common and of little diagnostic significance. It must be recognized that **multinucleation is a common phenomenon that may occur in benign and in malignant cells and, therefore, is of no diagnostic value, unless the configuration or arrangement of the nuclei is specific for a disease process.**

Other Nuclear Changes in Cancer Cells

In some malignant tumors, nonspecific nuclear abnormalities may occur that may be of diagnostic help. For example, in some thyroid carcinomas, malignant melanomas, and occasionally other cancers, **cytoplasmic intranuclear inclusions** appear as clear areas within the nucleus (**nuclear cytoplasmic invaginations, Orphan Annie nuclei**) (Fig. 7-19A). In electron microscopy, the clear zones contain areas of cytoplasm with cytoplasmic organelles, such as mitochondria (see Fig. 6-6). Nothing is known about the mechanism causing this nuclear abnormality, which, incidentally, can also occur in some benign cells, such as hepatocytes and ciliated bronchial cells. Another nuclear abnormality is **nuclear "creases," "grooves,"** or folds (Fig. 7-19B). The changes may appear as **dark, thin lines** within the nucleus or as linear densities with numerous short lateral processes, sometimes referred to as **"caterpillar nuclei"** or Anitschkow cells. These nuclear features have been observed in a **variety of normal cells,** such as squamous cells of the oral cavity, cornea, or uterine cervix, and in mesothelial cells (see appropriate chapters for further comments). Deli-

georgi-Politi (1987) observed numerous nuclear grooves in aspirated cells of thyroid carcinomas, an observation that has been confirmed many times. Subsequently, such nuclear changes have been observed in many different benign and malignant tumors, such as granulosa cell tumors of the ovary (Ehya and Lang, 1986) and ependymomas (Craver and McGarry, 1994), to name a few. In some tumors and conditions discussed throughout this book, the grooves are particularly numerous and their presence may be of diagnostic help (review in Ng and Collins, 1997). However, these nuclear changes should **never be considered as diagnostic of any entity** as concluded by Tahlan and Dey (2001).

Nucleolar Abnormalities

Nucleolar abnormalities are an important feature of cancer cells. The nucleoli are characterized by their eosinophilic center, surrounded by a border of nucleolus-associated chromatin (see Chap. 2). **The number and size of nucleoli in cancer cells is often increased and their configuration may be abnormal. Very large nucleoli (5 to 7 μm in diameter, macronucleoli) are, for all practical purposes, diagnostic of cancer** (Fig. 7-20). **Oddly, comma-shaped nucleoli,** that the late John Frost called **"cookie-cutter nucleoli,"** are fairly common in cancer cells. The reasons for this abnormality are unknown. **The abnormality in the shape of the nucleoli is a valuable diagnostic marker because it is rarely observed in repair reactions wherein the number and size of nucleoli can be substantially increased.**

It may be recalled that, in normal cells, nucleolus-organizing foci are found on terminal portions of chromosomes 13, 14, 15, 21, and 22, resulting in formation of up to 10 small nucleoli. Shortly after mitosis, the nucleoli merge to form usually one or two somewhat larger nucleoli. Because the nucleoli are the principal **centers of synthesis of nucleic acids,** their presence in the nuclei of normal cells reflects their protein requirement. Therefore, nearly all growing or metabolically active cells carry visible, albeit small nucleoli. **However, during regeneration of normal tissues (so-called repair reaction), when the need for cell**

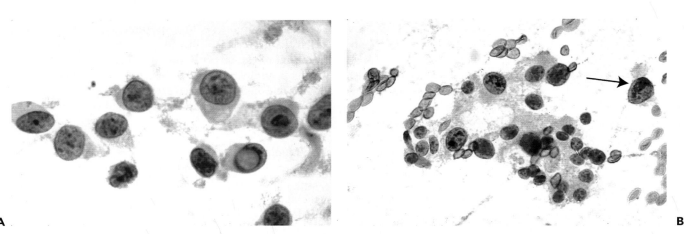

A   **B**

Figure 7-19 Intranuclear cytoplasmic inclusions (nuclear "holes") and nuclear grooves or creases. *A.* Intranuclear cytoplasmic inclusions. Note the sharp borders of the clear intranuclear space. Metastatic malignant melanoma to liver. *B.* Smear of a Hürthle cell tumor of thyroid. Nuclear folds or creases are seen as a diagonal line (*arrow*). (*A:* Oil immersion; *B:* high magnification.)

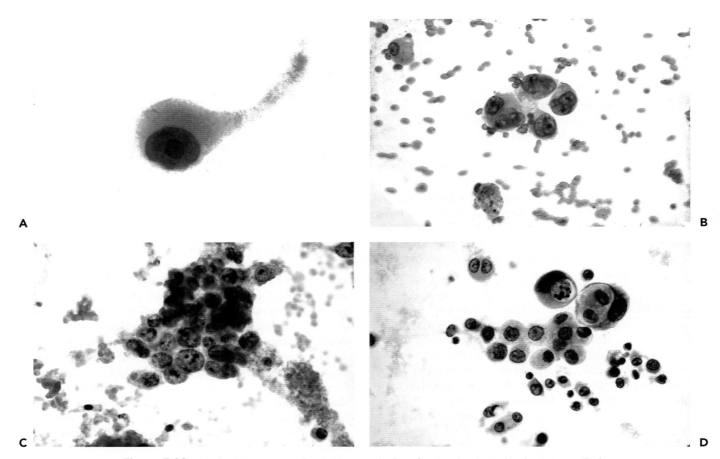

Figure 7-20 Nucleoli in cancer cells. *A.* Huge nucleolus of somewhat irregular shape in a cell of a malignant melanoma. *B.* Large, irregularly shaped and multiple nucleoli in cells of a spindle- and giant cell carcinoma of lung. *C.* Large, irregular nucleoli in a poorly differentiated tumor of anterior mediastinum. Cells of a metastatic gastric cancer. *D.* Large cancer cells of signet ring type are accompanied by smaller macrophages and still smaller leukocytes in pleural effusion. (*A:* Oil immersion.)

growth and, hence, protein synthesis is great, large, and sometimes multiple, nucleoli may be present.

Although abnormalities in the number and size of nucleoli in cancer cells were recorded by several observers in the 1930s (Haumeder, 1933; Schairer, 1935), the first objective data on the relationship of nucleoli to cancer were provided by Caspersson and Santesson (1942). Using ultraviolet spectrophotometry, these authors observed that there was a reciprocal relationship between the size of the nucleoli and the protein content of the cytoplasm of cancer cells. In cells located near blood vessels, the cytoplasm was rich in protein and contained small nucleoli **(Type A cells).** In cells distant from the blood vessels, the nucleoli were large and the amount of protein in the cytoplasm was small **(Type B cells).** It is logical that, in cancer cells with rapid growth and, therefore, high requirements for proteins, the nucleoli should be large and multiple. This was documented objectively by Long and Taylor (1956) in cells of **ovarian and endometrial cancers. The proportion of cancer cells with multiple nucleoli (up to five per cell), particularly in poorly differentiated tumors, was much larger than in benign ovarian tumors** and the differences were statistically significant.

The increase in the number of nucleoli in cancer cells

may be reflected in an **increase in the number of the nucleolar organizer sites (NOR).** These sites, which are constituted by open loops of DNA, can be revealed by **staining cells with silver salts (AgNOR).** After reduction of the silver salts to metallic silver the nucleolar organizer sites appear as black dots within the nucleus (Goodpasture and Bloom, 1975; review in Ruschaff et al, 1989). The assumption of such studies is that the **increase in the number of NORs per cell is indicative of a greater proliferation potential of the target tissue.** In general, cancer cells have a greater number of NORs than normal cells of the same origin. The method has been extensively applied to aspirated cell samples with questionable results (review in Cardillo, 1992).

The Nucleolini

Ultrastructural studies of nucleoli reveal the presence of two components—granular and fibrillar. The fibrillar component apparently corresponds to **small, round structures (nucleolini)** that may be observed within the nucleolus with the light microscope after staining with toluidine blue molybdate (Love et al, 1973). By the use of this method, it has been shown that the **nucleolini have a much greater variability in size and distribution (anisonucleolinosis)**

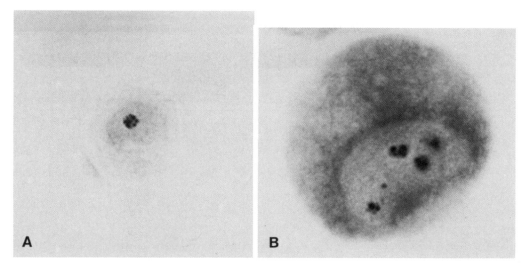

Figure 7-21 Nucleolini in a benign mesothelial cell (*A*) and a cell of metastatic adenocarcinoma (*B*) from a pleural fluid stained with toluidine blue molybdate. The small, even size of the nucleolini in the benign cell may be compared with the size variability in the malignant cell (anisonucleinosis). (Oil immersion.) (Courtesy of Dr. M. Takeda, Philadelphia, Pennsylvania.)

in cancer cells than in benign cells. These observations originally made on cells in tissue culture, have been extended to diagnostic human material by Love and Takeda et al (1974) (Fig. 7-21).

Cell Cycle and Mitoses

Cell Cycle

The principal characteristic of cancer cells is their uninhibited proliferation. **Clinically, the rate of proliferation of a cancer can be measured as doubling time of tumor volume,** using either clinical judgment or radiologic data. The doubling time may vary significantly from one cancer to another. There are two possible explanations for this phenomenon: (1) either the duration of the cell cycle is shortened, resulting in more frequent replication of the same cells, or (2) the number of cells undergoing mitosis is increased.

It is **commonly and erroneously assumed that the duration of the cell cycle** (time required for replication of the DNA, for the mitosis) **is much shorter in cancer cells than in normal cells. This is not true.** Both in the experimental systems and in humans, the **duration of the cell cycle in cancer cells is variable, very rarely shorter, and usually very much longer than normal.** Early studies by Clarkson et al (1965), and by others, documented that, in human cancers, cell cycle may be extended from the normal 18 hours to several days. Therefore, this mechanism cannot account for rapid growth of some malignant tumors. **Rather, it is the proportion of cells undergoing mitosis (mitotic rate) that is increased in cancer.**

Mitotic Rate

It has been observed, in experimental tumors, that the number of cells in mitosis increases substantially within hours or days after administration of a carcinogenic agent. Bertalanffy (1969) compared mitotic rates in normal, regenerat-

ing, and malignant cell populations in epidermal cell, mammary gland, and liver parenchyma in rats (Table 7-4). In general, **the mitotic rate of malignant tumors exceeded significantly the rate for normal tissues of origin.** However, the mitotic rate of regenerating or stimulated normal tissues (for instance, the breast in pregnancy or the regenerating liver after partial hepatectomy) could exceed the mitotic rate of cancer. There are, however, some significant differences. **The high mitotic rate of regenerating or stimulated benign tissues is a temporary phenomenon, followed by a return to normal values** once the reparative events have taken place or the stimulus has ceased. **In cancer, the high mitotic rate is usually a sustained phenomenon. In proliferating normal tissues, the mitotic rate usually matches the rate of cell loss. The mitotic rate in cancer is not offset by an equivalent cell loss.** The phenomenon of apoptosis, regulating normal cell growth, is reduced in cancer (see Chap. 6).

Although **mitotic counts** represent a method of assessing the proliferative potential of tissues and cells, the method is generally not reproducible and tedious. Another way to assess the proliferative potential of tumors is a determination of the proportion of proliferating cells by [3H]thymidine **incorporation,** the **estimation of cells in S-phase of the cycle** by flow cytometry or image analysis, or by determining the proportion of cells in a tumor expressing **proliferation cell nuclear antigen (PCNA), or reacting with the antibody Ki67.** Measuring the **incorporation of 5-bromodeoxyuridene (BRDU)** and replacing thymine in the DNA chain, is yet another way of determining DNA proliferation in cell populations (Gratzner, 1982; Rabinovitch et al, 1988). These issues are discussed in Chapters 46 and 47. In general, most malignant tumors show an increase in the proportion of proliferating cells when compared with normal tissue of the same origin, although there may be serious problems with the techniques and the interpretation of results.

TABLE 7-4	
COMPARISON BETWEEN 6-HOUR MITOTIC RATES OF NORMAL AND NEOPLASTIC CELL POPULATIONS	
Cell Population	**Mean 6-hr Percentage of Mitosis**
Epidermis (mouse)	
Normal	
Interfollicular and follicular wall epidermis	1.2–2.2
Hair matrix	29.8
Tumors	
Keratoacanthoma	3.4–6.5
Carcinoma	5.6
Mammary Gland (rat)	
Normal	
Virgin, lactation, involution	0.4–0.7
Pregnancy	0.4–4.4
Tumors	
Adenocarcinoma	0.4–8.4 (Ave. 2.2)
Liver (rat)	
Normal	0.02
Regeneration	0.7–16.2
Hepatoma	1.6–10.8

These data illustrate that the epidermal and mammary gland cancers proliferate faster than the normal cell populations of the same origin. Yet during some physiologic activities, the mitotic rate of normal cell populations may increase to exceed those of malignant tumors of the same origin (for instance: hair matrix or mammary gland during pregnancy). Similarly, mitotic activities of regenerating liver parenchyma may exceed that of a malignant hepatoma.
(Bertalanffy FD. *In* Fry R, Griem M, and Kirsten W (eds.). Normal and Malignant Cell Growth. New York, Springer, 1969.)

Abnormal Mitoses

Mitotic abnormalities have been recognized for many years as a common occurrence in malignant tumors. Boveri (1914) attempted to explain malignant growth as a consequence of mitotic abnormalities. The causes of mitotic abnormalities are not well understood.

Causes and Types of Mitotic Abnormalities

As originally proposed by Stubblefield (1968), it is thought today that the cause of mitotic abnormalities are disturbances in the formation of mitotic spindle (Zhou et al, 1998; Duesberg, 1999; Wilde and Zheng, 1999; Megee and Koshland, 1999; Kahana and Cleveland, 2001; Piel et al, 2001). The key to the abnormalities appears to be centrosome formation, which is governed by a complex of genes, among which p53 appears to play an important role (Fukasawa et al, 1996).

The mitotic abnormalities may be quantitative, qualitative, or both. The term **abnormal mitoses refers to mitotic figures with abnormal number or distribution of chromosomes or an excessive number of mitotic spindles,** hence, more than two mitotic poles (**multipolar mitoses**). The history of identification of mitotic and chromosomal abnormalities in cancer was summarized by Koller (1972), who also contributed a great deal of original work in this field. The following summary, modified from Koll-

er's work (1972), describes the principal abnormalities, illustrated in Fig. 7-22.

Defects in movement of chromosomes: Stickiness of chromosomes results in clumping or formation of metaphase bridges, preventing proper separation during metaphase.
Nondisjunction: Failure of separation of chromosomes during anaphase results in uneven division of the chromosomal complement between the daughter cells.
Chromosomal lag: Chromosomal lag reflects the failure of some chromosomes to join in the movement of chromosomes during ana-, meta-, or telophase. In such cells, some chromosomes remain at both poles of the spindle, whereas most chromosomes migrate to form the metaphase plate.
Abnormalities of the mitotic spindle: Such abnormalities result in multipolar mitoses with three, four or, rarely, more sets of centromeres (Fig. 7-23A). Perhaps the best known example of these abnormalities is the so-called **tripolar mitosis** (Dustin and Parmentier, 1953), often seen in carcinoma in situ of the uterine cervix, but not unique to this disease (Fig. 7-23B).
Abnormal number of chromosomes: The results of abnormalities of the mitotic spindle are either cells with **abnormal numbers of chromosomes** or gigantic tumor cells with numerous nuclei. The numerical abnormalities are more frequent than multipolar mitoses and are observed in **metaphases of cancer cells.** Excessive numbers of chromosomes are readily evident in metaphase rosettes and rarely require counting (Fig. 7-23C,D). Although tumor cells with an abnormal number of chromosomes may be viable, the fate of

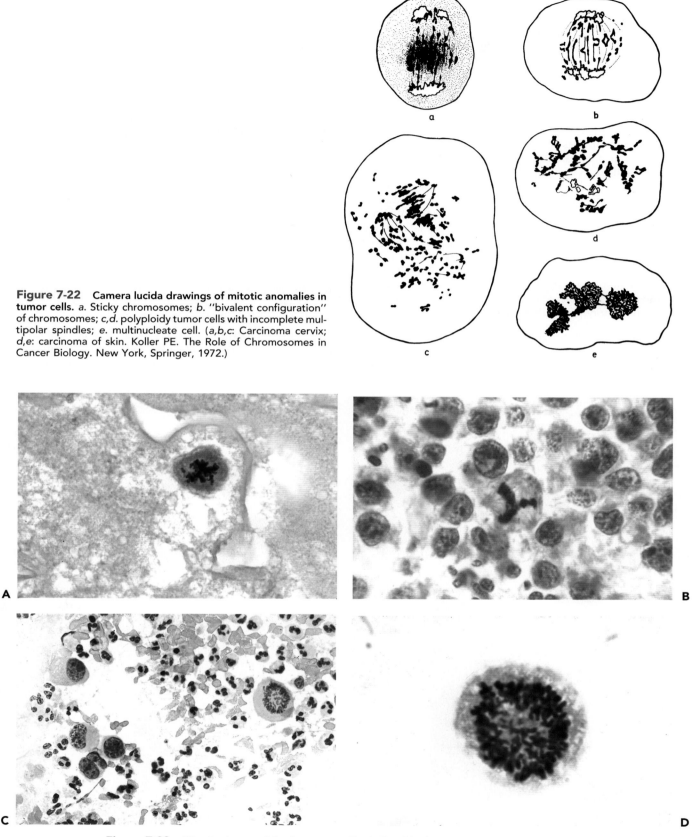

Figure 7-22   Camera lucida drawings of mitotic anomalies in tumor cells. *a.* Sticky chromosomes; *b.* "bivalent configuration" of chromosomes; *c,d.* polyploidy tumor cells with incomplete multipolar spindles; *e.* multinucleate cell. (*a,b,c:* Carcinoma cervix; *d,e:* carcinoma of skin. Koller PE. The Role of Chromosomes in Cancer Biology. New York, Springer, 1972.)

Figure 7-23   Mitotic abnormalities in cancer cells. *A.* Quadripolar mitosis, metastatic carcinoma to pericardial fluid. *B.* Tripolar mitosis, embryonal carcinoma, testis. *C.* Lung cancer, bronchial brush. Note a metaphase with numerous chromosomes next to cancer cells. *D.* Carcinoma of bladder, voided urine sediment with a tumor cell metaphase containing numerous chromosomes. (*A,B:* High magnification; *D:* oil immersion.) (*A* and *B* Courtesy of Dr. Carlos Rodriguez, Tucumán, Argentina.)

the monstrous caricatures of cells resulting from abnormal mitoses is uncertain. They probably represent evil-looking, but innocuous "gargoyles" of cancer, with no other future but ultimate death.

Mitoses in abnormal locations: Another abnormality observed in cancer is the presence of mitotic figures, whether morphologically normal or abnormal, in abnormal location. This is particularly applicable to situations **where the cancerous process is anatomically well-defined and polarized** as, for example, in squamous **carcinoma in situ**. In this disease (see Chap. 11), the presence of mitotic figures may be observed at all epithelial levels, whereas in normal epithelium, the mitotic activity is confined to the basal layer. Similarly, mitotic figures occurring within cancerous, mucus-secreting, glandular acini may be observed, whereas such activity is usually not obvious in mature glandular cells. It must be emphasized, however, that mitotic activity in abnormal location **may occur in benign tissues** as a result of reaction to injury or repair. In such instances, the mitoses usually occur in waves and then subside once the reparatory process has been completed.

Although, exceptionally, an abnormal mitosis may be encountered in the absence of cancer (see Fig. 6-9), it has been my experience that, **as a general rule, abnormal mitotic figures in cytologic material are associated with cancer and, therefore, constitute an important diagnostic clue.**

RECOGNIZING THE TYPE AND ORIGIN OF CANCER CELLS

Although the recognition of the malignant nature of cancer cells is based primarily on the nuclear features, the cytoplasmic features often reflect their origin and derivation of these cells. The issue is important because the recognition of cell derivation may be of significant diagnostic and clinical value, particularly in the classification of metastatic tumors of unknown origin. As a general principle, **cancer cells attempt, at all times, to mimic the tissue of origin with variable success and these attempts are expressed in the cytoplasm.** Thus, cancer cells of bronchial origin may mimic bronchial cells (Fig. 7-24A). Cancer cells of **squamous epithelial origin** often contain an abundance of **keratin filaments of high molecular weight;** this is reflected in **rigid polygonal shape** and intense **eosinophilic staining**

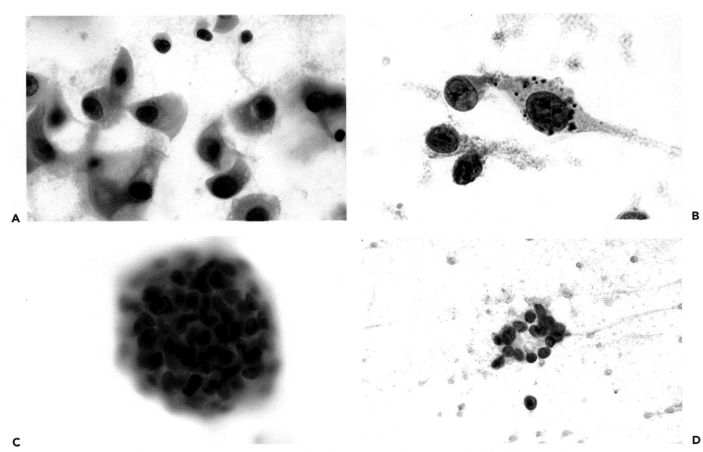

Figure 7-24   **Examples of differentiation of cancer cells.** *A.* Metastatic bronchogenic adenocarcinoma in pleural fluid. The cancer cells mimic bronchial epithelial cells. *B.* Metastatic malignant melanoma to liver. Melanin pigment granules in the cytoplasm are enhanced with Fontana-silver stain. *C.* Metastatic mammary adenocarcinoma in pleural fluid. The cells form a 3-dimensional spherical papillary cluster with evidence of mitotic activity. *D.* Lung brushings. Gland formation by cells of adenocarcinoma. (*B:* Oil immersion; *C:* high magnification.) (*B:* Courtesy of Prof. S. Woyke, Warsaw, Poland.)

of the cytoplasm, easily recognizable under the microscope. The formation of squamous "pearls," i.e., spherical structures composed of squamous cells surrounding a core of keratin, is commonly observed in squamous cancers (see Chaps. 11 and 20). The cytoplasm of cancer cells originating in the **glandular epithelium** may show evidence of **production** and **secretion of mucin** or related substances in the form of cytoplasmic vacuoles; such cells may also retain the **columnar configuration** of cells of the epithelium of origin. Cancer cells derived from **striated muscle** may display **cytoplasmic striations** and cells derived from pigment-producing malignant tumors, such as melanomas, may produce cytoplasmic deposits of **melanin pigment** (Fig. 7-24B).

It is not uncommon for differentiated cancer cells to form three-dimensional structures mimicking the structure of the tissue of origin. Thus, formation of **gland-like or tubule-like structures is fairly common in adenocarci-** nomas, as is the formation of spherical or oval three-dimensional clusters of cancer cells, mimicking the formation of papillary structures of the tumor observed in tissue sections (Fig. 7-24C,D). Leighton (1967) devised an experimental system of tissue culture wherein cancer cells may be observed to form three-dimensional structures mimicking the tissue of origin or its function, such as formation of melanin (Fig. 7-25).

In many cancer cells, however, the efforts at differentiation are stymied, resulting in cells that have very few or no distinguishing features under the light microscope. Such cells are classified as "**poorly differentiated**" or "**anaplastic**" (from Greek, *ana* = again and *plasis* = a moulding), suggesting a reversal to a more primitive, embryonic type of cell. Still, even **such cells may display features of sophisticated differentiation by electron microscopy or by immunostaining.** For example, cells derived from poorly differentiated tumors of the **nervous system,** such as neuro-

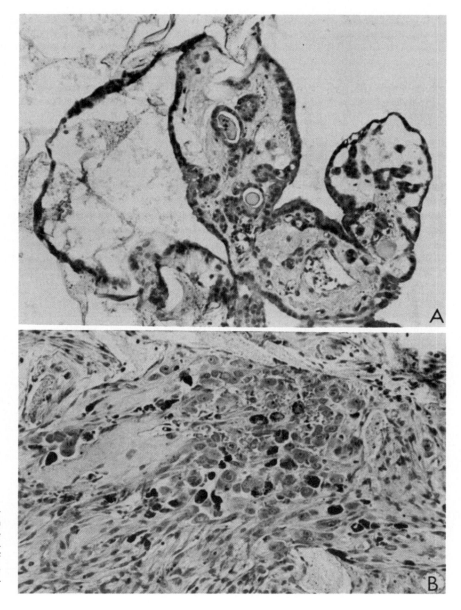

Figure 7-25 Growth pattern of human tumors on cellulose sponge matrix coated with fibrin. *A.* Papillary carcinoma of thyroid. Note formation of colloid-filled acini. *B.* Primary culture of fibroblasts with a secondary culture of malignant melanoma. Note pigment formation. (Courtesy of Dr. Joseph Leighton, Philadelphia, Pennsylvania.)

blastomas, may show ultrastructural evidence of formation of characteristic cell junctions (synapses), and of neurofibrils (see Chap. 40). Cells derived from tumors with **endocrine function** may show evidence of hormone formation in the form of the characteristic cytoplasmic vesicles in electron microscopy. The endocrine function may also be revealed by immunocytochemistry with antibodies to the endocrine granules in general or to the specific cell product. Many such examples could be given. Immunocytochemistry, discussed in detail in Chapter 45, may be applied in an attempt to determine the origin on undifferentiated cancer cells. An overview of the fundamental reagents is given in Table 7-5. The issue of cell differentiation in cancer is further complicated by the fact that **the expressions of differentiation may vary, not only from cell to cell within the same tumor, but may depend on the clinical presentation of the same tumor.** As an example, a poorly differentiated primary carcinoma of squamous or glandular lineage may become fully differentiated in a metastatic focus and vice versa; a well differentiated primary tumor may form poorly differentiated metastases. Further, a tumor that may appear to be of a single lineage in its primary presentation may form metastases showing two or sometimes more families of cancer cells. **In general, during the natural history of a cancer, recurrent or metastatic tumors tend to be less well differentiated than the primary but there are many exceptions to this rule.**

It is quite evident that the issues of cell differentiation in cancer are extremely complex and **depend on multiple genes** that may or may not be expressed in any given cancer cell. There is, at this time, essentially no factual information on the molecular biologic mechanisms that account for the differentiation of cancer cells. On the other hand, a great deal of work has been performed to explain the mechanisms

TABLE 7-5

CANCER CELL MARKERS*

Marker	Tumor Expression	Remarks
Oncofetal Antigens		
Carcinoembryonic antigen	Tumors of the gastrointestinal and respiratory tracts	Occasionally useful in diagnosis Used in monitoring of patients
Alphafetoprotein	Germ cell tumors of ovary and testis; primary hepatomas	Useful in diagnosis
Placental alkaline phosphatase Acid phosphatase Prostate specific antigen	Prostatic cancer	Useful in diagnosing stage and spread of tumor and in monitoring treatment
Hormones		
Hcg (human chorionic gonadotropin)	Tumors of placenta; germ cell tumors of testis, sometimes ovary	Useful in diagnosing and monitoring patients
Polypeptide hormones (calcitonin, gastrin, somatostatin, serotonin, parathyroid hormone, pituitary hormones)	Endocrine tumors of various organs: thyroid, pancreas, gastrointestinal, and respiratory tracts, adrenal medulla, pituitary	Useful in tumor identification and classification, sometimes in monitoring patients
Epitectin (Ca1), milk factor epithelial membrane antigen	Antigens without specificity	Recognize cancer cell epitopes—not reliable
Hormone receptors: estrogen, progesterone	Breast cancer Endometrial cancer	Guide to therapy Prognostic value still insecure
Growth factors, oncogene products, platelet-derived growth factor, insulin-like growth factor, nerve growth factor, epidermal growth factor	Widely distributed in many tumors	Have diagnostic value Prognostic value questionable except c-myc in neuroblastoma
Monoclonal antibodies recognizing specific organs or tumors (prostate, melanomas, ovarian tumors)	Various organs and tumors	Occasionally of diagnostic value
Monoclonal antibodies recognizing intermediate filaments	Widely distributed	Of value in diagnosis carcinoma vs sarcoma
Monoclonal antibodies recognizing stages of development of lymphocytes and their lineage (CDs, see Chap. 5)	Malignant lymphomas	Classification of lymphomas
Proliferation antigens	Ki67, PCNA (cyclin)	Possibly useful in tumor prognosis

* For further discussion see Chapter 45.

of differentiation occurring during embryonal life of multicellular animals, when germ cells are organized to form tissues and organs. The best known target of these studies is a small worm, *Caenorhabditis elegans,* which has been shown to carry 19,000 genes that have been sequenced. It is of interest that many genes that govern the embryonal development of the worm also occur in other multicellular organisms (Ruvkun and Hobert, 1998). It may be assumed that such developmental genes remain active in mature organisms and that they may be transmitted to cancer cells wherein they may be activated or inactivated according to circumstances about which nothing is known at this time. The proof that all genes are present in normal cells is provided by successful **animal cloning** using nuclei from mature cells inserted into the ovum.

MALIGNANCY-ASSOCIATED CHANGES

Under this name, Nieburgs et al (1967) described, many years ago, **changes observed in nuclei of leukocytes and epithelial cells in patients with cancer.** The changes were observed in cells that were either remote or adjacent to the site of cancer origin. The changes were classified as "orderly" with clear spherical areas in nuclear chromatin, or "disorderly," based on chromatin clumping. The orderly changes were observed in areas remote from the primary tumor and the disorderly changes were observed in cells adjacent to tumors.

The observations were revived by the observation that morphologically normal parabasal and intermediate squamous cells **in smears from patients with precancerous lesions of the uterine cervix** showed abnormal patterns of chromatin (Bibbo et al, 1981; Burger et al, 1981). These abnormalities could be measured and became the basis of an automated diagnostic system based on Feulgen-stained cells (Poulin et al, 1994). It is interesting that molecular biologic observations of morphologically normal epithelium, adjacent to cancer in various organs, may show genetic abnormalities. In practice, some degrees of nuclear atypia of benign epithelial cells may be observed in patients with various cancers, as will be discussed in appropriate chapter.

BIBLIOGRAPHY

Abercrombie M. Contact inhibition. The phenomenon and its biological implications. Natl Cancer Inst Monogr 26:249–277, 1967.
Abercrombie M, Ambrose EJ. Surface properties of cancer cells: A review. Cancer Res 22:525–548, 1962.
Agarwal V, Greenebaum E, Wersto R, Koss LG. DNA ploidy of spindle cell soft tissue tumors and its relationship to histology and clinical outcome. Arch Pathol Lab Med 115:558–562, 1991.
Akerman M, Dreinhofer K, Rydholm A, et al. Cytogenetic studies on fine-needle aspiration samples from osteosarcoma and Ewing's sarcoma. Diagn Cytopathol 15:17–22, 1996.
Albelda LM. Role of integrins and other cell adhesion molecules in tumor progression and metastases. Lab Invest 68:4–17, 1993.
Alvarez MR. Microfluorometric comparisons of chromatin thermal stability in situ between normal and neoplastic cells. Cancer Res 33:786–790, 1973.
Alvaro AS, Dalbagni G, Cordon-Cardo C, et al. Nuclear overexpression of p53 protein in transitional cell bladder carcinoma: A marker for disease progression. J Natl Cancer Inst 85:53–59, 1993.
Ashworth CT, Luibel FJ, Sanders E. The fine structure of nuclei in certain human malignant neoplasms. Am J Clin Pathol 34:9–20, 1960.
Atkin NB. Variant nuclear types in gynecologic tumors. Observations on squashes and smears. Acta Cytol 13:569–575, 1969.

Atkin NB. A high incidence of cells with a condensed (telophase) chromatin pattern in human tumors and carcinoma in situ. Acta Cytol 11:81–85, 1967.
Atkin NB. The relationship between the deoxyribonucleic acid content and the ploidy of human tumors. Cytogenetics 1:113–122, 1962.
Atkin NB, Baker MC. A nuclear protrusion in a human tumor associated with an abnormal chromosome. Acta Cytol 8:431–433, 1964.
Atkin NB, Mattison G, Baker MC. A comparison of the DNA content and chromosome numbers in fifty human tumours. Br J Cancer 20:87–101, 1966.
Atrighi FE, Hsu TC. Localization of heterochromatin in human chromosomes. Cytogenetics 10:81–86, 1971.
Bailar JC, Gornik HL. Cancer undefeated. N Engl J Med 336:1569–1574, 1997.
Barker BE, Sanford KK. Cytologic manifestations of neoplastic transformation in vitro. JNCI 44:39–63, 1970.
Barr ML, Bertram EG. A morphological distinction between neurons of the male and the female, and the behavior of the nucleolar satellite during accelerated nucleoprotein synthesis. Nature 163:676–677, 1949.
Baserga R. Multiplication and Division in Mammalian Cells. New York, Marcel Dekker, 1976.
Ben-Bassat H, Inbar M, Sachs L. Changes in the structural organization of the membrane in malignant cell transformation. J Membr Biol 6:183–194, 1971.
Bendich A, Vizoso AD, Harris RG. Intercellular bridges between mammalian cells in culture. Proc Natl Acad Sci USA 57:1029–1035, 1967.
Benedict W, Lerner SP, Zhou J, et al. Level of retinoblastoma protein expression correlates with p16 (MTS/INK4A/CDK2) status in bladder cancer. Oncogene 18:1197–1203, 1999.
Berenblum I. Carcinogenesis as a Biological Problem. New York, American Elsevier, 1974.
Bergers G, Javaherian K, Lo K-M, et al. Effects of angiogenesis inhibitors on multistage carcinogenesis in mice. Science 284:808–812, 1999.
Bernhard W. Electron microscopy of tumor cells and tumor viruses: Review. Cancer Res 18:491–509, 1958.
Bertalanffy FD. Comparison between the rates of proliferation of induced malignancies and their proliferation and their normal tissue of origin. In Fry RJM, Griem ML, Kristen WH (eds). Normal and Malignant Cell Growth. New York, Springer-Verlag, 1969.
Bibbo M, Bartels PH, Sychra JJ, Wied GL. Chromatin appearance in intermediate cells from patients with uterine cancer. Acta Cytol 25:23–28, 1981.
Bichsel VE, Liotta LA, Petricoin EF 3rd. Cancer proteomics: from biomarker discovery to signal pathway profiling. Cancer J 7:69–78, 2001.
Bishop JM. The molecular genetics of cancer. Science 235:305–311, 1987.
Bittner JJ. The cause and control of mammary cancer in mice. Harvey Lect 42:221–246, 1947.
Blackburn EH. Structure and function of telomeres. Nature 350:569–573, 1990.
Bodnar AG, Ouellette M, Frolkis M, et al. Extension of life-span by introduction of telomerase into normal human cells. Science 279:349–352, 1998.
Bohm N, Sandritter W. DNA in human tumors: A cytophotometric study. In Current Topics in Pathology, vol 6. New York, Springer-Verlag, 1975.
Bolodeoku J, Yoshida K, Sugino T, et al. CD44 expression in human breast cancer cell lines is related to oestrogen receptor (ER) status and confluency in vitro. Biochem Soc Trans 25:356S, 1997.
Borland RN, Partin AW, Epstein JI, Brendler CB. The use of nuclear morphometry in predicting recurrence of transitional cell carcinoma. J Urol 149:272–275, 1993.
Boshoff C, Weiss RA. Kaposi's sarcoma associated herpesvirus. Adv Cancer Res 75:57–86, 1998.
Boveri T. Zur Frage der Entstehung maligner Tumoren. Jena, Fischer, 1914.
Braunstein H, Stephens CL, Gibson RL. Secretory granules in medullary carcinoma of the thyroid. Arch Pathol 85:306–313, 1968.
Bunz F, Dutriaux A, Lengauer C, et al. Requirement for p53 and p21 to sustain G2 arrest after DNA damage. Science 282:1497–1500, 1998.
Burger G, Auettling U, Rodenacker K. Changes in benign cell population in cases of cervical cancer and its precursors. Anal Quant Cytol 3:261–271, 1981.
Busch H, Byvoet P, Smetana K. The nucleolus of the cancer cell: A review. Cancer Res 23:313–339, 1963.
Cairns J. Mutation selection and the natural history of cancer. Nature 255:197–200, 1975.
Cajulis RS, Frias-Hidvegi D. Detection of numerical chromosomal abnormalities in malignant cells in fine needle aspirates by fluorescence in situ hybridization of interphase nuclei with chromosome-specific probes. Acta Cytol 37:391–396, 1993.
Cajulis RS, Haines GK, Frias-Hidvegi D, McVary K. Interphase cytogenetics as an adjunct in the cytodiagnosis of urinary bladder carcinoma. A comparative study of cytology, flow cytometry and interphase cytogenetics in bladder washes. Anal Quant Cytol Histol 16:1–10, 1994.
Cajulis RS, Yu GH, Gokaslen ST, Hidvegi DE. Modfied interphase cytogenetics technique as an adjunct in the analysis of atypical cells in body fluids. Diagn Cytopathol 16:331–335, 1997.
Cardillo MR. Ag-NOR technique in fine needle aspiration cytology of salivary gland masses. Acta Cytol 36:147–151, 1992.
Caspersson T. Cell Growth and Cell Function: A Cytochemical Study. New York, WW Norton, 1950.
Caspersson T, Santesson L. Studies on protein metabolism in cells of epithelial tumors. Acta Radiol (Suppl) 46:1–105, 1942.
Chuaqui R, Vargas MP, Castiglioni T, et al. Detection of heterozygosity loss in microdissected fine needle aspiration specimens of breast carcinoma. Acta Cytol 40:642–648, 1996.

Clarkson B, Ota K, Ohkita T, O'Connor A. Kinetics of proliferation of cancer cells in neoplastic effusions in man. Cancer 18:1189–1213, 1965.

Collins FS. BRCA 1: Lots of mutations, lots of dilemmas. N Engl J Med 334:186–188, 1996.

Coman DR. Adhesiveness and stickness: Two independent properties of cell surface. Cancer Res 21:1436–1438, 1961.

Coman DR. Decreased mutual adhesiveness; property of cells from squamous cell carcinomas. Cancer Res 4:625–629, 1944.

Cossman J, Uppencamp M, Sundeen J, et al. Molecular genetics in the diagnosis of lymphoma. Arch Pathol Lab Med 112:117–127, 1988.

Couch FJ, DeShano ML, Blackwood A, et al. BRCA 1 mutations in women attending clinics that evaluate the risk of breast cancer. N Engl J Med 336:1409–1415, 1997.

Counter CM, Hirte HW, Bacchetti S, Harley CB. Telomerase activity in human ovarian carcinomas. Proc Natl Acad Sci USA 91:2900–2904, 1994.

Craver RD, McGarry P. Delicate longitudinal nuclear grooves in childhood ependymomas. Arch Pathol Lab Med 118:919–921, 1994.

Czerniak B, Chen R, Tuziak T, et al. Expression of ras oncogene p2l protein in relation to regional spread of human breast carcinomas. Cancer 63:2008–2013, 1989.

Czerniak B, Cohen GL, Etkin P, et al. Concurrent mutations of coding and regulatory sequences of the Ha-ras gene in urinary bladder carcinoma. Hum Pathol 23:1199–1204, 1992.

Czerniak B, Deitch D, Simmons H, et al. Ha-ras gene codon 12 mutation and ploidy in urinary bladder cancer. Br J Cancer 62:762–763, 1990.

Czerniak B, Herz F, Wersto RP, Alster P, et al. Quantitation of oncogene products by computer-assisted image analysis and flow cytometry. J Histochem Cytochem 38:463–466, 1990.

Czerniak B, Herz F, Wersto RP, Koss LG. Modification of Ha-ras Oncogene p21 expression and cell cycle progression in the human colonic cancer cell line HT-29. Cancer Res 47:2826–2830, 1987.

Czerniak B, Koss LG, Sherman A. Nuclear pores and DNA ploidy in human bladder carcinomas. Cancer Res 44:3752–3756, 1984.

Darzynkiewicz Z, Traganos F, Carter SP, Higgins PJ. In situ factors affecting stability of the DNA helix in interphase nuclei and metaphase Chromosomes. Exp Cell Res 172:168–179, 1987.

de Harven E. Ultrastructural studies on three different types of mouse leukemia: A review. *In* Tumors Induced by Viruses. New York, Academic Press, 1962, pp 183–206.

de la Chapelle A. Microsatellite instability. N Engl J Med 349:209–210, 2003.

de Lange T. Telomere capping: One strand fits all. Science 292:1075–1076, 2001.

de Lange T. Telomerase and senescence: Ending the debate. Science 279:334–335, 1998.

de Lange T, DePinho RA. Unlimited mileage from telomerase? Science 283:947–949, 1999.

de The G. Epidemiology of Epstein-Barr virus and associated diseases in man. *In* Rojzman B (ed). The Herpesviruses, vol. 1. New York, Plenum Press, 1982, pp 25–103.

Deligeorgi-Politi H. Nuclear crease as a cytodiagnostic feature of papillary thyroid carcinoma in fine-needle aspiration biopsies. Diagn Cytopathol 3:307–310, 1987.

Dhuldiner AR. Transgenic animals. N Engl J Med 334:653–655, 1996.

Diamond DA, Berry SJ, Umbright C, et al. Computerized image analysis of nuclear shape as a prognostic factor for prostatic cancer. Prostate 3:351–355, 1982.

Domagala W, Koss LG. Configuration of surfaces of cells in effusions by scanning electron microscopy. *In* Koss LG, Coleman DV (eds). Advances in Clinical Cytology. London, Butterworths, 1981, pp 270–313.

Domagala W, Kahan AV, Koss LG. The ultrastructure of surfaces of positively identified cells in the human urinary sediment: A correlative light and scanning electron microscopic study. Acta Cytol 23:147–155, 1979.

Domagala W, Koss LG. Configuration of surfaces of human cancer cell in effusions. A scanning electron microscope study of microvilli. Virch Archiv B (Zell Pathol) 26:27–42, 1977.

Duesberg P. Are centrosomes or aneuploidy the key to cancer? Science 284:2091–2092, 1999.

Dulbecco R. Transformation of cells in vivo by DNA-containing viruses. JAMA 190:721–726, 1964.

Dustin P, Parmentier R. Donnees experimentales sur la nature des mitoses anormales observés dans certains epitheliomas du col uterin. Gynecol Obstet 52:258–265, 1953.

Ehrich WE. Nuclear sizes in growth disturbances. With special reference to the tumor cell nuclei. Am J Path 192:772–790, 1936.

Ehya H, Lang WR. Cytology of granulosa cell tumor of the ovary. Am J Clin Pathol 85:402–405, 1986.

Epstein MA, Achong BG, Barr YM. Virus particles in cultured lymphoblasts from Burkitt's lymphoma. Lancet 1:702–703, 1964.

Esrig D, Elmajian D, Croshen S, et al. Accumulation of nuclear p53 and tumor progression in bladder cancer. N Engl J Med 331:1259–1264, 1994.

Esrig D, Spruck CHI, Nichols PW, et al. P53 nuclear protein accumulation correlates with mutations in the p53 gene, tumor grade, and stage in bladder cancer. Am J Pathol 143:1389–1397, 1993.

Fallenious AG, Auer GU, Carstensen JM. Prognostic significance of DNA measurements in 409 consecutive breast cancer patients. Cancer 62:331–341, 1988.

Fearon ER. Human cancer syndromes: Clues to the origin and nature of cancer. Science 278:1043–1050, 1997.

Fearon ER, Cho XR, Nigro JM, et al. Identification of a chromosome 18q gene that is altered in colorectal cancers. Science 247:49–56, 1990.

Fearon ER, Vogelstein B. A genetic model for colorectal tumorigenesis. Cell 61:759–767, 1990.

Feimesser R, Miyazaki I, Cheung R, et al. Diagnosis of nasopharyngeal carcinoma by DNA amplification of tissue obtained by fine-needle aspiration biopsy. N Engl J Med 326:17–21, 1992.

Fidler IJ, Hart MR. Biological diversity in metastatic neoplasms: Origins and implications. Science 217:998–1003, 1982.

Fidler IJ, Poste G. The cellular heterogeneity of malignant neoplasms: Implications for adjuvant chemotherapy. Semin Oncol 12:207–221, 1985.

Fitzgerald MG, MacDonald DJ, Krainer M, et al. BRCA germ-line mutations in Jewish and non-Jewish women with early-onset breast cancer. N Engl J Med 334:143–149, 1996.

Folkman J. Clinical applications of research on angiogenesis. N Engl J Med 331:1757–1763, 1995.

Folkman J, Klagsbrun M. Angiogenic factors. Science 235:442–447, 1987.

Fossel M. Telomerase and the aging cell. JAMA 279:1732–1735, 1998.

Frank TS. Hereditary cancer syndromes. Arch Pathol Lab Med 125:85–90, 2001.

Friedlander M, Brooks PC, Shaffer RW, et al. Definition of two angiogenic pathways by distinct alpha integrins. Science 270:1500–1502, 1995.

Friedwald WF, Rous P. The initiating and promoting elements in tumor production. J Exp Med 80:101–126, 1944.

Friend C, Pogo BG. The molecular pathology of Friend erythroleukemia virus strains. An overview. Biochem Biophys Acta 780:181–195, 1985.

Frisch M, Biggar RJ, Engels EA, Goedert JJ. Association of cancer with AIDS-related immunosuppression in adults. JAMA 285:1736–1745, 2001.

Fröstad B, Martinsson T, Tani E, et al. The use of fine-needle aspiration cytology in the molecular characterization of neuroblastoma in children. Cancer Cytopthol 87:60–68, 1999.

Fukasawa K, Choi T, Kuriyama R, et al. Abnormal centrosome amplification in the absence of p53. Science 271:1744–1747, 1996.

Futreal PA, Liu Q, Shattuck-Eidens D. BRCA1 mutation in primary breast and ovarian carcinoma. Science 266:120–122, 1994.

Gardner EJ. A follow-up study of a family group exhibiting dominant inheritance or a syndrome of intestinal polyps, osteomas, fibromas, and epidermal cysts. Am J Hum Genet 14:376–390, 1962.

Gavosto F, Pilieri A. Cell cycle of cancer cells in man. *In* Baserga R (ed). The Cell Cycle and Cancer. New York, Marcel Dekker, 1971.

Gehlsen KR, Dillner L, Engvall E, Ruoslahti E. The human laminin receptor is a member of the integrin family of cell adhesion receptors. Science 241:1228–1229, 1988.

Gerdes J, Li L, Schlueter C, et al. Immunochemical and molecular biologic characterisation of the cell proliferation-associated antigen that is defined by the monoclonal antibody Xi-67. J Immunol 133:1710–1715, 1984.

Gisselsson D, Bjork J, Hoglund M, et al. Abnormal nuclear shape in solid tumors reflects mitotic instability. Am J Pathol 158:199–206, 2001.

Gisselsson D, Pettersson L, Hoglund M, et al. Chromosomal breakage-fusion-bridge events cause genetic intratumor heterogeneity. Proc Natl Acad Sci USA 97:5357–5362, 2000.

Glassman AB. Cytogenetics, in situ hybridization and molecular approaches in the diagnosis of cancer. Ann Clin Lab Sci 28:324–329, 1998.

Goodpasture C, Bloom SE. Visualization of nuclear organizer regions in mammalian chromosomes using silver staining. Chromosoma 53:37–50, 1975.

Goodson S, Tarin D. Clinical implications of anomalous D44 gene expression in neoplasia. Front Biosc 2:E89–E109, 1998.

Gratzner HG. Monoclonal antibody to 5-bromo- and 5-iododeoxyuridine: A new reagent for detection of DNA replication. Science 218:474–475, 1982.

Gray JW, Mayall BH (eds). Monoclonal Antibodies against Bromodeoxyuridine. New York, AR Liss, 1985.

Greenblatt RM. Kaposi's sarcoma and human herpesvirus-8. Inf Dis Clin North Am 12:63–82, 1998.

Gryfe R, Kim H, Hsieh ETK, et al. Tumor microsatellite instability and clinical outcome in young patients with colorectal cancer. N Engl J Med 342:69–77, 2000.

Gura T. New kind of cancer mutation found. Science 277:1201–1202, 1997.

Haber DE. Telomeres, cancer, and immortality. N Engl J Med 332:955–956, 1995.

Hahn WC, Weinberg RA. Rules for making human tumor cells. N Engl J Med 347:1593–1603, 2002.

Hajdu SI, Bean MA, Fogh J, et al. Papanicolaou smear of cultured human tumor cells. Acta Cytol 18:327–332, 1974.

Hall JM, Lee MK, Newman B, et al. Linkage of early onset familial breast cancer to chromosome 17q21. Science 250:1684–1689, 1990.

Hall PA, Levison DA, Woods AL, et al. Proliferating cell nuclear antigen (PCNA) immunolocalization in paraffin sections: an index of cell proliferation with evidence of deregulated expression in some neoplasms. J Path 162:285–294, 1990.

Harris CC, Hollstein M. Clinical implications of the p53 tumor suppressor gene. N Engl J Med 329:1318–1327, 1993.

Haumeder E. Vergleichende Kern- und Nukleolenmessungen an verschiedenen Organengewebe mit besonder Berueksichtigung der malignen Tumorzellen. Z. Krebsforsch 40:105–116, 1933.

Hawley RS. Unresolvable endings: Defective telomeres and failed separation. Science 275:1441–1443, 1997.

Hayflick L. The cell biology of human aging. Sci Am 242:58–65, 1980.

Hayflick L. The limited in vitro lifetime of human diploid cell strains. Exp Cell Res 37:614–636, 1965.

He TC, Sparks AB, Rago C, Hermeking H, et al. Identification of c-MYC as a target of APC pathway. Science 281:1509–1512, 1998.

Heim S, Mitelman F. Cancer Cytogenetics, 2nd ed. New York, Alan Liss, 1995.

Herman JG, Baylin SB. Gene silencing in cancer in association with promoter hypermethylation. N Engl J Med 349:2042–2054, 2003.

Hinchcliffe EH, Li C, Thompson EA, et al. Requirement of Cdk-2 cyclin E activity for repeated centrosome reproduction in Xenopus egg extract. Science 283:851–854, 1999.

Hinchcliffe EH, Miller FJ, Cham M, et al. Requirement of a centrosomal activity for cell cycle progression through G_1 into S phase. Science 291:1547–1550, 2001.

Hofmann W, Schlag PM. BRCA1 and BRCA2: Breast cancer susceptibility genes. J Cancer Res Clin Oncol 126:487–496, 2000.

Holt JT, Thompson ME, Szabo C, et al. Growth retardation and tumour inhibition by BRCA 1. Natl Genetics 12:298–302, 1996.

Hopkins K. A surprising function for PTEN tumor suppressor. Science 282:1027–1030, 1998.

Housman D. Human DNA polymorphism. N Engl J Med 332:318–320, 1995.

Huang HJ, Yee JK, Shew JY, et al. Suppression of the neoplastic phenotype by replacement of the RB gene in human cancer cells. Science 242:1563–1566, 1988.

Hughes JH, Caraway NP, Katz RL. Blastic variant of mantle-cell lymphoma: Cytomorphologic, immunocytochemical, and molecular genetic features of tissue obtained by fine-needle aspiration biopsy. Diagn Cytopathol 19:59–62, 1998.

Ichikawa A, Kinishita T, Watanabe T, et al. Mutations of the p53 gene as a prognostic factor in aggressive B-cell lymphoma. N Engl J Med 337:529–534, 1997.

Inbar M, Ben-Bassat H, Sachs L. Membrane changes associated with malignancy. Nature 236:3–4, 1972.

Jacks T, Weinberg RA. The expanding role of cell cycle regulators. Science 280:1035–1036, 1998.

Juan G, Gruenewald S, Darzynkiewicz Z. Phosphorylation of retinoblastoma susceptibility gene protein assayed in individual lymphocytes during their mitotic stimulation. Exp Cell Res 239:104–110, 1998.

Kaelin WG Jr. Another p53 Doppelgaenger? Science 280:57–58, 1998.

Kahana JA, Cleveland DW. Some important news about spindle assembly. Science 291:1718–1719, 2001.

Kamel OW, Franklin WA, Ringus JC, Meyer JS. Thymidine labeling index and Ki-67 growth fraction in lesions of the breast. Am J Pathol 134:107–113, 1989.

Keesee SK, Marchese J, Meneses A, et al. Human cervical cancer-associated nuclear matrix proteins. Exper Cell Res 244:14–25, 1998.

Keinanen M, Griffin JD, Bloomfield CD, et al. Clonal chromosomal abnormalities showing multiple-cell-lineage involvement in acute myeloid leukemia. N Engl J Med 318:1153–1158, 1988.

Kiberts P, Marx J. The unstable path to cancer (preface to a series of articles on this topic). Science 297:543, 2002.

Kinzer KW, Vogelstein B. Landscaping the cancer terrain. Science 280:1036–1037, 1998.

Kinzer KW, Vogelstein B. Lessons from hereditary colorectal cancer. Cell 87:159–170, 1996.

Kirk KE, Harmon BP, Reichardt LK, et al. Block in anaphase chromosome separation caused by telomerase template mutation. Science 275:1478–1481, 1997.

Klein G, Klein E. Evolution of tumours and the impact of molecular oncology. Nature 315:190–195, 1985.

Knudson AG. Mutation and cancer: statistical study of neuroblastoma. Proc Natl Acad Sci USA 68:820–823, 1971.

Knudson AG, Meadows AT, Nichols WH, Hill R. Chromosomal deletion and neuroblastona. N Engl J Med 295:1120–1123, 1976.

Koller PS. The Role of Chromosomes in Cancer Biology. New York, Springer-Verlag, 1972.

Koss LG. Characteristics of chromosomes in polarized normal human bronchial cells provide a blueprint for nuclear organization. Cygogenet Cell Genet 82:230–237, 1998.

Koss LG. Human papillomavirus: passenger, driver, or both? (editorial). Human Path 29:309–310, 1998.

Koss LG. Automated cytology and histology: A historical perspective. Anal Quant Cytol Histol 2:369–374, 1987.

Koss LG. Analytical and quantitative cytology: A historical perspective. Anal Quant Cytol Histol 1:251–256, 1982.

Koss LG. Morphology of cancer cells. In Handbuch der allgemeinen Pathologie 6, Tumors I, 5th part. New York, Springer, 1974, pp 1–139.

Koss LG, Bartels PH, Bibbo M, et al. Computer discrimination between benign and malignant urothelial cells. Acta Cytol 19:378–391, 1975.

Koss LG, Czerniak B, Herz F, Wersto RP. Flow cytometric measurements of DNA, other cell components in human tumors: A critical appraisal. Hum Pathol 20:528–548, 1989.

Kovacs G. Observations on nuclear protrusions and the length of long arms of abnormal chromosomes in malignancy. Acta Cytol 26:247–250, 1982.

Kramer BS, Klausner RD. Grappling with cancer: Defeatism versus the reality of progress. N Engl J Med 337:931–934, 1997.

Kristoffersson U, Heim S, Heldrup J, et al. Cytogenetic studies of childhood non-Hodgkin lymphomas. Hereditas 103:77–84, 1985b.

Kristoffersson U, Olsson H, Akerman M, Mitelman F. Cytogenetic studies in non-Hodgkin lymphomas: results from fine-needle aspiration samples. Hereditas 103:63–76, 1985a.

Krontiris TG. Oncogenes. N Engl J Med 333:303–306, 1995.

Kunicka JE, Darzynkiewicz Z, Melamed MR. DNA in situ sensitivity to denaturation: A new parameter for flow cytometry of normal human colonic epithelium and colon carcinoma. Cancer Res 47:3942–3947, 1987.

Kurzrock R, Gutterman JV, Talpaz M. The molecular genetics of Philadelphia chromosome-positive leukemia. N Engl J Med 319:990–998, 1988.

Landon J, Ratcliffe JS, Rees LH, Scott AP. Tumour-associated hormonal products. J Clin Pathol 7(Suppl R Coll Pathol):127–134, 1974.

Lane DP. p53, guardian of the genome. Nature 358:15–16, 1992.

Langston AA, Malone KE, Thompson JD, et al. BRCA 1 mutations in a population-based sample of young women with breast cancer. N Engl J Med 334:137–142, 1996.

Lavin P, Koss LG. Effect of a single dose of cyclophosphamide on various organs in the rat. IV. Electron microscopic study of the renal tubes. Am J Path 62:169–180, 1971.

Leighton J. Human mammary cancer cell lines and other epithelial cells cultured as organoid tissue in lenticular pouches of reinforced collagen membranes. In Vitro Cell Dev Biol-Animal 33:783–790, 1997.

Leighton J. Invasive growth and metastasis in tissue culture systems. In Busch H (ed). Methods in Cancer Research, vol. 4. New York, Academic Press, 1967, pp 86–124.

Leppert M, Dobbs M, Scambler P, et al. The gene for familial polyposis coli maps to the long arm of chromosome 5. Science 238:1411–1413, 1987.

Levine AJ, Momand J, Finley CA. The P53 tumor suppressor gene. Nature 351:435–456, 1991.

Li FP, Fraumeni JF. Soft tissue sarcomas, breast cancer, and other neoplasms: A familial syndrome? Ann Int Med 21:747–752, 1969.

Li S, Tuck-Muller CM, Yan Q, et al. A rapid method for PCR amplification of DNA directly from cells fixed in Carnoy's fixative. Am J Med Genet 55:116–119, 1995.

Liotta LA. Tumor invasion and metastases: role of the extracellular matrix: Rhoads Memorial Award Lecture. Cancer Res 46:1–7, 1986.

Liotta LA, Rao CN, Barsky SH. Tumor invasion and the extracellular matrix. Lab Invest 49:636–649, 1983.

Liotta LA, Rao NC, Barsky SH, Bryant G. The laminin receptor and basement membrane dissolution: Role in tumour metastasis. Basement Membranes and Cell Movement (Ciba Foundation Symposium 108), 1984, pp 146–162.

Long ME, Taylor HC. Nucleolar variability in human neoplastic cells. Ann NY Acad Sci 63:1095–1106, 1956.

Love R, Soriano RZ. Correlation of nucleolini with fine nuclear constituents of cultured normal and neoplastic cells. Cancer Res 11:1030–1037, 1971.

Love R, Takeda M, Soriano RZ. Nucleolar structure in cancer and its diagnostic value. Ann Clin Lab Sci 4:131–138, 1974.

Lubinski J, Chosia M, Huebner K. Molecular genetic analysis in the diagnosis of lymphoma in fine needle aspiration biopsies: I. Lymphoma verus benign lymphoproliferation disorders. II. Lymphoma vs. nonlymphoid malignant tumors. Anal Quant Cytol Histol 10:391–398, 399–404, 1988.

Luke S, Shepelsky M. FISH. Recent advances and diagnostic aspects. Cell Vis 5:49–53, 1998.

Lynch HT, Lynch JF. The Lynch syndromes. Curr Opin Oncol 5:687–696, 1993.

Lynch HT, Smyrk T, Lynch JF. Overview of natural history, pathology, molecular genetics, and management of hereditary non-polyposis colorectal cancer (HNPCC-Lynch Syndrome). Int J Cancer 69:38–43, 1996.

Macieira-Coelho A, Ponten J, Philipson L. Inhibition of the division cycle in confluent cultures of human fibroblasts in vitro. Exp Cell Res 43:20–29, 1966.

Majzoub JA, Muglia LJ. Knockout mice. N Engl J Med 334:904–907, 1996.

Marx J. Possible function found for breast cancer genes. Science 376:531–532, 1997.

Marx J. Many gene changes found in cancer. Science 246:1386–1388, 1989.

Marx JL. The yin and yang of cell growth control. Science 232:1093–1095, 1986.

Marx JL. Tumors: A mixed bag of cells. Science 15:275–277, 1982.

McCormick D, Hall PA. The complexities of proliferating cell nuclear antigen. Histopathology 21:591–594, 1992.

McCutcheon M, Coman DR, Moore FB. Studies on invasiveness of cancer. Adhesiveness of malignant cells in various human carcinomas. Cancer 1:460–467, 1948.

Megee PC, Koshland D. A functional assay for centromere-associated sister chromatid cohesion. Science 285:254–256, 1999.

Mellors RC. Quantitative cytology and cytopathology: Nucleic acids and proteins in the mitotic cycle of normal and neoplastic cells. Ann NY Acad Sci 63:1177–1201, 1956.

Meyer JS, Bari WA. Granules and calcitonin-like activity in medullary carcinoma of the thyroid gland. N Engl J Med 278:523–529, 1968.

Miki Y, Shattuck-Eidens D, Futreal A, et al. A strong candidate for the breast and ovarian cancer susceptibility gene BRCA 1. Science 266:66–71, 1994.

Miles CP, Koss LG. Diagnostic traits of interphase human cancer cells with known chromosome patterns. Acta Cytol 10:21–25, 1966.

Miller GJ, Shikes AL. Nuclear roundness as a predictor of response to hormonal therapy of patients with stage D2 prostatic carcinoma. In Karr JP, Coffey DS, Gardner W (eds). Prognostic Cytometry and Cytopathology of Prostate Cancer. New York, Elsevier, 1988, pp 349–354.

Mitelman F. Catalogue of Chromosomal Aberrations in Cancer. New York, Wiley-Liss, 1991 (includes data on chromosomal aberrations in benign tumors).

Mitelman F, Mertens F, Johansson B. A breakpoint map of recurrent chromosomal rearrangement in human neoplasia. Nature Genet 15:417–474, 1997.

Morin PJ, Sparks AB, Korinek V, et al. Activation of beta-catenin-Tcf signaling in colon cancer by mutations in beta-catenin or APC. Science 275:1787–1790, 1997.

Moscona AA. Embryonic and neoplastic cell surfaces: Availability of receptors for concanavalin A, wheat germ agglutination. Science 171:905–907, 1971.

Mu XC, Brien TP, Ross JS, et al. Telomerase activity in benign and malignant cytologic fluids. Cancer CytoPathol 87:93–99, 1999.

Murray A, Hunt T. The Cell Cycle. New York, WH Freeman, 1993.

Nath J, Johnson KL. Fluorescence in situ hybridization (FISH): DNA probe production and hybridization criteria. Biotech Histochem 73:6–22, 1998.

Nemoto R, Kawamura H, Miyakawa I, et al. Immunohistochemical detection of proliferating cell nuclear antigen (PCNA/cyclin) in human prostate adenocarcinoma. J Urol 149:165–169, 1993.

Netland PA, Zetter BR. Organ-specific adhesion of metastatic tumor cells in vitro. Science 124:1113–1115, 1984.

Ng WK, Collins RJ. Diagnostic significance and possibly pitfalls of nuclear grooves in extrathyroid cytology. Diagn Cytopathol 16:57–64, 1997.

Nieburgs HE. Recent progress in the interpretation of malignancy associated changes (MAC). Acta Cytol 12:445–453, 1968.

Nieburgs HE, Goldberg AF. Changes in polymorphonuclear leukocytes as a manifestation of malignant neoplasia. Cancer 22:35–42, 1968.

Nieburgs HE, Parents AD, Perez V, Boudreau C. Cellular changes in liver tissue adjacent and distant to malignant tumors. Arch Pathol 80:262–272, 1965.

Nieburgs HE, et al. Malignancy associated changes (MAC) in blood and bone marrow cells of patients with malignant tumors. Acta Cytol 11:415–423, 1967.

Nielsen K, Colstrup H, Nilsson T, Gundersen HJG. Stereological estimates of nuclear volume correlated with histopathological grading and prognosis of bladder tumor. Virchows Arch B (Cell Pathol) 52:41–54, 1986.

Nilsson G, Wang M, Wejde J, et al. Reverse transcriptase polymerase chain reaction on fine needle aspirates for rapid detection of translocations in synovial sarcoma. Acta Cytol 42:1317–1324, 1998.

Nowell PC. The clonal evolution of tumor cell populations. Science 194:23–28, 1976.

Nowell PC, Hungerford DA. A minute chromosome in human chronic granulocytic leukemia. Science 132:1497–1498, 1960.

Nowinski WW. Fundamental Aspects of Normal and Malignant Growth. New York, Elsevier, 1960.

Oberling C, Bernhard W. The morphology of the cancer cell. In Brachet J, Mirski AEJ (eds). The Cell, vol 5. New York, Academic Press, 1961, pp 405–496.

Oktay MH, Oktay K, Hamele-Bena D, et al. Focal adhesion kinase as a marker of malignant phenotype in breast and cervical carcinomas. Hum Pathol 34: 240–245, 2003.

O'Neal L, Kipnis DM, Luse SA, et al. Secretion of various endocrine substances by ACTH secreting tumors: gastrin, melanotrophin, norepinephrine, serotonin, parathormone, vasopressin, glucagon. Cancer 221:1219–1232, 1968.

Oshiro Y, Chaturvedi V, Hayden D, et al. Altered p53 is associated with aggressive behavior of chondrosarcoma. A long term follow-up study. Cancer 83: 2324–2334, 1998.

Parsonnet J (ed). Microbes and Malignancy. Infection as a Cause of Human Cancer. New York, Oxford University Press, 1999.

Peifer M. Beta catenin as oncogene: the smoking gun. Science 275:1752–1753, 1997.

Pennisi E. The telomerase picture fills in. Science 276:528–529, 1997.

Piel M, Nordberg J, Euteneuer U, Bornens M. Centrosome-dependent exit of cytokinesis in animal cells. Science 291:1550–1553, 2001.

Pierce GB. Differentiation of normal and malignant cells. Fed Proc 29: 1248–1254, 1970.

Pierce GB, Wallace C. Differentiation of malignant to benign cells. Cancer Res 31:127–134, 1971.

Ponten J, Jensen F, Koprowski H. Morphological and virological investigation of human tissue cultures transformed with SV40. J Cell Comp Physiol 61: 145–163, 1963.

Porter KR, Thompson HP. A particulate body associated with epithelial cells cultured from mammary carcinoma of mice of milk factor strain. J Exper Med 88:15–85, 1948.

Poulin N, Harrison A, Palcic B. Quantitative precision of an automated image cytometric system for the measurement of DNA content and distribution in cells labelled with fluorescent nucleic acid stains. Cytometry 16:227–235, 1994.

Press MF, Pike MC, Chazin VR, et. al. HER2/neu expression in node negative breast cancer: direct tissue quantitation by computerized image analysis and association of overexpression with increased risk of recurrent disease. Cancer Res 53:4960–4970, 1993.

Rabinovitch PS, Kubbies M, Chen YC, et al. BrdU-Hoechst flow cytometry: a unique tool for quantitative cell cycle analysis. Exp Cell Res 174:309–318, 1988.

Rapin AMC, Burger MM. Tumor cell surfaces: General alterations detected by agglutinins. In Klein G, Weinhouse S (eds). Advances in Cancer Research, New York, Academic Press, 1974, pp 1–91.

Rather LJ. The Genesis of Cancer. A study in the History of Ideas. Baltimore MD, The Johns Hopkins University Press, 1978.

Rouch W. Putative cancer gene shows up in development instead. Science 276: 534–535, 1997.

Ruschoff J, Plate KH, Bittinger A, Thomas C. Nucleolar organizing lesions (NORs). Basic concepts and practical application in tumor pathology. Pathol Res Practice 185:878–885, 1989.

Ruvkun G, Hobert O. The taxonomy of developmental control in Caenorhabditis elegans. Science 282:2033–2041, 1998.

Sachs L. Cell differentiation and bypassing of genetic defects in the suppression of malignancy. Cancer Res 47:1981–1986, 1987.

Sallstrom JF, Juhlin R, Stenkvist B. Membrane properties of lymphatic cells in fine needle biopsies of lymphomas. 1. Cap formation after exposure to fluorescein conjugated concanavalin A. Acta Cytol 18:392–398, 1974.

Sanchez-Garcia I. Consequences of chromosomal abnormalities in tumor development. Annual Rev Genet 31:429–453, 1997.

Sandberg AA. The Chromosomes in Human Cancer and Leukemia, 2nd ed. New York, Elsevier, 1990.

Sandritter W, Carl M, Ritter W. Cytophotometric measurements of the DNA content of human malignant tumors by means of the Feulgen reactions. Acta Cytol 10:26–30, 1966.

Sarkis AS, Dalbagni G, Cordon-Cardo C, et al. Nuclear overexpression of p53 protein in transitional cell bladder carcinoma: a marker for disease progression. J Natl Cancer Inst 85:53–59, 1993.

Savino A, Koss LG. Evaluation of sex chromatin as a prognostic factor in carcinoma of the breast. A preliminary report. Acta Cytol 15:372–374, 1971.

Schafter PW. Centrioles of human cancer: Intercellular order and intercellular disorder. Science 164:1300–1303, 1969.

Schairer E. Kernmessungen und Chromosomenzahlungen an menschlichen Geschwülsten. Z Krebsforsch 41:1–38, 1935.

Schlott T, Nagel H, Ruschenburg I, et al. Reverse transcriptase polymerase chain reaction for detecting Ewing's sarcoma in archival fine needle aspiration biopsies. Acta Cytol 41:795–801, 1997.

Schnitt S, Livingston DM. Location of BRCA 1 in human breast and ovarian cells. Science 275:123–125, 1996.

Schraq D, Kuntz KM, Garber JE, Weeks JC. Decision analysis—effects of prophylactic mastectomy and oophorectomy on life expectancy among women with RBCA1 or BRCA2 mutations. N Engl J Med 336:1465–1471, 1997.

Segall JE, Tyerech S, Boselli L, et al. EGF stimulates lamellipod extension in metastatic mammary adenocarcinoma cells by an actin-dependent mechanism. Clin Exp Metastasis 14:61–72, 1996.

Service R. Slow DNA repair implicated in mutations found in tumors. Science 263:1374, 1994.

Shibata D, Reale MA, Levin P, et al. Protein and prognosis in colorectal cancer. N Engl J Med 335:1727–1732, 1996.

Shimkin MB. Contrary to Nature. Washington DC Department of Health, Education, and Welfare, Publication No. 76–720, 1976.

Shuldiner AR. Transgenic animals. N Engl J Med 334:653–655, 1996.

Silagi S. Control of pigment production in mouse melanoma cells in vitro. Evocation and maintenance. J Cell Biol 43:263–274, 1969.

Silagi S, Bruce SA. Suppression of malignancy and differentiation in melanotic melanoma cells. Proc Natl Acad Sci USA 66:72–78, 1970.

Slamon DJ, Godolphin W, Jones LA, et al. Protooncogene in human breast and ovarian cancer. Science 2:707–712, 1989.

Sobin LH, Wittekind C (eds). TNM classification of Malignant Tumors, 5th ed. Chichester (UK) and New York, John Wiley and UICC, 1997.

Spring-Mills E, Elias JJ. Cell surface differences in ducts from cancerous and noncancerous human breasts. Science 188:947–949, 1975.

Stanbridge EJ. Identifying tumor suppressor genes in human colorectal cancer. Science 247:12–13, 1990.

Stein GS, Montecino M, van Wijnen AJ, et al. Nuclear structure-gene expression interrelationships: Implications for aberrant gene expression in cancer. Cancer Res 60:2067–2076, 2000.

Stratton JF, Gayther S, Russell P, et al. Contribution of BRCA 1 mutation to ovarian cancer. N Engl J Med 336:1125–1130, 1997.

Sträuli P, Lindenmann R, Haemmerli G. Mikrokinematographische and electron mikroskopische Beobachtungen an Zelloberflächen und Zellkontakten der menschlichen Carcinom Zellkulturline HEP 2. Virchows Arch (B) 8: 143–161, 1971.

Struewing JP, Hartge P, Wacholder S, et al. The risk of cancer associated with specific mutations of BRCA 1, BRCA 2 among Ashkenazi Jews. N Engl J Med 336:1401–1408, 1997.

Stubblefield E. Centriole replication in a mammalian cell. In The Proliferation and Spread of Neoplastic Cells. Baltimore, Williams & Wilkins, 1968, pp 175–193.

Stubblefield E, Brinkley BR. Architecture and function of the mammalian centriole. In Warren KB (ed). Formation and Fate of Cell Organelles. New York, Academic Press, 1967, pp 175–218.

Syrjanen K, Gissmann L, Koss LG (eds). Papillomaviruses and Human Disease. Berlin, Heidelberg, New York, Springer-Verlag, 1987.

Tahlan A, Dey P. Nuclear grooves. How specific are they? Acta Cytol 45:48–50, 2001.

Takeichi M. Cadherin cell adhesion receptors as a morphogenetic regulator. Science 251:1455–1459, 1991a.

Takeichi M. Cadherin cell adhesion receptors as morphogenetic regulator. Science 251:1451–1455, 1991b.

Tardif CP, Partin AW, Qaqish B, Epstein JP, Mohler JL. Comparison of nuclear shape in aspirated and histologic specimens of prostatic carcinoma. Anal Quant Cytol Histol 14:474–482, 1992.

Tarin D, Matsumura Y. Deranged CD44 gene activity in malignancy. J Pathol 171:249–250, 1993.

Taubes G. Epidemiology faces its limits. Science 269:164–169, 1995.

Therman E, Sarto GE, Buchler DA. The structure and origin of giant nuclei in human cancer cells. Cancer Genet Cytogenet 2:9–18, 1983.

Todaro GJ, Lazar GK, Green H. The initiation of cell division in a contact inhibited mammalian cell line. J Cell Comp Physiol 66:325–333, 1965.

Tolles WB, Horvath WJ, Bostrom RC. A study of the quantitative characteristics of exfoliated cells from the female genital tract. Cancer 14:455–468, 1961.

Tomlinson I, Sasieni P, Bodmer W. Commentary: How many mutations in a cancer? Am J Pathol 160:755–758, 2002.

Trauth BC, Klas C, Peters AMJ, et al. Monoclonal antibody-mediated tumor regression by induction of apoptosis. Science 245:301–305, 1989.

Underwood JCE (ed). Pathology of the Nucleus. Berlin, Springer-Verlag, 1990.

van Dierendonck JH, Wijdman JH, Keijzer RA, et al. Cell-cycle related staining patterns of anti-proliferating cell nuclear antigen monoclonal antibodies: comparison with Brdu labelling and Ki-67 staining. Am J Path 138:1165–1172, 1991.

Varley JM, Evans DG, Birch JK. Li-Fraumeni syndrome: a molecular and clinical review. Br J Cancer 16:1–14, 1997.

Veltman JA, Hopman AH, Bot FJ, et al. Detection of chromosomal aberrations in cytologic brush specimens from head and neck squamous cell carcinoma. Cancer 81:309–314, 1997.

Vogelstein B, Fearon ER, Hamilton SR, et al. Genetic alterations during colorectal-tumor development. N Engl J Med 319:525–532, 1988.

Vogelstein B, Kinzler KW (eds). Genetic Basis of Human Cancer. New York, McGraw-Hill, 1998.

Wang SS, Esplin ED, Li JL, et al. Alterations of the PPP21RB gene in human lung and colon cancer. Science 282:284–287, 1998.

Warburg O. Ueber dem Stoffwechsel der Tumoren (Berlin, Springer 1926). Translated as: Metabolism of Tumors. London, Arnold Constable, 1930.

Weinstein IB. Addiction to oncogenes: The Achilles heal of cancer. Science 297:63–64, 2002.

Weinstein R, Pauli BU. Cell relationships in epithelia. In Koss LG, Coleman DV (eds). Advances in Clinical Cytology, vol. 1. London and Boston, Butterworth, 1981, pp 160–200.

Weinstein RS, Merk FB, Alroy J. The structure and function of intercellular junctions in cancer. Adv Cancer Res 23:24–89, 1976.

Weiss LM, Warnke RA, Sklar J, Cleary M. Molecular analysis of the t(14;18) chromosomal translocation in malignant lymphomas. N Engl J Med 317:1185–1189, 1987.

Wilde A, Zheng Y. Stimulation of microtubule aster formation and spindle assembly by the small GTPase ran. Science 284:1359–1362, 1999.

Williams GH, Romanowski P, Morris L, et al. Improved cervical smear assessment using antibodies against proteins that regulate DNA replication. Proc Natl Acad Sci USA 95:14932–14937, 1998.

Willman CL, Busque L, Griffith BB, et al. Langerhans cell histiocytosis (Histiocytosis X): A clonal proliferative disease. N Engl J Med 331:154–160, 1994.

Wolman SR. Applications of fluorescent in situ hybridization techniques in cytopathology. Cancer (CytoPathol) 81:193–197, 1997.

Wolman SR. Cytogenetics and cancer. Arch Pathol Lab Med 108:15–19, 1984.

Wu TC, Kuo TT. Detection of Epstein-Barr virus early RNA (EBER1) expression in thymic epithelial tumors by in situ hybridization. Human Path 24:235–238, 1993.

Yunis JJ, Frizzera G, Oken MM, et al. Multiple recurrent genomic defects in follicular lymphoma: A possible model for cancer. N Engl J Med 316:79–84, 1987.

Zetter BR. The cellular basis of site-specific tumor metastasis. N Engl J Med 322:605–612, 1990.

Zhou H, Kuang J, Zhong L, et al. Tumour amplified kinase STK15/BTAK induces centrosome amplification, aneuploidy and transformation. Nat Genet 2:189–193, 1998.

zur Hausen H. Human genital cancer: Synergism between two virus infections or synergism between a virus infection and initiating events? Lancet 2:1370–1372, 1982.

zur Hausen H, Villiers EM. Human papillomaviruses. Annu Rev Microbiol 48:427–447, 1994.

Diagnostic Cytology
of Organs

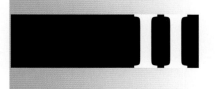

The Normal Female Genital Tract

ANATOMY

The female genital tract is composed of the vulva, the vagina, the uterus, the fallopian tubes, and the ovaries (Fig. 8-1).

Embryologic Note

The fallopian tubes, the uterus, and the adjacent part of the vagina are derived from two embryonal structures, the **müllerian ducts,** so named after Johannes Müller, a German anatomist of the early 19th century who first described them. The müllerian ducts fuse to become the uterus and the proximal vagina but remain separated to form the two oviducts (fallopian tubes). Imperfect fusion of the müllerian ducts results in formation of various degrees of duplication or subdivision of the uterus and the vagina, such as uterus septus and vagina septa. An excellent discussion of embryologic origin and congenital abnormalities of the female genital tract may be found in the book by Gray and Skandalakis (1972).

The Vulva

The vulva is the external portal of entry to the female genital tract. It is composed of two sets of **folds** or **labia** (from Latin, *labium* = lip; plural, *labia*), which frame both sides of the entrance to the vagina. The larger external folds, or **labia majora** (from Latin, *majus* = larger; plural, *majora*) are an ex-

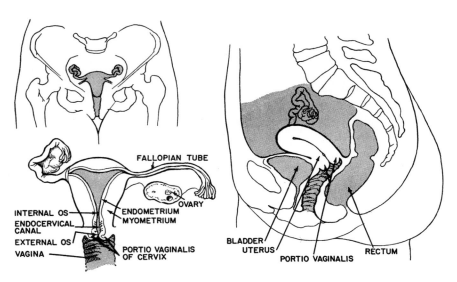

Figure 8-1 Schematic representation of the female genital tract in relation to bony structures (*upper left*); a coronal section (*lower left*); and a sagittal section showing the relationship to the bladder and the rectum (*right*).

tension of the skin. The smaller inner folds, or **labia minora** (from Latin, *minor* = lesser; plural, *minora*), form a transition between the skin and the vagina. The outer surfaces of the labia minora retain some features of the skin, such as the presence of sebaceous glands, whereas the inner surfaces blend with the vagina. Located anteriorly between the labia minora is the female counterpart of the penis, the **clitoris,** provided with a retractile, prepuce-like structure. Located about 1 cm behind the clitoris is the opening of the **urethra,** the terminal portion of the urinary tract.

The **lymphatic drainage** of the vulva is to the **inguinal lymph nodes,** which are the primary site of metastases in malignant tumors of the vulva.

The Vagina

In virgins, the entrance to the vagina is protected by a thin, perforated membrane, the **hymen.** The torn hymen persists in the form of small vestigial elevations at the entrance to the vagina. Just behind the vestigial hymen, on both sides of the posterior and lateral aspect of the vagina, there are two mucus-secreting glands, the glands of Bartholin or **Bartholin's glands.** During the childbearing age, the **adult vagina** is a canal, measuring approximately 10 cm in length, demarcated externally by the vulvar folds or labia, described above. The posterior end of the vagina is a blind pouch, the **cul-de-sac.** The anterior wall of the vagina, near the cul-de-sac, accommodates the uterine cervix. The area demarcated by the cervix and the blind end of the vaginal pouch is the **posterior vaginal fornix.** The fornix is quite deep and is the site wherein the secretions from the uterine glands, as well as exfoliated epithelial cells, accumulate. The wall of the vagina consists of three layers: the inner or mucosal layer of squamous epithelium, which shows transverse ridges or rugae. The mucosa is supported by a layer of smooth muscle. The thin outer serosal layer of the vagina is composed of connective tissue. The wall of the vagina is rich in lymphatic vessels. The **lymphatic drainage** of the anterior one-third of the vagina goes to the inguinal lymph nodes, whereas the posterior two-thirds drain into the pelvic lymph nodes.

Of importance are the **anatomic relationships of the vagina,** which are separated by thin connective tissue partitions or septa from the **rectum** posteriorly and the **bladder** anteriorly. Inflammatory processes and cancers of one of these organs may spread to the vagina and vice versa.

One of the rare but important congenital abnormalities of the vagina is **vagina septa,** in which the vagina, and possibly the uterus as well, is divided into two separate chambers. On occasion, this is of significance in tumor diagnosis, since cancer may be present in one part of the genital tract while the healthy part is being investigated with negative results.

The Uterus

The uterus is arbitrarily divided into two parts—**the body, or corpus, and the neck, or cervix.** The corpus and the cervix usually form an angle of 120°, with the corpus directed anteriorly. The body or corpus of the uterus is a roughly pyramidal organ, shaped like an inverted pear and flattened in the anteroposterior diameter. In the resting stage, it measures 4 to 7 cm in length and approximately the same at its widest point. The apex of the pyramid, which becomes the cervix, is directed downward, whereas the wide base, or **fundus,** is directed upward. The cervix is a tubular structure measuring approximately 4 cm in length and about 3 cm in diameter. Of its total length, about half is within the vagina and is called the **portio vaginalis** (also known as **ecto-** or **exocervix**); the rest is embedded within the vaginal wall and is continuous with the body of the uterus.

The bulk of the uterus is formed by smooth muscle, or the **myometrium,** which is capable of a manifold increase in size and weight during pregnancy. The muscle encloses the **uterine cavity,** described below, and is covered on its surface by a reflection of the peritoneum, known as the **uterine serosa.** The uterus is anchored in the pelvis by a series of bands of connective tissue, or ligaments, the most important being the posterior **round ligament,** and by folds or reflections of the peritoneum. Lateral folds, extending along the sides of the uterus and filled with loose connective tissue rich in lymphatics, are known as the broad ligaments forming the **left and the right parametrium** (plural, parametria).

The cervix has a very close anatomic relationship to the urinary bladder, which is anterior, and to both ureters, which run along the lateral walls of the cervix to reach the bladder. This anatomic arrangement explains the frequent involvement of the lower urinary tract by cervical cancer.

The Uterine Cavity

The thick, muscular walls of the uterus contain a cavity that, **within the cervix, is called the endocervical canal** and is continuous with the **endometrial cavity of the corpus.** The opening of the cervical canal into the vagina is referred to as the **external os** (from Latin, *os* = mouth). The point of transition of the endocervical canal into the endometrial cavity is known as the **internal os.** The endocervical canal is normally very narrow, measuring at the most 2 or 3 mm in diameter. The endometrial cavity follows the outline of the body of the uterus and is roughly conical, with the apex of the cone corresponding to the internal os and the base directed upward to the upper part, or **fundus,** of the uterine body. On each side of the triangular endometrial cavity, the horns, or the **cornua,** of the fundus are in communication with the **fallopian tubes,** or the oviducts. The lumen of the endometrial cavity in the resting stage is quite small, measuring only a few millimeters in the anteroposterior diameter. The endometrial cavity during pregnancy enlarges to harbor the fetus.

The Fallopian Tubes

The fallopian tubes (so named after Gabriello Fallopius, an Italian anatomist of the 16th century, who first described them), or the **oviducts,** measure between 8 and 12 cm in length and 3 and 5 mm in diameter. Their proximal ends are in direct continuation with the endometrial cavity, whereas their distal ends, with fingerlike **folds, or fimbriae,** open freely into the abdominal cavity, embracing the ovaries. The ova, released by the ovaries, find their way into the fallopian tubes, where they are fertilized by spermatozoa. The tubes are composed of three layers—the inner mucosal layer, followed by a layer of smooth muscle, and a serosal layer on the surface. A narrow canal, lined by the mucosa, is present throughout the entire length of the tube, thereby ensuring direct communication between the vagina and the abdominal cavity—a fact of some importance in the spread of infections and malignant tumors. The **histology** of the fallopian tubes is discussed in Chapter 15.

Ovaries

The ovaries are approximately ovoid structures, each measuring on the average 4 by 2 by 2 cm, located anatomically in the immediate vicinity of the abdominal or fimbriated end of the tubes, but not directly contiguous with the tubal lumens. In spite of this, the ova, formed in the ovary, find their way into the tubes and from there into the uterine cavity. The ovaries are loosely suspended, as are the tubes, by peritoneal folds. The histology of the ovaries is discussed in Chapter 15.

Adnexa and Lymphatic Drainage

The term **adnexa** or **uterine adnexa** is used to describe, as a single entity, the structures peripheral to the uterus, which consist of the fallopian tubes, ovaries, parametria, and regional lymph nodes. **The lymphatics of the uterus, the tubes, and the ovaries** are the tributaries of the pelvic and the aortic lymph nodes.

HISTOLOGY OF THE UTERUS

Cytologic examination of the female genital tract is based mainly on the study of epithelial cells, with cells of other derivation playing only a minor role. Three types of epithelia are present within the uterus and the vagina: (1) **the nonkeratinizing squamous epithelium** that lines the inner aspect of the labia minora of the vulva, the vagina, and the portio vaginalis of the cervix; (2) **the endocervical mucosa;** and (3) **the endometrium.** All these epithelia, but especially the endometrium and the squamous epithelium, are under hormonal influence. The **fullest development of these epithelia occurs during the childbearing age,** and our description will be based on their appearance at this time. Subsequently, the changes observed in prepubertal and postmenopausal women will be described. Further details on the histology of the vulva and vagina are provided in Chapter 15.

Nonkeratinizing Squamous Epithelium

Squamous epithelium of the female genital tract is of two different **embryologic origins.** The epithelium lining the inner aspect of the labia minora and contiguous with the adjacent vagina, presumably to the level of the cervix, originates from the urogenital sinus. The remainder of the vaginal epithelium and the squamous epithelium of the vaginal portio of the cervix are derived from the müllerian ducts by **transformation (metaplasia) of the original cuboidal epithelium into squamous epithelium.** This fact has considerable bearing on certain congenital, neoplastic, and drug-induced abnormalities in the vagina and the cervix. The original squamous epithelium, not derived from metaplasia, is sometimes referred to as **native squamous epithelium.**

The fundamental structure of the squamous epithelium is described in Chapter 5 (see Fig. 5-4). In the female genital tract, during sexual maturity, four layers or zones may be arbitrarily discerned and include the **bottom, or basal, layer,** which is the source of epithelial regeneration; the adjacent **parabasal zone,** imperceptibly blending with the **intermediate zone,** forming the bulk of the epithelial thickness; and the thin **superficial zone** (Fig. 8-2A). It is estimated that the process of squamous epithelial maturation

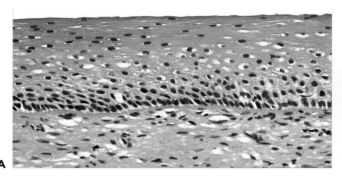
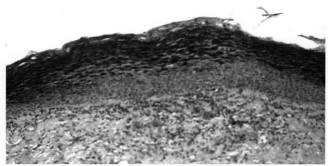

A   B

Figure 8-2 Normal squamous epithelium of the uterine cervix. *A.* Note the epithelial layers described in text and the absence of a keratin layer on the surface, which is composed of nucleated cells. *B.* The glycogen in the upper layers of the epithelium is documented by dark red stain with periodic acid-Schiff (PAS) reaction.

takes approximately 4 days. The process may be accelerated to 30 to 45 hours by the administration of estrogens. The mature **squamous epithelium of the cervix and vagina is rich in glycogen,** as documented by periodic acid–Schiff stain (Fig. 8-2B). Clinically, the presence of glycogen may be revealed by staining the squamous epithelium with Lugol's iodine solution, which, by binding with glycogen, stains the epithelium mahogany brown. This is the basis of **Schiller's test,** which serves to visualize nonstaining, pale areas of the epithelium suggestive of an abnormality that can be either benign or malignant.

The Epithelial Layers

The **basal, or germinative, layer** is composed of one row of small, elliptical cells, measuring approximately 10 μm in diameter. The vesicular nuclei, about 8 μm in diameter, commonly display evidence of active cellular growth, such as nucleoli or numerous chromocenters, and occasional mitoses. Under normal circumstances, the entire process of epithelial regeneration is confined to the basal layers; the remaining zones merely serving as stages of cell maturation.

The wide **midzone of the epithelium,** comprising the parabasal and intermediate layers, is composed of maturing squamous cells. As the maturation of the epithelium progresses toward the surface, the amount of cytoplasm per cell increases, whereas the sizes of the vesicular nuclei remain fairly constant, measuring about 8 μm in diameter. Arbitrarily, the two or three layers of smaller cells of the deeper portion of the midzone are designated as **parabasal layers.** The larger cells, adjacent to the superficial zone, form the **intermediate cell layers.** If further maturation is arrested under various circumstances, the midzone may form the surface of the squamous epithelium. The cells forming the bulk of the epithelium are bound to each other by well-developed desmosomal attachments or intercellular bridges (Fig. 8-3).

The **superficial zone** is composed of three or four layers of loosely attached cells that are still larger than intermediate cells. The nuclei of the cells forming the surface of the epithelium are considerably smaller and pyknotic, measuring about 4 μm in diameter. These cells are not capable of further growth. The most superficial cells of the squamous

epithelium are cast off the epithelial surface by a mechanism known as **desquamation or exfoliation.** The exfoliation either pertains to single squamous cells or to cell clusters. Within the clusters, the cells are still bound by desmosomes, as shown by electron microscopy (Dembitzer et al, 1976). The desquamation (exfoliation) of the squamous cells is related to **splitting of the desmosomal bonds** and, presumably, other cell attachments by an unknown mechanism (Fig. 8-4). It must be noted that, in vitro, the disruption of desmosomes among exfoliated squamous cells by either proteolytic enzymes or mechanical means, without destruction of the cells, is exceedingly difficult. Hence, one can only speculate either that specific enzyme systems become activated in the superficial layers of the epithelium or that intracytoplasmic changes occur that weaken the desmosomes and thereby allow the superficial cells to be dislodged, presumably by the pressure exercised by the growing epithelium.

The squamous epithelium is provided with an **immune apparatus,** represented by bone marrow–derived modified macrophages or **dendritic cells,** which are dispersed in the basal and central layers. Among the dendritic cells are the **Langerhans' cells,** characterized by clear cytoplasm and vesicular nucleus. With special staining procedures, the branching cytoplasm of these cells can be identified (Figueroa and Caorsi, 1980; Roncalli et al, 1988). In **electron microscopy,** the cells are characterized by the presence of typical **cytoplasmic tennis racquet–shaped granules, known as Birbeck's granules** (Younes et al, 1968). Edwards and Morris (1985) studied the distribution of the Langerhans' cells in the squamous epithelium of the various parts of the female genital tract and found the highest concentration in the vulva and the lowest in the vagina. The Langerhans' cells play an important role in the **immune functions of the squamous epithelium.**

The development of a **superficial horny keratin layer composed of anucleated, fully keratinized cells,** as observed in the epidermis of the skin (see Chap. 5), does not normally take place in the female genital tract but may occur under abnormal circumstances (see Chap. 10). On the other hand, in a variety of conditions (e.g., pregnancy, menopause, hormonal deficiency, inflammation), the squamous

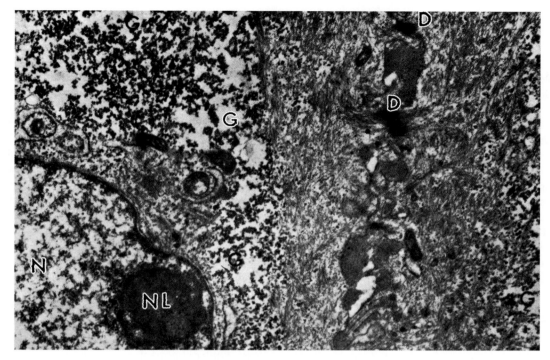

Figure 8-3   Squamous epithelium of human uterine cervix. Electron micrograph of portions of two adjacent squamous cells from epithelial midzone. There are numerous cytoplasmic filaments, many ending in desmosomes (D). Rich deposits of glycogen (G) are observed adjacent to the nucleus (N). The empty areas within the glycogen zone are due to partial dissolution of glycogen in the fixative (glutaraldehyde). A few vesicles are present between the nuclear membrane and the glycogen zone. A nucleolus (NL) is also noted. ($\times$9,000.)

epithelium may **fail to reach its full maturity.** In such cases, the surface of the squamous epithelium may be formed by intermediate or, sometimes, parabasal layers.

Basement Membrane and the Supporting Apparatus

Immediately underneath the basal layer of the epithelium, there is a thin band of hyaline material that is quite dense optically and is referred to as the **basement membrane;** it can also be found underneath the endocervical surface epithelium and glands (see Chap. 2). The significance of the basement membrane in determining invasion of a cancer is discussed in Chapters 11 and 12.

Beneath the basement membrane, there is a **connective tissue stroma,** containing variable numbers of **T and B lymphocytes,** with the highest concentration in the trans-

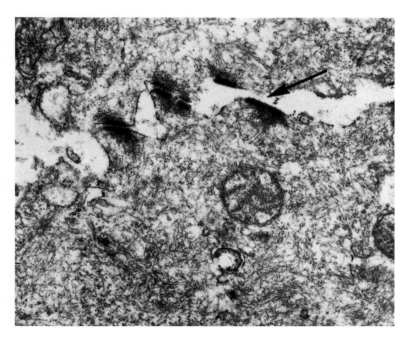

Figure 8-4   Electron micrograph of the superficial layer of the squamous epithelium of the vagina. Breakage of a desmosome (*arrow*) is shown next to two still intact desmosomes. ($\times$33,000.) (Photo by Dr. H. Dembitzer, Montefiore Hospital and Medical Center, New York, NY.)

formation zone (Edwards and Morris, 1985). Small, finger-like, **blood vessel–bearing** projections of connective tissue **(papillae)** supply the epithelium with nutrients.

Electron Microscopy

Transmission electron microscopy discloses a multilayer epithelium with cells bound to each other by numerous desmosomes. The cytoplasm is rich in glycogen and tonofibrils (see Fig. 8-3). In the most superficial epithelial layers, breakage of desmosomes is evident (Fig. 8-4) and accounts for spontaneous shedding of the superficial cells.

Scanning electron microscopy of the surface of the normal squamous epithelium discloses platelike arrangement of large squamous cells closely fitting with each other (Ferenczy and Richart, 1974). The surface of the cells is provided with a network of short uniform microridges. At the points of cell junctions, more prominent ridges may be noted (Fig. 8-5).

Endocervical Epithelium

The epithelial lining of the endocervical canal, and of the endocervical glands, is formed by a single layer of **mucus-producing tall columnar cells** with oval nuclei and clear cytoplasm, also known as **picket cells** (Fig. 8-6). The endocervical epithelium **participates in the events of the menstrual cycle,** described below, and this is reflected by the consistency of the endocervical mucus. During the **preovulatory phase of the cycle, the mucus is thick and readily crystallized;** it becomes **liquid just before and during the ovulation,** presumably to facilitate the entry of spermatozoa into the uterine cavity. Consequently, the appearance of the cytoplasm of the endocervical cells and the position of nuclei depends on the phase of the menstrual cycle. During the **proliferative phase,** the cytoplasm is opaque and the nuclei are centrally located (Fig. 8-6A). During the **secretory phase,** the transparent cytoplasm is bulging with accumulated mucus that pushes the flattened nuclei to the basal periphery of the cells (Fig. 8-6B). In such cells, the luminal surface is flat but may show tiny droplets or smudges, reflecting secretion of mucus. The **nuclei** of the normal endocervical cells are open (vesicular) and spherical, and measure approximately 8 μm in diameter. **Ciliated cells** are commonly present in the upper (proximal) segment of the endocervical canal, as confirmed in a careful study by Babkowski et al (1996). The nuclei of the ciliated cells are somewhat larger than those of nonciliated cells (see Figs. 8-19B and 8-20D). Located among the columnar cells at the base of the epithelium, adjacent to the basement membrane, there are small, triangular **basal, or reserve, cells.** These cells are very difficult to see in light microscopy of normal epithelium but have been clearly demonstrated by electron microscopy. Under abnormal circumstances, a hyperplasia of the reserve cells may be observed. The role of reserve cells as the cell of origin of squamous metaplasia of the endocervix is discussed in Chapter 10.

The endocervical glands are of the simple tubular branching type, and they may vary substantially in number and distribution. In some women, the normal glands may be situated deeply within the wall of the cervix, at a consider-

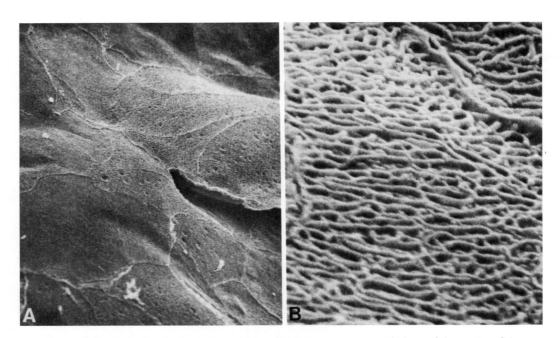

Figure 8-5   Scanning electron micrographs of mature squamous epithelium of the portio of the uterine cervix. A. Low-power view showing platelike, flat, superficial cells of various sizes. The points of junction of these cells are marked by ridges. A tear, suggestive of cell exfoliation, is seen on the right. B. Detail of the surface showing an interlacing network of microridges characteristic of mature squamous cells. In the right upper corner of the photograph, a more prominent ridge marks the point of junction with an adjacent superficial squamous cell. (A: High magnification; B: ×10,000.) (From Ferenczy A, Richart RM. Scanning electron microscopy of the cervical transformation zone. Am J Obstet Gynecol 115:151, 1973.)

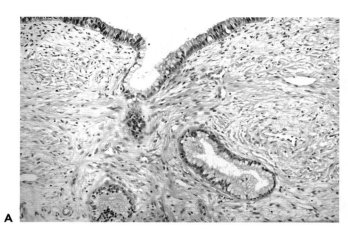
A

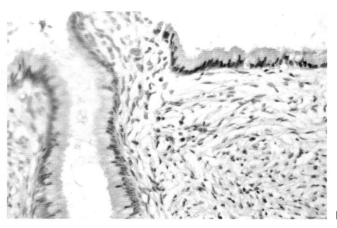
B

Figure 8-6 **Normal endocervix.** *A.* Typical columnar epithelium lining the surface of the endocervical canal and the endocervical glands. *B.* Higher power view of endocervical lining epithelium, composed of "picket cells" with clear cytoplasm, corresponding to the secretory phase of the menstrual cycle.

able distance from the surface; this distribution of endocervical glands is of importance in the diagnosis of extremely well-differentiated endocervical adenocarcinoma (see Chap. 12). The presence of glands underneath the squamous epithelium of the portio, in the area of the external os (transformation zone), is normal. The epithelium lining the glands is identical to the surface epithelium.

Electron Microscopy

Transmission electron microscopic studies of the endocervical epithelium reveal typical, mucus-secreting cells with secretory granules in the cytoplasm. On the luminal surface,

the cells are bound to each other by junctional complexes and, elsewhere, by desmosomes (Fig. 8-7). The basal reserve cells are readily observed at the base of the columnar endocervical cells.

Scanning electron microscopy shows that ciliated endocervical cells are more common than is generally estimated by light microscopy (Fig. 8-8).

Transformation Zone or the Squamocolumnar Junction

The area of the junction between the squamous and the endocervical epithelium is of considerable importance in

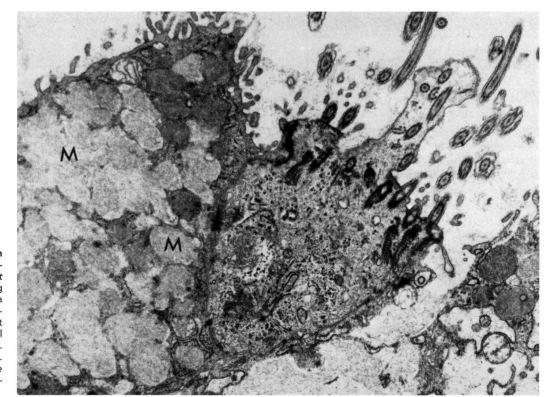

Figure 8-7 Electron micrograph of endocervical epithelium. At *left* there is a mucus-secreting cell, characterized by a large number of cytoplasmic granules (M); at *right* a ciliated epithelial cell is seen (see Fig. 8-8). (×13,000.) (Photo by Dr. H. Dembitzer, Montefiore Hospital and Medical Center, New York, NY.)

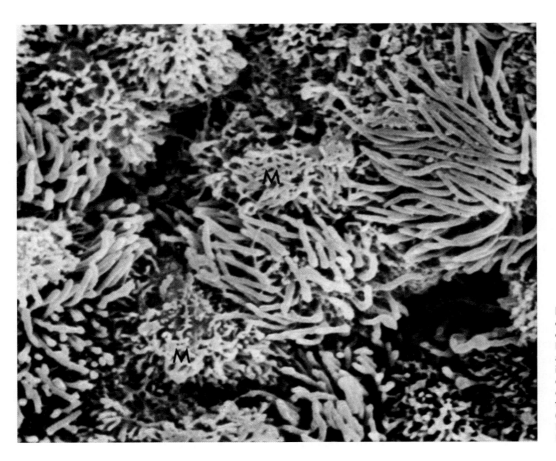

Figure 8-8 Scanning electron micrograph of endocervical epithelium. Numerous ciliated cells are next to mucus-secreting cells (M). The latter are characterized by a shaggy configuration of the surface (see Fig. 8-7). (×4,800.) (Courtesy of Dr. Ralph Richart, New York, NY.)

the genesis of carcinoma of the uterine cervix (see Chap. 11). In a normal, quiescent cervix, the transition between the two epithelial types is often sharp and is known as the **squamocolumnar junction,** now usually designated as **the transformation zone** (Fig. 8-9). The term **transformation zone** is based on colposcopic observations of adolescent and young women, documenting that the glandular epithelium of the cervix in the area of the squamocolumnar junction is undergoing constant metaplastic transformation into squamous epithelium. The events of transformation are sometimes reflected in cervical smears, showing side by side endocervical glandular cells and young metaplastic squamous cells.

The anatomic location of the transformation zone varies considerably and is age-dependent (Fig. 8-10). In **adolescents and young women,** the junction is usually located at the level of the external os, but may extend to the adjacent vaginal aspect of the uterine cervix. In the latter case, the area occupied by the endocervical epithelium on the surface of the cervix may be visible to the naked eye as a sharply demarcated red area, sometimes inappropriately called an **erosion,** but better designated as **eversion, ectropion, or ectopy.** The redness reflects the presence of blood vessels under the thin endocervical epithelium. The ectropion is a benign, self-healing condition, which, however, may mimic important lesions of the cervix. The cytologic presentation and clinical significance of the ectropion are discussed in Chapter 9.

With advancing age, the junction tends to move up

into the endocervical canal. At the time of the menopause, the junction is usually located within the endocervical canal and is hidden from view.

Because most of the initial precancerous changes in the uterine cervix occur within the transformation zone, this is an area of major importance in cervix cancer prevention (see Chap. 11). For this reason, much emphasis has been placed on sampling of the transformation zone by cervicovaginal smears (see comments on smear adequacy at the end of this chapter). It is evident that the transformation zone is more readily accessible in younger than in older women. For comments on cytology of the transformation zone, see below.

The Endometrium

The transition between the endocervical epithelium and the endometrium usually occurs at the level of the internal os. The transition between the large picket cells of the endocervical mucosa and the smaller cells of the endometrium is usually quite sharp.

The endometrium is essentially composed of layers of **surface epithelium composed of cuboidal cells,** forming simple **tubular glands, surrounded by stromal cells.** During the childbearing age, the endometrium undergoes **cyclic changes (menstrual cycle)** to prepare it for the implantation of the fertilized ovum, hence for pregnancy. The appearance of the glands and the stroma changes with the phase of the cycle, as described below. If the implantation

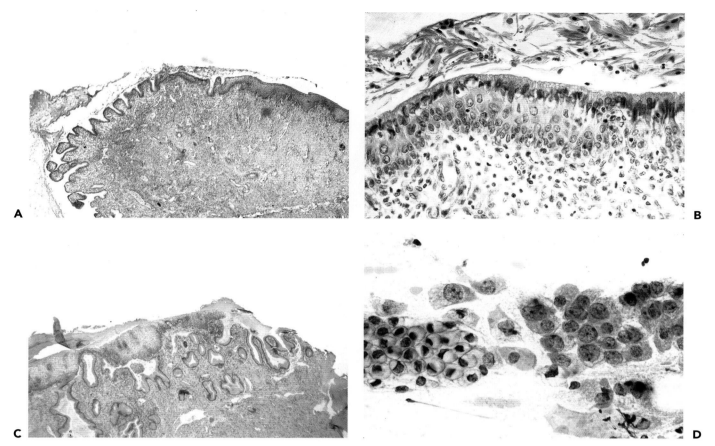

Figure 8-9   Transformation zone. *A.* Squamocolumnar junction in a cervix of a full-term infant girl. Note the border between the endocervical and squamous epithelium. *B.* Same child as in *A.* Higher magnification shows the process of squamous metaplasia in the endocervical canal. Squamous epithelium is beneath the surface layer of endocervical cells. *C.* Transformation zone in a young adult woman. Note the presence of endocervical glands beneath the level of squamous epithelium on left. *D.* A smear of the transformation zone in an adult young woman showing side-by-side secretory and nonsecretory (young metaplastic) endocervical cells.

does not occur, the endometrium is shed before the beginning of the next menstrual cycle. A detailed history of the cyclic changes and their hormonal background can be obtained elsewhere; for our purpose, only a brief summary is necessary.

The Endometrium During the Menstrual Cycle

The menstrual cycle is the result of a sequence of hormonal influences that, in a normal woman, follow each other with great regularity from puberty to menopause, except during pregnancy. It has been shown by Frisch and McArthur (1974) that a certain minimal body weight in relation to height is necessary for the onset and maintenance of the

menstrual activity. The ovarian hormones most directly responsible for the menstrual cycle are **estrogen,** produced by follicles that harbor ova, and **progesterone,** produced by corpus luteum that forms after expulsion of the ovum. The ovarian activity is regulated by hormones produced by the anterior lobe of the pituitary and the hypothalamus. A simple diagram summarizes the principal hormonal factors and their influence on the endometrium (Fig. 8-11).

Menstrual Bleeding

The beginning of the menstrual flow marks the **first day of the cycle.** It corresponds to disintegration and necrosis of the superficial portion of the endometrium, indicating

Figure 8-10   Transformation zone. The position of the transformation zone (squamocolumnar junction) varies according to age. In very young women and during the child-bearing age (20 to 50 years of age) the transformation zone is either in an exposed position (*left and center*) or at the external os. In postmenopausal women (*right*) the transformation zone is often located within the endocervical canal. It is evident that cytologic sampling of this epithelial target is much easier in younger women.

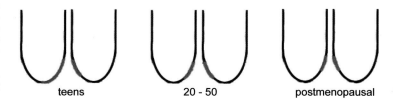

teens   20 - 50   postmenopausal

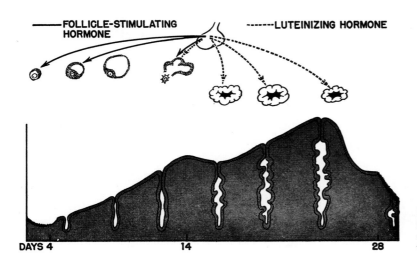

FOLLICLE-STIMULATING HORMONE

------LUTEINIZING HORMONE

DAYS 4   14   28

Figure 8-11 A diagrammatic and greatly simplified representation of the influence of anterior pituitary and ovarian functions on the cyclic growth and disintegration of endometrium.

the end of the activity of progestational hormones originating in the ovarian corpus luteum. The casting off of the endometrium usually takes 3 to 5 days and is accompanied by bleeding from the ruptured endometrial vessels.

Proliferative Phase

Endometrial necrosis is followed by regeneration and the onset of the growth or proliferative phase, during which the endometrium grows in thickness. This phase of endometrial growth is **under the influence of estrogens originating in the granulosa and the theca cells** of the ovarian follicles and, in essence, is a preparation for pregnancy. The **initial event** is the **regeneration of the surface epithelium** from residual endometrial glands. During this stage, the endometrial **surface epithelium** is composed of cuboidal to columnar cells with scanty cytoplasm and spherical, intensely

stained nuclei that show significant mitotic activity. Occasionally, larger cells with clear cytoplasm (helle Zellen of the Germans) are also present. Their significance is unknown.

The glands of the proliferative phase are formed by **invagination of the surface epithelium.** The glands are straight tubular structures lined by one or two layers of cuboidal, sometimes columnar, cells with scanty cytoplasm and intensely staining nuclei that show intense mitotic activity. The endometrial stroma in this stage is compact and formed by small cells (Fig. 8-12A). Single **ciliated cells** may be observed in proliferative endometrium, mainly on the surface.

Ovulation and the Secretory Phase

The release of the ovum from the ovarian follicle (ovulation) usually occurs between the 11th and 14th days of a 28-day

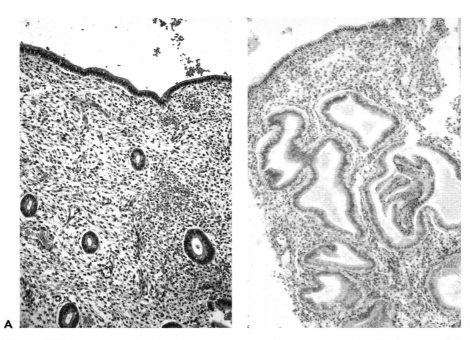

Figure 8-12 Histology of endometrium. *A.* Early proliferative phase. The glands are small, lined by cuboidal cells showing mitotic activity. *B.* Early secretory phase. The large, convoluted glands are lined by larger cells with subnuclear vacuoles.

menstrual cycle and signals the onset of the secretory phase. The ovarian corpus luteum, which replaces the follicle, begins to function by secreting progesterone, which stimulates the secretory activity of the cells lining the endometrial glands. **Secretory vacuoles,** composed mainly of **glycogen,** are formed, at first in subnuclear position, later shifting to a supranuclear one, closer to the lumen of the gland. At the same time, the straight tubular glands become more tortuous, and the surrounding **stromal cells** become larger and eosinophilic, resembling decidual cells (Fig. 8-12B). There is evidence that the actual process of secretion is of the apocrine type; that is, the apical portions of the glandular cells containing glycoproteins are cast off into the lumen of the gland. With the passage of time, the tortuosity of the glands and the vacuolization of the lining cells continue to increase and the stroma becomes loosely structured. Just before the beginning of the next menstrual flow, the glands acquire a **see-saw appearance** before collapsing, signaling the onset of the epithelial necrosis and the beginning of a new cycle.

Electron Microscopy

Transmission electron microscopic studies of human endometrium in various phases of the cycle were carried out by several investigators. In the proliferative phase, the glands are composed of columnar cells, some ciliated, resting on a basement membrane. These cells have no distinguishing features (Fig. 8-13). The secretory phase is accompanied by a rapid formation of **deposits of glycogen,** which is the chief product of the glandular cells. Accumulation of glycogen and glycoproteins in the secretory phase is accompanied by formation of large mitochondria with peculiar cristae arranged in parallel fashion (Fig. 8-14) (Gompel, 1962, 1964). **Scanning electron microscopic studies** disclosed some differences between the epithelium of the endometrial surface and that of the endometrial glands. The endometrial surface epithelium shows few cyclic changes. The cells produce cilia and show relatively little secretory activity during the secretory part of the cycle. The epithelium lining the endometrial glands during the proliferative phase shows an intense production of cilia and microvilli. During the secre-

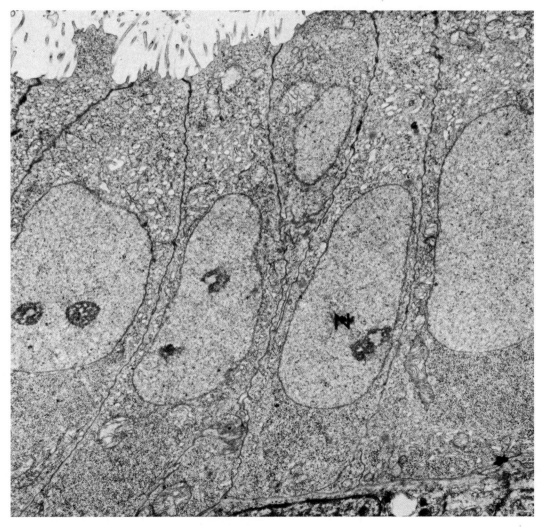

Figure 8-13 **Electron micrograph of proliferative endometrium.** View of an acinus of an endometrial gland showing cilia-forming columnar cells. The cytoplasm, although rich in a variety of organelles, shows no distinguishing features. The nuclei (N), some containing two nucleoli, are not remarkable. (×7,500.) (Courtesy of Prof. Claude Gompel, Brussels, Belgium.)

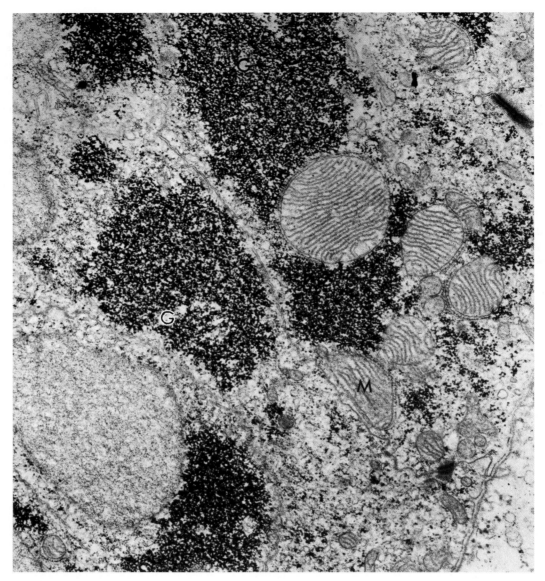

Figure 8-14 **Electron micrograph of secretory endometrium.** Glycogen deposit (G), seen as an accumulation of black granules, and large mitochondria (M) with parallel cristae are well in evidence. (×18,500.) (Courtesy of Prof. Claude Gompel, Brussels, Belgium.)

tory phase, the formation of cilia is inhibited, and, under the influence of progesterone, there is conversion of the glandular cells to the secretory function (Ferenczy, 1976; Ferenczy and Richart, 1973).

NORMAL CYTOLOGY OF THE UTERUS DURING CHILDBEARING AGE

Cells Originating from Normal Squamous Epithelium

Superficial Squamous Cells

During the childbearing age of a normal woman, the bulk of cells observed in cervicovaginal smears originate from the superficial zone of mature squamous epithelium. Although several varieties of cells may originate from the

surface of the squamous epithelium, the term **superficial squamous cells** is reserved for large **polygonal** cells possessing a **flat, delicate, transparent cytoplasm and small, dark nuclei, averaging about 4 μm in diameter** (Figs. 8-15A,B). The diameter of the superficial squamous cells is approximately 35 to 45 μm but somewhat smaller, or more often, larger cells may occur. The polygonal configuration of these cells reflects the rigidity of the cytoplasm, caused by the presence of numerous bundles of tonofibrils (intermediate filaments) seen in transmission electron microscopy (see previous). Scanning electron microscopy emphasizes the irregular configuration of these cells (Fig. 8-16). The flat surface, provided with microridges, shows a knoblike elevation of the spherical nucleus.

In well-executed Papanicolaou stains, **the cytoplasm** of the majority of the superficial cells stains predominantly **a**

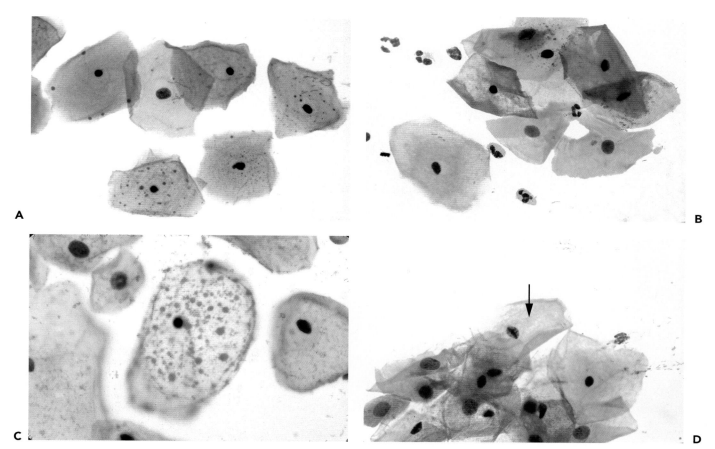

Figure 8-15 **Superficial and intermediate squamous cells.** *A.* Mature squamous cells with tiny, pyknotic nuclei, surrounded by a narrow clear zone. Some of the cells contain small, dark, brown cytoplasmic granules. *B.* Superficial and intermediate squamous cells, the latter with blue cytoplasm and larger, vesicular nuclei. *C.* ''Polka dot cell.'' A poorly preserved superficial squamous cell at higher magnification, showing brown granules of various sizes in the cytoplasm. *D.* Nuclear bar (*arrow*) in intermediate squamous cell.

delicate pink. This staining property reflects the chemical affinity of the cytoplasm for acid dyes such as eosin; hence, the term **eosinophilic,** or a less frequently used term, **acidophilic cytoplasm.** Dryness and exposure to air tend to enhance the eosinophilic properties of cells. The cytoplasm of the superficial cells may, at times, stain a pale blue, reflecting a slight affinity for basic dyes such as hematoxylin. Intense blue staining (cyanophilia) of the cytoplasm of superficial cells should not be seen in Papanicolaou stain, although it may be seen with other staining procedures such as the Shorr's stain (see Chap. 44).

Small, dark brown cytoplasmic granules are often visible, usually in a perinuclear location but, occasionally, they are also present in the periphery of the cytoplasm (see Fig. 8-15A). Masin and Masin (1964) documented that the granules contain lipids and that their presence is estrogen dependent. Occasionally, **larger, spherical, pale brown inclusions** of variable sizes may be observed in the cytoplasm of the superficial squamous cells, which have been named **polka-dot cells** (Fig. 8-15C). The nature of these inclusions is unknown. Some observers consider such cells to be an expression of human papillomavirus (HPV) (summary in DeMay, 1996). In our experience, such inclusions are un-

common and occur mainly in poorly preserved or degenerated squamous cells. The polka dot cells do not correspond to any known disease state, a view also shared by Schiffer et al (2001). Superficial squamous cells with **vacuolated cytoplasm, resembling fat cells,** have also been considered by some as reflecting HPV infection. In our experience, such cells are usually the result of treatment by radiotherapy or cautery (see Chap. 18).

The superficial squamous cells are the end-of-the-line dead cells and this is reflected in their small **nuclei,** which are **pyknotic,** that is, the nuclear material has become condensed and shrunken. A **narrow clear zone** often surrounds the condensed nucleus, indicating the area occupied by the nucleoplasm before shrinkage (see Fig. 8-15A,B). Sometimes the nuclear chromatin may be fragmented and broken into small granules, suggestive of **karyorrhexis** and, hence, **apoptosis** (see Chap. 6). Upon close inspection of such cells, minute detached fragments of nuclear material may be seen in the vicinity of the main nuclear mass. In phase microscopy, the pyknotic nuclei display a characteristic reddish hue.

Since complete maturity of the epithelium can rarely occur in the absence of estrogens, **nuclear pyknosis in ma-**

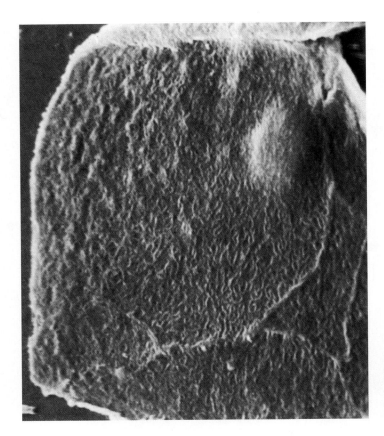

Figure 8-16 Scanning electron micrograph of a cluster of superficial squamous cells from the uterine cervix. The flat surface of the cells provided with microridges and a knoblike, elevated nucleus may be seen. More prominent ridges mark the cell junctions. (Approximately ×2,500.) (Courtesy of Dr. Ralph Richart, New York, NY.)

ture superficial cells constitutes morphologic evidence of estrogenic activity. This feature is of value in the analysis of hormonal status of the patient (see Chap. 9).

Intermediate Squamous Cells

The intermediate-type cells are of the same size as the superficial cells or somewhat smaller. Their cytoplasm is usually basophilic (cyanophilic) and occasionally somewhat more opaque in the Papanicolaou stain, although eosinophilic cells of this type may occur. The **chief difference between the superficial and the intermediate cells lies in the structure of the nucleus;** the nuclei of the intermediate cells measure about 8 μm in average diameter, are spherical or oval, with a clearly defined nuclear membrane surrounding a well-preserved homogeneous, faintly granular nucleoplasm. Chromocenters and sex chromatin may be observed within such nuclei. The term **vesicular nuclei** is applied to define this type of nuclear configuration.

It is not uncommon to observe in the nuclei of normal intermediate cells **nuclear grooves or creases** in the form of straight or branching dark lines (review in Payandeh and Koss, 2003). In some cases, **chromatin bars** with short lateral extensions (**caterpillar nuclei**), are observed along the longer axis of oval nuclei (Fig. 8-15D). Such bars are commonly observed in the nuclei of squamous cells in oral and conjunctival smears, discussed in Chapters 21 and 41. Kaneko et al (1998) suggested that the nuclear creases or bars represent an infolding of the nuclear membrane but the mechanism of their formation remains unknown. It has been documented that the presence or frequency of nuclear

grooves is not related to either inflammatory or neoplastic events (Payandeh and Koss, 2003).

A **variant of the intermediate** cells is the boat-shaped **navicular cell** (from Latin, *navis* = boat). These approximately oval-shaped cells store **glycogen in the form of cytoplasmic deposits** that stain yellow in Papanicolaou stain, and push the nucleus to the periphery (see Figs. 8-27B and 8-31A). The navicular cells are commonly seen in pregnancy and may be observed in early menopause (see below).

It must be emphasized that, under a variety of physiologic and pathologic circumstances (pregnancy, certain types of menopause, hormonal deficiencies, inflammation), the **squamous epithelium of the female genital tract may fail to reach full maturity.** In such cases, the intermediate, or sometimes even parabasal cells, form the epithelial surface and become the preponderant cell population in smears (see below and Chap. 9).

Physiologic Variations of the Superficial and Intermediate Squamous Cells

Cytoplasmic folding, often accompanied by **clumping** of cells is a normal phenomenon occurring during the last third of the menstrual cycle, prior to the onset of menstrual bleeding. Cytoplasmic folding may also occur during pregnancy (see below). Folding and clumping are often accompanied by lysis of the cytoplasm (cytolysis) caused by lactobacilli (see below; see also Fig. 8-31B).

The superficial and intermediate cells may form **tight whorls or "pearls"** in which the cells are concentrically arranged, in an onion-like fashion (Fig. 8-17A,B). The

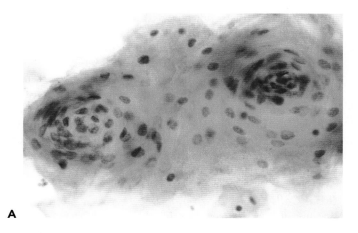

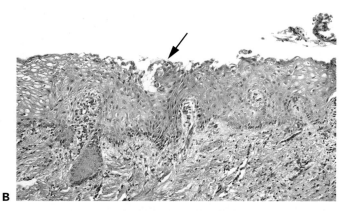

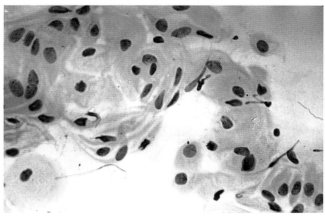

Figure 8-17 Benign squamous pearls and spindly squamous cells in cervical smear. *A.* Note the small nuclei in the whorls of keratin-forming cells. *B.* Cervix biopsy from the same patient showing pearl formation within the benign squamous epithelium (*arrow*). *C.* Spindly small intermediate squamous cells. Note normal nuclei.

whorls are often interpreted as reflecting estrogenic effect, but the proof of this is lacking. This must be differentiated from a similar arrangement of cells with abnormal nuclei, occurring in squamous carcinoma (see Chap. 11). An elongation of the intermediate cells, resulting in a **spindly shape,** has been observed at times (Fig. 8-17C). Such cells may somewhat resemble smooth-muscle cells (see Fig. 8-36). The identification of spindly squamous cells is facilitated in the presence of transitional forms of these cells, as shown in Figure 8-17C. Benign spindly squamous cells

must also be differentiated from similarly shaped cancer cells with abnormal nuclei (see Chap. 11).

Parabasal Cells

The parabasal squamous cells vary in size and measure from 12 to 30 μm in diameter. The nuclei are vesicular in type and similar to the nuclei of intermediate squamous cells. The frequency of occurrence and the **morphologic presentation** of parabasal squamous cells in cervicovaginal smears **depend on the technique of securing the sample.**

In vaginal pool smears obtained by a pipette or a blunt instrument, **spontaneously exfoliated parabasal cells occur singly and are usually round or oval in shape, with smooth cytoplasmic borders** (Fig. 8-18A). The cytoplasm is commonly basophilic (cyanophilic) and occasionally contains small vacuoles. Exposure to air and dryness may cause cytoplasmic eosinophilia. The **nuclei are usually bland and homogeneous.** This appearance of parabasal cells results from contraction of the cytoplasm following cell death and breakage of desmosomes that occurred prior to desquamation. Few cells of this type are seen in normal smears from women in their 20s and early 30s, but the number increases in women more than 35 years of age. Such cells may become the **dominant cell type in postmenopausal women** with epithelial atrophy (see below). In the presence of **inflammatory processes** within the vagina or the cervix with resulting damage to the superficial and intermediate layers of the squamous epithelium, the proportion of parabasal cells in smears **may increase substantially** (see Chap. 10).

In direct cervical scrapes and brush smears, the proportion of parabasal cells is much higher than in vaginal pool smears. Such cells are derived from areas of **immature squamous epithelium** and **areas of squamous metaplasia** of the endocervical epithelium in the transformation zone and the endocervical canal. For further discussion of squamous metaplasia (see Chap. 10). In cervical scrape smears, such cells are **trapped in streaks of endocervical mucus.** In preparations obtained by endocervical brushes and in preparations obtained from liquid fixatives, the relationship of parabasal cells to endocervical mucus is lost.

Parabasal cells forcibly dislodged from their epithelial setting by an instrument are often angular and have irregular polygonal shapes. Such cells occur singly, but often form flat clusters that vary in size from a few to several hundred cells. In clusters, such cells often form a **mosaic-like pattern,** in which the contours of the cells fit each other (Figs. 8-9D and 8-18B). The term **metaplastic cells** is often used to describe such cells, although their origin from squamous metaplasia is not always evident or secure. The reason for the angulated appearance of parabasal cells is the presence of intact desmosomes that bind the adjacent cells together. As the cytoplasm shrinks during the fixation process, the desmosomes are not affected and, consequently, the portions of the cytoplasm attached to the desmosomes stretch and become elongated, giving the cells an angulated appearance (see Fig. 8-18B). Thus, **the angulated appearance of the parabasal cells of "metaplastic" type, whether occurring singly or in clusters, is a useful fixation artifact.**

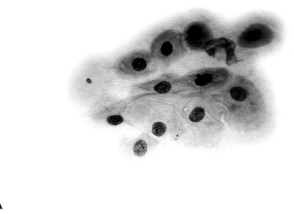

A

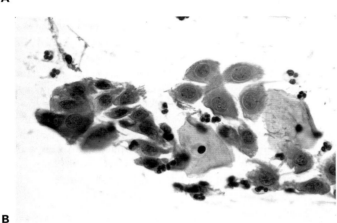

B

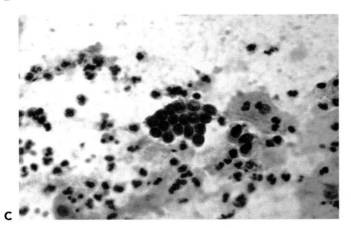

C

Figure 8-18   Parabasal and basal squamous cells. *A.* Parabasal cells from a cervicovaginal smear. Many of these small cells are spherical in shape, have a basophilic cytoplasm and spherical nuclei. *B.* Parabasal cells from a direct cervical sample. The angulated appearance of these cells suggests origin from the transformation zone. Such cells are usually classified as metaplastic. *C.* Basal cells in a brush specimen. A cohesive cluster of very small epithelial cells with very scanty cytoplasm and small nuclei of identical sizes. It may be assumed that these cells are basal squamous cells. The finding is uncommon.

The nuclei of parabasal cells, which measure about 8 μm in diameter, show a **fine network of chromatin, chromocenters,** and, occasionally, **very small nucleoli.** When compared with superficial or intermediate cells, the nuclei of parabasal cells occupy a much larger portion of the total cell volume and, therefore, give the erroneous impression of being larger. I have not observed mitotic figures among normal parabasal cells in smears.

The presence of parabasal cells in smears is of interest in defining an **"adequate cervical smear,"** which is often judged by the presence of "metaplastic" cells derived from the transformation zone and the endocervical canal (for further discussion of smear adequacy, see end of this chapter). It is evident that when the transformation zone is readily accessible to sampling, as in women of childbearing age, it will be better represented in the smears than in older women (see Figs. 8-9D and 8-10).

Basal Cells

Because of their protected status, the basal cells are practically never seen in smears. If present, it may be safely assumed that a pathologic process or vigorous brushing has damaged the upper layers of the squamous epithelium, resulting in the appearance of these very small round or oval cells, resembling miniature parabasal cells. Their very scanty cytoplasm is basophilic but may become eosinophilic in dry smears (Fig. 8-18C). The nuclei are of the same size as those of the parabasal cells but, because of the small size of the cells, appear to be larger. The nuclei display fine chromatin structure with chromatin granules and, occasionally, tiny round nucleoli. **The uncommon normal basal squamous cells should not be confused with small cancer cells that may be of similar size and configuration** (see Chap. 11).

Dendritic Cells and Langerhans Cells

These cells have never been identified by us in normal smears, although their presence in the histologic sections of the squamous epithelium has been well documented, as previously described.

Cells Originating from the Endocervical Epithelium

In **vaginal pool smears,** the endocervical cells are relatively uncommon and rarely well preserved. In **cervical smears** obtained by means of instruments, particularly endocervical brushes, the endocervical cells are usually numerous and well preserved. **When seen in profile, the endocervical cells are columnar** and measure approximately 20 μm in length and from 8 to 12 μm in width (Fig. 8-19A). Shorter cells, of plump, more cuboidal configuration may also occur. The columnar endocervical cells may occur singly but, quite often, they are seen as sheets of parallel cells, **arranged in a palisade** (Fig. 8-19B). When the endocervical cells are flattened on the slide and are seen "on end," they form **tight clusters or plaques,** wherein the cells form a tightly fitting mosaic resembling a **honeycomb.** In such plaques, the cell membranes form the partitions of the honeycomb and the centers are filled by clear cytoplasm surrounding the nuclei (Fig. 8-19A,C). The identification of such cells as endocervical is facilitated if columnar cells are present at the periphery of the cluster.

The cytoplasm of endocervical cells is either finely vacuolated or homogeneous and faintly basophilic or distended by clear, transparent mucus that is pushing the nuclei to-

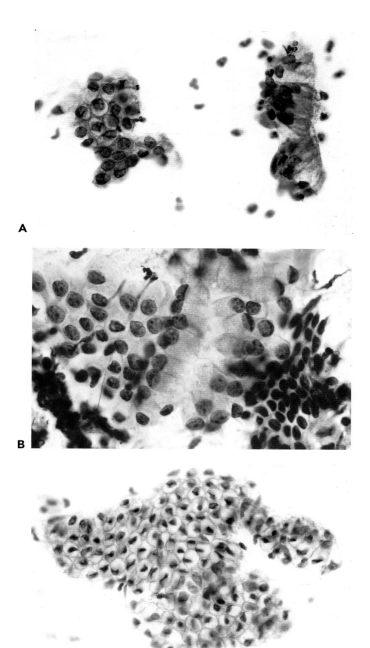

A

B

C

Figure 8-19 **Endocervical cells.** *A.* Two of the most characteristic presentations of endocervical cells in cervical smears are a strip of palisade-forming columnar cells with opaque cytoplasm and a cluster of such cells seen "on end," forming a "honeycomb pattern" wherein the borders of adjacent cells are clearly seen. In the palisading cluster, the surface of the cells is topped with a pink layer of mucus. *B.* Higher-power view of endocervical cells with clear cytoplasm. Some of the nuclei contain tiny nucleoli. *C.* A flat "honeycomb" cluster of endocervical cells with clear cytoplasm. The irregularly shaped nuclei show short, dense protrusions or "nipples."

ward the narrow end of the cell. Some such cells may become nearly spherical in shape because of cytoplasmic distention by mucus. On the surface of the mucus-containing cells, small droplets or smudges of mucus may be observed.

The nuclei are spherical or oval, vesicular in configuration, with delicate chromatin filaments, often showing chromocenters and very small nucleoli. The **nuclei may**

vary in size. The **dominant size of the nuclei is about 8 μm in diameter** but larger nuclei, up to 15 or 16 μm in diameter, are not uncommon. The variability of the nuclear sizes may reflect stages in cell cycle or other, unknown factors. **Multinucleated cells** may also occur (Fig. 8-20A). The fragile cytoplasm of the endocervical cells may disintegrate, with resulting **stripped, or naked, nuclei,** usually of spherical or somewhat elliptical configuration (Fig. 8-20B). These nuclei may also vary in size and may be difficult to recognize, unless they are similar to, or identical with, the nuclei of adjacent better-preserved endocervical cells. Small **intranuclear cytoplasmic inclusions** in the form of clear areas within the nucleus may occur in endocervical cells (Fig. 8-20B).

At the time of ovulation, and sometimes during the secretory (postovulatory) phase of the menstrual cycle, the nuclei of endocervical cells form **intensely stained, dark, nipple-like protrusions** of various sizes, up to 3 μm in length, that are an extension of the nucleus into the adjacent cytoplasm (see Figs. 8-19C and 8-20C). The protrusions appear mainly on the lumenal aspect of the nucleus, facing the endocervical lumen. Sometimes the protrusions are split in two. All stages of formation of the protrusions may be observed, ranging from a thickening of the nuclear membrane to protrusions growing in size. In nuclei with fully developed protrusions, the remainder of the nucleus is usually less dense and transparent, suggesting that there has been a shift of the chromatin to the protrusion. The mechanism of formation and the nature of the protrusions are the subject of a considerable debate. Taylor (1984) thought that the **protrusions occurred mainly in ciliated endocervical cells** and that their formation was the result of high ciliary activity. McCollum (1988) observed the protrusions in women receiving the long-term contraceptive drug medroxyprogesterone, during periods of amenorrhea, when the estrogenic activity was low. McCollum thought that the protrusions represented an **attempt at nuclear division arrested by progesterone and, therefore, consistent with events occurring at the onset of ovulation.** Zaharopoulos et al (1998) studied the protrusions by a number of methods, including electron microscopy, cytochemistry, and in situ hybridization of X chromosome. These investigators observed the presence of **nucleoli and single X chromosome within the protrusions** and reported findings suggestive of **formation of an abortive mitotic spindle** attached to the protrusion, thus providing support to McCollum's suggestion that the protrusion represents an attempt at mitotic division. Although further studies may shed some additional light on this very interesting phenomenon, it is quite certain that the protrusions **do not represent an artifact,** as has been suggested by Koizumi (1996). It is of note that **similar protrusions** may be occasionally observed in histologic sections of the endocervix during the secretory phase of the cycle **and in epithelial cells of various origins,** for example, in bronchial epithelial cells and in duct cells of the breast obtained by aspiration (see Chaps. 19 and 29). Zacharopoulos et al observed similar nuclear protrusions in occasional nonepithelial cells, suggesting that the phenome-

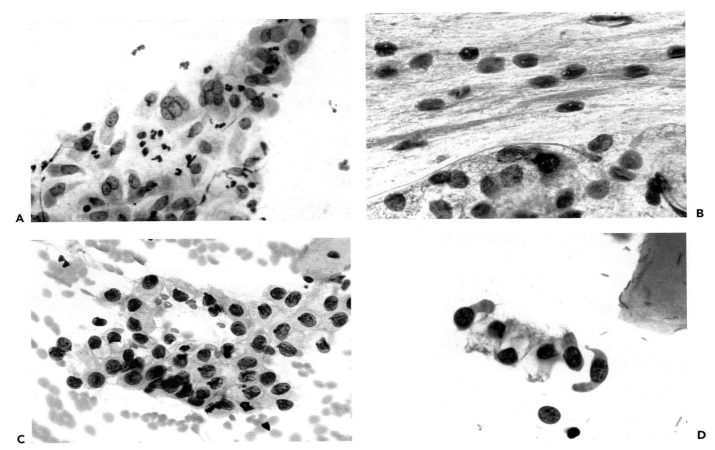

Figure 8-20   Nuclear variants of endocervical cells. *A.* Multinucleated cells. *B.* Stripped nuclei. Note intranuclear clear inclusions. *C.* Nipple-like projections and intranuclear vacuoles. *D.* Ciliated endocervical cells. The nuclei of these cells are often somewhat larger and stain darker than the nuclei of other endocervical cells. (*B:* High magnification.)

non is of a general nature and clearly worthy of further studies.

Ciliated Endocervical Cells

Endocervical cells showing recognizable **cilia, supported by a terminal plate,** are fairly frequent, particularly in brush specimens from the upper (proximal) segments of the endocervical canal. The nuclei of such cells are sometimes larger than average and somewhat hyperchromatic (Fig. 8-20D). The presence of the ciliated cells has been interpreted by some as evidence of **tubal metaplasia,** an entity that is discussed in Chapter 10.

Hollander and Gupta (1974) were the first to report the presence of **detached ciliary tufts** in cervicovaginal smears (Fig. 8-21A). This very rare event, occurring in about one-tenth of 1 percent of smears, cannot be correlated with time of cycle or age of patients. The ciliary tufts are fragments of ciliated endocervical cells, although sometimes their origin from the endometrium, or even the fallopian tubes, cannot be excluded. Next to detached ciliary tufts, remnants of the cell body with pyknotic nuclei may sometimes be observed (Fig. 8-21B). The phenomenon is similar to **ciliocytophthoria,** which was described by Papanicolaou in ciliated cells from the respiratory tract (see Chap. 19). So far, there is no evidence that the detached ciliary tufts in cervicovaginal

smears are related to a viral infection, which may be the cause of ciliocytophthoria in the respiratory tract, and the mechanism of their formation is not clear.

The tiny **basal cells** of the endocervical epithelium have never been identified by us with certainty in normal smears although, undoubtedly, they should occur in energetic endocervical brush specimens.

Endocervical Cells and the Menstrual Cycle

The changes in the consistency of the cervical mucus during the menstrual cycle were mentioned above and will be discussed again below in the assessment of ovulation in Chapter 9. It was suggested by Affandi et al (1985) that the morphology of the endocervical cells follows the events in the cell cycle. In the proliferative (preovulatory) phase, the cytoplasm of the endocervical cells in sheets is opaque and scanty and the nuclei are closely packed together. In the secretory (postovulatory) phase of the cycle, the cytoplasm is distended with clear mucus, the nuclei show degeneration (which, to this writer, appear to reflect the "nipple" formation described above), and, in cell sheets, are separated from each other by areas of clear cytoplasm. Affandi et al suggested that these differences in endocervical cell morphology in smears may be used to determine the occurrence of ovulation as reliably as endometrial biopsies. Affandi's observations have not been tested (see Chap. 9).

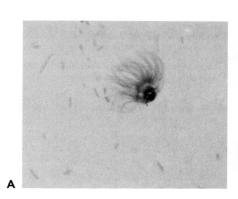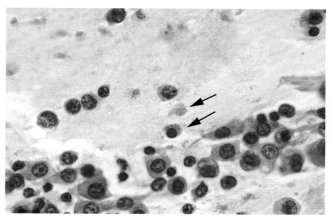

Figure 8-21 *A.* Detached ciliary tuft, cervical smear. *B.* Detached ciliated fragments of endocervical cells, next to residual cell fragments with pyknotic nuclei (*arrows*) (ciliocytophthoria). (*A:* Courtesy of Dr. David Hollander, Baltimore, MD; from Hollander DH, Gupta PK. Detached ciliary tufts in cervicovaginal smears. Acta Cytol 18:367, 1974.)

Cells of Normal Endometrium

The recognition and the presentation of endometrial cells vary according to the types of smears. By far, the best medium of analysis of the endometrial cells is the **vaginal smear,** which, unfortunately, has fallen out of fashion in recent years. The presence and the identification of endometrial cells in cervical smears, particularly those obtained by brush instruments, is less reliable and less frequent.

In cervical smears, the presence of endometrial cells during the childbearing age is closely related to the phases of the menstrual cycle. Such cells are common during the menstrual bleeding and for a few additional days as the endometrial cells are expelled from the uterine cavity. The upper limit of normal is the 12th day of the cycle. **The finding of endometrial cells in either vaginal or cervical smears, after the 12th day of the cycle, must be considered abnormal** (for further discussion of the clinical significance of this finding, see Chap. 13).

At the onset of the menstrual bleeding, sheets of small endometrial cells surrounded by blood and cell debris may be observed (Fig.8-22A). Easier to recognize are approximately **spherical or oval cell clusters** of variable sizes, wherein one can usually identify a **central core** made up of small, elongated, tightly packed **stromal cells** and, at the **periphery,** the much larger, vacuolated **glandular cells.** The latter are sometimes arranged in a rather orderly, concentric fashion around the core of stromal cells (Fig. 8-22B).

Endometrial stromal cells, not accompanied by glandular cells, are extremely difficult to identify during the first 3 or 4 days of the cycle. However, during the latter part of the menstrual flow, usually past the 5th or 6th day of the cycle, the endometrial stromal cells may be recognized as **small cells with phagocytic properties, resembling miniature macrophages,** often surrounding endometrial cells, singly and in clusters Fig. 8-22C,D). On close inspection, the small cells, about 10 to 12 μm in diameter, are of irregular shape, their cytoplasm is delicate, either basophilic or eosinophilic, and the small nuclei are spherical or kidney-shaped and bland. Miniscule particles of phagocytized material may be found in the cytoplasm. These cells may be so numerous that Papanicolaou referred to them as the **exodus.** The close relationship between endometrial cells and the miniature macrophages suggested to Papanicolaou that the latter may be of endometrial stromal origin. Supporting evidence for phagocytic properties of endometrial stromal cells in tissue culture was provided by Papanicolaou and Maddi (1958, 1959).

Endometrial cells at **mid-cycle** appear as **clusters of endometrial glandular cells,** not accompanied by stromal cells (Fig. 8-23A,B). Such clusters are usually less compact and the peripheral cells are often loosely attached and may become completely detached. These clusters offer a good opportunity to study **individual glandular endometrial cells,** which vary in size from 10 to 20 μm, have a basophilic cytoplasm, are round or elongated, and often contain one or more **cytoplasmic vacuoles** of variable sizes. The nuclei in such cells are spherical, inconspicuous, opaque or faintly granular, measuring about 8 to 10 μm in diameter, and are sometimes provided with very small nucleoli. The size of the normal nuclei should be no larger than the size of the nuclei of intermediate or parabasal squamous cells, which are commonly present in smears. The cytoplasmic vacuoles may displace and compress the nucleus to the periphery of the cell. In poorly preserved, degenerated cells, the vacuoles may sometimes be distended and conspicuous. Occasionally, the **vacuoles may be infiltrated by polymorphonuclear leukocytes.** The differentiation of single endometrial cells from small macrophages is, at times, difficult, if not impossible. However, macrophages, as a rule, do not form clusters. The role of macrophages in the diagnosis of endometrial abnormalities is discussed in Chapter 13. **Endometrial stromal cells at mid-cycle** are very difficult to recognize because of their small size, unless found in the company of larger, endometrial glandular cells. Occasionally, the stromal cells show mitotic activity (Fig. 8-23C).

Endometrium in Smears of Women Wearing Intrauterine Contraceptive Devices

As has been stated above, the presence of endometrium in cervicovaginal smears, after the 12th day of the cycle, is

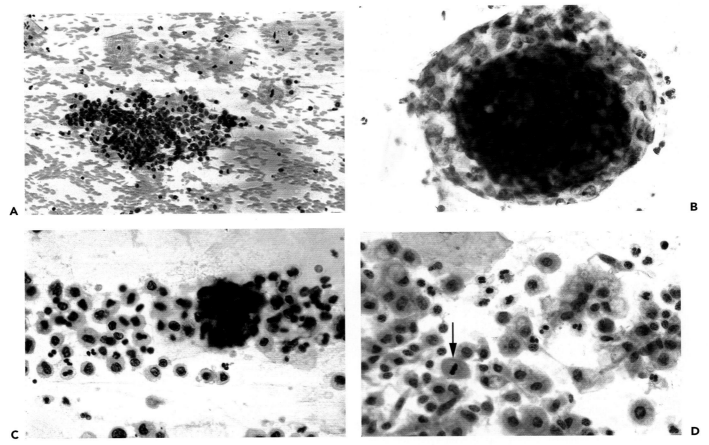

Figure 8-22 Endometrium in menstrual smears. *A.* Day 1 of bleeding: a cluster of endometrial cells in a background of blood, squamous cells, and debris. *B.* Day 6 of bleeding: typical spherical cluster of endometrial cells with the core formed by stromal cells and the periphery by poorly preserved large glandular cells. *C.* Exodus. Numerous small macrophages (modified stromal cells) surrounding a typical spherical cluster of endometrial cells. *D.* Exodus. Typical spread of small macrophages with vacuolated cytoplasm. Mitoses may occur, as shown in this photograph (*arrow*).

abnormal and must be a cause for concern. This matter is further discussed in Chapter 13 in reference to endometrial carcinoma. An important **exception to the rule** may be observed in wearers of intrauterine contraceptive devices (IUD), which may cause **endometrial shedding, predominantly at mid-cycle.** The clusters of endometrial glandular cells in smears are essentially similar in appearance to those shed during normal menstrual bleeding. Sometimes, however, the clusters are made up of cells with slightly atypical nuclei (Fig. 8-23D). The nuclei may be slightly hyperchromatic and granular but are generally of normal size. Knowledge of clinical history is essential in the correct interpretation of such findings. Other findings in IUD wearers are described in Chapter 13.

Endometrial Cells in Endocervical Brush Specimens

Vigorous brushing of the upper reaches of the endocervical canal may result in inadvertent sampling of the endometrium. As shown in Figure 8-24A, the recognition of endometrial cells under the scanning power of the microscope, may present significant difficulties. The endometrial cells may be **mistaken for cells of an endometrial adenocarcinoma,** particularly if they contain nucleoli (see Fig. 8-23B). The recog-

nition is easier if entire tubular glands are present (Fig. 8-24B). The most significant problems occur when thick sheets of endometrial cells (Fig. 8-24C,D) are observed. Clusters of small stromal cells may be **mistaken for malignant cells** derived from a small-cell type of high-grade squamous neoplastic lesion (HGSIL), as discussed and illustrated in Chapter 11. The differentiation of the endometrial cells from endocervical cells is usually based on cell size with the endometrial cells being much smaller. Also, the endometrial cells show much less variability in nuclear sizes and lack intranuclear cytoplasmic inclusions, which are fairly frequent in endocervical cells (see Fig. 8-20B).

Determination of Phases of the Menstrual Cycle in Endometrial Samples

Endometrial smears obtained by direct sampling are a cumbersome and not always reliable means of determining the stage of the cycle, although the task may be somewhat easier with adequate brushing and liquid fixation, wherein differences between the phases of the cycle can be observed, as described above. Still, a combination of cervicovaginal smears and endometrial biopsies is simpler and more informative. The use of direct endometrial samples in the diagnosis of early endometrial carcinoma is discussed in Chapter 13.

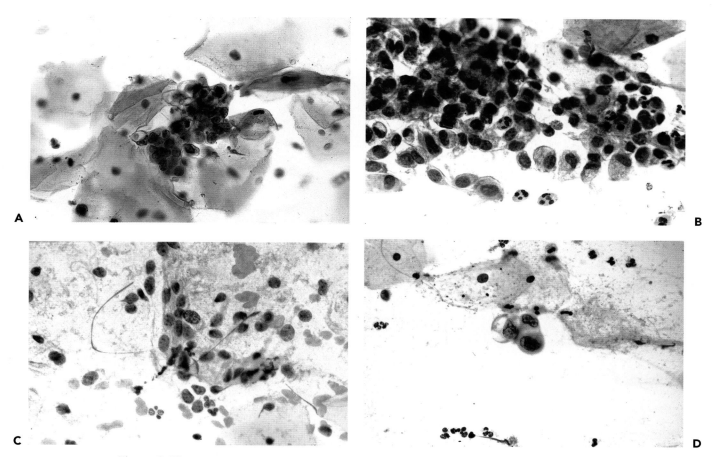

Figure 8-23 **Endometrial cells at mid-cycle.** *A.* A cluster of small endometrial glandular cells with vacuolated cytoplasm. Some of the nuclei show tiny nucleoli. In one cell, the accumulated secretions (glycogen) push the flattened nucleus to the periphery of the cell. *B.* Cluster of endometrial glandular cells showing vacuolated cytoplasm in an endocervical specimen. Tiny nucleoli may be observed in some cells. *C.* Endometrial stromal cells. Loose cluster of small cells, some with elongated pale cytoplasm. The somewhat elongated nuclei are finely granular. Such cells are difficult to identify, unless accompanied by endometrial glandular cells. *D.* Small cluster of endometrial glandular cells from a 27-year-old patient wearing an intrauterine contraceptive device (IUD). Note the clear vacuolated cytoplasm.

CYCLIC CHANGES IN CERVICOVAGINAL SMEARS

Diagnostic cytology, as we know it today, was the outgrowth of an investigation of hormonal changes of the vaginal epithelium by Stockard and Papanicolaou (1917). As has been stated above, the vaginal squamous epithelium depends on estrogens for maturation and the microscopic examination of changes, occurring in squamous cells, is the principle of hormonal cytology, discussed in detail in Chapter 9. The vagina of rodents is the ideal target of such investigations. The squamous epithelium undergoes significant and readily defined light microscopic changes during the phases of the menstrual cycle, described by Papanicolaou in smears obtained by means of a small glass pipette. His studies of the **menstrual cycle in vaginal smears of women** led to the incidental discovery of cancer cells, as described in Chapter 1. The cyclic changes in the vaginal squamous epithelium of the menstruating woman are much less striking than in rodents. In fact, in many women, the estimation of the time of the cycle, based on the appearance of the squamous cells is, at best, only approximate. As described in Chapter 9,

the most secure way to determine the cyclic changes is in a smear obtained by scraping the lateral wall of the vagina at some distance from the uterine cervix. Still, some information on the hormonal status of the woman can be obtained by studies of routine cervical smears. The ideal sequence of cyclic changes, described below, is not too frequent. Numerous factors, including inflammatory changes, may account for deviations from the normal cycle.

As has been described above in reference to the cyclic changes in the endometrium, the first part of the menstrual cycle until ovulation (days 1 to 12 or 13), is governed by estrogens. Following ovulation, the events in the cycle are governed by progesterone (see Fig. 8-11). The effect of these hormones is reflected in squamous cells in cervicovaginal smears. The changes are described for a cycle of 28 days duration.

Days 1 to 6

The first day of menstrual bleeding is customarily considered the first day of the cycle. During the first 5 days of the cycle, the smears are characterized by the presence of **blood, desquamated endometrial cells,** singly and in clusters, and

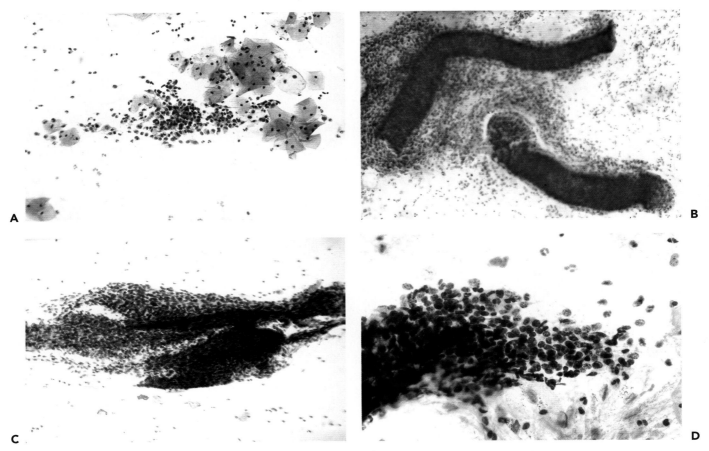

Figure 8-24 **Endometrial cells in endocervical brush specimens.** *A–C.* Typical presentation of endometrial cells at scanning magnification. In *A*, a cluster of glandular cells, also shown in Figure 8-23B. In *B*, typical endometrial tubular glands and stroma are easy to recognize. In *C*, a sheet of squashed endometrial glands. *D.* Higher-power view of the periphery of the cell cluster shown in *C*. The tiny endometrial stromal cells are much smaller and lack the cytoplasm of the endocervical cells (cfr. Fig. 8-19). These cells may be confused with neoplastic small cells from a high grade squamous intraepithelial neoplasia (see Chap. 12).

polymorphonuclear leukocytes. The **squamous cells of intermediate type dominate. Such cells form clumps** and their **cytoplasm is folded** and degenerated. On the 4th or 5th day, the squamous cells begin to show less clumping and a better cytoplasmic preservation.

Days 6 to 13 or 14

During the 6th and 7th days, there is a gradual disappearance of blood. **Endometrial cells** in well-preserved clusters, accompanied by large numbers of **small macrophages** (transformed stromal cells, **exodus**), may be observed up to the 10th or even 12th day (see Fig. 8-22C). From the 6th or 7th day on, the squamous cells are predominantly of the **basophilic intermediate variety with vesicular nuclei.** Gradually, the basophilic cells are **replaced by mature, flat eosinophilic superficial cells,** characterized by small pyknotic nuclei and transparent flat eosinophilic cytoplasm (see Fig. 8-15A,B). These cells predominate in vaginal smears at the time of ovulation, between the 12th and the 14th day. At this time, small **nipple-like nuclear protrusions may occasionally be seen in the endocervical cells** (see Fig. 8-20C). The **thick cervical mucus forms fern-like**

crystalline structures that vanish just prior to ovulation, when the mucus becomes liquid.

Days 14 to 28

Following ovulation, cytoplasmic folding may be noted in the superficial squamous cells. **The proportion of intermediate squamous cells gradually increases,** indicative of a reduced level of maturation of the squamous epithelium under the impact of progesterone. As the time of menstrual bleeding approaches, the intermediate cells **form clusters or clumps.** With the approach of menstrual bleeding, there is a marked increase in lactobacilli, resulting in **cytolysis** of the intermediate cells. The cytolysis results in "moth-eaten" cell cytoplasm, nuclei stripped of cytoplasm **(naked nuclei)** in a smear with a background of cytoplasmic debris **("dirty" type of smear)** (see Chap. 10). This appearance of the smear persists until the new cycle begins with the onset of the menstrual bleeding.

Cyclic Changes in Direct Endometrial Samples

Additional information pertaining to the status of the endometrium may be obtained by means of direct endometrial

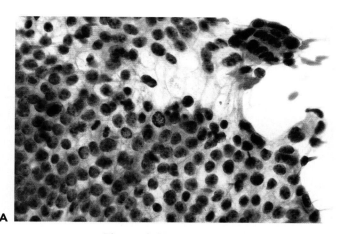

A

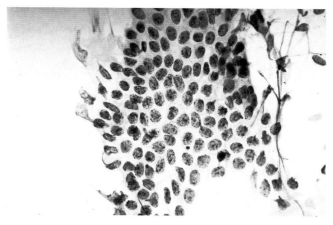

B

Figure 8-25   Direct endometrial smears in late proliferative (A) and secretory (B) phases of menstrual cycle. Both smears show glandular cells that are densely packed. Mitotic activity is evident in the proliferative phase (A); cells have more abundant cytoplasm in the secretory phase (B).

sampling by various methods (see Chap. 13). Some of the newer methods of endometrial sampling, such as collection of the material obtained by direct brushings in liquid media and processing of the material in the form of cytospins, have been described by Maksem and Knesel (1995). In ideal material, stages of cell cycle may be recognized.

In the **proliferative phase,** the **cuboidal glandular cells form honeycomb clusters,** characterized by spherical nuclei, varying somewhat in size. Small nucleoli and occasional **mitotic figures** may be observed (Fig. 8-25A). In good preparations, whole tubular glands and stroma may be observed. The **stroma** is composed of small spindly cells. During the **secretory phase,** the **glandular cells** are somewhat larger because of more abundant vacuolated cytoplasm (Fig. 8-25B). In good preparations, whole convoluted glands and somewhat **larger stromal cells** may be observed. The differentiation of the nuclei of the glandular cells from those of stromal cells is rarely possible. In fact, all the nuclei appear so similar that they very strongly suggest a common origin of both types of cells.

Determination of ovulation should never be attempted on direct endometrial samples. The method causes significant discomfort to the patient, it is costly, and not particularly accurate.

THE MENOPAUSE

The menopause is caused by the **cessation of cyclic ovarian function,** resulting in the arrest of menstrual bleeding. The onset of the menopause is rarely sudden, the changes are usually gradual and may stretch over a period of several years, with gradual reduction in duration and frequency of the menstrual flow. The age at which complete menopause occurs varies. As a part of a project on detection of occult, asymptomatic endometrial carcinoma (Koss et al, 1984), information was obtained on the age of onset of the menopause in 2063 women (Table 8-1). It may be noted that it is quite normal for 50% of the American women to continue menstruating

up to the age of 55 and even beyond. The significance of delayed menopause as a possible risk factor for endometrial carcinoma is discussed in Chapter 13.

Clinical and cytologic menopause do not necessarily coincide. Occasionally, a patient who is still menstruating regularly presents the cytologic image of early menopause. Conversely, at least 30% of the women who have entered their clinical menopause, may display a smear pattern reflecting varying degrees of ongoing hormonal activity and may even reveal some cyclic changes.

The most important manifestations of the menopause are associated with **reduced production of estrogen,** although other complex changes in the endocrine balance are known to occur. The **ovaries,** the principal source of estrogen, become scarred and hyalinized without any remaining evidence of ovogenic activity. Because of estrogen deficiency, there is a cessation of endometrial proliferation with resulting **endometrial atrophy.** The endometrium becomes very

TABLE 8-1		
ONSET OF MENOPAUSE IN A COHORT OF 2,063 NORMAL WOMEN*		
Age in Years at Onset of Menopause	**Number in Group**	**% of Cohort**
<39	43	2.0
40–44	138	6.7
45–49	789	38.2
50–55	1,031	50.0
≥55	62	3.0
	Total 2,063	99.9 (rounded to nearest decimal point)
* From Koss et al. Obst Gynec 64:1–11, 1984.		

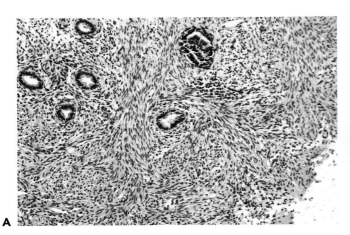
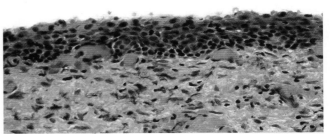

A   B

Figure 8-26 Postmenopausal atrophy of endometrium (*A*) and of squamous epithelium (*B*). *A.* Dispersed small glands in fibrotic stroma. *B.* The number of cell layers is reduced and there is lack of surface maturation.

thin. Scanty endometrial glands, some of which are enlarged and cystic, are seen within a depleted stroma (Fig. 8-26A).

Gradual estrogen depletion will also result in **gradual arrest of maturation of squamous epithelium,** with gradual loss of the superficial cell layers. In the final stages of atrophy, the surface of the squamous epithelium is composed of parabasal cells (Fig. 8-26B). The **endocervical epithelium** also shows evidence of atrophy; the columnar endocervical cells are often more cuboidal in shape, and their cytoplasm becomes opaque. A complicating factor in the evaluation of the menopausal cytology is the **cessation of the secretory activity of the endometrial and endocervical cells,** with resulting **dryness** of the lower genital passages, primarily the vagina. In smears, dryness **causes a number of artifacts,** similar to air drying of the smear, described below. In the absence of protective layers of the superficial squamous cells and because of dryness, the epithelium of the lower genital tract offers little resistance to bacterial invasion, resulting in vaginitis and cervicitis. In the presence of inflammation, the surface of the squamous epithelium becomes ragged and parabasal cells may be observed desquamating directly from the loose surface. The resulting **inflammatory changes** still further obscure the cytologic pattern, resulting in cell images that may mimic cancer. Indeed, recognition of cancer cells in atrophic postmenopausal smears may occasionally present substantial difficulties.

Basic Cytologic Patterns

Three basic cytologic patterns of the menopause may be differentiated—**early menopause, "crowded" menopause, and advanced or atrophic menopause.** The distribution of the patterns is shown in Table 8-2. A sharp separation of the three postmenopausal smear patterns is not always possible in practice, since one pattern may merge into another.

Early Menopause: Slight Deficiency of Estrogens

The smears are essentially those of the childbearing age, except for a **reduction in the proportion of superficial squamous cells.** The smears are composed predominantly of dispersed intermediate cells, occasionally showing cytolysis, and some large parabasal cells. These cells contain vesicular nuclei of normal size, about 8 μm in diameter. Because of a generally smaller size of the squamous cells, however, it may appear to a casual observer that the nuclei are diffusely enlarged. This

TABLE 8-2

VAGINAL SMEAR PATTERNS IN MENOPAUSE BASED ON EXAMINATION OF 1,100 CASES

Duration of Menopause	Estrogenic (Early Menopausal Pattern)	Intermediate ("Crowded" Pattern)	Atrophic
2–10 years 599 cases	21%	55%	24%
10 years or more 512 cases	14%	49%	37%

Stoll P. Vaginal smears in the menopause. Acta Cytol 4:148–150, 1960.

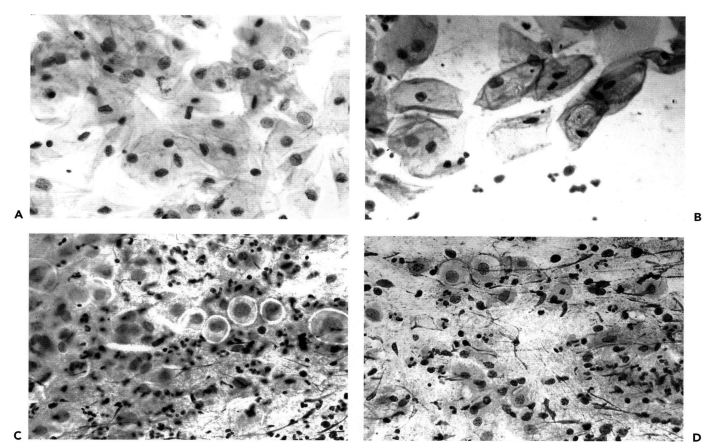

Figure 8-27 Cytologic patterns of menopause. *A.* "Crowded" menopause. The smear is composed of large parabasal cells forming clusters. *B.* Navicular cells in crowded menopause. Note the boat-shaped cells containing yellow deposits of glycogen that may push the nuclei to the periphery. *C.* Atrophic smear pattern—nuclear enlargement type. The smear is composed of parabasal cells with seemingly enlarged pale nuclei. However, the nucleocytoplasmic ratio is not altered. There are scattered inflammatory cells in the background. *D.* Atrophic smear pattern, eosinophilic-pyknotic type. The smear is composed of small parabasal cells with eosinophilic cytoplasm. Nuclear breakup is evident in several cells. Note filaments of DNA in the background.

smear pattern may be associated with diminishing, increasingly scanty menstrual flow or with cessation of menses. In many women, this smear pattern may persist for many years after the menopause and, perhaps, for life. It has been my impression that the smear patterns suggestive of persisting estrogen activity correlate positively with sexual activity of postmenopausal women. Women who lead an active sexual life after the menopause appear to be less likely to develop postmenopausal atrophy than sexually inactive women. This anecdotal observation has received ample support from a study by Leiblum et al (1983).

"Crowded" Menopause: Moderate Deficiency of Estrogens

This type of smear usually follows the smear of early menopause and is characterized by **thick, crowded clusters of intermediate and large parabasal cells** (hence, the name of this type of smear, proposed by Papanicolaou). The cells are well preserved and there is little, if any, dryness. Because of small size of the cells, their nuclei may appear to be relatively large but are of normal sizes (Fig. 8-27A). The cytoplasm frequently contains deposits of glycogen in the form of yellow deposits, similar to **navicular cells** observed in pregnancy (Fig. 8-27B).*

Atrophic or Advanced Menopause

The pattern of atrophic menopause appears to be invariably preceded by early or crowded menopause or both. There is always a stage of transition between the normal cycle and the advanced menopause, even if the latter was brought about by oophorectomy. The atrophic menopause represents a final stage of involution of the female genital tract.

---

* The cytologic pattern of pregnancy occurring late in life and early menopause may be similar. To separate the two entities, Wied recommended the administration of 5 mg of diethylstilbestrol daily for 4 days. If smears are reexamined on the 5th day, there will be a return to full maturation of squamous cells in women in the menopause, but there will be no effect on the smear pattern of the pregnant woman (see Fig. 9-6).

The **cytologic patterns** of the advanced atrophic menopause are influenced by **dryness of the genital tract and scarcity of recoverable cellular material,** resulting in preparations that contain relatively few cells. The dominant squamous cells are of the **parabasal type,** although it is not uncommon to see a few scattered, more mature cells, evidently corresponding to nonatrophic areas of the squamous epithelium. Two **main effects of dryness** may be observed. One is the **uniform enlargement of the parabasal cells,** accompanied by a characteristic uniform gray discoloration of the **enlarged opaque nuclei** (the **nuclear enlargement type;** Fig. 8-27C). The second pattern is marked **eosinophilia of the cytoplasm** accompanied by **nuclear pyknosis and break-up of nuclei or karyorrhexis** (the **eosinophilic-pyknotic type;** Fig. 8-27D). The two patterns may appear simultaneously. As a result of nuclear break-up, **basophilic filaments of DNA** are often seen in the background. In the smears of the eosinophilic pyknotic type, there may be a **striking variation in size and shape of squamous cells.** Sometimes perfectly normal superficial squamous cells may occur in such smears, next to small parabasal type cells (Fig. 8-28A). **Sheets of spindly squamous cells,** with elongated cytoplasm and relatively large and dark-staining nuclei, may make their appearance in atrophic smears, most likely an artifact of smear preparation (Fig. 8-28B). Such cell sheets may be mistaken for spindly cells of squamous carcinoma, even though their nuclei are not enlarged or otherwise abnormal (see Chap. 11).

The **endocervical cells in cervical smears, even if obtained by brushes, are usually scarce or absent.** When present, the **endocervical cells are smaller than during the childbearing age,** although their columnar or cuboidal configuration is still preserved. The nuclei, although of normal size, may appear somewhat hyperchromatic and the cytoplasm is scanty, opaque, and shows no evidence of secretory activity, except for an occasional vacuole.

As a consequence of extensive cell necrosis, **mono- or multinucleated macrophages,** often containing fragments of phagocytized material, are commonly observed in atrophic smears (Fig. 8-28C). **Multinucleated macrophages may also be found in normal endometrial samples** of postmenopausal women. These cells usually accompany scanty fragments of endometrial glands and sparse stromal cells, corresponding to atrophic endometrium of the menopause.

Round or oval **globules of inspissated blue-staining material, probably mucus,** about the size of parabasal squa-

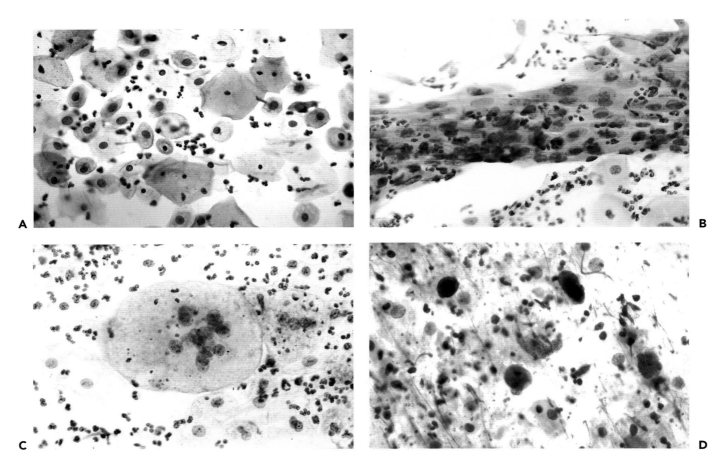

Figure 8-28 **Cytologic patterns of menopause.** *A.* Atrophic smear pattern with scattered mature superficial squamous cells. *B.* Spindly pattern of squamous cells—an artifact caused by dryness. Note normal nuclei. *C.* A foreign body giant cell in a postmenopausal atrophic smear. Note phagocytized cell debris in the cytoplasm. *D.* Blue or purple amorphous bodies, either inspissated mucus or degenerated parabasal cells, in postmenopausal atrophy.

mous cells, may appear in the late menopausal smears (Fig. 8-28D). Occasionally, the center of the globule is denser than the periphery and the structure may resemble a cell with a markedly hyperchromatic nucleus, **mimicking a cancer cell.** On close examination, the lack of actual structure within the globule is obvious and its true nature will be recognized. Such globules may, on rare occasion, be quite numerous in a vaginal smear and may result in an erroneous diagnosis of cancer. Some observers believe that the **blue globules** are not made up of inspissated mucus, but represent **degenerated small parabasal cells** (Ziabkowski and Naylor, 1976). This latter view is not sustained by convincing evidence. In any event, it is generally agreed that these structures are of no significance, except as a potential source of diagnostic error.

Because of loss of the protective superficial layers of squamous epithelium, **inflammatory processes** are commonly seen in smears of this type. **In the presence of vaginitis or cervicitis,** the background of the smear may contain **numerous leukocytes and cell debris** (see Fig. 8-27C). The inflammatory patterns will be described in detail in Chapter 10.

In some atrophic smears, **nuclear pyknosis** may be quite striking and may **mimic the hyperchromasia of cancer cells.** As is discussed in Chapter 11, the nuclei of cancer cells in postmenopausal women are usually very large, irregular and often markedly hyperchromatic, whereas the pyknotic nuclei of advanced menopause are usually enlarged only in proportion to the size of the cell, with retention of the normal nucleocytoplasmic ratio. Still, in some cases, to document the presence of cancer cells may require **administration of estrogen** that will normalize the atrophic cell population and enhance the abnormal appearance of cancer cells.

It has been the experience in this laboratory that the pronounced degenerative phenomena associated with atrophic menopause, resulting in cellular abnormalities, are usually observed in women whose vaginas have been free of outside contacts for prolonged periods of time. If the sampling is repeated within a few days, there is usually a striking improvement and sometimes there is a complete disappearance of abnormalities.

CYTOLOGY OF PREPUBERTAL FEMALES

Much of our knowledge of the cytologic patterns of vaginal smears in infants and children is derived from work by Fraenkel and Papanicolaou (1938) and Sonek (1967, 1969). The optimal method of study is a **vaginal smear** obtained by means of a very small pipette. **Urinary sediment** may sometimes be successfully used for the study of hormonal levels in a very small child (see urocytogram, discussed in Chap. 9).

In **newborn infants,** the squamous epithelium of the cervix and the vagina usually assumes the appearance of maturity under the influence of maternal hormones. The vaginal smears, or urinary sediments, in newborn infants are composed of superficial squamous cells comparable with those of women in the childbearing age (Fig. 8-29A). Within a few days after birth, the percentage of superficial cells drops in favor of small intermediate cells. This smear make-up changes within 2 weeks after birth by an increase in parabasal cells. After the 4th week of life, the smears are composed chiefly of parabasal cells (Fig. 8-29B). This smear type remains essentially unchanged until the approach of puberty, when there is a gradual maturation of the squamous epithelium of the genital tract. In the presence of an inflammatory process, the smear background may show leukocytes.

There are several **reasons for studying cell preparations from the prepubertal girl.**

The low squamous epithelium of the child, not unlike that of a postmenopausal woman, is susceptible to **infections.** A vaginal smear may be of assistance in the identification of the causative agent, such as *Trichomonas vaginalis.* Occasionally, it may be of interest to study the extent and the duration of the epithelial **response to hormonal medication** by vaginal smears. If the presence of an **ovarian tumor with endocrine activity** is suspected, the study of vaginal cytology is sometimes helpful in establishing the diagnosis. For instance, in the presence of feminizing tu-

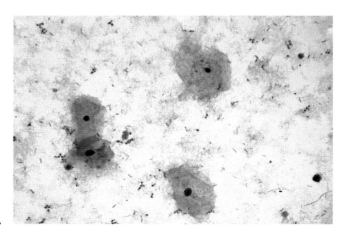

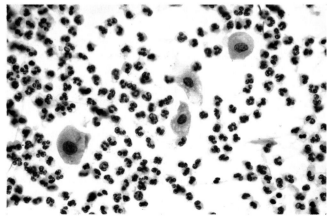

A   B

Figure 8-29 Cytology of prepubertal females. *A.* Newborn female. Urine sediment contains mature squamous cells, presumably of vaginal origin. *B.* Vaginal smear from a 7-year-old girl with vaginal discharge. The epithelial squamous cells are of small parabasal type—resembling a postmenopausal smear. Marked inflammatory exudate is present in the background.

mors, such as some of the granulosa cell tumors of the ovary, there may be maturation of squamous epithelium with a corresponding change in the smear pattern (see Chap. 15). A vaginal smear may also be helpful in the evaluation of various **endocrine disorders** (see Chap. 9).

PREGNANCY AND ABORTION

Pregnancy

Pregnancy constitutes a major physiologic upheaval in the life of a woman. The sequence of events in pregnancy is beyond the scope of this book and the readers are referred to other sources for a comprehensive review of this complex subject. This brief summary will stress those morphologic changes that may have an impact on cytology of the female genital tract.

Formation of Placenta

A detailed account of the formation of the human placenta may be found in the book by Boyd and Hamilton (1970). Through proliferation of the external cells of the embryonal *anlage*, a placenta is formed within a few days following implantation. The placental villi are initially lined by **trophoblastic cells;** the outer layer of large, multinucleated syncytial cells **(syncytiotrophoblasts)** and the inner layers of mononucleated **cytotrophoblasts** (also known as Langerhans' cells). By the 28th week of pregnancy, the cytotrophoblasts are reduced in number and the syncytial outer layer is the dominant lining of the villi. The placenta produces human **chorionic gonadotropin (hCG)** that can be used as a marker of cells derived from the placenta.

Formation of Decidua

The fertilization of the ovum takes place in the fallopian tube, whence the products of conception travel to the endometrial cavity, where the implantation takes place. At the site of the implantation, the cells of the endometrial stroma are transformed into **decidual cells,** which are **large, eosinophilic, polygonal cells, with round, vesicular nuclei.** The decidua, especially at the site of implantation of the ovum (decidua vera), carries the maternal vasculature, providing the fetus with necessary nutrients. Foci of **decidua may occur within the cervix,** where they may be confused with cancer in biopsy material (Fig. 8-30).

The Effects of Pregnancy on the Epithelia of the Cervix and Vagina

In histologic material, the cytoplasm of the **squamous epithelial cells** becomes markedly distended with glycogen, giving the cells a vacuolated appearance. The surface of the epithelium is often formed by intermediate squamous cells. There is usually some enlargement in the size of the **endocervical epithelial cells.** The endocervical glands are structurally more complex as a result of the elongation of the individual branches and are often filled with mucoid material (see Fig. 8-30). An eversion of the endocervix with the presence of a rim of endocervical tissue around the external os is frequent.

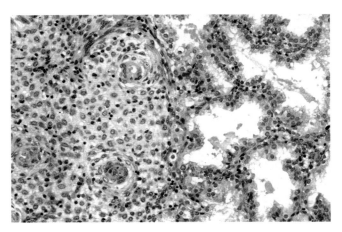

Figure 8-30   Decidual changes in the uterine cervix. The sheet of large, decidual cells in the cervical stroma may be mistaken for cancer. The endocervical glands are distended and filled with secretions.

Cytologic Manifestations of Pregnancy

Squamous Cells

The effects of pregnancy on the squamous epithelium are frequently, but not always, reflected in vaginal smears after the 2nd month. These changes are characterized by **clustering of intermediate squamous cells** and the predominance **of navicular cells, the latter** defined by yellow **cytoplasmic deposits of glycogen,** displacing the nuclei to the periphery, and sharply defined, accentuated borders (Fig. 8-31A). In the later stages of pregnancy, extensive **cytolysis** of squamous cell cytoplasm by lactobacilli is not uncommon (Fig. 8-31B).

Von Haam (1961) estimated that only 60% to 77% of pregnant women show the pattern of navicular cells. Furthermore, it has been pointed out above that early menopause may result in a smear pattern closely resembling pregnancy. Thus, the **presence of navicular cells is not diagnostic of pregnancy,** but the condition may be suspected when numerous such cells are present in smears from young women of childbearing age with a history of amenorrhea. The final diagnosis of pregnancy must be rendered by means other than a cytologic preparation.

Endocervical Cells

Endocervical cells may appear in somewhat increased numbers in cervical smears and may be larger than normal; the cytoplasm is often mucoid, and the nuclei are prominent, granular, and may show small nucleoli.

Uncommon Pregnancy-Related Findings

Trophoblastic Cells

Syncytiotrophoblasts are very rarely found in smears in normal pregnancy and are somewhat more frequent in smears preceding a spontaneous abortion. The cells are large, irregular, basophilic or eosinophilic, and contain a **variable number of large, often hyperchromatic homogeneous nuclei of uneven sizes** with a finely granular nuclear texture (Fig. 8-31C,D). Nearly identical cells may

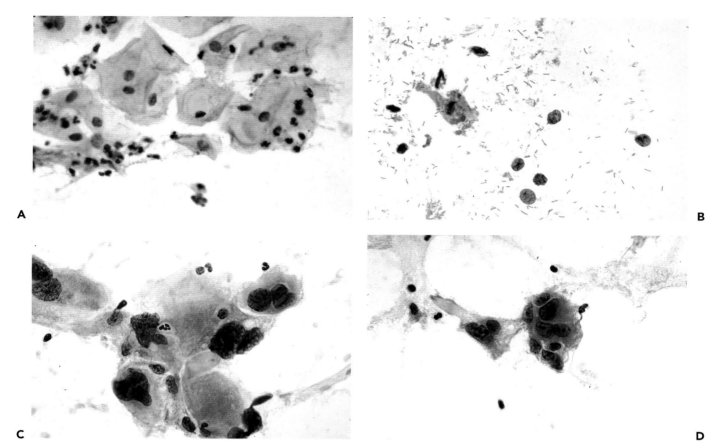

Figure 8-31 **Cytologic manifestations of pregnancy.** *A.* Navicular squamous cells, 2nd month of pregnancy. Note the deposits of yellow material, pushing the nuclei to the side of the cell. *B.* Cytolysis. The squamous cells are reduced to nuclei surrounded by wisps of cytoplasm. The change is caused by lactobacilli. *C,D.* Cytotrophoblasts. Abortion in a 29-year-old woman. The striking large cells contain multiple homogeneous nuclei of variable sizes (compare with cells of choriocarcinoma in Chap. 18).

be observed in **choriocarcinoma,** a malignant tumor derived from placental trophoblasts (see Chap. 18). Somewhat **similar multinucleated cells** may be seen in **herpes simplex infection** (see Chap. 10). It is questionable whether or not the mononucleated **cytotrophoblasts** may ever be correctly recognized in smears based on their morphology. Fiorella et al (1993) used a cocktail of **antibodies to human chorionic gonadotropin (hCG) and human placental lactogen** to identify syncytiotrophoblasts and cytotrophoblasts in smears during pregnancy. They could identify trophoblastic cells in 6 of 39 women and failed to observe any relationship of the presence of these cells with spontaneous abortion. It may be concluded from this study that cytotrophoblasts may sometimes occur in normal pregnancy but cannot be recognized without immunostaining. Frank and Bhat (1991) pointed out that **residual trophoblastic tissue may persist for several months after delivery and may be the source of abnormal cells** that may be confused with cancer.

Decidual Cells

Decidual cells may be identified in cervical smears on those rare occasions when decidual changes occur in the uterine cervix. These are **large mononucleated cells,** occurring singly or in clusters, with abundant eosinophilic or basophilic,

faintly vacuolated cytoplasm and prominent, centrally located **vesicular nuclei containing identifiable nucleoli** (Fig. 8-32). Occasionally, the **nuclei of the decidual cells may be dense and hyperchromatic,** particularly when derived from degenerating decidual tissue (Fig. 8-33). The decidual cells may be confused with cancer cells, as noted by Danos and Holmquist (1967), Schneider and Barnes (1981), and Pisharodi and Jovanoska (1995). Their recognition may be difficult in the absence of clinical history of pregnancy or amenorrhea and may require a biopsy for accurate diagnosis.

Arias-Stella Phenomenon

The abnormality, first described by Arias-Stella in 1954, is characterized by **large cells with large, hyperchromatic nuclei** located within the **endometrial gland lining in the presence of products of conception or in ectopic pregnancy.** Silverberg (1972) and Reyniak et al (1975) recorded the presence of Arias-Stella changes in endometrial glands, following curettage for interruption of pregnancy. The protruding large cells stand out among the normal endometrial cells (Fig. 8-34A). The great variability of the nuclear morphology was emphasized by Arias-Stella. Wagner and Richart (1968) reported that the Arias-Stella cells are polyploid (i.e., they contain a multiple of the normal amount of DNA). The mecha-

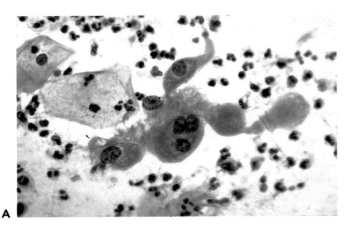

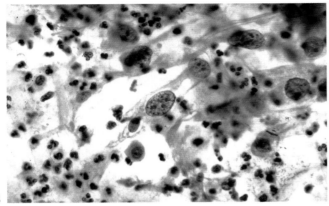

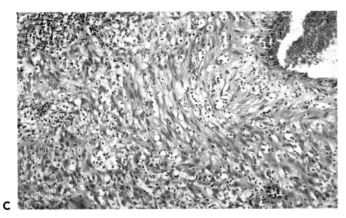

Figure 8-32 Decidual reaction, cervical smear, 41-year-old pregnant woman. *A,B.* Large cells of variable shapes with prominent nuclei containing conspicuous single or multiple nucleoli. *C.* Biopsy of a cervical polyp with decidual change in the stroma. (Case courtesy of Dr. N.W. Cunningham.)

nism of their formation is unclear. Similar abnormalities may be observed in histologic sections of the **endocervical epithelium** (Schneider, 1981) (Fig. 8-34B), **where they may be confused with an adenocarcinoma** (Cove, 1979). Schneider observed the endocervical Arias-Stella reaction in 9% of hysterectomy specimens obtained during pregnancy. **Similar changes may be observed in the endocervical epithelium in women receiving contraceptive hormones** with high progesterone content (see Chap. 18). The significance of such cell changes as a potential diagnostic pitfall in cytology was emphasized, notably by Albukerk (1974) and by Shrago

(1977) and by Benoit and Kini (1996). The exact identification of the highly abnormal and rare Arias-Stella cells in cytologic material is still a matter for some debate. Through the courtesy of Dr. Albukerk, I was privileged to examine some of his material. Arias-Stella cells appear in smears as **large cells with a single, large, somewhat hyperchromatic nucleus** and a finely vacuolated cytoplasm (Fig. 8-34C). In another case of a 29-year-old pregnant woman, we observed cells with large nuclei that were no longer present in postpartum smears (Fig. 8-34D). It was assumed that these were Arias-Stella cells. The cases recorded so far appear to be mainly related to ectopic pregnancy in which the products of conception do not prevent the shedding of such cells. Thus, the clinical history appears to be of critical diagnostic value in the assessment of such cells that otherwise may be readily mistaken for cancer cells.

Cytologic Assessment of Pregnancy at Term

During the 1950s, there was considerable interest in the application of the cytologic techniques in obstetrics, particularly with regard to the determination of pregnancy at term. With contemporary obstetrical techniques of fetal monitoring, the clinical value of these observations has diminished considerably. A brief account of the principal observations is appended for historical reasons.

In 1955, Lemberg-Siegfried and associates, and, in 1958 Lichtfus et al reported that pregnancy at term is characterized by the following cytologic changes:

- Rapid reduction in the number of clusters of intermediate squamous cells
- Increase in single superficial squamous cells with eosinophilic cytoplasm (increase in the eosinophilic index) or pyknotic nucleus (increase in the karyopyknotic index; for definitions of indices, see Chap. 9). Lichtfus et al cautioned that this evaluation is valid only if the smear has been obtained from the lateral wall of the vagina in the absence of infection and before the rupture of fetal membranes

Initially, these observations received wide support, particularly among European observers, but were subsequently seriously challenged. Abrams and Abrams (1962), Hindman et al (1962), Ruiz (1965), and Jing et al (1967) failed to observe the rapid transition of the prior-to-term pattern to the at-term pattern previously reported. In a very thorough study of serial smears obtained at weekly intervals from 135 antepartum patients, Abrams and Abrams failed to observe the at-term pattern in 66% of patients. In the remaining 34% of patients, the at-term pattern was observed but could not be correlated with the onset of labor. Since these authors meticulously followed the criteria of Lichtfus et al, it is clear that **the value of cytologic techniques in defining pregnancy at term is debatable.**

Rupture of Fetal Membranes

Rupture of fetal membranes results in spilling of **amniotic fluid** into the vagina. This fluid contains numerous **anucleated squamous cells** desquamated from the skin of the fetus (so-called vernix caseosa). Such cells may be found in the

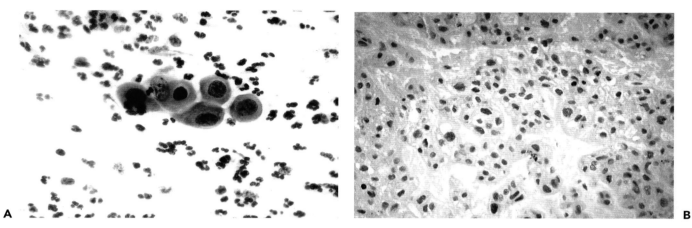

Figure 8-33 **Degenerating decidua in cervical smears.** *A.* Cells with hyperchromatic nuclei containing small nucleoli. *B.* Corresponding cervix biopsy showing degenerating decidua.

vaginal smear if it is obtained at the proper time. For further discussion of the cytology of amniotic fluid, see Chapter 26.

The Postpartum Period

During the postpartum period, there is often no evidence of estrogen activity and many women display an **atrophic** **smear pattern** with predominance of parabasal squamous cells. The views differ on the exact proportion of women with this smear pattern and the differences may be due to the techniques used. Butler and Taylor (1973), using a scrape smear of the lateral wall of the vagina, observed the atrophic pattern in only 28% of their population of postpartum women. McLennan and McLennan (1975), using a

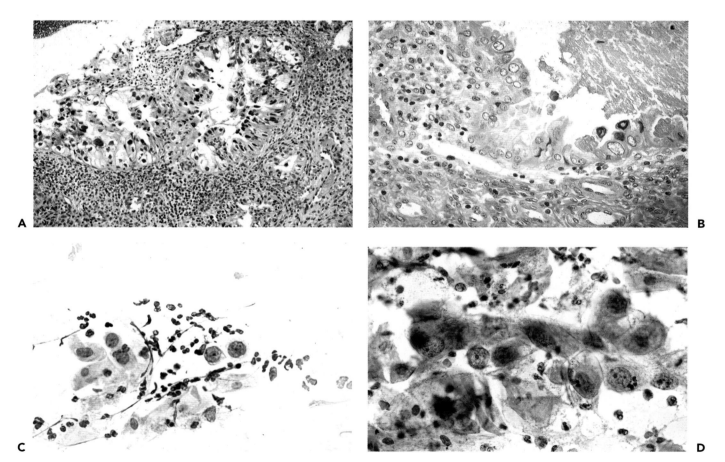

Figure 8-34 **Arias-Stella reaction in pregnancy.** Arias-Stella reaction in the endometrium (*A*) and the endocervix (*B*). Note scattered large cells with hyperchromatic nuclei in endometrial and endocervical glands. *C.* Isolated large cells in a cervical smear in a case of abortion presumed to be Arias-Stella cells. *D.* Several large cells in the smear of a 29-year-old, 7-month pregnant woman, presumed to be Arias-Stella cells. (*C:* Courtesy of Dr. Albukerk.).

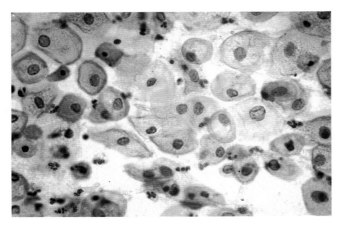

Figure 8-35 Postpartum smear, composed of navicular cells. (P stain; ×160.)

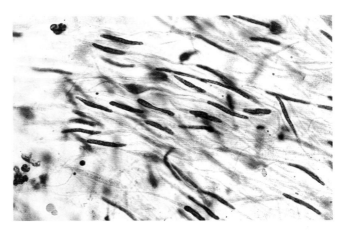

Figure 8-36 Smooth muscle cells in a cervical smear after abortion. Elongated cells with tapered cytoplasm and small central nuclei. (Oil immersion.)

mixed cervicovaginal smear 3 to 6 weeks postpartum, observed the atrophic pattern in 32% of nonlactating and 72% of lactating women. It must be noted that, **during lactation,** intermediate and large parabasal **cells of navicular type,** with large cytoplasmic glycogen deposits, may be observed (Fig. 8-35).

The return to normal cyclic patterns varies from patient to patient. In the great majority of patients, whether lactating or not, the cyclic pattern will be evident 6 months after delivery. Persistence of atrophic smear pattern, beyond 1 year after delivery, may indicate a serious endocrine disorder (see Chap. 9).

Alleged Pregnancy-Related Neoplastic Abnormalities

In the 1960s and 1970s, several articles, discussed in Chapter 11, attributed significant, cancer-like abnormalities of squamous and endocervical cells to pregnancy. The only cytologic changes characteristic of pregnancy are those described above. **Other disorders, particularly cytologic abnormalities consistent with precancerous lesions or cancer, are incidental to pregnancy** as recently reemphasized by Pisharodi and Jovanoska (1995) and by Michael and Esfahani (1997). To be sure, some of the cytologic findings, such as the presence of decidual cells, syncytiotrophoblasts, or Arias-Stella cells in smears, may be difficult to interpret and must be differentiated from manifestations of cancer, described in subsequent chapters of this book.

Cytology of Spontaneous Abortion

Although abortion is not, strictly speaking, a manifestation of normal events in the life of a woman, it appears appropriate to discuss it in conjunction with the events of normal pregnancy rather than elsewhere in this book. There are no cells diagnostic of abortion. A smear obtained during abortion may contain **navicular cells,** fresh blood, and inflammatory exudate. **Syncytiotrophoblastic cells** may be noted (see Fig. 8-31C,D). On the rarest occasions, **elongated, smooth mus-**

cle cells in smears (Fig. 8-36) will testify to trauma to the uterine wall. However, smooth muscle cells may also be derived from ulcerated submucous leiomyomas (fibroids), another very rare event (see Chap. 10).

Threatened Versus Inevitable Abortion

It is debatable whether cytologic techniques are of clinical value in distinguishing a threatened abortion from an inevitable abortion. Still, if an early pregnancy is associated with bleeding, it is occasionally possible to predict, in vaginal smears, whether or not an abortion is inevitable. A **preponderance of superficial squamous cells with pyknotic nuclei,** rather than the characteristic pattern of pregnancy consisting of intermediate and navicular cells, will usually indicate excessive estrogenic activity and may suggest the inevitability of an abortion. A study of the cells of the urinary sediment may be substituted for a vaginal smear. The information obtained from cytologic studies is of only relative value and should be used in conjunction with a careful clinical evaluation. Genetic studies on **fetal tissue from spontaneous abortions** (Carr, 1963; Szulman, 1965) demonstrated that, in many cases, the fetus carries **significant chromosomal abnormalities,** suggestive of major genetic defects. It appears probable that, in some cases at least, a spontaneous abortion is a natural defense against the birth of an abnormal child. The situation is different in habitual aborters, in whom a hormonal imbalance may exist.

THE NORMAL VAGINAL FLORA

The normal flora of the vagina varies from person to person, but *Lactobacillus* (bacillus Döderlein) is usually the preponderant organism. This organism is a **gram-positive slender rod** staining a pale blue by the Papanicolaou method. The bacterial rods may either be observed in the background of the smear (Fig. 8-37A) or may accumulate on the surface of squamous cells (Fig. 8-37B). The organism utilizes the **glycogen** contained in the cytoplasm of the intermediate and parabasal squamous cells and causes their

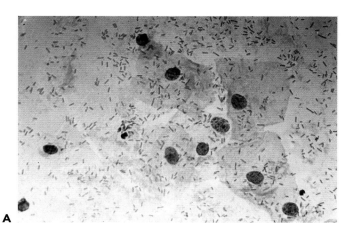
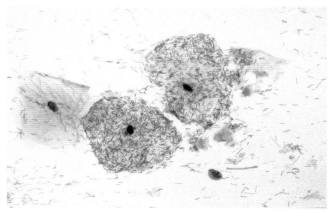

A   B

Figure 8-37   Lactobacilli (*b. vaginalis* or Döderlein bacilli) in cervicovaginal smears. *A,B.* Gram-positive rods of various length may occur in the background of the smears or on the surface of the squamous cells. See Figure 8-31B.

disintegration or cytolysis (see Fig. 8-31B). Fully mature superficial squamous cells are less likely to be cytolyzed, perhaps because of the presence of a firm cytoplasmic skeleton. *Lactobacillus* survives best at a vaginal pH of 5, which is maintained by glycolysis. For further discussion of lactobacilli, see Chapter 10.

CELLS OTHER THAN EPITHELIAL IN NORMAL SMEARS

Leukocytes

A variety of leukocytes may be observed in smears, even in the absence of inflammatory processes. Lymphocytes and polymorphonuclear leukocytes are frequently seen trapped in the cervical mucus. Plasma cells, which are very uncommon in smears, usually signify chronic inflammatory processes (see Chap. 10).

Macrophages (Histiocytes)

Small mononuclear macrophages are often seen during the late part of the menstrual bleeding (**exodus,** see above). The larger **mononucleated macrophages** are medium-sized cells (about 25 to 30 μm in diameter) with basophilic, often faintly vacuolated, cytoplasm that may contain fragments of phagocytized material. The nuclei are spherical or kidney-shaped with a finely granular chromatin and occasionally tiny nucleoli (Fig. 8-38A). Such cells are fairly common in cervical smears and may mimic endometrial or endocervical cells. The presentation and significance of such cells in vaginal smears in the diagnosis of endometrial cancer is discussed in Chapter 13. **Multinucleated macrophages** that may occur in smears are usually associated with the menopause, foreign bodies, or chronic inflammatory processes and are described above (see Fig. 8-28C) and discussed further in Chapter 10.

Spermatozoa and Cells of Seminal Vesicles

Spermatozoa are frequently observed in material from the female genital tract. Meisels and Ayotte (1976) recorded the presence of spermatozoa in nearly 10% of all smears of women between the ages of 25 and 40 and, with lesser frequency, in adult women of other age groups.

Well-preserved **spermatozoa** with the characteristic

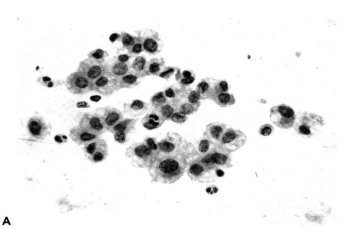
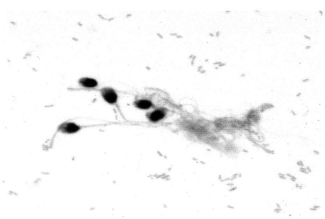

A   B

Figure 8-38   *A.* Sheets of macrophages with vacuolated cytoplasm. Note the relatively large nuclei of variable sizes. *B.* Spermatozoa in a cervicovaginal smear.

dense heads and thin, elongated flagella (tails) are readily identified (Fig. 8-38B). The head may be somewhat variable in size and configuration; it is most commonly egg-shaped and, in Papanicolaou stain, shows an uneven distribution of chromatin. The pole of the head attached to the flagellum usually appears somewhat denser than the opposite pole. This is very likely an artifact of fixation or preparation because, in material optimally fixed for light microscopy, the chromatin distribution is uniform throughout the head. The basic ultrastructure of the flagellum is similar to that of a cilium, described in Chapter 2. The energy required for the movement of the spermatozoon is provided by numerous mitochondria located along the flagellum. Degenerated spermatozoa or spermatozoa killed by spermicidal agents are also commonly observed in cytologic preparations from the female genital tract. The flagella are usually partially or completely destroyed and the heads are enlarged, but not uniformly so. In clusters, the degenerated spermatozoa appear as a collection of oval shaped nuclei of variable sizes with remnants of flagella attached to them.

Spermatozoa may be also phagocytized by macrophages. In such instances, the heads of spermatozoa may be observed within the cytoplasm of the macrophage, whereas the tails may be outside the cell (see Chap. 33; Fig. 33-6C).

Cells originating in **seminal vesicles** may also be observed in vaginal smears. Such cells, noted in about 10% of patients with spermatozoa, may have conspicuously **large, hyperchromatic nuclei** and are identifiable by the presence of **cytoplasmic granules of brown lipochrome pigment** (see Chap. 33). Spermatozoa and other cells of male origin may be identified in cervicovaginal material by fluorescent in situ hybridization (FISH) technique with probes to chromosomes X and Y (Roa et al, 1995). Such cells were detected in some women 3 weeks after coitus. These observations are of value in medicolegal cases (Collins et al, 1994).

ACELLULAR MATERIAL AND FOREIGN BODIES IN CERVICOVAGINAL SMEARS

Curschmann's Spirals

Coiled spirals of inspissated mucus with a dense core and translucent periphery, identical in appearance to Curschmann's spirals seen in sputum (see Chap. 19), may occasionally be observed in cervical or vaginal smears. Prolla (1974) reported finding such structures in six of 5,635 consecutive vaginal and cervical smears and pointed out that all six women were heavy cigarette smokers. He suggested that the vaginal-cervical Curschmann's spirals reflect a systemic effect of cigarette smoking. In an extensive study of this phenomenon, Novak et al (1984) observed Curschmann's spirals with a prevalence of 1 in 1,700 cervicovaginal smears and failed to note any relationship with smoking or extrinsic factors. Yet, in some cases at least, the possibility of extraneous origin of the spirals found in the vaginal pool must be considered. In one such case, a possible source was the sputum of an asthmatic sexual partner (Fig. 8-39). However, it is most likely

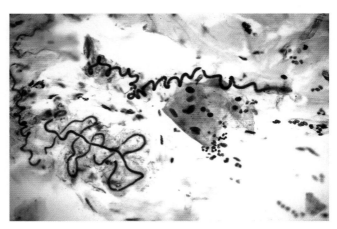

Figure 8-39   Curschmann's spirals in a cervicovaginal smear (see text).

that, in the majority of cases, the spirals are casts of inspissated endocervical mucus.

Contaminants

The normal cervicovaginal smears may contain a variety of contaminants. **Lubricating jellies, vaginal creams, or powders may obscure the smears** completely and render it useless. Small **polygonal refractile crystals,** frequently seen in smears, usually originate from sterile powders used for surgical gloves. Other crystals, rarely occurring in smears, are **hematoidin** crystals or cockleburrs (Hollander and Gupta, 1974; Capaldo et al, 1983) and **"crystalline bodies,"** probably inspissated cervical mucus, described by Zaharopoulos et al (1985). Occasionally, **pollen** and **plant cells** may occur (Avrin et al, 1972). Plant cells are described in Chapter 19. **Grains of pollen** may be particularly disturbing. The spherical or oval grains come in various sizes depending on the plant of origin, and some may mimic epithelial squamous cells by size and configuration (Fig. 8-40). Some pollens may have a dense central core that may mimic a cancer cell (Fig. 8-40B,C). Pollen grains are best recognized by a rigid, translucent external envelope, best seen in Figure 8-40D, and lack of structure in the central core.

Other contaminants, such as fungus of the family *Alternaria*, may be observed (see Chap. 19 for description). Other rare contaminants include **larval parts of carpet beetles** (Bechtold et al, 1985), as well as other arthropods, and various protozoa may be occasionally observed (Fig. 8-41). Undoubtedly, from time to time, still other contaminants will be reported. The so-called **ciliated bodies,** reported in cervical smears and initially thought to be parasites, represent detached tufts of ciliated endocervical cells, described above and shown in Figure 8-21.

Ova

Way and Dawson (1959) and Carvalho (1965) reported the finding of an ovum in the vaginal smear. Carvalho's ovum was a spherical structure surrounded by a peripheral zone, interpreted as zona pellucida, and a peripheral array

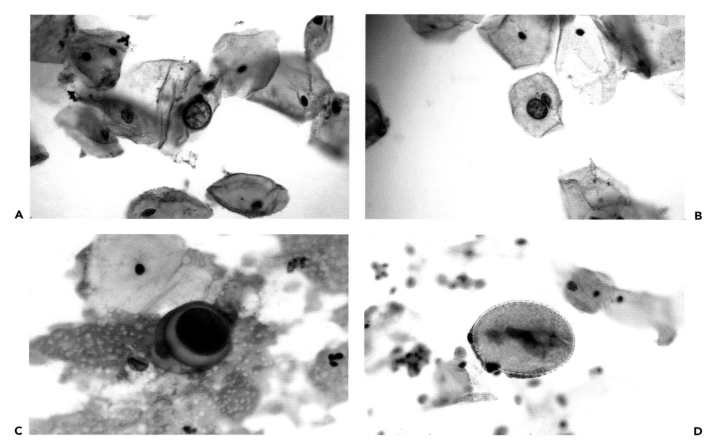

Figure 8-40   **Pollen in cervicovaginal smears.** *A–D.* Pollen grains of various sizes. Note the sharply demarcated translucent capsule. In *C*, the grain of pollen is phagocytized by a macrophage. *B* and *D* mimic cancer cells because of the dark center.

of cells, presumably the corona radiata. Unfortunately, the measurements of the ovum were not provided. Although the identity of Carvalho's ovum was questioned by Norman (1975), Wachtel and Wytcherly (1970), and by Benson (1972), a recent photograph by Greenebaum (1998), illustrating a human oocyte (ovum) derived directly from an ovarian cystic follicle, confirmed Carvalho's observations. Greenbaum's oocyte was about 150 μm in diameter, had a tiny, barely visible nucleus, and it was surrounded by a transparent, striated zona pellucida (the product of the ovum) and a layer of follicular cells (Fig. 8-42).

Benign Cells Originating in Adjacent Organs

Cells from adjacent organs may be observed in vaginal smears and in endocervical and endometrial aspirates. The significance of these observations in reference to cancer is discussed in the appropriate chapters. Occasionally, however, benign cells of extraneous origin may be of diagnostic importance. Cells originating in the urinary bladder and in the colon, when observed in gynecologic material, may indicate the presence of **vesicovaginal** or **rectovaginal fistula.** The identification of the **urothelial cells** of bladder origin may be difficult unless the multinucleated, large **umbrella cells** (see Chap. 22) are observed. Colonic cells, usually forming clusters or sheets of parallel cells, resemble en-

docervical cells, except for their larger size (Fig. 8-43A). Angeles and Saigo (1994) observed colonic cells in smears of 14 of 23 patients with rectovaginal fistula. Colon contents in the form of plant cells, characterized by a thick translucent cellulose membrane, may also be observed in such smears (Fig. 8-43B).

DEFINITION OF AN ADEQUATE CERVICOVAGINAL SAMPLE

The purpose of cytologic examination of the female genital tract is the detection of cancer and precancerous states, mainly of the uterine cervix. The question as to what constitutes an **adequate and representative cervicovaginal sample,** offering the best diagnostic opportunity, has been discussed for many years (see Koss and Hicklin, 1974). The issue has become important because the currently prevailing system of nomenclature, the Bethesda System (discussed in detail in Chap. 11), mandates the **reporting of inadequate samples** as a separate category. Severe medical and legal consequences may result from reporting such a sample as "negative" or "within normal limits," particularly in the presence of a precancerous lesion or cancer of the uterine cervix. The issue of sample adequacy was relatively simple, so long as **direct cervical smears** were the dominant mode

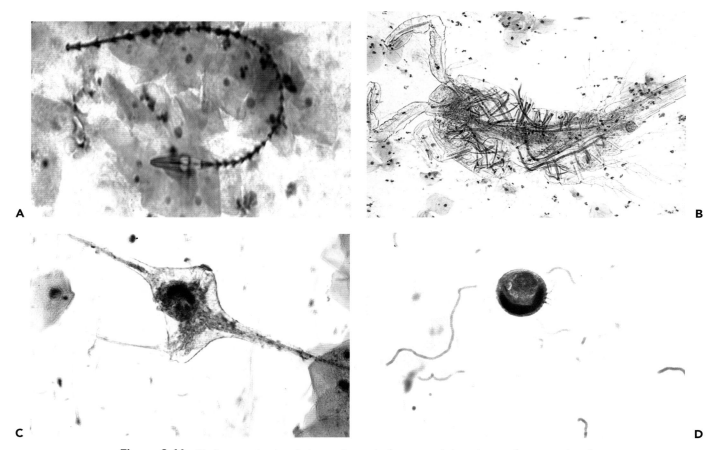

Figure 8-41 **Various contaminants in cervicovaginal smears.** *A.* Larval part of a carpet beetle larva. *B.* An arthropod, probably a louse. *C.* A flagellate of *ceratum* species. *D.* A high magnification of a water contaminant, probably a protozoon. Note cilia. (*A:* Courtesy of Dr. Jacques Legier; *B:* Courtesy of Dr. Ellen Greenebaum.)

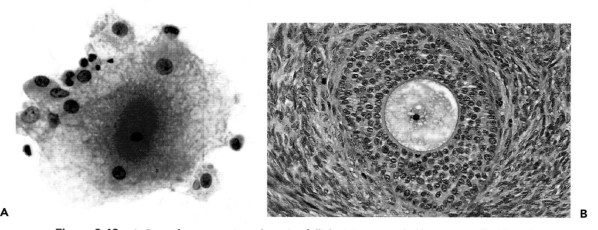

Figure 8-42 *A.* **Ovum from an aspirated ovarian follicle.** It is surrounded by a zona pellucida and a layer of follicular cells. Compare with histologic section of a similar oocyte and follicle (*B*). (Courtesy of Dr. Ellen Greenebaum, New York, NY. From Greenebaum E. Cytologic identification of oocytes in ovarian cyst aspirates. N Engl J Med 339:604, 1998.)

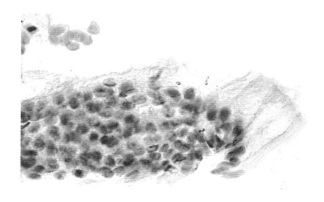

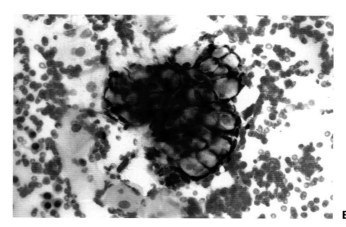

A

B

Figure 8-43   Cells from adjacent organs. *A.* Sheet of tall colonic cells with abundant cytoplasm in a cervicovaginal smear of a woman with vaginorectal fistula. *B.* A multinucleated structure, most likely distended goblet cells of rectal origin (rectovaginal fistula).

of examination, because the various components of the smear could be recognized. With the widespread use of **liquid monolayer, machine-generated preparations,** the issue became more complex.

Cervicovaginal Smears

A cervicovaginal smear should be representative of the squamous and endocervical epithelia of the uterine cervix, and include the transformation zone. A number of instruments, discussed in the Appendix to this chapter, have been introduced to improve the sampling of the uterine cervix. Therefore, **an adequate cervical smear should contain squamous cells from the vaginal portion of the uterine cervix, parabasal "metaplastic" cells, presumably derived from the transformation zone, and endocervical cells from the endocervical canal.** In practice, the composition of an adequate cervical smear **depends as much on the skill of the operator and the techniques used as on the age of the patient, because it depends on the location of the transformation zone.** As has been shown in Figure 8-10, the transformation zone in older women may be situated within the endocervical canal and will be much more difficult to sample than in a young woman. There is also some controversy as to the significance of endocervical cells. Mitchell and Medley (1992, 1993), careful Australian workers, consider the presence of columnar cells as indispensable in the assessment of a smear as adequate. Kurman and Solomon (1992) suggested that the **minimum presence of endocervical cells should be two clusters, each composed of at least 5 cells.** In the 2001 Bethesda System, this requirement has been modified to "at least 10 well-preserved endocervical or squamous metaplasia cells, singly or in clusters" (Solomon and Nayar, 2004). Other observers question whether the presence of endocervical cells is essential (Koss and Hicklin, 1974; Metcalf et al, 1994; Koss and Gompel, 1999; Birdsong, 2001). This writer considers **the presence of cervical mucus equally important evidence of smear adequacy as the presence of**

endocervical cells. The mucus, in the form of streaks containing cells desquamated from the endocervical canal, is an **invaluable diagnostic resource.** Unfortunately, with the use of endocervical brushes, which often require the removal of the plug of mucus from the external os, the presence of streaks of mucus can no longer be ascertained. The same is true of preparations of cervical cells collected in liquid samples. Therefore, the following **standards of smear adequacy are proposed for smears of women during the childbearing age:**

> An adequate smear must contain:
> Squamous cells from the portio of the uterine cervix
> Parabasal "metaplastic" cells
> A few endocervical cells or cervical mucus
> Smears of prepubertal girls or postmenopausal women need not contain either endocervical cells or cervical mucus.

As Koss and Hicklin observed in 1974, **any smear containing abnormal cells and requiring further action is by definition adequate,** regardless of whether the above criteria are fulfilled or not. The same authors also noted that the **diagnostic accuracy of routine cervical smears, regardless of technique, is not absolute. Therefore, a minimum of three consecutive cervical smears, at intervals of 6 to 12 months, should be obtained before the patient is considered free of disease. It was suggested that subsequent screening may take place at longer intervals every other or third year.** The current guidelines of the American Cancer Society are in agreement with these recommendations.

Liquid Preparations

It is the occasional failure of the cervical smear, with its legal consequences, that led to the current trend to replace them with **liquid preparation systems.** At the time of this writing (2004), two commercially available automated smear-equivalent processing systems have been approved by the Food and Drug Administration in the United States, ThinPrep (Cytyc Corp., Marlborough, MA) and SurePath

(TriPath Corp., Burlington, NC). Both systems **require that the sample be placed in a container with fixative and processed by a machine that deposits an aliquot of cells in small circular areas of the slide. The preparations are relatively free of blood and debris, thus facilitating and accelerating screening, but also modifying somewhat the morphology of the cells and, thus, requiring special training in interpretation of material.** The two systems appear to be somewhat more efficient in the discovery of cellular abnormalities, as discussed in Chapters 12 and 13. A significant benefit of collection in liquid fixative is the option of utilizing the **residual material for ancillary procedures,** such as the presence and typing of **human papillomavirus (HPV).**

Still, the issue of **adequacy of liquid preparations has not been solved.** Because these preparations use only a small aliquot of the entire sample, the figure of 5,000 well-preserved squamous cells per preparation was suggested as evidence of smear adequacy (Solomon and Nayar, 2004). Such a sample would contain only a very small number of abnormal cells and, therefore, requires intense screening, obviating the principal advantage of liquid processing. Only long-term follow-up of patients will determine the accuracy of these cancer detection systems.

APPENDIX

CLINICAL PROCEDURES IN GYNECOLOGIC CYTOLOGY

The successful practice of gynecologic cytology depends to a large extent on good quality material secured from the genital tract. Therefore, it is recommended that the simple guidelines discussed below be followed before the sampling takes place. **The patient should not douche for 24 hours before the genital smears are obtained. During the childbearing age,** smears should be obtained at **mid-cycle.** Smears obtained during menstrual bleeding may be difficult to interpret because of contamination with blood, endometrium, debris, and macrophages (histiocytes).

Prior to sampling, it is important to **secure the necessary materials** and lay them out on a suitable, conveniently located surface within the reach of the operator:

- **Instrument(s)** used to obtain smears
- **Clean microscopic glass slides** of good quality, preferably with frosted ends (0.96–1.06 mm in thickness) for preparation of smears
- Suitable **pencil for slides with frosted ends** or, if **plain slides** are used, a **diamond marker** for identification of slides. Each slide should be identified with **patient's name, date, and/or identifying number. If separate samples are obtained from different organs of the female genital tract, the slides must be appropriately identified by symbols, for example,** C = cervix, E =

endocervix, EN = endometrium. The **precise origin of each smear with the accompanying symbol must be noted on the laboratory form.**

- **Fixatives** (see below and Chap. 44)
- **Laboratory form** with clear identification of the patient and appropriate history. The minimum data required on each patient comprise:

  Date of procedure
  Name of physician or health facility submitting the sample
  Patient's name, address, and ID number, if any
  Sex and age
  Source and site of origin of the specimen with identifying symbols (see above)
  Method of collection
  Presumed clinical diagnosis
  Summary of prevailing symptoms
  Prior treatment, if any
  Prior cytology or histology
  Date of last menstrual period
  Contraceptive history
  Obstetric history

PREPARATION OF SMEARS

Every effort should be made to place as much of the material obtained as possible on the slide and to prepare a **thin, uniform smear.** Thick smears with overlapping cell layers are difficult or impossible to interpret. Considerable skill and practice are required to prepare excellent smears by a single, swift motion without loss of material or air drying.

Fixation of Smears

Immediate fixation of smears facilitates correct interpretations. Two types of fixatives are commonly used—fluid fixatives and spray fixatives. Both are described in detail in Chapter 44 and, hence, only a brief summary is required here.

Fixatives

For all practical purposes, **95% ethyl alcohol or equivalent is a suitable universal fixative for routine smears.** Liquid fixatives can be used in Coplin jars with covers. Also, a pipette filled with the fixative may also be used to **fix the smear placed on a hard surface** for 15 minutes or more, making sure to **replenish the fixative to prevent drying caused by evaporation.** The fixed slides may be placed in an appropriate cardboard or plastic container for shipment to the laboratory. Certain commercially available fixatives, particularly **CytoRichred** (TriPath Corp., Burlington, NC) has found many uses in preparation of endometrial smears, as discussed in Chapters 11 and 12 (Maksem and Knesel, 1995). The fixative preserves cells of diagnostic value while lysing erythrocytes.

Spray fixatives contain water-soluble polymers or plastics

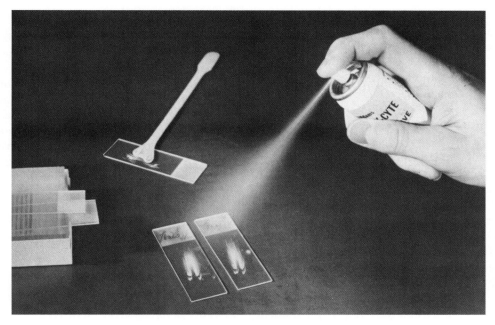

Figure 8-44 **Use of coating fixatives for smears of uterine cervix obtained with a wooden spatula.** Immediate application of fixative is essential. (Clay-Adams Inc., New York, NY.)

and are described in detail in Chapter 44. When correctly used, spray fixatives **protect the smears from drying** by forming an invisible film on the surface of the slides. If spray fixatives are selected (and they usually are easier to handle than liquid fixatives), they should be applied **immediately** after the process of smear preparation has been completed. Correct use of the spray fixatives calls for several precautions:

■ The spray must be **smooth and steady** and the operation of the nozzle must be checked before the smear is obtained.

■ The **distance between the nozzle of the spray and the smear to be sprayed must be about 10 to 12 inches (25 to 30 cm)**, as shown in Figure 8-44. If the spray is held too close to the smear, several mishaps commonly occur; the cells may be dislodged by the force of the spray, or the evaporation of the spray vehicle may freeze and irreversibly damage the cells. An artifact may also occur, inasmuch as normal squamous cells may acquire a perinuclear halo, rendering them similar to human papillomavirus-infected cells or koilocytes. If the nozzle is too far from the target, insufficient fixative will reach the surface.

■ **Smears coated with spray fixative are air dried** and placed in cardboard slide containers and forwarded to the laboratory.

■ Although there is no evidence at this time that the materials contained in the various spray preparations are harmful, it is advisable to protect the patient and the medical personnel from inhalation of the spray by using a face mask or by performing the spraying procedure under a protective glass plate or a laboratory hood.

Inexpensive liquid-coating fixatives may be prepared in the laboratory and used in lieu of spray fixatives. Carbowax fixative, described in Chapter 44, is an example. A few drops of this fixative are placed on the surface of the smear. After drying (5 to 10 minutes), the slides may be placed in slide containers for shipment to the laboratory.

COLLECTION OF MATERIAL FOR LIQUID PROCESSING AND "MONOLAYER" SMEARS

If processing by an **automated apparatus** is selected, the container with the company-recommended fixative should be available. The companies provide vials with fixatives accommodating collection devices or cell samples. For further discussion of these options, see Chapter 44.

SAMPLING SYSTEMS

Vaginal Smear

The original method, on which Papanicolaou and Traut based their initial observation in 1942, was the vaginal smear (see Chaps. 1, 11, and 13 for a detailed account of these events). Nowadays the procedure is rarely used, because it is **not efficient in the discovery of precancerous lesions of the uterine cervix** and requires time and skill in screening. The vaginal sample is often very rich in cells and difficult to interpret and, hence, not labor-effective.

The advantage of the vaginal smear lies chiefly in the **ease** with which it is obtained, even in the presence of an intact hymen. In **women past the age of 40,** the vaginal smear complements the cervical sample and may **contain important information pertaining to the endometrium, fallopian tubes, and the ovaries** and, occasionally, from **other, more distant sites** (see Chaps. 13 and 14). Therefore, in my judgment, it should be maintained in the armamentarium of cancer detection in older women. This smear is best obtained as the **first step in the gynecologic examination,** prior to introduction of the speculum. The patient is placed in a lithotomy position. The posterior fornix of the vagina is aspirated with the blunt end of a slightly curved **glass pipette** fitted with a rubber bulb. During aspiration, the end of the pipette should be gently moved from side to side to ensure a good sampling of cells. Alternately, a **tongue depressor or similar simple device** may be used to collect cells from the posterior vaginal fornix. The material is spread rapidly on a clean glass slide, which is fixed without delay. **A vaginal smear alone should never be considered as a sufficient cytologic sample in women with intact uteri and it must be accompanied by a cervical sample.**

The **vaginal smear for hormonal studies** should be obtained by scraping the **lateral wall of the vagina** at some distance from the cervix. These smears are reliable in the evaluation of the hormonal status of the woman in the absence of inflammation or hormonal treatment, as discussed in Chapter 9.

Cervical Smears

The cervical smear and its variants are utilized for diagnosis of precancerous lesions and cancer of the uterine cervix. Regardless of the instrument used, the cervical smear must be obtained **under direct vision after introduction of the unlubricated speculum.** If there are difficulties in introducing the speculum, a few drops of normal saline solution may be used to moisten it. **Several methods and instruments for securing cytologic material from the uterine cervix are available (Fig. 8-45). Although many are no longer used, they are generally much less expensive and more affordable in developing countries.**

Nonabsorbent Cotton Swab Smear

This inexpensive and simple mode of sampling the uterine cervix is no longer recommended because of loss of cells adhering to the cotton.

Cervical Scraper or Spatula

As initially proposed by Ayre (1947), a wooden tongue depressor, cut with scissors to fit the contour of the cervix,

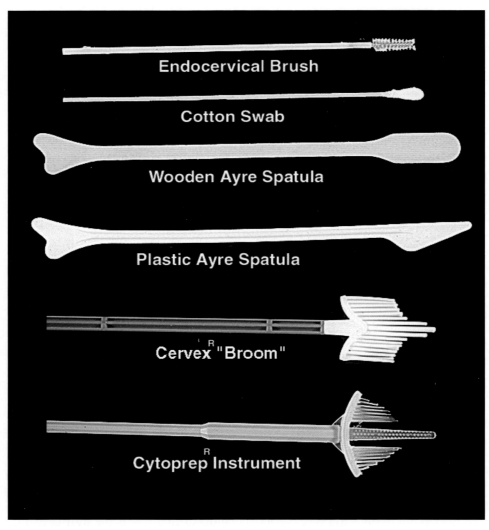

Figure 8-45 Instruments for sampling of the uterine cervix.

may be used. Commercial plastic scrapers are now widely available. The end of the scraper is U shaped, with one arm longer than the other. The scraper should fit the contours of the cervix, particularly the squamo-columnar junction, with the longer end introduced into the endocervical canal. The scraper is rotated 360° under pressure, the longer end being used as a pivot within the external os (see Fig. 1-4). The material is spread on a slide and fixed immediately. Abundant and diagnostically valuable material is obtained by this method. The method may occasionally be traumatic to the patient and may cause some minor bleeding.

Triple-Smear Method (VCE Smear)

Although now very rarely used, the method, described by Wied and Bahr (1959), advocates placing material from three sources (vagina, portio, and endocervix) on a single, specially prepared and etched glass slide. The method requires considerable dexterity on the part of the clinician to obtain material rapidly in order to avoid drying of smears.

Endocervical Brushes

Because of the insistence that an adequate cytologic sample must contain endocervical cells, several types of endocervical brushes for sampling of the cervix have been introduced. The advantage of these instruments was based on the concept that an adequate cervical smear must contain endocervical cells and that the brushes increase the yield of endocervical lesions, a concept supported by the Bethesda System (see above and Chap. 11). Such brushes must be introduced into the endocervical canal under visual control and gently rotated to provide adequate material. In the process, **the plug of cervical mucus, usually present at the external os, is displaced and lost**, although it is an important source of abnormal cells (see above and Chap. 11). Except in postmenopausal women with atrophy of the uterus, the endocervical brush yields endocervical cells in virtually all the smears, rendering them "adequate." However, in smears prepared from endocervical brushes, the thick clusters of endocervical cells, scraped from the endocervical surface, may be difficult to interpret. There is also evidence that many patients experience bleeding or spotting after the use of these instruments. **The endocervical brushes serve only for the sampling of the endocervix and must be supplemented with a scrape smear of the exocervix.**

Brushes Combining Endocervical and Exocervical Sampling

The prototype of such an instrument is the Cervex brush (Rovers Medical Devices, distributed by Therapak Corp. Irwindale, CA), which consists of a flat array of flexible plastic strips. The central strips are longer and, thus, enter the endocervical canal. Several rotations of the instrument ensure **sampling of the entire cervical epithelium with adequate representation of endocervical and squamous cells.** There are several **variants of the original Cervex brush,** one shown in Figure 8-45 (CytoPrep Inc., Eschen, Lichtenstein). These instruments have been recommended

as a single sample for use with the liquid collection for automated processing of samples.

Self-Administered Sampling of the Female Genital Tract

Vaginal Tampon

In the 1950s, a vaginal tampon, composed of compressed cotton enclosed in a nylon cover, the first self-administered device for cervical cancer detection, was developed by Draghi and tested by Brunschwig (1957) and by Papanicolaou (1954). Bader et al (1957) compared the performance of the tampon with simultaneously obtained vaginal and cervical smears in 2,691 asymptomatic patients. The quality of the smear, obtained by stamping the tampon on a microscopic slide, was judged to be **adequate** in about two-thirds of the patients. The tampon smears were considered negative in about half the patients with carcinoma in situ, diagnosed on cervical smears, and the device has never been accepted as a viable substitute of the direct cervical sample.

Self-Administered Pipette

Koch and Stakemann (1962) and Davis (1962) introduced a **self-administered pipette** for collection of cytologic material for purposes of cervix cancer detection that can be mailed to the patient, accompanied by a set of simple instructions. The disposable device consisted of a fixative-filled plastic bulb attached to a pipette. The patient inserts the pipette into the vagina and, by compressing the elastic bulb, expresses the fixative. The bulb is then released and the fixative, plus the collected cells, is aspirated back into the pipette. The pipette is sealed and mailed back to the laboratory. The fluid is spun down in a centrifuge and the sediment smeared on two or more slides. Residual material may be kept indefinitely. Davis considered 50 to 100 cells per low-power field as an adequate smear. The screening of this material was time-consuming because abnormal cells were few. In many ways, the material obtained by irrigation resembles a diluted vaginal smear. The device was evaluated by several independent observers with mixed results. Richart (1965) pointed out that irrigation smears failed to reveal 40% to 50% of early neoplastic lesions of the cervix. A similar result was reported by Muskett et al (1966) on a smaller group of carefully controlled patients. Reagan and Lin (1967), Mattingly et al (1967), Anderson and Gunn (1967), Carrow et al (1967), and Husain (1970) rendered reports ranging from highly skeptical to enthusiastic. It is generally considered that, unless the patient has no access to a more direct method of cytologic sampling, self-administered smears should not be recommended because of poor accuracy and because they deprive the patient of a clinical examination.

It is of interest that a **similar self-administered device was recently evaluated as a means of sample collection for analysis of human papillomavirus** (Wright et al, 2000).

Endometrial Sampling
The methods are described in Chapter 13.

BIBLIOGRAPHY

Abrams RY, Abrams J. Vaginal cytology during the final weeks of pregnancy. Acta Cytol 6:359–364, 1962.

Affandi MZ, Doctor V, Jhaveri K. The endocervical smear as a simple and quick method for determination of ovulation. Acta Cytol 29:638–641, 1985.

Albukerk J. False-positive cytology in ectopic pregnancy. [Letter] N Engl J Med 291:1142, 1974.

Alons-von Kordelaar JJ, Boon ME. Diagnostic accuracy of squamous cervical lesions studied in spatula-cytobrush smears. Acta Cytol 32:801–804, 1988.

Anderson WAD, Gunn SA. Premalignant and malignant conditions of the cervix uteri. Tissue validity study of the vaginal irrigation smear method. Cancer 20:1587–1593, 1967.

Angeles MA, Saigo PE. Cytologic findings in rectovaginal fistulae. Acta Cytol 38:373–376, 1994.

Arias-Stella J. Atypical endometrial changes associated with the presence of chorionic tissue. Arch Pathol 58:112–128, 1954.

Ashworth CT, Luibel FJ, Sanders E. Epithelium of normal cervix uteri. Studies with electron microscopy and histochemistry. Am J Obstet Gynecol 79:1149–1160, 1960.

Avrin E, Marquet E, Schwartz R, Sobel H. Plant cells resembling tumor cells in routine cytology. Am J Clin Pathol 57:303–305, 1972.

Ayre JE. Selective cytology smear for diagnosis of cancer. Am J Obstet Gynecol 53:609–617, 1947.

Babkowski RC, Wilbur DC, Rutkowski MA, et al. The effects of endocervical canal topography, tubal metaplasia, and high canal sampling on cytologic presentation of nonneoplastic endocervical cells. Am J Clin Pathol 105:403–410, 1996.

Bader GM, Simon TR, Koss LG, Day E. Study of detection-tampon method as screening device for uterine cancer. Cancer 10:332–337, 1957.

Bechtold E, Staunton CE, Katz SS. Carpet beetle larval parts in cervical cytology specimens. Acta Cytol 29:345–352, 1985.

Benoit JL, Kini SR. "Arias-Stella reaction"-like changes in endocervical glandular epithelium in cervical smears during pregnancy and postpartum states—a potential diagnostic pitfall. Diagn Cytopathol 14:349–355, 1996.

Benson PA. Human ovum-like structures in cervical smears. Acta Cytol 16:527–528, 1972.

Birdsong GG. Pap smear adequacy: Is our understanding satisfactory . . . or limited? Diagn Cytopathol 24:79–81, 2001.

Bonnilla-Musoles F, Hemandez-Yago J, Torres, JV. Scanning electron microscopy of the cervix uteri. Arch Gynaekol 216:91–97, 1974.

Boyd JD, Hamilton WJ. The Human Placenta. Cambridge UK. W Heffner and Sons, 1970.

Bredahl E, Koch F, Stakemann G. Cancer detection by cervical scrapings, vaginal pool smears and irrigation smears. A comparative study. Acta Cytol 9:189–193, 1965.

Brunschwig A. Detection of adenocarcinoma by tampon-smear method. Cancer 10:120–123, 1957.

Buntinx F, Essed GG, et al. Composition of cervical smears in patients with and without a cervical ectropion. J Clin Path 48:408–409, 1995.

Butler EB, Taylor DS. The postnatal smear. Acta Cytol 17:237–240, 1973.

Cabanne F, Michiels R, Mottot C, Bastien H. Ciliated bodies in gynecologic cytopathology: Parasite or cellular debris? Acta Cytol 19:407–410, 1975.

Capaldo G, LeGolvan DP, Dramczyk JE. Hematoidin crystals in cervicovaginal smears. Acta Cytol 27:237–240, 1983.

Carr DH. Chromosome studies in abortuses and stillborn infants. Lancet 2:603–606, 1963.

Carrow LA, Greene RR. Epithelia of pregnant cervix. Am J Obstet Gynecol 61:237–252, 1951.

Carrow LA, Hilker RR, Elesh RH, Eggum PR. Evaluation of the vaginal irrigation smear technique. Am J Obstet Gynecol 97:821–827, 1967.

Carvalho G. The presence of a human ovum in a vaginal smear. Report of a case. Acta Cytol 9:317–318, 1965.

Chandra K, Annousamy R, Azad M. An unusual finding in the vaginal smear. Acta Cytol 19:403, 1975.

Clendenin TM, Benirschke K. Chromosome studies in spontaneous abortions. Lab Invest 12:1281–1292, 1963.

Collins KA, Roa PN, Hayworth R, et al. Identification of sperm and non-sperm male cells in cervicovaginal smears using fluorescence in situ hybridization: application in alleged sexual assault cases. J Forensic Sci 39:1347–1355, 1994.

Cove H. The Arias-Stella reaction occurring in the endocervix in pregnancy. Recognition and comparison with adenocarcinoma of the endocervix. Am J Surg Path 3:607–612, 1979.

Dallenbach-Helweg G. Histopathology of the Endometrium. Berlin, Springer-Verlag, 1971.

Danos M, Holmquist ND. Cytologic evaluation of decidual cells: A report of two cases with false abnormal cytology. Acta Cytol 11:325–330, 1967.

Daunter B, Chantler EN, Elstein M. The scanning electron microscopy of human cervical mucus in the nonpregnant and pregnant states. Br J Obstet Gynaecol 83:738–743, 1976.

Davis HJ. The irrigation smear. A cytologic method for mass population screening by mail. Am J Obstet Gynecol 84:1017–1023, 1962.

Davis HJ. The irrigation smear. Accuracy in detection of cervical smear. Acta Cytol 6:459–467, 1962.

de Brux J, Bret J. Cells originating in ulcerated submucous myomas of uterus; so-called "vermiform bodies." Am J Clin Pathol 32:442–445, 1959.

Deckert JJ, Staten SF, Palermo V. Improved endocervical cell yield with cytobrush. J Fam Pract 26:639–641, 1988.

DeMay RM. The Art and Science of Cytopathology. Chicago, ASCP Press, 1996, pp 88–172.

Dembitzer HM, Herz F, Schreiber K, et al. The fine structure of exfoliated cervical and vaginal cells. Acta Cytol 20:243–248, 1976.

DeWaard F, Baanders-van Halewijn EA. Cross-sectional data on estrogenic smears in post-menopausal population. Acta Cytol 13:675–678, 1969.

DeWaard F, Pot H, Tonckens-Nanninga NE, et al. Longitudinal studies on the phenomenon of postmenopausal estrogen production. Acta Cytol 16:273–278, 1972.

Edwards JN, Morris HB. Langerhans' cells and lymphocyte subsets in the female genital tract. Br J Obstet Gynaecol 92:974–982, 1985.

Fayad MF. Vaginal cytology in clinically threatened abortion. J Obstet Gynaecol Br Commonw 70:39–45, 1963.

Feldman D, Romney SL, Edgcomb J, Valentine T. Ultrastructure or normal, metaplastic, and abnormal human uterine cervix: Use of montages to study the topographical relationship of epithelial cells. Am J Obstet Gynecol 150:573–688, 1984.

Ferenczy A. Studies on the cytodynamics of human endometrial regeneration. 1: Scanning electron microscopy. Am J Obstet Gynecol 124:64–74, 1976.

Ferenczy A. The surface ultrastructure of the human fallopian tube. A comparative morphophysiologic study. *In* Johari O (ed). Scanning Electron Microscopy in Advances in Biomedical Applications of the SEM, Chicago IIT. Research Institute, 1974, pp 613–622.

Ferenczy A, Richart RM. The Female Reproductive System. Dynamics of Scanning and Transmission Electron Microscopy. New York, John Wiley & Sons, 1974.

Ferenczy A, Richart RM. Scanning and transmission electron microscopy of the human endometrial surface epithelium. J Clin Endocrinol Metabol 36:99–108, 1973.

Ferenczy A, Richart RM. Scanning electron microscopy of the cervical transformation zone. Am J Obstet Gynecol 115:151–157, 1973.

Figueroa CD, Caorsi L. Ultrastructural and morphometric study of the Langerhans cell in the normal human exocervix. J Anat 90:669–682, 1980.

Fiorella RM, Cheng J, Kragel PJ. Papanicolaou smear in pregnancy. Positivity of exfoliated cells for human chorionic gonadotropin and human placental lactogen. Acta Cytol 37:451–456, 1993.

Fluhman CF. The Cervix Uteri and Its Diseases. Philadelphia, WB Saunders, 1961.

Frable WJ. Reflections on adequacy in cervical/vaginal cytology. Cancer Cytopathol 87:103–104, 1999.

Fraenkel L, Papanicolaou GN. Growth desquamation and involution of vaginal epithelium of fetuses and children with consideration of related hormonal factors. Am J Anat 62:427–451, 1938.

Frank TS, Bhat N, Noumoff JS, Yeh IT. Residual trophoblastic cells as a source of highly atypical cells in the postpartum cervicovaginal smear. Acta Cytol 35:105–108, 1991.

Frisch RE, McArthur JW. Menstrual cycles: Fatness as a determinant of minimum weight for height necessary for their maintenance or onset. Science 185:949–951, 1974.

Gibor Y, Garcia CJ, Cohen MR, Scommegna A. The cyclical changes in the physical properties of the cervical mucus and the results of the postcoital test. Fertil Steril 21:20–27, 1970.

Gompel C. Structure fine des mitochondries de la cellule glandulaire endometriale humaine au cours du cycles menstruel. J Microsc 3:427–436, 1964.

Gompel C. The ultrastructure of the human endometrial cell studied by electron microscopy. Am J Obstet Gynecol 84:1000–1009, 1962.

Gondos B, Marshall D, Ostergard DR. Endocervical cells in cervical smears. Am J Obstet Gynecol 114:833–834, 1972.

Gray SW, Skandalakis JE. Embryology for Surgeons. Philadelphia, WB Saunders, 1972.

Greenebaum E. Images in clinical medicine. Cytologic identification of oocytes in ovarian-cyst aspirates. N Engl J Med 339:604, 1998.

Gumley P. An unusual artifact found in cytologic preparations. Acta Cytol 20:192–193, 1976.

Hackermann M, Grubb C, Hill KR. The ultrastructure of normal squamous epithelium of the human cervix uteri. J Ultrastruct Res 22:443–457, 1968.

Hindman WM, Schwalenberg RR, Efstation TD. A study of vaginal smears in late pregnancy and pregnancy at term. Acta Cytol 6:365–369, 1962.

Hollander DH, Gupta PK. Detached ciliary tufts in cervico-vaginal smears. Acta Cytol 18:367–369, 1974.

Hollander DH, Gupta PK. Hematoidin cockleburrs in cervicovaginal smears. Acta Cytol 18:268–269, 1974.

Holmes EJ, Lyle WH. How early in pregnancy does the Arias-Stella reaction occur? Arch Pathol 95:302–303, 1973.

Holmquist ND, Danos M. The cytology of early abortion. Acta Cytol 11:262–266, 1967.

Hopman BC, Wargo JD, Werch SC. Cytology of vernix caseosa cells. Obstet Gynecol 10:656–659, 1957.

Husain OAN. The irrigation smear. Am J Obstet Gynecol 106:138–146, 1970.

Jing BJ, Kaufman RH, Franklin RR. Vaginal cytology for prediction of onset of labor. Am J Obstet Gynecol 99:546–550, 1967.

Johanisson E, Hagenfeldt K. Isolation and cytochemical properties of human endometrial cells. Karolinska Symp Res Methods Reprod Endocrinol 111: 81–108, 1971.

Johanisson E, Nilsson L. Scanning electron microscopic study of the human endometrium. Fertil Steril 23:613, 1972.

Jordan MJ, Bader G. New cannula for obtaining endometrial material for cytologic study. Obstet Gynecol 8:611–612, 1956.

Kaneko C, Shamoto M, Kobayashi TK. Nuclear grooves in vaginal cells [Letter]. Acta Cytol 42:823–824, 1998.

Koch F, Stakemann F. Irrigation smear: accuracy in gynecologic cancer detection. Dan Med Bull 9:127–131, 1962.

Koizumi JH. Nipple-like protrusions in endocervical and other cells: Further observations. Acta Cytol 40:519–528, 1996.

Koss LG. Vaginal Curschmann's spirals [Letter]. Ann Int Med 81:416, 1974.

Koss LG. Detection of carcinoma of the uterine cervix. JAMA 222:699–700, 1972.

Koss LG. Endocervical nuclear protrusions (nipples). Acta Cytol 4:49–50, 1960.

Koss LG, Gompel C. Introduction to Gynecologic Cytopathology with Histologic and Clinical Correlations. Baltimore, Lippincott, Williams & Wilkins, 1999.

Koss LG, Hicklin MD. Standards of adequacy of cytologic examination of the female genital tract. Conclusions of a study group on cytology. Obstet Gynecol 43:792–793, 1974.

Koss LG, Schreiber K, Oberlander SG, et al. Detection of endometrial carcinomas and hyperplasia in asymptomatic women. Obstet Gynecol 64:1–11, 1984.

Kurman RJ, Solomon D. The Bethesda System for Reporting Cervical/Vaginal Cytologic Diagnoses. New York, Springer, 1993.

Laverty C, Thurloe J. Endocervical cells and smear sample reliability. Lancet 337:741–742, 1991.

Leiblum S, Bachmann G, Ekkehard K, et al. Vaginal atrophy in the postmenopausal woman: The importance of sexual activity and hormones. JAMA 249: 2195–2198, 1983.

Lemberg-Siegfried S, Stamm O, de Wattevill H. Le frottis vaginal aux differents stades de la grossesse normale et pathologique. Presse Med 63:1558–1560, 1955.

Lencioni LJ, Amezaga LAM, Alonso C, et al. Urocytogram, pregnancy. II: Correlation with fetal condition at birth in high risk pregnancies. Acta Cytol 17: 125–127, 1973.

Lencioni LJ, Amezaga LAM, LoBianco VS. Urocytogram and pregnancy. I. Methods and normal values. Acta Cytol 13:279–287, 1969.

Lichtfus CJP. Vaginal cytology at the end of pregnancy. Acta Cytol 3:247–251, 1959.

Lichtfus C, Pundel JP, Gandar R. Le frottis vaginal a la fin de la grossesse. Gynécol Obstet (Paris) 57:380–398, 1958.

Liu W, Barrow MJ, Splitter MF, Kochis AF. Normal exfoliation of endometrial cells in premenopausal women. Acta Cytol 7:211–214, 1963.

Maksem JA, Finnemore M, Belsheim BL, et al. Manual method for liquid-based cytology: A demonstration using 1,000 gynecological cytologies collected directly to vial and prepared by a smear-slide technique. Diagn Cytopathol 25:334–338, 2001.

Maksem JA, Knesel E. Liquid fixation of endometrial brush cytology ensures a well-preserved, representative cell sample with frequent tissue correlation. Diagn Cytopath 14:367–373, 1995.

Marshall JC, Kelch RP. Gonadotropin-releasing hormone: Role of pulsatile secretion in the regulation of reproduction. N Engl J Med 315:1459–1468, 1986.

Masin F, Masin M. Lipid pattern in cervical and vaginal cells under hormonal stimulus. Acta Cytol 8:263–269, 1964.

Matoltsy AG, Matoltsy MN. The chemical nature of keratohyaline granules of the epidermis. J Cell Biol 47:593–603, 1970.

Mattingly RF, Boyd A, Frable WJ. The vaginal irrigation smear: a positive method of cervical cancer control. Obstet Gynecol 29:463–470, 1967.

McCollum SM. New observations on the significance of nipple-like protrusions in the nuclei of endocervical cells. Acta Cytol 32:331–334, 1988.

McLennan MT, McLennan CE. Hormonal patterns in vaginal smears from puerperal women. Acta Cytol 19:431–433, 1975.

Meisels A, Ayotte D. Cells from the seminal vesicles: Contaminants of the VCE smear. Acta Cytol 20:211–219, 1976.

Metcalf KS, Sutton J, Moloney MD, et al. Which cervical sampler? A comparison of four methods. Cytopathol 5:219–225, 1994.

Michael CW, Esfahani FM. Pregnancy related changes: A retrospective review of 278 cervical smears. Diagn Cytopathol 17:99–107, 1997.

Mintzer M, Curtis P, Resnick JC, Morrell D. The effect of the quality of Papanicolaou smears on the detection of cytologic abnormalities. Cancer Cytopathol 87:113–117, 1999.

Mitchell H, Medley G. Cellular differences between true-negative and false-negative Papanicolaou smears. Cytopathol 4:285–290, 1993.

Mitchell H, Medley G. Influence of endocervical status on cytological prediction of cervical intraepithelial neoplasia. Acta Cytol 36:875–880, 1992.

Moghissi KS, Syner FN, Borin B. Cyclic changes of cervical mucus enzymes related to the time of ovulation. II. Amino peptidase and esterase. Obstet Gynecol 48:347–350, 1976.

Moyer DL, Mishell DR. Reactions of human endometrium to the intrauterine device. II. Long-term effects on the endometrial histology and cytology. Am J Obstet Gynecol 111:66–80, 1971.

Müller Kobold-Wolterbeck AC, Beyer-Boon ME. Ciliocytophthoria in cervical cytology [Letter]. Acta Cytol 19:89–91, 1975.

Murphy EJ, Herbut PA. Uterine cervix during pregnancy. Am J Obstet Gynecol 59:384–390, 1950.

Muskett JM, Carter AK, Dodge OG. Detection of cervical cancer by irrigation smear and cervical scrapings. Brit Med J 2:341–342, 1966.

Naib ZM. Single trophoblastic cells as a source of error in the interpretation of routine vaginal smears. Cancer 14:1183–1185, 1961.

Nesbitt REL, Garcia R, Rome DS. The prognostic value of vaginal cytology in pregnancy. Obstet Gynecol 17:2–8, 1961.

Nieburgs HE. Comparative study of different techniques for diagnosis of cervical carcinoma. Am J Obstet Gynecol 72:511–515, 1956.

Nilsson O, Nygren KG. Scanning electron microscopy of human endometrium. Ups J Med Sci 773, 1972.

Noer T. The histology of the senile endometrium. Acta Pathol Microbiol Scand 51:193–203, 1961.

Norman JG. Example of a human ovum in a cervicovaginal smear. Fact or artifact? Med J Aust 2:827–828, 1975.

Novak PM, Kumar NB, Naylor B. Curschmann's spirals in cervicovaginal smears. Prevalence, morphology, significance, and origin. Acta Cytol 28: 5–8, 1984.

Noyes RW. Normal phases of the endometrium. In Norris HJ, Hertig AT, Abell MR (eds). The Uterus. Baltimore, Williams & Wilkins, 1973, pp 110–135.

Papanicolaou GN. Atlas of Exfoliative Cytology. Cambridge, MA, The Commonwealth Fund by Harvard University Press, 1954.

Papanicolaou GN. Cytological evaluation of smears prepared by tampon method for detection of carcinoma of uterine cervix. Cancer 7:1185–1190, 1954.

Papanicolaou GN. Epithelial regeneration in uterine glands and on surface of uterus. Am J Obstet Gynecol 25:30–37, 1933.

Papanicolaou GN. The sexual cycle in the human female as revealed by vaginal smears. Am J Anat 52(Suppl):519–637, 1933.

Papanicolaou GN, Maddi FV. Further observations on behavior of human endometrial cells in tissue culture. Am J Obstet Gynecol 78:156–173, 1959.

Papanicolaou GN, Maddi FV. Observations on behavior of human endometrial cells in tissue culture. Am J Obstet Gynecol 76:601–618, 1958.

Papanicolaou GN, Traut HF, Marchetti AA. The Epithelia of Women's Reproductive Organs; a Correlative Study of Cyclic Changes. New York, Commonwealth Fund, 1948.

Payandeh F, Koss LG. Nuclear grooves in normal and abnormal cervical smears. Acta Cytol 47:421–425, 2003.

Philipp E. Elektronenoptische Untersuchungen zur Sekretionsmorphologie am Epithel der Endocervix der Frau. Arch Gynakol 210:173–187, 1971.

Pisharodi LR, Jovanoska S. Spectrum of cytologic changes in pregnancy. A review of 100 abnormal cervicovaginal smears, with emphasis on diagnostic pitfalls. Acta Cytol 39:905–908, 1995.

Prolla JC. Curschmann spirals in cervical mucus [Letter]. Ann Intern Med 80: 674, 1974.

Pundel JP. Les Frottis Vaginaux Endocriniens. Paris, Masson et Cie, 1952.

Pundel JP, van Meensel F. Gestation et Cytolofie Vaginale. Paris, Masson et Cie, 1951.

Reagan JW, Lin F. An evaluation of the vaginal irrigation technique in the detection of uterine cancer. Acta Cytol 11:374–382, 1967.

Reyniak JV, Gordon M, Stone ML, Sedlis A. Endometrial regeneration after voluntary abortion. Obstet Gynecol 45:203–210, 1975.

Richart RM, Vaillant HW. The irrigation smear: false-negative rates in a population with cervical neoplasia. JAMA 192:199–202, 1965.

Rilke F, Alasio L. Detached ciliary tufts in cervico-vaginal smears [Letter]. Acta Cytol 20:189–190, 1976.

Roa PN, Collins KA, Geisinger KR, et al. Identification of male epithelial cells in routine postcoital cervicovaginal smears using fluorescence in situ hybridization. Application in sexual and molestation. Am J Clin Pathol 104:32–35, 1995.

Roncalli M, Sideri M, Giè P, Servida E. Immunophenotypic analysis of the transformation zone of the human cervix. Lab Invest 58:141–149, 1988.

Rubio CA. Two types of cells in the normal and atypical squamous epithelium of the cervix. II. Light microscopic study in human subjects. Acta Cytol 26: 121–125, 1982.

Rubio CA, Soderberg G, Grant CA, et al. The normal squamous epithelium of the human uterine cervix: A histological study. Pathol Eur 11:157–162, 1976.

Ruiz LM. Vaginal cytology during delivery. Acta Cytol 9:337–339, 1965.

Schiffer JD, Sandweiss L, Bose S. The "polka dot" cell (letter). Acta Cytol 45: 903–905, 2001.

Schmidt-Matthiesen HE. Das Normale Menschliche Endometrium. Stuttgart, Georg Thieme Verlag, 1963.

Schneider V. Arias-Stella reaction of the endocervix. Acta Cytol 25:224–228, 1981.

Schneider V, Barnes LA. Ectopic decidual reaction of the uterine cervix. Acta Cytol 25:616–622, 1981.

Schüller E. The epithelia of the uterine endocervix. Acta Cytol 3:333–337, 1959.

Selvaggi SM, Guidos BJ. Endocervical component: Is it determinant of specimen adequacy? Diagn Cytopathol 26:53–55, 2002.

Sengel A, Stoebner P. Ultrastructure de 1'endometre humain normal. III. Les cellules K. Z. Zellforsch 133:47–57, 1972.

Shrago SS. The Arias-Stella reaction. A case report of a cytologic presentation. Acta Cytol 21:310–313, 1977.

Silverberg SG. Arias-Stella phenomenon in spontaneous and therapeutic abortion. Am J Obstet Gynecol 112:777–780, 1972.

Singer A. The uterine cervix from adolescence to the menopause. Br J Obstet Gynaecol 82:81–99, 1975.

Solomon D, Davey D, Kurman R, et al. The 2001 Bethesda System. Terminology for reporting results of cervical cytology. JAMA 287:2114–2119, 2002.

Solomon D, Nayar R (eds). The Bethesda System for Reporting Cervical Cytology: Definitions, Criteria, and Explanatory Notes, 2nd ed. New York, Springer-Verlag, 2004.

Sonek M. Vaginal cytology in childhood and puberty. I. Newborn through puberty; II. Puberty. J Reprod Med 2:39–56; 198–208, 1969.

Sonek M. Vaginal cytology during puberty. Acta Cytol 11:41–50, 1967.

Stockard CR, Papanicolaou GN. The existence of a typical oestrus cycle in the guinea pig with a study of its histological and physiological changes. Am J Anat 22:225–283, 1917.

Stoll P. Vaginal smears in the menopause. Acta Cytol 4:148–150, 1960.

Stone DF, Sedis A, Stone ML, Turkel WV. Estrogenlike effects in the vaginal smears of postmenopausal women. Acta Cytol 11:349–352, 1967.

Szulman AE. Chromosomal aberrations in spontaneous human abortions. N Engl J Med 272:811–818, 1965.

Taylor R. Nippling of endocervical cell nuclei [Letter]. Acta Cytol 28:86–89, 1984.

Trimbos JB, Arenz NPW. The efficiency of the cytobrush versus cotton swab in the collection of endocervical cells in cervical smears. Acta Cytol 30: 261–263, 1986.

Valdes-Dapena MA. The development of the uterus in late fetal life, infancy and childhood. In Norris HJ, Hertig AT, Abell MR (eds). The Uterus. Baltimore, Williams & Wilkins, 1973.

Valente PT, Schantz D, Trabal JF. The determination of Papanicolaou smear adequacy using a semiquantitative method to evaluate cellularity. Diagn Cytopathol 7:576–580, 1991.

Van Leeuwen L, Jacoby H, Charles B. Exfoliative cytology of amniotic fluid. Acta Cytol 9:442–445, 1965.

von-Haam E. The cytology of pregnancy. Acta Cytol 5:320–329, 1961.

Vooijs GP, van der Graaf Y, Vooijs MC. The presence of endometrial cells in cervical smears in relation to the day of the menstrual cycle and the method of contraception. Acta Cytol 31:427–433, 1987.

Vooijs P, Elias A, van der Graaf Y, Poelen van der Bergh M. The influence of sample takers on the cellular composition of cervical smears. Acta Cytol 30: 251–257, 1986.

Wachtel E. Exfoliative Cytology in Gynaecological Practice. Washington DC, Butterworth, 1964.

Wachtel E, Wytcherley J. The egg that never was. Acta Cytol 14:1–2, 1970.

Waddell CA. The influence of the cervix on smear quality. I. Atrophy. An audit of cervical smears taken post-colposcopic for management of intraepithelial neoplasia. Cytopathology 8:274–281, 1997.

Wagner D, Richart RM. Polyploidy in the human endometrium with the Arias-Stella reaction. Arch Pathol 85:475–480, 1968.

Way S, Dawson N. A human ovum in a vaginal smear. J Obstet Gynaecol Br Emp 66:491, 1959.

White AJ, Buchsbaum HJ. Scanning electron microscopy of the human endometrium. I. Normal Gynecol Oncol 11:330–339, 1973.

Wied GL. Climacteric amenorrhea: Cytohormonal test for differential diagnosis. Obstet Gynecol 9:646–649, 1957.

Wied GL. Importance of site from which vaginal cytologic smears are taken. Am J Clin Pathol 25:742–750, 1955.

Wied GL, Bahr GF. Vaginal, cervical and endocervical cytologic smears on a single slide. Obstet Gynecol 14:362–367, 1959.

Wilbanks GD, Shingleton HM. Normal human cervical squamous epithelium in vitro: Fine structural differences from in vivo cells. Acta Cytol 14: 182–186, 1970.

Wright TC Jr, Denny L, Kuhn L, et al. HPV DNA testing of self-collected vaginal samples compared with cytologic screening to detect cervical cancer. JAMA 283:81–86, 2000.

Younes MS, Robertson EM, Bencosme SA. Electron microscope observations on Langerhans cells in the cervix. Am J Obstet Gynecol 102:397–403, 1968.

Zaharopoulos P, Wong J, Wen JW. Nuclear protrusions in cells from cytologic specimens. Mechanism of formation. Acta Cytol 42:317–329, 1998.

Zaharopoulos D, Wong JY, Edmonston G, Keagy N. Crystalline bodies in cervicovaginal smears. Acta Cytol 29:1035–1042, 1985.

Zaneveld LJD, Tauber PF, Port C, et al. Structural aspects of human cervical mucus. Am J Obstet Gynecol 122:650–654, 1975.

Ziabkowski TA, Naylor B. Cyanophilic bodies in cervicovaginal smears. Acta Cytol 20:340–342, 1976.

Cytologic Evaluation of Menstrual Disorders and Hormonal Abnormalities

9

PRINCIPLES

The established approach to the evaluation of ovarian function and endocrine disorders in the woman is based on serial biochemical analyses of hormones, such as estrogen, progesterone, luteinizing hormones and their metabolites (Albertson and Zinaman, 1987). More recently, the analysis of hormonal substances that participate in embryonal development of gonads has contributed still further to the clarification of endocrine disorders. For example, the measurements of the müllerian-inhibiting substance, a hormone that promotes the involution of the müllerian duct and thus enhances the development of male characteristics, allowed the discrimination between male children with a congenital absence of testes (anorchia) and undescended testes (Lee et al, 1997). In children suspected of other congenital abnormalities, molecular-genetic analyses may be performed. For example, in children with congenital adrenal hypoplasia, who may also display underdevelopment of gonads, a mutation of the responsible gene located on the X chromosome could be documented (Merke et al, 1999). Many additional such examples could be cited. In women who suffer from menstrual disorders and abnormalities of the ovarian cycle, the biochemical analyses can be effectively supplemented by the old-fashioned endometrial biopsies, or studies of endocervical mucus (Lotan and Diamant, 1978). In addition, the **cervicovaginal smear may sometimes provide useful information and has the advantage of being easy to obtain, rapidly evaluated, and inexpensive.** The cytologic approach is particularly valuable if laboratories specializing in endocrine analysis are not readily available. The **principle** of the cytologic hormonal analysis is simple. The degree of maturation of the squamous epithelium of the female genital tract depends on steroid hormones, mainly estrogen. Estrogen receptors are present in the squamous epithelium of the uterine cervix and vagina, particularly in the basal cells (Press et al, 1986; Kupryjanczyk and Moller, 1988), and are expressed more strongly during the proliferative phase of the cell cycle than during the secretory phase, accounting for the observed changes in epithelial maturation. Therefore, the **quantitative relationship of squamous cells of varying degree of maturity in a cervicovaginal smear may serve as an index of the hormonal status of the female. In some cases of congenital abnormalities, the analysis of sex chromatin bodies (Barr bodies) in the same smears may yield valuable information.**

It is beyond the scope of this book to discuss all the variants and metabolites of the steroid hormones. For the sake of simplicity, and because of their impact on cervicovaginal cytology, the key hormones and their activity to be discussed are estrogen, progesterone, and androgenic (masculinizing) hormones.

MECHANISMS OF FORMATION OF STEROID HORMONES

The main function of steroid hormones in the woman is to induce ovulation and prepare the uterus for pregnancy. The regularity with which this process occurs during the childbearing age of a normal woman is astounding and as yet not fully understood. As was summarized in Chapter 8 and Figure 8-18, the formation of steroid hormones by the ovary is governed by polypeptide hormones of pituitary origin (follicle-stimulating hormone [FSH] and luteinizing hormone [LH]). The ovary synthesizes the steroid hormones, which act on the endometrium, squamous epithelium, and other target cells in the uterus.

Mechanisms of Action of Pituitary Hormones on Ovarian Target Cells

The first sequence, which has for its purpose the formation in the ovary of various steroid hormones such as estrogen and progesterone from cholesterol, may be briefly summarized as follows:

■ Pituitary peptide hormone binds to the receptors on the membrane of ovarian cells with endocrine function, stimulating an increased activity of a common mediator, adenylate cyclase. Adenylate cyclase stimulates the synthesis of 3′5′-adenosine monophosphate (cyclic AMP or cAMP) from adenosine triphosphate (ATP).

■ cAMP activates the appropriate protein kinase leading to the formation of an enzyme, cholesterol esterase, and other enzymes involved in the biosynthesis of steroid hormones.

Mechanisms of Formation of Steroid Hormones in the Ovary

■ The cholesterol esterase leads to an increased accumulation of free cholesterol as a precursor for steroid biosynthesis.

■ Free cholesterol is transformed by enzymes into steroid hormones in the smooth endoplasmic reticulum of the appropriate ovarian cells. **Estrogen is produced by the follicular cells of the maturing ovarian follicles.** After ovulation, **progesterone is produced by cells of the corpus luteum.** For a recent review of the mechanisms of formation of steroid hormones in the pituitary and the gonads, see Adashi and Hennebold (1999).

Effect of Steroid Hormones on Target Cells

Ovarian steroids, such as estrogen and progesterone, interact with cells in the endometrium and the squamous epithelium of the cervix and vagina and the smooth muscle of the uterus. This sequence may be briefly summarized as follows:

■ The steroid hormone binds to a specific cytoplasmic receptor protein in the cells of the target organ and enters the cytoplasm. As has been recently reported, there are at least two types of estrogen receptors with complex patterns of function (McDonnell and Norris, 2002).

■ Steroid protein complex enters the nucleus and binds to the DNA specific receptor. Messenger RNA is formed.

■ Messenger RNA enters the cytoplasm, binds to ribosomes and leads to the synthesis of specific proteins, such as enzymes or structural proteins, that are expressed in the cytoplasm of the target cell.

Nuclear receptors for estrogen and progesterone have been identified and sequenced. Recent investigations shed light on the regulation of hormonal receptors in various target cells (McDonnell and Norris, 2002). This led to the development of specific antibodies that can be used to visualize the presence of these receptors in the nucleus by means of immunofluorescence or an immunocytochemical approach using the peroxidase-antiperoxidase reaction that forms visible precipitates. The precipitates can be measured by image analysis and related techniques (Bacus et al, 1988). This system of **steroid receptor identification and quantitation** has been extensively used in the assessment of mammary carcinoma (see Chap. 29), but its applicability to the cells of the female genital tract has been limited.

The effects of estrogen and progesterone on the endometrium and endometrial cells are discussed in Chapter 8. In this chapter, the effect of these and other hormones on the squamous epithelium of the female genital tract will be discussed.

THE EFFECT OF STEROID HORMONES ON SQUAMOUS EPITHELIUM OF THE FEMALE GENITAL TRACT

Smear Patterns

Naturally occurring **estrogen, or the parenteral administration of estrogen or its natural or synthetic substitutes** in adequate amounts, produces a rapid and complete maturation of the normal squamous epithelium of the female genital tract with a resulting preponderance of mature superficial squamous cells in smears. The effect takes place regardless of the prior hormonal status, **except during pregnancy.** Conversely, **complete atrophy of the squamous epithelium of the vagina and cervix may be equated with complete absence of estrogenic activity.** However, there are **no reliable data linking intermediate degrees of maturation of the squamous epithelium with the action of a specific hormone or hormones.** Thus, partial or incomplete maturation of the squamous epithelium may have various causes, such as an inadequate or low supply of estrogen and its derivatives; an effect of antagonistic hormones, such as progesterone or androgenic hormones; or the effect of some of the widely used estrogen agonists, such as tamoxifen; or to a combination of these and probably other factors. The fact that surgical castration does not necessarily lead to complete atrophy of the squamous epithelium strongly supports the possibility that **extragenital hormonal factors,** such as **adrenal hormones,** are capable of influencing the squamous epithelium of the genital tract of the female.

It is obvious, therefore, that the patterns of squamous cells should be interpreted cautiously in terms of endocrine status or therapeutic indications. Unfortunately, rigid diagnostic standards in this area of genital cytology are difficult to establish and, consequently, the literature is replete with contradictory statements. This is well illustrated by the problem of cytologic evaluation of pregnancy at term, discussed in Chapter 8. Nonetheless, in specific clinical situations, discussed below, endocrine cytology is a valuable guide to diagnosis and treatment.

Hormonal Cytology in Various Age Groups

Evaluation of the endocrine status of a menstruating woman **during the childbearing age** belongs among the most difficult tasks in diagnostic cytology. There is **considerable variation in the smear patterns from one patient to another,** even if matched for age and menstrual history. Furthermore, there is **considerable variation from cycle to cycle in the same patient.** Daily variations and even variations between simultaneously obtained smears may occur. **Even the mere effect of smear-taking may influence the pattern of the following smear** by increasing the vascularity of the epithelium.

However, hormonal evaluation of the smears may be of substantial assistance in situations associated with **amenorrhea or other significant disturbances of the menstrual cycle** and may be of value in determining the **time of ovulation** for **artificial insemination** or **in vitro fertilization** (see below).

Evaluation of the endocrine status in **prepubertal and postmenopausal patients** is an easier and more rewarding task than during the childbearing age. In a patient whose baseline smear shows complete atrophy, an increased maturation of the squamous epithelium is easy to assess. Still, even the procedure of smear-taking may reduce the dryness

of the vagina and result in a less atrophic smear pattern. In the absence of atrophy, some of the problems described above for women in the childbearing age may also preclude an accurate cytologic evaluation of hormonal effect.

The Influence of Factors Other Than Hormonal on Endocrine Evaluation of Smears

Several factors other than endogenous or exogenous hormones may influence the status of the squamous epithelium.

Inflammatory Processes

As is described in Chapter 10, inflammatory processes, particularly *Trichomonas vaginalis* infestation, may result in increased maturation of squamous cells in postmenopausal women. Histologic and colposcopic evidence suggests that increased vascularity of the epithelium may be a factor in this process. Other inflammatory processes, particularly coccal bacterial infections, may obscure the smear pattern because of pus formation. Therefore, **it is advisable to forego any attempts at estimation of maturation of squamous cells in the presence of a marked inflammatory process.**

Cancer

In postmenopausal women with **carcinoma of the uterine cervix or endometrium,** abnormally high levels of maturation of the squamous epithelium may be observed. Although in endometrial cancer this may represent a hormonal effect, in cervix cancer the effect is probably due to inflammation (Cassano et al, 1986).

Cytolysis

Cytolysis caused by *Lactobacillus* (the Döderlein bacillus) or related organisms may destroy squamous cells in sufficient numbers to preclude any reasonable estimation of level of maturation (see Chaps. 8 and 10). **The effects of hormones and other drugs** precluding the assessment of the hormonal status are discussed below.

Radiotherapy, Surgery and Other Interventions

Radiotherapy to the vagina or cervix exercises marked immediate and long-term effects on smear patterns, as discussed in Chapter 18. It is evident that radiotherapy, with its protracted and significant influence on the biology of the squamous epithelium, restricts the possibility of subsequent estimation of hormonal activity by smears. **Surgery, cauterization,** and other forms of treatment of diseases of the vagina or cervix also preclude proper hormonal evaluation **until the healing has become complete**—usually no fewer than 6 weeks after the procedure.

TECHNIQUES IN THE CYTOLOGIC EVALUATION OF THE HORMONAL STATUS

Vaginal Smears

Several conditions must be fulfilled before a successful hormonal evaluation of the squamous epithelium may be undertaken.

- There must be absence of inflammation or cytolysis.
- There must be no recent medication, either topical or systemic, especially with compounds known to affect the squamous epithelium of the lower genital tract.
- There must be no history of radiotherapy or recent surgery to the vagina or cervix.
- An adequate baseline investigation must have been performed in menstruating women. This should include daily smears during at least one and preferably two complete cycles, or their chronologic equivalent. In nonmenstruating patients, two or three smears may suffice.
- **The smears should be obtained from the proximal portion of the lateral wall of the vagina, care being taken to avoid contamination with material from the adjacent cervix.** Soost (1960), in an elaborate study, confirmed that this is the area of the vagina most accurately reflecting the hormonal status. The squamous epithelium of distal vagina or of the cervix shows a lesser response to hormonal stimulation.

Although **routine cervicovaginal smears are less accurate for purposes of hormonal evaluation,** their use cannot be unequivocally condemned because the patterns of maturation of squamous cells may provide useful information either in the presence of a marked estrogenic effect (dominance of mature squamous cells in smears) or complete absence thereof (atrophic smear pattern).

Urocytograms and Other Methods

A number of observers, starting with Papanicolaou (1948), and subsequently Lencioni et al (1969, 1972), Haour (1974), and O'Morchoe (1967), reported results of hormonal evaluation with the use of an **"urocytogram,"** which is the **evaluation of squamous cells in smears obtained from the sediment of voided urine.** It is not completely clear whether the squamous cells in the urinary sediment are a contaminant with cells of vaginal origin or whether they reflect the presence of squamous epithelium of vaginal type that may be observed in the bladder trigone of many women (see Chap. 22). The urinary sediment has the advantage of easy collection without the necessity of a gynecologic examination and is **particularly useful in the evaluation of some endocrine disorders in infants and children.**

Other methods of endocrine evaluation include smears obtained from the inner aspect of labia minora of the vulva, as suggested by Tozzini et al (1971).

In congenital disorders in which X chromosome may be affected, the evaluation of sex chromatin bodies is conveniently performed in vaginal smears just as in scrape smears of the oral mucosa. Although this is not the primary topic of this chapter, it must be mentioned here that **endometrial biopsies** offer important information on ovulation and disturbances of the menstrual cycle. For further discussion of this topic, see Chapter 13.

OBJECTIVE EVALUATION OF HORMONAL PATTERNS

The Indices of Squamous Cells

To confer numerical reproducibility upon hormonal evaluation, several indices defining the status of the squamous cells in a smear have been advocated.

The Karyopyknotic Index (KI)

The karyopyknotic index expresses the **percentile relationship of superficial squamous cells with pyknotic nuclei to all mature squamous cells.** Usually, 200 to 400 consecutive cells in three or four different fields on the smear are evaluated. According to Pundel (1966), in a normally menstruating woman, the peak of KI usually coincides with the time of ovulation and was estimated at 50% to 85%. Variation from patient to patient is considerable. Schneider et al (1977) found a statistically significant correlation between KI and plasma estradiol levels as measured by radioimmunoassays.

The Eosinophilic Index (EI)

The eosinophilic index expresses the **percentile relationship of mature squamous cells with eosinophilic cytoplasm to all mature squamous cells,** regardless of the status of the nucleus. The procedure is similar to that described for the karyopyknotic index. Often the simple **Shorr's stain** (see Chap. 44) is used in preference to Papanicolaou stain. Pundel (1966) reported that in a normal menstruating woman, the peak of EI coincides with the peak of KI and may reach 50% to 75% at the time of ovulation.

The Maturation Index (MI)

The maturation index, first described by the Czech investigator, Nykliček in 1951, expresses the maturation of the squamous epithelium as a **percentile relationship of parabasal cells to intermediate cells to superficial cells.** The count should be performed on single cells. Cell clusters must be avoided. For example, in a normal menstruating woman at the time of ovulation, an MI of 0:35:65 would indicate that the smear contained no parabasal cells, 35% of intermediate cells, and 65% of superficial cells. A postmenopausal patient with marked atrophy would have a MI of 90:10:0, indicating marked preponderance of parabasal cells. Reyniak et al (1971) found good correlation between the MI and endometrial biopsies for staging of the menstrual cycle. Estrogen-type smear corresponded to proliferative endometrium in 83% of cases, and the premenstrual type of smear corresponded to secretory endometrium in 88% of cases. On the other hand, Schneider et al (1977) found a poor correlation between MI and plasma estradiol levels.

The Maturation Value

Meisels (1967) suggested that a specific numerical value be attached to the three principal subgroups of the squamous cells—a value of 1.0 to superficial squamous cells, a value of 0.5 to intermediate cells, and a value of 0.0 to parabasal cells. The maturation value (MV) would be expressed by multiplying the percentage in each cell category by its assigned value. For example, the MV for the two patients discussed above under MI would be as follows:

Patient 1 with MI 0:35:65 (normal menstruating woman at time of ovulation)

$$0 \times 0 = 00.0$$
$$35 \times 0.5 = 17.5$$
$$65 \times 1.0 = \underline{65.0}$$
$$MV = \overline{82.5}$$

Patient 2 with MI 90:10:0 (woman with postmenopausal atrophy)

$$90 \times 0 = 0$$
$$10 \times 0.5 = 5$$
$$0 \times 1.0 = \underline{0}$$
$$MV = \overline{5}$$

This system gives a single figure from zero to 100 to express the hormonal status of the patient and, thus, offers advantages for computerized handling of data. **An MV of 100 indicates a pure population of superficial squamous cells, MV of zero indicates a pure population of parabasal cells.** For menstruating normal women, the MV is between 50 and 95; for women with varying degrees of atrophy of squamous epithelium, the MV is below 50.

Other Indices

The **folded-cell index** represents the relationship of mature superficial or intermediate squamous cells with folded cytoplasm to all mature squamous cells. The **crowded-cell index** represents the relationship of mature squamous cells lying in clusters of four or more cells to all mature squamous cells.

The reader is referred to several papers by Wied et al (1968, 1992) listed in the bibliography for additional information on the various indices.

Critique of Indices

In an extensive study, Cordoba (1964) pointed out that any indices based on a single smear are not reliable. Even several smears obtained on the same day yield an error of 20%, if 1,000 cells are evaluated. This critique is valid in my experience. Particularly vulnerable is the eosinophilic index, because it is known that even a short exposure to air may significantly increase the proportion of cells with eosinophilic cytoplasm. The most reasonable of the indices is the maturation index and its derivative, the maturation value, since it gives an idea of the make-up of the squamous epithelium. However, to obtain results that would withstand a critical statistical analysis, at least 500 single cells, dispersed in four quadrants of the smear, should be counted, surely a time-consuming procedure.

Alternative Ways of Reporting Hormonal Status

It has been my practice to base the evaluation of the maturation of the squamous epithelium on an **overall visual impression gained during the routine screening of smears.** Dr. George Wied has suggested the term **estimogram** for this procedure. This simplest of methods has not failed in revealing major abnormalities of smear patterns. By comparing the current smear pattern with original baseline smears, a good appreciation of changes in smear pattern may be gained. Small variations in smear pattern have no diagnostic meaning but may strongly influence the indices and thus give a false impression of hormonal "effects." The reporting of smears based on this overall visual impression is always given in reference to age, menstrual history, and possible clinical significance. Some examples follow:

- Patient age 35: "Midcycle smear pattern—consistent with functioning ovaries."
- Patient age 52: "Absence of maturation of squamous cells consistent with menopause."
- Patient age 25: "Absence of maturation of squamous cells—abnormal for age."
- Patient age 60: "High level of maturation of squamous cells not consistent with clinical menopause. It is assumed that this patient is not receiving estrogens or other drugs that may account for this smear pattern."

DETERMINATION OF THE TIME OF OVULATION FROM CERVICOVAGINAL SMEARS

A precise determination of the time of the ovulation is important in **artificial insemination** and in **in vitro fertilization,** which incidentally is also valuable in animal husbandry. Hormonal patterns of cervicovaginal smears were used as a guide for embryo transfer in in vitro fertilization with fair results (Bercovici et al, 1988). Boquoi and Hammerstein (1969) reported that vaginal hormonal cytology **correlated poorly** with hormonal patterns of urinary steroid hormone secretion in patients in whom **ovulation was induced with clomiphene citrate. The use of the cervicovaginal smears to establish the time of ovulation or the status of the endometrium has been of limited reliability** in the author's hands. Under the best of circumstances, the timing of the highest count of flat superficial squamous cells, reflecting the peak of estrogen activity just prior to ovulation, requires the analysis of two or more cycles. Furthermore, in some patients, particularly in those with disturbances of ovarian function, the ovulation pattern may not occur, or the change may be insignificant and difficult to assess. **It is, therefore, recommended that cytologic methods for estimation of ovulation or status of the endometrium be supplemented by other procedures, such as temperature curves and endometrial biopsies. The examination of endocervical mucus may also be of assistance.** Cyclic changes in the physicochemical properties of the cervical mucus have been known for a great many years. Prior to ovulation, the mucus tends to be viscous and when placed on a glass slide, form crystalline, **fern-like structures,** whereas at the time of and after ovulation, the mucus is more liquid and does not crystallize (see Chap. 8). Occasionally, crystallized mucus may be observed in cervical smears.

As discussed in Chapter 8, it has been suggested by Affandi et al (1985) that the **endocervical cells participate in the cyclic menstrual changes** and that their **morphology reflects the proliferative and secretory phases of the endometrium.** During the preovulatory proliferative phase of the cycle, the endocervical cell cytoplasm is opaque and the nuclei spherical. During the postovulatory secretory phase, the endocervical cells obtained on the 20th day of the cycle displayed abundant, clear cytoplasm and nuclear "distortion" or "nipples." If the ovulation has not taken place, the cytoplasm of the endocervical cells remains opaque, and the nuclear "nipples" do not appear. Although anecdotal observations support the concept, the method has not received critical evaluation.

CYTOLOGIC EVALUATION OF MENSTRUAL DISORDERS

Cytologic hormonal evaluation may be of assistance in the evaluation of **amenorrhea (cessation of menses),** in women who have never menstruated (**primary amenorrhea**) or who stopped menstruating at a young age after a period of normal menses (**secondary amenorrhea**). The most obvious cause of temporary secondary amenorrhea is **pregnancy,** which was discussed in Chapter 8. Hormonal cytology is of little help in the evaluation of abnormal bleeding, such as **meno- and metrorrhagias.**

Amenorrhea

In primary or secondary amenorrhea, a vaginal smear may be of value in determining **whether the disorder is due to an absence of ovarian function or to other factors.** A smear that **fails to show any evidence of maturation of squamous cells indicates an absence of ovarian activity.** This disturbance may be due to a **primary ovarian deficiency** or a **failure of the pituitary,** known as **Simmond's disease.** Patterns with partial maturation of squamous cells suggestive of some measure of ovarian activity, may also be associated with amenorrhea. On the other hand, **normal maturation of squamous epithelium indicates the presence of ovarian function** that is sometimes vested in undescended testes (see below). Disturbances of the menstrual cycle due to excessive activity of hormones with estrogenic effect will be discussed below.

Primary Amenorrhea

In many of the patients who have never menstruated, there is a **major congenital disorder of their reproductive apparatus. Some of these patients have a congenital absence of the uterus or a congenital deficiency of the pituitary gland. Others, although provided with female external genitalia and female secondary sex characteristics, may be either genetic males or have no genetic sex at all; in the cells of such patients, the sex chromatin (Barr body) will be absent.** Hence, in the cytologic investigation of

patients with primary amenorrhea, **the presence or absence of Barr bodies must be ascertained, together with the estimation of the level of maturation of the squamous epithelium.** The vaginal smear is an excellent medium, serving both purposes. Table 9-1 summarizes the pertinent cytologic findings in this group of patients.

Gonadal Dysgenesis: Turner's Syndrome

Patients with this congenital disorder have **only 45 chromosomes because one of the X chromosomes is absent.** This chromosomal pattern is designated as **XO** (see Chap. 4). The disorder is found with considerable frequency in spontaneously aborted products of conception. Most surviving patients are of short stature, have a short webbed neck, and their arms and forearms form a wide angle (known as *cubitus valgus*). The patients have a vagina and poorly developed female breasts. The uterus, if present, is rudimentary and the gonads are absent or represented by a band of fibrous tissue or streaks. Other congenital abnormalities, such as coarctation of the aorta, multiple pigmented nevi, and renal anomalies, may occur, as initially described by Turner (summary in Sanger, 1996). These patients do not menstruate. The cervicovaginal smears of such patients **fail to show any maturation of the squamous epithelium and thus mimic the pattern of epithelial atrophy of advanced menopause. Sex chromatin is absent.** This type of vaginal smear is unique and diagnostic of this disorder (Fig. 9-1).

Other Forms of Gonadal Dysgenesis

Variants of gonadal dysgenesis, such as XO-XY mosaicism or XX with gonadal streaks have been described in patients with female phenotype, a vagina, and occasionally an enlarged penis-like clitoris. The patients do not menstruate. The smear pattern and the presence of sex chromatin **depend on the karyotype.** In patients with XX karyotype, there may be some maturation of squamous cells and the sex chromatin is usually present. In mosaics, its presence is variable. In genetic males in whom rudimentary testes can be observed, the sex chromatin is absent.

TABLE 9-1

PERTINENT CYTOLOGIC FINDINGS IN PRIMARY AMENORRHEA

	Epithelial Maturation	Sex Chromatin
Turner's syndrome	Absent	Absent
Other forms of gonadal dysgenesis	Variable	Usually absent
Syndrome of feminizing testes	Present	Absent
Pituitary insufficiency	Variable	Present
Congenital absence of uterus	Normal	Present

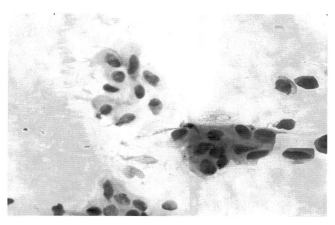

Figure 9-1 Turner's syndrome. Cervicovaginal smear in a 26-year-old woman with XO karyotype. Note absence of maturation of squamous cells and of sex chromatin (Barr) bodies.

The Syndrome of Feminizing Testes (Male Pseudohermaphroditism)

In this uncommon disorder, the patients are **genetic males** with 46 chromosomes (XY). The patients have either **undescended or partly descended testes, which produce female sex hormones** and accordingly induce both primary and secondary female sex characteristics, except for the **absence of the uterus and, hence, absence of menses**. A congenital error in testosterone biosynthesis has been documented in these patients. The cervicovaginal smears **fail to show any sex chromatin** but the level of maturation of the squamous epithelium is significantly better than that in gonadal dysgenesis, occasionally reaching full maturation (Rakoff, 1961). Because there is danger of the occurrence of a malignant tumor (seminoma) in the undescended testes, surgical ablation of the gonads is often performed in this condition. Subsequently, parenteral therapy with estrogens is used to supplant the removed source of hormones. **The cervicovaginal smear is an excellent means of following the effects of treatment on these patients.**

In passing, it must be noted that another **genetic abnormality in males, the Klinefelter's syndrome,** may also be recognized by cytologic techniques. **Smears of oral cavity** are an excellent medium of diagnosis of this chromosomal disorder by finding sex chromatin bodies, corresponding to the XXY karyotype (see Chap. 4).

Other Causes

Amenorrhea may also occur because of **congenital pituitary insufficiency.** Some of the patients with the classic clinical syndrome of **dwarfism** may show complete absence of maturation in the vaginal smears, but their sex chromatin pattern is normal. In other patients, primary amenorrhea may be due to the **absence of follicle-stimulating hormone (FSH) of the pituitary.** Such patients may appear clinically within normal limits. Their vaginal smears show variable degrees of maturation of the squamous cells; their sex chromatin pattern is normal. Amenorrhea resulting from **congenital absence of the uterus** results in vaginal smears compatible with ovarian function and a normal sex chromatin pattern. These and many other related disorders are caused by single-gene mutations (Adashi and Hennebold, 1999).

Secondary Amenorrhea

In the absence of pregnancy, secondary amenorrhea in a patient of childbearing age with an intact uterus indicates a **temporary or permanent arrest of normal ovarian function.** Except for iatrogenic castration, the value of the vaginal smear in the hormonal evaluation of secondary amenorrhea is far smaller than in primary amenorrhea. **Sex chromatin is present in all patients,** and the effects of various ovarian disorders are **unfaithfully mirrored in the maturation patterns of squamous cells.**

It is important to note that, in the presence of functioning ovaries, a prolonged absence of endometrial turnover may lead to endometrial carcinoma (see Chap. 13).

Disturbances of Ovulation (Polycystic Ovarian Disease, Stein-Leventhal Syndrome)

This group of patients shows a wide spectrum of clinical disorders with the common denominator being the **failure of release of the ovum from the maturing ovarian follicle.** As a result, the estrogen-producing follicles persist, becoming enlarged and cystic. In such patients, the postovulatory part of the cycle is usually absent: **there is no transformation of the follicle into a corpus luteum.** Consequently, the proliferative endometrium does not enter into the secretory phase or the secretory activity is focal or weak. The result of inadequate endometrial desquamation is **endometrial hyperplasia,** or an increase in the absolute amount of the endometrium, accompanied by various degrees of abnormality of endometrial glands and, in some cases, **endometrial carcinoma** (see Chap. 13). Ovarian stroma may show transformation into luteinized theca cells, which, in extreme cases, may be sufficiently extensive to be mistaken for an ovarian tumor (pseudothecoma of ovary, Koss et al, 1964). The accompanying amenorrhea may be intermittent or permanent and may be accompanied by episodes of heavy uterine bleeding or **metrorrhagia.**

In the group of patients with an ill-defined variant of this group of disorders, the **Stein-Leventhal** syndrome, fibrosis of the ovarian cortex may occur and was thought to be the cause of ovulatory disturbances. Indeed, a wedge resection of the ovaries may restore normal cyclic bleeding in some patients. However, many such cases show no evidence of cortical ovarian fibrosis.

The clinical setting of these disorders is fairly characteristic; periods of amenorrhea usually affect young women in their teens or early 20s. **Obesity, hirsutism, diabetes, and hypertension** are not infrequently observed and may occur either singly or in any combination. There is usually no biochemical evidence of either pituitary or adrenal disorders. The disturbance may be temporary, with a spontaneous return to normal, but more often it persists unless treated. The chief danger lies in the development of endometrial hyperplasia and **endometrial carcinoma.**

Cytology

In view of the arrest of ovulation, one would expect that the vaginal smears of patients with Stein-Leventhal syndrome would show a sustained high level of estrogenic activity. This has not been our experience, or the experience of Ra-koff (1961) or of Bamford et al (1965). The cases are too few and inadequately followed for a conclusive statement but, in general, the vaginal smears are composed of folded and clustered superficial and intermediate cells, thus resembling the postovulatory-type smears (see Chap. 8). Intracytoplasmic glycogenic deposits may occur and such smears may mimic the pattern observed in pregnancy.

Occasionally, however, especially in the presence of endometrial hyperplasia, a high level of estrogenic activity may be observed (see also Chap. 13). If sequential smears are taken over time, there is usually little variation in smear pattern. Pronounced cyclic variations are rarely seen and usually precede an episode of metrorrhagia.

Effects of Castration

The effects of castration, either surgical or radiation-induced, may be conveniently followed by vaginal smears. The effects of **surgical castration** are by no means uniform. In fact, complete atrophy of the squamous epithelium may not occur for several months or even years. Finkbeiner (un-published data) who observed numerous surgically castrated patients with breast cancer, noted that in some of them a drop in the level of maturation of squamous epithelium was followed within a few weeks by an improved maturation

(Fig. 9-2). This suggests that other sources of ovarian-like hormones, possibly the adrenal cortex, are able to step in to replace the missing ovaries. The effects of **radiation-induced castration** are still more variable and, not infrequently, the cytologic pattern may fail to reach the stage of complete epithelial atrophy. The cytologic evaluation here may be complicated by the effect of radiation on epithelial cells, described in Chapter 18.

OTHER DISORDERS WITH HORMONAL EFFECTS

Ovarian Tumors

Certain ovarian tumors, particularly the **granulosa cell tumors and the thecomas,** may produce estrogen-like substances. The resulting clinical disorders resemble those observed in disturbances of ovulation, as discussed above. The vaginal smear patterns are generally uninformative during the childbearing age. However, granulosa cell tumors may occur in all age groups and **the finding of a consistently high estrogenic effect in a prepubertal or postmenopausal woman warrants investigation of the ovaries.** High level of maturation of squamous cells after treatment of this tumor may be suggestive of a recurrence (see Chap. 15).

Ovarian tumors, usually classed as masculinizing **(arrhenoblastomas or Sertoli-Leydig cell tumors, hilar cell tumors, lipoid cell tumors),** are exceedingly rare. Little

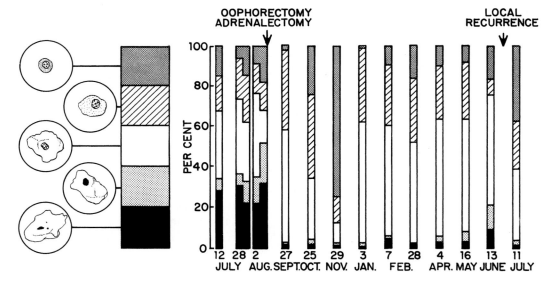

Figure 9-2 Diagrammatic representation of the differential cell count technique for hormonal evaluation of vaginal smears. From 200 to 400 cells are counted under high-dry magnification, enumerating the percentage of small parabasal, large parabasal, intermediate, precornified, and cornified cells as diagrammed. The *right-hand* portion of the diagram illustrates the clinical application of this method of endocrine evaluation in the follow-up care of patients with advanced breast cancer. This patient, a 61-year-old woman, who was 8 years postmenopausal, had recurrent inoperable breast cancer with multiple osseous and soft-tissue metastases. The individual bars represent a single day's smear pattern; the confluent bars are consecutive smears. The preoperative vaginal smears show a greater maturation of squamous cells than would ordinarily be expected in a patient of this endocrine status, suggesting that this tumor was growing in a relatively rich hormonal environment. Combined oophorectomy-adrenalectomy was followed by an excellent objective and subjective remission, with measurable regression of disease. The vaginal smear response to this procedure is shown. There was again a slight increase in vaginal smear maturation just before the appearance of recurrent disease, 10 months postoperatively. (Courtesy of Dr. John A. Finkbeiner.)

is known about the effect of these tumors on the vaginal smear. Rakoff (1961) reported the finding of an **atrophic smear type** in two patients with **arrhenoblastoma,** and a mixed population of squamous cells in a child with **"adrenal-like ovarian tumor"** (possibly a variant of granulosa cell tumor) and in a young woman with "lipoid cell tumor." Rakoff's studies occurred before the current nomenclature of the ovarian tumors was in place and, in the absence of histologic data, the tumors cannot be reclassified.

Precocious Puberty in Girls

In this uncommon disease affecting young girls and caused by a single-gene defect (Adashi and Hennebold, 1999), there is usually the association of **premature periodic vaginal bleeding and hyperplasia of breasts with a disease of the skeleton** (fibrous dysplasia) and **cafe-au-lait spots on the skin (McClure-Albright's syndrome)** (Figs. 9-3 and

9-4). Sequential vaginal smears disclose cyclic variation of the smear pattern, as shown in Figure 9-4A, corresponding to a cyclic function of the ovary.

Endometriosis

Endometriosis may sometimes lead to abnormal uterine bleeding. Although Schmidt and Christiaans (1965) claimed that endometriosis results in elevation of the maturation of squamous cells, when compared with normal for the time of the cycle, it has been our experience that there are no cytologic findings, whether quantitative or qualitative, that would permit the diagnosis of endometriosis in vaginal smears. For further discussion of cytologic findings in endometriosis, see appropriate chapters.

Galactorrhea

During the period of **normal lactation,** the vaginal smear pattern is that of the postpartum type (see Chap. 8). If

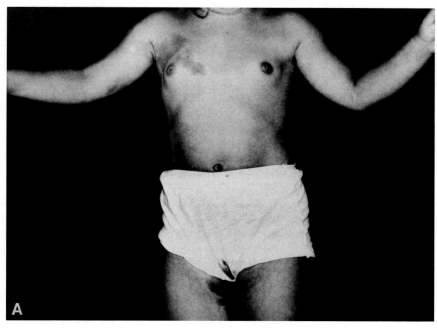

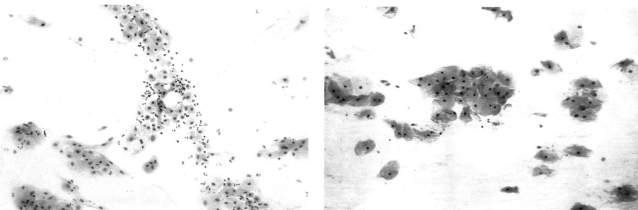

Figure 9-3 Case of precocious puberty, girl 3 years of age. *A.* Photograph shows enlarged breasts, café-au-lait skin spots, and evidence of vaginal bleeding. *B,C.* Patterns of vaginal smears obtained at an interval of 3 weeks. *B.* Normal smear pattern for age, with no evidence of maturation. *C.* Marked maturation with superficial squamous cells dominating.

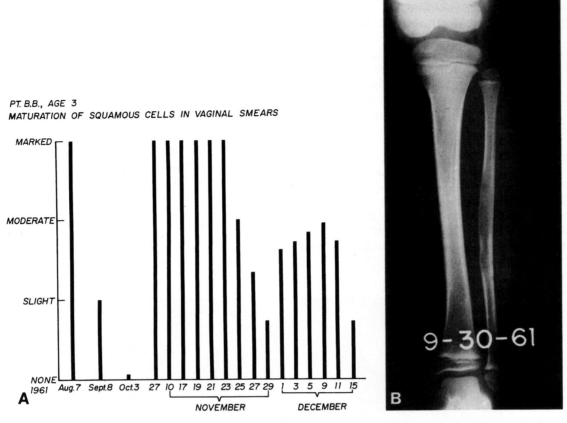

PT. B.B., AGE 3
MATURATION OF SQUAMOUS CELLS IN VAGINAL SMEARS

Figure 9-4 Same case as in Figure 9-3. *A.* Diagrammatic representation of sequential vaginal smears. A pattern of cyclic maturation is evident. *B.* Roentgenogram of a lesion affecting the left fibula of this child, which proved to be fibrous dysplasia.

normal lactation continues over a period of many months or years, it is usually accompanied by **amenorrhea** and a marked **atrophy of the squamous epithelium (Chiari-Frommel syndrome).** Occasionally, **galactorrhea** or milk formation may occur independently of pregnancy, and this may reflect a serious endocrine disorder, such as a **chromophobe adenoma of the pituitary** (see Chap. 29). In such instances, the **smear pattern may show moderate proliferation of the squamous epithelium,** even in the absence of documented estrogen or progesterone activity.

Hepatic Insufficiency

Patterns suggesting excessive levels of estrogens may also be noted in the presence of hepatic insufficiency. This is generally attributed to failure of the damaged liver cells to metabolize estrogens.

EFFECTS OF HORMONAL THERAPY ON THE SQUAMOUS EPITHELIUM

Estrogens

Except during pregnancy, parenteral or oral administration of estrogens and estrogen substitutes produces a **cytologic pattern of complete maturation of squa-**

mous epithelium. The effect is particularly evident in postmenopausal or prepubertal patients and may result in a striking and radical change of smear pattern, with a preponderance of single flat, superficial cells. Occasionally, very large squamous cells have been observed. Even the **administration of facial or vaginal creams containing estrogens may be reflected in the vaginal smears.** There is, however, **no direct quantitative relationship between the amount of the drug administered and the response of the squamous epithelium.** This relationship varies significantly from patient to patient. Some patients require large doses of estrogens to achieve full maturation of the squamous epithelium; others require very little drug. Once the full maturation of the squamous epithelium has been reached, further increases in the dosage of the drug will not be reflected in further changes in the smear pattern. The use of the vaginal smear as the sole guide in the therapeutic administration of estrogenic substances is probably not warranted.

If estrogen is withdrawn, its effect on the squamous epithelium may linger for some days or weeks but the stimulated **endometrium may break down** with resulting clinical spotting or bleeding (**withdrawal bleeding**). Clusters of endometrial cells may be observed in such smears (Fig. 9-5). The effect of estrogens on smear patterns in various conditions is summarized in Figure 9-6.

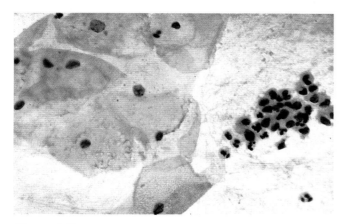

Figure 9-5 **Effect of estrogen.** Large, mature squamous cells in the cervicovaginal smear of a 70-year-old woman. A cluster of endometrial cells seen in the photograph was shed as the drug was being withdrawn (withdrawal bleeding).

There is considerable controversy about the value of **estrogen therapy used to alleviate the effects of the menopause.** On the one hand, this therapy is beneficial in preventing some of the common symptoms, such as hot flashes, and is perhaps useful in preventing osteoporosis. On the other hand, the drug may contribute to the development of endometrial hyperplasia and carcinoma, although this latter issue is by no means clear-cut (see Chap. 13). Further, the drug may contribute to the development of breast cancer (Clemons and Goss, 2002; Chlebowski et al, 2003). Still, it is preferable to use estrogens together with progesterone

in a form of cyclic therapy to prevent any untoward effects on the endometrium, but the value of this therapy in reference to coronary heart disease has been recently questioned (Manson et al, 2003). Still, the hormonal effects of the combined therapy may be monitored by cytology.

Other Hormones Influencing the Patterns of Squamous Epithelium

The response to a variety of hormones varies according to the menstrual status of the patient. **During the childbearing age** the administration of **progesterone or of androgens,** such as testosterone, may result in **some degree of suppression of maturation of the squamous epithelium, with intermediate cells** dominating the smear pattern. Intracytoplasmic glycogen deposits may be observed in such cells. The effect of androgens on smear patterns in various conditions is summarized in Figure 9-7.

In women with postmenopausal atrophy, whether spontaneous or iatrogenic, the administration of a variety of hormones, such as **progesterone, androgens, adrenal cortical steroids, or anterior pituitary hormones,** may bring about some measure of epithelial stimulation in most cases. Thus, cervicovaginal cytology is of a very limited value in assessing the effect of these drugs.

Contraceptive Medication

The cytologic effect of hormones administered for contraceptive purposes varies according to the make-up of the product. The commonly used drugs, composed of a mixture

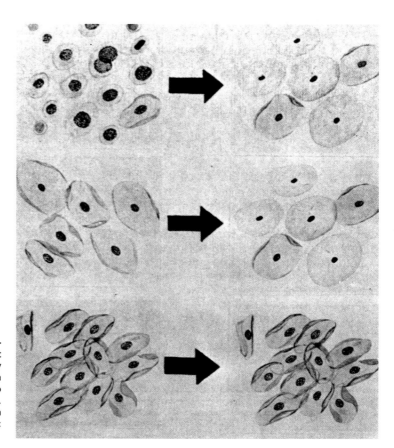

Figure 9-6 **Schematic representation of effects of estrogens on patterns of vaginal smears.** The effect is most striking in advanced atrophic menopause (*top*) and in early menopause (*center*), and results in full epithelial maturation with formation of squamous superficial cells. There is no effect on the smear pattern in normal pregnancy (*bottom*). (From Wied G. Hormonal evaluation of the patient through cytologic interpretation. Acta Unio Int Contra Cancrum 14: 277–285, 1958.)

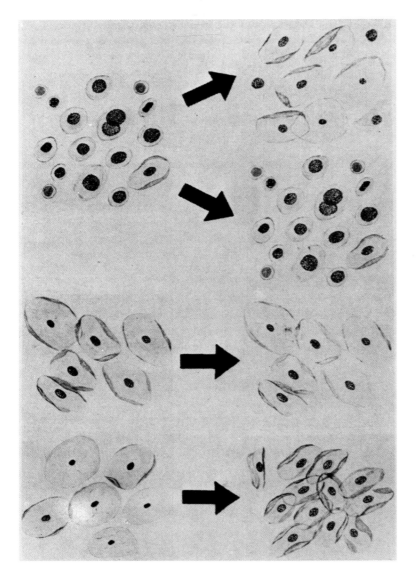

Figure 9-7 Schematic representation of the effects of parenterally administered androgens on patterns of vaginal smears. In advanced menopause (*top*) about 70% of women will show moderate epithelial maturation, whereas the drug will be without effect in 30% of cases. There is no noticeable drug effect on patterns of early menopause (*center*). During the childbearing age (*bottom*), there may be some arrest of epithelial maturation. (From Wied G. Hormonal evaluation of the patient through cytologic interpretation. Acta Unio Int Contra Cancrum 14:277–285, 1958.)

of estrogen and progesterone derivatives, may result in **some arrest of maturation of the squamous epithelium,** occasionally suggestive of a degree of epithelial atrophy. The effect of progesterone on endocervical cell morphology is discussed in Chapters 8 and 10.

The **long-term implanted contraceptive hormonal devices** usually contain progestogens (Johannisson, 1990). Valente et al (1998) described the long-term effect of one of these drugs (depot-medroxyprogesterone acetate) on young users, using the maturation value (MV). Many of the users developed amenorrhea, accompanied by **atrophic or postpartum patterns of smears** with significant lowering of the MV, when compared with control patients matched for age. Nothing is known about the hormonal effects of a new class of drugs, such as RU 486, that interfere with implantation of the ovum and thus effectively induce abortions (Baulieu, 1989).

Tamoxifen

This important **estrogen agonist** is now widely used in the treatment and prevention of carcinoma of the breast. Studies

by Eells et al (1990), Lahti et al (1994), and by Friedrich et al (1998) pertaining to the impact of the drug on the hormonal pattern of cervicovaginal smears in **postmenopausal women** indicated that these patients have an **increased maturation of the squamous epithelium.** In an elaborate study, Bertolissi et al (1998) studied karyopyknotic index (KI), the maturation index (MI), and the levels of hormone-binding globulin in 64 postmenopausal breast cancer patients receiving tamoxifen. Statistically significant increases in both indices and the globulin were observed in about 80% of the patients after 30 days of therapy and remained stable during the follow-up period of 12 months. This study confirmed that the drug induced an early and persistent estrogenic effect on the squamous epithelium of the lower genital tract. In a number of personally observed cases, the smear patterns were dominated by intermediate squamous cells. Thus, although the drug is an estrogen agonist, **it does not induce atrophy of the squamous epithelium or prevent its maturation. The effect of the drug is similar to that of steroid hormones other than estrogen,** as discussed above. Gill et al (1998) suggested that tamoxifen induces atypical benign changes in squamous cells.

TABLE 9-2

THE EFFECT OF DIGITALIS ON MATURATION OF SQUAMOUS EPITHELIUM IN POSTMENOPAUSAL WOMEN

Number of Patients	Length of Digitalis* Therapy	Maturation of Squamous Epithelium
20	>2 yr	Marked
3	<2 yr	Marked
3	<2 yr	Moderate
26	<2 yr	Atrophy
Controls { 4		Moderate
46		Atrophy

* As oral digitoxin 0.1–0.2 mg daily.
(Navab A, et al. Estrogen-like activity of digitalis. Its effect on the squamous epithelium of the female genital tract. JAMA 194:30–32, 1965.)

We have not seen such changes, and the full significance of this observation will require long-term controlled studies. The significance of tamoxifen in the **genesis of endometrial abnormalities and carcinoma** is discussed in Chapter 13. It is not clear whether or not tamoxifen is the cause of **vaginal adenosis,** as described by Genesan et al (1999). For further discussion of vaginal adenosis, see Chapter 14.

Drugs Other Than Hormones

The **antibiotic,** tetracycline, may be used to treat inflammatory conditions in the vagina. In the course of personal studies on carcinoma in situ of the cervix (see Chap. 11), it became apparent that **tetracycline vaginal suppositories have a marked desquamatory effect on the squamous epithelium** of the female genital tract. Smears from treated patients may contain sheets of desquamated squamous cells that are difficult to evaluate. At least 1 week, preferably longer, should be allowed to elapse after conclusion of treatment before the evaluation of the squamous epithelium is undertaken. It is quite likely that **other antibiotics** and perhaps **intravaginal medication** of any kind may influence patterns of maturation of squamous cells.

Studies by Britch and Azar (1963) and by Navab et al (1965) on the effects of **digitalis** on postmenopausal women revealed that this drug, if administered daily for 2 years or longer, has a marked influence on the maturation of the squamous epithelium. The results are summarized in Table 9-2. The manner in which digitalis, a compound biochemically related to steroids, affects the squamous epithelium of the vagina is unclear. **Gynecomastia in men,** also observed after digitalis therapy, may represent an allied phenomenon.

BIBLIOGRAPHY

Adashi EY, Hennebold JD. Single-gene mutations resulting in reproductive dysfunction in women. N Engl J Med 340:709–718, 1999.

Affandi MZ, Doctor V, Jhaveri K. The endocervical smear as a simple and quick method for determination of ovulation. Acta Cytol 29:638–641, 1985.

Albertson BD, Zinaman MJ. The prediction of ovulation and monitoring of the fertile period. Adv Contracept 3:263–290, 1987.

Bacus SS, Flowers JL, Press MF, et al. The evaluation of estrogen receptor in primary breast carcinoma by computer-assisted image analysis. Am J Clin Pathol 90:233–239, 1988.

Bamford SB, Mitchell GW Jr, Bardawil WA, Casin CM. Vaginal cytology in polycystic ovarian disease. Acta Cytol 9:332–337, 1965.

Batrinos ML, Eustratiades MG. Vaginal cytology in primary amenorrhea. Acta Cytol 16:376–380, 1972.

Baulieu EE. Contraception and other clinical applications of RU 486, an antiprogesterone at the receptor. Science 245:1351–1357, 1989.

Bercovici B, Lewin A, Rabinowitz R, et al. The cytology of vaginal, cervical and endometrial smears obtained at the time of embryo transfer during in vitro fertilization. Acta Cytol 32:789–793, 1988.

Bertolissi A, Cartei G, Turrin D, et al. Behavior of vaginal epithelial maturation and sex hormone binding globulin in post-menopausal breast cancer patients during the first year of tamoxifen therapy. Cytopathology 9:263–270, 1998.

Boquoi E, Hammerstein J. Discrepancies between colpocytology and urinary steroid hormone excretion in women treated with clomiphene citrate or gonadotropins for anovulatory sterility. Acta Cytol 13:332–346, 1969.

Britch CM, Azar HA. Estrogen effect in exfoliated vaginal cells following treatment with digitalis. Am J Obstet Gynecol 85:989–993, 1963.

Cassano PA, Saigo PE, Hajdu SI. Comparison of cytohormonal status of postmenopausal women with cancer to age-matched controls. Acta Cytol 30:93–98, 1986.

Castellanos H, O'Morchoe PJ, Yahia C, Sturgis SH. Urethral cytology in the diagnosis of secondary amenorrhea. JAMA 181:71–76, 1964.

Chan L, O'Malley BW. Mechanism of action of the sex steroid hormones. N Engl J Med 294:1322–1328; 1372–1381; 1430–1437, 1976.

Chlebowski RT, Hendrix SL, Langer RD, et al. Influence of estrogen plus progestin on breast cancer and mammography in healthy postmenopausal women: The Women's Health Initiative Randomized Trial. JAMA 289:3243–3253, 2003.

Clemons M, Goss P. Estrogen and the risk of breast cancer. N Engl J Med 344:276–285, 2002.

Cordoba F. Experimental evaluation of the "quantitative" differential count in exfoliative cytology. Acta Cytol 8:446–448, 1964.

Eells TP, Alpern HD, Grzywacz C, et al. The effect of tamoxifen on cervical squamous maturation in Papanicolaou stained cervical smears of postmenopausal women. Cytopathology 1:263–268, 1990.

Federman DD. Disorders of sexual development. N Engl J Med 277:351–360, 1967.

Fisher ER, Gregorio R, Stephan T, et al. Ovarian changes in women with morbid obesity. Obstet Gynecol 44:839–844, 1974.

Friedrich M, Mink D, Villena-Heinsen C, et al. The influence of tamoxifen on the maturation index of vaginal epithelium. Clin Exp Obstet Gynecol 25:121–124, 1998.

Genesan R, Ferryman SR, Wadell CA. Vaginal adenosis in a patient on Tamoxifen therapy. Cytopathology 10:127–130, 1999.

Gerald PS. Sex chromosome disorders. N Engl J Med 294:706–708, 1976.

German J, Vesell M. Testicular feminization in monozygotic twins with 47 chromosomes (XXY). Ann Genet 9:5–8, 1966.

Gill BL, Simpson JF, Somlo G, et al. Effect of tamoxifen on the cytology of the uterine cervix in breast cancer patients. Diagn Cytopathol 19:417–422, 1998.

Greenblatt RB, Dominquez H, Mahesh VB, Demos R. Gonadal dysgenesis intersex with XO/XY mosaicism. JAMA 188:221–224, 1964.

Gregg WI. Galactorrhea after contraceptive hormones. N Engl J Med 274:1430–1431, 1966.

Grumbach MM, Conte FA. Disorders of sexual differentiation. *In* Wilson JD, Foster DW (eds). Williams Textbook of Endocrinology, 7th ed. Philadelphia, WB Saunders, 1985, pp 312–401.

Haour P, Delacroix R. L'urocytogramme. Rev Fr Cytol Clin 4:35–39, 1974.

Heber KR. The effect of progestogens on vaginal cytology. Acta Cytol 19:103–109, 1975.

Hertz R, Odell WO, Ross GT. Diagnostic implications of primary amenorrhea. Ann Intern Med 65:800–820, 1966.

Hustin J, Van den Eynde J-P. Cytologic evaluation of the effect of various estrogens given in post-menopause. Acta Cytol 21:225–228, 1977.

Jackson RL, Dockerty MB. Stein-Leventhal syndrome: Analysis of 43 cases with special reference to association with endometrial carcinoma. Am J Obstet Gynecol 73:161–173, 1957.

Jensen EV, DeSombre ER. Estrogen-receptor interaction. Science 182:126–134, 1973.

Johannisson E. Effects on the endometrium, and endocervix following the use of local progestogen-releasing delivery systems. Center for Medical Research, The Population Council in New York, 1990.

Johnston WW, Goldston WR, Montgomery MS. Clinicopathologic studies in feminizing tumors of the ovary. III. The role of genital cytology. Acta Cytol 15:334–338, 1971.

Kendall B, Loewenberg LS. Testicular feminization. Report of 2 cases occurring in siblings. Obstet Gynecol 20:551–554, 1962.

Klinefelter HF Jr, Reifenstein EC Jr, Albright F. Syndrome characterized by gynecomastia, aspermatogenesis without aleydigism, and increased excretion of follicle-stimulating hormone. J Clin Endocrinol 2:615–662, 1942.

Koss LG, Pierce V, Brunschwig A. Pseudothecomas of ovaries. Cancer 17:76–85, 1964.

Kupryjanczyk J, Moller P. Estrogen receptor distribution in the normal and pathologically changed human cervix uteri: An immunohistochemical study with use of monoclonal anti-ER antibody. Int J Gynecol Pathol 7:75–85, 1988.

Lahti E, Vuopola S, Kauppila A, et al. Maturation of vaginal and endometrial epithelium in post-menopausal breast cancer patients receiving long-term tamoxifen. Gynecol Oncol 55:410–414, 1994.

Lee MM, Donahue P, Silverman BL, et al. Measurement of serum müllerian inhibiting substance in the evaluation of children with nonpalpable gonads. N Engl J Med 336:1480–1486, 1997.

Lencioni L. L'Uro-cytogramme. Diagnostic Cyto-Hormonal à Partir du Sédiment Urinaire, 3rd ed. Buenos Aires, Editorial Medica Panamericana, 1972.

Lencioni LJ, Staffieri JJ. Urocytogram diagnosis of sexual precocity. Acta Cytol 13:382–388, 1969.

Liu T, Liu S. The vaginal cytogram. JAMA 118:130–135, 1963.

Lotan Y, Diamant YZ. The value of simple tests in the detection of human ovulation. Int J Gynaecol Obstet 16:309–316, 1978.

Manson JE, Hsia J, Johnson KC, et al. Estrogen plus progestin and the risk of coronary heart disease. N Engl J Med 349:523–534, 2003.

McCusick VA, Clairborne RE. Medical Genetics. New York, HP Publishing Co, 1973.

McDonnell DP, Norris JD. Connections and regulation of the human estrogen receptor. Science 296:1642–1644, 2002.

McLennan MT, McLennan CE. Estrogenic status of menstruating and menopausal women assessed by cervico-vaginal smears. Obstet Gynecol 37:325–331, 1971.

Mehta PV. Study correlating endometrial biopsies and vaginal cytology in one hundred tubectomized women. Acta Cytol 19:330–333, 1975.

Meisels A. The maturation value. Acta Cytol 11:249, 1967.

Merke DP, Tajima T, Baron J, Cutler GB Jr. Hypogonadotropic hypogonadism in a female caused by an X-linked recessive mutation in the *DAX1* gene. N Engl J Med 340:1248–1252, 1999.

Metcalf MG. Use of small samples of urine to follow ovarian and placental changes in progesterone secretion. Am J Obstet Gynecol 117:1041–1045, 1973.

Mingeot R, Fievez C. Endocervical changes with the use of synthetic steroids. Obstet Gynecol 44:53–59, 1974.

Moghissi KS, Synder FN, Borin B. Cyclic changes of cervical mucus enzymes related to the time of ovulation. Am J Obstet Gynecol 125:1044–1048, 1976.

Moghissi KS, Snyder FN, Evans TN. A composite picture of the menstrual cycle. Am J Obstet Gynecol 114:405–418, 1972.

Moracci E, Berlingieri D. Hormonal evaluation of vaginal smears from artificial vagina. Acta Cytol 17:131–134 1973.

Morris JM. The syndrome of testicular feminization in male pseudohermaphrodites. Am J Obstet Gynecol 65:1192–1211, 1953.

Navab A, Koss LG, LaDue J. Estrogen-like activity of digitalis. JAMA 194:30–32, 1965.

Nykliček O. Importance of vaginal cytograms for diagnosis and therapy in the deficiency of oestrogenic hormones. Gynaecologia 131:173–178, 1951.

O'Malley BW, Means AR. Female steroid hormones and target cell nuclei. Science 183:610–620, 1974.

O'Malley BW, Schrader WT. The receptors of steroid hormones. Sci Am 234:32–43, 1976.

O'Morchoe PJ, O'Morchoe CCC. Method for urinary cytology in endocrine assessment. Acta Cytol 11:145–149, 1967.

Papanicolaou GN. Diagnosis of pregnancy by cytologic criteria in catheterized urine. Proc Soc Exp Biol Med 67:247–249, 1948.

Papanicolaou GN, Traut HF, Marchetti AA. The epithelia of women's reproductive organs; a correlative study of cyclic changes. New York, Commonwealth Fund, 1948.

Press MF, Nousek-Goebl NA, Bur M, Greene GL. Estrogen receptor localization in the female genital tract. Am J Pathol 123:280–292, 1986.

Pundel JP. Précis de Colpocytologie Hormonale. Paris, Masson et Cie, 1966.

Rakoff AE. Vaginal cytology of endocrinopathies. Acta Cytol 5:153–167, 1961.

Rakoff AE, Daley JG. Vaginal hormonal cytology. *In* Sunderman FW, Sunderman FW Jr (eds). Laboratory Diagnosis of Endocrine Diseases. St. Louis, WH Green, 1971.

Rakoff AE, Wachtel E, Wied G. Hormonal evaluation of patient through cytologic interpretation. Acta Unio Int Contra Cancrum 14:268–285, 1958.

Relkin R. Galactorrhea: A review. NY J Med 65:2800–2807, 1965.

Reyniak JV, Sedlis A, Stone D, Rimdusit P. Comparison of hormonal colpocytology with endometrial histology in gynecologic patients. Acta Cytol 15:329–333, 1971.

Saenger P. Turner's syndrome. N Engl J Med 335:1749–1754, 1996.

Schellhas HF. Malignant potential of the dysgenetic gonad. Part I. Obstet Gynecol 44:298–309, 1974.

Schellhas HF. Malignant potential of the dysgenetic gonad. Part II. Obstet Gynecol 44:455–462, 1974.

Schmidt ALC, Christiaans APL. The vaginal smear pattern in cases of endometriosis. Acta Cytol 9:247–250, 1965.

Schneider V, Friedrich E, Schindler AE. Hormonal cytology: A correlation with plasma estradiol, measured by radioimmunoassay. Acta Cytol 21:37–39, 1977.

Solomon C, Panagotopoulos P, Oppenheim A. The use of urinary sediment as an aid in endocrinological disorders in the female. Am J Obstet Gynecol 76:56–60, 1958.

Sonek M. Vaginal cytology in childhood and puberty. Part I. Newborn through prepuberty. J Reprod Med 2:39–56, 1968.

Sonek M. Vaginal cytology in childhood and puberty. Part II. Puberty. J Reprod Med 2:198–208, 1968.

Soost HJ. Comparative studies on the degree of proliferation of the vaginal and ectocervical epithelium in the hormonal evaluation of a patient by means of exfoliative cytology. Acta Cytol 4:199–209, 1960.

Stoll P, Ledermann O. Correlative studies of cytology in vaginal smears and endometrial histology during various phases of the menstrual cycle. Acta Cytol 6:307–309, 1962.

Sutherland EW. Studies on the mechanism of hormone action. Science 177:401–408, 1972.

Szulman AE. The significance of chromosomal abnormalities in spontaneous abortion. *In* Kistner WR, Behrman SJ (eds). Progress in Infertility. Boston, Little, Brown & Co, 1967.

Szulman AE. Chromosomal aberrations in spontaneous human abortions. N Engl J Med 272:811–818, 1965.

Teter J, Boczkowski K. Cytohormonal pattern and histologic studies in cases of pure gonadal dysgenesis. Acta Cytol 11:449–455, 1967.

Tozzini R, Sobrero AJ, Hoovis E. Vulvar cytology. Acta Cytol 15:57–63, 1971.

Tredway DR, Mishell DR Jr, Moyer DL. Correlation of endometrial dating with luteinizing hormone peak. Am J Obstet Gynecol 117:1030–1033, 1973.

Valente PT, Schantz HD, Trabal JF. Cytologic changes in cervical smears associated with prolonged use of depot-medroxyprogesterone acetate. Cancer 84:328–334, 1998.

Wachtel E. Exfoliative Cytology in Gynaecological Practice. Washington, DC, Butterworth, 1964.

Wachtel E, Plester JA. Hormonal assessment by vaginal cytology. J Obstet Gynaecol Br Emp 61:155–161, 1954.

Wied GL. Symposium on hormonal cytology. Acta Cytol 12:87–127, 1968.

Wied GL. Climacteric amenorrhea: Cytohormonal test for differential diagnosis. Obstet Gynecol 9:646–649, 1957.

Wied GL, Bibbo M, Keebler CM. Evaluation of the endocrinologic condition by exfoliative cytology. *In* Wied GL, Keebler CM, Koss LG, et al (eds). Compendium on Diagnostic Cytology. Tutorials of Cytology, 7th ed. Chicago, Tutorials of Cytology, 1992.

Wied GL, Davis ME. Comparative activity of progestational agents on the human endometrium and vaginal epithelium of surgical castrates. Ann NY Acad Sci 71:599–616, 1958.

Wied GL, del Sol JR, Dargan AM. Progestational and androgenic substances tested on highly proliferated vaginal epithelium of surgical castrates; I. Progestational substances. Am J Obstet Gynecol 75:98–111, 1958.

Wilson RA, Wilson TA. The fate of the nontreated post-menopausal woman: A plea for the maintenance of adequate estrogen from puberty to the grave. J Am Geriat Soc 9:347–362, 1963.

Benign Disorders of the Uterine Cervix and Vagina

10

NONINFLAMMATORY AND REACTIVE PROCESSES

In this chapter, a number of benign epithelial cytologic abnormalities is described. The knowledge of these abnormalities is essential in the practice of cytopathology because some of these changes must be differentiated from malignant processes. The abnormalities will be presented according to the epithelium of origin but in practice may be found side by side in the same cytologic preparation.

SQUAMOUS EPITHELIUM

Basal Cell Hyperplasia

This is a frequent finding in the biopsies of the cervix, as it is in other organs, such as the bronchus. On histologic examination, there is an **increase in the number of layers of small basal cells.** Consequently, the basal cells form one-fourth to one-third of the thickness of the squamous epithelium (see Fig. 6-11). However, there are **no nuclear abnormalities** and the maturation of the epithelium proceeds normally above the enlarged basal zone; hence, basal hyperplasia of squamous epithelium **cannot be detected in smears** unless there is a total loss of superficial cell layers or if the sample is obtained by energetic brushing. The etiology of the process is unknown but there is no evidence that it is related to cancer.

Leukoplakia

Leukoplakia (from Greek, *leukos* = white) is a clinical term describing a **white patchy discoloration of the squamous epithelium.** It is more common on the surface of the cervix than in the vagina. In most cases, it is a benign lesion caused by **abnormal keratinization of the mucosal surface.** It must be emphasized, however, that **keratinizing precancerous lesions of the uterine cervix and occasionally, keratinizing invasive carcinoma, may appear as clinical leukoplakia** (see Chap. 11).

Histology

In benign leukoplakia, the surface of the epithelium is covered by an **eosinophilic layer of keratin of variable thickness.** The keratinized layer is composed of anucleated cells, akin to those observed on the surface of the epidermis (Fig. 10-1A). The lesion may result from chronic trauma, prolapse of the uterus, pressure of a pessary, or previous cauterization of the cervix.

Cytology

Anucleated squamous cells **(squames),** of characteristic **pale yellow color** in Papanicolaou stain, are shed from the surface of the keratinized squamous epithelium (Fig. 10-1B). All stages of transition between mature nucleated squamous cells and the anucleated variety may be observed: There is a gradual change in the color of the cytoplasm from pink to yellow and the gradual disappearance of the nucleus. In the fully keratinized squames, **shadows of pre-existing nuclei can be observed.** Occasionally, brown cytoplasmic granules, akin to those seen in the normal superficial squamous cells, may be noted. The actual **frequency** of an-

ucleated squamous cells in cervicovaginal smears is low, estimated by Kern (1991) to be about 0.5%. In my opinion, the presence of anucleated squamous cells **should be noted in the report** because of the remote possibility that these cells may have originated from the surface of a squamous cancer, masquerading as leukoplakia. Such patients deserve a closer clinical look, although nearly all the lesions are benign. **In squamous carcinomas with features of leukoplakia, anucleated squamous cells are usually accompanied by cells with abnormal, hyperchromatic nuclei that allow an accurate diagnosis,** as discussed in Chapter 11.

Parakeratosis (Pseudoparakeratosis) of Squamous Epithelium

Histology

Occasionally, the surface of an otherwise normal squamous epithelium of the uterine cervix is lined by a few layers of very small nucleated squamous cells, instead of the usual large, mature squamous cells. This disorder is somewhat similar to the abnormalities occurring on the surface of the epidermis of the skin (for example, in psoriasis), which are referred to as **parakeratosis.** Therefore, this abnormality of the cervix epithelium was named *pseudoparakeratosis*.

Cytology

In cervical smears, large sheets of **irregularly-shaped, small squamous cells**, about 10 μm in diameter, with basophilic or eosinophilic cytoplasm, may be observed (Fig. 10-2A). The nuclei are spherical, of even sizes, often somewhat eccentric and usually pyknotic (Fig. 10-2B). The cause or the exact frequency of this **benign** abnormality is unknown. Voytek et al (1996) observed similar small cells in benign lesions but also in the presence of low- and high-grade squamous neoplastic lesions of the cervix. It is not certain whether this association is incidental. Still, the recognition of the pseudoparakeratotic cells as benign is sometimes very difficult because of their nuclear features. In case of doubt, colposcopy and biopsies of the cervix should be recommended. Frable (1994) included such cells among the **liti-**

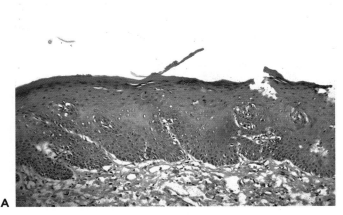

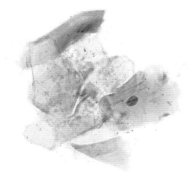

A

B

Figure 10-1   Leukoplakia of uterine cervix. *A.* Biopsy showing a layer of keratin on the surface. *B.* Cervical smear from the same case. The yellow or yellow-orange superficial squamous cells are either anucleated (anucleated squames) or show residual traces of nuclei.

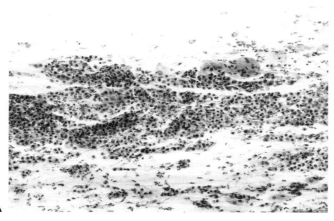
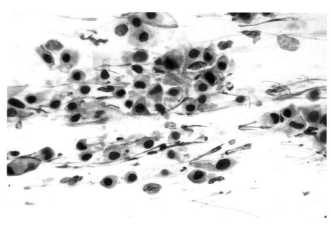

A   . B

Figure 10-2   Pseudoparakeratosis or parakeratosis. *A.* The cervical smear at survey magnification shows large sheets of very small squamous cells. *B.* At higher magnification, the spherical or slightly irregular cells have uniform, dark nuclei.

gation cells that are difficult to classify and may be the subject of a dispute as to their exact significance.

Somewhat similar cells were observed by Meisels and Fortin (1976) in **human papillomavirus (HPV) infection** and were named **dyskeratocytes.** Dyskeratocytes, as described and illustrated, are small **elongated, spindly cells** forming sheets with similar nuclear characteristics to pseudoparakeratotic cells described above. Meisels et al (1976) observed HPV virions in electron microscopy of dyskeratocytes. However, in pseudoparakeratosis, the underlying epithelium does not show any changes of papillomavirus infection and, therefore, the two entities may be similar but are possibly of different etiologies. (See Chap. 11 for further discussion of cytologic manifestations of human papillomavirus infection.)

ENDOCERVICAL EPITHELIUM

Basal Cell Hyperplasia

Histology

Proliferation of the small, basal endocervical cells, akin to the basal hyperplasia of squamous epithelium, may result from chronic inflammation or it may occur spontaneously. In tissue sections, **several layers of small, round cells are found beneath the columnar endocervical cells** (see Fig. 6-12).

Cytology

Basal cell hyperplasia is **rarely seen in cervical scrape smears.** However, with the use of **cervical brush instruments,** particularly after a vigorous brushing, basal cell hyperplasia may be seen from time to time in the form of **flat clusters of small, spherical or polygonal cells,** measuring about 10 μm in diameter. The cells have scanty cytoplasm and relatively large, **dense but regular nuclei, about 8 μm in diameter.** The nuclei vary somewhat in size and shape and **may show mitotic activity.** The recognition of the

basal endocervical cells is easier if well-differentiated columnar cells are attached to the periphery of such clusters (Fig. 10-3). The role of basal cell hyperplasia as a **step in squamous metaplasia** of the endocervical epithelium is discussed below.

The significance of basal cell hyperplasia of endocervical epithelium is in the **similarity of these small benign cells to small cancer cells.** The benign cells occur in flat clusters that are rarely dispersed. Also, the basal cells lack the nuclear features characteristic of cancer cells, described and discussed in Chapter 11. Errors of interpretation of such small cells may be twofold: **benign basal cells may be mistaken for cancer cells but, more often, the small cancer cells are mistaken for benign cells, sometimes with disastrous consequences for the patient.**

Squamous Metaplasia

Squamous metaplasia is a **replacement of normal endocervical epithelium by squamous epithelium** of varying degrees of maturity (see Fig. 6-12). This is a very frequent event that may be confined to a small area of the endocervix

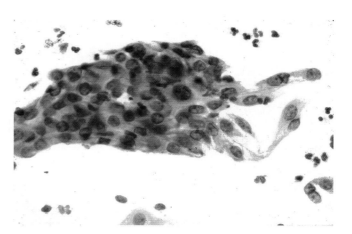

Figure 10-3   Basal cell hyperplasia of endocervix. A cluster of relatively small polygonal cells attached to well-differentiated endocervical cells.

or may be very extensive and involve the **surface epithelium and the glands.** Squamous metaplasia is a **normal, physiological event** during maturation of the female genital tract, notably in the epithelium of the transformation zone, as discussed in Chapter 8.

Pathogenesis

Electron microscopic studies, notably by Bonilla-Musoles and Barbera (1970) and by Philipp (1975), documented that the small **basal or reserve cells** of the endocervical epithelium have the dual potential of differentiating either into mucus-producing normal endocervical cells or into squamous cells, a view confirmed by Tsutsumi et al (1993). It is likely that **hormones,** notably estrogens, play a role in the origin of squamous metaplasia. However, because squamous metaplasia is often observed in biopsy material from cervices showing chronic inflammation, it has also been linked to **inflammatory processes.** Squamous metaplasia is also observed in the presence of intrauterine contraceptive devices and, therefore, may be a **reaction to mechanical pressure.** The precise mechanisms leading to squamous metaplasia must still be elucidated. There may be some **analogy between squamous metaplasia and the events occurring in the formation of the epidermis,** as proposed by Sun et al (see Chap. 2). Sun documented that the transformation of a simple cuboidal epithelium into mature epidermis of the skin is accompanied by a sequential activation of keratin genes of ever higher molecular weights (see Fig. 2-25). Still, keratin polypeptides in metaplastic epithelium appear to be unique and differ from cytokeratins normally present in the squamous epithelium of the cervix and those found in the endocervical epithelium (Gigi-Leitner et al, 1986).

The metaplastic epithelium occurring within the area of the **transformation zone (squamocolumnar junction)** is commonly **involved in initial neoplastic events** affecting the uterine cervix, as discussed in Chapter 11.

Histology

The earliest stages of squamous metaplasia can be identified as a focus of multiplication of the basal cells of the endocervical epithelium. As these small cells grow towards the surface and become larger, their **cytoplasm becomes eosinophilic and homogeneous** (Fig. 10-4A). The glandular epithelium may remain on the surface while the underlying squamous epithelium forms increasingly mature cells. In most cases, however, the glandular surface epithelium is cast off and the endocervical epithelium is replaced by squamous

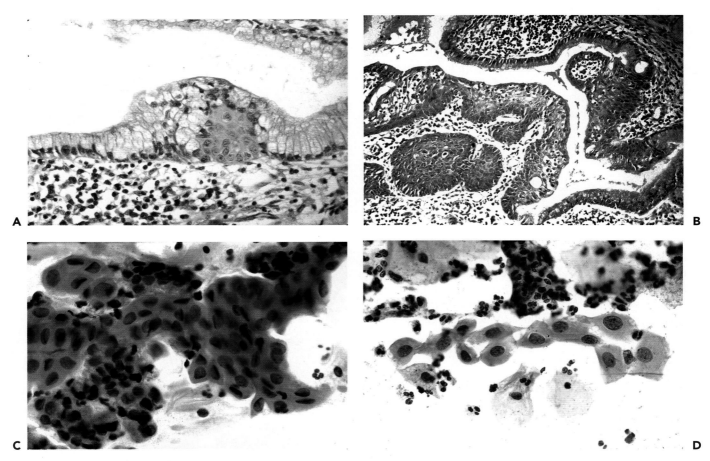

Figure 10-4   Squamous metaplasia of endocervix. *A.* A focus of squamous metaplasia undermining the endocervical glandular epithelium. *B.* Various stages of squamous metaplasia of the endocervix ranging from mature to immature manifestations of this process. *C.* A cluster of cells from a cervicovaginal smear corresponding to *B* and showing cohesive sheets of metaplastic cells. *D.* Sheets of metaplastic squamous cells showing the characteristic irregular configuration of the cytoplasm.

epithelium that may be either **mature, resembling the squamous epithelium of the vagina,** or **immature,** composed of **smaller squamous cells of intermediate or parabasal type** (Fig. 10-4B). The term *immature,* as used here, should not be confused with a malignant process. Various stages of transition between normal endocervical epithelium and mature metaplastic squamous epithelium may be observed. By special stains, **mucus may nearly always be demonstrated** in the cytoplasm of the metaplastic cells, indicating close relationship to the endocervical epithelium. Squamous metaplasia may replace the endocervical mucosa lining the **endocervical canal** or **endocervical glands.** Squamous metaplasia of endocervical glands may be discrete and focal, or diffuse. In extreme cases, one or several glands may be filled with squamous epithelium. If the metaplastic squamous epithelium is **immature, the finding may mimic a neoplastic process,** as discussed below under atypical metaplasia.

Cytology

Only immature squamous metaplasia can be identified in cytologic material because cells derived from mature metaplasia cannot be distinguished from normal squamous cells. Squamous metaplasia of the endocervical mucosa can be diagnosed **with certainty in cervical smears** if flat sheets of **polygonal parabasal squamous cells with basophilic or eosinophilic cytoplasm** are **contiguous with columnar endocervical cells** (Fig. 10-4C). Within the sheets, the metaplastic squamous cells usually form **clearly visible cell borders.** One surface of the sheets is often **flattened,** corresponding to the surface of the metaplastic epithelium. Occasionally, the clusters of metaplastic cells are **loosely structured** and are composed of **angulated squamous cells** (Fig. 10-4D). On close inspection, the distinct **flattening of the surface** of the cluster is evident and sometimes there are transitions toward well-formed, mucus-producing columnar endocervical cells.

The **cytoplasm** of the metaplastic cells is either **basophilic or eosinophilic** and may show **fine vacuoles** in which **mucus** can be demonstrated by special stain. Occasionally, the vacuoles can be large and may be **infiltrated with polymorphonuclear leukocytes.** The **nuclei** of the metaplastic cells are spherical, measuring on the average 8 μm in diameter, but may be larger. Within the nuclei, small **chromocenters and occasionally tiny nucleoli** may be observed. Rarely, **small spindly keratinized cells** with slender pyknotic nuclei may originate from the surface of squamous metaplastic epithelium.

Unfortunately, **metaplastic cells in their classical configuration in sheets are not always present in cell preparations, particularly those collected in a liquid medium and subsequently dispersed.** In such preparations, the **parabasal metaplastic squamous cells occur singly** and are usually characterized by **irregular, polygonal configuration with cytoplasmic processes, or spikes,** as commonly observed in parabasal cells removed from their epithelial setting. The **cytoplasmic processes are an artifact** occurring during smear preparation by **extensions of the cytoplasm at points of desmosomal junctions** with adjacent

cells. As the cells are being separated during smear preparation, the solid desmosomes resist rupture better than the elastic cytoplasm, which, as a consequence of mechanical stretching, becomes elongated at points of junction. Occasionally, one surface of these cells is flat, corresponding to the lining of the endocervical canal (see Fig. 10-8A).

As has been discussed in Chapter 8, the mere **presence of parabasal squamous cells in a cervicovaginal smear is not diagnostic of metaplasia.** Such cells may originate from the squamous epithelium of the vagina or the cervix under a variety of circumstances unrelated to metaplasia. The term **metaplastic cells** that has been suggested for parabasal cells, while picturesque, is not always scientifically sound.

Several attempts have been made to distinguish metaplastic cells from parabasal cells derived from native squamous epithelium by identification of keratins of various molecular weights. Thus, keratins 15, 16 and, occasionally, keratin 6 were observed in endocervical reserve cells and in squamous metaplasia (Smedts et al, 1993) whereas positive stain for keratin 17 was found useful in the differentization of metaplastic cells from normal parabasal cells (Martens et al, 1999).

Still, **if angulated parabasal cells are trapped in the endocervical mucus or if the sample has been removed directly from the transformation zone or the endocervical canal by an instrument, such cells may be considered as adequate evidence that the smear is representative of the endocervical epithelium undergoing squamous metaplasia.** The information on the value of such findings in liquid preparations as evidence of smear adequacy is not available. This issue is important in ensuring the adequacy of cervical smears, discussed in Chapter 8.

Atypical Squamous Metaplasia

Occasionally, the component cells of squamous metaplasia in tissue and smears show slight to severe abnormalities. The **slight changes** are **cell and nuclear enlargement or binucleation confined to a few cells within the cluster** (Fig. 10-5A). Although, in my experience, slight abnormalities of metaplastic cells are usually of no consequence to the patient and the biopsies in such cases disclose minimally atypical metaplasia, more severe changes, described below, often require further investigation of the patient.

More **severe changes** in metaplastic cells include **significant cellular and nuclear enlargement, variability in nuclear sizes, coarse granulation of chromatin and the presence of prominent nucleoli** (Fig. 10-5B–D). Some of these changes **may resemble "repair,"** discussed below. Because the precise identification of such changes is difficult, their classification as "metaplastic" or "endocervical" may depend on the preference of the observer. No doubt some of these abnormalities could be classified as **atypical squamous or endocervical cells of unknown significance (ASCUS or AGUS),** which will be discussed in detail in Chapter 11. On further investigation, many such patients

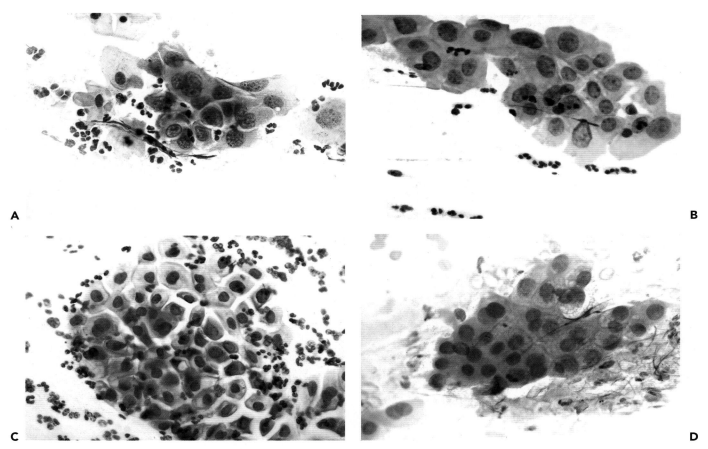

Figure 10-5 **Atypical squamous metaplasia.** *A.* A cohesive sheet of metaplastic endocervical cells showing nuclear enlargement and small nucleoli. *B.* A sheet of metaplastic cells showing significant nuclear enlargement. There was no evidence of a neoplastic lesion in this patient. *C.* A sheet of metaplastic endocervical cells showing variability in nuclear sizes. *D.* A sheet of metaplastic cells showing the "honeycomb" arrangement with clearly visible cell borders. The sizes of the nuclei are variable.

are subsequently shown to harbor precancerous lesions or even cancer **of either squamous or endocervical type.** Therefore, **patients with marked nuclear changes** (Fig. 10-5B–D) **should have the benefit of a close, careful follow-up, including colposcopy and biopsies of cervix,** particularly if, in addition to cell clusters, single abnormal cells are present in the smear. The role of testing for human papillomavirus in such cases is discussed in Chapter 11.

Tubal and Tubo-Endometrioid Metaplasia

Besides common squamous metaplasia, the endocervical epithelium occasionally shows **features of tubal or endometrial epithelium,** sometimes side by side. The condition has been labeled **metaplasia,** although in all probability, it represents a common variant of normal endocervical epithelium. As noted in Chapter 8 and described in detail by Babkowski et al (1996), **ciliated endocervical cells are invariably present in the upper, proximal reaches of the normal endocervical canal.**

Histology

In 1990, Suh and Silverberg described tubal metaplasia as a replacement of the normal epithelium, lining the endocer-

vical surface and glands, by **epithelium of tubal type,** composed of **columnar ciliated cells, clear secretory cells, and intercalated cells** (Fig. 10-6A). The secretory cells may show apocrine **snouts,** or small cytoplasmic projections, on their surfaces. The variant is common, as it was found in 31% of surgical specimens by Jonasson et al (1992). Some of the endocervical glands may also show the features of **endometrial epithelium,** occasionally accompanied by **endometrial stroma,** and thus suggestive of **endometriosis** (Oliva et al, 1995). The tubal or endometrial lining may form papillary projections and show cystic dilatation. All these features confer on the endocervical glands an unusual aspect that may vaguely resemble **precursor lesions of** endocervical adenocarcinoma, discussed in Chapter 12. However, the **cells lining the endocervical glands usually do not show any significant nuclear abnormalities** and are, therefore, consistent with benign lesions. However, personal experience shows that in some of these lesions, **the ciliated epithelium and adjacent endocervical glands may show marked abnormalities in the form of accumulation of small, highly abnormal cells with irregular, hyperchromatic nuclei, strongly suggestive of a small cell carcinoma.** This observation received strong support from work by Schlesinger and Silverberg (1999) who described several

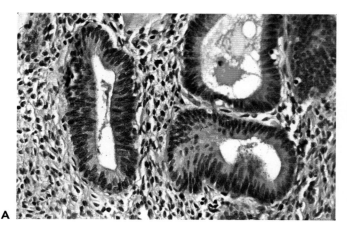

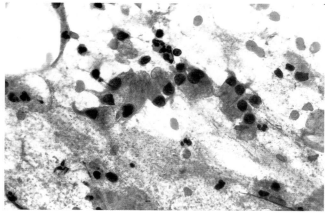

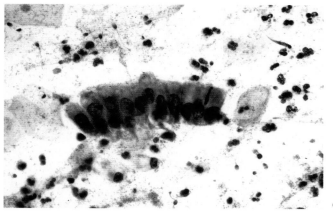

Figure 10-6   Tubal metaplasia. *A.* Biopsy of endocervix showing glands with ciliated surface and minor variability in nuclear sizes. *B.* Ciliated endocervical cells with somewhat hyperchromatic nuclei of even sizes. *C.* A sheet of endocervical cells from the upper reaches of the endocervical canal showing dark, somewhat enlarged nuclei of even sizes.

cases of endocervical carcinoma in situ of tubal type and stressed that the mere presence of ciliated epithelium does not guarantee that the lesion is benign.

Cytology of Tubal Metaplasia

With the widespread use of rigorous endocervical brushing techniques the presence of ciliated endocervical cells has become much more common in cervical smears than with the use of cervical scrapers. Thus "tubal metaplasia" became a recognized cytologic entity. In brush smears in some cases of tubal metaplasia, one can observe sheets of essentially normal ciliated endocervical cells with enlarged hyperchromatic nuclei (Fig. 10-6B,C). In some such cases, the nuclear abnormalities may be significant and the cells may be classified as **atypical glandular cells of unknown significance (AGUS),** requiring further investigation. Ducatman et al (1993) also claimed that one could recognize in smears the "peg cells," characterized by "dark and granular cytoplasm and elongated nuclei." We have not been able to identify such cells with certainty.

Cytologic Abnormalities in Tubal Metaplasia

Novotny et al (1992) claimed that tubal metaplasia may shed **abnormal cells** that can be **mistaken for cells derived from precursor lesions of endocervical adenocarcinoma.** These authors provided an elaborate table, listing the cytologic features of both types of lesions. This has not been my experience. As mentioned above, in

several cases seen in consultation in which smears contained **ciliated cells accompanied by small abnormal or suspicious cells, the corresponding biopsy material disclosed marked abnormalities of endocervical glands and adjacent endocervical epithelium, consistent with a malignant process.** Within the neoplastic epithelium, ciliated cells were occasionally present. These observations confirm that **cytologic abnormalities always have their counterpart in corresponding histologic material and are in keeping with the concept of carcinomas with ciliated cells, perhaps developing in tubal metaplasia,** as described by Schlesinger and Silverberg (1999). For further discussion of precancerous lesions of the endocervical epithelium, see Chapter 12.

Endometriosis

It has been mentioned above that Oliva et al (1995) observed the presence of endometrial stromal cells in areas of endometrioid metaplasia of the endocervix, consistent with the diagnosis of endometriosis. Similar observations were reported by Yeh et al (1993). No specific histologic or cytologic abnormalities were attributed by these authors to the histologic findings. However, Mulvany and Surtees (1999) reported that the **cervical brush smears in 7 of 10 cases of endometriosis located in the uterine cervix or vagina contained cells interpreted as consistent with endocervical adenocarcinoma, either invasive or in situ.** The cytologic abnormalities consisted of **nuclear hyperchromasia, large cohesive cell clusters, and the presence of mitotic activity and of necrotic cells, described as "apoptosis."** Similar observations were reported by Hanau et al (1997). The histologic findings in these cases disclosed various degrees of atypia in the glands which, in two cases, was "severe." Although Mulvany and Surtees did not classify the abnormalities as malignant, it is well known that endometrioid carcinomas may originate in the endometriotic glands (Koss, 1963; Brooks and Wheeler, 1977; Mostoufizadeh and Scully, 1980). These abnormalities must be considered in the differential diagnosis of endocervical adenocarcinoma.

Lesions Erroneously Classified as Metaplasia

There are few, if any, fields of microscopy that are as difficult to interpret as cervicovaginal cytopathology. The difficulty is compounded by the facts that many of the precancerous lesions of the uterine cervix have an unpredictable behavior and may require many years of follow-up until their true nature becomes evident, as discussed in Chapter 11. The interpretation of the cytologic material and of histologic patterns in **biopsy material** may be equally difficult and the separation of the **atypical metaplastic processes from true neoplasia may depend on the judgment, training, and experience of the observer.** Some investigators have suggested that human **papillomavirus typing** may help in the final classification of such difficult lesions (Crum et al, 1997) but this expensive technique is not always available and not necessarily reliable. It is, therefore, not surprising that under the **term of "metaplasia," several entities have been described in recent years that in the judgment of this writer are an erroneous and misleading misclassification of lesions that belong to the spectrum of precancerous lesions of the uterine cervix.**

Trivijitslip et al (1998) described a **papillary immature metaplasia (PIM),** a form of somewhat atypical metaplasia with formation of papillary folds. This abnormality was thought to represent an **immature form of condyloma of the uterine cervix epithelium** and was attributed by Mosher to infection with nononcogenic papillomaviruses types 6 and 11. Still, in a further study of PIM by Trivijitslip and Mosher (1998), **three of nine patients with PIM harbored a high-grade squamous intraepithelial lesion.** Thus, PIM should be included in the spectrum of precancerous events in the uterine cervix.

A particularly **dangerous concept** has been introduced into cervical cytology by Dressel and Wilbur (1992) under the term **atypical immature squamous metaplastic cells. Atypical metaplastic cells are small cancer cells that have some superficial similarity to metaplastic cells but differ markedly by the configuration of nuclei.** Such cells are described and discussed in Chapter 11. In an elaborate study, Geng et al (1999) confirmed the neoplastic nature of "atypical immature metaplasia." In 12 of 15 patients in whom the presence of human papillomavirus DNA was documented by polymerase chain reaction, a concurrent or subsequent diagnosis of a high-grade squamous epithelial lesion was established on biopsies. Park et al (1999) concluded that observer agreement in the differential diagnosis of this lesion from a high-grade neoplastic lesion was poor and not assisted by HPV typing.

Another misleading concept has been introduced by Egan and Russel (1997) under the name of **transitional (urothelial) cell metaplasia of the uterine cervix.** The entity was also described by Weir et al (1997) but was strenuously rejected by Koss (1998). In my judgment, many of the lesions described represent **intraepithelial neoplastic lesions of the uterine cervix undergoing atrophy** and occurring mainly in postmenopausal women. Harnden et al (1999) admitted that the so-called transitional metaplasia lacks the cardinal features of the urothelium. In many such cases, the cytologic and biopsy findings suggested a high-grade squamous intraepithelial lesion (HGSIL).

The entities inappropriately classified as **metaplasia** are discussed again in Chapter 11 together with other precancerous lesions of the cervix.

Microglandular Hyperplasia of Endocervical Glands

In 1967, Taylor et al reported that, in biopsies of patients receiving contraceptive hormones, a **marked proliferation of small endocervical glands** may be observed. The lesion may be polypoid and imitate an endocervical polyp or, in rare cases, adenocarcinoma of the cervix or endometrium (Young and Scully, 1989). Numerous other reports were published subsequent to Taylor's paper, generally attributing this lesion to contraceptive medication containing progesterone (recent summary in Candy and Abell, 2001). There is no doubt, however, that such lesions **may also be observed in the absence of contraceptive medication, in pregnant and postmenopausal women,** and, in about one-fourth of all cases, without an obvious cause at all.

Histology and Cytology

In tissue sections, microglandular hyperplasia consists of a grouping of well-formed endocervical glands of markedly variable sizes. The glands are lined by normal endocervical cells. The proliferation of smaller glands may deceptively suggest an invasion of the stroma and thus adenocarcinoma (Fig. 10-7A). Unusual histologic presentation of these lesions may include areas of solid growth and mucus-containing signet ring cells (Leslie and Silverberg, 1984; Young and Scully, 1989). In some such cases, the differentiation from endocervical or endometrial adenocarcinoma may cause problems. Clinical history and absence of mitotic activity and nuclear abnormalities are usually sufficient to reach the correct diagnostic conclusion.

On the other hand, some well-differentiated carcinomas may sometimes mimic microglandular hyperplasia. Nuclear abnormalities and mitotic activity are present in such lesions (Young and Scully, 1992). It has been suggested by Daniele et al (1993) and Alvarez-Santin et al (1999) that microglandular hyperplasia can be recognized in cervical brush smears by the presence of 2- and 3-dimensional fenestrated clusters of endocervical cells, some forming small, gland-like struc-

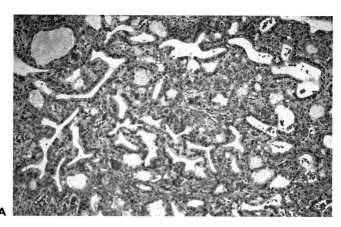
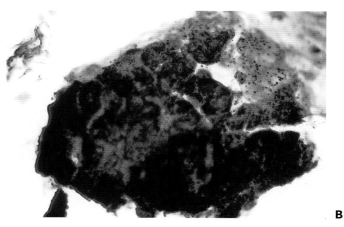

Figure 10-7   Microglandular hyperplasia. *A.* Section of endocervix showing numerous glands of uneven sizes and configuration, separated by fibrous stroma and lined by cuboidal cells of even sizes. *B.* A large complex fragment of endocervical epithelium in a brush specimen, conceivably reflecting microglandular hyperplasia.

tures (Fig. 10-7B). In order to secure such clusters, a very energetic brushing of the endocervix is required. **In our experience, there are no specific cytologic abnormalities that would allow a reproducible recognition of microglandular hyperplasia.** Some of the findings described are most likely artifacts caused by endocervical brushings (see below). However, some observers reported marked cytologic abnormalities associated with microglandular hyperplasia (Valente et al, 1994; Selvaggi and Haefner, 1997; Selvaggi, 2000). It is our judgment that, in such cases, the microglandular hyperplasia is an incidental biopsy finding. There is excellent evidence that the presence of **microglandular hyperplasia does not rule out the presence of precancerous intraepithelial lesions** of the cervix, as first pointed out by Nichols and Fidler (1971), or, for that matter, one of the rare cervical or endometrial **adenocarcinomas mimicking microglandular hyperplasia** (Young and Scully, 1992). Thus, the presence of atypical cells in smears calls for a careful investigation of the uterine cervix by methods discussed in Chapters 11 and 12, regardless whether or not microglandular hyperplasia is present.

Other Benign Abnormalities of Endocervical Glands

Tunnel clusters is an arrangement of endocervical glands forming small tubules or "tunnels" (Fluhmann, 1961A). A cystic form of this abnormality has been described (Segal and Hart, 1990).

Mesonephric hyperplasia is a proliferation of the remanents of Gartner (mesonephric) ducts usually located within the smooth muscle of the cervix (Ferry and Scully, 1990; Jones and Andrews, 1993).

Endocervicosis is a proliferation of histologically normal endocervical glands in an abnormal location, such as the outer rim of the uterine cervix or the urinary bladder (Young and Clement, 2000).

These lesions may be confused with endocervical adenocarcinoma in tissue sections. There is no systematic

study of the **cytologic presentation** of these benign lesions. Anecdotal evidence suggests that there are no specific cytologic abnormalities that would allow their recognition. The cytologic presentation of Gartner (mesonephric) duct carcinoma is described in Chapter 12.

ABNORMALITIES OF THE TRANSFORMATION ZONE. EVERSION OR ECTROPION ("EROSION") OF THE CERVIX

As discussed in Chapter 8, the squamous and endocervical types of epithelium usually meet within the **squamocolumnar junction or the transformation zone** of the uterine cervix. In some young women, the two epithelia meet on the surface of the vaginal portio of the cervix, outside of the external os. As a consequence, a **sharply circumscribed red patch appears on the vaginal portio of the cervix,** adjacent to the external os. The patch is lined by the delicate **endocervical glandular epithelium,** which is transparent. The visible vessels of the cervical stroma give the area the **red appearance** on visual inspection. Because to the naked eye the patch may mimic an ulcer, the **faulty clinical term of erosion** has been applied to the lesion. The correct term is **eversion or ectropion** (from Greek: *ek* = out, *trope* = a turning). The ectropion may occupy a small segment of the visible cervix or surround the external os (**circumoral erosion**). The importance of the ectropion is largely **clinical,** inasmuch as the red patch must be **differentiated from true ulceration of the cervix due to inflammation or to cancer.**

Histology and Cytology

The patch is lined by typical endocervical epithelium, sometimes forming papillary folds, containing a normal, occasionally hyperemic stroma (Fig. 10-8A). It is not uncommon to find a few normal endocervical glands in the area

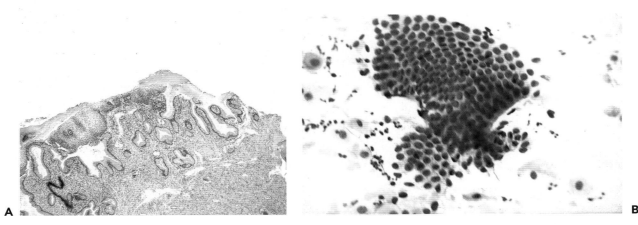

Figure 10-8 Eversion of endocervical mucosa. *A.* Histologic section showing the surface of the transformation zone lined by endocervical epithelium. Foci of squamous metaplasia are present. *B.* Sheet of normal endocervical cells characteristic of eversion in cervical smears.

of the ectropion. Direct cervical smears contain only **fragments of benign endocervical tissue and single columnar endocervical cells** (Fig. 10-8B). Because the delicate epithelium lining the area is readily damaged during the process of obtaining smears, fresh blood is often present in the cytologic specimen. If a portion or all of the everted endocervical mucosa has undergone squamous metaplasia, squamous cells of varying degrees of maturity will appear in smears. The cytologic picture is vastly different from inflammatory or neoplastic lesions that may also occur in this part of the cervix, as described below and in Chapter 11. The eversion requires no treatment because, with the passage of time, it will undergo squamous metaplasia.

REPAIR (FLORID SQUAMOUS METAPLASIA)

The term **repair** has been introduced into the field of gynecologic cytology by Bibbo et al (1971) and by Patten (1978). These authors described atypical cells of endocervical and squamous origin with a number of abnormal cytoplasmic and nuclear features in patients with recent past history of radiotherapy to the uterine cervix, recent hysterectomy, other clinical procedures, such as cautery or biopsy, past history of severe cervicitis (Bibbo et al, 1971), and "partial or complete destruction (of the epithelium) by infection and inflammation" (Patten, 1978). Thus, this is a very heterogeneous group of patients wherein many different factors may account for the cellular abnormalities. Most important, perhaps, histologic evidence of true repair of a damaged epithelium (i.e., epithelial regrowth over a defect) has not been provided by Bibbo and to a very limited extent by Patten.

The **concept of repair** is valid but only under well-defined circumstances, for example, after a conization of the uterine cervix or other documented form of epithelial injury. In the histologic material, **tongues of poorly formed, young epithelial cells bridging the defect caused by prior surgery**

may be observed (Fig. 10-9A). The mechanisms of "repair" or healing of a wounded epithelium are extremely complex (Singer and Clark, 1999) and have not been studied in the uterine cervix but probably resemble those in the skin.

Cytology

A smear obtained approximately 1 week after a procedure damaging the cervical epithelium may show some rather **characteristic cytologic features.** The smears show **flat sheets, composed of tightly fitting cells, generally resembling metaplastic cells** (Fig. 10-9B,C). The cells may **vary in size** and their cytoplasm may be vacuolated and infiltrated with polymorphonuclear leukocytes. Occasionally, the cells may show **bizarre, sometimes elongated configuration.** The **nuclei** of these cells also **vary in size, may show some degree of hyperchromasia, and, most importantly, contain one or more clearly visible nucleoli of variable sizes. Mitotic figures can be observed** (Fig. 10-9D). There are usually **few, if any, single cells** with similar characteristics. The background of the smear usually shows a great deal of fresh blood and inflammation.

The manifestations of repair may be particularly **difficult to interpret in smears of postmenopausal women with epithelial atrophy.** The nuclei of the epithelial cells are enlarged, of uneven sizes, and hyperchromatic, mimicking malignant lesions. Because the thin epithelial lining offers little protection, bundles of spindly cells representing cervical stroma, may be present. We observed such cells after cervical biopsies, conization, or energetic curettage. "Repair" reaction may occur **after surgical procedures,** as illustrated above, **as a reaction to chronic inflammatory events** or in the presence of a **foreign body or object in the endocervical canal.** For example, **intrauterine contraceptive devices** or **endocervical polyps** may be the cause of such abnormalities (see below). There remain, however, a number of patients in whom similar cell abnormalities may be observed in smears **in the absence of any known events that could account for the "repair."** It is likely that, in such patients, the cell abnormalities represent an **exuberant**

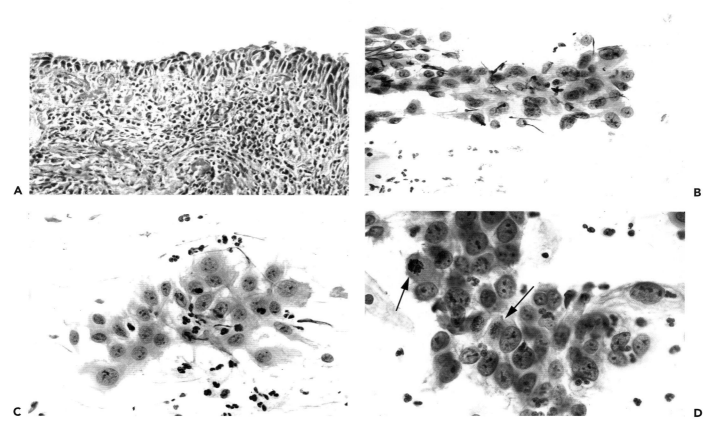

Figure 10-9 "Repair." *A.* The appearance of the cervical epithelium 4 days after a cone biopsy. The surface is lined by small, atypical epithelial cells. *B.* A sheet of epithelial cells from the same patient showing marked variability in sizes and configuration, corresponding to the young epithelium lining the surface of the cervical defect. *C.* Irregular flat sheets of endocervical or metaplastic cells showing prominent nucleoli. *D.* A cluster of endocervical cells showing marked variability in nuclear sizes and prominent nucleoli. Mitotics figure are present (*arrows*).

or **florid squamous metaplasia** of the endocervical epithelium.

The cytologic changes attributed to repair are similar to those occurring in inflammatory changes in the endocervical cells, described further on in this chapter, or in atypical squamous metaplasia, described above. The conspicuous atypia, such as shown in Figure 10-9D, **may reflect a neoplastic lesion, such as a high-grade squamous epithelial lesion or an endocervical adenocarcinoma. In such cases, however, the cell clusters are usually accompanied by single cells with similar morphologic features** (see Chaps. 11 and 12). Geirsson et al (1977) analyzed the features of the cells in repair and compared them with cells of adenocarcinoma. There was a significant overlap between the two lesions, particularly in reference to nucleolar abnormalities. It is virtually impossible to arrive at a conclusive cytologic diagnosis in such cases and **patients should be evaluated further by colposcopy and cervical and endocervical biopsies. The Bethesda System** of cervicovaginal smear classification, described in Chapter 11, calls for separation of **"typical" from "atypical" repair.** This proposition is not reasonable because the cytologic pattern of repair is atypical by definition. For example, Rimm et al (1996) observed that 25% of patients with "atypical repair"

pattern in smears harbored squamous intraepithelial lesions of low or high grade. Colgan et al (2001) reported that in a major survey of laboratories in the United States, **repair was the most common source of false-positive and false-negative smears**.

In the absence of supporting clinical or histologic evidence, **the concept of repair, although occasionally correct, is a dangerous one as it may mislead even an experienced observer. Cell abnormalities of considerable magnitude not based on secure clinical and histologic data must be investigated further, regardless of label.**

ENDOCERVICAL POLYPS

This common benign tumor may originate in any area of the endocervical canal. **Histologically,** a polyp is composed of a central connective tissue stalk lined by gland-forming endocervical mucosa. Squamous metaplastic epithelium may replace portions of the outer lining and may extend to the glands. Inflammation of varying type and intensity is often observed in the stroma. Very uncommonly, cervix cancer may start in a polyp.

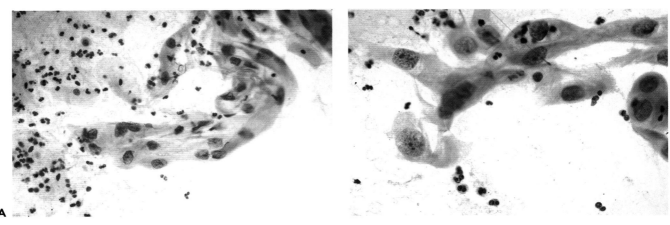

Figure 10-10 Repair reaction caused by an endocervical polyp. *A,B.* Marked abnormalities of metaplastic squamous cells with very large nuclei and bizarre cell shapes.

An **endocervical polyp cannot be recognized in cervical smears,** except for the rare events when a fragment of polyp may be observed (Ngadiman and Yang, 1995). Still, polyps may **cause nonspecific atypias of squamous and endocervical cells.** Small, **keratinized squamous cells** with fairly large pyknotic nuclei may be occasionally observed in cervical smears corresponding to areas of somewhat atypical squamous metaplasia on the surface of the polyp. In rare instances, the pressure of the polyp on adjacent endocervical epithelium may cause a **florid repair reaction** (Fig. 10-10A,B). Upon removal of the polyp, the cytologic abnormalities promptly disappear. Nevertheless, this uncommon occurrence represents a potentially important source of cytologic error.

EFFECTS OF INTRAUTERINE CONTRACEPTIVE DEVICES (IUD)

Sagiroglu and Sagiroglu (1970) documented that intrauterine contraceptive devices produce a chronic inflammatory reaction in the endometrium, resulting in the presence of leukocytes and macrophages in uterine lavage and in smears obtained directly from IUDs after removal. These authors suggested that the principal contraceptive effect of these devices is related to the presence of macrophages, which are capable of phagocytosis of spermatozoa. The effect of IUDs on the **endometrial cytology** and smear pattern has been discussed in Chapter 8 and is discussed again in reference to endometrial pathology in Chapter 13.

Endocervical Epithelium

The mechanical effect of IUD on endocervical epithelium may result in the shedding of columnar **endocervical cells with distended, vacuolated cytoplasm.** Occasionally, the vacuoles may be infiltrated by polymorphonuclear leukocytes, thus mimicking cells of endometrial adenocarcinoma (see Chap. 13). The cells may be similar to those observed in some instances of squamous metaplasia, described above. The pressure of the IUD on the endocervical epithelium

may also result in **florid squamous metaplasia or the "repair reaction,"** as shown in Figures 10-9 and 10-10. Although Sagiroglu and Sagiroglu (1970) observed innumerable macrophages in smears obtained directly from IUDs after removal, there is no evidence that the population of these cells is significantly increased in routine cervical or vaginal samples of women wearing IUDs.

Other Findings

An important finding in women wearing IUDs is the presence of bacteria, *Actinomyces*, discussed in detail in the second part of this chapter and observed mainly in women wearing devices made of plastic for 3 or more consecutive years without replacement. The presence of *amoebae* in smears of IUD users was described by Arroyo and Quinn (1989) and by DeMoraes-Ruehsen et al (1980).

An occasionally disturbing finding in cervical smears from such patients is **amorphous debris that are sometimes calcified** (Fig. 10-11A–C) and occasionally form **small, concentrically calcified spherical bodies, akin to psammoma bodies.** The latter may be surrounded by macrophages (Fig. 10-11D). Schmidt et al (1980, 1982, 1986) has shown, by electron microscopy, that the calcified debris in IUD wearers represents fragments of plastic. There are usually few problems with the identification of the calcified debris. However, because psammoma bodies are commonly associated with ovarian and sometimes endometrial cancer (see Chaps. 13 and 15), the presence of debris mimicking psammoma bodies **calls for a precautionary examination of the patient after removal of the IUD.** The most commonly applied procedure is ultrasound of the pelvic organs.

A number of studies, beginning with the study by Melamed et al (1969) and subsequently repeatedly confirmed (Boyce et al, 1972; Ory et al, 1975; Sandmire et al, 1976) noted that **women using oral contraceptives or wearing IUD were at a higher risk of neoplastic cervical lesions than women using barrier contraceptives,** such as a diaphragm. These differences may be caused by exposure to human papillomaviruses, as discussed in Chapter 11. There-

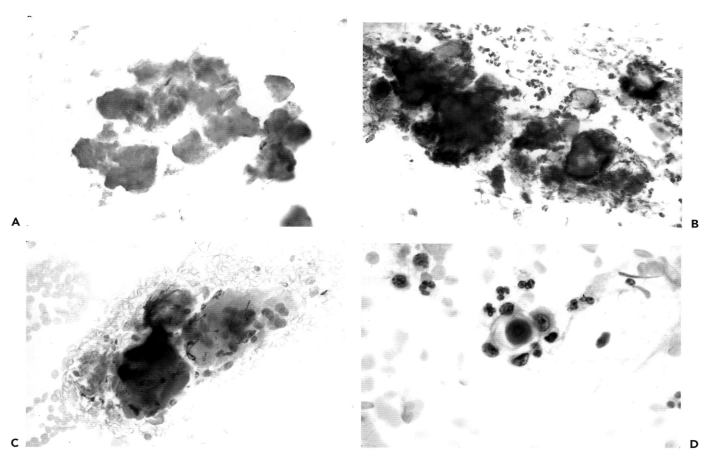

Figure 10-11 **Effects of intrauterine contraceptive devices (IUD).** *A,B.* Calcified debris characteristic of this condition. *C.* Calcified debris with a foreign body giant cell. *D.* A very small calcified fragment with concentric calcification, surrounded by macrophages, shown under high magnification. This structure, although very small, was similar to a psammoma body. There was no evidence of neoplasm on careful examination.

fore, the screening and evaluation of smears from patients wearing IUDs must be thorough and careful, and any abnormalities that cannot be clearly attributed to the device itself should be further evaluated and investigated.

CHANGES INDUCED BY ENDOCERVICAL BRUSHES

The widespread use of endocervical brush instruments had for its purpose securing cells from the endocervical canal to insure adequacy of sampling. However, rigorous use of these instruments may also result in cytologic abnormalities that may cause difficulties of interpretation. The resulting smear may contain **thick clusters of endocervical cells, sometimes of complex configuration (such as loose peripheral cells, a phenomenon known as "feathering") that may mimic changes attributed to endocervical carcinoma** (Fig. 10-12A–C). It is possible that some of the cellular changes attributed to various abnormalities of the uterine endocervix, such as tubal metaplasia or microglandular hyperplasia are actually brush-induced artifacts. These clusters may persist in liquid preparations and may also cause prob-

lems of interpretation. **The fundamental principle of cytopathology requires that all cell abnormalities in smears must find their counterpart in histologic material. Lesions incidentally found in histologic material are not necessarily the source of cytologic abnormalities and vice versa, without appropriate documentation.**

Wilbur (1995) also pointed out that endocervical brushings present the observer with numerous difficult-to-interpret cell images that may be mistaken for various neoplastic lesions. Babkowski et al (1996) pointed out that **the most complex cell clusters** are derived from the upper reaches of the endocervical canal and may be associated with tubal metaplasia (see above). Such clusters are occasionally too dense or too complex to interpret as normal and may either lead to unnecessary biopsies or result in a request for additional sampling. If the additional sampling is performed **before the brush-induced injury to the cervical epithelium has healed** (6 to 12 weeks), the resulting atypia of **repair** may cause additional interpretative difficulties (Fig. 10-12D). In my experience, the **interpretation of thick, 3-dimensional endocervical cell clusters should be conservative, unless the smear also contains abnormal cells singly or in small clusters that are easier to evaluate.** It is rare for a neoplastic

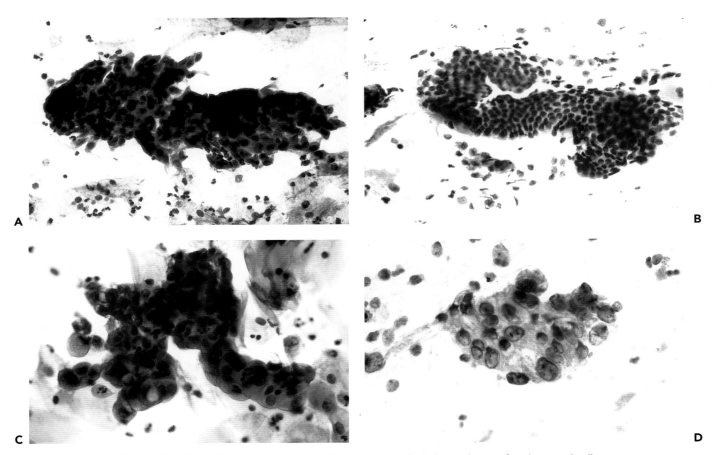

Figure 10-12 Artifacts induced by brushes. *A.* A very thick, large cluster of endocervical cells difficult to analyze. *B.* A very large sheet of endocervical cells difficult to interpret. *C.* Thick clusters of endocervical cells with "feathering" mimicking the appearance of endocervical adenocarcinoma. *D.* Marked endocervical repair reaction in a smear obtained 2 weeks after previous brushing.

lesion to occur in the form of tightly knit clusters of endocervical cells, without some ancillary evidence of disease, as discussed in the appropriate chapters.

Another consequence of rigorous brushings is the presence of normal **endometrial cells** in the sample. Such small cells, when seen in the endocervical sample may be **mistaken for small cancer cells.** This issue is discussed further in Chapter 8.

In general, the endocervical brush instruments, hailed as an important advance in cervicovaginal cytology because they insure sampling of the endocervical canal, are also a source of potential diagnostic errors.

INFLAMMATORY PROCESSES OF THE FEMALE GENITAL TRACT

INFLAMMATORY AGENTS

Inflammatory processes within the female genital tract may be caused by infections with a variety of microorganisms and parasites or by physical and chemical agents. Sometimes the causes of the inflammation remain unknown as in Behçet's

disease (Sakane et al, 1999). In this chapter, the basic mechanism of inflammation and diseases caused by bacterial, fungal, viral, and parasitic agents will be described. The physical and chemical agents are discussed in Chapter 18. Most of the organisms responsible for inflammatory processes may be recognized in Papanicolaou-stained smears although, occasionally, special stains or procedures may be required for identification. The principal infectious agents are as follows:

Bacterial agents
  Cocci and coccoid bacteria
    Gram-positive cocci: species of *Streptococcus* and *Staphylococcus*
    Gram-negative cocci: *Gonococcus*
    Gardnerella vaginalis (Haemophilus vaginale or *vaginalis)*
    Diphtheroids
    Calymmatobacterium granulomatis Donovan *(granuloma inguinale)*
    Mycoplasma and *Ureaplasma*
    Chlamydia trachomatis
  Acid-fast organisms: *Mycobacterium tuberculosis, Mycobacterium avium*
  Actinomyces
  Spirochaeta pallida (syphilis)

Organisms that are normally saprophytic but may be associated with infections:

Lactobacillus (Döderlein bacillus) and Leptothrix

Other uncommon bacterial agents

Fungal agents

Candida species: C. albicans (monilia), C. glabrata (Torulopsis glabrata)

Aspergillus species

Coccidioidomycosis

Paracoccidioidomycosis

Cryptococcus species

Blastomyces

Viral agents

Herpesvirus types I, II, VIII

Cytomegalovirus

Human polyomavirus

Measles

Adenovirus

Molluscum contagiosum (vulva)

Human papillomavirus, various types (see Chap. 11)

Other rare viruses

Parasitic infections and infestations

Protozoa

Trichomonas vaginalis

Entamoeba histolytica

Entamoeba gingivalis

Balantidium coli

Helminths (worms)

Schistosoma haematobium, S. mansoni, S. japonicum

Filariae

Intestinal worms

Enterobius vermicularis (pinworm)

Trichuris trichiura (whipworm)

Teniae (flat worms)

T. solium (intermediate host: swine)

T. saginata (intermediate host: cattle)

T. echinococcus (intermediate host: dog)

Other uncommon parasites

Trypanosomiasis

With the spread of the **acquired immunodeficiency syndrome (AIDS),** in which normal immune defenses of the human body are reduced or abolished, unusual organisms (not listed above) may be encountered.

MECHANISMS OF INFLAMMATION

The female genital tract is a common site of inflammatory processes that may involve the **vulva, vagina, uterine cervix, endometrium** and spread to organs located in the bony pelvis, such as the **fallopian tubes, ovaries, and parametria.** Many, although not all, of the agents causing inflammation may be sexually transmitted (Borchardt and Noble, 1996).

The **predisposing factors** are: not fully mature squamous epithelium of the vagina and cervix, such as that seen in prepubertal girls or in menopausal women; injury to the endocervical canal, especially during pregnancy or delivery; or trauma of any kind. The variations of the **vaginal acidity (pH)** are also significant. Alkaline pH, such as observed

during the menstrual flow, favors the growth of the common parasite, Trichomonas vaginalis, which does not prosper in an acid pH of less than 5. Other microorganisms have other pH requirements.

Three **basic pathways of infection** of the genital tract are recognized:

1. **Direct invasion** of the genital tract by pathogens, often sexually transmitted
2. Spread of an infectious process **from an adjacent organ**
3. **Blood-borne** infections

Regardless of the pathway or the causative organism, all infectious processes may lead to an acute or chronic inflammatory reaction. Although any component of the female genital tract can be affected by an inflammatory process, **certain agents may favor one type of tissue to another.** For example, Trichomonas vaginalis infestation affects mainly the squamous epithelium of the vagina, cervix, and urethra. Many **pus-producing bacteria,** such as staphylococci and streptococci, find favorable conditions for survival in the **endocervical canal,** whence the infection may spread into the endocervical glands. From the cervix, the infectious agents may ascend the endocervical canal and reach the **endometrium, the fallopian tubes, and thence the pelvic organs, causing pelvic inflammatory disease.** Other organisms may have a different behavior pattern, as will be discussed below. Because the epithelial changes accompanying inflammation may result in considerable cytologic atypias, they are reported in some detail.

Sequence of Events in Inflammatory Processes

An inflammatory process is a complex reaction of the living tissue to various forms of injury that may be caused by a variety of agents, many of them listed above. An excellent summary of the current state of knowledge pertaining to mechanisms of inflammation can be found in a paper by Luster (1998). Only a simple summary of the key events is provided here.

Acute Inflammation

The first event in an acute inflammatory process is injury to the tissue. The common cause of injury is pathogenic organisms or physical and chemical agents. The injury causes **cell death** or **necrosis** which **attracts polymorphonuclear leukocytes,** principally neutrophils, that invade the affected tissue exiting from the dilated **regional capillary vessels.** This function is governed by chemotactic agents known as **chemokines** (Luster, 1998). The role of the neutrophils is to phagocytize, neutralize and destroy the agent(s) causing cell death. There are several consequences of this initial sequence of events. The **capillary vessels** may be injured and blood may seep into the affected area. The neutrophils often die while performing the initial defensive role and release into the surrounding tissues a number of proteolytic enzymes that damage the tissues further, **increasing the area of necrosis.** The second echelon of defenses is vested in **B and T lymphocytes and in macro-**

phages, which enter the area of injury. The macrophages are activated to phagocytize the debris and eliminate the damages. In **some parasitic infestations, eosinophilic leukocytes** may play a key role.

There are several possible **outcomes of the initial, acute inflammatory process:**

- The injurious agent is eliminated, the inflammatory process is contained and healing commences, heralded by activation of **stromal fibroblasts.** The fibroblasts will provide the **collagen** necessary to replace the necrotic, injured tissue, resulting in the formation of a **scar.**
- The acute inflammatory process continues with resulting increased necrosis and formation of **purulent exudate or pus.** Pus is a semiliquid mixture of blood serum, necrotic neutrophils, macrophages and debris derived from the injured tissue. Accumulation of pus within a limited area of tissue results in an **abscess** that may be contained within a **connective tissue capsule** formed by fibroblasts. A breakdown of an abscess towards an open surface results in an **ulcer.** Healing of an abscess usually requires drainage of the pus, followed by a connective tissue growth into the area occupied by the abscess and formation of a scar.
- The acute inflammation may subside and become **chronic.**

Chronic Inflammation

Chronic inflammation is characterized by reduction in the population of polymorphonuclear leukocytes in favor of **lymphocytes** and **macrophages,** often accompanied by **activation of fibroblasts** and new growth of **capillary vessels** into the affected area. In some cases, the process may be designated as **granulation tissue,** because, when located on the surface of an organ, it may be visible to the naked eye as a red granule (see below).

There are several **forms of chronic inflammation.** Some of them are designated as **specific** because of the characteristic changes caused by the nature of the invading microorganism. For example, the infection with **mycobacterium**

tuberculosis, results in **granulomatous inflammation,** which forms a recognizable pattern of abnormalities (granulomas, to be described below). Other chronic inflammatory processes are **nonspecific,** i.e., without features that would allow the identification of the causative organism. Chronic inflammation may have major consequences on cytologic patterns in cervicovaginal smears.

Acute Inflammatory Processes in the Uterine Cervix and Vagina

Histology of Acute Cervicitis and Vaginitis

Of these two organs, the uterine cervix is more often affected than the vagina and is more often sampled by biopsy. The **dominant feature** of acute inflammatory processes in the cervix is the presence of a **dense inflammatory infiltrate,** composed mainly of neutrophils in the stroma of the organ. Dilated capillary vessels with margination of leukocytes are usually observed. Focal necrosis and pus formation may occur.

Changes in Squamous Epithelium

The response of the squamous epithelium to injury is particularly common in *Trichomonas vaginalis* infestations but may also be caused by other inflammatory agents. The first event in inflammation is a **vascular response.** The normally small connective tissue plugs, or **papillae,** that carry the capillary vessels supplying the squamous epithelium with blood, become markedly elongated. The capillary vessels within the papillae become distended with blood, followed by **margination and migration of polymorphonuclear leukocytes** resulting in acute papillitis (Fig. 10-13A). The entire epithelium may become permeated by polymorphonuclear leukocytes. Marked accumulation of fluid **(edema)** in between the epithelial cells is sometimes noted. The squamous epithelium may shed loosely attached layers of superficial cells, leading to **epithelial erosion.** This may be followed by **necrosis** of some part or the entire epithelial thickness which, combined with an inflammatory infiltrate, results in a formation of a **crater: an ulcer.** Purulent exudate

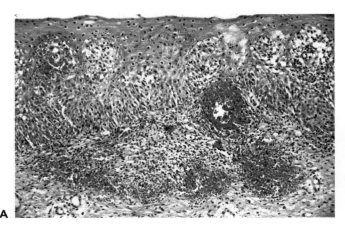
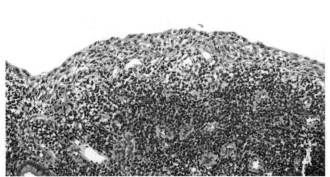

A   **B**

Figure 10-13 **Histology of severe cervicitis.** *A.* Acute inflammatory reaction involving the squamous epithelium and characterized by marked dilatation of capillary vessels. The patient had trichomoniasis. *B.* Severe cervicitis showing damaged surface of the squamous epithelium and thick inflammatory infiltrate involving the stroma and the epithelium.

may coat the necrotic surface (Fig. 10-13B). Inflammatory changes affecting the epithelium of the vagina have a similar histologic pattern.

The Endocervix

The stroma of the endocervix is infiltrated with polymorphonuclear leukocytes and shows other changes described above. Primary necrosis of the endocervical mucosa is uncommon. The endocervix may be coated by a thin layer of pus, but the structures mainly affected are the **endocervical glands,** wherein the acute inflammatory changes and sometimes **abscess formation** may occur. The acute inflammatory processes may cause substantial changes in the endocervical glandular cells: swelling, enlargement, and necrosis of these cells may occur.

Cytology of Acute Cervicitis and Vaginitis

In the presence of an acute inflammation, the smears have a "dirty" appearance, caused by inflammatory exudate (Fig. 10-14A,B). The exudate is composed of a **mixture of polymorphonuclear leukocytes, necrotic cells or cell debris, necrotic cells, and clumps of bacteria** in a background of proteinaceous material and **lysed or fresh blood.** Care must be taken **not to confuse the physiologic presence of scattered polymorphonuclear leukocytes** in premenstrual and menstrual smears and in smears of the mucus plug of the cervix with an acute inflammatory process. In acute inflammation, the squamous cells may display marked **cytoplasmic eosinophilia,** involving the normally basophilic squamous cells of the intermediate and parabasal type (Fig. 10-14C). This feature of the squamous cells is particularly evident in ***Trichomonas vaginalis*** infestation.

During the childbearing age, an **increase in the population of parabasal squamous cells** is a frequent alteration of the cervical smear pattern in acute inflammation that, in extreme cases, may suggest a low level of estrogenic activity and may even mimic the pattern of post-menopausal atrophy (Figs. 10-14D and 10-15). The **sources** of the parabasal cells are superficial erosions and ulcerations of the squamous epithelium, resulting in the exposure of the deeper epithelial layers.

In postmenopausal women with a basically atrophic

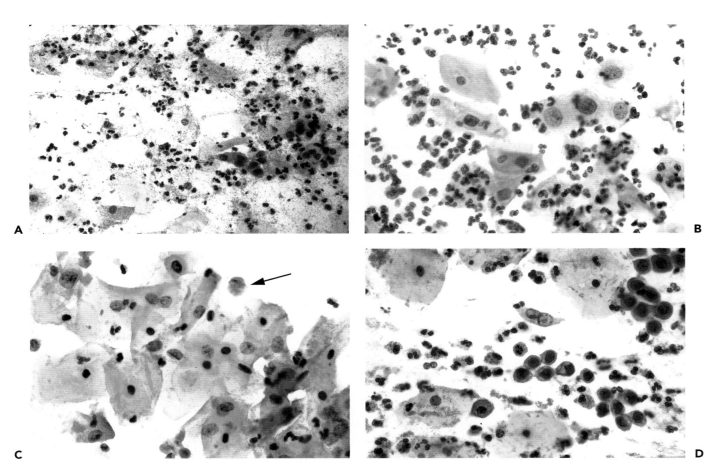

Figure 10-14   Various manifestations of inflammatory reaction in cervicovaginal smears. *A.* Typical smear pattern in acute cervicitis. The background contains polymorphonuclear leukocytes and necrotic cell debris. Squamous cells and a small cluster of degenerating parabasal cells may be observed. *B.* Atypia of squamous cells in cervicitis caused by *Trichomonas* infestation. Note nuclear enlargement and pallor caused by impending necrosis of the squamous cells. The background is typical of an acute inflammatory reaction. *C.* Marked eosinophilia of squamous cells in a case of *Trichomonas* infestation. A single parasite may be seen in the field of vision (*arrow*). *D.* Marked increase in the population of parabasal squamous cells in a young woman with severe trichomonas cervicitis.

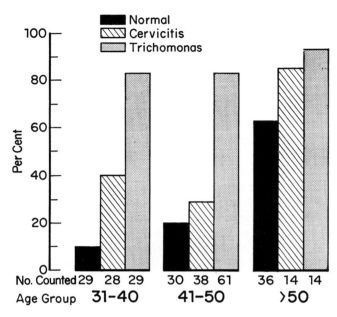

Figure 10-15   A graphic demonstration of the increase of parabasal cells in cervical smears in nonspecific cervicitis and in cervicitis due to *Trichomonas*. The figures were obtained by counting 200 consecutive single cells in cervical smears. The figures immediately underneath the bars indicate the number of smears evaluated in each category. A marked increase in parabasal cells is noticeable, especially in the younger patients. These differences are of no diagnostic value in postmenopausal patients. (From Koss LG, Wolinska WH. *Trichomonas vaginalis* cervicitis and its relationship to cervix cancer. Cancer 12:1171–1193, 1959.)

smear pattern, **an acute inflammation may have two effects.** The first is an **increased maturation of the squamous epithelium** with reappearance of intermediate and even superficial squamous cells (see Fig. 10-15). The reason for this phenomenon is in all probability an increased blood supply to the squamous epithelium that is noticeably present in *Trichomonas* infestation. As discussed in Chapter 9, one should not attempt to estimate the level of estrogenic activity in smears in the presence of a marked inflammation. The second effect of acute inflammation may be an **increase in cell necrosis and, hence, cell debris which, combined** with the phenomena of naturally occurring cell damage in advanced atrophy discussed in Chapter 8, may make the interpretation of such smears particularly difficult.

The presence of a marked inflammatory exudate and cell necrosis may also occur in advanced cancers of the cervix and the endometrium. Therefore, careful screening of such smears is mandatory.

Cytologic Atypias in Acute Inflammation

Depending on the etiology of an inflammatory lesion, cytologic changes may affect the squamous cells, the endocervical cells, or both cell types. For reasons of clarity, the changes will be described separately for the various categories of cells.

Squamous Cells

Acute inflammation affecting the squamous epithelium of the vagina and the ectocervix may bring about **necrosis of superficial, intermediate, and parabasal cells.** Some-

what **enlarged, blown-up homogeneous nuclei** without any nuclear structure may be noted (see Figs. 10-14A and Fig. 16A). Nuclear **pyknosis,** often associated with **break-up of chromatin** (karyorrhexis or apoptosis), is often present. The affected nuclei are quite dark and appear somewhat irregular because of fragments of chromatin protruding into the cytoplasm (see Figs. 10-14D and 10-16C). The lack of internal structure in the pyknotic nucleus and the preservation of a normal nucleocytoplasmic ratio are important to note in order to avoid any confusion with neoplastic changes. The pyknotic nuclei are often surrounded by **narrow clear cytoplasmic zones (halos)** (Fig. 10-16B) **which should not be confused with large perinuclear clear zones characteristic of koilocytosis,** described in Chapter 11. Binucleation, as well as slight cellular enlargement, may occur.

Necrosis and shedding of the superficial layers of the squamous epithelium, often observed during acute inflammation, result in an **increase** in the proportion of **parabasal cells** in smears of young women (see above and Fig. 10-15). In cervical smears, the parabasal cells occur singly or in **aggregates or plaques** composed of cells with **cytoplasmic processes** of various lengths. Such cells are of irregular shapes and, when in plaques, give the appearance of a jigsaw puzzle (see Fig. 10-4D). The term **"metaplastic cells"** is usually applied to such clusters, although their origin from squamous metaplasia is not always secure or evident. For further discussion of squamous metaplasia, see above. In well-preserved parabasal cells, the cytoplasm is chiefly basophilic; the density of the stain is often greater in the perinuclear area. Fine, **small cytoplasmic vacuoles** may be noted. The nuclei may appear somewhat enlarged; numerous **chromocenters and occasionally single small nucleoli** may be noted. Nuclear **pyknosis and karyorrhexis (apoptosis)** may also occur in parabasal cells (Fig. 10-16C). Binucleation or even multinucleation may occur.

Endocervical Cells

Acute endocervicitis may produce a **striking enlargement of the endocervical cells and their nuclei. Conspicuous cytoplasmic vacuoles,** sometimes infiltrated by polymorphonuclear leukocytes, may be observed (Fig. 10-17A). **Multinucleated endocervical cells** may occur. **Pyknotic nuclei are uncommon but bare nuclei** stripped of cytoplasm are often observed. The correct identification of such nuclei is facilitated by comparison with well-preserved endocervical cells. The **most conspicuous nuclear changes** consist of the presence of numerous **chromocenters** and one or more quite large and **conspicuous nucleoli** (Fig. 10-17B). **Mitotic figures** may occur. Similar findings occur in "repair," discussed above. Such findings are often disconcerting to the observer and the **differentiation of such cell abnormalities from those occurring in precancerous lesions or adenocarcinoma is at times very difficult** (see Chap. 12, where such mistakes are discussed). The presence of single abnormal cells favors a neoplastic process, but there are exceptions to the rule.

A final diagnostic decision as to the nature of endocervical cell changes cannot always be made on smears.

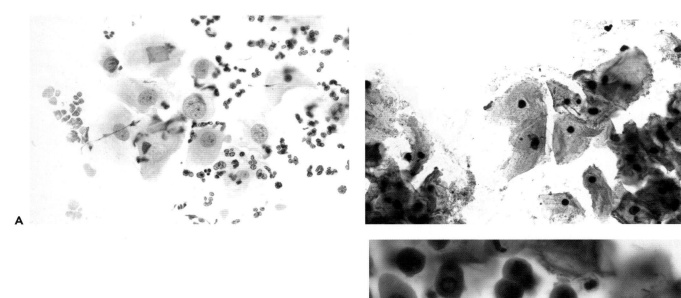

Figure 10-16 **Squamous epithelial cell abnormalities associated with severe cervicitis.** *A.* Nuclear pallor and enlargement indicative of impending cell necrosis. *B.* Prominent perinuclear halos common in trichomonas infestation. *C.* Hyperchromasia of parabasal cells, some showing nuclear fragmentation or apoptosis under high magnification.

While the absence of single abnormal cells speaks strongly in favor of a benign process, follow-up of such patients, which should include **colposcopy and biopsy,** is often indicated.

Chronic Inflammatory Processes

Chronic inflammatory processes of a minor degree are exceedingly common in the female genital tract and **produce few, if any, specific morphologic changes in epithelial cells.** The smears may show evidence of **benign abnormalities such as squamous metaplasia and repair, although their relationship to inflammatory processes is not always evident.** These conditions are discussed above. The only constant evidence of chronic inflammation is the presence of **lymphocytes, occasional plasma cells, and macrophages** in the background of the smear.

Macrophages (Histiocytes)

In the description of the menstrual cycle, it was noted that great numbers of small macrophages (**exodus**) may be found

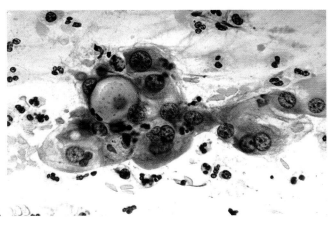

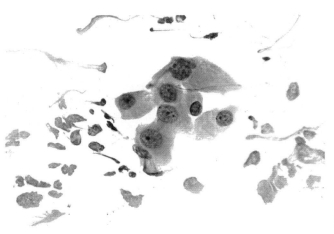

Figure 10-17 **Abnormalities of endocervical cells commonly seen in inflammation.** *A.* Marked vacuolization of cytoplasm. *B.* The presence of prominent nucleoli.

in cervicovaginal smears toward the end of the menstrual bleeding. In chronic inflammation, **mononucleated macrophages** occur commonly and are usually quite a bit larger than their "menstrual" counterpart (see Fig. 8-22A,B). They are characterized by a very finely **vacuolated, lacy cytoplasm, often containing ingested debris** and a rather **characteristic nucleus.** The latter is oval or bean-shaped and has a prominent nuclear membrane that stands out readily against the delicate bluish cytoplasm. Within the nucleus, there are a few sharply defined **chromocenters** and a few thin threads of chromatin. Occasionally, it is difficult to differentiate small macrophages from parabasal cells originating from squamous metaplasia of the endocervix. **Rarely, mitotic figures may be observed** in macrophages in smears. Nasiell (1961) pointed out that the mononucleated macrophages may be mistaken for cancer cells and that the differential diagnosis is based on evidence of phagocytic activity.

As described in Chapter 8, **multinucleated macrophages** are frequently observed in smears of postmenopausal women and may achieve very large sizes, even in the absence of inflammation (see Fig. 8-28C). However, in nonspecific chronic inflammatory processes in women of all ages, multinucleated macrophages may occur, sometimes in large numbers. A special type of multinucleated macrophages with peripheral placement of nuclei **(Langhans' cells)** may be observed in specific inflammatory processes such as tubercu-

losis (see below). The multinucleated macrophages **may show abnormal nuclear features such as nuclear enlargement and hyperchromasia that may mimic a malignant tumor.** This is particularly evident in the presence of **granulation tissue** (see below). The significance of macrophages (histiocytes) in the diagnosis of endometrial carcinoma is discussed in Chapter 13.

Granulation Tissue and Atypical Macrophages

Following a disruption of the epithelial surface and exposure of the underlying connective tissue, and usually as a consequence of a chronic inflammation, surgery or radiotherapy, the repair of the epithelial defect is preceded by formation of granulation tissue which may be visible on the **surface of the organ as a granulated red protrusion,** accounting for the name of the lesion (Singer and Clark, 1999). The granulation tissue is exposed to trauma and it bleeds easily as a consequence of rich vascularization. The identification of granulation tissue is of particular diagnostic importance after surgery or radiotherapy because it may be clinically mistaken for persisting or recurrent malignant tumor.

Histology. The granulation tissue consists of an **exuberant proliferation of fibroblasts, accompanied by formation of numerous young capillaries and by a marked inflammatory infiltrate consisting of** leukocytes, lymphocytes, and macrophages of the mono- and multinucleated type.

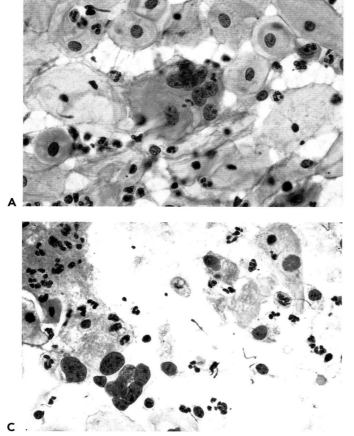

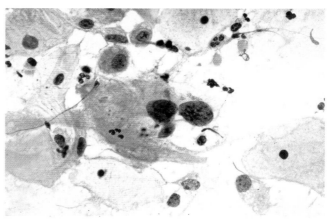

Figure 10-18 Nuclear abnormalities in atypical macrophages in a patient with granulomatous reaction in the uterine cervix. *A.* A multinucleated macrophage with nuclei of variable sizes. *B,C.* Very large hyperchromatic nuclei derived from macrophages.

Cytology. Smears obtained from granulation tissue are characterized by a marked inflammatory exudate. Leukocytes of various types are commonly seen in the background of smears. **Poorly preserved epithelial cells,** occasionally elongated **fibroblasts,** and numerous **macrophages** arepresent. The latter cells occasionally contain **multiple, highly abnormal, enlarged, and hyperchromatic nuclei** (Fig. 10-18A,B). A breakdown of these highly abnormal macrophages may result in the presence of isolated, **large hyperchromatic nuclei** that, for all intents and purposes, mimic nuclei of cancer cells (Fig. 10-18C). The differentiation of such cells or nuclei from cancer cells is based on **finding transition forms between clearly benign multinucleated macrophages and the rather uncommon, highly atypical, forms.** It is sometimes of value in the **differential diagnosis between atypical multinucleated macrophages and multinucleated cancer cells** to notice the **placement of nuclei,** which, in the macrophages, tend to be located at the periphery of the cell, whereas in the cancer cells they tend to be more centrally located, although there are many exceptions to this rule. Evidence of **phagocytic activity** is also in favor of macrophages, although it may occasionally be observed

in cancer cells as well. In case of doubt, a biopsy may be necessary.

Unusual Forms of Chronic Cervicitis

Follicular Cervicitis

This is an uncommon benign disorder wherein formation of **mature lymph follicles occurs in the subepithelial location in the uterine cervix** (see Fig. 10-19D). Roberts and Ng (1975) observed that follicular cervicitis is significantly more common in postmenopausal women, although it may occur in women of all age groups and menstrual status. Clinically, the disorder may be observed as pinhead-size white or gray elevations on the surface of the cervix. If the epithelium of the cervix is ulcerated or if the lymphoid tissue is forcibly removed by scraping, **clusters of lymphocytes may be observed in cervical smears.** The pathogenesis and full clinical significance of follicular cervicitis is not understood. There have been several observations linking follicular cervicitis with an infection with *Chlamydia trachomatis.* To what extent, if any, follicular cervicitis reflects

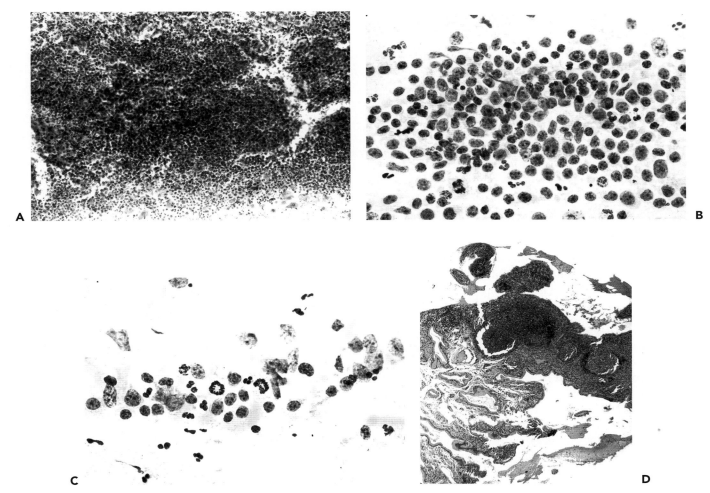

Figure 10-19 Follicular cervicitis. *A.* The presence of a large deposit of lymphocytes in the smear of the cervix is characteristic of this disorder. *B,C.* High-power views of lymphocytic population. In *C,* mitotic activity in follicle center cells may be noted. *D.* Biopsy of cervix showing deposits of lymphocytes.

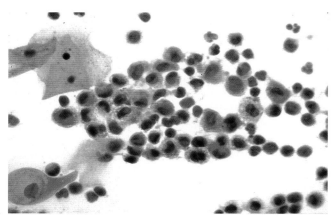

Figure 10-20   An accumulation of plasma cells in a cervicovaginal smear.

a general disorder of the immune system is not known at the time of this writing.

Cytology

In smears, the disorder is characterized by the presence of **pools of lymphocytes** which, in most cases, can be identified as such under low power of the microscope (Fig. 10-19A).

The diagnosis becomes more difficult if the lymph follicles are broken up. The smear then displays a **mixture of lymphocytes and large, follicle center cells,** the latter derived from the germinative centers of the lymph follicles (Fig. 10-19B). The follicle center cells have the appearance of mononucleated **large lymphocytes with a delicate, vacuolated cytoplasm and large vesicular nuclei, occasionally provided with one or more prominent nucleoli.** The follicle center cells may show **numerous mitoses** (Fig. 10-19C). Small macrophages with evidence of phagocytic activity may also be present. The diagnosis is based usually on smear pattern and the monotonous aspect of the benign lymphocytes. The **differential diagnosis comprises malignant lymphoma and leukemia** involving cervix or vagina. In both these disorders, the malignant lymphoid cells are dispersed and there is little evidence of clustering of lymphocytes.

Plasma Cell Cervicitis

Qizilbash (1974) reported a case of what appears to be an extremely rare disorder of the cervix, characterized by the presence of **plasma cells of varying degrees of maturity.** The plasma cells infiltrated the cervical stroma and were observed in the cervical smears. Some of the plasma cells were multinucleated and bizarre. There was no evidence of generalized plasma cell myeloma. It must be pointed out that plasma cells are a common component of the cell population infiltrating the uterine cervix **in chronic cervicitis** of bacterial origin and may find their way into cervical smears (Fig. 10-20). We have also observed **plasma cells in smears in an occasional case of microglandular hyperplasia,** as discussed above.

SPECIFIC INFECTIONS OF THE CERVIX AND THE VAGINA

Bacterial Infections

Normal Bacterial Flora

Although the dominant organism in the normal female genital tract is *Lactobacillus* (see Chap. 8), comprehensive studies by Ohm and Galask (1975), Roupas et al (1985), and Bibbo and Wied (1997) have shown that the bacterial flora of the vagina also contains small properties of other **aerobic and anaerobic microorganisms.** Although some of these organisms are considered to be pathogenic, their mere presence within the vagina or cervix is usually harmless. Many of the bacterial agents may be identified in cytologic preparations. The principal species, the diseases caused by them, and their effect on cervicovaginal smears will be described below.

Lactobacillus (Döderlein), Also Known as Bacillus vaginalis (B. vaginalis)

As described in Chapter 8, *Lactobacillus* is the normal inhabitant of the lower genital tract. Lactobacilli are **aerobic, gram-positive rods.** In genital smears stained with Papanicolaou stain, *Lactobacillus* organisms are identified as **slender basophilic rods of various lengths** distributed on cell surface and in smear background (see Fig. 8-37). The frequency of occurrence of *Lactobacillus* as the principal vaginal microorganism varies with the population studied. In patients with good vaginal hygiene, approximately 50% harbor this microorganism. In clinic populations attended by women with poor vaginal hygiene and high levels of sexual exposure, this figure drops significantly to approximately 20% or less.

Lactobacilli ferment cytoplasmic glycogen and, therefore, cause **cytolysis** of glycogen-containing squamous cells described in Chapter 8 (see Fig. 8-31B). The most mature superficial squamous cells and the parabasal cells are often spared. Therefore, **cytolysis is mainly observed in situations in which intermediate cells predominate, to wit: the premenstrual phase of the menstrual cycle, pregnancy, and early menopause.** The moth-eaten appearance of the cytoplasm of the intermediate squamous cells and the presence of isolated nuclei remaining after lysis of the cytoplasm by the bacteria are characteristic of this condition. Cytolysis is seldom observed in postmenopausal women with an atrophic smear pattern. It is a matter for some debate whether *Lactobacillus* is ever responsible for inflammatory states. Occasionally, **clear vaginal discharge** apparently due to excessive glycolysis may be observed.

Gardnerella vaginalis (Previously Known as Corynebacterium vaginale and Haemophilus vaginalis)

This **anaerobic organism** is encountered in about 6% of women of childbearing age and causes vaginitis and cervicitis in some of them. The organism is a Gram-negative or Gram-variable short rod that, in Papanicolaou stain, stains dark blue. The organism tends to **accumulate on the surfaces of squamous epithelial cells,** giving them a peculiar and rather uniquely diagnostic appearance of a **"clue cell"**

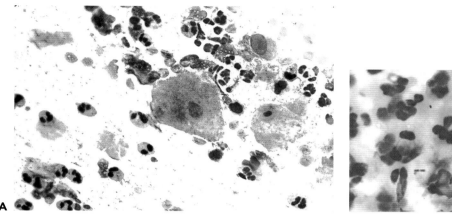
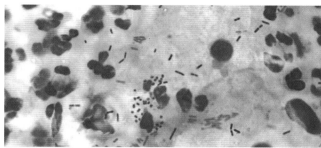

Figure 10-21   **Changes caused by inflammatory reaction.** *A.* "Clue cell." The surface of the squamous cell is obscured by a large accumulation of bacilli. *B.* Gonorrhea. Intracytoplasmic accumulation of diplococci may be noted. The background also shows lactobacilli. (*B*, Gram stain, oil immersion.)

(Gardner and Dukes, 1955; Gardner and Kaufman, 1969; Dunkelberg, 1965). In some cases, the **entire surface of the cell is obscured by the *Gardnerella;*** in most instances, only a part of the cell surface is covered by the microorganism (Fig. 10-21). The same small microorganisms in variable numbers are usually observed in the background. There is no cytolysis. It must be pointed out, however, that **lactobacilli may also accumulate on the surfaces of squamous cells** (see Fig. 8-37B). However, the **lactobacilli appear as distinct rods, whereas in the clue cells, the surface is hazy and the individual *Gardnerella* organisms cannot be clearly discerned.** Gardner and Kaufman emphasized that in the presence of mixed infections with pyogenic bacteria or *Trichomonas vaginalis,* the clue cells often cannot be identified. The organisms play an important role in **bacterial vaginosis,** described below.

Diphtheroids

Short rods, arranged in the form of **"Chinese characters"** with a terminal clublike thickening, have been described in a small percentage of vaginal and cervical smears by Leppäluoto (1974). The staining is uneven and the thickened end is darker than the body of the rod. The pathogenicity of this organism has not been established.

Corynebacterium diphtheriae

True **diphtheria** of the vagina is exceedingly rare. The causative organism resembles morphologically the diphtheroids described above. In contrast with the diphtheroids *C. diphtheriae* causes a **necrotizing inflammation of the vaginal epithelium** similar to that observed in the nasopharynx.

Gram-Positive Cocci

A large variety of Gram-positive cocci may be observed in cervicovaginal smears. The organisms cannot be specifically classed without identification by culture. **Staphylococci** and **streptococci** are the common varieties with *Staphylococcus epidermidis,* the most common variant (Ohm and Galask, 1975). Most cocci appear as **clusters or chains of very small, round or oval organisms, staining dark blue or gray in Papanicolaou stain,** usually occupying the background of the smear, with few organisms superimposed on

the surfaces of the squamous cells. In extreme cases, the background of the smear appears **"dirty"** because it is filled with cocci. The gram-positive cocci may be the cause of **pyogenic infections** of the female genital tract and are an important cause of **pelvic inflammatory disease.** The cocci are frequently associated with other organisms and with *Trichomonas vaginalis* (Gardner and Kaufman, 1969).

Gram-Negative Cocci

Neisseria gonorrhoeae (N. gonorrhoeae) or gonococcus is the causative organism of **acute and chronic gonorrhea,** the most common of all sexually transmitted diseases. The organism is a **Gram-negative diplococcus** that is an **intracellular parasite.** It may be observed in Papanicolaou-stained material adhering to the surface or in the cytoplasm of intermediate and parabasal squamous cells as **tiny coffee-bean organisms arranged in pairs** (Fig. 10-21B). Heller (1974) observed the organisms mainly in cells from squamous metaplasia of the endocervical canal, but I have repeatedly seen gonococci in squamous cells apparently originating in mature squamous epithelium. Oil immersion is required for identification of gonococci in cervical smears. Morphologic separation of *N. gonorrhoeae* from other species of *Neisseria,* notably the very important *N. meningitidis,* is not possible and it is advisable to confirm the diagnosis by culture.

During the acute stage of gonorrhea, acute purulent **urethritis,** both in man and in woman, is a nearly universal manifestation of infection. While in men the disease is usually symptomatic, it may be completely asymptomatic in women. Litt et al (1974) emphasized that in children and adolescents, gonorrheal **vaginitis** may be more common than in adult women. In women, the disease may cause cervicitis, endocervicitis, and inflammation of Bartholin's glands and may spread via the fallopian tube to the pelvic organs and cause **tubo-ovarian abscesses** or even acute peritonitis. Gonorrhea may cause **acute arthritis,** usually limited to a single joint.

Neither acute nor chronic gonorrhea cause specific cytologic abnormalities. The smear pattern is that of an acute or chronic cervicitis or vaginitis.

Mobiluncus *Species*

These curved, Gram-variable anaerobic bacteria, sometimes described as **boomerang-shaped,** may aggregate on the surfaces of squamous cells. The organisms are present in a small percentage of normal women but are nearly universally observed in women with bacterial vaginosis, described below.

Mycoplasma *and* Ureaplasma

Mycoplasma, previously known as pleuropneumonia-like organism (PPLO), is the **smallest free-living organism.** It causes **atypical pneumonias** and may cause immune disturbances such as formation of cold-agglutinins. Its role as an infectious agent in the female genital tract has been investigated by Gregory and Payne (1970) and by Leppäluoto (1972). *Mycoplasma hominis*, type I, has been identified in 30% of asymptomatic women and **in 92% of women with sexually transmitted diseases.** There are no known cytologic changes attributable to *Mycoplasma*; however, the organism participates in bacterial vaginosis.

A related microorganism, *Ureaplasma urealyticum*, may also be documented by culture in 37% of normal women and 56% of women with known infection (Roupas et al, 1985). No documented cytologic abnormalities are associated with this organism.

Bacterial Vaginosis

Bacterial vaginosis is the **most frequent cause of vaginitis and cervicitis** during the childbearing age. The disorder is caused by profound **changes in the vaginal flora,** normally dominated by lactobacteria, in favor of a **mixed bacterial flora dominated by G. vaginalis, Mobiluncus species, mycoplasma, and a large variety of other organisms, mainly Gram-negative rods** (Hill, 1993). Sobel (1997) discussed the chemical changes occurring in this disorder to explain the dominant symptom, the **"fish-smelling" vaginal discharge.** The principal change is in increased alkalinity of the vaginal milieu with elevation of pH. Many women with this disorder are asymptomatic, others may experience pruritus. **Risk factors** include intrauterine contraceptive devices (IUDs) and pregnancy but quite often no risk factors are apparent. Besides personal discomfort, the significance of bacterial vaginosis is in its **association with preterm delivery of low-birth-weight infants** (Hillier et al, 1995).

Cytology

The cervicovaginal smears in bacterial vaginosis show a characteristic **"dirty"** appearance, caused by presence of innumerable organisms, many covering the surfaces of squamous cells. The **"clue" cells,** caused by *G. vaginalis* and described above, are usually well evident, but other microorganisms, such as the comma-shaped *Mobiluncus* species may also aggregate on cell surfaces. Clearly, the value of the cervicovaginal smear in the diagnosis of bacterial vaginosis is limited. Schnadig et al (1989) aptly referred to this disorder as "clues, commas, and confusion." The treatment must be based on clinical and bacteriologic data.

Tuberculosis

Tuberculosis of the female genital tract is, as a general rule, a **manifestation of disseminated disease.** There is no evidence that the genital tract can be the primary portal of entry. The most common manifestations of genital tuberculosis are tuberculous **salpingitis** and **endometritis,** but occasionally, though rarely in the Western world, the infection may involve the **uterine cervix** and, exceptionally, the vagina (Sutherland, 1985). The onset of AIDS has contributed to a marked increase in pulmonary tuberculosis, but so far there is no evidence that this has led to an increase in genital tuberculosis. The acid-fast mycobacterium tuberculosis cannot be identified in Papanicolaou stain. However, the presence of **tuberculous granulomas** can be occasionally recognized in cytologic preparations. As described in Chapters 19 and 31, the granulomas are nodular structures composed of modified macrophages resembling epithelial cells **(epithelioid cells)** and **multinucleated giant cells** with nuclei arranged at the periphery **(Langhans' cells).** A central area of necrosis (so-called **caseous necrosis**) is often present in the center of the granulomas.

Cytology

The smear pattern is that of chronic inflammation, wherein the epithelioid cells and Langhans' cells can sometimes be recognized. The epithelioid cells **have the approximate size of endocervical cells, are elongated, often carrot-shaped, pale-staining, eosinophilic, or cyanophilic cells with single round or oval finely stippled nuclei, occasionally containing small nucleoli.** The cytoplasm is usually finely vacuolated. The epithelioid cells sometimes form **approximately spherical clusters,** corresponding to the tubercles. Single epithelioid cells are difficult to identify in contrast to the large **Langhans'-type giant cells with peripheral nuclei** (Fig. 10-22). Fragments of amorphous eosinophilic material, corresponding to the central necrotic portions of the tubercle, round out the picture. The cytologic presentation of pulmonary tuberculosis is discussed in Chapter 19.

Although a number of communications pertaining to tuberculosis of the uterine cervix have emphasized the descriptive aspects of the cytologic presentation, the diagnosis is not easy. The identification of epithelioid cells in cervical and vaginal smears is difficult, and the **differentiation of Langhans' cells from other forms of the common multinucleated macrophages is very difficult** for all practical intents and purposes. It would be particularly **inadvisable to suspect any woman with multinucleated macrophages in smears of harboring tuberculosis.** Thus, although the disease is still fairly common in the developing countries, in the industrialized countries it will remain a cytologic curiosity with most diagnoses rendered retrospectively after the histologic or microbiologic diagnosis has been established. Baum et al (2001) documented that polymerase chain reaction (PCR) may be helpful in the diagnosis of this disease.

Mycobacterium avium-intracellulare *Complex*

As a consequence of the infection with human immunodeficiency virus **(HIV)** and acquired immunodeficiency syndrome **(AIDS),** a large number of previously very rare opportunistic infections have come to light, among them the acid-fast *Mycobacterium avium* (summaries in Perfect, 1988 and Lifson et al, 1994). The bacterium may lead to the formation of granulomas, similar to those seen in tuber-

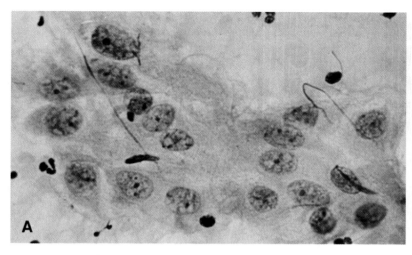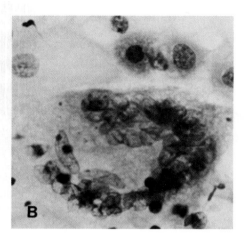

Figure 10-22   **Tuberculosis of the cervix (cervical smear).** *A.* Sheet of epithelioid cells characterized by a pale, faintly vacuolated, elongated cytoplasm and round or oval nuclei. The latter are finely stippled and contain small nucleoli. *B.* Large multinucleated Langhans' giant cell with peripherally placed nuclei. (High magnification.) (Courtesy of Dr. K.A. Misch, London, UK; from Misch KA, et al. Tuberculosis of the cervix: Cytology as an aid to diagnosis. J Clin Pathol 29:313–316, 1976.)

culosis, but quite often the organisms are phagocytized by large macrophages with vacuolated cytoplasm that do not form any organized structures, hence the name of the complex (see Chap. 19). To our knowledge, this organism has not been observed in cervicovaginal smears but is discussed in Chapter 31.

Granuloma venereum (Granuloma inguinale)

This is a sexually transmitted disease affecting mainly the skin and subcutaneous tissue of external genitalia in both sexes. **Ulcerative lesions** may affect the penis, vagina and uterine cervix (Fig. 10-23A). The disease is caused by Gram-negative, **bacillary encapsulated bodies (*Calymmatobacterium granulomatis*, or Donovan bodies)** that may be numerous in the cytoplasm of large, vacuolated "foamy" macrophages. They are best seen in Gram stain under oil immersion. The bipolar bodies, measuring about 1 to 2 μm in length, have been compared with tiny "closed safety pins" (Fig. 10-23B).

Actinomyces

This group of bacterial organisms that is sometimes difficult to classify on culture may be occasionally observed in the female genital tract. Gupta et al (1976) first pointed out the **association of this organism with the use of intrauterine contraceptive devices (IUDs)** and identified some of the organisms as ***Actinomyces israeli,*** which are known as human pathogens. In cervicovaginal smears, the organisms appear as a **central "ball" of basophilic filaments, with single, slender filaments spreading peripherally, sometimes surrounded by inflammatory exudate** (Fig. 10-24A,B). **Special stains, such as Brown and Brenn, may be required to document the club-shaped tips of the filaments** (Fig. 10-24C). **The finding of *Actinomyces* in cervicovaginal smears is a strong indication that the patient is a wearer of an IUD,** even if this history is not provided by the clinician.

Although in most instances, ***Actinomyces*** infection is harmless to the patient, there are several documented cases

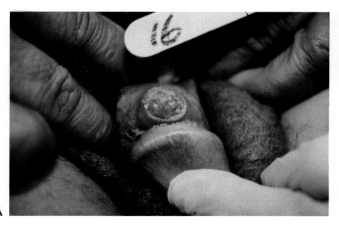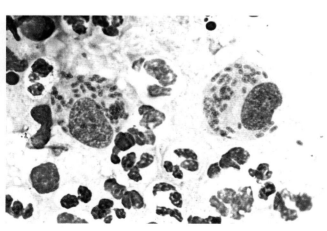

A   B

Figure 10-23   **Granuloma inguinale.** *A.* Typical ulceration of penis. *B.* Donovan bodies. Note large macrophages containing numerous intracytoplasmic "safety pin"-like inclusions. (Oil immersion.)

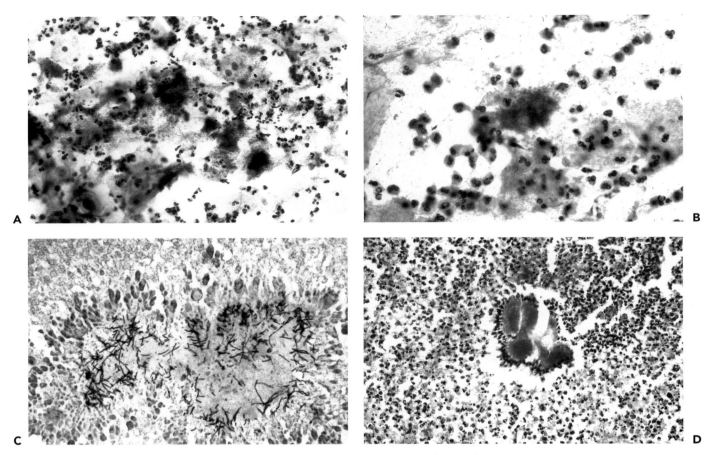

Figure 10-24   Actinomycosis in cervicovaginal smears. *A,B.* Colonies of actinomyces in a cervicovaginal smear from a woman who was a long-term IUD wearer. The colonies are composed of tangles of filaments which appear as bluish structures in the background of the smear. *C.* Structure of an actinomycotic deposit seen in Brown-Brenn stain. The clublike thickening of the periphery of the filaments is well seen. *D.* Tubo-ovarian abscess in a 49-year-old IUD wearer who had not changed her device for 13 years. The large colony of actinomyces surrounded by inflammatory reaction are shown.

of **pelvic inflammatory disease occurring mainly in women whose IUD has not been changed for 3 or more years.** These women can develop **pelvic abscesses** that may lead to sterility or even death of the patient (Fig. 10-24D). Subcutaneous abscesses may also occur, wherein the characteristic **"sulfur granules"** or grossly visible small yellow spheres of fungus, can be observed.

An interesting rare finding in the differential diagnosis of actinomycosis was described in six patients by Bhagavan et al (1982). These are eosinophilic radiate structures, mimicking granules of ***Actinomyces,*** but composed of glycoproteins and lipids that may be calcified. The structures, which stain with Ziehl-Neelsen's stain for acid-fast organisms, were named ***pseudoactinomycotic radiate granules*** and were thought to represent a reaction to microorganisms or foreign bodies, repeatedly described in the past as the ***Splendore-Hoeppli phenomenon.*** It must be noted that only three of the six patients reported by Bhagavan were IUD users, and the granules were observed in tissues and not in smears.

For further discussion of cytologic findings in IUD wearers see above.

Leptothrix

There appears to be considerable controversy as to the identity of long, curving, filamentous organisms known as ***Leptothrix vaginalis.*** Rosebury (1962) identified two such organisms: a form of *Lactobacillus* (*Leptotrichia*) identical with *Leptothrix buccalis*, and a bacterium of the family of *Actinomyces* (*Bacterionema*), both of a similar morphologic appearance. According to Bibbo et al (1997), the *Actinomyces* type of organism is identifiable because of larger size and occasional branching. **Leptothrix is most commonly observed in conjunction with vaginal trichomoniasis** (see below). Bibbo et al (1997) observed this association in 95% of 1,300 consecutive genital smears with **Leptothrix.** Occasionally, association with fungi and other infectious agents was noted. The reason for this association is not known.

Chlamydia (Bedsonia)

These small, gram-negative microorganisms are the **agents of a variety of acute and chronic inflammatory disorders, such as inclusion conjunctivitis, trachoma, lymphogranuloma venereum, nonspecific urethritis, salpingitis, vaginitis, and cervicitis.** Screening of women for occult cervical **chlamydia** infection was shown as an effective means of prevention of pelvic inflammatory disease (Scholes et al, 1996). The organisms are obligate intracellular parasites and are transmitted by personal contact. The first description of the cytologic presentation of this organism was by Naib (1970) in conjunctival smears of newborns and their mothers' genital tract. Gupta et al (1979) analyzed in considerable detail the cytologic presentation of the *Chlamydia* infection that can be observed in cervicovaginal smears. In the cytoplasm of squamous, metaplastic, and endocervical cells, the organism forms **tiny elementary coccoid bodies surrounded by narrow clear zones.** In the later stages of infection, the affected cells display one or more, sharply circumscribed, readily visible, **clear cytoplasmic vacuoles with a central acidophilic or basophilic inclusion—representing a condensation of the microorganisms** (Fig. 10-25A,B). Shiina (1985), in an elaborate study of inclusions in chlamydial infection, named the largest inclusions **"nebular inclusions,"** to differentiate them from smaller inclusions, a terminology also accepted by Henry et al (1993).

The cells containing *Chlamydia* may be somewhat atypical or multinucleated (Fig. 10-25C). Still, it must be stressed that **the presence of *Chlamydia* infection does not rule out the simultaneous presence of neoplastic lesions.** Patients with significant cellular abnormalities should have the benefit of further workup.

The original description of the morphologic manifestations of *Chlamydia* infection has been repeatedly challenged, notably by Shafer et al (1985), who compared the results of cytologic findings with culture of the microorganism. The presence of large vacuoles containing central inclusions (see Fig. 10-25B) could not be correlated with positive cultures. On the other hand, in several women with positive cultures, no cytologic abnormalities of the type described above could be observed. The unreliability of morphologic recognition of *Chlamydia* was also emphasized by Vinette-Leduc et al (1997).

Because the infection with *Chlamydia trachomatis* is of major clinical significance, the consensus is that **the identification of this agent should always be confirmed by culture,** which also requires considerable care and optimal conditions for success (Kellog, 1989). Antibodies to *Chlamydia* have been developed. Fluorescence microscopy, using a labeled antibody, can be used as a screening procedure with a high degree of accuracy when compared with results of culture (Lindner et al, 1986). More recently, polymerase chain reaction, enzyme immunoassays, and ligase chain reaction using urine have been shown to be reliable in the diagnosis of this infection (Vinette-Leduc et al, 1997; Gaydos et al, 1998).

Chlamydia infection may also be associated with follicular cervicitis (see above).

Syphilis

This disease is caused by a sexually transmitted spirochete, **Treponema pallidum.** The disease which starts with an ulcerated localized lesion, the chancre, usually located on the genitalia, and subsequently becomes generalized, may cause inflammatory changes in the cervix that may mimic cervical cancer (Gutmann, 1995). The pattern of the **cervicovaginal smears** in Gutmann's cases showed only **non-**

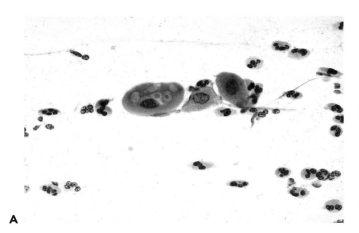

A

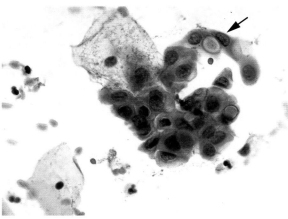

B

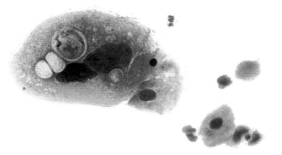

C

Figure 10-25 Chlamydia infection. *A.* Small encapsulated primary bodies may be seen in the cytoplasm of the affected cell. *B.* Large cytoplasmic inclusion with an eosinophilic center (*arrow*). *C.* Multinucleated giant cell with several large cytoplasmic inclusions.

specific inflammation but the diagnosis could be established by the identification of the spirochetes in the granulomatous lesion in the biopsy.

Fungal Infections

Candida glabrata (Moniliasis)

This family of fungal infections comprises two common organisms, **Candida albicans** and **Torulopsis glabrata (jointly referred to as monilia).** These are the most common pathogenic fungal agents observed in the female genital tract. Diabetes, pregnancy, and the use of antibacterial antibiotic agents that change the make-up of the vaginal flora are frequently associated with moniliasis. **Monilia** may also appear in patients with impaired leukocyte functions, in patients receiving immunosuppressive drugs and **may be the first manifestation of AIDS.** The infection may cause a **thick, milky vaginal discharge associated with intense itching and discomfort.**

Like most fungi of the family of Cryptococcaceae, **Candida albicans** and **Torulopsis glabrata** appear in two forms in smears: the **yeast form (conidia)** and the **fungus form (pseudohyphae).** The **conidia** appear as **small, encapsulated, round, or oval organisms** (Fig. 10-26A). The capsule is inconspicuous. Budding may be noted in the form of smaller oval structures attached to one pole of the conidium. The **fungus form** is made up of long, thin filaments consisting of **elongated, bamboo-like spores. Usually, the spores are not surrounded by a capsule and, therefore, are designated as pseudohyphae** (see Fig. 10-26B).

Schnell and Voigt (1976) documented by electron microscopy that the fungus spores may be intracellular and located within the cytoplasm of squamous epithelial cells, wherein they can also multiply.

Cytology

In spite of the intracytoplasmic penetration, the fungus does not appear to cause any serious injury to the epithelial lining of the cervix or the vagina but there may be complicating inflammatory phenomena. Neither the histologic nor the cytologic findings are specific or impressive. In the majority of cases, there are **no significant changes in smear patterns except for the presence of the fungus.** In other instances, there may be a mild inflammation affecting the squamous epithelium and the endocervix. **It must be stressed that secure identification of the fungi is usually not possible on the strength of morphologic examination alone.** Cultural and serologic data should be obtained for species diagnosis. Reports of cytologic atypias associated with this infection most likely reflect incidental abnormalities (Heller and Hoyt, 1971; Miguel et al, 1997).

Other Fungi

Occasionally, fungi other than **Candida** and **Torulopsis** are encountered in routine cytologic material. Their exact identification must rest on cultural characterization.

Coccidioidomycosis of the female genital tract has been reported (Saw et al, 1975). A case of **Paracoccidioides brasiliensis** was reported by Sheyn et al (2001). We also observed a case of **paracoccidioidomycosis** in the cervicovaginal smear of an asymptomatic 38-year-old woman. This fungus is mainly observed in Brazil and may cause pulmonary disease (see Chap. 19). The organism is spherical, brown, measuring from 10 to 60 μm in diameter, and is recognized by teardrop-shaped multiple buds resulting in the very characteristic "ship's wheel" appearance (Fig. 10-27A).

Cysts of **Toxoplasma** have been reported in cervicovaginal smears by Dominguez and Giron (1976), San Cristobal and Roset (1976), and Wasylenko et al (1991). A case of **blastomycosis,** identified in cervical smears, apparently transmitted to the patient from her husband with a prostatic infection, was reported by Dryer et al (1983).

We observed several examples of **Aspergillosis,** mainly in women wearing IUDs (Fig. 10-27B–D). In patients with AIDS, the fungus **Cryptococcus neoformans** may be observed, sometimes forming the unusual pseudohyphae rather than the common spherical spores with a mucoid capsule (Anandi et al, 1991). For further comments on this fungus, see Chapters 19 and 27. There are several additional published examples of uncommon fungus infections of the female genital tract, some cited in the bibliography. The clinical significance of these infections is uncertain and depends on whether the involvement of the genital tract is a

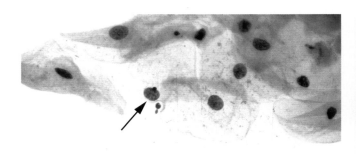

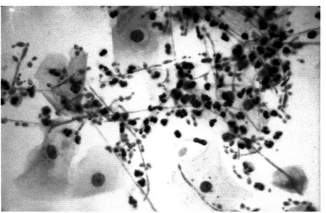

A   **B**

Figure 10-26   Moniliasis. *A.* The budding yeast form of the fungus *(arrow). B.* Pseudohyphae.

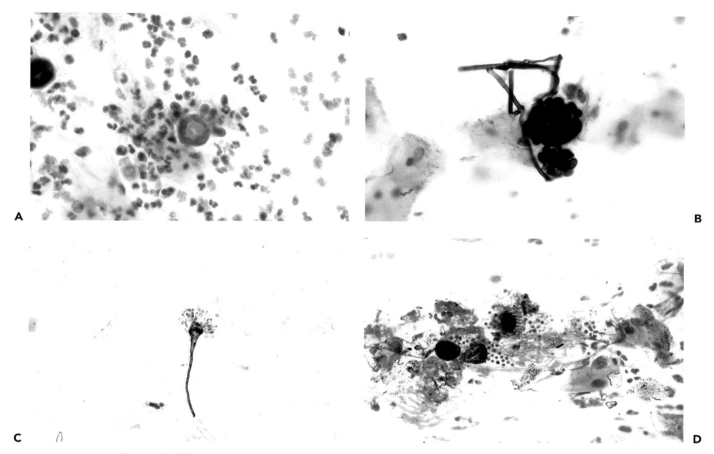

Figure 10-27 **Various fungal infections.** *A.* Paracoccidioidomycosis. The fungus is surrounded by spores that mimic a ship's steering wheel. *B–D.* Various forms of aspergillosis. *B* shows filaments and *C* and *D* fruiting heads of the fungus.

localized event or a manifestation of systemic disease, particularly in AIDS. The specific fungi are discussed again in several chapters, in reference to organs and organ systems where they are commonly encountered.

Viral Infections

Genital Herpes (Herpes Simplex Genitalis)

This is an important and common viral infection of the female genital tract, usually caused by **herpes simplex virus (HSV)** type II, whereas the perioral herpes (the common cold sores) is usually caused by HSV type I. The two types of herpesvirus cannot be distinguished morphologically but vary in their cultural and serologic characteristics. The frequency of the genital herpes varies according to the population studied from 0.09 to 0.9 per 1,000. Women in low socioeconomic brackets are more frequently affected than women from economically favored population groups. Jordan et al (1972) found a statistically significant increase in African Americans, when compared with American Indians, Hispanic Americans, and white women residents of the same region.

It was documented that nearly 40% of newly acquired HSV type II and two-thirds of HSV type I infections are asymptomatic (Langenberg et al, 1999). This observation has been first reported by cytology laboratories where the telltale cytologic evidence of herpesvirus infection has been observed in asymptomatic patients.

Clinically, **small vesicles** with clear content or, later, **superficial erosions** on the vulva or the penis characterize the genital herpes virus infection. The erosions may be painful. The vesicles are difficult to see in the vagina or on the cervix; however, the **erosions on the cervix may mimic cancer.** The disease is **chronic,** inasmuch as recurrences are common. It is generally thought that the virus **persists in ganglion cells** and becomes reactivated under a variety of circumstances. Obara et al (1997) were able to document the presence of viral DNA in human spinal ganglia by polymerase chain reaction (PCR) and in situ hybridization. A vaccine of moderate efficacy in women (but not in men) has been recently tested (Stanberry et al, 2002).

Histology

Regardless of viral type, the histologic and cytologic abnormalities of cells, characteristic of the common HSV infections are similar. The disease affects more commonly the squamous epithelium of the skin, vagina, and cervix than the endocervical epithelium.

On the skin and vulva, the disease begins as inflammatory nodules that lead to blister or vesicle formation by separation of layers of epidermis (Fig. 10-28). The center of the blister is filled with fluid. The epithelial cells lining

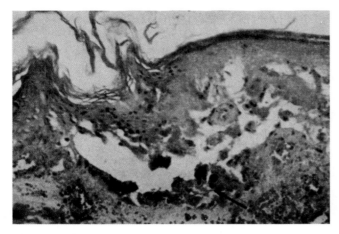

Figure 10-28 Herpetic vesicle—skin. The presence of large intranuclear inclusions and multinucleated cells with degenerating dark nuclei is evident at the margin of the vesicle (*arrow*).

the blisters show changes characteristic of herpesvirus infection that are better seen in cytologic preparations.

Cytology

The cytologic changes induced by herpesvirus are very characteristic and their identification in cervicovaginal smears is usually easy. In the **early stages of the disease, there is a moderate to marked nuclear enlargement in squamous or endocervical cells,** accompanied by a peculiar, faintly basophilic and opaque **homogenization of the nuclear contents, known as the "ground-glass" nuclei** (Fig. 10-29A). Occasionally, the homogenization is preceded or accompanied by nuclear vacuolization. This appearance of the nuclei is caused by an invasion of the nucleus by the virus, easily documented by electron microscopy. The herpes virions, composed of a capsule and a central electron-dense core, measure about 150 nm in diameter, are concentrated mainly in the nucleus, although cytoplasmic particles and membrane budding are a part of the picture. The virus causes **nuclear multiplication, resulting in crowding, and**

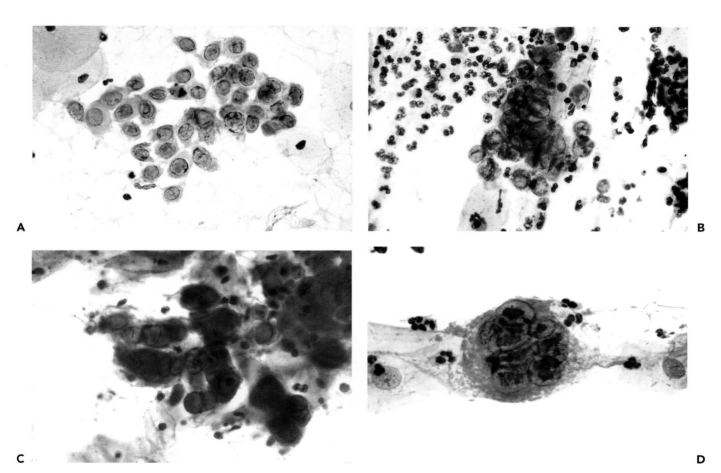

A

B

C

D

Figure 10-29 Herpesvirus infection. *A.* Early stage of viral infection. Enlarged and homogeneous "ground glass" nuclei in endocervical cells. *B.* A formation of a multinucleated giant cell with "ground glass" nuclei and nuclear molding. *C.* Multinucleated giant cells with "ground glass" nuclei and nuclear molding next to a cell with intranuclear viral inclusion. *D.* Higher magnification showing intranuclear viral inclusions forming in a multinucleated giant cell. The eosinophilic inclusions are surrounded by clear halo.

molding of the adjacent "ground-glass" nuclei, leading to the formation of multinucleated, often very large cells (occasionally well over 60 μm in diameter; Fig. 10-29B, C). The homogeneous inclusions **become condensed** and finally are localized in the center of the nuclei as **large eosinophilic inclusions,** significantly larger than any nucleolus. The inclusions are surrounded by a **clear area within the nucleoplasm** (Fig. 10-29D). Takeda (1969) documented the presence of herpes virions in the inclusions by electron microscopy. Experimental data (Teplitz et al, 1971) documented that intranuclear inclusions are a late event in the course of herpesvirus infection in vitro.

In the final stages of the infection, nuclear degeneration may set in, occasionally resulting in formation of **bizarre, sometimes hyperchromatic nuclear masses due to nuclear fusion.** Occasionally, **pearl-like structures, imitating squamous carcinoma, may be observed** (Fig. 10-30). The identity of the bizarre cells in smears can be established by finding the characteristic ground-glass nuclei or nuclear inclusions in adjacent cells, or by use of additional techniques, described below. Ng et al (1970) proposed that certain morphologic differences may be observed between primary and recurrent herpetic infection. In the primary infection, there was a preponderance of multinucleated cells and few cells with eosinophilic inclusions; the opposite was observed for recurrent dis-

ease. Vesterinen et al (1977), in a careful study, failed to confirm Ng's findings and found no cytologic differences between primary and recurrent infections.

The **differential diagnosis of herpetic cervicitis** in cervicovaginal smears must include the very uncommon **trophoblastic syncytial cells** seen in pregnancy (see Chap. 8) and, in cases of extreme abnormalities, **squamous cancer.** In such cases, the absence of more classical evidence of herpes is crucial in the differential diagnosis. In difficult cases, the mophologic suspicion of herpesvirus infection can be confirmed by **other techniques.** Stenkvist and Brege (1975) first applied **immunofluorescent techniques for the diagnosis of herpesvirus keratitis,** but the technique is also applicable to cervicovaginal smears. More recently, techniques of **in situ hybridization of viral DNA** (Tomita et al, 1991; Kobayashi et al, 1993), and **polymerase chain reaction** (Shibata, 1992; Slomka, 1998) have been applied to the diagnosis of this disease. Marshall et al (2001) reported that the results of the PCR techniques were more sensitive and took less time than viral culture.

It must be noted that **the presence of herpes does not rule out the presence of precancerous lesions or cancer of the uterine cervix.** In fact, we observed occasional cases where **the presence of herpes obscured and delayed the diagnosis of a cancerous lesion.** Longatto-Filho et al

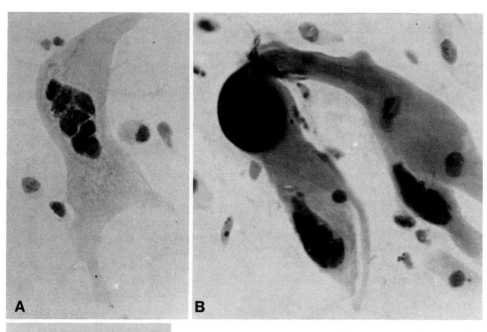

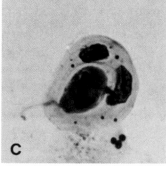

Figure 10-30 **Cervical smears.** Herpetic cervicitis. A few examples of exceptionally bizarre squamous cells resulting from infection with herpes simplex virus. *A.* Multinucleation. *B.* The huge degenerated nuclear mass undoubtedly represents the result of fusion of smaller nuclei that may still be observed in the two adjacent cells. *C.* Note the squamous pearl-like arrangement of cells. Elsewhere in these smears, clear-cut evidence of herpes was evident. (*A–C,* High magnification.) (Case courtesy of Dr. V. Palladino, Meadowbrook Hospital, East Meadow, NY.)

(1990) noted the presence of herpetic infection in **smears of women after radiotherapy for cervical cancer.**

Genital herpesvirus infection in the woman has **important clinical implications.** The disease may be **transmitted to the fetus** during vaginal delivery with resulting disastrous infection resulting in major abnormalities (Florman et al, 1973). Type II herpesvirus has been implicated as a possible causative agent in carcinoma of the uterine cervix (see Chap. 11).

Cytomegalovirus

Cytomegalovirus is a virus of the **herpesvirus family,** so named because it forms very large inclusions in the affected cells. Even before the onset of AIDS, Morse et al (1974) recorded serologic evidence of **cytomegalovirus infection in the female genital tract** in women attending a venereal disease clinic. Surprisingly, the frequency of cytomegalovirus was similar to that of herpesvirus. Cytomegalovirus was associated in several instances with the presence of condylomata acuminata involving the vulva and sometimes the uterine cervix. The characteristic cytomegalic inclusions were, however, identified in smears of only 1 of 12 patients. Several observations of **cytomegalovirus in endocervical epithelium** are on record (Huang and Naylor, 1993; Henry-Stanley et al, 1993). Wenckebach and Curry (1976) observed three instances of cytomegalovirus infection in material from uterine curettage. In patients with AIDS, widespread cytomegalovirus infections are frequent and the **characteristic large intranuclear inclusions, accompanied by smaller satellite inclusions in the nucleus and the cytoplasm** may be observed in cervicovaginal smears. Hunt et al (1998) observed rod-shaped laminal satellite cytoplasmic inclusions. The reader will find further comments and illustrations in Chapters 19 and 22.

Herpesvirus of Unknown Type

We observed a case of herpesvirus infection in a cervicovaginal smear of a 31-year-old woman with AIDS. The virus caused **very large, homogeneous intranuclear inclusions** in squamous and endocervical cells (Fig. 10-31). Our initial impression was that the inclusions were of polyomavirus type but the electron microscopy of the viral inclusions was typical of a herpesvirus infection. The virions, filling the nuclei, had a typical core and capsule (Fig. 10-31C).

Dr. Yuan Chang of Columbia University College of Physicians and Surgeons, the discoverer of herpesvirus type VIII, examined some material from this patient and could not match it with any known viruses of the herpes family. Unfortunately, the material was insufficient for sequencing of viral DNA and the type of the virus remains unknown at this time.

Other Viruses

Occasionally, *human polyomavirus,* which forms **homogeneous nuclear inclusions in urothelial cells,** commonly observed in the urinary sediment (discussed in detail in Chap. 22), has also been observed in vaginal smears, particularly during pregnancy (Wachtel, 1977).

Measles

The measles virus is usually transmitted among children but occasionally affects adults. The disease is characterized morphologically by hyperplasia of lymphoid tissues and by formation of **giant cells with numerous, up to 100, nuclei,** known as **Warthin-Finkeldey cells.** A case of measles cervicitis with these cells in smears and a molecular biologic confirmation of the disease were described by Heiman et al (1992).

Nonviral Inclusions

Occasionally, **eosinophilic cytoplasmic inclusions** may be observed in endocervical cells. These inclusions are of no diagnostic significance and closely resemble those observed in the bronchial cells (see Chap. 19) and in urothelial cells (see Chap. 22).

Parasitic Infections and Infestations

Trichomonas vaginalis

Infestation of the lower genital tract of the female with protozoon, *Trichomonas vaginalis,* is exceedingly common. Trussell (1947) estimated that at least 20% to 25% of adult women harbor the parasite and this estimate has not changed with the passage of time. It is generally accepted that **the male is the carrier of the parasite and that the infection is transmitted by sexual contact.** Gardner et al (1986) could document the presence of *Trichomonas* in the prostate by means of specific antisera. Kean and Wolinska (1956) have shown that *Trichomonas* frequently invades the urethra, which is thus a source of reinfection. Generally, patients with gynecologic symptoms, such as discharge or itching, have a higher incidence of infestation than do asymptomatic examinees. **The mere presence of *Trichomonas* in the genital tract of women is not synonymous with inflammation.** About 10% of infected women seem to suffer no ill effects from the presence of the parasite; however, an inflammatory process may occur in such patients with relative facility. The majority of women with inflammatory disease due to *Trichomonas* experience spontaneous healing and freedom of symptoms on repeated occasions. The exact mechanism that brings about the capricious clinical course of infestation with *Trichomonas* is not clear. The rise in the vaginal and cervical pH, just prior to and during the menstrual period, favors growth of the parasite. Experimental work by Weld and Kean (1956) suggests that tissue injury may be an important factor in survival of *Trichomonas vaginalis.*

Histology

Study of biopsies of the uterine cervix in the course of *Trichomonas* cervicitis suggests that the **parasite is capable of directly attacking the squamous epithelium,** which responds initially with **dilatation of capillary vessels** in epithelial papillae, followed by papillitis, edema, erosion of the superficial layers, and necrosis. The **"strawberry cervix"** observed clinically corresponds to a marked distention of the superficial blood vessels and focal hemorrhages as seen in histologic material (see Fig. 10-13A).

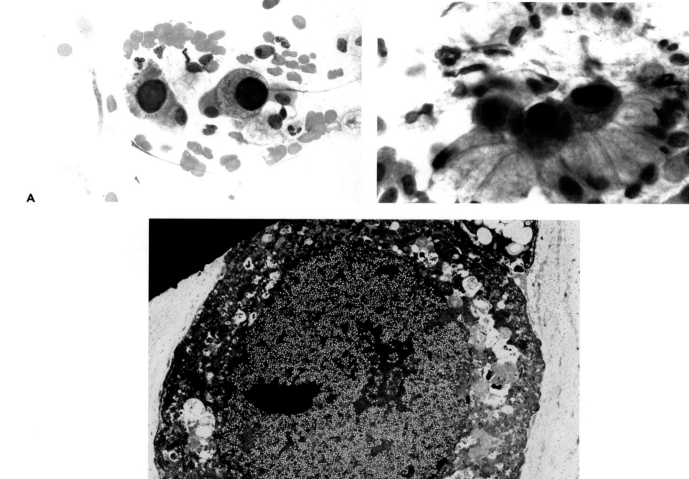

Figure 10-31 **Infection with herpesvirus of unknown type described in text.** *A,B.* Very large homogeneous intranuclear inclusions in squamous cells (*A*) and endocervical cells (*B*). *C.* Electron micrograph of the affected nucleus showing viral particles, nearly completely replacing the nuclear chromatin. The inset (×103,000) shows the typical structure of herpesvirus virions with a central core and a capsule. (*C:* Courtesy of Dr. Karen Weidenheim, Montefiore Medical Center. *Inset:* Courtesy of Dr. Jan Orenstein, George Washington University.)

Kolstad (1964), using colposcopy, confirmed the existence of a specific vascular pattern in the squamous epithelium of the cervix in *Trichomonas* infestation. Kolstad spoke of **"double-crested capillaries,"** which to his mind were diagnostic of the disease. The mechanisms of the interaction of *Trichomonas* with the squamous epithelium and the capillary vessels are unknown at the time of this writing.

Recognition

The identification of the parasite is essential before the diagnosis can be established with assurance and treatment instituted. The best way to recognize the parasite is the **"hanging drop"** technique in which a drop of vaginal secreta is placed on a slide and examined under the microscope. The flagellated parasites will be readily recognized as mobile structures rapidly criss-crossing the visual field. Wendel et al (2002) reported that culture and polymerase chain reaction in vaginal fluid have a higher sensitivity and specificity than "hanging drop" method in the recognition of the parasite. These methods, however, require a delay of several hours or days and add significantly to the cost.

In Papanicolaou-stained smears, the protozoa appear as **gray-green round or elliptical structures,** varying in size from 8 to 20 μm (Fig. 10-32A,B). Recognition of the **ec-centrically located round nucleus** is helpful in the diagnosis. **Flagella,** in the form of filaments on one pole of the parasite, are seen only in well-preserved material. The parasite must be distinguished from particles of inspissated mucus and degenerating cellular material. Okuyama et al (1998) and Wendel et al (2002) identified the presence of *Trichomonas* **by polymerase chain reaction** in DNA obtained from cervicovaginal smears.

The size of the *Trichomonas* organism is unrelated to its pathogenicity. Large *Trichomonas,* sometimes with multiple nuclei and flagella, appear when growth conditions are unfavorable; small sizes prevail when the growth conditions are favorable (D. Hollander, personal communication, 1976). Giant forms of this organism have been occasionally reported which are clearly a very rare event. **Filamentous bacteria of the genus *Leptothrix* are often found in smears in association with *Trichomonas*** (Fig. 10-32C). Synchronous infection with *Trichomonas* and *monilia* may be observed (Fig. 10-32D).

Cytology

As discussed above in the general description of inflammatory changes, Trichomoniasis is a prototype of cervicitis because it may induce changes in **smear pattern and cell**

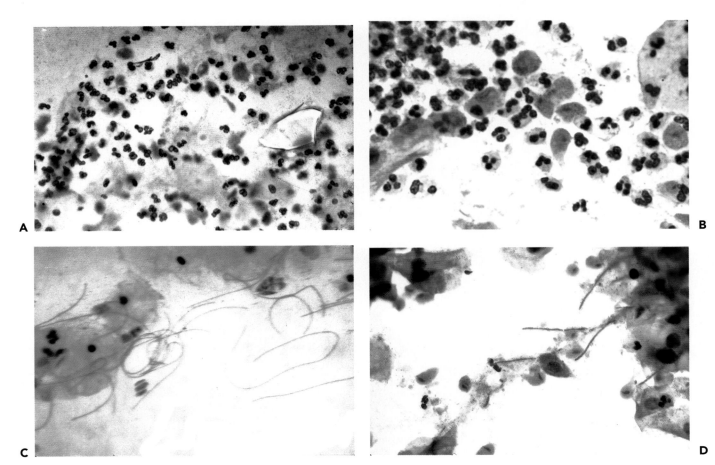

Figure 10-32 Trichomoniasis. *A.* The presence of gray-green parasites may be observed in the background of the inflammatory smear. *B.* High-power view of the parasite showing the typical gray-green tint and poorly preserved nuclei. The flagella cannot be seen in this preparation (see also Fig. 10-14C). *C.* Leptothrix. The filamentous bacterium commonly accompanies *Trichomonas* infestation. *D.* Synchronous infection with *Trichomonas* and *monilia.* Both organisms can be readily recognized in the smear.

configuration. Based on these features, an experienced observer may suggest *Trichomonas vaginalis* infestation, even if the parasite cannot be identified. Perhaps the most common change is **marked eosinophilia** observed in superficial, intermediate and larger parabasal squamous cells (see Fig. 10-14C). **Enlarged perinuclear clear zones or halos** in superficial cells are another common feature (see Fig. 10-16B). The halos surround the entire nucleus in a regular fashion and must be distinguished from the larger and asymmetrical clear zones of koilocytes, discussed in Chapter 11. In younger women with severe inflammatory reaction with necrosis of the superficial layers of the squamous epithelium, the smear may be dominated by parabasal cells, whereas in postmenopausal women, epithelial maturation can occur, presumably because of increased blood flow (see Fig. 10-15). However, it must be stressed that at least 20% of women, bearers of *Trichomonas,* have no symptoms whatever and the finding of the parasite in cervicovaginal smears is purely incidental.

Other changes that may be observed are nuclear pallor and enlargement, suggestive of **cell necrosis** (see Fig. 10-16A) and occasionally **apoptosis** (see Fig. 10-16C). Abnormalities of endocervical cells, such as cell enlargement, cytoplasmic vacuolization (see Fig. 10-17), presence of visible nucleoli and florid squamous metaplasia ("repair") may also occur.

Many years ago, some observers suggested that *Trichomonas* infestation may produce cytologic changes simulating cancer. This is most emphatically not the case. The question of whether patients with *Trichomonas* infestation are more prone to develop cervix cancer than other women has been answered in the negative (Koss and Wolinska, 1959). However, it should be emphasized that patients with all forms of cervix cancer, including carcinoma in situ, have a higher incidence of *Trichomonas* infestation than the normal population. Therefore, the presence of *Trichomonas* in a smear does not rule out the presence of a synchronous precancerous lesion or cancer of the uterine cervix.

Other Protozoa

Uncommon protozoa found in cervical smears include *Vorticella* [Hermann and Deininger (1963), San Cristobal et al (1976)] and *Entamoeba histolytica.* The latter, in the form of **cysts and trophozoites (amoebae),** is seen predominantly in countries where amebic colitis is common. In Papanicolaou stain, the **trophozoites** are round or oval basophilic structures of variable sizes, averaging 15 to 20 μm in diameter but occasionally larger. The **nucleus** is usually eccentric, round, and provided with a central karyosome. The **cytoplasm** contains ingested red blood cells (**erythrophagocytosis**) (Fig. 10-33). Unless erythrocytes are identified, the diagnosis should be rendered with extreme caution. DeTorres and Benitez-Bribiesca (1973) suggested periodic acid-Schiff stain and acid-phosphatase stain for secure identification. These authors also point out that, in countries with high prevalence of amebiasis, the parasite may cause lesions of the vulva and cervix, clinically resembling carcinoma.

DeMoraes-Ruehsen et al (1980) described the presence of amebae, resembling *Entamoeba gingivalis,* in the genital tracts of users of **intrauterine contraceptive devices.**

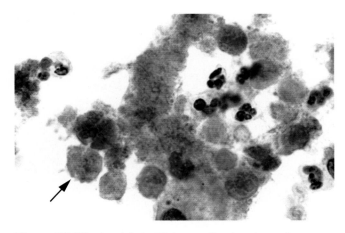

Figure 10-33 **Amebiasis.** High magnification shows the organisms as a spherical structure with poorly preserved nuclei (*arrow*). Erythrophagocytosis is not evident. (Oil immersion.)

A case of **Chagas' disease** affecting the cervix was reported by Concetti et al (2000) in a woman with AIDS. The intracellular parasite, *Trypanosoma cruzi,* could be recognized in multinucleated giant cells, containing the characteristic reproductive form of the parasite, known as amastigotes. It is likely that this disorder will be observed in cervicovaginal smears in countries where the Chagas' disease is endemic, such as Peru.

The protozoon, *Balantidium coli,* is usually the cause of an intractable diarrhea. Several cases of balantidial vaginitis have been recorded (Berry, 1976). The **trophozoites** are very large (from 50 to 80 μm in length and from 40 to 60 μm in width) and are provided with a pellicle, bearing short cilia. At one end of the trophozoite, there is an indentation or a cytosome. A large nucleus is usually visible (Berry, 1976). A cyst form of the parasite has also been described. The identification of the large parasite in Papanicolaou stain is easy (Fig. 10-34).

Helminthic Infections (Worms)

Schistosomiasis (Bilharziasis)

Three important organisms cause diseases in humans: *Schistosoma haematobium, Schistosoma mansoni,* **and** *Schistosoma japonicum.* All three organisms are flukes, with a complex natural history, with man as the final host. Two of these, *S. haematobium* and *S. mansoni,* can affect the female genital tract. Freshwater snails are the intermediate host for these parasites. From the snails, the motile forms of the organisms, the **cercariae,** are released in water, penetrate human skin, causing "swimmers' itch," and establish themselves in various organs. *S. haematobium* usually lodges in lymphatics of the pelvic organs, mainly the urinary bladder, whereas *S. mansoni* establishes itself primarily in the liver and the lower gastrointestinal tract. The **cercariae become mature worms.** The female worms release the characteristic ova, whence larval forms (**miracidia**) hatch and are released into water in urine or feces. In suitable surroundings the miracidia find the intermediate host (snails) and the cycle recommences. For a detailed account of the life cycle of schistosomes, the reader is referred to the book by Jordan and Webbe

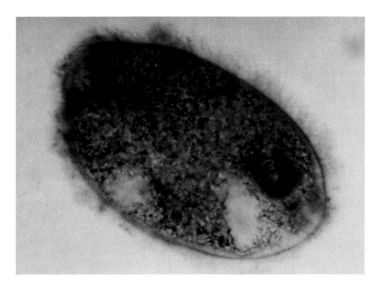

Figure 10-34 *Balantidium coli*, **vaginal smear.** Very large trophozoite with ciliated pellicle. Note the large nucleus and, at the opposite pole, a cytosome. (×600.) (Photo courtesy of the late Dr. Ann V. Berry, Johannesburg, South Africa.)

(1969) and to the outstanding contributions by the late Anne Berry (1966, 1971, 1976).

S. haematobium is found principally in Africa, whereas **S. mansoni** is found in Africa, South America, and the Caribbean. As a consequence of jet-age movement of people across the continents, such infections may now be seen in all geographic locations. Both **S. haematobium and S. mansoni** **may invade the lymphatics of the uterus and deposit ova in the stroma of the uterine cervix** (Fig. 10-35A). Clinically, the lesions of the uterine cervix due to schistosomiasis may imitate cancer. The identification of the parasites is based on **recognition of ova** and larval stages (miracidia) in the cervicovaginal smears.

In Papanicolaou-stained material, the **ova** of both species

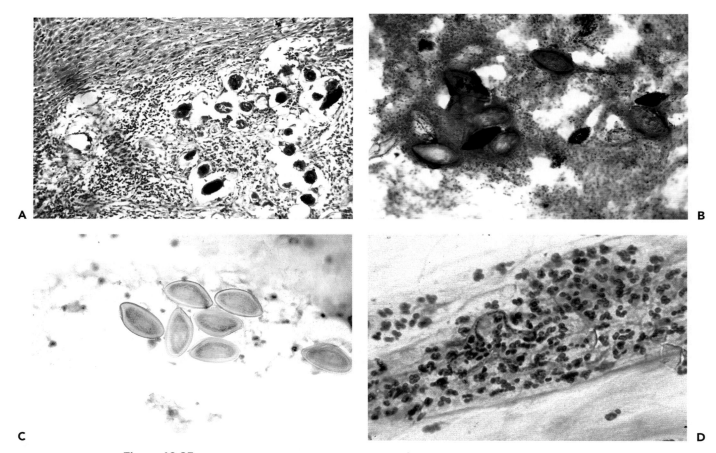

Figure 10-35 Parasites. *Schistosoma haematobium* in tissue (*A*) and in vaginal/cervical smear (*B*). The terminal spine of the ova is well seen. *C. Enterobius* (pin worm) ova. The typical polar operculum may be observed. *D.* Filaria (*Mansonella*) in a cervicovaginal smear.

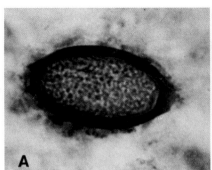
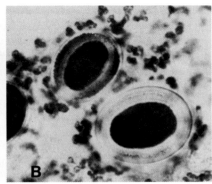

Figure 10-36 Vaginal smears. Ovum of *Trichuris trichiura* (A) and ova of *Taenia* (B). (Photos courtesy of the late Dr. Ann V. Berry, Johannesburg, South Africa.)

have a **thick, semitranslucent shell provided with a spine.** The **spine is usually terminal in *S. haematobium*** and **lateral in *S. mansoni*.** The ova average about 140 μm in length and 60 to 70 μm in width. Smaller and larger sizes may be observed (Fig. 10-35B).

The **miracidia are boat-shaped organisms,** that in general configuration, resemble the ova, except for the absence of the shell. The miracidia may show active movement and, therefore, may show variable shapes and sizes. For the detail of anatomy of the miracidia, the reader is referred to Berry's papers. The **smear background in schistosomiasis** usually shows purulent exudate with an admixture of **eosinophilic leukocytes,** a common component of tissue reactions to parasites.

Intestinal Parasites: Nematodes (Roundworms) and Cestodes (Tapeworms)

Ova of various intestinal parasites may be observed in vaginal and cervical smears (Berry, 1976). It must be stressed that while these findings are uncommon in the developed countries, they are frequent in the developing countries. **Ova of *Enterobius vermicularis* (pinworm)** are perhaps the most frequent finding: the ova measure about 50 × 25 μm, stain yellow in Papanicolaou stain, and have a refringent, translucent, thick membrane, one edge of which is folded. A larva may be observed within the ovum (Fig. 10-35C). Occasionally, free larvae have been observed (San Cristobal and DeMundi, 1976).

In tropical countries, ***Trichuris trichiura* (whipworm)** may be observed. The brown ova are of approximately the same size as those of *Enterobius* but are provided with a trans-lucent knob on both poles (Fig. 10-36A). There is so far no record of ova of ***Ascaris lumbricoides*** in genital smears.

The flat worms, ***Taenia solium, Taenia saginata, and Taenia echinococcus,*** also play a role in diagnostic cytology. The round, brown eggs, about 35 μm in diameter, have a radially striated shell and have been observed in smears from the female genital tract (Fig. 10-36B). The reader is referred to Chapters 19, 25, and 29 for further comments on echinococcosis.

Strongyloides stercoralis, another intestinal parasite, usually observed in pulmonary specimens, has been observed in a cervicovaginal smear by Murty et al (1994). For a full description of this parasite and its life cycle see Chapter 19.

Filariae

The extent of worldwide spread of various forms of filariasis is enormous. For the most part, the tiny, **thread-like worms** invade humans through insect bites, multiply in blood, and then settle in various organs, often blocking lymphatics of subcutaneous tissue. For the fine points of morphologic differential diagnosis among the various species and for the geographic distribution of filariae, the reader is referred to other sources (e.g., Ash and Spitz *Atlas*, 1945).

There are several recorded instances of various species of filariae observed in the smears from the female genital tract: ***Wuchereria bancrofti*** (Chandra et al, 1975), ***Onchocerca volvulus*** (DeBorges, 1971), and ***Dipetalonema perstans*** (Sharma et al, 1971). All filariae share the slender worm-like appearance with filiform end and measure from 1 to 4 cm in length (see Figs. 10-35D and 10-37).

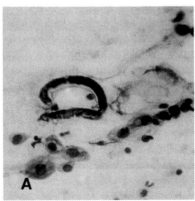
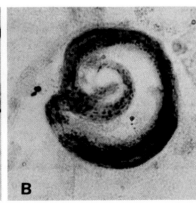

Figure 10-37 Filaria (*Onchocerca volvulus*) in vaginal smears. (Oil immersion.) (Courtesy of Dr. Rosa de Borges, Caracas, Venezuela.)

Arthropods (Insects)

Occasionally arthropods, such as water fleas or mites, or parts thereof, may be observed in vaginal smears. Bechtold et al (1952) pointed out that **carpet beetle hairs,** resembling serrated brown arrows, are a fairly common finding (see Chap. 8).

BIBLIOGRAPHY

Alvares-Santin C, Sica A, Rodriguez M, et al. Microglandular hyperplasia of the uterine cervix. Cytologic diagnosis in cervical smears. Acta Cytol 43: 110–113, 1999.

Alvarez F, Brache V, Fernandez E, et al. New insights on the mode of action of intrauterine contraceptive devices in women. Fertil Steril 49:768–773, 1988.

An SH. Herpes simplex virus infection detected on routine gynecologic cell specimens. Acta Cytol 13:354–358, 1969.

Anandi V, Babu PG, John JJ. *Cryptococcus neoformans* of unusual morphology in a patient with AIDS. Mycoses 34:377–379, 1991.

Angrish K, Verma K. Cytologic detection of tuberculosis of the uterine cervix. Acta Cytol 25:160–162, 1981.

Arroyo G, Quinn JA Jr. Association of amoebae and actinomyces in an intrauterine contraceptive device user. Acta Cytol 33:298–300, 1989.

Ash JE, Spitz S. Pathology of Tropical Diseases: An Atlas. Philadelphia, WB Saunders, 1945.

Babkowski RC, Wilbur DC, Rutkowski MA, et al. The effect of endocervical canal topography, tubal metaplasia, and high canal sampling on the cytologic presentation of nonneoplastic endocervical cells. Am J Clin Pathol 105:403–410, 1996.

Barter JF, Orr JW, Holloway RW, et al. Psammoma bodies in a cervicovaginal smear associated with an intrauterine device: A case report. J Reprod Med 32:147–148, 1987.

Baum SE, Dooley DP, Wright J, et al. Diagnosis of culture-negative female genital tract tuberculosis with peritoneal involvement by polymerase chain reaction. J Reprod Med 46:929–932, 2001.

Bechtold E, Reicher NB. Relationship of *Trichomonas* infestations to false diagnoses of squamous carcinoma of cervix. Cancer 5:442–457, 1952.

Bechtold E, Staunton CE, Katz SS. Carpet beetle larval parts in cervical cytology specimens. Acta Cytol 29:345–352, 1985.

Bennett BD, Bailey JM, Gardner WA. Immunocytochemical identification of trichomonads. Arch Pathol Lab Med 103:247–249, 1979.

Bergogne-Berezin E, Slim A, Benhamou G. Septicemie à torulopsis glabrata. Sem Hop Paris 52:147–151, 1976.

Bergsjo P, Koller O, Kolstad P. The vascular pattern of *Trichomonas vaginalis* cervicitis. Acta Cytol 7:292–294, 1963.

Bernal JN, Martinez MA, Dabancens A. Evaluation of proposed cytomorphologic criteria for the diagnosis of *Chlamydia trachomatis* in Papanicolaou smears. Acta Cytol 33:309–313, 1988.

Bernstine JB, Rakoff AE. Vaginal Infections, Infestations, and Discharges. New York, Blakiston, 1953.

Berry A. A cytopathological and histopathological study of bilharziasis of the female genital tract. J Pathol Bacteriol 91:325–338, 1966.

Berry A. Evidence of gynecologic bilharziasis in cytologic material. A morphologic study for cytologists in particular. Acta Cytol 15:482–498, 1971.

Berry A. Multispecies schistosomal infections of the female genital tract detected in cytology smears. Acta Cytol 20:361–365, 1976.

Bertini B, Hornstein M. The epidemiology of trichomoniasis and role of this infection in the development of carcinoma of the cervix. Acta Cytol 14: 325–332, 1970.

Bhagavan BS, Gupta PK. Genital actinomycosis and intrauterine contraceptive devices. Hum Pathol 9:567–578, 1978.

Bhagavan BS, Ruffier J, Shinn B. Pseudoactinomycotic radiate granules in the lower female genital tract: Relationship to the Splendore-Hoeppli phenomenon. Hum Pathol 13:898–904, 1982.

Bhambhani S, Das DK, Singh V, Luthra UK. Cervical tuberculosis with carcinoma in situ: A cytodiagnosis [Letter]. Acta Cytol 29:87–88, 1985.

Bibbo M, Keebler CM, Wied GL. The cytologic diagnosis of tissue repair in the female genital tract. Acta Cytol 15:133–137, 1971.

Bibbo M, Wied GL. Inflammatory reactions and microbiology of the female genital tract. *In* Wied GL, Bibbo M, Keebler CM, et al (eds). Compendium on Diagnostic Cytology, 8th ed. Chicago, Tutorials of Cytology, 1997, pp 68–75.

Blank H, Burgoon CF, Baldridge GD, et al. Cytologic smears in diagnosis of herpes simplex, herpes zoster and varicella. JAMA 146:1410–1412, 1951.

Blank H, Rake GW. Viral and Rickettsial Diseases of the Skin, Eye and Mucous Membranes of Man. Boston, Little, Brown & Co, 1955.

Bonilla-Musoles F, Barbera E. Die Bipotenz der Reservezellen; electronmikroskopische Uutersuchung der indirekten Metaplasie. Z Gebh Gynak 173: 79–88, 1970.

Borchardt KA, Noble MA (eds). Sexually Transmitted Diseases. Boca Raton, FL, CRC Press, 1996.

Boyce JG, Lu T, Nelson JH Jr, Joyce D. Cervical carcinoma and oral contraception. Obstet Gynecol 40:139–146, 1972.

Brooks JJ, Wheeler JE. Malignancy arising in extragonadal endometriosis. Cancer 40:3065–3073, 1977.

Brown JR. Human actinomycosis. Hum Pathol 4:319–330, 1973.

Brown S, Senekjian EK, Montag AG. Cytomegalovirus infection of the uterine cervix in a patient with acquired immunodeficiency syndrome. Obstet Gynecol 71:489–491, 1988.

Brunham RC, Paavonen J, Stevens CE, et al. Mucopurulent cervicitis—the ignored counterpart in women of urethritis in men. N Engl J Med 311:1–6, 1984.

Buckner SB, Mikel U. Unusual and giant forms of *Trichomonas vaginalis*. Acta Cytol 27:549–550, 1983.

Candy MD, Abell MR. Progestogen-induced adenomatous hyperplasia of the uterine cervix. JAMA 203:323–326, 2001.

Cano RJ, Beck MA, Grady DV. Detection of *Gardnerella vaginalis* on vaginal smears by immunofluorescence. Can J Microbiol 29:27–32, 1983.

Carvalho G, Kramer WM, Kay S. The presence of *Leptothrix* in vaginal smears. Acta Cytol 9:244–246, 1965.

Cederqvist L, Eliasson G, Lindell L, Stormby L. Nuclear inclusion bodies in vaginal smears from patients with vaginal discharge. Acta Cytol 49:13–16, 1970.

Chandra K, Annousamy R. An unusual finding in the vaginal smears [Letter]. Acta Cytol 19:403–404, 1975.

Ciotti RA, Sondheimer SJ, Nachamkin I. Detecting *Chlamydia trachomatis* by direct immunofluorescence using a cytobrush sampling technique. Genitourin Med 64:245–246, 1988.

Coleman DV. A case of tuberculosis of the cervix. Acta Cytol 13:104–107, 1969.

Colgan TJ, Woodhouse SL, Styer PE, et al. Reparative changes and the false-positive/false-negative Papanicolaou test. Arch Pathol Lab Med 125: 134–140, 2001.

Concetti H, Retegui M, Perez G, Perez H. Chagas' disease of the cervix uteri in a patient with acquired immunodeficiency syndrome. Hum Pathol 31: 120–122, 2000.

Corey L, Spear PG. Infections with herpes simplex viruses (two parts). N Engl J Med 314:686–691, 749–757, 1986.

Crum CP, Cibas ES, Lee KR. Pathology of Early Cervical Neoplasia. New York, Churchill Livingstone, 1997.

Dabancens A, Prado R, Larraguibel R, Zanartu J. Intraepithelial cervical neoplasia in women using intrauterine devices and long-acting injectable progestogens as contraceptives. Am J Obstet 119:1052–1056, 1974.

Daling JA, Weiss NS, Metch BJ, et al. Primary tubal infertility in relation to the use of an intrauterine device. N Engl J Med 312:937–941, 1985.

Daniele E, Nuara R, Morello V, et al. Microglandular hyperplasia of the uterine cervix: Histopathological evaluation, differential diagnosis and review of the literature. Pathologica 85:607–635, 1993.

De Boer A, de Boer F, Van der Merwe JV. Cytologic identification of Donovan bodies in granuloma inguinale. Acta Cytol 28:126–128, 1984.

De Peralta VMN, Purslow MJ, Kini SR. Endometrial cells of the "lower uterine segment" (LUS) in cervical smears obtained by endocervical brushings. A source of potential diagnostic pitfall. Diag Cytopathol 12:263–271, 1995.

DeBorges R. Findings of microfilarial larval stages in gynecologic smears. Acta Cytol 15:476–478, 1971.

DeMoraes-Ruehsen M, McNeill RE, Frost JK, et al. Amebae, resembling *Entamoeba gingivalis* in genital tract of IUD users. Acta Cytol 24:413–420, 1980.

DeTorres EF, Benitez-Bribiesca L. Cytologic detection of vaginal parasitosis. Acta Cytol 17:252–257, 1973.

DiBerardino MA, Hoffner NJ, Etkin LD. Activation of dormant genes in specialized cells. Science 224:946–952, 1984.

Dominguez A, Giron JJ. Toxoplasma cysts in vaginal smears. Acta Cytol 20: 268–270, 1976.

Dorman SA, Danos LM, Wilson DJ, et al. Detection of chlamydial cervicitis by Papanicolaou stained smears and culture. Am J Clin Pathol 79:421–425, 1983.

Dougherty CM. Cervical cytology and sequential birth control pills. Obstet Gynecol 36:741–744, 1970.

Dressel DM, Wilbur DC. Atypical immature squamous metaplastic cells in cervical smears: Association with high grade squamous epithelial lesions and carcinoma of the cervix (abstr.) Acta Cytol 36:630, 1992.

Drusin LM, Singer C, Valenti AJ, Armstrong D. Infectious syphilis mimicking neoplastic disease. Arch Int Med 137:156–160, 1977.

Dryer ML, Young TL, Kattine AA, Wilson DD. Blastomycosis in a Papanicolaou smear. Report of a case with a possible venereal transmission. Acta Cytol 27:285–287, 1983.

Ducatman BS, Wang HH, Jonasson JG, et al. Tubal metaplasia: a cytologic study with comparison to other neoplastic and non-neoplastic conditions of the endocervix. Diagn Cytopathol 9:98–103; discussion 103–105, 1993.

Duggan MA, Pomponi C, Kay D, Robboy SJ. Infantile chlamydial conjunctivitis. A comparison of Papanicolaou, giemsa and immunoperoxidase staining methods. Acta Cytol 30:341–346, 1986.

Dunkelberg WE Jr. Diagnosis of *Hemophilus vaginalis* vaginitis by Gram-stained smears. Am J Obstet Gynecol 91:998–1000, 1965.

Dunkelberg WE Jr, Skaggs R, Kellogg DS Jr. A study and new description of *Corynebacterium vaginale* (*Haemophilus vaginalis*). Am J Clin Pathol 53: 370–377, 1970.

Dunlop EMC, Garner A, Darougar S, et al. Colposcopy, biopsy, and cytology results in women with chlamydial cervicitis. Genitourin Med 65:22–31, 1989.

Egan AJM, Russel P. Transitional (urothelial) cell metaplasia of the uterine cervix: morphologic assessment of 31 cases. Int J Gynecol Pathol 16:89–98, 1997.

Ferenczy A, Richart RM. Female Reproductive System: Dynamics of Scan and Transmission Electron Microscopy. New York, John Wiley & Sons, 1974.

Ferry JA, Scully RE. Mesonephric remnants, hyperplasia, and neoplasia in the uterine cervix: a study of 49 cases. Am J Surg Pathol 14:1100–1111, 1990.

Fink CG, Thomas GH, Allen JM, Jordan JA. Metaplasia in endocervical tissue maintained in organ culture: an experimental model. J Obstet Gynaecol Br Commonw 80:169–175, 1973.

Florman AL, Gershon AA, Blackett PR, Nahmias AJ. Intrauterine infection with herpes simplex virus. JAMA 225:129–132, 1973.

Fluhmann CF. Focal hyperplasia (tunnel clusters) of the cervix uteri. Obstet Gynecol 17:206–214, 1961.

Fluhmann CF. The Cervix Uteri and Its Diseases. Philadelphia, WB Saunders, 1961.

Fornari ML. Cellular changes in the glandular epithelium of patients using IUCD. A source of cytologic error. Acta Cytol 18:341–343, 1974.

Frable WJ. Litigation cells: definition and observations on a cell type in cervical vaginal smears not addressed by the Bethesda System. Diagn Cytopathol 11:213–215, 1994.

Gall SA, Bourgeois CH, Maguire R. The morphologic effects of oral contraceptive agents on the cervix. JAMA 207:2243–2247, 1969.

Gardner HL, Dukes CD. *Haemophilus vaginalis* vaginitis: a newly defined specific infection previously classified as "nonspecific" vaginitis. Am J Obstet Gynecol 69:962–976, 1955.

Gardner HL, Kaufman RH. Benign Diseases of the Vulva and Vagina. St. Louis, CV Mosby, 1969.

Gardner WA, Culberson DE, Bennett BD. *Trichomonas vaginalis* in the prostate gland. Arch Pathol Lab Med 110:430–432, 1986.

Gaydos CA, Howell MR, Pare B, et al. *Chlamydia trachomatis* infections in female military recruits. N Engl J Med 339:739–744, 1998.

Geerling S, Nettum JA, Lindner LE, et al. Sensitivity and specificity of the Papanicolaou-stained cervical smear in the diagnosis of *Chlamydia trachomatis* infection. Acta Cytol 29:671–675, 1985.

Geirsson G, Woodworth FE, Patten SF Jr, Bonfiglio TA. Epithelial repair and regeneration in the uterine cervix: I. Analysis of the cells. Acta Cytol 21:371–378, 1977.

Geng L, Connolly DC, et al. Atypical immature metaplasia (AIM) of the cervix: is it related to high-grade squamous intraepithelial lesion (HSIL)? Hum Pathol 30:345–351, 1999.

Giampolo C, Murphy J, Benes S, et al. How sensitive is the Papanicolaou smear in the diagnosis of infections with *Chlamydia trachomatis*? Am J Clin Pathol 80:844–849, 1983.

Gigi-Leitner O, Geiger B, Levy R, Czernobilsky B. Cytokeratin expression in squamous metaplasia of the human uterine cervix. Differentiation 31:191–205, 1986.

Goldman RL, Bank RW, Warren NE. Cytomegalovirus infection of the cervix: An "incidental" finding of possible clinical significance. Report of a case. Obstet Gynecol 34:326–329, 1969.

Govan AD, Black WP, Sharp JL. Aberrant glandular polypi of the uterine cervix associated with contraceptive pills: Pathology and pathogenesis. J Clin Pathol 22:84–89, 1969.

Gregory JE, Payne FE. Cervical cytology and mycoplasma in two populations. Acta Cytol 14:434–438, 1970.

Grimes DA. Deaths due to sexually transmitted diseases: The forgotten component of reproductive mortality. JAMA 255:1727–1729, 1986.

Gupta PK. Intrauterine contraceptive devices: Vaginal cytology, pathologic changes, and clinical implications. Acta Cytol 26:571–613, 1982.

Gupta PK, Hollander DH, Frost JK. Actinomycetes in cervicovaginal smears: An association with IUD usage. Acta Cytol 20:295–297, 1976.

Gupta PK, Lee EF, Erozan YS, et al. Cytologic investigations of Chlamydia infection. Acta Cytol 23:315–320, 1979.

Gutmann EJ. Syphilitic cervicitis simulating stage II cervical cancer: Report of two cases with cytologic findings. Am J Clin Pathol 104:643–647, 1995.

Hanau C, Begley N, Bibbo M. Cervical endometriosis: A potential pitfall in the evaluation of glandular cells in vaginal smears. Diagn Cytopathol 16:274–280, 1997.

Handsfield HH, Jasman LL, Roberts PL, et al. Criteria for selective screening for *Chlamydia trachomatis* infection in women attending family planning clinics. JAMA 255:1730–1734, 1986.

Hare MJ, Taylor-Robinson D, Cooper P. Evidence for an association between *Chlamydia trachomatis* and cervical intraepithelial neoplasia. Br J Obstet Gynecol 89:489–492, 1982.

Harnden P, Kennedy W, Andrew AC, Southgate J. Immunophenotype of transitional metaplasia of the uterine cervix. Int J Gynecol Pathol 18:125–129, 1999.

Harnekar AB, Leiman G, Markowitz S. Cytologically detected chlamydial changes and progression of cervical intraepithelial neoplasias. A retrospective case-control study. Acta Cytol 29:661–664, 1985.

Harrison HR, Phil D, Costin M, et al. Cervical *Chlamydia trachomatis* infection in university women: Relationship to history, contraception, ectopy, and cervicitis. Am J Obstet Gynecol 153:224–251, 1985.

Hart WR, Prins RP, Tsai JC. Isolated coccidioidomycosis of the uterus. Hum Pathol 7:235–239, 1976.

Heiman A, Scanlon R, Gentile J, et al. Measles cervicitis. Report of a case with cytologic and molecular biologic analysis. Acta Cytol 36:727–730, 1992.

Heller C, Hoyt V. Squamous cell changes associated with the presence of candida sp. in cervical-vaginal Papanicolaou smears. Acta Cytol 15:379–384, 1971.

Heller CJ. *Neisseria gonorrhoeae* in Papanicolaou smears. Acta Cytol 18:338–340, 1974.

Henderson SR. Pelvic actinomycosis associated with an intrauterine device. Obstet Gynecol 41:726–732, 1973.

Henry MR, de Mesy Jensen KL, Skoglund CD, Armstrong DW. Chlamydia trachomatis in routine cervical smears. A microscopic and ultrastructural analysis. Acta Cytol 37:343–352, 1993.

Henry-Stanley MJ, Stanley MW, et al. Cytologic diagnosis of cytomegalovirus in cervical smears. Diagn Cytopathol 9:364–365, 1993.

Hermann GI, Deininger JT. Vorticella, an unusual protozoa (sic!) found on endocervical smear (letter to the editor). Acta Cytol 7:129–130, 1963.

Heyderdahl TD. Type I and type II herpes virus and abnormal cervical cytology. J Irish Med Assoc 67:445–447, 1974.

Highman WJ. Cervical smears in tuberculous endometritis. Acta Cytol 16:16–20, 1971.

Hill GB. The microbiology of bacterial vaginosis. Am J Obstet Genecol 169:450–454, 1993.

Hillier SL, Nugent RP, Eschenbach DA, et al. Association between bacterial vaginosis and preterm delivery of low-birth-weight infant. N Engl J Med 333:1737–1742, 1995.

Hollander DH. Colonial morphology of *Trichomonas vaginalis* in agar. Parasitology 62:826–828, 1976.

Hook EW, Marra CM. Acquired syphilis in adults. N Engl J Med 326:1060–1069, 1992.

Huang JC, Naylor B. Cytomegalovirus infection in the cervix detected by cytology and histology. Diagn Cytopathol 4:237–241, 1993.

Hunt JL, Baloch Z, Judkins A, et al. Unique cytomegalovirus intracytoplasmic inclusions in ectocervical cells on a cervical/endocervical smear. Diagn Cytopathol 18:110–112, 1998.

Hunter CA Jr, Long KR. Vaginal pH in normal women and in patients with vaginitis. Am J Gynecol 75:872–874, 1958.

Jirovec O, Petru M. *Trichomonas vaginalis* and trichomoniasis. *In* Dawes B (ed). Advances in Parasitology, vol 6. New York, Academic Press, 1968, pp 117–188.

Jonasson JG, Wang HH, Antonioli DA, Ducatman DS. Tubal metaplasia of the uterine cervix. A prevalence study in patients with gynecologic pathologic findings. Int J Gynecol Pathol 11:89–95, 1992.

Jones MA, Andrews J, Tarraza HM. Mesonephric remnant hyperplasia of the cervix. A clinicopathologic analysis of 14 cases. Gynecol Oncol 49:41–47, 1993.

Jones MC, Buschmann BO, Dowling EA, Pollock HM. The prevalence of *Actinomyces*-like organisms in cervicovaginal smears of 300 IUD wearers. Acta Cytol 23:282–286, 1979.

Jordan P, Webbe G. Human Schistosomiasis. London, Wm. Heinemann, 1969.

Jordan SW, Evangel E, Smith NL. Ethnic distribution of cytologically diagnosed herpes simplex genital infections in a cervical cancer screening program. Acta Cytol 16:363–365, 1972.

Kean BH, Wolinska WH. Urethral trichomoniasis: Cytologic study. Am J Clin Pathol 26:1142–1144, 1956.

Kearns PR, Gray JE. Mycotic vulvovaginitis. Obstet Gynecol 22:621–625, 1963.

Kellog JA. Clinical and laboratory considerations of culture vs. antigen assays for detection of *Chlamydia trachomatis* from genital specimens. Arch Pathol Lab Med 113:453–460, 1989.

Kern SB. Significance of anucleated squames in Papanicolaou-stained cervicovaginal smears. Acta Cytol 35:89–93, 1991.

Khilnami PH, Powar HS. Detection of microfilaiae in cervical cytology [Letter]. Acta Cytol 36:451–452, 1992.

Kirloskar J, Tulasi P, Vasantha CC. Tuberculosis of cervix (a study of 23 cases). J Obstet Gynaecol 18:709–712, 1968.

Kiviat NB, Paavonen JA, Brockway J, et al. Cytologic manifestations of cervical and vaginal infections. I. Epithelial and cellular changes. JAMA 253:989–996, 1985.

Kleger B, Prier JE, Rosato DJ, McGinnis AE. Herpes simplex infection of the female genital tract. Am J Obstet Gynecol 102:745–748, 1968.

Kobayashi TK, Okamoto H, Yakushiji M. Cytologic detection of herpes simplex virus DNA in nipple discharge by in situ hybridization. Diagn Cytopathol 9:296–299, 1993.

Kolstad P. The colposcopical picture of *Trichomonas* vaginitis. Acta Obstet Gynecol Scand 43:388–398, 1964.

Koss LG. Miniature adenoacanthoma arising in an endometriotic cyst in an obturator lymph node. Report of first case. Cancer 16:1369–1372, 1963.

Koss LG. Transitional cell metaplasia of the uterine cervix—a misnomer [Letter to Editor]. Am J Surg Pathol 22:774–775, 1998.

Koss LG, Wolinska WH. *Trichomonas vaginalis* cervicitis and its relationship to cervical cancer: Histocytological study. Cancer 12:1171–1193, 1959.

Kyriakos M, Kempson RL, Konikov NF. A clinical and pathologic study of endocervical lesions associated with oral contraceptives. Cancer 22:99–110, 1968.

Langenberg AGM, Corey L, Ashley RL, et al. A prospective study of new infections with herpes simplex virus type 1 and type 2. N Engl J Med 341:1432–1438, 1999.

Langlinais PC. *Enterobius vermicularis* in a vaginal smear. Acta Cytol 13:40–47, 1969.

Laverty CR, Russell P, Black J, et al. Adenovirus infection of the cervix. Acta Cytol 21:114–117, 1977.

Le Van L, Novotny D, Dotters DJ. Distinguishing tubal metaplasia from endocervical dysplasia on cervical Papanicolaou smears. Obstet Gynecol 78:974–976, 1991.

Lebreuil G, Erny R, Sudan N, et al. Endométrite à cytomegalovirus. Arch Anat Pathol 21:155–160, 1973.

Leppäluoto PA. A cytologic evaluation of the relationship of coitus and vaginal mycoplasma. J Reprod Med 9:35–39, 1972.

Leppäluoto PA. The etiology of the cocci type "Streptokokkentyp" vaginal smear [Letter to the Editor]. Acta Cytol 15:211–215, 1971.

Leppäluoto PA. The occurrence of vaginal diphtheroids in Papanicolaou smears. Acta Cytol 18:362–366, 1974.

Leslie KO, Silverberg SG. Microglandular hyperplasia of the cervix: Unusual clinical and pathological presentations and their differential diagnosis. Prog Surg Pathol 5:95–11, 1984.

Lewis JF, Alexander JJ. Isolation of Neisseria meningitidis from the vagina and cervix (abstr). Am J Clin Pathol 61:216–217, 1974.

Lifson AR, Olson R, Roberts MG, et al. Severe opportunistic infections in AIDS patients with late-stage disease. J Am Board Fam Pract 7:288–291, 1994.

Lindner E, Geerling S, Nettum JA, et al. Identification of Chlamydia in cervical smears by immunofluorescence: Technic, sensitivity, and specialty. Am J Clin Pathol 85:180–185, 1986.

Lindner LE, Geerling S, Nettum JA, et al. The cytologic features of Chlamydia cervicitis. Acta Cytol 29:676–682, 1985.

Litt IF, Edberg SC, Finberg L. Gonorrhea in children and adolescents: A current review. J Pediatr 85:595–607, 1974.

Longatto-Filho A, Maeda MY, Oyafuso MS, et al. Herpes simplex virus in postradiation cervical smears. A morphologic and immunocytochemical study. Acta Cytol 34:652–656, 1990.

Louria VB, Greenberg SM, Molander DW. Fungaemia caused by certain nonpathogenic strains of the family Cryptococcaceae. Report of two cases due to Rhodotorula and Torulopsis glabrata. N Engl J Med 263:1281–1284, 1960.

Luster AD. Chemokines-chemotactic cytokines that mediate inflammation. N Engl J Med 338:436–445, 1998.

Mardh PA, Stormby N, Westrom L. Mycoplasma and vaginal cytology. Acta Cytol 15:310–315, 1971.

Mariano M, Spector WG. Formation and properties of macrophage polykaryons (inflammatory giant cells). J Pathol 113:1–19, 1974.

Marks M, Langston C, Eickhoff TC. Torulopsis glabrata. An opportunistic pathogen in man. N Engl J Med 283:1131–1135, 1970.

Marshall DS, Linfert DR, Draghi A, et al. Identification of herpes simplex virus genital infection: Comparison of a multiplex PCR assay and traditional viral isolation techniques. Mod Pathol 14:152–156, 2001.

Martens J, Baars J, Smedts F, et al. Can keratin 8 and 17 immunohistochemistry be of diagnostic value in cervical cytology? A feasibility study. Cancer 87:87–92, 1999.

McCracken AW, D'Agostino AN, Brucks AB, et al. Acquired cytomegalovirus infection presenting as viral endometritis. Am J Clin Pathol 61:556–560, 1974.

McIndoe WA, Churchouse MJ. Herpes simplex of the lower genital tract in the female. Aust NZ J Obstet Gynaecol 12:14–23, 1972.

McLachlan JA, Newbold RR. Reproductive tract lesions in male mice exposed prenatally to diethylstilbestrol. Science 190:991–992, 1975.

Meisels A. Microbiology of the female reproductive tract as determined in the cytologic specimen. III. In the presence of cellular atypias. Acta Cytol 13:64–71, 1969.

Meisels A, Fortin R. Condylomatous lesions of the cervix and vagina. I. Cytologic patterns. Acta Cytol 20:505–509, 1976.

Meisels A, Fortin R. Genital tuberculosis cytologic detection. Acta Cytol 19:79–81, 1975.

Melamed MR, Koss LG, Flehinger BJ, et al. Prevalence rates of uterine cervical carcinoma in situ for women using the diaphragm or contraceptive oral steroids. Br Med J 3:195–200, 1969.

Memik F. Trichomonads in pleural effusion. JAMA 204:211–212, 1968.

Meyer R. Ueber Epidermoidalisierung (Ersatz des Schleimepithels durch Plattenepithel) an der portio vaginalis uteri nach Erosion, an Cervicalpolypen und in der Cervical-schleimhaut; ein Beitrag zur Frage der Stäuckchendiagnose und des precancerosen Stadiums. Zentralbl Gynäkol 47:946–960, 1923.

Miguel NL, Lachowicz CM, Kline TS. Candida-related changes and ASCUS—A potential trap. Diagn Cytopathol 16:83–86, 1997.

Minkowitz S, Koffler D, Zak FG. Torulopsis glabrata septicemia. Am J Med 34:252–255, 1963.

Misch KA, Smithies A, Twomey D, et al. Tuberculosis of the cervix: Cytology as an aid to diagnosis. J Clin Pathol 29:313–316, 1976.

Morse AR, Coleman DV, Gardner SD. An evaluation of cytology in the diagnosis of herpes simplex virus infection and cytomegalovirus infection of the cervix uteri. J Obstet Gynaecol Br Commonw 81:393–398, 1974.

Mostoufizadeh M, Scully RE. Malignant tumors arising in endometriosis. Clin Obstet Gynecol 23:951–963, 1980.

Mulvany NJ, Surtees V. Cervical/vaginal endometriosis with atypia: A cytohistopathologic study. Diagn Cytopathol 21:188–193, 1999.

Munguia H, Franco E, Valenzuela P. Diagnosis of genital amebiasis in women by the standard Papanicolaou technique. Am J Obstet Gynecol 94:181–188, 1966.

Murty DA, Luthra UK, Schgal K, Sodhani P. Cytologic detection of Strongyloides stercoralis in a routine cervicovaginal smear. Acta Cytol 38:223–225, 1994.

Naib ZM. Cytology of TRIC agent infection of the eye of the unborn infants and their mothers' genital tract. Acta Cytol 14:390–395, 1970.

Naib ZM, Nahmias AJ, Josey WE. Cytology and histopathology of cervical herpes simplex infection. Cancer 19:1026–1031, 1966.

Nasiell M. Histiocytes and histiocytic reaction in vaginal cytology. A survey of the risks of false positive diagnosis. Cancer 14:1223–1225, 1961.

Navarro M, Furlani B, et al. Cytologic correlates of benign versus dysplastic abnormal keratinization. Diagn Cytopathol 17:447–451, 1997.

Ng ABP, Reagan JW, Lindner E. The cellular manifestations of primary and recurrent herpes genitalis. Acta Cytol 14:124–129, 1970.

Ngadiman S, Yang GH. Adenomyomatous lower uterine segment and endocervical polyps in cervicovaginal smears. Acta Cytol 39:643–647, 1995.

Nichols TM, Fidler HK. Microglandular hyperplasia in cervical cone biopsies taken for suspicious and positive cytology. Am J Clin Pathol 56:424–429, 1971.

Novotny DB, Maygarden SJ, Johnson DE, Frable WJ. Tubal metaplasia. A frequent potential pitfall in the cytologic diagnosis of endocervical glandular dysplasia on cervical smears. Acta Cytol 36:1–10, 1992.

Nowakovsky S, McGrew EA, Medak H, et al. Manifestations of viral infections in exfoliated cells. Acta Cytol 12:227–236, 1968.

Nucci MR, Ferry JA, Young RH. Ectopic prostatic tissue in the uterine cervix: A report of four cases and review of ectopic prostatic tissue. Am J Surg Pathol 24:1224–1230, 2000.

Obara Y, Furuta Y, Takasu T, et al. Distribution of herpex simplex virus types 1 and 2 genomes in human spinal ganglia by PCR and in situ hybridization. J Med Virol 52:135–142, 1997.

O'Hara CM, Gardner WA, Bennett BD. Immunoperoxidase staining of Trichomonas vaginalis in cytologic material. Acta Cytol 24:448–451, 1980.

Ohm MJ, Galask RP. Bacterial flora of the cervix from 100 prehysterectomy patients. Am J Obstet Gynecol 122:683–687, 1975.

Okuyama T, Takahashi R, Mori M, et al. Polymerase chain reaction amplification of Trichomonas vaginalis DNA from Papanicolaou-stained smears. Diagn Cytopathol 19:437–440, 1998.

Oliva E, Clement PB, Young RH. Tubal and tubo-endometrioid metaplasia of the uterine cervix. Am J Clin Pathol 103:618–623, 1995.

Ory HW, Jenkins R, Byrd JY, et al. Cervical neoplasia in residents of a low-income housing project: An epidemiologic study. Am J Obstet Gynecol 123:275–277, 1975.

Pandit AA, Khilnani PH, Powar HS. Detection of microfilariae in cervical cytology [Letter]. Acta Cytol 36:451–452, 1992.

Park JJ, Genest DR, Sun D, Crum CP. Atypical immature metaplastic-like proliferations of the cervix: Diagnostic reproducibility and viral (HPV) correlates. Hum Pathol 30:1161–1165, 1999.

Paryani SG, Arvin AM. Intrauterine infection with varicella-zoster virus after maternal varicella. N Engl J Med 314:1542–1546, 1986.

Patten SF Jr. Diagnostic Cytopathology of the Uterine Cervix, 2nd ed. New York, S Karger, 1978.

Perfect JR. Mycobacterium avium-intracellulare complex infections in the acquired immunodeficiency syndrome. J Electr Microsc Tech 8:105–113, 1988.

Philipp E. Elektronenmikroskopische Untersuchungen an der sogenannten Reservezelle am Zylinderepithel der menschlichen cervix uteri. Arch Gynecol 218:295–311, 1975.

Plaut A. Human infection with Cryptococcus glabratus: Report of case involving uterus and fallopian tube. Am J Clin Pathol 20:377–380, 1950.

Qizilbash AH. Chronic plasma cell cervicitis. A rare pitfall in gynecological cytology. Acta Cytol 18:198–200, 1974.

Rhoads JL, Wright C, Redfield RR, Burke DS. Chronic vaginal candidiasis in women with human immunodeficiency virus infection. JAMA 257:3015–3107, 1987.

Rimm DL, Gmitro S, Frable WJ. Atypical reparative changes on cervical/vaginal smears may be associated with dysplasia. Diagn Cytopathol 14:374–379, 1996.

Roberts TH, Ng AB. Chronic lymphocytic cervicitis: cytologic and histopathologic manifestations. Acta Cytol 19:235–243, 1975.

Roongpisuthipong A, Grimes DA, Haagu A. Is the Papanicolaou smear useful for diagnosing sexually transmitted diseases? Obstet Gynecol 69:1–5, 1987.

Rosebury T. Microorganisms Indigenous to Man. New York, McGraw-Hill, 1962.

Ross L. Incidental finding of cytomegalovirus inclusions in cervical glands. Am J Obstet Gynecol 95:956–958, 1966.

Roupas A, Wyss R, Anner R. Prévalence de sept microorganismes dans les secretions vaginales anormales (vaginite). Schweiz Med Wochenschr 115:1454–1460, 1985.

Sagiroglu N, Sagiroglu E. The cytology of intrauterine contraceptive devices. Acta Cytol 14:58–64, 1970.

Sakane T, Takeno M, Suzuki N, Inaba G. Behçet's disease. N Engl J Med 341:1284–1299, 1999.

San Cristobal A, DeMundi A. Enterobius vermicularis larvae in vaginal smears. Acta Cytol 20:190–192, 1976.

San Cristobal A, Roset S. Toxoplasma cysts in vaginal and cervical smears. Acta Cytol 20:285–286, 1976.

San Cristobal A, Roset S, Blay C. Finding of ciliated protozoa genus Vorticella on cervical and endocervical smears. Acta Cytol 20:387–389, 1976.

Sandmire HF, Austin SD, Bechtel RC. Carcinoma of the cervix in oral contraceptive steroid and IUD users and nonusers. Am J Obstet Gynecol 125:339–345, 1976.

Saw EC, Smale LE, Einstein H, Huntington RW. Female genital coccidioidomycosis. Obstet Gynecol 45:199–202, 1975.

Schlesinger C, Silverberg SG. Endocervical carcinoma in situ of tubal type and its relation to atypical tubal metaplasia. Int J Gynecol Pathol 18:1–4, 1999.

Schmidt WA. IUD's, inflammation, and infection: Assessment after two decades of IUD use. Hum Pathol 13:878–881, 1982.

Schmidt WA, Bedrossian CWM, Ali V, et al. Actinomycosis and intrauterine contraceptive devices. The clinicopathologic entity. Diagn Gynecol Obstet 2:165–177, 1980.

Schmidt WA, Schmidt KL. Intrauterine device (IUD) associated pathology: A review of pathogenic mechanisms. Scan Electron Microsc 11:735–756, 1986.

Schnadig VJ, Davie KD, Shafer SK, et al. The cytologist and bacterioses of the vaginal-ectocervical area: Clues, commas and confusion. Acta Cytol 33:287–297, 1989.

Schnell JD, Voigt WH. Are yeasts in vaginal smears intracellular or extracellular? Acta Cytol 20:343–346, 1976.

Scholes D, Stergachis A, Heidrich FE, et al. Prevention of pelvic inflammatory disease by screening for cervical chlamydial infection. N Engl J Med 334:1362–1366, 1996.

Segal GH, Hart WR. Cystic endocervical tunnel clusters: a clinicopathologic study of 29 cases of so-called adenomatous hyperplasia. Am J Surg Pathol 14:895–903, 1990.

Selvaggi SM. Microglandular hyperplasia of the uterine cervix: Cytologic diagnosis in cervical smears [Letter]. Acta Cytol 44:480–481, 2000.

Selvaggi SM, Haefner HK. Microglandular cervical hyperplasia and tubal metaplasia: pitfalls in the diagnosis of adenocarcinoma in cervical smears. Diagn Cytopathol 16:168–173, 1997.

Shafer MA, Beck A, Balin B, et al. *Chlamydia trachomatis*: Important relationships to race, contraception, and lower genital tract infection in Papanicolaou smears. J Pediatr 104:141–146, 1984.

Shafer M-A, Chew KL, Kromhout LK, et al. Chlamydial endocervical infections and cytologic findings in sexually active female adolescents. Am J Obstet Gynecol 151:765–771, 1985.

Sharma SD, Zeigler O, Trussell RR. A cytologic study of *dipetalonema perstans* in cervical smears. Acta Cytol 15:479–481, 1971.

Sheyn I, Mira JL, Thompson MB. Paracoccidioides brasiliensis in a postpartum Pap smear. A case report. Acta Cytol 45:79–81, 2001.

Shibata D. PCR diagnostics of herpes-virus group infections. Ann Med 24:221–224, 1992.

Shiina Y. Cytomorphologic and immunocytochemichal studies of chlamydial infection in cervical smears. Acta Cytol 29:683–691, 1985.

Siapco B, Kaplan BJ, Bernstein GS, Moyer DL. Cytodiagnosis of *Candida* organisms in cervical smears. Acta Cytol 30:477–480, 1986.

Simmons PD, Vosmik F. Cervical cytology in non-specific genital infection. An aid to diagnosis. Br J Venereol Dis 50:313–314, 1974.

Singer AJ, Clark RAF. Cutaneous wound healing. N Engl J Med 341:738–746, 1999.

Sivin I. IUDs are contraceptives, not abortifacients: A comment on research and belief. Stud Fam Plann 20:355–359, 1989.

Slomka MJ, Emery L, Munday PE, et al. A comparison of PCR with virus isolation and direct antigen detection for diagnosis and typing of genital herpes. J Med Virol 55:177–183, 1998.

Smedts F, Ramaekers F, Leube RE, et al. Expression of keratins 1, 6, 15, 16, and 20 in normal cervical epithelium, squamous metaplasia, cervical intraepithelial neoplasia, and cervical carcinoma. Am J Pathol 142:403–412, 1993.

Sobel JD. Vaginitis. N Engl J Med 337:1896–1903, 1997.

Stanberry LR, Spruance SL, Cunningham AL, et al. Glycoprotein-D-adjuvant vaccine to prevent genital herpes. N Engl J Med 347:1652–1661, 2002.

Stango S, Whitley RJ. Medical intelligence. Current concepts. Herpesvirus infections of pregnancy. Part I. Cytomegalovirus and Epstein-Barr virus infections. N Engl J Med 313:1720–1774, 1985.

Stenkvist EO, Brege KG. Application of immunofluorescent technique in the cytologic diagnosis of human herpes simplex keratitis. Acta Cytol 19:411–414, 1975.

Stern E, Clark VA, Coffelt CF. Contraceptives and dysplasia: Higher rate for pill choosers. Science 169:497–498, 1970.

Stern E, Longo LD. Identification of herpes simplex virus in a case showing cytological features of viral vaginitis. Acta Cytol 7:295–299, 1963.

Stowell SB, Wiley CM, Powers CM. Herpesvirus mimics. A potential pitfall in endocervical brush specimens. Acta Cytol 38:43–50, 1994.

Suh KS, Silverberg SG. Tubal metaplasia of the uterine cervix. Int J Gynecol Pathol 9:122–128, 1990.

Sutherland AM. Gynaecological tuberculosis: analysis of a personal series of 710 cases. Aust NZJ Obstet Gynaecol 25:203–207, 1985.

Sweet RL, Gibbs RS. Infectious Diseases of the Female Genital Tract. Baltimore, Williams & Wilkins, 1985.

Takeda M. Virus identification in cytologic and histologic material by electron microscopy. Acta Cytol 13:206–209, 1969.

Tam MR, Stamm WE, Handsfield HH, et al. Culture-in-dependent diagnosis of *Chlamydia trachomatis* using monoclonal antibodies. N Engl J Med 310:1146–1150, 1984.

Taylor HB, Irey NS, Norris HJ. Atypical endocervical hyperplasia in women taking oral contraceptives. JAMA 202:637–639, 1967.

Tenjin Y, Yamamoto K, Sugishita T, Igarashi Y. Basic studies on repair, especially histology, cytology, and microspectrophotometry of DNA content. Acta Cytol 23:245–251, 1979.

Teplitz RL, Valco Z, Rundall T. Comparative sequential cytologic changes in following in vitro infection with herpes virus types I and II. Acta Cytol 15:455–459, 1971.

Thomas DB. Relationship of oral contraceptives to cervical carcinogenesis. Obstet Gynecol 40:508–518, 1972.

Tomita T, Chiga M, Lenahan M, Balachandran N. Identification of herpes simplex virus infection by immunoperoxidase and in situ hybridization methods. Virch Arch A, Pathol Anat Histopathol 419:99–105, 1991.

Trager W. Some aspects of intracellular parasitism. Intracellular protozoa enter host cells in subtle ways and escape the cell's digestive processes. Science 183:269–273, 1974.

Trivijitsilp P, Mosher R, Sheets EE, et al. Papillary immature metaplasia (immature condyloma) of the cervix: A clinicopathological analysis and comparison with papillary squamous carcinoma. Hum Pathol 29:641–648, 1998.

Trussell RE. *Trichomonas vaginalis* and Trichomoniasis. Springfield, IL, Charles C Thomas, 1947.

Tsutsumi K, Sun Q, Yasumoto S, et al. In vitro and in vivo analysis of cellular origin of cervical squamous metaplasia. Am J Pathol 143:1150–1158, 1993.

Tweeddale DN, Scott RC, Fields MJ, et al. Giant cells in cervicovaginal smears. Acta Cytol 12:298–304, 1968.

Valdivieso M, Luna M, Bodey GP, et al. Fungemia due to *Torulopsis glabrata* in the compromised host. Cancer 38:1750–1756, 1976.

Valente PT, Schantz HD, Schultz M. Cytologic atypia associated with microglandular hyperplasia. Diagn Cytopathol 10:326–321, 1994.

Vesterinen E, Purola E, Saksela E, Leinikki P. Clinical and virological findings in patients with cytologically diagnosed gynecologic herpes simplex infections. Acta Cytol 21:199–205, 1977.

Vinette-Leduc D, Yazdi HM, Jessamine P, Peeling RW. Reliability of cytology to detect chlamydia infection in asymptomatic women. Diagn Cytopathol 17:258–261, 1997.

Voytek TM, Kannan V, Kline TS. Atypical parakeratosis: a marker for dysplasia? Diagn Cytopathol 15:288–291, 1996.

Wachtel E. Detection of Papova virus in a vaginal aspirate [Letter to Editor]. Acta Cytol 21:489–490, 1977.

Walton BC, Bacharach T. Occurrence of trichomonads in the respiratory tract: Report of three cases. J Parasitol 49:35–38, 1963.

Wasylenko M, Racela L, Papasian CJ, Watanabe I. *Toxoplasma gondii* in cervical smears [Letter]. Acta Cytol 35:145–146, 1991.

Weir MM, Bell DA. Transitional cell metaplasia of the cervix: a newly described entity in cervical smears. Diagn Cytopathol 18:222–226, 1998.

Weir MM, Bell DA, Young RH. Transitional cell metaplasia of the uterine cervix and vagina: an underrecognized lesion that may be confused with high-grade dysplasia: A report of 59 cases. Am J Surg Pathol 21:510–517, 1997.

Weld JT, Kean BH. Experimental ocular trichomoniasis: Pathologic observations. Am J Pathol 32:1135–1145, 1956.

Wenckebach GFC, Curry B. Cytomegalovirus infection of the female genital tract. Arch Pathol Lab Med 100:609–612, 1976.

Wendel KA, Erbelding EJ, Gaydos CA, Rompalo AM. Trichomonas vaginalis polymerase chain reaction compared with standard diagnostic and therapeutic protocols for detection and treatment of vaginal trichomoniasis. Clin Infect Dis 35:576–580, 2002.

Wied GL. Interpretation of inflammatory reactions in vagina cervix, and endocervix by means of cytologic smears. Am J Clin Pathol 28:233–242, 1957.

Wied GL, Bibbo M. Microbiologic classification on the cellular sample. Management of patients with vaginal infection. J Reprod Med 9:1–16, 1972.

Wilbur DC. Endocervical glandular atypia: a "new" problem for the cytologist. Diagn Cytopathol 13:463–469, 1995.

Wilkinson E, Dufour DR. Pathogenesis of microglandular hyperplasia of the cervix uteri. Obstet Gynecol 47:189–195, 1976.

Williamson JD, Silverman JF, Mallak CT, Christie JD. Atypical cytomorphological appearance of *Cryptococcus neoformans*: a report of five cases. Acta Cytol 40:363–370, 1996.

Wolinska WH. Value of prepared culture medium in diagnosis of *Trichomonas vaginalis*. Am J Obstet Gynecol 77:306–308, 1959.

Wolinska WH, Melamed MR. Herpes genitalis in women attending planned parenthood of New York City. Acta Cytol 14:239–242, 1970.

Wong JY, Zaharopoulos P, Dinh TV. Diagnosis of herpes simplex virus in routine smears by an immunoperoxidase technique. Acta Cytol 29:701–704, 1985.

Worth AJ, Boyes DA. A case control study into possible effects of birth control pills on preclinical carcinoma of the cervix. J Obstet Gynaecol Br Commonw 79:673–679, 1972.

Yeh I-T, Bronner M, Le Volsi VA. Endometrial metaplasia of the uterine cervix. Arch Pathol Lab Med 117:734–735, 1993.

Young RH, Clement PB. Endocervicosis involving the uterine cervix: a report of four cases of a benign process that may be confused with deeply invasive endocervical adenocarcinoma. Int J Gynecol Pathol 19:322–328, 2000.

Young RH, Clement PB. Pseudoneoplastic lesions of the uterine cervix. Semin Diagn Pathol 8:234–249, 1991.

Young RH, Scully RE. Atypical forms of microglandular hyperplasia of the cervix simulating carcinoma. A report of five cases and review of the literature. Am J Surg Pathol 13:50–56, 1989.

Young RH, Scully RE. Uterine carcinomas simulating microglandular hyperplasia. A report of six cases. Am J Surg Pathol 16:1092–1097, 1992.

Squamous Carcinoma of the Uterine Cervix and Its Precursors

11

NATURAL HISTORY, EPIDEMIOLOGY, ETIOLOGY, AND PATHOGENESIS

Carcinoma of the uterine cervix and its precursors belong to the best studied forms of human cancer. In this chapter, only cancers and precancerous lesions with the origin in, or characteristics of, squamous epithelium will be discussed. The term **squamous carcinoma** has been in general use to describe these lesions. The alternate term **epidermoid carcinoma** will be used to describe lesions with limited formation of keratin. **Adenocarcinomas** and related lesions are discussed in Chapter 12.

It has been repeatedly documented that invasive carcinoma of the uterine cervix, regardless of type, **develops from precursor lesions or abnormal surface epithelium,** which, in its classic form, is known as **carcinoma in situ** (International Stage O). The precursor lesions do not produce any specific alterations of the cervix visible to the naked eye. Therefore, before the introduction of cervicovaginal cytology and colposcopy, these lesions were a rarity and their discovery was incidental in biopsies of the cervix and in hysterectomy specimens. Since the introduction of mass screening by smears, and with accumulated experience, it has been shown that these lesions are quite common. The investigations of the precursor lesions is facilitated by the accessibility of the cervix to clinical examination and inspection by the colposcope and the ease of cytologic and histologic sampling that could be subjected, not only to microscopic scrutiny, but also to cytogenetic and molecular biologic analysis. Although considerable progress has been made in the understanding of the natural history of these lesions, there are still many areas of ignorance requiring further clarification.

The assumption of **the prevention programs of cancer of the uterine cervix** is that **the precursor lesions may be identified in cervicovaginal preparations and eradicated, thus preventing the occurrence of invasive cancer.** The success of these programs has been confirmed because, over the past half century, the rate of invasive cancer of the uterine cervix has been reduced by about 70% in the United States and other developed countries (summaries in Koss, 1989; Cannistra and Niloff, 1996). In developing countries, however, cancer of the cervix remains a common disease with a high mortality rate.

The first part of the chapter is devoted to epidemiology, etiology, pathogenesis, and natural history of precursor lesions and squamous cancer of the uterine cervix. The cytology and histopathology of these lesions are discussed in Part 2.

HISTORICAL PERSPECTIVE

The identification of invasive carcinoma of the uterine cervix as a distinct disease, different from other tumors of the uterus, was significantly enhanced with the introduction of uterine biopsies by Ruge and Veit in 1877. The histologic features of invasive squamous cancer were well known toward the end of the 19th century and were illustrated in a number of textbooks, such as that by Amann, published in 1897. In fact, Amann also recognized the component cells of squamous carcinoma (Fig. 11-1) but neither he nor his contemporaries addressed the issue of the origin of invasive cancer. The credit for this contribution goes to W. Schauenstein, a gynecologist from Graz, Austria, who published, in 1908, a remarkable paper pointing out the striking similarity between the histologic patterns of cancerous sur-

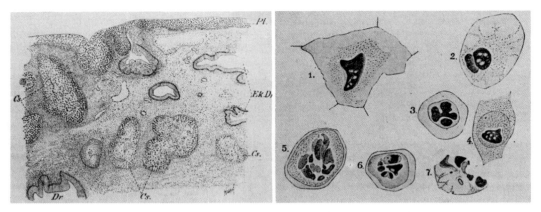

Figure 11-1 Facsimile of drawings of a cervical carcinoma and cancer cells, derived from Amann's book on gynecologic histology, which appeared in 1897. The tissue lesion that was diagnosed as "carcinoma of cervix originating from squamous epithelium" would undoubtedly be classified today as a carcinoma in situ with extension to endocervical glands. Note the remarkably accurate drawings of "pyknotic cancer cells." (JF Bergman, publisher, Wiesbaden, Germany.)

face epithelium (Krebsbelag in the original German) and superficially infiltrating squamous cancer of the cervix. He expressed the opinion that the abnormal surface epithelium deserved the name of cancer because it was the source of origin of infiltrating carcinoma (Fig. 11-2).

Pronai in 1909 and Rubin in 1910 supported Schauenstein's observations by additional examples. The matter was also dealt with in considerable detail in a large book by Schottländer and Kermauner, published in 1912, which contains a detailed analysis of several hundred cases of uterine cancer. In reference to cancer of the uterine cervix, Schottländer and Kermauner coined the term **carcinoma in situ** to describe the cancerous epithelium on the surface of the uterine cervix and considered this lesion to be malignant. Although, in the American literature, the term "carci-

noma in situ" is often attributed to the pathologist A.C. Broders of the Mayo Clinic, who published a paper on this topic in 1932, he was not the first person to use this term. Numerous synonyms, such as **preinvasive carcinoma, intraepithelial carcinoma, precancerous epithelium, Bowen's disease of the cervix, and squamous or epidermoid carcinoma without evidence of invasion,** have been used intermittently in the literature for many years to describe and discuss this lesion. The critical issue of whether such epithelial abnormalities may be recognized as cancerous in the absence of an invasive component was the subject of numerous controversies in the first decades of the 20th century, first addressed by Rubin in 1910. In the 1920s and 1930s, two German gynecologic pathologists, Walter Schiller and Robert Meyer (both of whom escaped to the United States to avoid Hitler's racial laws) wrote extensively on the subject of interpretation of cervical biopsies and concluded that precancerous intraepithelial lesions were indeed precursors of invasive cervical cancer and could be so identified under the microscope. Still, **because the behavior of the precancerous lesions has been shown to be unpredictable** and not necessarily leading to invasive cancer, the controversy was not put to rest. With the onset of the 21st century, there are few observers who use the term "carcinoma in situ." Most of them favor other terms, such as **dysplasia, cervical intraepithelial neoplasia (CIN), and squamous intraepithelial lesions (SIL) of low (LGSIL) and high-grade (HGSIL),** to be defined and discussed below.

In 1925, a German gynecologist, Hinselmann, realized that the naked eye was not sufficiently keen to detect inconspicuous alterations of the cervical epithelium caused by early cancer and devised a magnifying instrument—**the colposcope**—that allowed the inspection of the **vascular changes on the surface of the cervix** at magnifications up to 20 times. Hinselmann supplemented the colposcopic investigation with cervical biopsies. As related by Limburg (1956), Hinselmann had much difficulty in trying to convince the conservative German pathologists that the precur-

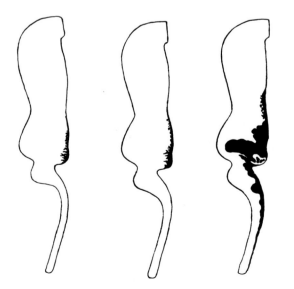

Figure 11-2 Facsimile of a drawing from the paper of **Schauenstein,** published in 1908, which served as a basis for his statement that the various forms of cervical cancer "show only quantitative and not qualitative differences." The two lesions on the left are carcinomas in situ. (From Arch Gynaecol 85:576–616, 1908.)

sor lesions discovered by colposcopy were malignant. To avoid controversies he devised a system of classification of the lesions into four groups (**Rubriks**), thus avoiding the term cancer. Unfortunately, the **Rubriks** included a variety of findings ranging from simple metaplasias to carcinomas in situ; thus, this method of classification has not found much following. The **Rubriks** are reminiscent of Papanicolaou's **"Classes,"** a system of diagnosis applied to cervicovaginal smears many years later and discussed below.

In trained hands, the colposcope proved to be a very useful instrument, which has been extensively used in Europe and, with a delay of several decades, has also been adopted in the United States. It is of historical interest that the resistance to colposcopy in the United States was based on the notion that "no American woman will stay still long enough to be colposcoped," as related to me many years ago by a senior gynecologist. The principal current **application of colposcopy is in the localization and biopsies of epithelial abnormalities detected by cytology.**

The introduction of **cervicovaginal cytology,** as a means of detection of precancerous lesions of the uterine cervix, has been another milestone in the study of cancer of the uterine cervix (Babès, 1928; Papanicolaou, 1928; Viana, 1928). The method has played a central role as a tool of prevention of cervix cancer. As narrated in Chapter 1 of this book, Dr. George N. Papanicolaou's name is synonymous with the cytologic method of cervix cancer diagnosis and detection, and his contributions have been honored by the common term, **Pap smear.** Events leading to the recognition of **human papillomavirus (HPV)** as an important factor in the genesis of cancer of the uterine cervix are described below.

EPIDEMIOLOGY

In 1842, an Italian physician, Rigoni-Stern, examined the death records of the city of Verona for the years 1760 to 1839 and pointed out that **cancer of the uterus was much more frequent among married women and widows than among unmarried women and nuns.** He made a number of other fundamental observations and is considered to be the father of cancer epidemiology. The term **cancer of the uterus,** used by Rigoni-Stern, undoubtedly comprised a large proportion of cancers of the uterine cervix, which was then, and remained for another century, by far the most common malignant disease of the uterus until the cancer detection systems took hold in the 1960s. Rigoni-Stern's paper appears to be the first recorded reference to what has been subsequently termed **"marital" or "sexual" events** that play a major role in epidemiology of squamous carcinoma of the cervix. Two epidemiologic factors play a major role in the genesis of this disease. These are:

- **Young age at first intercourse**
- **Promiscuity or multiplicity of sexual partners**

It has been documented that women who begin their sexual life in their teens, who have multiple sexual partners, or who are multiparous at an early age, are at a greater risk for cancer of the cervix than women who begin their sexual

activity later in life and are monogamous or have only few partners. This disease is extremely rare among nuns but common among prostitutes (Dunn, 1953; Wynder, 1954; Towne, 1955; Kaiser and Gilliam, 1958; Taylor et al, 1959; Pereira, 1961; Roitkin, 1962, 1973; Nix, 1964; Christopherson and Parker, 1965; Martin, 1967; Barron and Richart, 1971; Kessler et al, 1974). Pridan and Lilienfeld (1971) pointed out that, although cancer of the uterine cervix is rare among Jewish women, it may be observed either in promiscuous women or women whose *husbands* were promiscuous. As briefly discussed in Chapter 10, women using intrauterine contraceptive devices or hormonal contraception are at a higher risk for development of cervical cancer precursors than women using the diaphragm, or whose partners use condoms, again suggesting that a direct contact between the sexes is a factor in carcinoma of the cervix. **Thus, the pattern of occurrence of carcinoma of the uterine cervix is, in many ways, similar to that of a sexually transmitted disease, suggesting that a sex-related transfer of a factor or factors triggers the cancerous events.**

RISK FACTORS

Sexually Transmitted Diseases

A great many sexually transmitted disease agents were, at one time or another, considered as possible triggers of cancer of the cervix, including **syphilis** (Levin et al, 1942) and ***Trichomonas vaginalis*** (De Carnieri and DiRe, 1970). With effective treatment of syphilis by antibiotics, this disease ceased to be considered to be a suspect agent. In an extensive study, Koss and Wolinska (1959) ruled out Trichomoniasis as a candidate agent. Association of subtypes of ***Chlamydia trachomatis*** with cervical squamous carcinoma was discussed as a possible risk factor by Antilla et al (2001).

Spermatozoa, Smegma, and Cigarette Smoking

In 1968, Coppleson and Reid proposed that **spermatozoa** may penetrate the endocervical cells, change their genetic make-up (genome), and thus trigger cancerous proliferation. This theory received little attention until further observations by Bendich et al (1974, 1976) and by Higgins (1975), who pointed out that **mammalian spermatozoa** may indeed penetrate cultured mammalian cells in vitro and significantly **modify their morphology, growth characteristics, and genome.** Thus, this suggestion, which has been revived again in a paper by Singer et al (1976), is deserving of further investigation.

The role of **smegma** as a possible carcinogenic agent was linked to the absence of circumcision in marital partners of women developing cervical cancer. There is no objective supportive evidence that this theory is valid, as summarized by Terris et al (1973).

Several epidemiologic studies pointed out that **cigarette smoking** is a possible risk factor in cancer of the cervix

(Leyde and Broste, 1989; Slattery et al, 1989; Cocker et al, 1992; Daling et al, 1996). The finding of metabolites of tobacco carcinogens in cervical mucus (Philips et al, 1990; Prokopczyk et al, 1997) suggests that the relationship does not only pertain to lifestyle but may, in fact, have a biochemical basis. DNA damage in cervical epithelium related to tobacco carcinogens has been reported (Simons et al, 1995). Ho et al (1998) observed some synchrony between cigarette smoking, human papillomavirus type 16, and the occurrence of high-grade precursor lesions of the uterine cervix.

Immune deficiencies, as a consequence of infection with human immunodeficiency virus (HIV), acquired immunodeficiency syndrome (AIDS), immunosuppression after organ transplant or chemotherapy for cancer, are also risk factors for cervix cancer, to be discussed below in reference to human papillomavirus infection.

VIRAL AGENTS

During the last 30 years of the 20th century, several sexually transmitted viruses were considered as possible agents involved in the genesis of cancer of the uterine cervix. The two most important agents are herpesvirus type 2 and human papillomavirus (HPV).

Herpesvirus Type 2 (HSV-2)

The proponents of the HSV-2, a variant of herpesvirus discussed in Chapter 10, as the transmissible biologic agent triggering carcinoma of the uterine cervix, pointed out that the virus is sexually transmitted and ubiquitous and that women with antibodies to HSV-2 have a higher incidence of precancerous lesions of the cervix than controls (Adam et al, 1971; Nahmias et al, 1974). Aurelian et al (1971) isolated the virus from cervical cancer cells grown in vitro. The expression of the viral genome could be demonstrated in cervical cancer cells by immunofluorescence (Aurelian, 1974). Centifano et al (1972) demonstrated the virus in the male genitourinary tract, a possible source of infection. Wentz et al (1975) produced carcinoma of the cervix in mice with HSV-2.

The studies of antibodies to HSV-2 in various population groups, which first suggested a relationship of this virus to carcinoma of the cervix, were not consistent. In a review of this evidence, Kessler (1974) pointed out that the serologic methods used by the various investigators were quite variable and may have accounted for the observed differences. Subsequent studies, notably a much cited paper by Vonka et al (1984), failed to confirm the differences in serologic positivity between women with and without precancerous lesions or cancer of the uterine cervix. At the time of this writing (2004), there is little enthusiasm for the role of HSV-2 as a causative factor of cancer of the uterine cervix. On the other hand, the possibility that HSV-2 infection plays an indirect role in the pathogenesis of these lesions as a co-factor in human papillomavirus infection has been suggested (zur Hausen, 1982; Daling et al, 1996).

Human Papillomaviruses (HPVs)

In 1933, Shope and Hurst demonstrated that skin papillomas in wild cottontail rabbits could be transmitted from animal to animal by a cell-free extract, leading to the assumption that this disease was caused by a virus. The domestic rabbit was generally resistant to this infection, although, in some animals, the infection produced skin cancer (Rous and Beard, 1935). In 1940, Rous and Kidd documented that the virus (by then named **papillomavirus**) could produce invasive and metastatic skin cancers in domestic rabbits pretreated with tar. Thus, the **Shope papillomavirus was thought to be a co-carcinogenic agent, usually requiring the presence of another initiating agent, to produce a malignant tumor** in a species of animals other than the species of origin.

Many animal papillomaviruses are known today; they are generally species-specific and usually produce **benign lesions of the skin or subcutaneous tissues.** The bovine papillomavirus is thought to be a contributory factor in bladder tumors in cows.

In reference to the uterine cervix, the occurrence of invasive cancer (Hisaw and Hisaw, 1958) and of carcinoma in situ and related precancerous lesions in monkeys (*Macaca* species) was reported (Sternberg, 1961; Hertig et al, 1983). One such lesion is illustrated in Figure 11-3. It is of interest, therefore, that **papillomavirus type RhPV-1 has been observed in penile and cervix cancers in rhesus monkeys** (Kloster et al, 1988; Ostrow et al, 1995). Summaries of studies on animal papillomaviruses may be found in a contribution by Sundberg (1987) and in the IARC (International Association for Research on Cancer) monograph on Human Papillomaviruses (1995).

Early Observations in Humans

Human papillomaviruses (**HPVs** or **"wart viruses"**) have been suspected for many years as the cause of ordinary **skin warts** and of the common wart-like skin lesions known as **venereal warts** or *condylomata acuminata,* often simply designated as **"condylomas."** *Condylomata acuminata* generally occur on external genitalia, the perineum, and the

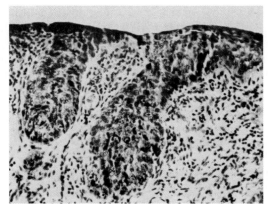

Figure 11-3 Carcinoma in situ observed in the cervix of a monkey, *Macaca mulatta.* (From Sternberg SS. In situ carcinoma of the cervix in a monkey [*Macaca mulatta*]. Am J Obstet Gynecol 82: 96–98, 1961.)

perianal region (the latter most commonly seen in homosexual males, but, occasionally, also observed in women and children), where they form multiple, pedunculated or sessile, cauliflower-like excrescences surfaced by thick folds of squamous epithelium (Fig. 11-4); such lesions may also occur in the vagina and, rarely, on the uterine cervix. Similar flat, moist lesions, known as *condylomata lata,* occurring on external genitalia, are associated with secondary syphilis.

The viral origin of *condylomata acuminata* received strong additional support when **viral particles were observed in the nuclei of squamous epithelial cells** by electron microscopy (Dunn and Ogilvie, 1968; Oriel and Alameida, 1970). Studies of veterans returning from the Korean War, and of their spouses, have shown that *condylomata acuminata* is a sexually transmitted disease that takes several months to develop (Oriel, 1971). This was the first evidence that **HPVs can cause a disease in humans.**

In 1956, Koss and Durfee coined the term **koilocytotic atypia** (from Greek, *koilos* = a hollow and *kytos* = cell) to describe, in cervicovaginal smears, peculiar **large squamous cells with enlarged, hyperchromatic nuclei and a large clear perinuclear clear zone or halo, known today as koilocytes** (see Fig. 11-6D). It has been shown subsequently, by electron microscopy, that the nuclei of koilocytes contain mature viral particles, whereas the **clear cytoplasmic zones (halos)** represent **a collapse of the cytoplasmic filaments or cytoplasmic necrosis** (see Fig. 11-6A) caused by the viral infection (Shokri Tabibzadeh et al, 1981; Meisels et al, 1983, 1984). For a detailed analysis of koilocytes in cervicovaginal cytologic material, see Part 2 of this chapter. The presence of these cells in smears was shown by Koss and Durfee to **correlate with histologic abnormalities of squamous epithelium resembling skin warts and, hence, named "warty lesions"** (see Fig. 11-4B). An association of koilocytes, or warty lesions with bona fide carcinoma in situ, was observed in 18 of 40 cases and in 9 of 53 invasive carcinomas. Koilocytes were also observed in two "squamous papillomas" of the cervix that today would be classified as condylomas.

Such cells were previously described in 1949 and in several subsequent publications by a major contributor to cervical cytology, J. Ernest Ayre, who variously named them **"precancer cell complex," "halo cells,"** or **"nearocarcinoma"** (early cancer). In a very few poorly documented anecdotal cases, Ayre reported a progression of this cytologic pattern to carcinoma of the cervix. **In 1960, Ayre proposed that the "halo cells" may be caused by a not further defined viral infection.**

In December 1976 and January 1977, Meisels and Fortin, from Canada, and Purola and Savia, from Finland, simultaneously published papers linking condylomas and similar precancerous lesions of the uterine cervix with "wart virus" (since renamed **human papillomavirus or HPV**). The **common denominator of these lesions** was the presence of **"halo cells" or koilocytes.** The first confirmations of the association of some precancerous lesions of the uterine cervix with a viral infection were published in 1978 by Laverty et al from Australia and in 1979 by Torre et al from Italy, who observed, by electron microscopy, viral particles consistent with a papillomavirus in precancerous cervical lesions.

In a critically important paper, Kreider et al (1985) reported the induction of koilocytosis in fragments of normal human squamous epithelium by HPV type 11 in nude mice, thus confirming the role of HPV in the formation of this cell alteration. Subsequently, the presence of viruses of the papillomavirus family in precancerous lesions and invasive cancer of the uterine cervix was confirmed by a variety of techniques (see below).

The initial cytologic, histologic, and clinical studies confirmed that **the presence of koilocytes and, hence, HPV infection, was common in women with precancerous lesions of the uterine cervix, particularly in bearers of flat, wart-like lesions, soon renamed "flat condylomas"** (Purola and Savia, 1977; Meisels and Morin, 1983). In young women, age 20 or less, nearly all precancerous cervical lesions had a morphologic configuration suggestive of HPV infection (Syrjänen, 1979). In subsequent years, these studies were significantly expanded, confirming the relationship between the precancerous lesions and manifestations of HPV infection in thousands of women.

It was also reported in the first edition of this book in

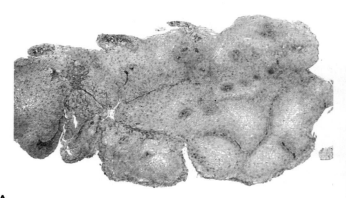

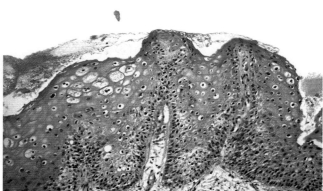

A   B

Figure 11-4   Condylomata. Condyloma of anus (*A*) and of the vulva (*B*). For detailed description of structure, see text. Note epithelial folds in *A*.

1961 (and in subsequent editions), that **the cytologic features of the uncommon large condylomas on the surface of the uterine cervix in very young women show marked similarities with precursor lesions of cervical cancer.** For description of these findings, see Part 2 of this chapter.

Subsequently, other minor cytologic abnormalities, such as parakeratosis, formation of **squamous "pearls," binucleation, slight enlargement of nuclei in squamous cells, and karyorrhexis** were also considered as secondary landmarks of HPV infection. These abnormalities are discussed in Chapter 10. In the experience of this writer, these changes are not specific and may occur under a variety of circumstances, not necessarily related to HPV infection, in agreement with Tanaka et al (1993).

Molecular Biology

While the initial morphologic observations were being pieced together, substantial work was going on in several laboratories of molecular virology to identify and characterize papillomaviruses and clarify their role as possible oncogenic agents. Unfortunately, HPVs are very finicky and, so far, there is no tissue culture system to support their growth in vitro. Hence, the initial evidence had to be gathered by molecular cloning of viral DNA in plasmids and by Southern type analysis of viral DNA (Gissmann and zur Hausen, 1976; zur Hausen, 1976). For description of the plasmid technique and of the Southern blot analysis, see Chapter 3.

These studies led to the identification of a few common types of HPVs (6, 11, and 16) and their fundamental structure.

The HPVs are **small, circular, double-stranded DNA viruses, each strand being composed of approximately 7,900 nucleotides.** Only one of the two DNA strands is transcribed. The genetic organization of the viruses is usually presented as a single strand of DNA in the form of **"open reading frames" (ORFs) or genes,** containing messages for protein formation (Fig. 11-5). There are seven early (E) ORFs, ensuring the replication of the genetic machinery of the virus, and two late (L) ORFs inscribing capsular proteins. The protein products of ORF 1 and 2 reproduce the viral genome; ORF 2 regulates the transcription of the viral genome, whereas ORFs E6 and E7 play a role in cell transformation (see below).

Classification

There are more than 70 types of HPV with several more types still not identified (Table 11-1). **The types differ from each other by 50% or more in nucleotide homology and are sequentially numbered by an international agreement, starting with type 1.** Several types of HPV, that can be designated as **mucosal (anogenital) HPVs,** are observed in neoplastic lesions of the uterine cervix and other organs of the lower female genital tract. The introduction of the **polymerase chain reaction (PCR)** contributed sig-

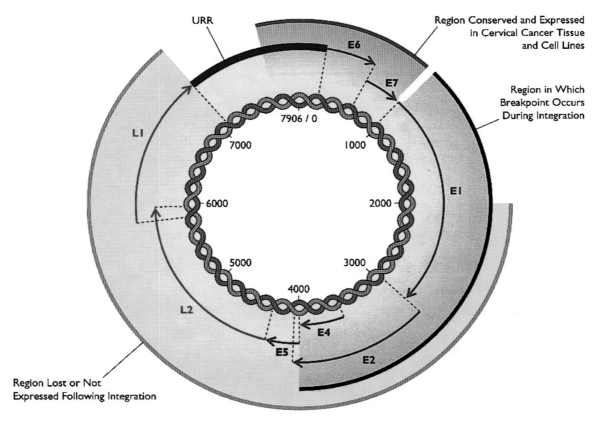

Figure 11-5   Structure of HPV. The drawing shows double-stranded DNA composed of approximately 7,900 nucleotides (center ring) and the position of open reading frames (ORFs) E1–E7 and L1 and L2 (outer rings). The function of the reading frames is discussed in text. (Courtesy of Dr. Robert Burk, Albert Einstein College of Medicine, Bronx, NY.)

TABLE 11-1

PRINCIPAL TYPES OF MUCOSAL (ANOGENITAL) TYPES OF HPV*

HPV Type	Origin of cloned genome
HPV-6	Condyloma acuminatum
HPV-11	Laryngeal papilloma
HPV-16[†]	Cervical carcinoma
HPV-18[†]	Cervical carcinoma
HPV-31[†]	CIN
HPV-33[†]	Cervical carcinoma
HPV-34	Bowen's disease
HPV-35[†]	Cervical carcinoma
HPV-39[†]	Penile intraepithelial neoplasia
HPV-40	Penile intraepithelial neoplasia
HPV-42	Vulvar papilloma
HPV-43	Vulvar hyperplasia
HPV-44	Vulvar condyloma
HPV-45[†]	CIN
HPV-51[†]	CIN
HPV-52[†]	CIN
HPV-53[‡]	Normal cervical mucosa
HPV-54	Condyloma acuminatum
HPV-55	Bowenoid papulosis
HPV-56[†]	CIN, cervical carcinoma
HPV-58[†]	CIN
HPV-59[†]	VIN
HPV-61	VaIN
HPV-62	VaIN
HPV-64	VaIN
HPV-66[‡]	Cervical carcinoma
HPV-67	VaIN
HPV-68[†]	Genital lesion
HPV-69[†]	CIN
HPV-70	Vulvar papilloma

* Since 1994, additional types of HPV were identified as high-risk types 26, 73, 77, 82, and several others, not yet numbered (Muñoz et al., 2003).
† High risk.
‡ Probable high risk.
CIN: cervical intraepithelial neoplasia; VIN: vulvar intraepithelial neoplasia; VaIN: vaginal intraepithelial neoplasia.
Modified from IARC Monograph, Vol. 64, Human papillomaviruses. Lyon, France, 1995, with permission.

nificantly to the identification of new HPV types and their presence in various lesions. By the use of this technique, minute amounts of viral DNA extracted from lesions could be amplified and analyzed in vitro by Southern blotting (Shibata et al, 1988; Nuovo, 1990; Nuovo et al, 1990, 1991; Bauer et al, 1991). For description of the principles of these techniques, see Chapter 3. Credits for the identification of various types of HPV are given in papers by Lorincz et al (1992) and de Villiers (2001). A novel classification system of papillomaviruses based on taxonomy was published recently by de Villiers et al (2004).

Depending on the **frequency of occurrence in invasive cancer of the uterine cervix,** the genital HPVs were initially classified as "low risk," "intermediate risk," and "high risk"

types (Lorincz et al, 1992). The current trend is to recognize only two groups, **low-risk** and **high-risk or oncogenic viruses.** The latest classification, proposed by Muñioz et al (2003) and based on 11 case-controlled studies from 9 countries, lists 15 viral types as **high-risk** (16, 18, 31, 33, 35, 39, 45, 51, 52, 56, 58, 59, 68, 73, and 82), three as **probable high-risk** types (26, 53, and 66) and 12 as **low-risk types** (6, 11, 40, 42, 43, 44, 54, 61, 70, 72, 81, and CP6108).

The most common "oncogenic" types of HPV are 16 and 18. HPV type 16 is most often observed in invasive squamous carcinomas, whereas HPV type 18 appears to have a predilection for lesions derived from the endocervical epithelium, such as small-cell carcinomas and adenocarcinomas (for discussion of these lesions, see below and Chapter 12). Type 18 and, to a lesser degree, type 16 were also identified in several cell lines derived from invasive cancers of the uterine cervix, such as HeLa, Caski, and C4-1. The distribution of HPV types in the genital tract of normal women, women with cytologic atypias, precursor lesions, and invasive cancer of the uterine cervix is shown in Table 11-2, based on a very large study by Lorincz et al (1992).

The frequency of occurrence of other oncogenic types in invasive cancer is provided by Muñoz et al (2003). A few additional points must be stressed: in a small subgroup of cervix cancer, multiple viral types were identified. In a very small number of women, **cancers were associated with the "low-risk" types 6 and 11.** In all, 90.7% of 1,918 women with cervical cancer were shown to harbor HPV DNA.

In a control cohort of 1,928 women without cervical cancer 13.4% harbored HPV DNA, mainly of high risk type. Muñoz et al calculated the **risk ratio** of cervical cancer in women infected with any type of HPV at 158 times the rate observed in women not carriers of the virus.

Life Cycle

The life cycle of HPVs takes place **in the nuclei of squamous epithelial cells** and depends on the mechanisms of epithelial maturation about which little is known. The viruses achieve their **full maturity only in the nuclei of cells forming the superficial layers of the squamous epithelium** and this phenomenon is known as a **permissive infection. The koilocytes are an expression of permissive infection with HPV because their nuclei are filled with mature viral particles or virions.** Electron microscopic studies of the infected nuclei have shown that the mature virions measure about **50 nm in diameter,** have an **icosahedral,** that is having 20 faces, **protein capsule,** and usually form crystalline arrays (Fig. 11-6).

In **lower layers of the squamous epithelium and in other types of epithelia, the viruses do not achieve full maturity and their presence can only be detected by their DNA (occult or latent infection).**

An important difference of presentation of HPV was observed between most precancerous lesions and invasive cancer (and the cell lines derived therefrom). **In precancerous lesions, the virus is usually episomal, that is, not**

TABLE 11-2

DISTRIBUTION OF VARIOUS TYPES OF HUMAN PAPILLOMAVIRUS IN CERVICAL SPECIMENS IN A COHORT OF 2,627 WOMEN FROM SEVERAL STUDIES*

HPV types*	Distribution of Viral Types					
	Normal cervix[†]	Atypia of unknown significance	LGSIL	HGSIL	Invasive cancer	Total
None	1,465	206	115	33	16	1,835
Low risk (6/11,42–44)	14	13	76	11	0	114
Intermed. risk (31,33,35,51,52,58)	23	9	45	49	12	138
High risk (16,18,45,56)	31	22	106	153	117	429
Unknown type[‡]	33	20	35	15	8	111
TOTAL	1,566	270	377	261	153	2,627

Percentage Distribution of Intermediate and High Risk HPV				
Normal cervix[†] N = 1,566	Atypia of unknown significance N = 270	LGSIL N = 377	HGSIL N = 261	Invasive cancer N = 153
3.4%	11.5%	40.0%	77.3%	84.3%

* HPV by Southern blot.
[†] Most had negative cytology and colposcopy.
[‡] Since this study was published in 1992, several of the "unknown" types of HPV have been identified as intermediate or high risk types 26, 39, 59, 68, 69, 73, 77, and 82.
LGSIL = low grade squamous intraepithelial lesions; HGSIL = high grade squamous intraepithelial lesions.
(Modified from Lorincz et al. Obstet Gynecol 79:328–337, 1992, with permission.)

integrated into cellular DNA but behaving as an independent plasmid, capable of its own life cycle, without the participation of host cell DNA. In invasive cancer, cell lines derived therefrom, and in some precancerous lesions of high-grade, truncated sequences of viral DNA are integrated into cellular DNA (Fig. 11-7) and their life cycle depends on the life cycle of the host cells.

Role of Open Reading Frames E6 and E7 in Carcinogenesis

In the search for a possible carcinogenic function of HPV, it has been documented that the proteins of the open reading frames E6 and E7 from the high-risk HPV types 16 and 18 react with proteins regulating the events in cell cycle. Thus, the E6 protein reacts with p53, which is one of the key regulatory genes governing the transcription of DNA in the G_1 phase of the cell cycle and leads to its degradation (Chen et al, 1993). E7 protein reacts with the Rb gene, which governs the orderly transition of cells from G_1 to G_2 phase of the cell cycle and leads to its degradation (Fig. 11-8). The reactions require intermediate molecules, including ubiquitins. Loss of the open reading frame E2 that has a regulatory function is probably important in this sequence of events (Dowhanick et al, 1995). It has been fairly universally assumed that this relationship of the E6 and E7 proteins contributes to events leading to carcinoma of the uterine cervix (summaries in Shah and Howley, 1992; Howley, 1995; Munger et al, 1992). In experimental systems, the activation of E6 and E7 genes proved to be important in immortalization of normal human squamous cells in culture by HPV types 16 or 18 (De Palo et al, 1989;

Woodworth et al, 1989; Montgomery et al, 1995). The E6 and E7 genes are usually well preserved and, perhaps, even enhanced in the integrated viral DNA, possibly contributing to the malignant transformation (Einstein et al, 2002).

In this context, it is important to note that other DNA viruses, such as adenovirus and simian virus 40 (SV 40), interact with p53 and Rb genes more efficiently than HPV but are not carcinogenic in humans. Thus, additional mechanisms must be operational to explain the carcinogenic role of HPV (Lazo, 1999).

HPV in Precursor Lesions and Cancer of the Uterine Cervix

The earliest study documenting the presence of HPVs in a neoplastic lesion of the cervix were based on electron microscopy of biopsies of the cervix, cited above, and extended to corresponding cells in smears by Meisels et al (1983). By this technique, only the mature virions of unknown type can be demonstrated in the nuclei of the affected cells (see Fig. 11-6). Another technique suitable for demonstration of mature virions was based on an antibody to common antigen contained in capsids of bovine papillomavirus (Jenson et al, 1980). Using an immunologic technique on tissue sections of precursor lesions, it was shown that the presence of mature virions was generally limited to the nuclei of cells in the upper layers of the squamous epithelium, notably the nuclei of koilocytes (Fig. 11-9A). A positive reaction with the nuclei of cells of the basal layer was exceptional. This technique was applied to abnormal cells in smears by Jean Gupta et al (1983), but provided no information on latent infection.

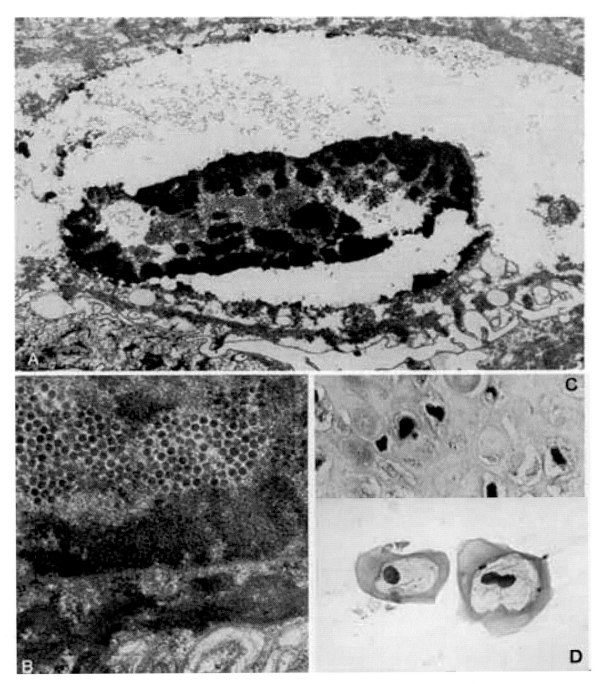

Figure 11-6   **Light and electron microscopic presentation of koilocytes.** The light microscopic appearance of these cells is shown in *D*. Note the enlarged single or double nuclei and the sharply demarcated perinuclear clear zone surrounded by a narrow rim of cytoplasm. *A,B.* Electron micrographs of koilocytes from a cervical smear. In *A*, an array of viral particles is present in the nucleus and there is a near-complete destruction of the perinuclear cytoplasm, accounting for the perinuclear "cavity" in light microscopy. In *B*, the crystalline array of viral particles, each measuring approximately 50 nm in diameter. *C.* Immunoperoxidase-labeled HPV antibody reaction (black stain) in nuclei of a histologic section of a vulvar condyloma, treated with a broad spectrum antibody to papillomaviruses. (*A:* ×5,590; *B:* ×44,200.)

To identify latent infection and to determine the relationship of specific viral types to human disease, molecular hybridization techniques were required. The general principle is based on **hybridization homology between a known DNA sequence and the unknown target DNA** (see Chap. 3 for a description of the basic principles of these

techniques). An essential first step was the unraveling of the molecular structure of the viruses of various types, leading to the production of **type-specific DNA probes** (zur Hausen, 1976; Gissmann et al, 1983). The hybridization techniques can be used under *stringent* or *nonstringent* conditions. The nonstringent conditions may reveal the presence of viral

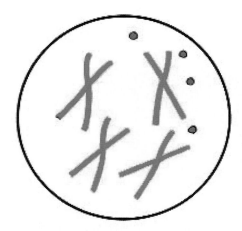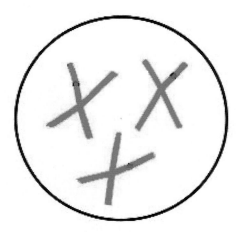

Nonintegrated plasmid form
(independent reproduction), seen
mainly in precancerous lesions

Integrated form (reproduction
linked to host cell), seen
mainly in invasive cancer and
corresponding cell lines

Figure 11-7   **Schematic representation of nonintegrated and integrated human papillomavirus DNA (red dots).**

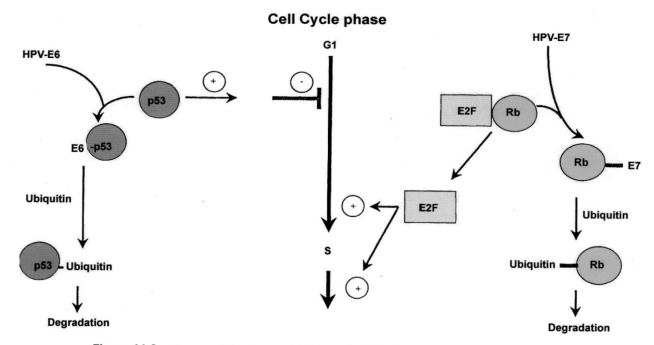

Figure 11-8   **Diagram of the impact of HPV proteins E6 and E7 on various stages of cell cycle.** The protein E6 interacts with p53 affecting the GI stage of the cell cycle. Protein E7 reacts with retinoblastoma (Rb) gene and, thus, with the terminal phase of G_1 and the beginning of S phase of the cell cycle. Ubiquitin mediates degradation of both tumor expressor proteins, thus facilitating the expression of genes needed for completion of cell cycle. (Courtesy of PA Lazo. The molecular genetics of cervical carcinoma. Br J Cancer 80:2008–2018, 1999.)

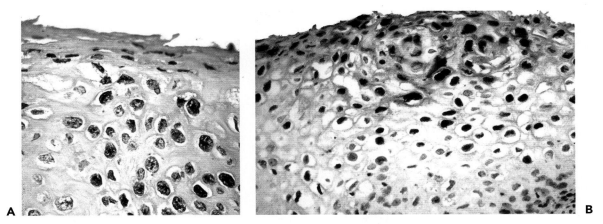

Figure 11-9   *A.* Anal condyloma stained with immunoperoxidase-labeled antibody to broad spectrum capsular antigen of HPV. The dark nuclei contain viral particles. *B.* In situ hybridization of a low-grade squamous intraepithelial lesion of cervix with a probe to HPV type 16. The dark brown–stained nuclei contain viral DNA.

DNA of several related viral types. Under stringent conditions, only one specific viral type will be demonstrated.

Southern blotting technique remains the "gold standard" of such studies because of its sensitivity and specificity. The technique can be applied to liquid samples collected from the cervix or vagina of patients or to DNA extracted from specific lesions. It was **assumed that the viral type in the liquid sample corresponded to the viral type present in the lesion.** By this technique, initial information could be obtained on the presence of various types of HPV in DNA extracted from various lesions, such as invasive cancer. The technique also provided information on the relationship of the viral DNA to the genomic DNA, that is, whether the viral DNA was episomal or integrated, but provided no information on the distribution of viral DNA in lesions.

In situ hybridization of tissue sections with probes to various types of HPV provides information on the distribution of specific types of viral DNA in histologically identified specific lesions (Fig. 11-9B). The probes can be labeled with either radioactive compounds, requiring lengthy exposure and development of photographic plates, or with biotin for a rapid microscopic visualization of the positive immune reaction. An imaginative application of the in situ hybridization technique is the use of **antisense RNA probes,** which hybridize to mRNA produced by the virus and, hence, reveal active viral transcription (Stoler and Broker, 1986). A relatively simple **dot blot hybridization** technique can be used for screening of cell samples suspended in a liquid medium. The latter technique allows synchronous analysis of multiple samples. Cell DNA is placed (spotted) onto a nitrocellulose membrane, denatured by heat, and hybridized with viral DNA labeled with a radioactive probe under stringent conditions.

The identification of viral presence is facilitated by **polymerase chain reaction (PCR),** to amplify small amounts of DNA extracted from cells or tissues. Probes to most viral types are now commercially available and the procedure has been automated. Most recent studies describing the relationship of HPV with cervical cancer are based on this technique. **PCR** may also be used **in situ** in cells and tissues with markedly increased sensitivity (Nuovo et al, 1991; Bernard et al, 1994) but the technique is difficult and prone to errors. Most recently, a **hybrid capture technique** has been developed to document the presence of the virus in liquid samples obtained from the female genital tract (Lörincz, 1996). The principles of the technique are described in the legend to Figure 11-10. The test has been automated with apparently reliable results. It was approved by the Food and Drug Administration (FDA) in 2003 as an ancillary test for evaluation of precancerous lesions of the uterine cervix (see Part 2 of this chapter for further discussion of this topic).

The **sensitivity of these techniques varies significantly.** Common capsid antigen has low sensitivity and requires a fairly massive presence of mature virions to be positive. Southern blotting may give a positive signal with a small number of viral copies. Dot blotting, used as a screening test, has moderate sensitivity. The in situ hybridization techniques with DNA probes are less sensitive than Southern blotting and require from 10 to 50 copies of viral DNA for the signal to reveal the presence of the virus. In situ hybridization with RNA probes is more sensitive. With the use of the PCR, a single copy of the virus can be detected. Hybrid capture technique appears to have a sensitivity similar to Southern blotting.

Evidence Supporting the Role of HPV as a Carcinogenic Agent

Over the past decade, the literature on this topic has grown exponentially and only a very brief summary of the salient facts can be given here. **The presence of high-risk (including intermediate-risk) HPVs has been documented in nearly all invasive cancers and in 50% to 90% of precancerous lesions** (Lorincz et al, 1992; zur Hausen, 1994; Bosch et al, 1995; Fahey et al, 1995; Howley, 1995; Shah and Howley, 1995; Kleter et al, 1998; Lazo, 1999; Burk, 1999; Muñoz et al, 2003). The highest figures, published since 1990, were based on PCR, which allowed for the

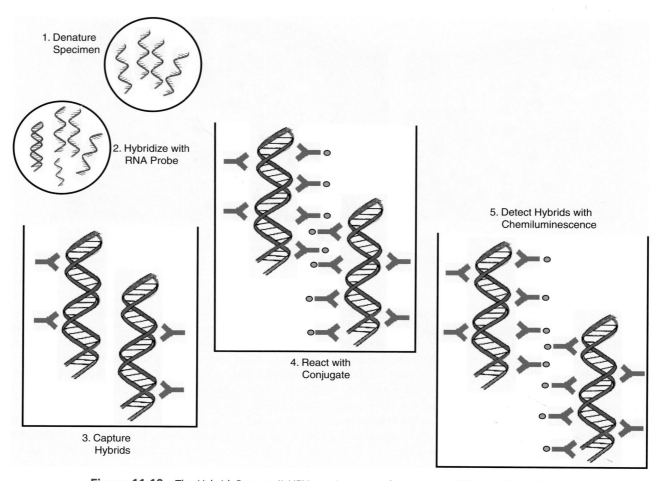

1. Denature Specimen

2. Hybridize with RNA Probe

3. Capture Hybrids

4. React with Conjugate

5. Detect Hybrids with Chemiluminescence

Figure 11-10 The Hybrid Capture II HPV test is a second-generation DNA test that relies on signal amplification to achieve high sensitivity. Specimens are treated with a denaturant to break up cell DNA to form single-stranded DNA. Then HPV-specific RNA probes are added and hybridization is allowed to proceed. If there is a specific HPV type in the specimen, its genomic DNA will form an RNA-DNA hybrid. These hybrids are captured on a microplate well and reacted with an alkaline phosphatase monoclonal antibody conjugate specific for RNA-DNA hybrids. Unbound molecules are removed by washing, and the hybrid conjugates are detected by chemiluminescence produced by the dephosphorylation of a dioxetane-based substrate. The test has been approved by the FDA as an ancillary method of screening for carcinoma of the uterine cervix. (Courtesy of Dr. Attila Lörincz, Digene Corp., Gaithersburg, MD 20878; modified.)

detection of minute amounts of viral DNA in target tissues or cells. It is generally thought that integration of HPV into the cell genome and the affinity of the oncoproteins E6 and E7 for the p53 and Rb regulatory proteins are the triggers leading to the multiple genetic abnormalities that are the hallmark of cancer. In 1995 **a committee of experts** convened by the IARC, **declared HPV 16 to be a carcinogenic agent** and HPV types 18 and 31 as probable carcinogenic agents (see IARC Monograph 1995 for a detailed analysis of the published data). Latest classification by IARC team was discussed above (Muñoz et al, 2003).

Initial studies of patients suggested that the mere presence of HPV was a risk factor for the development of cancer of the cervix. Subsequent studies in women with normal cervicovaginal smears gave inconsistent results, ranging from 0 in virgins (Fairley et al, 1992) to 47% (ter Meulen et al, 1992) in various populations from several continents (for summary, see IARC Monograph 1995 and Muñoz et al, 2003). **Follow-up of patients,** with or without cytologic

abnormalities, suggested that women carriers of **HPVs, particularly of the high-risk type, are at risk for developing intraepithelial precursor lesions, some of which are high-grade** (de Villiers et al, 1992; Koutsky et al, 1992; Schlecht et al, 2001). Burk (1999) estimated that women carriers of the virus were three times as likely to develop precancerous lesions as women free of virus.

With the introduction of the sensitive PCR method of virus detection, in a number of studies of various populations of healthy young women in the United States, it has been shown that **the presence of HPV, mainly of high-risk type, could be documented in nearly half of them** (Bauer et al, 1991). The proportion of women carriers of high-risk HPV increased with the number of sexual partners, reaching 100% in those with 10 sexual partners (Lay et al, 1991). **Clearly, only a tiny fraction of these women would be likely to develop cancer of the cervix. Serologic methods** of immunotesting for the past or current infection with HPV have also been conducted, searching for antibodies to viral capsids (Kirnbauer et al, 1994; Viscidi et al, 1997; Rudolf et al, 1999). The method appears to be efficient in identifying people exposed to the virus (usually type 16), but its clinical value has not been proven.

It was subsequently documented that, **in most young women, the presence of the virus is transient and of no apparent clinical significance.** Ho et al (1998) documented that **the dominant type of virus may change with each test.** Moscicki et al (1998) followed 618 women positive for HPV; in 70% of them, the presence of the virus could no longer be documented after 24 months. In women with persisting infection, only 12% developed precursor lesions. **Normal pregnant women** are frequent carriers of HPV. Depending on the trimester of pregnancy, 30% to 50% of women showed evidence of HPV infection, half of them of the high-risk type (Schneider et al, 1987). Rando et al (1989) reported that the proportion of women with HPV DNA rose from about 21% in the first trimester of pregnancy to 46% in the third trimester. Thus, **the presence of the virus in pregnant women is transient and is related to somewhat lowered immunity occurring during pregnancy.**

Because the proportion of normal women carriers of the virus is extremely high, **a new theory had to be constructed, to wit, that only persisting infections with viruses of high-risk type lead to precancerous lesions and, by implication, to invasive cancer.** Several follow-up studies, notably by Ho et al (1995); Walboomers et al (1995); Moscicki et al (1998); Chua and Hjerpe (1996); and Wallin et al (1999), presented persuasive evidence that women with persisting infection with a high-risk type HPV were at risk for the development of high-grade lesions and, by implication, invasive cancer of the cervix. Perhaps the most interesting prospective studies were conducted in the Netherlands (Remmink et al, 1995; Nobbenhuis et al, 1999). In the Remmink study 342 women with cytologic diagnosis of "Pap IIIb," a suspicious smear suggestive of some form of intraepithelial neoplasia, were followed for about 16 months. Every 3 to 4 months, the women were examined by colposcopy (without biopsies) and HPV DNA testing for 27 "high risk" types was performed by using the PCR method. At the start of the follow-up, 62% of the women were HPV-positive. At the conclusion of the study 19 women (5.6% of the cohort) who were HPV positive throughout the study, progressed to CIN III, occupying two or more quadrants of the cervix. In the Nobbenhuis study, 353 women with a cytologic diagnosis of mild, moderate, or severe dyskaryosis and, hence, some form of "dysplasia," were followed, as in the Remmink study, for a period of over 5 years. Thirty three (9.3%) of the cohort developed a high-grade precursor lesion (CIN III) occupying three or more quadrants of the uterine cervix, all having been HPV positive throughout the study period. The conclusions of the Dutch studies stated that women with **persisting infection with a high-risk HPV** were those most likely to develop an extensive high-grade neoplastic lesion. At the time of this writing (2004), it is the consensus of the investigators that persisting infection with a high-risk HPV causes cervical cancer (Manos et al, 1999; Stoler,

2000; Schlecht et al, 2001). **Still, cancer of the uterine cervix is, at best, a rare complication of HPV infection, as recently confirmed by the Dutch investigators who were among the most active promoters of the HPV-cancer relationship** (Helmerhorst and Meijer 2002).

An important, although indirect, confirmation of the role of HPV 16 in carcinogenesis of the uterine cervix has been the development of a **vaccine,** first in mice (Balmelli et al, 1998) and then in humans. In preliminary trials, the vaccine has been shown to be protective of HPV-associated precancerous abnormalities (Koutsky et al, 2002).

Unresolved Questions

- **It is evident that the presence of HPV, even in the high-risk type, in the genital organs of a woman, does not constitute evidence of a precancerous event or cancer.** Studies of persisting infection with high-risk HPV, summarized above, do not address the question why some women have a persisting HPV infection and most do not, why only a small percentage of the women with persisting infection will develop precancerous lesions, nor does it address the question of what percentage of women with CIN III will progress to invasive cancer. In my view (LGK), this algorithm represents a simplistic explanation of a very complex problem and raises many questions that have not been addressed to date.

- **The frequency of documented viral presence diminishes with age.** It is highest in teenagers and in women in the third decade of life, but becomes much lower in the fourth and subsequent decades. **Yet, invasive cancer of the uterine cervix has its peaks in the fourth and fifth decades of life,** hence, the conclusion that **the virus must remain latent for many years and yet remain active to induce the multiple molecular genetic changes that are a prerequisite of invasive disease.** Virtually nothing is known about these events.

- **There are no specific associations of HPV types with precursor lesions of cervix cancer.** All HPV types, whether low-, intermediate-, or high-risk, occur in precursor lesions, regardless of their morphologic configuration and classification as either low-grade or high-grade (see Table 11-2). Thus, **the severity of the abnormality in a precursor lesion cannot be correlated with viral type.** The end point, usually invasive cancer of the cervix, but not always, correlates with high-risk viral types but it represents only a very small fraction of infected women.

- **The behavior of intraepithelial precursor lesions, whether high- or low-grade, is insecure.** Although many of them, particularly the low-grade lesions, may regress or persist without progression, some other lesions of identical morphologic configuration may progress to invasive cancer, as is discussed later on in this chapter. **In the absence of long-term prospective follow-up studies of the precursor lesions, their insecure behavior has not been correlated with viral types.** In attempting to explain the mechanisms controlling the behavior of these lesions, Kadish et al (1997) have suggested that the immune response in the patients' cervical stroma may be the decisive factor accounting for this behavior. Kobayashi et al (2002) observed the presence of lymphoid aggregates in the stroma of the cervix in the presence or absence of neoplastic lesions but failed to correlate the findings with behavior. In keeping with the viral persistence theory, discussed above, it has been suggested that women who get rid of their virus may have regressing lesions, but such a study has not been conducted to date.

- **The mechanisms of viral transmission.** It is generally assumed that HPV is transmitted between sexual partners. In support of this thesis, it has been shown that **the presence of HPV in sexually active young women increases with the number of sexual partners, reaching 100% in women with 10 partners** (Ley et al, 1991). However, tracing the virus to male partners has proven to be difficult. Initial studies of penile lesions in male partners of women with precancerous lesions of the uterine cervix suggested that in 50% to 70% of the males, inconspicuous lesions on the skin on the shaft of the penis, detected with a colposcope, may be the source of the infection (Barrasso et al, 1987). In a subsequent communication in a French journal (1993), Barrasso et al reduced this figure to 35% to 40% of males. In a study by Baken et al (1995) using PCR, the **presence of any type of HPV in both sexual partners occurred in only about half of the couples and matching viral types were relatively uncommon;** a complex analysis was used to show that the limited concordance was statistically significant. Castellsqué et al (2002) reported that circumcision in males has a protective effect on males and their female partners. It is beyond the scope of the present work to cite additional references on this topic and the reader is referred to the IARC Monograph (1995) for additional reading. At the time of this writing, **the source of the viral infection is not clear in many female patients with neoplastic lesions of the uterine cervix.**

- Further, the presence of HPV sequences in carcinomas of the **cornea, larynx, esophagus,** and **lung,** discussed below, strongly suggest that **sexual mode of transmission is not the only mechanism of activation of HPV** which has great **affinity for squamous cancer of many organs.**

- **Mechanism of infection.** It is currently assumed that the infection of the epithelium with HPV occurs at the level of the basal layer of the squamous epithelium of the cervix, this being the only part of the epithelium capable of mitotic activity necessary to induce epithelial transformation. There are many aspects of this assumption that have not been proven. For example, it is not known whether mature virions or sequences of viral DNA are capable of infecting the target epithelium. It is not known whether receptors exist on the surfaces of the target cells to capture the virus and to facilitate the transfer of viruses into the cell interior. It is not known how the viruses travel across the cytoplasm to reach the nucleus.

- Therefore, the **carcinogenic role of the virus can only**

take place under certain conditions that favor its persistence. Little is known about these **risk factors** but one of them may be the **immunodeficiency.** The first study to this effect was a report from this laboratory on four immunodeficient female patients (three of them with **Hodgkin's disease**) who developed multifocal HPV-related precancerous lesions in their genital tracts, which in one of them progressed to invasive cancer. The presence of the virus in the precancerous lesions was documented by electron microscopy in all four patients (Shokri-Tabibzadeh et al, 1984). A similar observation was made by Katz et al (1987) in a larger group of patients with Hodgkin's disease. **Immunosuppressed organ-transplant recipients** also show a high rate of cutaneous warts and cervical carcinoma in situ (Baltzer et al, 1993; also see Chapter 18). A high frequency of viral infection and precancerous lesions is observed in immunosuppressed women, particularly women infected with human immunodeficiency virus (HIV) and women with **AIDS** (Schrager et al, 1989; Feingold et al, 1990; Maiman et al, 1990, 1993; Klein et al, 1994; Sun et al, 1997; Palefsky et al, 1999; Ellenbrock et al, 2000). We have observed evidence of HPV infection in **female children** treated with chemotherapy (see Fig. 18-7A) and in **women past the age of 80 or even 90.**

- It has been proposed (Koss, 1989, 1998) that **a nonsexual mode of viral infection may exist** and that the infection may occur at birth and remain latent and not detectable until the virus is activated under circumstances related to the onset of sexual activity. The **presence of HPV in neoplastic lesions of many organs other than the genital tract is in favor of this concept.** Galloway and Jenison (1990) and Jenison et al (1990) observed high rates of serologic positivity, as evidence of past infection, in normal adults and in children, using antibodies to fusion proteins of HPV. In subsequent studies, using antibodies to capsids of HPV type 16, seropositivity was limited to some patients with documented past or current infection (Carter et al, 1996). The possibility of **viral transmission at birth** was investigated by Sedlacek et al (1989) by studying nasopharyngeal material in newborn infants. In 15 of 45 infants, the presence of viral DNA could be documented by Southern blotting. Also 2 of 13 amniotic fluid samples contained HPV DNA. **Perinatal transmission of the virus** was also studied by Tseng et al (1998) and by Tenti et al (1999). In both studies, from 22% to 30% of the infants were shown to carry the virus, although the long-term significance of this observation is still under debate. However, a prospective study by Watts et al (1998) considered the risk of perinatal transmission of the virus as very low.

- **Assuming that a nonsexual mode of viral transmission does exist,** the activation at the onset of sexual activity would have to be explained. The possible role of **spermatozoa** as a carcinogenic agent has been discussed above and is deserving of further investigation. Another possible risk factor that has not been investigated so far is the possibility that the amount of exposure may be important; a **"superinfection"** with a massive number

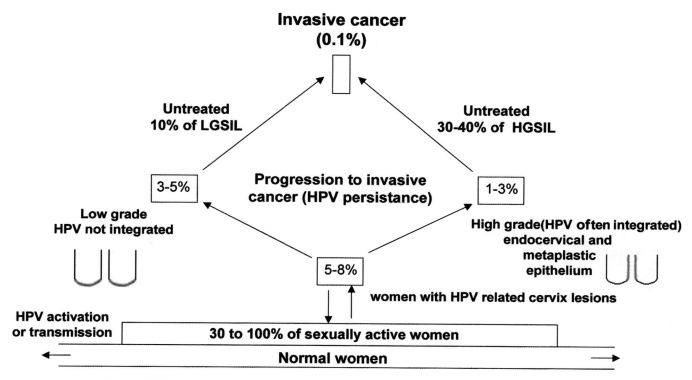

Figure 11-11 Diagram summarizing the probable sequence of events leading from the very common human papillomavirus infection to the rare invasive cancer of the uterine cervix. Two patterns of disease are recognized. The untreated low-grade squamous intraepithelial lesions (LGSIL, *left*) infrequently progress to invasive cancer. The progression of untreated high-grade intraepithelial lesions (HGSIL, *right*) is more common but still far from certain. The figures are approximate and reflect the writer's preferences and concepts.

of virions may be significant, especially in very young teenagers who were shown to be particularly susceptible to this infection (Hein et al, 1977). Zur Hausen (1982) also speculated on the possible role of **synchronous infection with herpesvirus type 2**. Ho et al (1998) speculated that cigarette smoking may be a risk factor (see above).

There is no doubt that HPV is associated with precancerous and cancerous lesions of the female genital tract and that behavioral factors play a role in the development of these lesions. To paraphrase Pagano's comment on the role of Epstein-Barr virus in nasopharyngeal carcinoma (1992): *Is the HPV a "passenger," a "driver," or both?* (cited by Koss 1998). Several issues of importance have been discussed above. A possible sequence of events in the relationship of HPV to precancerous and cancerous lesions of the uterine cervix is shown in Figure 11-11.

HPV Testing for Triage and Diagnosis of Precancerous Lesions of the Uterine Cervix

Within the recent years, numerous papers have been published describing the results of HPV testing as a means of detection and characterization of precancerous lesions of the uterine cervix. The initial observations pertaining to the prognostic significance of persistence of the virus have been cited above. The use of HPV testing, usually by the Hybrid

Capture technique, discussed above, was investigated among others by Vassilakos et al (1998), Sherman et al (1998), Manos et al (1999), Cox et al (1999), Denny et al (2000), Schiffman et al (2000), Wright et al (2000), and Zuna et al (2001).

All observers agree that the testing is possible and reliable when performed on residual cells from liquid cytologic samples but **vary widely in assessment of the utility of the test** as a method of cancer detection. The most important argument against this application of HPV testing is the very large number of false positive tests in sexually active young women (Clavel et al, 1999; Bishop et al, 2000; Davey and Armenti, 2000; Koss, 2000; Cuzick, 2000).

Although the performance of the cervicovaginal cytology is labor intensive and, therefore, costly, whereas HPV testing could be automated, the utility of the test as a cancer detection tool replacing the Pap smear is a saving of doubtful value.

The application of HPV testing in the assessment of atypical squamous or glandular cells of unknown significance (ASC-US, AGUS) is discussed in Part 2 of this chapter.

HPV in Organs Other Than the Uterine Cervix

Most HPV types are observed in **skin lesions;** several were identified in a rare hereditary skin disorder, sometimes leading to skin cancer, known as **epidermodysplasia verruci-**

formis (Orth, 1986). **Bowenoid papulosis, usually a self-limiting disease of the anogenital skin** occurring as brown papules, mainly in young sexually active people, was shown to be associated with HPV type 16; this disorder is now considered a source of viral transmission between sexual partners.

Anal lesions, which are similar to the lesions of the uterine cervix, will be discussed in Chapter 14. The occurrence of condylomas on the **penis** is well known. A lesion of the shaft of the penis, which is intermediary between a condyloma and a low-grade squamous cancer, known as the **giant condyloma of Buschke-Loewenstein, usually contains HPV 6.** Invasive squamous cancer of the penis, rare in the developed countries, but fairly common in Latin America and in Africa, often contains HPV 16. However, **the presence of high-grade precancerous lesions, either on the shaft of the penis or in the penile urethra, has not been well documented,** an issue of importance in epidemiology of HPV (see above). **Squamous carcinomas in situ (Bowen's disease) and invasive squamous cancers of the vulva were shown to contain several viral types, including 6, 11, and 16.** The references pertaining to these lesions will be found in the appropriate chapters and in the IARC Monograph (1995).

Several studies linked **oral cancer** with various types of HPV, particularly types 6 and 16 (Maden et al, 1992). For further discussion, see Chapter 21. **Laryngeal papillomatosis,** an uncommon chronic disorder of the larynx, observed mainly in children (juvenile form) but occasionally in adults, has been shown to be associated with **HPV types 6 and 11** (Mounts et al, 1982; Steinberg et al, 1983; Lele et al, 2002). It is likely that the juvenile form of laryngeal papillomatosis may be the result of contamination of the infant with the virus at birth, during passage through the vaginal canal. Byrne et al (1986) have shown that the **laryngeal lesions may become malignant** and form **metastases containing HPV type 11,** an observation confirmed on four additional patients by Lele et al (2002). Condylomas of the **urinary bladder** were shown to contain HPV types 6 and 11 (Del Mistro et al, 1988; see Chapter 22). Precancerous lesions and cancer of the **conjunctiva and the cornea of the eye** (McDonell et al, 1989) **and carcinomas of the esophagus in China** (Chen et al, 1994) have been shown to contain HPV type 16 (see Chapter 24). Another candidate for the observation with HPV is squamous cancer of the lung (Syrjänen et al, 1989; Papadopoulou et al, 1998), although this association requires further confirmation. It is evident that, in most of these situations, sexual transmission of the virus is extremely unlikely.

SEQUENCE OF MORPHOLOGIC EVENTS IN THE DEVELOPMENT OF CERVIX CANCER

Over the years, many attempts have been made to establish a logical sequence of morphologic events in the genesis of invasive cancer of the uterine cervix. A progression of intraepithelial lesions from slight to marked to invasive cancer has been postulated (Cain and Howell 2000). Unfortunately, the reality defies such simplistic schemes. As is set forth below, **although a transformation of the initial low-grade lesions to high-grade lesions may occur, it is a relatively uncommon event. Most high-grade lesions develop independently in adjacent segments of endocervical epithelium.** The sequence of events is illustrated in Figure 11-12. The behavior of precancerous lesions is discussed below.

Initial Events: Low-Grade Squamous Intraepithelial Lesions (LGSIL)

The initial events in carcinogenesis of the uterine cervix occur in **most, but not all, cases** within the **squamous epithelium** in the area of the **squamocolumnar junction** or **transformation zone** (Fig. 11-12A). Ferenczy and Richart (1974) have shown, by scanning electron microscopy, that the surface configuration of the squamous epithelium of the transformation zone is characterized by smaller cells lacking the microridges characteristic of mature squamous epithelium (Fig. 11-13). It is not known whether this feature is of significance in carcinogenesis.

The earliest morphologically identifiable precancerous tissue lesions **(LGSIL, or mild dysplasia)** are characterized by **enlarged and hyperchromatic nuclei, and the presence of normal and abnormal mitoses, occurring at various levels of the reasonably orderly squamous epithelium** (Figs. 11-12B, 11-14). In **some of these lesions, the abnormal nuclei are surrounded by a clear cytoplasmic zone (koilocytes)** that provide morphologic evidence of a **permissive human papillomavirus infection with a variety of viral types** (see Fig. 11-9B). **In some cases, the squamous epithelium is thickened, folded, and provided with a superficial layer of keratinized cells.** Such lesions resemble a wart or a *condyloma acuminatum* and, therefore, are sometimes referred to as a **"flat condyloma,"** a term that is no longer recommended (see Fig.11-4 and Part 2 of this chapter).

The early neoplastic events may also take place outside of the transformation zone, either on the native squamous epithelium of the uterine portio or in the endocervical epithelium. The lesions on the native squamous epithelium are identical to those occurring in the transformation zone, described above. The early neoplastic events occurring in endocervical epithelium are difficult to recognize or classify and are generally known as **atypical squamous metaplasia,** discussed in Chapter 10 and again further on in this chapter.

Studies of populations of women with multiple cytologic screenings show that, after elimination of all precursor lesions, the predominant **new lesions** observed in such women are the low-grade squamous lesions described above (Melamed et al, 1969) (Fig. 11-15). **The incidence of these lesions** is approximately **5 to 6 per 1,000 women's years. The prevalence depends on the type of population**

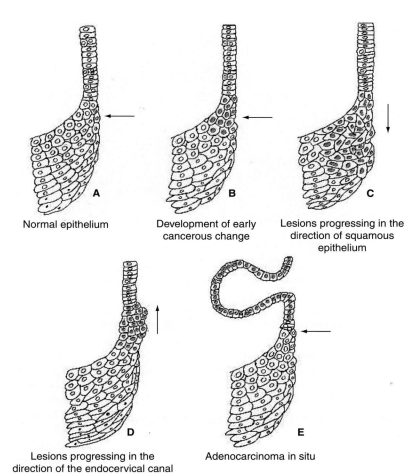

Normal epithelium

Development of early cancerous change

Lesions progressing in the direction of squamous epithelium

Figure 11-12   **Sequence of events in the development of precancerous lesions of the uterine cervix.** *A.* Normal cervix. Horizontal arrow indicates transformation zone (TZ). *B.* Early neoplastic events (red dots) occurring in the TZ (horizontal arrow). *C.* Lesion progressing from the transformation zone to squamous epithelium of the outer cervix, resulting in low-grade squamous intraepithelial lesion (LGSIL; arrow down). These lesions may sometimes progress to squamous carcinoma. *D.* Lesion progressing from the TZ in the direction of endocervical canal (arrow up), resulting in high-grade intraepithelial lesions (HGSIL). *E.* Development of endocervical adenocarcinoma (TZ; horizontal arrow). Events depicted in *C–E* may be synchronous. (Drawing by Prof. Claude Gompel, Brussels, Belgium.)

Lesions progressing in the direction of the endocervical canal

Adenocarcinoma in situ

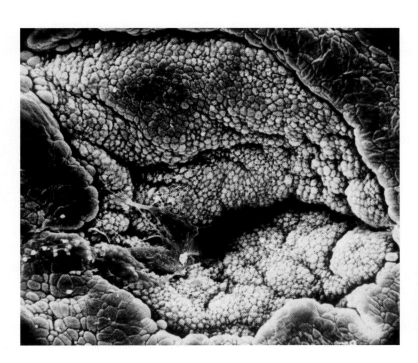

Figure 11-13   **Scanning electron micrograph of the transformation zone.** The mature squamous epithelium forms a ridge around the central zone (transformation zone), wherein the component squamous cells are much smaller. The external os is seen as a comma-shaped opening. (×220.) (Courtesy of Drs. A. Ferenczy and R.M. Richart, New York, NY.)

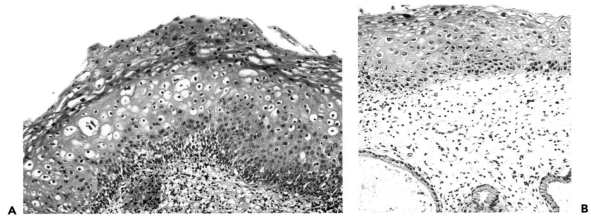

Figure 11-14 Low-grade squamous intraepithelial lesions (LGSILs) of the uterine cervix. *A.* The similarity of the lesion with condylomas shown in Figure 11-4B is striking. Also note the superficial layers of keratinized cells. *B.* The squamous epithelium is of normal thickness but shows nuclear abnormalities and koilocytes in the upper epithelial layers.

studied and ranges from 1 to 5%, occasionally somewhat **higher.** Although most initial lesions are generally **first observed in young women or even adolescents** (Hein et al, 1977), **they may also be observed in older women, even after the menopause.**

High-Grade Squamous Intraepithelial Lesions (HGSIL)

There is excellent evidence that most cases of HGSIL **develop in the endocervical epithelium, either within the transformation zone or in the endocervical canal, as confirmed by mapping studies** (see Fig. 11-12C,D). **The HGSIL may be adjacent to LGSIL** (Fig. 11-16A) **or occur in the absence of LGSIL, as a primary event** (Fig. 11-16B).

There are **three principal histologic patterns of** HGSIL.

About 60 to 70% of these **lesions mimic squamous metaplasia and are characterized by medium size cancer cells, about the size of metaplastic cells, showing enlarged, hyperchromatic nuclei throughout the epithelium of variable thickness that shows moderate to marked disturbance of layering** (Fig. 11-16C).

In about 15 to 20% of cases, the neoplastic process is derived **from the basal or reserve cells of the endocervical epithelium** and results in **lesions composed of crowded small cancer cells with scanty cytoplasm** (Fig. 11-16B,D). **Adenocarcinomas of the endocervix probably share the same origins with high-grade lesions of this type** (see Fig. 11-12E and Chapter 12).

High-grade squamous lesions of metaplastic and small cell type **frequently extend to endocervical glands** (Fig. 11-16D). **This extension should not be considered as evidence of invasion.** In such lesions, **human papillomavirus infection is usually occult** and the documentation of the

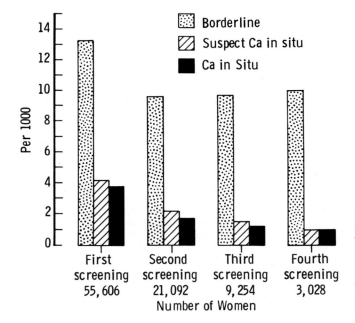

Figure 11-15 Results of several sequential annual cytologic screenings with histologic confirmation. The lesions are divided into three groups; borderline (consistent with mild to moderate [low-grade] dysplasia, or CIN I), suspicious (consistent with high-grade dysplasia, or CIN II), and carcinoma in situ (corresponding to CIN III). It may be noted that with the elimination of the more severe lesions the prevalence of the borderline lesions remains essentially unchanged year after year. (From Koss LG. Significance of dysplasia. Obstet Gynecol 13:873–888, 1970.)

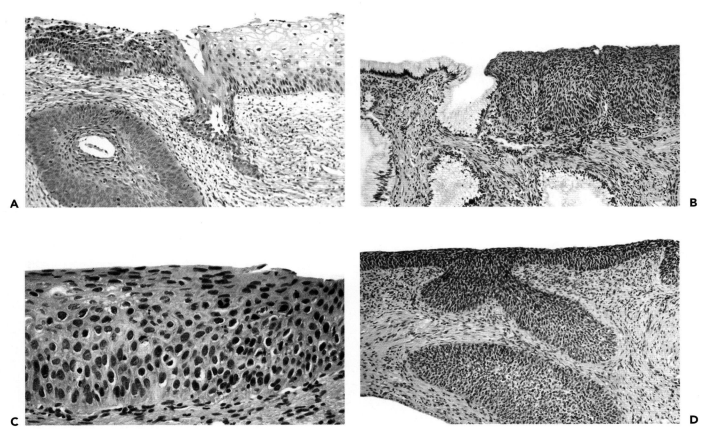

Figure 11-16 High-grade squamous intraepithelial lesions (HGSIL) of the uterine cervix. *A.* Shows the presence of a low-grade lesion on the right and of a high-grade lesion on the left. The latter extends into the adjacent endocervical gland. *B.* HGSIL composed of medium-size cells in the endocervical canal. *C.* HGSIL mimicking squamous metaplasia of the endocervix. Note nuclear abnormality, mitotic figures and disorderly arrangement of cells. *D.* Small cell HGSIL extending into endocervical glands.

presence of the virtual DNA requires hybridization or other molecular techniques.

The third, currently least frequent histologic pattern of HGSIL, is the **high-grade lesion of squamous type,** known as either **keratinizing carcinoma in situ or keratinizing dysplasia that usually retains many morphologic features of the squamous epithelium of origin** (Fig. 11-17A). These lesions **develop in LGSIL** that, for reasons unknown, progress to HGSIL. **Such lesions are usually located on the outer portion of the cervix, may spread to the adjacent vagina, and may retain the features of the permissive human papillomavirus infection, such as koilocytosis.** It is uncommon for these lesions to extend to the endocervical glands.

All **high-grade lesions,** regardless of type, contain **abundant mitoses at all levels of the epithelium, some of which are abnormal, such as** the so-called **tripolar mitoses** (Fig. 11-17B). In some of these lesions, the malignant epithelium shows **two sharply demarcated layers** (Fig. 11-17C). Usually, the top layer is composed of larger, better differentiated cells than the bottom layer. The mechanism of this event is unknown. HGSIL may sometimes **coat the endometrial** surface (Fig. 11-17D). This is a very uncom-

mon event, usually associated with invasive cancer elsewhere in the cervix.

In histologic material, the different patterns of precursor lesions may be present on the same cervix side-by-side. The differences in the epithelium of origin and anatomic location of the intraepithelial lesions are reflected in histology and cytology of these lesions and may have considerable bearing on the interpretation and classification of biopsies and cervicovaginal smears.

The prevalence of high-grade squamous lesions varies according to the population studied from 0.5% to 3% and, hence, is generally much lower than that of the low-grade lesions.

Also, the high-grade lesions are usually **observed in women who are somewhat older than those with low-grade lesions and younger than women with invasive carcinoma.** The peak of prevalence falls between 25 and 40 years of age (Melamed et al, 1969). The age difference between women with high-grade lesions and those with invasive cancer has been variously estimated at 6.6 to 20 years. In other words, one can expect a latency period of several years until a precursor lesion becomes invasive, thus increasing the chance of its discovery by a systematic screening.

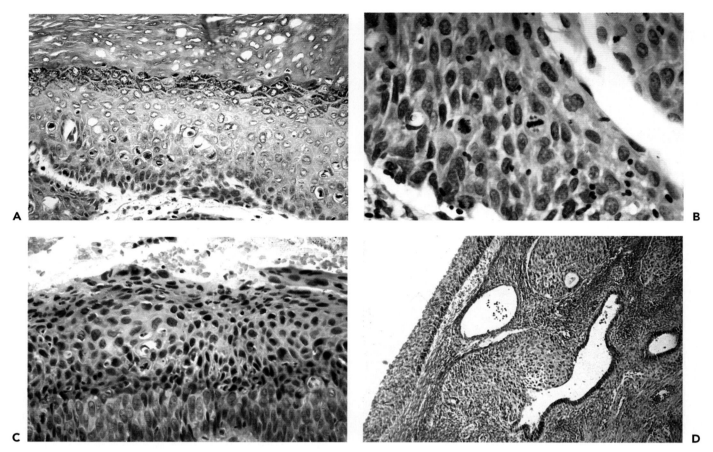

Figure 11-17 High-grade squamous intraepithelial lesions (HGSIL). *A.* Note the marked formation of keratin on the epithelial surface. *B.* High magnification view of HGSIL showing a tripolar mitotic figure. *C.* Two-layer arrangement of HGSIL. As is common in these lesions, the upper part is composed of larger, better differentiated cells than the lower part of the lesion. *D.* HGSIL coating the surface of endometrial cavity. Elsewhere, this tumor was invasive.

Mapping Studies of Precursor Lesions

Extensive mapping studies by Foote and Stewart (1948) (Figs. 11-18–11-21), Przybora and Plutowa (1959), Bangle (1963), Burghardt and Holzer (1972), and Burghardt (1973) confirmed that **keratinizing squamous high-grade lesions are usually located on the outer surface of the cervix** (corresponding to the location of the low-grade lesions), whereas the **high-grade lesions of the endocervical (metaplastic) type, composed of cells of medium sizes, are located in the transformation zone and the endocervical canal. However, lesions composed of small cells are usually confined to the endocervical canal.** The summary of these observations is shown in Figure 11-21.

Behavior of Precursor Lesions

Follow-up studies of precursor lesions, regardless of histologic type, **have shown that the behavior of these lesions is unpredictable. Many of these lesions, particularly of the low-grade type, may vanish without treatment or after biopsies. Other precursor lesions may persist without major changes for many years and may undergo atrophy after the menopause,** in keeping with the atrophy of normal epithelia of the female genital tract. **On the other**

hand, invasive cancer may follow any type of precursor lesion, although it is much more likely to develop from high-grade lesions. However, epidemiologic data strongly suggest that invasive cancer is a relatively rare event, occurring in only approximately 10% of the intraepithelial precursor lesions (Koss et al, 1963; Östör, 1993; Herbert and Smith, 1999). An example of the behavior patterns of a precursor lesion is shown in Figure 11-22. Regardless of these considerations, because most invasive cancers are derived from high-grade lesion, it is the consensus among gynecologists that the high-grade lesions represent a clear and present danger to the patients and, therefore, should be treated. **Prognostic factors** under current investigation are discussed below.

Behavior and Staging of Invasive Carcinoma

Intraepithelial precursor lesions, regardless of degree of histologic or cytologic abnormality, do not endanger the life of the patient because they are not capable of producing metastases. **The onset of danger is related to invasion, which occurs when the cancerous process breaks out of the epithelial confines through the basement membrane into the stroma of the uterine cervix.** The biologic circum-

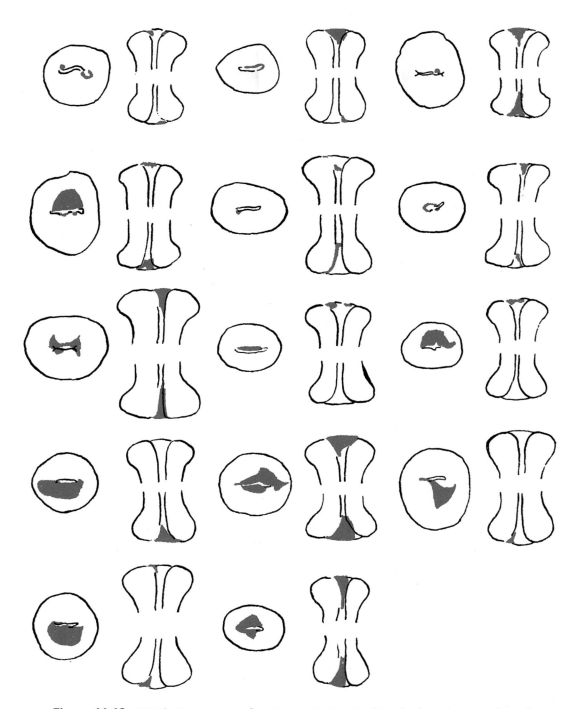

Figure 11-18 Distribution pattern of carcinomas in situ involving both portio vaginalis and endocervical canal. (From Foote FW Jr, Stewart FW. The anatomical distribution of intraepithelial epidermoid carcinomas of the cervix. Cancer 1:431–440, 1948.)

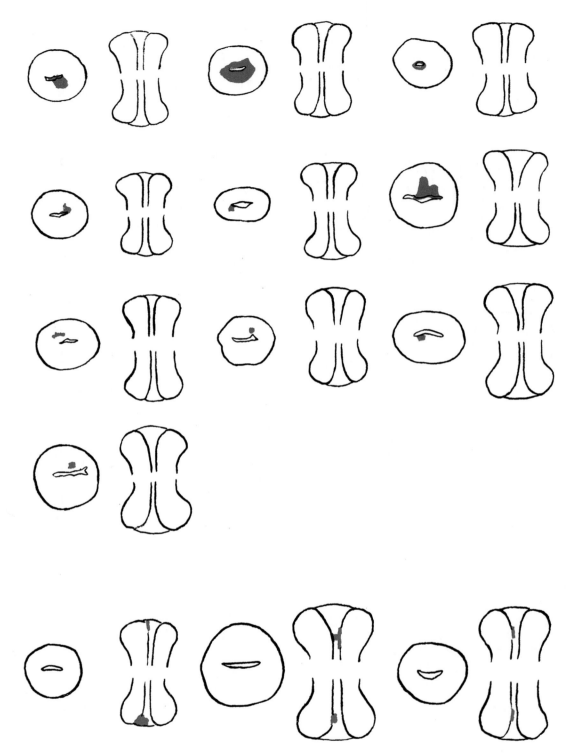

Figure 11-19 **Carcinoma in situ.** (*Top*) Distribution of carcinomas in situ limited to portio vaginalis. (*Bottom*) Distribution pattern of carcinomas in situ limited to endocervical canal. (From Foote FW Jr, Stewart FW. The anatomical distribution of intraepithelial epidermoid carcinomas of the cervix. Cancer 1:431–440, 1948.)

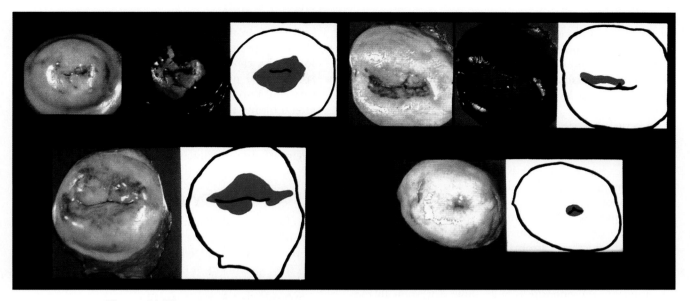

Figure 11-20 Four illustrations that demonstrate how visual examination can give faulty impressions of the distribution or even the presence of carcinoma in situ of the cervix. The actual extent of the lesions is shown in red in the line drawings. Two of the cervices have been painted with Lugol's solution. (From Foote FW Jr, Stewart FW. The anatomical distribution of intraepithelial epidermoid carcinomas of the cervix. Cancer 1:431–440, 1948.)

stances accounting for invasion are not clear and the many hypotheses are discussed in Chapter 7.

It has been known for many years that the prognosis of carcinoma of the uterine cervix depends on the stage of the disease. The current staging by the International Federation of Gynecologists (FIGO) is shown in Table 11-3. Stage I is subdivided into stage IA1 (no grossly visible tumor), stage IA2 (grossly visible and measurable tumor less than 1 cm in diameter) and stage IB, describing larger lesions confined to the cervix.

Any cancer of the cervix that extends beyond the anatomic boundaries of the surface epithelium or the basement membrane of the endocervical glands must be considered invasive.

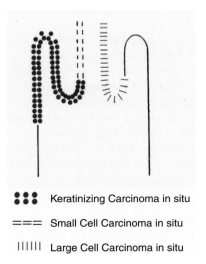

●●● Keratinizing Carcinoma in situ

=== Small Cell Carcinoma in situ

||||| Large Cell Carcinoma in situ

Figure 11-21 The prevailing anatomic distribution of the three types of carcinoma in situ.

TABLE 11-3	
STAGING OF CARCINOMA OF THE UTERINE CERVIX	
Stage 0	Intraepithelial precancerous lesions (dysplasia, cervical intraepithelial neoplasia, low- and high-grade squamous intraepithelial lesions, carcinoma in situ)
Stage I	Carcinoma limited to cervix
	Stage IA – Invasive carcinoma identified microscopically
	IA1 – Microinvasive carcinoma (invasion <3 mm)
	IA2 – Microinvasive carcinoma not larger than 7 mm horizontally and 5 mm vertically*
	Stage IB – Lesion larger than stage IA2 whether or not visible
	IB1 <4 cm
	IB2 >4 cm
Stage II	Extension beyond the cervix (uterus, upper 2/3 of vagina, parametria)
	IIA – no obvious parametrial involvement
	IIB – obvious parametrial involvement
Stage III	Extension to pelvic wall or lower 1/3 of vagina
Stage IV	**IVA** – extension to adjacent organs
	IVB – metastatic spread

* Measured from base of epithelium, either surface or glands.

Invasion of the cervical stroma occurs in stages. The earliest stage of invasion is defined as **microinvasive carcinoma (stage IA), a lesion with invasion limited to 3 mm. Lesions with invasion greater than 3 mm must be considered as fully invasive cancer.** The histologic and cytologic patterns of these lesions are discussed in Part 2 of this chapter.

In actual practice, it is sometimes exceedingly **difficult to determine the anatomic boundaries on which the diagnosis of early invasion is based.** For example, the epithelium of the endocervical glands may be destroyed by cancer, leaving one quite helpless in deciding where the basement membrane of the glands is located. Precursor lesions occurring in squamous epithelium may produce "dips" surrounded by the basement membrane without actually invading the underlying stroma. Another difficulty may be due to inadequate sampling by biopsy and a precursor lesion may prove to be invasive in additional histologic material. Occasionally, the opposite is true: some distortion in the biopsy material may suggest invasion, whereas the surgical specimen will disclose only a precursor lesion. Studies of tenascin, a glycoprotein of the stroma of the uterine cervix, suggested an increased expression of this protein in microinvasive carcinoma (Iskaros and Koss 2000). **In debatable cases, as a rule of thumb, in the absence of clear-cut invasion in ample diagnostic material, the lesion may be considered as a precursor lesion and treated accordingly.**

The histologic and cytologic features of fully invasive cancer of the cervix are discussed in Part 2 of this chapter. Regardless of the histologic patterns and grade of invasive cancer, the **clinical stage of the disease is the most important prognostic yardstick.** In this respect, it must be noted that the errors in clinical staging may be considerable. Even with the availabilty of modern radiologic techniques, lymph node metastases may not be discovered prior to surgery. For example, among the 115 cases of Stage I cervix cancers, there were 19 cases (16.5%) with clinically unsuspected lymph node metastases (Sidhu et al, 1970).

HISTOLOGIC AND CYTOLOGIC TERMINOLOGY OF PRECURSOR LESIONS

Historical Overview

During the first half of the 20th century, all incidentally discovered intraepithelial lesions were universally known as **"carcinoma in situ"** or equivalent name and were treated by hysterectomy. As a consequence of cytologic screening and the first population studies conducted in the 1950s in the United States, it was noted that the precursor lesions differed from invasive cancer in several respects.

■ The precursor lesions occurred generally in women several years younger than those with invasive cancer.
■ The rate of discovery of the precancerous lesions was much higher than the calculated risk of developing invasive carcinoma in the same population, suggesting that not all of the precancerous lesions progressed to invasive cancer within the lifetime of the patient.
■ Untreated precursor lesions did not necessarily progress to invasive cancer within a period of months or years.
■ Some of the precancerous lesions "disappeared" (i.e., they could no longer be found in the uteruses removed after a biopsy that showed a precancerous lesion).
■ There were marked cytologic and histologic differences among the various precursor lesions with regard to the degree of abnormality and cell configuration.

The Concept of "Dysplasia"

These observations led to attempts to separate, on cytologic and histologic grounds, the intraepithelial lesions with good prognosis (i.e., those unlikely to progress to invasive cancer) from "true" precursors of cancer of the uterine cervix, i.e., **carcinoma in situ.** This resulted in the introduction of the term **"dysplasia,"** first suggested by a pathologist, William Ober, to Papanicolaou who used this term, in a paper published in 1949, to discuss lesions with low malignant potential. As the first results of follow-up of precursor lesions became available, James Reagan et al reintroduced, in 1953, the term **dysplasia or atypical hyperplasia** to describe biopsy-documented precursor lesions with benign, or at least noninvasive, behavior. For purposes of comparison, Reagan selected carcinomas in situ made up of small cells. All carcinomas in situ were treated but the "atypical hyperplasias" were followed. The conclusions of this paper were carefully worded and reflected considerable diagnostic uncertainty. Although 35 of 65 lesions classed as "dysplasia" or "atypical hyperplasia" disappeared, many after biopsies, the remaining lesions remained unchanged, and one progressed to invasive cancer. Subsequent writings by Reagan and his colleagues, notably Stanley Patten (1962), further emphasized the **concept of dysplasia as a neoplastic intraepithelial lesion of uncertain prognosis, to be contrasted with carcinoma in situ, an obligate precursor of invasive cancer.** Patten (1978) subdivided dysplasia into three types: **keratinizing (pleomorphic), nonkeratinizing, and metaplastic,** each category **further subdivided into mild, moderate, and severe.**

The concept of **dysplasia** suggested that there are **two categories of intraepithelial lesions** in the uterine cervix: **carcinoma in situ,** an obligate precursor lesion of invasive cancer of the cervix, and **dysplasia,** an ill-defined but essentially "less malignant" abnormality.

The diagnostic system **dysplasia-carcinoma in situ** was formalized in 1962 as "An International Agreement on Histological Terminology for the Lesions of the Uterine Cervix," published in *Acta Cytologica* 6:235–236, 1962. The following definitions were offered:

"Carcinoma in Situ: Only those cases should be classified as carcinoma *in situ* which, in the absence of invasion, show as surface lining an epithelium in which, throughout its whole thickness, no differentiation takes place."
"Dysplasia: All other disturbances of differentiation of

the squamous epithelial lining of surface and glands are to be classified as dysplasia. They may be characterized as of high or low degree. . . ."

Many observers, including the famous surgical pathologist, Arthur Purdy Stout (1957) and this writer (1978), **objected to these definitions** as entirely too narrow, particularly in reference to the claim that any lesion that showed surface differentiation was a "dysplasia" and not a carcinoma in situ and, therefore, was not capable of invasion. Nonetheless, the term "dysplasia" proved nearly irresistible to the practicing pathologists and gynecologists who embraced it with enthusiasm. The advantage of this term was quite apparent: for pathologists, the term was vague enough to lift the burden of establishing a diagnosis of a carcinoma in situ, then requiring immediate treatment, and for the gynecologists, it provided a choice of therapies ranging from "do nothing" to hysterectomy, with a number of intermediate procedures. In fact, as precursor lesions were being observed **in organs other than the uterine cervix,** the term **dysplasia** was also adopted to describe these lesions.

It has been the assumption of many clinicians that the pathologists were able to distinguish among the various levels of dysplasia and separate these lesions from carcinoma in situ, and that this distinction was of prognostic value. This assumption is not accurate. Several diagnostic surveys documented lack of consistency among knowledgeable pathologists in the classification of precursor lesions of the cervix (Siegler, 1956; Cocker et al, 1968; Seybolt and Johnson, 1971; Ismail et al, 1989, 1990; Robertson et al, 1989). It has been recently proposed that **typing for human papillomavirus (HPV) may serve as an aid to classification of precursor lesions** (Sherman et al, 1994; Crum et al, 1997). Although the results of these studies, besides their cost, are not fully persuasive, the issue is not without merit and it is further discussed in Part 2 of this chapter.

The Concept of Cervical Intraepithelial Neoplasia

Follow-up studies by Richart and Barron (1969) confirmed the views previously expressed by Koss et al (1963) that, regardless of morphologic appearance, all precancerous intraepithelial abnormalities of the uterine cervix are capable of progression to invasive cancer, albeit with a low frequency for the better differentiated (low-grade) lesions and a higher frequency for poorly differentiated (high-grade) lesions. Richart suggested the name **cervical intraepithelial neoplasia (CIN)** for these lesions. In order to satisfy the requirements of cytologic and histologic reporting, Richart initially suggested that the lesions be graded from I to IV. Grade I corresponded to morphologically lesser lesions and grade IV to classic carcinomas in situ. Subsequently, **the number of grades of CIN was reduced to three, and still more recently to two, "low-grade" and "high-grade" CIN** in keeping with the Bethesda System of nomenclature, to be discussed below.

Cytologic Nomenclature

Papanicolaou's Classes

The initial classification of cervicovaginal smears was proposed by Papanicolaou who formulated a series of guidelines of smear interpretation in **five classes:**

Class I. Absence of atypical or abnormal cells.
Class II. Atypical cytology but no evidence of malignancy.
Class III. Cytology suggestive of, but not conclusive for, malignancy.
Class IV. Cytology strongly suggestive of malignancy.
Class V. Cytology conclusive for malignancy.

The system of classes was generally well received and it is still in use in many laboratories in many countries, although the significance of "classes" was often modified to fit the requirements of the laboratories in their contacts with clinicians. Papanicolaou himself was not fully satisfied with the system, particularly with Classes II and III, because they offered little diagnostic flexibility. In the years 1952–1958, when this writer had the privilege of working with him, Papanicolaou used plus and minus signs, added to the class, to express more precisely his diagnostic opinion. For example, Class II +, or III − were used to define cervicovaginal smears. To my knowledge, Papanicolaou has never published these observations.

The Bethesda System

With the passage of time, it became apparent that the histologic and cytologic nomenclatures should be similar, if not identical, to facilitate the exchange of information among investigators and laboratories. Starting with the first edition of this book (1961), it was advocated that cytologic diagnosis should reflect, whenever possible, the histologic nature of the underlying lesions. In December 1988, a committee of experts, convened under the auspices of the National Cancer Institute (United States) in Bethesda, Maryland, proposed a system of diagnostic guidelines for the interpretation of the cervicovaginal smears.

The Bethesda System (modified in 2001) was officially accepted by the federal authorities in the United States in a series of rules governing the performance of the laboratories and incorporated in 1988 into the amendment to the Clinical Laboratory Improvement Act **(CLIA 88),** passed by the United States Congress (for the complete text of the Bethesda System, see Appendix at the end of Part 2 of this chapter). Several features of the Bethesda System will be discussed elsewhere in this book. **The cytologic features of the precursor lesions of squamous carcinomas of the uterine cervix were divided into two groups:**

- **Low-grade squamous intraepithelial lesions (LGSIL),** corresponding to histologic patterns in which the fundamental structure of the epithelium of origin (usually the squamous epithelium) is reasonably well preserved (see Fig. 11-14). LGSIL includes, under the same umbrella, lesions variously known as mild or slight dysplasia, flat condylomas, CIN I, with or without features of condyloma.

TABLE 11-4

COMPARATIVE CYTOLOGIC AND HISTOLOGIC NOMENCLATURE OF PRECURSOR LESIONS AND SQUAMOUS CARCINOMA OF THE UTERINE CERVIX

	No evidence of disease	Atypia not further defined	Low-grade lesions	High-grade lesions	Invasive cancer
Papanicolaou	Class I	Class II	Class III	Class IV	Class V
The Bethesda System	Within normal limits	ASC-US AGUS	LGSIL	HGSIL	Cancer
Reagan and Patten			Mild dysplasia*	Moderate and severe dysplasia, carcinoma in situ	Cancer
Richart original			CIN I	CIN II and III	Cancer
Richart modified			CIN low grade	CIN high grade	Cancer

*AGUS is no longer recommended (see Part 2 of this chapter).

- **High-grade squamous intraepithelial lesions (HGSIL),** corresponding to histologic lesions in which the epithelium of origin is replaced by highly abnormal smaller cells. HGSIL includes lesions variously known as moderate and severe dysplasia and carcinoma in situ, CIN II, III (see Figs. 11-16 and 11-17).

This binary system of smear classification, which is consistent with the developments in histologic nomenclature, proved to be easier to use and is probably better reproducible than other diagnostic approaches.

Table 11-4 summarizes the prevailing classification systems of precursor lesions of the uterine cervix.

FOLLOW-UP STUDIES OF PRECURSOR LESIONS OF CARCINOMA OF THE UTERINE CERVIX

Recent observations on the role of human papillomavirus in the genesis of cervical cancer, several of which were cited above, have led to a number of follow-up studies of untreated precursor lesions in the belief that HPV typing may provide a better guide to behavior of these lesions than morphologic assessment. Such studies, that may put the lives of patients into serious jeopardy, have been undertaken with limited, if any, regard of past experiences with these lesions. For this reason, a summary of "old" studies is provided for the interested reader. These studies, which were conducted without the "informed consent," either because it was not required or because the investigator did not believe in the malignant potential of precursor lesions, could not be implemented today because of risk to patients.

Earliest Studies

The concept of carcinoma in situ as a precursor lesion of invasive cervical cancer received initial support from comparative histologic studies of patterns of invasive carcinoma and the surface alterations of the epithelium accompanying invasive cancer (Schauenstein, 1907). In fact, in suitable histologic material, the invasive component of superficially invasive carcinomas can always be traced to the surface epithelium which may vary in appearance and occasionally shows only trivial abnormalities rather than a high-grade precursor lesion. Additional support for the role of carcinoma in situ as a formative stage of cervical cancer was received from observations made prior to 1952. Several dozen cases were published in which biopsies of the uterine cervix, obtained anywhere from 2 to 16 years prior to the occurrence of invasive carcinoma, showed patterns of carcinoma in situ (summary in Stoddard 1952).

Prospective studies of precursor lesions of the uterine cervix carry with them substantial risk to the health of patients because of the danger of developing invasive carcinoma. Therefore, some of the most important data were accumulated during the 1950s and early 1960s before the threat to patients was fully understood. Thus, in the Abraham Flexner lecture of 1953, the well-known Swedish gynecological radiotherapist, Dr. Hans L. Kottmeier, said this about carcinoma in situ of the uterine cervix: "Many surgeons and gynecologists are of the opinion that patients having so-called carcinoma in situ should always be referred for treatment. This has not been proved." In support of his doubt, Kottmeier presented a series of 59 patients with carcinoma in situ, followed at the Radiumhemmet in Stockholm without treatment. At the time of the Flexner lecture, only eight of these patients (13.5%) had developed invasive carcinoma after 2 to 10 years of observation. With the passage of time, Kottmeier was forced to change his mind. In a personal communication (to LGK), dated August 2, 1968, he stated that, out of a group of 34 patients with untreated carcinoma in situ, followed for periods of 20 years or more 25 (73%) developed invasive cancer of the cervix. Three patients developed invasive carcinoma within less than two years and possibly the lesion had been overlooked on initial examination. In the remaining 22 patients, invasive cancer was observed after a follow-up period varying from 5 to 21 years.

Another classical series of observations was published by Petersen of Copenhagen (1955), who shared Kottmeier's doubts as to the significance of intraepithelial precursor lesions. In a remarkable study stretching over a period of more than ten years, Petersen was able to follow, without major treatment 127 women whose cervical biopsies disclosed lesions classified into two groups, as "epithelial hyperplasia with nuclear abnormalities" and "borderline cases." Although the supporting photographic evidence is scanty, it appears that Petersen's group of "epithelial hyperplasia with nuclear abnormalities" represented low-grade lesions in which the features of cancer were not well developed; in the group designated by him as "borderline cases," the lesions probably would have been classified today as a high-grade lesion (CIN III or carcinoma in situ). Yet, 34 patients (26.8%) from both groups, developed invasive cervix cancer with only a slight percentile preference for the more abnormal patterns. Petersen also documented that not all of the lesions progressed to carcinoma; at the end of three years of observation the abnormal epithelium apparently disappeared in 30 patients and remained stationary in 50 patients, regardless of the initial biopsy findings. It is also worth emphasizing that Petersen did not consider superficial electrocautery leaving no visible scars, or application of silver nitrate to the cervix as treatment, although these procedures may have contributed to the regressions of some of the lesions. Petersen concluded the paper by stating that **"the methods used (histological assessment of biopsies of the cervix) have not been able to distinguish 'genuine' from 'false' precancerosis."**

Another study from Copenhagen by Lange (1960), later updated by Sorenson et al (1964), gave similar results: 18 of 83 patients (22%) with "epithelial hyperplasia with nuclear abnormalities" (or low-grade lesions), and 6 of 17 (35%) "borderline cases" (or high-grade lesions), developed invasive carcinoma within five years.

These initial studies provide ample evidence that **some high-grade lesions, such as carcinomas in situ, but also lower grade precursor lesions, if untreated, will progress to invasive carcinoma of the uterine cervix in a substantial proportion of patients and that the risk to the patients increases with the passage of time.** On the other hand, it became equally evident that **some of these lesions will either regress without treatment or persist without changes.** Because of poor histologic documentation, the older studies shed limited light on the prognostic value of various histologic patterns encountered in the precursor lesions. This led to the Memorial Hospital study, supervised by competent pathologists, which is summarized below.

Personal Observations on Behavior of Untreated Precursor Lesions

In a prospective study of carcinoma in situ and related lesions conducted at the Memorial Hospital for Cancer (now the Memorial-Sloan Kettering Cancer Center) between 1952 and 1963, 93 patients with precancerous lesions of the cervix were followed without treatment for periods ranging from seven months to eleven years (Koss et al, 1963). A few patients with untreated lesions, observed prior to 1952, were also included in the study. At the onset of the study, all patients were asymptomatic and of childbearing age. The lesions, detected by cytology, were classified into two groups according to the degree of **histologic abnormality: the group of "carcinoma in situ,"** comprising classical carcinomas in situ and lesions with various degrees of surface maturation that other observers could classify as moderate or severe dysplasia. The second **group of "borderline lesions"** comprised epithelial abnormalities that would be classified today as "low-grade." The emphasis in the study was on a minimum of disturbance of the cervical lesions; therefore, cytology was used extensively as a method of follow-up after the initial diagnosis was established by biopsy. Additional biopsies were obtained only if there was a clinical or cytologic indication that the lesion was changing in character (Fig. 11-22). Douches and vaginal

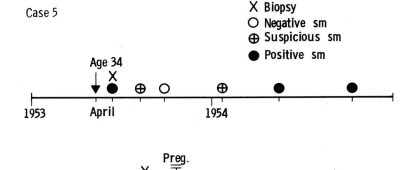

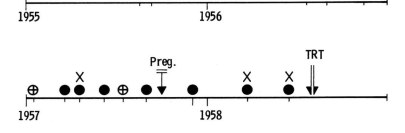

Figure 11-22 Diagrammatic representation of follow-up of a 34-year-old patient with carcinoma in situ. The time that elapsed from the initial cytologic diagnosis until treatment by conization of the cervix was more than 5 years. The patient delivered two children vaginally while under observation. Note the occasional cytologic negativity in spite of persistence of the lesion. *Single arrow* indicates the beginning of follow-up; *double arrow* indicates treatment. (Same case as in Fig. 11-25.) (From Koss LG, et al. Some histological aspects of behavior of epidermoid carcinoma in situ and related lesions of the uterine cervix. Cancer 16:1160–1211, 1963.)

TABLE 11-5

PATTERNS OF BEHAVIOR OF LESIONS OF CERVICAL EPITHELIUM

Behavior	Carcinoma in Situ		Borderline Lesions		Total	
	No.	%	No.	%	No.	%
Disappeared*	17	25.4	10	38.5	27	29
Persisted	41	61.2	4	15.4		
Progressed to carcinoma in situ	0		11	42.3		
Progressed to questionable invasion	5	7.5	0		66	71
Progressed to invasive carcinoma	4	5.9	1	3.8		
Total	67		26		93	

* See Table 11-6.
(Koss LG, et al. Some histological aspects of behavior of epidermoid carcinoma in situ and related lesions of uterine cervix. A long-term prospective study. Cancer 16:1160–1211, 1963.)

tetracycline or trichotine (an antiparasitic agent) suppositories were used in some patients as the only interim treatment. If there was any clinical, histologic, or cytologic suspicion of a possible invasion, or if the lesion showed no signs of regression after several years of follow-up, the patients were treated by hysterectomy.

Sixty-seven patients with high-grade lesions and 26 patients with low-grade lesions were evaluated. The observations are summarized in Tables 11-5 and 11-6.

High-Grade Lesions

In spite of all the precautions outlined above, four of the patients with carcinoma in situ developed superficial but frank invasive cancer after 16 months to 4½ years of follow-up. In an additional five patients, the possibility of microscopic invasion could not be ruled out in serial sections because the lesions produced "dips" into the stroma. The lesions remained relatively stationary in 41 patients for periods varying from one to ten years. Often, however, **there were significant changes in the histologic appearance of the lesion.** The changes were unpredictable and suggested either an increase or a decrease in the degree of abnormalities. Corresponding changes were noted in smears (Fig. 11-23). Seventeen of the 67 patients, or one quarter, showed total regression of the lesion, documented by a negative cytologic follow-up of at least three years' duration. Shorter follow-up proved unreliable and lesions were observed that "recurred" after an "absence" of two years.

An analysis of the effects of the biopsies suggests that **even a small biopsy may cause a regression of a focus of carcinoma in situ** (Figs. 11-24 and 11-25). It is unlikely that the biopsies, per se, removed the entire lesion, particularly when it was present in two or more quadrants of the cervix. It appears more reasonable to assume that regenerating epithelium may dislodge and replace fragments of abnormal epithelium (Fig. 11-26). It is also evident that **new lesions may develop in adjacent, previously normal areas of the cervical epithelium,** as shown in Figures 11-24 and 11-25. It is of note that, **in some patients, the regression of the lesion occurred after treatment with vaginal suppositories of tetracycline and Trichotine,** possibly because of a desquamative effect of these drugs on the cervical epithelium.

TABLE 11-6

DISAPPEARING LESIONS

	Carcinoma in Situ	Borderline Lesions
Biopsy	6	7
Terramycin	7	2
Trichotine	2	0
Spontaneous	2	1
Total	17	10

(Koss LG, et al. Some histological aspects of behavior of epidermoid carcinoma in situ and related lesions of uterine cervix. A long-term prospective study. Cancer 16:1160–1211, 1963.)

Borderline or Low-Grade Lesions

Of the 26 patients with a low-grade (borderline) lesion 11 developed a high-grade lesion 4 remained stationary, and 10 lesions regressed, either spontaneously or following biopsies or vaginal suppositories. It was assumed that, because of their exposed position on the surface of the cervix, these lesions were generally easier to eradicate than carcinoma in situ. One patient, who refused therapy, developed an invasive cancer 13 years after biopsy (Fig. 11-27).

It must be stressed that **cytology was not always reliable** as a tool of follow-up. As shown in Figure 11-22, negative smears were observed repeatedly throughout the follow-up period even though in some patients there was synchronous

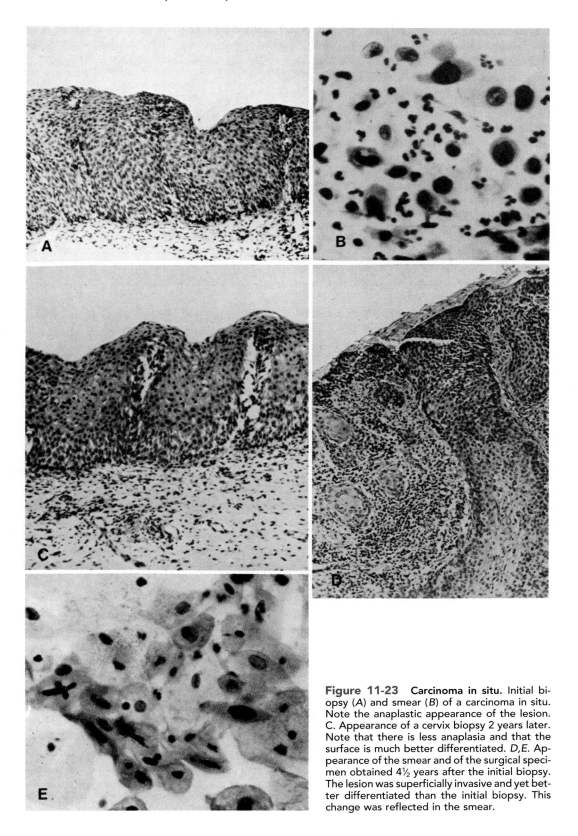

Figure 11-23   Carcinoma in situ. Initial biopsy (*A*) and smear (*B*) of a carcinoma in situ. Note the anaplastic appearance of the lesion. C. Appearance of a cervix biopsy 2 years later. Note that there is less anaplasia and that the surface is much better differentiated. *D,E.* Appearance of the smear and of the surgical specimen obtained 4½ years after the initial biopsy. The lesion was superficially invasive and yet better differentiated than the initial biopsy. This change was reflected in the smear.

Pt. C.M.

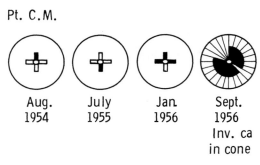

| Aug. 1954 | July 1955 | Jan. 1956 | Sept. 1956 Inv. ca in cone |

Figure 11-24 **Diagrammatic representation of serial biopsies of the cervix** obtained on a 39-year-old patient. By careful designation of the areas of the biopsy, it was possible to ascertain the effect of biopsies on carcinoma in situ. Each square represents a biopsied area; the black squares represent biopsies with carcinoma in situ. Note that the 12-o'clock area, which showed tumor on the initial biopsy, was "cured" 11 months later; at that time the tumor appeared in the 6-o'clock area. Six months later the tumor was present in the 3-, 9-, and 12-o'clock areas but had disappeared from the 6-o'clock area. At the time of conization 9 months later, the tumor had regrown in all four quadrants of the cervix.

biopsy evidence that the lesion was present in the cervix epithelium at the time the smear was obtained. Thus, **this study casts serious doubt on the reliability of the smears as a follow-up procedure.**

These studies clearly established that, **under uniform conditions of observation, the level of histologic abnormality of the intraepithelial precancerous lesions may vary with the passage of time and is of limited prognostic value.** Lesions classed either as high-grade or as low-grade, hence the entire histologic spectrum of lesions comprising the cervical intraepithelial neoplasia, **disclosed a capricious and unpredictable behavior that was significantly influenced by minor diagnostic or therapeutic procedures.** Sufficient numbers of these lesions, regardless of epithelial make-up, progressed to invasive carcinoma, **confirming the potentially malignant nature of all precursor lesions.** Of signal importance, in view of the current trends to consider low-grade lesions as innocuous, was the progression of these lesions to higher grade of intraepithelial abnormalities or, in a patient lost to follow-up for several years, to invasive cancer.

Pt. E. B.

Pregnant   Pregnant

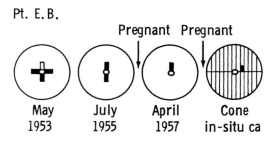

| May 1953 | July 1955 | April 1957 | Cone in-situ ca |

Figure 11-25 **Diagram representing the shifting position of carcinoma in situ after biopsies.** This patient was 34 years old at the time of the initial biopsy and succeeded in establishing a family while under observation (see diagram in Fig. 11-22). Note especially that the last biopsy obtained shortly before conization removed most of the tumor so that only a small area of carcinoma in situ was noted in the cone. There was no trace of cancer in the 6- and 9-o'clock areas of the cone as was observed in the first set of biopsies.

Other Studies

A confirmation of the conclusions of the personal studies summarized above was provided by Richart (1967) who followed, by cytology and colpomicroscopy, a group of 557 women with varying degrees of "dysplasia" for an average period of 36 months. Admission to the study was based on three consecutive abnormal smears; hence, these patients may have represented a select population of women at risk. The study was interrupted after three patients with "mild dysplasia" developed invasive carcinoma. Only 6% of the lesions disappeared spontaneously. In the remaining patients, the lesions either persisted without change or progressed to higher levels of dysplasia and, in 18 women, to carcinoma in situ. **The patterns of cytologic or histologic abnormalities was of no prognostic value, even among the low-grade lesions (mild dysplasia), which led Richart to the conclusion that all of these lesions constitute a spectrum of abnormalities for which the term cervical intraepithelial neoplasia (CIN)** was suggested (see above).

Important evidence in the assessment of "dysplasia" and, hence, lesions with only slight or moderate abnormalities as a step in the genesis of carcinoma of the cervix, was provided by Stern and Neely (1963). In 94 cases of dysplasia, the rate of new carcinomas in situ was 106 per 1,000 (as compared with the new population rate of 5.1/1,000), and the rate of invasive carcinoma was 11 per 1,000 (compared with the new population rate of 1.5/1,000). In a subsequent study (1964), these same authors observed that **women with dysplasia had a 1,600 times greater chance of developing carcinoma in situ and 100 times greater chance of developing invasive cancer than women without disease of the cervix epithelium.**

There are two much cited Swedish studies on mild and moderate dysplasia (Nasiell et al, 1983, 1986). In the 555 women with mild dysplasia, followed without treatment for up to 12 years (mean follow-up 39 months), 342 lesions (62%) regressed; 122 lesions (22%) persisted unchanged; 91 lesions (16%) progressed to severe dysplasia or carcinoma in situ; and 2 progressed to invasive cancer. The 2 invasive cancers were observed in women who failed to appear for a follow-up examination (Nasiell et al, 1986). Biopsies, performed in 76 patients (14%), failed to influence the outcome. The regression was observed in 167 women for more than 1 year and in 175 women for less than 1 year. The behavior of the lesions was not age related. In a study of 894 women with moderate dysplasia, followed without treatment for up to 12 years (mean 78 months) and reported in 1983 (Nasiell et al, 1983), the lesions disappeared in 483 patients (54%), persisted unchanged in 140 patients (16%), and progressed to carcinoma in situ and beyond in 271 patients (30%). In the last group, 3 developed invasive cancer. In this group of patients, biopsies contributed to regression of the lesions. In patients age 51 or older, fewer lesions progressed and the time of progression was longer than in younger women. These authors observed long periods of negative cytology in many of the patients with persisting or progressing lesions. Nasiell et al (1983) estimated the risk of carcinoma in situ or invasive cancer for patients with mild dysplasia at 500 times and for

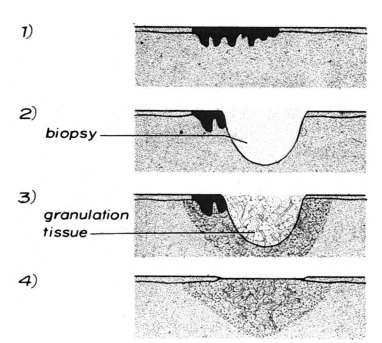

1)

2)

biopsy ——

3)

granulation
tissue ——

4)

Figure 11-26 Schematic representation of a possible mechanism involved in eradication of areas of carcinoma in situ (in black). It is assumed that fragments of residual carcinoma in situ may be cast off during the inflammatory and reparative processes following biopsy. (From Koss LG, et al. Some histological aspects of behavior of epidermoid carcinoma in situ and related lesions of the uterine cervix. Cancer 16:1160–1211, 1963.)

patients with moderate dysplasia at 2,000 times greater than for women without lesions. These studies are summarized in Figure 11-28.

A number of other reports are summarized in Table 11-7. Varga (1966), reporting a follow-up study of 78 untreated patients with dysplasia, observed carcinoma in situ in 39 of them and invasive carcinoma in 11. Thus, progression of "dysplasia" to an identifiable form of cancer was observed in 64% of patients, one of the highest figures reported. Villa Santa (1971) reported on two groups of patients with an ini-tial diagnosis of "dysplasia" established on punch biopsies of the cervix. In a group of 297 patients in whom immediate conization of the cervix was performed, the tissue study revealed carcinoma in situ in 66 patients (22.2%), microinvasive carcinoma in 12 patients (4%), and fully invasive carcinoma in 7 patients (2.4%). There was an additional group of 63 patients in whom, for various reasons, conization was delayed for periods from 2 to 115 months. In this group 10 patients (15.8%) developed carcinoma in situ and 13 patients (20.6%) invasive carcinoma, 3 of which were microinvasive.

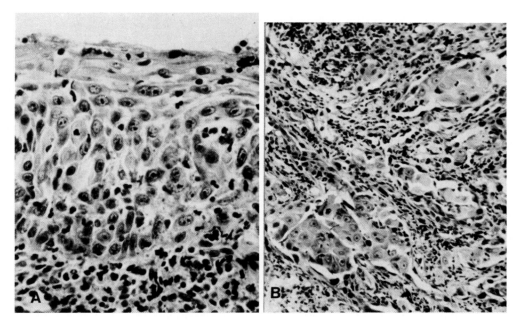

Figure 11-27 A borderline lesion of the cervix observed in a biopsy obtained in 1946 because of "abnormal smear." *A.* Note the nuclear abnormalities and the very satisfactory epithelial stratification. This patient refused treatment and was seen elsewhere 13 years later with a frank invasive carcinoma of the cervix (*B*). (*B:* Courtesy of Dr. Harry Zimmerman, New York, NY.)

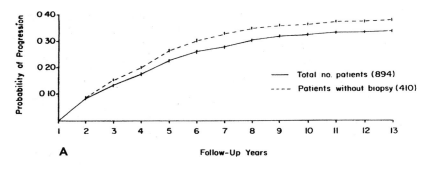

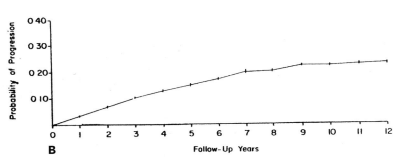

Figure 11-28 Results of long-term follow-up without treatment and probability of progression of 894 patients with moderate dysplasia (*A*) and 555 patients with mild dysplasia (*B*) of the uterine cervix epithelium. In *A*, the probability of progression of moderate dysplasia (CIN II) to CIN III or invasive carcinoma is approximately 30% for all patients and somewhat higher (about 35%) for the 410 patients observed without biopsies. In *B*, the probability of progression is only slightly less for the patients with mild dysplasia (CIN I). Apparently, cervix biopsies had no impact on this group of women. (*A:* Redrawn from Nasiell K, et al, 1983. *B:* Redrawn from Nasiell K, et al, 1986.)

Gad (1976), in a small but important study, reported follow-up data on 13 patients with "severe dysplasia" and 17 patients with carcinoma in situ, not treated except for initial biopsy. Two of the 13 patients with severe dysplasia and 7 of the 17 patients with carcinoma in situ developed invasive cervical cancer, and 2 died of the disease.

In a study of severe dysplasia (Westergaard and Norgaard, 1981), progression to carcinoma in situ and invasive carcinoma was observed in 57% of 49 patients who underwent biopsy but were otherwise untreated, whereas no recurrent disease was observed in 38 patients treated by conization.

The results of a long-term follow-up study of a cohort of 2,279 patients with cytologic "dyskaryosis" and, hence, precursor lesions below the level of carcinoma in situ, were provided as a personal communication by David Boyes of Vancouver, British Columbia, Canada, where one of the best cervix cancer prevention programs was instituted in 1950. A spontaneous regression of the cytologic abnormalities was observed in 32% of patients. Among 1,550 patients with persisting cytologic abnormalities, 44% developed carcinoma in situ, and 5% developed invasive carcinoma of the uterine cervix.

Two other important studies were performed in the United Kingdom. In 1978, Kinlen and Spriggs could trace 52 British patients with abnormal smears who had neither a biopsy nor further treatment. After several years (mean 5.2 years), 19 patients were found to be free of lesions, 20 patients had some form of precancerous lesion ("dysplasia" or carcinoma in situ) on biopsy, 3 patients developed a microinvasive carcinoma, and 10 had fully invasive cancer. In a subsequent paper, Spriggs and Boddington (1980) reviewed the smears of 28 of these patients, 17 with regression and 11 with progression to invasive cancer. They supplemented this small series with 35 smears from untreated patients from the files of their laboratory, 25 of whom "re-

gressed" and 10 of whom "progressed" to invasive cancer. The review of the cytologic material revealed that, in patients whose lesions regressed, the dominant smear pattern was that of low-grade lesions (mild dysplasia, CIN I). Of 36 women with smear patterns suggestive of high-grade lesions (CIN II, III), 15 regressed and 21 progressed to invasive cancer. The average rate of invasive cancer in the eligible patient groups listed in Table 11-7 was 4.4%.

Additional important data on the natural history of carcinoma in situ were the result of skepticism as to the true nature of this disorder in New Zealand (Green 1969, 1970; Green and Donovan, 1970). The results of 5 to 28 years follow-up of a cohort of 948 women with biopsy-documented carcinoma in situ, but no further treatment, were described by McIndoe et al (1984). A great many of these women had a "cone biopsy" of the cervix either at the onset or during the follow-up period. The patients were divided into two groups; there were 817 patients with "normal" cytologic follow-up and 131 patients with continuing cytologic abnormalities. Twelve patients in the first group (1.5%) and 29 patients in the second group (22%) developed invasive cancer either of the cervix or of vaginal vault. Thus, diagnostic conization did not prevent the development of invasive cancer.

The unfortunate results of this study created a great deal of upheaval and led to the introduction of strict guidelines of cervix cancer detection and treatment in New Zealand (Jones, 1991).

Östör (1993) performed a meta-analysis based on a large number of follow-up papers and concluded that for CIN I, the cumulative rate of regression was 57%, rate of persistence 32%, rate of progression to CIN III was 11%, and to invasive cancer 1%. The figures for CIN II were: regression 43%, persistence 35%, progression to CIN III 22%, and to invasive cancer 5%. The figures for CIN III were: regression 32%, persistence 56%, and progression to inva-

TABLE 11-7

EARLY STUDIES ON BEHAVIOR OF PRECURSOR LESIONS FOLLOWED WITHOUT TREATMENT

Author/ year	Type of lesion	No. of pts.	Duration of follow-up	Regression	Persistence	Progression to high-grade lesions	Development of inv. ca	Comments
Varga 1966	"Dysplasia"	78	Several yrs.			39 (50%)	11 (14.1%)	
Richart 1967	"Mild dysplasia"	557	3 yrs.	33 (6%)			3 (0.5%)	Study interrupted as dangerous to patients
Fox 1968	Mild or Mod. Severe dysplasia	125 15		50 (40%) 0	51 (40%) 6	24 (20%) 9		
Hall and Walton 1968	Mild or Mod. Severe dysplasia	172 24		88 (51%) 5 19%	56 (32.5%) 11 (48%)	28 (16.5%) 8 (33%)		
Villa Santa 1971	"Dysplasia" on punch biopsy	Immed. treatment 297	2–115 months			66 (22.2%)	12 microinvasive 4 invasive (6.4%)	
		Treatment delayed 63				10 (15.8%)	3 microinvasive 10 invasive (20.6%)	
Gad 1976	Severe dysplasia	13	Variable	9	12		2 (30%)	
	Carcinoma in situ	17	Variable				7 (41.1%)	
Boyes 1978‡	"Dyskaryosis"	2,279	Variable	729 (32%)	737 (32.3%)	684 (30.0%)	83 (3.6%)	Closely surveyed population
Kinlen and Spriggs	"Dyskaryosis"	52	Mean 5.2 years	19 (36.5%) mainly low grade	20 (38.4%)		3 microinvasive 10 invasive (25%)	
Westergaard Norgaard 1981	"Severe dysplasia"	38 treated 49 untreated	Mean 47.6 months	16 (32.7%)		Microinvasive Ca included 28 (57.1%)		

* See text.
† See text for detailed analysis.
‡ Personal communication.

sive cancer about 12%. Unfortunately, in this study, as in many other studies of precursor lesions, the precise diagnoses could not be verified.

Although there are some important numerical differences among the studies cited, they all confirm the basic behavior patterns of the precursor lesions. **Regardless of grade of abnormality, these lesions may regress, remain the same, or progress to invasive cancer.** A diagrammatic summary of these events is shown in Figure 11-29. Although low-grade lesions are more likely to regress and less likely to progress to CIN III or invasive cancer than high-grade lesions, their presence puts the patients at a significant risk for

future neoplastic events, including invasive cancer. These observations are particularly pertinent because of current recommendations that allow for conservative follow-up of low-grade lesions (Kurman et al, 1994). It still remains to be documented, by a long-term prospective study, whether the presence of high-risk human papillomavirus is the main factor accounting for the behavior of precancerous lesions, as has been advocated by some observers (see above). **Conservative follow-up of precursor lesions, regardless of grade, should never be done unless the patient is fully and carefully informed about the risks and perils of this approach.**

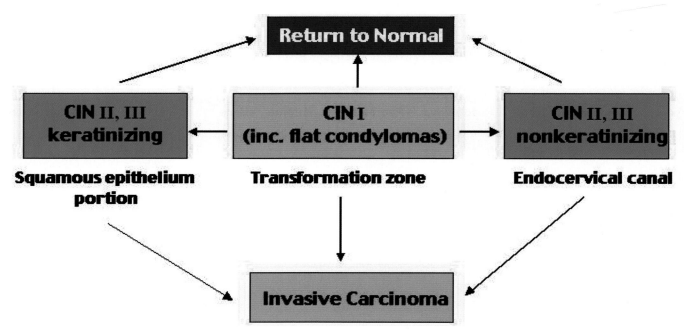

Figure 11-29 Diagrammatic presentation of the sequence of events in carcinogenesis of the uterine cervix. The diagram indicates that as the disease "progresses," adjacent segments of cervical epithelium become involved. Any one of the precancerous lesions may disappear (return to normal) or progress to invasive cancer. The latter event is more likely to occur with CIN II or III than with CIN I. CIN, cervical intraepithelial neoplasia.

THE SEARCH FOR OBJECTIVE PROGNOSTIC PARAMETERS IN PRECURSOR LESIONS

The unpredictable behavior of precursor lesions of cancer of the uterine cervix has led to a large number of studies to predict the future behavior of these lesions.

Human Papillomavirus Typing

This issue was discussed at length above in reference to human papillomavirus. Briefly, persistent infection with a high risk virus is considered a risk factor for high-grade intraepithelial lesion and, by implication, invasive cancer of the uterine cervix. The practical considerations of HPV typing will be discussed in Part 2 of this chapter.

Immunochemistry

Blood Group Antigens

Davidsohn and Kovarik (1969), using a red cell adherence test, observed that the blood group isoantigens A, B, H, present in the normal epithelia, cannot be detected in carcinomas of the uterine cervix. The loss of isoantigens was progressive from "dysplasia" to carcinoma in situ to invasive and metastatic carcinoma, as evidence of progressive tumor dedifferentiation. These results were confirmed by Bonfiglio and Feinberg (1976) but not by Lill et al (1976). Lindgren (1986), using monoclonal antibodies, observed a relationship of **blood group antigen expression** to **5 year survival and, hence, prognosis,** which was better in the antigen-positive group than in the antigen-negative group. As the interest in

the expression of blood group antigens waned, there have been no recent studies on the clinical value of this approach.

Other Antigens

With the use of cytochemical and histochemical techniques (see Chapter 45), a number of tumor markers and embryonic antigens were studied in cervical cancer and its precursors. Thus, the presence of **carcinoembryonic antigen (CEA)** and its distribution in tissue were studied, among others, by van Nagell et al (1982) and Bychkov et al (1983). The CEA was expressed by a large proportion of precancerous lesions and invasive epidermoid carcinomas and by all endocervical adenocarcinomas. **Alpha-fetoprotein (AFP)** expression was seen by Bychkov in only one case of a glassy carcinoma (see Chapter 12). **Human chorionic gonadotropin (hCG)** was not expressed by any of the precancerous lesions or carcinomas studied by Bychkov. Epithelial membrane antigen **(EMA)** is strongly expressed by abnormal squamous cells from precancerous lesions, as reported by Moncrieff et al (1984).

Oncogenes

Oncogene expression in invasive carcinoma was studied with an antibody to p21 *ras* **oncogene** product by Sagae et al (1989) and Hayashi et al (1991). The studies were of limited prognostic value. **p53 mutation** was observed as a late event in cervical cancer of no prognostic value (Bremer et al, 1995). The expression of p63 (a homologue of p53) was studied in a wide variety of cervical cancers (Wang et al, 2001). Nearly all squamous cell carcinomas were strongly positive for this protein, whereas adenocarcinomas and a subset of neuroendocrine carcinomas were negative. A number of genes involved in **apoptosis** have been studied in cervical cancer precursors and in invasive cancer but the published data are contradictory and do not appear to be of prognostic value at this time. Studies of **erB-2** expression had limited value (Hale et al, 1992). **Epidermal growth factor** expression was studied by several observers with debatable results (Berchuk et al, 1990; Chapman et al, 1992).

Loss of retinoblastoma (Rb) gene was a common event in small-cell carcinomas of cervix (Harrington et al, 1999). The finding did not correlate with type of HPV, even though the interaction of E7 protein of HPV16 with Rb gene has been repeatedly confirmed (Boyer et al, 1996; Chetty et al, 1997).

Further possibilities of molecular studies have been suggested by Chuakai et al (1999) who documented that mRNA of good quality can be extracted from cells in archival cervicovaginal smears.

DNA Synthesis and Proliferation Indices

Studies with tritiated thymidine, a labeled precursor of DNA, carried out by Moricard and Cartier (1964), pointed out that DNA synthesis in normal squamous epithelium is confined to the basal layer, whereas, in neoplastic epithelium, evidence of DNA synthesis may be found throughout the epithelial thickness. Similar studies conducted by Rubio and Lagerlöf (1974) on various precursor lesions documented that low-grade lesions showed less DNA synthesis than classic carcinoma in situ. These observations were confirmed in more recent times by other techniques. Al-Saleh et al (1995) reported that the distribution of **nuclear proliferation antigens, Ki-67,** was confined to the basal layers in normal and metaplastic epithelium. In low-grade precursor lesions, the nuclear proliferation was also seen in intermediate epithelial layers, but some overlap occurred with squamous metaplasia. In high-grade precursor lesions, however, the antigen expression could be observed throughout the epithelial thickness. The density of Ki-67 expression was higher in lesions associated with intermediate- and high-risk HPVs than in lesions associated with the low-risk HPVs, types 6 and 11. Using the **proliferating cell nuclear antigen (PCNA),** Mittal et al (1993) reported similar results.

Because HPV interferes with cell cycle (see above), Keating et al (2001) studied the expression of **cell-cycle–associated proteins** as surrogate biomarkers. **Ki67, cyclin E, p16^{INK4}** were assessed by immunochemistry. The study had for its purpose a clarification of criteria for cervical lesions ranging from metaplasia to HGSIL because of diagnostic disagreements among the participating expert pathologists. Although predictably higher staining levels were associated with HGSIL than other lesions, several of the benign lesions also had weak expressions of these proteins. In spite of an enthusiastic endorsement of these costly and cumbersome techniques by the authors of this paper, their practical value requires further studies.

Skylberg et al (2001) studied aberration of centrosomes in CIN lesions by immunofluorescence to **tubulin,** the enzyme necessary for formation of mitotic spindle. An **increased number of centrosomes** (predictive of abnormal

mitoses) was observed in LGSIL, HGSIL, and invasive cancer when compared with normal epithelium.

Predictably, **mitotic counts** also indicated that the frequency of mitoses is higher in high-grade than in low-grade lesions (Tanaka, 1986). Further, the presence of **abnormal mitotic figures** was common in lesions associated with HPV 16 (Crum et al, 1984). There is no evidence that these observations can be used for prognostic purposes.

Telomerase expression was found to be universal in neoplastic lesions but confined to the basal layers in normal epithelium (Frost et al, 2000).

Along similar lines, Williams et al (1998) used **antibodies to proteins regulating DNA replication** to recognize cancer cells in cervicovaginal smears.

DNA Quantitation

Early studies by Mellors et al (1952), Reid and Singh (1960), Atkin (1964), O. Caspersson (1964), Sandritter (1964), and others demonstrated, by microspectrophotometric methods, that many (but not all) cells derived from precursor lesions of carcinoma of the cervix show increased DNA content. Subsequently, other techniques, such as Feulgen cytophotometry and flow cytometry were used on histologic and cytologic material in the search for data of prognostic significance. The results of numerous studies were contradictory and failed to produce data of value (Brandão, 1969; Grundmann et al, 1961; Sacks et al, 1972). The likely reason for the inconsistency of the results was demonstrated by Fu et al (1981), who showed that precursor lesions could be either diploid, polyploid, or aneuploid. Fu postulated that the aneuploid lesions (regardless of grade) were more likely to persist or progress, but the significance of this observation has not been independently confirmed. Perhaps the most significant of these studies was presented by Hanselaar et al (1988), who studied DNA distribution in carcinoma in situ (CIN III) with or without adjacent invasive cancer. In this carefully constructed retrospective study in 20 patients with CIN III, adjacent to invasive cancer, both lesions had an identical DNA pattern, suggesting that the two lesions were related. In 8 patients, all younger than 35 years of age, both lesions were diploid. In 12 patients older than 50, both lesions were polyploid in two cases or aneuploid in 10 cases. Of the 19 CIN III lesions without adjacent invasive cancer 2 were diploid, 7 polyploid, and 10 aneuploid. In personal unpublished studies of precancerous lesions, all CIN I, II, III lesions had at least some cells with hyperdiploid and hypertetraploid DNA values, regardless of the type of HPV present. **The presence of HPV DNA in the nuclei of precursor lesions may have a major impact on these measurements,** as documented by Chacho et al (1990). There is no adequate evidence that **DNA ploidy measurements are of any value as a prognostic factor in precursor lesions and cancer of the uterine cervix.**

Cytogenetic Studies

Integration of HPV DNA in some precursor lesions and in most invasive cancers of the uterine cervix has led to speculations about the impact of these events on the genome of the affected cells, and specifically on chromosomal abnormalities (summary in Lazo, 1999). Yet, it has been shown many years ago by conventional cytogenetic techniques that such abnormalities may also occur in precursor lesions wherein HPV DNA is presumably not integrated into the host DNA. Spriggs et al (1962) were the first to demonstrate numerical chromosomal abnormalities and the presence of marker chromosomes in precursor lesions, observations confirmed by Boddington et al (1965), Spriggs et al (1971), Kirkland (1966, 1967), Jones et al (1968), and Granberg (1971). In general, these workers suggested that the level of abnormalities increased with the degree of morphologic abnormalities. Boddington et al (1965) stated that "extensive chromosome rearrangement takes place in precancerous epithelium, often for years before the onset of (invasive) carcinoma." Invasive cervical cancers fell into two groups: those with normal or nearly normal chromosomal component (**diploid range tumors**) and **aneuploid tumors** with increased number of chromosomes; the latter fell into the triploid-tetraploid group and tetraploid group (Wakonig-Vartaaja et al, 1965, 1971; Atkin and Baker, 1982, 1984; Atkin, 1984). It is clear that the tumors in the diploid range are not necessarily free of subtle chromosomal abnormalities that cannot be captured by the techniques used to date. Meisner (1996) used fluorescent in situ hybridization (FISH) technique for chromosomes 11 and X. Cells with an elevated number of signals (3 or higher) were observed more often in HGSIL than in LGSIL.

Recent studies, using the technique of **comparative genomic hybridization (CGH),** disclosed high levels of genomic instability and one characteristic finding, **a gain in the short arm of chromosome 3** as one of the landmarks of invasive carcinoma of the uterine cervix. This change was observed in tumors with and without documented presence of high-risk HPV DNA (Heselmeyer et al, 1996, 1997). Hidalgo et al (2000) correlated the presence of human papillomavirus type 18 with chromosomal abnormalities in 12 micro-dissected invasive carcinoma and 12 cell lines. Deletion of the short arm of chromosome 3 and gain in the long arm of the same chromosome were observed in invasive cancer. These findings were at variance with Helsemeyer's work but were confirmed by Guo et al (2001), who reported a **deletion of chromosome 3p** as the most common lesion in cervical cancer. Using the CGH technique on cells isolated from cervicovaginal smears by microdissection, Aubele et al (1998) documented the presence of abnormalities affecting from 6 to 9 different chromosomes in various forms of dysplasia. It remains to be seen whether these data are of practical value. Dellas et al (1999) studied invasive cervical carcinomas stage 1B by CGH. Deletion of the short arm of chromosome 9 ($-9p$) was associated in a statistically significant fashion with lymph node metastases. Losses of the short arm of chromosome 1 ($-11p$) and of the long arm of chromosome 18 ($-8q$) were associated with poor prognosis in the absence of metastases. This study, if confirmed, may prove to be of clinical value.

Some of the more conventional cytogenetic observations were of diagnostic significance: My co-workers, Forni and Miles (1966), **demonstrated large size and increase in number of sex chromatin in abnormal cells exfoliating from precursor lesions.** These findings were confirmed by Naujoks (1969) and Nishiya et al (1981), who correlated the increase in the number of sex chromatin bodies with increased DNA ploidy. Uyeda et al (1966) and Atkin and Brandão (1968) observed, in smears and tissues of precursor lesions, **unusually shaped nuclei with protrusions associated with very long marker chromosomes.** A similar observation was made by Brandão (1987) in koilocytosis.

Clonality Analysis

It is generally assumed that normal tissues are polyclonal (i.e., express paternal and maternal chromosomes), whereas **cancers** are derived from a single transformed cell and are, therefore, **monoclonal,** expressing only one set of genes. For the uterine cervix, it has been documented, by a variety of approaches, that most LGSIL lesions are polyclonal, whereas HGSIL, invasive cancer are, for the most part, monoclonal (Enomoto et al, 1994; Park et al, 1996; Choi et al, 1997; Guo et al, 1998). El Hamidi et al (2003) microdissected abnormal cells from archival cervicovaginal smears and correlated clonality with behavior. Monoclonal pattern was observed in all CIN III lesions and most CIN II lesions. Some CIN II lesions and all CIN I lesions were polyclonal. All patients with monoclonal pattern (and high-risk HPV) had recurrences despite treatment.

It is obvious, at the time of this writing (2004), that the search for prognostic parameters will continue and may ultimately provide us with reliable tools of clinical value.

CYTOLOGIC PATTERNS AND HISTOLOGIC CORRELATION

Some years after the introduction of cervicovaginal cytology, it became evident that morphologic features of neoplastic cells in smears could be correlated, not only with invasive cancer, but also with precursor lesions of various types, grades, and clinical significance. These observations led to a much better understanding of natural history of carcinoma of the uterine cervix, narrated in Part 1 of this chapter. The differences among cells derived from invasive cancer and from various precursor lesions are sometimes subtle but recognizable and applicable to the practice of cervical cytopathology. As discussed at length in Chapter 7, **cancer cells can be recognized by their marked nuclear abnormalities and classified according to their cytoplasmic features.** The recognition of **precursor lesions** was based on the concept of **dyskaryosis** (from Greek, *dys* = abnormal and *karion* = nucleus) introduced by Papanicolaou (1949). **Dyskaryotic cells differ from cancer cells by their well-differentiated, mature cytoplasm and lesser, although variable, levels of nuclear abnormalities.** Because dyskaryotic cells were often associated with tissue lesions classified as "dysplasia," the term **"dysplastic cells"** is now in current usage in the United States. In the United Kingdom, however, the term "dyskaryosis," classified as to degree of abnormality, is the official form of cytologic diagnosis of cervicovaginal samples. In this text, the two terms are synonymous and are used side-by-side.

The cells seen in cervical samples originate from the surface of the epithelial lesion. If the epithelial surface is composed of large, mature, albeit abnormal squamous cells, the cervical sample will contain mainly superficial or intermediate squamous cells with various levels of nuclear abnormalities. Quite often, the abnormal nuclear features of such cells can be better appreciated in the cell samples than in corresponding histologic sections. If the epithelial surface is composed of less mature, smaller cells, this will also be reflected in the cervical sample. Although, in most cervical smears and corresponding liquid preparations, the neoplastic abnormalities are reasonably well characterized and readily recognized, there are many diagnostic pitfalls that are discussed at length in this chapter. The endless variety of abnormal cytologic patterns that may be encountered is sometimes a humbling experience in terms of the observer's ability to deliver at all times a precise and final diagnostic statement on a cytologic sample.

The introduction of liquid methods of cell collection and processing has not rendered the recognition and interpretation of cell abnormalities any easier than the traditional direct smears. Testing for human papillomavirus (see Part 1 and the closing pages of this chapter) has not rendered cervicovaginal cytology obsolete.

CLASSIFICATION AND MORPHOLOGIC FEATURES OF NEOPLASTIC CELLS IN CERVICOVAGINAL SMEARS

For didactic purposes, the cell changes in cervicovaginal material may be classified into three categories with **increasing degree of abnormality:**

- **Karyomegaly:** nuclear enlargement in otherwise normal-appearing cells
- **Dysplastic (dyskaryotic) cells:** slight to marked nuclear abnormalities in well-differentiated cells, easily classified as either squamous or glandular
- **Cancer cells:** marked abnormalities of the nucleus and the cytoplasm

This subdivision is artificial inasmuch as these categories of abnormalities frequently overlap and because individual cells may defy this classification.

Nuclear Enlargement, or Karyomegaly, a Component of ASC-US

The term **karyomegaly** (from Greek, *karyon* = nucleus and *megalos* = large) was proposed by Papanicolaou (1949) to describe **enlargement of nuclei occurring in superficial, intermediate, or large parabasal squamous with morphologically normal cytoplasm,** resulting in a somewhat in-

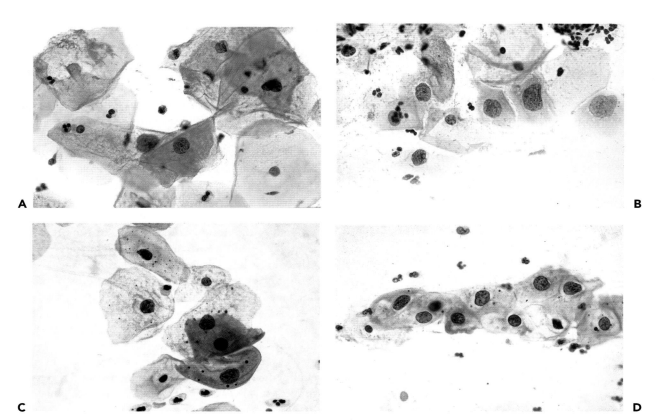

Figure 11-30 **Karyomegaly and dysplastic/dyskaryotic intermediate and parabasal squamous cells.** *A.* Karyomegaly in intermediate squamous cells with large, somewhat hyperchromatic nuclei. *B.* Karyomegaly in large parabasal cells. *C.* Dysplastic (dyskeratotic) intermediate squamous cells. Note greater nuclear hyperchromasia when compared with *A. D.* Dysplastic (dyskeratotic) large parabasal cells. Note irregular nuclear contour.

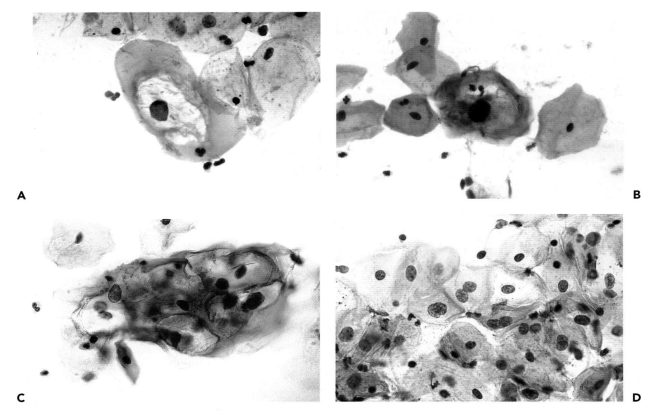

Figure 11-31   Koilocytes and pseudokoilocytes. *A.* Large squamous cell with the characteristic features of koilocytes, that is enlarged hyperchromatic nucleus and large, sharply demarcated perinuclear clear zone. *B.* Koilocyte from a liquid preparation (ThinPrep). *C.* A cluster of smaller koilocytes from another liquid preparation (SurePath). *D.* Squamous cells with cytoplasmic clearing but without nuclear abnormalities or sharply demarcated halos. These cells should not be mistaken for koilocytes.

creased nucleocytoplasmic ratio. The **cytoplasm** of the affected cells may show **normal folding or cytolysis** during the second half of the menstrual cycle (see Chapter 8). **Karyomegaly** occurring in **small parabasal squamous cells is usually accompanied by more pronounced nuclear abnormalities.** In the 2001 Bethesda System, **karyomegaly is included in the category of atypical squamous cells of unknown significance or ASC-US.**

Karyomegaly and similar abnormalities of **endocervical cells** are classified in the 2001 Bethesda System as **"atypia of glandular cells of unknown significance"** (previous **AGUS**), are discussed further on in this chapter and in Chapter 12. I have never been persuaded that karyomegaly may be observed in endometrial cells (see Chapter 13).

In karyomegaly of squamous cells, the enlarged nuclei are of normal, spherical shape with smooth nuclear membranes. The nuclei may be transparent, but are more often opaque or somewhat hyperchromatic (Fig. 11-30A,B). Karyomegaly with significant nuclear hyperchromasia blends with cell changes observed in dysplastic (dyskaryotic) cells (see below).

Karyomegaly represents an abnormality of the nuclear structure. It has been proposed that karyomegaly represents the **earliest, but reversible, nuclear change** in human papillomavirus (HPV) infection (Stoler 2003). The presence of HPV in the nuclei of karyomegalic cells may be documented by in situ hybridization.

Kurman and Solomon (1994) suggested that **nuclei enlarged "two and a half to three times"** above the size of normal nuclei of intermediate squamous cells may qualify as karyomegaly or ASC-US. This definition should not be taken as an absolute requirement because, in routine work, the sizes of the nuclei are not measured. Still, only **conspicuous nuclear enlargement** may qualify as karyomegaly. The **increase** in nuclear sizes is **best verified by comparing the nuclear size of an atypical cell with the nuclear size of adjacent normal cells. The term karyomegaly should be limited by the number of such cells in the preparation.** In our experience, a preparation containing more than 6 to 8 karyomegalic superficial or intermediate squamous cells **should be classified as low-grade squamous intraepithelial neoplasia (LGSIL).** The diagnosis of a neoplastic lesion is easier if karyomegaly is observed **in the company of other abnormal cells,** notably dysplastic (dyskaryotic) cells, particularly koilocytes (see below).

Karyomegaly must be differentiated from slight **nuclear enlargement occurring in inflammatory and regenerative processes,** described in Chapter 10. If slight nuclear enlargement **affects a large proportion of squamous cells in a smear, it is unlikely to be neoplastic and may be caused by technical problems in smear preparation or fixation, early menopause, or effects of therapy, such as radiotherapy.**

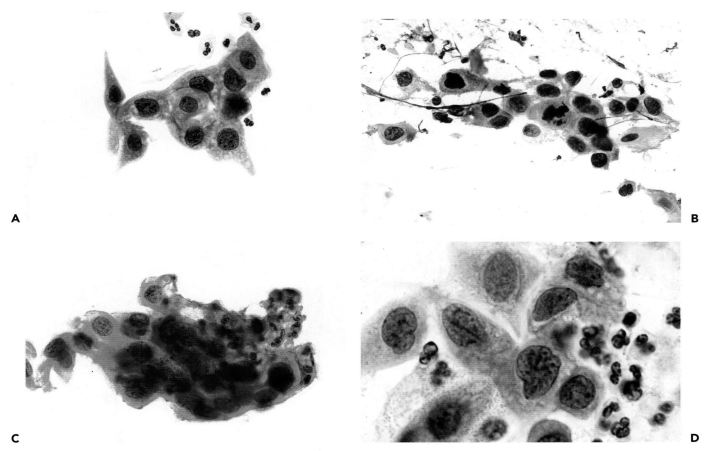

Figure 11-32 Dysplastic (dyskaryotic) parabasal squamous cells. *A.* Cohesive cell cluster mimicking metaplastic cells, except for nuclear enlargement, hyperchromasia, and irregular contours. One cell is columnar in shape. *B.* Loosely structured cluster with similar nuclear features and eosinophilic cytoplasm. *C.* Cluster of similar cells in ThinPrep. Note loss of detail in the large, hyperchromatic nuclei. *D.* Oil immersion view of nuclei of parabasal dysplastic cells to document coarse granulation of chromatin, irregular nuclear shapes, and a nuclear "crease."

Diagnostic Significance of Karyomegaly

In the past, the term **atypia** was often used to describe karyomegaly limited to a few cells. This term has been replaced in the 2001 Bethesda System by **ASC-US.** The outcome of ASC-US or karyomegaly is variable. In most cases, the abnormality is transient and will not be found in subsequent smears. Personal experience suggests, however, that **patients with "atypia" or karyomegaly are at an increased risk for future neoplastic events** (see also discussion of atypical smears later in this chapter). In some cases, colposcopy and biopsy will disclose a low-grade squamous intraepithelial lesion (LGSIL) but sometimes even a high-grade squamous neoplastic lesion (HGSIL) or, in rare cases, **invasive cancer,** as will be documented below. **Testing for human papillomavirus to triage patients with ASC-US** is described in the closing pages of this chapter. Briefly, the test has a **high negative predictive value.** Patients testing negative for the virus are not likely to develop neoplastic lesions but the fate of patients testing positive is much less secure.

Dysplastic (Dyskaryotic) Cells

Regardless of size, such cells, observed mainly in **precursor lesions of squamous carcinoma** of the uterine cervix, **are** characterized by enlargement and other nuclear abnormalities, occurring in otherwise well differentiated squamous and endocervical cells** (Figs. 11-30C,D to 11-36).

The nuclear enlargement within cells with a relatively normal cytoplasm results in an **increased nucleocytoplasmic (N/C) ratio;** this change is more readily observed in larger, rather than smaller cells. In some cells, **the nuclear enlargement is identical to that observed in karyomegaly** (see Fig. 11-30C,D).

Other nuclear abnormalities pertain to nuclear staining, texture, and configuration. The intensity of nuclear staining may vary from **relatively slight hyperchromasia** to **markedly hyperchromatic nuclei.** The nuclei may be **dark and homogenous** (see Fig. 11-32A,B) or show **an abnormal chromatin texture in the form of coarse clumping of chromatin,** commonly associated with a **thickening of the nuclear membrane** and **nuclear creases or folds** (see Fig. 11-32D). **The nuclei also display an irregular contour** in the form of **small indentations, notches or spikes,** visible under the high power of the microscope (see Fig. 11-30D). Irregularly shaped nuclei **with finger-like projections** (presumably caused by long marker chromosomes) may occur (Atkin and Brandão, 1968). Nuclear break-up or apoptosis is common (Fig. 11-

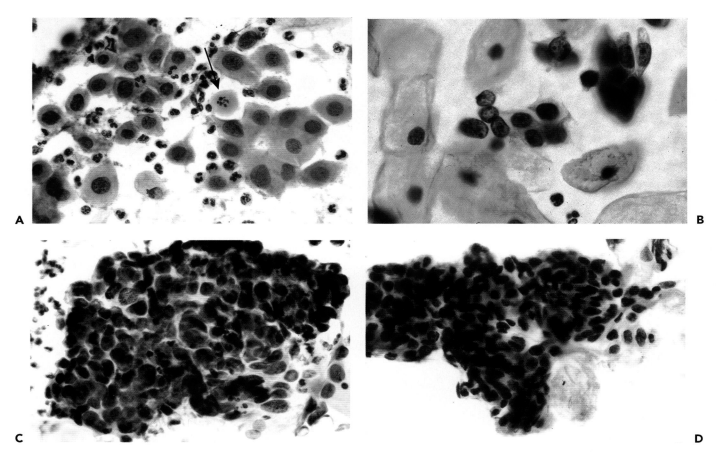

Figure 11-33 **Parabasal dysplastic (dyskaryotic) squamous cells.** *A.* Loosely structured cluster of parabasal cells with abnormal nuclei. The cytoplasm is either basophilic or eosinophilic, the latter suggestive of squamous lineage. In the center, a cell with apoptotic nucleus (*arrow*). *B.* A cluster of similar cells in SurePath. *C, D.* Thick clusters of abnormal parabasal cells in a direct smear (*C*) and in a ThinPrep (*D*). The nuclear detail is sharper in *C.* Such clusters are sometimes referred to as "syncytia," an inaccurate term (see text).

33A). **Enlarged and multiple, sometimes irregular, nucleoli may be observed, usually in cells of endocervical rather than squamous origin** (see Fig. 11-34D). **Multinucleated dysplastic (dyskaryotic) cells occur from time to time** (Fig. 11-36C). The nuclei in such cells are usually hyperchromatic but relatively small.

The presence of two or more inactivated X chromosomes **(sex chromatin or Barr bodies),** in the form of approximately triangular dense fragments of chromatin attached to the nuclear membrane, may be occasionally noted under the high power of the microscope (see Fig. 11-36D). This finding is of diagnostic value as it **indicates an abnormal chromosomal component and is therefore almost unequivocal evidence** of a neoplastic change (Forni and Miles, 1966; Nishiya et al, 1981). Barr bodies are difficult to identify in cells with coarsely clumped chromatin. For further discussion of Barr bodies, see Chapters 4, 8, 9, and 29.

In some dysplastic (dyskaryotic) cells, the nuclei show the characteristic abnormalities of nuclear contour and the presence of nucleoli, but **hyperchromasia may be absent** (see Fig. 11-34D). The term **pale dyskaryosis** describing this

phenomenon is found in the British literature (summaries in Smith and Turnbull, 1997; Coleman and Evans, 1999).

Nature of Nuclear Abnormalities

The nuclear abnormalities in dysplastic (dyskaryotic) cells are similar to those occurring in cancer cells, though less pronounced. The possible **role of E6 and E7 human papillomavirus genes in generating such changes** was discussed in Part 1 of the chapter and was recently summarized by Stoler (2003). It is, therefore, interesting to note that **similar nuclear abnormalities occur in precancerous lesions and cancer of organs other than the uterine cervix, where the role of the virus remains enigmatic or unproved.** Further, similar changes can be observed in cervical smears and tissues of mice treated with **methylcholanthrene,** a known carcinogenic agent (von Haam and Scarpelli, 1955). The mitotic inhibitor, **podophyllin,** applied to the human cervix prior to hysterectomy, results in somewhat similar abnormalities (Saphir et al, 1959; Kaminetzky and McGrew, 1961). As early as 1958, I observed cytologic abnormalities, similar to dyskaryosis, in patients treated with

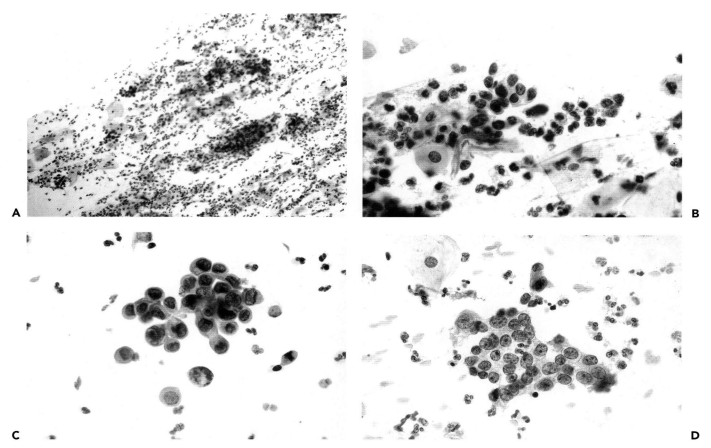

Figure 11-34   Cells from a small-cell carcinoma in situ (CIN III). *A.* An overview of a smear showing multiple clusters of small cancer cells, which may be readily overlooked on screening. *B,C.* Examples of tiny cancer cells, some showing coarse chromatin pattern and cytoplasmic vacuolization. *D.* A cluster of small cancer cells with pale nuclei and visible nucleoli (so-called pale dyskaryosis).

cytotoxic chemotherapeutic agents (for further discussion of this topic, see Chapter 18).

These data strongly suggest that dyskaryosis represents a major upheaval of the nuclear chromatin and DNA, which is either transient, perhaps because the affected cells die out, or may be the precursor of important neoplastic lesions that, in some cases, may lead to invasive cancer. Much additional research will be required to explain the nature and the unpredictable behavior of these cell abnormalities.

Classification
The squamous dysplastic cells may be classified as superficial, intermediate (usually combined in the same category), parabasal, and small parabasal or basal. This classification has diagnostic significance. The most common and important variant of intermediate dysplastic squamous cells is **koilocytosis.**

Koilocytes
As defined by Koss and Durfee in 1956, **koilocytes are mature squamous cells, usually of the intermediate type, characterized by abnormal, enlarged and hyperchromatic, single, double or, rarely, multiple nuclei surrounded by large, sharply demarcated perinuclear clear zones or halos. The nuclei are usually smudged and ho-**

mogeneous (see Fig. 11-31A,B). The clear zones are sharply demarcated at their periphery and are surrounded by a residual rim of the cytoplasm. **Koilocytes may be larger than normal superficial squamous cells and may occur singly or in clusters,** the latter particularly well seen in some types of liquid preparations (see Fig. 11-31C). **The presence of nuclear abnormalities, regardless how slight, is essential for the recognition of koilocytes.**

The koilocytes are **pathognomonic of a permissive human papillomavirus (HPV) infection.** In the nuclei of such cells, mature virions can be documented by electron microscopy (see Fig. 11-6), by reaction with broad-spectrum antibody to viral capsular proteins (see Fig. 11-9), and by in situ hybridization with DNA probes to viral DNA (see Fig. 11-10). Koilocytosis is **not HPV-type dependent,** as it may be caused by any type of HPV virus, whether "low-," or "high-" risk (see Part 1 of the chapter). Other minor cell changes, sometimes attributed to HPV infection, such as **pseudoparakeratosis** or **karyorrhexis,** are not reliable as evidence of viral presence (Tanaka et al, 1993).

Koilocytes are dead cells, victims of HPV infection. The perinuclear "cavity" represents a zone of cytoplasmic necrosis, which is demarcated at the periphery by an accumulation of residual cytoplasmic fibrils (see Fig. 11-6). Recher (1984), using scanning electron microscopy, confirmed that

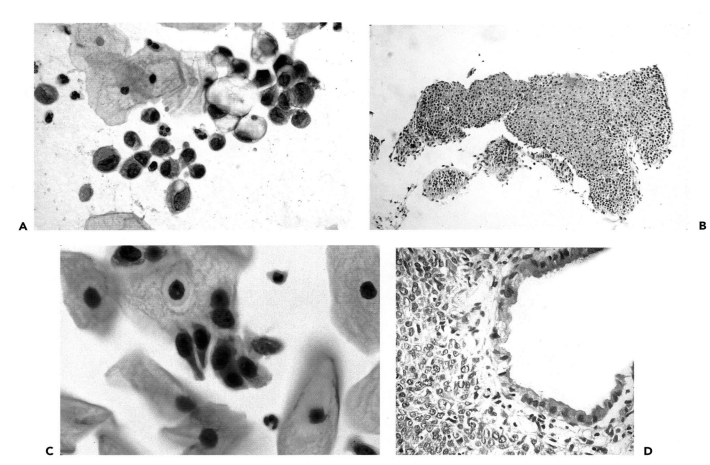

Figure 11-35 Dysplastic (dyskaryotic) squamous cells derived from the endocervical canal. *A.* A cluster of very small cancer cells with vacuolated cytoplasm, distended by mucus. This feature is characteristic of small-cell carcinomas derived from the endocervical canal, shown in *B. C.* Dysplastic endocervical cells. Note the columnar configuration and enlarged, hyperchromatic nuclei. *D.* Endocervical gland with atypical lining adjacent to a high-grade squamous intraepithelial lesion (HSIL).

the "halo" portion of koilocytes was depressed, indicating a collapse of the cytoplasmic filaments.

The **nature of the nuclear abnormalities** in koilocytes has not been conclusively settled. Lucia et al (1984) and Chacho et al (1990) reported that, in contrast to normal squamous cells, some of the nuclear DNA in koilocytes is not digestible by deoxyribonuclease (DNase, type I). In fact, Lucia et al suggested that this nuclear feature is, per se, diagnostic of HPV infection, as previously suggested by Williams (1961). These observations suggest that the **nuclear abnormalities in koilocytes may, in part, be caused by the presence of viral DNA, and in part, by repackaging of cellular DNA caused by viral infection.** Thus, **measuring the DNA content in koilocytes** and other cells infected with HPV, either by image analysis using Feulgen stain or by flow cytometry, **is most likely inaccurate.** It is unknown why some of the koilocytes are larger than normal squamous cells of similar type.

Koilocytes **must be differentiated from inflammatory cell changes,** such as seen in infection with *Trichomonas vaginalis* and occasionally other organisms, which may cause **slight nuclear abnormalities and narrow perinuclear clear zones** (see Fig. 10-16). Occasionally, intermediate squamous cells, **without obvious nuclear abnormalities,**

may display large perinuclear clear zones, similar to those seen in koilocytosis, but not as sharply demarcated at their periphery (see Fig. 11-31D). Such cells may be difficult to classify and are sometimes considered as "atypias of squamous cells of unknown significance" (ASC-US). In my experience, such cytoplasmic "atypias" have limited clinical significance and usually disappear spontaneously. **An artifact mimicking koilocytes** has been reported in ThinPrep preparations from women receiving **oral contraceptives** (Morrison et al, 2000). These authors attributed the change to pressure induced alteration of glycogen.

Diagnostic Significance. Koilocytes are seen predominantly in low-grade squamous intraepithelial lesions (LGSIL) with features of HPV infection. However, such cells **may also be observed in some high-grade squamous lesions (HGSILs) and even in invasive squamous cancers,** as documented below.

Superficial and Intermediate Dysplastic (Dyskaryotic) Squamous Cells

These cells originate in the squamous epithelium of the cervix and vagina. They **differ from koilocytes** by the **absence of the perinuclear "cavitation"** but share with them

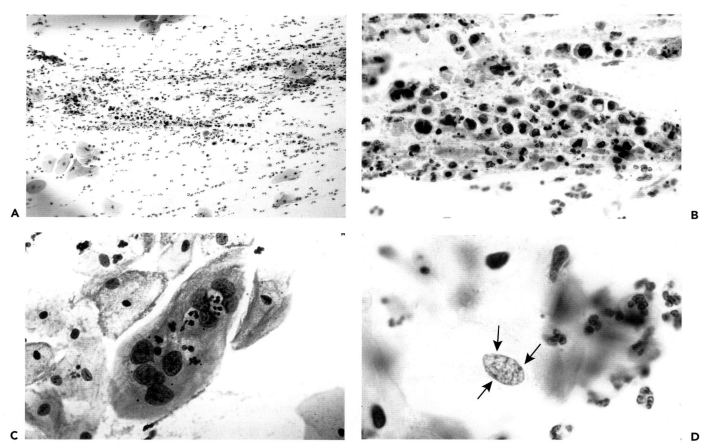

Figure 11-36   Trapping of cancer cells in streaks of endocervical mucus. *A, B.* Smear containing numerous cancer cells obtained by a scraper. Note the sheets of malignant cells. *C.* Multinucleated dysplastic (dyskaryotic) cells. Note the large size of hyperchromatic nuclei. *D.* Triple sex chromatin bodies (Barr bodies) in a high-grade cervical intraepithelial neoplasia shown under high magnification (*arrows*).

their size which is equal to, or occasionally larger than, their normal counterparts (see Fig. 11-30C). The **homogeneous cytoplasm is usually thin and transparent but may be opaque, eosinophilic, or basophilic.** In some women of childbearing age, the cytoplasm of the intermediate cells may follow cyclic changes. **The nuclei are, by definition, enlarged and may show variable degrees of abnormality, ranging from hyperchromasia to more complex abnormalities described above.**

Parabasal Dysplastic (Dyskaryotic) Cells

These **smaller squamous cells** may be derived either from the surface of lesions of squamous epithelium or from lesions mimicking squamous metaplasia, located in the endocervical canal. The cells vary in diameter from 20 to 12 μm in size and may closely resemble **normal parabasal or metaplastic squamous cells** by their configuration and the staining qualities of their relatively scanty, **basophilic or eosinophilic cytoplasm** (see Fig. 11-32). Although the basophilic cytoplasm of such cells may appear to be perfectly normal, some abnormalities of configuration, in the form of **irregular cell contour** or **molding of the cytoplasm** of adjacent cells, may be observed (see Fig. 11-32A). The cells

with eosinophilic cytoplasm resemble small squamous cancer cells (see Fig. 11-32B).

The enlarged, usually hyperchromatic nuclei of these cells show the classical marked abnormalities of nuclear size, shape, and configuration, as described above. It warrants repeating that in some cells of this type, **the chromatin may be pale and the recognition is based mainly on abnormalities of chromatin configuration, nuclear shape, and the presence of nucleoli (pale dyskaryosis)** (see Fig. 11-34D).

The parabasal dyskaryotic cells, particularly of smaller sizes, may appear **singly or in sheets and tight clusters** (see Figs. 11-32 and 11-33). In direct cervical smears, such cells may be trapped in the endocervical mucus and form **strings or files** that are extremely characteristic (see Fig. 11-36A,B). **This relationship is lost in specimens collected in liquid media. In tight clusters,** sometimes referred to as "**syncytia,**" the identity of the cells may be difficult to recognize (see Fig. 11-33C,D). The term **syncytia** is catchy but faulty, because these cells do not merge and have retained their identity. At the periphery of such clusters, the classical nuclear abnormalities may be recognized. Usually the tight clusters are accompanied by detached single dysplastic cells, which are much easier to recognize.

Small Parabasal and Basal Dysplastic Cells (Small Cancer Cells)

As a rule, these cells originate from the abnormal epithelium of the endocervical canal and **virtually always reflect the presence of an important and potentially dangerous neoplastic lesion.** The classification of these cells as either **"dysplastic cells"** or as **"small cancer cells"** is semantic and a matter of personal preference. **These diagnostically very important small cells,** about 10 to 15 μm in diameter, have clearly abnormal nuclei and very **scanty cytoplasm that is usually basophilic,** and may **form vacuoles** (see Figs. 11-34B,D, 11-35A). The cells occur **singly or form small, loosely structured clusters. Tightly knit clusters or "syncytia" may sometimes occur** (see Fig. 11-34C). The full appreciation of the **nuclear abnormalities** requires high magnification that will disclose abnormal nuclear contour and coarse granulation of the chromatin (see Fig. 11-32D).

The recognition and classification of these small cancer cells is one of the great challenges of cervical cytology, as they are one of the **main sources of false-negative diagnostic errors. The single small cells may be overlooked on screening; the clusters may be mistaken for inflammatory cells, endometrial cells, or a host of other small cells** (see Fig. 11-34A). Close attention to nuclear abnormalities is necessary to prevent errors.

Dysplastic (Dyskaryotic) Endocervical Cells

These cells originate in the epithelium of endocervical type. They are relatively **uncommon and often difficult to recognize,** particularly in thick cell clusters obtained with endocervical brushes (see Chapter 10). By definition, these are **columnar endocervical cells with enlarged nuclei that are either hyperchromatic or relatively pale,** and often contain **large nucleoli** (see Fig. 11-35C). It is a matter of semantics whether the small cancer cells with mucin-containing cytoplasmic vacuoles should also be classified as endocervical (see Fig. 11-35A), although they always originate in lesions of the endocervical canal. **Dysplastic endocervical cells** may be observed in high-grade squamous epithelial lesions (see Fig. 11-35B) or in adjacent benign, but atypical, endocervical glands (see Fig. 11-35D). This accounts for the high rate of squamous neoplastic lesions observed in smears with atypias of glandular cells (formerly AGUS; see discussion below). Similar abnormalities may also occur in the **early stages of endocervical adenocarcinoma,** discussed in Chapter 12. Occasionally, **endometrial cells may mimic endocervical cells and vice versa,** as discussed at length in Chapter 13. The diagnostic reproducibility in the morphologic recognition of these abnormalities of glandular cells is low (Simsir et al, 2003).

Benign abnormalities of endocervical cells occurring in **inflammation, pregnancy, hormone-induced changes or "repair,"** may mimic endocervical cell dyskaryosis. These benign abnormalities were discussed in Chapter 10 and will be brought up again in Chapter 12.

Diagnostic Significance of Dysplastic (Dyskaryotic) Cells

Depending on the size and type of these cells, they reflect **various types of precursor lesions and sometimes inva**sive cancer of the cervix. The correlation of cell patterns with types of lesions is discussed below.

CANCER CELLS

Cancer cells, whether derived from invasive cancer or high-grade precursor lesions, usually display significant **nuclear and cytoplasmic abnormalities.** Still, many of the cancer cells are **differentiated,** that is they retain a clear-cut tissue identity with cytoplasmic features, corresponding to either squamous or glandular epithelium. If the origin of cancer cells is not evident, the cells should be classified as **undifferentiated cancer cells.**

This **classification of cancer cells is arbitrary** and its purpose didactic. Transitional cell forms exist between dysplastic and differentiated cancer cells and between differentiated and undifferentiated cancer cells. For this reason, it is often impossible to classify accurately a single cell, nor would such a procedure be essential or desirable. As will be pointed out repeatedly, **most cytologic diagnoses are established on *patterns* of abnormal cells, rather than on single cells.**

Differentiated Cancer Cells

Cancer Cells of Squamous Origin

Squamous cancer cells are characterized by an extraordinary **variety of cell shapes** and formation of **abundant keratin.** These cells have a **characteristic bright orange, or occasionally yellow, cytoplasm that is thick and dense and lacks the transparent qualities of normal squamous or superficial dyskaryotic (dysplastic) cells** (Fig. 11-37A). This cytoplasm does not follow the cyclic changes that are sometimes observed in dyskaryotic cells. The **size of keratinized cancer cells** varies from very large, comparable with or larger than normal superficial squamous cells, to as small as small parabasal cells. Their shape varies from round or polyhedral to spindly, to irregular and bizarre. The **nuclei** of such cells are usually **hyperchromatic, coarsely granular, and of irregular shape** and frequently undergo pyknosis, giving them a dense, **"drop of India ink"** appearance. The **nuclear sizes are variable** and may vary from conspicuous enlargement to nearly normal. In some of these cells, the **nuclei may become pale** and, in final stages of keratinization, may **disappear** altogether, submerged by overgrowth of keratin. Such **anucleated squames of bizarre shapes** (see Fig. 11-37B) are diagnostically as important as the nucleated squamous cancer cells, but must be differentiated from benign squames, found in innocuous leukoplakia (see Chapter 10).

"Tadpole" cells (cells with a tail or caudate cells) are fairly uncommon cells observed mainly in **invasive squamous cancer of the cervix** and, occasionally, also in **high-grade squamous precursor lesions.** They are elongated, club-shaped cells of variable sizes, with one broad and one narrow end. The usually spherical, or somewhat irregular, hyperchromatic **single or multiple nuclei** are eccentrically

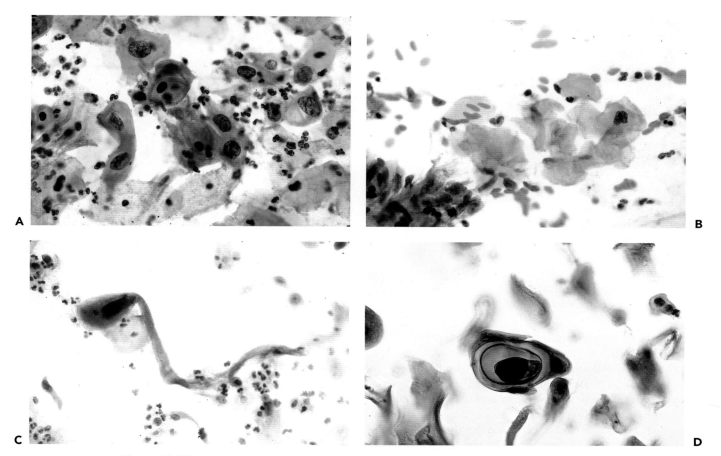

Figure 11-37 Keratinizing squamous cancer cells. *A.* Malignant squamous cells of variable sizes with large hyperchromatic nuclei. *B.* Keratinized nucleated and anucleated cells. *C.* A so-called tadpole cell with large nucleus forming the head and long, thin cytoplasmic tail. *D.* Squamous pearl wherein the component cells have large hyperchromatic nuclei.

located within the broad area of the cytoplasm (see Fig. 11-37C). The degree of cytoplasmic keratinization is variable.

Spindly squamoid cells occur most often in invasive epidermoid cancers of the cervix but may also be observed in keratinized high-grade precursor lesions. These cells are elongated and **needle-shaped** and vary in length from 10 to 40 μm (see Fig. 11-51C). Keratinization is not always evident and, thus, the cytoplasm may be either eosinophilic or basophilic. Elongated filaments **(Herzheimer's fibrils)** may be sometimes observed within the cytoplasm of spindly cells (Potter, 1978). The nuclei are nearly always elongated, hyperchromatic, and large for the size of the cell. **Nuclear abnormalities must be observed before such cells are classified as malignant, because benign spindly squamous cells, smooth muscle cells and fibroblasts, may occasionally occur in cervical smears.** The spindly squamoid cells may be the only cancer cells in cervical smears that will allow the correct cytologic classification of a poorly differentiated carcinoma as squamous or epidermoid type.

Squamous "pearls" are **concentrically arranged clusters of squamous cancer cells** that resemble similar clusters of benign squamous cells described in Chapter 10. The difference between the benign and malignant "pearls" is in the configuration of the **nuclei,** which, in the cancerous pearl, are **enlarged and hyperchromatic** (Fig. 11-37D). In

the **center** of the cancerous pearl, one may occasionally observe a **deposit of keratin** that stains orange or yellow in Papanicolaou stain. The pearls are usually observed in invasive squamous cancers but, occasionally, may be encountered in high-grade squamous precursor lesions.

Cancer Cells of Endocervical Glandular Origin

The differences between dysplastic and cancerous endocervical cells are trivial (compare Fig. 11-35 with Fig. 11-38). These cells are usually of **columnar configuration** and their basophilic cytoplasm is either homogeneous or contains one large or several smaller **cytoplasmic vacuoles,** wherein **mucin** may be demonstrated by special stains (see Fig. 11-38). As mentioned above, mucus vacuole formation may also occur in small squamous dysplastic or cancer cells of endocervical origin (see Figs. 11-34C and 11-35A). In such cells, the **nuclei** are **large** and are often **eccentric.** In larger cancer cells, **nuclear hyperchromasia** and coarsely filamentous chromatin are less frequent than in squamous cancer cells, but **large, eosinophilic nucleoli** are often present. **Nuclear pyknosis,** so characteristic of keratinized cells of squamous origin, **is generally absent. Papillary, spherical cell clusters** may occur in adenocarcinomas of the cervix (see Chap. 12).

Other glandular cancer cells in cervicovaginal material

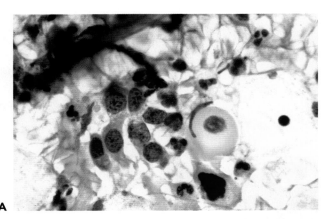 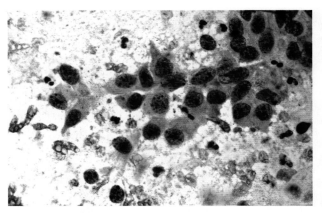

A   B

Figure 11-38 Glandular cancer cells. *A,B.* Columnar cancer cells with vacuolated cytoplasm and enlarged hyperchromatic nuclei with visible nucleoli, derived from the endocervical epithelium.

may be derived from endometrial, ovarian, or metastatic carcinomas and are described in Chapters 13, 16, and 17.

Diagnostic Significance of Differentiated Cancer Cells

Although by definition, the cancer cells should reflect the presence of an invasive carcinoma, this is not always the case. Such cells **may also occur in precursor lesions, particularly of squamous type.** It is also important to emphasize that **glandular cancer cells may be shed from squamous or epidermoid cancers of the cervix involving the endocervical canal** (see Fig. 11-35A,B) **and are, therefore, important evidence of anatomic location of the lesion.** Such cells may also be derived from **atypical, but noncancerous, endocervical glands adjacent to high-grade lesions** (see Fig. 11-35C,D). This point will be brought up again in discussing the cytologic presentation of the various forms of cervical cancer.

Undifferentiated Cancer Cells

These cells are, in a way, the embodiment of cancer and represent, in a classic fashion, the **cytoplasmic and nuclear characteristics of malignant cells.** For all practical purposes, they are always derived from invasive cancer. Their **cytoplasm,** although varying in amount, is **generally scanty,** predominantly **basophilic,** and fails to display any features that would enable one to classify the cells according to the tissue of origin (Fig. 11-39A,B). The cells may **vary in size from very small ones, about 10 μm in diameter or even less,** to occasional **gigantic multinucleated forms** (see Fig. 11-41C). Their shape varies considerably, but most of the cells are approximately spherical or oval. The **nuclei** display all the changes attributable to cancer cells, such as a relatively **large size, hyperchromasia, irregular contour, coarsely filamentous chromatin, prominent nucleoli, and frequently mitotic activity** (Fig. 11-39D). However, **large, pale, homogeneous nuclei** occur from time to time in cancer cells in **invasive squamous cancer.** There is nearly always a marked reversal of the nucleocytoplasmic ratio in favor of the nucleus. Cytoplasmic fragility and degeneration

result in cell **debris** or in isolated **"naked"** nuclei. Nuclear necrosis and karyorrhexis (apoptosis) are common.

Undifferentiated cancer cells may form **large clusters, wherein the classical features of cancer cells are absent because of poor preservation of the cells.** A careful examination of such clusters under high power of the microscope will often disclose the presence of **large nucleoli within the poorly preserved, often pale, large nuclei.** In such cases, it is highly advisable to **search for single cancer cells with more classical features.** Undifferentiated cancer cells are usually accompanied by debris, fresh and lysed or fibrinated blood, and leukocytes—all constituting evidence of necrosis and inflammation accompanying advancing or advanced cancer, and sometimes referred to as **"cancer diathesis."**

IMPACT OF COLLECTION OF CERVICAL SAMPLES IN LIQUID MEDIA ON MORPHOLOGY OF CELLS

The basis of a correct cytologic diagnosis of neoplastic abnormalities of the epithelium of the uterine cervix is the assessment of the relationship of various types of abnormal cells to each other. **At all times, the pattern of abnormalities is more significant than abnormalities of individual cells** and a careful **synthesis of the cytologic evidence** is required before a diagnosis can be rendered. Unfortunately, with the use of **liquid media** for collection of cell samples and automated processing, the **pattern of lesions, seen in direct smears, particularly the entrapment of abnormal cells in the endocervical mucus** (see Fig. 11-36A,B), **is lost and the diagnosis must be based on assessment of individual cells or cell clusters.** This disadvantage is compensated by **reduction or absence of obscuring blood and inflammatory debris.** In our experience with the **SurePath** (TriPathology Imaging, Inc., Burlington, NC), **the quality of the preparations, the distribution and dispersion of cells, and the morphologic details of normal and abnormal cells are outstanding and comparable to routine smears** (see Figs. 11-31C and 11-35C). **In the ThinPrep**

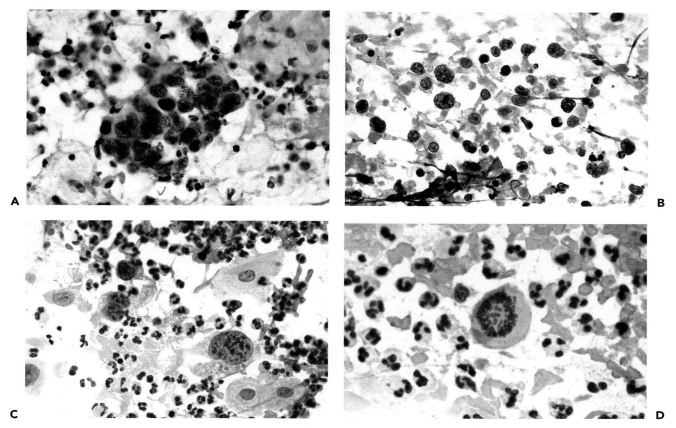

Figure 11-39   Undifferentiated cancer cells. *A.* A thick cluster of cancer cells derived from an invasive cancer. *B.* Dispersed stripped nuclei of cancer cells of variable sizes. *C.* A very large single cancer cell. *D.* High magnification showing an abnormal mitotic figure in a malignant cell.

System (Cytyc Corporation, Boxborough, MA), **the cell distribution is sometimes uneven, there is some shrinkage of cells, and the crispness of the nuclear structure is not as sharp as in routine smears** (see Figs. 11-32C and 11-33D). The ThinPrep System requires considerable training and experience in the interpretation of these preparations.

Incidentally, one of the much touted advantages of liquid preparations, namely the spread of cells as a **monolayer, is not correct. Often, thick clusters of cells obtained by brushing (including endocervical, endometrial, dysplastic, or cancer cells), are not dispersed and are in a different plane of vision than the single cells forming the background** (see Figs. 11-31C, 11-32C, and 11-33D). The results reported with the liquid systems are discussed in the closing pages of this chapter.

CORRELATION OF CYTOLOGIC AND HISTOLOGIC PATTERNS OF SQUAMOUS PRECURSOR LESIONS OF THE UTERINE CERVIX

One of the important features of cervicovaginal cytology is that the **type of abnormal cells and the degree of cell-** **and nuclear abnormalities may be reasonably correlated with the type of lesion present in the uterine cervix.** As discussed in the opening pages of this chapter, **the smears reflect the degree of maturation of the epithelium of origin.** Thus, **the presence of large, superficial dysplastic (dyskaryotic) squamous cells, particularly koilocytes, suggests a lesion with a mature surface, which, in most cases, is a low-grade squamous intraepithelial lesion (LGSIL). The presence of smaller dysplastic (dyskaryotic) squamous (or sometimes glandular) cells will reflect a lesion with a surface composed of immature smaller cells and, hence, a high-grade lesion (HGSIL), often located within the endocervical canal. Although cells showing the highest degree of nuclear and cytoplasmic abnormality and classified as cancer cells are observed mainly in invasive cancer, they may also occur in high-grade precursor lesions. The border between smaller dysplastic (dyskaryotic) cells and cancer cells is often blurred and the designation of these cells in either category depends on the preference of the observer.**

The relationship of various cell types and the corresponding histologic lesions is illustrated in a diagram, in which the proportions of dysplastic (dyskaryotic) cells of various types and cancer cells in a cervical sample are plotted against the degree of tissue abnormality (Fig. 11-40). Borrowing

Cytologic Diagnosis of Epidermoid Cancer and Related Lesions

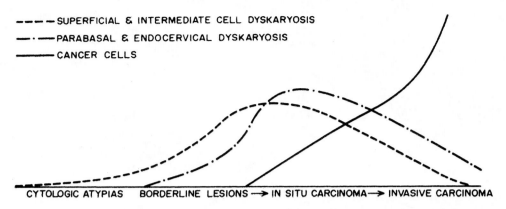

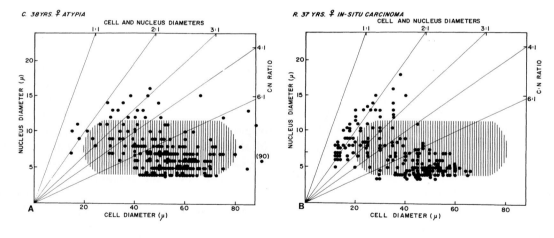

Figure 11-40 A diagrammatic and greatly simplified representation of the interrelation of types of abnormal cells in various lesions of the epithelium of the uterine cervix. This diagram has no bearing on the number of abnormal cells present, which is largely dependent on the techniques used. Some emphasis has been put on the fact that the patterns of some of the low-grade borderline lesions and of carcinomas in situ may overlap. The same is true of some in situ and early invasive cancers.

an expression from the field of hematology, the increase in the less mature dysplastic (dyskaryotic) cells and cancer cells represents a "shift to the left," corresponding to the increasing degree of abnormality in histologic preparations. This is also illustrated in a series of diagrams representing the distribution patterns of various types of abnormal cells in

the lesions of the epithelium of the cervix. There is an increase in small cells and in the nucleocytoplasmic ratio in high-grade squamous intraepithelial lesions, carcinoma in situ (HGSIL), and invasive cancer when compared with the patterns of a low-grade lesion (Fig. 11-41). Supporting evidence for this concept was provided by Reagan et al

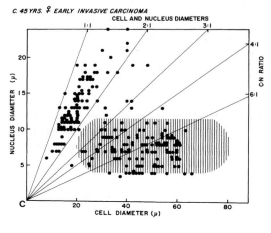

Figure 11-41 Diagrams demonstrating the differences in the sizes of abnormal cells in a case of borderline atypia (low-grade lesion) (*A*); a case of carcinoma in situ (*B*); and a case of invasive carcinoma (*C*). The oval shaded area in the center represents the field of distribution of normal cells. Note the gradual shift of abnormal cells toward the left side of the diagram corresponding to a gradually diminishing cytoplasmic : nuclear ratio. The very large cells in the right field of *A* represent superficial cell dyskaryosis, which may sometimes be associated with cellular enlargement. (From Koss LG, Durfee GR. Unusual patterns of squamous epithelium of uterine cervix; cytologic and pathologic study of koilocytotic atypia. Ann NY Acad Sci 63:1245–1261, 1956. Diagrams prepared by Airborne Instruments Laboratories, Mineola, NY.)

TABLE 11-8

MEASUREMENTS OF CELL AREA

	Normal	Dysplasia	In Situ Cancer	Invasive Cancer
Cases	50	100	100	100
Total cells measured	2,500	5,000	10,000	5,000
Cell				
Diameter in μm	44.93 $\pm$ 4.28	36.81 $\pm$ 5.59	20.85 $\pm$ 3.16	16.85 $\pm$ 2.94
Area in μm^2	1,604.15 $\pm$ 312.35	1,087.59 $\pm$ 311.00	352.51 $\pm$ 115.78	229.49 $\pm$ 82.81
Nucleus				
Diameter in μm	6.75 $\pm$ 1.20	14.52 $\pm$ 1.57	11.67 $\pm$ 1.652	9.78 $\pm$ 1.59
Area in μm^2	36.51 $\pm$ 13.31	167.20 $\pm$ 38.20	109.38 $\pm$ 33.04	77.04 $\pm$ 26.57
Relative nuclear area*	2.32% $\pm$ 84	16.45% $\pm$ 4.35	31.96% $\pm$ 6.040	34.44% $\pm$ 6.77

* All areas represent means/case and were computed on the basis of measured dimensions except for invasive cancer, which is based on planimetry. See legend to Table 11-9.

(1952, 1957) who, using **planimetry,** calculated the **nuclear and cellular diameters** of abnormal cells in low-grade lesions (dysplasia), high-grade lesions (represented by carcinomas in situ), and invasive carcinomas of the uterine cervix. **A gradual decrease in cell size with a synchronous increase in the nucleocytoplasmic ratio and the occurrence of aberrant cell types were recorded with increasing severity of the tissue lesions** (Tables 11-8 and 11-9). Figure 11-42 illustrates the distribution of abnormal cell types in squamous precursor lesions of the uterine cervix according to the epithelium of origin.

Johannisson et al (1966) **documented that the number and type of abnormal cells in a cervical scrape smear could be correlated with size and type of lesion,** confirming a common experience of cytopathologists, namely that a well-taken smear showing a small number of abnormal cells, usually corresponds to a small lesion, whereas a smear with a large number of abnormal cells usually indicates a lesion of large size. The cytologic recognition of various types of precancerous intraepithelial lesions is discussed below.

It must be stressed that, quite often, the correlation of the cytologic and histologic patterns of lesions is far from perfect. Knowledge of such pitfalls is important as it may prevent errors of interpretation.

Protruding Papillary Squamous Lesions of the Cervix

Condylomata Acuminata ("Condylomas")

The natural history of *condylomata acuminata,* or venereal warts, occurring on external genitalia, was discussed in Part 1 of the chapter in conjunction with the role of human papillomavirus (HPV) in the genesis of these lesions. **Large condylomas,** visible with the naked eye and similar to those observed on the external genitalia, are **uncommon on the**

TABLE 11-9

CELL CONFIGURATION*

	Normal (%)	Dysplasia (%)	In Situ Cancer (%)	Invasive Cancer (%)
Number of cells	11,000	5,000	10,000	10,000
Type of cell				
Polyhedral	94.81	52.68	8.19	2.05
Round	.95	20.58	52.63	45.98
Oval	2.81	21.02	31.41	30.53
Ellipsoidal	1.21	4.00	1.67	.54
Irregular	.21	.20	4.08	5.17
Elongate	.01	1.50	1.76	15.08
Tadpole	.00	.02	.26	.65
Isodiametric	95.76	73.26	60.82	48.03
Nonisodiametric	4.24	26.74	39.18	51.97

* Tables 11-8 and 11-9 indicate the variation of cell characteristics in normal cervix, dysplasia (synonymous with low-grade lesions as used in the present work), and in situ and invasive carcinoma of the cervix. Note the increase in the relative nuclear area and the increase in irregular cell shapes as the lesions progress to invasive carcinoma.
(Reagan JW, Hamonic MJ, and Wentz WB. Analytical study of the cells in cervical squamous-cell cancer. Lab Invest 6:241–250, 1957.)

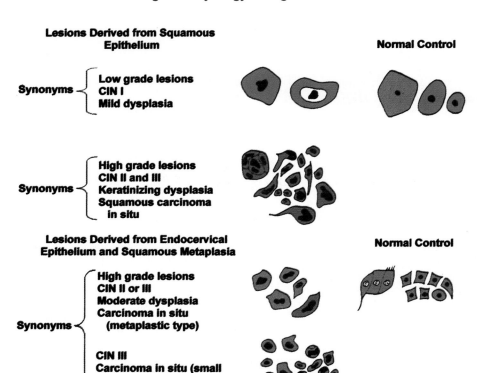

Figure 11-42 Diagrammatic representation of principal cell types occurring in squamous intraepithelial precursor lesions of the uterine cervix (SIL). The lesions were classified according to epithelium of origin as low-grade (LGSIL) and high-grade (HGSIL). The cell types in the drawing follow the text. Normal controls are on right. Top row: superficial dysplastic (dyskaryotic) squamous cells and koilocytes. Second row: keratin-forming dysplastic (dyskaryotic) or cancer cells. Third and fourth rows: dysplastic (dyskaryotic) or cancer cells of medium and small sizes.

uterine cervix and rarely require a cytologic diagnosis. Still, occasionally, cytologic samples are obtained. **The cytologic presentation of these lesions differs from the more common, flat lesions.** I have observed several such cases in young women.

Histology

The lesions in their classic form are composed of a central stalk of connective tissue lined by thick squamous epithelium arranged in numerous papillary folds (Fig. 11-43A). Toward the surface, the epithelium is characterized by the presence of koilocytes, in the form of cells with enlarged single or double hyperchromatic nuclei, surrounded by a clear perinuclear zone (Fig. 11-43B). Mitotic activity may be intense. A few layers of small, keratinized cells are commonly seen on the surface of these lesions. The **presence of HPV** may be documented in the nuclei of koilocytes by the use of the common HPV capsular antigen (see Fig. 11-9A) or by in situ hybridization with specific HPV type DNA (see Fig. 11-9B). In the perirectal condylomas studied by us, the dominant HPV types were **6 or 11** but, occasionally, **types 16 or 18** have been observed (Vallejos et al, 1987).

The studies of patterns of distribution of glucose-6-phosphate dehydrogenase suggest multicellular origin of these lesions, contrary to monocellular (clonal) origin of cervix cancer (Friedman and Fialkow, 1976). Jagella and Stegner (1974) studied **DNA distribution** in 50 condylomas and found aneuploid DNA values in several such lesions. Other observers claimed that the DNA content of condylomas is "polyploid." In our own studies, virtually all such lesions had an abnormal, aneuploid DNA pattern (Vallejos et al, 1987).

Cytology

The **cytologic presentation** of large cervical condylomata in direct smears may be alarming. Besides cells showing moderate levels of nuclear atypia, the lesions may shed **large, highly abnormal squamous cells,** showing **marked nuclear enlargement and hyperchromasia** (Fig. 11-43C,D). Occasionally, concentric arrangement of squamous cells or **"squamous pearls"** may be noted. Sheets of **small, spindly squamous cells with hyperchromatic nuclei,** derived from the surface of the lesions, may also occur. Classical **koilocytes,** with large hyperchromatic, sometimes smudged, single or double nuclei, are usually present but **rarely constitute the majority population in the wart-like lesions.**

Clinical Significance

The clinical significance of the protruding, wart-like lesions of the cervix **is somewhat obscure. At least some of these lesions may recur after treatment and may be accompanied or followed by flat precursor lesions (CIN) or even invasive cancer, justifying their inclusion among precancerous lesions.** The **practical conclusions** based on these considerations suggest that the cytologic abnormalities caused by *condylomata acuminata* must receive the same clinical attention as other precancerous lesions of the uterine cervix. Prudence suggests that these patients should have the benefit of a colposcopic examination of the cervix and of the vagina. **All persisting lesions are deserving of biopsy and further treatment must depend on the histologic findings.**

Solitary Squamous Papilloma

It is not known whether **the rare solitary squamous papillomas of the cervix,** occurring mainly in patients below

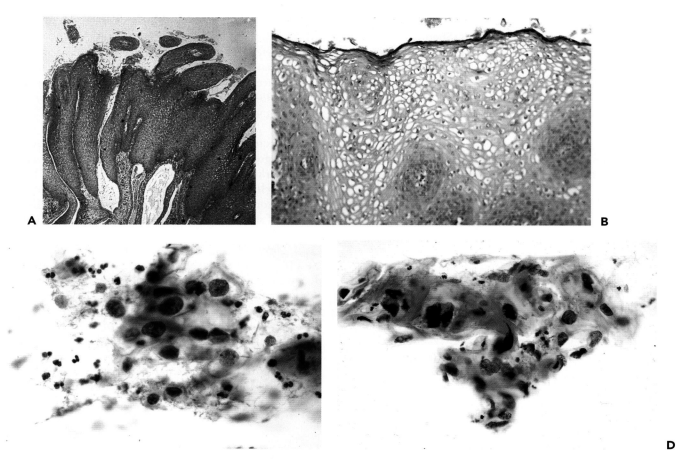

Figure 11-43 **Condyloma of cervix.** *A.* The characteristic surface of a condylomatous lesion with clogs of keratin on the surface. *B.* Surface epithelium of a condyloma showing marked koilocytosis. *C, D.* Cytology of a condylomatous lesion in a 17-year-old woman. Note the marked nuclear abnormalities and the presence of koilocytes.

the age of 40, are related to *condylomata acuminata* or constitute a distinct and different lesion. Histologically, solitary squamous papillomas of the cervix are structurally similar to a *condylomata acuminata,* but the surface squamous epithelium shows only slight deviation from normal (Kazol and Long, 1958). Koilocytes are absent. Because of the rarity of these lesions, their relationship to HPV is unknown. However, unless widely excised, these lesions have a tendency to recur, and at least some of them are ultimately capable of invasive growth. A case of this type was reported by Marsh (1952). Goforth (1952) reported two such cases with adjacent carcinoma in situ. I have also observed a few such cases, **followed many years later by invasive squamous cancer.** Squamous papillomas should not be confused with **papillary (warty) and verrucous squamous carcinomas of the cervix,** discussed below, and similar lesions of the vagina, discussed in Chapter 14.

FLAT PRECURSOR LESIONS

Low-Grade Squamous Intraepithelial Lesions (LGSILs)

Synonyms: **mild dysplasia, cervical intraepithelial neoplasia (CIN), grade I (with or without features of human papillomavirus infection), "flat condylomas."**

Histology

As briefly discussed in Part 1 of the chapter, the low-grade precancerous lesions of the uterine cervix occur **mainly on the squamous epithelium of the transformation zone and in the adjacent squamous epithelium of the outer (vaginal) aspect of the uterine cervix.** These lesions are characterized by a relatively slight disturbance of the structure and maturation of the squamous epithelium. The squamous epithelium can be of **normal thickness** (Fig. 11-44B) **or thickened,** the latter feature being most conspicuous in the so-called "flat condyloma" variant of the lesion (see Fig. 11-45B,D). **These lesions may extend to adjacent endocervical glands in the transformation zone and to the epithelium of the vagina. Nuclear abnormalities in the form of nuclear enlargement and hyperchromasia** may be scattered throughout all layers of the epithelium, but are often **most conspicuous in the upper one-third,** particularly in the presence of koilocytes. The **surface** of many of these lesions shows a few layers of **small keratinized cells, so-called "dyskeratocytes"** (Meisels, 1984). **Mitotic activity** is commonly present in the lower one-third, occasionally extending to the middle, very rarely to upper layers of the epithelium. Abnormal mitoses may occur. As has been discussed above, **all types of HPV** may be associated with these lesions (see Table 11-4). Hence, HPV typing as an adjunct to cytology that has been proposed as an "objective" system of classification of these lesions (Sherman et al, 1994) should be applied with caution, if at all, in this group of patients, particularly if they are less than 30 years of age. For further discussion of HPV typing as an adjunct to cytology, see Part 1 of the chapter and further comments below.

The **most common error** in the histologic diagnosis of these lesions is **normal squamous epithelium rich in glycogen,** wherein normal intermediate and superficial squamous cells may show large clear cytoplasm, **mistaken for koilocytes. Such epithelia do not show nuclear abnormalities, an essential feature of low-grade lesions.** Pirog et al (2002) proposed that positive immunostaining for a marker for cell proliferation (**MIB antibody**) is helpful in separating the normal from abnormal epithelia.

Cytology

The **background of the smears** is often clear and free of inflammation. Corresponding to the histologic picture, the **dominant abnormal cells in the cervical smears, derived from the relatively mature surface of the epithelial lesion, belong to the category of superficial and intermediate dysplastic (dyskaryotic) cells** (Figs. 11-44A,C and 11-45C). **Koilocytes, singly and in clusters,** occur in a great many of these cases, confirming the close relationship of

the low-grade lesions with permissive HPV infection (Fig. 11-45A,B). Some observers proposed that, in the presence of koilocytes, it is possible to establish a diagnosis of **human papillomavirus infection,** suggestive of viral presence in the absence of histologic abnormalities. As shown by Abadi et al (1998), this is not the case and the cytologic or histologic diagnosis of "human papillomavirus infection" is not helpful.

Also commonly observed in such smears are **clusters or dense aggregates of small, usually spindly squamous cells with markedly eosinophilic cytoplasm and small, pyknotic nuclei, "so-called" dyskeratocytes** (Fig. 11-46A,C), derived from the surface of the epithelium (Fig. 11-46B,C). **Sheets of such cells** may be observed in liquid preparations from LGSIL.

In samples from some low-grade lesions, the **superficial and intermediate dysplastic (dyskaryotic) cells and koilocytes** are accompanied by **smaller, parabasal dysplastic (dyskaryotic) squamous cells** (see Fig. 11-32A,B). The classification of the material as to low- or high-grade squamous lesions depends on the **proportion of the smaller cells.** If only a few smaller dysplastic (dyskaryotic) cells are present, the lesion should still be judged to be low-grade. If the **population of the smaller dyskaryotic cells is 10% or more of the abnormal cells, it becomes likely that the**

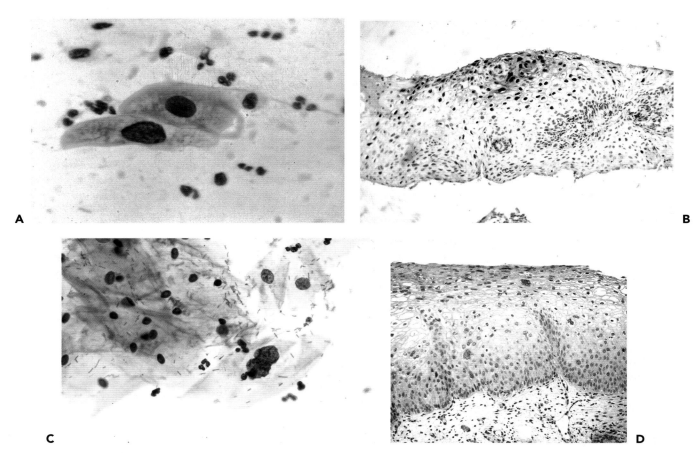

A   **B**   **C**   **D**

Figure 11-44   Low-grade squamous intraepithelial lesions (LGSILs). *A.* Large intermediate dyskaryotic cells corresponding to biopsy shown in *B. B.* In situ hybridization of the biopsy with HPV 16. Note the dark nuclei showing evidence of HPV in the upper regions of the epithelium. *C.* A multinucleated dyskaryotic cell corresponding to low-grade CIN shown in *D.* Similar multinucleated cells may be observed in the epithelium.

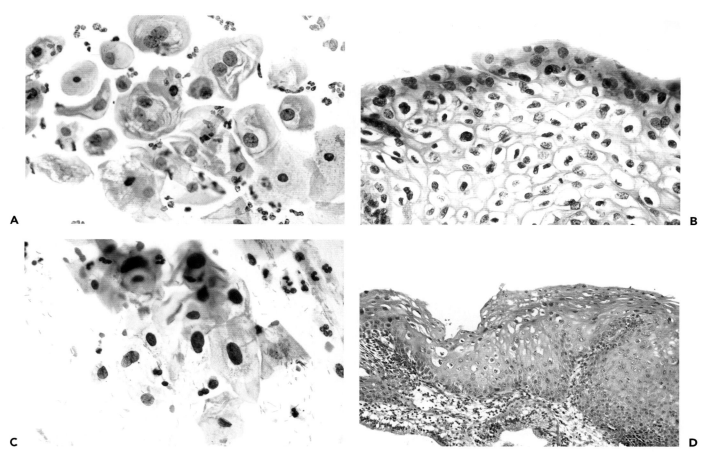

Figure 11-45 **Low-grade squamous intraepithelial lesions with koilocytes.** *A.* Numerous koilocytes in one field of a cervical smear corresponding to the tissue biopsy shown in *B. B.* A low-grade intraepithelial lesion with koilocytes. *C.* A cluster of large dysplastic intermediate squamous cells corresponding to the tissue biopsy shown in *D. D.* A low-grade lesion that extended into the endocervical glands.

low-grade lesion is accompanied by a high-grade lesion in the adjacent epithelium. In some liquid preparations, the two populations of cells can be better visualized than in conventional smears.

While koilocytes characteristically occur in low-grade lesions, they may also be found in smears of keratinized carcinoma in situ (keratinizing dysplasia) and, occasionally, in invasive squamous cancer. Thus, Allerding (1985) observed koilocytes in 25% of earlier smears of patients with biopsy-documented carcinoma in situ. **Further, koilocytes derived from a low-grade lesion may obscure the presence of high-grade lesions (HGSIL) located in an adjacent epithelial segment.** These views received strong support in an analysis of koilocytotic atypia by Lee et al (1997). **In some patients, koilocytosis may precede a high-grade lesion, or even invasive cancer, by several years** (Fig. 11-47).

Superficial dysplastic cells may also occur in or precede high-grade lesions. In the example shown in Figure 11-48A,B, superficial dysplastic (dyskaryotic) cells corresponded to a **two-tier neoplastic lesion,** with the bottom part of the epithelium formed by a high-grade lesion. In the case illustrated in Figure 11-48C,D, scanty superficial cell dysplasia (dyskaryosis) corresponded to a high-grade lesion in the biopsy.

Clinical Significance

As has been repeatedly emphasized in Part 1 of the chapter and above, the behavior of the low-grade lesions is unpredictable. Many of these lesions **disappear** spontaneously or after a biopsy (Fig. 11-49) but may also persist or progress. There is evidence that some **LGSILs are extremely fragile and, therefore, susceptible to minimal therapeutic handling, perhaps even to cytologic sampling.** However, **neither cytologic nor the histologic patterns of abnormality permit prognostication in any individual case; hence, the patients must have long-term follow-up, as they are prime candidates for further abnormalities.**

Kurman et al (1994) recommended that patients with LGSIL should either have the benefit of a colposcopic examination or close cytologic surveillance. If the latter is chosen, experience has shown that at least 3 years of completely negative cytologic follow-up is necessary before the patient may be declared to be free of disease (Koss et al, 1963).

HPV typing, discussed in the closing pages of this chapter, is, at the time of this writing (2004), the most widely used prognostic test, which, unfortunately, is not reliable in women below the age of 30 in whom LGSIL is most often observed. Still, Matsuura et al (1998) claimed that disappearance vs. persistence and progression of LGSIL cor-

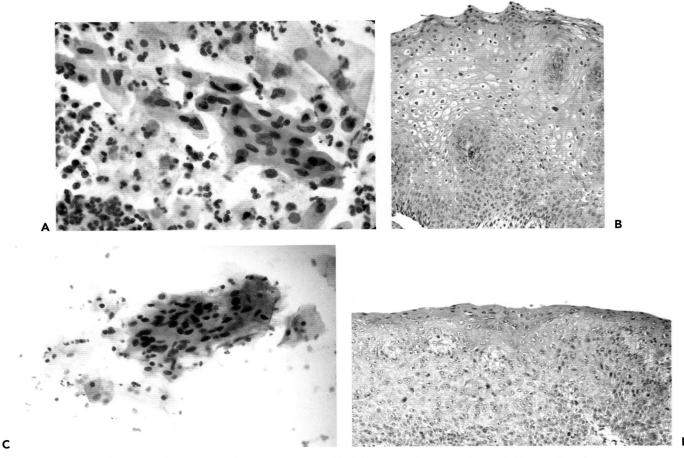

Figure 11-46   Low-grade squamous intraepithelial lesions with dyskeratocytes. *A.* Cluster of keratinizing superficial cells, commonly observed in, but not diagnostic of, low-grade lesion shown in *B. B* shows a low-grade squamous intraepithelial lesion with koilocytes. Note the keratinized cells on the surface. *C.* A small cluster of densely packed, small squamous cells described by Meisels as "dyskeratocytes." *D.* A low-grade lesion with koilocytes showing surface keratinization corresponding to *C.*

related with the presence or absence of HPV. Molecular and genetic approaches so far failed to establish a reliable and simple set of parameters applicable to routine cytologic or histologic samples. In an elaborate recent study, Kruse et al (2004) reported that lesions with a high level of expression of proliferation antigen Ki67 were more likely to progress than lesions with low values.

High-Grade Squamous Intraepithelial Lesions (HGSILs)

Synonyms: **moderate dysplasia, marked (severe) dysplasia, carcinoma in situ, cervical intraepithelial neoplasia (CIN) grades II, III, "atypical condylomas."**

High-grade squamous intraepithelial lesions show **a variety of histologic and cytologic patterns that may cause diagnostic controversy, even among competent observers.** One of the benefits of the Bethesda System was the introduction of a **binary system of classification** of the precancerous lesions of the cervix (low- and high-grade), replacing three or even four subdivisions that were not reproducible.

The easiest to define is a lesion with severe abnormalities throughout the epithelial thickness, known as **carcinoma in situ.** This writer has searched in vain for an objective and reproducible definition of the term **moderate dyspla-**

sia, orCIN II, which some observers include with low-grade and some with high-grade lesions. It is obviously a subjective diagnosis that may depend, to a large extent, on the training and experience of the pathologist. A number of lesions with moderate nuclear changes and some surface differentiation of the neoplastic epithelium, some illustrated in this chapter, could be so classified. For example, low-grade lesions shown in Figures 11-44D and 11-45D could be reclassified as CIN II or moderate dysplasia. Keratin-forming high-grade lesions (see Fig. 11-47D) could also be classified as CIN II, so could the lesions shown in Figures 11-48D and 11-52D. The significance of this lesion is illustrated in Figure 11-56, showing its transition into invasive cancer. Hence, the precise cytologic or histologic definition of the lesion is of limited value, **so long as the lesion is recognized** and included in the group of precancerous lesions, requiring further investigation and treatment. Regardless of morphology, nearly all lesions belonging to the HGSIL group harbor persisting infection with a high risk human papillomavirus (see Table 11-2).

There are very few cases of a high-grade lesion that have an identical histologic or cytologic presentation. However, **the population of abnormal cells in individual cases is**

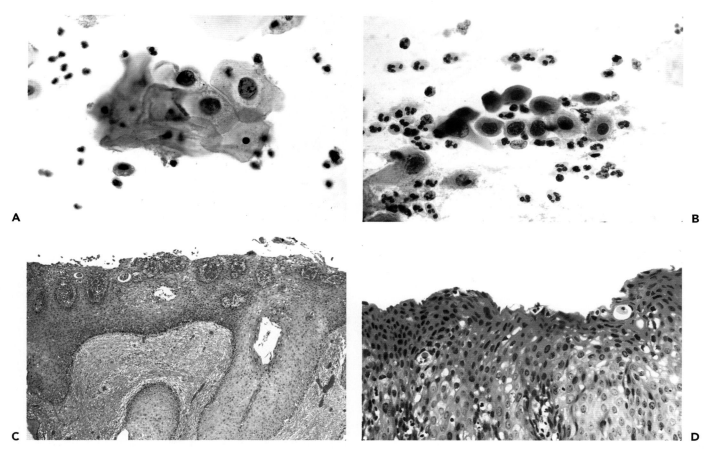

Figure 11-47 Dysplastic (dyskaryotic) intermediate squamous cells with halos (koilocytes), corresponding to a high-grade lesion observed 4 years later. *A.* Dyskaryosis of intermediate cells. *B.* Small cancer cells observed on a smear obtained 4 years later. *C.* Tissue biopsy obtained after the second smear shows carcinoma in situ (CIN III) with extension to endocervical glands. *D.* Shows details of the surface of the lesion.

often remarkably uniform. Marked variability of cell configuration is more consistent with invasive cancer.

For didactic purposes, the high-grade lesions may be divided into three principal morphologic groups, illustrated in Figure 11-16:

- **Keratin-forming lesions** derived from and retaining the characteristics of squamous epithelium
- **Lesions derived from endocervical epithelium,** often retaining features of squamous metaplasia
- **Lesions derived from reserve cells,** usually of endocervical origin, characterized by small cancer cells, sometimes with endocrine features

These subtypes of high-grade lesions are not necessarily homogeneous and oftentimes **several patterns may be observed side by side within the same cervix.** However, this **classification is reproducible, to a significant extent, in cervical smears and it does provide guidance to the location of the lesion,** either on the uterine portio or in the endocervical canal.

High-Grade Keratinizing Squamous Intraepithelial Lesions

Synonyms: **keratin-forming carcinoma in situ, keratinizing or pleomorphic dysplasia, moderate dysplasia, severe dysplasia, CIN grade II or III.**

As may be seen from the number of synonyms, this is a group of lesions that presents considerable difficulties in diagnosis and classification. The lesions are **located primarily on the squamous epithelium of the portio of the cervix and occasionally have a keratinized surface and, hence, may clinically resemble benign leukoplakia.** These lesions are sometimes "warty" and may resemble squamous papilloma. An association of these lesions with condylomas was reported by McLachlin et al (1995). Transitions between low- and high-grade keratinizing lesions may also be observed (Fig. 11-50B).

Most high-grade lesions of this type represent a **transformation of low-grade squamous intraepithelial lesions** and are precursor lesions of well differentiated, keratinized invasive cancer of the cervix or vagina. It cannot be ruled out, however, that some of these lesions may develop de novo in squamous epithelium. Although, to my knowledge, no statistical evaluation of the frequency of these lesions has been performed, it has been my experience that these lesions have become much less common in the United States in recent years, possibly as a consequence of detection and treatment of low-grade lesions. The keratinizing precursor lesions of the uterine cervix and the corresponding well-differentiated invasive squamous cancer are still common in countries without an effective cancer-detection program.

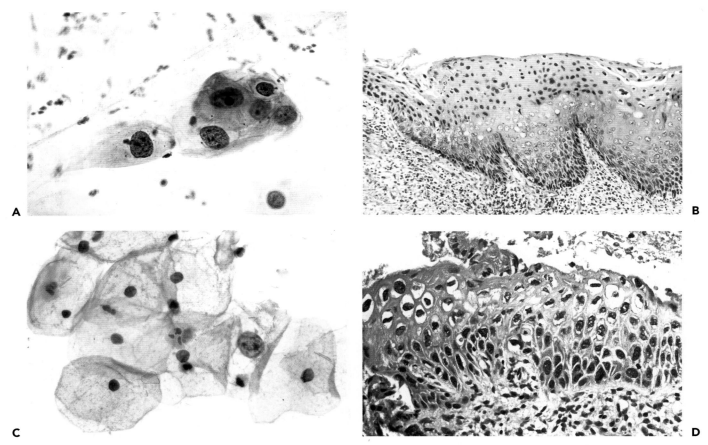

Figure 11-48 Low-grade lesions in smears with high-grade squamous lesions (HGSIL) in tissue biopsies. *A.* Dysplastic (dyskaryotic) intermediate squamous cells corresponding to biopsies shown in *B. B* shows a two-layer lesion with the high-grade component forming the bottom segment. *C.* An intermediate dyskaryotic cell in Pap smear corresponding to a HGSIL in the tissue biopsy shown in *D.*

Histology

These lesions are nearly always derived from, and located on, the squamous epithelium of the vaginal aspect of the uterine cervix. The epithelium is usually thickened **and is composed of squamous cancer cells with markedly enlarged, usually hyperchromatic nuclei, arranged in disor-** **derly layers. Mitoses, often abnormal, can be observed throughout the cancerous epithelium. Layers of keratin of variable thickness are present on the surface of the lesions which still retain the over-all configuration of the squamous epithelium of origin** (Figs. 11-50D, 11-51D). These lesions may **extend to the lower end of the**

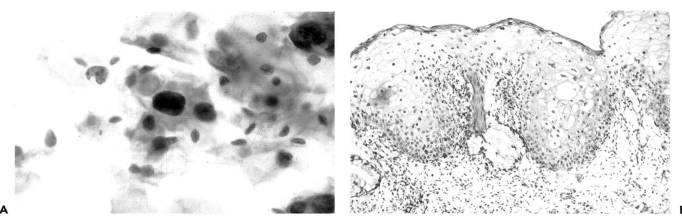

Figure 11-49 **Disappearing low-grade lesion in a 17-year-old woman.** *A.* Severe dyskaryosis of intermediate cells corresponding to the tissue biopsy of a low-grade lesion shown in *B.* The lesion disappeared after the biopsy and long-term follow-up was negative.

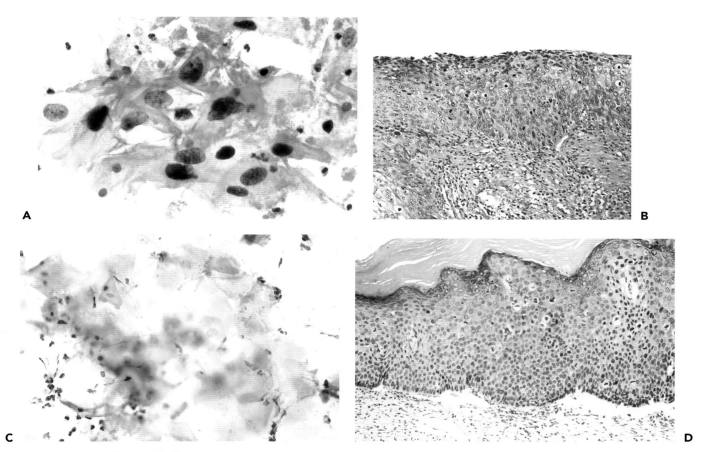

Figure 11-50 **High-grade squamous intraepithelial lesion.** *A.* Group of keratinized squamous cancer cells showing large, dark nuclei, corresponding to biopsy shown in *B.* Note the presence of cells with clear perinuclear zones reminiscent of koilocytes. *B.* The lesion is a combination of low and high-grade with keratinized surface. *C.* Anucleated squamous material corresponding to tissue lesions shown in *D* that shows squamous high-grade CIN with keratinized surface.

endocervical canal but more often spread to the vagina (see Chap. 14).

In biopsy material, the lesions **are frequently underestimated** because, under the low power of the microscope, they may be mistaken for **benign leukoplakia,** or, because of the relatively orderly arrangement of the epithelium, considered to be **a "dysplasia" or a low-grade lesion.** Such material should be studied under **a high-power lens to identify the cytologic abnormalities described above. The lesions are fully capable of progression to invasive cancer.**

Cytology

The **smear background** shows considerable inflammation. Associated **trichomoniasis is common.** The presence of blood and marked necrosis may be indicative of invasive cancer. The dominant feature is usually the presence of **keratin-forming cancer cells of a variety of shapes with abundant orange or yellow opaque, thick cytoplasm,** accounting for the term "pleomorphic dysplasia" (Patten 1972) (Figs. 11-50 and 11-51). **Tadpole (caudate) cells** (see Fig. 11-37C), **spindly squamous cancer cells** (see Fig. 11-51C), and **squamous "pearls"** made up of cancer cells (see Fig. 11-37D) may be observed in such smears. The

nuclei of such cells, although enlarged and of irregular shape, are often pyknotic and not amenable to a detailed microscopic analysis (India ink nuclei) (see Fig. 11-50A). Some of the cancer cells may sometimes appear as mere **"ghosts,"** in which the nucleus has been partially or completely replaced by keratin. **Anucleated keratin material from the surface of the lesion** may accompany the ghost cells (see Fig. 11-50C). In fact, **the differential diagnosis between benign leukoplakia, which also sheds anucleated squames** (see Chap. 10), **and keratinizing cancer of the cervix, is best accomplished by a cytologic sample.** The samples may also contain **nonkeratinized, dysplastic cells and koilocytes,** the latter suggestive of origin of the abnormality in a low-grade lesion (see Fig. 11-50A).

In some of these lesions, the cytologic evidence may be limited to a few atypical squamous cells. It must also be noted that, in this group of lesions, the cytologic differentiation of noninvasive precursors from invasive, keratin-forming squamous cancer may be impossible, as recently confirmed by Levine et al (2003).

Clinical Significance

Because of the **possibility that an invasive cancer may be present,** an adequate **colposcopic evaluation and biopsies**

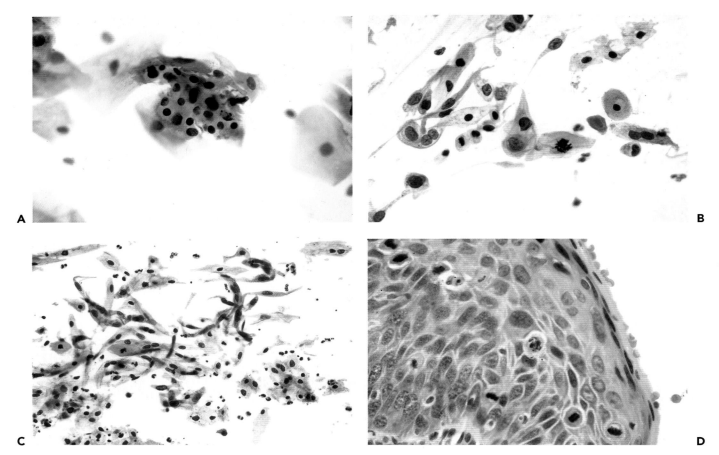

Figure 11-51 Various manifestations of a keratinizing high-grade squamous intraepithelial lesion. *A.* A cluster of small squamous cells with dark, enlarged nuclei. *B.* Single squamous cells with large, hyperchromatic nuclei. *C.* Spindly squamous cells. *D.* Corresponding biopsy of a high-grade lesion with keratinized surface. Note the presence of tripolar mitoses.

of cervix are particularly important for this group of lesions and must include the adjacent vagina.

Intraepithelial Lesions with Features of Squamous Metaplasia

Synonyms: **moderately well-differentiated or intermediate type of carcinoma in situ, large- or medium-size cell carcinoma in situ, moderate or severe dysplasia, CIN grade II or III.**

Histology

This is, by far, the most common form of high-grade lesion, **usually straddling the transformation zone, and involving the adjacent squamous and endocervical epithelia. The extension of the process into endocervical glands is common and should not be mistaken for invasive cancer.** The cytologic and histologic appearance of the lesions is variable, which accounts for the many synonyms.

The neoplastic epithelium is of **variable thickness,** usually comprising 10 to 20 layers of cells, but it sometimes may be composed of only three or four layers of small cells. In such cases, the lesion may be difficult to recognize and one must pay close attention to the nuclear features of component cells. The very thin epithelium may reflect **loss of**

upper epithelial layers because of fragility of these lesions. These cases are reminiscent of the **"clinging" form of carcinoma in situ of the bladder,** discussed in Chapter 23. The over-all histologic pattern and anatomic distribution of the epithelial lesions often bears considerable resemblance to squamous metaplasia of the endocervical epithelium. The neoplastic epithelium is **composed of medium-sized cancer cells arranged in disorderly layers.** On close inspection, the cells have **large, irregularly shaped, hyperchromatic nuclei and scanty basophilic cytoplasm** (see Figs. 11-52C, 11-53B,D, 11-54D). **In some lesions, the component cells retain squamous features, are somewhat larger, and have eosinophilic cytoplasm.** Some of these lesions show **two or three layers of small, keratinized cells with pyknotic nuclei** on the surface (see Fig. 11-52D). **Mitotic activity, including abnormal mitotic figures,** is usually quite evident. **These lesions are often accompanied by atypia of endocervical epithelium lining the adjacent glands** (see Fig. 11-35D).

Some of these lesions are composed of two layers of malignant cells of different morphology (see Fig. 11-48B). The mechanisms of this arrangement are not understood but it is likely that one type of lesion is growing underneath and undermining the older abnormal surface epithelium.

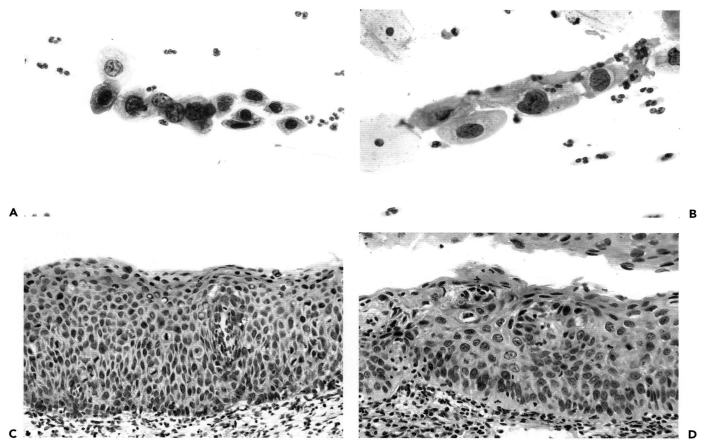

Figure 11-52 High-grade squamous intraepithelial lesion of the "so-called" metaplastic type. *A,B.* Parabasal malignant squamous cells with marked nuclear enlargement and hyperchromasia. Note the general similarity of these cells to benign metaplasia, except for marked nuclear abnormalities. *C.* The tissue lesion corresponding to smear pattern shown in *A* and *B. D.* Another biopsy example of this type of lesion with keratin formation on the surface.

Differential Diagnosis Between HGSIL of Metaplastic Type with Atypical or Immature Squamous Metaplasia

Atypical or immature metaplasia **is an ill-defined histologic entity that is either benign, neoplastic *ab initio,* or may be a step in the development of high-grade lesions of metaplastic type.** One such lesion, named **papillary immature metaplasia** (PIM) and often containing HPV types 6 and 11, was thought to represent an early stage of formation of condyloma (Crum et al, 1996).

The lack of diagnostic reproducibility among competent observers was vividly illustrated in a paper by Park et al (1999). These authors attempted to use human papillomavirus typing to solve the problems of classification with limited success. On the other hand, Geng et al (1999) reported **progression of 13 of 16 patients with "atypical immature metaplasia" to HGSIL.** The progression was more frequent in HPV-positive than in HPV-negative patients. Such lesions have been observed by us during the long-term followup of cervical neoplasia, reported in Part 1 of the chapter and in recent years.

The histologic differential diagnosis between atypical metaplasia and HGSIL may be very difficult. The **principles in the histologic classification of these lesions can** be summarized as follows: **if, on close inspection, the epithelium shows formation of desmosomes (intracellular bridges) and the component cells show no conspicuous nuclear abnormalities, the odds are that the lesion is benign. If the cells show variation in nuclear sizes, crowd each other and do not form visible desmosomes, the lesion is most likely malignant.** Some such lesions may become invasive (see Fig. 11-56A,B). The **cytologic material may provide an answer in difficult cases:** in the presence of cells with malignant nuclear features, the lesions are malignant. If the cytology shows merely metaplastic cells with relatively slight nuclear abnormalities, as described in Chapter 10, the identity of the lesions is uncertain and a follow-up should be instituted.

Cytology

In general, this group of lesions is characterized by a fairly monotonous population of **moderately sized parabasal, dysplastic (dyskaryotic) or cancer cells with marked nuclear abnormalities,** occurring singly and in clusters (see Figs. 11-52A,B and 11-54). **Not all such cells have hyperchromatic nuclei (pale dyskaryosis)** and their identification may be challenging. The cytoplasm of the abnormal cells is predominantly basophilic. However, in every sample,

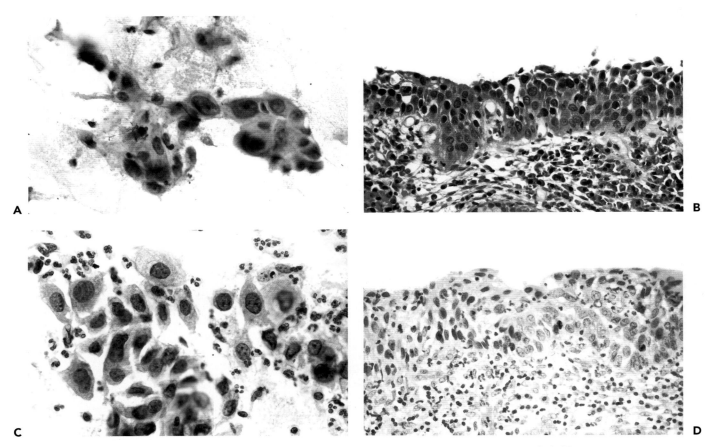

Figure 11-53   The smear pattern and histology of a high-grade squamous intraepithelial lesion located in the endocervical canal. *A,B.* An example of HGSIL with keratinization of component cells. *A.* Medium-sized cancer cells with keratinized cytoplasm. *B.* The corresponding tissue lesion. *C.* Columnar cancer cells that could be interpreted as endocervical adenocarcinoma. *D.* The corresponding tissue lesion.

some or most cells show the eosinophilic cytoplasm, characteristics of squamous cancer cells that may not be evident in the corresponding biopsy (see Fig. 11-53A,B). In some instances, **cancer cells of endocervical type with large nucleoli** may be observed, sometimes mimicking to perfection the cytologic presentation of endocervical adenocarcinoma (see Fig. 11-53C,D).

As illustrated in Figure 11-36A,B, **streaks of dysplastic cells,** trapped in endocervical mucus, may be observed in **direct cervical smears.** This diagnostically very helpful feature is no longer present in liquid cell collection systems. Still, in our experience, with good liquid preparations using the SurePath System (TriPathology Imaging, Burlington, NC), the abnormal cells stand out because of nuclear enlargement and hyperchromasia and retain the fine features of nuclear chromatin (Fig. 11-54).

Because the parabasal dysplastic (dyskaryotic) cells may bear considerable resemblance to benign metaplastic squamous cells, some observers have redescribed these cells as **"atypical immature squamous metaplastic cells"** (Dressel and Wilbur, 1992; Sheils and Wilbur, 1997), while acknowledging that such cells reflect the presence of high-grade lesions in most cases. Sherman et al (1999) used this

term to designate smears as "atypical, rule out high-grade lesions." In my judgment, **this term is highly misleading** and merely confuses the issues. In some patients, the **atypical metaplastic cells in smears may be followed by clear-cut dysplastic or malignant cells,** leading to a biopsy diagnosis of HGSIL (Fig. 11-55).

Clinical Significance

It is generally assumed that HGSIL of the metaplastic type is a precursor of invasive cancer, composed of medium-sized cells. **It is of note that invasive carcinomas derived from such lesions may show a much greater degree of keratin formation than the precursor lesions.** By consensus, HGSIL should be treated after the lesion has been localized by colposcopy and appropriate biopsies, although it is known that some such lesions can disappear or not progress for many years (see Part 1 of the chapter). The issue of HPV typing as a prognostic parameter will be discussed at the end of this chapter.

High-Grade Lesions Composed of Small Cells

Synonyms: small-cell squamous (epidermoid) carcinoma, carcinoma in situ, CIN grade III.

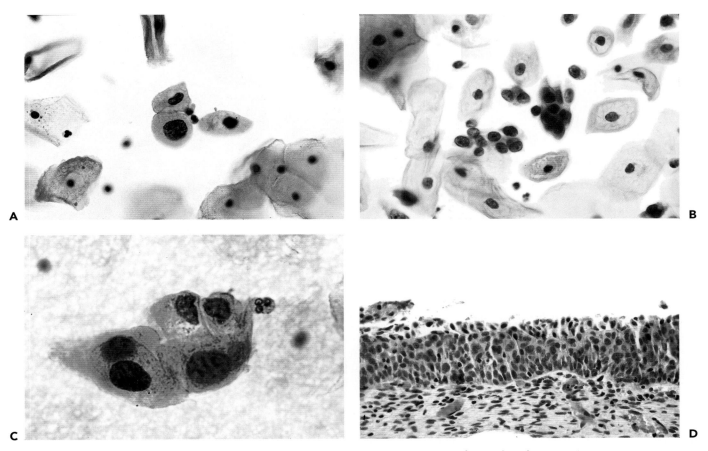

Figure 11-54 High-grade squamous intraepithelial lesion (HGSIL) from a liquid preparation (SurePath). *A,B.* Scattered small malignant cells, singly and in clusters. Note the excellent quality of nuclear stain. *C.* High power view of large cells with hyperchromatic nuclei. Note the irregular nuclear outline and coarse arrangement of chromatin. *D.* Corresponding HGSIL of "metaplastic" type.

Histology

This group of intraepithelial lesions, derived from reserve or basal cells of the endocervical epithelium, is **composed of small malignant cells. The lesions replace the epithelium lining the endocervical canal and frequently extend to endocervical glands** (Figs. 11-57D, 11-58D). The lesion may extend to the transformation zone and be identified by colposcopy. In many instances, however, **the lesion is beyond the reach of the colposcope** and, therefore, represents a diagnostic challenge to the clinician and the pathologist. Because the initial colposcopy may be negative, **delays in securing biopsies are common. Endocervical curettage,** which is often used for diagnosis, may result in tiny fragments of tumor that are sometimes difficult to interpret or are overlooked. In many cases, **repeated biopsies or diagnostic conization may be required** to secure the diagnosis, a procedure that is sometimes reluctantly undertaken by the gynecologist, and only if the follow-up smears remain positive and the pathologist insists on further diagnostic procedure. Not uncommonly, the lesion is accompanied by **abnormalities of endocervical epithelium and glands that have the features of adenocarcinoma in situ** (see Fig. 11-53C and Chapter 12). The small-cell lesion is the **precursor of invasive cancer composed of small- or me-**dium-sized cells that may have endocrine features. Because of the problems with cytologic detection of these lesions, they are often discovered in invasive stage and are thought to have rapid progression (see below).

Cytology

This group of lesions, corresponding to the "classic" carcinoma in situ, is characterized primarily by **very small cancer cells with scanty, often barely visible, usually basophilic, rarely eosinophilic cytoplasm,** occurring singly and in clusters (Figs. 11-57 through 11-59). The single, dispersed cancer cells **have relatively large, hyperchromatic, coarsely granular nuclei that usually show irregularity of contour. Cells with "pale" nuclei may also occur ("pale dyskaryosis")** (see Fig. 11-35C). In some cases, **large nucleoli** may be observed, but this is not a common finding. Because the cells are very small (10 to 15 μm in diameter), an examination under the **high power of the microscope** is often needed for the recognition of the nuclear abnormalities (see Figs. 11-57C, 11-58C). The small cancer cells may show **mucus-containing cytoplasmic vacuoles, confirming their kinship with endocervical epithelium** (see Fig. 11-35A).

Equally important for the diagnosis is the presence of

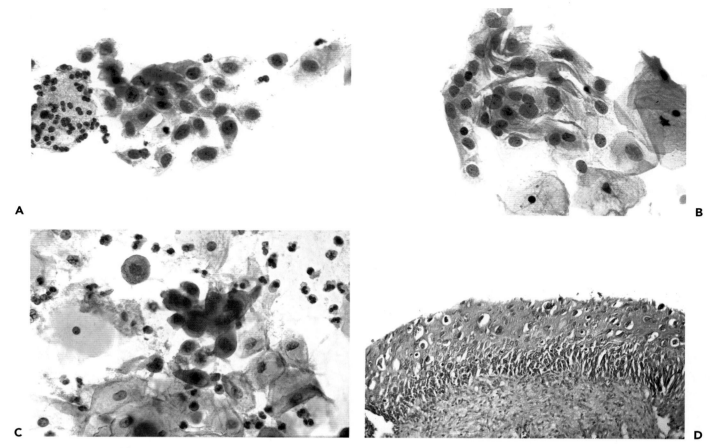

Figure 11-55 Atypical metaplastic cells preceding HGSIL. *A.* Metaplastic cells with nuclear abnormalities. *B.* Cells with similar characteristics forming a cluster. *C.* Small cancer cells observed one year later. *D.* Biopsy obtained after second smear, showing a HGSIL.

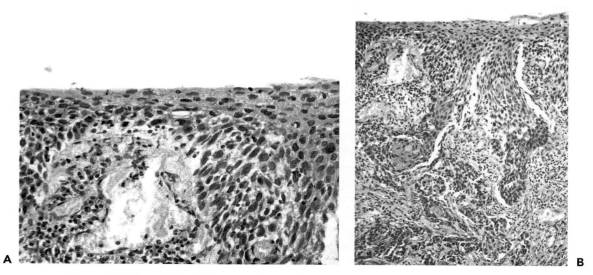

Figure 11-56 HGSIL with features of metaplasia *(A)* with microinvasion *(B)*. Histologic appearance of a microinvasive high-grade lesion with well differentiated.

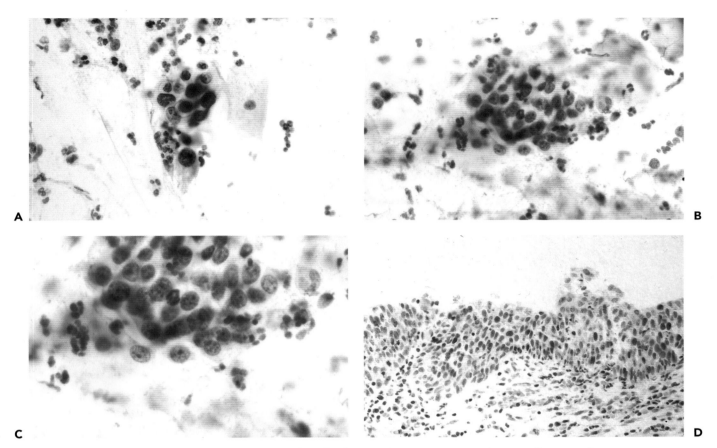

Figure 11-57   HGSIL composed of small cells. *A,B.* Clusters ("syncytia") of very small cancer cells easily overlooked on screening. *C.* High-power view of the cluster shown in *B* to document coarse chromatin pattern and the presence of nucleoli. *D.* Tissue lesion corresponding to *A–C,* showing a small-cell HGSIL that extended into endocervical glands.

tightly knit cell clusters, sometimes incorrectly referred to as "syncytia" (see Figs. 11-57B,C, 11-58A, and 11-59B). The number of clusters depends on the technique of cytologic sampling; in smears obtained by cervix scraper, the clusters may be few but, with the use of an endocervical brushing instrument, clusters are usually numerous. The recognition of the nature of the clusters may also require the use of the **high power** of the microscope. If the centers of the clusters are too dense for analysis, the **periphery will virtually always disclose the characteristic nuclear features of the small cancer cells.**

It must be stressed that this type of high-grade lesion is, **by far, the most difficult cervix lesion to identify in cytologic preparations,** if the observer is unaware of the small size and microscopic characteristics of cancer cells. Errors occur when such cells are **mistaken for leukocytes, plasma cells, small macrophages (histiocytes), small clusters of benign metaplastic or endometrial cells.** The last error may occur in brush specimens, when the instrument is inserted too deeply into the endocervical canal. Other sources of error include **atypical lymphocytes,** such as observed in **follicular cervicitis** (see Chap. 10), cells of **malignant lymphoma,** or metastatic cancer composed of small

cells (see Chap. 17). Mitchell and Medley (1995), in a careful comparative study, documented that the small-cell malignant lesions are the **main cause of false-negative smears.** Small-cell lesions, missed on screening or misinterpreted, are **the most common reason for legal cases against laboratories.** In several personally observed cases, the failure to identify the small cancer cells led to invasive cancer within a few years.

The diagnostic dilemmas are not necessarily limited to cytologic presentation. Biopsies may also be the cause of diagnostic delays. A case in point is the patient shown in Figure 11-59, whose cytologic diagnosis of small-cell carcinoma (Fig. 11-59A,B) resulted in a first biopsy showing herpetic cervicitis (Fig. 11-59C), which was accepted as the cause of an erroneous cytologic interpretation. One year later, after another positive smear, the biopsy was repeated, disclosing a superficially invasive squamous carcinoma (Fig. 11-59D). We also observed cases with small fragments of carcinomas, either missed in the biopsy material or misinterpreted as "metaplasia," particularly in scanty endocervical curettings.

Similar small malignant cells may be observed in the so-called **tubal metaplasia.** As discussed in Chapter 10,

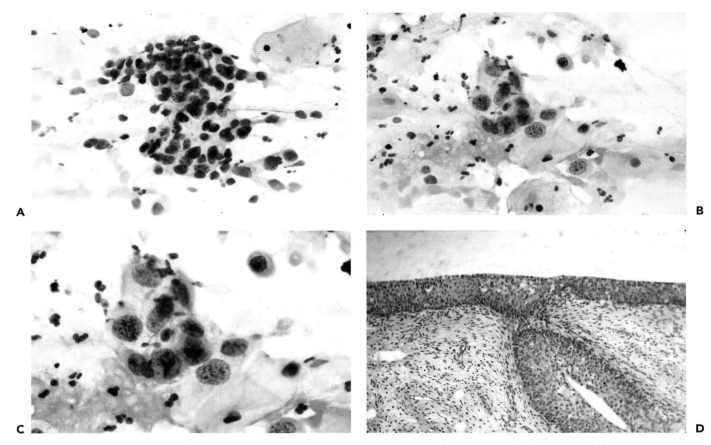

Figure 11-58   HGSIL composed of small cells. *A,B.* Clusters of tiny cancer cells that are easily mistaken for leukocytes or endometrial cells or may be entirely overlooked on screening. *C.* Cluster shown in *B* under high magnification to document granularity of chromatin and the presence of nucleoli. *D.* The histologic features of the corresponding tissue lesion composed of small cells with extension to endocervical glands.

the presence of such cells strongly suggests the presence of a **malignant process involving the ciliated epithelium** (Fig. 11-60).

Mixed Types of High-Grade Squamous Intraepithelial Lesions

Clear-cut cytologic identification of the three principal types of high-grade lesions is not always possible. **Intermediate and mixed forms may occur. The presence of dysplastic (dyskaryotic) squamous cells of the superficial and intermediate variety,** next to the small cancer cells, is **suggestive of a simultaneous involvement of the transformation zone and of the squamous epithelium of the portio by a lesion composed of larger cells that may be either low- or high-grade.** Another important and not unusual combination is that of an **epidermoid carcinoma in situ and endocervical adenocarcinoma,** to be discussed in Chapter 12.

RAPIDLY PROGRESSING PRECANCEROUS LESIONS

Within recent years, sporadic observations were reported on rapidly evolving invasive carcinomas of the uterine cervix,

usually developing in young women within a year or two after a negative cervical smear (summary in Hildesheim et al, 1999). Consequently, several observers suggested that, in some women, invasive cancer of the cervix develops rapidly, without going through a detectable precancerous stage. In my judgment and experience, this concept is not correct. Provided that prior cytologic samples were reasonably adequate, review of the previous "negative" cytologic samples **nearly always** reveal at least a few abnormal cells. Quite often, there is substantial evidence of a precursor lesion or cancer that was either missed on screening or misinterpreted. **Although it may be true that some precancerous lesions of the uterine cervix, such as a small-cell carcinoma in situ, may have a relatively short evolution of perhaps 5 years, they are usually detectable in cervical cytologic samples for some years before invasion occurs.** This has been documented in a multi-institutional study of high-grade lesions wherein it has been shown that cancer cells were present in a substantial proportion of previously "negative" smears (Koss et al, 1997). Several other papers and evidence addressing the issue of "false-negative" smears in women developing high-grade lesions or invasive cancer are discussed below. Similar observations were reported by Wain et al (1992) who denied the existence of "rapid onset

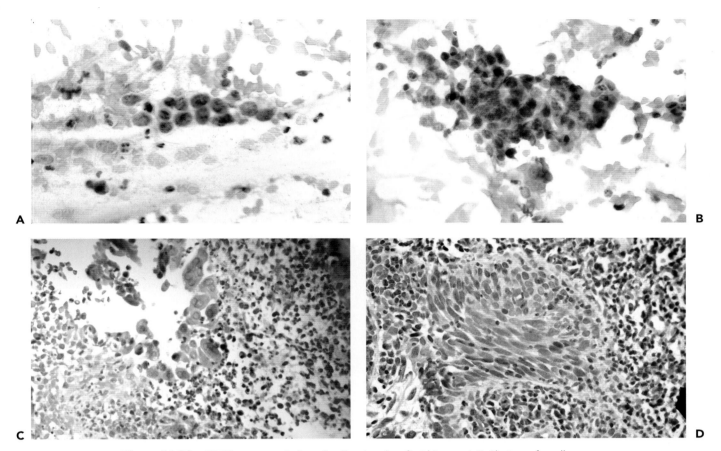

Figure 11-59   HGSIL composed of small cells missed on first biopsy. *A,B.* Clusters of small cancer cells observed in the original smear. *C.* Endocervical biopsy showing herpetic endocervicitis with ulceration. This was followed by another positive smear and another biopsy one year later. The second biopsy (*D*) showed invasive squamous carcinoma.

cancer" by finding cancer cells on review of previous "negative" smears.

INTERVAL CANCERS

A concept similar to "rapidly progressing lesions" is **interval cancers,** that is, carcinomas of the uterine cervix, occurring after a negative screening result. Mitchell et al (1990) reported on 138 such patients developing invasive cancer of the cervix within 36 months after one or more negative cervical smears. On review of the negative smears, all but 11.9% showed either evidence of cytologic abnormality or suboptimal sampling (absence of endocervical or metaplastic cells). Thus, the concept of **"interval cancer" is not**

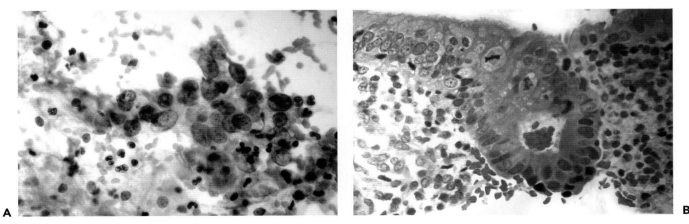

Figure 11-60   A malignant lesion arising in a focus of tubal metaplasia of the endocervix. *A.* The smear pattern composed of medium-sized cancer cells. *B.* Endocervical biopsy with a striking number of mitotic figures.

valid in most cases, as it is caused, as the "rapid onset cancer," by **failures of the screening system.**

SPECIAL CYTOLOGIC PRESENTATIONS OF SQUAMOUS INTRAEPITHELIAL LESIONS

Cytolysis

Extensive cytolysis caused by *Lactobacillus* (Döderlein) (see Chaps. 8 and 10) may **destroy the cytoplasm of the abnormal cells** to the point where the nuclei of such cells are surrounded only by a narrow rim of residual frayed cytoplasm (see Fig. 11-66). Cytolysis is most commonly observed during pregnancy but may also occur in a nonpregnant woman (Fig. 11-61). **The cells most commonly affected are intermediate squamous dysplastic (dyskaryotic) cells, although occasionally, larger, more mature squamous cancer cells may be so affected.** The cytologic diagnosis may prove very difficult under these circumstances and is based mainly on **comparison of nuclear sizes and degree of nuclear hyperchromasia** between normal and abnormal nuclei.

Postmenopausal Atrophy

Most lesions observed in this age group are **high-grade intraepithelial squamous lesions** (HGSIL) or invasive carcinoma. As discussed in Chapter 8, the interpretation of atrophic smears is a common source of diagnostic difficulty. Atrophy of the vaginal and cervical epithelia and the resulting changes in cell pattern caused by dryness have a major impact on neoplastic cells. **The crisp appearance of the well-preserved dysplastic or cancer cells is often lost and the cells appear enlarged and smudgy. Their nuclei, flattened and spread over a larger area, lose some or all of their hyperchromasia and appear relatively pale, and often their internal structure is no longer discernible** (Fig. 11-62). The diagnosis is reached mainly by careful comparison of the abnormal cells with adjacent dry, but normal, squamous cells and an **assessment of the relative nuclear hyperchromasia and altered nucleocytoplasmic ratio.** Using a readily recognized landmark (such as a polymorphonuclear leukocyte) to compare with abnormal cells, is also helpful in estimating the degree of cellular and nuclear enlargement. In most such cases, a careful review of the entire preparation will usually reveal a few well-preserved cancer cells, clinching the diagnosis.

Rarely, LGSILs may occur in postmenopausal women, sometimes at age 80 or even 90. Cytologic samples in such cases may display **koilocytes** and, hence, the features of the permissive human papillomavirus (HPV) infection (Fig. 11-63). It is not known whether the presence of active viruses represents a newly acquired infection, somewhat unlikely but not impossible, in patients of any age, or a persistence or a reactivation of an old, occult infectious process, as discussed in Part 1 of the chapter. In keeping with my experience, Rader et al (1999) reported that, in women age 55 or older, low-grade squamous neoplastic lesions of the cervix **are relatively uncommon and may be represented in smears only by atypical cells** (ASCUS).

Occasionally, a **markedly atrophic benign smear with extreme degree of cell distortion** (including the presence of elongated, spindly squamous cells) **may suggest the presence of cancer, even to an experienced observer** (see Chap. 8). Under these circumstances, a **comparison of nuclear sizes among the epithelial cells** is necessary. If the nuclear sizes of the suspect cells are identical or closely similar to those of other, clearly benign cells, the diagnosis of carcinoma is not warranted. If some of the suspect cells in the smear show considerable nuclear enlargement and hyperchromasia, the possibility of a malignant lesion may be entertained. An atrophic smear may also contain the **benign "blue bodies"** (see Chap. 8), which may imitate cancer cells to perfection.

In spite of the accumulated experience, there are situations where lingering doubts will persist as to whether an atrophic smear is benign or contains cells suspicious of cancer. In such uncommon cases, there are several approaches available. Perhaps the simplest solution is to refer the patient for **colposcopic evaluation and possible biopsies.** Alter-

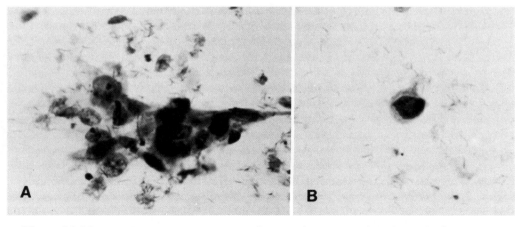

Figure 11-61   *A,B.* Carcinoma in situ in cervical smear of a patient in the 8th month of pregnancy. Note the extensive cytolysis.

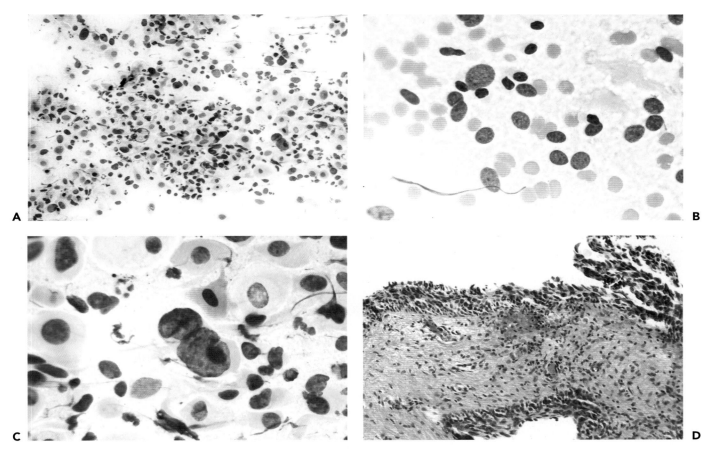

Figure 11-62   **HGSIL in an atrophic smear, compared with a negative smear.** *A.* Negative smear with pattern of atrophy and some nuclear enlargement, shown in *B. C.* Malignant cells in an atrophic smear, characterized by very large, flattened, and semitransparent nuclei. Compare with *B. D.* Tissue lesion corresponding to *C* showing a HGSIL.

nately, the patient may be given a **short course of estrogens** and the smear repeated after restoration of the epithelium, as discussed in Chapter 9. This latter procedure carries with it the risk of a false-negative second smear in the presence of an important lesion, as will be set forth below. The role of **HPV testing** in such situations has not been determined but may perhaps be useful (see below).

Interpretation of Biopsies in Postmenopausal Women

High-grade precursor lesions may present a problem of recognition, not only in cytologic samples, but also in biopsies. **Most of the high-grade lesions in biopsies are morphologically identical to those seen in young women. In a number of such cases, however, the lesions undergo**

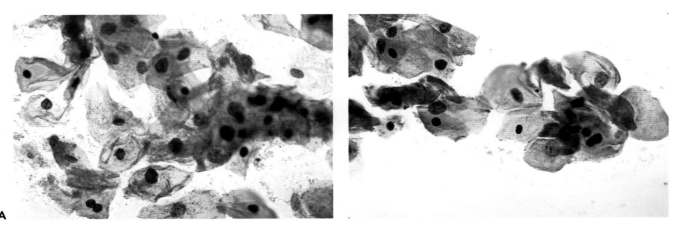

Figure 11-63   *A,B.* **Dysplastic (dyskaryotic) cells and koilocytes** in a smear from a woman age 90 receiving estrogens. The smear with estrogenic pattern contains several koilocytes with enlarged dark nuclei and perinuclear halos.

atrophy, in keeping with the general atrophic status of the epithelia of the lower genital tract. In such women, the smears may contain fairly well-preserved and recognizable dysplastic (dyskaryotic) and cancer cells, whereas the tissue biopsies show effects of atrophy. In some cases, only fragments of atrophic CIN may be observed (Fig. 11-64). In other cases with clearly positive smears, the atrophic malignant epithelium in biopsies mimics squamous metaplasia (Fig. 11-65). The spacing of the abnormal nuclei increases and there is no nuclear overlap, usually observed in younger women. The atrophy may even extend to endocervical glands (Fig. 11-65D). We have also observed cases of HGSIL in postmenopausal women wherein the smear contained strips and fragments of malignant epithelium removed by energetic sampling. The biopsies in such cases may show only denuded surface or small fragments of atrophic malignant epithelium difficult to interpret and considered a "crushing artifact." Such events may be interpreted as "false-positive smears" (see below).

Some epithelial abnormalities occurring predominantly in postmenopausal women with suspicious cytologic findings were described in histologic material as transitional cell metaplasia (Egan and Russel, 1997; Weir et al, 1998). In these lesions, the characteristic features of the urothelium, discussed at length in Chapter 22, have not been documented, beyond a vague morphologic similarity. In biopsies of such lesions, the nuclear abnormalities are evident but are not striking and there is some flattening of the surface, vaguely reminiscent of the urothelium. On further search, more classical high-grade lesions usually can be identified either on recuts or in adjacent segments of the epithelium. In my experience, the "transitional cell metaplasia" represents atrophic HGSIL in most, if not all, cases. As is shown in Figure 11-66, these lesions are capable of progression to invasive cancer. Interestingly, the smears in such cases may or may not show atrophic changes but virtually always show abnormal cells. For comments on vaginal lesions in postmenopausal women with atrophic smears, see Chapter 14.

Pregnancy

The cytologic diagnosis of squamous intraepithelial lesions in pregnancy may represent a challenge, for reasons discussed and illustrated in Chapters 8 and 10. Abnormalities caused by the presence of decidual cells, the Arias-Stella phenomenon, or florid, atypical squamous metaplasia may be mistaken for malignant processes. On the other hand, pregnancy, which nearly always places the woman under the care of a physician, is a particularly beneficial time to search for cervical cancer. This is especially true of multiparae, who were shown on several epidemiologic

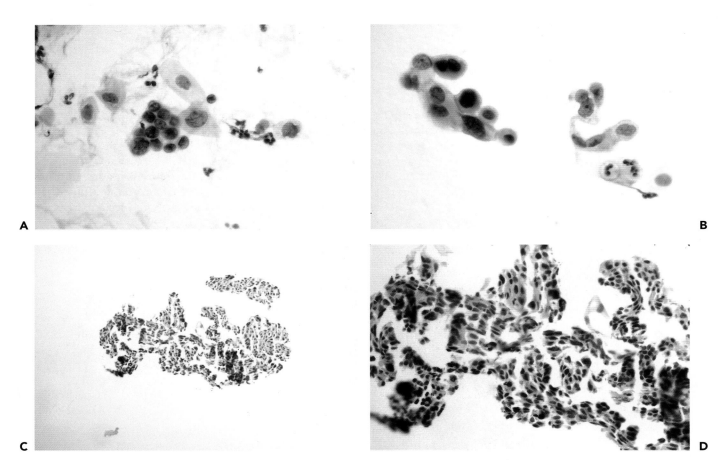

A B C D

Figure 11-64 High-grade CIN in an 84-year-old woman with marked atrophy of the malignant epithelium. *A,B.* Small clusters of cancer cells. *C,D.* The corresponding biopsy fragment with marked atrophy of the fragmented high-grade lesion.

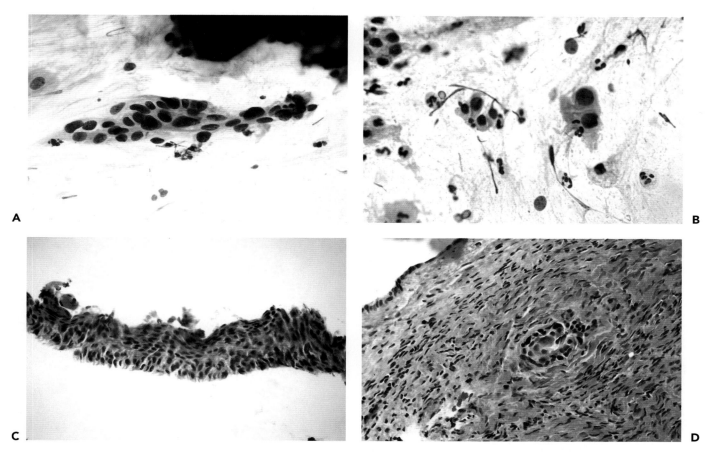

Figure 11-65 Another example of a HGSIL occurring in a postmenopausal woman with epithelial atrophy. *A,B.* Clusters of cancer cells. *C.* A strip of atrophic CIN that may be mistaken for metaplasia. *D* shows that the atrophy extended to the endocervical glands.

surveys to be more apt to develop cervical cancer than nulliparae.

In the 1950s, several observers reported that precursor lesions, diagnosed by biopsy as carcinomas in situ during pregnancy, could not be found postpartum, leading to the suggestion that these lesions were not "true" in situ cancers but "an epithelial alteration associated with pregnancy and similar to in situ carcinoma" (Schleifstein, 1950; Nesbitt and Hellman, 1952). Subsequently, Marsh and Fitzgerald (1956), Greene and Packham (1958) and many others, demonstrated that **carcinoma in situ (HGSIL), observed during pregnancy, is identical to lesions in nonpregnant women.** Personal observations support these latter views. In some patients with precancerous lesions followed for several years, pregnancy occurred while the patient was under observation (Koss et al, 1963). There was no substantial regression of the lesions (see Fig. 11-27), a view shared by Boutselis (1972). In a major review by Hacker et al (1982), the similarity of the precursor lesions and of invasive cancer in pregnant and nonpregnant women was confirmed. Coppola et al (1997) observed persisting CIN II or III in 20 of 25 women post-partum. Inexplicably, a paper by Yost et al (1999) revived the old controversy. These authors, reporting on 153 pregnant patients, observed regression of about 70% of precancerous lesions after delivery.

In my judgment, **the association of precursor lesions of cervical cancer with pregnancy is purely coincidental.** It is entirely consistent with our present knowledge of behavior of precancerous lesions, to believe that biopsies of the cervix, the trauma of delivery, or instrumentation may well account for the disappearance of some of these lesions. Because pregnant women are immunosuppressed to some extent, the high frequency of transient HPV infection (with subsequent recovery) may account for some of these observations (see Part 1 of the chapter).

Conservative approach to the evaluation and treatment of precursor lesions observed during pregnancy was stressed in a major contribution from Sweden by Hellberg et al (1987). Jain et al (1997) considered progression of LGSIL to HGSIL to be unusual during pregnancy and also advocated conservative approach to treatment.

Although **the treatment of precursor lesions can usually be postponed until post-partum, in rare cases, I observed a rapid progression of such lesions to invasive cancer** (Fig. 11-67). **Therefore, if conservative approach is chosen, a very careful surveillance of pregnant patients with abnormal smears and biopsies is advocated.**

Lesions in Teenagers

Sexually active adolescent girls and very young women may harbor precancerous lesions of the uterine cervix

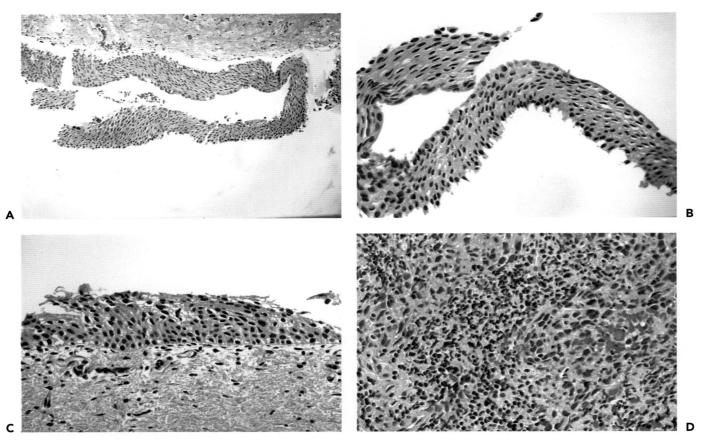

Figure 11-66 Examples of atrophic malignant epithelium mimicking the so-called transitional cell metaplasia. *A,B.* Sheets of atrophic epithelium with minimal nuclear abnormality. *C.* Adjacent fragments of epithelium showing atrophic CIN. *D.* A focus of invasive carcinoma adjacent to *C.* (Case courtesy of Dr. C.M. Lombard, Los Altos, CA.)

and occasionally invasive carcinoma. The prevalence of histologically confirmed precancerous lesions in young patients varied from 2.7 per 1,000 to as high as 24.3 per 1,000 (Table 11-10) and, to my knowledge, has not changed in recent years. Studies of sexually active young women strongly suggest that this group of women often harbor an active **HPV infection** of low- and high-risk types that **is usually transient** (see Part 1 of the chapter). **Thus, HPV testing of this group of patients is not reliable and should not be used to identify patients at high risk. The discovery of precancerous lesions and cancer in this group must rest on cytologic and histologic findings.** Other sexually transmitted diseases, such as trichomoniasis, gonorrhea, and herpes, may be uncovered in such patients.

In a study performed in our laboratories at Montefiore Medical Center, biopsy-confirmed cytologic abnormalities suggestive of CIN grade I or II were observed in 14 (3.4%) of the 403 delinquent girls ages 12 to 16, detained in custody of law-enforcement, who agreed to be tested. Twelve of the 14 abnormal smears contained koilocytes, hence, evidence of permissive human papillomavirus infection (Hein et al, 1977). It was of particular interest that the period of sexual activity preceding CIN was exceedingly short, only a few months in some girls and less than two years in others, again consistent with HPV infection. No follow-up infor-

mation could be obtained on these patients. Rader et al (1997) also reported a high rate of "dysplasia" in young women with cytologic diagnosis of ASC-US.

Lesions in Immunodeficient Women

Infection with human immunodeficiency virus (HIV 1) and AIDS are additional risk factors for very young women. Maiman et al (1990, 1991) reported a high rate of cervical lesions, and even invasive cancer, in very young patients with impaired immunity caused by these conditions and resulting in an altered CD4 to CD8 lymphocyte ratio. Similar observations were reported by Feingold et al (1990), Wright et al (1994), and Ellenbrock et al (2000).

MICROINVASIVE CARCINOMA

Definition and Clinical Data

Microinvasive carcinoma was initially defined by the International Federation of Gynecologists (FIGO) as a clearly invasive epidermoid carcinoma of the uterine cervix in which the depth of invasion of the stroma did not exceed 5 mm. Subsequent careful studies by Van Nagell (1983) established that

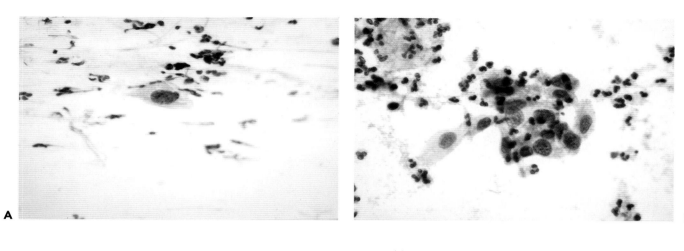

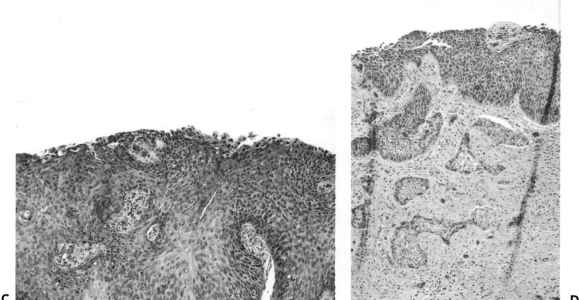

Figure 11-67 **Progression of HGSIL to invasive carcinoma during pregnancy.** *A.* Smear obtained during the second month of pregnancy showing a few scattered dysplastic cells. *B.* Smear obtained during the 4th month of pregnancy showing a cluster of cancer cells. *C.* Biopsy obtained immediately following the smear shown in *B* showing a well-differentiated HGSIL. There was no evidence of invasion. *D.* The patient received a Caesarean section in the seventh month of pregnancy. At that time, cervical biopsies showed an invasive carcinoma.

lesions with invasion deeper than 3 mm were capable of metastases. Hence, the current definition of microinvasive carcinoma, recommended by the Society of Gynecologic Oncologists, is **invasive cervical cancer with depth of stromal invasion not greater than 3 mm** (Fig. 11-68). I feel that the above definition is deficient because it does not address the issue of the volume of microinvasion. **If the invasion is limited to one or two tongues of cancerous tissue penetrating into the stroma,** metastases do not occur. If, however, there are **multiple points of penetration into the stroma, even if the invasion is limited to 2 mm, metastases to pelvic lymph nodes occasionally may be observed** and the lesion must be considered and treated as an occult invasive carcinoma of the cervix. Ng and Reagan (1969) reported that unicentric invasion in microinvasive carcinoma was observed in only 7.5% of cases.

The decision as to **whether or not a precancerous lesion is invasive** is sometimes very difficult in biopsy material, particularly when dealing with lesions with "pushy" borders. Several studies from our laboratories examined potentially useful markers to determine invasion in SIL (squamous intraepithelial lesion). Thus, Iskaros and Koss (2000) studied the expression of the **matrix protein tenascin** and suggested that its increased expression may be suggestive of invasion. Oktay et al (2003) studied **focal adhesion kinase (FAK)** with similar results. In the cases studied by Oktay, the expression of human papillomaviruses type 16 or 18 was not related to the expression of FAK.

Microinvasive carcinoma is generally asymptomatic, does not produce visible changes on the surface of the cervix and, therefore, its discovery is incidental to the search for precursor lesions. Ng and Reagan reported that

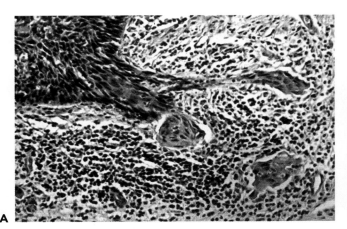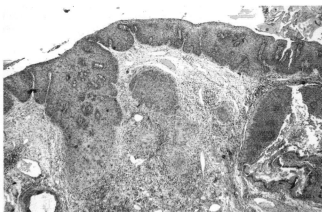

Figure 11-68   *A,B.* **Examples of microinvasive carcinoma.**

the average age at the time of discovery of microinvasive carcinoma is 6 years less than for fully invasive cancer. By serial or step sectioning of tissue blocks with precursor lesions, a number of **unsuspected microinvasive carcinomas** may be uncovered, ranging from 4.7% (Killackey et al, 1986), to 6% (Fidler and Boyes, 1959), to 8.4% (Ng and Regan, 1969). Such lesions are generally **considered to be of biologic interest rather than practical importance** because they can be successfully treated by LEEP (loop electrosurgical excise procedure) conization.

Cytology

In 1972, Ng et al suggested that a cytologic diagnosis of microinvasive epidermoid carcinoma of the uterine cervix can be made with a high degree of accuracy. These observers reported the following cytologic criteria of microinvasion based on a study of 52 patients:

- Presence of inflammation and necrosis ("tumor diathesis") in two-thirds of the cases
- Occurrence of most (75%) malignant cells in aggregates ("syncytia")
- Irregular distribution of nuclear chromatin in 50% of the cancer cells
- Presence of prominent nucleoli in 20% of the cancer cells

The same authors performed a planimetric study of cancer cells in microinvasive carcinoma, compared with cells from carcinoma in situ and fully invasive carcinoma. A number of features including cell area, nuclear area, several nuclear descriptors, and the total number of nucleoli per cell were intermediate between the two other lesions.

Subsequent studies were conflicting as to whether cytologic features are reliable in separating microinvasive carcinoma from a high-grade precursor lesion or invasive cancer. Thus, Rubio (1974) was unable to confirm Ng's data, whereas Nguyen (1984) was in partial agreement. In a more recent study of cervical smears in 28 patients with microinvasive carcinomas from the Netherlands, 2 lesions were missed, 3 were diagnosed as LGSIL (CIN I or II), 15 as HGSIL (CIN III), and 8 as "carcinoma" (Kok et al, 2000). There are no studies of this topic using liquid collection method.

Microinvasive carcinomas, in which the invasion is confined to one or two tongues of cancerous tissue invading the stroma, particularly those originating from low-grade lesions, are extremely unlikely to shed specific cell types suggestive of early invasion. **The lesions, with multiple foci of superficial invasion, may occasionally show smear patterns that are intermediate between a high-grade lesion (HGSIL) and invasive carcinoma. Such smears often contain a large number of dysplastic (dyskaryotic) and cancer cells, corresponding to a large lesion, and evidence of necrosis and inflammation.** One can also encounter, in such smears, **bizarre cell forms and a relatively large number of cancer cells with prominent nucleoli,** especially if the lesion is of endocervical derivation. For many years now, smears of this type have been classified in our laboratories as "squamous" or "epidermoid carcinoma—cannot rule out invasion," presumably an equivalent statement to Ng's "microinvasive carcinoma." The histologic findings in such cases were variable; about half of the patients harbored HGSIL without invasion, whereas in the remaining cases, varying degrees of invasion, including rare fully invasive carcinomas, were observed. Thus, in my experience, **the cytologic concept of microinvasive carcinoma has limited validity in the day-to-day practice of diagnostic cytology.**

INVASIVE SQUAMOUS CARCINOMA

Clinical Data and Indications for Cytologic Sampling

The **prognosis of invasive cancer of the uterine cervix** depends on **stage** of the disease (see Table 11-3). The prognostic significance of tumor **grade** is less secure, although high-grade tumors are likely to be more aggressive. Invasion of lymphatics, metastases to regional lymph nodes, and invasion of blood vessels, may occur in all types of cervical cancer and is considered to be of **unfavorable prognostic significance.** A prognostically **favorable** feature in stage I tumors is the presence of **lymphocytic infiltrate** in the stroma (Sidhu et al, 1970). Because women with low stages of the disease have a much better chance of survival than those with more advanced carcinomas, the discovery of the lesion in the earliest possible time is important to the patient. Hagmar et al (1995) correlated prognosis with types of human papillomaviruses; patients with HPV types 18 or 33 had a poorer prognosis and shorter survival than patients harboring other high-risk types of the virus.

Contrary to precursor lesions, which are usually not evident on visual speculum examination and require colposcopic identification, **advanced invasive cancers** of the uterine cervix usually produce **grossly visible changes** in the form of ulceration or a tumor of the cervix. Application of cytologic techniques to the diagnosis of clinically obvious invasive carcinoma is a diagnostic luxury since these lesions **should be diagnosed by biopsy.** However, many women are now first seen by family physicians or nurse-practitioners who may not have the same familiarity with the clinical presentation of invasive cancer as trained gynecologists. Consequently, some invasive cancers may pass unrecognized on clinical examination. **In such situations, listening to the patient is very important:** many women with early invasive cancer report bleeding, spotting, or dyspareunia. Still, **some invasive cancers, particularly those of low stage with intact surface and those originating in the endocervical canal, may fail to produce obvious gross changes and may be unrecognized,** even by an expert eye. An "erosion" or a reddened cervix bleeding on touch, often with some discharge, may be observed, and the diagnosis

of **"cervicitis"** or **"friable cervix"** is rendered. In these situations, a cytologic sample may prove to be life-saving by establishing the initial diagnosis **but, as is common in invasive cancer, the method may fail, resulting in a further diagnostic delay.** In many of the legal cases on behalf of women with severe damage to their health or even loss of life caused by cancer of the cervix, failure to biopsy the relatively inconspicuous abnormalities was followed by a failure of cytologic examination.

Adenocarcinomas and their variants are discussed in Chapter 12.

Histology

Invasive squamous cancer generally follows the patterns of the precursor lesions and may be classified histologically into three main groups:

■ **Well-differentiated (grade I), pearl-forming, keratinizing squamous carcinoma** (Fig. 11-69A). Keratin formation is the dominant feature of these tumors, which are otherwise composed of typical squamous cancer cells. As is the case with keratin-forming precursor lesions, most of these cancers **originate in the surface squamous epithelium of the cervix** and are preceded by low-

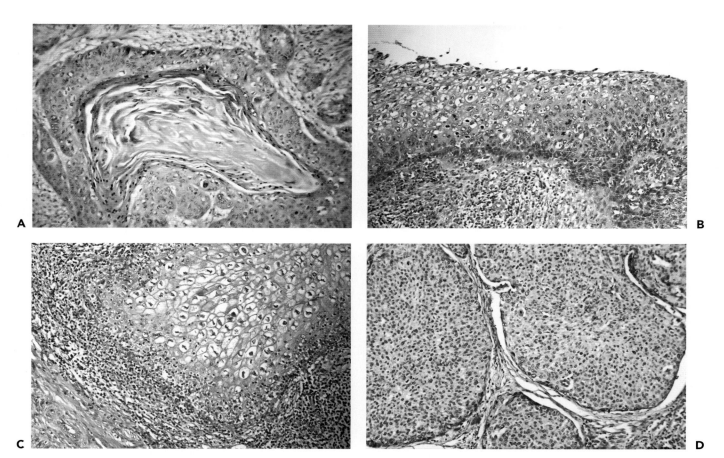

Figure 11-69   Invasive squamous carcinomas of cervix. *A.* Well differentiated carcinoma (grade I) with formation of large keratin deposits. *B,C.* High-grade squamous intraepithelial lesion with numerous koilocytes with transition to invasive carcinoma of similar configuration. *D.* Grade II squamous cancer.

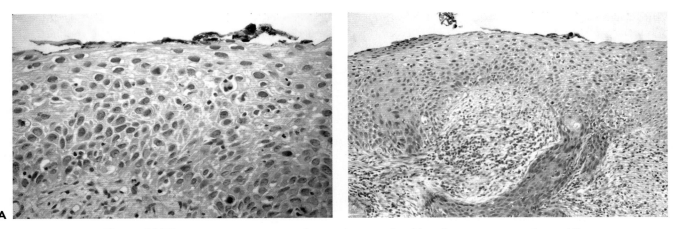

Figure 11-70 **Invasive squamous carcinoma.** An example of invasive squamous carcinoma (*A*) derived from a nearly normal surface epithelium (*B*).

grade precursor lesions. In some of these tumors, conspicuous koilocytes may be observed (Fig. 11-69B,C). Occasionally, invasive squamous cancers may originate in **quasi-normal squamous epithelium** (Fig. 11-70). Morrison et al (2001), in describing such rare lesions, noted their aggressive behavior and lack of association with human papillomavirus. A rare variant of squamous cancer is the **verrucous carcinoma** that may grossly resemble giant condylomata acuminata of Löwenstein-Buschke type of penile lesions (see Part 1 of the chapter). These tumors, which very rarely metastasize but may be deeply invasive, show only slight nuclear abnormalities (Fig. 11-71D) and have a relatively benign course after treatment (Morrison et al, 2001).

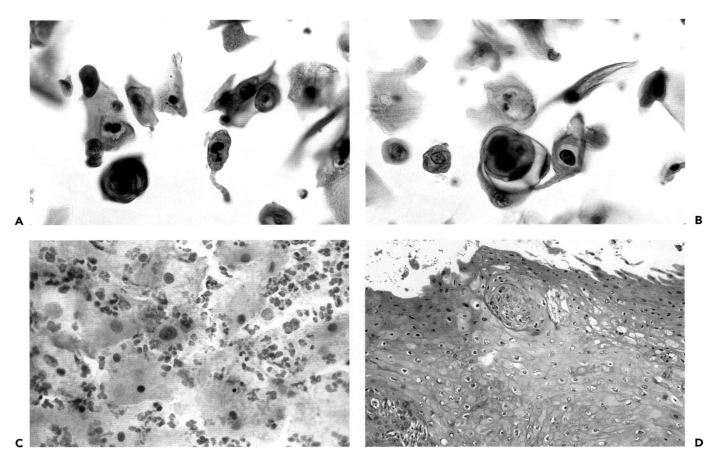

Figure 11-71 **Invasive squamous carcinoma.** *A,B.* Extraordinary variety of squamous cancer cells in a SurePath. *C,D.* Verrucous carcinoma of cervix. *C* shows atypical squamous cells that are characteristic of this disorder. The abnormality is limited to nuclear enlargement with slight hyperchromasia. *D* shows a biopsy of the cervical lesion with markedly keratinized surface.

- Medium-sized cell squamous (epidermoid) carcinoma, grade II, derived from high-grade lesions of metaplastic type (Fig. 11-72D). **The tumors are composed of sheets of cancer cells of relatively monotonous appearance but often contain foci of keratinizing squamous cancer, not evident in the precursor lesion** (see Fig. 11-67).
- Small cell carcinoma, grade III, derived from precursor lesions composed of small cells (Fig. 11-73D). The cancer cells are either arranged in nests separated by connective tissue septa or diffusely infiltrate the stroma. Some of these tumors have **endocrine function,** which is occasionally reflected in the formation of **rosette-like structures.** Still, electron microscopy and immunochemistry are required to establish their identity. In rare cases, the tumors may be **hormone-producing.** Thus, Kothe et al (1990) reported such a tumor secreting **antidiuretic hormone.** Iemura et al (1991) reported a case of **Cushing's syndrome** caused by a small-cell cervical carcinoma secreting ectopic adrenocorticotropin hormone. In a recently reported case, **hypoglycemia** was observed in a young patient with an insulin-secreting cervical carcinoma (Seckl et al, 1999). Watanabe et al (2000) re-

ported a case secreting **granulocyte-colony stimulating factor** in a 70-year-old woman with marked leukocytosis. Herrington et al (1999) reported that, in many tumors of this type, there is a loss of retinoblastoma (Rb) gene expression. Invasive squamous carcinomas may be either **"pure,"** composed of cells of only one type, or **"mixed,"** containing several types of cancer side by side. For example, **focal keratinization** with pearl formation and **focal gland formation** may occur in medium- or small-cell cancers. Some of the invasive cancers may show **unusual patterns,** discussed in Chapter 17.

Some of the **difficulties in cytologic recognition of invasive squamous cancer** were illustrated by a study of 43 such lesions from the Netherlands. Seven of the smears were considered to be negative on screening, 6 were reported as low-grade lesions, 15 as high-grade lesions, and only 15 smears were reported as invasive cancer. On review, 4 of the missed smears consisted only of inflammatory exudate, necrotic debris, and blood, in which no cancer cells could be identified. In three remaining missed cases, the evidence of cancer was very scanty and limited to a few cancer cells hidden in exudate. The classical features of invasive cancer

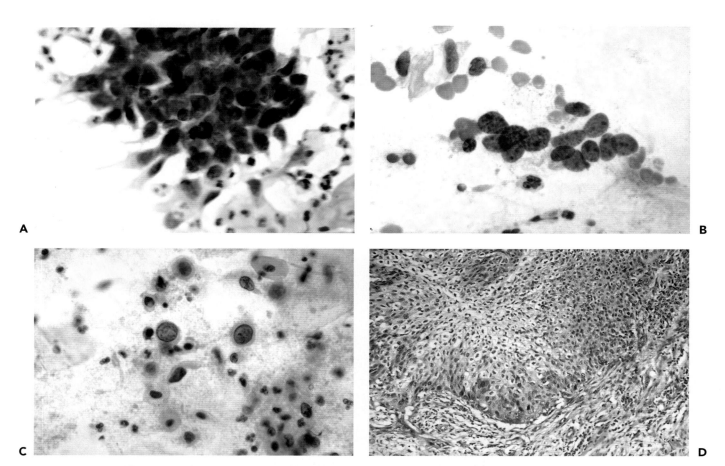

Figure 11-72 Invasive squamous carcinoma represented by medium-sized cancer cells. *A.* The dense cluster is composed of cancer cells of medium size. At the periphery of the cluster, some of the cancer cells are of columnar shape, an indication of endocervical origin. Note nuclear abnormalities. *B.* High magnification to show "naked" large cancer cell nuclei from an invasive carcinoma composed of medium-sized cells. *C.* Scattered cancer cells of medium size corresponding to the invasive carcinoma shown in *D.*

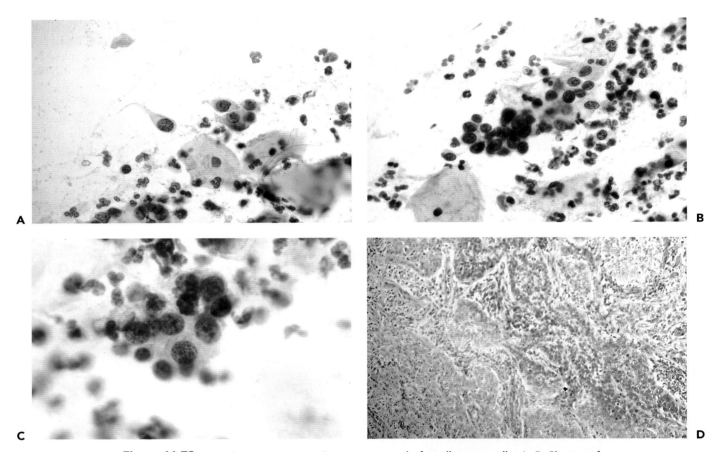

Figure 11-73   **Invasive squamous carcinoma composed of small cancer cells.** *A, B.* Clusters of tiny cancer cells easily overlooked on screening. *C.* A high-power view of one of the clusters showing irregular nuclear contour and granulation of chromatin. *D.* Tissue pattern corresponding to *A–C.*

were absent in most smears diagnosed as precursor lesions (Kok et al, 2000). Similar observations were reported by Levine et al (2003).

Cytology

The cytologic diagnosis of invasive squamous carcinoma is **often more difficult** than that of precursor lesions, because the preparations may **contain necrotic material, blood, and debris,** obscuring the often poorly preserved cancer cells. The term **"cancer diathesis"** has been applied to such features, which are a reflection of necrosis of the surface of invasive tumor. In such instances, a careful examination of the preparation with frequent use of a high-power objective may be necessary to avoid errors of omission. **Not all invasive cancers show "cancer diathesis," particularly those in early stages without surface necrosis.** In such instances, the cell sample may be difficult to interpret as invasive tumor.

Dysplastic (dyskaryotic) cells, including koilocytes, may be present in cytologic preparations from invasive squamous carcinomas and are sometimes the only evidence of disease. These cells are derived from areas of precursor lesions on the margin of invasive cancer but may also originate from the surface of a well-differentiated invasive keratinizing carcinoma. However, the predominant abnor-

mal cells are **differentiated and undifferentiated cancer cells,** displaying marked aberrations of the nucleus and the cytoplasm (see Figs. 11-72, 11-73; see also Figs. 11-37 to 11-39). This heterogeneous population of cancer cells is very characteristic of invasive cervical cancer (see Tables 11-8 and 11-9). **Cell necrosis, apoptosis, and aberrant mitotic figures may also be observed** in cytologic preparations (see Fig. 11-39D).

Another common feature of cytologic presentation of invasive cancer is the presence of **large sheets of cells or fragments of tumor** removed from the fragile surface, which are often too thick for a detailed microscopic study (see Fig. 11-72A). Nuclei stripped of cytoplasm (**"naked nuclei"**) are not uncommon (see Fig. 11-72B). In some cases, the large nuclei of cancer cells may be pale, bland, vesicular, and sometimes contain a single visible nucleolus (see Fig. 11-72C). The **large fragments of tumor should never be ignored or dismissed** but, rather, should be carefully examined, especially at their periphery (see Figs. 11-33C,D and 11-72A).

The cytologic identification of the three principal patterns of invasive carcinoma in smears is sometimes possible but is of limited clinical value. However, certain basic differences in cell types may be observed.

- **Keratinizing (squamous) carcinomas** shed mainly differentiated, keratinized, squamous cancer cells, some of which may closely resemble dysplastic (dyskaryotic) cells. Koilocytes may be present. In such tumors, squamous "pearls," spindly cancer cells, tadpole cells, and other bizarre cell types are common (see Fig. 11-37).

- **Keratinized debris (anucleated squames) may dominate the smear pattern** (see Fig. 11-39B). The extraordinary **diversity of cell types and shapes** can be very well documented in liquid preparations such as SurePath (see Fig. 11-71A,B).

It is sometimes very difficult to separate cytologically invasive carcinomas of this type from their noninvasive precursors in the absence of "cancer diathesis" because the cell populations may be so similar. Similar observations were reported by Levine et al (2003).

- The rare **verrucous squamous carcinomas** of the cervix may be **extremely difficult to recognize in the cytologic sample.** The squamous cancer cells are often very well differentiated and mimic normal squamous cells, except for some cytoplasmic keratinization and nuclear enlargement and pyknosis (see Fig. 11-71C). Cases of this tumor type shedding obvious cancer cells were reported by Fentanes de Torres and Mora (1981) and by Barua and Matthews (1983).
- The extremely rare squamous carcinomas derived from quasi-normal surface epithelium cannot be recognized in cytologic preparations.
- **The intermediate type of invasive carcinoma** often combines the features of all types of cancer cells. In some of these lesions, **dysplastic (dyskaryotic) cells of parabasal type, and medium-sized keratinized cancer cells predominate.** In other lesions, **undifferentiated cancer cells of medium sizes, singly and in clusters, form the bulk of the population of abnormal cells** (see Fig. 11-72). "Naked" cancer cell nuclei showing coarse chromatin patterns are fairly common (see Fig. 11-72B). In the majority of lesions, there is a mixture of various cell types side-by-side.
- **Small cell carcinomas** usually shed a relatively monotonous population of undifferentiated, small malignant cells, occurring singly or in small clusters (Fig. 11-73). Small columnar-shaped cancer cells are not an unusual finding (Fig. 11-73A). Such cells may display cytoplasmic vacuoles and, when numerous, the sample can be misclassified as adenocarcinoma. In the endocrine variant of this tumor, arrangement of cancer cells in rosettes may be occasionally observed but this is a very rare finding.
- As is the case with high-grade precursor lesions of small cell type, this type of invasive carcinoma causes the greatest difficulties of recognition because of the small size of the abnormal cells, sometimes obscured by blood and debris. This problem was illustrated in a paper by Zhou et al (1998) in which the cervical smears in 7 of 12 such lesions were reported as negative. On review, cancer cells were found in 2 of the 7 negative smears. The issue is discussed further below in reference to accuracy of cervical samples.

ATYPICAL SQUAMOUS OR GLANDULAR CELLS OF UNKNOWN SIGNIFICANCE: THE LEGACY OF THE BETHESDA SYSTEM

Ever since the introduction of cytologic screening over half a century ago, it has been known that there are daily instances in practice when a cervicovaginal preparation contains a few cells with relatively slight nuclear or cytoplasmic abnormalities that are difficult or impossible to interpret accurately. In the past, the term **atypia** sometimes accompanied by a comment guiding the clinician in further investigation of the patient, Papanicolaou's class II or, rarely, class III diagnoses, were used in such instances. Regardless of the system of reporting, such diagnoses created problems of clinical handling and caused anxiety in patients. In most such instances, the problem could be resolved one way or another by follow-up smears or sometimes by colposcopy and biopsies.

It must be stressed that some precursor lesions or invasive cervical cancer may be very difficult to recognize in smears with **extensive inflammation and necrosis** and may be represented by only a few abnormal cells. Some of these difficulties have been reduced by the use of liquid systems of processing.

In the original, 1991 Bethesda System, these terms have been replaced by the terms **atypical squamous cells of unknown significance (ASC-US)** and **atypical glandular cells of unknown significance (AGUS),** thus condemning the term "atypical smear" and Papanicolaou's classification to the heap of history. It was suggested, in reference to the ASC-US diagnoses, that a preference should be expressed as to whether the smear pattern was probably benign (reactive) or probably malignant. **It seems contradictory to the definition of "cells of *unknown* significance" to be further classified as either probably benign or possibly malignant.** In fact, Malik et al (1999), among others, found the subdivision of ASC-US in low-and high risk groups to be of limited value. Still, the concept of ASC-US and AGUS was accepted as "national standard" in the United States by the governmental agency, Centers for Disease Control in Atlanta, Georgia.

The 2001 Bethesda System modified these recommendations. **ASCUS** was subdivided into two categories: **(1) atypical squamous cells of undetermined significance (ASC-US) and (2) atypical squamous cells, cannot exclude high-grade squamous intraepithelial lesion (ASC-H)** (Sherman et al, 2004; Solomon et al, 2002; Solomon and Nayar, 2004). The ASC-H classification replaces the very useful **old term "suspicious,"** for smears with a small number of abnormal cells that, in the opinion of the cytopathologist, were insufficient for a diagnostic conclusion and required further clarification. **No separate provisions were made in the 2001 Bethesda System for ASC-US samples suggestive of, or suspicious of, LGSIL, apparently in the erroneous belief that such lesions can always be recognized or that they are harmless manifestations of HPV infection.** It was suggested that such cases should be included in the ASC-US category (Sherman et al, 2004). Pirog et al (2004) reported that elimination of the category ASC-US-reactive improved the performance of her laboratory.

The **AGUS** category was abolished and replaced with **"atypical glandular cells of endocervical, endometrial, or unknown origin"** that are either not further specified (NOS) or accompanied by a comment (Covell et al, 2004).

The term **ASC-US** was defined by Kurman and Solomon in 1993 as the presence of **intermediate squamous cells with nuclear enlargement 2½ to 3 times above that of a normal cell,** corresponding to the definition of **karyomegaly,** discussed in the early part of this chapter (see Fig. 11-30). The term **AGUS** was vaguely defined as **"changes in the endocervical cells that are intermediate between benign abnormalities and cancerous changes."** The latter abnormalities are discussed above in reference to squamous lesions located in the endocervical canal, and again in reference to precursor lesions of adenocarcinoma in Chapter 12. The old definition of AGUS did not mention cells of endometrial origin, discussed in Chapter 13.

Kurman and Solomon suggested in 1993 that the rate of ASC-US in a laboratory should not be higher than 2 to 3 times the rate of SIL. The source of this statement is not clear. However, in a survey of a large number of laboratories conducted by the College of American Pathologists, the rate of ASC-US was 2.8%, whereas the rate of SIL was 2.0% (Davey et al, 1996). In a subsequent survey, the rate of ASC-US rose to 5% (Davey et al, 2000).

As discussed in reference to karyomegaly, the definition of ASC-US, as proposed by Kurman and Solomon, is difficult to apply because it is subjective and limited to large squamous cells. For example, the presence of 6 or more such cells may indicate the presence of a squamous neoplastic lesion, usually LGSIL. The terms **ASC-L or "suspicious," are lacking in the Bethesda System. This is important inasmuch as significant lesions may be hiding behind the relatively insignificant cell abnormalities, as documented above.** Further, karyomegaly is not the only abnormality of note that may be difficult to interpret.

The term **ASC-H,** as illustrated by Sherman et al (2004), apparently pertains to **small dysplastic (dyskaryotic) cells** that should have been recognized as malignant (see Fig. 11-34) and to **metaplastic cells with enlarged nuclei** that may be the precursor of high-grade lesions (see Fig. 11-38). To be sure, in some cases, particularly in liquid preparations resulting in dispersion of such cells, the firm diagnosis cannot be established and requires further follow-up. The old term "suspicious" or class III smears corresponded to such findings.

Few events in the history of diagnostic cytology have had an impact as marked as the introduction of the terms ASC-US and AGUS. Dozens of papers have been published on this subject, mainly documenting that the **definitions are too vague to be universally accepted** and are not reproducible (Schiffman and Solomon, 2003; Confortini et al, 2003). Smith et al (2000) reported that a review of the Bethesda System Atlas by Solomon and Kurman (1993), by a panel of pathologists, did not improve the reproducibility or accuracy of classification of ASC-US. In fact, the **terminology has contributed significantly to the cost of cancer detection** by proposing expensive solutions, such as HPV testing (see below) that, so far, have not been shown to improve the detection system and reduce the mortality from cervix cancer in a documented fashion.

There are several reasons for the diagnosis of atypical smears, or its current Bethesda System equivalents. **Probably the most common cause for these diagnoses lies in the observer's lack of experience, timidity, or inability to identify accurately the cytologic patterns.** Sherman et al (2003) reported that among 171 women with documented CIN III or cancer 123 or 72% had initial smears classified as ASC-US, strongly suggesting that either the screening or the interpretation of this material was faulty. Zonky et al (1999) noted that 77% of high-grade lesions and invasive cancer were found after "minor" smear abnormalities. The term is also used as a **defensive measure** to avoid a potential legal entanglement (Austin 2003). In 2003, Schiffman and Solomon estimated 2 million cervical preparations will be classified as ASC-US in the United States.

There are instances, however, in which the diagnosis is justified because of cell changes that are difficult to classify. Some sources of atypical smears encountered over the years are listed below.

Abnormalities That Could Be Classified as ASC-US

- Karyomegaly: moderate or marked nuclear enlargement without marked hyperchromasia, limited to a few intermediate or large parabasal squamous cells (see discussion of karyomegaly in the opening pages of the second part of this chapter)
- Cytoplasmic vacuolization in intermediate squamous cells, suggestive, but not diagnostic, of koilocytosis (see Fig. 11-31D)
- Pattern of advanced atrophy of the cervix and vagina, particularly in the presence of "blue bodies," mimicking cancer cells (see Chap. 8)
- Inflammatory events, resulting in slight nuclear enlargement and pyknosis and slight irregularities of nuclear shape, such as observed in severe infestation with *Trichomonas vaginalis* or in herpetic infections (see Chap. 10)
- Metaplastic squamous cells with enlarged nuclei (see Chap. 10)
- Pattern of abnormal keratinization of squamous cells

Abnormalities That Could Be Classified as Atypical Endocervical Cells (Former AGUS)

- Endocervical cells with nuclear enlargement, slight hyperchromasia and enlarged nucleoli (see also Chaps. 10 and 12)
- Acute inflammatory and reactive phenomena in the epithelium of the endocervix, resulting in patterns of "repair" or florid metaplasia (see Chap. 10)
- Atypical, florid metaplasia (see Chap. 10)
- Thick clusters of endocervical cells (brush effect), difficult to classify (see Chap. 8)

What Should *Not* Be Classified as ASC-US or AGUS?

Over the years, we have seen a number of cervical smears diagnosed as "atypia," ASC-US, or AGUS, that did not merit this classification because they represented definitive lesions. Some of these findings were:

- A significant number of cells with karyomegaly (more than six in my experience) or related well-differentiated dysplastic superficial or intermediate squamous cells— such smears should be diagnosed as LGSIL
- Heavily keratinized squamous cells with somewhat enlarged, pyknotic nuclei that usually represent a keratin-forming malignant process
- Small dysplastic (dyskaryotic) cells, sometimes mimicking metaplastic cells, which should be classified as HGSIL
- Dense clusters ("syncytia") of small or large dysplastic (dyskaryotic) cells or cancer cells that represent a HGSIL or even invasive cancer

There are also benign abnormalities, discussed in Chapters 8 and 10, that may mimic a malignant lesion. Chief among them are:

- Pregnancy changes (see Chap. 8)
- Atrophic smears with atypia caused by dryness or containing "blue bodies"

Follow-up Studies of ASC-US, AGUS, or "Atypical Smears"

Before the introduction of the terms ASC-US and AGUS, there were several **follow-up studies** of patients with **atypical smears.** As early as 1976, Melamed and Flehinger reported a follow-up study of 1,973 women attending the Planned Parenthood clinics in New York City with "atypias" of squamous cells in cervicovaginal smears. The "atypias" were defined as **abnormalities of squamous cells not attributable to inflammation, yet not sufficient to establish the diagnosis of a neoplastic lesion.** The results documented that **"atypia" was a risk factor in the development of precancerous lesions of the cervix.** The probability of a neoplastic event in these women was calculated at 5 to 10 times higher than for women with negative smears. Women with **two sequential atypical smears had an approximately 10 times higher probability of subsequent CIN.**

The limited clinical value of the term **atypia** was brought sharply into focus by several older clinical studies. Scott (1964) and Nyirjesy (1972) recognized that hiding behind this terminology was a broad variety of important neoplastic events such as CIN, and occasionally, invasive cancer. Benedet et al (1976) reported that, among 320 patients with "Class II" smears (a numerical equivalent of benign atypia) there were 135 (42%) "dysplasias" of various degrees and 83 (25%) carcinomas in situ. Jones et al (1987) found 25% of CIN in 236 patients with diagnosis of "atypical" smears. Frisch et al (1987, 1990) pointed out that 12% of cervical smears from 200 young college students, diagnosed as "inflammatory epithelial changes," concealed CIN. The unifying theme of these studies was that **a substantial proportion of women, ranging from 12% to 25%, with a cytologic diagnosis of "atypia" or "inflammatory changes," harbor precancerous lesions or invasive cancer of the uterine cervix that can be detected by colposcopy and biopsies.**

Since the introduction of the Bethesda System, numerous papers reported the results of follow-up studies of patients with the cytologic diagnosis of ASC-US; in nearly all of them, some of the patients were shown to harbor squamous neoplastic lesions, usually of low-grade (70% to 95%) but some of high-grade, or even invasive cancers (Sidawy and Tabbara, 1993; Davey et al, 1994; Selvaggi and Haefner, 1995; Williams, 1997; Sidawy and Solomon, 1997). There are **significant differences in the percentage of HGSIL, invasive cancer reported in recent years from different laboratories.** The range is from none (Gonzales et al, 1996), 1% to 2% (Kobelin et al, 1998; Ettler et al, 1999; Malik et al, 1999; Sherman et al, 1999) to 9% or more (Kaufman, 1996; Auger et al, 1997; Nyirjersy et al, 1998; Raab et al, 1999). Rader et al (1999) pointed out that diagnosis of **ASC-US** in women age 55 or older is relatively uncommon (1.8% of 8,175 smears) but may also lead to the discovery of neoplastic lesions, ranging from LGSIL to invasive cancer, albeit in a lesser proportion than in younger women. In a very large Norwegian study of more than 500,000 women with 7 years of follow-up, Nygaard et al (2003) reported that women with ASC-US were 15 to 30 times more likely than normal women to develop a CIN III or invasive cancer of the cervix. Dvorak et al (1999) recommended an aggressive follow-up for women with ASC-US or LGSIL because of the large number of high-grade lesions hiding behind these diagnoses.

The disparities of the results from the various centers may be a reflection on the **population studied, definition and usage of the term ASC-US, the performance of the laboratory, and its philosophy of reporting "non-normal" material.** Some of these differences may be based on divergent interpretation of biopsies that varies from observer to observer and from laboratory to laboratory (Grenko et al, 2000).

It is of interest that the **high-grade lesions, observed in patients with ASC-US, are often very small in size and of questionable clinical significance** (Pinto et al, 2002; Sherman et al, 2003). Figure 11-74A summarizes the findings in ASC-US.

The AGUS category was abolished in the 2001 Bethesda System because of a very high rate of malignant events in this group of patients, summarized in Figure 11-74B, courtesy of Dr. Mary Sidawy. Although the abnormal cells were of endocervical type, the frequency of **SIL was significantly higher than that of adenosarcomas,** as previously discussed in this chapter. Bose et al (1994) reported 17 LGSIL, 18 HGSIL in 44 women whose smears were diagnosed as AGUS. Lee et al (1995) reported that the diagnosis of "severe glandular atypia" corresponded, in 26% of patients, to an endocervical adenocarcinoma and, in 53% of patients, to HGSIL. In patients diagnosed as

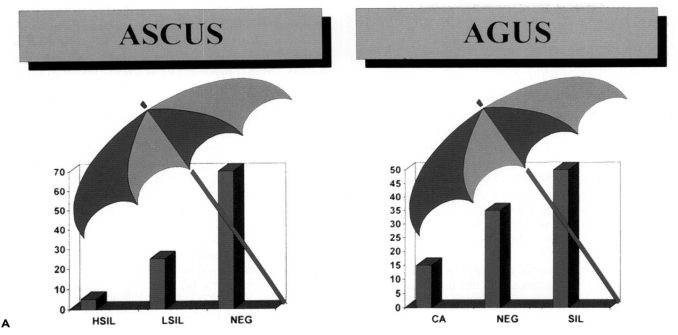

Figure 11-74 *A.* A diagrammatic drawing showing the proportion of high-grade lesions in smears designated as ASC-US. The number of high-grade malignant lesions is small. *B.* A diagrammatic drawing showing the outcome of smears diagnosed as AGUS. The number of malignant lesions is much higher than in the ASC-US series. (Courtesy of Dr. Mary Sidawy, Washington, DC.)

"mild glandular atypia," follow-up studies disclosed 2.5% adenocarcinoma in situ, 35% of HGSIL, 2.5% of LGSIL, with the remaining cases showing no significant lesions. Samsir et al (2003) reported that there is a very limited consensus among competent observers in classifying atypical glandular cells. **A particularly unfortunate diagnosis of AGUS is based on the finding of "atypical metaplasia," which, in most cases, represents a high-grade squamous lesion of endocervical origin, as discussed above.** For further discussion of AGUS as a precursor lesion of endocervical adenocarcinoma, see Chapter 12.

It is evident that the diagnoses of ASC-US, AGUS, or the equivalent term, **atypical smears,** is widely used but **should be avoided at all cost. In many such instances, a careful rescreening of the preparation or a consultation with a competent colleague may be helpful in eliciting a definitive diagnosis of either a benign lesion, CIN, or even invasive cancer.**

Still, in every laboratory, there is a **small residue of adequate cervical preparations that cannot be definitively classified because of scarcity of abnormal cells or because of cell changes that are difficult to interpret, that can justifiably be reported as ASC-US or AGUS.** Pitman et al (2002) reported that the abolition of AGUS would lead to a loss of about one-half of HGSILs. The current clinical approaches to the handling of such patients, including HPV typing, are discussed below.

REPRODUCIBILITY OF CYTOLOGIC DIAGNOSES IN CERVICAL SAMPLES

The interpretation of cytologic pattern in adequate cervical smears is often a major problem. There is a similarity here with mammography, another test based on visual assessment (Elmore et al, 1994). As has been documented in early studies by Seybolt and Johnson (1971), Koss (1982), Yobs et al (1985, 1987), Klinkhamer et al (1988), and others, **the reproducibility of cytologic diagnosis among various otherwise competent observers is low.**

The situation has not changed in recent years. Stoler and Schiffman (2001) observed only moderate reproducibility in the interpretation of liquid preparations (kappa value 0.46, 1 being complete agreement). Renshaw et al (2003), based on a very large number of responses from practicing pathologists, observed that the reproducibility of diagnoses was somewhat better for benign smear patterns and low-grade squamous lesions (LSIL) than for high-grade lesions (HGSIL) and invasive cancers. In 2004, Renshaw et al analyzed these results further and noted that the cell patterns in some invasive cancers were interpreted as "reparative," particularly in the presence of *Trichomonas* infestation. The problem lies often in philosophic approach to smear interpretation that separates the "conservative" from "aggressive" observers. Although the criteria for classification of cytologic samples may be verbalized and the key findings illustrated, as was done in the preceding pages, **the application of these principles depends on the training, experience, and talent of the observer.** Further, the infinite variety of morphologic patterns that may be observed in cervical samples often defies the classical standards of diagnosis. **The cytologic patterns that are most often underestimated are those of keratin-forming lesions, small-cell carcinomas, and invasive carcinomas of various types.** Also, smears containing only a few abnormal dysplastic (dyskaryotic) cells, as is often the case, are often undercalled and placed in the category of ASC-US.

The **reproducibility of diagnoses by the same observer** at various time intervals is also low. This was documented in an unpublished study by Wied, who submitted the same set of cervical smears to a group of expert cytopathologists (including this writer) at 6 month intervals. Quite often, on the second review, the observers disagreed with their own prior diagnosis. It is generally easier to achieve reasonable consistency of diagnoses among members of the same group than among different laboratories.

CORRELATION OF BIOPSIES WITH CYTOLOGIC PATTERNS

Although biopsies have been often considered to be the "gold standard" against which the cytologic diagnoses should be measured, this is often not the case. To be sure, errors in the assessment of cytologic samples do occur but there is evidence that, **in a significant proportion of cases, biopsy sampling and the interpretation of tissue patterns are often inaccurate and not necessarily superior to cytology.** Tritz et al (1995) reported discrepancies between cytologic and histologic diagnoses in 69 (11%) of 615 patients with a cytologic diagnosis of a neoplastic abnormality. **The most common source of error was inappropriate biopsy that missed the lesion in 51%, followed by faulty biopsy interpretation that occurred in 13% of the discordant cases.** Similar observations were reported by Joste et al (1995), Rasbridge and Nayagam (1995) and Stoler and Schiffman (2001).

Jones and Novis (1996) studied the **correlation of diagnoses** rendered on cervical **smears with biopsies** in 348 American laboratories. In 22,439 paired smears and biopsies, the **sensitivity of cytologic findings** was 89.4%, **specificity** 64.8% and **predictive value** of positive cytology 88.9%. It was noted that the knowledge of results of cytology improved the accuracy of biopsy interpretation. There is also **extensive documentation** that the interpretation of biopsies **may vary from one observer to another.** In a classical study, Siegler (1956) selected 20 biopsies of the uterine cervix, showing fairly classical carcinoma in situ (HGSIL) to 25 pathologists. Approximately half of the diagnoses were missed by the participants, with some failing to recognize any of the lesions. Although the study was conducted before widespread use of cervical smears and may be, in part, explained by limited exposure of pathologists to these lesions, the observations were confirmed in later years by Holmquist et al (1967), Cocker et al (1968), and Robertson et al (1989). These problems persist until today (year 2005). In a recent study of difficult-to-interpret biopsies showing "atypical immature metaplastic proliferations," the diagnostic concordance between two observers working in the same laboratory as to the benign or malignant nature of these lesions was, at best, mediocre (Park et al, 1999). Grenko (2000) also reported lack of agreement among experienced pathologists in the interpretation of cervical biopsies.

There are **several situations where a biopsy can be misinterpreted or the lesion missed.** These are listed below:

- Inadequate sampling of the cervix by inexperienced colposcopists. This is particularly important when the lesion is located in the endocervical canal.
- Interpretation of endocervical curettings, wherein tiny fragments of a high-grade lesion are readily overlooked.
- Interpretation of endometrial curettings containing fragments of a squamous malignant lesion, derived from the uterine cervix, that are either overlooked or sometimes interpreted as decidual reaction.
- Interpretation of biopsies in postmenopausal women may also cause difficulties, particularly when the fragments of CIN are atrophic. As has been stated above, the term "transitional cell metaplasia" is a misnomer in the interpretation of atrophic CIN lesions in this group of patients.
- An important source of errors is inadequate training in the interpretation of cervical biopsies which is prevalent among pathologists who have no experience with cytology of the cervix or those who were instructed that the interpretation of intraepithelial neoplastic lesions of the cervix should be conservative in order to avoid unnecessary treatment. Many of these observers use the term "dysplasia" and strenuously avoid the use of terms such as high-grade lesion, CIN III, or carcinoma in situ.

ACCURACY OF CERVICAL SAMPLES IN THE DETECTION OF SQUAMOUS LESIONS

Preceding its introduction as a mass-screening procedure, the effectiveness of cervicovaginal cytology **as a means of detection of precancerous lesions and early cancer of the uterine cervix had never been tested in a double blind study** (Koss 1989). **The performance of the system has been judged by its effectiveness, based on epidemiologic studies, showing that the rate of invasive cancers among screened women fell by about 75%.** Because the majority of women who developed invasive cancer of the uterine cervix had no previous screening, **it has been assumed by many clinicians and by the lay public that the "Pap smear" had a high degree of accuracy.**

Further, the assumption that careful analysis of smear patterns **in satisfactory cytologic material** allows a precise **classification of the underlying precursor lesion has been incorporated into the Bethesda System.** Regrettably, this is not the case, because **the margin of error in such assessments may be substantial,** as has been repeatedly documented by a careful correlation of cytologic diagnoses with histologic material and will be illustrated below.

As early as 1964, Navratil from Graz, Austria, reported smear failure in 15% of precancerous lesions diagnosed by colposcopy. Hill (1966) reported from the same clinic that cervical smears failed in 59 (7%) of 838 cases of precancerous lesions of the cervix. A startling indictment of cytology as the tool for cervical cancer detection was presented from Sweden by Rylander (1976), who reported the Stockholm experience for the years 1968 through 1974. Of the 179 women with invasive cervical cancer, 143 had the benefit of early competent cytologic examination. In 64 (44%) of the 144 women, earlier smears were reported as "negative." In 13 of these patients, invasive cervix cancer occurred within 1 year, in 23 within 2 years, in 17 within 3 years, and in 11 within 4.5 years after the negative smear. Thus, it is likely that at least some of these patients had precancerous lesions or early cancer at the time of screening. Because Stockholm's laboratories enjoyed an excellent reputation, Rylander's publication should have elicited a major outcry but it did not. These European reports were ignored in the US because the competence of the cytology laboratories was unknown.

However, the review of the American literature from the years 1970–1983 clearly shows that failures of the cervical smears as a case-finding procedure were also recognized in the United States. Thus, Figge et al (1970), Gunn and Gould (1973), Shulman et al (1974), and Fetherstone (1983) reported that cervical smears failed in recognizing a substantial proportion of precancerous lesions or invasive cancer diagnosed by biopsy. The accuracy of the cervix cancer detection system was questioned by Foltz and Kelsey (1978). Again, these reports were ignored.

However, the issue was brought into sharp focus when an investigative journalist, Walt Bogdanicz, reported in the *Wall Street Journal* on November 2, 1987, that young women were dying of cervix cancer because of laboratory errors. He received a Pulitzer prize for his reporting. Perhaps because of the type of readership that the *Wall Street Journal* enjoys, Bogdanicz's report resulted in a flurry of legislative activity in the Congress of the United States, "to protect the American women from bad laboratories." The resulting legislation, enacted in 1988, is the Amendment to the Clinical Laboratory Improvement Act, known as CLIA 88, which put the performance of the laboratories processing cervicovaginal material under Federal jurisdiction. The practical issues pertaining to laboratory operation, resulting from CLIA 88 are discussed in Chapter 44.

The Bogdanicz report also elicited the interest of attorneys representing women whose injuries (and sometimes death from invasive cancer of the uterine cervix), were allegedly caused by misinterpretation of cervical smears. Subsequently, a flurry of legal proceedings against pathologists and laboratories took place, sometimes with substantial monetary penalties assessed by juries. All these events led to a thorough re-examination of laboratory performance in cervicovaginal cytology, casting new light on the effectiveness of cervicovaginal cytology. **It became rapidly apparent that errors of omission (false-negative smears) and, to a much lesser extent, errors of commission (false-positive smears) occur in virtually every laboratory of cytology,** although the rate of these errors may vary significantly among them. The detection and classification of cytologic abnormalities in cervicovaginal material, whether in the form of direct smears or material prepared from liquid samples, belongs to the most **difficult human tasks.** In an average laboratory, at least 90% of preparations show no findings of note and require no further action. Therefore, only a relatively small proportion of cytologic samples contain abnormal cells that may be few in number, small in size,

difficult to interpret or obscured by benign cells, blood, inflammatory exudate or debris. The identification of such cells or cell clusters under screening power of the microscope requires a high level of undivided attention of the screener, which is difficult to maintain over a period of many hours of work. Further, the decision whether the observed abnormalities are of benign or malignant nature may also cause substantial problems.

ERRORS IN THE INTERPRETATION OF CYTOLOGIC SAMPLES

False-Negative Smears

Numerous papers have been published at the end of the 20th century examining the rate and causes of false-negative smears. Only a few key contributions will be analyzed. An important early study by van der Graaf et al (1987) was based on a second review of **prior negative smears** in 555 women (out of a total screened population of 165,185 women) who 3 years later were shown to have biopsy-documented moderate or severe dysplasia, carcinoma in situ or invasive cancer. On review 12.3% of the smears were considered inadequate, 58.3% were found to be "atypical," and **29.3% of the smears contained missed evidence of "dysplasia" or "carcinoma in situ."** The study did not address the issue of the sources of errors, whether caused by **faulty sampling, screening, or interpretation, but it did document that the performance of a reputable laboratory is fraught with considerable error. The manner in which this error is assessed is important.** If the error were to be calculated as a percentage of smears missed in the entire screened population of 165,185 women, it becomes minuscule. If, however, the error is calculated as a proportion of lesions missed, as shown in Table 11-10, it becomes substantial. **The only meaningful way of presenting data on false-negative smears is as a percentage of biopsy-documented abnormalities.**

There were several studies showing that there is a **substantial false-negative rate** (20% to 30%) of cervicovaginal smears in patients with biopsy-documented invasive carcinomas of the uterine cervix (Troncone and Gupta, 1995; Tabbara and Sidawy, 1996; Bergeron et al, 1997; Kok et al, 2000). All these studies documented that approximately three-quarters of the previously negative smears showed, on review, some degree of cytologic abnormality. Relatively few of these false-negative smears showed evidence of HGSIL (20% in the Bergeron study). Most of these **"false-negative" smears showed either evidence of LGSIL or of ASCUS.**

Mitchell and Medley (1995) and O'Sullivan et al (1998) noted that the **small size of cancer cells and their scarcity in smears** are major sources of false-negative smears. Fewer than 200 abnormal cells in a preparation is an important source of diagnostic errors. Montes et al (1999) considered the presence of "atypical metaplastic cells" as the source of diagnostic difficulty in negative smears of women who subsequently developed HGSIL. These cells were discussed above.

TABLE 11-10

RELATIVE INCIDENCE OF HISTOLOGICALLY CONFIRMED PRECANCEROUS LESIONS OF THE CERVIX IN YOUNG WOMEN IN 8 STUDIES

Author	Year	Population Studied (All patients below the age of 20)	Rate of "Other than Negative" Cytology	Rate of Histologically Confirmed Precancerous Lesions (Dysplasia and Carcinoma in Situ)
Ferguson	1961	2,300	33.4/1,000	14.3/1,000
Kaufman et al.	1970	10,246	29.4/1,000	4.8/1,000
Wallace and Slankard	1973	7,520	6.7/1,000	5.8/1,000
Snyder et al.	1976	27,508	8.9/1,000	2.7/1,000
Fields et al.	1976	33,641	42/1,000	Unknown*
Personal data (Hein et al.)[†]	1977	403[†]	35/1,000	3.4/1,000 (mainly LGSIL)
Rader et al.	1997	630	10/1,000 (ASCUS)	5/1,000
Moscicki et al.	2001	605 (496 HPV positive)	Unknown	21/1,000 (LGSIL only in HPV positive women)

* Only a few of 58 patients with cytologic suspicion of a precancerous lesion were referred for diagnosis. Seven dysplasias and four carcinomas in situ were confirmed and treated.
[†] Girls, ages 12 to 16, mean 15.

An authoritative review, encompassing 312 laboratories of cytology in the United States that volunteered for this survey, was presented by Jones (1995). On rescreening of 3,762 smears in women who developed biopsy-documented high-grade intraepithelial lesions or invasive cancer, about **10% of smears were false-negative. If the diagnoses of ASCUS or AGUS were included as diagnostic mistakes, the error rate rose to about 20%.** An analysis of the sources of errors disclosed several components, such as **adequacy of sampling, accuracy of screening, and adequacy of interpretation.** These will be discussed in sequence.

Adequacy of the Cervical Sample as a Source of False-Negative Results

The definition of an adequate cytologic sample was provided in Chapter 8. Briefly, such material should contain cells **representative of the exo- and endocervix but is age-related.** The interpreters of the Bethesda System, Kurman and Solomon (1994), defined **an adequate smear as a smear with "at least 10% of the slide surface covered by well preserved and visualized squamous cells and at least two clusters of five endocervical cells representing the transformation zone and the endocervical epithelium." These minimal criteria are clearly arbitrary and are not applicable to postmenopausal women with atrophy** (see Chap. 8). For smears not meeting these minimal criteria, the Bethesda System offers the option of considering the cervical sample as either **unsatisfactory (rejected) or examined and found unsatisfactory** for whatever reason.

Specimen adequacy in liquid preparations is rather poorly defined. Solomon et al (2002) suggested that 5,000 well preserved squamous cells per preparation constitute an adequate liquid sample. The scientific evidence supporting this statement was not cited. The presence of endocervical cells in such preparations, as a criterion of adequacy, was not specifically discussed.

Several papers addressed the issue of **inadequate material** as a source of false negative errors, based on review of earlier "negative" smears in women developing high-grade lesions or carcinoma. Gay et al (1985), van der Graaf et al (1987), Sherman and Kelly (1992), Davey et al (1994), Mitchell and Medley (1995), and Kok et al (2000) observed that **some "false-negative" cervical smears contained no abnormal cells.** The rate of such smears varied from one laboratory to another but the average was about 10% to 12%. Most such smears were considered to be **sampling errors. This is not necessarily correct; adequate samples can also be false negative, apparently because some lesions do not shed abnormal cells.** Richart (1964) estimated that 1.4% of precancerous lesions fall into this category. During the follow-up studies of precursor lesions and reported in detail in Part 1 of the chapter (Koss et al, 1963), some patients with known intraepithelial lesions had interval smears free of abnormal cells (see Fig. 11-22). The reasons for these observations are not clear and may be related to the adhesiveness of the cells within the abnormal epithelium. Rubio and Lagerlöf (1975) suggested that energetic douching or cleansing of the cervix prior to sampling may account for some of these events. However, regardless of cause, the absence of abnormal cells in a cytologic preparation **cannot always be blamed on the smear taker.**

Ransdell et al (1997) reported that 16% of sequential patients with "unsatisfactory" smears were shown, on follow-up, to harbor a neoplastic lesion.

Unusual Presentation of Abnormal Cells

Poorly preserved, inadequately fixed or stained material may be the cause of false negative smears. Another, less common, source of error is caused by the excessive zeal of clinicians who remove **fragments of precancerous lesions or invasive cancer** by energetic sampling. These fragments, sometimes true **minibiopsies,** may be very difficult to interpret in smears or liquid preparations and are sometimes **ignored or considered to be fragments of benign endocervical or endometrial epithelium.** Lesions composed of medium or small cancer cells are usually the source of such fragments. In most cases, the fragments are accompanied by a scattering of other abnormal cells, occurring singly or in small clusters, leading to the correct diagnosis, but sometimes the single cells are absent and a lesion is missed on screening. In my experience, this occurs more often in postmenopausal women with fragile atrophic epithelial lesions (see above).

Boon et al (1993, 1994) reported the use of a **confocal microscope** to study the thick cell clusters. This costly and difficult-to-use instrument allows the inspection of component cells, layer by layer, and allows recognition of nuclear abnormalities.

Accuracy of Screening

The detection and classification of cytologic abnormalities in cervicovaginal material, whether in the form of direct smears or material prepared from samples collected in a liquid medium, belongs among the most **difficult human tasks.** In an average laboratory, at least 90% of preparations show no findings of note and require no further action. Therefore, only a relatively small proportion of cytologic samples contain abnormal cells that may be few in number, small in size, and obscured by benign cells, blood, inflammatory exudate or debris. The identification of such cells or cell clusters under screening power of the microscope requires a high level of undivided attention of the screener that is difficult to maintain over a period of many hours of work. Further, the decision whether the observed abnormalities are of benign or malignant nature may also cause substantial problems.

Early personal experience with a large population of Planned Parenthood clients, conducted in the 1960s (Melamed et al, 1969), disclosed a first-smear miss rate of about 30% of precursor lesions that were diagnosed on subsequent smears obtained within 6 to 12 months. Because, at that time, the issue of false-negative smears was not urgent, only an aliquot of the original first smears was reviewed. Substantial cytologic abnormalities, missed on screening, were

found in nearly all of these smears. The observations were not published.

Several recent studies addressed the question of screening errors. The results of a **second review of smears** of women considered to be at **"high risk"** performed at Montefiore Medical Center is shown in Table 11-11 (Koss, 1993). The procedure is described below. It may be noted that approximately 25% of all smears were reviewed and that, in this population, the **average screening error** for the years 1989–1992, **as a percentage of abnormal smears, was 3.9%. These errors were prevented by rescreening.** Jones (1995), in a large American study, reported that faulty screening accounted for 74.8% of the errors on 544 smears reported as "negative." Sherman and Kelly (1992), Hatem and Wilbur (1995), and Mitchell and Medley (1995) reported that the **most important common denominator of false-negative smears was the small-cell lesion. Single small cancer cells and dense clusters were most likely to be overlooked or misinterpreted on screening.** This has also been our experience. Other causes of errors leading to false-negative smears are shown in Table 11-12. **Poor recognition of keratinized abnormal squamous cells and underestimation of the significance of clusters of atypical metaplastic cells, sometimes classified as "repair," are of special significance.**

Errors of Interpretation

This issue is rarely addressed in the literature because accurate data are difficult to come by. In the Jones study (1995), **135 of 195 (69.2%) of false-negative smears, initially considered as "benign atypia," were misinterpreted** by the pathologists. Duggan and Brasher (1999) documented that, in 449 cervical smears diagnosed as LGSIL, about 7% were undercalled and 12.5% were overcalled, for an overall 80% accuracy rate for 14 Canadian laboratories. Errors of screening and interpretation accounted for most mistakes. Anecdotal evidence suggests that pathologists, without prior special training and supervised experience in cytopathology of the female genital tract, are most likely to misinterpret the evidence. One of the **essential ingredients** in the interpretation of cervical cytologic material is **time.** The interpretation of a difficult preparation may require 10 or 15 minutes of careful review of the evidence and its analysis, a true

TABLE 11-11

RESULTS OF PROSPECTIVES RESCREENING OF CERVICOVAGINAL SMEARS FOR 1989–1991

Year	Total of smears	Total rescreened (%)	Total suspicious/ positive smears (%)	False-negative (%)*
1989	14,851	2,822 (19)	495 (100)	13 (2.6)
1990	13,837	4,245 (30.7)	532 (100)	19 (3.6)
1991	14,433	3,307 (22.9)	666 (100)	34 (5.1)
Total	43,121	10,374 (24.0)	1,693 (100)	66 (3.9)

* Calculated as percentage of all suspicious/positive smears.
(From Koss LG. Cancer 71:1406–1422, 1993, with permission.)

TABLE 11-12

COMMON SOURCES OF FALSE-NEGATIVE CERVICAL SMEARS

Problem	Solution
Nuclear enlargement in a few intermediate squamous cells (Fig. 12-1).	Either a LGSIL or ASC-US, depending on the number of such cells
Heavily keratinized nucleated squamous cells, regardless of degree of nuclear abnormality	Consider keratinized squamous neoplastic lesion (either in situ or invasive)
Metaplastic cells with nuclear enlargement and nucleoli	Repair reaction, atypical metaplasia, or HGSIL, depending on the severity of the nuclear abnormality and configuration of cell clusters
Endocervical cells with large nuclei and nucleoli	Repair reaction, HGSIL located in endocervical canal, or endocervical neoplasia (see Chap. 12)
Cytolysis with isolated large nuclei	Could be LGSIL with cytolysis; search for well-preserved dyskaryotic cells
Smears obscured by blood or heavy inflammatory exudate	Careful screening is required. Invasive carcinoma must be ruled out
Dense clusters of small or very small cells, mimicking leukocytes	Consider small-cell carcinoma; look for single small cancer cells
Fragments of necrotic tissue in smears; not otherwise interpretable	Consider the possibility of invasive carcinoma; search for abnormal nuclei and nucleoli
Thick clusters of endocervical cells in brush specimens	Could be brush artifact. Search for isolated atypical cells; do not repeat such smears
"Pale dyskaryosis"	for 3 months

SIL, squamous intraepithelial lesion; HG, high grade; LG, low grade; ASC-US, atypia of squamous cells of unknown significance.

luxury in the medical climate that requires cost-controlled efficiency on the part of the laboratory personnel.

False-Positive Cytologic Samples

False-positive cervicovaginal samples are relatively uncommon but may be the cause of considerable anxiety in patients and their caretakers. There are two situations when such events occur: **a sample showing clear evidence of a malignant lesion is not confirmed by biopsies, and misinterpretation of a benign process by the cytopathologists.**

■ **Lack of confirmation of a neoplastic lesion by biopsies may have multiple causes,** which were discussed above in reference to correlation of biopsies with cervical samples. The most common cause is **inadequate biopsy** of the uterine cervix. In such cases, the procedure **requires a review of the cytologic sample and of the biopsies, preferably by a second expert observer.** Sometimes the review of the original biopsy material (and recuts) will solve the dilemma because a lesion will be found. If the biopsy review fails to reveal a lesion and **the review of the smear confirms the original opinion, additional sampling of the uterine cervix that may require a conization are indicated.** If, as it sometimes happens, these precautionary common sense procedures fail to reveal a lesion, further **follow-up of the patient by additional**

cytologic procedures is mandatory. Sometimes, several years of follow-up may be required before the presence of a lesion is documented. Anderson and Jones (1997) documented patients with abnormal smears and initial lack of confirmation by biopsy require long follow-up to discover occult neoplastic lesions. In some cases, the neoplastic lesions may be located **in the vagina or the endometrium or may even sometimes represent a metastatic cancer.**

■ **Removal of the entire lesion by energetic brushings** has been observed, resulting in **biopsies with denuded surface.** Another source of error may be **postmenopausal atrophy** in which the **atrophic lesion** is not recognized or considered to be a "crush artifact" as we have repeatedly observed (see above).

■ **True false-positive reports are usually based on misinterpretation of the evidence in the cytologic sample. The most important causes** of such errors are listed in Table 11-13. A second review of such cell samples by a second observer and a correlation with clinical data is mandatory in such cases.

Finally, there is a residue of patients in whom no evidence of disease will be found on long-term follow-up. It is likely that, in such cases, a small focus of disease has been destroyed during the bioptic procedures or that the lesion regressed.

TABLE 11-13

COMMON SOURCES OF FALSE-POSITIVE CERVICAL SMEARS

Findings	Solution
Clusters of endocervical cells with large nuclei and nucleoli	Repair or endocervical neoplasia. Search for single abnormal cells—if present consider neoplasia
Single endocervical cells with large hyperchromatic nuclei, no nucleoli	The patient may be pregnant (Arias-Stella cells) or receiving contraceptive medication with high progesterone content (see Chap. 18)
Ciliated endocervical cell with atypical nuclei	Tubal metaplasia, or rare carcinomas
Atrophic smear with isolated large, dark structures	The so-called "blue bodies" (see Chap. 8)
Atrophic smear with markedly enlarged nuclei in a few squamous cells	Could be atrophy or SIL. Short course of estrogen therapy may solve the problem
Intermediate squamous cells with perinuclear halo, no significant nuclear enlargement	Trichomoniasis (search for parasite) or poorly developed koilocytosis (ASC-US) [search for other evidence of HPV infection]
Multinucleated cells with pyknotic nuclei	Herpes. Search for more classical cell changes (see Chap. 10)
Large squamous cells with cytoplasmic or nuclear vacuoles	Clinical history, radiotherapy, or chemotherapy (see Chap. 18)
Large, dense clusters of endocervical cells with frayed edges	May be brush artifact or endocervical lesion (see Chap. 13)
Clusters of endometrial cells, particularly in brush specimens	May be mistaken for carcinoma. Check menstrual history and estrogen level

SIL, squamous intraepithelial lesion; ASC-US, atypia of squamous cells of unknown origin; HPV, human papillomavirus.

FAILURES OF CERVICAL SAMPLES AS A FOLLOW-UP PROCEDURE

It is customary in many laboratories to suggest that the cervical smear be repeated to confirm a prior ASCUS, AGUS, or "atypical" smear. Studies of patients from Planned Parenthood of New York City conducted from 1967 to 1970 (Melamed et al, 1969) required that a suspicious or positive cervical smear be followed by biopsies or diagnostic conizations of the cervix. As a routine procedure, a second smear was obtained just prior to conization. **In approximately 40% of patients with histologically proven carcinoma in situ, the second smear, usually obtained within 3 months or less after the original diagnosis, showed no evidence of abnormal cells.** Similar anecdotal observations were recorded by Nyirjesy (1972), Rylander (1976), and Rubio (1974). Follow-up studies of precursor lesions (Koss et al, 1963) also documented that repeat smears are often negative in the presence of biopsy-documented lesions. A study by Wheelock and Kaminski (1989) also pointed out that at least 40% of "repeat" smears obtained prior to colposcopy failed to reflect the underlying CIN. The issue was studied extensively by Bishop et al (1997) **who pointed out that the sensitivity of repeat cervical smears was low until 120 days have elapsed between smears,** in keeping with prior observations (Koss 1989).

Several important **conclusions of clinical significance** can be reached as a consequence of these observations:

- Follow-up cytologic sampling, within less than 4 months after the original equivocal smear, may result in false-negative smears in a large proportion of patients.
- Short-term follow-up by cytology may be highly misleading; a negative sample, or even two, does not necessarily indicate that the lesion has regressed. A minimum of 3 negative smears over a period of at least 2 years is required before the patient can be assured that she is free of disease.
- The patients should be referred for colposcopy on the strength of the highest cytologic diagnosis, which is often obtained in the first sample.

ATTEMPTS TO IMPROVE THE RESULTS OF SCREENING OF CERVICAL SMEARS

Sampling Instruments

Papanicolaou's early work in cervical cancer detection was based on examination of vaginal pool samples in which the evidence of cytologic abnormalities was much diluted. The lesions were discovered because of painstaking and time-consuming screening and search for single abnormal cells, often hidden among the multitude of benign cells. The instruments currently available for sampling are described in the Appendix to Chapter 8. With the introduction of the cervical spatula and, hence, direct cervical smears by Ayre in 1947, the task of screening became easier because of a greater concentration of abnormal cells in the targeted sample and less contamination with benign cells. It was soon documented that even the cervical smears failed to uncover a certain proportion of precancerous lesions or invasive cancer (see above). Hence, the search began for an ideal sampling device that, with a minimum of screening effort, would provide the most accurate cytologic diagnosis. To improve the sampling procedure, a number of **endocervical brushes and brush instruments, combining sampling of exo- and endocervix, were introduced** (see Fig. 8-45). Several early observers, notably Vooijs et al (1985), Boon et al (1986, 1989), and Deckert et al (1988) provided evidence that, in the presence of endocervical cells secured by brushes, the rate of detection of precancerous lesions of squamous and endocervical type rose. These observations led to a more precise definition of adequacy of the samples, discussed in Chapter 8 and above. However, the use of these instruments is not always totally harmless. Some of the problems that may occur after vigorous brushings are as follows:

■ **Energetic brushing** may cause bleeding.

■ **Spreading the sticky material** on a slide may be difficult, resulting in thick clusters of endocervical cells that may be difficult to interpret (see Fig. 10-12). Such clusters may have frayed edges and may mimic "feathering," a feature observed in some endocervical adenocarcinomas (see Chap. 12).

■ **Repetition of such smears** within a few days or weeks after the original sampling may result in a repair reaction that may also cause problems of interpretation difficult to interpret (see Fig. 10-9). Some of the problems associated with slide preparation and interpretation of brush samples have been solved by placing brushes in liquid fixative for processing (see below).

■ **Vigorous sampling** of the upper reaches of the endocervical canal may yield endometrial cells or cells derived from tubal metaplasia that may cause significant difficulties of interpretation (see Chap. 10).

Use of Two Synchronous Smears

Sedlis et al (1974) were the first to study the yield of two cervical smears obtained one after another and independently evaluated on a large cohort of more than 17,000 women. These observers noted that the **failure rate of detection of high-grade lesions was about 25%, either in the first, or in the second set of smears.** Subsequently, several observers, notably Shulman et al (1975), Davis et al (1981), Beilby et al (1982), and others, confirmed that the addition of a second cervical smear increases the yield of cytologic diagnoses of CIN by about 20%. Unfortunately, this relatively simple procedure adds to the costs of screening

and, therefore, found little following in the days of managed care. Still, this is an effective screening system, less expensive than liquid-based cell collection.

Second Review of Smears on High-Risk Patients

In 1989, Mr. Paul Elgert, who was then the Chief Cytotechnologist at Montefiore Medical Center, instituted a quality control measure based on **second review of all cervical smears from "high risk" examinees.** For each patient, a computer print-out of past history or current clinical data were obtained. **Patients referred by clinics for sexually transmitted disease, patients infected with human immunodeficiency virus (HIV), patients with AIDS, and patients with a past history of cytologic or biopsy abnormalities were considered to be "high risk."** All "negative" smears from such patients were reviewed by a second competent observer. The results of a 3-year study, shown in Table 11-11, documented a surprisingly large number of screening errors (3.9% of abnormal smears) that were uncovered by this measure. Because a very high percentage (about 25%) of patients seen at the Montefiore Medical Center fall into the "high risk" category this percentage may be lower in laboratories in different geographic locations. **Nonetheless, the smears from this group of patients contain nearly all of the significant neoplastic lesions. Five-year follow-up of the high risk patients revealed only three biopsy-documented HGSILs that were missed on screening, for an error rate of less than 0.3% of abnormal smears (unpublished data).** The method was adopted by a large laboratory in Paris, France with equally good results (Bergeron and Fagnani, 1995). The cost of the implementation of this technique is the cost of rescreening about 15% of the preparations, somewhat higher than the mandated rescreening rate of 10%. However, **the method is much more efficient at case finding than random selection of preparations for the mandatory quality control.** For further comments on quality control, see Chapter 44.

Five-Year Rescreening

Centers for Disease Control established a set of rules governing cervical cancer screening, discussed in Chapter 44. One provision of these rules, pertinent to this text, is the requirement that all available negative smears, obtained within 5 prior years on patients with biopsy-documented HGSIL or invasive cancer, must be reviewed. Allen et al (1994) identified 44 such patients with 80 smears, of which 14 were reclassified as ASC-US or AGUS (6 cases) and 3 patients in each category as LGSIL, HGSIL. These authors considered the rescreening rule as an effective quality-control measure. Similar experience was reported by Sidawy (1996).

Thirty-Second Rapid Rescreening

This rescreening method was developed in the United Kingdom. The principle of the method is a rapid review of the smear along one horizontal, vertical and diagonal line, the combined review not lasting more than 30 seconds. The initial studies suggested a marked improvement in the recognition of abnormal smears and prevention of false-negative results (Baker and Melcher, 1991; Faraker, 1993; Dudding, 1995). Coleman and Evans (1999) considered the results as flawed and suggested that the sensitivity of the rapid review on smears with known abnormalities was between 76% and 80% (Baker et al, 1997). It was noted that, because of the rapidity of the screening process, malignant cells in the track of screening were not recognized, strongly suggesting that **adequate time** is important in the evaluation of cytologic abnormalities.

NEW TECHNIQUES OF CERVIX CANCER DETECTION

As a consequence of legal proceedings following the publication of Bogdanicz's article, numerous commercial companies attempted to improve the yield of the conventional cervicovaginal smear. The principal three approaches to this problem were:

- **Improved methods of cell collection in liquid media and preparation of "monolayer" smears**
- **Automated screening of smears**
- **Testing for human papillomavirus (HPV)**

There is no doubt that the combination of these three new techniques will **reduce the false-negative error rate,** but it can be anticipated that the **number of false-positive alarms and cost to the society will be greatly increased** (recent summaries in Vassilakos et al, 1998; Sherman et al, 1998; Manos et al, 1999; Bishop et al, 2000; Austin, 2003; Limaye et al, 2003).

Liquid Preparations

Starting about 1995, a number of commercial companies introduced systems of cytologic sample collection in a liquid fixative, followed by either **reverse filtration** or **sedimentation,** resulting in a "monolayer" preparation wherein the cells are deposited on the slide within **a small circle.** The staining and screening of these preparations are the same as for direct smears. The details of the techniques are described in Chapter 44. The first system to be approved by the FDA was the ThinPrep method of processing (Cytyc Corp., Boxborough, MA), followed by the AutoCyte Prep; now marketed as SurePath (TriPath Imaging, Burlington, NC). The number of papers on this topic is very large and only a few can be cited here.

The fundamental paper by Lee et al (1997) that was the basis of the approval of the ThinPrep method of processing encompassed 6 laboratories, three within academic hospitals and 3 commercial screening centers. The "split sample" method was used, allowing a comparison between a routine smear and the liquid preparation method. An analysis of the data shows a clear advantage of liquid preparations for the screening centers but little, if any, obvious benefit for the academic laboratories, particularly in the detection of HGSIL or invasive cancer. Ferenczy et al (1996) noted that the ThinPrep preparations had a slightly greater sensitivity and specificity when compared with conventional smears but that the difference was statistically not significant. In marked contrast was the study by Papillo et al (1998) which described an increase in the number of biopsy-documented cases of SIL, particularly LGSIL, with a concomitant reduction in debatable diagnoses. A summary of published data by Austin and Ramzy (1998) also emphasized the diagnostic benefits of the liquid collection systems. Bergeron et al (2001), using AutoCyte Prep reported an increased sensitivity and lowered specificity in patients with high-grade CIN, documented by biopsies. An important study from Costa Rica by Hutchinson et al (1999) documented that the ThinPrep method had heightened the sensitivity but significantly lowered the specificity when compared with conventional smears. These features of this paper were emphasized by Koss (2000). Selvaggi and Guidos (2000) noted that the adequacy of the liquid preparations, not unlike that of conventional smears, depended greatly on the collection instruments and the skills of the provider.

The liquid preparations offer certain advantages and disadvantages. **The most important advantages are:**

- Ease of handling by providers
- Reduction in the proportion of inadequate smears, caused by blood or inflammation
- An increase in the number of cell abnormalities when compared with routine smears; this increase varies markedly from one laboratory to another
- Reduction in screening time, resulting in greater efficiency of the cytotechnologists who can handle a larger number of preparations
- Opportunity to use the residual sample for additional testing, including molecular studies for the presence of infectious agents, such as human papillomavirus (see below)

The disadvantages are:

- Adjustment to modified morphologic images
- Multilayering, resulting in different planes of vision for cell clusters compared with dispersed cells, requiring adjustment of focusing
- Difficulties in the interpretation of dense clusters of cells
- Lowered specificity of diagnoses
- High cost

Klinkhamer et al (2003) reviewed and analyzed the available literature on the AutoCyte Prep, SurePath, and Thin-Prep systems and concluded that the ThinPrep system had a **higher sensitivity** for the detection of squamous precancerous lesions and a **reduced rate of ASC-US.** Similar conclusions were reached by Negri et al (2003). With tissue diagnosis as the end point, Chacho et al (2003) reported occasional failure of the ThinPrep system in the diagnosis of invasive carcinomas. The benefits of liquid cytology are predictably greater for laboratories with a very large volume of cervicovaginal samples than for academic laboratories. **The most important benefit of liquid samples is the option of molecular analysis of the residual material for the presence of human papillomavirus and other infectious organisms.**

Automated Screening

A number of semi-automated and fully automated devices have been manufactured and some became available for primary screening and quality control rescreening of routine cervical smears in the 1990s. The principles of these devices are discussed in Chapter 46.

The device extensively studied in our laboratories was the **Papnet System,** manufactured by Neuromedical Systems, Inc., Suffern, New York, a company that no longer exists. The device, based on neural net, performed rather well in capturing images of abnormal cells in conventional cervicovaginal smears with resulting decrease in false-negative diagnoses (Koss et al, 1994 and 1997). Several examples of images generated by the Papnet System can be found in this book, particularly in Chapter 24.

An automated image analysis system known as **Focal Point** (previously known as AutoPap, manufactured by Tri-Pathology Imaging, Inc., Burlington, NC) has been approved by the FDA for primary screening of conventional and liquid (SurePath) cervical samples in low-risk women. Up to 25% of samples designated by the machine as "no further review" need not be rescreened manually. The system has been favorably reviewed by Colgan et al (1997), Bibbo and Howthorne (1999), and Vassilakos et al (2002). A **location guide,** known as Slide Wizzard, has been added to the Focal Point system. It determines the location of abnormal cells on the slide. This system has also received favorable reviews from several investigators (Lee et al, 1998; Chang et al, 2002; Wilbur et al, 2002). The devices are particularly useful in laboratories with a very high volume of cervicovaginal preparations.

HPV Testing as an Adjunct to Cytology

The principles of HPV identification and typing and its role in the genesis of carcinoma of the cervix are discussed at length in Part 1 of the chapter. Briefly, it is assumed that the virus is sexually transmitted, but the evidence supporting this hypothesis is weak because only a small proportion of male partners of women with precursor lesions or invasive cancer harbor the virus and because the same type of virus was very rarely identified in the two partners (Franceschi et al, 2002). The presence of the virus can be documented in a very large proportion of sexually active women. In women below the age of 35 and during normal pregnancy, the rate of **transient infections** documented by polymerase chain reaction (PCR) is very high and may reach 100% in some groups. Although women harboring high risk viruses are at an increased risk of developing precursor lesions or carcinoma of the cervix, epidemiologic data strongly suggest that only a **very small fraction** of these women will develop the disease. There is good evidence that only women with **persisting presence of a high risk virus, documented by two or more tests,** are at risk (Ho et al, 1995; Walboomers et al, 1995; Remmink et al, 1995; Chua and Hjerpe, 1996; Wallin et al, 1999; Nobbenhuis et al, 1999) but, again, they constitute only a small fraction of infected women. In other words, **cervical cancer is a rare complication of infection with oncogenic HPV** (Helmerhorst and Meijir, 2002; Schiffman and Castle, 2003).

An important technologic step in HPV DNA identification and typing was the development of the **Hybrid Capture 2 System** (Digene Corp., Gaithersburg, MD) that is applicable to residual material in liquid samples collected for cytology. The principles of the system are shown in Figure 11-10. Two kits are available, one to detect the presence of low risk HPVs, and the other to detect the presence of high risk viruses. In 2003, the FDA approved the **high-risk kit for testing of patients with ASC-US, regardless of age,** and, in **women age 30 or older** as an **adjunctive screening test** with, or without, a synchronous cell sample. It is the assumption of this approval that the HPV test will offer a **triage option** between women at low or no risk and women deserving further investigation and possibly treatment (see below).

Besides the Hybrid Capture 2 System, other approaches to HPV testing on a large scale are being explored, including several variants of the PCR. **Real time quantitative PCR** appears to be promising (Hubbard, 2003). Undoubtedly, with the passage of time, other testing systems will be developed.

An important development in the history of HPV testing was the **triage study of atypical squamous cells of unknown significance/low-grade squamous intraepithelial lesion (ALTS study),** sponsored by the National Cancer Institute (Schiffman and Adrianza, 2000). The initial results, pertaining to 642 women with LGSIL, were published in the *Journal of the National Cancer Institute* (2000) as an anonymous paper entitled, "Human papillomavirus testing . . . etc." Because 81.4% of the 642 women tested positive for high-risk HPV, it was concluded that the **test offered no triage options and was, therefore, of a very limited value for women with LGSIL.**

In a subsequent publication, Solomon et al (2001) reported on 3,488 women with ASC-US from several participating institutions who were assigned to one of the three arms of the study:

- Immediate colposcopy
- High-risk HPV triage before colposcopy
- Follow-up by cervical smears

The prevalence of HGSIL (CIN 3) in the entire group was 5.1%. The most important conclusion of this paper was that **a negative HPV determination had a very high negative predictive value of about 99%.** In other words, a woman whose genital tract did not harbor documented HPV had a minimal likelihood of developing a HGSIL within the duration of the trial (2 years). On the other hand, although **HPV testing, based on a single initial determination, had a higher sensitivity than cytology, it also had low specificity and high false-positive value, particularly in women below the age of 30.** Stoler and Schiffman (2001) cast yet another shadow on the ALTS study by pointing out that, among the participating institutions, the interobserver **reproducibility of cytologic and histologic diagnoses was low** (kappa value about 0.40, 1 being perfect agreement). Based on the results of the study,

Herbst et al (2001) cautioned that the value of HPV testing should be viewed with caution. Kim et al (2002) calculated that the cost of HPV testing compared favorably with other procedural options, except reclassification of ASC-US as normal.

In a subsequent publication by the ASC-US LSIL Triage Study (ALTS) Group (2003), the cumulative value of CIN 3 in the same group of women was raised to between 8% to 9% and a single HPV test for high risk viruses had predictably higher sensitivity than a single cytologic examination. **After two cytologic examinations, however, the sensitivity of the two tests was equal.** A review by Cuzick (2000) noted that the **specificity** of HPV typing for HGSIL, cancer was **much lower than that of conventional cytology,** resulting in twice the number of women referred for colposcopy. **Clearly, a positive HPV test will stigmatize a great many women who have no documented lesions, all in the name of finding all CIN 3 that could be missed on a single cytologic examination.** As was pointed out above, the **high-grade lesions** discovered in ASC-US patients **are usually small** and not likely to progress to invasive carcinoma (Pinto et al, 2002; Sherman et al, 2003). The issue will be discussed again in reference to follow-up and treatment of ASC-US.

Several possible scenarios of application of HPV DNA analysis have been considered:

- **HPV typing of all women as a replacement for cervical cytology as a screening system for detection of precancerous lesions and early cancer.** Viral typing on a large scale, particularly if performed only once, will select a large proportion of younger women with transient infections who are not at risk for cancer of the uterine cervix. Therefore, this proposal cannot be seriously considered.

- HPV testing can be used as an ancillary test to cytology in women over the age of 30. The benefits of this approach, approved by the FDA, are not evident as yet. In order to seek out women at high risk of HGSIL, persistence of the oncogenic virus will have to be demonstrated. This would require two or more costly tests at a suitable time interval. Again, women testing positive for HPV in the absence of a documented lesion, will be stigmatized and anxious with untold social consequences.

  Wright et al (2000) promoted the idea of HPV **testing on self obtained samples** from underprivileged women who had no access to cytologic screening. Neither the cost of this enterprise nor access of these women to further care were seriously contemplated. Goldie et al (2001) predictably reported that the effectiveness of HPV testing was higher than direct visual inspection **in the developing countries** but its cost was also higher. These considerations are not applicable to the industrialized societies.

- **HPV typing, as a guide to colposcopy and treatment, only after cytologic evidence of CIN.** The eligibility for colposcopy will be limited to women showing persisting infection with a high-risk HPV type (Nobbenhuis et al, 1999). For a number of reasons discussed in Part 1 of the chapter, this proposal presents a high risk to the patients because of the high failure rate of cytologic screening.

- **HPV typing of women with equivocal cytologic abnormalities (ASC-US) to identify patients at risk for progression of the lesions** (Sherman et al, 1994; Manos et al, 1999, ALTS studies cited above). The high **negative predictive value** of these studies was documented in the ALTS studies but the **specificity of positive results is questionable.** Some of the published data pertaining to the **specificity of HPV testing** are highly **misleading** because they are based on specificity of the test in the presence of HGSIL. To be sure, nearly all women with biopsy-documented CIN II or III will harbor high risk HPV (Lörincz and Richart, 2003). However, if the test is applied to a larger population of women of all ages, most of the younger, transient carriers of high-risk HPV will not develop documented disease. Lonky et al (2003) noted a 39.3% false-positive HPV test rate in women with ASC-US. As Lörincz and Richart (2003) appropriately state, HPV testing offers a **protection against potential litigation.** In the Manos paper, HPV typing compared favorably with the results of follow-up smears, but at a much higher cost. Several newer papers examined the management strategies of ASC-US using the Hybrid Capture System compared with cytology, with generally favorable results (Bergeron et al, 2000; Solomon et al, 2001; Wright et al, 2002; Wright and Schiffman, 2003; Lörincz and Richart, 2003). Sarode et al (2003) examined the effect of **reflex testing** on all patients with ASC-US, and observed that 91% of HGSIL were HPV positive (2% for low risk viruses). Levi et al (2003) also addressed the issue of **reflex testing** for women with ASC-US, reported that clinicians do not pay much attention to the cytology report and refer patients with positive high risk HPV test to colposcopy.

- **HPV typing may, perhaps, be of value in the interpretation of biopsies of lesions difficult to classify** (Crum et al, 1997; Park et al, 1999). The results of these interesting studies are not persuasive because of the low specificity of HPV typing.

As discussed in a thoughtful editorial by Crum (1998), with increasing sensitivity of the methods of HPV detection, such as described by Kleter et al (1998), the frequency of positive results also increases, reducing the specificity of the test and confusing still further the value of HPV testing as a public health measure. Wright and Schiffman (2003) also cautioned about the downside of HPV testing.

HPV Vaccines

An apparently successful trial of a human HPV vaccine was reported by Koutsky et al (2002).

Application of HPV Testing to Clinical Practice

A series of recommendations for handling of patients with abnormal cytology were adopted at a National Consensus Conference in Bethesda, MD, in 2001 (Solomon et al, 2002; Wright et al, 2002). These recommendations were formalized as guidelines by the American Society for Colposcopy and Cervical Pathology (ASCCP). The society summarized these recommendations in a series of algorithms pertaining to various levels of cytologic abnormality (Cox, 2003). These recommendations that incorporate HPV testing as an important step in the management of patients are summarized in Figure 11-75.

ASC-US (Atypical Smears)

The management options include:

- **Follow-up by smears 6 months later**
- **HPV testing: if negative**—return to routine screening schedule (the screening interval could be extended to 3 years) and **if positive**—refer to colposcopy
- In some laboratories, the HPV testing is "**reflex**" and is automatically performed on any ASC-US cytology results
- **Postmenopausal women with atrophy** may require estrogen therapy before repeat smears or may be referred for colposcopy or HPV testing without delay

ASC-H (Suspicious Smears)

The management options are as follows:

- **Colposcopic examination**
- If no lesion is seen, refer the patient for follow-up, HPV testing and cytology (every 6 to 12 months, possibly followed by **diagnostic conization**)

LGSIL

The management options are as follows:

- **Colposcopic examination**
- HPV testing has been shown to be of no diagnostic or prognostic value
- In **postmenopausal women**, estrogen therapy may be of value before colposcopy
- **In adolescents, a conservative (wait and see) approach may be adopted**

HGSIL

- **Colposcopic examination with biopsies**
- If colposcopy is negative and, on review, the cytologic diagnosis is confirmed, a **diagnostic conization** is indicated

BIOPSY CONFIRMATION OF CONCLUSIVE CYTOLOGIC EVIDENCE OF NEOPLASTIC LESIONS

The evidence has been presented in the preceding pages to show that the spectrum of neoplastic events in the uterine cervix comprises lesions ranging from low-grade CIN lesions (LGSIL, mild dysplasia, CIN grade I) to invasive carcinoma. It has been emphasized that **the cytologic presenta-**

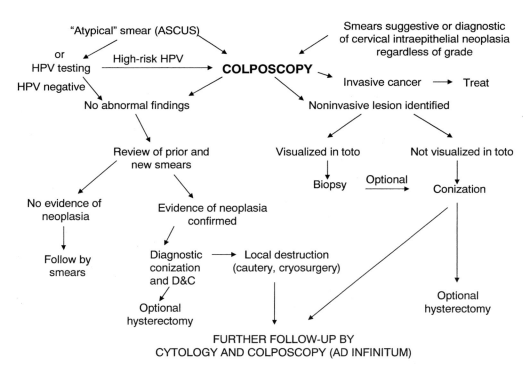

Figure 11-75 Diagnostic and therapeutic choices available to women with abnormal cervical cytology. The sequence of events in this diagram attempts to include all diagnostic and therapeutic options. Colposcopy and biopsies of the cervix remain the pivotal diagnostic procedures, leading to therapeutic decisions. Testing for HPV, which may be "reflex" (i.e., performed on all samples reported as ASC-US) to "selective" (i.e., limited to high-risk patients), is a step added to the list of diagnostic options. Although this approach increases the number of early neoplastic events discovered, its long-term impact on morbidity and mortality from cancer of the cervix remains to be proven.

tion may be, at times, misleading and show a pattern of abnormalities that may be much below the level of the histologic abnormality. Therefore, in my judgment and experience, any patient with cytologic abnormalities suggestive, or diagnostic, of a neoplastic lesion of the uterine cervix, regardless of results of HPV testing, should be referred for colposcopic evaluation and for possible biopsies of abnormal areas. This referral must take place on the basis of the first abnormal smear because of the very high failure rate of "confirmatory" smears, as outlined in the preceding paragraphs. The recommended procedures in handling patients with abnormal smears are shown in Figure 11-75.

It must be stressed that the option of cytologic follow-up, instead of colposcopy for patients with low-grade lesions, is judged to be acceptable because of the high rate of disappearance of these lesions (Kurman et al, 1994). In fact, smears in many women with this disorder will revert to normal (Alanen et al, 1994). This conservative approach may be used so long as the practitioner and the patient are aware of the caveats pertaining to the failure of smears in the accurate assessment of the lesion and as a follow-up procedure, and the failure of the patients to present themselves for follow-up examination. Clearly, the patient must be informed about the findings and their significance and should consent to the conservative approach after a careful explanation of the options. Colposcopy and biopsy, followed by conservative treatment of the lesions, are clearly safer for the patient than cytologic follow-up that must be extended for a minimum of 3 years. As discussed above, there is limited evidence that HPV testing is useful in these patients.

COLPOSCOPY AND CERVICOGRAPHY

The **colposcope** is a stereoscopic magnifying instrument allowing an inspection of the uterine cervix at magnifications from 4 to 20 times. The inspection of the cervix is helped by application of a weak solution (2% to 3%) of acetic acid, which dissolves mucus. The instrument also allows the inspection of the remaining areas of the portio and of the adjacent vagina. The areas of neoplastic epithelial changes, ranging from low-grade lesions (LGSIL, mild dysplasia) to HGSIL or carcinoma in situ, are characterized by vascular abnormalities. The patterns of the visible vascular changes have received various descriptive terms, such as "mosaic" or "punctation." The inspection may also reveal white zones of surface keratinization or "leukoplakia."

Stafl (1981) introduced a variant of colposcopy, **cervicography,** based on color photographs of the cervix obtained with a special apparatus, the cerviscope, and evaluated by an expert. Patients with abnormalities observed in the photographs are requested to return for colposcopy. Ferris et al (2001) reported that cervicography was of moderate value in detecting high-grade lesions in women with ASC-US or LGSIL. Schneider et al (2002) reported that for neoplastic lesions, the sensitivity of cervicography was 64% and specificity 94%.

Colposcope-Guided Biopsies of Cervix

Experienced colposcopists claim that they can identify varying degrees of epithelial abnormality and early invasion with only a small margin of error. Nevertheless, it is mandatory and prudent to confirm the visual impression by colposcopic biopsies, which have the advantage of being obtained under visual control and, hence, directly from the abnormal epithelium. Colposcopic biopsies are an office procedure, usually not requiring any anesthesia. Occasionally, the colposcopic biopsies are very small and therefore, difficult to handle in the laboratory and sometimes very shallow—a point of some importance if the suspicion of invasive carcinoma cannot be settled in a decisive manner.

Nevertheless, there are circumstances when even the most expert use of the colposcope and of the colposcopic biopsy will not preclude the necessity of additional investigative procedures, such as endocervical curettage or a diagnostic conization.

USE OF SPECIAL PROCEDURES TO INCREASE THE ACCURACY OF BIOPSIES OF THE CERVIX

Schiller's Iodine Test

In the absence of a grossly visible lesion, painting the cervix (or the vagina) with a solution of iodine (Schiller's test) may assist in localizing epithelial abnormalities. Normal squamous epithelium is rich in glycogen, which combines with iodine to form a **mahogany-brown stain.** If there is an epithelial defect from whatever cause, the defect area remains unstained or poorly stained. Schiller's iodine test provides only a very general guidance in the search for areas to be biopsied (see Fig. 11-20). Certain keratinizing cancers of the portio may contain glycogen and stain with iodine. On the other hand, benign abnormalities, such as eversion of the endocervical mucosa or leukoplakia, may fail to stain with iodine. Schiller's test gives no information on the status of the endocervix. Richart (1964) carefully evaluated the Schiller test by means of a colpomicroscope and found that about one-quarter of the patients with known carcinoma in situ and nearly one-half of the patients with other forms of cervical intraepithelial neoplasia failed to display significant abnormality with this test. Rubio and Thomassen (1976) confirmed Richart's observations in a study of 87 patients with precancerous intraepithelial lesions and 100 normal women serving as controls. The study, which was carefully controlled, revealed a high percentage of false-positive and false-negative staining. Most important, Schiller's test proved unreliable in detecting or rejecting areas of precancerous abnormalities at the surgical margin of the conization specimen. Thus, Schiller's test can only be considered as **a poor substitute for colposcopy** in the detection of precancerous lesions and should be used as a guide to biopsies only if colposcopy is not available.

Toluidine Blue Stain

Richart (1963) advocated the use of 1% aqueous solution of toluidine blue for delineation of precancerous lesions and carcinoma in situ in vivo. The method is as follows: The cervix is cleaned with a mucolytic solution, prepared by adding a 1% solution of acetic acid to a 1 oz. (30-ml) cup, the bottom of which has been covered by Caroid powder. Following cleansing, the cervix is dried with cotton balls. The solution of toluidine is then applied with a cotton-tipped applicator. After several minutes, the excess stain is blotted with cotton. The cervix is then washed again with the 1% acetic acid solution; the nonneoplastic epithelium of the cervix becomes decolorized or contains only a faint residuum of stain, whereas the **areas of neoplasia retain a royal-blue stain.** Inflammatory areas and endocervical columnar epithelium (such as eversions) may retain the stain but stain blue-black.

Because toluidine blue is a nuclear stain, the staining reaction correlated with nuclear density. Accordingly, the intensity of the positive (royal-blue) stain reflected, to some degree, the nuclear density of the underlying lesion and was less intense in low-grade lesions (dysplasia) than in high-grade lesions, including fully developed carcinoma in situ. The test has also been applied to oral lesions (see Chap. 21).

Endocervical Curettage (EEC) and Endometrial Curettage

This procedure allows the sampling (scraping) of the endocervical canal with a small curet without resorting to conization. In my experience, the samples are often fragmented and difficult to interpret, particularly in deciding whether or not an invasion has occurred. **It must be stressed that, occasionally, important tissue evidence of cervical neoplastic events, including invasive cancer, may be found in material from *endometrial curettage,* which always should be inspected with care.**

Diagnostic Conization

This consists of a surgical removal of a conical segment of cervical tissue with the base comprising the transformation zone, the adjacent ectocervical tissue, and the apex, extending into the endocervical canal, preferably all the way to the internal os. The procedure, requiring anesthesia, may be carried out by means of a scalpel (cold knife conization), a laser beam, or a cautery loop (LEEP). Diagnostic conization is required when:

- **No lesion is visible on colposcopic examination** in the presence of definitely abnormal cytology; thus, the lesion is presumably located within the endocervical canal, which cannot be inspected by the colposcope.
- **Only a part of the lesion is visible to the colposcopist,** and there is evidence of extension into the endocervical canal, beyond the reach of the colposcope.
- **The original biopsies raise the question of invasion,** which cannot be definitely settled in the material available.
- **The evidence in the original colposcopic biopsies** is not in keeping with the cytologic evidence. For example, if cytology is consistent with a fully developed invasive

carcinoma and the colposcopic biopsy shows only a trivial epithelial atypia, conization should be performed.
- **The findings of endocervical curettage,** particularly in reference to the presence of invasive cancer, must be clarified.

Diagnostic conization should not be undertaken lightly because the procedure may result in short- and long-term complications (see below). A very close cooperation between the gynecologist and the pathologist is suggested before deciding on diagnostic conization and its scope. **The cytologic sample may often give a very good indication of the location of the lesion and, thus, may guide the gynecologist as to the manner in which the procedure should be carried out. Thus, a lesion composed only of large squamous dysplastic (dyskaryotic) and keratinized cancer cells is presumably located on the portio of the cervix. In such cases, a relatively shallow conization, encompassing the transformation zone and the squamous epithelium of the vaginal portio of the cervix, but not necessarily the entire endocervical canal, should be carried out. On the other hand, if cytologic evidence suggests a lesion located in the endocervical canal, the conization should reach the internal os but need not include all of the squamous epithelium of the portio.**

Regardless of the type of biopsy, certain common rules should apply. Preparation of the cervix prior to biopsy should be very gentle. Any vigorous scrubbing of the surface of the cervix may result in removal of valuable tissue evidence. The cervix biopsy or biopsies should be obtained preferably in a manner that yields information concerning the geographic distribution and the extent of the lesion. Thus, **if multiple colposcopic biopsies are obtained, each should be preserved in a separate bottle of fixative with precise indication of its site of origin, preferably in form of a diagram.**

TREATMENT OF PRECANCEROUS CERVICAL LESIONS

Until the relatively recent understanding of the natural history of intraepithelial precancerous lesions of the cervix, their relatively slow evolution, and low level of progression to invasive cancers, the standard therapy for these lesions was hysterectomy with a resection of the cuff of the adjacent vagina. In some instances, even radiotherapy was used.

Since the 1970s, the tendency has been to apply more conservative approaches to treatment **once invasive carcinoma has been ruled out.** In the absence of invasion, none of the intraepithelial lesions endangers the life of the patient. All lesions may be treated in a manner most consistent with the well-being of the patient and preferably with preservation of the reproductive functions. The latter is particularly important for women who nowadays may delay childbirth until a later age. The principal modes of therapy in chronological order are:

- Conization, either by scalpel (cold knife) or, more recently, by laser beam
- Cautery

- Cryosurgery
- Laser pulverization
- Large loop electrosurgical excision of the transformation zone (LLETZ)
- **Radiotherapy is not indicated for the treatment of CIN**

All these modes of therapy have the advantage of avoiding hysterectomy, hence, preserving the reproductive function. All of these procedures have certain advantages and disadvantages.

Cold knife conization provides the pathologist with a generous sample of tissues and is the most secure way to rule out invasive cancer. Jordan et al (1964) emphasized that the removal of tissue in such cases **must include all of the endocervical canal, including the internal os,** because less extensive procedures are apt to leave behind foci of carcinoma in situ or even invasive carcinoma, a point also emphasized by Ferguson and Demick (1960), Anderson et al (1980) stressed that the extension of neoplastic lesions into endocervical glands in histologic sections may reach 3.8 mm or, occasionally, even more. Thus, accounting for 20% shrinkage of tissue, **the depth of the conization must be about 6 mm.** Burghardt and Holzer (1980) emphasized the need for a careful histologic examination of the conization material by step sections to rule out invasive cancer. Luesley et al (1985) reported on **complications of cold-**

knife conization performed on 915 patients—in 13% there was **hemorrhage,** in 17% **stenosis of the endocervical canal,** and in 4% either **infertility or abnormal pregnancy.**

Neither hysterectomy nor cold-knife conization for precursor lesions guarantee cure. Kolstad and Klem (1976) reported on 1,122 patients with carcinoma in situ treated by conization. The recurrence rate was 2.3% for carcinoma in situ and 0.9% for unexpectedly discovered small invasive carcinomas. After hysterectomy, there were 1.2% recurrent carcinomas in situ and 2.1% invasive cancers. Bjerre et al (1976) reported treatment failure in 13% of patients treated by conization. Among 186 patients treated by hysterectomy 8 developed invasive cancers. Thus, all patients must have the benefit of follow-up for at least 5 years.

The selected results of treatment of CIN by cautery, cryosurgery, and laser are shown in Table 11-14. It may be noted that a failure of treatment occurred in all of the series, regardless of mode of therapy, ranging from a low of 2.7% to a high of nearly 20% in an early study by Creasman et al (1973). With accumulated experience, the treatment failure rate is probably between 3% and 5%. It is of interest that the treatment failure was independent of the grade of abnormality (where reported) and was just as likely to happen with CIN I as with CIN

TABLE 11-14

RESULTS OF CONSERVATIVE TREATMENT OF CIN

Authors	Treatment Mode	Total Number of Patients Treated	Failure Rate	Remarks
Benedet et al. (1987)	Various	1,675	5%–7% regardless of grade of CIN	81 lesions recurred: 2 CIN I, 16 CIN II, 63 CIN III
Creasman et al. (1973)	Cryosurgery	75	48.5% after one treatment, 18.7% after 2 treatments	
Levine et al. (1985)	Cryosurgery	279	2.9%–5.7% regardless of grade	After subsequent conization, the failure rate was from 0.7% to 2.7%
Anderson (1982)	Laser vaporization	441	23.6% after 1 treatment, 2% after 2nd treatment	
Hatch et al. (1981)	Cryosurgery	772	Persistence 10%–20%; recurrence 3.2%–3.8%, regardless of grade of CIN	
Chanen et al. (1983)	Coagulation diathermy	1,864	2.7% after single treatment	Cost-effective
Deigen et al. (1986)	Cautery	776	10%–11% after 1 treatment	No anesthesia, cost-effective
Baggish (1986)	Laser excisional conization	120	Not reported	Same results with both methods
	Laser vaporization	100		
Hanau and Bibbo (1997)	LEEP	162 (121 with follow-up)	33% LGSIL	LGSIL most common followed by HGSIL

III, supporting the concept that the size and location of the lesion are more important than the morphologic grade of abnormality.

The large loop electrosurgical excision of the transformation zone (LEEP or LLETZ), initially proposed by Cartier of Paris, is based on thin wire loop electrodes of various sizes that can be used to excise the transformation zone and the affected segment of the cervix, with a reasonably good preservation of tissues. Low-voltage electrodiathermy current is used for the excision, which is, at the same time, of diagnostic and therapeutic value. Therapeutic successes in about 95% of patients have been reported (Minucci et al, 1991; Wright et al, 1991; Luesley, 1992). The method is not without problems and cervical stenosis has been reported as a complication of the procedure (Dunn et al, 2004). Sadler et al (2004) noted that LEEP, laser cone procedures were a **risk factor** for preterm delivery. The interpretation of the histologic evidence provided by LLETZ, may also present problems because of tissue destruction (Montz et al, 1993).

Follow-up of Treated Patients

All patients with CIN, regardless of mode of therapy, require follow-up by colposcopy and cytology. Regardless of therapeutic procedure, the healing of the cervix takes a minimum of 6 weeks. During this period, cytologic abnormalities caused by treatment and the healing process may be observed (see Chap. 18). **If the smear, obtained 6 weeks or more after treatment, shows cells with neoplastic changes, these must be considered as evidence of a persisting or recurring lesion.**

The efficacy of a single smear in detecting persisting or recurrent CIN is not particularly high, probably on the order of 25% (23% in Falcone and Ferenczy's experience). Therefore, **at least three sets of post-treatment smears must be obtained to rule out the presence of a lesion.** It must be stressed that the **recurrent lesion may occur in the vagina,** after eradication of the cervical disease.

Testing for high-risk HPV may be useful in this regard. **Patients with persisting presence of a high-risk virus are at risk for recurrent lesions** (Chua and Hjerpe, 1997; Schiffman et al, 2003).

LABORATORY PROCESSING OF CERVICAL BIOPSIES AND CONIZATION SPECIMENS

Cervical Biopsies

Each biopsy should be processed individually and **embedded "on edge."** Because of the fragility of the epithelial lesions, which may readily become detached from the main part of the specimen, **filtering the fixation fluid is advisable and all fragments of tissues, thus obtained, should be embedded.**

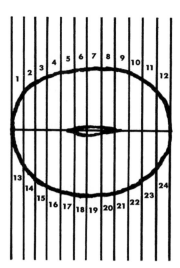

Figure 11-76 Diagram of the method of processing the uterine cervix as devised by Foote and Stewart. The cervix is split horizontally, and each half is cut into a series of numbered blocks. A diagram accompanies the specimen so that an accurate designation of the distribution of carcinoma is possible. (From Foote FW, Stewart FW. Anatomical distribution of intraepithelial epidermoid carcinomas of cervix. Cancer 1:431–440, 1948.)

Conization Specimens

The exact geographic designation of the areas involved by a precancerous lesion may be of direct value to the patient. Thus, if the margins of the excised specimen are occupied by tumor, further therapy may be necessary. Unless the entire specimen is investigated, a focus of invasion may be overlooked. Therefore, a **systematic approach to the investigation of all tissue specimens of cervical origin is essential.** The surgeon can be of help in the laboratory processing of cervical cones *by designating a predetermined point, for instance, the 12 o'clock area, by a stitch.*

Method of Foote and Stewart (1949)

This method was used in mapping studies of the precursor lesions of the uterine cervix, illustrated in Figure 11-76 and it has proven to be very useful to this day. After splitting the cervical cone (or the cervix in cervical amputation and hysterectomy specimens) horizontally, the anterior and posterior halves are cut vertically into a series of blocks not thicker than 5 mm. Each block is numbered, marked as to the surface that has to be cut, and put into a separate container. A diagram of the cervix is prepared, indicating the area of origin of each block. A map of the distribution of lesions on the cervix can be created.

PROGRAMS OF CERVIX CANCER DETECTION AND PREVENTION

The epidemiologic factors associated with carcinoma of the uterine cervix were discussed in the opening pages of this chapter. The data pertaining to the events in cancer of the uterine cervix were collected as a consequence of population screening based on cervicovaginal smears. The screening systems are either based on voluntary participation of women (so-called **opportunistic screening**), as in the United States, or within the framework of programs organized by state-supported health care systems, as in Iceland, Finland, Sweden, the United Kingdom, and the Netherlands. The state-organized programs usually offer cytologic services to women within defined age groups (for example from 25 to 45), and at defined time intervals (for example, every 3 to 5 years), likely to yield the greatest benefits as determined by epidemiologists (Geirson, 1986; Hakama 1978, 1988). The women are reminded of screening intervals and the results are computerized for analysis. For example, the program in the Netherlands, with screening at 5-year intervals, resulted in **stabilization** but not reduction of cervix cancer (Siemens et al, 2004). Marshall (1965, 1968) documented that if the screening is performed on a regular basis within a closed community, invasive cancer of the cervix can be eliminated. Unfortunately, such ideal conditions do not prevail in larger screening programs, all of which have shown a reduction in the rate of invasive cancer but none of which has so far succeeded in complete elimination of a theoretically preventable disease (Koss, 1989). Perhaps the most successful program has been conducted in British Columbia, Canada, where the rate of invasive cancer of the cervix dropped from 28.4 per hundred thousand at the onset of the program in 1955 to 4.0 in 1987 (Table 11-15). The program, originally conceived and described by Fidler et al in 1962 and 1968, updated by Boyes et al in 1981, and by Anderson et al in 1988, served as a prime example of cervix cancer detection systems. Information of value can be obtained from **incidence and prevalence rates** of precursor lesions in a given population.

Discovery Rates in Newly Screened Populations (Prevalence Rates)

Primary screening of large populations revealed that from 5 to 20 women per 1,000 have an occult precancerous lesion or carcinoma of the cervix. **The discovery rate is in reverse ratio to the economic status,** with the highest rate among the economically underprivileged group (Christopherson and Parker, 1969). **Prevalence of a lesion does not indicate its duration prior to discovery.** It merely indicates the total number of lesions present in a given population at a given time. Some of the lesions may have been present for 10 or more years and some for a few months or weeks only. Thus, the prevalence tells nothing about the incidence rate at which these lesions are formed de novo.

Discovery Rates in Returning Populations (Incidence Rates)

To establish true incidence rates for carcinoma of the cervix, a given population of women, previously thoroughly investigated and found free of lesions of the cervix, has to be re-examined at specified intervals. It may be assumed that all lesions found in such a group represent new lesions and, thus, true frequency of new occurrence may be established. The results of early population surveys (Christopherson et al, 1962, 1969, 1977) indicate that the initial screening resulted in a significant reduction in the prevalence of precursor lesions and invasive carcinoma. However, the very high rate of "dysplasia" in returning populations, about 50% of the original prevalence rate, **strongly suggested that the original screening was not effective and that true incidence rates may require repeated screening over a period of several years.** This has been documented in repeated screenings of the population in a study by Melamed et al (1969). The study documented that, after three screenings, the true constant incidence rate of new lesions is about 5% for low-grade squamous lesions (LGSIL, mild dysplasia, CIN grade I).

Duration of Precancerous Lesions Before Onset of Invasive Cancer and Probability of Invasion

By determining the age differences among cohorts of women with various lesions of the uterine cervix, an attempt can be made to determine the approximate duration of the stages in the development of cancer of the cervix. For example, if the average age of women with a LGSIL is 22 years of age, HGSIL 29 years, and invasive cancer 40, it can be speculated that 7 years are required for a low-grade lesion to "progress" to a high-grade lesion and 11 years are required for a high-grade lesion to progress to invasive cancer. In fact, the issue is much more complex, because the ideal sequence of events is practically never seen. Further, the frequency of precancerous events is vastly in excess of the observed rate of invasive cancer. **Thus, the complex issues of carcinogenesis in the uterine cervix model cannot be explained based on purely epidemiologic data.** Some of the other risk factors, including the role of HPV infection, have been discussed in Part 1 of the chapter.

TABLE 11-15			
CLINICAL INVASIVE SQUAMOUS CARCINOMA OF THE CERVIX: INCIDENCE IN BRITISH COLUMBIA			
Year	Population in Thousands Over Age 20	Total Cases	Incidence per 100,000
1955	422.9	120	28.4
1960	486.4	96	19.7
1965	543.2	80	14.7
1970	664.4	82	12.3
1975	805.5	70	8.7
1980	912.9	63	6.9
1985	1,063.1	68	6.4
1987	1,085.7	44	4.0

(Courtesy of Dr. George H. Anderson, Vancouver, B.C., Canada)

Guidelines for Cervix Cancer Detection

The most recent guidelines for detection of precancerous lesions and carcinoma of the uterine cervix, established by a committee of experts, were published by the American Cancer Society in 2002 (Saslow et al, 2002).

- The **start of screening** should be approximately 3 years after the onset of vaginal intercourse but not later than age 21.
- **The screening can be discontinued** at age 70, after three consecutive negative cervical cytology results within a 10-year period.
- **Screening after medical hysterectomy** (with removal of the cervix) **for benign disease** is not recommended. Women with history of CIN II, III should continue screening until three consecutive normal cytology results have been secured over a 10-year period.
- **Screening intervals.** Young women should be screened annually (or every 2 years using liquid-based cytology).

The **frequency** of most effective screening is also being debated. Patients past the age of 30, testing negative for high risk HPV, or patients who had three negative cervical smears may safely be screened every 3 years with a minimal risk of developing cervix cancer (Sawaya et al, 2003).

New Technologies

- **Liquid cytology.** Because of greater sensitivity, a 2-year interval between screening is permissible (*the statement does not address the issue of lower specificity—author's comment*).
- **HPV testing.** The frequency of combined cytology-HPV testing should **NOT** be done more often than 3 years. Counseling of patients about HPV infection is mandatory.

Additional Recommendations

Women should be educated that a pelvic examination is not equal to a Pap smear *[the opposite statement that the Pap smear is not an adequate diagnostic modality in the presence of abnormal clinical findings was not included (author's comment)]*.

APPENDIX—THE 2001 BETHESDA SYSTEM

The Bethesda System (The NCI Terminology and Classification of Cervical / Vaginal Cytology). Developed and approved at the National Cancer Institute Workshop on Terminology for Cervical / Vaginal Cytology, December 12–13, 1988; modified 1991 (JAMA, 267:1892, 1992, and 2001) (Solomon et al, 2002).

ORGANIZATION OF THE NEW TERMINOLOGY AND CLASSIFICATION

It is recommended that laboratory reports address each of the following elements:

- **Specimen type** (Pap smear, liquid-based, other)
- **A statement on the adequacy of the specimen** for diagnostic evaluation
- **A general categorization** of the diagnosis (*within normal limits or other*)
- **Descriptive diagnosis,** using the following terminology and classification.

Specimen Adequacy

- Satisfactory for evaluation (note presence/absence of endocervical/transformation zone component)
- Unsatisfactory for evaluation . . . (specify reason)
- Specimen rejected/not processed (specify reason)
- Specimen processed and examined, but unsatisfactory for evaluation of epithelial abnormality because of (specify reason)

GENERAL CATEGORIZATION (OPTIONAL)

- Negative for intraepithelial lesion or malignancy
- Epithelial cell abnormality
- Other

INTERPRETATION/RESULTS

- Negative for intraepithelial lesion or malignancy
- Organisms
- Trichomonas vaginalis
- Fungal organisms morphologically consistent with *Candida* species
- Shift in flora suggestive of bacterial vaginosis
- Bacteria morphologically consistent with *Actinomyces* species
- *Cellular changes consistent with herpes simplex virus*
- Other non-neoplastic findings (Optional to report; list not comprehensive)
- Reactive cellular changes associated with inflammation (includes typical repair)
- Radiation
- Intrauterine contraceptive device
- Glandular cells status posthysterectomy
- Atrophy

EPITHELIAL CELL ABNORMALITIES

Squamous Cell

- Atypical squamous cells (ASC) of undetermined significance (ASC-US)
- Cannot exclude HSIL (ASC-H)
- Low-grade squamous intraepithelial lesion (LSIL) *encompassing* human papillomavirus/mild dysplasia/cervical intraepithelial neoplasia (CIN) 1

- High-grade squamous intraepithelial lesion (HSIL) *encompassing* moderate and severe dysplasia, carcinoma in situ; CIN 2 and CIN 3
- Squamous cell carcinoma

Glandular Cell

- Atypical glandular cells (AGC) (specify endocervical, endometrial, or not otherwise specified)
- Atypical glandular cells, favor neoplastic (specify endocervical or not otherwise specified)
- Endocervical adenocarcinoma in situ (AIS)
- Adenocarcinoma
- Other (list not comprehensive)
- Endometrial cells in a woman ≥40 years of age

Comment

The key to successful practice of gynecologic cytopathology (and tissue pathology) is excellent communications between the laboratories and the gynecologists or other practitioners interested in their patients. Many a difficult diagnostic problem, in a cytologic sample or in a biopsy, can be resolved by a discussion with the clinician. Bits of valuable information, not included in the brief summary submitted with the laboratory request, may have a major impact on the diagnosis and recommendations in reference to further handling of the patient's problem.

BIBLIOGRAPHY

Abadi MA, Ho GYF, Burk RD, et al. Stringent criteria for histological diagnosis of koilocytosis fail to eliminate overdiagnosis of human papillomavirus infection and cervical intraepithelial neoplasia grade 1. Hum Pathol 29: 54–59, 1998.

Abdul-Karim FW, Fu YS, Reagan JW, Wentz WB. Morphometric study of intraepithelial neoplasia of the uterine cervix. Obstet Gynecol 60:210–214, 1982.

Adachi A, Fleming I, Burk RD, et al. Women with immunodeficiency virus infection and abnormal Papanicolaou smears: A prospective study of colposcopy and clinical outcome. Obstet Gynecol 81:372–377, 1993.

Ahlgren M, Ingemarsson I, Lindberg LG, Nordqvist RB. Conization as treatment of carcinoma in situ of the uterine cervix. Obstet Gynecol 46:135–140, 1975.

Alanen KW, Elit LM, Molinaro PA, McLachlin CM. Assessment of cytologic follow-up as the recommended management for patients with atypical squamous cells of undetermined significance or low-grade squamous intraepithelial lesions. Cancer Cytopathol 84:5–10, 1998.

Allen KA, Zaleski S, Cohen MB. Review of negative Papanicolaou tests. Is the retrospective 5-year review necessary? Am J Clin Pathol 101:19–21, 1994.

Allerding TJ, Jordan SW, Boardman RE. Association of human papillomavirus and Chlamydia infection with incidence of cervical neoplasia. Acta Cytol 29:653–660, 1985.

Alons-van Kordelaar JJM, Boon ME. Diagnostic accuracy of squamous cervical lesions studied in spatula-cyto-brush smears. Acta Cytol 32:801–804, 1988.

Al-Saleh W, Delvenne P, Greimers R, et al. Assessment of Ki-67 antigen immunostaining in squamous intraepithelial lesions of the uterine cervix. Am J Clin Pathol 104:154–160, 1995.

Amann JA, Jr. Kurzgefasstes Lehrbuch der mikroskopisch-gynakologischen Diagnostik. Wiesbaden, Germany, JF Bergmann, 1897.

Anderson ES, Thorup K, Larsen G. The results of cryosurgery for cervical intraepithelial neoplasia. Gynecol Oncol 30:21–25, 1988.

Anderson GH, Boyes DA, Benedet JL, et al. Organization and results of the cervical cytology screening programme in British Columbia 1955–85. Br Med J 296:975–978, 1988.

Anderson MB, Jones BA. False positive cervicovaginal cytology. A follow-up study. Acta Cytol 41:1697–1700, 1997.

Anderson MC. Treatment of cervical intraepithelial neoplasia with the carbon dioxide laser: Report of 543 patients. Obstet Gynecol 59:720–725, 1982.

Anderson W, Frierson H, Barber S, et al. Sensitivity and specificity of endocervical curettage and the endocervical brush for the evaluation of the endocervical canal. Am J Obstet Gynecol 159:702–707, 1988.

Anttila T, Saikku P, Koskela P, et al. Serotypes of Chlamydia trachomatis and risk for development of cervical squamous cell carcinoma. JAMA 285:47–51, 2001.

Arends MJ, Wyllie AH, Bird CC. Papillomaviruses and human cancer. Hum Pathol 21:686–698, 1990.

ASCUS-LSIL Triage Study (ALTS) Group. Results of a randomized trial on the management of cytology interpretations of atypical squamous cells of undetermined significance. Am J Obstet Gynecol 188:1383–1392, 2003.

ASCUS-LSIL Triage Study (ALTS) Group. A randomized trial on the management of low-grade squamous intraepithelial cytology interpretations. Am J Obstet Gynecol 188:1393–1400, 2003.

ASCUS-LSIL Triage Study (ALTS) Group. Human papillomavirus testing for triage of women with cytologic evidence of low-grade squamous intraepithelial lesions: Baseline from a randomized trial. The Atypical Squamous Cells of Undetermined Significance/Low-Grade Squamous Intraepithelial Lesions Triage Study (ALTS) Group. J Natl Cancer 92:397–402, 2000.

Ashworth CT, Stembridge VA, Luibel FJ. A study of basement membranes of normal epithelium, carcinoma in situ, and invasive carcinoma of uterine cervix utilizing electron microscopy and histochemical methods. Acta Cytol 5:369–382, 1961.

Atkin NB. Prognostic value of cytogenetic studies of tumors of the female genital tract. In: Koss LG, Coleman DV (eds). Advances in Clinical Cytology, vol 2. New York, Masson, 1984, pp 103–121.

Atkin NB. The desoxyribonucleic acid content of malignant cells in cervical smears. Acta Cytol 8:68–72, 1964.

Atkin NB, Baker MC. Nonrandom chromosome changes in carcinoma of the cervix uteri. II. Ten tumors in the triploid-tetraploid range. Cancer Genet Cytogenet 13:189–207, 1984.

Atkin NB, Baker MC. Nonrandom chromosome changes in carcinoma of the cervix uteri. I. Nine near diploid tumors. Cancer Genet Cytogenet 7: 209–222, 1982.

Atkin NB, Baker MC. Possible differences between the karyotypes of preinvasive lesions and malignant tumours. Br J Cancer 23:329–336, 1969.

Atkin NB, Brandão HJS. Evidence for the presence of a large marker chromosome in histological sections of a carcinoma in situ of the cervix uteri. J Obstet Gynecol Br Commonw 75:211–214, 1968.

Atkin NB, Richards BM. Clinical significance of ploidy in carcinoma of cervix: Its relation to prognosis. Br Med J 2:1445–1446, 1962.

Atkin NB, Richards BM, Ross AJ. The desoxyribonucleic acid content of carcinoma of the uterus. An assessment of its possible significance in relation to histopathology and clinical course, based on data from 165 cases. Br J Cancer 13:773–787, 1959.

Attwood ME, Woodman CBJ, Luesley D, Jordan JA. Previous cytology in patients with invasive carcinoma of cervix. Acta Cytol 29:108–110, 1985.

Aubele M, Zitzelsberger H, Schenck U, et al. Distinct cytogenetic alterations in squamous intraepithelial lesions of the cervix revealed by laser-assisted microdissection and comparative genomic hybridization. Cancer 84: 375–379, 1998.

Auersperg N, Erber H, Worth A. Histologic variation among poorly differentiated invasive carcinomas of the human uterine cervix. JNCI 51:1461–1477, 1973.

Auersperg N, Wakonig-Vaartaja T. Chromosome changes in invasive carcinomas of the uterine cervix. Acta Cytol 14:495–501, 1970.

Auger M, Charbonneau M, Arseneau J. Atypical squamous cells of undetermined significance. A cytohistologic study of 52 cases. Acta Cytol 41: 1671–1675, 1997.

Aurelian L. Persistence and expression of the herpes simplex virus type 2 genome in cervical tumor cells. Cancer Res 34:1126–1135, 1974.

Aurelian L, Schumann B, Marcus RL, Davis HJ. Antibody to HSV-2 induced tumor specific antigens in serums from patients with cervical carcinoma. Science 181:161–163, 1973.

Aurelian L, Strandberg JD, Melendez LV, Johnson LA. Herpesvirus type 2 isolated from cervical tumor cells grown in tissue culture. Science 174: 704–706, 1971.

Austin RM. The detection of precancerous cervical lesions can be significantly increased. Who cares and who should know? Arch Pathol Lab Med 127: 143–145, 2003a.

Austin RM. Human papillomavirus reporting. Minimizing patient and laboratory risk. Arch Pathol Lab Med 127:973–977, 2003b.

Austin RM, Ramzy I. Increased detection of epithelial cells abnormalities by liquid-based cytology preparations. A review of accumulated data. Acta Cytol 42:178–184, 1998.

Ayre JE. Role of the halo cell in cervical cancerogenesis: A virus manifestation in premalignancy? Obstet Gynecol 17:175–182, 1960.

Ayre JE. Regression of cervical carcinoma in situ following Aureomycin; further report. South Med J 45:915–921, 1952.

Ayre JE. The vaginal smear: "Precancer" cell studies using a modified technique. Am J Obstet Gynecol 58:1205–1219, 1949.

Ayre JE, Ayre WB. Progression from "precancer" state to early carcinoma of cervix within 1 year; combined cytologic and histologic study with report of case. Am J Clin Pathol 19:770–778, 1949.

Babès A. Le diagnostique du cancer du col utérin par les frottis. Presse Méd 36: 451–454, 1928.

Baggish MS. A comparison between laser excisional conization and laser vaporization for the treatment of cervical intraepithelial neoplasia. Am J Obstet Gynecol 155:39–44, 1986.

Bajardi F. Koexistenz nervaler Proliferate mit frühen epithelialen Neoplasien und benignen Ektopien der Cervix uteri. Gynäkol Geburtshilfliche Rundsch 35:188–193, 1995.

Bajardi F. Histogenesis of spontaneous regression of cervical intraepithelial neoplasias. Cancer 54:616–619, 1984.

Baken LA, Koutsky LA, Kuypers J, et al. Genital human papillomavirus infection among male and female sex partners: Prevalence and type-specific concordance. J Infect Dis 171:429–432, 1995.

Baker A, Melcher DH. Rapid cervical cytology screening. Cytopathology 2: 299–301, 1991.

Baker RW, Wadsworth J, Brugal G, Coleman DV. An evaluation of rapid review as a method of quality control of cervical smears using the AxioHOME microscope. Cytopathology 8:85–95, 1997.

Balmelli C, Roden R, Potts A, et al. Nasal immunization of mice with human papillomavirus type 16 virus-like particles elicits neutralizing antibodies in mucosal secretions. J Virol 72:8220–8229, 1998.

Barasso R, Aynaud O. L'examen du partenaire masculin des femmes avec lesions a HPV. Bilan de six ans de depistage (Examination of the male partner of women with HPV lesions: Summary of six years of detection). Lettre du Gynecologue (Paris) 181:3–6, 1993.

Barber HRK, Jones W. Lymphadenectomy in pelvic exenteration for recurrent cervix cancer. JAMA 215:1945–1949, 1971.

Barber HRK, O'Neil WH. Recurrent cervical cancer after treatment by a primary surgical program. Obstet Gynecol 337:165–172, 1971.

Barrasso R, De Brux J, Croissant O, Orth G. High prevalence of papillomavirus-associated penile intraepithelial neoplasia in sexual partners of women with cervical intraepithelial neoplasia. N Engl J Med 317:916–923, 1987.

Barron BA, Richart RM. Statistical model of the natural history of cervical carcinoma. II. Estimates of the transition time from dysplasia to carcinoma in situ. JNCI 45:1025–1030, 1970.

Barron BA, Richart RM. A statistical model of the natural history of cervical carcinoma based on a prospective study of 557 cases. JNCI 41:1343–1353, 1968.

Barua R, Matthews CD. Verrucous carcinoma of the uterine cervix. A case report. Acta Cytol 27:540–542, 1983.

Bauer HM, Ting Y, Greer CE, et al. Genital human papillomavirus infection in female university students as determined by a PCR-based method. JAMA 265:472–477, 1991.

Bendich A, Borenfreund E, Sternberg SS. Penetration of somatic mammalian cells by sperm. Science 183:857–859, 1974.

Bendich A, Borenfreund E, Witkin SS, et al. Information transfer and sperm uptake by mammalian somatic cells. Progr Nucleic Acid Res Mol Biol 17: 43–75, 1976.

Benedet JL, Miller DM, Nickerson KG, Anderson GH. The results of cryosurgical treatment of cervical intraepithelial neoplasia at one, five, and ten years. Am J Obstet Gynecol 157:268–273, 1987.

Berchuck A, Rodriguez G, Karmel A, et al. Expression of epidermal growth factor receptor and HER-2/neu in normal and neoplastic cervix, vulva, and vagina. Obstet Gynecol 76:381–387, 1990.

Berg JW, Bader GM. Present potential of exfoliative cytology in detection of cervix cancer. Cancer 11:758–764, 1958.

Bergeron C, Bishop J, Lemarie A, et al. Accuracy of thin-layer cytology in patients undergoing cervical cone biopsy. Acta Cytol 45:519–524, 2001.

Bergeron C, Debaque H, Ayivi J, et al. Cervical smear histories of 585 women with biopsy-proven carcinoma in situ. Acta Cytol 41:1676–1680, 1997.

Bergeron C, Fagnani F. Individual cytotechnologist performance and quality control. Acta Cytol 39:274–275, 1995.

Bergeron C, Jeannel D, Poveda J-D, et al. Human papillomavirus testing in women with mild cytologic atypia. Obstet Gynecol 95:821–827, 2000.

Bernard C, Mougin C, Bettinger D, et al. Detection of human papillomavirus by in-situ polymerase chain reaction in paraffin embedded cervical biopsies. Mol Cell Probes 8:337–343, 1994.

Bibbo M, Bartels PH, Sychra JJ, Wied GL. Chromatin appearance in intermediate cells from patients with uterine cancer. Acta Cytol 25:23–28, 1981.

Bishop JW, Hartinger JS, Pawlick GF. Time interval effect on repeat cervical smear results. Acta Cytol 41:269–276, 1997.

Bishop JW, Marshall CJ, Bentz JS. New technologies in gynecologic cytology. J Reprod Med 45:701–719, 2000.

Bjerre B, Johansson S. Invasive cervical cancer in a cytologically screened population. Acta Obstet Gynecol Scand 62:569–574, 1983.

Black, Capt. PE, Brown EA. Spontaneous regression of carcinoma of the cervix. Report of a case. J Maine Med Assoc 50:358–361, 1959.

Boddington MM, Spriggs AI, Wolfendale MR. Cytogenetic abnormalities in carcinoma-in-situ and dysplasias of the uterine cervix. Br Med J 16:154–158, 1965.

Bogdanicz W. Lax laboratories. The Pap test misses much cervical cancer through lab's errors. Wall Street J Nov:2, 1987.

Bohm JW, Krupp PJ, Lee FYL, Batson HWK. Lymph node metastasis in microinvasive epidermoid cancer of the cervix. Obstet Gynecol 48:65–67, 1976.

Bonfiglio TA, Feinberg MR. Isoantigen loss in cervical neoplasia. Arch Pathol Lab Med 100:307–310, 1976.

Boon ME, Alons-van Kordelaar JJ, Rietveld-Scheffers PE. Consequences of the introduction of combined spatula and cytobrush sampling for cervical cytology. Improvements in smear quality and detection rates. Acta Cytol 30: 264–270, 1986.

Boon ME, de Graaff-Guilloud JC, Rietveld WJ. Analysis of five sampling methods for the preparation of cervical smears. Acta Cytol 33:843–848, 1989.

Boon ME, Kok LP, Sutedja G, Dutrieux RP. Confocal sectioning of thick, otherwise undiagnosable cell groupings in cervical smears. Acta Cytol 37:40–48, 1993.

Boon ME, Schut JJ, Benita EM, Kok LP. Confocal optical sectioning and three-dimensional reconstruction of carcinoma fragments in Pap smears using sophisticated image data processing. Diagn Cytopathol 10:268–275, 1994.

Bosch MMC, Rietveld-Scheffers PEM, Boon ME. Characteristics of false-negative smears tested in the normal screening situation. Acta Cytol 36:711–716, 1992.

Boschann HW. Gynakologische Zytodiagnostik fur Klinil und Praxis, 2 ed. Berlin, deGruyter, 1973.

Bose S, Kannan V, Kline TS. Abnormal endocervical cells: Really abnormal? Really endocervical? Am J Clin Pathol 101:708–713, 1994.

Boutselis JG. Intraepithelial carcinoma of the cervix associated with pregnancy. Obstet Gynecol 40:657–665, 1972.

Boutselis JG, Ullery JC, Charme L. Diagnosis and management of stage 1A (microinvasive) carcinoma of the cervix. Am J Obstet Gynecol 110:984–989, 1971.

Boyce JG, Fruchter RG, Nicastri AD, et al. Vascular invasion in stage I carcinoma of the cervix. Cancer 53:1175–1180, 1984.

Boyer SN, Wazer DE, Band V. E7 protein of human papillomavirus-16 induces degradation of retinoblastoma protein through the ubiquitin-proteasome pathway. Cancer Res 56:4620–4624, 1996.

Boyes DA, Fidler KH, Lock DR. Significance of in situ carcinoma of the uterine cervix. Br Med J 1:203–205, 1962.

Boyes DA, Worth AJ, Anderson GH. Experience with cervical screening in British Columbia. Gynecol Oncol 12:S143–S156, 1981.

Boyes DA, Worth AJ, Fidler HK. The results of treatment of 4389 cases of preclinical cervical squamous carcinoma. J Obstet Gynecol Br Commonw. 77:769–780, 1970.

Brandão HJS. Possible evidence for the presence of a large marker chromosome in histologic sections of cervical koilocytotic atypia and other mitotic abnormalities (in Portuguese). J Bras Ginec 97:83–85, 1987.

Brandão HJS. DNA content in epithelial cells of dysplasias of the uterine cervix. Histologic and microspectrophotometric observations. Acta Cytol 13: 232–237, 1969.

Brandsma JL, Steinberg BM, Abramson AL, Winkler B. Presence of human papillomavirus type 16 related sequences in verrucous carcinoma of the larynx. Cancer Res 46:2185–2188, 1986.

Bremer GL, Tieboschb AT, van der Putten HW, et al. p53 tumor suppressor gene protein expression in cervical cancer: relationship to prognosis. Eur J Obstet Gynecol Reprod Biol 63:55–59, 1995.

Bremond A, Frappart L, Migaud C. Study of 68 microinvasive carcinomas of the cervix uteri. J Gynecol Obstet Biol Reprod 14:1025–1031, 1985.

Brescia RJ, Jenson AB, Lancaster WD, Kurman RJ. The role of human papillomaviruses in the pathogenesis and histologic classification of precancerous lesions of the cervix. Hum Pathol 17:552–558, 1986.

Broders AC. Carcinoma in situ contrasted with benign penetrating epithelium. JAMA 99:1670–1674, 1932.

Broker TR, Botchan M. Papillomaviruses: Retrospectives and prospectives. Cancer Cells/DNA Viruses, Cold Spring Harbor Lab 4:17–36, 1986.

Buckley CH, Herbert A, MacKenzie EFD, et al. Borderline nuclear changes in cervical smears: Guidelines on their recognition and management. J Clin Pathol 47:481–492, 1994.

Burghardt E. Early Histological Diagnosis of Cervical Cancer (translated by EA Friedman). Stuttgart, G Thieme, 1973.

Burghardt E, Holzer E. Treatment of carcinoma in situ: Evaluation of 1609 cases. Obstet Gynecol 55:539–545, 1980.

Burghardt E, Holzer E. Die Lokalisation des pathologischen Cervixepithels. IV. Epithelgrenzen. Letzte Cervixdruse. Schlussfolgerungen. Arch Gynäkol 212: 130–150, 1972.

Burk RD. Human papillomavirus and the risk of cervical cancer. Hosp Pract 34:103–111, 1999.

Burk RD, Kadish AS, Calderin S, Romney SL. Human papillomavirus infection of the cervix detected by cervicovaginal lavage and molecular hybridization: Correlation with biopsy results and Papanicolaou smear. Am J Obstet Gynecol 154:982–989, 1986.

Buxton EJ, Luesley DM, Wade-Evans T, Jordan JA. Residual disease after cone biopsy: Completeness of excision and follow-up cytology as predictive factors. Obstet Gynecol 70:529–532, 1987.

Bychkov V, Rothman M, Bardawil WA. Immunocytochemical localization of carcinoembryonic antigen (CEA), alpha-fetoprotein (AFP), and human chorionic gonadotropin (CG) in cervical neoplasia. Am J Clin Pathol 79: 414–420, 1983.

Byrne JC, Tsao M-S, Fraser RS, Howley PM. Human papillomavirus-11 DNA in a patient with chronic laryngotracheobronchial papillomatosis and metastatic squamous-cell carcinoma of the lung. N Engl J Med 317:873–878, 1987.

Cain JM, Howett MK. Preventing cervical cancer. Science 288:1753–1754, 2000.

Calore EE, Cavaliere MJ, Calore NM. Squamous intraepithelial lesions in cervical smears of human immunodeficiency virus-seropositive adolescents. Diagn Cytopathol 18:91–92, 1998.

Campion MJ, McCance DJ, Cuzick J, Singer A. Progressive potential of mild cervical atypia: Prospective cytological, colposcopic and virological study. Lancet 2:237–240, 1986.

Campion MJ, Singer A, Clarkson PK, McCance DJ. Increased risk of cervical neoplasia in consorts of men with penile condylomata acuminata. Lancet 1:943–946, 1985.

Cannistra SA, Niloff JM. Cancer of the uterine cervix. N Engl J Med 334: 1030–1038, 1996.

Cannizzaro LA, Dürst M, Mendez MJ, et al. Regional chromosome localization of human papillomavirus integration sites near fragile sites, oncogenes, and cancer chromosome breakpoints. Cancer Genet Cytogenet 33:93–98, 1988.

Caorsi I, Figueroa CD. Langerhans' cells in squamous exocervical carcinoma: A quantitative and ultrastructural study. Ultrastr Pathol 7:25–40, 1984.

Carmichael JA, Clarke DH, Moher D, et al. Cervical carcinoma in women aged 34 and younger. Am J Obstet Gynecol 154:264–269, 1986.

Carter JJ, Koutsky LA, Wipf GC, et al. The natural history of human papillomavirus type 16 capsid antibodies among a cohort of university women. J Infect Dis 174:927–936, 1996.

Cartier R. Practical Colposcopy, 2 ed. Paris, Laboratoire Cartier, 1984, pp 139–156.

Caspersson O. Quantitative cytochemical studies on normal, malignant, premalignant, and atypical cell populations from the human uterine cervix. Acta Cytol 7:45–60, 1964.

Castellsaque X, Bosch X, Muñoz N, et al. Male circumcision, penile human papillomavirus infection, and cervical cancer in female partners. N Engl J Med 346:1105–1112, 2002.

Ceccini S, Iossa A, Ciatto S, et al. Routine colposcopic survey of patients with squamous atypia. Acta Cytol 34:778–780, 1990.

Cellier KM, Kirkland JA, Stanley MA. Statistical analysis of cytogenetic data in cervical neoplasia. JNCI 44:1221–1230, 1970.

Centifano YM, Drylie DM, Deardourff SL, Kaufman HE. Herpesvirus type 2 in the male genitourinary tract. Science 178:318–319, 1972.

Chacho MS, Eppich E, Wersto RP, Koss LG. Influence of human papilloma virus on DNA ploidy determination in genital condylomas. Cancer 65:2291–2294, 1990.

Chacho MS, Mattie ME, Schwartz PE. Cytohistologic correlation rates between conventional Papanicolaou smears and ThinPrep cervical cytology: A comparison. Cancer Cytopathol 99:135–140, 2003.

Chang AR, Lin WF, Chang A. Can technology expedite the cervical cancer screening process? A Hong Kong experience using the AutoPap Primary Screening System with location-guided screening capability. Am J Clin Pathol 117:437–443, 2002.

Chang F, Syrjänen S, Shen Q, et al. Human papillomavirus (HPV) DNA in esophageal precancer lesions and squamous cell carcinoma from China. Papilloma virus workshop, Heidelberg, Abstract 351, 1990.

Chapman WB, Lorincz AT, Willett GD, et al. Epidermal growth factor receptor expression and the presence of human papilloma virus in cervical squamous intraepithelial lesions. Int J Gynecol Path 11:221–226, 1992.

Chaudhuri S, Koprowska I, Rowinski J. Different agglutinability of fibroblasts underlying various precursor lesions of human uterine cervical carcinoma. Cancer Res 35:2350–2354, 1975.

Chen TM, Chen C-A, Hsieh C-Y, et al. The state of p53 in primary human cervical carcinomas and its effect in human papillomavirus—immortalized human cervical cells. Oncogene 8:1511–1518, 1993.

Cherry CP, Glucksmann A. Histology of carcinomas of the uterine cervix and survival rates in pregnant and non-pregnant patients. Surg Gynecol Obstet 113:763–776, 1961.

Chetty R, Bramdev A, Aguirre-Arteta A, et al. Relation between retinoblastoma and p53 proteins in human papillomavirus 16/18 positive and negative cancers of the uterine cervix. J Clin Pathol 50:413–416, 1997.

Christopherson WM, Broghamer W. Progression of experimental cervical dysplasia in the mouse. Cancer 14:201–204, 1961.

Christopherson WM, Lundin FE, Jr, Mendez WM, Parker JE. Cervical cancer control. Cancer 38:1357–1366, 1976.

Christopherson WM, Mendez WM, Ahuja EM, et al. Cervix cancer control in Lousiville, Kentucky. Cancer 26:29–38, 1970.

Chua KL, Hjerpe A. Human papillomavirus analysis as a prognostic marker following conization of the cervix uteri. Gynecol Oncol 66:108–113, 1997.

Chua KL, Hjerpe A. Persistence of human papillomavirus (HPV) infections preceding cervical carcinoma. Cancer 77:121–127, 1996.

Chua KL, Wiklund F, Lenner P, et al. A prospective study on the risk of cervical intra-epithelial neoplasia among healthy subjects with serum antibodies to HPV compared with HPV DNA in cervical smears. Int J Cancer 68:54–59, 1996.

Chuaqui R, Cole K, Cuello M, et al. Analysis of mRNA quality in freshly prepared and archival Papanicolaou samples. Acta Cytol 43:831–836, 1999.

Clauss J, Beric B. Über das Mikrokarzinom am Collum uteri. Oncologia 11:23–41, 1958.

Clavel C, Masure M, Bory J-P, et al. Hybrid capture II-based human papillomavirus detection, a sensitive test to detect in routine high-grade cervical lesions: A preliminary study on 1518 women. Br J Cancer 80:1306–1311, 1999.

Clavel C, Zerat L, Binninger I, et al. DNA content measurement and in situ hybridization in condylomatous cervical lesions. Diagn Mol Pathol 1:180–184, 1992.

Cocker J, Fox H, Langley FA. Consistency in the histological diagnosis of epithelial abnormalities of the cervix uteri. J Clin Pathol 21:67–70, 1968.

Coker AL, Rosenberg AJ, McCann MF, et al. Active and passive cigarette smoke exposure and cervical intraepithelial neoplasia. Cancer Epidemiol Biomarkers Prev 1:349–356, 1992.

Coleman DV, Evans DMD. Biopsy Pathology and Cytology of the Cervix. London, Arnold, 1999, pp 446.

Confortini M, Carozzi F, Dalla Palma P, et al. Interlaboratory reproducibility of atypical squamous cells of undetermined significance report: a national survey. Cytopathology 14:263–268, 2003.

Coppleson LW, Brown B. Estimation of the screening error rate from the ob-served detection rates in repeated cervical cytology. Am J Obstet Gynecol 119:953–958, 1974.

Coppleson M. The origin and nature of premalignant lesions of the cervix uteri. Int J Gynaecol Obstet 8:539–550, 1970.

Coppleson M, Reid B. The etiology of squamous carcinoma of the cervix. Obstet Gynecol 32:432–436, 1968.

Coppola A, Sorosky J, Casper R, et al. The clinical course of cervical carcinoma in situ diagnosed during pregnancy. Gynecol Oncol 67:162–165, 1997.

Coste J, Cochand-Priollet B, de Cremoux P, et al. Cross sectional study of conventional cervical smear, monlayer cytology and human papillomavirus DNA testing for cervical cancer screening. Br Med J 326:733, 2003.

Covell JL, Wilbur DC, Guidos B, et al. Epithelial Abnormalities: Glandular. In: Solomon and Nayar (eds). The Bethesda System for Reporting Cervical Cytology. New York, Springer, 2004, pp 123–156.

Cox JT. Role of human papillomavirus testing in the American Society for Colposcopy and Cervical Pathology guidelines for the management of abnormal cervical cytology and cervical cancer precursors. Arch Pathol Lab Med 127:950–958, 2003.

Cox JT. Management of atypical squamous cells of undetermined significance and low-grade squamous intraepithelial lesion by human papillomavirus testing. Best Pract Res Clin Obstet Gynaecol 15:715–741, 2001.

Cox JT, Herbst AL, Kinney W, et al. Advanced technologies in cervical cancer screening, ASCCP Biennial Meeting 1998. J Lower Genital Tract Dis 3: S8–S28, 1999.

Cox JT, Lorincz AT, Schiffman MH, et al. Human papillomavirus testing by hybrid capture appears to be useful in targeting women with a cytologic diagnosis of atypical squamous cells of unknown significance. Am J Obstet Gynecol 172:946–954, 1995.

Cox JT, Schiffman M, Solomon D, et al. Prospective follow-up suggests similar risk of subsequent cervical intraepithelial neoplasia grade 2 or 3 among women with cervical intraepithelial neoplasia grade 1 or negative colposcopy and direct biopsy. Am J Obstet Gynecol 188:1406–1412, 2003.

Cramer DW. The role of cervical cytology in the declining morbidity and mortality of cervical cancer. Cancer 34:2018–2027, 1974.

Creasman WT, Clarke-Pearson DL, Ashe L, et al. The abnormal Pap smear. What to do next. Cancer 48:515–522, 1981.

Creasman WT, Weed JC, Jr, Curry SL, et al. Efficacy of cryosurgical treatment of severe cervical intraepithelial neoplasia. Obstet Gynecol 41:501–506, 1973.

Crombach G, Scharl A, Vierbuchen M, et al. Detection of squamous cell carcinoma antigen in normal squamous epithelia and in squamous cell carcinomas of the uterine cervix. Cancer 63:1337–1342, 1989.

Crum CP. Detecting every genital papilloma virus infection. What does it mean? (Commentary). Am J Pathol 153:1667–1671, 1998.

Crum CP, Cibas ES, Lee KR. Pathology of Early Cervical Neoplasia. New York, Churchill Livingstone, 1997.

Crum CP, Ikenberg H, Rochart RM, Gissmann L. Human papillomavirus types 16 and early cervical neoplasia. N Engl J Med 310:880–883, 1984.

Crum CP, Mitao M, Levine RU, Silverstein S. Cervical papillomaviruses segregate within morphologically distinct precancerous lesions. J Virol 54:675, 1985.

Cuzick J. Human papillomavirus testing for primary cervical cancer screening. JAMA 283:108–109, 2000.

Daling JR, Madeleine MM, McKnight B, et al. The relationship of human papillomavirus-related cervical tumors to cigarette smoking, oral contraceptive use, and prior herpes simplex virus type 2 infection. Cancer Epidemiol, Biomarkers and Prev 5:541–548, 1996.

Daling JR, Weiss NS, Hislop TG, et al. Sexual practices, sexually transmitted diseases, and the incidence of anal cancer. N Engl J Med 317:933–937, 1987.

Davesa SS. Descriptive epidemiology of cancer of the uterine cervix. Obstet Gynecol 63:605–612, 1984.

Davey DD, Naryshkin S, Nielsen ML, Kline TS. Atypical squamous cells of undetermined significance: interlaboratory comparison and quality assurance monitoring. Diagn Cytopathol 11:390–396, 1994.

Davey DD, Nielsen ML, Naryshkin S, et al. Atypical squamous cells of undetermined significance. Current laboratory practices of participants in the College of American Pathologists interlaboratory comparison program in cervicovaginal cytology. Arch Pathol Lab Med 120:440–444, 1996.

Davey DD, Woodhouse S, Styer P, et al. Atypical epithelial cells and specimen adequacy. Current laboratory practices of participants in the College of American Pathologists Interlaboratory Comparison Program in Cervicovaginal Cytology. Arch Pathol Lab Med 124:203–211, 2000.

Davidsohn I, Kovarik S. Isoantigens A, B, H in benign and malignant lesions of the cervix. Arch Pathol 87:306–314, 1969.

Davidsohn I, Ni LY. Immunocytology of cancer. Acta Cytol 14:276–282, 1970.

De Brux J, Orth G, Croissant O, et al. Lesions condylomateuses du col utérin; evolution chez 2466 patients. Bull Cancer (Paris) 70:410–422, 1983.

de Villiers EM. Taxonomic classification of papillomaviruses. Papillomavirus Rep 12:57–63, 2001.

de Villiers EM, Fauquet C, Broker TR, et al. Classification of papillomaviruses. Virology 324:17–27, 2004.

de Villiers EM, Lavergne D, Chang F, et al. An interlaboratory study to determine the presence of human papillomavirus DNA in esophageal carcinoma from China. Int J Cancer 81:225–228, 1999.

de Villiers EM, Wagner D, Schneider A, et al. Human papillomavirus DNA in women without and with cytologic abnormalities: Results of a 5-year follow-up study. Gynecol Oncol 44:33–39, 1992.

de Villiers EM, Wagner D, Schneider A, et al. Human papillomavirus infections in women with and without abnormal cervical cytology. Lancet 2:703–706, 1987.

DeCarneri I, DiRe F. Vaginal trichomoniasis and precancerous states of the cervix: A preliminary report. J Obstet Gynaecol Br Commonw 77: 1016–1018, 1970.

Degefu S, O'Quinn AG, Lacey CG, et al. Verrucous carcinoma of the cervix: A report of two cases and literature review. Gynecol Oncol 25:37–47, 1986.

Del Mistro A, Braunstein JD, Hawler M, Koss LG. Identification of human papillomavirus types in male urethral condylomata acuminata by in situ hybridization. Hum Pathol 18:936–940, 1987.

Dellas A, Torhorst J, Jiang F, et al. Prognostic value of genomic alterations in invasive cervical squamous cell carcinoma of clinical stage IB detected by comparative genomic hybridization. Cancer Res 59:3475–3479, 1999.

Dickinson L. Evaluation of the effectiveness of cytologic screening for cervical cancer. III. Cost-benefit analysis. Mayo Clin Proc 47:550–555, 1972.

Dickinson L, Mussey ME, Kurland LT. Evaluation of the effectiveness of cytologic screening for cervical cancer. II. Survival parameters before and after inception of screening. Mayo Clin Proc 47:545–549, 1972.

Dickinson L, Mussey ME, Soule EH, Kurland LT. Evaluation of the effectiveness of cytologic screening for cervical cancer. I. Incidence and mortality trends in relation to screening. Mayo Clin Proc 47:534–544, 1972.

Diddle AW, Watts J. Cervical carcinoma in women under 30 years of age. Am J Obstet Gynecol 84:745–748, 1962.

DiPaolo JA, Woodworth CD, Popescu NC, et al. Induction of human cervical squamous cell carcinoma by sequential transfection with human papillomavirus 16 DNA, viral Harvey ras. Oncogene 4:395–399, 1989.

Douglass LE. Odorico Viana and his contribution to diagnostic cytology. Acta Cytol 14:544–549, 1970.

Douglass LE. A further comment on the contributions of Aurel Babès to cytology and pathology. Acta Cytol 11:217–224, 1967.

Dowhanick JJ, McBride AA, Howley PM. Suppression of cellular proliferation by the papillomavirus E2 protein. J Virol 69:7791–7799, 1995.

Dudding N. Rapid rescreening of cervical smears: An improved method of quality control. Cytopathology 6:95–99, 1995.

Duggan MA, Brasher PMA. Accuracy of Pap tests reported as CIN I. Diagn Cytopathol 21:129–136, 1999.

Dunn AEG, Ogilvie NM. Intranuclear virus particles in human genital wart tissue: Observations on the ultrastructure of the epidermal layer. J Ultrastruct Res 22:282–295, 1968.

Dunn JE, Crocker DW, Rube IF, et al. Cervical cancer occurrence in Memphis and Shelby County, Tennessee, during 25 years of its cervical cytology screening program. Am J Obstet Gynecol 150:861–864, 1984.

Dunn JE, Jr, Martin PL. Morphogenesis of cervical cancer. Findings from San Diego County Cytology Registry. Cancer 20:1899–1906, 1967.

Dunn MR. Prevalence of carcinoma in cervical stumps. Am J Obstet Gynecol 82:83–87, 1961.

Dunn TS, Killoran K, Wolf D. Complications of outpatient LLETZ procedures. J Reprod Med 49:76–78, 2004.

Dürst M, Croce CM, Gissmann L, et al. Papillomavirus sequences integrate near cellular oncogenes in some cervical carcinomas. Proc Natl Acad Sci USA 84: 1070–1074, 1987.

Dürst M, Gissmann L, Ikenberg H, zur Hausen H. A papillomavirus DNA from a cervical carcinoma and its prevalence in cancer biopsy samples from different geographic regions. Proc Natl Acad Sci USA 80:3812–3815, 1983.

Dvorak KA, Finnemore M, Maksem JA. Histology correlation with atypical squamous cells of undetermined significance (ASCUS) and low-grade squamous intraepithelial lesion (LSIL) cytology diagnoses: An argument to ensure ASCUS follow-up that is as aggressive as that for LSIL. Diagn Cytopathol 21:292–295, 1999.

Dyson N, Howley PM, Munger K, Harlow E. The human papillomavirus-16 E7 oncoprotein is able to bind to the retinoblastoma gene product. Science 243:934–937, 1989.

Egan AJM, Russell P. Transitional (urothelial) cell metaplasia of the uterine cervix: Morphological assessment of 31 cases. Int J Gynecol Pathol 16: 89–98, 1997.

El Hamidi A, Kocjan G, Du M-Q. Clonality analysis of archival cervical smears. Correlation of monoclonality with grade and clinical behavior of cervical intraepithelial neoplasia. Acta Cytol 47:117–123, 2003.

Ellerbrock TV, Chiasson MA, Bush TJ, et al. Incidence of cervical squamous intraepithelial lesions in HIV-infected women. JAMA 283:1031–1037, 2000.

Elmore JG, Wells CK, Lee CH, et al. Variability in radiologists' interpretation of mammograms. N Engl J Med 331:1493–1499, 1994.

Erickson CC, Evertt BE, Jr, Graves LM, et al. Population screening for uterine cancer by vaginal cytology; preliminary summary of results of first examination of 108,000 women and second testing of 33,000 women. JAMA 162: 167–173, 1956.

Ettler HC, Joseph MG, Downing PA, et al. Atypical squamous cells on undetermined significance: A cytohistological study in a colposcopy clinic. Diagn Cytopathol 21:211–216, 1999.

Evander M, Edlund K, Gustafsson A, et al. Human papillomavirus infection is transient in young women: A population-based cohort study. J Infect Dis 171:1026–1030, 1995.

Evans DMD, Shelley G, Cleary B, Baldwin Y. Observer variations and quality control of cytodiagnosis. J Clin Pathol 27:945–950, 1974.

Falcone T, Ferenczy A. Cervical intraepithelial neoplasia and condyloma: An analysis of diagnostic accuracy of posttreatment follow-up methods. Am J Obstet Gynecol 154:260–264, 1986.

Faraker CA. Rapid review. Cytopathology 9:71–76, 1998.

Faraker CA. Partial rescreening of all negative smears: An improved method of quality assurance in laboratories undertaking cervical cytology. Cytopathology 4:47–50, 1993.

Feingold AR, Vermund SH, Burk RD, et al. Cervical cytologic abnormalities and papillomavirus in women infected with human immunodeficiency virus. J Acquir Immune Defic Syndr 3:896–903, 1990.

Feinstein AR, Sosin DM, Wells CK. The Will Rogers phenomenon: Stage migration and new diagnostic techniques as a source of misleading statistics for survival in cancer. N Engl J Med 312:1604–1608, 1985.

Fennell RH Jr. Carcinoma in situ of uterine cervix: report of 113 cases. Cancer 9:374–384, 1956.

Fennell RH, Jr. Carcinoma in situ of cervix with early invasive changes. Cancer 8:302–309, 1955.

Fentanes de Torres E, Mora A. Verrucous carcinoma of the cervix uteri. Acta Cytol 25:307–309, 1981.

Ferenczy A, Mitao M, Nagai N, et al. Latent papillomavirus and recurring genital warts. N Engl J Med 313:784–788, 1985.

Ferenczy A, Richart R. Scanning electron microscopy of the cervical transformation zone. Am J Obstet Gynecol 115:151–157, 1973.

Ferenczy A, Richart RM. Female Reproductive System: Dynamics of Scan and Electron Microscopy. New York, John Wiley & Sons, 1974.

Ferenczy A, Robitaille J, Franco E, et al. Conventional cervical cytology smears vs. ThinPrep smears. A paired comparison study on cervical cytology. Acta Cytol 40:1136–1142, 1996.

Ferguson JH. Positive cancer smears in teenage girls. JAMA 178:365–368, 1961.

Ferguson JH, Demick PE. Diagnostic conization of the cervix. N Engl J Med 262:13–16, 1960.

Ferris DG, Schiffman M, Litaker MS. Cervicography for triage of women with mildly abnormal cervical cytology results. Am J Obstet Gynecol 185: 939–943, 2001.

Fetherstone WC. False negative cytology in invasive cancer of the cervix. Clin Obstet Gynecol 23:929–937, 1983.

Fidler HK, Boyd JR. Occult invasive squamous carcinoma of cervix. Cancer 13: 764–771, 1960.

Fidler HK, Boyes DA. Patterns of early invasion intra-epithelial carcinoma of the cervix. Cancer 12:673–680, 1959.

Fidler HK, Boyes DA, Auersperg N, Lock DR. The cytology program in British Columbia. I. An evaluation of the effectiveness of cytology in the diagnosis of cancer and its application to the detection of carcinoma of the cervix. Can Med Assoc J 86:779–784, 1962.

Fidler HK, Boyes DA, Lock DR, Auersperg N. The cytology program in British Columbia. II. The operation of the cytology laboratory. Can Med Assoc J 86:823–830, 1962.

Fidler HK, Boyes DA, Worth AJ. Cervical cancer detection in British Columbia. J Obstet Gynaecol Br Commonw 75:392–404, 1968.

Fields C, Restivo RM, Brown MC. Experience in mass Papanicolaou screening and cytologic observations of teenage girls. Am J Obstet Gynecol 124: 730–734, 1976.

Figge DC, Bennington JL, Schweid AI. Cervical cancer after initial negative and atypical vaginal cytology. Am J Obstet Gynecol 108:422–428, 1970.

Figge DC, Creasman WT. Cryotherapy in the treatment of cervical intraepithelial neoplasia. Obstet Gynecol 62:353–358, 1983.

Figueroa CD, Caorsi I. Ultrastructural and morphometric study of the Langerhans cell in the normal human exocervix. J Anat 90:669–682, 1980.

Fishman WH, Mitchell GW, Jr, Borges PRF, et al. Enzymorphology of cancer of the cervix: β-glucuronidase, α-naphthylesterase, alkaline phosphatase, acid phosphatase, and reduced diphosphopyridine nucleotide (DPNH) diaphorase. Cancer 16:118–125, 1963.

Fluhmann FC. The Cervix Uteri and Its Diseases. Philadelphia, WB Saunders, 1961.

Foote FW, Jr, Stewart FW. Anatomical distribution of intraepithelial epidermoid carcinomas of cervix. Cancer 1:431–440, 1948.

Foote FW, Li KYY. Smear diagnosis of in situ carcinoma of cervix. Am J Obstet Gynecol 56:335–339, 1948.

Foraker AG, Reagan JW. Nuclear mass and allied phenomena in normal exocervical mucosa, squamous metaplasia, atypical hyperplasia, intraepithelial carcinoma, and invasive squamous cell carcinoma of uterine cervix. Cancer 12: 894–901, 1959.

Forni A, Miles CP. Sex chromatin abnormalities in carcinoma of the cervix uteri. Acta Cytol 10:200–204, 1966.

Fox CH. Time necessary for conversion of normal to dysplastic cervical epithelium. Obstet Gynecol 31:749–754, 1968.

Franceschi S, Castellsague X, Dal Maso L, et al. Prevalence and determinants of human papillomavirus genital infection in men. Br J Cancer 86:705–711, 2002.

Friedell GH, Hertig AT, Younge PA. Problem early stromal invasion in carcinoma in situ of uterine cervix. Arch Pathol 66:494–503, 1958.

Frisch LE. Inflammatory atypia: Subsequent cervical intraepithelial neoplasia explained by cytologic underreading. Acta Cytol 31:869–872, 1987.

Frisch LE, Parmar H, Buckley LD, Chalem SA. Colposcopy of patients with cytologic inflammatory epithelial changes. Acta Cytol 34:133–135, 1990a.

Frisch LE, Parmar H, Buckley LD, Chalem SA. Improving the sensitivity of cervical cytologic screening. A comparison of duplicate smears and colposcopic examination of patients with cytologic inflammatory epithelial changes. Acta Cytol 34:136–139, 1990b.

Frost M, Bobak JB, Gianani R, et al. Localization of telomerase hTERT protein and hTR in benign mucosa, dysplasia, and squamous cell carcinoma of the cervix. Am J Clin Pathol 114:726–734, 2000.

Fu YS, Hall TL. DNA ploidy measurements in tissue sections. Anal Quant Cytol 7:90–95, 1985.

Fuchs PG, Girardi F, Pfister H. Human papillomavirus DNA in normal, metaplastic, preneoplastic and neoplastic epithelia of the cervix uteri. Int J Cancer 41:41–45, 1988.

Fukushima M, Okagaki T, Twiggs LB, et al. Histological types of carcinoma of the uterine cervix and the detectability of human papillomavirus DNA. Cancer Res 45:3252–3255, 1985.

Futoran RJ, Nolan JF. Stage I carcinoma of the uterine cervix in patients under 40 years of age. Am J Obstet Gynecol 125:790–797, 1976.

Gad C. The management and natural history of severe dysplasia and carcinoma in situ of the uterine cervix. Br J Obstet Gynecol 83:554–559, 1976.

Gale RE, Wainscoat JS. Clonal analysis using X-linked DNA polymorphisms. Br J Hematol 85:2–8, 1993.

Galloway DA. Papillomavirus capsids: a new approach to identify serological markers of HPV infection (Editorial). JNCI 86:474–475, 1994.

Galloway DA, Jenison SA. Characterization of the humoral immune response to genital papillomaviruses. Mol Biol Med 7:59–72, 1990.

Galvin GA, Jones HW, Jr, TeLinde RW. Clinical relationship of carcinoma in situ and invasive cervical cancer. JAMA 149:744–748, 1952.

Gard PD, Fields MJ, Noble EJ, Tweeddale DN. Comparative cytopathology of squamous carcinoma in situ of the cervix in the aged. Acta Cytol 13:27–35, 1969.

Garden JM, O"Banion MK, Shelnitz LS, et al. Papillomavirus in the vapor of carbon dioxide laser-treated verrucae. JAMA 259:1199–1202, 1988.

Gardner HL, Kaufman RH. Condylomata acuminata. Clin Obstet Gynecol 8:938–945, 1965.

Gay JD, Donaldson LD, Goellner JR. False-negative results in cervical cytology studies. Acta Cytol 29:1043–1046, 1985.

Geirson G. Organization of screening in technically advanced counties: Iceland. *In:* Hakama M, Miller AB, Day NE (eds). Screening for Cancer of the Uterine Cervix. Lyons, France, International Agency for Research on Cancer, 1986, pp 239–250.

Genest DR, Cean B, Lee KR, et al. Qualifying the cytologic diagnosis of "atypical squamous cells of undetermined significance" affects the predictive value of a squamous intraepithelial lesion on subsequent biopsy. Arch Pathol Lab Med 122:338–341, 1998.

Geng L, Connolly DC, Isacson C, et al. Atypical immature metaplasia (AIM) of the cervix: Is it related to high-grade squamous intraepithelial lesion (HSIL)? Hum Pathol 30:345–351, 1999.

Ghoussoub RA, Rimm DL. Degree of dysplasia following diagnosis of atypical squamous cells of undetermined significance is influenced by patient history and type of follow-up. Diagn Cytopathol 17:14–19, 1997.

Gilbert EF, Palladino A. Squamous papillomas of the uterine cervix. Review of the literature and report of a giant papillary carcinoma. Am J Clin Pathol 46:115–121, 1966.

Giles JA, Deery A, Crow J, Walker P. The accuracy of repeat cytology in women with mildly dyskaryotic smears. Br J Obstet Gynaecol 96:1067–1070, 1989.

Gissmann L, Dürst M, Oltersdorf T, von Knebel Doieberitz M. Human papillomaviruses and cervical cancer. *In:* Steinberg BM, Brandsma JL, Taichmann LB (eds). Cancer Cells. Cold Spring Harbor NY, Cold Spring Harbor Laboratory, 1987, pp 275–324.

Gissman L, Ikenberg H, zur Hausen H. A papillomavirus DNA from a cervical carcinoma and its prevalence in cancer biopsy samples from different geographic regions. Proc Natl Acad Sci USA 80:3812–3815, 1983.

Gissmann L, Schneider A. Human papillomavirus DNA in preneoplastic and neoplastic genital lesions. *In:* Peto R, zur Hausen H (eds). Viral Etiology of Cervical Cancer: Banbury Report 21. Cold Spring Harbor NY, Cold Spring Harbor Laboratory 1986 pp 217–224.

Gissmann L, Wolnik L, Ikenberg H, et al. Human papillomavirus types of 6 and 11 sequences in genital and laryngeal papillomas and in some cervical cancers. Proc Natl Acad Sci USA 80:560–563, 1983.

Gissmann L, zur Hausen H. Human papillomaviruses DNA. Physical mapping and genetic heterogeneity. Proc Natl Acad Sci USA 73:1310–1313, 1976.

Goff BA, Atanasoff P, Brown E, et al. Endocervical glandular atypia in Papanicolaou smears. Obstet Gynecol 79:101–104, 1992.

Goforth JL. Polyps and papillomas of the cervix uteri. Texas J Med 49:81–86, 1953.

Goforth JL. Squamous cell papilloma of the cervix uteri. South Med J 49:921–926, 1952.

Goldberger SB, Rosen DJ, Fejgin MD, et al. An unusually aggressive verrucose carcinoma of the uterine cervix. Acta Obstet Gynecol Scand. 67:369–371, 1988.

Goldie SJ, Kuhn L, Denny L, et al. Policy analysis of cervical cancer screening strategies in low-resource settings. Clinical benefits and cost-effectiveness. JAMA 285:3107–3115, 2001.

Goldstein MS, Shore B, Gusberg SB. Cellular immunity as a host response to squamous carcinoma of the cervix. Am J Obstet Gynecol 111:751–755, 1971.

Gondos B, Townsend DE, Ostergard DR. Cytologic diagnosis of squamous dysplasia of the cervix. Am J Obstet Gynecol 110:107–110, 1971.

Graham JB, Meigs JV. Recurrence of tumor after total hysterectomy for carcinoma in situ. Am J Obstet Gynecol 64:1159–1162, 1952.

Granberg I. Chromosomes in preinvasive, microinvasive and invasive cervical carcinoma. Hereditas 68:165–218, 1971.

Green GH. Cervical carcinoma in situ. Aust NZJ Obstet Gynaecol 10:41–48, 1970.

Green GH. Invasive potential of cervical carcinoma in situ. Int J Gynaecol Obstet 7:157, 1969.

Green GN, Donavan JW. The natural history of cervical carcinoma in situ. J Obstet Gynecol Br Commw 77:1–9, 1970.

Greene RR, Peckham BM. Preinvasive cancer of the cervix and pregnancy. Am J Obstet Gynecol 75:551–564, 1958.

Grenko RT, Abendroth CS, Frauenhoffer EE, et al. Variance in the interpretation of cervical biopsy specimens obtained for atypical squamous cells of undetermined significance. Am J Clin Pathol 114:735–740, 2000.

Griffin NR, Dockey D, Lewis FA, Wells M. Demonstration of low frequency of human papillomavirus DNA in cervical adenocarcinoma and adenocarcinoma in situ by the polymerase chain reaction and in situ hybridization. Int J Gynecol Pathol 10:36–43, 1991.

Groben P, Reddick R, Askin F. The pathologic spectrum of small cell carcinoma of the cervix. Int J Gynecol Pathol 4:42–57, 1985.

Grubb C, Janota I. Non-neoplastic surface epithelium continuous with invasive cervical carcinoma. Neoplasm 16:215–221, 1969.

Grundmann E, Hillemanns HG, Rha K. Cytophotometrische Untersuchungen am menschlichen Portioepithel während der Krebsentwicklung. I. Das Verhalten von Kernvolumen und Desoxyribonucleinsäure. Z Krebsforsch 64:390–402, 1961.

Grüssendorf-Conen E-I, Deutz FJ, de Villiers EM. Detection of human papillomavirus-6 in primary carcinoma of the urethra in men. Cancer 60:1832–1835, 1987.

Grüssendorf-Conen E-I. Papillomavirus-induced tumors of the skin: Cutaneous warts and epidermodysplasia verruciformis. *In:* Syrjänen K, Gissmann L, Koss LG (eds). Papillomaviruses and Human Diseases. New York, Springer-Verlag, 1987, pp 158–181.

Guido R, Schiffman M, Solomon D, et al. Postcolposcopy management strategies for women referred with low grade squamous intraepithelial lesions or human papillomavirus DNA-positive atypical squamous cells of undetermined significance: A 2 year prospective study. Am J Obstet Gynecol 188:1401–1405, 2003.

Gunn SA, Gould TC. Reliability of negative gynecological cytological findings. JAMA 223:326, 1973.

Guo Z, Thunberg U, Sallstrom J, et al. Clonality analysis of cervical cancer on microdissected archival materials by PCR-based X-chromosome inactivation approach. Int J Oncol 12:1327–1332, 1998.

Guo Z, Wu F, Asplund A, et al. Analysis of intratumoral heterogeneity of chromosome 3p deletions and genetic evidence of polyclonal origin of cervical squamous carcinoma. Mod Pathol 14:54–61, 2001.

Gupta J, Gendelman HE, Naghashfar Z, et al. Specific identification of human papillomavirus type in cervical smears and paraffin sections by in situ hybridization with radioactive probes: A preliminary communication. Int J Gynecol Pathol 4:211–218, 1985.

Gupta JW, Gupta PK, Shah KV, Kelly DP. Distribution of human papillomavirus antigen in cervico-vaginal smears and cervical tissues. Int J Gynecol Pathol 2:160–170, 1983.

Hacker NF, Berek JS, Lagase LD, et al. Carcinoma of the cervix associated with pregnancy. Obstet Gynecol 59:735–746, 1982.

Hagmar B, Christensen JJ, Johansson B, et al. Implications of human papillomavirus type for survival in cervical squamous cell carcinoma. Int J Gynecol Cancer 5:341–345, 1995.

Hajdu SI, Adelman HC. Anatomic distribution and grading of carcinoma in situ of the cervix. Cancer 19:1466–1472, 1966.

Hakama M. Trends in the incidence of cervical cancer in the Nordic counties. *In:* Magnus K (ed). Trends in Cancer Incidence, Causes and Practical Implications. Stockholm, Hemisphere Publishing Corp 1988, pp 279–292.

Hakama M. Mass screening for cervical cancer in Finland. *In:* Miller AB (ed). Screening in Cancer: A report of a UICC International Workshop, Toronto, April 1978. International Union Against Cancer, 1978, pp 93–107.

Hakama M. Louhivuori K. A screening programme for cervical cancer that worked. Cancer Surv 7:403–416, 1988.

Hale RJ, Buckley CH, Fox H, et al. Prognostic value of cerB-2 expression in uterine cervical carcinoma. J Clin Pathol 45:594–596, 1992.

Hall JE, Boyce JG, Nelson JH. Carcinoma in situ of the cervix uteri. A study of 409 patients. Obstet Gynecol 34:221–225, 1969.

Hall JE, Walter L. Dysplasia of the cervix. A prospective study of 206 cases. Am J Obstet Gynecol 100:662–667, 1968.

Hamperl H, Kaufmann C, Ober KG. Histologische Untersuchungen an der cervix schwangerer Frauen; die Erosion und das carcinoma in situ. Arch Gynecol 184:181–280, 1954.

Hanau CA, Bibbo M. The case for cytologic follow-up after LEEP. Acta Cytol 41:731–736, 1997.

Handy VH, Wieben E. Detection of cancer of the cervix: A Public Health approach. Obstet Gynecol 25:348–355, 1965.

Hanselaar AG, Vooijs GP, Mayall BH, et al. DNA changes in progressive cervical intraepithelial neoplasia. Anal Cell Pathol 4:315–324, 1992.

Hanselaar AGJM, Vooijs GP, Oud PS, et al. DNA ploidy patterns in cervical intraepithelial neoplasia grade III, with and without synchronous invasive squamous cell carcinoma: Measurements in nuclei isolated from paraffin-embedded tissue. Cancer 62:2537–2545, 1988.

Hare MJ, Taylor-Robinson D, Cooper P. Evidence for an association between *Chalmydia trachomatis* and cervical intraepithelial neoplasia. Br J Obstet Gynecol 89:489–492, 1982.

Harnekar AB, Leiman G, Markowitz S. Cytologically detected chlamydial changes and progression of cervical intraepithelial neoplasias. A retrospective case-control study. Acta Cytol 29:661–664, 1985.

Hawthorn RJ, Murdoch JB, MacLean AB, MacKie RM. Langerhans' cells and subtypes of human papillomavirus in cervical intraepithelial neoplasia. Br Med J 297:643–646, 1988.

Hayashi Y, Hachisuga T, Iwasaka T, et al. Expression of ras oncogene product and EGF receptor in cervical squamous cell carcinomas and its relationship to lymph node involvement. Gynecol Onc 40:147–151, 1991.

Hein K, Schreiber K, Cohen MI, Koss LG. Cervical cytology: The need for routine screening in sexually active adolescent. J Pediatr 91:123–126, 1977.

Held E. Das Oberflachencarcinom (nicht invasives atypisches Plattenepithel). Arch Gynäkol 183:322–364, 1953.

Hellberg D, Axelsson O, Gad A, Nilsson S. Conservative management of the abnormal smear during pregnancy. Acta Obstet Gynecol Scand 66:195–199, 1987.

Helmerhorst TJM, Meijer CJLM. Cervical cancer should be considered as a rare complication of oncogenic HPV infection rather than a STD. Int J Gynecol Cancer 12:235–236, 2002.

Henry MJ, Stanley MW, Cruikshank S, Carson L. Association of human immunodeficiency virus-induced immunosuppression with human papillomavirus infection and cervical intraepithelial neoplasia. Am J Obstet Gynecol 160:352–353, 1989.

Herbert A, Smith JAE. Cervical intraepithelial neoplasia grade III (CIN III) and invasive cervical carcinoma: Tthe yawning gap revisited and the treatment of risk. Cytopathology 10:161–170, 1999.

Herbst AL, Pickett KE, Follen M, Noller KL. The management of ASCUS cervical cytologic abnormalities and HPV testing: a cautionary note. Obstet Gynecol 98:849–851, 2001.

Herrington CS, Graham D, Southern SA, et al. Loss of retinoblastoma protein expression is frequent in small cell neuroendocrine carcinoma of the cervix and is urelated to HPV type. Hum Pathol 30:906–910, 1999.

Hertig AT. Early concepts of dysplasia and carcinoma in situ (a backward look at a forward process). Obstet Gynecol Surv 34:795–803, 1979.

Hertig AT, MacKey JJ, Feeley G, Kampschmidt K. Dysplasia of the lower genital tract in the female monkey, *Macaca fascicularis*, the crab-eating macaque from South-east Asia. Am J Obstet Gynecol 145:968–980, 1983.

Heselmeyer K, Macville M, Schroeck E, et al. Advanced-stage cervical carcinomas are defined by recurrent pattern of chromosomal aberrations revealing high genomic instability and a consistent gain of chromosome arm 3q. Genes, Chromos. Cancer 19:233–240, 1997.

Heselmeyer K, Schroeck E, du Manoir S, et al. Gain of chromosome 3q defines the transition from severe dysplasia to invasive carcinoma of the uterine cervix. Proc Natl Acad Sci USA 93:479–484, 1996.

Hessling JJ, Raso DS, Schiffer B, et al. Effectiveness of thin-layer preparations vs. conventional Pap smears in a blinded, split-sample study. Extended cytologic evaluation. J Reprod Med 46:880–886, 2001.

Hidalgo A, Schewe C, Petersen S, et al. Human papilloma virus status and chromosomal imbalances in primary cervical carcinomas and tumour cell lines. Eur J Cancer 36:542–548, 2000.

Higgins PJ, Borenfreund E, Bendich A. Appearance of foetal antigens in somatic cells after interaction with heterologous sperm. Nature 257:488–489, 1975.

Hildesheim A, Hadjimichael O, Schwartz PE, et al. Risk factors for rapid-onset cervical cancer. Am J Obstet Gynecol 180:571–577, 1999.

Hildesheim A, Schiffman MH, Gravitt PE, et al. Persistence of type-specific human papillomavirus infection among cytologically normal women. J Infect Dis 169:235–240, 1994.

Hills E, Laverty CR. Electron microscopic detection of papilloma virus particles in selected koilocytic cells in a routine cervical smear. Acta Cytol 23:53–56, 1979.

Hinselmann H. Verbesserung der aktiven Ausgestaltung der Gefässe beim jungen Portikarzinom als neues diffrential diagnostisches Hilfsmittel. Zbl Gynäk 72, 1733–1925.

Hirschowitz L, Raffle AE, Mackenzie EFD, Hughes AO. Long term follow-up of women with borderline cervical smear test results: Effects of age and viral infection on progression to high grade dyskaryosis. Br Med J 304:1209–1212, 1992.

Hisaw FL, Hisaw FL, Jr. Spontaneous carcinoma of cervix uteri in monkey (*Macaca mulatta*). Cancer 11:810–816, 1958.

Ho GYF, Bierman MD, Beardsley L, et al. Natural history of cervicovaginal papillomavirus infection in young women. N Engl J Med 338:423–428, 1998.

Ho GYF, Burk RD, Klein S, et al. Persistent genital human papillomavirus infection as a risk factor for persistent cervical dysplasia. J Natl Cancer Inst 87:1365–1371, 1995.

Ho GYF, Kadish AS, Burk RD, et al. HPV 16 and cigarette smoking as risk factors for high-grade cervical intraepithelial neoplasia. Int J Cancer 78:281–285, 1998.

Hoeg K, Roger V. Dysplasia, carcinoma in situ, and invasive carcinoma of the cervix uteri in previously screened women. Scand J Clin Lab Invest 22:173–180, 1968.

Hollingworth T, Barton S. The natural history of early cervical neoplasia and cervical human papillomavirus infection. Cancer Surv 7:519–527, 1988.

Hollinshead AC, Lee O, Chretien PB, et al. Antibodies to herpesvirus nonvirion antigens in squamous carcinomas. Science 182:713–715, 1973.

Holmquist ND, McMahan CA, Williams OD. Variability in classification of carcinoma in situ of the uterine cervix. Arch Pathol 84:334–345, 1967.

Holzer E, Burghardt E. Die Lokalisation des pathologischen Cervixepithels. II. Aufsteigende Überhäutung, Plattenepithelmetaplasie und basale Hyperplasie. Arch Gynecol 210:395–415, 1971.

Howard LH, Jr, Erickson CC, Stoddard LD. Study of incidence and histogenesis of endocervical metaplasia and intraepithelial carcinoma; observations on 400 uteri removed for noncervical disease. Cancer 4:1210–1223, 1951.

Howe DT, Vincenti AC. Is large loop excision of the transformation zone (LLETZ) more accurate than colposcopically directed punch biopsy in the diagnosis of cervical intraepithelial neoplasia? Br J Obstet Gynaecol 98:588–591, 1991.

Howley PM. Role of human papillomaviruses in human cancer. Cancer Res 51 (suppl):5019–5022, 1991.

Hrushovetz SB. Two-wavelength Feulgen cytophotometry of cells exfoliated from the uterine cervix. Acta Cytol 13:583–594, 1969.

Hubbard RA. Human papillomavirus testing methods. Arch Pathol Lab Med 127:940–945, 2003.

Hudson E, Hewerston S, Jansz C, Gordon H. Screening hospital patients for uterine cervical cancer. J Clin Pathol 36:611–615, 1983.

Hulka BS. Cytologic and histologic outcome following an atypical cervical smear. Am J Obstet Gynecol 101:190–199, 1968.

Husain OAN, Butler EB. A Colour Atlas of Gynaecological Cytology. London, Wolfe, 1989.

Hutchinson ML, Zahniser DJ, Sherman ME, et al. Utility of liquid-based cytology for cervical carcinoma screening. Cancer (Cancer Cytopathol) 87:48–55, 1999.

Iemura K, Sonoda T, Hayakawa A, et al. Small cell carcinoma of the uterine cervix showing Cushing's syndrome caused by ectopic adrenocorticotropin hormone production. Jpn J Clin Oncol 21:293–298, 1991.

International Agency for Research on Cancer: Human Papillomaviruses. Monograph 64, Lyon, France, 1995.

International Committee on Histological Definitions (1961) (Editorial). Acta Cytol 6:235–236, 1962.

Isaacs JH. Verrucous carcinoma of the female genital tract. Gynecol Oncol 4:259–269, 1976.

Iskaros BF, Koss LG. Tenascin expression in intraepithelial neoplasia and invasive carcinoma of the uterine cervix. Arch Pathol Lab Med 124:1282–1286, 2000.

Ismail SM, Colclogh AB, Dinnen JS, et al. Observer variation in histopathological diagnosis and grading of cervical intraepithelial neoplasia. Br Med J 298:707–710, 1989.

Ismail SM, Colclogh AB, Dinnen JS, et al. Reporting cervical intraepithelial neoplasia: intra- and interpathologist variation and factors associated with disagreement. Histopath 16:371–376, 1990.

Jafari K. False-negative Pap smears in uterine malignancy. Gynecol Oncol 6:76–82, 1978.

Jain AG, Higgins RV, Boyle MJ. Management of low-grade squamous intraepithelial lesions during pregnancy. Am J Obstet Gynecol 177:298–302, 1997.

Jakobsen A. Prognostic impact of ploidy level in carcinoma of the cervix. Am J Clin Oncol 7:475–480, 1984.

Jakobsen A, Kristensen PB, Poulsen HK. Flow cytometric classification of biopsy specimens from cervical intraepithelial neoplasia. Cytometry 4:166–169, 1983.

Jakobsen A, Nielsen KV, Ronne M. DNA distribution and chromosome number in human cervical carcinoma. Anal Quant Cytol 5:13–18, 1983.

James GK, Kalousek DK, Auersperg N. Karyotypic analysis of two related cervical carcinoma cell lines that contain human papillomavirus type 18 DNA, express divergent differentiation. Cancer Genet Cytogenet 38:53–60, 1989.

Jenison SA, Yu X, Valentine JM, et al. Evidence of prevalent genital-type human papillomavirus infections in adults and children. J Infect Dis 162:60–69, 1990.

Jenson AB, Rosenthal JR, Olson C, et al. Immunocological relatedness of papillomaviruses from different species. JNCI 64:495–500, 1980.

Johannesson G, Geirsson G, Day N. The effect of mass screening of cancer in Iceland 1965–74 on the incidence and morality of cervical carcinoma. Int J Cancer 21:418–425, 1978.

Johannisson E, Kolstad P, Soderberg G. Cytologic, vascular, and histologic patterns of dysplasia, carcinoma in situ and early invasive carcinoma of the cervix. Acta Radiol 258:(Suppl), 1966.

Johnson JE, et al. Increased rate of SIL detection with excellent biopsy correlation after implementation of direct-to-vial ThinPrep liquid-based preparation of cervicovaginal specimens at a university medical center. Acta Cytol 42:1242–1243, 1998.

Johnson LD, Hertig AT, Hinman CH, Easterday CL. Pre-invasive cervical lesions in obstetric patients. Obstet Gynecol 16:133–145, 1960.

Johnson LD, Nickerson RJ, Easterday CL, et al. Epidemiologic evidence for the spectrum of change from dysplasia through carcinoma in situ to invasive cancer. Cancer 22:901–914, 1968.

Johnston WW, Myers B, Creasman WT, Owens SM. Cytopathology and the management of early invasive cancer of the uterine cervix. Obstet Gynecol 60:350–353, 1982.

Jones BA. Rescreening in gynecologic cytology. Rescreening of 3762 previous cases for current high-grade squamous intraepithelial lesions and carcinoma. A College of American Pathologists Q-Probes study of 312 institutions. Arch Path Lab Med 119:1097–1103, 1995.

Jones BA, Novis DA. Cervical biopsy-cytology correlation. A College of American Pathologists Q-Probes study of 22,439 correlations in 348 laboratories. Arch Pathol Lab Med 120:523–531, 1996.

Jones DE, Creasman WT, Dombroski RA, et al. Evaluation of the atypical Pap smear. Am J Obstet Gynecol 157:544–549, 1987.

Jones HW, Jr, Davis HJ, Frost JK, et al. The value of the assay of chromosomes in the diagnosis of cervical neoplasia. Am J Obstet Gynecol 102:624–639, 1968.

Jones HW, Katayama KP, Stafl A, Davis HJ. Chromosomes of cervical atypia, carcinoma in situ, and epidermoid carcinoma of the cervix. Obstet Gynecol 30:790–805, 1967.

Jones RW. Reflections on carcinoma in situ. NZ Med J 104:339–341, 1991.

Jordan JA, Williams AE. Scanning electron microscopy in the study of cervical neoplasia. J Obstet Gynecol Br Commonw 78:940–946, 1971.

Jordan MJ, Bader GM, Day E. Carcinoma in situ of the cervix and related lesions. An 11-year prospective study. Am J Obstet Gynecol 89:160–182, 1964.

Jordan MJ, Bader GM, Day E. Rational approach to management of atypical lesions of cervix. Am J Obstet Gynecol 72:725–739, 1956.

Jordan SW, Key CR. Carcinoma of the cervix in South-western American Indians: Results of a cytologic detection program. Cancer 47:2523–2532, 1981.

Joste NE, Crum CP, Cibas ES. Cytologic/histologic correlation for quality control in cervicovaginal cytology. Experience with 1,582 paired cases. Am J Clin Pathol 103:32–34, 1995.

Kadish AS, Burk RD, Kress Y, et al. Human papillomaviruses of different types in precancerous lesions of the uterine cervix: Histologic, immunocytochemical and ultrastructural studies. Hum Pathol 17:384–392, 1986.

Kadish AS, Hagan RJ, Ritter DB, et al. Biologic characteristics of specific human papillomavirus types predicted from morphology of cervical lesions. Hum Pathol 23:1262–1269, 1992.

Kadish AS, Ho GYF, Burk RD, et al. Lymphoproliferative responses to human papillomavirus (HPV) type 16 proteins E6 and E7: outcome of HPV infection and associated neoplasia. JNCI 89:1285–1293, 1997.

Kamentsky LA, Derman H, Melamed MR. Ultraviolet absorption in epidermoid cancer cells. Science 142:1580–1583, 1963.

Kamentsky LA, Melamed MR, Derman H. Spectro-photometer: New instrument for ultrarapid cell analysis. Science 150:630–631, 1965.

Kaminetzky HA, McGrew EA. The effect of podophyllin on the human endocervix. Obstet Gynecol 18:255–258, 1961.

Kaminski PF, Sorosky JI, Wheelock JB, Stevens CW Jr. The significance of atypical cervical cytology in an older population. Obstet Gynecol 73:13–15, 1989.

Katz RL, Veanattukalathil S, Weiss KM. Human papilloma virus infection and neoplasia of the cervix and anogenital region in women with Hodgkin's disease. Acta Cytol 31:845–854, 1987.

Kaufman RH. Atypical squamous cells of undetermined significance and low-grade squamous intraepithelial lesion: diagnostic criteria and management. Am J Obstet Gynecol 175:1120–1128, 1996.

Kaufman RH, Burmeister RE, Spjut HJ. Cervical cytology in the teenage patient. Am J Obstet Gynecol 108:515–519, 1970.

Kaufman RH, Leeds LT. Cervical and vaginal cytology in the child and adolescent. Pediatr Clin North Am 19:547–559, 1972.

Kaufman RH, Strama T, Norton PK, Conner JS. Cryosurgical treatment of cervical intraepithelial neoplasia. Obstet Gynecol 42:881–886, 1973.

Kazol HH, Long JP. Squamous cell papillomas of the uterine cervix. A report of 20 cases. Cancer 11:1040–1059, 1958.

Keating JT, Cviko A, Riethdorf S, et al. Ki-67, cyclin E, p16^{INK4} are complimentary surrogate biomarkers for human papilloma virus-related cervical neoplasia. Am J Surg Pathol 25:884–891, 2001.

Keebler CM, Wied GL. The estrogen test: An aid in differential cytodiagnosis. Acta Cytol 18:482–493, 1974.

Kehar U, Wahi PN. Cytologic and histologic behavior patterns of the premalignant lesions of the cervix in experimentally induced cervical dysplasia. Acta Cytol 11:1–15, 1967.

Kennedy AW, Salmieri SS, Wirth SL, et al. Results of the clinical evaluation of atypical glandular cells of undetermined significance (AGUS) detected on cervical cytology screening. Gynecol Oncol 63:14–18, 1996.

Kern G, Nolens JP. Langzeitbeobachtungen von dysplastischem und gesteigert atypischem Epithel. Arch Gynkol 207:67, 1969.

Kessler II. Perspectives on the epidemiology of cervical cancer with special reference to the herpes virus hypothesis. Cancer Res 34:1091–1110, 1974.

Killackey MA, Jones WB, Lewis JL, Jr. Diagnostic conization of the cervix: Review of 460 consecutive cases. Obstet Gynecol 67:766–770, 1986.

Kim JJ, Wright TC, Goldie SJ. Cost-effectiveness of alternative triage strategies for atypical squamous cells of undetermined significance. JAMA 287:2382–2390, 2002.

Kinderman G, Jabusch HP. The spread of squamous cell carcinoma of the uterine cervix into the blood-vessels. Arch Gynecol 212:1–8, 1972.

Kinlen LJ, Spriggs AI. Women with positive cervical smears but without surgical intervention. A follow-up study. Lancet 2:463–465, 1978.

Kirkland JA. Chromosomal and mitotic abnormalities in preinvasive and invasive carcinomas of the cervix. Aust NZ J Obstet Gynaecol 6:35–39, 1966.

Kirkland JA. Carcinoma in situ—diagnosis and prognosis. J Obstet Gynaecol Br Commonw 70:232–243, 1963.

Kirkland JA, Stanley MA, Cellier KM. Comparative study of histologic and chromosomal abnormalities in cervical neoplasia. Cancer 20:1934–1952, 1967.

Kirnbauer R, Hubbert NL, Wheeler CM, et al. A virus-like particle enzyme-linked immunosorbent assay detects serum antibodies in a majority of women infected with human papillomavirus type 16. JNCI 86:494–499, 1994.

Kivlahan C, Ingram E. Papanicolaou smears without endocervical cells. Are they inadequate? Acta Cytol 30:258–260, 1986.

Kiyabu MT, Shibata D, Arnheim N, et al. Detection of human papillomavirus in formalin-fixed, invasive squamous carcinomas using the polymerase chain reaction. Am J Surg Pathol 13:221–224, 1989.

Kjaer SK, de Villiers EM, Haugaard BJ, et al. Human papillomavirus, herpes simplex virus and cervical cancer incidence in Greenland and Denmark. A population-based cross-sectional study. Int J Cancer 41:518–524, 1988.

Kjaer SK, van den Brule AJC, Bock JE, et al. Human papillomavirus: the most significant risk determinant of cervical intraepithelial neoplasia. Int J Cancer 65:601–606, 1996.

Kjaergaard J, Poulsen EF. Scanning electron microscopy of cotton swab smears from ectocervix. A methodological study. Acta Cytol 21:68–71, 1977.

Klein RS, Ho GYF, Vermund SH, et al. Risk factors for squamous intraepithelial lesions on Pap smear in women at risk for human immunodeficiency virus infection. J Infect Dis 170:1404–1409, 1994.

Kleter B, van Doorn, L-J, ter Schegget J, et al. Novel short-fragment PCR assay for highly sensitive broad-spectrum detection of anogenital human papillomaviruses. Am J Pathol 153:1731–1739, 1998.

Kling TG, Buchsbaum HJ. Cervical carcinoma in women under twenty-one years of age. Obstet Gynecol 42:205–208, 1973.

Klinkhamer PJ, Meerding WJ, Rosier PF, Hanselaar AG. Liquid-based cervical cytology. Cancer 99:263–271, 2003.

Klinkhamer PJ, Vooijs GP, de Haan AFJ. Intraobserver and interobserver variability in the diagnosis of epithelial abnormalities in cervical smears. Acta Cytol 32:794–800, 1988.

Kloster BE, Manias DA, Ostrow RS, et al. Molecular cloning and characterization of the DNA in two papillomaviruses from monkeys. Virology 166:30–40, 1988.

Kobayashi A, Darragh T, Herndier B, et al. Lymphoid follicles are generated in high-grade cervical dysplasia and have differing characteristics depending on HIV status. Am J Pathol 160:151–164, 2002.

Kok MR, Boon ME, Schreiner-Kok PG, Koss LG. Cytological recognition of invasive squamous cancer of the uterine cervix: Comparison of conventional light-microscopical screening and neural network-based screening. Hum Pathol 31:23–28, 2000.

Kolstad P. Cytological mass screening of a defined population. Acta Obstet Gynecol 48 (Suppl 3):50–57, 1969.

Kolstad P, Klem V. Long-term followup of 1121 cases of carcinoma in situ. Obstet Gynecol 48:125–129, 1976.

Kolstad P, Stafl A. Atlas of Colposcopy, ed 2. Baltimore, University Park Press, 1977.

Komorowski RA, Clowry LJ, Jr. Koilocytotic atypia of the cervix. Obstet Gynecol 47:540–544, 1976.

Koprowska I, Bogacz J, Pentikas C, Stypulkowski W. Induced cervical carcinoma of the mouse. A quantitative cytologic method for evaluation of the neoplastic process. Cancer Res 18:1186–1190, 1958.

Korn AP, Judson PL, Zaloudek CJ. Importance of atypical glandular cells of uncertain significance in cervical cytologic smears. J Reprod Med 43:774–778, 1998.

Koss LG. Human papillomavirus testing as a screening tool for cervical cancer (Letter to Editor). JAMA 283:2525, 2000.

Koss LG. Utility of liquid-based cytology for cervical carcinoma screening. Letter. Cancer (Cancer Cytopathol) 90:67–68, 2000.

Koss LG. Human papillomavirus—passenger, driver, or both? (Editorial). Hum Pathol 29:309–310, 1998.

Koss LG. Error rates in cervical cancer screening: causes and consequences. *In:* Franco E, Monsonego J (eds). New Developments in Cervical Cancer Screening and Prevention. Oxford, Blackwell Science, 1997, pp 163–168.

Koss LG. Performance of cytology in screening for precursor lesions and early cancer of the uterine cervix. *In:* Franco E, Monsonego J (eds). New Developments in Cervical Cancer Screening and Prevention. Oxford, Blackwell Science, 1997, pp 147–150.

Koss LG. Cervical (Pap) smear—New directions. Cancer 71:1406–1412, 1993.

Koss LG. The Papanicolaou test for cervical cancer detection. A triumph and a tragedy. JAMA 261:737–743, 1989.

Koss LG. From koilocytosis to molecular biology: The impact of cytology on concepts of early human cancer. Modern Pathol 2:526–535, 1989.

Koss LG. Current concepts of intraepithelial neoplasia in the uterine cervix (CIN). Appl Pathol 5:7–18, 1987.

Koss LG. Cytologic and histologic manifestations of human papillomavirus infection of the female genital tract and their clinical significance. Cancer 60:1942–1950, 1987.

Koss LG. Cytologic evaluation of the uterine cervix: Factor influencing its accuracy. Pathologist 36:401–407, 1982.

Koss LG. Pathogenesis of carcinoma of the uterine cervix. *In:* Dallenbach-Hellweg G (ed). Cervical Cancer. Current Topics in Pathology, vol 70. New York, Springer, 1981, pp 112–142.

Koss LG. The attack on the annual 'Pap smear.' Acta Cytol 24:181–183, 1980.

Koss LG. Dysplasia. A real concept or a misnomer? Obstet Gynecol 51:374–379, 1978.

Koss LG. Precancerous lesions of the uterine cervix in pregnancy. CA—A Journal for Physicians 24:141–143, 1974.

Koss LG. Detection of carcinoma of the uterine cervix (Editorial). JAMA 222:699–700, 1972.

Koss LG. Significance of dysplasia. Clin Obstet Gynecol 13:873–888, 1970.

Koss LG. Concept of genesis and development of carcinoma of the cervix. Obstet Gynecol Surv 24:850–860, 1969.

Koss LG, Durfee GR. Cytological changes preceding appearance of in situ carcinoma of uterine cervix. Cancer 8:295–301, 1955.

Koss LG, Durfee GR. Unusual patterns of squamous epithelium of the uterine cervix; cytologic and pathologic study of koilocytotic atypia. Ann NY Acad Sci 63:1245–1261, 1956.

Koss LG, Melamed MR, Daniel WW. In situ epidermoid carcinoma of cervix and vagina following radiotherapy for cervix cancer. Cancer 14:353–360, 1961.

Koss LG, Stewart FW, Foote FW, et al. Some histological aspects of behavior of epidermoid carcinoma in situ and related lesions of uterine cervix. A long-term prospective study. Cancer 16:1160–1211, 1963.

Koss LG, Wolinska WH. Trichomonas vaginalis cervicitis and its relationship to cervical cancer; histocytological study. Cancer 12:1171–1193, 1959.

Kothe MJC, Prins JM, de Wit R, et al. Small cell carcinoma of the cervix with inappropriate antidiuretic hormone secretion. Case report. Br J Obstet Gynaecol 97:647–648, 1990.

Kottmeier HL. Erfahrungen des Radiumhemmet, Stockholm, mit der Behandlung des Oberflachen-carcinoms und des Fruhinvasiven carcinoms der Cervix. Verh Dtsch Ges Gynakol 37:332–342, 1968.

Koutsky LA, Ault KA, Wheeler CM, et al. A controlled trial of a human papillomavirus type 16 vaccine. N Engl J Med 347:1645–1651, 2002.

Koutsky LA, Holmes KK, Critchlow CW, et al. A cohort study of the risk of cervical intraepithelial neoplasia grade 2 or 3 in relation to papillomavirus infection. N Engl J Med 327:1272–1278, 1992.

Kovi J, Tillman RL, Lee SM. Malignant transformation of condyloma acuminatum. Am J Clin Pathol 61:702–710, 1974.

Kreider JW, Howett MK, Wolfe SA, et al. Morphological transformation in vivo of human uterine cervix with papillomavirus from condylomata acuminata. Nature 317:639–641, 1985.

Kristensen GB, Skyggebjerg KD, Holund B, et al. Analysis of cervical smears obtained within three years of the diagnosis of invasive cervical cancer. Acta Cytol 35:47–50, 1991.

Kruse A-J, Baak JPA, Helliesen T, et al. Evaluation of MIB-1-positive cell clusters as a diagnostic marker for cervical intraepithelial neoplasia. Am J Surg Pathol 26:1501–1507, 2002.

Kruse A-J, Skaland I, Janssen EA, et al. Quantitative molecular parameters to identify low-risk and high-risk early CIN lesions: Role of markers of proliferative activity and differentiation and Rb availability. Int J Gynecol Pathol 23:100–109, 2004.

Kulda J, Honigberg BM, Frost JK, Hollander DH. Pathogenicity of Trichomonas vaginalis. Am J Obstet Gynecol 108:908–918, 1970.

Kurman RJ, Henson DE, Herbst AL, et al. Interim guidelines for management of abnormal cervical cytology. JAMA 271:1866–1869, 1994.

Kurman RJ, Shiffman RM, Lancaster WD, et al. Analysis of individual human papillomavirus types in cervical neoplasia: A possible role for type 18 in rapid progression. Am J Obstet Gynecol 159:293–296, 1988.

Kurman RJ, Solomon D. The Bethesda System for Reporting Cervical/Vaginal Cytologic Diagnoses. New York, NY, Springer-Verlag, 1994, pp 30–43.

Kurtycz D, Nunez M, Arts T, et al. Use of fluorescent in situ hybridization to detect aneuploidy in cervical dysplasia. Diagn Cytopathol 15:46–51, 1996.

Lange P. Clinical and histological studies on cervical carcinoma. Acta Pathol Microbiol Scand (Suppl 143) 50:1–79, 1960.

Laverty CR, Russell P, Hills E, Booth N. The significance of non-condyloma wart virus infection of the cervical transformation zone: A review with discussion of two illustrative cases. Acta Cytol 22:195–201, 1978.

Layde PM, Broste SK. Carcinoma of the cervix and smoking. Biomed Pharmacother 43:161–165, 1989.

Lazo PA. The molecular genetics of cervical carcinoma. Br J Cancer 80:2008–2018, 1999.

Lee JSJ, Kuan L, Oh S, et al. A feasibility study of the AutoPap system location-guided screening. Acta Cytol 42:221–226, 1998.

Lee KR, Asfaq R, Birdsong GG, et al. Comparison of conventional Papanicolaou smears and a fluid-based, thin-layer system for cervical cancer screening. Obstet Gynecol 90:278–284, 1997.

Lee KR, Manna EA, St. John T. Atypical endocervical glandular cells: Accuracy of cytologic diagnosis. Diagn Cytopathol 13:202–208, 1995.

Lee KR, Minter LJ, Crum CP. Koilocytotic atypia in Papanicolaou smears. Reproducibility and biopsy correlations. Cancer Cytopathol 81:10–15, 1997.

Leham MH, Benson WL, Kurman RJ, Park RB. Microinvasive carcinoma of the cervix. Obstet Gynecol 48:571–578, 1976.

Lele SM, Pou AM, Ventura K, et al. Molecular events in the progression of recurrent respiratory papillomatosis to carcinoma. Arch Pathol Lab Med 126:1184–1188, 2002.

Lerch V, Okagaki T, Austin JH, et al. Cytologic findings in progression of anaplasia (dysplasia) to carcinoma in situ: A progress report. Acta Cytol 7:183–186, 1963.

Levi AW, Kelly DP, Rosenthal DL, Ronnett BM. Atypical squamous cells of undetermined significance in liquid-based cytologic specimens: results of reflex human papillomavirus testing and histologic follow-up in routine practice with comparison of interpretive and probabilistic reporting methods. Cancer 99:191–197, 2003.

Levin ML, Kress LC, Goldstein H. Syphilis and cancer. NY State J Med 42:1713–1745, 1942.

Levine L, Lucci JA. 3rd, Dinh TV. Atypical glandular cells: New Bethesda Terminology and Management Guidelines. Obstet Gynecol Surv 58:399–406, 2003.

Levine PH, Elgert PA, Mittal K. False-positive squamous cell carcinoma in cervical smears: Cytologic-histologic correlation in 19 cases. Diagn Cytopathol 28:23–27, 2003.

Levine RU, Crum CP, Herman E, et al. Cervical papillomavirus infection and intraepithelial neoplasia: A study of male sexual partners. Obstet Gynecol 64:16–20, 1984.

Ley C, Bauer HM, Reingold A, et al. Determinants of genital human papillomavirus infection in young women. JNCI 83:997–1003, 1991.

Lie AK, Isaksen CV, Skarsvag S, Haugen OA. Human papillomavirus (HPV) in high-grade cervical intraepithelial neoplasia (CIN) detected by morphology and polymerase chain reaction (PCR)—a cytohistologic correlation of 277 cases treated by laser conization. Cytopathology 9:112–121, 1998.

Lill PH, Norris HJ, Rubenstone AI, et al. Isoantigens ABH in cervical intraepithelial neoplasia. Am J Clin Pathol 66:767–774, 1976.

Limaye A, Connor AJ, Huang X, Luff R. Comparative analysis of conventional Papanicolaou tests and a fluid-based thin-layer method. Arch Pathol Lab Med 127:200–204, 2003.

Limburg H. Die Fruhdiagnose des Uteruscarcinoms; Histologie, Kolposkopie, Cytologie, biochemische Methoden, ed 3. Stuttgart, Georg Thieme, 1956.

Linden G, Henderson BE. Genital-tract cancers in adolescents and young adults. N Engl J Med 286:760–1972.

Lindgreen J, Wahlstrom T, Sappala M. Tissue CEA in premalignant epithelial lesions and epidermoid carcinoma of the uterine cervix: Prognostic significance. Int J Cancer 23:448–453, 1979.

Lindgren A, Stendahl U, Brodin T, et al. Blood group antigen expression and prognosis in squamous cell carcinoma of the uterine cervix. Anticancer Res 6:255–258, 1986.

Liu W. Positive smears in previously screened patients (certain cytologic findings of public health importance). Acta Cytol 11:193–198, 1967.

Livingstone 1997.

Lonky NM, Felix JC, Naidu YM, Wolde-Tsadik G. Triage of atypical squamous cells of undetermined significance with hybrid capture II: Colposcopy and histologic human papillomavirus correlation. Obstet Gynecol 101:481–489, 2003.

Lonky NM, Sadeghi M, Tsadik GW, Petitti D. The clinical significance of the poor correlation of cervical dysplasia and cervical malignancy with referral cytologic results. Am J Obstet Gynecol 181:560–566, 1999.

Lorincz AT. Hybrid Capture method for detection of human papillomavirus DNA in clinical specimens. Pap Report 7:1–5, 1996.

Lorincz AT, Lancaster WD, Kurman RJ, et al. Characterization of human papillomaviruses in cervical neoplasias and their detection in routine clinical screening. In: Peto R, zur Hausen H (eds). Viral Etiology of Cervical Cancer: Banbury Report 21. Cold Spring Harbor NY, Cold Spring Harbor Laboratory, 1986, pp 225–237.

Lorincz AT, Reid R, Jenson B, et al. Human papillomavirus infection of the cervix: Relative risk associations of 15 common anogenital types. Obstet Gynecol 79:328–337, 1992.

Lorincz AT, Richart RM. Human papillomavirus DNA testing as an adjunct to cytology in cervical screening programs. Arch Pathol Lab Med 127:959–968, 2003.

Lorincz AT, Schiffman MH, Jaffurs WJ, et al. Temporal associations of human papillomavirus infection with cervical cytologic abnormalities. Am J Obstet Gynecol 162:645–651, 1990.

Lorincz AT, Temple GF, Kurman RJ, et al. Oncogenic association of specific human papillomavirus types with cervical neoplasia. JNCI 79:671–677, 1987.

Lucia HL, Livolsi VA, Loweel DM. A histochemical method for demonstrating papilloma virus infection in paraffin-embedded tissue. Am J Clin Pathol 82:589–593, 1984.

Luesley D. Advances in colposcopy and management of cervical intraepithelial neoplasia. Curr Opin Obstet Gynecol 4:102–108, 1992.

Luesley DM, McCrum A, Terry PB, et al. Complications of cone biopsy related to the dimensions of the cone and the influence of prior colposcopic assessment. Br J Obstet Gynaecol 92:158–164, 1985.

Luibel FJ, Sanders E, Ashworth C Tg. Electron microscopic study of carcinoma in situ and invasive carcinoma of cervix uteri. Cancer Res 20:357–361, 1960.

Lynge E, Poll P. Incidence of cervical cancer following negative smear. A cohort study from Maribo county, Denmark. Am J Epidemiol 124:345–352, 1986.

Macnab JCM, Walkinshaw SA, Cordiner JW, Clements JB. Human papillomavirus in clinically and histologically normal tissue of patients with genital cancer. N Engl J Med 315:1052–1058, 1986.

Maden C, Beckman AM, Thomas DB, et al. Human papillomaviruses, herpes simplex viruses, and the risk of oral cancer in men. Am J Epidemiol 135:1093–1102, 1992.

Maier RC, Schultenover SJ. Evaluation of the atypical squamous cell Papanicolaou smear. Int J Gynecol Pathol 5:242–248, 1986.

Maiman MA, Fruchter RG, DiMaio TM, Boyce JG. Superficially invasive squamous cell carcinoma of the cervix. Obstet Gynecol 72:399–403, 1988.

Maiman M, Fruchter R, Guy L, et al. Human immunodeficiency virus infection and invasive cervical carcinoma. Cancer 71:402–406, 1993.

Maiman M, Fruchter RG, Serur E, et al. Human immunodeficiency virus infection and cervical neoplasia. Gynecol Oncol 38:377–382, 1990.

Makino S, Sasaki MS, Fukushima T. Preliminary notes on the chromosomes of human chorionic lesions. Proc Japan Acad 39:54–58, 1963.

Malek RS, Goellner JR, Smith TF, et al. Human papillomavirus infection and intraepithelial, in situ, and invasive carcinoma of the penis. J Urol 42:159–170, 1993.

Malik SN, Wilkinson EJ, Drew PA, et al. Do qualifiers of ASCUS distinguish between low- and high-risk patients? Acta Cytol 43:376–380, 1999.

Mandelblatt J, Gopaul I, Wistreich M. Gynecological care of elderly women. Another look at Papanicolaou smear testing. JAMA 256:367–371, 1986.

Manias DA, Ostrow RS, McGlennen RC, et al. Characterization of integrated human papillomavirus type 11 DNA in primary and metastatic tumors from a renal transplant recipient. Cancer 49:2514–2519, 1989.

Manos MM, Kinney WK, Hurley LB, et al. Identifying women with cervical neoplasia: Using human papillomavirus DNA testing for equivocal Papanicolaou results. JAMA 281:1605–1610, 1999.

Marcuse PM. Incipient microinvasive carcinoma of the uterine cervix. Morphology and clinical data of 22 cases. Obstet Gynecol 37:360–367, 1971.

Marsh MR. Papilloma of cervix. Am J Obstet Gynecol 64:281–291, 1952.

Marsh M, Fitzgerald PJ. Carcinoma in situ of human uterine cervix in pregnancy; prevalence and postpregnancy persistence. Cancer 9:1195–1207, 1956.

Marshall CE. A ten-year cervical-smear screening programme. Lancet 1026–1029, 1968.

Marshall CE. Effect of cytologic screening on the incidence of invasive carcinoma of the cervix in a semi-closed community. Cancer 18:153–156, 1965.

Martin PL. How preventable is invasive cervical cancer? Am J Obstet Gynecol 113:541–548, 1972.

Marx JL. The annual Pap smear: An idea whose time has gone? Science 205: 177–178, 1979.

Masin M, Masin F. Cytophotometric data on fluorochromed cervical cells. JNCI 27:311–331, 1961.

Matsuura Y, Kawagoe T, Toki N, et al. Low grade cervical intraepithelial neoplasia associated with human papillomavirus infection. Long-term follow-up. Acta Cytol 42:625–630, 1998.

McCance DJ, Kalache A, Ashdown K, et al. Human papillomavirus types 16 and 18 in carcinomas of the penis from Brazil. Int J Cancer 37:55–59, 1986.

McDonnell JM, Mayr AJ, Martin WJ. DNA of human papillomavirus type 16 in dysplastic and malignant lesions of the conjunctiva and cornea. N Engl J Med 320:1442–1446, 1989.

McGrew EA, Kaminetzky HA. The genesis of experimental cervical epithelial dysplasia. Am J Clin Pathol 35:538–545, 1961.

McIndoe WA, McLean MR, Jones RW, Mullins PR. The invasive potential of carcinoma in situ of the cervix. Obstet Gynecol 64:451–458, 1984.

McKenna H, Fraser M, Silverstone H. Squamous papilloma of the cervix uteri. A two-year prospective cytological study. Med J Aust 2:304–306, 1975.

McLachlin CM, Sheets E, Crum CP. High-grade cervical intraepithelial neoplasia: Frequency and significance of coexisting condyloma. J Surg Pathol 1: 165–172, 1995.

McLachlin CM, Tate J, Zitz J, et al. Human papillomavirus type 18 and low grade squamous intraepithelial lesions of the cervix. Am J Pathol 144:141, 1994.

McNutt NS, Weinstein RS. Carcinoma of the cervix: Deficiency of nexus intercellular junctions. Science 165:597–599, 1969.

Meisner L. Use of fluorescent in situ hybridization to detect aneuploidy in cervical dysplasia. Diagn Cytopathol 15:46–51, 1996.

Meisels A, Fortin R. Condylomatous lesions of the cervix and vagina. I. Cytologic patterns. Acta Cytol 20:505–509, 1976.

Meisels A, Fortin R, Roy M. Condylomatous lesions of the cervix: II. Cytologic, colposcopic and histopathologic study. Acta Cytol 21:379–390, 1977.

Meisels A, Morin C, Casa-Cordero M. Lesions of the uterine cervix associated with papillomavirus and their clinical consequences. In Koss LG, Coleman DV (eds). Advances in Clinical Cytology, vol. 2. New York, Masson, 1984, pp 1–31.

Meisels A, Roy M, Fortier M, et al. Human papillomavirus infection of the cervix: The atypical condyloma. Acta Cytol 25:7–16, 1981.

Melamed MR, Flehinger BJ. Non-diagnostic squamous atypia in cervico-vaginal cytology as a risk factor for early neoplasia. Acta Cytol 20:108–110, 1976.

Melamed MR, Koss LG, Flehinger BJ, et al. Prevalence rates of uterine cervical carcinoma in situ for women using the diaphragm or contraceptive oral steroids. Br Med J 3:195–200, 1969.

Melkert PWJ, Hopman E, van den Brule AJC, et al. Prevalence of HPV in cyto-morphologically normal cervical smears, as determined by polymerase chain reaction, is age-dependent. Int J Cancer 53:919–923, 1993.

Mellors RC, Glassman A, Papanicolaou GN. A microfluorometric scanning method for the detection of cancer cells in smears of exfoliated cells. Cancer 5:458–468, 1952.

Mellors RC, Keane JF, Papanicolaou GN. Nucleic acid content of the squamous cancer cell. Science 116:265–269, 1952.

Melnick JL, Adam E, Rawls WE. The causative role of herpesvirus type 2 in cervical cancer. Cancer 34:1375–1385, 1974.

Meyer R. Basis of histological diagnosis of carcinoma; with special reference to carcinoma of cervix and similar lesions. Surg Gynecol Obstet 73:14–20, 1941.

Meyer R. Die histologischen Grundlagen der Karzinomdiagnose. In: Berichte aus wissenschaftlichen Gesellschaften; 90. Versammlung der Gesellschaft deutscher Naturforscher und Ärzte in Hamburg. Zentralbl Gynäkol 52: 2792–2796, 1928.

Meyer R. Die pathologische Anatomie der Gebärmutter. In: Henke F, Lubarsch O (eds). Handbuch der speziellen pathologischen Anatomie und Histologie. Bd 7. T1. 1. Berlin, Springer, 1930, pp 1–624.

Miller AB, Lindsay J, Hill GB. Mortality from cancer of the uterus in Canada and its relationship to screening for cancer of the cervix. Int J Cancer 17: 602–612, 1976.

Miller BE, Copeland LJ, Hamberger AD, et al. Carcinoma of the cervical stump. Gynecol Oncol 18:100–108, 1984.

Minucci D, Cinel A, Insacco E. Diathermic loop treatment for CIN, HPV lesions. A follow-up of 130 cases. Eur J Gynaecol Oncol 12:385–393, 1991.

Mitchell H, Medley G, Giles G. Cervical cancers diagnosed after negative results on cervical cytology: perspective in the 1980s. Br Med J 300:1622–1626, 1990.

Mitchell H, Medley G. Differences between Papanicolaou smears with correct and incorrect diagnoses. Cytopathology 6:368–375, 1995.

Mittal KR, Demmopoulos RI, Goswami S. Proliferating cell nuclear antigen (cyclin) expression in normal and abnormal cervical squamous epithelia. Am J Surg Pathol 17:117–122, 1993.

Mittal KR, Miller HK, Lowell DM. Koilocytosis preceding squamous cell carcinoma in situ of uterine cervix. Am J Clin Pathol 87:243–245, 1987.

Moncrieff D, Ormerod MG, Coleman DV. Immunocytochemical staining of cervical smears for the diagnosis of cervical intraepithelial neoplasia. Anal Quant Cytol 6:201–205, 1984.

Montes MA, Cibas ES, DiNisco SA, Lee KR. Cytologic characteristics of abnormal cells in prior "normal" cervical/vaginal Papanicolaou smears from women with high grade squamous intraepithelial lesions. Cancer 87:56–59, 1999.

Montgomery KD, Tedford KL, McDougall JK. Genetic instability of chromosome 3 in HPV-immortalized and tumorigenic human keratinocytes. Genes Chromos Cancer 14:97–105, 1995.

Montz FJ, Holschneider CH, Thompson LD. Large loop excision of the transformation zone: Effect on the pathologic interpretation of resection margins. Obstet Gynecol 81:976–982, 1993.

Morell ND, Taylor JR, Snyder RN, et al. False-negative cytology rates in patients whom invasive cervical cancer subsequently developed. Obstet Gynecol 60: 41–45, 1982.

Morris HHB, Gatter KC, Sykes G, et al. Langerhans cells in human cervical epithelium: Effects of wart virus infection on intraepithelial neoplasia. Br J Obstet Gynaecol 90:412–420, 1983.

Morrison C, Catania J, Wakely P Jr, Nuovo GJ. Highly differentiated keratinizing squamous cell cancer of the cervix. A rare, locally aggressive tumor not associated with human papillomavirus or squamous intraepithelial lesions. Am J Surg Pathol 25:1310–1315, 2001.

Morrison C, Prokorym P, Piquero C, et al. Oral contraceptive pills are associated with artifacts in ThinPrep Pap smears that mimic low-grade squamous intraepithelial lesions. Cancer 99:75–82, 2003.

Moscicki A-B, Hills N, Shiboski S, et al. Risks for incident human papillomavirus infection and low-grade squamous intraepithelial lesion development in young females. JAMA 285:2995–3002, 2001.

Moscicki AB, Palefsky J, Smith G, et al. Variability of human papillomavirus DNA testing in a longitudinal cohort of young women. Obstet Gynecol 82: 578–585, 1993.

Moscicki AB, Shiboski S, Broering J, et al. The natural history of human papillomavirus infection as measured by repeated DNA testing in adolescent and young women. J Pediatr 132:277–284, 1998.

Munger K, Scheffner M, Huibregtse JM, Howley PM. Interactions of HPV E6 and E7 oncoproteins with tumour suppressor gene products. Cancer Surv 12:197–217, 1992.

Muñoz N, Bosch FX, de Sanjose S, et al. Epidemiologic classification of human papillomavirus types associated with cervical cancer. N Engl J Med 348: 518–527, 2003.

Murphy JF, Allen JM, Jordan JA, Williams AE. Scanning electron microscopy of normal and abnormal exfoliated cervical squamous cells. Br Obstet Gynaecol 82:44–51, 1975.

Murphy MW, Fu YS, Lancaster WD, Jenson AB. Papillomavirus structural antigen in condyloma acuminatum of the male urethra. J Urol 130:84–85, 1983.

Murphy WM, Coleman SA. The long-term course of carcinoma in situ of the uterine cervix. Cancer 38:957–963, 1976.

Mussey E, Decker DG. Management of patients with abnormal cervical cytology findings during pregnancy. Obstet Gynecol 26:556–559, 1965.

Mussey E, Soule EH, Welch JS. Microinvasive carcinoma of the cervix. Am J Obstet Gynecol 104:738–744, 1969.

Myllynen L, Karjalainen O. Accuracy of the diagnosis in suspected intraepithelial neoplasia of the cervix. Ann Chir Gynaecol 73:45–49, 1984.

Nahmias AJ, Naib ZM, Josey WE. Epidemiological studies relating genital herpetic infection to cervical carcinoma. Cancer Res 34:1111–1117, 1974.

Naib ZM, Masukawa N. Identification of condyloma acuminata (sic) cells in routine vaginal smears. Obstet Gynecol 18:735–738, 1961.

Nasiell K, Nasiell M, Vaclavinkova V. Behavior of moderate cervical dysplasia during long-term follow-up. Obstet Gynecol 61:609–614, 1983.

Nasiell K, Naslund I, Auer G. Cytomorphologic and cytochemical analysis in the differential diagnosis of cervical epithelial lesions. Anal Quant Cytol 6: 196–200, 1984.

Nasiell K, Roger B, Nasiell M. Behavior of mild cervical dysplasia during long term follow-up. Obstet Gynecol 67:665–669, 1986.

National Cancer Institute Workshop. The 1988 Bethesda System for Reporting Cervical/Vaginal Cytological Diagnosis. JAMA 262:931–934, 1989.

Naujoks H. Sex chromatin in exfoliated cells of cervical carcinoma in situ. Acta Cytol 13:634–636, 1969.

Naujoks H, Leppien G, Rogosaroff-Fricke R. Negativerzytologischer Abstrich bei Carcinoma in situ der Cer uteri. Geburtshilfe Frauenheilkd 36:570–575, 1976.

Navratil E. Colposcopy. In: Gray LA (ed). Dysplasia, Carcinoma In Situ and Micro-invasive Carcinoma of the Cervix Uteri. Springfield, IL, Charles C Thomas, 1964, pp 228–283.

Negri G, Menia E, Egarter-Vigl E, et al. ThinPrep versus conventional Papanicolaou smear in the cytologic follow-up of women with equivocal cervical smears. Cancer Cytopathol 99:342–345, 2003.

Nelson JH, Jr, Averette HE, Richart RM. Cervical intraepithelial neoplasia (dysplasia and carcinoma in and early invasive cervical carcinoma. CA Can J Clin 3:157–179, 1989.

Nelson JH, Jr, Hall JE. Detection, diagnostic evaluation, and treatment of dysplasia and early carcinoma of the cervix. Cancer 20:150–163, 1970.

Ng ABP, Reagan JW. Microinvasive carcinoma of the uterine cervix. Am J Clin Pathol 52:511–529, 1969.

Ng ABP, Reagan JW, Lindner EA. The cellular manifestations of microinvasive squamous cell carcinoma of the uterine cervix. Acta Cytol 16:5–13, 1972.

Nieburgs HE, Stergus I, Stephenson EM, Harbin BL. Mass screening of total female population of county for cervical carcinoma. JAMA 164:1546–1551, 1957.

Nindl I, Zahm DM, Meijer CJLM, et al. Human papillomavirus detection in high-grade squamous intraepithelial lesions: comparison of hybrid capture assay with a polymerase chain reaction system. Diagn Microbiol Infect Dis 23:161–164, 1995.

Nishiya I, Ishizaki Y, Sasaki M. Nuclear DNA content and the number of Barr bodies in premalignant and malignant lesions of the uterine cervix. Acta Cytol 25:407–411, 1981.

Nobbenhuis MAE, Walboomers JMM, Helmerhorst TJM, et al. Relation of human papillomavirus status to cervical lesions and consequences for cervical-cancer screening: A prospective study. Lancet 354:20–25, 1999.

Nodskov-Pedersen S. Degree of malignancy of cancer involving the cervix uteri, judged on the basis of clinical stage, histology, size of nuclei, and content of DNA. Acta Pathol Microbiol Scand A79:617–628, 1971.

Noumoff JS. Atypia in cervical cytology as a risk factor for intraepithelial neoplasia. Am J Obstet Gynecol 156:628–631, 1987.

Nuovo GJ, Blanco JS, Leipzig S, Smith D. Human papillomavirus detection in cervical lesions nondiagnostic for cervical intraepithelial neoplasia: Correlation with Papanicolaou smear, colposcopy, and occurrence of cervical intraepithelial neoplasia. Obstet Gynecol 75:1006–1011, 1990.

Nuovo GJ, Cottral S, Richart RM. Occult human papillomavirus infection of the uterine cervix in postmenopausal women. Am J Obstet Gynecol 160:340–344, 1989.

Nuovo GJ, Hochman HA, Eliezri YD, et al. Detection of human papillomavirus DNA in penile lesions histologically negative for condylomata. Am J Surg Pathol 14:829–836, 1990.

Nuovo GJ, Mac Connell P, Forde A, Delvenne P. Detection of human papillomavirus DNA in formalin fixed tissue by in situ hybridization after amplification by polymerase chain reaction. Am J Pathol 139:847–854, 1991.

Nuovo GJ, Pedemonte BM. Human papillomavirus types and recurrent cervical warts. JAMA 263:1223–1226, 1990.

Nyeem R, Wilkinson EJ, Groover LJ. Condylomata acuminata of the cervix: Histopathology and association with cervical neoplasia. Int J Gynecol Pathol 1:246–257, 1982.

Nygard JF, Sauer T, Skjeldestad FE, et al. CIN 2/3 and cervical cancer after an ASCUS Pap smear. A 7-year prospective study of the Norwegian population-based, coordinated screening program. Acta Cytol 47:991–1000, 2003.

Nyirjesy I. Atypical or suspicious cervical smears. An aggressive diagnostic approach. JAMA 222:691–693, 1972.

Nyirjesy I, Billingsley FS, Forman MR. Evaluation of atypical and low-grade cervical cytology in private practice. Obstet Gynecol 92:601–607, 1998.

O'Connor DP, Bennett MA, Murphy GM, et al. Do human papillomaviruses cause cancer? Curr Diagn Pathol 3:123–125, 1996.

O'Leary JJ, Landers RJ, Chetty R. Review. In situ amplification in cytological preparations. Cytopath 8:148–160, 1997.

O'Sullivan JP. Observer variation in gynaecological cytopathology. Cytopathology 9:6–14, 1998.

O'Sullivan JP, A'Hern RP, Chapman PA, et al. A case-control study of true-positive versus false-negative cervical smears in women with cervical intraepithelial neoplasia (CIN) III. Cytopathology 9:155–161, 1998.

Odell LD, Merrick FW, Ortiz R. A comparison between negative, slightly atypical and suspicious cervical smears and colposcopic observations. Acta Cytol 12:305–308, 1968.

Oktay MH, Oktay K, Hamele-Bena D, et al. Focal adhesion kinase as a marker of malignant phenotype in breast and cervical carcinomas. Hum Pathol 34:240–245, 2003.

Old JW, Jones DG. Squamous carcinoma in situ of the uterine cervix. III. A long-term follow-up of 23 unsuspected cases of 6- to 10-year duration without interim treatment. Cancer 18:1622–1630, 1965.

Oota K. Histopathological study of "carcinoma in situ" especially of uterine cervix. Acta Pathol Jpn 5 (Suppl):349–380, 1955.

Oriel JD. Genital and anal papillomavirus infections in human males. In: Syrjänen K, Gissmann L, Koss LG (eds). Papillomaviruses and Human Disease. New York, Springer-Verlag, 1987, pp 182–196.

Oriel JD. Natural history of genital warts. Br J Vener Dis 47:1–13, 1971.

Oriel JD, Alameida JD. Demonstration of virus particles in human genital warts. Br J Vener Dis 46:37–42, 1970.

Orth G. Epidermodysplasia verruciformis: A model for understanding the oncogenicity of human papillomaviruses. In: Evered D, Clark C (eds). Papillomaviruses. New York, John Wiley & Sons, 1986, pp 157–168.

Osband R, Jones WN. Carcinoma in situ in pregnancy. Am J Obstet Gynecol 83:599–606, 1962.

Ostergard DR, Gondos B. The incidence of false negative cervical cytology as determined by colposcopically directed biopsies. Acta Cytol 15:292–293, 1971.

Ostergard DR, Nieberg RK. Evaluation of abnormal cervical cytology during pregnancy with colposcopy. Am J Obstet Gynecol 134:756–758, 1979.

Östör AG. Natural history of cervical intraepithelial neoplasia. A critical review. Int J Gynecol Pathol 12:186–192, 1993.

Östör AG, Fortune DW, Davoren RAM. Diagnosis of cervical epithelial abnormalities from "routine" uterine curettings. Pathology 12:23–30, 1980.

Ostrow RS, Coughlin SM, McGlennen RC, et al. Serological and molecular evidence of rhesus papillomavirus type 1 infection in tissues from geographically distinct institutions. J Gen Virol 76:293–299, 1995.

Palefsky JM, Minkoff H, Kalish LA, et al. Cervicovaginal human papillomavirus infection in human immunodeficiency virus-1 (HIV)-positive and high-risk HIV-negative women. JNCI 91:226–236, 1999.

Papadopoulou K, Labropoulou V, Davaris P, et al. Detection of human papillomaviruses in squamous cell carcinomas of the lung. Virch Arch 433:49–54, 1998.

Papanicolaou GN. Atlas of Exfoliative Cytology. Cambridge, Harvard University Press, 1954 (Supplement I, 1956; Supplement II, 1960).

Papanicolaou GN. Cytologic diagnosis of uterine cancer by examination of vaginal and uterine secretions. Am J Clin Pathol 19:301–308, 1959.

Papanicolaou GN. Survey of actualities and potentialities of exfoliative cytology in cancer diagnosis. Ann Intern Med 31:661–674, 1949.

Papanicolaou GN. New cancer diagnosis. Proc. of the 3rd Race Betterment Conference. Battle Creek, Michigan, 1928, pp 528–530.

Papanicolaou GN, Traut HF. Diagnosis of Uterine Cancer by the Vaginal Smear. New York, Commonwealth Fund, 1943.

Papillo H, Zarka MA, St. John TL. Evaluation of the ThinPrep Pap test in clinical practice. A seven-month 16,314 case experience in northern Vermont. Acta Cytol 42:203–208, 1998.

Park JJ, Genest DR, Sun D, Crum CP. Atypical immature metaplastic-like proliferations of the cervix: diagnostic reproducibility and viral (HPV) correlates. Hum Pathol 30:1161–1165, 1999.

Park SJ, Chan PJ, Seraj IM, King A. Denaturing gradient gel electrophoresis screening of the BRCA1 gene in cells from precancerous cervical lesions. J Reprod Med 44:575–580, 1999.

Park TW, Richart RM, Sun XW, Wright TCJ. Association between human papillomavirus type and clonal status of cervical squamous intraepithelial lesions. JNCI 88:355–358, 1996.

Patten SF. Diagnostic Cytology of the Uterine Cervix,. 2nd ed. Basel, S Karger, 1978.

Peckham B, Greene RR. Follow-up on cervical epithelial abnormalities. Am J Obstet Gynecol 74:804–815, 1957.

Pereyra AJ. Relationship of sexual activity to cervical cancer: Cancer of the cervix in a prison population. Obstet Gynecol 17:154, 1961.

Perez CA, Zivnuska F, Askin F, et al. Prognostic significance of endometrial extension from primary carcinoma of the uterine cervix. Cancer 35:1493–1504, 1975.

Peterson O. Precancerous changes of cervical epithelium in relation to manifest cervical carcinoma; clinical and histological aspects. Acta Radiol 127:1–168, 1955.

Pfister H, Fuchs PG. Papillomaviruses: Particles, genome organisation and proteins. In: Syrjänen K, Gissmann L, Koss LG (eds). Papillomaviruses and Human Disease. New York, Springer-Verlag 1987, pp 1–18.

Philipp E. Elektronenmikroskopische Untersuchungen uber die sogenannten Reservezellen am Zylinderepithel der menschlichen Cervix uteri. Arch Gynäkol 218:295–311, 1975.

Phillips DH, Hewer A, Malcolm AD, et al. Smoking and DNA damage in cervical cells (Letter). Lancet 335:417, 1990.

Pickel H, Burghardt E. Die Lokalisation des beginnend invasiven Krebswachstums an der Cervix. Arch Gynecol 215:187–198, 1973.

Pilleron JP, Durand JC, Hamelin JP. Location of lymph node invasion in cancer of the uterine cervix: Study of 140 cases treated at the Curie Foundation. Am J Obstet Gynecol 119:453–457, 1974.

Piloti S, Rilke F, De Palo G, et al. Condylomata of the uterine cervix and koilocytosis of cervical intraepithelial neoplasia. J Clin Pathol 34:532–541, 1981.

Pinto AP, Tuon FF, Torres LF, Collaco LM. Limiting factors for cytopathological diagnosis of high-grade squamous intraepithelial lesions: a cytohistological correlation between findings in cervical smears and loop electrical excision procedure. Diagn Cytopathol 26:15–18, 2002.

Pirisi L, Creek KE, Doniger J, Di Paolo JA. Continuous cell lines with altered growth and differentiation properties originate after transfection of human keratinocytes with human papillomavirus type-16 DNA. Carcinogenesis 9:1573–1579, 1988.

Pirog EC, Baergen RN, Soslow RA, et al. Diagnostic accuracy of cervical low-grade squamous intraepithelial lesions is improved with MIB-1 immunostaining. Am J Surg Pathol 26:70–75, 2002.

Pirog EC, Erroll M, Harigopal M, Centeno BA. Comparison of human papillomavirus DNA prevalence in atypical squamous cells of undetermined significance subcategories as defined by the original Bethesda 1991 and the new Bethesda 2001 systems. Arch Pathol Lab Med 128:527–532, 2004.

Pitman MB, Cibas ES, Powers CN, et al. Reducing or eliminating use of the category of atypical squamous cells of undetermined significance decreases the diagnostic accuracy of the Papanicolaou smear. Cancer 96:128–134, 2002.

Piver MS, Chung WS. Prognostic significance of cervical lesion size and pelvic node metastases in cervical carcinoma. Obstet Gynecol 46:507–510, 1975.

Porreco R, Penn I, Droegemueller W, et al. Gynecologic malignancies in immunosuppressed organ homograft recipients. Obstet Gynecol 45:359–364, 1975.

Prasad R, Kaufman RH, Mumford DM. Distribution of isozyme patterns in cervical dysplasia. Obstet Gynecol 43:665–667, 1973.

Pridan H, Lilienfeld AM. Carcinoma of the cervix in Jewish women in Israel (1960–67). An epidemiological study. J Med Sci Israel 7:1465–1470, 1971.

Pronai K. Zur Lehre von der Histogenese und dem Wachsthum des Uteruscarcinoms. Arch Gynäkol 89:596–607, 1909.

Przybora LA. Incipient invasion of cervical cancer: Morphological aspects of carcinogenesis in 74 cases. Gynaecologia 160:69–86, 1965.

Przybora LA, Plutowa A. Histological topography of carcinoma in situ of cervix uteri. Cancer 12:263–277, 1959.

Purola E, Savia E. Cytology of gynecologic condyloma acuminatum. Acta Cytol 21:26–31, 1977.

Quizilbash AH. Papillary squamous tumors of the uterine cervix. A clinical and pathologic study of 21 cases. Am J Clin Pathol 61:508–520, 1974.

Raab S, Isacson C, Layfield LJ, et al. Atypical glandular cells of undetermined significance. Cytologic criteria to separate clinically significant from benign lesions. Am J Clin Pathol 104:574–582, 1995.

Raab SS, Bishop S, Zaleski S. Long-term outcome and relative risk in women with atypical squamous cells of undetermined significance. Am J Clin Pathol 112:57–62, 1999.

Raab SS, Geisinger KR, Silverman JF, et al. Interobserver variability of a Papanicolaou smear diagnosis of atypical glandular cells of undetermined significance. Am J Clin Pathol 110:653–659, 1998.

Rader AE, Lazebnik R, Arora CD, et al. Atypical squamous cells of undetermined significance in the pediatric population. Implications for management and comparison with the adult population. Acta Cytol 41:1073–1078, 1997.

Rader AE, Rose PG, Rodriguez M, et al. Atypical squamous cells of undetermined significance in women over 55. Comparison with the general population and implications for management. Acta Cytol 43:357–362, 1999.

Raffle AE, Alden B, Mackenzie EFD. Detection rates for abnormal cervical smears: What are we screening for? Lancet 345:1469–1473, 1995.

Rando RF, Lindheim S, Hasty L, et al. Increased frequency of detection of human papillomavirus deoxyribonucleic acid in exfoliated cervical cells during pregnancy. Am J Obstet Gynecol 161:50–55, 1989.

Ransdell JS, Davey DD, Zaleski S. Clinicopathologic correlation of the unsatisfactory Papanicolaou smear. Cancer Cytopathol 81:139–143, 1997.

Rasbridge SA, Nayagam M. Discordance between cytologic and histologic reports in cervical intraepithelial neoplasia. Results of a one-year audit. Acta Cytol 39:648–653, 1995.

Rawls WE, Gardner HL, Kaufman RL. Antibodies to genital herpesvirus in patients with carcinoma of the cervix. Am J Obstet Gynecol 107:710–716, 1970.

Reagan JW, Bell BA, Neuman JL, et al. Dysplasia in uterine cervix during pregnancy. An analytical study of cells. Acta Cytol 5:17–29, 1961.

Reagan JW, Hamonic MJ. Cellular pathology in carcinoma in situ; cytopathological correlation. Cancer 9:385–402, 1956.

Reagan JW, Hamonic MJ. Dysplasia of the uterine cervix. Ann NY Acad Sci 63:1236–1244, 1956.

Reagan JW, Hamonic MJ, Wentz WB. Analytical study of the cells in cervical squamous-cell cancer. Lab Invest 6:241–250, 1957.

Reagan JW, Hicks DJ, Scott RB. Atypical hyperplasia of uterine cervix. Cancer 8:42–52, 1955.

Reagan JW, Moore RD. Morphology of malignant squamous cell; study of 6,000 cells derived from squamous cell carcinomas of uterine cervix. Am J Pathol 28:105–127, 1952.

Reagan JW, Patten SF, Jr. Dysplasia; basic reaction to injury in uterine cervix. Ann NY Acad Sci 97:662–682, 1962.

Reagan JW, Seidemann IL, Saracusa Y. Cellular morphology of carcinoma in situ and dysplasia or atypical hyperplasia of uterine cervix. Cancer 6:224–235, 1953.

Reagan JW, Wentz WB. Changes in desquamated cells in carcinogenesis. Arch Pathol 67:287–292, 1959.

Reagan JW, Wentz WB. Changes in mouse cervix antedating induced cancer. Cancer 12:389–395, 1959.

Reagan JW, Wentz WB, Machicao N. Induced cancer of the cervix uteri in mouse. Arch Pathol 60:451–456, 1955.

Recher L. Scanning electron microscopy of koilocytotic atypia. Acta Cytol 28:516–517, 1984.

Reid R, Crum CP, Herschman VR. et al. Genital warts and cervical cancer. III. Subclinical papillomavirus infection and cervical neoplasia are linked by a spectrum of continuous morphologic and biologic change. Cancer 53:943–953, 1984.

Reid R, Stanhope R, Herschman BR, et al. Genital warts and cervical cancer. IV. A colposcopic index for differentiating subclinical papillomaviral infections from cervical intraepithelial neoplasia. Am J Obstet Gynecol 149:815–823, 1984.

Remmink AJ, Walboomers JMM, Helmerhorst TJM, et al. The presence of persistent high-risk HPV genotypes in dysplastic cervical lesions is associated with progressive disease: natural history up to 36 months. Int J Cancer 61:306–311, 1995.

Renshaw AA, Davey DD, Birdsong GG, et al. Precision in gynecologic cytologic interpretation. A study from the College of American Pathologists interlaboratory comparison program in cervicovaginal cytology. Arch Pathol Lab Med 127:1413–1420, 2003.

Renshaw AA, Dubray-Benstein B, Cobb CJ, et al. Cytologic features of squamous cell carcinoma in ThinPrep slides. Evaluation of cases that performed poorly versus those that performed well in the College of American Pathologists interlaboratory comparison program in cervicovaginal cytology. Arch Pathol Lab Med 128:403–405, 2004.

Reuter B, Schenck U. Investigation of the visual cytoscreening of conventional gynecologic smears. II. Analysis of eye movement. Anal Quant Cytol Histol 3:210–218, 1986.

Richards BM, Atkin NB. The differences between normal and cancerous tissues with respect to the ratio of DNA content to chromosome number. Acta Un Int Cancr 16:124–128, 1960.

Richardson AC, Lyon JB. The effect of condom use on squamous cell cervical intraepithelial neoplasia. Am J Obstet Gynecol 140:909–913, 1981.

Richart RM. The natural history of cervical intraepithelial neoplasia. Clin Obstet Gynecol 10:748–784, 1967.

Richart RM. Influence of diagnostic and therapeutic procedures on the distribution of cervical intraepithelial neoplasia. Cancer 19:1635–1638, 1966.

Richart RM. Evaluation of the true false negative rate in cytology. Am J Obstet Gynecol 89:723–726, 1964.

Richart RM. The growth characteristics in vitro of normal epithelium, dysplasia, and carcinoma-in-situ of the uterine cervix. Cancer Res 24:662–669, 1964.

Richart RM. A radioautographic analysis of cellular proliferation in dysplasia and carcinoma in situ of the uterine cervix. Am J Obstet Gynecol 86:925–930, 1963.

Richart RM, Barron BA. A follow-up study of patients with cervical dysplasia. Am J Obstet Gynecol 105:386–393, 1969.

Richart RM, Lerch V, Barron BA. A time-lapse cinematographic study in vitro of mitosis of normal human cervical epithelium, dysplasia, and carcinoma in situ. JNCI 39:571–577, 1967.

Richart RM, Ludwig AS. Alterations in chromosome and DNA content in gynecologic neoplasms. Am J Obstet Gynecol 104:463–471, 1969.

Richart RM, Nuovo GJ. Human papillomavirus DNA in situ hybridization may be used for the quality control of genital tract biopsies. Obstet Gynecol 75:223–226, 1990.

Richart RM, Wilbanks GD. The chromosome in human intraepithelial neoplasia; a review. Cancer 26:60–74, 1966.

Rietveld WJ, Boon ME, Meulman JJ. Seasonal fluctuations in the cervical smear detection rates for (pre) malignant changes and for infections. Diagn Cytopathol 17:452–455, 1997.

Rigoni-Stern: Fatti statistici relativi alle malattie cancerose che servirono di base alle poche cose dette dal dott. Gior Servire Progr Path Therap 2:507–517, 1842.

Ritter DB, Kadish AS, Vermund SH, et al. Detection of human papillomavirus deoxyribonucleic acid in exfoliated cervicovaginal cells as a predictor of cervical neoplasia in a high-risk population. Am J Obstet Gynecol 159:1517–1525, 1988.

Robboy SJ, Keh PC, Nickerson RJ, et al. Squamous cell dysplasia and carcinoma in situ of the cervix and vagina after prenatal exposure to diethylstilbestrol. Obstet Gynecol 51:528–535, 1978.

Robboy SJ, Noller KL, O'Brien P, et al. Increased incidence of cervical and vaginal dysplasia in 3,980 diethylstilbestrol-exposed young women. JAMA 252:2979–2983, 1984.

Roberston AJ, Anderson JM, Swansonbeck J, et al. Observer variability in histopathological reporting of cervical biopsy specimens. J Clin Pathol 42:231–238, 1989.

Roitkin ID. A comparison review of key epidemiological studies in cervical cancer related to current searches for transmissible agents. Cancer Res 33:1353–1367, 1973.

Roitkin ID. Relation of adolescent coitus to cervical cancer risk. JAMA 179:486–491, 1962.

Rombach JJ, Cranendonk R, Velthuis FJJM. Monitoring laboratory performance by statistical analysis of rescreening cervical smears. Acta Cytol 31:887–894, 1987.

Ronnett BM, Manos MM, Ransley JE, et al. Atypical glandular cells of undetermined significance (AGUS): cytopathologic features, histopathologic results, and human papillomavirus DNA detection. Hum Pathol 30:816–825, 1999.

Rosenfeld WD, Rose E, Vermund SH, et al. Follow-up evaluation of cervicovaginal human papillomavirus infection in adolescents. J Pediatr 121:307–311, 1992.

Rosenfeld WD, Vermund SH, Wentz SJ, Burk RD. High prevalence rate of human papillomavirus infection and association with abnormal Papanicolaou smears in sexually active adolescents. Am J Dis Child 143:1443–1447, 1989.

Rous P, Beard JW. The progression to carcinoma of virus-induced rabbit papillomas (Shope). J Exp Med 62:532–548, 1935.

Rous P, Kidd JG. The activation, transforming and carcinogenic effects of the rabbit papillomavirus (Shope) upon implanted tar tumors. J Exp Med 71:787–812, 1940.

Rowson KEK, Mahy BWJ. Human papova (wart) virus. Bact Rev 31:110–131, 1967.

Rubin IC. Pathological diagnosis of incipient carcinoma of uterus. Am J Obstet 62:668–676, 1910.

Rubio CA, Biberfeld P. The basement membrane of the uterine cervix in dysplasia and squamous carcinoma: An immunofluorescent study with antibodies to basement membrane antigen. Acta Pathol Microbiol Scand 83:744–748, 1975.

Rubio CA, Kranz I. The exfoliating cervical epithelial surface in dysplasia, carcinoma in situ and invasive squamous carcinoma. Acta Cytol 20:144–150, 1976.

Rubio CA, Lagerløf B. Proliferating and nonpenetrating compartments in cervical dysplasia and carcinoma in situ. Acta Pathol Microbiol Scand 83:191, 1975.

Rubio CA, Lagerløf B. Who is responsible for the false negative smear? (letter to the editor). Acta Cytol 19:319, 1975.

Rubio CA, Lagerløf B. Studies on the histogenesis experimentally induced cervical carcinoma. Acta Pathol Microbiol Scand A82:153–160, 1974.

Rubio CA, Lagerlöf B. Autoradiographic studies dysplasia and carcinoma in situ in cervical cones. Acta Pathol Microbiol Scand A82:411–418, 1974.

Rubio CA, Soderberg G, Einhorn N. Histological and follow-up studies in cases of micro-invasive carcinoma of the uterine cervix. Acta Pathol Microbiol Scand A82:397–410, 1974.

Rubio CA, Soderberg G. Carcinoma in situ and microinvasive carcinoma of the cervix. Lancet 2(7621):639–640, 1969.

Rubio CA. Two types of cells in the normal and atypical squamous epithelium of the cervix. II. Light microscopic study in human subjects. Acta Cytol 26: 121–125, 1982.

Rubio CA. False negatives in cervical cytology: Can they be avoided? (letter to the editor). Acta Cytol 25:199–202, 1981.

Rubio CA. The cervical epithelial surface. III. Scanning electron microscopic study in atypias and invasive carcinoma in mice. Acta Cytol 20:375–380, 1976.

Rubio CA. The false positive smear (letter to the editor). Acta Cytol 19:212–213, 1975.

Rubio CA. Cytologic studies in cases with carcinoma in situ and microinvasive carcinoma of the uterine cervix. Acta Pathol Microbiol Scand A82:161–168, 1974.

Rubio CA. The frequency and topographical distribution of carcinoma in situ with buds in the uterine cervix. Acta Pathol Microbiol Scand A82:605–612, 1974.

Rudolf MP, Nieland JD, DaSilva DM, et al. Induction of HPV16 capsid protein-specific human T cell responses by virus-like particles. Biol Chem 380: 335–340, 1999.

Ruge C, Veit J. Anatomische Bedeutung der Erosion am Scheidentheil. Zentralbl F Gynaekol 1:17–19, 1877.

Rylander E. Cervical cancer in women belonging to a cytologically screened population. Acta Obstet Gynecol Scand 55:361–366, 1976.

Sachs H, Stegner H-E, Bahnsen J. Cytophotometrische Untersuchungen an Epitheldysplasien des Collum. Arch Gynäkol 212:97–129, 1972.

Sadeghi SB, Hsieh EW, Gunn SW. Prevalence of cervical intraepithelial neoplasia in sexually active teenagers and young adults. Am J Obstet Gynecol 148: 726–729, 1984.

Sadler L, Saftlas A, Wang W, et al. Treatment for cervical intraepithelial neoplasia and risk of preterm delivery. JAMA 291:2100–2106, 2004.

Sagae S, Kuzumaki N, Hisada T, et al. Ras oncogene expression and invasive squamous cell carcinomas of the uterine cervix. Cancer 63:1577–1582, 1989.

Sall S, Rini S, Pineda A. Surgical management of invasive carcinoma of the cervix in pregnancy. Am J Obstet Gynecol 118:1–5, 1974.

Sandritter W, Cramer H, Mondorf W. Zur Kresidiagnostic an vaginalen Zellausstrichen mittles cytophotometrischer Messungen. Arch Gynäkol 192: 293–303, 1960.

Sandritter W. Cytophotometrische Untersuchungen am Portiocarcinom und seinen Vorstufen. Verh Dtsch Ges Pathol 48:34–43, 1964.

Saphir O, Leventhal ML, Kline TS. Podophyllin-induced dysplasia of cervix uteri: Its histologic resemblance to carcinoma in situ. Am J Clin Pathol 32: 446–456, 1959.

Sarode VR, Werner C, Gander R, et al. Reflex human papillomavirus DNA testing on residual liquid-based (TPPT) cervical samples: focus on age-stratified clinical performance. Cancer 99:149–155, 2003.

Saslow D, Runowicz CD, Solomon D, et al. American Cancer Society guideline for the early detection of cervical neoplasia and cancer. CA Cancer J Clin 52:342–362, 2002.

Sawaya GF, McConnell KJ, Kulasingam SL, et al. Risk of cervical cancer associated with extending the interval between cervical-cancer screenings. N Engl J Med 349:1501–1509, 2003.

Sawchuk WS, Weber PJ, Lowy DR, Dzubow LM. Infectious papillomavirus in the vapor of warts treated with carbon dioxide laser or electrocoagulation: Detection and protection. J Am Acad Dermatol 21:41–49, 1989.

Scapier J, Day E, Durfee GR. Intraepithelial carcinoma of cervix; cytohistological and clinical study. Cancer 5:315–323, 1952.

Scarpelli DG, von Haame E. Experimental carcinoma of uterine cervix in mouse; gross and histopathologic study. Am J Pathol 33:1059–1073, 1957.

Schafer A, Friedmann W, Mielke M, et al. The increased frequency of cervical dysplasia-neoplasia in women infected with the human immunodeficiency virus is related to the degree of immunosuppression. Am J Obstet Gynec 164:593–599, 1991.

Schauenstein W. Histologische Untersuchungen uber atypisches Plattenepithel an der Portio und an der Innenfläche der Cervix uteri. Arch Gynäkol 85: 576–616, 1908.

Scheffner M, Munger K, Byrne JC, Howley PM. The state of the p53 and retinoblastoma genes in human cervical carcinoma cell lines. Proc Natl Acad Sci USA 88:5523–5527, 1991.

Scheffner M, Werness BA, Huibregtse JM, et al. The E6 oncoprotein encoded by human papillomavirus types 16 and 18 promotes the degradation of p53. Cell 63:1129–1136, 1990.

Schenck U, Reuter B, Vohringer P. Investigation of the visual cytoscreening of conventional gynecologic smears. I. Analysis of slide movement. Anal Quant Cytol Histol 8:35–45, 1986.

Schiffman M, Adrianza ME. ASCUS-LSIL Triage Study. Design, methods and characteristic participants. Acta Cytol 44:726–742, 2000.

Schiffman M, Castle PE. Human papillomavirus. Epidemiology and public health. Arch Pathol Lab Med 127:930–934, 2003.

Schiffman M, Herrero R, Hildesheim A, et al. HPV DNA testing in cervical cancer screening. Results from women in a high-risk province of Costa Rica. JAMA 283:87–93, 2000.

Schiffman M, Solomon D. Findings to date from the ASCUS-LSIL triage study (ALTS). Arch Pathol Lab Med 127:946–949, 2003.

Schiller W. Uber Frühstadien des Portiocarcinoms und ihre Diagnose. Arch Gynäkol 133:211–283, 1928.

Schiller W. Untersuchungen zur Entstehung der Geschwülste. I. Collumcarcinom des Uterus. Virchows Arch Pathol Anat 263:279–367, 1927.

Schlecht NF, Kulaga S, Robitaille J, et al. Persistent human papillomavirus infection as a predictor of cervical intraepithelial neoplasia. JAMA 286: 3106–3114, 2001.

Schleifstein J. Changes in uterine cervix associated with pregnancy and epidermoid carcinoma in situ. NY J Med 50:2795–2801, 1950.

Schneider A, de Villiers E-M, Schneider V. Multifocal squamous neoplasia of the female genital tract: Significance of human papillomavirus infection of the vagina after hysterectomy. Obstet Gynecol 70:294–298, 1987.

Schneider A, Hotz M, Gissmann L. Increased prevalence of human papillomaviruses in the lower genital tract of pregnant women. Int J Cancer 40:198–201, 1987.

Schneider A, Kraus H. The "suspicious" gynecologic smear. Acta Cytol 29: 795–799, 1985.

Schneider A, Meinhardt G, Kirchmayr R, Schneider V. Prevalence of human papillomavirus genomes in tissues from the lower genital tract as detected by molecular in situ hybridization. Int J Gynecol Pathol 10:1–14, 1991.

Schneider A, Sawada E, Gissmann L, Shah K. Human papillomavirus in women with a history of abnormal Papanicolaou smears and in their male partners. Obstet Gynecol 69:554–562, 1987.

Schneider DL, Burke L, Wright TC. Can cervicography be improved? An evaluation with arbitrated cervicography interpretations. Am J Obstet Gynecol 187: 15–23, 2002.

Schneider V. CIN prognostication: Will molecular techniques do the trick? (Editorial) Acta Cytol 47:115–116, 2003.

Schneider V, Kay S, Lee HM. Immunosuppression: High risk factor for the development of condyloma acuminata and squamous neoplasia of the cervix. Acta Cytol 27:220–224, 1983.

Schottlander J, Kermauner F. Zur Kenntnis des Uteruskarzinoms; monographische Studie uber Morphologie. Entwicklung, Wachstum nebst Beiträgen zur Klinik der Erkrankung. Berlin, S Karger, 1912.

Schrager LK, Friedland GH, Maude D, et al. Cervical and vaginal squamous cell abnormalities in women infected with human immunodeficiency virus. J AIDS 2:570–575, 1989.

Schulman H, Cavanagh D. Intraepithelial carcinoma of the cervix. The predictability of residual carcinoma of the uterus from microscopic study of the margins of the cone biopsy specimen. Cancer 14:795–800, 1961.

Schulman H, Ferguson JH. Comparison of the behavior of intra-epithelial carcinoma of the cervix in the pregnant and the nonpregnant patient. Am J Obstet Gynecol 84:1497–1501, 1962.

Schwarz E. Papillomavirus infections and cancer. In: Syrjänen K, Gissmann L, Koss LG (eds). Papillomaviruses and Human Disease. New York, Springer-Verlag, 1987, pp 443–466.

Schwarz E, Freese UK, Gissmann L, et al. Structure and transcription of human papillomavirus sequences in cervical carcinoma cells. Nature 314:111–114, 1985.

Schweid AI, Smith MR, Figge DC. Symmetrical epithelial reactions in cervices of didelphic uteri: A field response. Acta Cytol 12:406–409, 1968.

Scipiades EJ, Stevenson KS. Uber die Latenzperiode des beginnenden Collum-Carcinoms und die Dauer seiner Symptomfreiheit. Arch. Gynäkol. 167: 416–464, 1938.

Scott JW. Stereocolposcopic Atlas of the Uterine Cervix. Kendall, FL, Zephyr, 1971.

Seckl MJ, Mulholland PJ, Bishop AE, et al. Hypoglycemia due to an insulin-secreting small-cell carcinoma of the cervix. N Engl J Med 341:733–736, 1999.

Sedlacek TV, Cunnane M, Carpiniello V. Colposcopy in the diagnosis of penile condyloma. Am J Obstet Gynecol 154:496–496, 1986.

Sedlacek TV, Lindheim S, Eder C, et al. Mechanism for human papillomavirus transmission at birth. Am J Obstet Gynecol 161:55–59, 1989.

Sedlis A, Walters AT, Balin H, et al. Evaluation of two simultaneously obtained cervical cytological smears. Acta Cytol 18:291–296, 1974.

Sedlis A. Cervical dysplasia: Diagnosis, prognosis and management. In: Progress in Gynecology, vol 6. New York, Grune & Stratton, 1975, pp 559–581.

Selvaggi SM. Cytologic detection of condylomas and cervical intraepithelial neoplasia of the uterine cervix with histologic correlation. Cancer 58: 2076–2081, 1986.

Selvaggi SM, Guidos BJ. Specimen adequacy and the ThinPrep Pap test: The endocervical component. Diagn Cytopathol 23:23–26, 2000.

Selvaggi SM, Haefner HK. Reporting of atypical squamous cells of undetermined significance on cervical smears. Is it significant? Diagn Cytopathol 13:352–356, 1995.

Seybolt JF, Johnson WD. Cervical cytodiagnostic problems: A survey. Am J Obstet Gynecol 109:1089–1103, 1971.

Shah KV, Howley PM. Papillomaviruses. In: Lennette EH (ed). Laboratory Diagnosis of Viral Infection, 2nd ed. New York, Marcel Dekker, 1992.

Sheils LA, Wilbur DC. Atypical squamous cells of undetermined significance. Stratification of the risk of association with, or progression to, squamous intraepithelial lesions based on morphologic subcategorization. Acta Cytol 41:1065–1072, 1997.

Sherman ME, Abdul-Karim FW, Berek JS, et al. Atypical squamous cells. In:

Solomon and Nayar (eds). The Bethesda System for Reporting Cervical Cytology. New York, Springer, 2004, pp 67–87.

Sherman ME, Friedman HB, Busseniers AE, et al. Cytologic diagnosis of anal intraepithelial neoplasia using smears and Cytyc ThinPreps. Mod Pathol 8: 270–274, 1995.

Sherman ME, Kelly D. High grade squamous intraepithelial lesions and invasive carcinoma following the report of three negative Papanicolaou smears: Screening failures or rapid progression. Mod Pathol 5:337–342, 1992.

Sherman ME, Lorincz AT, Scott DR, et al. Baseline cytology, human papillomavirus testing, and risk for cervical neoplasia: a 10-year cohort analysis. JNCI 95:46–52, 2003.

Sherman ME, Mendoza M, Lee KR, et al. Performance of liquid-based, thin-layer cervical cytology: Correlation with reference diagnoses and human papillomavirus testing. Mod Pathol 11:837–843, 1998.

Sherman ME, Schiffman M, Cox JT, et al. Effects of age and human papilloma viral load on colposcopy trial data from the randomized Atypical Squamous Cells of Undetermined Significance/Low-Grade Squamous Intraepithelial Lesion Triage Study (ALTS). JNCI 94:102–107, 2002.

Sherman ME, Schiffman MH, Lorincz AT, et al. Toward objective quality assurance in cervical cytopathology: correlation of cytopathologic diagnoses with detection of high-risk human papillomavirus types. Am J Clin Pathol 101: 182–187, 1994.

Sherman ME, Schiffman MH, Strickler H, Hildesheim A. Prospects for a prophylactic HPV vaccine: Rationale and future implications for cervical cancer screening. Diagn Cytopathol 18:5–9, 1998.

Sherman ME, Tabbara SO, Scott DR, et al. "ASCUS, rule out HSIL": Cytologic features, histologic correlates, and human papillomavirus detection. Mod Pathol 12:335–342, 1999.

Sherman ME, Wang SS, Tarone R, et al. Histopathologic extent of cervical intraepithelial neoplasia 3 lesions in the atypical squamous cells of undetermined significance low-grade squamous intraepithelial lesion triage study: Implications for subject safety and lead-time bias. Cancer Epidemiol Biomarkers Prev 12:372–379, 2003.

Shibata D, Fu YS, Gupta JW, et al. The detection of human papillomavirus in normal and dysplastic tissues by the polymerase chain reaction. Lab Invest 59:555–559, 1988.

Shield PW, Cox NC. The sensitivity of rapid (partial) review of cervical smears. Cytopathology 9:84–92, 1998.

Shingleton HM, Richart RM, Wiener J, Spiro D. Human cervical intraepithelial neoplasia: Fine structure of dysplasia and carcinoma in situ. Cancer Res 28: 695–706, 1968.

Shingleton HM, Wilbanks GD. Fine structure of human cervical intraepithelial neoplasia in vivo and in vitro. Cancer 33:981–989, 1974.

Shokri-Tabibzadeh S, Koss LG, Molnar J, Romney S. Association of human papillomavirus with neoplastic processes in genital tract of four women with impaired immunity. Gynecol Oncol 12:S129–S140, 1981.

Shope RE. Serial transmission of virus of infectious papillomatosis in domestic rabbits. Proc Soc Exp Biol Med 32:830–832, 1934.

Shope RE, Hurst EW. Infectious papillomatosis of rabbits. J Exp Med 58: 607–624, 1933.

Shulman JJ, Hontz A, Sedlis A, et al. The Pap smear. Take two. Am J Obstet Gynecol 121:1024–1028, 1975.

Shulman JJ, Leyton M, Hamilton R. The Papanicolaou smear. An insensitive case-finding procedure. Am J Obstet Gynecol 120:446–451, 1974.

Sidawy MK, Solomon D. Pitfalls in diagnostic cytology. In: Koss LG, Linder J (eds). Errors and Pitfalls in Diagnostic Cytology. Baltimore, Williams & Wilkins, 1997.

Sidawy MK, Tabbara SO. Reactive changes and atypical squamous cells of undetermined significance in Papanicolaou smears. Diagn Cytopathol 9: 423–427, 1993.

Sidhu GS, Koss LG, Barber HRK. Relation of histologic factors to the response of stage I epidermoid carcinoma of the cervix to surgical treatment: Analysis of 115 patients. Obstet Gynecol 35:329–338, 1970.

Siegler EE. Microdiagnosis of carcinoma in situ of the uterine cervix. A comparative study of pathologists' diagnoses. Cancer 9:463–469, 1956.

Siemens FC, Boon JM, Kuypers JC, Kok LP. Population-based cervical screening with a 5-year interval in the Netherlands. Stabilization of the incidence of squamous cell carcinoma and its precursor lesions in the screened population. Acta Cytol 48:348–354, 2004.

Sigurdsson K, Adalsteinsson S, Tulinius H, Ragnarsoon J. The value of screening as an approach to cervical cancer control in Iceland 1964–1986. Int J Cancer 43:1–5, 1989.

Sillman F, Boyce J, Fruchter R. The significance of atypical vessels and neovascularization in cervical neoplasia. Am J Obstet Gynecol 139:151–159, 1981.

Silverstone H. Squamous papilloma of the cervix uteri. A two year prospective cytological study. Med J Aust 2:304–306, 1975.

Simon NL, Gore H, Shingleton HM, et al. Study of superficially invasive carcinoma of the cervix. Obstet Gynecol 68:19–24, 1986.

Simsir A, Hwang S, Cangiarella J, et al. Glandular cell atypia on Papanicolaou smears: interobserver variability in the diagnosis and prediction of cell of origin. Cancer 99:323–330, 2003.

Singer A. The uterine cervix from adolescence to the menopause. Br J Obstet Gynaecol 82:81–99, 1975.

Singer A, Reid BL, Coppleson M. A hypothesis: The role of a high-risk male in the etiology of cervical carcinoma. A correlation of epidemiology and molecular biology. Am J Obstet Gynecol 126:110–115, 1976.

Siracky J. Sex chromatin in cancer of the uterine cervix. Acta Cytol 11:486–487, 1967.

Skapier J. Diagnosis of preinvasive carcinoma of cervix. Surg Gynecol Obstet 89:405–410, 1949.

Skapier J. Evaluation of cytologic test in early diagnosis of cancer: 2 year survey of routine use of smear technique. Am J Obstet Gynecol 58:366–375, 1949.

Skyldberg B, Fujioka K, Hellstrom A-C, et al. Human papillomavirus infections, centrosome aberration, and genetic stability in cervical lesions. Mod Pathol 14:279–284, 2001.

Slater DN. Review. Sensitivity of primary screening by rapid review: 'To act or not to act on the results, that is the question.' Cytopathology 9:77–83, 1998.

Slattery ML, Robison LM, Schuman KL, et al. Cigarette smoking and exposure to passive smoke are risk factors for cervical cancer. JAMA 261:1593–1598, 1989.

Slawson DC, Bennett JH, Herman JM. Follow-up Papanicolaou smear for cervical atypia: Are we missing significant disease? A HARNET study. J Fam Pract 36:289–293, 1993.

Smith AE, Sherman ME, Scott DR, et al. Review of the Bethesda System atlas does not improve reproducibility of accuracy in the classification of atypical squamous cells of undetermined significance smears. Cancer 90:201–206, 2000.

Smith JW, Townsend DE, Sparkes RS. Genetic variants of glucose-6-phosphate dehydrogenase in the study of carcinoma of the uterine cervix. Cancer 28: 529–532, 1971.

Smith KHS, Bostrom SG, Galey WT. Correlation between Pap smears and cervical biopsies in an Air Force colposcopy clinic. J Reprod Med 30:681–684, 1985.

Smith PA, Turnbull LS. Invited Review. Small cell and 'pale' dyskaryosis. Cytopathology 8:3–8, 1997.

Snyder RN, Ortiz Y, Willie S, Cove JKJ. Dysplasia and carcinoma in situ of the uterine cervix: Prevalence in very young women (under age 22). Am J Obstet Gynecol 124:751–756, 1976.

Solomon D, Davey D, Kurman R, et al. The 2001 Bethesda System: terminology for reporting results of cervical cytology. JAMA 287:2114–2119, 2002.

Solomon D, Nayar R (eds). The Bethesda System for Reporting Cervical Cytology, 2nd ed. New York, Springer, 2004.

Solomon D, Schiffman M, Tarone R. Comparison of three management strategies for patients with atypical squamous cells of undetermined significance: Baseline results from a randomized trial. JNCI 93:293–299, 2001.

Soofer SB, Sidawy MK. Reactive cellular change. Is there an increased risk for squamous intraepithelial lesions? Cancer Cytopath 81:144–147, 1997.

Soost HJ, Bocknuhl B, Zock H. Results of cytologic mass screening in the Federal Republic of Germany. Acta Cytol 26:445–452, 1982.

Sorenson HM, Peterson O, Nielsen J, et al. The spontaneous course of premalignant lesions of the vaginal portion of the uterus. Acta Obstet Gynecol Scand 43(Suppl 7):103–104, 1964.

Spitzer M, Krumholz BA, Seltzer VL. The multicentric nature of disease related to human papillomavirus infection of the female lower genital tract. Obstet Gynecol 73:303–307, 1989.

Sprenger E, Hilgarth M, Schaden M. A followup of doubtful findings in cervical cytology by Fuelgen-DNA-cytophotometry. Beitr Pathol 152:58–65, 1974.

Sprenger E, Moore GW, Naujoks H, et al. DNA content and chromatin pattern analysis on cervical carcinoma in situ. Acta Cytol 17:27–31, 1973.

Spriggs AI. Follow-up of untreated carcinoma-in-situ of cervix uteri. Lancet 2: 599–600, 1971.

Spriggs AI, Boddington MM. Progression and regression of cervical lesions: Review of smears from women followed without initial biopsy or treatment. J Clin Pathol 33:517–525, 1980.

Spriggs AI, Boddington MM, Clarke CM. Carcinoma-in-situ of the cervix uteri: Some cytogenetic observations. Lancet 1:1383–1384, 1962.

Spriggs AI, Bowey CE, Cowdell RH. Chromosomes of precancerous lesions of the cervix uteri. New data and a review. Cancer 27:1239–1254, 1971.

Stafl A. Cervicography: A new method for cervical cancer detection. Am J Obstet Gynecol 139:815–825, 1981.

Stafl A, Friedrich EG, Jr, Mattingly RF. Detection of cervical neoplasia: Reducing the risk of error. Clin Obstet Gynecol 16:238–260, 1973.

Stafl A, Mattingly RF. Colposcopic diagnosis of cervical neoplasia. Obstet Gynecol 41:168–176, 1973.

Stafl A, Mattingly RF. Isoantigens ABO in cervical neoplasia. Gynecol Oncol 1: 26–35, 1972.

Stanley MA, Kirkland JA. Chromosome and histologic patterns in preinvasive lesions of the cervix. Acta Cytol 19:142–147, 1975.

Stenkvist B, Bergstrom R, Eklund G, Fox CH. Papanicolaou smear screening and cervical cancer. What can you expect? JAMA 252:1423–1426, 1984.

Stern E. Epidemiology of dysplasia. Obstet Gynecol Surv 24:711–723, 1969.

Stern E, Dixon WJ. Cancer of the cervix. A biometric approach to etiology. Cancer 14:153–160, 1961.

Stern E, Neely PM. Dysplasia of the uterine cervix: Incidence of regression, recurrence, and cancer. Cancer 17:508–512, 1964.

Stern E, Neely PM. Carcinoma and dysplasia of the cervix. A comparison of rates for new and returning populations. Acta Cytol 7:357–361, 1963.

Sternberg SS. Carcinoma in situ of cervix in monkey (Macaca mulatta). Report of case. Am J Obstet Gynecol 82:96–98, 1961.

Stewart FW. Factors influencing curability of cancer. In: Proceedings of the Third National Cancer Conference. Philadelphia, JB Lippincott, 1957, pp 62–73.

Stewart HL, Dunham LJ, Casper J, et al. Human papillomavirus infection in women infected with the human immunodeficiency virus. N Engl J Med 337:1343–1349, 1997.

Stoler MH. Human papillomavirus biology and cervical neoplasia. Implications for diagnostic criteria and testing. Arch Pathol Lab Med 127:935–939, 2003.

Stoler MH. Human papillomavirus and cervical neoplasia: A model for carcinogenesis. Int J Gynecol Pathol 19:16–28, 2000.

Stoler MH, Broker TR. In situ hybridization detection of human papillomavirus DNAs and messenger RNAs in genital carcinomas and a cervical carcinoma. Hum Pathol 17:1250–1258, 1986.

Stoler MH, Mills SE, Gersell DJ, Walker AN. Small-cell neuroendocrine carcinoma of the cervix. A human papillomavirus type 18-associated cancer. Am J Surg Pathol 15:28–32, 1991.

Stoler MH, Schiffman M. Interobserver reproducibility of cervical cytologic and histologic interpretations: realistic estimates from the ASCUS-LSIL Triage Study Group. JAMA 285:1500–1505, 2001.

Stoll P, Jaeger J, Dallenbach-Hellweg G. Gynakologische Cytologie. Berlin, Springer, 1969.

Stout AP. Observations on biopsy diagnosis of tumors. Cancer 10:912–921, 1957.

Strang P, Lindgren A, Stendahl U. Comparison between flow cytometry and single cell cytophotometry for DNA content analysis of the uterine cervix. Acta Radiol [Oncol] 24:337–341, 1985.

Sun X-W, Kuhn L, Ellerbrock TV, et al. Human papillomavirus infection in women infected with the human immunodeficiency virus. N Engl J Med 337:1343–1349, 1997.

Sundberg JP. Papillomavirus infections in animals. In Syrjänen K, Gissmann L, Koss LG (eds). Papillomaviruses and Human Diseases. New York, Springer-Verlag, 1987, pp 40–103.

Syrjänen HK, Heinonen UM, Kauraneimi T. Cytologic evidence of the association of condylomatous lesions with dysplastic and neoplastic changes in the uterine cervix. Acta Cytol 25:17–22, 1981.

Syrjänen K, Gissmann L, Koss LG (eds). Papillomaviruses and Human Disease. New York, Springer-Verlag, 1987.

Syrjänen K, Mantyjarvi R, Saarkoski S, et al. Factors associated with progression of cervical human papillomavirus (HPV) infections into carcinoma in situ during a long-term prospective follow-up. Br J Obstet Gynaecol 95:1096–1102, 1988.

Syrjänen K, Nurmi T, Mäntyjärvi R, et al. HLA types in women with cervical human papillomavirus (HPV) lesions prospectively followed up for 10 years. Cytopathology 7:99–107, 1996.

Syrjänen KJ, Syrjänen SM. Human papillomavirus (HPV) typing as an adjunct to cervical cancer screening. Cytopathology 10:8–15, 1999.

Syrjänen K, Syrjänen S, Kellokoski J, et al. Human papillomavirus (HPV) type 6 and 16 DNA sequences in bronchial squamous cell carcinomas demonstrated by in situ DNA hybridization. Lung 167:33–42, 1989.

Szulman AE. The histological distribution of the blood group substances in man as disclosed by immunofluorescence: II. The H-antigen and its relation to A, B antigens. J Exp Med 115:977–996, 1962.

Tabbara SO, Sidawy MK. Evaluation of the 5-year review of negative cervical smears in patients with high grade squamous intraepithelial lesions. Diagn Cytopathol 15:7–10, 1996.

Taft PD, Adams LR. Flow cytofluorimetry in routine diagnostic cytology. Am J Clin Pathol 72:533–539, 1979.

Tanaka T. Proliferative activity in dysplasia, carcinoma in situ and microinvasive carcinoma of uterine cervix. Path Res Pract 181:531–539, 1986.

Tanaka H, Chua KL, Lindh E, Hjerpe A. Patients with various types of human papillomavirus: Covariation and diagnostic relevance of cytological findings in Papanicolaou smears. Cytopathology 4:273–283, 1993.

Tanaka H, Sato H, Sato N, et al. Adding HPV 16 testing to abnormal cervical smear detection is useful for predicting CIN 3: A prospective study. Acta Obstet Gynecol Scand 83:497–500, 2004.

Taylor RS, Carroll BE, Lloyd JW. Mortality among women in 3 Catholic religious orders with special reference to cancer. Cancer 12:1207–1225, 1959.

Tenti P, Zappatore R, Migliora P, et al. Perinatal transmission of human papillomavirus from gravidas with latent infections. Obstet Gynecol 93:475–479, 1999.

Terris M, Wilson F, Nelson JH, Jr. Relation of circumcision to cancer of the cervix. Am J Obstet Gynecol 117:1056–1066, 1973.

Therman E, Denniston C, Nieminen U, et al. X chromatin, endomitoses, and mitotic abnormalities in human cervical cancers. Cancer Genet Cytogenet 16:1–11, 1985.

Timonen S, Nieminen U, Kauraniemi T. Mass screening for cervical carcinoma in Finland. Ann Chir Gynaecol Fenn 63:104–112, 1974.

Tolles WF, Horvath WJ, Bostrom RC. A study of the quantitative characteristics of exfoliated cells from the female genital tract. I. Measurement methods and results. Cancer 14:437–454, 1961.

Toon PG, Arrand J, Wilson LP, Sharp DS. Human papillomavirus infection of the uterine cervix of women without cytological signs of neoplasia. Br Med J 293:1261–1264, 1986.

Torre GD, Pilotti S, De Palo G, Rilke F. Viral particles in cervical condylomatous lesions. Tumori 64:549–553, 1978.

Towne JE. Carcinoma of the cervix in nulliparous and celibate women. Am J Obstet Gynecol 69:606–613, 1955.

Townsend DE, Richart RM, Marks E, et al. Invasive cancer following outpatient evaluation and therapy for cervical disease. Obstet Gynecol 57:145–149, 1981.

Tritz DM, Weeks JA, Spires SE, et al. Etiologies for non-correlating cervical cytologies and biopsies. Am J Clin Pathol 103:594–597, 1995.

Troncone G, Gupta PK. Cytologic observations preceding high grade squamous intraepithelial lesions. Acta Cytol 39:659–662, 1995.

Tseng CJ, Liang CC, Soong YK, Pao CC. Perinatal transmission of human papil-

lomavirus in infants: Relationship between infection rate and mode of delivery. Obstet Gynecol 91:92–96, 1998.

Tweeddale DN. Cytopathology of cervical squamous carcinoma in situ in postmenopausal women. Acta Cytol 14:363–369, 1970.

Tweeddale DN, Langenbach SR, Roddick JW, Holt ML. The cytopathology of microinvasive squamous cancer of the cervix uteri. Acta Cytol 13:447–454, 1969.

Uyeda CK, Davis HJ, Jones HW Jr. Nuclear protrusions and giant chromosome anomalies in cervical neoplasia. Acta Cytol 10:331–334, 1966.

Vallejos H, Del Mistro A, Kleinhaus S, et al. Characterization of human papilloma virus types in condylomata acuminata in children by in situ hybridization. Lab Invest 56:611–615, 1987.

Van der Graff Y, Vooijs GP, Gaillard HLJ, Go DMDS. Screening errors in cervical cytology smears. Acta Cytol 31:434–438, 1987.

Van Herik M, Decker DG, Lee RA, Symmonds RE. Late recurrence in carcinoma of the cervix. Am J Obstet Gynecol 108:1183–1186, 1970.

van Leeuwen AM, Ploem-Zaaijer JJ, Pieters WJ, et al. The suitability of DNA cytometry for the prediction of the histological diagnosis in women with abnormal cervical smears. Br J Obstet Gynaecol 103:359–365, 1996.

van Nagell JR, Hudson S, Gay EC, et al. Carcinoembryonic antigen in carcinoma of the uterine cervix. Antigen distribution in primary and metastatic tumors. Cancer 49:379–383, 1982.

van Nagell JR, Roddick JW, Lowin DM. The staging of cervical cancer: Inevitable discrepancies between clinical staging and pathologic findings. Am J Obstet Gynecol 110:973–978, 1971.

van Nagell JR Jr, Greenwell N, Powell DF, et al. Microinvasive carcinoma of the cervix. Am J Obstet Gynecol 145:981–991, 1983.

Varangot J, Nuovo V, Vassy S. Recherches sur le diagnostic des cancers génitaux féminins par les frottis vaginaux; le diagnostic des lésions épithéliomateuses du col utérin au cours de la gestation. Gynécol. Obstét. 54:261–293, 1955.

Varga A. The relationship of cervical dysplasia to in situ and invasive carcinoma of the cervix. Am J Obstet Gynecol 95:759–762, 1966.

Vassilakos P, Carrel S, Petignat P, et al. Use of automated primary screening on liquid-based, thin-layer preparations. Acta Cytol 46:291–295, 2002.

Vassilakos P, de Marval F, Muñoz M, et al. Human papillomavirus (HPV) DNA assay as an adjunct to liquid-based Pap test in the diagnostic triage of women with an abnormal Pap smear. Int J Gynaecol Obstet 61:45–50, 1998.

Viana O. La diagnosi precoce del cancro uterino mediante lo stricio. Clin Obstet 30:781–793, 1928.

Villa L L, Franco E L. F. Epidemiologic correlates of cervical neoplasia and risk of human papillomavirus infection in asymptomatic women in Brazil. JNCI 81:332–340, 1989.

Viscidi RP, Kotloff KL, Clayman B, et al. Prevalence of antibodies to human papillomavirus (HPV) type 16 virus-like particles in relation to cervical HPV infection among college women. Clin Diagn Lab Immunol 4:122–126, 1997.

Vogel A, Glatthaar E. Weitere elektronenmikroskopische Untersuchungen am Portiokarzinom. Oncologia 11:138–147, 1958.

von Haam E. Dyskaryotic cells in experimentally produced carcinoma of uterine cervix (letter to the editor). Acta Cytol 2:19–21, 1958.

von Haam E, Scarpelli DG. Experimental carcinoma of cervix: Comparative cytologic and histologic study. Cancer Res 15:449–455, 1955.

Vonka V, Kanta J, Hirsch I, Zavadova H. Prospective study on the relationship between cervical neoplasia and herpes simplex type-2 virus. II. Herpes simplex type-2 antibody prevalence in sera taken at enrollment. Int J Cancer 33:61–66, 1984.

Vooijs PG, Elias A, van der Graff Y, Velig S. Relationship between the diagnosis of epithelial abnormalities and the composition of cervical smears. Acta Cytol 29:323–328, 1985.

Vooijs PG, van der Graff Y, Elias AG. Cellular composition of cervical smears in relation to the day of the menstrual cycle and the method of contraception. Acta Cytol 31:417–426, 1987.

Voytek TM, Kanna V, Kline TS. Atypical parakeratosis. A marker for dysplasia? Diagn Cytopathol 15:288–291, 1996.

Wagner D, de Villiers EM, Gissmann L. Detection of various papilloma virus types in cytologic smears of precancerous conditions and cancers of the uterine cervix. Geburtshilfe Fraunheilkd. 45:226–231, 1985.

Wagner D, Ikenberg H, Boehm N, Gissmann L. Identification of human papillomavirus in cervical swabs of deoxyribonucleic acid in situ hybridization. Obstet Gynecol 64:767–772, 1984.

Wagner D, Sprenger E, Merkle D. Cytophotometric studies in suspicious cervical smears. Acta Cytol 20:366–371, 1976.

Wain GV, Farnsworth A, Hacker NE. Cervical carcinoma after negative Pap smears: Evidence against rapid onset cancers. Int J Gynecol Cancer 2:318–322, 1992.

Wakonig-Vaartaja R, Hughes DT. Chromosomal anomalies in dysplasia, carcinoma-in-situ, and carcinoma of the cervix uteri. Lancet 2:756–759, 1965.

Wakonig-Vaartaja R, Kirkland JA. A correlated chromosomal and histopathologic study of preinvasive lesions of the cervix. Cancer 18:1101–1112, 1965.

Walboomers JMM, Husman AM, Snijders PJF, et al. Human papillomavirus in false negative archival cervical smears: Implications for screening for cervical cancer. J Clin Pathol 48:728–732, 1995.

Walboomers JMM, Jacobs MV, Manos MM, et al. Human papillomavirus is a necessary cause of invasive cervical cancer worldwide. J Pathol 189:12–19, 1999.

Walkinshaw SA, Dodgson J, McCance DJ, Duncan ID. Risk factors in the development of cervical intraepithelial neoplasia in women with vulval warts. Genitourin Med 64:316–320, 1988.

Wall RL. Didelphic uterus with carcinoma in situ of both cervices. Am J Obstet Gynecol 76:803–806, 1958.

Wallace DL, Slankard JE. Teenage cervical carcinoma in situ. Obstet Gynecol 41:697–700, 1973.

Wallin K-L, Wiklund F, Angstrom T, et al. Type-specific persistence of human papillomavirus DNA before the development of invasive cervical cancer. N Engl J Med 341:1633–1638, 1999.

Walz WW. Colpomicroscopy: Basic outlines, techniques, application, diagnostics. J Reprod Med 12:207–210, 1974.

Wang SE, Ritchie MJ, Atkinson BF. Cervical cytology smear false negative fraction: Reduction in a small community hospital. Acta Cytol 41:1690–1696, 1997.

Wang T-Y, Chen F-F, Yang Y-C, et al. Histologic and immunophenotypic classification of cervical carcinomas by expression of the p53 homologue p63: A study of 250 cases. Hum Pathol 32:479–486, 2001.

Watanabe A, Wachi T, Omi H, et al. Granulocyte colony-stimulating factor-producing small-cell carcinoma of the uterine cervix: Report of a case. Diagn Cytopathol 23:269–274, 2000.

Watanabe S, Kanda T, Yoshike K. Human papillomavirus type 16 transformation of primary human embryonic fibroblasts requires expression of open reading frames E6 and E7. J Virol 63:965–969, 1989.

Watts DH, Koutsky LA, Holmes KK, et al. Low risk of perinatal transmission of human papillomavirus: Results from a prospective cohort study. Am J Obstet Gynecol 178:365–373, 1998.

Way S. Microinvasive carcinoma of the cervix. Acta Cytol 8:14–15, 1964.

Weir MM, Bell DA. Transitional cell metaplasia of the cervix: A newly described entity in cervicovaginal smears. Diagn Cytopathol 18:222–226, 1998.

Weir MM, Bell DA, Young RH. Transitional cell metaplasia of the uterine cervix and vagina: An under-recognized lesion that may be confused with high grade dysplasia: A report of 59 cases. Am J Surg Pathol 21:510–517, 1997.

Wells M, Griffiths S, Lewis F, Bird CC. Demonstration of human papillomavirus types in paraffin processed tissue from human anogenital lesions by in-situ DNA hybridization. J Pathol 152:77–82, 1987.

Wells M, Robertson S, Lewis F, Dixon MF. Squamous carcinoma arising in a giant peri-anal condyloma associated with human papillomavirus types 6 and 11. Histopathology 12:319–323, 1988.

Wentz WB, Reagan JW. Survival in cervical cancer with respect to cell type. Cancer 12:384–388, 1959.

Wentz WB, Reagan JW, Heggie AD. Cervical carcinogenesis with herpes simplex virus, type 2. Obstet Gynecol 46:117–121, 1975.

Werness BA, Levine AJ, Howley PM. Association of human papillomavirus types 16 and 18 E6 proteins with p53. Science 248:76–69, 1990.

Westergaard L, Norgaard M. Severe cervical dysplasia: Control by biopsies or primary conization? A comparative study. Acta Obstet Gynecol Scand 60:549–554, 1981.

Wheeler JD, Hertig AT. Pathologic anatomy of carcinoma of uterus. I. Squamous carcinoma of cervix. Am J Clin Pathol 25:345–375, 1955.

Wheelock JB, Kaminski PF. Value of repeat cytology at the time of colposcopy for the evaluation of CIN 1 Pap smears. J Reprod Med 34:815–817, 1989.

Wied GL, Legoretta G, Mohr D, Rauzy A. Cytology of invasive cervical carcinoma and carcinoma in situ. Ann NY Acad Sci 97:759–766, 1962.

Wied GL, Messina AM, Rosenthal E. Comparative quantitative DNA measurements on Feulgen-stained cervical epithelial cells. Acta Cytol 10:31–37, 1966.

Wielenga G, Old JW, von Haam E. Squamous carcinoma in situ of the uterine cervix. II. Topography and clinical correlations. Cancer 18:1612–1621, 1965.

Wilbanks GD, Campbell JA. In vitro observations of sex chromatin in cells from the human uterine cervix. Acta Cytol 15:297–302, 1971.

Wilbanks GD, Richart RM, Terner JV. DNA content of cervical intraepithelial neoplasia studied by two wavelength Feulgen cytophotometry. Am J Obstet Gynecol 98:792–799, 1967.

Wilbanks GD. Tissue culture in early cervical neoplasia. Obstet Gynecol Surv 24:804–837, 1969.

Wilbanks GD, Richart RM. Fluorescence of cervical intraepithelial neoplasia induced by tetracycline and acridine orange. Am J Obstet Gynecol 106:726–730, 1970.

Wilbanks GD, Richart RM. Postpartum cervix and its relation to cervical neoplasia: A colposcopic study. Cancer 19:273–276, 1966.

Wilbur DC, Bonfiglio TA, Stoler MH. Continuing of human papillomavirus (HPV) type between neoplastic precursors and invasive cervical carcinoma: An in situ hybridization study. Am J Surg Pathol 12:182–186, 1988.

Wilbur DC, Parker EM, Foti JA. Location-guided screening of liquid-based cervical cytology specimens. Am J Clin Pathol 118:399–407, 2002.

Wilczynski SP, Bergen S, Walker J, et al. Human papillomaviruses and cervical cancer: Analysis of histopathologic features associated with different viral types. Hum Pathol 19:697–704, 1988.

Willcox F, de Somer ML, Roy JV. Classification of cervical smears with discordance between the cytologic and/or histologic ratings. Acta Cytol 31:883–886, 1987.

Williams AE, Jordan JA, Allen JM, Murphy JF. The surface ultrastructure of normal and metaplastic cervical epithelia and of carcinoma in situ. Cancer Res 33:504–513, 1973.

Williams G, Stoeber K. Clinical applications of a novel mammalian cell-free DNA replication system. Br J Cancer 80:20–24, 1999.

Williams GH, Romanowski P, Morris L, et al. Improved cervical smear assessment using antibodies against proteins that regulate DNA replication. Proc Natl Acad Sci USA 95:14932–14937, 1998.

Williams MC. Histochemical observations of verruca vulgaris. J Invest Dermatol 37:279–282, 1961.

Williams ML, Rimm DL, Pedigo MA, Frable WJ. Atypical squamous cells of undetermined significance: Correlative histologic and follow-up studies from an academic medical center. Diagn Cytopathol 16:1–7, 1997.

Winkler B, Crum CP, Fujii T, et al. Koilocytotic lesions of the cervix. The relationship of mitotic abnormalities to the presence of papillomavirus antigens and nuclear DNA content. Cancer 53:1081–1087, 1984.

Witkin SS, Korngold GC, Bendich A. Ribonuclease-sensitive–DNA-synthesizing complex in human sperm heads and seminal fluid. Proc Natl Acad Sci 72:3295–3299, 1975.

Wolff JP, Lacour J, Chassagne D, Berend M. Cancer of the cervical stump: A study of 173 patients. Obstet Gynecol 39:10–16, 1972.

Woodruff JD, Peterson WF. Condylomata acuminata of the cervix. Am J Obstet Gynecol 75:1354–1361, 1958.

Woodworth CD, Doniger J, DiPaolo JA. Immortalization of human foreskin keratinocytes by various human papillomavirus DNAs corresponds to their association with cervical carcinoma. J Virol 63:159–164, 1989.

Wright RC, Schiffman M. Adding a test for human papillomavirus DNA to cervical-cancer screening. N Engl J Med 348:489–490, 2003.

Wright TC, Cox JT, Massad S, et al. 2001 Consensus guidelines for the management of women with cervical intraepithelial neoplasia. Am J Obstet Gynecol 189:295–304, 2003.

Wright TC, Gagnon S, Ferenczy A, Richart RM. Excising CIN lesions by loop electrosurgical procedure. Contemp OB/GYN, March 1991, 57–73.

Wright TC Jr, Cox JT, Massad LS, et al. 2001 Consensus guidelines for the management of women with cervical cytological abnormalities. JAMA 287:2120–2129, 2002.

Wright TC Jr, Denny L, Kuhn L, et al. HPV DNA testing of self-collected vaginal samples compared with cytologic screening to detect cervical cancer. JAMA 283:81–86, 2000.

Wright TC Jr, Ellerbrock TV, Chiasson MA, et al. Cervical intraepithelial neoplasia in women infected with human immunodeficiency virus: Prevalence, risk factors, and validity of Papanicolaou smears: New York Cervical Disease Study. Obstet Gynecol 84:591–597, 1994.

Wright TC Jr, Schiffman M, Solomon D, et al. Interim guidance for the use of human papillomavirus DNA testing as an adjunct to cervical cytology for screening. Obstet Gynecol 103:304–309, 2004.

Wynder EL, Cornfield J, Schroff PD, Doraiswami KR. A study of environmental factors in carcinoma of cervix. Am J Obstet Gynecol 68:1016–1052, 1954.

Yee C, Krishnan-Hewlett I, Baker CC, et al. Presence and expression of human papillomavirus sequences in human cervical carcinoma cell lines. Am J Pathol 119:361–366, 1985.

Yobs AR, Plott AE, Hicklin MD, et al. Retrospective evaluation of gynecologic cytodiagnosis: II. Interlaboratory reproducibility as shown in rescreening large consecutive samples of reported cases. Acta Cytol 31:900–910, 1987.

Yobs AR, Swanson RA, Lamotte LC, Jr. Laboratory reliability of the Papanicolaou smear. Obstet Gynecol 65:235–244, 1985.

Yost NP, Santoso JT, McIntire DD, Iliya FA. Postpartum regression rates of antepartum cervical intraepithelial neoplasia II, III lesions. Obstet Gynecol 93:359–362, 1999.

Youkeles L, Forsythe AB, Stern E. Evaluation of Papanicolaou smear and effect of sample biopsy in follow-up of cervical dysplasia. Cancer 36:2080–2084, 1976.

Young LS, Bevan IS, Johnson MA, et al. The polymerase chain reaction: A new epidemiological tool for investigating cervical human papillomavirus infection. Br Med J 298:14–18, 1989.

Young NA, Naryshkin S, Atkinson BF, et al. Interobserver variability of cervical smears with squamous cell abnormalities: A Philadelphia study. Diagn Cytopathol 11:352–357, 1994.

Younge PA, Hertig AT, Armstrong D. Study of 135 cases of carcinoma in situ of cervix at Free Hospital for Women. Am J Obstet Gynecol 58:867–895, 1949.

Zhou C, Hayes MM, Clement PB, Thomson TA. Small cell carcinoma of the uterine cervix: Cytologic findings in 13 cases. Cancer 84:281–288, 1998.

Zuna RE, Moore W, Dunn ST. HPV DNA testing of the residual sample of liquid-based Pap test: Utility as a quality assurance monitor. Mod Pathol 14:147–151, 2001.

zur Hausen H. Papillomaviruses in human cancer. Appl Pathol 5:19–24, 1987.

zur Hausen H. Intracellular surveillance of persisting viral infections. Lancet 2:489–491, 1986.

zur Hausen H. Human genital cancer: Synergism between two virus infections or synergism between a virus infection and initiating events? Lancet 2:1370–1372, 1982.

zur Hausen H. Condylomata acuminata and human genital cancer. Cancer Res 36:794, 1976.

Adenocarcinoma and Related Tumors of the Uterine Cervix

12

EPIDEMIOLOGY

Adenocarcinomas derived from the endocervical epithelium constitute approximately 10% to 15% of all invasive cancers of the cervix. There is suggestive evidence that the **frequency** of endocervical adenocarcinoma may be **on the rise** (Kjaer and Brinton, 1993). It is possible that a better recognition of this group of lesions combined with a reduction in the rate of invasive squamous cancer may account for some of the increase. The increased frequency may be limited to geographic regions: a marked increase has been observed in Australia, United Kingdom and Norway, whereas none has been observed in Italy (Debate, 1999). In the United States, there is some evidence of increase in young women (Peters et al, 1986; Schwartz and Weiss, 1986; Horowitz et al, 1988). The disease occurs in adult women of all ages but is most common in women in their late 40s or early 50s.

Dallenbach-Hellweg (1981) proposed a possible relationship between endocervical adenocarcinoma and long-term use of oral contraceptives containing progesterone. Peters et al (1986), Jones and Silverberg (1989), Brinton et al (1990), and Ursin et al (1994) found some evidence in support of this concept. Because of a possible association of *all* forms of carcinoma of the cervix with the use of oral contraceptives (see Chap. 10), the selective increase of adenocarcinomas in this group of patients has not been documented in a persuasive fashion. Horowitz et al (1988) and Parazzini et al (1988) failed to observe significant epidemiologic differences between women with squamous carcinoma of the cervix and those with adenocarcinoma of the cervix. In fact, the **coexistence of precancerous squamous lesions or invasive squamous cancer may be observed in nearly one half of patients with endocervical adenocarcinoma, suggesting a common denominator for these lesions.** This common denominator may be **human papillomaviruses, particularly types 16 and 18,** which are frequently observed in endocervical neoplastic lesions (Wilczynski et al, 1988; Tase et al, 1989; Fransworth et al, 1989; Nielson et al, 1990; Duggan et al, 1995; Iwasawa et al, 1996; Riethdorf et al, 2002) (for discussion of the human papillomavirus, see Chap. 11). Endocervical adenocarcinoma may also be synchronous with endometrial cancer (Friedell and McKay, 1953) and with ovarian carcinoma (Livolsi et al, 1983).

SEQUENCE OF NEOPLASTIC EVENTS

It is generally assumed that the sequence of events in the development of endocervical adenocarcinoma of the uterine cervix is similar to squamous carcinoma, described in the preceding chapter. Theoretically at least, minor morphologic abnormalities of endocervical epithelium, variously termed as "atypia" or "dysplasia," should precede the development of the true precursor lesions—the adenocarcinomas in situ—which, in turn, should lead to microinvasive and fully invasive cancers. The term **endocervical carcinoma in situ,** first introduced by Friedell and McKay (1953), has been enshrined in the 2001 Bethesda System of reporting (see Chap. 11). Documenting the sequence of neoplastic events in the endocervix poses problems because, except for its lowest segment, the endocervical canal cannot be visualized by colposcopy and, therefore, cytologic sampling cannot be targeted. Also, in spite of numerous efforts, the morphologic recognition of sequential abnormalities of the endocervical cells is much more difficult than in squamous cells (Lee et al, 2000). The issue is complicated still further by the fact that at least half of endocervical adenocarcinoma is associated with squamous or epidermoid neoplasia in various forms that may have common cytologic features with endocervical neoplasia. To simplify the discussion of a difficult topic, this chapter will begin with a discussion of histology and cytology of invasive endocervical adenocarcinoma, followed by a discussion of precursors.

INVASIVE ENDOCERVICAL ADENOCARCINOMA

Several elaborate systems of classification of endocervical adenocarcinoma have been proposed and recently summarized (Zaino, 2000; Young and Clement, 2002). Because the prognosis of these tumors depends more on stage of disease than histologic presentation (Berek et al, 1984; Kilgore et al, 1988), the simplest classification is their subdivision into common and less common or rare types of tumors.

Among the common types are:

- Adenocarcinoma mimicking normal endocervical glands
- Mucus-producing adenocarcinomas
- Endometrioid carcinomas
- Poorly differentiated carcinomas
- Synchronous adenocarcinoma and squamous carcinoma

Less common or rare are:

- Adenosquamous carcinoma
- Villoglandular papillary adenocarcinomas
- Adenoma malignum (minimal deviation adenocarcinoma)
- Glassy-cell carcinoma
- Mucoepidermoid carcinomas
- Clear-cell carcinoma (see Chap. 14)
- Extremely rare adenocarcinomas

Common Types of Well-Differentiated Adenocarcinoma

Histology

Tumors Mimicking Endocervical Glands

The tumors infiltrate the stroma of the cervix and **form glands similar to normal endocervical glands,** although the glands vary in size and have irregular configuration. Papillary projections, on the surface of the tumor and within the malignant glands, are fairly common. The malignant glands are lined by one or more layers of tumor cells that are either columnar or cuboidal in shape, have an opaque, granular cytoplasm, and show significantly enlarged, hyperchromatic, coarsely granular nuclei, sometimes provided with large nucleoli (Fig. 12-1A). Histologic diagnosis of the well-differentiated endocervical adenocarcinomas may occasionally cause **diagnostic problems** because the glands may be mistaken for normal endocervical tissue, particularly in scanty biopsies or endocervical curettage material.

A number of **benign variants or benign abnormalities** of the endocervical glands may be mistaken for adenocarcinoma. **Microglandular hyperplasia,** occurring mainly in women with progesterone exposure, **endocervical tunnel clusters, mesonephric hyperplasia,** and **endocervicosis** were discussed in Chapter 10. They all have, in common, formation of glandular structures lined by bland benign cuboidal or columnar cells and, regardless of other opinions, are not recognizable in cytologic preparations, contrary to endocervical adenocarcinoma. Thus, cytologic samples may be of significant help in the interpretation of small biopsies of cervix.

A very rare lesion termed **microcystic endocervical adenocarcinoma** mimics benign lesions of the endocervix but the cysts are lined by clearly malignant cells. In some of these patients, malignant cells may be observed in cervical smears but the precise type of lesion cannot be established (Tambouret et al, 2000).

Although many observers consider all adenocarcinomas derived from endocervical glands as mucinous or mucus-producing, it has been my experience that there is little evidence of mucus production in the most common adenocarcinomas wherein it is usually confined to a few scattered cells. Therefore, endocervical adenocarcinomas with a substantial component of mucus-producing cells, are separated out. This subdivision is of value in the interpretation of cytologic findings.

Mucus-Producing Adenocarcinomas

In these tumors, a substantial proportion of cells lining the glands resemble goblet- or intestinal cells, characterized by markedly distended clear cytoplasm filled with mucus (Fig. 12-1B). **Some of these tumors may mimic intestinal cancers** because of the presence of occasional **Paneth cells** with cytoplasmic granules. **Signet-ring types of** cancer cells may sometimes occur.

Endometrioid Type of Carcinomas

These tumors form glands lined by one or more cuboidal cancer cells, mimicking a similar tumor of endometrial origin (Fig. 12-1C). Mucus production in the tumor cells is either absent or very limited. The nuclear features of the

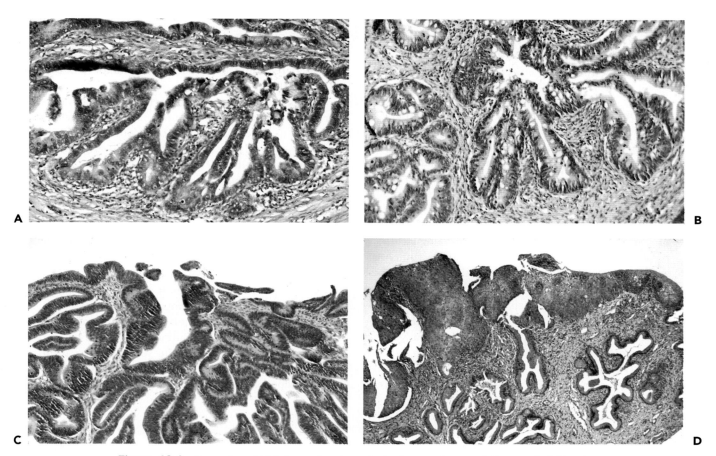

Figure 12-1 **Examples of histology of endocervical adenocarcinoma.** *A.* Tumor mimicking the structure of normal endocervical glands. *B.* Tumor with marked mucin secretions. *C.* Tumor mimicking endometrial carcinoma. *D.* Synchronous presence of a high-grade squamous intraepithelial lesion (HGSIL) and endocervical adenocarcinoma.

tumors are similar to those of the adenocarcinoma of endocervical type, described above. For a detailed morphologic description of endometrioid carcinomas, see Chap. 13. Some of the endocervical lesions may be traced to foci of endocervical endometriosis. Others probably represent a histologic variant of endocervical adenocarcinoma. In some cases, curettage may be required to determine the origin of the tumor in the endocervix or the endometrium.

As mentioned, **these three dominant tumor types are associated with either precursor lesions (CIN) or invasive squamous carcinomas which occur in about 50% of cases** (Fig. 12-1D). The impact of this association on cytology will be discussed later in this chapter.

Cytology

Cytologic presentation of endocervical adenocarcinoma has been influenced by the widespread use of endocervical brushes. A large number of papers, many cited in this text, described and analyzed the abnormalities of endocervical cells in minute details that allegedly led to a more precise assessment of the sequence of neoplastic events in the endocervix. Following the example of Rosenthal et al (1982), Van Aspert-van Erp et al (1995, 1997), in a series of elaborate studies, analyzed at great length numerous visual and computer-generated features of endocervical cells in **"endocervical columnar cell intraepithelial neoplasia" (ECCIN)**,

ranging from mild to moderate to severe atypia, endocervical adenocarcinoma in situ, and invasive adenocarcinoma. When the numerous criteria established in these studies were tested for reproducibility, only a few of them proved to be of practical diagnostic value. They were **essentially the same abnormalities of endocervical cells that have been previously recognized as consistent with adenocarcinoma.** Unfortunately, the analysis of abnormalities of the endocervical cells is further complicated by benign atypias occurring in these cells, discussed in Chapter 10 and later in this chapter. If the endocervical brush-induced sampling artifacts are added to the mix, it becomes evident that the topic of abnormalities of endocervical cells may be extremely complex and the elaborate studies have been of limited value in the practice of cytopathology. ThinPrep liquid preparations of cervical samples have a significant effect on morphology of endocervical cells. **The nuclei are generally smaller (shrunken) and the nucleoli** are often evident in benign cells (Johnson and Rahemtulla, 1999; Selvaggi, 2002).

Cells of Well-Differentiated Invasive Endocervical Adenocarcinoma

It is virtually impossible to separate the three main types of endocervical adenocarcinoma from each other in cytologic preparations, although, occasionally, mucus-producing adenocarcinomas may shed cells suggestive of this tumor type (see below). In the cervical material, the **smear background often shows blood, necrosis, and cell debris.**

In samples obtained by either cervical scrapers or endocervical brushes, the following features may be observed:

- The **dominant cancer cells** are usually **columnar**, although often larger or smaller than normal endocervical cells. They have **opaque and granular or clear cytoplasm** and abnormal nuclei. The **nuclear changes** comprise **enlargement, hyperchromasia, coarse granulation of chromatin** and sometimes large, **irregular, and multiple nucleoli** (Figs. 12-2A and 12-3A).
- The cancer cells often form **spherical or oval clusters of superimposed cancer cells,** corresponding to tumor papillae (Figs. 12-2B,C and 12-3B). At the periphery of such clusters, the columnar configuration of the component cells may be observed. On careful focusing, gland formation within the clusters can be observed.
- In yet other cases, **mitotic figures** and **apoptotic breakup of nuclei** may occur (Fig. 12-4A). Occasionally, large malignant cells, without distinguishing features, may be noted (Fig. 12-4B,C).
- The cancer cells are often arranged in **parallel clusters** **(palisading)**, reflecting the arrangement of the tumor cells on the surface epithelium (Fig. 12-5A).
- They may be **arranged around a central lumen (rosettes),** reflecting the tendency of the tumor cells to form glands (Fig. 12-5B).
- Approximately spherical "**signet ring**" cancer cells are characteristic of mucus-producing adenocarcinoma. Such cells have a **large, peripheral nucleus** and a **cytoplasm** with a large, **mucus-containing single vacuole or several smaller vacuoles** (Fig. 12-5C).
- It is not uncommon to observe, in cervical smears of **endocervical adenocarcinomas, a few dysplastic (dyskaryotic) or cancer cells of squamous type.** These reflect abortive forms of squamous carcinoma, which may be associated with endocervical adenocarcinoma (see below). Very rarely, similar findings may be observed in **adenoacanthomas of the endometrium** (see Chap. 13).
- **In samples obtained by endocervical brushes,** additional features of such tumors can be noted:
- **Large, complex clusters of tumor cells** are often removed from the fragile surface of the tumor. Sometimes capillary vessels can be seen coursing through the cluster (Fig. 12-6A). Again, **the search for columnar shape of the component cells and gland forma-**

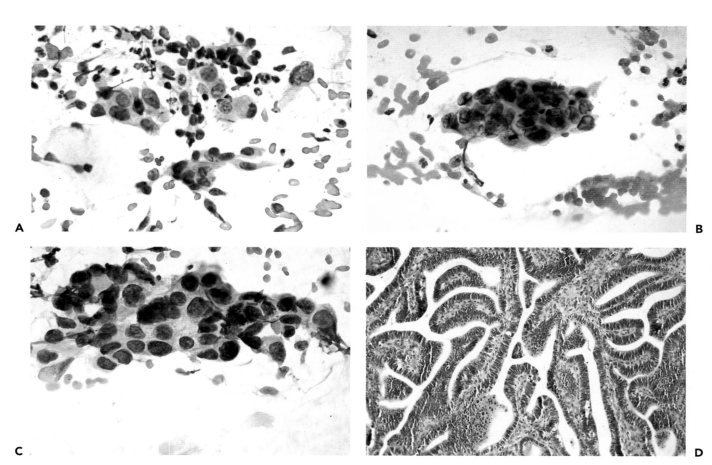

A   **B**   **C**   **D**

Figure 12-2   Endocervical adenocarcinoma. *A–C.* Cancer cells, either dispersed or forming tight papillary clusters. The elongated columnar configuration of some of the cancer cells is particularly evident in *A. D.* Tissue lesion corresponding to *A–C,* showing a well-differentiated endocervical adenocarcinoma.

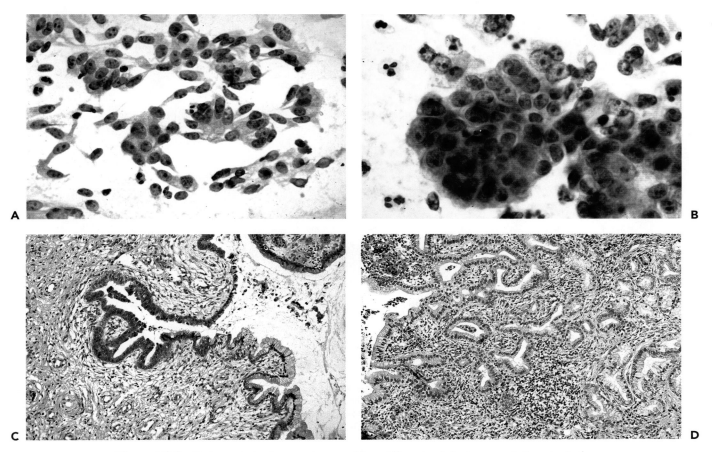

Figure 12-3 Endocervical adenocarcinoma with a different cytologic presentation. In *A*, the cancer cells mimic normal endocervical cells, except for nuclear enlargement and hyperchromasia. *B* shows a papillary cluster of cancer cells which are much larger than those shown in *A* and shows significant nuclear and nucleolar abnormalities. *C,D*. Tissue sections corresponding to *A* and *B*. In *C*, a clear transition between normal and cancerous endocervical epithelium is shown. *D* shows the invasive component of the tumor.

tion within the cluster are the essential prerequisites of diagnosis.

- Isolated "naked" nuclei of malignant cells are more common in brush than in scrape specimens and may be quite numerous (Fig. 12-6B). Some of these nuclei may appear quite bland and pale (Fig. 12-6C).

- "Feathering" of cells on the surface of the cluster is less common, although this feature has been strongly emphasized in the literature. The term, introduced by Ayer et al (1987), pertains to clusters, wherein the peripheral cancer cells are approximately perpendicular to the long axis of the cluster, thus having some resemblance to a feather (Fig. 12-7B,C). It is essential to verify that the **nuclear features of the component cells are those of a malignant tumor because, on rare occasions, this cell arrangement may also occur with benign endocervical cells** and cells from other organs, such as the bronchus (Fig. 12-7D).

- It is of historic interest that, in **adenocarcinoma of the endocervix, the malignant cells will be found primarily in the direct cervical sample, whereas those of endometrial (and tubal or ovarian) origin will be found primarily in the vaginal pool smears** which, nowadays,

are unfortunately very rarely obtained. These differences cannot be recognized in liquid preparations.

Poorly Differentiated Endocervical Adenocarcinomas

Histology

These tumors are usually observed in advanced stages of disease as grossly visible tumors of the cervix. Their derivation from either the endocervical or endometrioid adenocarcinomas or, for that matter, poorly differentiated squamous (epidermoid) type of cancer may be difficult to determine. The tumor cells grow in **solid sheets,** wherein only occasional gland formation may be observed (Fig. 12-7).

Cytology

Poorly differentiated adenocarcinomas may be difficult to recognize because of **necrotic debris and blood** that are usually present in such preparations and may obscure cancer cells. The cancer cells derived from such tumors **may retain some of the features of a well-differentiated carcinoma, notably the columnar shape of the cells and the spherical clustering.** In many such cases, however, the cancer cells are **of spherical or irregular configuration, vary in size,**

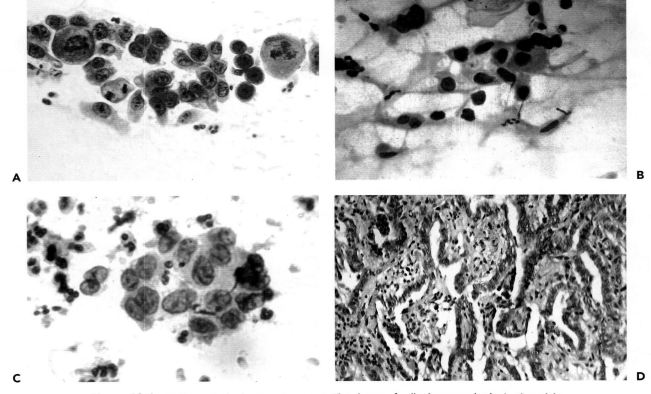

Figure 12-4   Endocervical adenocarcinoma. *A.* The cluster of cells shows marked mitotic activity. *B.* Scattered cancer cells, some with columnar configuration. *C.* A papillary cluster of poorly differentiated cells with large nuclei and nucleoli. *D.* Tissue section corresponding to *C* showing invasive well-differentiated adenocarcinoma.

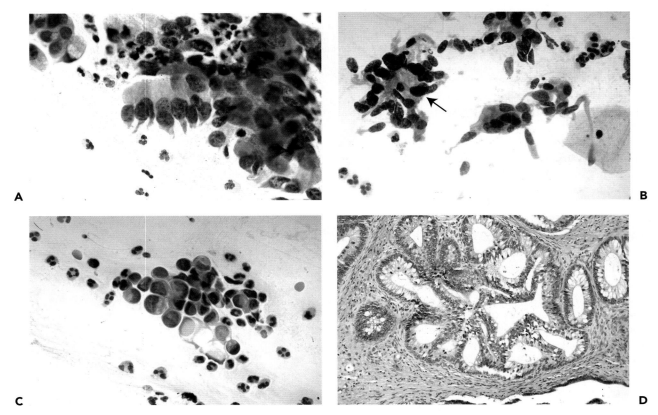

Figure 12-5   Endocervical adenocarcinoma. *A.* The smear shows palisading of columnar cancer cells, usually attributed to adenocarcinoma in situ. *B.* Columnar cells forming a rosette (*arrow*). *C.* Signet ring cancer cells. *D.* Tissue section corresponding to *B* and *C* showing invasive mucus-producing adenocarcinoma of the endocervix.

400

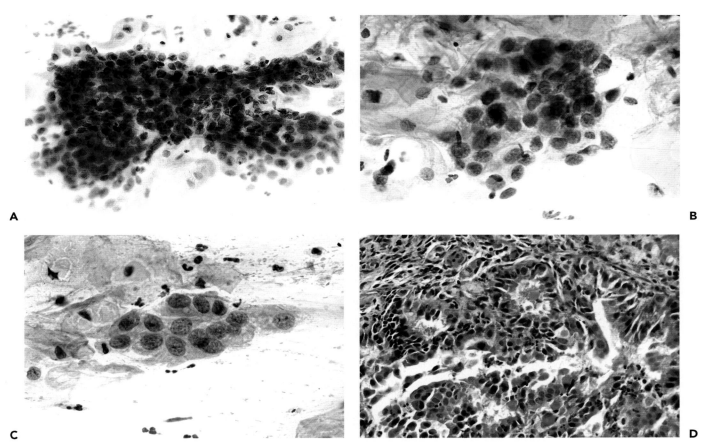

Figure 12-6   Poorly differentiated endocervical adenocarcinoma in a brush specimen. *A.* A large, compact cluster of cancer cells. *B.* Isolated "naked" nuclei of cancer cells. *C.* Cancer cells with bland nuclei forming clusters. *D.* Invasive adenocarcinoma.

and have the characteristic nuclear features of advanced cancer, to wit, **irregular shape, coarse chromatin arrangement and large nucleoli.** In some cases, however, **hyperchromasia may be absent and the large nuclei may be pale** (see Fig. 12-6C). The cytoplasm is scanty and, therefore, the **nucleocytoplasmic ratio** is modified in favor of the nucleus. Abnormal mitotic figures may be observed. In such cases, **the diagnosis of cancer is usually evident but the precise cytologic diagnosis of an adenocarcinoma may be difficult to establish and usually requires histologic evidence.**

Microinvasive Adenocarcinoma

Histology

Using criteria applicable to the definition of microinvasive squamous carcinoma, Christopherson et al (1979) were apparently the first to apply this concept to cervical adenocarcinoma. Tumors infiltrating the cervical stroma to the depth of 5 mm or less were designated as microinvasive endocervical adenocarcinomas. The term was used by Bousfield et al (1980) in a large series of cases without further definition. Betsill and Clark (1986) defined this entity as tumors infiltrating to the depth of 2 mm or less. Mulvany and Östör (1997) described 24 cases classified as microinvasive adenocarcinoma with invasion of 5 mm or

less. In such cases, **small malignant glands or solid nests of cancer cells are seen in the cervical stroma, outside of the normal boundaries of the cancerous surface epithelium or glands.** However, as previously discussed, the depth of distribution of normal endocervical glands varies from patient to patient and so do the boundaries. Such tumors virtually never form metastases.

It is our judgment that the diagnosis of **microinvasive endocervical carcinoma is very difficult to establish, is not reproducible, and, in any event, it is of questionable practical value,** because the prognosis of surgically treated endocervical microinvasive adenocarcinoma appears to be as favorable as that of carcinoma in situ, as documented by Betsill and Clark (1986), Östör et al (1997), and Mulvany and Östör (1997).

Cytology

Despite elaborate descriptions by Bousfield et al (1980) and Ayer et al (1988) from the same laboratory, it is doubtful that the cytologic identification of microinvasive carcinoma is possible in a reliable and reproducible fashion. In 12 of the 40 cases so classified, Mulvany and Östör (1997) observed more pleomorphic nuclei, coarse chromatin pattern, karyorrhexis and cell detritus and, hence, findings consistent with invasive adenocarcinoma described above.

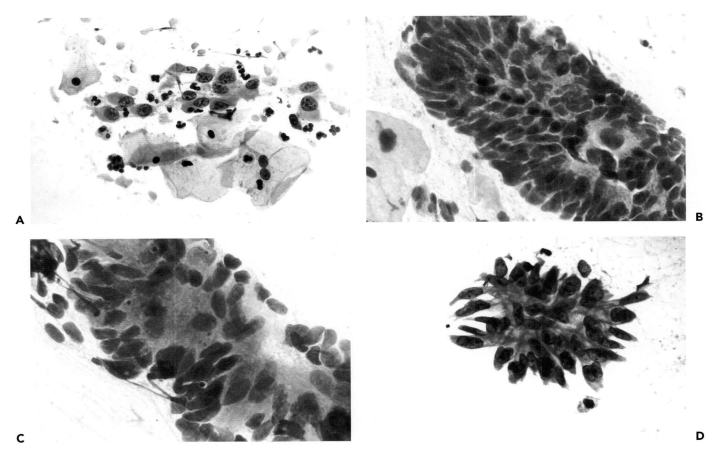

Figure 12-7 **Other cytologic features of adenocarcinoma.** *A.* Cells of endocervical adenocarcinoma mimicking the so-called repair. *B.* The so-called feathering of cancer cells which is a useful brush-induced diagnostic artifact. *C.* Higher magnification of feathering in *B. D.* Feathering of normal endocervical cells in a brush specimen. (*B,C:* Courtesy of Dr. M. Zaman, New York Medical College, Valhalla, NY.)

PRECURSOR LESIONS OF INVASIVE ENDOCERVICAL ADENOCARCINOMA

Endocervical Adenocarcinoma In Situ

It is logical to expect that invasive endocervical adenocarcinomas are preceded by a cancerous change in the endocervical epithelium and glands. By definition, **adenocarcinoma in situ is a malignant transformation of surface and endocervical gland epithelium in its normal anatomic setting.** There are major individual differences in the distribution of endocervical glands and, **in some women, normal glands may be found in the depth of the cervical stroma.** When such deeply seated glands show malignant changes, **it is sometimes difficult to state with certainty whether an adenocarcinoma is still in situ or whether an invasion has taken place. In most such cases, it is prudent to err on the conservative side.**

Histology

The affected **epithelium lining the endocervical canal and the adjacent endocervical glands** is composed of **columnar, less often cuboidal, cancer cells that are usually larger than normal endocervical cells** (Figs. 12-

8C,D, 12-9D, 12-10C,D). The size and configuration of the cancer cells is best assessed in cases wherein there is a clear-cut **transition of normal to cancerous epithelium within the same or adjacent glands** (Figs. 12-9D and 12-10D). In some of the glands, "bridges" of cancer cells criss-crossing the lumen may be observed (Fig. 12-9D), as is also the case in other ductal carcinomas such as the breast (see Chap. 29). The epithelium of some adenocarcinomas in situ contains **Paneth cells** with cytoplasmic granules, suggestive of intestinal differentiation. Although the malignant epithelium may be formed by a **single, fairly orderly layer of cuboidal or columnar cells,** similar to the normal endocervix, **in many areas the cancer cells form two or three layers and short papillary projections.** Nuclear crowding may be particularly evident at the tips of the papillae.

In the cancerous epithelium, the nuclei are enlarged, of irregular contour, hyperchromatic, and sometimes coarsely granular. In some cells, **readily visible nucleoli are present** but this is rarely the dominant feature of these cells. **Mitotic figures are often evident in the cancerous epithelium and are an important diagnostic feature because mitoses are rare in normal endocervical epithelium** (Fig. 12-8D). Biscotti and Hart (1998) pointed out that

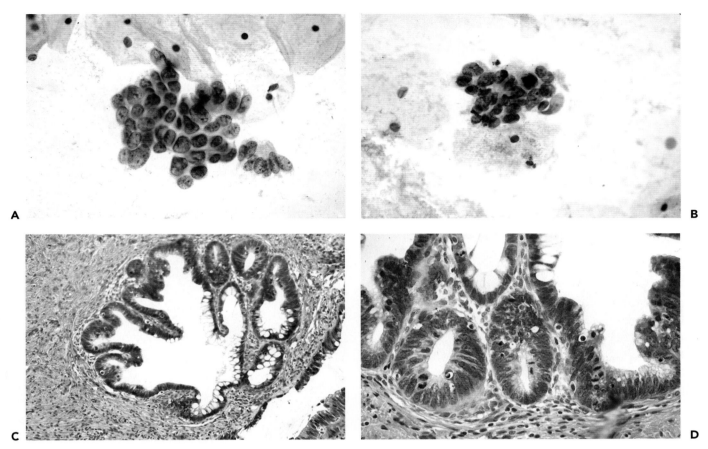

Figure 12-8 **Endocervical adenocarcinoma in situ.** *A.* A cluster of cancer cells showing some peripheral palisading. *B.* Cancer cells forming small rosettes. *C,D.* Corresponding tissue lesion showing in situ transformation of endocervical glands *(C)* and surface epithelium *(D).* Note numerous mitoses in *D.*

the presence of **apoptotic bodies** (i.e., nuclear necrosis with coarse fragmentation of chromatin; see Chap. 6), within the malignant epithelium, is characteristic of this disorder.

The configuration of carcinoma in situ is similar in nearly all cases, although Jaworski et al (1988) classified two cases as **"endometrioid carcinoma in situ,"** because of absence of mucus production in the lesions. **In a large proportion of cases, endocervical adenocarcinomas in situ are accompanied by preinvasive lesions of squamous type** (CIN) or even invasive squamous carcinoma (see below).

Natural History

There are few reports in the literature about progression of endocervical carcinoma in situ to invasive carcinoma. In the case reported by Büttner and Kyank (1973), 11 years elapsed before invasive carcinoma developed. Boddington et al (1976) reviewed prior cervical smears in 13 women who developed endocervical adenocarcinoma. In six of these patients, prior cytologic abnormalities were observed over a period of several years, leading to the conclusion that adenocarcinomas have an evolution extending over two to eight years. On retrospective review, Boon et al (1981) observed adenocarcinoma in situ that was not recognized in biopsies obtained three to seven years before the development of invasive adenocarcinoma. Lee and Flynn (2000)

estimated that the progression of adenocarcinoma in situ to invasive cancer requires approximately 5 years.

Personal observations also point to a long developmental period in the natural history of these lesions. This information is anecdotal, based generally on cases in which a cytologic diagnosis of adenocarcinoma was followed by **endocervical curettage in which evidence of adenocarcinoma was not recognized,** some years prior to the development of invasive tumor. The most **common source of biopsy error was the presence of strips of mucus-forming epithelium which, in spite of nuclear abnormalities, were thought to represent benign endocervical epithelium** (see Fig. 12-11). Because of the life-threatening nature of endocervical adenocarcinoma, no follow-up studies of untreated adenocarcinoma in situ have been conducted and none should be contemplated. However, in follow-up studies of several personally observed patients treated for adenocarcinoma in situ by conization, it was noted that these patients were prone to the development of other neoplastic events in the cervix in the form of recurrent adenocarcinoma or squamous precursor lesions (CIN).

Cytology

Adenocarcinoma in situ of the cervix has been recognized in the Bethesda System 2001 as a separate cytologic cate-

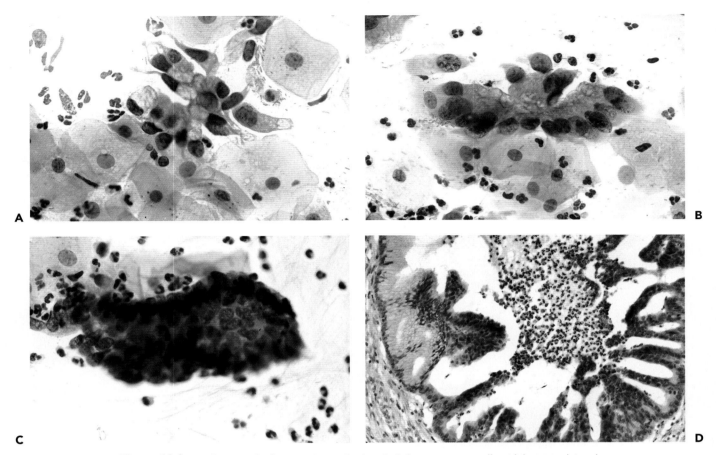

Figure 12-9 **Endocervical adenocarcinoma in situ.** *A.* Columnar cancer cells with large nuclei and nucleoli. *B.* A fragment composed of palisading endocervical cancer cells. *C.* A thick papillary cluster of cancer cells. *D.* The tissue lesion corresponding to *A–C*. Note sharp transition between normal and malignant epithelium.

gory. The cytologic presentation of this entity has been extensively discussed in the literature (Qizilbash, 1975; Betsill and Clark, 1986; Ayer et al, 1987, 1988; Lee et al, 1991, 1997; Keyhani-Rofagha et al, 1995; Biscotti et al, 1997; Cangiarella and Chhieng, 2003; Chhieng and Cangiarella, 2003). In some of the pertinent papers, the smear patterns of this lesion have been compared, on the one hand, with invasive adenocarcinoma and, on the other hand, with benign abnormalities of endocervical cells. The difficulties of cytologic diagnosis of adenocarcinoma in situ have been previously emphasized (Boon et al, 1981; Luesley et al, 1987; Di Tomasso et al, 1996; Lee et al, 1997). Renshaw et al (2004), in an elaborate study of performance of practicing pathologists, reported that the cytologic recognition of this entity was significantly lower than that of other important precancerous lesions or cancer. It is quite evident that there is no unanimity on the reproducible features of this lesion and, therefore, this description is based mainly on personal experience.

The cytologic presentation of an endocervical adenocarcinoma in situ is that of a well-differentiated invasive endocervical adenocarcinoma with several added features:

■ **The background of the cytologic preparation is usually free of necrosis and cell debris, although a few** leukocytes and blood may be present. In our experience, this feature is valuable in separating an adenocarcinoma in situ from invasive cancer (see Figs. 12-8A,B and 12-10A).

■ **In some cases, fairly slender, dispersed columnar cells with nuclear enlargement and moderate hyperchromasia may be observed** (see Figs. 12-8A, 12-9A, 12-10A). Such cells are less common in invasive adenocarcinoma.

■ **The nuclear abnormalities observed in the columnar or cuboidal malignant cells vary and are sometimes less marked than in invasive cancer:** although the nuclei are enlarged and hyperchromatic, they do not always display coarse granulation of chromatin. **Large, prominent nucleoli are uncommon** (see Figs. 12-8A,B and 12-9A).

■ **Compact, spherical clusters of malignant cells and fragments of abnormal endocervical glands** are fairly frequent (see Figs. 12-9C and 12-10B).

■ **Cell palisading and "rosette" formation are fairly common** (see Figs. 12-8B and 12-9B). **These features occur more often in adenocarcinoma in situ than in invasive cancer.**

■ **Signet ring cells and "naked" enlarged and hyperchromatic nuclei are rare.** We have not observed the "**apoptotic bodies**" reported in tissue sections.

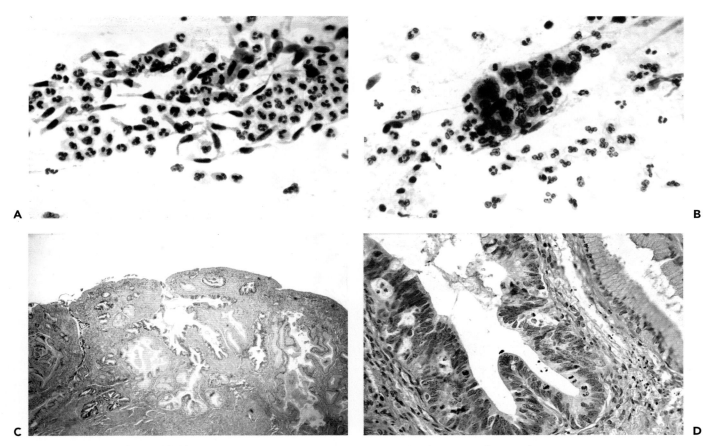

Figure 12-10 **Endocervical adenocarcinoma in situ.** *A.* The dominant cells are columnar cancer cells with somewhat enlarged hyperchromatic nuclei. *B.* A small papillary cluster of endocervical cancer cells. *C,D.* Tissue sections corresponding to *A* and *B* and showing the contrast between normal and cancerous endocervical glands.

■ Changes observed in brush specimens are rarely of value in separating adenocarcinoma in situ from invasive cancer. Large, complex clusters of endocervical cells and "feathering" are observed in both types of lesions, but also as a brushing artifact with benign endocervical cells (see Fig. 12-7).

■ Occasionally, ciliated abnormal cells may be present. Although such cells occur mainly in tubal metaplasia, discussed in Chapter 10, their presence does not necessarily indicate a benign lesion if the nuclear features of such cells suggests a malignant transformation. Endocervical adenocarcinomas with ciliated cells have been described (Schlesinger and Silverberg, 1999).

A number of observers (Bousfield et al, 1980; Betsill and Clark, 1986; Ayer et al, 1987; Pacey et al, 1988; Laverty et al, 1988; Di Tomasso et al, 1996) attempted to classify endocervical adenocarcinomas in situ into well-differentiated and poorly differentiated types, based on the level of nuclear abnormality. In our experience, this subclassification is not reproducible and is not of clinical significance since it does not lead to different prognostic or therapeutic conclusions. **In general, the cytologic diagnosis of an adenocarcinoma is usually fairly easy, but the determination whether the lesion is still in situ or invasive is much more difficult.** The custom in our departments is to em-

phasize that **the lesion is "possibly" or "probably" a carcinoma in situ.** Bai et al (2000) claimed that the yield of glandular lesions of the endocervix was increased using the ThinPrep technique but this issue is contentious (Cangiarella and Chhieng, 2003).

Endocervical Gland Atypia or Dysplasia

Based on experience with squamous lesions of the uterine cervix, it has been postulated that endocervical adenocarcinoma in situ is preceded by lesser degrees of abnormality that may, perhaps, be recognized in cytologic and histologic samples of the uterine cervix.

The term **endocervical dysplasia** was introduced by Alva and Lauchlan (1975), who described slight histologic abnormalities of endocervical epithelium that may have preceded an adenocarcinoma in situ. Bousfield et al (1980) used this term to describe cytologic findings not supported by histologic observations although, in two of the three such cases, the initial cytologic diagnosis was adenocarcinoma, not confirmed on biopsy. Brown and Wells (1986), in a review of histology, proposed the term **possibly pre-malignant cervical glandular atypia,** describing changes in endocervical glands accompanying high grade squamous lesions, as shown in Figure 12-3. Wakefield and Wells (1985)

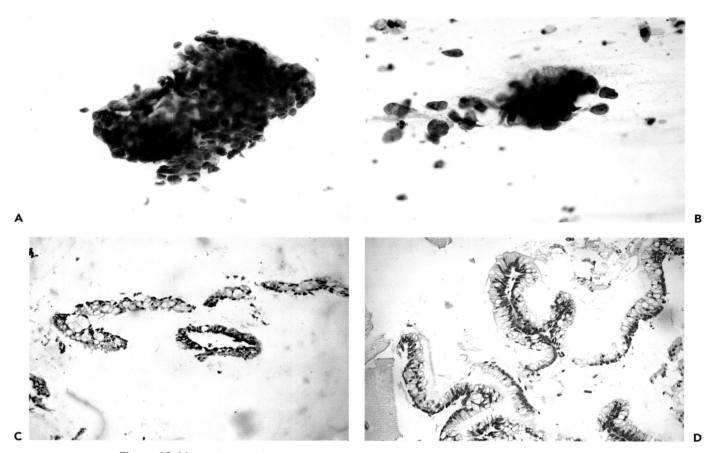

Figure 12-11   Endocervical adenocarcinoma missed on biopsy. *A,B.* Clusters of cancer cells diagnosed as adenocarcinoma. *C.* A biopsy fragment interpreted as normal endocervical gland. *D.* A subsequent biopsy, obtained 1 year later, showing fragments of well-differentiated endocervical adenocarcinoma.

observed, in such glands, **changes in the composition of endocervical mucus** with increase in sialomucins, similar to those observed in colonic adenocarcinoma. The change can be demonstrated by staining the cells with Alcian blue (pH 2.5) which is negative with normal mucins but positive in the presence of sialomucins. Lee et al (2000) attempted to identify the "dysplastic" lesions with HPV testing and proliferation index with debatable results. In a recent review, Young (2002) qualified these abnormalities as "nebulous" and this writer agrees.

Relatively minor abnormalities of cells lining the endocervical glands may be observed, usually at the **periphery of adenocarcinoma in situ,** or sometimes in **glands adjacent to high grade squamous lesions** (see Fig. 11-35D). **Slight nuclear enlargement and hyperchromasia, sometimes accompanied by irregularly shaped or angular nuclei,** are a common feature of such glands. **Mitoses** may be occasionally observed. Such changes in endocervical cells are **not specific** as they may also occur in a variety of benign events (described in Chap. 10).

Ioffe et al (2003) proposed three criteria to separate "glandular dysplasia" from either benign or clearly malignant noninvasive glandular lesions. These were: nuclear atypia, stratification of cells and the sum of mitosing and apoptotic cells in selected glands. By scoring these three

parameters on a scale from 1 to 3 and adding the results, it was proposed that values 0 to 3 represented a benign lesion, scores 4 to 5 glandular dysplasia, and scores 6 to 9 an adenocarcinoma in situ. The **scoring system** was tested by the authors who reported a good agreement among observers. The value of this proposal must be independently tested.

Because most of these lesions are excised by biopsy, there are no follow-up studies known to us that could clarify the prospective significance of such lesions which we prefer to classify as **"nonspecific atypias of endocervical epithelium"** or glands. Occasionally, such changes are observed **in incidental biopsies of the endocervix** and may sometimes cause diagnostic problems, requiring additional biopsies to determine whether or not the lesion is malignant or, perhaps, adjacent to an adenocarcinoma or even a high grade squamous lesion. In **some of these patients, a squamous lesion or an endocervical adenocarcinoma is ultimately recognized.** The term **dysplasia,** applied to these changes, is not helpful because it does not provide therapeutic guidelines to the clinician. The reproducibility of these diagnoses is doubtful. Lee and Crum et al (2000), using proliferative index and HPV testing, concluded that most of these minor atypias are not precursors of carcinoma.

The 1988 Bethesda System initially recognized the difficulty to classify abnormalities of endocervical cells as **atypical glandular cells of unknown significance (AGUS).** The term has been abolished in the 2001 Bethesda System because of a very large proportion of neoplastic lesions of the uterine cervix that were recognized on colposcopy and biopsies of the cervix (Jackson et al, 1996; Korn et al, 1998; Chhieng et al, 2000; Reuss et al, 2001; Meath et al, 2002; Hammoud et al, 2002). As discussed in Chapter 11, perhaps the most surprising outcome of the AGUS smears was **the high frequency of high-grade squamous intraepithelial lesions (HGSIL) discovered in these women, whereas adenocarcinomas were relatively uncommon,** constituting less than 10% of the lesions found in biopsies of the cervix. An effort to subdivide AGUS into "favor reactive" or "favor neoplastic" was of limited value (Siziopikou et al, 1997; Moriarty and Wilbur, 2003; Cangiarella and Chhieng, 2003). Raab et al (1998) noted that the reproducibility of the AGUS category of diagnoses was very poor among experienced cytopathologists. This was amply confirmed on a more recent study by Simsir et al (2003). As emphasized in Chapter 11, **high grade squamous lesions, located in the endocervical canal, often shed columnar cancer cells, similar to those seen in endocervical carcinomas.**

Cytology

In my experience, there are no specific cell features that would reproducibly identify the atypical endocervical glands, as predictive of an adenocarcinoma. However, it appears appropriate to describe here the nonspecific changes that may be observed in cytologic material.

Atypia of Endocervical Cells

Such abnormalities may be observed in scrape smears and in endocervical brush specimens. The minimal abnormalities in the endocervical cells of potential diagnostic significance are **nuclear enlargement and hyperchomasia of various degrees in otherwise well-formed, but often enlarged columnar endocervical cells,** occurring either singly or in small cohesive clusters (Fig. 12-12A–C). **Coarse granulation of chromatin and irregular nuclear contour are occasionally observed, but nucleoli are absent or small.** Some of these clusters may show parallel arrangement or **palisading** of endocervical cells, when derived from the surface epithelium (Fig. 12-12C). Such cells were described in Chapter 11 as karyomegaly or dyskaryosis (dysplasia) of endocervical cells but may also occur in cervicitis with negative follow-up (Fig. 12-12D). It is presumed that karyomegaly of endocervical cells corresponds to the term of **"endocervical-columnar cell dysplasia"** (Bousfield et al, 1980) or **"endocervical columnar cell intraepithelial neoplasia of mild or moderate grade,"** a term coined by van Aspert-van Erp et al (1995).

Some of these abnormalities may be classified as **atypical endocervical cells,** discussed in Chapter 11 and above. Their **diagnostic significance is not always clear, because such cell changes represent a common denominator of a broad spectrum of lesions, some of which are benign and some malignant** (Selvaggi and Haefner, 1997). However, the malignant lesions can be **an adenocarcinoma, a**

squamous precursor lesion of endocervical derivation, or both. In an occasional biopsy, it is possible to trace the origin of such cells to **atypical epithelium in endocervical glands,** usually adjacent to the transformation zone and commonly observed in high grade squamous epithelial lesions (see Fig. 12-12D and Chap. 10).

Among the benign lesions, it must be noted that **similar and usually transient abnormalities of endocervical cells may occur:**

- In "repair," or in florid metaplasia of the endocervical epithelium (see Chap. 10)
- In single endocervical cells for a variety of reasons, such as tubal metaplasia or inflammation
- During normal pregnancy
- In women wearing intrauterine contraceptive devices **(IUDs)** (see Chap. 10)
- In women receiving contraceptive medication with a high progesterone content (see Chap. 10)

The finding of endocervical cell dyskaryosis, not otherwise accompanied by more conspicuous cell changes, is relatively uncommon, but it is **deserving of a most careful clinical examination, combined with colposcopy, endocervical biopsies or curettage** to rule out incipient carcinoma.

Attempts to Separate Preneoplastic From Nonneoplastic Abnormalities of Endocervical Cells

Because of **limits of morphology** in predicting the future behavior of endocervical cell atypias, several attempts have been proposed to identify women at risk. The chief approach was based on HPV testing, discussed at some length in Chapter 11. Perhaps the most important study cited was the **ALTS study** (Solomon et al, 2001) which documented a **very high negative predictive value** of HPV testing, i.e., extremely low probability that women testing negative for HPV will develop a neoplastic lesion of the cervix. The study failed to demonstrate that the presence of HPV did necessarily lead to neoplastic events. On the other hand, Ronnett et al (1999) reported that testing for high risk HPV types in women with the diagnosis of AGUS **accurately identified the carriers of HGSIL and endocervical adenocarcinoma.** Riethdorf et al (2002) and Negri et al (2003) used the **cyclin-dependent kinase inhibitor (a tumor suppressor gene)** p16^{INK4A} as a marker for HPV-encoded transcription of E6 and E7 open reading frames. The stain was negative or weakly positive in a number of benign controls and strongly positive in adenocarcinoma in situ. A number of caveats about the specificity of the reaction and its applicability to cytologic samples robbed this observation of practical value. Still, Negri et al (2003) reported **strong expression of this gene in neoplastic endocervical cells** in liquid samples.

Several authors used the **antibody MIB 1** directed against the **proliferation antigen Ki-67,** a marker for mitotically active cells, to separate benign changes from endocervical neoplasia (McCluggage et al, 1995; Cina et al, 1997; Lee et al, 2000; Pirog et al, 2001). The results were equivocal. Lesions with fewer than 10% nuclei staining were usu-

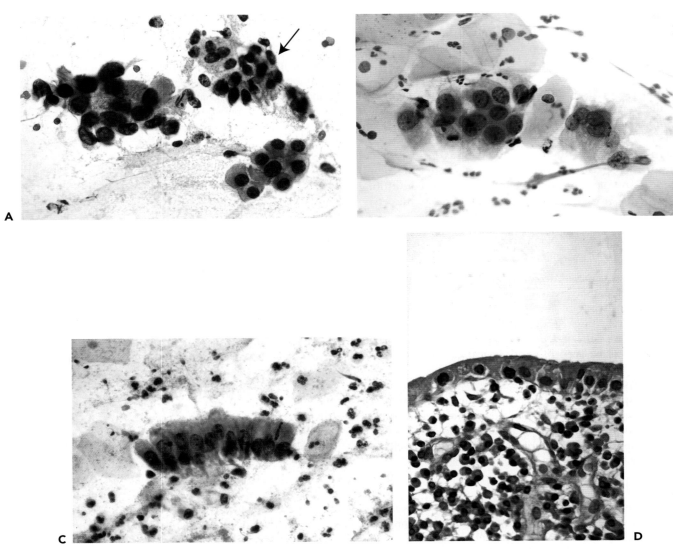

Figure 12-12   Examples of atypical endocervical cells, some of which may be the precursor lesions of endocervical adenocarcinoma. *A.* Two clusters of endocervical cells with enlarged hyperchromatic nuclei compared with normal endocervical cells in the same field (*arrow*). The follow-up of this patient was negative. *B.* A cluster of endocervical cells with markedly enlarged, somewhat hyperchromatic nuclei. The follow-up on this patient was negative. *C.* A cluster of palisading endocervical cells with slight nuclear enlargement. The follow-up on this patient was negative. *D.* Biopsy of endocervix corresponding to *C* shows surface epithelium with enlarged dark nuclei. There was no evidence of carcinoma in this case.

ally benign and lesions with over 50% of positive nuclei were usually malignant. HPV testing of the lesions with over 10% positive nuclei allowed additional triage of the lesions. The method appears to be effective on both low and high ends of the spectrum but is insecure in cases of microglandular hyperplasia, tubal metaplasia, and in patients with recent biopsies (Lin et al, 2000; Pirog et al, 2001).

Biscotti and Hart (1998) and Moritani et al (2002) observed that **mitotic index** and the presence of **cells showing apoptosis** were characteristic of malignant glandular lesions and were helpful in separating them from a broad spectrum of benign disorders. Unfortunately, mitoses and apoptosis may not be evident in the cytologic samples and are, therefore, of limited practical value.

SYNCHRONOUS ADENOCARCINOMA AND SQUAMOUS CARCINOMA

Synchronous association of squamous (epidermoid) and adenocarcinoma is a common event that occurs in about half of the glandular lesions (Ayer et al, 1987). **Both lesions may be in situ, one of them may be in situ and the other invasive, or both of them may be invasive.** Each tumor appears to be leading an independent existence and maintains its behavior pattern, with the adenocarcinoma apparently capable of earlier distant metastases than epidermoid carcinoma. As has been mentioned in the introductory remarks to this chapter, the two types of lesions may have a common denominator in the form of human papillomavirus infection, mainly types 16 and 18.

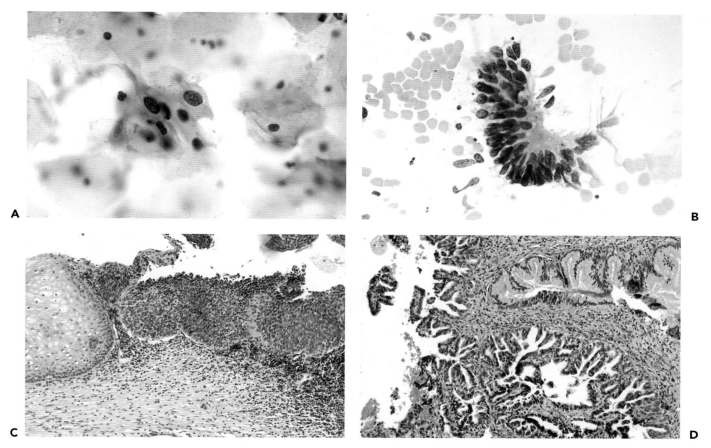

Figure 12-13 **Coexisting squamous and adenocarcinoma.** *A.* A cluster of dysplastic squamous cells. *B.* Endocervical cancer cells arranged in a form of a palisade. *C.* The HGSIL coexisting with endocervical adenocarcinoma shown in *D.* Both lesions were focally invasive.

Cytology

The coexisting adenocarcinomas and squamous carcinomas may shed cells of both tumor types side by side. In many instances, however, **the squamous malignant cells conceal or precede the presence of adenocarcinoma.** In several personally observed cases, **the disease began as a dyskaryosis (dysplasia) of superficial squamous cells,** followed without treatment, and culminated in the development of squamous and adenocarcinoma several years later (Fig. 12-13). In many instances, the adenocarcinoma will be a surprise diagnosis in biopsies (Fig. 12-14).

BEHAVIOR AND PROGNOSIS OF THE COMMON TYPES OF ENDOCERVICAL ADENOCARCINOMA

Adenocarcinomas originating within the endocervical canal **may remain clinically occult for long periods of time, unless detected by a cytologic sample or an incidental biopsy.** Fully developed invasive adenocarcinomas are sometimes bulky and may produce clinical symptoms of spotting, bleeding, or discharge. The tumors rarely occur before the age of 30, but otherwise can occur at any age, most often between the ages of 50 to 60. The **prognosis**

of endocervical adenocarcinoma is **stage dependent** (Berek et al, 1984; Kilgore et al, 1988). For staging of cervical carcinomas, see Table 11-3.

For stage 0 tumors (carcinoma in situ and microinvasive carcinomas), the survival after surgical treatment is close to 100%. **Cure of endocervical adenocarcinoma in situ** can be achieved with cold knife conization procedure or a large electron loop excision (LLETZ procedure) but, in many instances, this treatment will be followed by a hysterectomy (Betrand et al, 1987). Hopkins et al (1988) suggested that all these patients should be treated by hysterectomy and lymph node evaluation. Personal experience suggests that women treated conservatively for early stage disease are prone to develop new neoplastic lesions of the cervix with the passage of time and, therefore, should be carefully followed.

For higher stage lesions, the 5-year survival depends on tumor size, grade of differentiation, and depth of invasions (Berek et al, 1984; Kilgore et al, 1988). For high-stage, high-grade lesions, particularly those with spread beyond the uterine cervix, the survival is low. The behavior of the advanced adenocarcinomas is often much more aggressive than that of epidermoid carcinoma of similar stage, and distant metastases may be observed at the time of the initial clinical diagnosis (Saigo et al, 1986; Weiss and Lucas, 1986; Kilgore et al, 1988; Drescher et al, 1989). On the other

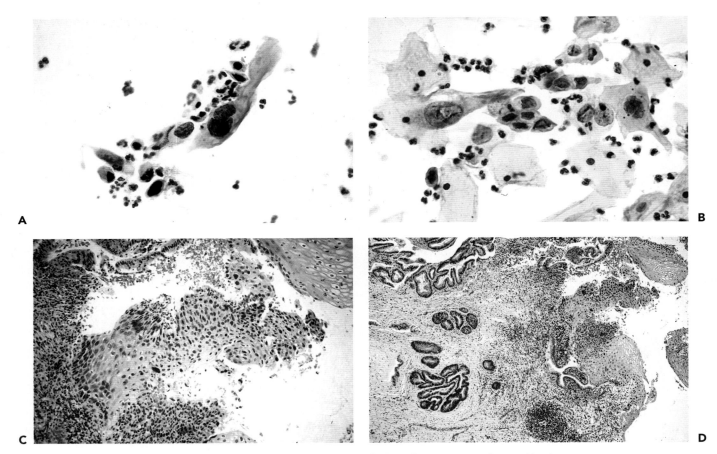

Figure 12-14   An example of adenocarcinoma which, in the smear, was obscured by the pattern of a high grade squamous lesion. *A,B.* Cancer cells of squamous type. *C.* Fragment of HGSIL. *D.* Underlying endocervical adenocarcinoma.

hand, Grigsby et al (1988) reported equal survival for both tumor types in their series of cases.

LESS COMMON TYPES OF ENDOCERVICAL ADENOCARCINOMA

Adenosquamous Carcinoma

These uncommon tumors combine the elements of adenocarcinoma and squamous carcinoma with varying degrees of differentiation (Fig. 12-15A,B). We have seen patients in whom the two patterns were individually represented in separate metastatic foci (Fig. 12-15C,D). The prognosis of these tumors is apparently less favorable than that of classical types of well-differentiated carcinomas (Fu et al, 1982; Gallup et al, 1985).

The cytology of these tumors is identical to that of coexisting adenocarcinoma and squamous carcinoma, described above and shown in Figures 12-13 and 12-14. Either squamous to adenocarcinoma patterns, or a combination of both, may be found in cytologic samples.

Papillary Villoglandular Carcinomas

This relatively uncommon form of endocervical adenocarcinoma has been recognized mainly in women under 40 years

of age (Young and Scully, 1989; Jones et al, 1993). Similar tumors may have been reported as **"villous adenoma"** of the cervix with an invasive component (Alvaro and Nogales, 1988). Clinically, the tumors may mimic a **friable endocervical polyp.** This tumor type, even when deeply invasive, appears to have a very favorable prognosis: as of 1993, no metastases have been reported (Jones et al, 1993). The association of this tumor type with a high grade squamous epithelial lesion (carcinoma in situ) has been reported by Young and Scully (1989).

Histology

On the **surface, the tumor forms delicate, slender, sometimes branching, papillary projections,** lined either by a single or stratified layers of cuboidal or columnar cancer cells, surrounding a connective tissue core often showing a marked inflammatory infiltrate (Fig. 12-16 A,B). The epithelial lining may contain mucin-producing cells or even goblet cells. The infiltrating portions of the tumors show well-formed, branching glands. The level of cytologic abnormality in the epithelial lining is modest with only slight nuclear enlargement and very rare mitoses.

Cytology

The key cytologic feature of these uncommon tumors is the presence of **numerous, tightly cohesive multilayered**

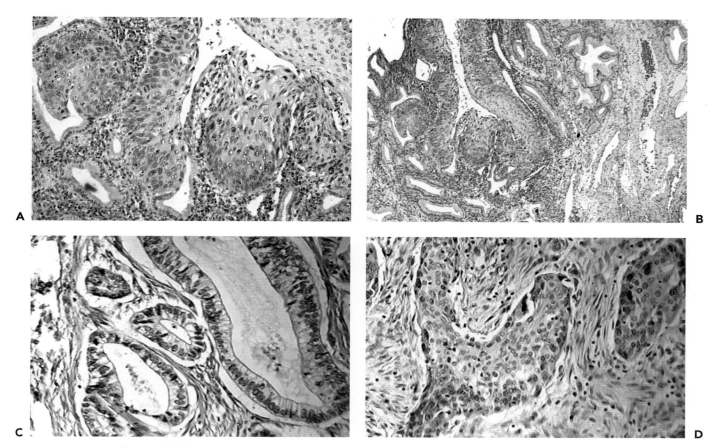

Figure 12-15 *A,B.* **Example of adenosquamous carcinoma combining the elements of squamous and adenocarcinomas.** *C,D.* Pelvic node metastases from an adenosquamous carcinoma of the cervix, showing two distinct patterns. In *C*, the tumor was a clear cut adenocarcinoma. In *D*, the tumor was a squamous cancer.

clusters of endocervical cells. The clusters are either **spherical,** with flattened cells at the periphery, corresponding to papillae of the tumor, or **irregularly shaped,** lined by columnar cells. The **nuclei** within the clusters are **somewhat enlarged** and **hyperchromatic** but these features can only be recognized by comparison with normal endocervical cells which are absent in these preparations (Fig. 12-16C,D). **Except for their large number and irregular configuration, the cell clusters may be readily mistaken for clusters of normal endocervical cells** obtained by brushing. Single cancer cells or rosettes have been reported as a rare event by Ballo et al (1996). The same authors reported that only 1 of 11 smears was initially diagnosed as endocervical adenocarcinoma; other diagnoses rendered comprised a wide spectrum of benign and malignant lesions. On review, however, 9 of 11 smears contained the features of papillary villoglandular lesions. The difficulties with the recognition of this tumor were confirmed in reports by Novotny and Ferlisi (1997) and Chang et al (1999).

Serous Adenocarcinoma

These are very uncommon high grade tumors of the endocervix, mimicking the serous carcinoma of the ovary and similar tumors of the endometrium, and composed of cuboidal malignant cells with high nucleocytoplasmic ratio and marked nuclear abnormalities (Zhou et al, 1998) (also see Chaps. 13 and 17). We have not observed such tumors in our cytologic material and, to our knowledge, only one such case has been briefly reported (Nguyen, 1997).

Minimal Deviation Carcinomas (Adenoma Malignum)

Histology

Adenoma malignum is a rare form of endocervical adenocarcinoma, characterized by a **proliferation of very well differentiated, mucus-producing endocervical glands, closely resembling normal glands.** In their fully developed form, these tumors show an invasion of the cervical stroma by mucus-producing glands that vary in size yet show few, if any, cellular or nuclear abnormalities in gland lining (Fig. 12-17C,D). Mitotic activity is very low. The presence of **Paneth cells and cells with endocrine granules** has been reported in the lining of the endocervical glands (Fetissof et al, 1985). At the time of diagnosis, the entire thickness of the cervix is usually invaded by tumor so that the malignant nature of the lesion is beyond doubt. McKelvey and Goodlin, who first de-

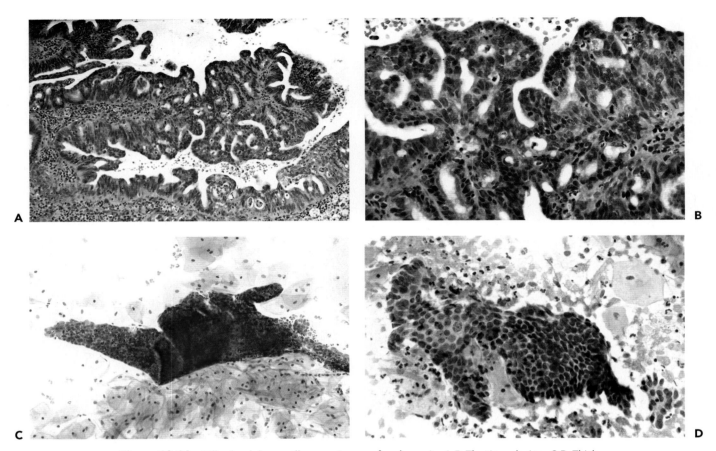

Figure 12-16 Villoglandular papillary carcinoma of endocervix. *A,B.* The tissue lesion. *C,D.* Thick cohesive clusters of endocervical cells which, at higher magnification, failed to show any nuclear abnormalities. (*C,D:* Courtesy Dr. Mary Sidawy, George Washington University, Washington, DC.)

fined the lesion in 1963, pointed out the **exceptional diagnostic difficulties in identifying the lesion in cervical biopsies** because of the unwillingness of the pathologists to entertain the diagnosis of cancer on debatable evidence. Thus, **many of these tumors remain undiagnosed in the early stages until there is obvious clinical evidence of cancer,** sometimes with metastases. In 1969, Kese reported the association of this unusual tumor with **Peutz-Jeghers syndrome,** the latter consisting of skin pigmentation and hematomatous polyps in the gastrointestinal tract. Gallager et al (1971), Gloor et al (1978), McGowan et al (1980), and Kaku et al (1985) also reported such cases. Another association of adenoma malignum is with **ovarian tumors of sex cord type** with annular tubules (Young et al, 1982). Only some of the adenoma malignum-type lesions show these associations, but it is advisable to keep these complications in mind at the time of diagnosis. Gilks et al (1989) failed to identify any immuno-histologic features of diagnostic value in these rare tumors with poor prognosis.

Cytology

The cells desquamating from adenoma malignum closely **resemble benign endocervical cells in shape and manner of exfoliation in clusters.** However, in our experience, **the cells and their nuclei are somewhat larger than normal and the clusters tend to be multilayered and crowded.**

The clusters rarely allow a diagnosis, but the background of the smears often contains **detached, single tumor cells that are more spherical and have large but pale nuclei, provided with large, spherical or sometimes irregularly-shaped nucleoli** (Fig. 12-17A,B). Essentially similar findings were reported by Szyfelbein et al (1984) in three patients, two with Peutz-Jeghers syndrome.

The accurate cytologic diagnosis of this type of tumor is very difficult, matching the difficulty of the histologic diagnosis. As is often the case with cells derived from endocervical neoplasia, the differential diagnosis includes cells seen in acute endocervicitis, florid squamous metaplasia or repair, and cells from other forms of endocervical adenocarcinoma. Granter and Lee (1996) reviewed the cytologic findings in seven patients. In only one case did the cervical smear lead to biopsy diagnosis. On review, cells similar to reactive endocervical cells were observed in five patients. The cytologic suspicion of disease must be confirmed by histologic evidence, which, as stated above, may be deceptive and difficult to interpret.

Mesonephric Carcinomas (Carcinomas Derived From Gartner's Duct)

Histology

These very rare cancers originate in the remnants of the wolffian ducts that are found in the ovaries, the tubes, the

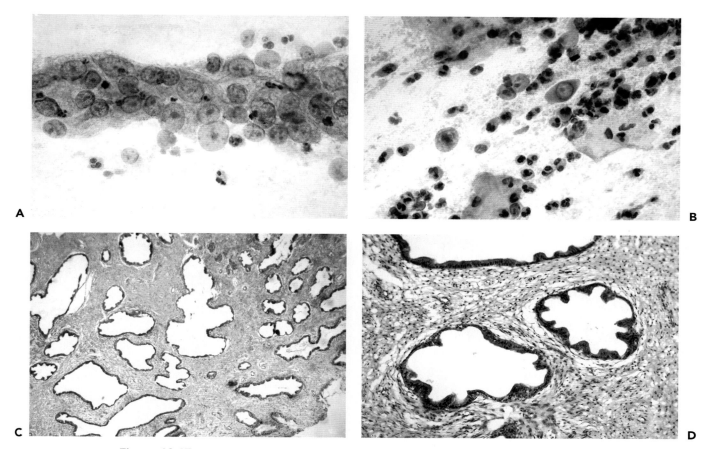

Figure 12-17 Adenoma malignum (minimal deviation adenocarcinoma). *A.* A large cluster of endocervical cells with large nuclei and visible nucleoli. *B.* A scattering of single cells with similar features. *C.* The invasive pattern of the lesion. *D.* The make-up of glands which closely resemble normal endocervical glands.

stroma of the cervix, and vagina. They are characterized by proliferation of glandular structures of varying sizes, sometimes with small papillary projections. The component cells of these tumors are often large, with clear cytoplasm, and protrude from the gland lining in "hobnail" fashion.

These tumors have many similarities with vaginal and cervical carcinomas associated with diethylstilbestrol (DES) (discussed in Chap. 14). Gartner duct tumors are usually observed in adult women but occur also in adolescents. Because of their protected location within the stroma of the cervix, the diagnosis is often delayed until the tumor breaks into the lumen of the endocervical canal, although the prognosis appears to be somewhat better than that of endocervical adenocarcinoma. Several subtypes of these very rare tumors have been identified but this classification is irrelevant to this text (Ferry and Scully, 1990; Clement et al, 1995; Silver et al, 2001).

Cytology

Because these tumors originate in the body of the cervix, they are not accessible to cytologic sampling until they reach the surface of the endocervical canal. We have observed one such case in a 14-year-old girl many years ago. The cytologic presentation was that of an adenocarcinoma (Fig. 12-18A). Welsh et al (2003) observed abnormal endocervical cells in

several patients with **remnants** or **hyperplasia of mesonephric ducts.**

However, there is some evidence that Gartner duct carcinoma may also have a long silent history prior to clinical manifestation of disease. This is illustrated in Fig. 12-18B–D. The original smear, obtained 4 years before the second, was interpreted as showing changes consistent with acute cervicitis or "repair" (Fig. 12-18B). The changes in the second smear (Fig. 12-18C), this time accompanied by spotting, were considered sufficient to warrant a biopsy, which revealed a Gartner duct carcinoma still confined to the lateral wall of the grossly normal cervix but involving the endocervical canal (Fig. 12-18D).

Mucoepidermoid Carcinomas

These very rare tumors mimic the well differentiated variant of mucoepidermoid tumors of the salivary glands and are, therefore, discussed separately from adenosquamous carcinomas (see above).

Histology

Occasional tumors of the cervix **composed of solid cords of eosinophilic epidermoid cells contain isolated, large, mucus-producing cells** (Fig. 12-19C,D). Sometimes, well formed glands, lined by a mixture of squamous and mucus-

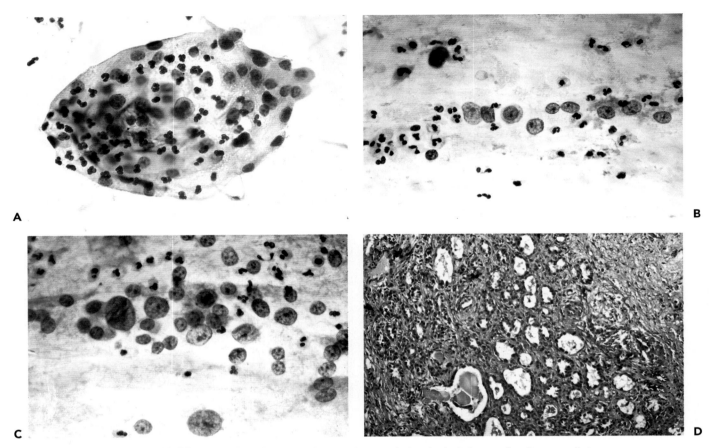

Figure 12-18 **Examples of Gartner duct carcinoma.** *A.* A spherical cluster of malignant cells in a smear from a 14-year-old girl. *B,C.* Cytologic patterns of Gartner duct carcinoma from another patient, initially misinterpreted as "endocervicitis" or repair. *D.* Gartner duct carcinoma diagnosed by biopsy 4 years after the smears shown in *B* and *C* were obtained.

producing cells, may be observed within such tumors. Hamperl and Hellweg (1957) pointed out that some mucus formation may be demonstrated in most epidermoid cancers of the cervix; however, the presence of single, large cells with mucus-distended cytoplasm is typical of mucoepidermoid carcinoma.

Cytology

There is no recorded experience pertaining to the cytologic presentation of these tumors. In a personally observed case courtesy of Dr. David Clark, the dominant abnormalities in the cervical smears were large, well-formed atypical endocervical cells with prominent nucleoli, more consistent with reactive atypia than an endocervical adenocarcinoma (Fig. 12-19A). Atypical squamous cells, singly or in small clusters, were also present (Fig. 12-19B). This evidence was insufficient for diagnosis of carcinoma but led to a diagnostic cervical biopsy (Fig. 12-19C,D).

Glassy-Cell Carcinomas

Histology

In 1956, Glucksmann and Cherry described a **radiotherapy-resistant variant of mucoepidermoid carcinoma** of the uterine cervix, composed of **sheets of large cancer cells with "ground-glass" appearance of the cytoplasm and**

infrequent droplets of mucicarmine positive material (Fig. 12-20C,D). **The tumors also may form squamous "pearls." The presence of large nuclei with particularly large nucleoli was noted.** Littman et al, in 1976, revived the term "glassy cell carcinoma" and generally confirmed the descriptions by Glucksmann and Cherry.

Although these tumors are uncommon and poorly defined, they nonetheless elicited a large number of publications, particularly in the 1980s, that is disproportionate to the frequency and clinical significance of this lesion. There are a few such cases reported in the American literature (Maier and Norris, 1982; Pak et al, 1983; Tamimi et al, 1988). The tumors, even in stage IB, have a poor prognosis, with only about 50% of patients having 5-year survival (Lotocki et al, 1992).

Cytology

It is a matter for considerable debate whether the glassy cell carcinoma is deserving of a separate classification or whether it is a minor and rare variant of poorly differentiated squamous carcinoma of endocervical origin. Nonetheless, glassy cell carcinomas shed large **cancer cells with faintly granular, delicately vacuolated cytoplasm and large vesicular nuclei with remarkably large, irregular eosinophilic nucleoli** (Fig. 12-20A,B). In Papanicolaou stain, **the large, usually single nucleoli stand out as large, pink intranu-**

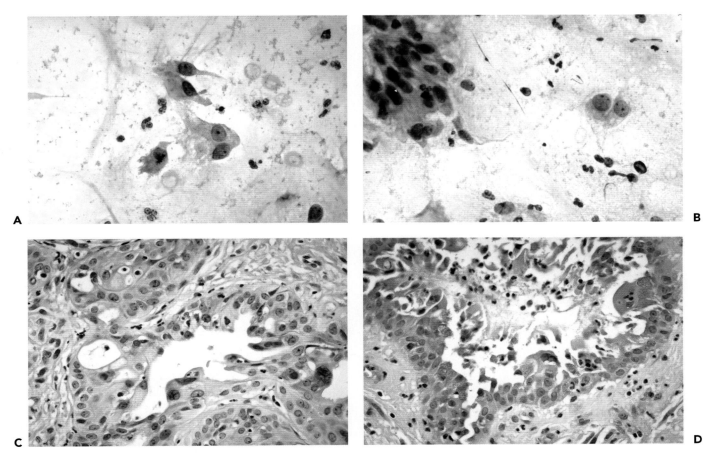

Figure 12-19   Mucoepidermoid carcinoma of endocervix. *A.* Scattered endocervical cells with minimally enlarged nuclei. *B.* A small cluster of endocervical cells with minimally enlarged nuclei. *C,D.* Histologic pattern of the lesion which was, in every way, similar to lesions of salivary glands. (*D:* Mucicarmine stain.)

clear bodies and may be mistaken for inclusions of herpesvirus or Reed-Sternberg cells in Hodgkin's disease (see Chaps. 10 and 31).

Pak et al (1983) reported a substantial number of false-negative smears in patients with glassy cell carcinoma wherein cancer cells with the characteristic nucleolar enlargement were found on review in 4 of 12 samples. Nunez et al (1985) and Chung et al (2000) also confirmed the presence of unusually large nucleoli as a characteristic feature of glassy cell carcinoma.

Very Rare Tumors

Clear-cell carcinomas are usually associated with vaginal adenosis and clear cell carcinoma of the vagina (discussed in Chap. 14).

Adenoid cystic carcinoma, adenoid basal carcinoma (epithelioma), lymphoepithelioma and other unusual tumors of the uterine cervix are discussed in Chapter 17.

DIFFERENTIAL DIAGNOSIS. ENDOCERVICAL ADENOCARCINOMA VERSUS OTHER TUMOR TYPES

■ In the presence of clusters of small malignant cells, without distinguishing features, similar to those oc-

curring in high grade squamous lesions of endocervical origin, it is not possible to separate an adenocarcinoma from a squamous cancer of endocervical origin on cytologic preparations. Still, it is advisable to suggest that the tumor, whatever its type, is likely to be located in the endocervical canal.

■ **Poorly differentiated squamous (epidermoid) high grade precursor lesions originating in the endocervical canal, may sometimes be represented in smears by large, columnar cancer cells** (see Figs. 11-35 and 11-53).

■ It may be difficult to separate an **endocervical from endometrial adenocarcinoma, though the latter is usually composed of smaller cancer cells** (see Chap. 13). Several histochemical approaches have been tried. Thus, Cohen et al (1982) proposed that **carcinoembryonic antigen (CEA) and mucin** are expressed in endocervical adenocarcinoma but not in endometrial carcinoma. A subsequent study by Cooper et al (1987) failed to confirm these findings. The issue was revived recently, again with insecure results (McCluggage et al, 2001; Kamoi et al, 2002). It is evident that, in such cases, careful clinical history and adequate histologic sampling cannot be replaced by other laboratory methods.

■ **Metastatic adenocarcinoma, particularly of colonic or-**

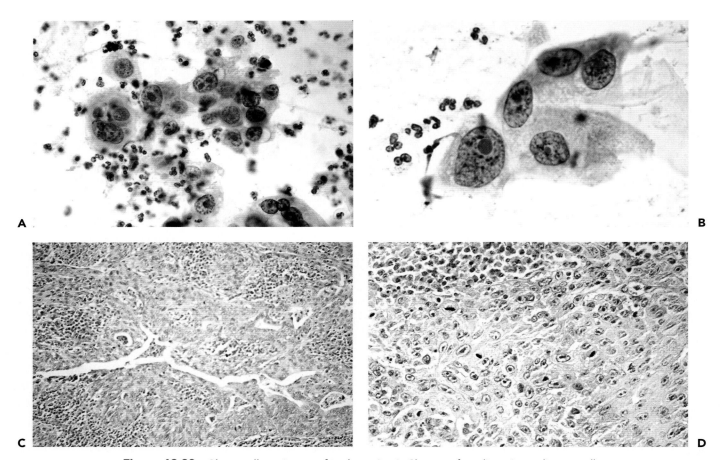

Figure 12-20 **Glassy cell carcinoma of endocervix.** *A.* Clusters of medium-size malignant cells with exceptionally large nucleoli. *B.* A high-power view of these cells, again to demonstrate the exceptionally large size of nucleoli. *C.* Infiltrating glassy cell carcinoma showing focal glandular differentiation. *D.* Higher power view of the tumor, again to document the large size of the nucleoli.

igin, that shed large columnar cancer cells may mimic endocervical adenocarcinoma (see Chap. 17).

■ It has been reported that **abnormal cells observed in tubal and tubo-endometrioid metaplasia, and particularly in endometriosis, may mimic cells of adenocarcinoma** (see recent review by Cangiarella and Chhieng, 2003). This issue has been discussed at length in Chapters 10 and 11. It is my judgment that, **in most such cases, the abnormal cells reflect a significant abnormality of premalignant or malignant nature that may be observed in the upper reaches of the endocervical canal.**

■ The main points of differential diagnosis of adenocarcinoma of the cervix are shown in Tables 12-1 and 12-2.

ACCURACY OF CYTOLOGIC DIAGNOSIS OF ENDOCERVICAL ADENOCARCINOMA

The diagnosis of adenocarcinoma of the endocervix may cause substantial difficulties, either because the subtle changes in the endocervical cells are mistaken for benign events or, because in many cases, adenocarcinoma is obscured by an adjacent neoplastic squamous lesion.

In 1985, Saigo et al reported on 58 patients with endocervical adenocarcinoma, 18 of who were asymptomatic, with a remarkable diagnostic accuracy of 91%. These results appear to be unmatched. There are few recent surveys of diagnostic accuracy based on contemporary techniques (endocervical brushings, liquid preparations). Hayes et al (1997) reported the cytologic findings on 131 patients with histologically documented adenocarcinomas of various stages, including adenocarcinoma in situ (AIS) but excluding minimal deviation tumors. In 18 patients, the smears showed no abnormalities whatsoever. In 46 cases, only a HGSIL was detected. In the remaining cases, significant abnormalities were observed, as described above in this chapter. Most importantly, perhaps, **the authors were unable to separate AIS from invasive adenocarcinoma,** in keeping with the writer's experience.

Soofer and Sidawy (2000) reported that women with smears diagnosed as "reactive cell changes" were more likely to develop squamous intraepithelial lesions than negative controls. No adenocarcinomas were found in this study. Selvaggi (2002) reported on similarities and differences between AIS and HGSIL with endocervical gland involvement in liquid-based cytology. She noted that "cell polarity" was maintained in AIS and lost in HGSIL. Rosettes and palisading were observed in AIS but not in HGSIL. Most other

TABLE 12-1

BENIGN CYTOLOGIC ABNORMALITIES THAT CAN BE MISTAKEN FOR ENDOCERVICAL ADENOCARCINOMA

Condition	Most Characteristic Single Feature	Compared With Adenocarcinoma
"Repair" (Chap. 10)	*Flat* sheets of endocervical cells with large nucleoli; normal nucleocytoplasmic ratio	Multilayered sheets in spherical (papillary) configuration. Large nucleoli uncommon
Acute or chronic endocervicitis or IUD wearers or pregnancy (Chaps. 8 and 10)	Enlarged, usually single endocervical cells with enlarged, slightly hyperchromatic nuclei and nucleoli; see repair above	Clinical history is important. Similar cells may occur in adenocarcinoma – search for other evidence of disease, otherwise classify as endocervical cell atypia (AGUS)
Tuboendometrial metaplasia (Chap. 10)	Ciliated cells. If there are nuclear abnormalities, a malignant process cannot be ruled out	Rare ciliated cells may occur in brush specimens
Benign endometrium in brush specimens (Chaps. 8 and 14)	Usually a tight cluster of uniform small cells, sometimes whole fragments of endometrium. If nuclear abnormalities are present, endometrial or endocervical neoplastic abnormalities cannot be ruled out	Usually the cells of endocervical carcinoma are of variable sizes, larger and of columnar or cuboidal shape

features of cancer cells, including the presence of abnormal columnar cells, were common to both lesions. Other surveys (Kristensen et al, 1991; Krane et al, 2001) disclosed a high rate of false negative diagnoses in 30% to 50% of cases. Negri et al (2003) proposed that **immunostaining with an antibody to the tumor suppressor gene p16^{INK4A}** is helpful in the diagnosis of adenocarcinoma in liquid prepara-

tions. Lack of reproducibility of cytologic diagnoses, among experienced observers in benign and malignant endocervical cell samples, was recently emphasized in a study by Simsir et al (2003). The role of human papillomavirus testing in identification of endocervical cancer is insecure at this time (Cangiarella and Chhieng, 2003).

In summary, precise cytologic diagnosis of endocervical

TABLE 12-2

MALIGNANT LESIONS THAT CAN BE MISTAKEN FOR ENDOCERVICAL ADENOCARCINOMA

Differential Diagnosis	Distinguishing Features
High grade squamous lesions originating in endocervical epithelium (Chap. 11)	May have identical presentation to endocervical adenocarcinoma. Histologic study is essential
Endometrial carcinoma (Chap. 13)	Usually the cells of endometrial carcinoma are smaller and of spherical configuration
Endometrial adenoacanthoma or adenosquamous carcinoma (Chap. 13)	May have very similar presentation to endocervical adenosquamous carcinoma. Histologic study is essential
Metastatic cancer (Chap. 17)	Clinical history is essential. Metastatic colonic carcinoma may mimic endocervical adenocarcinoma (large, columnar, mucus-producing cancer cells). Other metastatic cancers are usually composed of smaller cells.

adenocarcinoma is fraught with difficulties which have been reported from a large number of laboratories from several countries. The difficulties in separating benign reactive endocervical changes from adenocarcinoma and the presence of squamous neoplastic lesions obscuring the presence of adenocarcinoma are the principal culprits. It follows that aggressive clinical follow-up of patients with atypical endocervical cells may result in a better diagnostic performance. Moriarty and Wilbur (2003) recently expressed the hope that molecular markers may be helpful in this regard.

BIBLIOGRAPHY

Alva J, Lauchlan SC. The histogenesis of mixed cervical carcinomas. The concept of endocervical columnar-cell dysplasia. Am J Clin Pathol 64:20–25, 1975.

Alvaro T, Nogales F. Villous adenoma and invasive adenocarcinoma of the cervix. Int J Gynecol Pathol 7:96–97, 1988.

Andersen ES, Arffmann E. Adenocarcinoma in situ of the uterine cervix: A clinico-pathologic study of 36 cases. Gynecol Oncol 35:1–7, 1989.

Ayer B, Pacey F, Greenberg M, Bousfield L. The cytologic diagnosis of adenocarcinoma *in situ* of the cervix uteri and related lesions. I. Adenocarcinoma *in situ*. Acta Cytol 31:397–411, 1987.

Ayer B, Pacey F, Greenberg M. The cytologic diagnosis of adenocarcinoma in situ of the cervix uteri and related lesions. II. Microinvasive adenocarcinoma. Acta Cytol 32:318–324, 1988.

Baggish M, Woodruff JD. Adenoid basal lesions of the uterine cervix. Obstet Gynecol 37:807–819, 1971.

Bai H, Sung CJ, Steinhoff MM. ThinPrep Pap Test promotes detection of glandular lesions of the endocervix. Diagn Cytopathol 23:19–22, 2000.

Ballo MS, Silverberg SG, Sidawy MK. Cytologic features of well-differentiated villoglandular carcinoma of the cervix. Acta Cytol 40:536–540, 1996.

Benitez E, Rodriguez HA, Rodriguez-Cuevas H, Chavez GB. Adenoid cystic carcinoma of the uterine cervix. Report of a case and review of 4 cases. Obstet Gynecol 33:757–762, 1969.

Berek JS, Hacker NF, Fu YS, et al. Adenocarcinoma of the uterine cervix: Histologic variables associated with lymph node metastasis and survival. Obstet Gynecol 65:46–52, 1984.

Betrand M, Lickrish GM, Colgan TJ. The anatomic distribution of cervical adenocarcinoma in situ: Implications for treatment. Am J Obstet Gynecol 157:21–25, 1987.

Betsill WL, Clark AH. Early endocervical glandular neoplasia. I. Histomorphology and cytomorphology. Acta Cytol 30:115–126, 1986.

Biscotti CV, Hart WR. Apoptotic bodies: a consistent morphologic feature of endocervical adenocarcinoma in situ. Am J Surg Pathol 22:434–439, 1998.

Biscotti CV, Gero MA, Toddy SM, et al. Endocervical adenocarcinoma in situ: An analysis of cellular features. Diagn Cytopathol 17:326–332, 1997.

Bittencourt AL, Guimaraes JP, Barbosa HS, et al. Adenoid cystic carcinoma of the uterine cervix: Report of six cases and review of the literature. Acta Med Port Y1:697–706, 1979.

Boddington MM, Spriggs AI, Cowdell RH. Adenocarcinoma of the uterine cervix: Cytological evidence of a long preclinical evolution. Br J Obstet Gynaecol 83:900–903, 1976.

Boon ME, Baak JPA, Kurver PJH, et al. Adenocarcinoma in-situ of the cervix. An underdiagnosed lesion. Cancer 48:768–773, 1981.

Boon ME, Kirk RS, Rietveld-Scheffers PEM. The morphogenesis of adenocarcinoma of the cervix—a complex pathological entity. Histopathology 5:565–577, 1981.

Bousfield L, Pacey F, Young Q, et al. Expanded cytologic criteria for the diagnosis of adenocarcinoma *in situ* of the uterine cervix and related lesions. Acta Cytol 24:283–296, 1980.

Brainard JA, Hart WR. Adenoid basal epitheliomas of the uterine cervix: A reevaluation of distinctive cervical basaloid lesions currently classified as adenoid basal carcinoma and adenoid basal hyperplasia. Am J Surg Pathol 22:965–975, 1998.

Brinton LA, Reeves WC, Brenes MM, et al. Oral contraceptive use and risk of invasive cervical cancer. Int J Epidemiol 19:4–11, 1990.

Brown LJ, Wells M. Cervical glandular atypia associated with squamous intraepithelial neoplasia: A premalignant lesion? J Clin Pathol 39:22–28, 1986.

Buttenberg D, Stoll P. Cyto- and histomorphology of carcinoma of the Gartnerian duct. Acta Cytol 4:344–346, 1960.

Büttner HH, Kyank H. Adenocarcinoma in situ der Cervix uteri nach 11 Jahren gefolgt von invasivem Adenocarcinom. Z Krebsforsch 80:197–200, 1973.

Cangiarella JF, Chhieng DC. Atypical glandular cells—An update. Diagn Cytopathol 29:271–279, 2003.

Capraro VJ, Chen CM, Quebral R, Bartels J. Mesonephroma of the cervix. Report of a case. Obstet Gynecol 36:861–864, 1970.

Chang SH, Maddox WA. Adenocarcinoma arising within cervical endometriosis and invading the adjacent vagina. Am J Obstet Gynecol 110:1015–1017, 1971.

Chang WC, Matisic JP, Zhou C, et al. Cytologic features of villoglandular adenocarcinoma of the uterine cervix. Comparison with typical endocervical adenocarcinoma with a villoglandular component and papillary serous carcinoma. Cancer Cytopathol 87:5–11, 1999.

Chhieng DC, Cangiarella JF. Atypical glandular cells. Clin Lab Med 23:633–657, 2003.

Chhieng DC, Elgert PA, Cangiarella JF, Cohen J-M. Clinical significance of atypical glandular cells of undetermined significance. A follow-up study from an academic medical center. Acta Cytol 44:557–566, 2000.

Christopherson WM, Nealon N, Gray LA Sr. Noninvasive precursor lesions of adenocarcinoma and mixed adenosquamous carcinoma of the cervix uteri. Cancer 44:975–983, 1979.

Chung J-H, Koh J-S, Lee S-S, Cho K-J. Glass cell carcinoma of the uterine cervix. Cytologic features and expression of estrogen and progesterone receptors. Acta Cytol 44:551–556, 2000.

Cina SJ, Richardson MS, Austin RM, Kurman RJ. Immunohistochemical staining for Ki-67 antigen, carcinoembryonic antigen, and p53 in the differential diagnosis of glandular lesions of the cervix. Mod Pathol 10:176–180, 1997.

Clark AH, Betsill JWL. Early endocervical glandular neoplasia. II. Morphometric analysis of the cells. Acta Cytol 30:127–134, 1986.

Clement PB, Young RH, Keh P, et al. Malignant mesonephric neoplasms of the uterine cervix: A report of eight cases, including four with a malignant spindle cell component. Am J Surg Pathol 19:1158–1171, 1995.

Cohen C, Shulman G, Budgeon LR. Endocervical and endometrial adenocarcinoma: An immunoperoxidase and histochemical study. Am J Surg Pathol 6:151–157, 1982.

Cooper P, Russell G, Wilson B. Adenocarcinoma of the endocervix: A histochemical study. Histopathology 11:1321–1330, 1987.

Costa MJ, Kenny MB, Naib ZM. Cervicovaginal cytology in uterine adenocarcinoma and adenosquamous carcinoma. Acta Cytol 35:127–134, 1991.

Cullimore JE, Luesley DM, Rollason TP, et al. A prospective study of conization of the cervix in the management of cervical intraepithelial glandular neoplasia (CIGN) - a preliminary report. Br J Obstet Gynaecol 99:314–318, 1992.

Dallenbach-Hellweg G. Structural variations of cervical cancer and its precursors under the influence of exogenous hormones. *In* Dallenbach-Hellweg G (ed). Cervical Cancer. Current Topics in Pathology, vol 70. New York, Springer, 1981, pp 143–170.

Daroca PJ, Durandhar HN. Basaloid carcinoma of the uterine cervix. Am J Surg Pathol 4:235–239, 1980.

Debate, 1999: Glandular lesions of the cervix. Moderator: R Barasso (Paris, France). Participants: M Coppleson (Sydney, Australia), G Di Palo (Milan, Italy), PA Lapointe (Montreal, Canada). International Federation for Cervical Pathology and Colposcopy Newsletter, 1999.

De La Maza LM, Thayer BA, Naeim F. Cylindroma of the uterine cervix with peritoneal metastases: Report of a case and review of the literature. Am J Obstet Gynecol 112:121–125, 1972.

Deligdisch L, Escay-Martinez E, Cohen CJ. Endocervical carcinoma: A study of 33 patients with clinical-pathological correlation. Gynecol Oncol 18:326–333, 1984.

Di Tomasso JP, Ramzy I, Mody DR. Glandular lesions of the cervix. Validity of cytologic criteria used to define reactive changes, glandular intraepithelial lesions, and adenocarcinoma. Acta Cytol 40:1127–1135, 1996.

Drescher CW, Hopkins MP, Roberts JA. Comparison of the pattern of metastatic spread of squamous cell cancer and adenocarcinoma of the uterine cervix. Gynecol Oncol 33:340–343, 1989.

Duggan MA, McGregor E, Benoit JL, et al. The human papillomavirus status of invasive cervical adenocarcinoma: A clinicopathological and outcome analysis. Human Pathol 26:319–325, 1995.

Duk JM, Aalders JG, Fleuren GJ, et al. Tumor markers CA 125, squamous cell carcinoma antigen, and carcinoembryonic antigen in patients with adenocarcinoma of the uterine cervix. Obstet Gynecol 73:661–668, 1989.

Ferry JA, Scully RE. "Adenoid cystic" carcinoma and adenoid basal carcinoma of the uterine cervix: A study of 28 cases. Am J Surg Pathol 12:134–144, 1988.

Ferry JA, Scully RE. Mesonephric remnants, hyperplasia, and neoplasia in the uterine cervix: A study of 49 cases. Am J Surg Pathol 14:1100–1111, 1990.

Fetissof F, Berger G, Dubois MP, et al. Female genital tract and Peutz-Jeghers syndrome: An immunohistochemical study. Int J Gynecol Pathol 4:219–229, 1985.

Fluhmann C. The glandular structures of the cervix uteri. Surg Gynecol Obstet 106:715–723, 1958.

Fransworth A, Laverty C, Stoler MH. Human papillomavirus messenger RNA expression in adenocarcinoma in situ of the uterine cervix. Int J Gynecol Pathol 8:321–330, 1989.

Friedell GH, McKay DG. Adenocarcinoma in situ of endocervix. Cancer 6:887–897, 1953.

Fu Y-S, Reagan JW, Hsiu JG, et al. Adenocarcinoma and mixed carcinoma of the uterine cervix. I. A clinicopathologic study. Cancer 49:2650–2570, 1982a.

Fu Y-S, Reagan JW, Fu AS, Janiga KE. Adenocarcinoma and mixed carcinoma of the uterine cervix. II. Prognostic value of nuclear DNA analysis. Cancer 49:2571–2577, 1982b.

Fu YS, Hall TL, Berek JS, et al. Prognostic significance of DNA ploidy and morphometric analyses of adenocarcinoma of the uterine cervix. Anal Quant Cytol Histol 9:17–24, 1987.

Gallager HS, Simpson CB, Ayala AG. Adenoid cystic carcinoma of the uterine cervix. Cancer 27:1398–1402, 1971.

Gallup DG, Harper RH, Stock RJ. Poor prognosis in patients with adenosquamous cell carcinoma of the cervix. Obstet Gynecol 65:416–422, 1985.

Gilks CB, Young RH, Aguirre P, et al. Adenoma malignum (minimal deviation adenocarcinoma) of the uterine cervix: A clinicopathologic and immunohistochemical analysis of 26 cases. Am J Clin Pathol 13:717–729, 1989.

Gloor E. Un cas de syndrome de Peutz-Jeghers associé a un carcinome mammaire bilateral, a un adénocarcinome ducol utérin et a des tumeurs des cordons sexuels a tubules annelés bilaterales dans les ovaires. Schweiz Med Wochenschr 108:717–721, 1978.

Gloor E, Hurlimann J. Cervical intraepithelial glandular neoplasia (adenocarcinoma in situ and glandular dysplasia). A correlative study of 23 cases with histologic grading, histochemical analysis of mucins, and immunohistochemical determination of the affinity for four lectins. Cancer 58:1272–1280, 1986.

Glucksmann A, Cherry CP. Incidence, histology and response to radiation of mixed carcinomas (adenoacanthomas) of the uterine cervix. Cancer 9:971–979, 1956.

Goodman HM, Buttlar CA, Niloff JM, et al. Adenocarcinoma of the uterine cervix: Prognostic factors and patterns of recurrence. Gynecol Oncol 33:241–247, 1989.

Gordon HW, McMahon NJ, Agliozzo CM, et al. Adenoid cystic (cylindromatous) carcinoma of the uterine cervix: Report of two cases. Am J Clin Pathol 58:51–57, 1972.

Grafton WD, Kamm RC, Cowley LH. Cytologic characteristics of adenoid cystic carcinoma of the cervix uteri. Acta Cytol 20:164–166, 1976.

Granter SR, Lee KR. Cytologic findings in minimal deviation adenocarcinoma (adenoma malignum) of the cervix. A report of seven cases. Am J Clin Pathol 105:327–333, 1996.

Grayson W, Taylor LF, Cooper K. Adenoid cystic and adenoid basal carcinoma of the uterine cervix: Comparative morphologic, mucin, and immunohistochemical profile of two rare neoplasms of putative "reserve cell" origin. Am J Surg Pathol 23:448–458, 1999.

Greeley C, Schroeder S, Silverberg SG. Microglandular hyperplasia of the cervix: A true "pill" lesion? Int J Gynecol Pathol 14:50–54, 1995.

Grigsby PW, Perez CA, Kuske RR, et al. Adenocarcinoma of the uterine cervix: Lack of evidence for a poor prognosis. Radiother Oncol 12:289–296, 1988.

Hammoud MM, Haefner HK, Michael CW, Ansbacher R. Atypical glandular cells of undetermined significance (AGUS): Histologic findings and proposed management. J Reprod Med 47:266–270, 2002.

Hamperl H, Hellweg G. On mucoepidermoid tumors of different sites. Cancer 10:1187–1192, 1957.

Hart WR, Norris HJ. Mesonephric adenocarcinomas of the cervix. Cancer 29:106–113, 1972.

Hayes MM, Matisic JP, Chen CJ, et al. Cytologic aspects of uterine cervical adenocarcinoma, adenosquamous carcinoma and combined adenocarcinoma-squamous carcinoma: appraisal of diagnostic criteria for in situ versus invasive lesions. Cythopathol 8:397–408, 1997.

Hellweg G. Uber Schleimbildung in Plattenepithelcarcinomem, insbesondere an der Portio uteri (mucoepidermoidecarcinome). Z Krebsforsch 61:688–715, 1956–1957.

Hildesheim A, Hadjimichael O, Schwartz PE, et al. Risk factors for rapid-onset cervical cancer. Am J Obstet Gynecol 180:571–577, 1999.

Hopkins MP, Roberts JA, Schmidt RW. Cervical adencarcinoma in situ. Obstet Gynecol 71:842–844, 1988.

Hopkins MP, Schmidt RW, Roberts JA, Morley GW. The prognosis and treatment of stage I adenocarcinoma of the cervix. Obstet Gynecol 72:915–921, 1988.

Horowitz IR, Jacobson LP, Zucker PK, et al. Epidemiology of adenocarcinoma of the cervix. Gynecol Oncol 31:25–31, 1988.

Hurl WG, Silverberg SG, Frable WJ. Adenocarcinoma of the cervix: Histopathologic and clinical features. Am J Obstet Gynecol 129:304–315, 1977.

Ioffe OB, Sagae S, Moritani S, et al. Proposal of a new scoring scheme for the diagnosis of noninvasive endocervical glandular lesions. Am J Surg Pathol 27:452–460, 2003.

Ireland D, Hardiman P, Monaghan JM. Adenocarcinoma of the uterine cervix: A study of 73 cases. Obstet Gynecol 65:65–82, 1985.

Iwasawa A Nieminen P, Lehtinen M, et al. Human papillomavirus DNA in uterine cervix squamous cell carcinoma and adenocarcinoma detected by polymerase chain reaction. Cancer 77:2275–2279, 1996.

Jackson SR, Hollingworth TA, Anderson MC, et al. Glandular lesions of the cervix—Cytological and histological correlation. Cytopathol 7:10–16, 1996.

Jaworski RC, Pacey NF, Greenberg ML, Osbor RA. The histologic diagnosis of adenocarcinoma in situ and related lesions of the cervix uteri. Adenocarcinoma in situ. Cancer 61:1171–1181, 1988.

Johnson JE, Rahemtulla A. Endocervical glandular neoplasia and its mimics in ThinPrep Pap tests. A descriptive study. Acta Cytol 43:369–375, 1999.

Jones MA, Tarraza HM. Mesonephric remnant hyperplasia of the cervix: A clinicopathologic analysis of 14 cases. Gynecol Oncol 49:41–47, 1993.

Jones MW, Silverberg SG. Cervical adenocarcinoma in young women: Possible relationship to microglandular hyperplasia and use of oral contraceptives. Obstet Gynecol 117:464–468, 1989.

Jones MW, Silverberg SG, Kurman RJ. Well-differentiated villoglandular adenocarcinoma of the uterine cervix: A clinicopathologic study of 24 cases. Int J Gynecol Pathol 12:1–7, 1993.

Kagan AR, Nussbaum H, Chan PYM, Ziel HI. Adenocarcinoma of the uterine cervix. Am J Obstet Gynecol 117:464–468, 1973.

Kaku T, Hachisuga T, Toyoshima S, et al. Extremely well-differentiated adenocarcinoma ("adenoma malignum") of the cervix in a patient with Peutz-Jeghers syndrome. Int J Gynecol Pathol 4:266–273, 1985.

Kamoi S, AlJubory MI, Akin M-R, Silverberg SG. Immunohistochemical stain-

ing in the distinction between primary endometrial and endocervical adenocarcinomas: Another viewpoint. Int J Gynecol Pathol 21:217–223, 2002.

Kese G. Adenocarcinoma cervicis uteri bei einer 28 jahrigen Frau mit Peutz-Jeghers-Syndrom. Zentralbl Gynäkol 91:215–218, 1969.

Keyhani-Rofagha S, Brewer S, Prokorym P. Comparative cytologic findings of in situ and invasive adenocarcinoma of the uterine cervix. Diagn Cytopathol 12:120–125, 1995.

Kilgore LC, Soong SJ, Gore H, et al. Analysis of prognostic features in adenocarcinoma of the cervix. Gynecol Oncol 31:137–153, 1988.

King LA, Talledo OE, Gallup DG, et al. Adenoid cystic carcinoma of the cervix in women under age 40. Gynecol Oncol 31:26–30, 1989.

Kjaer SK, Brinton LA. Adenocarcinoma of the uterine cervix: The epidemiology of an increasing problem. Epid Rev 15:486–498, 1993.

Korn AP, Judson PL, Zaloudek CJ. Importance of atypical glandular cells of uncertain significance in cervical cytologic smears. J Reprod Med 43:774–778, 1998.

Koss LG. Pathogenesis of carcinoma of the uterine cervix. In: Dallenbach-Hellweg G (ed). Cervical Cancer. Current Topics in Pathology, vol 70. Berlin Heidelberg–New York, Springer, 1981, pp 112–142.

Krane JF, Granter SR, Trask CE, et al. Papanicolaou smear sensitivity for the detection of adenocarcinoma of the cervix: A study of 49 cases. Cancer 25:8–15, 2001.

Kristensen GB, Skyggebjerg K-D, Holund B, et al. Analysis of cervical smears obtained within three years of the diagnosis of invasive cervical cancer. Acta Cytol 35:47–50, 1991.

Larraza-Hernandez O, Molberg KH, Lindberg G, et al. Ectopic prostate tissue in the uterine cervix. Int J Gynecol Pathol 16:291–293, 1997.

Lauchlan SC, Penner DW. Simultaneous adenocarcinoma in situ and epidermoid carcinoma in situ. Report of 2 cases. Cancer 20:2250–2254, 1967.

Laverty CR, Farnsworth A, Thurloe J, Bowditch R. The reliability of a cytological prediction of cervical adenocarcinoma in situ. Aust NZ J Obstet Gynaecol 28:307–312, 1988.

Lee KR, Flynn CE. Early invasive adenocarcinoma of the cervix. Cancer 89:1048–1055, 2000.

Lee KR, Manna EA, Jones MA. Comparative cytologic features of adenocarcinoma in situ of the uterine cervix. Acta Cytol 35:117–126, 1991.

Lee KR, Minter LJ, Granter SR. Papanicolaou smear sensitivity for adenocarcinoma in situ of the cervix. A study of 34 cases. Am J Clin Pathol 107:30–35, 1997.

Lee KR, Sun D, Crum CP. Endocervical intraepithelial glandular atypia (dysplasia): A histopathologic, human papillomavirus, and MIB-1 analysis of 25 cases. Hum Pathol 31:656–664, 2000.

Lewis TLT. Collid (mucus secreting) carcinoma of the cervix. J Obstet Gynaecol Br Commonw 78:1128–1132, 1971.

Lin CT, Tseng CJ, Lai CH, et al. High-rish HPV DNA detection by Hybrid Culture II. An adjunctive test for mildly abnormal cytologic smears in women > or = 50 years of age. J Reprod Med 45:345–350, 2000.

Littman P, Clement PB, Henriksen B, et al. Glassy cell carcinoma of the cervix. Cancer 37:2238–2246, 1976.

LiVolsi VA, Merino MJ, Schwartz PE. Coexistent endocervical adenocarcinoma and mucinous adenocarcinoma of ovary: A clinicopathologic study of four cases. Int J Gynecol Pathol 1:391–402, 1983.

Lotocki RJ, Krepart GV, Paraskevas M, et al. Glass cell carcinoma of the cervix: A bimodal treatment strategy. Gynecol Oncol 44:254–299, 1992.

Luesley DM, Jordan JA, Woodman CBJ, et al. A retrospective review of adenocarcinoma-in-situ and glandular atypia of the uterine cervix. Br J Obstet Gynaecol 94:699–703, 1987.

Mackles A, Wolfe SA, Neigus I. Benign and malignant mesonephric lesions of cervix. Cancer 11:292–305, 1958.

Maier RC, Norris HJ. Coexistence of cervical epithelial neoplasia with primary adenocarcinoma of the endocervix. Obstet Gynecol 56:361–364, 1980.

Maier RC, Norris HJ. Glassy cell carcinoma of the cervix. Obstet Gynecol 60:219–224, 1982.

Mazur MT, Battifora HA. Adenoid cystic carcinoma of the uterine cervix: Ultrastructure, immunoflourescence, and criteria for diagnosis. Am J Clin Pathol 77:494–500, 1982.

McCluggage WG, Maxwell P, McBride HA, et al. Monoclonal antibodies Ki-67 and MIB1 in the distinction of tuboendometrial metaplasia from endocervical adenocarcinoma and adenocarcinoma in situ in formalin-fixed material. Int J Gynecol Pathol 14:209–221, 1995.

McCluggage WG, Sumathi VP, McBride HA, Patterson A. A panel of immunohistochemical stains, including carcinoembryonic antigen, vimentin, and estrogen receptor, aids the distinction between primary endometrial and endocervical adenocarcinomas. Int J Gynecol Pathol 21:11–15, 2001.

McGowan L, Young RH, Scully RE. Peutz-Jeghers syndrome with "adenoma malignum" of the cervix. A case report of two cases. Gynecol Oncol 10:125–133, 1980.

McKelvey JL, Goodlin RR. Adenoma malignum of the cervix. A cancer of deceptively innocent histological pattern. Cancer 16:549–557, 1963.

Meath AJ, Carley ME, Wilson TO. Atypical glandular cells of undetermined significance: Review of final histologic diagnoses. J Reprod Med 47:249–252, 2002.

Melnick PJ, Lee LE Jr, Walsh HM. Endocervical and cervical neoplasms adjacent to carcinoma in situ. Am J Clin Pathol 28:354–376, 1957.

Michael H, Grawe L, Kraus FT. Minimal deviation endocervical adenocarcinoma: Clinical and histologic features, immunohistochemical staining for carcinoembryonic antigen, and differentiation from confusing benign lesions. Int J Gynecol Pathol 3:261–276, 1984.

Moriarty AT, Wilbur D. Those gland problems in cervical cytology: Faith or fact? Observations from the Bethesda 2001 Terminology Conference. Diagn Cytopathol 28:171–174, 2003.

Moritani S, Ioffe OB, Sagae S, et al. Mitotic activity and apoptosis in endocervical glandular lesions. Int J Gynecol Pathol 21:125–133, 2002.

Mullins JD, Hilliard GD. Cervical carcinoid (argyrophyl cell carcinoma) associated with an endocervical adenocarcinoma: A light and ultrastructural study. Cancer 47:785–790, 1981.

Mulvany N, Östör A. Microinvasive carcinoma of the uterine cervix. A cytopathologic study of 40 cases. Diagn Cytopathol 16:430–436, 1997.

Mulvany NJ, Surtees V. Cervical/vaginal endometriosis with atypia: A cytohistopathologic study. Diagn Cytopathol 21:188–193, 1999.

Nagakawa S, Yoshikawa H, Onda T, et al. Type of human papillomavirus is related to clinical features of cervical carcinoma. Cancer 78:1935–1941, 1996.

Negri G, Egarter-Vigl E, Kasal A, et al. p16^{INK4a} is a useful marker for the diagnosis of adenocarcinoma of the cervix uteri and its precursors. An immunohistochemical study with immunocytochemical correlations. Am J Surg Pathol 27:187–193, 2003.

Nielson AL. HPV type 16/18 in uterine cervical adenocarcinoma in situ and adenocarcinoma: A study by in situ hybridization with biotinylated DNA probes. Cancer 65:2588–2593, 1990.

Nguyen G. Papillary serous adenocarcinoma of cervix [Letter]. Diagn Cytopathol 16:548–550, 1997.

Nguyen G, Jeannot AB. Exfoliative cytology of in situ and microinvasive carcinoma of the uterine cervix. Acta Cytol 28:461–467, 1984.

Novotny DB, Ferlisi P. Villoglandular adenocarcinoma of the cervix: Cytologic presentation. Diagn Cytopathol 17:383–387, 1997.

Nucci MR, Clement PB, Young RH. Lobular endocervical gland hyperplasia: A report of 13 cases and comparison with adenoma malignum. Am J Surg Pathol 23:886–891, 1999.

Nucci MR, Ferry JA, Young RH. Ectopic prostate tissue in the uterine cervix: A report of four cases and review of ectopic prostatic tissue. Am J Surg Pathol 24:1224–1230, 2000.

Nunez C, Abdul-Karin FW, Somrak TM. Glassy-cell carcinoma of the uterine cervix: Cytopathologic and histopathologic study of five cases. Acta Cytol 29:303–309, 1985.

Ostor AG, Pagano R, Davoren RAM. Adenocarcinoma in situ of the cervix. Int J Gynecol Pathol 3:179–190, 1984.

Ostor A, Rome R, Quinn M. Microinvasive adenocarcinoma of the cervix: A clinicopathologic study of 77 women. Obstet Gynecol 89:88–93, 1997.

Pacey F, Ayer B, Greenberg M. The cytologic diagnosis of adenocarcinoma in situ of the cervix uteri and related lesions. III. Pitfalls in diagnosis. Acta Cytol 32:325–330, 1988.

Pak HY, Yokota SB, Paladugu RR, Agliozzo CM. Glassy cell carcinoma of the cervix: Cytologic and clinicopathologic analysis. Cancer 52:307–312, 1983.

Parazzini F, La Vecchia C, Negri E, et al. Risk factors for adenocarcinoma of the cervix: A case-control study. Br J Cancer 57:201–204, 1988.

Paulsen SM, Hansen KC, Nielsen VT. Glassy-cell carcinoma of the cervix: Case report with a light and electron microscopy study. Ultrastruct Pathol 1:377–384, 1980.

Peters RK, Chao A, Mack TM, et al. Increased frequency of adenocarcinoma of the uterine cervix in young women in Los Angeles county. J Natl Cancer Inst 76:423–428, 1986.

Pirog EC, Isacson C, Szabolcs MJ, et al. Proliferative activity of benign and neoplastic endocervical epithelium and correlation with HPV DNA detection. Int J Gynecol Pathol 21:22–26, 2001.

Prempree T, Villasanta U, Tang C-K. Management of adenoic cystic carcinoma of the uterine cervix (cylindroma). Cancer 46:1631–1635, 1980.

Qizilbash AH. In-situ and microinvasive adenocarcinoma of the uterine cervix. A clinical, cytologic and histologic study of 14 cases. Am J Clin Pathol 64:155–170, 1975.

Raab SS, Geisinger KR, Silverman JF, et al. Interobserver variability of a Papanicolaou smear diagnosis of atypical glandular cells of undetermined significance. Am J Clin Pathol 110:653–659, 1998.

Raab SS, Isacson C, Layfield LJ, et al. Atypical glandular cells of undetermined significance. Cytologic criteria to separate clinically significant from benign lesions. Am J Clin Pathol 104:574–582, 1995.

Raab SS, Snider TE, Potts SA, et al. Atypical glandular cells of undetermined significance. Diagnostic accuracy and interobserver variability using select cytologic criteria. Am J Clin Pathol 107:299–307, 1997.

Ramzy I, Yuzpe AA, Hendelman. J. Adenoid cystic carcinoma of the uterine cervix. Obstet Gynecol 45:679–683, 1975.

Renshaw AA, Mody DR, Lozano RL, et al. Detection of adenocarcinoma in situ of the cervix in Papanicolaou tests. Arch Pathol Lab Med 128:153–157, 2004.

Reuss E, Price J, Koonings P. Atypical glandular cells of undetermined significance. Subtyping as a predictor of outcome. J Reprod Med 46:701–705, 2001.

Riethdorf L, Riethdorf S, Lee KR, et al. Human papillomavirus, expression of p16^{INK4A} and early endocervical glandular neoplasia. Hum Pathol 33:899–904, 2002.

Ronnett BM, Manos MM, Ransley JE, et al. Atypical glandular cells of undetermined significance (AGUS): Cytopathologic features, histopathologic results, and human papillomavirus DNA detection. Hum Pathol 30:816–825, 1999.

Rosen Y, Dolan TE. Carcinoma of the cervix with cylindromatous features believed to arise in mesonephric duct. Cancer 36:1739–1747, 1975.

Rosenthal DL, McLatchie C, Stern E, et al. Endocervical columnar cell atypia coincident with cervical neoplasia characterized by digital image analysis. Acta Cytol 26:115–120, 1982.

Roth LM, Hornback NB. Clear-cell adenocarcinoma of the cervix in young women. Cancer 34:1761–1768, 1974.

Rotkin ID. Etiology and epidemiology of cervical cancer. In: Dallenbach-Hellweg G (ed). Cervical Cancer. Current Topics in Pathology, vol 70. New York, Springer, 1981, pp 81–110.

Rutledge FN, Galakatos AE, Wharton JT, Smith JP. Adenocarcinoma of the uterine cervix. Am J Obstet Gynecol 122:236–245, 1975.

Ryden SE, Silverman EM, Goldman RT. Adenoid cystic carcinoma of the cervix presenting as a primary bronchial neoplasm. Am J Obstet Gynecol 120:846–847, 1974.

Sachs H, Wurthner K. Zytologische, histologiche und zytofotometrische Befunde eines Adenocarcinoma in situ der cervix uteri. Geburtshilfe Frauenheilkd 32:846–849, 1972.

Saigo PE, Cain JM, Kim WS, et al. Prognostic factors in adenocarcinoma of the uterine cervix, Cancer 57:1584–1593, 1986.

Saigo PE, Wolinska WH, Kim WS, Hajdu SI. The role of cytology in the diagnosis and follow-up of patients with cervical adenocarcinoma. Acta Cytol 29:785–794, 1985.

Schlesinger C, Silverberg SG. Endocervical carcinoma in situ of tubal type and its relation to atypical tubal metaplasia. Int J Gynecol Pathol 18:1–4, 1999.

Schwartz SM, Weiss NS. Increase incidence of adenocarcinoma of the cervix in young women in the United States. Am J Epidemiol 124:1045–1047, 1986.

Segal GH, Hart WR. Cystic endocervical tunnel clusters: A clinicopathologic study of 29 cases of so-called adenomatous hyperplasia. Am J Surg Pathol 14:895–903, 1990.

Selvaggi SM. Cytologic features of high-grade squamous intraepithelial lesions involving endocervical glands on ThinPrep cytology. Diagn Cytopathol 26:181–185, 2002.

Selvaggi SM, Haefner HK. Microglandular endocervical hyperplasia and tubal metaplasia: Pitfalls in the diagnosis of adenocarcinoma on cervical smears. Diagn Cytopathol 16:168–173, 1997.

Shingleton HM, Groe H, Bradley DH, Soong SJ. Adenocarcinoma of the cervix. I. Clinical evaluation and pathologic features. Am J Obstet Gynecol 139:799–814, 1981.

Silver SA, Devouassoux-Shisheboran M, Mezzetti TP, Tavassoli FA. Mesonephric adenocarcinomas of the cervix. A study of 11 cases with immunohistochemical findings. Am J Surg Pathol 25:379–387, 2001.

Simsir A, Hwang S, Cangiarella J, et al. Glandular cell atypia on Papanicolaou smears: Interobserver variability in the diagnosis and prediction of cell of origin. Cancer 99:323–330, 2003.

Siziopikou KP, Wang HH, Abu-Jawdeh G. Cytologic features of neoplastic lesions in endocervical glands. Diagn Cytopathol 17:1–7, 1997.

Sneeden VD. Mesonephric lesions of cervix; practical means of demonstration and suggestion of incidence. Cancer 11:334–336, 1958.

Solomon D, Schiffman M, Tarone R. ALTS Study Group: Comparison of three management strategies for patients with atypical squamous cells of undetermined significance: baseline results from a randomized trial. J Natl Cancer Inst 93:293–299, 2001.

Soofer SB, Sidawy MK. Atypical glandular cells of undetermined significance: clinically significant lesions and means of patient follow-up. Cancer 90:207–214, 2000.

Steeper TA, Wick MR. Minimal deviation adenocarcinoma of the uterine cervix ("adenoma malignum"): An immunohistochemical comparison with microglandular endocervical hyperplasia and conventional endocervical adenocarcinoma. Cancer 58:1131–1138, 1986.

Szyfelbein WM, Young RH, Scully RE. Adenoma malignum of cervix. Cytologic findings. Acta Cytol 28:691–698, 1984.

Tabon H, Dave H. Adenocarcinoma in situ of the cervix. Clinicopathologic observations of 11 cases. Int J Gynecol Pathol 7:139–151, 1988.

Tambouret R, Bell DA, Young RH. Microcystic endocervical adenocarcinomas: A report of eight cases. Am J Surg Pathol 24:369–374, 2000.

Tamimi HK, Ek M, Hesla J, et al. Glassy cell carcinoma of the cervix redefined. Obstet Gynecol 71:837–841, 1988.

Tamini HK, Figge DC. Adenocarcinoma of the uterine cervix. Gynecol Oncol 13:335–344, 1982.

Tase T, Okagaki T, Clark BA, et al. Human papillomavirus DNA in adenocarcinoma in situ, microinvasive adenocarcinoma of the uterine cervix, and coexisting cervical squamous intraepithelial neoplasia. Int J Gynecol Pathol 8:8–17, 1989.

Tase T, Okagaki T, Clark BA, et al. Human papillomavirus DNA in glandular dysplasia and microglandular hyperplasia: Presumed precursors of adenocarcinoma of the uterine cervix. Obstet Gynecol 73:1005–1008, 1989.

Tateishi R, Wada A, Hayakawa K, et al. Argyrophil cell carcinomas (apudomas) of the uterine cervix. Virchows Arch [A] 366:257–274, 1975.

Teter J. A comparative cytological and histological study of an endocervical Gartner duct carcinoma. In the case of a prepubertal girl. Acta Pathol Microbiol Scand 80:39–47, 1972.

Ulbright TM, Gersell DJ. Glassy cell carcinoma of the uterine cervix. Cancer 51:2255–2263, 1983.

Ursin G, Peters RK, Henderson BE, et al. Oral contraceptive use and adenocarcinoma of cervix. Lancet 344:1390–1394, 1994.

Van Aspert-van Erp AJM, van't Hof-Grootenboer BE, et al. Endocervical columnar cell intraepithelial neoplasia. I. Discriminating cytomorphologic criteria. II. Grades of expression of cytomorphologic criteria. Acta Cytol 39:1199–1215, 1216–1236, 1995.

Van Aspert-van Erp AJM, vant't Hof-Grootenboer BE, et al. Identifying cytologic characteristics and grading endocervical columnar cell abnormalities. A study aided by high-definition television. Acta Cytol 41:1659–1670, 1997.

Van Dinh T, Woodruff JD. Adenoid cystic and adenoid basal carcinomas of the cervix. Obstet Gynecol 65:705–709, 1985.

Vandrie DM, Puri S, Upton RT, Demeester LJ. Adenosquamous carcinoma of the cervix in a woman exposed to diethylstilbestrol in utero. Obstet Gynecol 61:84S–87S, 1983.

Van Velden DJJ, Chuang JT. Cylindromatous carcinoma of the uterine cervix. A case report. Obstet Gynecol 39:17–21, 1972.

Wakefield A, Wells M. Histochemical study of endocervical glycoproteins throughout the normal menstrual cycle and adjacent to cervical intraepithelial neoplasia. Int J Gynecol Pathol 4:230–239, 1985.

Weiss RJ, Lucas WE. Adenocarcinoma of cervix. Cancer 57:1996–2001, 1986.

Wells M, Brown LJR. Glandular lesions of the uterine cervix: The present state of our knowledge. Histopathology 10:777–792, 1986.

Welsh T, Fu YS, Chan J, et al. Mesonephric remnants or hyperplasia can cause abnormal Pap smears: A study of three cases. Int J Gynecol Pathol 22: 121–126, 2003.

Wilczynski SP, Walker J, Liao SY, et al. Adenocarcinoma of the cervix associated with human papillomavirus. Cancer 62:1331–1336, 1988.

Woyke S, Domagala W, Olszewski W. Mesonephroma of the uterine cervix: Submicrobial study and comparison with fine structure of endocervical adenocarcinoma. Virchows Arch [A] 355:29–40, 1972.

Young RH. Simple clefts, complex problems: Reflections on glandular lesions of the uterine cervix. Int J Gynecol Pathol 21:212–216, 2002.

Young RH, Clement PB. Endocervical adenocarcinoma and its variants: Their morphology and differential diagnosis. Histopathology 41:185–207, 2002.

Young RH, Scully RE. Villoglandular papillary adenocarcinoma of the uterine cervix. A clinicopathologic analysis of 13 cases. Cancer 63:1773–1779, 1989.

Young RH, Scully RE. Minimal-deviation endometrioid adenocarcinoma of the uterine cervix: A report of five cases of a distinctive neoplasm that may be misinterpreted as benign. Am J Surg Pathol 17:660–665, 1993.

Young RH, Welch WR, Dickersin GR, Scully RE. Ovarian sex cord tumor with annular tubules. Review of 74 cases including 27 with Peutz-Jeghers syndrome and four with adenoma malignum of the cervix. Cancer 50: 1384–1402, 1982.

Zaino RJ. Glandular lesions of the uterine cervix. Mod Pathol 13:261–274, 2000.

Zaino RJ, Nahhas WA, Mortel R. Glassy carcinoma of the uterine cervix. Arch Pathol Lab Med 106:250–254, 1982.

Zhou C, Gilks CB, Hayes M, Clement PB. Papillary serous carcinoma of the uterine cervix: A clinicopathologic study of 17 cases. Am J Surg Pathol 22: 113–120, 1998.

Proliferative Disorders and Carcinoma of the Endometrium

13

With a marked decrease in the rate of invasive cancer of the uterine cervix, cancer of the endometrium has become **the most common cancer of the female genital tract diagnosed in the United States, with the second highest mortality rate after ovary.** The death rate from endometrial carcinoma increased substantially between the years 1990 and 2000 (Greenlee et al, 2000). A major increase in the rate of endometrial cancer has also been observed in other countries, such as Japan (Sato et al, 1998) and Canada (Byrne, 1990). Therefore, the primary goal of diagnostic cytology of the endometrium should be the **diagnosis of clinically unsuspected endometrial carcinoma of low stage and, hence, amenable to cure.** In a study of a large group of asymptomatic women, it has been documented by Koss et al (1981, 1984) that **approximately 8 per 1,000 peri- and postmenopausal women harbor such lesions.** The study is described in detail further on in this chapter. Prior to this work, *primary* cytologic diagnosis of *occult endometrial carcinoma* was rarely reported, particularly when compared with the wealth of material on the uterine cervix. Twenty-two of 102 endometrial cancers, diagnosed in cervicovaginal smears, occurred in asymptomatic women (Koss and Durfee, 1962). In a series of 285 endometrial carcinomas reported by Reagan and Ng (1973), there were only 18 cases with primary diagnosis by cytology. Only a few additional cases may be found in the older case reports, including some illustrated in Papanicolaou's *Atlas* (1954). It is quite evident that detection of early endometrial carcinoma has not reached the level of interest equal to detection of mammary or cervical cancer. For whatever reasons, this important disease has been neglected by the society.

Endometrial cytology belongs to the most difficult areas of morphology. There are two main reasons for it:

■ **The difficulties with obtaining a representative sample of the endometrium**
■ **The difficulties in the interpretation of the cytologic evidence and the recognition of normal and abnormal cells of endometrial origin**

This chapter is dedicated to the description of endometrial cytology in health and disease, compared with histologic observations.

CYTOLOGY OF ENDOMETRIUM IN HEALTH AND BENIGN CONDITIONS

Routine Cervicovaginal Samples

The recognition of normal glandular and stromal endometrial cells in **routine cervicovaginal samples** plays a critical role in the diagnosis of endometrial abnormalities. Therefore, a brief recall of commonly observed cytologic findings is summarized here.

Normal Findings

Childbearing Age
As described and illustrated in Chapter 8, glandular and stromal endometrial cells are normally found in routine cervicovaginal samples during **menstrual bleeding** and for 2 to 3 days thereafter. As a rule, **the finding of endometrial cells, regardless of morphology, after the 12th day of the cycle (considering the first day of bleeding as the first day of the cycle) must be considered abnormal.** Depending on the clinical situation (e.g., patient's age, clinical history, risk

factors for endometrial cancer; see discussion below), **the patient may be deserving of follow-up or further investigation,** although, in most such women, no significant lesions are found and the endometrial cells are most likely a variant of normal shedding.

In endocervical brush specimens, normal endometrial cells, derived from the lower uterine segment (LUS) of the endometrial cavity, may be observed, regardless of day of cycle, and should not be a cause for alarm, although incidental endometrial abnormalities may sometimes be recognized in such samples (see below). De Peralta-Venturino et al (1995) and Heaton et al (1996) stressed that material obtained from LUS may contain large fragments of endometrial glands and stroma that may be mistaken for carcinomas of endometrial or endocervical origin and benign entities, such as **endometriosis.**

Menopause
In postmenopausal women, the presence of endometrial cells in routine smears must be considered, a priori, abnormal and calls for further investigation of the endometrium.

Benign Conditions and Disorders

Pregnancy
Endometrial cells are practically never seen in normal pregnancy. The **decidual cells** and particularly the large **Arias-Stella cells with dark, polyploid nuclei, either derived from the endometrium or the endocervix,** both discussed and illustrated in Chapter 8, may be mistaken for endometrial cancer cells in cervicovaginal material. **Pregnancy does not rule out endometrial cancer.** On the rarest occasion, we have observed **normal pregnancy occurring in women with endometrial carcinoma** documented by prior biopsy and confirmed postpartum. A similar case was described by Kowalczyk et al (1999) who also summarized the very scanty literature on this topic. Apparently, normal implantation of the ovum may occur under these circumstances. Also on record are several cases of normal pregnancies occurring in women with documented endometrial hyperplasia (Kurman et al, 1985).

Intrauterine Contraceptive Devices
As has been described in Chapters 8 and 10, the wearers of intrauterine contraceptive devices (IUDs) may shed endometrial cells at midcycle. Occasionally, such cells have a **vacuolated cytoplasm and poorly preserved nuclei that may appear to be somewhat enlarged and slightly hyperchromatic and that may be** mistaken for cells of an adenocarcinoma (Fig. 13-1). Sometimes, the cervicovaginal smears may also contain **inflammatory cells and macrophages,** creating a cytologic background, not unlike that seen in endometrial carcinoma (see below). The young age of most wearers of IUDs is usually against this latter diagnosis. Another potential source of error is the presence of **endocervical "repair" caused by IUD, in which the reactive endocervical cells may be mistaken for abnormal endometrial cells** (see Chapter 10; and comments below).

An important **histologic** finding in wearers of the IUD

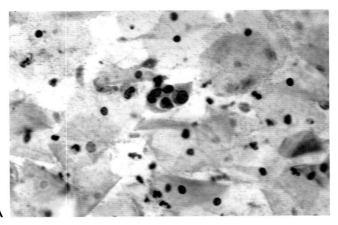

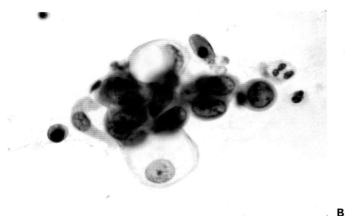

A

B

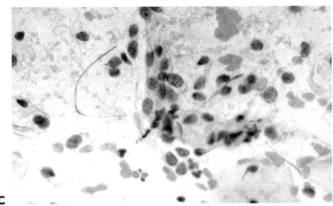

C

Figure 13-1 Benign endometrial cells in cervicovaginal smears. *A.* A small cluster of endometrial cells, difficult to identify at this magnification. *B.* High-power view of a cluster of endometrial cells in an IUD wearer. It may be noted that several of the cells have vacuolated cytoplasm. *C.* A small cluster of endometrial stromal cells showing mitotic activity. These cells are extremely difficult to recognize in routine material.

is the presence of **small, round foci (morulae) of squamous cells in** the superficial layers of the endometrium, presumably a form of squamous metaplasia, induced by the mechanical effect of the devices. Lane et al (1974) suggested that this abnormality is transient, although evidence of reversal of this process is poor. These abnormalities are very rarely seen and **should not be mistaken for an endometrioid carcinoma with squamous component or an adenoacanthoma** (see below).

Signet-Ring Cells

Iezzoni and Mills (2001) described 5 symptomatic patients in whom routine endometrial tissue samples contained aggregates of **benign signet ring cells** with small nuclei. The authors traced these cells to decidualized stromal cells. There is no record of such cells in cytologic samples.

Endometrial Metaplasia

Johnson and Kini (1996) described the presence of atypical endometrial cells in the presence of eosinophilic, papillary, squamous and tubal metaplasia of the endometrium. Five of seven patients were postmenopausal and three had abnormal bleeding. The nature of this observation is questionable and it cannot be excluded that some of the patients had a poorly defined neoplastic process.

Exogenous Hormones

Contraceptive Hormones

Women receiving this medication occasionally bleed or spot and shed **endometrium at mid-cycle (breakthrough**

bleeding) until the dosage is adjusted. Long-term usage of these agents may result in **decidua-like changes** in endometrial stroma, followed by **atrophy;** neither of these conditions is known to cause endometrial shedding. Abnormalities of nuclei of **endocervical cells** may occur **in women receiving progesterone-rich contraceptive agents** (see Chapter 10). Accurate clinical history is helpful in preventing errors but, in some cases, may require biopsies for clarification.

Steroid Hormones

In patients receiving **steroid hormones, particularly estrogens,** two important cytologic changes may be observed.

■ In postmenopausal women, the **level of maturation of the squamous cells may increase** (see Chapter 9), resulting in a smear pattern that is sometimes seen in endometrial hyperplasia and early endometrial carcinoma (see below).
■ The patients may shed endometrial cells during medication and, particularly, immediately after withdrawal of estrogens **(withdrawal bleeding). In the absence of clinical data in postmenopausal women, the presence of endometrial cells may cause an unnecessary alarm.** The potential carcinogenic effects of **estrogens and tamoxifen** are discussed below, in conjunction with epidemiology of endometrial carcinoma.

For further comments on effects of steroid hormones, see Chapter 9.

Regenerating Endometrium

Following a curettage or other form of trauma to the endometrium, the healing of the endometrial defect leads to an **intensive proliferation of the surface epithelium, followed by formation of endometrial glands by invagination of the surface epithelium. In histologic sections, the surface epithelium is composed of large cells of variable sizes with hyperchromatic nuclei, sometimes with large nucleoli, and with numerous mitoses. In endometrial aspiration smears,** the large and poorly preserved endometrial glandular cells have a **vacuolated cytoplasm, sometimes infiltrated with polymorphonuclear leukocytes and enlarged hyperchromatic nuclei** (Fig. 13-2). These cells may be mistaken for cancer cells. In this situation, it is advisable to wait until after a normal menstrual bleeding has taken place (usually about 6 weeks after the procedure) before attempting to judge the status of the endometrium.

Inflammatory Lesions

Purulent endometritis resulting from bacterial infection may follow childbirth or abortion. The cervicovaginal smears may disclose **pus and debris.** Smears obtained by direct **endometrial sampling** show acute inflammation and necrosis. Fragments of endometrial glands with degenerated, blown-up cells may be difficult to distinguish from cells of necrotizing endometrial carcinoma. The differential diagnosis may have to rest on clinical history and histologic evidence.

Chronic nonspecific endometritis is an uncommon condition in which there is an infiltration of the endometrium by lymphocytes, plasma cells, and macrophages, sometimes with atrophy of the glands. The condition is virtually never recognized in cytologic samples.

Tuberculosis of the Endometrium

A resurgence of tuberculosis in patients with immune deficiency caused by AIDS has revived interest in this disease in the developed countries. The disease is common in the developing world.

Histology

Advanced tuberculosis of the endometrium may be associated with a **marked disruption of the endometrial gland pattern. Atypical glandular proliferation may be very**

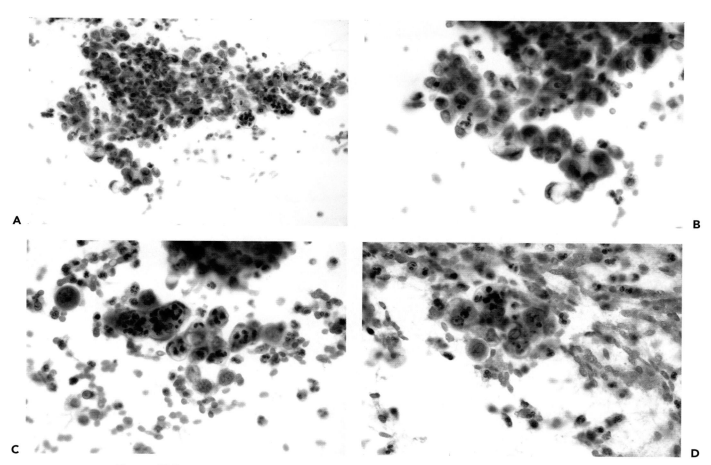

Figure 13-2   Regenerating endometrium 3 days after curettage. All four photographs from the same 20-year-old patient. *A.* A large cluster of endometrial cells, some showing vacuolization. *B.* A cluster of endometrial cells with hyperchromatic nuclei, some showing nucleoli and cytoplasmic vacuoles. *C.* In addition to the features described for *B,* the cytoplasm of many of the vacuolated cells is populated by polymorphonuclear leukocytes. *D.* Another example of regenerating endometrial cells in the background of blood and inflammatory reaction.

marked and misleading to the point of suggesting a carcinoma. Only the presence of **granulomas** identifies the condition. The diagnosis should be confirmed by demonstration of tubercle bacilli. The clinical presentation of endometrial tuberculosis is not helpful because the symptoms, such as metrorrhagia, may suggest cancer clinically.

Cytology

The abnormalities of the endometrial glands are also reflected in cervicovaginal smears. Sheets of **large endometrial glandular cells of uneven size and with pronounced nuclear hyperchromasia may suggest endometrial cancer** (Fig. 13-3). In such cases, the differential diagnosis between tuberculosis and endometrial carcinoma may prove to be extremely difficult, if not impossible, on cytologic grounds. To our knowledge, **neither epithelioid cells nor Langhans'-type giant cells** have been so far identified in endometrial material as they have been in cervical smears (see Chap. 10). The presence of **multinucleated histiocytes in**

the cervicovaginal smears is of no diagnostic value in the diagnosis of tuberculosis.

Sarcoidosis

This granulomatous disease of unknown etiology may affect the endometrium (Chalvardijian, 1978; Skehan and McKenna, 1986; Elstein et al, 1994). **Noncaseating granulomas,** characteristic of this disorder, are observed in histologic material but, so far, have not been observed in cytologic material. For a description of cytologic presentation of pulmonary sarcoidosis, see Chapter 19.

Viral Endometritis

Astin and Askin (1975) and Wenckebach and Curry (1976) described endometritis due to **cytomegalovirus.** The tissue showed evidence of chronic inflammation and formation of lymphocytic deposits, in addition to large cells containing the characteristic viral inclusions. Wenckebach and Curry confirmed the diagnosis by electron microscopy. Duncan et al (1989) described a case of **necrotizing endometritis**

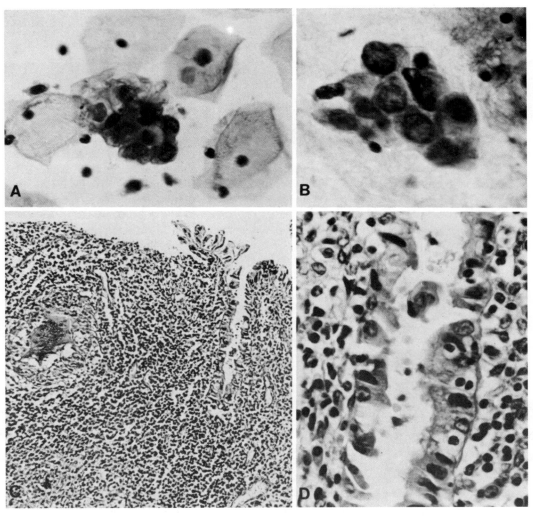

Figure 13-3 A case of endometrial tuberculosis. Abnormal endometrial cells in the vaginal pool smear (A) and in an endometrial aspiration (B). Note the hyperchromatic nuclei and the scanty cytoplasm. The histologic sections of the endometrium under low power (C) and high power (D) disclose atypical endometrial glands as the source of cellular abnormalities. Note the tubercle in C. (Tissue section from Dr. Jacob M. Ravid.)

associated with herpesvirus infection. Neither of these viral infections of the endometrium have been reported in cytologic writing.

Other Inflammatory Disorders

A case of **malacoplakia** was described by Thomas et al (1978). For further comments on histologic and cytologic presentation of malacoplakia, see Chapter 22.

Cytologic Atypias Associated With Endometriosis

Several observers reported that brush samples in cases of endocervical or transformation zone endometriosis may contain abnormal glandular cells that may mimic either an endocervical or an endometrial carcinoma (Hanau et al, 1997; Mulvany and Surtees, 1999; Lundeen et al, 2002).

The abnormalities allegedly caused by endometriosis were illustrated in Figure 11-35C, as examples of atypical glandular cells of unknown significance. In the judgment of this writer, cytologic diagnosis of endometriosis cannot be established. The changes described are most likely brush-artifacts with inadequate correlation with histologic findings.

Endometrial Abnormalities Associated With Uterine Leiomyomas

Leiomyomas are by far the most common benign tumors of the uterine corpus. The tumors, composed of bundles of smooth muscle and connective tissue, richly supplied with blood vessels, are often multiples and may reach large sizes. Hemorrhagic necrosis or infarction are known complications of leiomyomas. Many women with benign leiomyomas of the uterus experience episodes of **abnormal uterine bleeding.** The bleeding is attributed to various causes, such as the inability of the uterus to contract because of interference of leiomyoma with myometrial functions, or to submucosal position of the leiomyoma, causing focal ulceration of the endometrium. Objective evidence for these events is conspicuously absent. However, there is evidence that, at least in some women, the bleeding may be caused by **endometrial hyperplasia,** which is present in about 50% of women with leiomyomas (Deligdisch and Loewenthal, 1970). Both these disorders (hyperplasia and leiomyomas) may have a common denominator, namely, hormonal imbalance due to preponderance of estrogens. In such cases, the **cytologic presentation is similar to other forms of endometrial hyperplasia** (see below).

ENDOMETRIAL POLYPS

Benign endometrial polyps may occur in any adult woman but are more common in the fifth decade of life and are a known cause of abnormal uterine bleeding and endometrial shedding. The tumors may originate in any part of the endometrial cavity and may vary in diameter from a few millimeters to several centimeters. The polyps, which may be single or multiple, may be broad-based or pedunculated and sometimes may protrude through the external os of the uterine cervix. **Atypia of endometrial glands is common in polyps and may account for abnormalities of endometrial cells in direct endometrial samples** (see below). Also, **endometrial carcinomas may originate in polyps.** The uncommon **mesodermal mixed tumors** of endometrium may **originate in or mimic endometrial polyps** (see Chapter 17).

Histology

The benign polyps consist of a stroma resembling normal endometrial stroma intermingled with connective tissue that is sometimes hyalinized. The polyps are sometimes richly vascularized, with vessels present near the surface. The epithelial surface lining usually resembles proliferative endometrium but, in polyps originating in the lower uterine segment, it is occasionally composed of columnar cells, resembling normal endocervical lining. Occasionally, the epithelial cells are ciliated. Endometrial glands of variable sizes and shapes are present within the stroma. The epithelial lining of the glands is usually nonsecretory in type and does not participate in the cyclic changes. **Atypical endometrial glands,** lined by cells with enlarged nuclei and nucleoli mimicking glands observed in atypical hyperplasia, are fairly common in polyps (Fig 13-4D).

Cytology

An accurate cytologic diagnosis of an endometrial polyp is impossible in cervicovaginal samples. Occasionally, **clusters or single endometrial cells** are noted during the secretory phase of the cycle when endometrial cells should not be present, or in postmenopausal women (Fig. 13-4A–C). In postmenopausal women, the cytologic findings may be mistaken for an endometrial carcinoma. This error is **unavoidable.** Abnormalities mimicking carcinoma are also observed in **direct endometrial samples,** as described in detail below.

Large, protruding **polyps, pressing on the endocervical epithelium, may elicit a florid squamous metaplasia or "repair"** reaction (see Chapter 10). **Endometrial carcinomas, originating in polyps, have the same cytologic presentation as primary endometrial cancer** (see below).

Atypical polypoid adenomyoma is a rare and presumably benign type of endometrial polyp wherein markedly atypical proliferation of endometrial glands may occur (summary in Young et al, 1986). The possibility that these lesions represent an early stage of a mesodermal mixed tumor cannot be ruled out (see Chapter 17). There is no information on their cytologic presentation.

ENDOMETRIAL ADENOCARCINOMA

As described in the opening paragraphs of this chapter, endometrial carcinoma is, at the time of this writing (2004), the most common form of genital cancer. Partridge et al (1996) observed that the mortality rate from this disease is high and that advancing age, minority status, and low in-

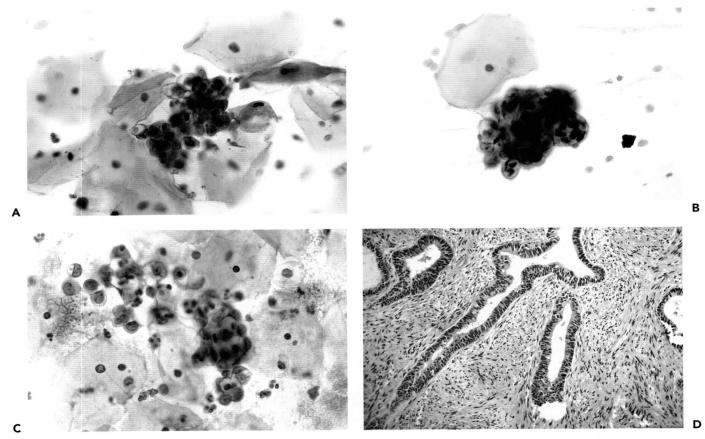

Figure 13-4 **Endometrial polyp in a markedly obese 56-year-old woman.** *A,B.* Clusters of endometrial cells against a background of high maturation of squamous cells. *C.* Large, endometrial cells with markedly vacuolated cytoplasm, granular nuclei, and occasional nucleoli. The endometrial cells show cytoplasmic and nuclear features consistent with endometrial adenocarcinoma. *D.* Endometrial polyp in the same patient.

come had a negative impact on survival. These authors deplored the absence of acceptable early detection systems. Such systems do exist, as narrated below, but their implementation and societal acceptance are thoroughly lagging when compared with carcinoma of the uterine cervix and female breast.

Some of the reasons for a marked increase in the rate of this disease are discussed here.

Epidemiology

The constant growth and disintegration of the endometrium during the menstrual cycles of the childbearing age constitute a terrain that is not favorable to neoplastic growth and accounts for the rarity of endometrial cancer in women prior to menopause. **The absence of cyclic desquamation after the menopause or an arrest of endometrial turnover because of hormonal imbalance are important risk factors in the formation of endometrial carcinomas and their precursor lesions.** Examples of naturally occurring conditions leading to hormonal imbalances are the **Stein-Leventhal syndrome** and similar disorders of ovulation (see Chapter 9) or **estrogen-producing ovarian tumors (granulosa cell tumors and thecomas).** Endometrial carcinoma has also been observed in the presence of ovarian dysfunc-

tion associated with masculinizing features (Koss et al, 1964).

Risk Factors

Exogenous Estrogens

In the late 1960s and in the 1970s, a statistically significant increase in the rate of endometrial carcinoma has been observed in many institutions throughout the United States. Smith et al, Ziel and Finkle simultaneously pointed out in 1975 that **widespread administration of conjugated and nonconjugated exogenous estrogens** to alleviate menopausal symptoms and prevent osteoporosis **was statistically associated with this increase.** Mack et al (1976) calculated the risk ratio for endometrial carcinoma in estrogen users when compared with nonusers at 8.0 times, and for conjugated estrogens at 5.6 times; these investigators also demonstrated a dose-related effect on endometrial carcinoma. In a study by a writers group for the PEPI Trial (1996), the administration of unopposed estrogens was shown to cause endometrial hyperplasia and occasional adenocarcinoma. The effect could be prevented by the administration of progesterone. Exogenous estrogens have been shown to be associated with endometrial carcinoma, even in the absence of ovarian function, for example in ovarian agenesis (Gray et al, 1970; Cutler et al, 1972) or in Sheehan's syndrome (Reid and Shirley, 1974).

Although the evidence is substantial that estrogens may cause endometrial carcinoma, it has been shown that such lesions observed in estrogen-treated patients are usually **fully curable, low-grade and low-stage cancers** (Robboy et al, 1982). Horwitz and Feinstein (1978) addressed this issue and reported on the status of peripheral endometrium in a case control study of 233 postmenopausal women, 112 of whom had endometrial carcinoma. Peripheral, simple endometrial hyperplasia was more commonly observed with grade 1 cancer among estrogen users than in cancer of higher grades among nonusers of estrogen. The authors concluded that **"it was likely that many otherwise asymptomatic tumors might have remained undetected except for the manifestations of the estrogen-related comorbid condition" (hyperplasia).** The observation was repeated by Horwitz et al (1981) who proposed that the effect of estrogens on endometrium is indirect: the drugs cause endometrial hyperplasia and, hence, uterine bleeding that leads to curettages and results in incidental discovery of small foci of early endometrial cancer. In fact, in our own study of occult endometrial carcinomas, estrogen treatment has not been shown to be a risk factor except for women with lower than average weight. It was hypothesized that this observation may perhaps be explained by the inability of this group of women to store the estrogens in their subcutaneous fat, resulting in more direct action on the endometrium (Koss et al, 1984; see below). The use of either estrogen therapy or estrogens combined with progesterone, also **increases the risk of breast cancer** (Colditz et al, 1995; Schairer et al, 2000) (see Chap. 29).

Tamoxifen

Tamoxifen is a steroid agent best characterized as an estrogen agonist or estrogen-receptor modulator, which blocks estrogen receptors in a variety of tissues and is now extensively used for **prevention and treatment of breast cancer** (summary in Osborne, 1998). The drug has several side effects affecting the female genital tract and, specifically, the endometrium.

- It induces maturation of squamous cells in postmenopausal women with atrophic genital tract (Athanassiadou et al, 1992; Abadi et al, 2000).
- It has a stimulatory effect on the endometrium and has been recognized as a **cause of abnormal endometrial proliferative processes, including polyps, hyperplasias, and carcinoma** (Silva et al, 1994; Assikis and Jordan, 1995; Barakat, 1996; Fisher et al, 1994). The risk appears to be greater for obese women (Bernstein et al, 1999). Sporadic cases of mesodermal mixed tumors were also observed (Bouchardy et al, 2002; Wysowski et al, 2002; Wickerham et al, 2002). Common sense would suggest that the status of the endometrium should be determined in all women prior to tamoxifen therapy.

Measuring the thickness of the endometrium by ultrasound is a favored method of follow-up of patients receiving tamoxifen and other hormones (Achiron et al, 1995; Levine et al, 1995; Hann et al, 1997). It has been suggested that endometrial thickness of 8 mm or more should trigger an endometrial investigation by biopsy or curettage. Langer et al (1997), using the thickness of 5 mm as a trigger for endometrial biopsies in women receiving estrogen replacement therapy, noted that at this level of endometrial thickness, the technique has a very poor positive predictive value but a high negative predictive value for important endometrial disorders.

Cytologic Observations in Tamoxifen Users

The information on the use of cytologic techniques to determine the status of the endometrium in tamoxifen-treated patients is scarce. Yet, anecdotal evidence based on personal observations of a few patients by endometrial sampling has shown that, **after a few years of medication, significant nuclear abnormalities may occur in glandular endometrial cells, that differ significantly from patterns of endometrial hyperplasia or carcinoma and most likely represent tamoxifen-induced endometrial atypia** (Fig. 13-5). Abadi et al (2000), in a study encompassing a small number of patients treated with tamoxifen, some of whom devel-

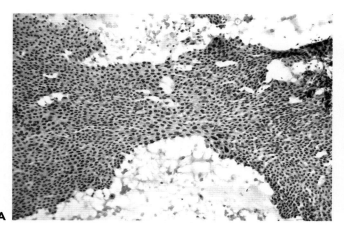
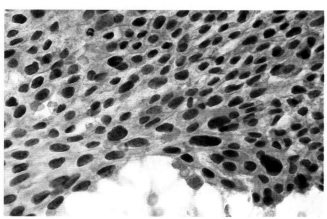

A **B**

Figure 13-5 Endometrial atypia associated with Tamoxifen. Endometrium in a 69-year-old woman receiving Tamoxifen for 5 years. Marked nuclear abnormalities of endometrial surface epithelium are seen under scanning (A) and higher (B) magnifications in an endometrial aspirate.

oped endometrial carcinoma, noted that **the presence of endometrial cells and an increase in macrophages in cervicovaginal smears,** correlated in a statistically significant fashion with endometrial cancer.

Other Hormones

Endometrial carcinoma has been observed in approximately 0.05% of women treated with a variety of hormones for carcinoma of the breast (Hoover et al, 1976). **Hormonal contraceptive agents** usually cause endometrial atrophy. It is not known, at this time, whether these agents may also contribute to the genesis of endometrial cancer, although a few such cases have been recorded (Silverberg and Makowski, 1975).

Radiotherapy

Malignant tumors of the endometrium (carcinomas and occasionally mesodermal mixed tumors) have been observed in patients who received a **curative dose of radiation for invasive carcinoma of the uterine cervix** (Fehr and Prem, 1974).

Clinical Risk Factors

Carcinoma of the endometrium has been traditionally thought to be associated with **diabetes, obesity, hypertension, a past history of abnormal menses, and late menopause** (Wynder et al, 1966; Elwood et al, 1977). Our own epidemiologic studies of asymptomatic women with occult carcinoma failed to confirm these observations (Koss et al, 1984) but this cohort may have differed from symptomatic women who have been the common target of such studies. The only statistically significant factor in the Koss study was **delayed onset of menopause** (see Table 13-8). The full extent of the clinical epidemiology of the disease is deserving of further studies comparing symptomatic with asymptomatic patients.

Clinical Symptoms: Application of Cytologic Techniques

The principal clinical symptom associated with endometrial carcinoma is abnormal bleeding. Endometrial carcinoma is rare in women below the age of forty. **Any woman 40 years of age or older who shows clinical evidence of abnormal uterine bleeding for which no obvious cause can be found by obstetrical history or on clinical examination, should be, a priori, suspected of harboring endometrial cancer.** A diagnostic workup, at least an endometrial biopsy, but preferably an endometrial curettage, should be obtained without delay. **Cytology should not be used as a diagnostic weapon in obvious clinical situations unless a curettage cannot be performed.** However, **endometrial cancers may produce no symptoms whatever or only insignificant symptoms (such as discharge or spotting)** that are not readily elicited on routine questioning of the patient. **Such lesions may be discovered by cytologic techniques, and their diagnosis constitutes the chief application of cytology to the detection of endometrial cancer.**

CLASSIFICATION OF ENDOMETRIAL CARCINOMAS AND THEIR PRECURSORS

It is generally assumed that endometrial carcinoma is preceded by a series of molecular-genetic and morphologic modification of structure and configuration of endometrial epithelium and glands. **Two pathways** of disease have been advocated (Sherman, 2000). For the common **endometrioid type of endometrial carcinoma,** the precursor lesion is known as **endometrial hyperplasia.** For the relatively uncommon **serous carcinoma,** the precursor lesion has been named **intraepithelial carcinoma.**

Histologic make-up of endometrial cancer may have considerable bearing on cytologic diagnosis because tumors of high grade with marked nuclear abnormalities are much easier to recognize than very well differentiated low grade tumors with relatively trivial nuclear changes. The classification of endometrial carcinomas and their precursor lesions, modified from the WHO classification (Scully et al, 1994), is shown below.

- **Endometrioid carcinoma**
- **Villoglandular carcinoma**
- **Endometrioid carcinoma with squamous differentiation (adenoacanthoma, adenosquamous carcinoma)**
- **Squamous carcinoma**
- **Precursor lesions of endometrioid carcinoma–endometrial hyperplasia**
- **Simple proliferative hyperplasia**
- **Atypical hyperplasia, carcinoma in situ (Hertig)**
- **Serous (papillary serous) carcinoma**
- **Intraepithelial carcinoma**
- **Rare type of carcinomas**

Endometrioid Carcinoma

Histology

As the name indicates, this malignant tumor is characterized by a **disorderly proliferation of the endometrial glands resulting in a grotesque image of the endometrium.** These tumors are usually **primary in the endometrium** but may also develop in **endometrial polyps** and in foci of **endometriosis that** may be located in a variety of primary sites, including the ovary and even the regional lymph nodes (Koss, 1963). The cancerous glands **vary in size and configuration,** are often **crowded,** and adjacent to each other without intervening endometrial stroma. Papillary projections into the lumen of the glands is not uncommon (Fig. 13-6A). The cancerous glands are lined by **cells that are larger than normal,** usually cuboidal but sometimes columnar (tall-cell carcinoma) in configuration. The nuclei of these cells vary from **simple enlargement and slight hyperchromasia** in low grade tumors to markedly **enlarged, sometimes hyperchromatic nuclei** in high grade tumors. **A characteristic feature of cells of endometrioid carcinoma is the presence of clearly visible nucleoli.** The number and size of the nucleoli also vary with tumor type, with one or two small nucleoli present in well differentiated tumors, when compared with up to four larger nucleoli in

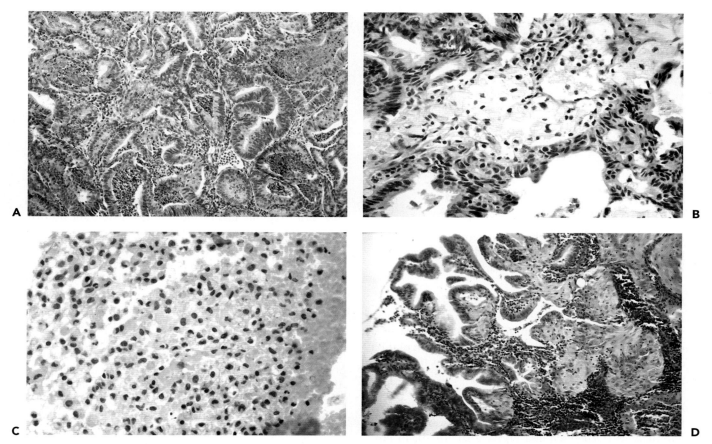

Figure 13-6 Various histologic aspects of endometrioid carcinoma. *A.* Grade II adeno-carcinoma. *B.* A cluster of large macrophages in the stroma of an adenocarcinoma. *C.* Another cluster of macrophages in the stroma of another endometrioid carcinoma. *D.* Adenoacanthoma.

high grade tumors (Long et al, 1958). The degree of nuclear abnormalities is the basis for nuclear grading that is thought to be of prognostic value. The frequency of mitotic figures varies.

The **stroma** separating the cancerous glands may occasionally show rather remarkable changes in the form of clusters of very **large macrophages,** first described by Dubs in 1923 (Fig. 13-6B,C). Rarely, concentric, often calcified protein secretions **(psammoma bodies)** may be formed by some of these tumors (Parkash and Carcangiu, 1997).

The degree of architectural differentiation of endometrial cancer may vary considerably and is of prognostic significance. Some tumors present only a **slight deviation from the normal endometrial pattern (grade I carcinomas, sometimes referred to as adenoma malignum);** at the other extreme, there is a **grade III carcinoma,** presenting as a nearly **solid growth of cancer cells** in sheets with only an occasional attempt at gland formation. Most of the endometrial cancers fall somewhere between the two extremes and are graded II.

Villoglandular carcinoma is an uncommon variant of endometrioid carcinoma, characterized by formation of slender papillary fronds on the surface of the tumor (see Fig. 13-17B). The tumor cells are similar to those of a well-differentiated endometrioid cancer.

Endometrioid Carcinomas With Squamous Component (Adenoacanthomas and Adenosquamous Carcinomas)

In 25% to 40% of endometrial adenocarcinomas, depending on sampling, a squamous epithelial component may be observed. **The histologic appearance of the squamous component may vary from deceptively benign to frankly malignant** epidermoid or squamous cancer (Fig. 13-6D). The term **adenoacanthoma** has now been dismissed but I still find it useful in describing tumors with the histologically benign squamous component. The tumor type with malignant squamous component is usually classified as **adenosquamous carcinoma.** There is little doubt, however, that, regardless of its degree of differentiation and microscopic appearance, **the squamous component in adenoacanthomas is malignant and even capable of metastases.** We observed several cases in which the metastatic foci in the lungs were represented solely by the "benign" squamous component. The malignant nature of the squamous component has been confirmed by comparative genomic hybridization studies performed in this laboratory, that documented the presence of chromosomal abnormalities similar to those occurring in cancerous glands (Baloglu et al, 2000).

In fact, in our experience, **the occurrence of squamous "metaplasia" in material from endometrial curettings** should always be viewed with suspicion, as it may represent fragments of low-grade adenoacanthoma. There is no known prognostic difference between endometrial adenocarcinomas with or without the squamous component (Marcus, 1961; Pokoly, 1970), although an unfavorable prognosis has been recorded for patients with adenosquamous carcinoma treated by radiotherapy (Ng et al, 1973). Pure **squamous cancers of the endometrium may occur, though rarely,** and usually in older women (Peris et al, 1958; White et al, 1973; Houissa-Vuong et al, 2002).

Precursor Lesions of Endometrioid Carcinoma: Endometrial Hyperplasia

It is commonly thought that endometrioid carcinoma is preceded by precursor stages of endometrial carcinoma known as **endometrial hyperplasia** of various types.

Risk Factors

Hyperplasia, which occurs mainly in premenopausal women, is caused by a **hormonal imbalance** in favor of estrogens and may result from **disturbances of ovulation,** such as the **Stein-Leventhal syndrome,** in which the estrogenic phase is not followed by a progesterone phase. Hormone-producing ovarian tumors, such as **theca or granulosa cell tumors,** may also produce endometrial hyperplasia. Simple hyperplasia may also be **associated with leiomyomas** (Deligdisch and Loewenthal, 1970). In postmenopausal women, administration of unopposed exogenous estrogens is a known cause of hyperplasia (the Writing Group for the PEPI Trial, 1996).

Clinical Features

The essential clinical feature of endometrial hyperplasia, regardless of type, is a **period of amenorrhea followed by uterine bleeding that may be excessive in amount (menorrhagia) or irregular (metrorrhagia).** In some patients, the bleeding may be fairly cyclic in character, whereas in others it is very irregularly spaced.

Histology

Although current textbooks and atlases of gynecologic pathology (e.g., Silverberg and Kurman, 1992) offer a variety of terms to describe various forms of endometrial hyperplasia, according to the configuration of the glands and the level of abnormalities in the epithelial lining, a simple classification is used here. **Three forms of endometrial hyperplasia** can be distinguished:

- Simple proliferative hyperplasia (endometrial hyperplasia with simple tubular glands without nuclear abnormalities)
- Cystic hyperplasia, which is probably a variant of simple hyperplasia
- Atypical hyperplasia (endometrial hyperplasia with nuclear abnormalities)

This classification disregards the configuration of the glands, but experience has shown that **in most hyperplasias** with nuclear abnormalities, the endometrial glands are abnormally configured.

Simple Proliferative Hyperplasia

Simple endometrial hyperplasia is an abnormality of endometrial growth in which the **equilibrium between the proliferative and the desquamative processes is disturbed in favor of the proliferative phase.** In this form of endometrial hyperplasia, the pattern of the endometrium is characterized primarily by an **increase in the number of tubular endometrial glands or their cross-sections per low-power field.** The glands are separated from each other by endometrial stroma. Often, the glands show slight **variability in size and irregular shapes** and thus differ from the normal, tubular proliferating glands, which appear round in cross-section (Fig. 13-7A,B). The **epithelial cells lining the hyperplastic glands** tend to pile up and are often arranged in a somewhat disorderly fashion (loss of polarity). Under high power of an optical microscope and, even more so, by scanning electron microscopy, **cilia are commonly observed on the surfaces of the endometrial glandular cells,** a feature normally associated with the estrogenic phase of endometrial proliferation (see Chapter 8). **Mitotic activity** may take place at all levels of the epithelium. The size of the nuclei reflects phases of the cell cycle. Most nuclei are of normal size. Occasionally, however, the nuclei are **slightly enlarged, reflecting late phases of cell cycle, and contain small nucleoli, changes that may also be observed in normal endometrium in proliferative phase.**

Simple proliferative hyperplasias **do not show any chromosomal abnormalities by comparative genetic hybridization** and, therefore, must be considered as a benign disorder (Baloglu et al, 2000). These lesions are **polyclonal by molecular techniques, whereas malignant lesions are usually monoclonal** (Mutter et al, 2000).

Clinical Significance. In many premenopausal women, the restoration of the ovulatory cycle by hormonal manipulation has resulted in the return to a normal endometrial pattern (the Writing Group for the PEPI Trial, 1996). Return to normal may also be expected after removal of estrogen-producing ovarian tumors. Yet, in rare cases, proliferative hyperplasia of long duration may become associated with atypical hyperplasia and endometrial carcinoma. Whether these are coexisting incidental events, as advocated by Horwitz et al (1981) or reflect some, as yet unknown, common pathway among these lesions, cannot be stated at this time.

Cystic Hyperplasia (Swiss Cheese Hyperplasia)

This disorder is seen mainly in peri- and postmenopausal women, although it may occasionally occur in premenopausal women. **The endometrial glands are of variable sizes but most are markedly dilated and cystic.** Their lumina are either empty or filled with amorphous material and debris. The epithelial lining of the glands is quite variable and may be separated into active and inactive forms. When the disease is observed **in premenopausal women, the gland lining is usually "active" and resembles that**

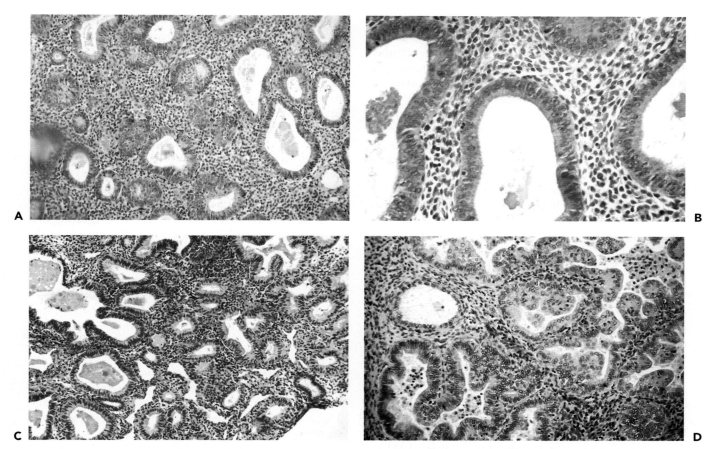

Figure 13-7   Endometrial hyperplasia and Hertig's carcinoma in situ. *A,B.* Simple endometrial hyperplasia with cystic dilatation of glands. The epithelium of these glands is often ciliated. *C.* Complex (atypical) hyperplasia in which the glands are numerous, crowded, and of unequal size and irregular configuration. *D.* A form of atypical endometrial hyperplasia in which the glands form papillary projections lined by tall cells with eosinophilic cytoplasm. This lesion, named **carcinoma in situ,** was observed by Hertig et al (1949) in endometrial curettage specimens obtained some years before the development of an endometrioid carcinoma.

of simple proliferative hyperplasia, described above. **In postmenopausal women, the gland lining is "inactive," consisting of a single layer of cuboidal cells without any evidence of proliferative activity.** In the latter situation, the disease must be differentiated from cystic atrophy of the endometrium (see Chap. 8).

It is likely that cystic hyperplasia represents an end stage of involution of the simple proliferative endometrial hyperplasia. The association of this form of hyperplasia with endometrial adenocarcinoma is uncommon, but I have repeatedly observed such lesions side by side.

Atypical Hyperplasia

Atypical or adenomatous hyperplasia is defined by an increase in the number of endometrial glands of various sizes and variable configuration per low-power field, usually associated with nuclear abnormalities in cells of the glandular epithelium (Fig. 13-7C). The atypical glands are separated from each other by endometrial stroma, although "back to back" glands, without intervening stroma, are also seen.

The epithelial cells in most of these lesions are similar to cancer cells because they are frequently enlarged, have

enlarged nuclei with prominent nucleoli, and show intense mitotic activity at all levels of the epithelium. As in endometrioid carcinomas, the **stroma may show accumulation of large macrophages.**

In an important retrospective study by Hertig et al (1949), the precursors of endometrioid carcinoma were classified as **endometrial carcinoma in situ,** to be differentiated from the newly established entity, **endometrial intraepithelial carcinoma (EIC),** the precursor lesion of the serous-papillary carcinoma. **Endometrial carcinoma in situ is a form of atypical hyperplasia** that was observed in prior endometrial biopsies and curettage material in women who subsequently developed endometrioid carcinomas. This lesion was characterized by endometrial glands of variable, irregular configuration, **lined with large, usually columnar cells with eosinophilic cytoplasm,** forming either single or multiple layers. Papillary proliferation and bridging of the lumen of the gland by proliferating epithelial cells may be observed. **The nuclei,** which occupy variable positions in relation to the lumen, **are enlarged, vesicular, and usually contain visible nucleoli.** The degree of cell abnormality is better appreciated if the gland lumen contains desquamated cells; these often show nuclear hyperchromasia and large nucleoli (Fig. 13-7D).

Comparative genomic hybridization disclosed that the atypical hyperplasia, even with trivial nuclear abnormalities, shares with endometrioid carcinoma a number of chromosomal abnormalities and, therefore, should be considered a precancerous lesion or an early stage of endometrioid carcinoma (Baloglu et al, 2000). It is not surprising, therefore, that in many instances the histologic differentiation of atypical hyperplasia from early carcinoma is a matter of dispute among competent pathologists. In fact, photographs of the two lesions in various publications could often be substituted for one another. One could repeat verbatim the statement regarding the differential diagnosis of precancerous lesions of the cervix, that "every debatable case could become a 'shopping slide,'" ultimately handled by ablation of the uterus, not out of knowledge, but out of desperation. The famous saying *"kein Karzinom aber besser heraus"* (not a carcinoma but better take it out), attributable to a German gynecologist, Halban (cited by Novak, 1956), pertains to atypical hyperplasia. Some observers proposed the term **endometrial intraepithelial neoplasia (EIM), to encompass atypical hyperplasia and well differentiated endometrioid carcinomas** (Sherman and Brown, 1979; Fox and Buckley, 1982), a term that reflects the realities of the situation. The term has been revived recently by an Endometrial Collaborative Group that included 19 gynecologic pathologists from several countries by adding molecular biologic criteria (Mutter et al, 2000). **Monoclonality and instability of microsatellites, were the principal molecular abnormalities linking EIM to endometrial carcinoma.**

The relationship of simple proliferative hyperplasia to atypical hyperplasia is not clear and one cannot rule out the possibility that the benign form may sometimes be transformed into the malignant form.

The differential diagnosis of endometrial hyperplasia in curetted material includes endometrial polyps, artifacts produced by dull curettes, secretory endometrium in the premenstrual stage showing see-saw appearance of endometrial glands, and the glands of the endometrial basal layer, which are often somewhat dilated and irregular in shape.

Role of Hyperplasia in the Genesis of Endometrial Carcinoma

Evidence for progression of atypical hyperplasia to carcinoma of the endometrium is relatively poor because most of these lesions cause symptoms and are treated, at least by curettage and hormonal manipulation, but not infrequently by hysterectomy. At the time of this writing (2004), few patients with these abnormalities are left untreated. The evidence of progression is based on older studies. A frequently cited study is that by Gusberg and Kaplan (1963) in which a group of patients with "adenomatous hyperplasia" were prospectively followed; several of them (about 10%) developed endometrial cancer. Anecdotal evidence of progression of endometrial hyperplasia to carcinoma was also provided by Foster and Montgomery (1965). In a retrospective study of 170 patients, Kurman et al (1985) classified hyperplasias according to the degree of nuclear abnor-

mality. Carcinoma developed in only 2 of 122 patients without significant cytologic atypia and in 11 of 48 women (23%) with "atypical" glands. The "progression" also depended on the complexity of the glandular pattern with "simple" lesions less likely to progress than "complex" lesions. Many of the lesions illustrated in the Kurman paper as "atypical complex hyperplasia" could be classified by other observers as a well-differentiated endometrioid carcinoma. Further, even though none of these patients were initially treated by hysterectomy, most received some form of treatment such as hormonal manipulation, curettage, or both. Hence, the rate of development of invasive cancer in untreated patients could be much higher.

However, **there is substantial evidence suggesting that endometrial hyperplasia is not a mandatory stage in the development of endometrioid carcinoma (or other types of endometrial cancer) that may also develop de novo, particularly in postmenopausal women.** The search for occult endometrial cancer (Koss et al, 1981, 1984) strongly suggested this possibility (see below). In an older contribution, Greene et al (1959) observed peripheral hyperplasia in only 10 of 120 cases of endometrial carcinomas. These authors expressed the view that, **"some (and probably the minority) of endometrial carcinomas are preceded by or possibly induced in or developed from areas of endometrial hyperplasia."** These observations are particularly valuable because they were published in 1959, before widespread use of hormones obscured endometrial pathology.

Based on a case control study, cited above, Horwitz and Feinstein (1978) proposed that **"endometrial hyperplasia and carcinoma may represent separate expressions of endometrial pathology, which may occur side by side, but do not necessarily follow each other. It is further suggested that the so-called atypical hyperplasia, a lesion most likely to 'progress' to invasive carcinoma, does in fact represent a low-grade endometrial carcinoma. The two lesions can only be separated from each other by a series of intricate and generally nonreproducible morphologic criteria."** Still, endometrial hyperplasia of whatever type must be construed as a warning sign that an endometrium is not cycling or not cycling properly and, therefore, is susceptible to neoplastic events. With luck and skill, the cytologic diagnosis of occult endometrial hyperplasia is sometimes possible either in cervicovaginal smears or in direct endometrial samples.

It has been reported that hormonal manipulation of atypical hyperplasia with progesterone and related drugs may occasionally restore the cycling endometrial pattern (the Writing Group for the PEPI Trial, 1996). Yet, in our experience, these drugs are rarely, if ever, curative of the disease. There is little doubt, however, that the presence of these abnormalities puts the untreated patient at risk for the development of endometrial carcinoma, although the degree of risk cannot be estimated in any individual patient.

Serous (Papillary Serous) Carcinoma

About 10% of endometrial cancers that are similar to ovarian tumors of comparable configuration have been recognized many years ago as tumors with poor prognosis, capable of forming metastases, even if diagnosed in early stages (Chen et al, 1985). The tumors are composed of **large malignant cells, often forming papillary structures** that may contain **psammoma bodies** (Spjut et al, 1964; Factor, 1974). It must be stressed, however, that psammoma bodies may also occur in endometrioid carcinoma, in benign endometria, and endometrial polyps in the absence of cancer. Quite often, the tumors infiltrate the myometrium as poorly formed glands or solid strands of tumor cells. **Mutation of p53 gene** occurs in the primary tumor and its metastases (Baergen et al, 2001).

Precursor Lesions of Serous Carcinoma

Recent studies of this group of tumors traced their origin to **malignant changes in the surface endometrium** and adjacent glands that has been labeled **endometrial intraepithelial carcinoma** (Fig.13-8A,B), **and which is characterized by expression of mutated protein p53** (Sherman et al, 1992, 1995, 2000). On the surface, the lesion is composed of a single or double layer of large cancer cells with large nuclei and nucleoli, sometimes in a palisade arrangement. Adjacent glands show similar changes. Mitotic activity is abundant. The proponents of EIC avoided the use of the term **endometrial carcinoma in situ,** an abnormality

of **endometrial glands,** described by Hertig et al (1949) as a precursor lesion of endometrioid carcinoma, discussed above. It has been proposed that the genesis of serous endometrial carcinoma follows a different pathway from endometrioid carcinoma and is unrelated to endometrial hyperplasia (Sherman et al, 1992, 1995, 2000).

Rare Histologic Variants of Endometrial Carcinoma

Endometrial carcinomas may show evidence of secretory activity **(secretory carcinomas)** that may be a mucin-like substance **(mucinous carcinomas).** Such tumors should be differentiated from endocervical carcinoma. Some endometrial tumors are composed of "clear" cells, i.e., cells with transparent cytoplasm, showing cell arrangement not unlike that seen in similar tumors of the uterine cervix and vagina **(clear cell carcinomas; Fig. 13-8C).** Other rare types of endometrial cancer include **carcinomas with argyrophilic cells** (Ueda et al, 1979; Aguirre et al, 1984), **small cell (oat cell) type** (Paz et al, 1984), carcinoma with "**glassy cell features**" (Arends et al, 1984), **carcinoma with ciliated cells** (Hendrickson and Kempson, 1983; Gould et al, 1986; Maksem, 1997) and **carcinoma with giant cells,** resembling osteoclasts (Fig. 13-8D) (Jones et al, 1991).

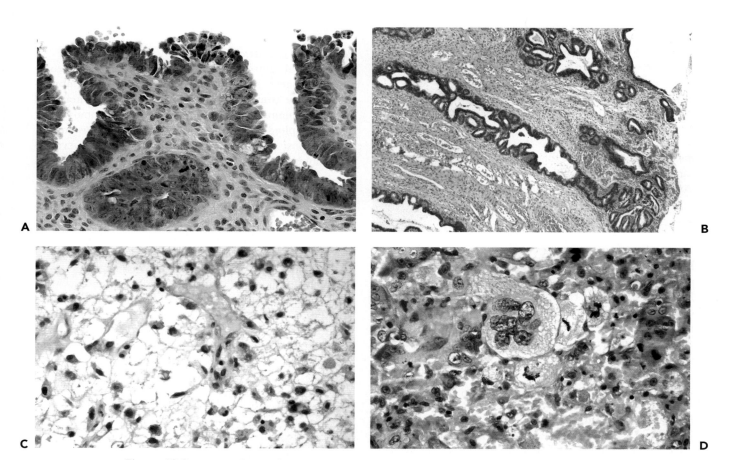

Figure 13-8 **Various forms of endometrial carcinoma.** *A.* An example of intraepithelial carcinoma on the endometrial surface, notable for the expression of mutated p53 gene. *B.* Extension of the intraepithelial carcinoma to endometrial glands (hysterectomy specimen). *C.* An example of clear cell carcinoma. *D.* An example of endometrial adenocarcinoma with multinucleated giant cells. (*A,B:* courtesy of Dr. Robert Kurman, Johns Hopkins, Baltimore, MD.)

Occasionally, endometrial carcinomas are composed in part of spindly malignant cells (**spindle cell carcinomas or carcinosarcomas**). The differential diagnosis of these tumors with mesodermal mixed tumors is discussed in Chapter 17.

Staging and Prognosis

Endometrial carcinoma is staged according to the spread of the disease. In **stage I,** the disease is confined to the corpus, subdivided into **Ia** (depth of uterine canal less than 8 cm) and **Ib** (depth of uterine canal 8 cm or more). **Stage II** disease indicates involvement of corpus *and* cervix. **Stage III** indicates extension beyond the uterus but still confined within the bony pelvis, and **stage IV** indicates spread to the bladder and/or rectum, or evidence of distant metastases. Tambouret et al (2003) pointed out that extension of endometrial carcinoma to the uterine cervix may have a deceptively benign appearance in histologic sections. The role of **peritoneal washings** in staging of endometrial cancer is discussed in Chapter 16. Staging may also include **histologic grade (G) of the lesion,** discussed above, with G1 indicating a well-differentiated carcinoma, G3 poorly differentiated cancer, and G2 cancer of an intermediate grade. Poor prognosis of serous carcinoma, regardless of stage, has been mentioned above.

The results of treatment are by no means spectacular; only stage I G1 lesions respond well and offer a nearly 100% 5-year cure. For all stages and grades, the 5-year survival rate is only about 65%, and this figure has not changed much over the years (Frick et al, 1973; Prem et al, 1979; Robboy and Bradley, 1979; Partridge et al, 1996). More recent figures, based on a very large cohort of women in Norway, reported 5-year survival for all stages at 78% and 10-year survival at 67% (Abeler et al, 1992). The survival was stage dependent, with best results reported for stage I disease, and the poorest for stage IV. Hence, endometrial carcinoma is a serious, often misunderstood, disease and its early detection is a worthwhile undertaking.

Other Features of Prognostic Significance

Tumor Ploidy

DNA ploidy measurements have been shown to be of prognostic value in endometrial carcinoma (Atkin, 1984; Iverson and Laerum, 1985; Iverson and Utaaker, 1988; and others). It has been documented that tumors with approximately diploid DNA content have a better prognosis than aneuploid tumors. In general, well-differentiated endometrioid carcinomas have a diploid DNA content but occasionally higher grade tumors are also in the diploid range of measurements.

Morphometric Studies

Baak et al (1988) reported that combined architectural and nuclear morphometric features in tissue sections were a more accurate predictor of behavior of endometrial hyperplasia than nuclear features alone. This elaborate study requiring costly instrumentation and dedicated personnel is not likely to be of practical value in the laboratory.

Steroid Receptors

These studies have documented the presence of estrogen and progesterone receptors in most endometrial carcinomas and in some metastases (Ehrlich et al, 1981; Kauppila et al, 1982; Creasman et al, 1985; Utaaker et al, 1987). Lower-stage, better-differentiated tumors appear to have higher levels of both receptors and better prognosis than the receptor-negative tumors. The presence of receptors in metastases may be used as a guide in hormonal manipulation and treatment of disseminated disease.

Molecular Studies

The presence of **mutated p53 protein** in serous carcinoma and, to a much lesser extent, in advanced endometrioid carcinomas, has been documented by Bur et al (1992) and by Sherman et al (1995). The presence of mutated p53 may be an expression of the documented poor prognosis of serous carcinoma. **Epidermal growth factor (EGF) expression** was extensively studied in endometrial cancer with conflicting results. While some investigators found the increased expression of this factor to be correlated with stage and grade of the disease (Battaglia et al, 1989), others failed to confirm these findings (Reynolds et al, 1990; Nyholm et al, 1993; Jassoni et al, 1994). It is of interest that Jassoni et al recorded the highest expression of EGF in adenoacanthomas. Cell cycle regulators, such as **proteins related to the Rb gene,** are down-regulated in atypical hyperplasia and adenocarcinoma (Susini et al, 2001).

Molecular Genetic Studies

Baloglu et al (2001) have shown by the technique of comparative genetic hybridization that **chromosomal abnormalities are common in endometrioid carcinomas and in their squamous component.** Excess of chromosome 1 (at least triploidy), and gains and losses of chromosome 10, are the most common features, confirming direct cytogenetic observations. The reader is referred to the article cited for a detailed analysis of these abnormalities.

It has been documented that **endometrial cancers (and some atypical hyperplasias) are monoclonal in reference to chromosome X,** i.e., the tumors contain two X chromosomes, both of either maternal or paternal origin, whereas benign tissues and lesions are polyclonal, i.e., contain one chromosome each of maternal and paternal origin (summary in Mutter et al, 2000). It has also been observed that a subset of endometrial carcinomas show **microsatellite instability,** i.e., a change in the size of repetitive DNA sequences, known as microsatellites (Reisinger et al, 1993; Duggan et al, 1994). It remains to be seen whether these observations are of prognostic significance.

CYTOLOGIC PRESENTATION OF ENDOMETRIAL CARCINOMAS IN ROUTINE CERVICOVAGINAL SAMPLES

General Appearance

The **smears** from fully developed endometrial carcinomas are often characterized by the **presence of inflammation, necrotic material, and fresh and old (fibrinated) blood**

(Fig. 13-9). The latter may be observed in asymptomatic patients in the absence of clinical evidence of bleeding and may confer upon the smear a peculiar yellow-orange discoloration. The finding is more common in vaginal pool smears than in cervical samples. Such smears must be carefully screened for evidence of endometrial cancer, particularly in perimenopausal or postmenopausal patients. In **liquid samples,** this background **may be lost.**

Hormonal Pattern

In advanced cancer, the hormonal pattern is not distinctive and is of little diagnostic help, even though high maturation of squamous cells may be observed occasionally in a postmenopausal patient. Patients with *early* stages of endometrial carcinoma are more likely to display excellent maturation of squamous cells (Fig. 13-10A).

Recognition of Endometrial Cancer Cells

Endometrial cancer cells, usually accompanied by leukocytes and macrophages, **are often poorly preserved, concealed by blood and debris** and are difficult to identify

under the scanning power of the microscope (see Fig. 13-9A). Therefore, the cytologic evidence of disease is often very scanty. The finding of endometrial cancer cells **in cervicovaginal smears** usually indicates the presence of **a fully developed endometrial carcinoma which may be occult.** When interrogated, most patients report a history of spotting.

Cells of endometrial adenocarcinoma occur **singly and in clusters of various sizes. Their appearance varies in keeping with the degree of tumor differentiation.** Reagan and Ng (1973) used planimetry in the evaluation of cells of endometrial adenocarcinoma, and pointed out that the number of malignant cells in smears, the size of such cells, the size of their nuclei, and the degree of nucleolar abnormalities increase in proportion to the degree of histologic abnormality of the parent tumor. In our experience, high degrees of cytologic abnormalities in smears usually, though not always, correspond to fully invasive tumors.

Well-Differentiated Carcinomas

Single Cancer Cells

In such tumors, the single cancer cells are often **inconspicuous and small,** measuring from 10 to 20 μm in diameter

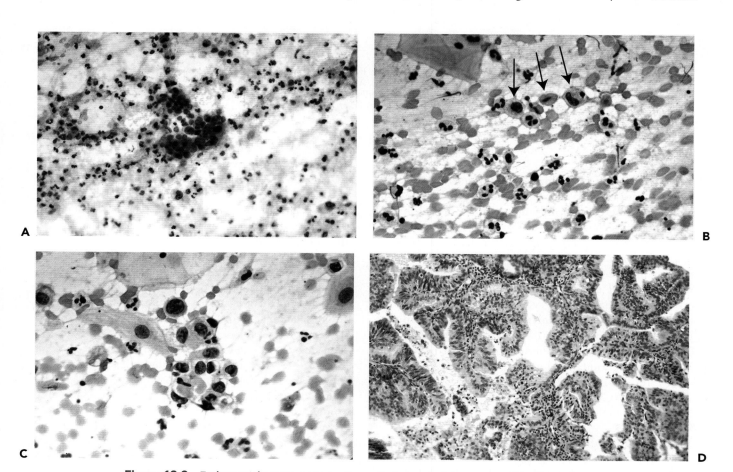

Figure 13-9 **Endometrial carcinoma in cervicovaginal smears.** *A.* Low-power view of two clusters of endometrial cells against a background of marked inflammation. *B.* Higher power view of some of the inconspicuous small cancer cells (*arrows*) and macrophages. Note a mature squamous cell in the background. *C.* A cluster of cancer cells of various shapes and sizes. Some of the cells are cuboidal. The nuclear abnormalities consist of enlargement, coarse granulation, and the presence of nucleoli. *D.* Papillary endometrioid carcinoma corresponding to smears shown in *A–C.*

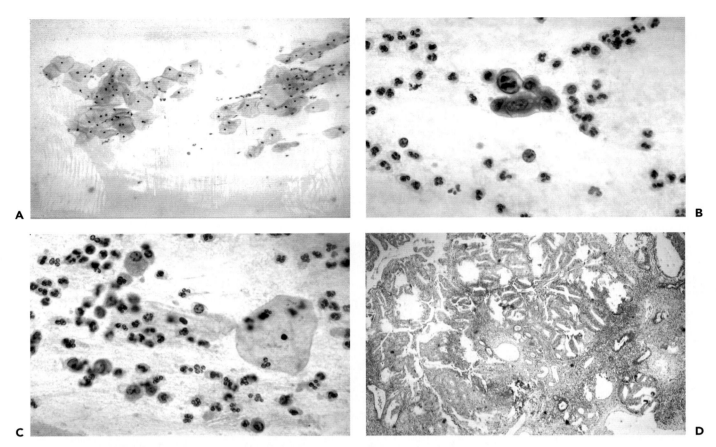

Figure 13-10 **Endometrial adenocarcinoma in cervicovaginal smears.** *A.* The smear pattern shows very high maturation of squamous cells. *B.* A cluster of endometrial cancer cells, one showing vacuolated cytoplasm and one showing nuclear enlargement. *C.* Numerous macrophages in a vaginal pool smear from the same patient. *D.* Endometrioid carcinoma grade II.

and, hence, are about the size of small parabasal squamous cells (see Figs. 13-9B,C and 13-10C). The cells are usually roughly **spherical, cuboidal or columnar.** Their **cytoplasm is bluish or slate gray in color, very delicate, and poorly outlined. Cytoplasmic vacuoles** are commonly present but vary in size and may be small and inconspicuous or occupy much of the cytoplasm. In the latter instance, the cells often assume the **signet-ring appearance** with the nucleus in eccentric position. Some of these cancer cells **resemble small macrophages.** As is common in mucus-producing tumor cells, the cytoplasmic vacuoles are sometimes **infiltrated with polymorphonuclear leukocytes** that may obscure the details of cell structure (Fig. 13-11C). **The nuclei are usually spherical, somewhat hyperchromatic, finely granular and often, but not always, contain small, but clearly visible nucleoli** (see Figs. 13-9C, 13-10B, 13-11A–C).

Cell Clusters

Well-differentiated endometrioid adenocarcinoma is easier to identify if the cancer cells occur in clusters. The clusters may be small and made up of only a few cells (Figs. 13-9C and 13-10B) or they may be larger. The clusters are often obscured by fresh or fibrinated blood and necrotic debris. The **cells forming the small clusters are often cuboidal or columnar in shape** and are characterized by somewhat

granular spherical nuclei, usually provided with small but **clearly discernible nucleoli** (see Fig. 13-11B). Sometimes, the cancer cells form **rosette-like clusters** (see Fig.13-11B). In larger clusters, which are sometimes of spherical (papillary) configuration, the small cancer cells are usually piled up, one on top of the other, and their identity may be difficult to establish.

The greatest **challenge** in cytology of well-differentiated endometrial carcinoma is the **identification and recognition** of endometrial origin of the often inconspicuous small cells, let alone their diagnostic significance. The **interpretation** of such preparations is often extremely difficult, particularly in the absence of symptoms.

In many such tumors, there are no detectable cytologic abnormalities at all and only **morphologically normal endometrial cells,** singly and in clusters, are observed. This finding is **particularly important in postmenopausal women.** In one of the very few papers dealing with cytology of **well differentiated (low-grade) endometrial carcinomas,** Gu et al (2001) observed that only 43% of 44 such patients had abnormal cervicovaginal samples, when compared with 72% (23 of 32) for high grade lesions (see below).

The **most important point of differential diagnosis** of clusters of endometrial cancer cells is **with atypical endocervical cells.** The endometrial cells are usually smaller than

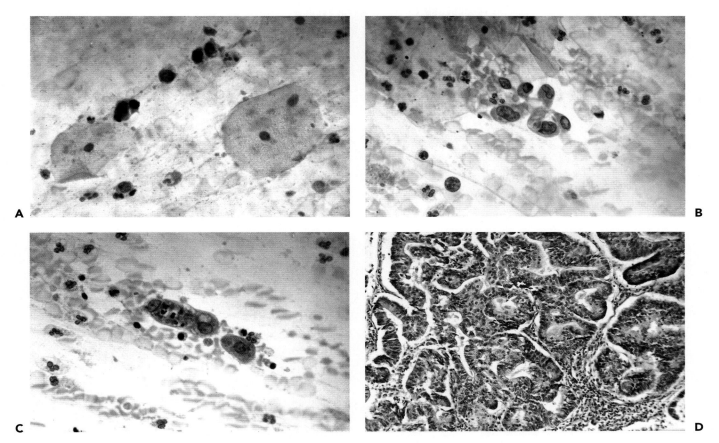

Figure 13-11 **Occult endometrial adenocarcinoma diagnosed in cervicovaginal smears.** *A.* A string of small cancer cells with hyperchromatic nuclei and very scanty cytoplasm against a background of high maturation of squamous cells. *B.* A cluster of very characteristic endometrial cells, some of columnar configuration, all showing enlarged granular nuclei, some containing nucleoli. *C.* Isolated poorly preserved endometrial cells, one with cytoplasm unfiltrated by neutrophiles. *D.* Asymptomatic endometrioid carcinoma, grade II, found in this patient.

endocervical cells and their cytoplasm is pale, scanty, and not sharply demarcated, whereas the cytoplasm of endocervical cells is usually more abundant and crisply outlined. Still, when the endometrial cells are of columnar shape, the distinction may be very difficult. Clinical history may help: endometrial cancer cells are most often encountered in perior postmenopausal women whereas the atypical endocervical cells occur mainly in younger age groups. Exceptions to these rules, however, occur quite often.

High-Grade (Poorly Differentiated) Endometrial Carcinomas

Single Cells

Single cells of high-grade endometrioid carcinomas (and papillary-serous carcinomas, as emphasized by Wright et al, 1999) are much easier to recognize. The **cancer cells are large, measuring from 15 to 30 μm in diameter, and are usually provided with large, granular or homogeneous nuclei, often containing large, sometimes multiple nucleoli** (Fig. 13-12). Less often the nuclei are finely granular or even clear. **Enlarged and multiple nucleoli are an important diagnostic feature of the endometrial cancer cells in high grade tumors.** The nucleoli may not be visible in poorly preserved dark nuclei but usually stand out in better preserved cells. Long et al (1958) found a direct correlation

between the number and the size of the nucleoli and tumor differentiation: In poorly differentiated tumors the number and the size of the nucleoli per nucleus were larger than in well-differentiated carcinomas.

The **cytoplasm** of the endometrial cancer cells is often distended by **vacuoles** of variable sizes. It may also be infiltrated with polymorphonuclear leukocytes. Sometimes, very bizarre cancer cells may be observed (Fig. 13-13A,B). The derivation of such cells may be difficult to establish.

Cell Clusters

In their most **conspicuous and classic form, the clusters are of oval or round papillary configuration and are made up of clearly malignant cells with scanty, frayed, basophilic cytoplasm and large, hyperchromatic nuclei** (Fig. 13-13C,D). The size of the component cells in clusters may vary and is related to the grade of the tumor. In relatively well-differentiated endometrial carcinomas, the cancer cells are generally smaller than in high-grade, poorly differentiated tumors. In all tumor grades, however, **conspicuous nuclear abnormalities are present: there is nuclear enlargement, nuclear hyperchromasia of varying degrees, and the presence of visible, occasionally large, sometimes multiple, and often irregularly shaped nucleoli.** The clusters are usually accompanied by single, clas-

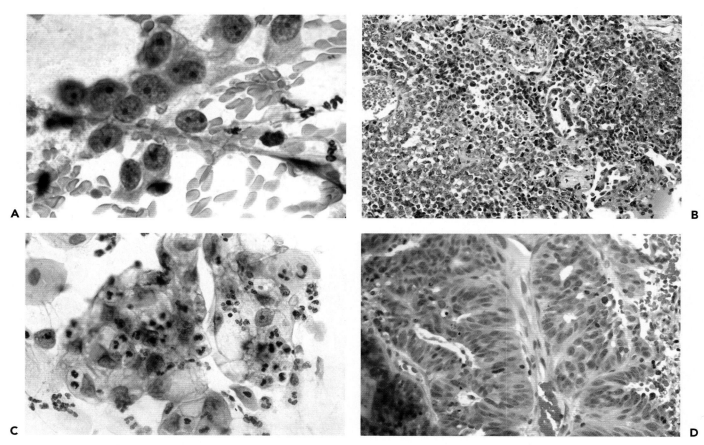

Figure 13-12   High grade endometrial carcinoma in cervicovaginal smears. *A.* A cluster of large cancer cells at higher magnification to show markedly enlarged nuclei and irregular nucleoli. The smear background shows blood and mature squamous cells. *B.* High-grade, poorly differentiated tumor corresponding to *A. C.* Endometrial cancer cells showing large nuclei with prominent nucleoli and vacuolated cytoplasm, occasionally infiltrated by neutrophiles. *D.* Endometrial carcinoma corresponding to *C.*

sic cancer cells elsewhere in the preparation. Similar clusters may reflect ovarian or tubal carcinomas (see Chap. 15).

The presence of **psammoma bodies** in cases of endometrioid or serous carcinoma has been reported by Spjut et al (1964), Factor (1974), and Parkash and Carcangiu (1997). This finding is rare in cytologic preparations of carcinomas of the endometrium and much more common in ovarian cancer (see Chap. 15).

Macrophages (Histiocytes) in the Diagnosis of Endometrial Carcinoma

In our original contribution on the subject of endometrial carcinoma (Koss and Durfee, 1962), it was pointed out that, in **vaginal pool smears,** the presence of **macrophages (or of endometrial cancer cells mimicking macrophages)** is of help in the recognition of endometrial disease (Fig. 13-14). These observations were subsequently **re-examined** by various observers in **cervical smears** with negative results (Zucker et al, 1985; Nguyen et al, 1998; Tambouret et al, 2001). **We have repeatedly emphasized that the finding of macrophages in cervical smears is of no diagnostic value and that the negative results of these studies could**

be fully anticipated. Still, **macrophages and macrophage-like cells** may accompany cells of endometrial adenocarcinoma but rarely tumor cells of other origins (see Figs. 13-11C and 13-14C). These cells have a delicately vacuolated cytoplasm and a round or kidney-shaped, occasionally eccentric nucleus. They may vary considerably in size. The origin of these cells appears to be endometrial stroma, which often contains islands of similar cells in histologic sections, as described above (see Fig. 13-6B,C). **Macrophages of this type may be, at times, the only evidence of endometrial cancer,** particularly in postmenopausal patients, **but are not diagnostic of this disease.** Still, their presence may lead the experienced observer to call for additional investigation of the endometrium. These observations were recently confirmed by Wen et al (2003). These authors reported that the presence of macrophages alone, in the absence of endometrial cells in cervicovaginal smears, led to the diagnosis of endometrial pathology (mainly polyps, but also carcinomas) in several patients.

Cells of Adenoacanthoma and Adenosquamous Carcinoma

It is sometimes possible to diagnose adenoacanthoma or adenosquamous carcinoma on cytologic evidence. In such

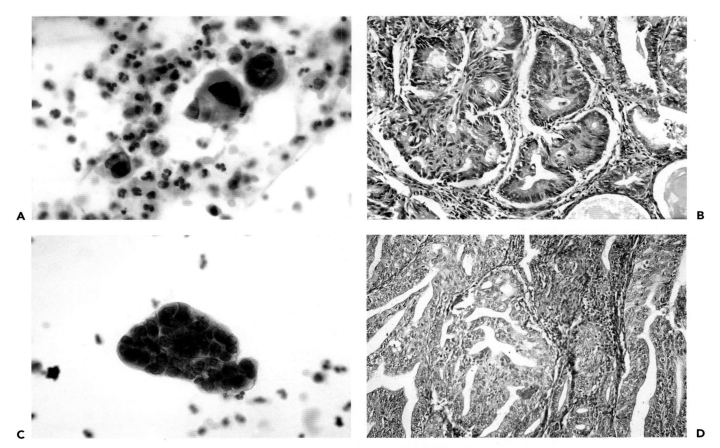

Figure 13-13   Various cytologic presentations of endometrial carcinoma. *A.* Very large, poorly differentiated tumor cells. Such cells are rarely found in endometrial cancer. *B.* Moderately differentiated, but focally markedly atypical, endometrioid carcinoma corresponding to *A. C.* Vaginal pool smear showing a papillary cluster of cancer cells that could be of endometrial, ovarian, or tubal origin. *D.* Endometrial carcinoma corresponding to *C.*

cases, the preparations contain **cells of endometrial adenocarcinoma and atypical or frankly malignant squamous cells** (Figs. 13-15 and 13-16). Usually, the squamous cells **differ somewhat from cells of cervical squamous carcinoma;** their cytoplasm is sometimes **deeply keratinized,** and they tend to be **round or oval and lack the irregularity of shape seen in cervical cancer** (Fig. 13-15C). Buschmann et al (1974) referred to some such cells as **"keratin bodies."** In extreme cases, fragments of keratin may be seen. The configuration of malignant squamous cells does not always provide a clue to the nature of the endometrial tumor. **Thus, squamous cancer cells may be observed either in adenosquamous carcinoma or in low grade adenoacanthoma.** The latter cases confirm the malignant nature of the seemingly benign "metaplastic" squamous component. Baloglu et al (2001) studied the foci of squamous differentiation in one such lesion by **comparative genomic hybridization and observed in it chromosomal abnormalities consistent with endometrioid carcinoma, thus confirming that the squamous component is an integral part of the malignant tumor.**

Rare Types of Endometrial Carcinomas

We have observed examples of superficial **villoglandular carcinoma.** The lesion shed papillary cell clusters composed

of large cells with abundant eosinophilic cytoplasm and large, pale nuclei with visible nucleoli (Fig. 13-17A,B). We also observed a case of the very rare **clear cell carcinoma.** The large tumor cells with clear cytoplasm formed glandular structures, diagnostic of adenocarcinoma (Fig. 13-17C,D). The tumor type came as a surprise.

Praca et al (1998) described a case of the extremely rare **neuroendocrine small cell carcinoma** of the endometrium. The cytologic pattern of small malignant cells could not be distinguished from similar tumors of the uterine cervix.

Tumor Typing in Cytologic Samples

Although well-differentiated endometrioid carcinomas have a reasonably characteristic cytologic presentation, described above, **the precise histologic type of endometrial carcinoma can rarely be established in cytologic material. High grade endometrioid carcinomas, their variants, and serous-papillary carcinomas shed similar cells.**

When endometrial adenocarcinomas shed **papillary cell clusters,** the differential diagnosis must comprise **adenocarcinomas of the fallopian tube and ovary and adenocarcinomas of other origins metastatic to the female genital tract.** If only **single, large cancer cells** are present in the

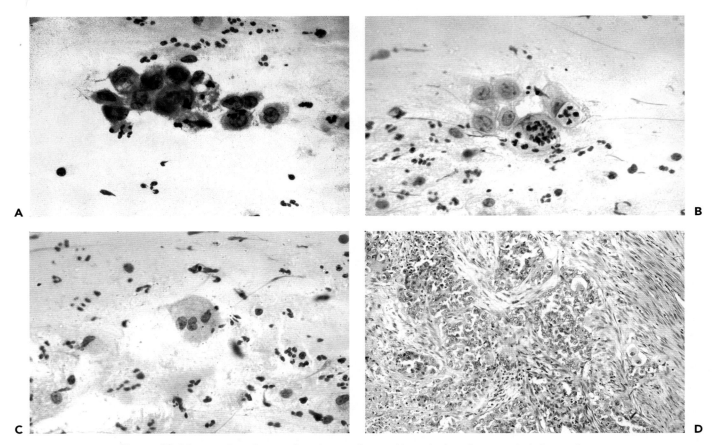

Figure 13-14 Occult endometrial carcinoma observed in vaginal pool smears. *A.* A cluster of endometrial cancer cells showing large granular nuclei and occasional nucleoli. *B.* Poorly preserved small endometrial cancer cells, some with the vacuolated cytoplasm infiltrated by neutrophiles. *C.* Multinucleated macrophages shown in the same smear. The presence of macrophages is of interest only **in vaginal smears** (see text). *D.* Endometrial carcinoma with marked stromal reaction.

cytologic sample, **the differential diagnosis should include other cancers, such as a poorly differentiated squamous (epidermoid) carcinoma and other poorly differentiated primary or metastatic tumors.** Tissue evidence and immunohistochemistry may solve the problem in some, but not necessarily all, the cases.

Although the adenoacanthomas and adenosquamous carcinomas of the endometrium have a characteristic presentation, described above, they still have to be differentiated from coexisting endocervical adenocarcinoma and epidermoid carcinoma and adenosquamous carcinomas of the endocervix. The squamous component of all these lesions may be similar or identical but there is a difference in the configuration of the cells of endometrial and endocervical adenocarcinomas (see Chap. 12).

Efficacy of Cytologic Diagnosis

In our experience, about 65% of all cases of endometrial adenocarcinoma may be diagnosed in the now rarely used **vaginal smears** (Koss and Durfee, 1962). The **cervical smears** will yield a positive diagnosis in about 25% of cases. Nonetheless, the cytologic suggestion or diagnosis of endometrial carcinoma may be of diagnostic assistance if clinical symptoms of endometrial cancer are inadequately reported

by the patient or improperly interpreted by the physician. In such patients, the cytologic diagnosis of endometrial carcinoma may come as a surprise to the clinical provider but requires further investigation with beneficial diagnostic and therapeutic results (Table 13-1).

The cytologic presentation of endometrial adenocarcinoma in direct endometrial samples is described below.

Pitfalls

- **Menstrual smears.** As repeatedly mentioned, endometrial cells and cell clusters may be found in cervicovaginal smears until the 12th day of the cycle, hence for several days after the cessation of the clinical bleeding. Therefore, one should **abstain from making the diagnosis of endometrial carcinoma in menstruating patients.**
- **Intrauterine contraceptive devices** may result in endometrial shedding, particularly at mid-cycle.
- **Effects of hormonal medication.** One of the most important pitfalls in evaluation of the endometrium in postmenopausal women is the effect of hormones. **All hormones,** whether estrogen, progesterone, androgens, or corticosteroids, **may stimulate endometrial growth** to varying degrees, resulting in **shedding of endometrial**

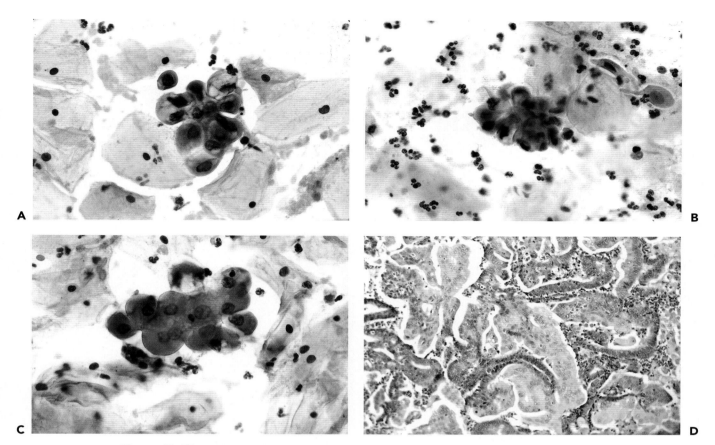

Figure 13-15 **Endometrial adenoacanthoma in cervicovaginal smears in a 68-year-old woman.**
A. Endometrial cancer cells with vacuolated cytoplasm. *B.* A papillary rosette-like cluster of endometrial cancer cells. *C.* Endometrial cancer cells surrounding spherical, extremely well-differentiated squamous cells. *D.* Tissue section corresponding to *A–C* showing an endometrioid carcinoma with well-differentiated squamous component.

cells. If the pattern of the cervicovaginal smear is atrophic prior to therapy, any of these hormones but especially estrogens (and other **drugs, such as Tamoxifen and digitalis**), may produce improved maturation of the squamous cells (see Chap. 18). These effects have been observed by us even after administration of beauty creams with hormones. **Withdrawal bleeding,** particularly after the use of estrogens, may produce the perfect picture of endometrial carcinoma: high maturation of squamous cells, presence of endometrium and blood. Similar findings may be observed in women wearing IUDs (see above).

■ In material from patients receiving **contraceptive hormones with high progestin content, single endocervical cells with enlarged, hyperchromatic nuclei, may appear,** rendering the differential diagnosis very difficult (see Chaps. 10 and 18). The only way to avoid the pitfalls of these iatrogenic situations is to obtain an accurate history of medications and to insist on histologic confirmation of any cytologic suspicion of endometrial carcinoma.

■ **Endometrial polyps** may shed atypical endometrial cells that may be mistaken for cancer. Other disorders of endometrium that may mimic carcinoma are **chronic inflammatory processes,** particularly tuberculosis, re-

generating endometrium, and **Arias-Stella cells** (see Chap. 8). Ehrman (1975) described two cases of postmenopausal women with cytologic findings suggestive of endometrial carcinoma, caused by atypical endometrial lining overlying **foci of stromal breakdown.** Ehrman pointed out that similar abnormalities may occur during normal menstrual bleeding and that the nuclei of endometrial epithelial cells may be very large and contain conspicuous nucleoli.

CYTOLOGIC DIAGNOSIS OF ENDOMETRIAL HYPERPLASIA IN ROUTINE CYTOLOGIC SAMPLES

Most patients with endometrial hyperplasia, regardless of type, are symptomatic and offer few opportunities for a cytologic diagnosis. Occasionally, however, there occurs an asymptomatic (or minimally symptomatic) patient in whom the diagnosis of hyperplasia may be attempted in routine smears. Much of the confusion in the literature pertaining to the cytologic diagnosis of endometrial hyperplasia is caused by lack of correlation of the cytologic findings with histology. The findings differ according to the histologic patterns of the

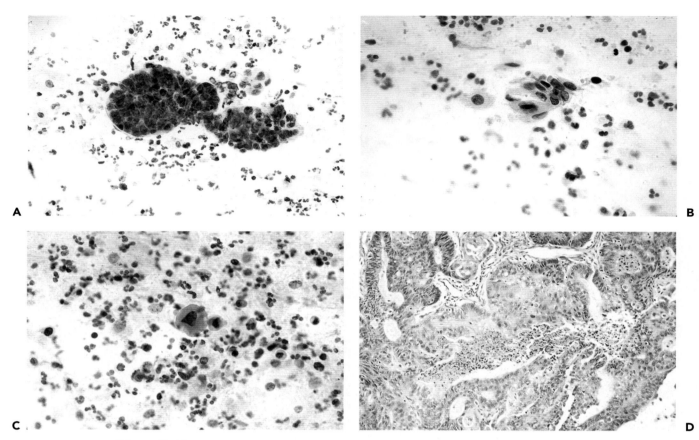

Figure 13-16 **Endometrial adenoacanthoma.** *A.* Two large papillary clusters of endometrial cancer cells. *B,C.* Isolated, well-differentiated squamous cancer cells in the same smear. *D.* Adenoacanthoma corresponding to *A–C.*

lesions. The only feature that these disease states may have in common is the hormonal pattern in smears.

Hormonal Pattern

Premenopausal Women

Sequential vaginal smears in women with endometrial hyperplasia may show a fairly constant pattern of maturation of squamous cells *without the customary cyclic variations.* The maturation is not necessarily very high and may remain moderate for long periods of time. **The assessment of the hormonal status in a single cervicovaginal smear may be highly misleading.** Only multiple smears repeated over several cycles may provide this information (see Chap. 9).

Postmenopausal Women

In these patients, there is usually a pattern of good maturation of squamous epithelium. As has been emphasized before, **such findings in postmenopausal patients are not necessarily abnormal** and only a constant, very high level of maturation of squamous cells **in the absence of medication of any type** may be considered unusual.

Endometrial Cells

Simple Proliferative and Cystic Hyperplasia

In the rare asymptomatic patients with simple proliferative or cystic endometrial hyperplasia, there is limited sponta-

neous shedding of endometrial cells, except during episodes of bleeding. In routine cytologic preparations, the **cells shed from hyperplastic endometrial glands resemble normal endometrial cells in size and appearance.** Rarely, there is slight nuclear enlargement and hyperchromasia and small nucleoli can be visualized (see Fig. 10-18A,B). In several personally observed **premenopausal patients** who did not wear IUDs, the possibility of endometrial hyperplasia could be suggested because of the presence of morphologically normal endometrial cells past the 12th day of the cycle.

In **postmenopausal patients, the finding of endometrial cells in routine smears may indicate either a hyperplasia** *or* **a carcinoma, and the cytologic diagnosis of hyperplasia should not be attempted.** All such patients should be investigated by biopsy or curettage.

Atypical Hyperplasia

The cells shed from **atypical endometrial hyperplasia cannot be differentiated from cells of a well-differentiated endometrioid carcinoma, described above.** In several such personally observed cases, the diagnosis of atypical hyperplasia was established in histologic material and could be, as always, a matter for some dispute (Fig. 13-18C,D).

These observations were confirmed by Ng, Reagan, and Cechner (1973) who studied the cell patterns and features of endometrial cells in endocervical aspiration smears of 116 women with various forms of endometrial hyperplasia and

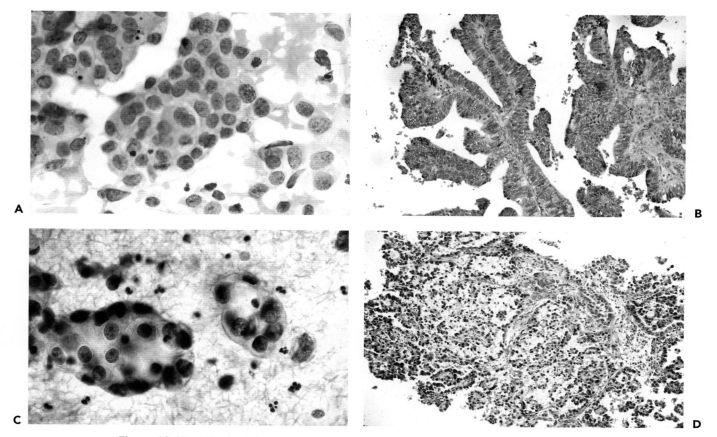

Figure 13-17   Villoglandular and clear cell carcinomas. *A.* A large papillary cluster of well-differentiated endometrial cancer cells with large nucleoli. *B.* In the tissue section corresponding to *A,* the typical villoglandular pattern of an endometrial cancer. *C.* Papillary clusters of large cells with clear cytoplasm, large nuclei, and nucleoli, corresponding to the tissue section of a clear cell endometrial carcinoma shown in *D.*

endometrial carcinoma in situ, as defined by Hertig et al (1949), and observed that the degree of cytologic abnormality was related to the severity of histologic abnormality.

Endometrial Lesions in Endocervical Brush Specimens

Although the endocervical brushes were not designed to sample the endometrium, vigorous brushing may reach the lower segments of the uterine cavity. As has been discussed in Chapter 8, benign endometrial cells may be found in such samples and constitute a known source of diagnostic

error. **Occasionally, however, the endocervical sample contains evidence of an endometrial lesion.** An example of markedly atypical endometrial hyperplasia discovered in an endocervical brush specimen is shown in Figure 13-19.

CYTOLOGY OF DIRECT ENDOMETRIAL SAMPLES

Instruments

Over the years, many instruments have been introduced for purposes of direct endometrial sampling. Some of the

TABLE 13-1		
ENDOMETRIAL ADENOCARCINOMA IN SYMPTOMATIC PATIENTS: VAGINAL SMEARS ONLY		
Total Cases	**Positive**	**No Diagnosable Cancer**
63 (100%)	40 (63.5%)*	23 (37.1%)

* In 8 cases, cytology contributed significantly to speedy diagnosis. (Koss LG, Durfee GR. Cytologic diagnosis of endometrial carcinoma. Result of ten years of experience. Acta Cytol 6:519–531, 1962.)

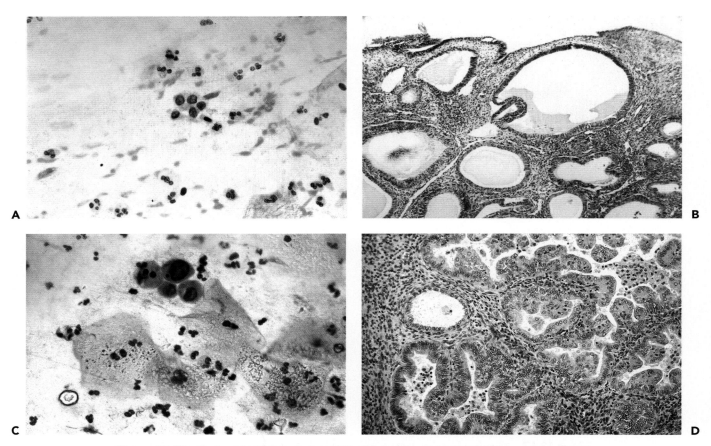

Figure 13-18   Endometrial hyperplasia and Hertig's carcinoma in situ. *A.* A cluster of small endometrial cells corresponding to cystic hyperplasia shown in *B. C.* A cluster of abnormal endometrial cells, one with large nucleus, corresponding to the classical Hertig's carcinoma in situ shown in *D.* The cells in *A* are benign in configuration. The cells in *C* could be classified as endometrial carcinoma.

instruments were to replace an endometrial biopsy or even curettage in symptomatic or "high-risk" patients. Other instruments were proposed as "screening" tools for the detection of occult carcinoma or hyperplasia. The goal of all these instruments was to secure an adequate sample of the endometrium, without causing much discomfort to the patient.

The first such device, with which the writer had personal experience, was a simple endometrial aspiration cannula, introduced by the late Dr. Michael Jordan in the 1950s. The cannula was used as an office instrument on high-risk patients and led to the discovery of a number of occult endometrial hyperplasias and carcinomas (Jordan et al, 1956; also see below). Numerous sampling instruments were subsequently introduced, among them the endometrial brush (Johnsson and Stormby, 1968), Gravlee's negative-pressure jet wash (Gravlee, 1969), an endometrial "pistol" (Bouchardy et al, 1987), Mendhosa cannula (Jimenez-Ayala et al, 1975), Matsubuchi apparatus (Inoue et al, 1983) and others, listed in the bibliography. Two instruments, Isaacs' endometrial sampler and Mi-Mark cannula, were used by us in a large study of endometrial cancer detection in asymptomatic women (Koss et al, 1981, 1984). More recently, a number of thin, plastic sampling instruments were introduced, the Endopap Sampler (Bistoletti et al, 1988) and

the Tao brush (Tao, 1993; Maksem and Knesel, 1995; Maksem, 2000). The instruments cause less discomfort to the patients. A number of newer small biopsy devices are currently on the market (for a detailed discussion of these devices see Mishell and Kaunitz, 1998) and appear to give satisfactory results with only a moderate degree of discomfort to the patients.

The initial testing of all these instruments was usually performed on symptomatic women, prior to endometrial biopsy or curettage. Not surprisingly, the initial reports usually presented the performance of the instrument in glowing terms, often claiming an accuracy of 100% or close to it, in the diagnosis of endometrial cancer and hyperplasia. On subsequent scrutiny, however, the performance was usually less successful and many of these instruments are no longer produced. The key issue, namely the discovery of asymptomatic endometrial cancer, was rarely addressed.

As an example, we had considerable experience with the **Gravlee Jet Wash.** The ingeneous instrument was designed to obtain endometrial samples by washing the endometrium with a stream of normal saline, under negative pressure that prevented the fluid from entering the fallopian tubes or the peritoneal cavity (Kanbour et al, 1974). The fluid, containing endometrial fragments and cells, was centrifuged; the button was embedded in paraffin for histologic processing;

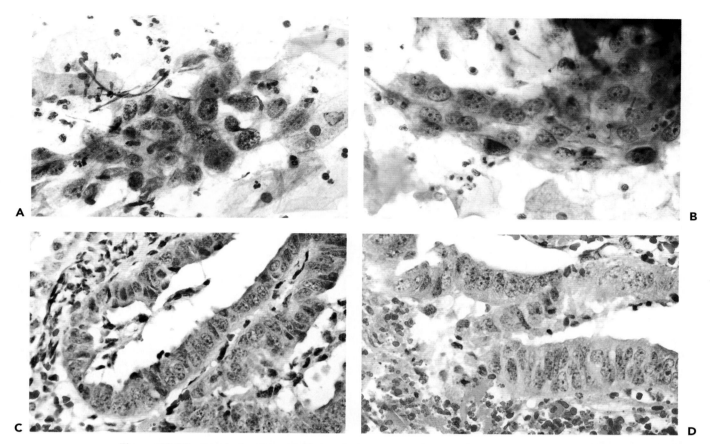

Figure 13-19 Atypical endometrial hyperplasia recognized in an endocervical brush specimen. *A,B.* Clusters of endometrial cells with markedly enlarged nuclei and nucleoli. The original diagnosis on the smear was that of an endometrial carcinoma. *C,D.* The tissue lesion corresponding to the cytology shown in *A* and *B* shows markedly atypical hyperplastic glands (complex hyperplasia). There was no conclusive evidence of endometrial carcinoma.

and the supernatant was examined by cytologic techniques. Initially, very high accuracy in the diagnosis of endometrial carcinoma was recorded by So-Bosita et al (1970), Bibbo et al (1974), and Lukeman (1974). However, when this technique was applied to a group of 303 unselected consecutive patients by Rodriques et al (1974), there was a substantial failure rate in the diagnosis of endometrial carcinoma (4 out of 8 cases) and an even higher failure rate for various forms of endometrial hyperplasia. Only advanced, symptomatic endometrial cancers with friable tissue could be diagnosed by this method. The jet of saline was apparently unable to remove sufficient diagnostic material from cohesive target tissue. To our knowledge, the cumbersome method is no longer used.

The **processing** of the endometrial samples can be performed either by **direct endometrial smears,** by the **cell block technique,** or by a combination of the two methods. Maksem and Knesel (1995) advocated the **collection of the endometrial samples in a liquid fixative** (CytoRich Fixative System, TriPath Inc) and processing of the sediment in a Hettich cytocentrifuge.

The **direct endometrial smears** are much easier and faster to prepare than cell blocks **but more difficult to interpret. The interpretation of the tissue patterns in cell blocks or microbiopsies is much easier, although the preparation is time-consuming.**

We had extensive experience with the cell block technique, beginning in the 1960s, when the late Dr. Virginia Pierce and this writer conceived of a histologic method of investigation of the endometrium. The procedure, based on a **simple suction-aspiration of the endometrium via a cannula,** was well tolerated by patients, and resulted in small tissue fragments processed by the cell block technique. The method, applied to several hundred patients, gave excellent quality of preparations, was very rapid, and resulted in a number of important, sometimes unsuspected diagnoses.

The Mi-Mark and Isaacs instruments were used in the search for occult carcinoma in a large cohort of asymptomatic women (see below). A **combination of direct smears and cell blocks** was used. The **procedure** was as follows: after preparation of a direct smear, the material still attached to the sampler was first carefully retrieved with a thin forceps; additional fragments were retrieved by shaking and washing the instrument in **Bouin's fixative,** prior to processing as cell blocks. Bouin's fixative was selected as offering the optimal preservation of the tissue fragments. Multiple sections of the cell block must be examined. The combination of the two procedures, admittedly time-consuming and costly, gave satisfactory results. A diagram of the procedure is shown in Figure 13-20.

PREPARATION OF ENDOMETRIAL MATERIAL
FOR MICROSCOPIC STUDY

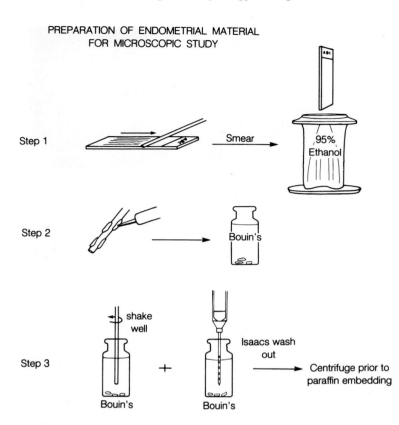

Figure 13-20 Method of endometrial sampling, combining the use of direct endometrial smears with cell block technique, used in the search for occult endometrial carcinoma in asymptomatic women. The two instruments used in this study were Mi-Mark and Isaacs.

Interpretation

Adequacy of Samples

Except in women with complete atrophy of the endometrium (usually past the age of 55), the smears should contain at least five or six clusters of endometrial epithelial cells to be judged adequate.

Composition of Smears

The summary of cytologic findings that follows is a composite of the early experience with several hundred samples obtained with Jordan's cannula prior to 1970 and on data from over 4,000 direct endometrial smears examined in the 1980s during the search for occult endometrial carcinoma and hyperplasia, described below. Some material, processed by liquid fixation in CytoRich and centrifugation, graciously made available by Dr. John Maksem from Mercy Hospital Medical Center, Des Moines, Iowa, was also included in the review. The analysis of direct endometrial samples is facilitated by **accurate clinical information, including the age of the patient, obstetrical and menstrual history and clinical symptoms, if any.**

Key Features

The interpretation of the microscopic findings requires knowledge of the many aspects of benign endometrial cytology and sources of error.

The key features that should be investigated are:

- **Number and cellular make-up of epithelial clusters**
- **Cohesiveness of epithelial cell clusters**

- **Nuclear abnormalities,** mainly enlargement and the presence of **readily visible nucleoli** in endometrial epithelial cells

Cycling Endometrium

Except in the presence of marked inflammation or a necrotic carcinoma, the smears usually have a clean background. Blood is invariably present, unless eliminated by processing. In menstruating women, the endometrial samples usually contain **numerous clusters of epithelial and stromal cells.**

Benign epithelial glandular cells, derived from the superficial layers of the endometrial lining and adjacent glands, **appear mainly as flat, cohesive "honeycomb" type of sheets, wherein cell borders can be clearly seen, or as three-dimensional, tubular structures, reflecting endometrial glands** (Fig. 13-21A,B). In the flat clusters, **the nuclei, measuring about 7 to 8 μm in diameter, comparable in size to the nuclei of parabasal squamous cells, are open (vesicular) and sometimes faintly granular.** The appearance of the epithelial cells and their nuclei varies somewhat with the phase of the menstrual cycle.

In the proliferative phase, the epithelial cells have scanty, basophilic cytoplasm. There is some **variability of nuclear sizes,** accounted for by various stages of cell cycle in proliferating cells. Tiny, single **nucleoli** and occasional **mitotic figures** can be observed (Fig. 13-21B). In some cases, there is a **breakdown of clusters,** probably an artifact of smear preparation: in the dispersed cells, the variability of nuclear sizes can be better appreciated. Exceptionally, **ciliated glandular cells** can be observed. Their provenance from the endometrium or the endocervix cannot be ascertained.

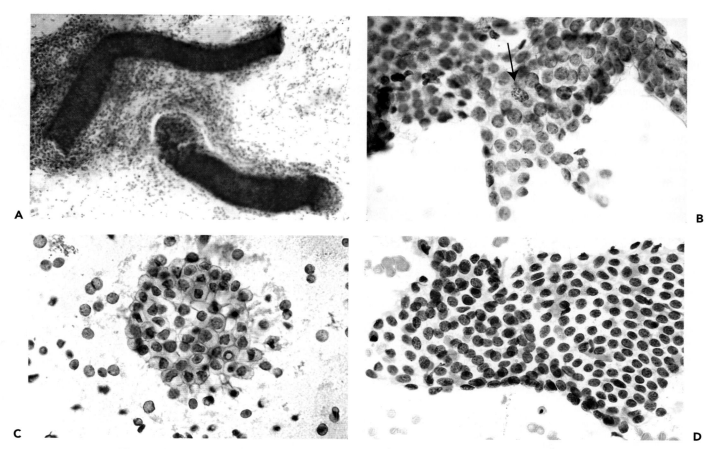

Figure 13-21   Normal endometrium in direct endometrial samples. *A.* Normal endometrial tubular glands. *B.* A sheet of endometrial cells in proliferative phase. The cells form a cohesive cluster wherein mitoses may be noted (*arrow*). *C.* Loosely structured cluster of endometrial cells with vacuolated cytoplasm, corresponding to the secretory phase. *D.* Atrophic endometrium. The sheet of endometrial cells shows spacing between nuclei, characteristic of atrophy.

In the early secretory phase, the epithelial cells are usually larger because of increased volume of cytoplasm that is often vacuolated. At the edge of cell clusters, columnar cells with clear cytoplasm may be observed (Fig. 13-21C). Similar features may be observed in dispersed cells. The **nuclei** are usually **monotonous in size and** do not show either nucleoli or mitotic activity. In **late secretory endometrium,** the endometrial cells usually occur in **thick clusters,** sometimes in tubular or glandular configuration. At the periphery of the clusters, columnar epithelial cells with clear cytoplasm may resemble endocervical cells.

Endometrial Stromal Cells

In menstruating women, regardless of the stage of cell cycle, or in proliferating endometrium from whatever cause, the **stromal cells** appear in the background **as numerous, small, spindly "naked" nuclei,** sometimes surrounded by a very narrow rim of cytoplasm. In late secretory endometrium or under the influence of hormones, the stromal cells may become **larger, with a more abundant cytoplasm, reflecting decidual changes** that may occur under such circumstances. Tao (1995) reported that the configuration of stromal cells is helpful in assessing the stage of the menstrual cycle but, in my experience, this feature is difficult to assess.

Timing of Ovulation

Although differences could be observed between proliferative and secretory endometria, it has been our judgment that direct endometrial cytologic samples are ***not*** the proper tool for timing of ovulation. Endometrial biopsies, study of endocervical mucus, body temperature, and hormonal determination, as described in Chapter 9, are easier to interpret and better-suited methods for this purpose. It must be mentioned that Tao (1995) reported adequate results of endometrial dating, using his instrument, the Tao brush.

Atrophic Endometrium

In **postmenopausal women with endometrial atrophy, the number of clusters of epithelial cells is small,** sometimes limited to three or four small clusters. In smears of this type, the endometrial epithelial cells usually form **flat, well-spread clusters,** wherein the cells show a distinct honeycomb-type arrangement. The epithelial cells and their nuclei are generally smaller than those in the proliferative or secretory endometrium (Fig. 13-21D). The **stromal cells** are sparse. **Mono- and multinucleated macrophages** are occasionally observed in such smears (see Chap. 8). Changes in the cytologic pattern in this group of women should always suggest the possibility of a neoplastic disorder and warrant careful scrutiny of such material (see below).

Endometrial Adenocarcinoma

The diagnosis of endometrial carcinoma in direct endometrial samples can be established by the presence of **enlarged endometrial epithelial (glandular) cells with enlarged nuclei, wherein reside clearly visible large, usually single, nucleoli.** The cytoplasm is usually scanty, basophilic, and sometimes vacuolated. The cancer cells may **be dispersed and occur singly** or may form **clusters,** that are either **flat or multilayered,** the latter of **papillary configuration.** The **flat clusters** are usually **loosely structured, sometimes forming "rosettes," often with detached cancer cells at their periphery. The multilayered clusters appear as dark, oval, spherical or irregular structures that are, per se, abnormal,** even if their cellular make-up may be difficult to study, except at their periphery. By comparing cytologic findings with endometrial tissue samples, it could be documented that similar cells are found in the lumens of cancerous glands (Figs. 13-22 to 13-24).

Nuclear Abnormalities

As mentioned above, the most conspicuous nuclear changes are **nuclear enlargement, hyperchromasia, and the presence of large nucleoli.** In some cases, however, there is the **absence of nuclear hyperchromasia, resulting in granu**lar, **pale nuclei with visible nucleoli, that stand out as pink dots that vary in size and configuration, ranging from small and spherical to large and irregular, the latter usually seen in high grade cancers (Fig. 13-22B).**

In high grade carcinomas, the nuclear abnormalities are conspicuous (Fig. 13-24). However, during the extensive search for occult endometrial carcinoma, it became evident that, **in some cases of endometrial cancer, the nuclear enlargement is only slight and the nucleoli are small (Fig. 13-23C,D).** Yet, subsequent histologic evidence has shown that all or nearly all of the minimally abnormal cells had to be derived from cancerous endometrium that was lining the entire surface of the endometrial cavity.

Nuclear Grading

In 1995, Zaino et al introduced the concept of nuclear grading as a prognostic factor in endometrioid adenocarcinoma. Small, spherical nuclei were graded as I, whereas large, irregularly shaped nuclei with large nucleoli were graded III, grade II being intermediate between the two. Maksem (2000) applied the system to direct endometrial samples. However, the results of the study were not completely convincing because high grade nuclear abnormalities were occasionally observed in the absence of documented

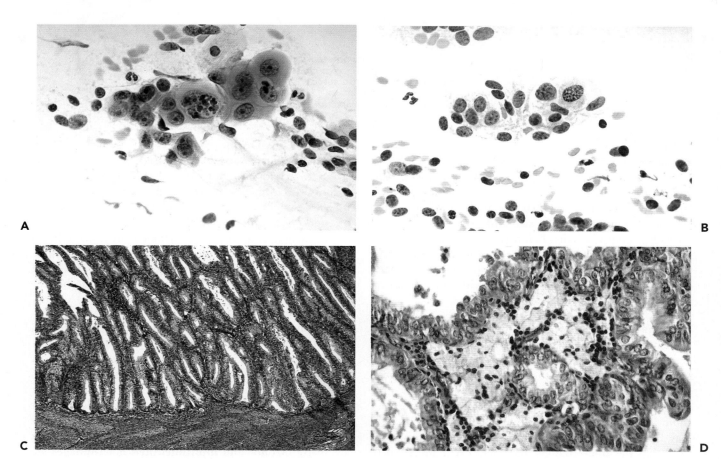

Figure 13-22 Occult endometrial carcinoma diagnosed on direct endometrial sample. *A.* A cluster of malignant endometrial cells showing large nuclei and prominent, irregular nucleoli. *B.* A cluster of endometrial, glandular cells showing marked granularity of the nuclei and the presence of small nucleoli. *C.* The endometrium showed a low-grade endometrial carcinoma which focally contained nests of large macrophages shown in *D.*

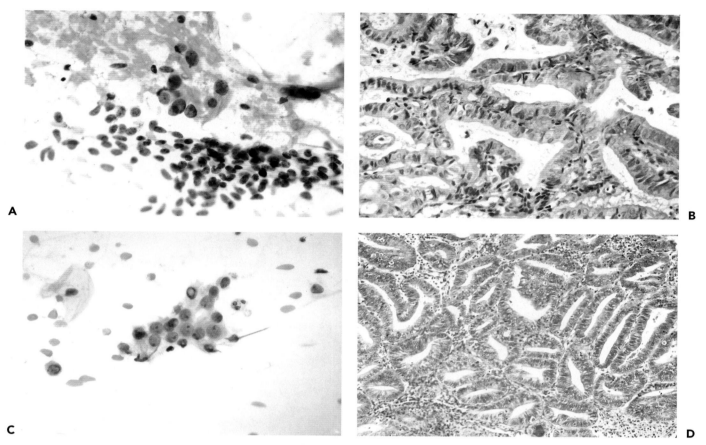

Figure 13-23   Occult endometrial adenocarcinomas discovered on direct sampling. *A.* A papillary cluster of endometrial cancer cells with enlarged nuclei, visible nucleoli, and vacuolated cytoplasm. Next to this cluster, there is a sheet of spindly endometrial stromal cells. Note the difference in nuclear sizes. *B.* Well-differentiated endometrial adenocarcinoma corresponding to *A. C.* A cluster of inconspicuous endometrial cancer cells showing only slight deviation from normal. The nuclei are somewhat enlarged and granular, containing tiny nucleoli. *D.* Section of well-differentiated endometrial carcinoma corresponding to *C.*

cancer, possibly representing small foci of endometrial atypia that escaped histologic scrutiny. The clinical significance of Maksem's observations is unknown at this time.

Unusual Findings

Occasionally, the **endometrial cancer cells are mixed with atypical squamous cells,** leading to a diagnosis of an **adenoacanthoma.** In such cases, it is important to rule out a cervical lesion of a similar cellular make-up (see Chap. 11). Unusual findings include **ciliated carcinoma and endometrial intraepithelial carcinoma,** both described by Maksem (1997, 1998). Infiltration of cancer cells by polymorphonuclear leukocytes may be conspicuous (see Figs. 13-24C and 13-27C).

Diagnosis of Endometrial Carcinoma in Various Age Groups

In **menstruating women,** the diagnosis of endometrial carcinoma in direct endometrial samples is **difficult** because the evidence may be scanty and may be obscured by a large number of clusters of benign endometrial epithelial cells.

The **diagnosis is easier in postmenopausal women.**

Endometrial cancer cells, singly or in clusters, as described above, **are much easier to recognize against the sparse cellular background.** In the extensive search for occult endometrial carcinoma (see below), it became evident that the **mere presence of abundant clusters or sheets of endometrial cells in a postmenopausal woman was an important warning sign of possible pathologic changes, even in the absence of conspicuous nuclear abnormalities.**

Endometrial Hyperplasia

The recognition of endometrial hyperplasia in direct endometrial smears is fraught with difficulty. This was recognized already during the early experience with Jordan's cannula and enhanced still further during the search for endometrial abnormalities in asymptomatic women. As a general rule, the endometrial samples in hyperplasia are **rich in cells and cell clusters.** This finding is **significant only in postmenopausal women** in whom, in my experience, hyperplasia is a relatively uncommon finding **and cannot be differentiated from a carcinoma.**

It is virtually impossible to establish the diagnosis of **proliferative, simple hyperplasia in endometrial samples.** The

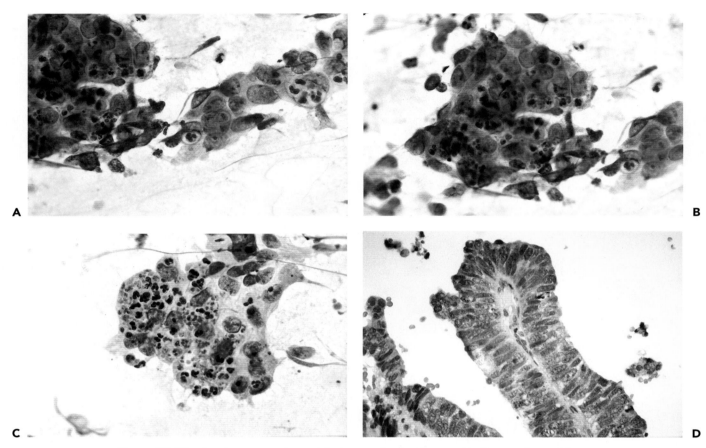

Figure 13-24   Occult serous endometrial adenocarcinoma diagnosed in direct endometrial sample. *A,B.* Large clusters of endometrial cancer cells with markedly enlarged nuclei and prominent nucleoli. *C.* Cancer cells with cytoplasm densely infiltrated by polyps. *D.* Fragment of endometrial papillary serous carcinoma corresponding to *A–C.*

pattern of smears is that of benign endometrium, occasionally with a slight nuclear enlargement and some evidence of mitotic activity in epithelial cells. The recognition of **atypical hyperplasia** is almost equally difficult in either premenopausal or postmenopausal patients. The only finding of note, observed several times in the large endometrial study, was *cohesive* **sheets of epithelial endometrial cells with moderately enlarged nucleoli** (Fig. 13-25A,B). The differentiation of such clusters from a well-differentiated carcinoma (or **endometrial polyps** that may have an identical presentation) is impossible on cytologic grounds alone. The difficulty persists, even if the cytologic samples are supplemented by cell blocks. Occasionally, the diagnosis **cannot be proved,** either on biopsies or curettages, even after extensive follow-up (Fig. 13-25C,D). Such findings may represent transient or tiny abnormalities of the endometrium.

Our difficulties with the diagnosis of endometrial hyperplasia are by no means unique. Thus, Meisels and Jolicoeur (1985), using a device known as the "Endo-pap" endometrial sampler, diagnosed only one half of 207 cases of hyperplasia using a number of complex criteria. Unfortunately, their paper failed to address the issues of type of hyperplasia and the clinical setting in which the diagnosis was established (symptoms and age of patients). In a large review of endometrial cytology, Mencaglia (1987) also admitted a large number of failures in the cytologic diagnosis of hyperplasia.

Sources of Error in Direct Endometrial Samples: Endocervical Cells vs. Endometrial Cells

The most important **source of diagnostic difficulty in direct endometrial samples is the separation of endometrial from endocervical cells.** In our own studies, numerous endometrial biopsies were obtained, based on a mistaken belief that the atypical endocervical cells represented an endometrial lesion. In general, the **endocervical cells are larger and have more abundant, sharply demarcated cytoplasm** than endometrial cells. A nuclear protrusion (nipple) often found in endocervical cells at midcycle (see Chap. 8) has not been observed by us in endometrial cancer cells although such changes may be observed in normal endometrium.

The difficulties are compounded if the endocervical cells in the endometrial samples show abnormalities such as large nucleoli that may be present in acute or chronic cervicitis and in florid metaplasia or repair. The latter may be caused by an endometrial or endocervical polyp and may be readily confused with endometrial carcinomas. Occasionally, **chronic cervicitis with papillary configuration of epithelium (papillary endocervicitis)** may shed cell fragments mimicking papillary endometrial carcinoma (Fig. 13-26). Another feature of

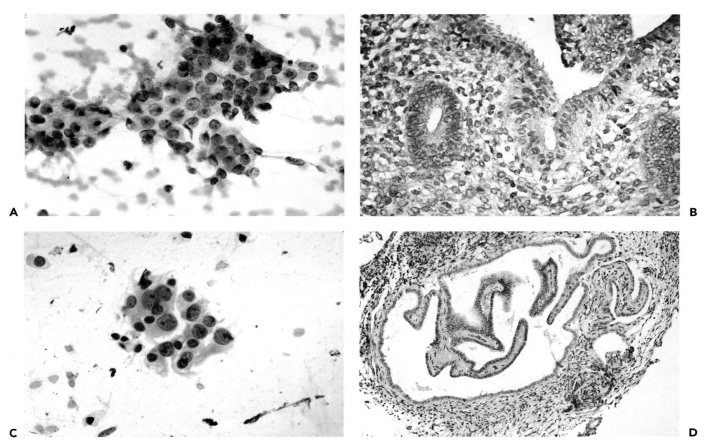

Figure 13-25 Endometrial hyperplasia in direct samples. *A.* A cluster of endometrial cells with large nuclei and prominent nucleoli in a 53-year-old woman. These cells mimic endometrial cancer cells. *B.* Fragment of endometrial curettage corresponding to (*A*) showing slight atypia of endometrial glands. *C.* Markedly atypical clusters of endometrial cells, some showing large nuclei and prominent nucleoli. Extensive investigation of the endometrium failed to reveal any evidence of carcinoma or hyperplasia, except for the papillary lesion shown in *D*.

endocervical cells, namely the presence of occasional **enlarged, hyperchromatic nuclei (karyomegaly), such as observed in the presence of CIN** or **endocervical adenocarcinoma** (see Chaps. 11 and 12), may also be mistaken for an endometrial process.

OCCULT ENDOMETRIAL CARCINOMA

As yet, no method of screening for endometrial carcinoma has been devised, combining the ease of application with low cost and high reliability, comparable to the cytologic screening for precancerous lesions of the uterine cervix. Routine cytologic examination of **vaginal pool smears,** as originally advocated by Papanicolaou, serves a very useful purpose in this regard as discussed below. Regrettably, the method has been abandoned as a routine procedure because its efficiency in the diagnosis of cervical lesions is low. It must be stressed that **routine cervical smears are essentially useless for endometrial cancer detection,** except in the rare cases of fully developed cancers in asymptomatic women, usually because of stenosis of the cervical canal. As has been stated above, **endocer-**

vical brush specimens may occasionally provide evidence of an endometrial lesion.

Vaginal Pool Smears

The **vaginal pool smears, obtained by a glass pipette or another instrument,** are very easy to obtain with no discomfort to the patients. **In our judgment, a properly obtained and fixed vaginal smear should be part of every gynecologic examination in all women past the age of 50 and in those younger women whose history or symptomatology may suggest an endometrial abnormality.** The search for asymptomatic endometrial carcinoma is facilitated in **vaginal smears** if the following categories of patients are scrutinized with particular care:

- Smears of postmenopausal patients with high maturation of squamous cells of unexplained etiology
- Smears of any patient in the fifth decade of life or older who has a history of abnormal bleeding or staining, or microscopic evidence thereof
- Smears displaying evidence of marked necrosis and containing macrophages in menopausal or postmenopausal patients. **It must be stressed, once again, that the pres-**

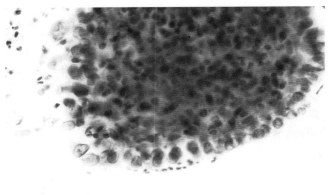

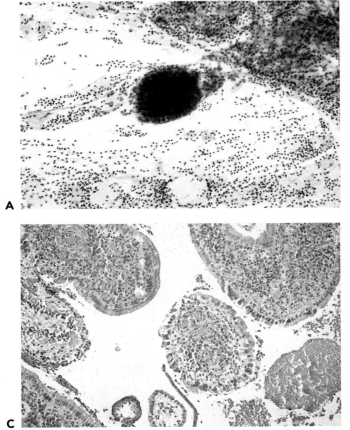

Figure 13-26 Clusters of endocervical cells from a case of papillary cervicitis, mimicking endometrial carcinoma. *A,B.* A dense cluster of glandular cells (*A*) which, on close inspection (*B*), shows columnar cells at the periphery. *C.* The corresponding tissue lesion showing papillary cervicitis.

ence of macrophages in *cervical* smears has no bearing on the status of the endometrium.

The cytologic presentation of asymptomatic endometrial carcinoma is usually inconspicuous and calls for a systematic, often tedious and time-consuming search of the vaginal smear **for endometrial cells, regardless of morphologic appearance. The background of vaginal smears** is sometimes free of blood and debris. More commonly, fresh blood and/or amorphous, yellow-orange (in Papanicolaou stain) areas of old fibrinated blood may be observed. There is frequently **excellent maturation of squamous cells, regardless of menopausal status or time of cycle.**

The **endometrial cancer cells** in asymptomatic endometrial carcinoma **in vaginal smears** are usually **small, inconspicuous, and sometimes only slightly larger than normal endometrial cells** (Fig. 13-27). There are **three cytoplasmic features** that may assist in the identification of such cells:

- **Columnar shape** of small endometrial cells is observed in lesions of the lower uterine segment, although most such cells are approximately spherical or cuboidal
- The presence of **cytoplasmic vacuoles**
- The **infiltration of the cytoplasm by polymorphonuclear leukocytes.** This feature is not specific and may also be observed in degenerating, mucus-producing benign cells of either endocervical or endometrial origin, but it should trigger further investigation.

The **nuclei of the small endometrial cancer cells are larger than the nuclei of the parabasal or intermediate squamous cells** usually present in the field. They are generally finely granular and provided with conspicuous, although not necessarily very large single nucleoli. Rarely, the nuclei are **hyperchromatic and provided with large nucleoli,** usually reflecting the presence of a high grade tumor. Inadequate clinical follow-up of such patients may result in advanced cancer diagnosed at a later date.

The endometrial cancer cells are easier to identify when occurring in **clusters** that are usually small and rarely made up of more than a dozen cells. The clusters may be **flat, sometimes forming small rosette-like structures, or are multilayered, irregular or papillary** in configuration. The cells in clusters are usually round or oval, have a clear, sometimes vacuolated cytoplasm, and relatively **large, opaque, finely granular or somewhat hyperchromatic nuclei and often small nucleoli.** Sometimes, the manner of cluster formation of endometrial cancer cells closely resembles normal endometrium.

It must be emphasized that, in early endometrial carcinoma, **the shedding of cancer cells may be intermittent** and that a negative smear may immediately follow a positive smear and vice versa. **Thus, it is important to insist on further clarification of any abnormal cytologic finding, by endometrial biopsy or curettage, risking at times a false alarm.** It is equally important to insist on long-term follow-up if histologic confirmation of carci-

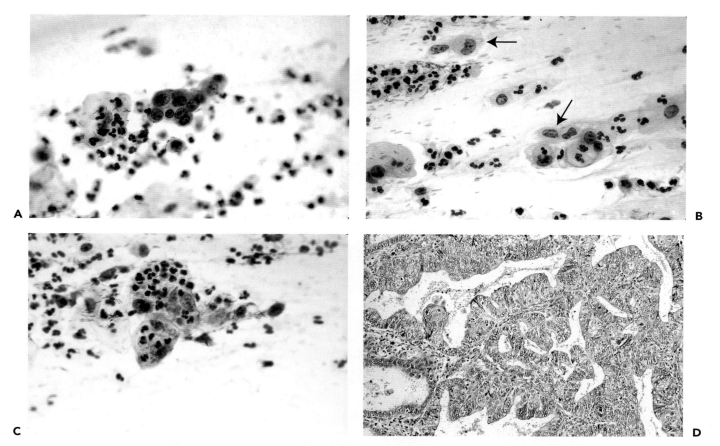

Figure 13-27   **Occult endometrial adenocarcinoma diagnosed in vaginal pool smears 4 years before histologic diagnosis.** *A–C.* Various aspects of endometrial cancer cells forming clusters (*A*), dispersed (*B*), and cells with the cytoplasm densely infiltrated by neutrophiles in *C. D.* The corresponding well-differentiated endometrial carcinoma observed 5 years after the cytologic diagnosis of carcinoma.

noma is not immediately forthcoming (Fig. 13-27). **Special care must be exercised in patients with stenosis of the endocervical canal in whom an endometrial biopsy may be difficult or impossible to obtain as an office procedure.**

Results

Table 13-2 summarizes the relationship of clinical symptomatology to histologic lesions in 102 cases of endometrial adenocarcinoma reported by Koss and Durfee in 1962. The diagnosis in all of the 22 asymptomatic patients and in 17 patients with slight symptoms (such as brownish discharge or history of spotting but no frank bleeding), a total of 39 cases, was made by **vaginal pool smear** cytology and subsequently confirmed by histology. In this study, 12 of the 22 patients with asymptomatic endometrial carcinoma were still menstruating; their average age was 6 years less than that of fully symptomatic patients. The latter findings are summarized in Table 13-3. It may be noted that not all of the patients with early lesions were asymptomatic and not all of the patients with advanced lesions were symptomatic. Among the asymptomatic patients there were also several invasive endometrioid cancers. It must be noted that, in three patients, a major delay in clinical diagnosis occurred. At the time of histologic diagnosis, advanced carci-

noma was present (see Fig. 13-27). This experience, repeatedly confirmed since the publication of this paper, points out that the evolution of endometrial carcinoma is slow in many cases, offering ample opportunity to diagnose the disease in its early stages.

Endometrial Minibiopsies (Cell Block Technique)

The method of endometrial investigation that was conceived in the 1960s by Dr. Virginia Pierce and this writer to supplement or replace vaginal smears was briefly described above. The procedure, based on a simple suction-aspiration of the endometrium via a small caliber metal cannula attached to a syringe, was inexpensive and reasonably well tolerated by the patients. The tiny tissue fragments were processed by the cell block technique. The method, applied to several hundred patients, gave excellent quality of preparations, was rapid, and resulted in a number of important, sometimes unsuspected diagnoses of endometrial carcinoma (Fig. 31-28).

The procedure was not tested on asymptomatic women and, therefore, its value as a detection method of occult endometrial carcinoma is unknown.

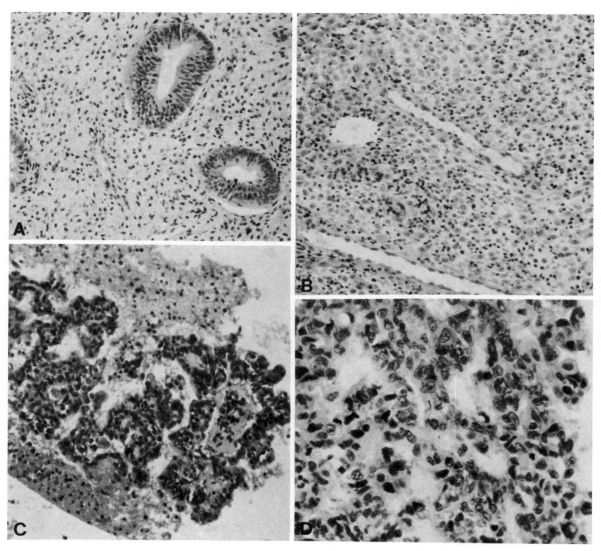

Figure 13-28   Microbiopsies of endometrium obtained by the Pierce method described in text.
A. Somewhat atypical proliferative endometrium. *B.* Decidual reaction in endometrial stroma (the effect of contraceptive hormones). *C,D.* Unsuspected endometrial adenocarcinoma.

SYSTEMATIC SEARCH FOR ENDOMETRIAL CARCINOMA AND HYPERPLASIA IN ASYMPTOMATIC WOMEN

Under a contract with the National Cancer Institute, USA, a major program of endometrial cancer detection was undertaken by the writer and his colleagues between January 1979 and June 1982 (Koss et al, 1981, 1984). The purposes of the program were as follows:

- To determine by direct endometrial sampling and conventional cytologic methods whether occult endometrial carcinoma is a detectable disease in asymptomatic women age 45 and above
- To identify the optimal methods of screening for occult endometrial carcinoma
- To determine the prevalence and incidence of occult endometrial carcinoma and hyperplasia and the relationship of these entities to each other

- To identify, by epidemiologic study, high-risk groups to facilitate future screening efforts

The patients were recruited to this study by advertising, visits to local churches and temples, and talks to groups of women. The services were offered free of charge. The conditions of acceptance to the project were age 45 or older, intact uterus, no history or evidence of abnormal vaginal bleeding or spotting, and the willingness to sign an informed consent after explanation of the procedure. To satisfy the epidemiologic aspects of this study, a detailed questionnaire, pertaining to the pertinent medical history, was obtained on each examinee by a trained social worker. Each woman's weight, height, and blood pressure were measured before gynecologic examination and breast palpation, also a part of the services offered to the volunteers.

In all, 2,586 women were enrolled in the study, each receiving a full initial examination; of these, 1,567 women were examined for a second time 1 year later, and 187 were screened for a third time, two years after the initial examina-

TABLE 13-2

HISTOLOGIC LESIONS IN CARCINOMA OF THE ENDOMETRIUM

| | In Situ Adenocarcinoma | Adenocarcinoma with Only Superficial Invasion of Myometrium | Advanced Adenocarcinoma | Radiation Prior to Hysterectomy | | Diagnosis on Biopsy, Curettage, or Submitted Slide Only |
				No Residual Cancer	Residual Cancer	
Asymptomatic (22 cases) 100%	7 (31.8%)	5	2*	3	2	3
Slight symptoms (17 cases)† 100%	2 (12%)	4	4‡	3	1	3
Symptomatic (63 cases) 100%	4 (0.6%)§	16	26	3	3	11

* Histologic diagnosis and treatment delayed 4 years in 1 case.
† Carcinoma suspected clinically in 5 cases only.
‡ Histologic diagnosis and treatment delayed 5 years in 1 case. Os stenosed in second case.
§ In 2 cases also polyps and hyperplasia.
(Koss LG, Durfee GR. Cytologic diagnosis of endometrial carcinoma. Result of ten years of experience. Acta Cytol 6:519–531, 1962.)

tion. The age distribution of the primary examinees and the returnees is shown in Table 13-4. It may be noted that the cohort included 2.3% of women between the ages of 40 and 45 who could not be excluded from the study for social reasons.

At the time of the initiation of this project, there were two promising commercially available endometrial sampling devices: the Mi-Mark and the Isaacs' instruments. The Mi-Mark, invented by Milan and Markley, was a two-part plastic instrument, comprising a uterine sound and a helical sampling spatula, 3.5 mm in diameter. The Isaacs' instrument consisted of a malleable, perforated metal suction cannula, 2 mm in diameter, provided with an adjustable cervical obturator and attached to a syringe. The instruments were assigned by a computer program to insure random distribution. Either instrument could be introduced into the uterine cavity of about 93% of asymptomatic examinees without anesthesia, although the success rate was somewhat higher and the level of discomfort less with the Isaacs' instrument because of its smaller diameter. The method of pro-

cessing by direct smears and by cell blocks is shown in Figure 13-20. Besides the direct endometrial sampling, each woman received a lateral scrape smear of the vaginal wall (to determine the level of maturation of squamous cells), a vaginal pool smear, and a cervical scrape and cotton swab smears. An endocervical aspiration smear, obtained by means of a commercially available device, proved quite useless and was discontinued after the first 1,000 examinations.

The study yielded a number of important observations, summarized in several prior publications (Koss et al, 1981, 1984). The study has, so far, been unique, has not been duplicated, and may serve as a model for future studies of this type. For this reason, the key results of this study are reported.

Age at Onset of Menopause

There were 2,061 postmenopausal women enrolled in the study. As shown in Table 13-5, the study revealed that the **normal American woman may menstruate to the age of 55 years.** A small group of women is apparently capable of normal menstruation to the age of 59 (3% of the sample). There was epidemiologic evidence that the late menstruating women were at an increased risk for endometrial carcinoma (see below). The same table also shows other data of significance in the epidemiologic study (see below).

Occult Endometrial Carcinoma

Table 13-6 shows the prevalence and incidence of endometrial carcinomas in this cohort of women. The **prevalence** was defined as all cancers diagnosed on the first screening or coming to light within one year after the first screening. The **incidence,** expressed in women years, included all can-

TABLE 13-3

AVERAGE AGE OF PATIENTS WITH ENDOMETRIAL CARCINOMAS

Asymptomatic (22 patients)	Slight Symptoms (17 patients)	Symptomatic Patients (63 patients)
52.0 years	56.5 years	58.1 years

(Koss LG, Durfee GR. Cytologic diagnosis of endometrial carcinoma: Result of ten years of experience. Acta Cytol 6:519–531, 1962.)

TABLE 13-4

AGE DISTRIBUTION OF 2,586 PRIMARY EXAMINEES AND 1,567 RETURNEES

	Primary Examinees		Returnees	
Age	Number of Patients	Percentage of Sample	Number of Patients	Percentage of Samples
40–44	61	2.36	8	0.51
45–49	532	20.57	277	17.68
50–54	574	22.19	384	24.51
55–59	535	20.69	338	21.57
60–64	388	15.00	229	14.61
65–69	248	9.59	173	11.04
70–74	167	6.46	101	6.45
75–79	64	2.47	41	2.62
80–90	17	0.66	16	1.02
Total	2,586	100.00	1,567	100.00

(Koss LG, et al. Detection of endometrial carcinoma and hyperplasia in asymptomatic women. Obstet Gynecol 64:1–11, 1984.)

cers diagnosed on the second or third screening or coming to light thereafter. The term, **women-years,** indicates the likelihood of developing a disease process calculated per 1,000 years of women's life, following an episode, in this case, 1 year after the first screening.

There were 16 endometrial carcinomas discovered on first screening and two missed on screening and observed in women who became symptomatic within the 12 months following the first screening, for a **prevalence rate of 7 in 1,000.** Another carcinoma was diagnosed on the second screening; two additional cancers, missed on screening, were observed after the second screening in women who became symptomatic, for an **incidence rate of 1.7 per 1,000 women years.**

Table 13-7 shows the pathologic findings in the 17 endometrial carcinomas discovered by screening. All cases were

TABLE 13-5

EPIDEMIOLOGIC PROFILE OF 2,586 PRIMARY EXAMINEES

	No. of Women	Percentage
Age at Onset of Menopause		
39 or younger	43	2.90
40–44	138	6.70
45–49	788	38.23
50–55	1,029	49.93
56–59	62	3.01
Not recorded	1	0.05
Total	2,061	100.00
Other Data*		
Nulliparity†	204	7.88
Use of estrogen	565	21.84
Use of contraceptives	335	12.95
Hypertension	538	20.80
Diabetes	104	4.02
History of cancer	115	4.44

* Percentages for Other Data are of total population.
† Remaining women had from one to six children.
(Koss LG et al. Detection of endometrial carcinoma and hyperplasia in asymptomatic women. Obstet Gynecol 64:1–11, 1984.)

TABLE 13-6

PREVALENCE AND INCIDENCE RATES OF HISTOLOGICALLY PROVEN ENDOMETRIAL CARCINOMA AND HYPERPLASIA

	Prevalence	Incidence/ Women Years
No. of examinees	2,586	1,754*
Occult carcinomas	16†	1
Missed carcinomas	2‡	2†
Total carcinomas	18	3
Rate per 1,000 women	6.96/1,000	1.71/1,000
Hyperplasia	17	3
Polyps with hyperplasia	4	0
Total	21	3
Rate per 1,000 women	8.12	1.71/1,000

* Second and subsequent annual clinic visits. Additional follow-up through doctors' office was obtained in about 20 additional women.
† One patient was diagnosed on second screening. On review the original material was suspicious.
‡ See text.
(Koss LG, et al. Detection of endometrial carcinoma and hyperplasia in asymptomatic women. Obstet Gynecol 64:1–11, 1984.)

TABLE 13-7				
PATHOLOGIC FINDINGS IN 17 PATIENTS* WITH OCCULT CARCINOMA OF ENDOMETRIUM				
Uterus of normal size	14	Myometrial invasion		
Enlarged	2	None	5	
Size unknown	1	Superficial†	3	
(radiotherapy only)				17
		Deep	4	
		Unknown (radiotherapy alone or before hysterectomy)	5	
Histologic type of tumor				
Adenocarcinoma (9),				
Adenoacanthoma (8)				
Grade 1	6	Accompanying hyperplasia		
Grade 2	8	Focal	5	
Grade 3	1	Extensive	1‡	
Too scanty to grade	2			

* 16 prevalence, 1 incidence.
† One with carcinoma of left ovary, metastatic or primary.
‡ On estrogen therapy of long duration.
(Koss LG, et al. Detection of endometrial carcinoma and hyperplasia in asymptomatic women. Obstet Gynecol 64 : 1–11, 1984; with permission.)

in stage 1A although, in four patients, there was deep invasion of the myometrium.

Occult Endometrial Hyperplasia

As shown in Table 13-6, the **rate of occult hyperplasias, including endometrial polyps, was approximately equal to the rate of occult carcinomas.** There may be some minor bias in the study, inasmuch as symptomatic women (hence, possibly including those with hyperplasia) were excluded. However, no more than three women were excluded from the study and referred for further care because of a history of symptoms; thus the rate of endometrial hyperplasias was exceedingly low. On the assumption, based on studies of Gusberg and Kaplan (1963), that about 10% of hyperplasias become associated with cancer, the observed rate of hyperplasias was much below the expected rate, casting serious doubts on the relationship of hyperplasia to endometrial cancer. In the 12 hysterectomy specimens from patients with endometrial carcinoma, examined without prior radiotherapy (see Table 13-7), focal hyperplasia was present in five and extensive hyperplasia was found in only one uterus, in a woman receiving long-term estrogen therapy. In six uteri, there was no evidence of hyperplasia adjacent to carcinoma.

Risk Factors
Obesity
Because obesity is classically considered a risk factor in endometrial carcinoma, the status of our examinees was determined by an index of obesity, known as the **Quetelet index.** This index takes into account, not only the weight, but also the height of the person, by a formula shown in Figure 13-29. The distribution of the Quetelet index and the distribution of 21 endometrial carcinomas within the Quetelet groups are also shown in this figure, taking into account the history of estrogen therapy. It may be noted that endometrial **carcinomas in women receiving estrogen therapy occurred more often in the group of slender women** with low Quetelet indices; although the difference was below statistical significance, it showed an interesting trend, discussed above.

Other Risk Factors
A statistical evaluation of risk factors in occult endometrial carcinoma, performed by Dr. Martin Lesser, is shown in Table 13-8. Among the several factors listed, only one, namely **late onset of menopause,** proved to be statistically valid. In other words, women whose menstrual activity ceases before the age of 50 appear to be protected from endometrial cancer. **Diabetes,** classically considered a risk factor for endometrial carcinoma, did not prove to be so in this study. **Hormonal level,** as determined by maturation of squamous cells in scrape smears of the lateral vaginal wall, **was not helpful in this study.** Contrary to the prior observations suggesting that a high level of maturation of squamous cells was a common event in the vaginal pool smears of patients with occult endometrial carcinoma (see above), this was not the case in this cohort of patients. The 17 postmenopausal patients with endometrial carcinoma had, for the most part, a pattern of postmenopausal atrophy.

Thus, this study failed to reveal a specific high-risk group of women who should be selected for screening for occult endometrial cancer. Although menopause delayed past the

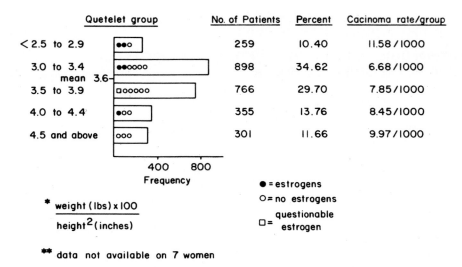

Figure 13-29 Distribution of 21 occult endometrial carcinomas according to Quetelet (obesity) index, calculated for a screened population of 2,579 women (data on seven women were not available).

age of 50 appeared to be a risk factor, this event was observed in nearly 80% of our population (see Table 13-4).

The Performance of Sampling Methods in the Discovery of Occult Endometrial Carcinoma

Direct endometrial smears, the cell blocks of direct endometrial samples, and the vaginal smears contributed to the discovery of 17 cases of occult endometrial carci- **noma.** Direct endometrial sampling proved to be the most efficacious part of the diagnostic system, having established the diagnosis in 16 cases. In one case, the endometrial smear alone was positive and, in one case, only the cell block. In the remaining 14 cases, both the endometrial smear and the cell block showed evidence of disease. In the 17th case, a 71-year-old woman **with cervical stenosis preventing endometrial sampling, the vaginal pool smear was positive.** This patient had a deeply infiltrating stage IA carci-

TABLE 13-8

ASSESSMENT OF RISK FACTORS IN 2,579 WOMEN

Factor	No. of Women	No. of Carcinomas	Rate/1,000	Odds Ratio	P Value
Race					
White	2,031	18	8.8	1.65 : 1	NS
Nonwhite	555	3	5.4		
Parity					
Nulliparity	204	2	9.8	1.07 : 1	NS
Parous	2,382	19	8.0		
Onset of menopause					
≤ 49 yr	969	5	5.1		
50–55 yr	1,030	14	13.5		P < 0.04
56 yr	62	2	32.3		
Obesity					
Quetelet index > 3.4	1,422	12	8.4	1.09 : 1	NS
Quetelet index ≤ 3.4	1,157	9	7.7		
Quetelet index > 4.4	301	3	9.9	1.26 : 1	NS
Quetelet index ≤ 4.4	2,278	18	7.9		
Estrogen					
Yes	565	6	10.6	1.31 : 1	NS
No	2,021	15	7.4		

* P value, Mantel-Haenszel test; for "onset of menopause" Mantel's extension procedure.
NS = not significant. Risk factors for diabetes and hypertension (not shown) were NS.
(Koss LG, et al. Detection of endometrial carcinoma and hyperplasia in asymptomatic women. Obstet Gynecol 64 : 1–11, 1984; with permission.)

noma. It is of interest that, in four other patients, the vaginal pool smears also showed evidence of endometrial carcinoma. In all, **5 of the 17 occult carcinomas (or nearly one-third of the cases) could have been diagnosed by vaginal smear alone.**

Other Findings

There were several unanticipated incidental findings in the study: there were **two cases of ovarian carcinoma and one case of tubal carcinoma.** One ovarian cancer was recognized in an endometrial smear and was initially mistaken for an endometrial carcinoma. The other ovarian cancer was observed in a vaginal pool smear. The tubal carcinoma was observed in the endometrial sampling and in the vaginal pool smear.

There were also 22 cases of **cervical intraepithelial neoplasia, including three classical carcinomas in situ** recognized in the screened population, all suggesting that the postmenopausal women do not receive the proper gynecologic care that they deserve. There were also **four mammary carcinomas** identified by palpation of the breasts, a part of the examination offered in this study.

It is our belief that the study offered **new vistas on the need for care for the postmenopausal woman.** It is regrettable that the study had to be discontinued after 4 years for lack of funding.

Other Studies

Currently, some attempts are in progress to perform endometrial sampling on asymptomatic women by the **Tao brush** (Maksem, 2000). The results of this study, conducted on 113 patients, although not correlated with clinical data, suggest that the method may be successfully used in the diagnosis of occult cancers of the endometrium.

Rare lesions of the endometrium are discussed in Chapter 17.

BIBLIOGRAPHY

Abadi MA, Barakat RR, Saigo PE. Effects of tamoxifen on cervicovaginal smears in patients with breast cancer. Acta Cytol 44:141–146, 2000.

Abate SD, Edwards CL, Vellios F. A comparative study of the endometrial jet-washing technic and endometrial biopsy. Obstet Gynecol 43:118–122, 1972.

Abeler VM, Kjerstad KE, Berle E. Carcinoma of the endometrium in Norway: a histopathological and prognostic survey of a total population. Int J Gynecol Cancer 2:9–22, 1992.

Achiron R, Lipitz S, Sivan E, et al. Changes mimicking endometrial hyperplasia in postmenopausal, tamoxifen-treated women with breast cancer: a transvaginal Doppler study. Ultrasound Obstet Gynecol 6:116–120, 1995.

Aguirre P, Scully RE, Wolfe HJ, DeLellis RA. Endometrial carcinoma with argyrophilic cells: A histochemical and immunohistochemical analysis. Hum Pathol 210:210–217, 1984.

Alberhasky RC, Connelly PJ, Christopherson WM. Carcinoma of the endometrium. IV. Mixed adenosquamous carcinoma. A clinical-pathological study of 68 cases with long-term follow-up. Am J Clin Pathol 77:655–664, 1982.

Anderson DG, Eaton CJ, Galinkin LJ, et al. The cytologic diagnosis of endometrial adenocarcinoma. Am J Obstet Gynecol 125:376–380, 1976.

Anderson WA, Taylor PT, Fechner RE, Pinkerton JAV. Endometrial metaplasia associated with endometrial adenocarcinoma. Am J Obstet Gynecol 157:579–602, 1987.

Arends JW, Willebrand D, Dekoning Gans HJ, et al. Adenocarcinoma of the endometrium with glassy-cell features—immunohistochemical observations. Histopathol 8:837–839, 1984.

Armenia CS. Sequential relationship between endometrial polyps and carcinoma of the endometrium. Obstet Gynecol 30:524–529, 1967.

Assikis VJ, Jordan VC. Gynecologic effects of tamoxifen and the association with endometrial cancer. Int J Gynecol Obstet 49:241–257, 1995.

Athanassiadou PP, Kyrkou KA, Antoniades LG, Athanassiades PH. Cytologic evaluation of the effect of tamoxifen in premenopausal and postmenopausal women with primary breast cancer by analysis of the karyopyknotic indices of vaginal smears. Cytopathol 3:203–208, 1992.

Atkin NB. Prognostic value of cytogenetic studies of tumors of the female genital tract. In Koss LG, Coleman DV (eds). Advances in Clinical Cytology, vol 2. New York, Masson, 1984, pp 103–121.

Baak JPA, Nauta J, Wisse-Brekelmans E, Bezemer P. Architectural and morphometrical features together are more important prognosticators in endometrial hyperplasias than nuclear morphometrical features alone. J Pathol 154:335–341, 1988.

Badib AO, Kurohara SS, Vongtama VY, et al. Biologic behavior of adenocanthoma of endometrium. Am J Obstet Gynecol 106:205–209, 1970.

Baergen RN, Warren CD, Isacson C, Ellenson LH. Early uterine serous carcinoma: Clonal origin of extrauterine disease. Int J Gynecol Pathol 20:214–219, 2001.

Baggish MS, Woodruff JD. The occurrence of squamous epithelium in the endometrium. Obstet Gynecol Surv 22:69–115, 1967.

Baloglu H, Cannizzaro LA, Jones J, Koss LG. Atypical endometrial hyperplasia shares genomic abnormalities with endometrioid carcinoma by comparative genomic hybridization. Hum Pathol 32:615–622, 2001.

Bamford DS, Hall EW, Newman MR. The Isaac endometrial cell sampler. An evaluation in 100 patients with postmenopausal bleeding. Acta Cytol 28:101–104, 1984.

Barakat RR. Tamoxifen and endometrial neoplasia. Clin Obstet Gynecol 39:629–640, 1996.

Battaglia F, Scambia G, Panici PB, et al. Epidermal growth factor expression in gynecological malignancies. Gynecol Obstetr Investig 27:42–44, 1989.

Berg JW, Durfee GR. Cytological presentation of endometrial carcinoma. Cancer 11:158–172, 1958.

Bernstein L, Deapen D, Cerhan JR, et al. Tamoxifen therapy for breast cancer and endometrial cancer risk. J Natl Cancer Inst 91:1654–1662, 1999.

Berry AV, Livni NM, Epstein N. Some observations on cell morphology in the cytodiagnosis of endometrial carcinoma. Acta Cytol 13:530–533, 1969.

Bibbo M, Reale FR, Azizi F, et al. Assessment of three sampling techniques to detect endometrial carcinoma and its precursors. A preliminary report. Acta Cytol 23:353–359, 1979.

Bibbo M, Rice AM, Wied GL, Zuspan FP. Comparative specificity and sensitivity of routine cytologic examinations and the Gravlee Jet Wash technic for diagnosis of endometrial changes. Obstet Gynecol 43:253–256, 1974.

Bistoletti P, Hjerpe A, Mollerstrom G. Cytologic diagnosis of endometrial cancer and preinvasive endometrial lesions. A comparison of the Endo-Pap sampler with fractional curettage. Acta Obstet Gynecol Scand 67:343–345, 1988.

Blumenfeld W, Holly EA, Mansur DL, King EB. Histiocytes and the detection of endometrial adenocarcinoma. Acta Cytol 29:317–322, 1985.

Boon ME, Luzzatto R, Brucker N, et al. Diagnostic efficacy of endometrial cytology with the Abradul cell sampler supplemented by laser scanning confocal microscopy. Acta Cytol 40:277–282, 1996.

Bouchardy C, Vassilakos P, Riotton G. Endometrial cytohistology by the pistol–aspiration technique. Obstetr Gynecol 70:389–393, 1987.

Bouchardy C, Verkooijen HM, Fioretta G, et al. Increased risk of malignant Müllerian tumor of the uterus among women with breast cancer treated by tamoxifen. J Clin Oncol 20:4403, 2002.

Bowey CE, Spriggs AI. Chromosomes of human endometrium. J Med Genet 4:91–95, 1967.

Bur ME, Perlman C, Edelman L, et al. p53 expression in neoplasms of the uterine corpus. Am J Clin Pathol 98:81–87, 1992.

Buschmann C, Hergenrader M, Porter D. Keratin bodies. A clue in the cytological detection of endometrial adenocanthoma. Report of two cases. Acta Cytol 18:297–299, 1974.

Byrne AJ. Endocyte endometrial smears in the cytodiagnosis of endometrial carcinoma. Acta Cytol 34:373–381, 1990.

Cassano PA, Saigo PE, Hajdu SI. Comparison of cytohormonal status of postmenopausal women with cancer to age-matched controls. Acta Cytol 30:93–98, 1986.

Chalvardjian A. Sarcoidosis of the female genital tract. Am J Obstet Gynecol 132:78–80, 1978.

Chamlian DL, Taylor HB. Endometrial hyperplasia in young women. Obstet Gynecol 36:659–666, 1970.

Chang YC, Craig JM. Vaginal smear assessment of estrogen activity in endometrial carcinoma. Obstet Gynecol 21:170–174, 1963.

Charles D. Endometrial adenocanthoma. A clinicopathological study of 55 cases. Cancer 18:737–750, 1965.

Chatfield WR, Bremner AD. Intrauterine sponge biopsy. A new technique to screen for early intrauterine malignancy. Obstet Gynecol 39:323–328, 1972.

Chen JL, Trost DC, Wilkinson EJ. Endometrial papillary adenocarcinomas: Two clinicopathological types. Int J Gynecol Pathol 4:279–288, 1985.

Christopherson WM, Alberhasky RC, Connelly PJ. Carcinoma of the endometrium: I. A clinicopathologic study of clear-cell carcinoma and secretory carcinoma. Cancer 49:1511–1523, 1982.

Christopherson WM, Mendez WM, Parker JE, Lundin FE, Jr, Ahuja EM. Carcinoma of the endometrium: A study of changing rates over a 15-year period. Cancer 27:1005–1008, 1971.

Cohen CJ, Gusberg SB, Koffler D. Histologic screening for endometrial cancer. Gynecol Oncol 2:279–286, 1974.

Colditz GA, Hankinson SE, Hunter DJ, et al. The use of estrogens and progestins and the risk of breast cancer in postmenopausal women. N Engl J Med 332:1589–1593, 1995.

Costa MM, Einhorn N, Sjovall K, et al. Endometrial carcinoma diagnosed by the Gynoscann method. Acta Obstet Gynecol Scand 65:473–475, 1986.

Creasman WT, Soper JT, McCarty KS Jr, et al. Influence of cytoplasmic steroid receptor content on prognosis of early stage endometrial carcinoma. Am J Obstet Gynecol 151:922–932, 1985.

Crow J, Gordon H, Hudson E. An assessment of the MiMark endometrial sampler technique. J Clin Pathol 33:72–80, 1980.

Crum CP, Richart RM, Fenoglio CM. Adenocanthosis of the endometrium. A clinicopathologic study in premenopausal women. Am J Surg Pathol 5:15–20, 1981.

Curran WJ Jr, Whittington R, Peters AJ, Fanning J. Vaginal recurrences of endometrial carcinoma: The prognostic value of staging by a primary vaginal carcinoma system. Int J Radiat Oncol Biol Phys 15:803–808, 1988.

Curtin CT, Mitchell V, Curtin E. Cytology of primary squamous carcinoma of the endometrium. Acta Cytol 27:313–316, 1983.

Cutler BS, Forbes AP, Ingersoll FM, Scully RE. Endometrial carcinoma after stilbestrol therapy in gonadal dysgenesis. N Engl J Med 287:628–631, 1972.

Dallenbach FD, Rudolph GG. Foam cells and estrogen activity of the human endometrium. Arch Gynak 217:335–347, 1974.

Dallenbach-Hellweg G. Adenomatöse Hyperplasien von Korpusendometrium und Endozervix. Fortschr Med 94:256–263, 1976.

Dallenbach-Hellweg G, Weber J, et al. Zur Differentialdiagnose adenomatöser Endometrium-hyperplasien junger Frauen. Arch Gynecol 210:303–320, 1971.

De Peralta-Venturino MN, Purslow MJ, Kini SR. Endometrial cells of the "lower uterine segment" (LUS) in cervical smears obtained by endocervical brushings: a source of potential diagnostic pitfall. Diagn Cytopathol 12:263–268, 1995.

Dehner LP, Askin FB. Cytomegalovirus endometritis. Report of a case associated with spontaneous abortion. Obstet Gynecol 45:211–214, 1975.

Deligdisch L, Holinka CF. Endometrial carcinoma: Two diseases? Cancer Detect Prev 10:237–246, 1987.

Deligdish L, Loewenthal M. Endometrial changes associated with myomata of the uterus. J Clin Pathol 23:676–680, 1970.

DePetrillo AD, DiSaia PJ, Morrow CP, Townsend DE. Gravlee Jet Washer effectiveness as performed by obstetric/gynecologic paramedical personnel. Am J Obstet Gynecol 117:371–374, 1973.

Dowling EA, Gravlee LC, Hutchins KE. A new technique for the detection of adenocarcinoma of the endometrium. Acta Cytol 13:496–501, 1969.

Dubs I. Xanthomzellenbildung in der Uterusschleimhaut bei Funduskarzinom. Zentralbl Allg Pathol 34:145, 1923.

Duggan BD, Felix JC, Muderspach LI, et al. Microsatellite instability in sporadic endometrial carcinoma. J Natl Cancer Inst 86:1216–1221, 1994.

Duncan DA, Varner RE, Mazur MT. Uterine herpesvirus infection with multifocal necrotizing endometritis. Hum Pathol 20:1021–1024, 1989.

Ehrlich CE, Young PCM, Cleary RE. Cytoplasmic progesterone and estradiol receptors in normal, hyperplastic, and carcinomatous endometria: Therapeutic implications. Am J Obstet Gynecol 141:539–546, 1981.

Ehrman RL. Atypical endometrial cells and stromal breakdown. Two case reports. Acta Cytol 19:465–469, 1975.

Elstein M, Woodcock A, Buckley CH. An unusual case of sarcoidosis. Br J Obstet Gynaecol 101:452–453, 1994.

Elwood JM, Cole P, Rothman KJ, Kaplan SD. Epidemiology of endometrial cancer. J Natl Cancer Inst 59:1055–1060, 1977.

Evans LH, Martin JD, Hahnel R. Estrogen receptor concentration in normal and pathological human uterine tissues. J Clin Endocrinol Metab 38:23–32, 1974.

Factor SM. Papillary adenocarcinoma of the endometrium with psammoma bodies. Arch Pathol 98:201–205, 1974.

Farhi DC, Nosanchuk J, Silverberg SG. Endometrial adenocarcinoma in women under 25 years of age. Obstet Gynecol 68:741–745, 1986.

Fechner RE, Kaufman RH. Endometrial adenocarcinoma in Stein-Leventhal syndrome. Cancer 34:444–452, 1974.

Fehr PE, Prem KA. Malignancy of the uterine corpus following irradiation therapy for squamous cell carcinoma of the cervix. Am J Obstet Gynecol 119:685–692, 1974.

Ferenczy A. The ultrastructural dynamics of endometrial hyperplasia and neoplasia. In Koss LG, Coleman DV (eds). Advances in Clinical Cytology, vol. 1. London, Butterworths, 1981, pp 1–43.

Ferenczy A, Gelfand M. The biologic significance of cytologic atypia in progestogen-treated endometrial hyperplasia. Am J Obstet Gynecol 160:126–131, 1989.

Ferenczy A, Richart RM. Scanning electron microscopy of hyperplasia and neoplastic endometria. In Johari O (ed). Scanning Electron Microscopy, Part III. Proceedings of the Workshop on Scanning Electron Microscopy in Pathology. Chicago, Research Institute, 1973, pp 613–620.

Ferenczy A, Richart RM, Agate FJ Jr, et al. Scanning electron microscopy of the human endometrial surface epithelium. Fertil Steril 23:515–521, 1972.

Fisher B, Constantino JP, Redmond CK, et al. Endometrial cancer in tamoxifen-treated breast cancer patients: Findings from the National Surgical Adjuvant Breast and Bowel project (NASBP) B-14. J Natl Cancer Inst 86:527–537, 1994.

Foster LN, Montgomery R. Endometrial carcinoma. A review of prior biopsies. Am J Clin Pathol 43:26–38, 1965.

Frick HC, Munnell EW, Richart RM, et al. Carcinoma of the endometrium. Am J Obstet Gynecol 115:663–676, 1973.

Geisinger KR, Kute ET, Marshall RB, et al. Analysis of the relationships of the ploidy and cell cycle kinetics to differentiation and the female sex steroid hormone receptors in adenocarcinoma of the endometrium. Am J Clin Pathol 85:536–541, 1986.

Gompel C. Aspects cytologiques du carcinome du corps uterin. Bruxelles Med 33:504–515, 1953.

Gordon J, Reagan JW, Finkle WD, Ziel HK. Estrogen and endometrial carcinoma. An independent pathology review supporting original risk estimate. N Engl J Med 297:570–571, 1977.

Gore H. Hyperplasia of the endometrium. In Norris HJ, Hertig AT, Abell MR (eds). The Uterus. Baltimore, Williams & Wilkins, 1973, pp 255–275.

Gould PR, Li L, Henderson DW, et al. Cilia and ciliogenesis in endometrial adenocarcinomas. An ultrastructural analysis. Arch Pathol Lab Med 110:326–330, 1986.

Graham R. The diagnostic accuracy of vaginal smears for detection of endometrial carcinoma. Acta Cytol 2:579, 1958.

Granberg I, Gupta S, Joelsson I, Sprenger E. Chromosome and nuclear DNA study of a uterine adenocarcinoma and its metastases. Acta Pathol Microbiol Scand 82:1–6, 1974.

Grattarola R, Secreto G, Recchione C, Castellini W. Androgens in breast cancer. II. Endometrial adenocarcinoma and breast cancer in married postmenopausal women. Am J Obstet Gynecol 118:173–178, 1974.

Gravlee LC Jr. Jet-irrigation method for the diagnosis of endometrial adenocarcinoma. Its principle and accuracy. Obstet Gynecol 34:168–173, 1969.

Gray PH, Anderson CT Jr, Munnell EW. Endometrial adenocarcinoma and ovarian agenesis. Report of a case. Obstet Gynecol 35:513–518, 1970.

Greene RR, Roddick JW Jr, Milligan M. Estrogens, endometrial hyperplasia, and endometrial carcinoma. Ann NY Acad Sci 75:586–600, 1959.

Greenlee RT, Murrey T, Bolden S, Wingo PA. American Cancer Society Cancer Satistics, 2000. CA Cancer J Clin 50:7–33, 2000.

Gu M, Shi W, Barakat RR, et al. Pap smears in women with endometrial carcinoma. Acta Cytol 45:555–560, 2001.

Gusberg SB. Precursors of corpus carcinoma; estrogens and adenomatous hyperplasia. Am J Obstet Gynecol 54:905–927, 1947.

Gusberg SB, Kaplan AL. Precursors of corpus cancer. IV. Adenomatous hyperplasia as stage 0 carcinoma of the endometrium. Am J Obstet Gynecol 87:662–676, 1963.

Hameed K, Morgan DA. Papillary adenocarcinoma of endometrium with psammoma bodies. Histology and fine structure. Cancer 29:1326–1335, 1972.

Hanau CA, Begley N, Bibbo M. Cervical endometriosis: a potential pitfall in the evaluation of glandular cells in cervical smears. Diagn Cytopathol 16:274–280, 1997.

Hann LE, Giess CS, Bach AM, et al. Endometrial thickness in tamoxifen-treated patients: correlation with clinical and pathologic findings. Am J Roentgenol 168:657–661, 1997.

Heaton RB Jr, Harris TF, Larson DM, Henry MR. Glandular cells derived from direct sampling of the lower uterine segment in patients status post-cervical cone biopsy. A diagnostic dilemma. Am J Clin Pathol 106:511–516, 1996.

Hecht EL. Cytologic approach to uterine carcinoma; detection, diagnosis, and therapy. Am J Obstet Gynecol 64:81–90, 1952.

Hecht EL. Endometrial aspiration smear; research status and clinical value. Am J Obstet Gynecol 71:819–833, 1956.

Hendrickson MR, Kempson RL. Ciliated carcinoma—a variant of endometrial adenocarcinoma: A report of 10 cases. Int J Gynecol Pathol 2:1–12, 1983.

Hendrickson MR, Kempson RL. Endometrial epithelial metaplasias: Proliferations frequency misdiagnosed as adenocarcinoma: Report of 89 cases and proposed classification. Am J Surg Pathol 4:525–542, 1980.

Hendrickson MR, Kempson RL. Endometrial epithelial metaplasias: Proliferations frequency misdiagnosed as adenocarcinoma—report of 89 cases and proposed classification. Am J Surg Pathol 4:525–542, 1980.

Hendrickson MR, Kempson RL. Non-neoplastic metaplasias: Epithelial and mesenchymal musical chairs. In Surgical Pathology of the Uterine Corpus. Philadelphia, WB Saunders, 1980.

Hertig AT, Sommers SC. Genesis of endometrial carcinoma. I. Study of prior biopsies. Cancer 2:946–956, 1949.

Hertig AT, Sommers SC, Bengloff H. Genesis of endometrial carcinoma. III. Carcinoma in situ. Cancer 2:964–971, 1949.

Highman WJ. Cervical smears in tuberculous endometritis. Acta Cytol 16:16–20, 1972.

Hoffman MS, Cavanagh D, Walter TS, et al. Adenocarcinoma of the endometrium and endometrioid carcinoma of the ovary associated with pregnancy. Gynecol Oncol 32:82–85, 1989.

Hoover R, Fraumeni JF Jr, Everson R, Myers MH. Cancer of the uterine corpus after hormonal treatment for breast cancer. Lancet 2:885–887, 1976.

Horwitz RI, Feinstein AR. Alternative analytic methods for case-control studies of estrogens and endometrial cancer. N Engl J Med 299:1089–1094, 1978.

Horwitz RI, Feinstein AR, Horowitz SM, Robboy SJ. Necropsy diagnosis of endometrial cancer and detection-bias in case/control studies. Lancet 2:66–68, 1981.

Horwitz RI, Feinstein AR, Vidone RA, et al. Histopathologic distinctions in the relationship of estrogens and endometrial cancer. JAMA 246:1425–1427, 1981.

Houissa-Vuong S, Catanzano-Laroudie M, Baviera E, et al. Primary squamous cell carcinoma of the endometrium: Case history, pathologic findings, and discussion. Diagn Cytopathol 27:291–293, 2002.

Iezzoni JC, Mills SE. Nonneoplastic endometrial signet-ring cells. Vacuolated decidual cells and stromal histiocytes mimicking adenocarcinoma. Am J Clin Pathol 115:249–255, 2001.

Inoue Y, Ikeda M, Kimura K, et al. Accuracy of endometrial aspiration in the diagnosis of endometrial cancer. Acta Cytol 27:477–481, 1983.

Isaacs JH, Ross FH. Cytologic evaluation of the endometrium in women with postmenopausal bleeding. Am J Obstet Gynecol 131:410–415, 1978.

Iverson OE, Laerum OD. Ploidy disturbances in endometrial and ovarian carcinomas. A review. Anal Quant Cytol Histol 7:327–336, 1985.

Iverson OE, Utaaker ES. DNA ploidy and steroid receptors as predictors of disease course in patients with endometrial carcinoma. Acta Obstet Gynecol Scand 67:531–537, 1988.

Jassoni VM, Santini D, Amadori A et al. Epidermal growth factor receptor expression and endometrial cancer histotypes. In Buletti C, Gurpide E, Flamigni C (eds). The Human Endometrium, vol 734. New York, Ann NY Acad Sci, 1994, pp 298–305.

Jeffrey JF, Krepart GV, Lotocki RJ. Papillary serous adenocarcinoma of the endometrium. Obstet Gynecol 67:670–674, 1986.

Jimenez-Ayala M, Vilaplana E, Becerro de Bengoa C, et al. Endometrial and endocervical brushing techniques with a Medhosa Cannula. Acta Cytol 19: 557–563, 1975.

Johannisson E. Effects on the Endometrium, Endo- and Endocervix Following the Use of Local Progestogen-Releasing Delivery Systems. Center for Medical Research, The Population Council, New York, 1990.

Johannisson E, Engstrom L. Cytological diagnosis of endometrial disorders with a brush technique. Acta Obstet Gynecol Scand 50:141–148, 1971.

Johannisson E, Parker RA, Landgren B-M, Diczfalusy E. Morphometric analysis of the human endometrium in relation to peripheral hormone levels. Fertil Steril 38:564–571, 1982.

Johnson TL, Kini SR. Endometrial metaplasia as a source of atypical glandular cells in cervicovaginal smears. Diagn Cytopathol 14:25–31, 1996.

Johnsson JE, Stormby NG. Cytological brush technique in malignant disease of the endometrium. Acta Obstet Gynecol Scand 47:38–51, 1968.

Jones MA, Young RH, and Scully RE. Endometrial adenocarcinoma with a component of giant cell carcinoma. Int J Gynecol Pathol 10:260–270, 1991.

Jordan MJ, Bader GM, Namazie AS. Comparative accuracy of preoperative cytologic and histologic diagnosis in endometrial lesions. Obstet Gynecol 7: 646–653, 1956.

Kanbour A, Klionsky B, Cooper R. Cytohistologic diagnosis of uterine jet wash preparations. Acta Cytol 18:51–58, 1974.

Kauppila A, Jujansuu E, Vihko R. Cytosol estrogen and progesterone receptors in endometrial carcinoma treated with surgery, radiotherapy, and progestin: Clinical correlates. Cancer 50:2157–2162, 1982.

Kay S. Clear-cell carcinoma of the endometrium. Cancer 10:124–130, 1957.

Keubler DL, Nikrui N, Bell DA. Cytologic features of endometrial papillary serous carcinoma. Acta Cytol 33:120–126, 1989.

Khosla T, Lower CR. Indices of obesity derived from body weight and height. Br J Prev Soc Med 21:122, 1967.

Koss LG. Miniature adenocanthoma arising in an endometriotic cyst in an obturator lymph node. Report of first cases. Cancer 16:1369–1372, 1963.

Koss LG. Early diagnosis of uterine and ovarian carcinoma. 10th International Cancer Congress. Oncol Proc 4:211–220, 1970.

Koss LG. (Panelists: Cramer D, Ferenczy A, Gurpide E, Reagan JW, Siiteri PK, Sommers SC.) Recent advances in endometrial neoplasia. Acta Cytol 24: 478–493, 1980.

Koss LG, Durfee GR. Cytologic diagnosis of endometrial carcinoma. Result of ten years of experience. Acta Cytol 6:519–531, 1962.

Koss LG, Pierce V, Brunschwig A. Pseudothecomas of ovaries: A syndrome of bilateral ovarian hypertrophy with diffuse luteinization, endometrial carcinoma, obesity, hirsutism, and diabetes mellitus. Report of 2 cases. Cancer 17:76–85, 1964.

Koss LG, Schreiber K, Moussouris H, Oberlander SG. Endometrial carcinoma and its precursors: Detection and screening. Clin Obstet Gynecol 25:49–61, 1982.

Koss LG, Schreiber K, Oberlander SG, et al. Screening of asymptomatic women for endometrial cancer. Obstet Gynecol 57:681–691, 1981.

Koss LG, Schreiber K, Oberlander SG, et al. Detection of endometrial carcinoma and hyperplasia in asymptomatic women. Obstet Gynecol 64:1–11, 1984.

Kowalczyk CL, Malone J Jr, Peterson EP, et al. Well-differentiated endometrial adenocarcinoma in an infertility patient with later conception. A case report. J Reprod Med 44:57–60, 1999.

Kreiger N, Marrett LD, Clarke EA, et al. Risk factors for adenomatous endometrial hyperplasia: A case-control study. Am J Epidemiol 123:291–301, 1986.

Kurman RJ, Norris HJ. Evaluation of criteria for distinguishing atypical endometrial hyperplasia from well-differentiated carcinoma. Cancer 49:2549–2559, 1982.

Kurman RJ, Scully RE. Clear cell carcinoma of the endometrium. An analysis of 21 cases. Cancer 37:872–882, 1976.

Kurman RJ, Kaminsky PF, Norris HJ. The behavior of endometrial hyperplasia. A long-term study of "untreated" hyperplasia in 170 patients. Cancer 56: 403–412, 1985.

Kusuyama Y, Yoshida M, Imai H, et al. Secretory carcinoma of the endometrium. Acta Cytol 33:127–130, 1989.

Lane ME, Dacalos E, Sobrero AJ, Ober WB. Squamous metaplasia of the endometrium in women with an intrauterine contraceptive device: Follow up study. Am J Obstet Gynecol 119:693–697, 1974.

Langer RD, Pierce JJ, O'Hanlan KA. et al. Transvaginal sonography compared with endometrial biopsy for the detection of endometrial disease. N Engl J Med 337:1792–1798, 1997.

Larson DM, Copeland LJ, Gallager HS, et al. Primary squamous-cell carcinoma of the endometrium. Acta Obstet Gynecol Scand 66:181–182, 1981.

Levine D, Gosink BB, Johnson LA. Changes in endometrial thickness in endometrial thickness in postmenopausal women undergoing hormone-replacement therapy. Radiol 197:603–608, 1995.

Liggins GC, Way J. Comparison of prognosis of adeno–acanthoma and adenocarcinoma of corpus uteri. J Obstet Gynaecol Br Commonw 67:294–296, 1960.

Liu CT. A study of endometrial adenocarcinoma with emphasis on morphologically variant types. Am J Clin Pathol 57:562–573, 1972.

Liu W, Barrow MJ, Spitler MF, Kochis AF. Normal exfoliation of endometrial cells in premenopausal women. Acta Cytol 7:211–214, 1963.

Long ME, Doko F, Taylor HC Jr. Nucleoli and nucleolar ribonucleic acid in nonmalignant and malignant human endometria. Am J Obstet Gynecol 75: 1002–1014, 1958.

Lukeman JM. An evaluation of the negative pressure "Jet Washing" of the endometrium in menopausal and post-menopausal patients. Acta Cytol 18: 462–471, 1974.

Lundeen SJ, Horwitz CA, Larson CJ, Stanley MW. Abnormal cervicovaginal smears due to endometriosis: A continuing problem. Diagn Cytopathol 26: 35–40, 2002.

MacDonald PC, Siiteri PK. The relationship between the extraglandular production of estrone and the occurrence of endometrial neoplasia. Gynecol Oncol 2:259–263, 1974.

Mack TM, Pike MC, Henderson BE, et al. Estrogens and endometrial cancer in a retirement community. N Engl J Med 294:1262–1267, 1976.

Maksem JA. Ciliated cell adenocarcinoma of the endometrium diagnosed by endometrial brush cytology and confirmed by hysterectomy: case report detailing a highly efficient cytology collection and processing techniques. Diagn Cytopathol 16:78–82, 1997.

Maksem JA. Perfomance characteristics of the Indiana University Medical Center Endometrial sampler (Tao Brush) in an outpatient office setting, first year's outcomes: recognizing histological patterns in cytologic preparations of endometrial brushings. Diagn Cytopathol 22:186–195, 2000.

Maksem JA, Knesel E. Liquid fixation of endometrial brush cytology ensures a well-preserved, representative cell sample with frequent tissue correlation. Diagn Cytopathol 14:367–373, 1995.

Maksem JA, Lee SS. Endometrial intraepithelial carcinoma diagnosed by brush cytology and p53 immunostaining, and confirmed by hysterectomy. Diagn Cytopathol 19:78–82, 1998.

Malone JJM, Rutledge FN. Prognostic factors in stage II endometrial carcinoma. Cancer 60:1358–1361, 1987.

Marcus SL. Adenocanthoma of the endometrium: Report of 24 cases and a review of squamous metaplasia. Am J Obstet Gynecol 81:259–267, 1961.

Mazur MT. Atypical polypoid adenomyomas of the endometrium. Am J Surg Pathol 5:473–482, 1981.

McBride JM. Pre-menopausal cystic hyperplasia and endometrial carcinoma. J Obstet Gynaecol Br Emp 66:288–296, 1959.

McKenna TJ. Pathogenesis and treatment of polycystic ovary syndrome. N Engl J Med 318:558–562, 1988.

Meisels A, Jolicoeur C. Criteria for the cytologic assessment of hyperplasias in endometrial samples obtained by the Endopap endometrial sampler. Acta Cytol 29:297–302, 1985.

Mencaglia L. Endometrial cytology: six years of experience. Diagn Cytopathol 3:185–190, 1987.

Mishell DR Jr, Kaunitz AM. Devices for endometrial sampling. A comparison. J Reprod Med 43:180–184, 1998.

Morse AR. The value of endometrial aspiration in gynaecological practice. In Koss LG, Coleman DV (eds). Advances in Clinical Cytology, vol 1. London, Butterworths, 1981, pp 44–63.

Moyer DL, Mishell DR. Reactions of human endometrium to the intrauterine foreign body. II. Long-term effects on the endometrial histology and cytology. Am J Obstet Gynecol 111:66–80, 1971.

Mulvany NJ, Surtees V. Cervical/vaginal endometriosis with atypia: A cytohistopathologic study. Diagn Cytopathol 21:188–193, 1999.

Mutter GL, Baak JPA, Crum CP, et al. Endometrial precancer diagnosis by histopathology, clonal analysis, and computerized morphometry. J Pathol 190: 462–469, 2000.

Nahhas WA, Lund CJ, Rudolph JH. Carcinoma of the corpus uteri. A 10-year review of 225 patients. Obstet Gynecol 38:564–570, 1971.

Nakano KK, Schoene WC. Endometrial carcinoma with a predominant clear-cell pattern with metastases to the adrenal, posterior mediastinum, and brain. Am J Obstet Gynecol 122:529–530, 1975.

Ng ABP. The cellular detection of endometrial carcinoma and its precursors. Gynecol Oncol 2:162–179, 1974.

Ng ABP, Reagan JW, Cechner RL. The precursors of endometrial cancer. A study of their cellular manifestations. Acta Cytol 17:439–448, 1973.

Ng ABP, Reagan JW, Hawliczek S, Wentz BW. Significance of endometrial cells in the detection of endometrial carcinoma and its precursors. Acta Cytol 18:356–361, 1974.

Ng ABP, Reagan JW, Storaasli JP, Wentz WB. Mixed adenosquamous carcinoma of the endometrium. Am J Clin Pathol 59:765–781, 1973.

Nguyen TN, Bourdeau J-L, Ferenczy A, Franco EL. Clinical significance of histiocytes in the detection of endometrial adenocarcinoma and hyperplasia. Diagn Cytopathol 19:89–93, 1998.

Norris HJ, Becker RL, Mikel UV. A comparative morphometric and cytophotometric study of endometrial hyperplasia, atypical hyperplasia, and endometrial carcinoma. Hum Pathol 20:219–223, 1989.

Novak ER. Postmenopausal endometrial hyperplasia. Am J Obstet Gynecol 71: 1312–1321, 1956.

Nuovo V. The cell type in vaginal smears of patients with ovarian or endometrial carcinoma. Acta Cytol 4:119–120, 1960.

Nyholm HCJ, Nielsen AL, Ottesen B. Expression of epidermal growth factor receptors in human endometrial carcinomas. Int J Gynecol Pathol 12: 241–245, 1993.

Osborne CK. Tamoxifen in the treatment of breast cancer. N Engl J Med 339: 1609–1618, 1998.

Padubidri V, Baijal L, Prakash P, Chandra K. The detection of endometrial tuberculosis in cases of infertility by endometrial aspiration cytology. Acta Cytol 24:319–324, 1980.

Palermo VG. The detection of endometrial adenocarcinoma using the Endopap endometrial cytology sampler. Acta Cytol 26:738, 1982.

Palermo VG, Blythe JG, Kaufman RH. Cytologic diagnosis of endometrial adenocarcinoma using the Endopap sampler. Obstet Gynecol 65:271–275, 1985.

Pang S, Softness B, Sweeney WJ, New MI. Hirsutism, polycystic ovarian disease, and ovarian 17-ketosteroid reductase deficiency. N Engl J Med 316: 1295–1301, 1987.

Papanicolaou GN. Atlas of Exfoliative Cytology. Cambridge, MA, Harvard University Press for the Commonwealth Fund, 1954.

Parkash V, Carcangiu ML. Endometrioid adenocarcinoma with psammoma bodies. Am J Surg Pathol 21:399–406, 1997.

Partridge EE, Shingleton HM, Menck HR. The national cancer data base report on endometrial cancer. J Surg Oncol 61:111–123, 1996.

Paz RA, Frigerio B, Sundblad AS, Eusebi V. Small-cell (oat cell) carcinoma of the endometrium. Arch Pathol Lab Med 109:270–272, 1985.

PEPI Trial. Effects of hormone replacement therapy on endometrial histology in postmenopausal women. The Postmenopausal Estrogen/Progestin Interventions (PEPI) Trial. The Writing Group for the PEPI Trial. JAMA 275: 370–375, 1996.

Peris LA, Jernstrom P, Bowers PA. Primary squamous-cell carcinoma of uterine corpus; report of case and review of literature. Am J Obstet Gynecol 75: 1019–1026, 1958.

Pokoly T. A comparison of the clinical behavior of uterine adenocarcinomas and adenoacanthomas. Am J Obstet Gynecol 108:1080–1084, 1970.

Praca D, Keyhani-Rofagha S, Copeland L, Hameed A. Exfoliative cytology of neuroendocrine small cell carcinoma of the endometrium. A report of two cases. Acta Cytol 42:978–982, 1998.

Prem KA, Adcock LL, Okagaki T, Jones TK. The evolution of a treatment program for adenocarcinoma of the endometrium. Am J Obstet Gynecol 133: 803–813, 1979.

Prichard KI. Screening for endometrial cancer: Is it effective? [editorial]. Ann Intern Med 110:177–179, 1989.

Rascoe RR. Endometrial aspiration smear in diagnosis of malignancy of the uterine corpus. Am J Obstet Gynecol 87:921–925, 1963.

Reagan JW, Ng ABP. The cells of uterine adenocarcinoma, 2nd ed. Baltimore, Williams & Wilkins, 1973.

Reid DE, Shirley RL. Endometrial carcinoma associated with Sheehan's syndrome and stilbestrol therapy. Am J Obstet Gynecol 119:264–266, 1974.

Reisinger JI, Berchuck A, Kohler MF, et al. Genetic instability of microsatellites in endometrial carcinoma. Cancer Res 53:5100–5103, 1993.

Reynolds RK, Talavera F, Roberts JA, et al. Characterisation of epidermal growth factor receptor in normal and neoplastic human endometrium. Cancer 66:1967–1974, 1990.

Robboy SJ, Bradley R. Changing trends and prognostic features in endometrial cancer associated with exogenous estrogen therapy. Obstet Gynecol 54: 269–277, 1979.

Robboy SJ, Miller AW III, Kurman RJ. The pathologic features and behavior of endometrial carcinoma associated with exogenous estrogen administration. Pathol Res Pract 174:237–256, 1982.

Rodriques A, Rubin A, Koss LG, Harris J. Evaluation of endometrial jet wash technique (Gravlee) in 303 patients in a community hospital. Obstet Gynecol 43:392–399, 1974.

Rose PG. Endometrial carcinoma. N Engl J Med 335:640–649, 1996.

Sachs H, Wamtach EV, Wurthner K. DNA content of normal, hyperplastic and malignant endometrium, determined cytophotometrically. Arch Gynecol 217:349–365, 1974.

Sagiroglu N. Phagocytosis of spermatozoa in the uterine cavity of woman using intrauterine device. Int J Fertil 16:1–15, 1971.

Sagiroglu N, Sagiroglu E. The cytology of intrauterine contraceptive devices. Acta Cytol 14:58–64, 1970.

Salm R. The incidence and significance of early carcinomas in endometrial polyps. J Pathol 108:47–53, 1972.

Sano ME. The cytology antedating overt endometrial carcinoma. A preliminary report. Acta Cytol 13:523–529, 1969.

Sato S, Matsunaga G, Konno R, Yajima A. Mass screening for cancer of the endometrium in Miyagi Prefecture, Japan. Acta Cytol 42:295–298, 1998.

Schafer G, Marcus RS, Kramer EE. Postmenopausal endometrial tuberculosis. Am J Obstet Gynecol 112:681–687, 1972.

Schairer C, Lubin J, Troisi R, et al. Menopausal estrogen and estrogen-progestin replacement therapy and breast cancer risk. JAMA 283:485–491, 2000.

Schneider J, Bradlow HL, Strain G, et al. Effects of obesity on estradiol metabolism: Decreased formation of nonuterotropic metabolites. J Clin Endocrinol Metab 56:973–978, 1983.

Scully RE, Poulson H, Sobin LH. International histologic classification and histologic typing of female genital tract tumors. Berlin, Springer Verlag, 1994.

Segadal E, Iversen OE. Endoscan, a new endometrial sampler. Br J Obstet Gynecol 90:266–271, 1983.

Sherman AI. Chromosome constitution of endometrium. Obstet Gynecol 34: 753–766, 1969.

Sherman AI, Brown S. The precursors of endometrial carcinoma. Am J Obstet Gynecol 135:947–954, 1979.

Sherman AI, Woolf RB. Endocrine basis for endometrial carcinoma. Am J Obstet Gynecol 77:233–242, 1959.

Sherman ME. Theories of endometrial carcinogenesis: A multidisciplinary approach. Mod Pathol 13:295–308, 2000.

Sherman ME, Bitterman P, Rosenshein NB, et al. Uterine serous carcinoma. A morphologically diverse neoplasm with unifying clinicopathologic features. Am J Surg Pathol 16:600–610, 1992.

Sherman ME, Bur ME, Kurman RJ. p53 in endometrial cancer and its putative precursors: evidence for diverse pathways in tumorigenesis. Hum Pathol 26: 1268–1274, 1995.

Silva EG, Tornos CS, Follen-Mitchell M. Malignant neoplasms of the uterine corpus in patients treated for breast carcinoma: the effects of tamoxifen. Int J Gynecol Pathol 13:248–258, 1994.

Silverberg SG. Adenomyomatosis of endometrium and endocervix. Am J Clin Pathol 64:192–199, 1975.

Silverberg SG. Significance of squamous elements in carcinoma of the endometrium: A review. In Fenoglio CM, Wolff M (eds). Progress in Surgical Pathology, vol. IV. New York, Masson Publishing, 1982, pp 115–136.

Silverberg SG, Bolin MG, DeGiorgi LS. Adeno-acanthoma and mixed adeno-squamous carcinoma of the endometrium: A clinicopathologic study. Cancer 30:1307–1314, 1972.

Silverberg SG, Giorgi LS. Clear cell carcinoma of the endometrium. Cancer 31: 1127–1140, 1973.

Silverberg SG, Makowski EL. Endometrial carcinoma in young women taking oral contraceptive agents. Obstet Gynecol 46:503–506, 1975.

Silverberg SG, Mullen D, Faraci JA, et al. Primary squamous cell carcinoma of the endometrium. Gynecol Oncol 31:454–461, 1988.

Silverberg SG, Kurman RJ. Tumors of the Uterine Corpus and Gestational Trophoblastic Disease in Atlas of Tumor Pathology (Series 3, vol 3). Washington, DC: Armed Forces Institute of Pathology, 1992.

Skaarland E. Nuclear size and shape of epithelial cells from the endometrium: Lack of value as a criterion for differentiation between normal, hyperplastic, and malignant conditions. J Clin Pathol 38:502–506, 1985.

Skehan M, McKenna P. Sarcoidosis of the endometrium: A case presentation. Irish J Med Sci 154:213, 1986.

Smith DC, Prentice R, Thompson DJ, Herrmann WL. Association of exogenous estrogen and endometrial carcinoma. N Engl J Med 293:1164–1167, 1975.

So-Bosita JL, Lebherz TB, Blair OM. Endometrial jet washer. Obstet Gynecol 36:287–293, 1970.

Soslow RA, Pirog E, Isacson C. Endometrial intraepithelial carcinoma with associated peritoneal carcinomatosis. Am J Surg Pathol 24:726–732, 2000.

Speert H. Premalignant phase of endometrial carcinoma. Cancer 5:927–944, 1952.

Spiegel GW. Endometrial carcinoma in situ in postmenopausal women. Am J Surg Pathol 19:417–432, 1995.

Spjut HJ, Kaufman RH, Carrig SS. Psammoma bodies in the cervicovaginal smear. Acta Cytol 8:352–355, 1964.

Stanley MA. Chromosome constitution of human endometrium. Am J Obstet Gynecol 104:99–103, 1969.

Stovall TG, Solomon SK, Ling FW. Endometrial sampling prior to hysterectomy. Obstet Gynecol 73:405–409, 1989.

Susini T, Massi D, Paglierani M, et al. Expression of the retinoblastoma-related gene Rb2/p130 is downregulated in atypical endometrial hyperplasia and adenocarcinoma. Hum Pathol 32:360–367, 2001.

Sutherland JV. Endometrial carcinoma: Clinical-pathologic comparison of cases in post-menopausal women receiving and not receiving exogenous estrogens. Cancer 45:3018–3026, 1980.

Swingler GR, Cave DG, Mitchard P. Diagnostic accuracy of the MiMark endometrial cell sampler in 101 patients with postmenopausal bleeding. Br J Obstet Gynecol 86:816–818, 1979.

Symonds D, Reed T, Didolkar S, Graham R. AGUS in cervical endometriosis. J Reprod Med 42:39–43, 1997.

Szulman AE. Histology of endometrial carcinoma including some cytogenetical considerations. In Lewis GC Jr, Wentz WB, Jaffe RM (eds). New Concepts in Gynecological Oncology. Philadelphia, FA Davis, 1966, pp 225–228.

Tambouret R, Bell DA, Centeno BA. Significance of histiocytes in cervical smears from peri/postmenopausal women. Diagn Cytopathol 24:271–275, 2001.

Tambouret R, Clement PB, Young RH. Endometrial endometrioid adenocarcinoma with a deceptive pattern of spread to the uterine cervix. A manifestation of stage IIB endometrial carcinoma liable to be misinterpreted as an independent carcinoma or a benign lesion. Am J Surg Pathol 27:1080–1088, 2003.

Tao, LC. Cytopathology of the endometrium. Direct intrauterine sampling. Chicago, ASCP Press, 1993.

Tao LC. Cytomorphologic appearances of normal endometrial cells during different phases of the menstrual cycle: a cytologic approach to endometrial dating. Diagn Cytopathol 13:95–102, 1995.

Tavassoli FA, Krauss FT. Endometrial lesions in uteri resected for atypical endometrial hyperplasia. Am J Clin Pathol 70:770–779, 1978.

TeLinde RW, Jones HW Jr, Galvin GA. What are earliest endometrial changes to justify diagnosis of endometrial cancer? Am J Obstet Gynecol 66: 953–969, 1953.

Thomas W, Sadeghhieh B, Fresco R, et al. Malacoplakia of the endometrium, a probable cause of postmenopausal bleeding. Am J Clin Pathol 69:637–641, 1978.

Torres JE, Holmquist ND, Danos ML. The endometrial irrigation smear in the detection of adenocarcinoma of the endometrium. Acta Cytol 13:163–168, 1969.

Tseng PY, Jones HW. Chromosome constitution of carcinoma of the endometrium. Obstet Gynecol 33:741–752, 1969.

Ueda G, Yamasaki M, Masaki I, Kurachi KA. Clinicopathologic study of endometrial carcinomas with argyrophil cells. Gynecol Oncol 7:223–232, 1979.

Underwood PB Jr, Kellett MP, et al. The Gravlee Jet Washer: Can it replace the diagnostic curettage? Am J Obstet Gynecol 117:201–209, 1973.

Utaaker E, Iverson OE, Sakaarland E. The distribution and prognostic implications of steroid receptors in endometrial carcinomas. Gynecol Oncol 28: 89–100, 1987.

Valicenti JF, Jr, Priester SK. Psammoma bodies of benign endometrial origin in cervicovaginal cytology. Acta Cytol 21:550–552, 1977.

Van der Putten HWHM, Baak JPA, et al. Prognostic value of quantitative pathologic features and DNA content in individual patients with stage 1 endometrial adenocarcinoma. Cancer 63:1378–1387, 1989.

Varangot J, Granjon A, Nuovo V, Vassy S. Detection and diagnosis of carcinoma of endometrium by vaginal and endometrial smears. Am J Obstet Gynecol 68:474–479, 1954.

Vassilakos P, Wyss R, Wenger D, Riotton G. Endometrial cytohistology by aspiration technic and by Gravlee Jet Washer. Obstet Gynecol 45:320–324, 1975.

Veneti SZ, Kyrkou KA, Kittas CN, Perides AT. Efficacy of the Isaacs endometrial cell sampler in the cytologic detection of endometrial abnormalities. Acta Cytol 28:546–554, 1984.

Von Luedinghausen M, Anastasiadis P. Anatomic basis of endometrial cytology. Acta Cytol 28:555–562, 1984.

Wachtel E, Gordon H, Wycherley J. The cytological diagnosis of endometrial pathology using a uterine aspiration technique. J Obstet Gynecol Br Commonw 80:164–168, 1973.

Wagner D, Richart RM, Terner JY. Deoxyribonucleic acid content of presumed precursors of endometrial carcinoma. Cancer 20:2067–2077, 1967.

Warhol MJ, Rice RH, Pinkus GS, Robboy SJ. Evaluation of squamous epithelium in adenoacanthoma and adenosquamous carcinoma of the endometrium: Immuno-peroxidase analysis of involucrin and keratin localization. Int J Gynecol Pathol 3:82–91, 1984.

Wen P, Abramovich CM, Wang N, et al. Significance of histiocytes on otherwise normal cervical smears from postmenopausal women: A retrospective study of 108 cases. Acta Cytol 47:135–140, 2003.

Wenckebach GFC, Curry B. Cytomegalovirus infection of the female genital tract. Arch Pathol Lab Med 100:609–612, 1976.

White AJ, Buchsbaum HJ. Scanning electron microscopy of the human endometrium. I. Normal. Gynecol Oncol 11:330–339, 1973.

White AJ, Buchsbaum HJ. Scanning electron microscopy of the human endometrium. II. Hyperplasia and adenocarcinoma. Gynecol Oncol 2:1–8, 1974.

White AJ, Buchsbaum HJ, Macasaet MA. Primary squamous cell carcinoma of the endometrium. Obstet Gynecol 41:912–919, 1973.

Wickerham DL, Fisher B, Wolmark N, et al. Association of tamoxifen and uterine sarcoma. J Clin Oncol 20:2758–2760, 2002.

Wolfe B and Mackles A. Malignant lesions from benign endometrial polypi. Obstet Gynecol 20:542–550, 1962.

Wolfson WL. Histologic and cytologic correlation of endometrial wreath. Acta Cytol 27:63–64, 1983.

Wright CA, Leiman G, Burgess SM. The cytomorphology of papillary serous carcinoma of the endometrium in cervical smears. Cancer 87:12–18, 1999.

Wynder EL, Escher GC, Mantel N. An epidemiological investigation of cancer of the endometrium. Cancer 19:489–520, 1966.

Wysowski DK, Honig SF, Beitz J. Uterine sarcoma associated with tamoxifen use. N Engl J Med 346:1832–1833, 2002.

Yazigi R, Piver MS, Blumenson L. Malignant peritoneal cytology as prognostic indicator in Stage I endometrial cancer. Obstet Gynecol 62:359–362, 1983.

Young RH, Treger T, Scully RE. Atypical polypoid adenomyoma of the uterus. A report of 27 cases. Am J Clin Pathol 86:139–145, 1986.

Zaino RJ, Kurman, RJ Diana KL, Morrow CP. The utility of revised International Federation of Gynecology and Obstetrics histologic grading of endometrial adenocarcinomas using a defined nuclear grading system: a Gynecologic Oncology group study. Cancer 75:81–86, 1995.

Zheng W, Khurana R, Farahmand S, et al. P53 immunostaining as a significant adjunct diagnostic method for uterine surface carcinoma, precursor of uterine papillary serous carcinoma. Am J Surg Pathol 22:1463–1473, 1998.

Ziel HK, Finkle WD. Increased risk of endometrial carcinoma among users of conjugated estrogens. N Engl J Med 293:1167–1170, 1975.

Zucker PK, Kasdon EJ, Feldstein ML. The validity of Pap smears parameters as predictors of endometrial pathology in menopausal women. Cancer 56: 2256–2263, 1985.

Diseases of the Vagina, Vulva, Perineum, and Anus

THE VAGINA

Normal Cytology

Except for the mucus-secreting Bartholin's glands, discussed below, the vagina is lined by squamous epithelium that is identical to that lining the outer surface of the uterine cervix. Normal cytology consists of squamous cells and their variants, identical to those described in Chapter 8.

Benign Abnormalities

Inflammatory Disorders

The inflammatory disorders and their causes, observed in the vagina, are generally the same as in the uterine cervix (see Chap. 10). **Ulceration of the vaginal epithelium** may occur under a variety of circumstances, such as the presence of a pessary. Wilbur et al (1993) described vaginal ulcers in a rare disorder of unknown etiology, **the Behçet's disease.** In the case described, **abnormal squamous cells, mimicking cancer,** were observed in cervicovaginal smears. Cases of **malakoplakia** of the vagina were reported by Lin et al (1979) and by Chalvardjian et al (1985). For further discussion of this rare disorder, see Chapter 22.

Melanosis of vagina, i.e., accumulation of melanin in the epithelium, is a very uncommon benign condition that may mimic a malignant melanoma (Karney et al, 2001). Malignant melanoma is discussed in Chapter 17.

Infections and Hormonal Status

The responses of the vaginal squamous epithelium to events in the normal menstrual cycle and under the impact of hormonal medication are discussed in Chapters 8 and 9. The susceptibility of the vagina to infectious agents depends on the hormonal status of the squamous epithelial lining: **absence of epithelial maturation before puberty and after the menopause favors the proliferation of infectious agents** (see Chap. 10).

Posthysterectomy Glandular Cells

Glandular cells **of endocervical type have been observed in vaginal smears after hysterectomy** (Bewtra, 1992; Tambouret et al, 1998). The origin of these cells is not clear but the authors postulated **focal glandular metaplasia** or **adenosis,** occurring in the vaginal epithelium after treatment by radiotherapy or 5-fluorouracil (for further discussion of vaginal adenosis, see below.)

Fistulous Tracts

Fistulous tracts between the vagina and an adjacent organ, such as **the rectum (recto-vaginal fistula), or the bladder (vesicovaginal fistula),** may result in the presence of epithelial cells of urothelial or intestinal origin in vaginal smears.

In **rectovaginal fistulae,** the tall, columnar, **mucus-producing colonic epithelial cells** may be recognized in cervicovaginal smears because of their large size and columnar configuration. These cells usually occur in compact sheets or clusters with basal nuclei and smooth luminal epithelial surface. The differential diagnosis is with vaginal adenosis (see below) and with endocervical or endometrial benign or malignant cells, which are usually smaller. The endocervical-type cells that have sometimes been observed in vaginal smears **in posthysterectomy patients** may also be confused with colonic cells. The colonic cells are often accompanied by bowel contents in the form of fecal material, often containing indigested **muscle or vegetable fibers and plant cells** originating in the colon (see Chap. 8). Because the nuclei of the plant cells are large and dark they may be mistaken for cancer cells. For further discussion of plant cells and their identification in sputum, see Chapter 19.

In **vesicovaginal fistulae,** the multinucleated, **large urothelial umbrella cells,** derived from the epithelium of the bladder, can **sometimes be identified in cervicovaginal smears.** These cells can be mistaken for cancer cells (see Chap. 22 for a detailed description of these cells).

Foreign Bodies

A variety of foreign material and foreign bodies, described in Chapter 8, may be found in the vagina and, hence, in cervicovaginal smears.

Benign Tumors and Tumorous Conditions

Except for **condylomata acuminata** and **vaginal adenosis** (to be discussed below), benign tumors and tumorous conditions are infrequent in the vagina and of very limited significance in diagnostic cytology. **Endometriosis, cysts or benign tumors of Gartner ducts,** and very uncommon benign tumors, **such as leiomyomas or rhabdomyomas,** occur in the wall of the vagina, do not produce any perceptible abnormalities in the vaginal epithelium and, hence, cannot be recognized cytologically, except by aspiration biopsy.

Vaginal and Cervical Adenosis

Natural History

A synthetic compound with estrogen-like effect, **diethylstilbesterol (DES),** was extensively used for prevention of abortions and other complications of pregnancy during the late 1940s and early 1950s. About 20 years later, it became apparent that the use of this drug adversely affected the offspring of the patients so treated.

In some of the **male offspring,** cysts of the epididymis and abnormal spermatogenesis were observed, a finding of limited cytologic significance (Gill et al, 1976). In the **female offspring, vaginal and cervical adenosis** has been observed, a disorder caused by **a replacement of vaginal squamous epithelium by glandular epithelium,** that on inspection appear as **red patches in the upper reaches of the vagina and adjacent cervix.** In about 40% of the affected females, there are also abnormalities in the gross configuration of the vagina and the cervix, described as **ridges. Most importantly, adenocarcinomas and squamous carcinomas and precursor lesions were observed in a small subset of females with vaginal adenosis.** These lesions are discussed below.

It has been shown by Sonek et al (1976) that DES administered between the seventh and eighth weeks of pregnancy resulted in 100% of adenosis in the offspring; if the drug was administered later during pregnancy, the frequency of adenosis was reduced but remained at about 70%.

Although there has been considerable speculation as to the mechanism of formation of adenosis, the evidence currently available strongly suggests that DES inhibits the transformation of the müllerian cuboidal epithelium into squamous epithelium that normally takes place during the last stages of the fetal life. A similar mechanism, although on a very limited scale, must be evoked in reference to cervical eversion or ectropion (see Chapter 10). Thus, **adenosis may be conceived as a very large eversion of the endocervical epithelium,** affecting the outer portions of the uterine cervix and the adjacent vagina. This has been confirmed by ultrastructural studies (Fenoglio et al, 1976). Experimentally, adenosis can be induced in mice by estrogen treatment (Forsberg, 1976). Vaginal adenosis was also reproduced in the female offspring of the monkey, *Cebus apella,* exposed to DES during pregnancy (Johnson et al, 1981).

It is of interest, though, that exposure to **DES is not a mandatory event in vaginal adenosis.** Robboy et al (1986) reported 41 patients with this disorder who had no DES exposure. Adenosis of the vagina has also been observed **after treatment with 5-fluorouracil and carbon dioxide laser,** usually for extensive condylomas of the vulva and vagina (Sedlacek et al, 1990; Goodman et al, 1991; Bernstein et al, 1983). A case of vaginal adenosis in a patient on **Tamoxifen therapy** was reported by Ganesan et al (1999).

Histology

In adenosis, areas of **proximal vagina and adjacent outer rim of the uterine cervix are lined by mucus-producing glandular epithelium, usually of the endocervical type,** replacing the normal squamous epithelium. Occasionally, the epithelium resembles that of the **endometrium or the fallopian tubes.** The glandular epithelium also forms tubular glands of endocervical type in the lamina propria that may reach the muscularis (Fig. 14-1A,B).

All changes commonly observed in the endocervical epithelium may be observed in adenosis: **tubal metaplasia, squamous metaplasia,** and **malignant transformation leading to adenocarcinoma, epidermoid carcinoma and its precursor lesions, or both.**

With the discontinuation of the use of DES for prevention of obstetrical difficulties, adenosis has become a rare disorder, limited to those few women, daughters of DES-exposed mothers, now in their 50s or 60s, and the rare

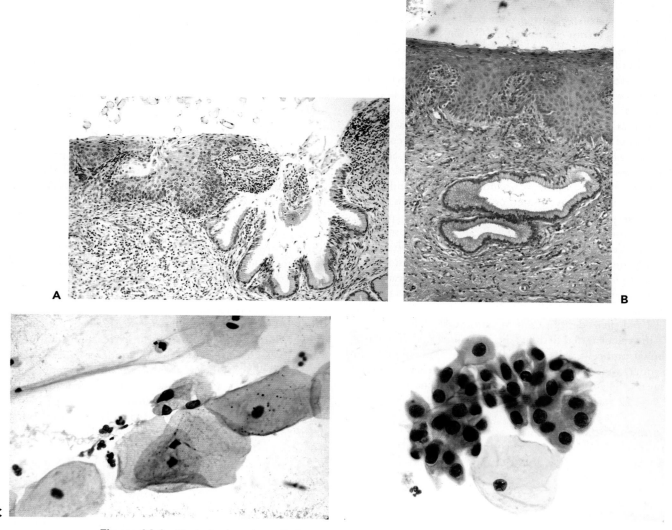

Figure 14-1 **Vaginal adenosis.** *A.* Endocervical type epithelium lining the surface of the vagina. *B.* Residual endocervical type glands underneath the squamous epithelium lining the vagina. *C.* Vaginal scrape smear containing scattered endocervical type cells next to squamous cells. *D.* Scrape of adenosis. The dominant cells are parabasal cells from squamous metaplasia.

women who develop it spontaneously or after treatment (see above). Nonetheless, for the sake of completeness, we have retained the description of the cytologic manifestations of this disorder.

Cytology

The purpose of cytologic examination of the vagina in children and women at risk is to determine the **presence of adenosis and of malignant changes, if any, by noninvasive methods.** Unfortunately, in uncomplicated adenosis, the cytologic techniques are not very efficient because the glandular epithelium does not desquamate easily. The best method is based on **direct scrapes of the lesions under visual control;** this approach is applicable only to adult women. In children and virginal adolescents, **a vaginal pool smear** obtained by a small pipette is the only method available.

Vaginal Pool Smears

Adenosis is characterized by **mucus-secreting columnar endocervical cells** of various sizes, occurring singly or in clusters, **or endocervical cells showing transition to squamous metaplasia** (Fig. 14-1C,D). The diagnosis is possible because the finding of normal endocervical cells in vaginal smears is otherwise exceptional. The finding of small squamous cells ("metaplastic cells"), unless in company of columnar mucus-secreting cells, is of a very limited diagnostic value because such cells may also originate in normal squamous epithelium. The efficacy of diagnosis of adenosis in vaginal pool smears is low.

Direct Scrape Smears From Areas of Adenosis

This is the sampling method of choice in adult women at risk. Bibbo et al (1975) advocated taking **four separate scrape smears from the four quadrants of the proximal vagina.** This may be supplemented by direct smears of the outer portio of the uterine cervix, preferably under visual control. **Prior to cytologic sampling, the accumulated mucus should be removed with a gauze sponge.**

Direct vaginal scrape smears from cases of adenosis contain either **secure or presumptive evidence of disease.** Secure evidence of disease is either the presence of glandular cells of endocervical type or glandular cells showing transition to squamous metaplasia. The presence of small squamous cells, singly or in clusters ("metaplastic cells"), cannot be considered as secure evidence of adenosis. Other cell types listed by Bibbo et al (1975), such as anucleated squamous cells or dyskaryotic squamous cells (dysplastic cells), have no specificity whatsoever for adenosis. Applying these criteria to Bibbo's series of 66 patients with known adenosis, the cytologic diagnosis of this disorder could be securely established in nine patients and a presumptive diagnosis of adenosis based on "metaplastic cells" in an additional 33 patients. The **limited value of cytology in the diagnosis of uncomplicated adenosis** was also emphasized by Robboy et al (1986), who could establish the diagnosis of adenosis in only 22% of 575 such patients.

Confirmation of the Cytologic Diagnosis of Adenosis
This is best accomplished by colposcopy. The colposcopist can clearly identify the extent of adenosis and, more important perhaps, examine the large and sometimes multiple transformation zones for evidence of possible neoplastic lesions. If colposcopy is not available, Schiller's test will disclose iodine-negative areas of glandular mucosa within the vagina and the outer cervix.

Clinical Significance

Melnick et al (1987) estimated the **risk of adenocarcinoma at 1 case per 1,000 women** with adenosis through the age of 34 years. The peak incidence was at 19 years of age but tumors have been observed in children as young as 7 and in women age 30 (Herbst and Bern, 1981). Tuboendometrial type of epithelium appears to be the most common source of adenocarcinomas (Robboy et al, 1982, 1984). By far more common in adenosis are the **precursor lesions of squamous cancer in the vagina and the adjacent cervix** (see below).

Follow-up of many thousands of patients with adenosis disclosed the very high probability of **self healing. The glandular epithelium undergoes squamous metaplasia which becomes mature** and identical to normal squamous epithelium. Thus, unless there is evidence or suspicion of malignant transformation, it appears safe to observe these patients without treatment. Adenocarcinomas and premalignant or malignant squamous lesions observed in patients with adenosis are discussed below.

Malignant Tumors

The most common primary malignant tumors of the vagina are **carcinomas of squamous derivation and type.** Since the appearance of adenosis on a large scale, increased attention has been devoted to **adenocarcinomas** associated with this disorder. Primary adenocarcinomas, in the absence of adenosis, are very uncommon, although they have been repeatedly observed. **Rare tumors,** including **malignant melanomas, sarcomas,** and metastatic tumors to the vagina are discussed in Chapter 17. **Postradiation carcinoma in situ** (dysplasia) of the vagina is discussed in Chapter 18.

Squamous Carcinoma

Invasive squamous carcinomas of the vagina and their precursor lesions are usually observed in women past the age of 40. In approximately 50% of these patients, there is evidence of a **synchronous or metachronous squamous carcinoma of the uterine cervix** that may be invasive or in situ (Kanbour et al, 1974; Murad et al, 1975; Lee and Symmonds, 1976). Bell et al (1984) also observed vaginal cancer in several patients after hysterectomy for allegedly benign disease. Norris et al (1970) reported a case of vaginal squamous carcinoma in an infant.

Association of vaginal carcinomas with other malignant tumors of the female genital tract may also occur. We have personally observed synchronous or metachronous tumors of the vagina, vulva, and occasionally of the endometrium, tube, and ovary. Thus, the presence of a vaginal carcinoma should automatically trigger the search for other malignant lesions. Conversely, **follow-up of patients with carcinoma or precancerous states of the epithelium of the uterine cervix and the vulva must include periodic examinations of the vagina.**

Observations pertaining to the possible role of **human papillomavirus (HPV)** in the genesis of cervical carcinoma are also applicable to squamous carcinomas of the vagina and vulva (see Chap. 11). The proof of viral presence in the relatively uncommon vaginal lesions is not nearly as extensive as for the cervical and vulvar squamous carcinomas and their precursor lesions. Still, there is no doubt that the vaginal neoplastic disorders follow the pattern of cervical disease and share identical cytologic, histologic, and biologic backgrounds (Okagaki et al, 1984).

Histology

Most squamous carcinomas of the vagina are keratin-producing, both on the surface of the epithelium of origin and within the invasive and metastatic foci. Occasionally, such lesions have thick layers of keratin on their surfaces and may bear considerable similarity to the warty (verrucous) carcinomas of various organs (Fig. 14-2). The tendency to keratin formation is also observed in precancerous lesions (see below). **Nonkeratinizing (epidermoid) carcinomas of the vagina made up of medium-size cells or small cells may also occur** (Fig. 14-3). Small cell carcinomas with endocrine features were described by Albores-Saavedra et al (1972) and by Chafe (1989). In a case reported by Colleran et al (1997), the tumor was shown to be secreting ACTH and causing a Cushing's syndrome.

The term **microinvasive carcinoma of the vagina** was discussed by Peters et al (1985), based on experience with six patients with invasion up to 2.5 mm in whom the results of surgical treatment by partial or total vaginectomy were uniformly good. **In our experience, however, even superficially invasive vaginal carcinomas are capable of forming metastases. Two territories of lymph nodes may be involved: carcinomas of the distal third of the vagina usually form metastases to the inguinal lymph nodes; carcinomas of the proximal third may metastasize to pelvic lymph nodes; carcinomas of the middle third may metastasize to either or both of these two groups of**

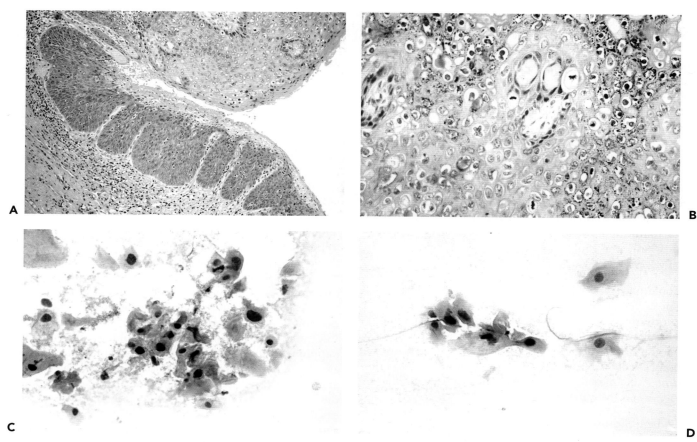

Figure 14-2 **Keratinizing squamous carcinoma of the vagina.** *A.* Keratinized carcinoma in situ from which well-differentiated squamous carcinoma shown in *B* was derived. *C,D.* Various aspects of small squamous cancer cells in a vaginal smear.

lymph nodes. The reasons for the very aggressive behavior of carcinomas of the vagina are not clear. Presumably, the lack of a thick muscularis and the abundance of lymphatics in the vaginal wall account for the striking differences in behavior when compared with the superficially invasive carcinomas of the uterine cervix (see Chap. 11).

We have also observed a case of a bulky **vaginal tumor with features of pseudosarcoma.** On the surface of the lesion, there was a squamous carcinoma in situ. The stroma of the tumor was composed of spindly cells mimicking a sarcoma with focal differentiation into an invasive squamous carcinoma (Fig. 14-4). This tumor was identical to the uncommon tumors of this type observed in the esophagus and adjacent organs described in Chapter 25.

Squamous Carcinoma In Situ and Related Lesions (Vaginal Intraepithelial Neoplasia; VAIN)

Carcinomas in situ and noninvasive epithelial lesions with lesser degrees of abnormality ("dysplasias") have been grouped as **vaginal intraepithelial neoplasia (VAIN)** that can be graded I, II, III as initially proposed for similar lesions of the uterine cervix (see Chap. 11). Although the Bethesda nomenclature (see Chap. 11) has not been extended to the vagina, it appears reasonable to classify **VAIN I as low-grade lesions** (mild dysplasia with features of condyloma) (Fig. 14-5) and **VAIN II and III as high-grade lesions.** This suggestion gained support from a study by

Sherman and Paull (1993) who documented better reproducibility of diagnoses, using the binary system. Logani et al (2003) reported that most of the precancerous lesions of the vagina contain high risk HPV, contrary to vulvar lesions. These authors also noted that staining with proliferation antigen M1B1 helps in distinguishing benign from potentially malignant epithelial changes.

The **clinical appearance** of these lesions depends on the level of keratinization: **the heavily keratinized lesions appear as white patches (leukoplakia),** whereas the **poorly differentiated (epidermoid) lesions with limited keratin formation may appear as red areas** in the vagina (Hummer et al, 1970).

Predictably, **the low-grade lesions resemble structurally normal squamous epithelium,** except for the presence of nuclear enlargement, hyperchromasia, and mitotic activity (Fig. 14-5). In the presence of **koilocytes, the lesions are identical to the so-called flat condylomas observed on the surface of the uterine cervix** (see Chap. 11). Keratin deposits are often present on the surface. The **low-grade lesions** may occur as **multiple condylomas that form small elevations of the vaginal epithelium (condylomatous colpitis) and are often associated with similar lesions on the vulva;** although these lesions are difficult to eradicate, they are not considered threatening to the patient. They have been observed in children, presumably as a consequence of sexual abuse. More important is the **single low-**

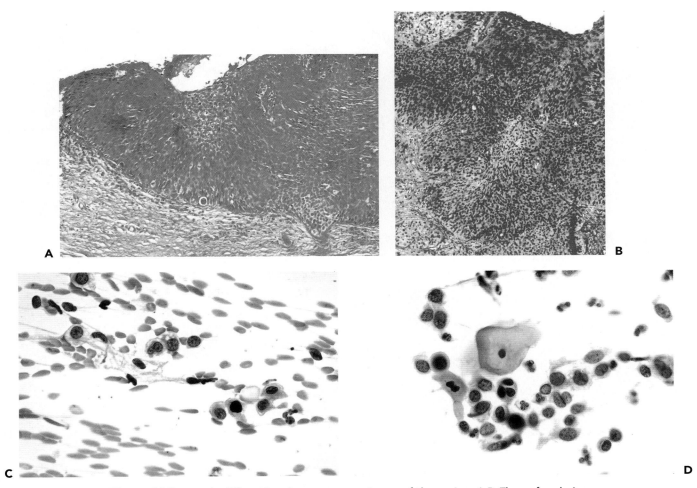

Figure 14-3   Poorly differentiated squamous carcinoma of the vagina. *A,B.* The surface lesion (*A*), which became invasive (*B*). *C,D.* Small cancer cells in vaginal smears.

grade lesion. Although many of these lesions may disappear, presumably spontaneously or after treatment, there is at least some evidence, based on personal experience, that the **vaginal low-grade lesion may progress to invasive cancer more rapidly and more frequently than similar lesions in the uterine cervix.** This observation has received support from a follow-up study of untreated VAIN by Aho et al (1991) who also observed the progression of a low grade lesion to invasive cancer.

The **high-grade lesions fall into two groups: keratin-forming lesions, that may show remarkable similarity to low-grade lesions** except for the presence of abnormal cells throughout the thickness of the epithelium (see Fig. 14-2A); and **nonkeratinizing lesions that are similar to high-grade lesions of the endocervical canal,** composed of smaller malignant cells and show little or no keratin formation on the surface (see Fig. 14-3A). Anecdotal evidence has been accumulated that these lesions, particularly the classical carcinoma in situ, have the ability to progress to invasive squamous cancer (Rutledge, 1967; Benedet and Sanders, 1984; Aho et al, 1991), although the frequency of progression remains unknown because few of these lesions are followed without treatment.

Cytology

The customary source of diagnosis of vaginal carcinoma is the smear obtained by aspiration of the vaginal pool. Occasionally, however, cancer cells of vaginal origin may be observed in cervical smears.

If cervical and/or vaginal smears contain evidence of squamous carcinoma or a related precancerous lesion and there is no evidence of disease in the uterine cervix, the vagina must be investigated. Direct scrape smears of the vaginal wall may be used initially to confirm the diagnosis. On occasions when there is no visible mucosal abnormality, we have recommended **mapping smears,** i.e., taking multiple, separately labeled smears from separate vaginal sites to identify the source of the abnormal cells for biopsy.

Invasive Carcinoma

Invasive keratinizing epidermoid carcinomas of the vagina closely resemble invasive squamous carcinomas of the uterine cervix. Most tumors shed relatively **highly differentiated squamous cancer** cells of various sizes with thick, yellow or orange cytoplasm (see Fig. 14-2). Keratin "pearls" of malignant type and bizarre cell types (tadpole cells, spindly cells) are common. **Koilocytes** may be observed, sug-

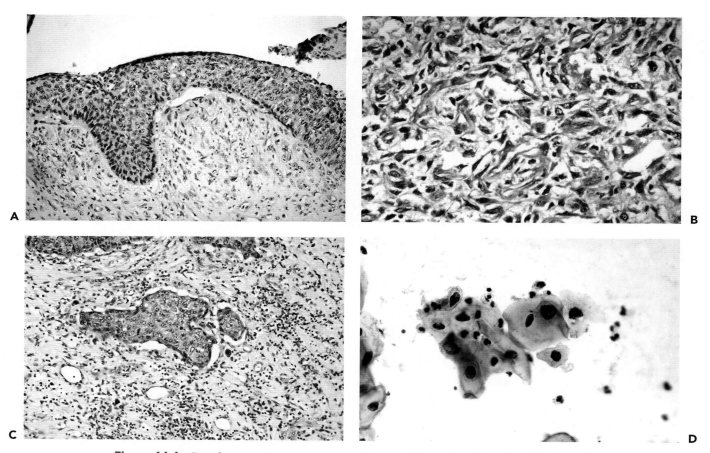

Figure 14-4 **Pseudosarcomatous squamous carcinoma of the vagina.** The polypoid lesion with smooth surface was clinically protruding into vaginal lumen. *A.* Squamous carcinoma in situ on the surface of a tumor composed of spindly cells, shown in *B. C.* Focus of squamous differentiation in the invasive spindly component of the tumor. *D.* A vaginal pool smear from a similar case showing well-differentiated squamous cancer cells.

gesting the origin of such lesions from "flat condylomas." Necrosis, which is so commonly present in invasive cancer of the cervix, is often absent. Inflammation and trichomoniasis are commonly observed.

Invasive nonkeratinizing carcinomas are made up of smaller cancer cells with less evidence of keratin formation (see Fig. 14-3). Occasionally, only small, undifferentiated cancer cells are present. Other features of such smears are similar to those described above.

Cytologic findings in a case of **small-cell neuroendocrine carcinoma** of vagina were described by Ciesla et al (2001). Numerous small cancer cells, some with nuclear molding, were observed and illustrated.

Precursor Lesions of Vaginal Squamous Carcinoma (VAIN)

Low-Grade Lesions (VAIN Grade I, Mild Dysplasia, Flat Condylomas)

The cytologic presentation of these lesions, shown in Figure 14-5D, consists of **superficial and intermediate dyskaryotic (dysplastic) squamous cells and koilocytes,** characterized by a delicate, transparent cytoplasm and enlarged, irregular, hyperchromatic nuclei, often surrounded by a clear zone. The underlying tissue abnormality (Fig. 14-5B) is very

similar to that of low-grade lesions occurring on the uterine cervix (see Chap. 11).

High-Grade Lesions (Carcinoma In Situ, VAIN Grade II or III)

Precursor lesions of epidermoid carcinoma often follow, or are synchronous with, similar lesions of the uterine cervix, most often the keratin-forming type. **Two types of high-grade lesions (carcinoma in situ) may be observed in the vagina.** The uncommon **small cell type** is characterized by the presence of small cancer cells, occurring singly or in clusters (see Fig. 14-3C,D). These lesions and their cytologic presentation usually follow and are akin to the "classic" small cell carcinoma in situ of the uterine cervix (see Chap. 11).

More common are the **keratin-forming** high grade lesions (keratinizing carcinomas in situ (Fig. 14-6). These lesions shed dyskaryotic (dysplastic) and **squamous cancer cells of variable sizes,** some with opaque, thick, keratinized cytoplasm and large pyknotic nuclei. **Koilocytes** with a wide perinuclear clear zone are commonly present. The tissue, however, may disclose a high-grade lesion capable of invasion, showing residual evidence of a condyloma (Fig. 14-6D). These lesions are **clear examples of malig-**

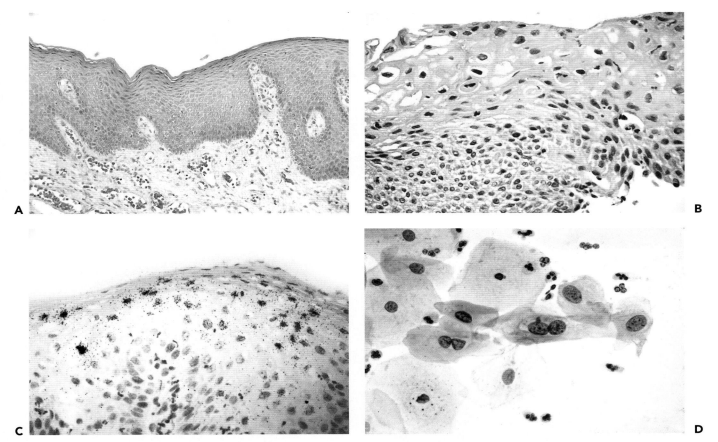

Figure 14-5   Low-grade condylomatous-type lesion of the vagina in a child. *A,B.* Low and higher magnification views of the lesion which consists of thickened, folded squamous epithelium with numerous koilocytes in the upper layers. *C.* In situ hybridization of the same lesion with antibodies to HPV 11. The black nuclei show positive reaction. *D.* Vaginal smear from a similar lesion showing well differentiated dyskaryotic (dysplastic) intermediate squamous cells, one of which shows perinuclear halos consistent with koilocytosis.

nant transformation of low-grade (condylomatous) lesions that may be particularly dangerous in the vagina. One should not be misled by the presence of koilocytes into believing that the lesion will disappear without treatment.

High-grade VAIN lesions are not infrequently observed in postmenopausal women with atrophic smear pattern. As was discussed in Chapter 11 in reference to similar lesions of the uterine cervix, the recognition of cancer cells in dry, atrophic smears may be fraught with difficulty, particularly because the feature of nuclear hyperchromasia is not readily evident in dry cancer cells spread on the slide. **In such smears, the *nuclear size* and the *nucleocytoplasmic ratio*** become the principal criteria of recognition of cancer cells: the nuclei are substantially larger than those of benign squamous cells in the same smears, and the nucleocytoplasmic ratio is altered in favor of the nucleus. Reviving the epithelium with estrogen may be quite helpful in the diagnosis.

It is quite evident that there are significant cytologic similarities between the low-grade lesion shown in Figure 14-5 and the high-grade keratin-forming lesion shown in Figure 14-6. The difference lies in the cytoplasm which, in

many cells derived from the high-grade lesion, is heavily keratinized and opaque whereas it is more transparent and delicate in the low-grade lesion.

Cytologic assessment of the type of histologic abnormalities, which may be carried out with reasonable accuracy in the uterine cervix, is rarely possible with vaginal lesions. The **cytologic presentation of vaginal low-grade lesions, carcinoma in situ, and invasive carcinoma may overlap significantly.** The presence or the absence of necrosis is of limited diagnostic help.

Because of the potentially highly malignant behavior of these lesions, **any cytologic evidence of a neoplastic process in the vaginal epithelium, regardless of the degree of cytologic abnormality, must be followed by an attempt to localize and destroy the lesion** before metastases set in. Colposcopy, or, if unavailable, Schiller's test or mapping smears (see above), will help in localizing the disease and in obtaining histologic evidence. If the lesion is still confined to the epithelium, surgical excision, carbon dioxide laser treatment, or chemotherapy with 5-fluorouracil ointment, may prove curative, although the treatment may lead to formation of vaginal adenosis (see above).

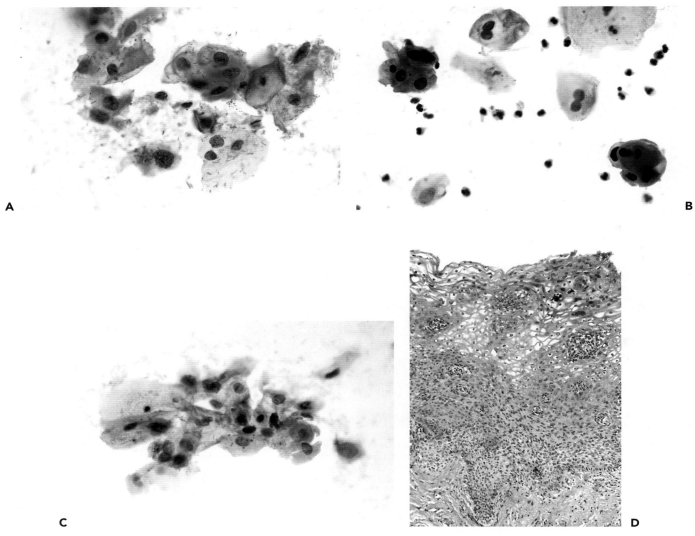

Figure 14-6   Well-differentiated squamous carcinoma of the vagina. *A–C.* Vaginal smears containing well differentiated dyskaryotic (dysplastic) cells, some with perinuclear halos indicative of koilocytosis. *D.* The histologic appearance of an invasive squamous carcinoma from the same case.

Vaginal Adenosis and Squamous Carcinoma and Its Precursors

In discussing the nature of adenosis (see above), it has been pointed out that the presence of endocervical tissue in the vagina greatly increased the size of the transformation zone. Because of the important role that the transformation zone plays in the genesis of epidermoid carcinoma of the uterine cervix (see Chap. 11), it has been anticipated by us in early editions of this book that squamous carcinoma and its precursors will be encountered with increasing frequency in adenosis. These observations were amply confirmed. Thus, Stafl et al (1974), Bibbo et al (1975), and Fetherston (1975) observed several instances of dysplasia and epidermoid carcinoma in situ in the vagina adjacent to adenosis. The incidence of these lesions was estimated by Robboy et al (1984) at 15.7 per 1,000 person-years of follow-up, approximately double the rate of an unexposed population. Most of these lesions can be identified by cytologic sampling of the vagina and adjacent cervix (see Fig. 14-9). Two cases of invasive squamous carcinoma occurring in adenosis were reported by Veridiano et al (1976).

Adenocarcinoma of the Vagina

Adenocarcinomas of the vagina, otherwise very rare, assumed new importance in the generation of women afflicted with DES-induced vaginal adenosis (Barber and Sommers, 1974; Robboy et al, 1976). **Adenocarcinoma occurring in adenosis affected girls and very young women, often in their teens, many of whom are initially asymptomatic.** Cytologic examination may serve a dual purpose: as a means of detection of adenocarcinoma or as a follow-up procedure after treatment of the lesion.

Taft et al (1974) summarized their experience with 95 cases from the registry of these tumors maintained at the Massachusetts General Hospital in Boston, Massachusetts. In 11 asymptomatic patients, **the tumors were detected by cervicovaginal cytology.** The smears were positive or suspicious in 43 of 55 patients with prior positive biopsies.

In three patients, vaginal smears served as the first indication of local recurrence after treatment. Thus, cytologic evaluation plays an important role in the diagnosis and management of these patients.

Histology

Adenocarcinomas originating in adenosis are, in many ways, similar to endocervical adenocarcinomas and to adenocarcinomas of Gartner duct origin (see Chap. 12). The neoplastic glands are lined by cuboidal and sometimes columnar cells, often protruding into the lumen in hobnail fashion (Figs. 14-7D and 14-8D). Because the cytoplasm of many of these cells is transparent, the term **clear cell carcinoma or mesonephric carcinoma** is often used to describe these tumors. Occasionally, the tumors resemble the endometrial type of adenocarcinoma and are then associated with foci of adenosis resembling endometrial glands or endometriosis. In all tumors, foci of solid growth may be observed.

The origin of the tumors can be traced to the glandular surface epithelium; more often, however, the lesion originates from the deep glands. It is theoretically predictable that an adenocarcinoma in situ must exist in adenosis, but such a lesion has not yet been described.

A very rare **adenocarcinoma of intestinal type** of the vagina, derived from an adenoma, was described by Mudhar et al (2001) who also reviewed the literature. We have not seen a tumor of this type.

Cytology

Adenocarcinoma originating in adenosis may involve the vagina and, in about 40% of the cases, the adjacent cervix. If the uterine cervix is involved, the cervical scrape smear is very efficient in the diagnosis of the tumor. If only the vagina is involved, the cervical smear will fail to reveal tumor in many cases. Thus, the **importance of a vaginal pool smear** in young women, particularly those at risk for adenosis and adenocarcinoma, cannot be sufficiently emphasized. Direct scrape smears of the vaginal wall in patients with high risk for adenosis have been discussed above. Such smears, although not particularly efficient in the diagnosis of benign adenosis, are very helpful in the diagnosis of vaginal adenocarcinoma.

In their classic form, the well-preserved cells of vaginal adenocarcinoma appear as **polygonal or columnar cancer cells singly and in clusters** (Fig. 14-7A,B). The cells vary in size and measure from 20 to 30 μm in their largest dimensions. The **cytoplasm is delicate, transparent, and**

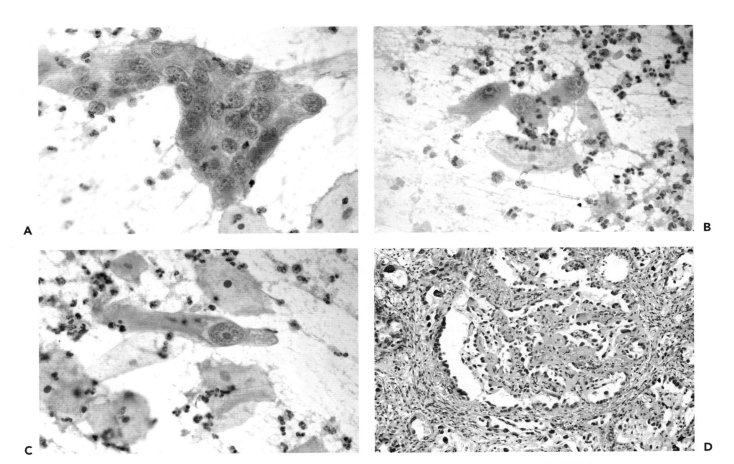

Figure 14-7 **Cytologic presentation of adenocarcinoma of vagina in a young girl.** *A–C.* Various aspects of the vaginal smear. *A.* Sheet of cancer cells with large nuclei and nucleoli. In *B* and *C*, the cells are elongated and have a vague similarity to endocervical cancer cells. *D.* corresponding tissue lesion shows an invasive adenocarcinoma derived from adenosis. (Case courtesy of Dr. Priscilla Taft, Massachusetts General Hospital, Boston, MA.)

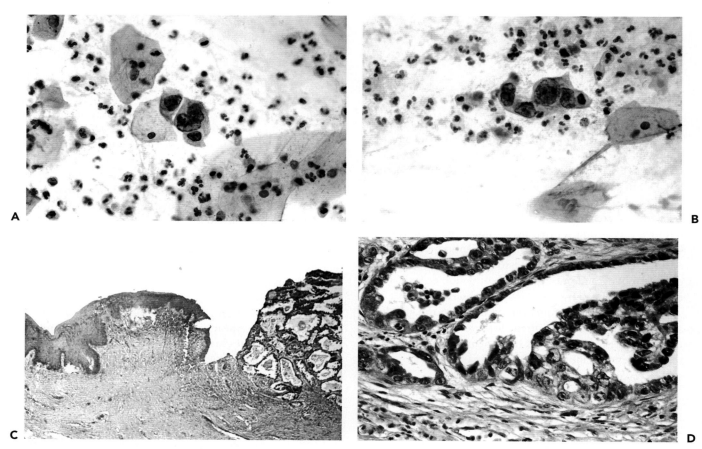

Figure 14-8 Adenocarcinoma of the vagina in a young woman. *A,B.* Relatively small cancer cells resembling a squamous rather than a glandular lesion. *C.* Focus of adenocarcinoma of the vagina adjacent to normal vaginal squamous epithelium. *D.* Details of the tumor composed of convoluted and papillary glands. Note the "hobnail" arrangement of tumor cells. (Case courtesy of Dr. Priscilla Taft, Massachusetts General Hospital, Boston, MA.)

generally basophilic, sometimes studded with small vacuoles. The large nuclei appear finely granular. The nucleoli vary in size and may be very large in some cancer cells. In most cases, however, when the tumor cells are less well preserved, the characteristic features described above may not be present. In such situations, clusters of **small cancer cells without distinguishing features** are commonly seen (Fig. 14-8A,B). Origin from an adenocarcinoma may be suspected if the cytoplasm is vacuolated and infiltrated with polymorphonuclear leukocytes or if the clusters have papillary configuration and the cells have large nucleoli. **In many instances, the identification of tumor type may not be possible on cytology alone.** Taft et al (1974) pointed out the similarity of this cytologic presentation with that of epidermoid carcinoma. **Very bizarre, large cancer cells** that may be occasionally observed (Fig. 14-7C) may suggest a sarcoma.

The smears in vaginal adenocarcinoma contain a large admixture of squamous cells of vaginal origin that may partly obscure the evidence of cancer. Also if there is adjacent residual adenosis, in the vagina or in the adjacent cervix, benign cells of endocervical type may confuse the cytologic picture. In ulcerated tumors, evidence of inflammation and necrosis is usually present. Although the accurate diagnosis of vaginal carcinoma may not always be possible on cytologic evidence, **any significant cytologic abnormality in a young girl or woman warrants a careful colposcopic examination of the vagina.** While much less common now than when DES was prescribed during pregnancy, occasional instances of adenosis still occur and adenocarcinomas associated with adenosis are fully capable of metastasis.

Tumor Variants

As in the uterine cervix, we have observed a **coexisting adenocarcinoma and epidermoid carcinoma in situ in adenosis.** In this instance, the smear pattern was that of a low-grade squamous lesion and no cells of adenocarcinoma were present. Tissue evidence disclosed an epidermoid carcinoma in situ lining the surface of vaginal adenosis and, in the depth of the vaginal wall, an invasive adenocarcinoma (Fig. 14-9). A case of invasive **adenosquamous carcinoma** was described by Vandrie et al (1983).

Prognostic Factors

Fu et al (1979) attempted to establish the prognosis of the epidermoid and glandular lesions associated with DES exposure by measuring the **DNA content** of the component cells. These authors postulated that lesions of diploid or polyploid make-up have a higher chance of regression than

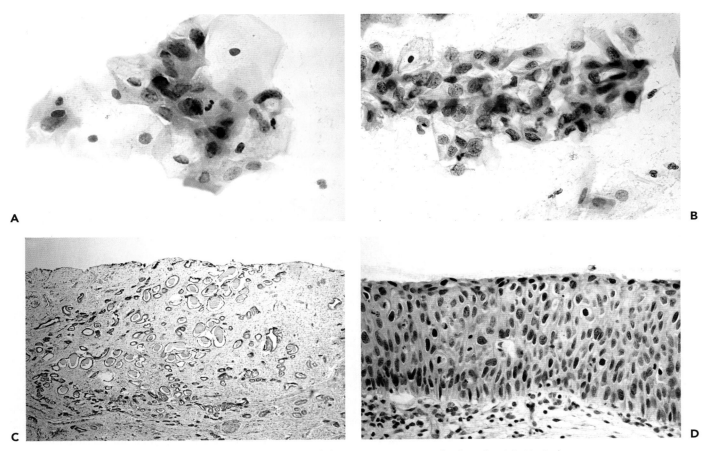

Figure 14-9   Epidermoid carcinoma of the vagina in a case of adenosis. *A,B.* Vaginal smear containing medium-size squamous cancer cells. *C.* An overview of the vaginal lesion showing numerous glands, consistent with adenosis and possibly an early adenocarcinoma. *D.* Surface abnormality in this case showing a high-grade squamous carcinoma in situ.

aneuploid lesions. As noted in Chapter 11 in reference to the uterine cervix, such measurements have limited value in the presence of permissive infection with HPV that modifies the DNA measurements (Chacho et al, 1990).

Uncommon tumors of the vagina are discussed in Chapter 17.

Lesions of the Neovagina

Neovagina or an artificial vagina may be constructed in women with congenital absence of vagina (Belleannée et al, 1998) or after surgical removal of vagina for a variety of reasons. The artificial vagina, whether constructed from skin grafts or an intestinal loop, usually becomes lined with squamous epithelium that may display a normal hormonal pattern. It is of particular interest that **squamous carcinoma** (summary in Rotmensch et al, 1983; Belleannée et al, 1998) or **vaginal intraepithelial neoplasia,** as reported by Lathrop et al (1985), may also be observed in neovaginas. The possibility that HPV infection may be a factor in such rare events was supported by the presence of koilocytes in vaginal smears of the patient described by Belleannée et al (1998).

Adenocarcinomas have also been observed in neovaginas **constructed from segments of the intestine** (Ritchi,

1929; Lavand'Homme, 1938). No recent reports of this very rare complication could be found.

Tumors of Bartholin's Glands

Tumors of the Bartholin's glands, located near the intruitus in the posterior wall of the vagina, are generally not accessible to routine cytologic sampling except by needle aspiration. Thus, Bartholin's gland **hyperplasias, adenomas, and cysts** have no known cytologic presentation in routine smears (Koenig and Tavassoli, 1998). Two cases of **malakoplakia** have been described (Paquin et al, 1986). For a detailed description of the pathology and cytology of this disease, see Chapter 22. However, the very rare **carcinomas of Bartholin's glands may break through the gland capsule into the vagina and occasionally yield malignant cells in cervicovaginal material.** Several such cases were reported (De Mauro et al, 1986). **Adenocarcinoma and adenoacanthoma,** morphologically similar to carcinoma of the endometrium, are the most common types of malignant tumors. Several cases of **adenoid cystic carcinoma** have been described (Copeland et al, 1986) and one has been diagnosed on needle aspiration smears by Frable and Goplerud (1975). Cytologic presentation of adenoid cystic carcinomas is discussed in Chapter 32. A case of **squamous**

carcinoma, diagnosed in a vaginal smear, was reported by Gupta et al (1977). Other, very rare disorders such as **metastatic renal carcinoma** (Leiman et al, 1986) have been reported.

VULVA AND PERINEUM

Although the perineum is rarely the target of direct cytologic examinations, many of the vulvar lesions, discussed below, may also affect the adjacent perineum.

Histology

As discussed in Chapter 8, **the vulva** is composed of two sets of labia. There are basic structural differences between the epithelia of the vulvar external labia majora and the internal labia minora. The **labia majora** are lined by epidermis of the skin and contain the accessory apparatus thereof: hair, sebaceous glands, and sweat glands of the eccrine and apocrine type. The **labia minora** is an organ of transition between the skin of labia majora and the epithelium of the vagina. The squamous epithelium is not keratinized, resembles the lining of the vagina, and is free of hair; however, the subcutaneous tissue contains numerous sebaceous glands. The general configuration of the vulva depends on the **hormonal status** of the woman: it undergoes varying degrees of atrophy after the menopause. However, the epidermis of the labia majora does not show any cyclic changes. It is not known whether the epithelium of the inner surfaces of labia minora follows the cyclic changes occurring in the vagina (see Chap. 9).

The perineum is lined by skin.

Cytologic Sampling

It is generally considered that superficial scrape or cotton swab smears of the vulva have limited diagnostic value and that an energetic scraping with a wood or metal spatula is required to obtain a meaningful sample of cells. Dennerstein

(1968) and Nauth (1986) recommended a **vigorous scrape of the vulvar lesions, if necessary, after removal of the layer of keratin** and claimed excellent diagnostic results in vulvar cancer.

Normal Cytology

Smears of normal **labia majora** are **uniformly composed of anucleated squames and a minor population of nucleated superficial squamous cells.** Smears from **labia minora** more closely resemble vaginal smears and are **composed of nucleated squamous cells of various degrees of maturity.** Inflammatory cells are uncommon under normal circumstances.

Inflammatory Diseases

Herpes Genitalis

Herpes is commonly observed on the vulva and the clinical lesions are usually quite painful. Small vesicles filled with clear fluid or small, superficial ulcerations that are observed after the rupture of the vesicles are characteristic of the disease. Scrape smears of the lesions usually reveal the characteristic changes, described in Chap. 10.

Molluscum Contagiosum

A highly contagious pox virus causes pale, elevated and umbilicated lesions on the skin of the vulva. The lesions are composed of **large squamous cells filled with viral particles, coalescing to form large cytoplasmic inclusions that push the nucleus of the cell to the periphery (molluscum bodies).** The molluscum bodies can be readily recognized in scrape smears of the lesions (Fig. 14-10).

Moniliasis of the vulva occurs mainly during pregnancy, in AIDS patients, and in diabetics. The fungus may be identified in scrape smears (see Chap. 10).

Other inflammatory diseases are usually sexually transmitted, such as **lymphogranuloma venereum** (caused by *Chlamydia trachomatis*) or **granuloma inguinale** (caused by *Calymmatobacterium granulomatis*) which may be observed on the vulva. The cytologic presentation of these disorders is described in Chapter 10.

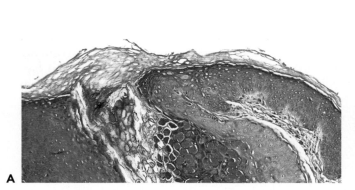
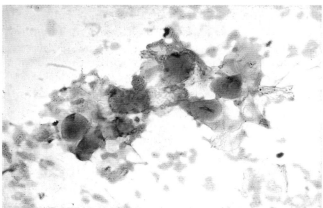

A

B

Figure 14-10 **Molluscum contagiosum of the vulva.** *A.* Classical histologic aspect of this lesion with crevices filled with pox virus-containing cells. *B.* A scrape smear showing the particles of pox virus filling the entire cytoplasm of cells and pushing the nuclei to the periphery.

A variety of benign skin disorders may also be observed. Of particular cytologic interest is **pemphigus vulgaris.** The vesicles, upon rupture, may yield the characteristic **Tzanck cells,** mimicking cancer, described in Chapters 19 and 21. Also of note is **vulvar involvement in Crohn's disease** in the form of ulcers (Freidrich, 1983; Holohan et al, 1988).

Lichen Sclerosus

This is a skin disorder of unknown etiology, affecting the vulva and the adjacent perineum. The disease has two forms: an **atrophic form** in which the squamous epithelium becomes thin and is accompanied by hyalinization of the underlying dermis, and a **hypertrophic form** in which the squamous epithelium is thickened (Ridley et al, 1989). It is thought that this disorder is a part of the spectrum of **"vulvar dystrophies"** that apparently predispose women to carcinoma of vulva. Van Hoeven et al (1997) described **cytologic findings** in a group of 29 patients with lichen sclerosus, six of whom had synchronous squamous carcinoma, either in situ or invasive. Besides the customary anucleated squames and nucleated squamous cells, these authors observed **elongated parabasal squamous cells** and, in some cases, atypical cells which, however, were insufficient for diagnosis of a malignant tumor in all but one case.

Benign Tumors

Except for condylomata acuminata (see below), benign tumors such as **granular cell myoblastoma, sweat gland adenoma, hidradenoma papilliferum** (Virgili et al, 2000), **ectopic breast tissue or fibroadenomas of mammary type** (Prasad et al, 1995) are usually subcutaneous in location and thus not accessible to cytologic sampling, except by aspiration biopsy.

Condylomata Acuminata

These are the most common benign tumors of the vulva, known to be caused by a sexually transmitted infection with human papillomavirus (HPV), usually types 6 and 11 but occasionally other types as well (see Chap. 11). The presence of HPV in condylomata acuminata can be documented with the use of the common viral antigen or by in situ hybridization with viral DNA of specific type under stringent conditions, as shown in Figure 14-15C, which documents the presence of a permissive infection with HPV type 11. Viral DNA is located mainly in the upper layers of the epithelium containing koilocytes. In two studies of condylomas from this laboratory, one conducted in children with anal lesions, and the other on penile condylomas in adults, the principal types of HPV observed were 6 and 11 but there were sporadic cases in which HPV 16 and 18 could also be demonstrated (Vallejos et al, 1987; Del Mistro et al, 1987) (see Chap. 11).

The wart-like tumors are usually multiple and may also involve adjacent areas of the skin, such as the perineum and the perianal area (Fig. 14-5C). Some lesions of this type grow to large sizes and **may show invasive and destructive growth.** It is often a matter of preference as to whether to classify such lesions as **giant condylomas or as verrucous squamous carcinomas.** They are usually associated with HPV type 11 and may also occur on the shaft of the penis, where they are known as **giant condylomas of Buschke-Löwenstein.**

Condylomata acuminata have traditionally been considered a benign disorder, although **recurrent condylomas and their progression to squamous carcinoma in situ** (Fig. 14-11B) **and to invasive squamous carcinoma have been recorded repeatedly** (Fig. 14-11C,D).

Many condylomas respond to treatment with the antimitotic agent, **podophyllin,** or the antiviral agent, **interferon.** The lesions can be removed by surgical resections or by **laser.** Unfortunately, at least 20% of the patients fail to respond fully to these forms of treatment. Based on studies of immunologic events in response to HPV infection, an **immune-response modifier, imiquimod,** was isolated first from tissues of experimental animals, then in humans (Coleman et al, 1994). Imiquimod induces a number of cytokines and acts as an anti-viral and anti-tumor agent (Imbertson et al, 1998; Tyring et al, 1998). Clinical experience in patients with anogenital condylomas showed a 50% response rate to 5% imiquimod cream (Aldara, 3M Pharmaceuticals, St. Paul, MN) (Edwards et al, 1998). One can anticipate that, in the future, other immunotherapeutic agents will become available that will prove to be more effective in the treatment of condylomas.

Histology of condylomas was discussed in Chapter 11. Suffice it to add that the presence of koilocytes in the upper layers of the epithelial lining is a common feature of these lesions. Few condylomas require **cytologic diagnosis,** but some of the flat forms of this disease may be so investigated, particularly in the **anal area** (see below). The cytologic presentation of flat condylomas of the cervix, dominated by koilocytes, is discussed in Chapter 11. Ward et al (1994) considered condylomas as a risk factor for cervical neoplasia and recommended cervical cytology and colposcopy as a routine procedure in such patients.

Malignant Tumors

Squamous Carcinomas

Squamous carcinomas are by far the most common malignant tumors of the vulva, usually involving the interior aspect of the labia majora but occasionally labia minora and the introitus. These tumors, and their precursors, are usually seen in women ages 40 to 60 (Jones et al, 1994). Within the last two decennia of the 20th century, a clear increase in younger women has been observed (Sturgeon et al, 1992; Joura et al, 2000). Vulvar cancer has also been observed in immunodeficient patients (Serraino et al, 1999). An invasive cancer of the vulva in a 12-year-old girl with HIV infection has been reported by Giaquinto et al (2000). Squamous carcinomas can be roughly divided into two groups, though intermediate-type lesions may occur:

- **Carcinomas with marked surface keratinization, akin to most squamous carcinomas of the skin and occurring mainly on labia majora. Verrucous carcinomas are a variant of these tumors. Koilocytosis is frequently**

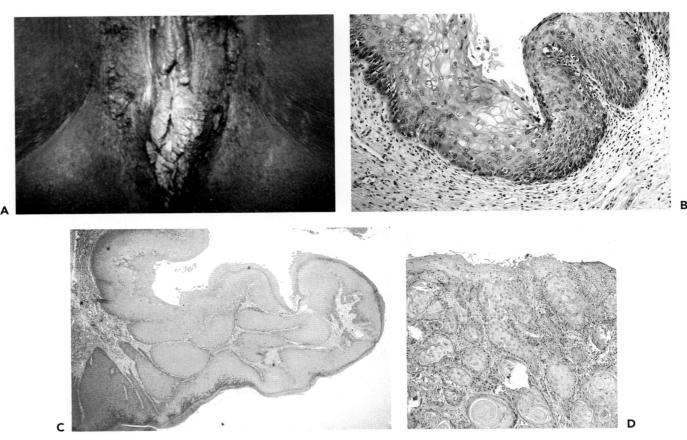

Figure 14-11 **Condylomas of vulva.** *A.* The clinical aspect of the disease showing numerous wart-like structures surrounding the vulva. *B.* Histologic features of the surface epithelium of a lesion shown in *A. C.* Vulvar condyloma observed in 1962 and treated by local excision. *D.* Invasive squamous carcinoma in the same area of the vulva observed in 1969.

observed in these tumors, suggesting origin from condylomas (Dvoretsky et al, 1984).

■ The relatively uncommon, **highly malignant, poorly differentiated carcinomas composed of small cells, and often growing in solid sheets, mimicking basal cell carcinoma of the skin. Such lesions, also referred to as basaloid carcinomas, occur mainly on labia minora.**

The information on HPV in vulvar carcinomas is contradictory. The presence of HPV sequences has been documented in some invasive carcinomas and in nearly all carcinomas in situ. Although HPV types 6 and 11 have been shown to be associated with some vulvar carcinomas of verrucous type (see Chap. 11), subsequent studies suggested that the oncogenic types of HPV, namely types 16 and rarely 18, are associated with some but not all tumors (Toki et al, 1991). In a recent study, Logani et al (2003) observed prevalence of low risk HPV in these lesions, contrary to similar lesions in the vagina.

Cytogenetic studies of vulvar carcinomas disclosed a pattern of chromosomal abnormalities very similar to squamous cancer of the uterine cervix (Jee et al, 2001). Losses of the short arms of chromosomes 3 and 4 and gain in the long arm of chromosome 3 were also described in the uterine cervix (see Chap. 11).

Microinvasive Squamous Carcinoma

Microinvasive squamous carcinoma of the vulva is poorly defined. It is a matter of debate whether a depth of invasion of 1 or 3 mm is an acceptable criterion. Dvoretsky et al (1984) favored the depth of 3 mm as the best standard. Although the outcome of very superficially invasive carcinoma of the vulva is usually favorable (Wharton et al, 1974), there are sufficient cases on record of superficially invasive vulvar carcinoma with metastases to inguinal lymph nodes to consider such lesions as potentially lethal and deserving of aggressive treatment (Jafari and Cartnick, 1976; Nakao et al, 1974; Chu et al, 1982).

Cytology

Invasive squamous carcinomas are **warty or ulcerated,** or both, and most are identified clinically. Occasionally, however, **kraurosis vulvae,** extensive **herpetic vulvitis or another ulcerative process may imitate vulvar carcinoma and vice versa.** In such situations, a scrape smear may help in establishing the diagnosis. It must be pointed out that the rare low-grade verrucous carcinomas of the vulva may have a thick layer of keratin on the surface and may not yield any identifiable cancer cells, unless the keratinized layer is removed.

Smears from invasive squamous carcinomas are often

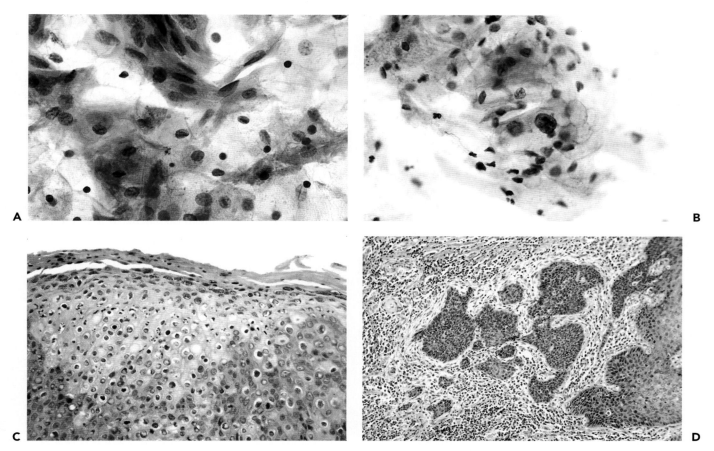

Figure 14-12   Invasive carcinoma of vulva with a smear pattern suggestive of condyloma. *A.* Spindly dyskaryotic (dysplastic) cells. *B.* Cells with features of koilocytes. *C.* Biopsy of vulva corresponding to *A* and *B* showing a lesion of squamous epithelium of the vulva with numerous koilocytes. *D.* Invasive squamous carcinoma of vulva adjacent to the lesion shown in *C.*

partly obscured by inflammation and necrosis. Well-preserved cancer cells of squamous type are sparse and sometimes difficult to identify among anucleated squames. Quite often, only well differentiated dyskaryotic (dysplastic) cells may be observed with a cytologic pattern similar to condylomas (Fig. 14-12). The cytologic diagnosis of carcinoma of the vulva **may be difficult to establish** (Kashimura et al, 1993). **Therefore, the presence of atypical squamous cells with enlarged nuclei should lead to a request for a tissue biopsy risking, at times, a false alarm.** It may be noted that ulcerative lesions of the vulva, such as ulcers and herpetic vulvitis, may also yield atypical squamous cells. Tissue biopsy may be required to settle the diagnosis.

Predisposing Conditions

Atrophy of the vulvar skin, often associated with intense itch **(kraurosis vulvae),** excessive keratinization of vulvar skin (appearing as white lesions or **leukoplakia**), and **lichen sclerosus** are considered to be conditions predisposing to squamous carcinoma. Kraurosis vulvae shows atrophy of the epidermis, accompanied by an inflammatory infiltrate. In leukoplakia, the surface epithelium is covered with thick layers of keratin. Lichen sclerosus has been discussed above. The term **"vulvar dystrophy"** has been proposed to encom-

pass a variety of lesions, including lichen sclerosus, allegedly preceding vulvar carcinoma (Friedrich, 1976). Sagerman et al (1996) studied the distribution of HPV in 41 cases of **"vulvar dystrophy,"** 19 accompanying invasive squamous carcinoma and 22 not associated with cancer. Interestingly, the presence of HPV types 16 and 18 occurred in only 3 of 19 "dystrophies" accompanying cancer and in 12 of 22 of the lesions not associated with cancer. As the likelihood of progression of "dystrophies" to carcinoma is very small, this study, if confirmed, casts an uncertain light on the role of HPV in vulvar cancer.

Carcinoma In Situ of the Vulva (Bowen's Disease) and Related Lesions (Vulvar Intraepithelial Neoplasia; VIN)

Histology

Precancerous epithelial lesions of the vulva are now considered as a family of lesions known as vulvar intraepithelial neoplasia (VIN), which may be graded from I to III, as is the case for the cervical lesions (CIN) and vaginal lesions (VAIN). Alternately, the lesions can be classified as **low-grade and high-grade VIN.** One can consider **condylomata acuminata as low-grade lesions, keeping in mind their occasional role as a stepping stone to invasive squamous carcinoma.** Hart (2001) separated the vulvar lesions into two groups: the classic Bowenoid VIN of different grades and a rare, extremely well differentiated variant that he called "simplex" or "differentiated type."

The high-grade VIN may be subdivided into two types of lesions, corresponding to invasive squamous cancer:

■ The keratinizing variant, also known as Bowen's disease because of its resemblance to the identical lesion of the skin and to keratin-forming lesions (keratinizing carcinoma in situ) of the cervix and vagina. The epithelium of the vulva is thickened and its surface is usually lined by a layer of keratin or by several layers of keratinized cells that may deceptively suggest a benign wart-like lesion. Occasionally, a **wart-like configuration of these lesions** may be observed. Scattered throughout the thickness of the abnormal epithelium are **cells with enlarged, hyperchromatic nuclei.** Some of these are very large. Mitotic activity is observed at all levels of the epithelium. Raju et al (2003) described a **pagetoid variant** of carcinoma in situ, containing large cells with clear cytoplasm, mimicking Paget's disease (see below).

■ **Occasionally, high-grade VIN, particularly when located on labia minora, may be composed of small cancer cells and show little evidence of keratin formation on the surface.** Such lesions correspond to classical carcinomas in situ that are identical with poorly differentiated precancerous lesions of the vagina or the cervix.

Cytology

Most high-grade VIN are readily visible as either a "red" or a "white" lesion and the diagnosis should be established by biopsy. Occasionally, however, the clinical differential diagnosis between an inflammatory lesion, such as ulcerated herpetic lesions, a flat condyloma, a high-grade VIN, or an invasive carcinoma cannot be made and a scrape smear of the vulva is obtained.

Vulvar smears are often dry and the cells are distorted. Therefore, the interpretation of such material must be painstaking and careful. **In the presence of even a few squamous cells with large nuclei, further investigation by biopsy should be suggested.** Even in well-preserved material, the cytologic presentation may be inconspicuous and the neoplastic lesion may be represented by a **few keratinized squamous cells with enlarged, hyperchromatic nuclei, in a setting of anucleated squames. This is particularly important in the recognition of keratinizing precursor lesions or cancer, particularly verrucous carcinoma.**

Poorly differentiated carcinomas of the vulva and their precursor lesions are uncommonly seen. The cells correspond to poorly differentiated carcinomas of the vagina or cervix (see Fig. 14-3 and Chap. 11).

There is no information on the cytologic presentation of microinvasive carcinoma.

Paget's Disease

Natural History and Histology

Paget's disease presents as an area of vulvar redness, sometimes associated with oozing of serous fluid from its surface. Actual ulceration is uncommon but may occur. This disorder, occurring in women above 40 years of age, must be considered in the differential diagnosis of inflammatory lesions, carcinoma in situ, and superficial malignant melanoma (see Chap. 17).

Similar to Paget's disease of the breast (see Chap. 29), the vulvar disease is associated with an **infiltration of the epidermis by large cells with clear cytoplasm and enlarged nuclei (Paget's cells).** Large nucleoli may be present. Paget's cells may occur singly or in clusters, occasionally forming gland-like structures. Paget's cells may be spread along the ducts of sweat glands as well as hair shafts and hair follicles (Fig. 14-13C). Paget's disease of the vulva may spread to the perineum and even the perianal area, and, less commonly, the vagina. The cytoplasm of Paget's cells contains glycogen and mucin-like material that **stains intensely with mucicarmine,** a simple laboratory reaction helpful in the differential diagnosis from other lesions, particularly malignant melanoma.

It has been shown that some cases of Paget's disease of the vulva, like its breast equivalent, are associated with an underlying carcinoma of sweat glands, although the latter is sometimes very inconspicuous and difficult to identify (Koss et al, 1968). In many instances, however, **no underlying carcinoma can be found;** the pathogenesis of this type of Paget's disease is unknown. It should be noted that Paget's cells form desmosomal attachments to normal epithelial cells, a feature that appears to be unique to this disease (Koss and Brockunier, 1969). It is noteworthy that **metastatic carcinoma of the bladder to the vagina may mimic Paget's disease** (Koss, 1985; see Chap. 23). **Vulvar Paget's disease,** caused by spread of **bladder cancer,** was also reported by Wilkinson and Brown (2002). Staining with Uroplakin III antibody confirmed the urothelial origin of this disorder (Brown and Wilkinson, 2003).

The prognosis of Paget's disease depends on the depth of invasion and the presence of an underlying sweat gland carcinoma: if the latter is large, metastases to inguinal lymph nodes often occur. Still, even Paget's disease, without demonstrable underlying cancer, is often difficult to control, even by extensive surgical excision, and recurrences and spread to adjacent organs may occur. In an elaborate study of 21 cases, Crawford et al (1999) were unable to find any factors of predictive value.

Cytology

The diagnosis of Paget's disease of the vulva is usually based on biopsies. In fortuitous cases, in a scrape smear of the vulva or the adjacent vagina, **large, malignant cells with clear cytoplasm and enlarged, slightly hyperchromatic nuclei may be observed** (see Fig. 14-13). The cytologic findings are similar to those in mammary Paget's disease (see Chap. 29). The findings are not specific but the diagnosis may be suspected in an appropriate clinical setting. It is of note that **squamous cells in smears from Paget's disease may also show some nuclear atypia.** This feature, combined with the scarcity of cancer cells, may suggest a squamous carcinoma rather than Paget's disease. Few cases of Paget's disease with cytologic findings have been reported in the literature (Bennington et al, 1966; Masukawa and

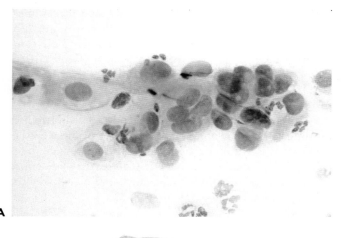

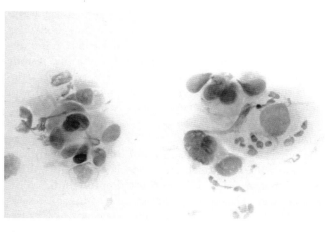

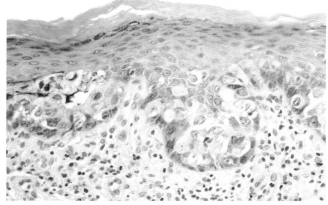

Figure 14-13   Paget's disease of the vulva. *A,B.* Air-dried scrape smears of the surface of the lesion. Note cells with large nuclei and eosinophilic cytoplasm. The identity of the lesion shown in *C* cannot be recognized in these smears.

Friedrich, 1978; Costello et al, 1988; Castellano Megias et al, 2002). They added very little to the above description.

A case of **Paget's disease of the penis,** secondary to a sweat gland carcinoma, was described by Mitsudo et al (1981).

Bowenoid Papulosis

This disorder is characterized by **multiple, raised, pigmented (tan or brown) lesions of the skin of the genital area,** observed mainly in young male and female patients. The lesions are **histologically similar to Bowen's disease** but differ in behavior, inasmuch as they often disappear spontaneously and **do not progress to invasive cancer.** The presence of **HPV type 16** has been universally noted in these lesions, which are thought to constitute an important source of infection. The reason for behavioral differences between Bowen's disease and bowenoid papulosis is obscure at the time of this writing (2004). There is no information on the cytologic presentation of these lesions.

Other Tumors

The labia majora of the vulva may be the site of malignant tumors affecting the skin. We have observed a few **basal cell carcinomas** mistaken for other entities and, therefore, examined by scrape smears. Clusters of small, uniform, spindly cells with peripheral cells arranged perpendicularly to the main cell mass (palisading) are characteristic of this tumor. For further discussion of cutaneous tumors, see Chapter 34. A mamary **ductal carcinoma in situ,** derived

from the vulva, was described by Castro and Deavers (2001). **Mammary carcinomas** derived from supernumerary breasts have also been described (Rose et al, 1990). Malignant melanomas and other uncommon tumors of the vulva are discussed in Chapter 17.

Male Partners of Patients With Vulvar Disorders

In principle, all male partners of women with condylomas or other forms of a permissive HPV infection should be examined because many of them will also be carriers of HPV and some may have **penile lesions** (Gross et al, 1985; Barrasso et al, 1987). Although visible penile lesions (**condylomas, bowenoid papulosis, carcinoma in situ, erythroplasia of Queyrat**) should be treated, there is no unanimity as to whether a colposcopic examination of the skin of the penis with laser treatment of minor skin abnormalities is warranted.

ANUS

Basic Concepts

As a corollary to the cytologic diagnosis of vulvar lesions, it has been observed that **precancerous lesions and cancers of the anus may be amenable to cytologic examination.** Patients at a high risk of neoplastic anal lesions are men and women engaging in receptive anal intercourse (Law et al, 1991), immunosuppressed patients infected with human immunodeficiency virus, patients with AIDS, organ transplant recipients (summary in Palefsky et al, 1994; Frisch et al, 1997; Sillman et al, 1997; Goldie et al, 1999; Ryan et al, 2000). The presence of **human papillomavirus of various types appears to be the common denominator of the anal lesions** (Lowhagen et al, 1999; Palefsky, 1999). HPV type 16, particularly the HPV 16PL variant, appear to be associated with high-grade lesions (Frisch et al, 1997; Xi et al, 1998).

Anatomy and Histology

The outer aspects of the anus, and immediately adjacent portion of the anal canal, are lined by **squamous epithelium.** A narrow band of **"transitional epithelium,"** composed of several layers of small cells and having some resemblance to the urothelium (described in detail in Chapter 22), separates the squamous epithelium from the rectal mucosa. The **rectal mucosa** resembles the mucosa of the colon and is composed of tall, columnar, mucus-secreting cells, forming tubular crypts. For an excellent review of anatomy of this region, see Ryan et al (2000).

Benign Disorders

Disregarding vascular disorders such as hemorrhoids that are commonly observed, important diseases of the anus occur in men and women who practice anal sexual intercourse (Law et al, 1991). Infections with herpesvirus, Epstein-Barr virus, and human papillomavirus are more common in homosexual men than in women (Jacobs, 1976; Moscicki et al, 1999). Infection with HIV and resulting AIDS are significant additional risk factors (Hillemanns et al, 1996; Palefsky et al, 1998; Lowhagen et al, 1999).

The most common of these disorders is condylomata acuminata that may occur on the perianal squamous epithelium but also within the anal canal. These lesions are morphologically identical to vulvar condylomas, described above. In patients with AIDS, condylomas may be the site of **Kaposi's sarcomas** (Fig. 14-14A,B).

Malignant Lesions

Malignant lesions of the anus and their precursors (anal intraepithelial neoplasia, or AIN) resemble in many ways the lesions of the uterine cervix: **lesions derived from the squamous epithelium are well differentiated squamous carcinomas, some containing koilocytes in their surface epithelium and, hence, displaying features of condylomas,** in this example associated with Kaposi's sarcoma (Fig. 14-14C). Their precursor lesions resemble flat condylomas.

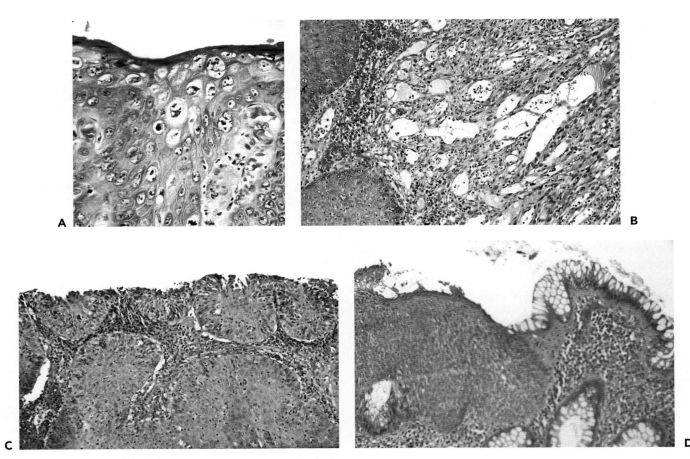

Figure 14-14   Anal lesions. *A.* Condyloma-like disease of squamous epithelium (*A*) with an underlying Kaposi's sarcoma (*B*) in a patient with AIDS. *C.* A poorly differentiated anal squamous carcinoma. *D.* A basaloid carcinoma of the anus.

The highly malignant poorly differentiated carcinomas are derived from the "transitional epithelium" and resemble basaloid carcinomas or nonkeratinizing squamous (epidermoid) cancers (Fig. 14-14D). Their precursor lesions resemble squamous (epidermoid) nonkeratinizing high grade lesions derived from the epithelium of the endocervical canal (see Chapter 11). The terms **low-grade anal intraepithelial neoplasia (LGAIN)** and **high-grade anal intraepithelial neoplasia (HGAIN)** have been proposed to describe the precursor lesions of anal carcinoma (Lacey et al, 1999).

Palefsky et al (1990, 1998) observed that, in homosexual men with advanced AIDS, the anal neoplasia may develop over a short period of time. The same author (1999) noted that effective antiviral therapy does not lead to regression of the neoplastic lesions.

Cytology

Methods

Moistened cotton swabs or plastic scrapers can be used to secure cell samples from the anus (Haye et al, 1988). It is unresolved whether the "adequate" sample must also contain glandular cells of the rectal mucosa. According to Sher-

man et al (1995) and Darragh et al (1997), such cells are more readily found in samples collected in liquid fixative than in conventional smears. Palefsky et al (1997) observed that the absence of such cells did not affect the sensitivity of the procedure.

Normal Anus

Smears of normal anus are identical to normal vulvar scrape smears and contain mainly anucleated and nucleated squamous cells. In specimens obtained from the anal canal, tall, columnar, mucus-producing rectal cells may be observed.

Inflammatory Disorders

Herpes genitalis may be observed in anal smears (Jacobs, 1976). There is no record of other identifiable infectious organisms known to us. For cytologic features of herpesvirus, see Chapter 10.

Precursor Lesions (AIN)

Low-Grade Lesions

Superficial squamous dyskaryotic (dysplastic) cells and koilocytes are the dominant cell types in perianal and anal condylomas (Fig. 14-15). These may be accompanied by

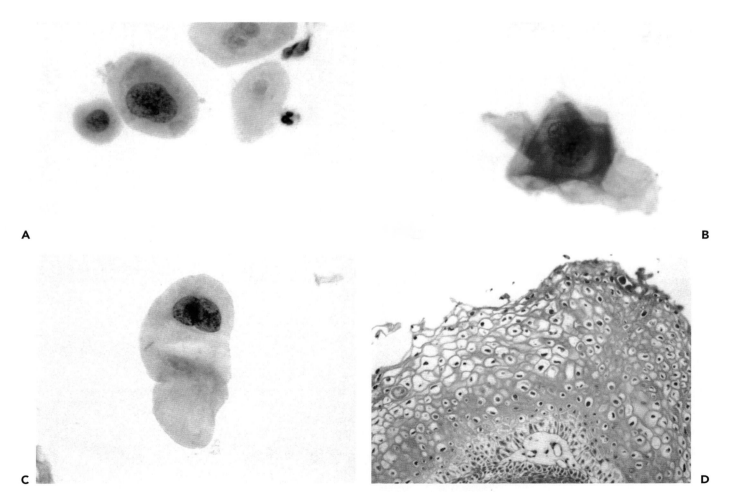

Figure 14-15 **Low-grade squamous intraepithelial anal lesion (AIN I).** *A–C.* Various aspects of dyskaryotic (dysplastic) cells showing enlarged nuclei in an anal scrape smear. In one of the fields, there is a multinucleated cell with a perinuclear halo. *D.* The histologic aspect of the condylomatous lesion, the source of cells shown in *A–C.* (Courtesy of Dr. Oscar Lin, Memorial Sloan-Kettering Cancer Center, New York, NY.)

somewhat atypical squamous cells with enlarged nuclei. Smaller malignant squamous cells, similar to those observed in **high-grade lesions** derived from the endocervical epithelium, are characteristic of the high grade anal lesions (see Fig. 14-3). Scholefield et al (1998) observed a better reproducibility of diagnoses among pathologists with high-grade lesions than low-grade lesions.

Invasive Cancer

Invasive carcinomas of the anus, whether well or poorly differentiated, are morphologically identical to similar lesions of the vulva and vagina, described above. An example of a high-grade invasive carcinoma is shown in Figure 14-16.

Follow-Up of Cytologic Abnormalities

Colposcopy of the anus (anoscopy) followed by biopsies appears to be the method of choice to confirm cytologic abnormalities (Lacey et al, 1999).

Value of Anal Cytology

Anal cytology has now been accepted as a screening tool for anal neoplasia. The sensitivity of anal cytology (about 40% to 70% of the lesions, depending on the authors) is much greater than its specificity which appears to be about 40%. Palefsky et al (1997) emphasized the need for biopsy confirmation of abnormal findings. This **suggests that anoscopy and biopsies should be performed as a follow-up procedure of cytologic atypias, even in the absence of specific cytologic diagnosis** (De Ruiter et al, 1994). In one of the early papers on this subject, Sonnex et al (1991) compared the effectiveness of cytology, anoscopy, and in situ hybridization in the search for evidence of HPV infection and pointed out that anoscopy was more effective in the discovery of AIN than cytology. During the intervening years and improvement in sample collection, processing and interpretation the results have become more reliable. Perhaps the greatest value of anal cytology is in **situations when anoscopy is negative and cytology is suggestive or diagnostic of a neoplastic lesion.** Seven such cases were reported by Surawicz et al (1995).

Goldie et al (1999) studied the clinical- and cost-effectiveness of cytologic screening of homosexual and bisexual men infected with HIV. They concluded that the procedure is beneficial, cost effective, and comparable to other clinical preventive interventions.

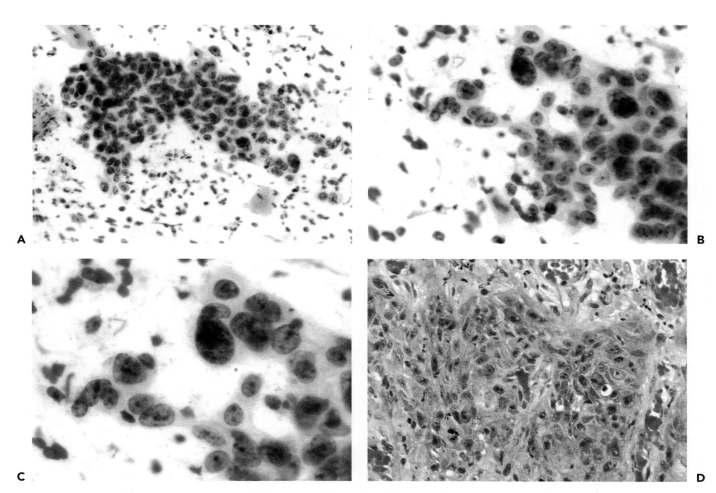

Figure 14-16. **Squamous cell carcinoma of anus.** *A,B,C.* Anal scrape smear with clusters of small cancer cells with large nuclei and prominent nucleoli at increasing magnifications from *A* to *C*, corresponding to the biopsy shown in *D.* (Courtesy of Dr. Oscar Lin, Memorial Sloan-Kettering Cancer Center, New York, NY.)

BIBLIOGRAPHY

Abell MR, Gosling JRG. Intraepithelial and infiltrative carcinoma of vulva, Bowen's type. Cancer 14:318–329, 1961.

Aho M, Vesterinen V, Meyer B, et al. Natural history of vaginal intraepithelial neoplasia. Cancer 68:195–197, 1991.

Albores-Saavedra J, Poucell S, Rodriguez-Martinez HA. Primary carcinoid of the cervix. Pathologica 10:185–193, 1972.

Anderson ES. Primary carcinoma of the vagina: A study of 29 cases. Gynecol Oncol 33:317–320, 1989.

Andreasson B, Bock JE. Intraepithelial neoplasia in the vulvar region. Gynecol Oncol 21:300–305, 1985.

Baltzer J, Zander J. Primary squamous cell carcinoma of the neovagina. Gynecol Oncol 35:99–103, 1989.

Barber HR, Sommers SC. Vaginal adenosis, dysplasia, and clear cell adenocarcinoma after diethyl stilbestrol treatment in pregnancy. Obstet Gynecol 43:645–652, 1974.

Barraso R, de Brux H, Crissani O, Orth G. High prevalence of papillomavirus-associated penile intraepithelial neoplasia in sexual partners of women with cervical intraepithelial neoplasia. N Engl J Med 317:916–923, 1987.

Beckmann AM, Daling JR, Sherman KJ, et al. Human papillomavirus and anal cancer. Int J Cancer 43:1042–1049, 1989.

Beckmann AM, Kiviat NB, Daling JR, et al. Human papillomavirus type 16 in multifocal neoplasia of the female genital tract. Int J Gynecol Pathol 7:39–47, 1988.

Bell J, Sevin BU, Averette H, Nadji M. Vaginal cancer after hysterectomy for benign disease: value of cytology screening. Obstet Gynecol 64:699–702, 1984.

Belleannée G, Brun JL, Trouette H, et al. Cytologic findings in neovagina created by Vecchietti's technique for treating vaginal aplasia. Acta Cytol 42:945–948, 1998.

Benedet JL, Sanders BH. Carcinoma in situ of the vagina. Am J Obstet Gynecol 148:695–700, 1984.

Bennington JL, Smith DC, Sigge DC. Detection of cells from extra-mammary Paget's disease of the vulva in a vaginal smear. Report of a case. Obstet Gynecol 27:772–775, 1966.

Bergeron C, Naghashfar Z, Canaan C, et al. Human papillomavirus type 16 in intraepithelial neoplasia (Bowenoid papulosis) and coexistent invasive carcinoma of the vulva. Int J Gynecol Pathol 6:1–11, 1987.

Bernstein SG, Voet RL, Lifshitz S, Buchsbaum HJ. Adenoid cystic carcinoma of Bartholin's gland. Case report and review of the literature. Am J Obstet Gynecol 147:385–390, 1983.

Bewtra C. Columnar cells in post-hysterectomy vaginal smears. Diagn Cytopathol 8:342–345, 1992.

Bibbo M, Ali I, Al-Nageeb M, et al. Cytologic findings in female and male offspring of DES treated mothers. Acta Cytol 19:568–572, 1975.

Bivens MD. Primary carcinoma of vagina: Report of 46 cases. Am J Obstet Gynecol 65:390–399, 1953.

Bornstein J, Kaufman RH, Adam E, Adler-Storthz K. Human papillomavirus associated with vaginal intraepithelial neoplasia in women exposed to diethylstilbestrol in utero. Obstet Gynecol 70:70–75, 1987.

Bornstein J, Kaufman RH, Adam E, Adler-Storthz K. Multicentric intraepithelial neoplasia involving the vulva: Clinical features and association with human papillomavirus and herpes simplex virus. Cancer 62:1601–1604, 1988.

Bornstein J, Lova Y, Lurie M, Abramovici H. Development of vaginal adenosis following combined 5-fluorouracil and carbon dioxide laser treatment for diffuse vaginal adenomatosis. Obstetr Gynecol 81:896–898, 1993.

Bottles K, Lacey CG, Goldberg J, et al. Merkel cell carcinoma of the vulva. Obstet Gynecol 63:61S–65S, 1984.

Boutselis JG. Intraepithelial carcinoma of the vulva. Am J Obstet Gynecol 113:733–738, 1972.

Brand E, Fu YS, Lagasse LD, Berek JS. Vulvovaginal melanoma: Report of seven cases and literature review. Gynecol Oncol 33:54–60, 1989.

Breen JL, Neubecker RD, Greenwald E, Gregori CA. Basal cell carcinoma of the vulva. Obstet Gynecol 46:122–129, 1975.

Brooks JJ, LiVolsi VA. Liposarcoma of the vulva. Am J Obstet Gynecol 156:73–75, 1987.

Brown HM, Wilkinson EJ. Uroplakin-III to distinguish primary vulvar Paget disease from Paget disease secondary to urothelial carcinoma. Hum Pathol 33:545–548, 2002.

Buscema J, Woodruff JD, Parmley TH, Genadry R. Carcinoma *in situ* of the vulva. Obstet Gynecol 55:225–230, 1980.

Caglar H, Tamer S, Hreshchyshyn MH. Vulvar intra-epithelial neoplasia. Obstet Gynecol 60:346–349, 1982.

Carson LF, Twiggs LB, Okagaki T, et al. Human papillomavirus DNA in adeno-squamous carcinoma and squamous cell carcinoma of the vulva. Obstet Gynecol 72:63–67, 1988.

Carter ER, Salvaggio AT, Jarkowski TL. Squamous cell carcinoma of the vagina following vaginal hysterectomy for intraepithelial carcinoma of the cervix. Am J Obstet Gynecol 82:401–404, 1961.

Castellano Megias VM, Ibarrola de Andres C, et al. Cytology of extramammary Paget's disease of the vulva. A case report. Acta Cytol 46:1153–1157, 2002.

Castro CY, Deavers M. Ductal carcinoma in-situ arising in mammary-like glands of the vulva. Int J Gynecol Pathol 20:277–283, 2001.

Chacho MS, Eppich E, Wersto RP, Koss LG. Influence of human papilloma virus on DNA ploidy determination in genital condylomas. Cancer 65:2991–2994, 1990.

Chafe W. Neuroepithelial small cell carcinoma of the vagina. Cancer 64:1948–1951, 1989.

Chalvardjian A, Picard L, Shaw R, et al. Malacoplakia of the female genital tract. Am J Obstet Gynecol 138:391–394, 1980.

Chalvardjian A, Carydis B, Cohen S. Cytologic diagnosis of extravesical malacoplakia. Diagn Cytopathol 1:216–220, 1985.

Chamlian DL, Taylor HB. Primary carcinoma of Bartholin's gland. Obstet Gynecol 39:489–494, 1972.

Chang SH, Maddox WA. Adenocarcinoma arising within cervical endometriosis and invading the adjacent vagina. Am J Obstet Gynecol 110:1015–1017, 1971.

Cho D, Buscema J, Rosenshein NB, Woodruff JD. Primary breast cancer of the vulva. Obstet Gynecol 66:79S–81S, 1985.

Chu J, Tamini HK, Ek M, Figge DC. Stage I vulvar cancer: Criteria for microinvasion. Obstet Gynecol 59:716–719, 1982.

Chung AF, Woodruff JM, Lewis JL Jr. Malignant melanoma of the vulva: Report of 44 cases. Obstet Gynecol 45:638–646, 1975.

Ciesla MC, Guidos BJ, Selvaggi SM. Cytomorphology of small-cell (neuroendocrine) carcinoma on ThinPrep$^{(R)}$ cytology as compared to conventional smears. Diagn Cytopathol 24:46–52, 2001.

Coates JB III, Hales JS. Granular cell myoblastoma of the vulva. Obstet Gynecol 41:796–799, 1973.

Coleman N, Birley HD, Renton AM, et al. Immunological events in regressing genital warts. Am J Clin Pathol 102:768–774, 1994.

Colleran KM, Burge MR, Crooks LA, Dorin RI. Small cell carcinoma of the vagina causing Cushing's syndrome by ectopic production and secretion of ACTH: A case report. Gynecol Oncol 65:526–529, 1997.

Collins CG, Roman-Lopez JJ, Lee FYL. Intraepithelial carcinoma of the vulva. Am J Obstet Gynecol 108:1187–1191, 1970.

Committee on Terminology. New nomenclature for vulvar disease. Obstet Gynecol 47:122–124, 1976.

Copeland LJ, Cleary K, Sneige N, Edwards CL. Neuroendocrine (Merkel cell) carcinoma of the vulva: A case report and review of the literature. Gynecol Oncol 22:367–378, 1985.

Copeland LJ, Sneige N, Gershenson DM, et al. Adenoid cystic carcinoma of the Bartholin gland. Obstet Gynecol 67:115–120, 1986.

Costello TJ, Wang HH, Schnitt SJ, et al. Paget's disease with extensive involvement of the female genital tract initially detected by cervical cytosmear. Arch Pathol Lab Med 112:941–944, 1988.

Cox SM, Kaufman RH, Kaplan A. Recurrent carcinoma in situ of the vulva in a skin graft. Am J Obstet Gynecol 155:177–179, 1986.

Crawford D, Nimmo M, Clement PB, et al. Prognostic factors in Paget's disease of the vulva: A study of 21 cases. Int J Gynecol Pathol 18:351–359, 1999.

Creasman WT, Gallager HS, Rutledge F. Paget's disease of the vulva. Gynecol Oncol 3:133–148, 1975.

Crowdon WA, Fu YS, Lebherz TB, et al. Pruritic vulvar squamous papillomatosis: Evidence for human papillomavirus etiology. Obstet Gynecol 66:564–568, 1985.

Crowther ME, Shepherd JH, Fisher C. Verrucous carcinoma of the vulva containing human papillomavirus-11: Case report. Br J Obstet Gynaecol 95:414–418, 1988.

Crum CP. Vulvar intraepithelial neoplasia: The concept and its application. Hum Pathol 13:187–189, 1982.

Crum CP, Braun LA, Shah KV, et al. Vulvar intraepithelial neoplasia: Correlation of nuclear DNA content and the presence of a human papilloma virus (HPV) structural antigen. Cancer 49:468–471, 1982.

Crum CP, Fu YS, Levine RU, et al. Intraepithelial squamous lesions of the vulva: Biologic and histologic criteria for the distinction of condylomas from vulvar intraepithelial neoplasia. Am J Obstet Gynecol 144:77–83, 1982.

Crum CP, Liskow A, Petras P, et al. Vulvar intraepithelial neoplasia (severe atypia and carcinoma in situ). A clinicopathologic analysis of 41 cases. Cancer 54:1429–1434, 1984.

Cruz-Jimenez PR, Abell MR. Cutaneous basal cell carcinoma of vulva. Cancer 36:1860–1868, 1975.

Cuyler WK, Kaufmann LA, Palumbo L, Carter B. Cytologic studies in malignant lesions of vagina. I. Primary squamous cell carcinoma. Surg Gynecol Obstet 96:115–117, 1953.

Daling JR, Weiss NS, et al. Sexual practices, sexually transmitted diseases, and the incidence of anal cancer. N Engl J Med 317:973–977, 1987.

Darragh TM, Jay N, Tupkelewicz BA, et al. Comparison of conventional cytologic smears and ThinPrep preparations from the anal canal. Acta Cytol 41:1167–1170, 1997.

De Mauro JM, Skolom J, Wallach RC, Rorat E. Cytologic diagnosis of Bartholin's gland adenocarcinoma. Acta Cytol 30:491–493, 1986.

De Ruiter A, Carter P, Katz DR, et al. A comparison between cytology and histology to detect anal intraepithelial neoplasia. Genitourin Med 70:22–25, 1994.

Del Mistro A, Braunstein JD, Halwer M, Koss LG. Identification of human papillomavirus types in male urethral condylomata acuminata by in situ hybridization. Hum Pathol 18:936–940, 1987.

Dennerstein GJ. The cytology of the vulva. J Obstet Gynecol Br Commonw 75:603–609, 1968.

Deppisch LM. Cysts of the vagina. Classification and clinical correlations. Obstet Gynecol 45:632–637, 1975.

DiPaola GR, Gomez-Rueda N, Arrighi L. Relevance of microinvasion in carcinoma of the vulva. Obstet Gynecol 45:647–649, 1975.

Dodson MG, O'Leary JA, Averette HE. Primary carcinoma of Bartholin's gland. Obstet Gynecol 35:578–584, 1970.

Downey GO, Okagaki T, Ostrow RS, et al. Condylomatous carcinoma of the vulva with special reference to human papillomavirus DNA. Obstet Gynecol 72:68–73, 1988.

Dreyfuss W, Neville WE. Buschke-Lowenstein tumors (giant condyloma acuminata). Am J Surg 90:146–150, 1955.

Duckler L. Squamous cell carcinoma developing in an artificial vagina. Obstet Gynecol 40:35–38, 1972.

Duray PH, Merino MJ, Axiotis C. Warty dyskeratoma of the vulva. Int J Gynecol Pathol 2:286–293, 1983.

Dvoretsky PM, Bonfiglio TA, Helmkamp BF, et al. The pathology of superficially invasive, thin vulvar squamous cell carcinoma. Int J Gynecol Pathol 3:331–342, 1984.

Edwards L. Imiquimod in clinical practice. Australa H Dermatol 39:S14–S16, 1998.

Fenn ME, Morley GW, Abell MR. Paget's disease of vulva. Obstet Gynecol 38:660–670, 1971.

Fenoglio CM, Ferenczy A, Richart RM, Townsend D. Scanning and transmission electron microscopic studies of vaginal adenosis and the cervical transformation zone in progeny exposed in utero to diethylstilbestrol. Am J Obstet Gynecol 126:170–180, 1976.

Fetherston WC. Squamous neoplasia of vagina related to DES syndrome. Am J Obstet Gynecol 122:176–181, 1975.

Forsberg JG. Estrogen-induced adenosis of vagina and cervix in mice. Am J Pathol 84:669–672, 1976.

Fowler WC, Jr, Schmidt G, Edelman DA, et al. Risks of cervical intraepithelial neoplasia among DES-exposed women. Obstet Gynecol 58:720–724, 1981.

Foye G, Marsh MR, Minkowitz S. Verrucous carcinoma of the vulva. Obstet Gynecol 34:484–488, 1969.

Frable WJ, Goplerud DR. Adenoid cystic carcinoma of Bartholin's gland. Diagnosis by aspiration biopsy. Acta Cytol 19:152–153, 1975.

Frable WJ, Smith JH, Perkins J, Foley C. Vaginal cuff cytology: Some difficult diagnostic problems. Acta Cytol 17:135–140, 1973.

Freidrich EG Jr. Reversible vulvar atypia: A case report. Obstet Gynecol 39:173–181, 1972.

Friedrich EG Jr. Vaginitis. Am Fam Physician 28:238–242, 1983.

Friedrich EG Jr, Wilkinson EJ, Steingraeber PH, Lewis JD. Paget's disease of the vulva and carcinoma of the breast. Obstet Gynecol 46:130–134, 1975.

Friedrich J. New nomenclature for vulvar disease. Obstet Gynecol 47:122–124, 1976.

Frisch M, Glimelius B, van den Brule AJC, et al. Sexually transmitted infection as a cause of anal cancer. N Engl J Med 337:1350–1358, 1997.

Fu YS, Lancaster WD, Richart RM, et al. Cervical papillomavirus infection in diethylstilbestrol-exposed progeny. Obstet Gynecol 61:59–62, 1983.

Fu YS, Reagan JW, Richart RM, Townsend DE. Nuclear DNA and histologic studies of genital lesions in diethylstilbestrol-exposed progeny. I. Intraepithelial squamous abnormalities. Am J Clin Pathol 72:503–514, 1979.

Fu YS, Reagan JW, Richart RM, Townsend DE. Nuclear DNA and histologic studies of genital lesions in diethylstilbestrol-exposed progeny. II. Intraepithelial glandular abnormalities. Am J Clin Pathol 72:515–520, 1979.

Gad A, Eusebi V. Rhabdomyoma of the vagina. J Pathol 115:179–181, 1975.

Gallup DG, Morley GW. Carcinoma in situ of the vagina: A study and review. Obstet Gynecol 46:334–336, 1975.

Ganesan R, Ferryman SR, Waddell CA. Vaginal adenosis in a patient on Tamoxifen therapy: a case report. Cytopathol 10:127–130, 1999.

Gardner HL, Kaufman RH. Benign Diseases of the Vulva and Vagina. St. Louis, CV Mosby, 1969.

Giaquinto C, Del Mistro A, De Rossi A, et al. Vulvar carcinoma in a 12-year-old girl with vertically acquired human immunodeficiency virus infection. Pediatrics 106:E57, 2000.

Gill WB, Schmacher GFB, Bibbo M. Structural and functional abnormalities in the sex organs of male offspring of mothers treated with diethylstilbestrol (DES). J Reprod Med 16:147–153, 1976.

Gilson MD, Dibona DD, Knab DR. Clear cell adenocarcinoma in young females. Obstet Gynecol 41:494–500, 1973.

Gold JH, Bossen EH. Benign vaginal rhabdomyoma: A light and electron microscopic study. Cancer 37:2283–2294, 1976.

Goldie SJ, Kuntz KM, Weinstein MC, et al. The clinical effectiveness and cost-effectiveness of screening for anal squamous intraepithelial lesions in homosexual and bisexual HIV-positive men. JAMA 281:1822–1829, 1999.

Goodman A, Zukerberg LR, Nikrui N, Scully RE. Vaginal adenosis and clear cell carcinoma after 5-fluorouracil treatment for condylomas. Cancer 68:1628–1632, 1991.

Gray LA, Christopherson WM. In situ and early invasive carcinoma of the vagina. Obstet Gynecol 34:226–230, 1969.

Greenwalt P, Barlow JJ, Nasca PC, Burnett WS. Vaginal cancer after maternal treatment with synthetic estrogens. N Engl J Med 285:390–392, 1971.

Gross G. Lesions of the male and female external genitalia associated with human papillomaviruses. In Syrjanen K, Gissmann L, Koss LG (eds). Papillomaviruses and Human Diseases. Berlin-Heidelberg-New York, Springer-Verlag, 1987, pp 197–234.

Gross G, Hagedom M, Ikenberg H, et al. Bowenoid papulosis. Presence of human papillomavirus (HPV) structural antigens and of HPV 16-related DNA sequences. Arch Dermatol 121:858–863, 1985.

Gross G, Wagner D, Hauser-Braimer N, et al. Bowenoid papulosis and carcinoma in situ of the cervix uteri in sex partners. An example of the transmissibility of HPV-16 infection. Hautarzt 36:465–469, 1985.

Guarner J, Cohen C. Vulvar Paget's disease: Cytologic and immunohistologic diagnosis of a case. Acta Cytol 32:727–730, 1988.

Guillet GY, Braun L, Masse R, et al. Bowenoid papulosis: Demonstration of human papillomavirus (HPV) with anti-HPV immune serum. Arch Dermatol 120:514–516, 1984.

Gunning JE, Ostergard DR. Value of screening procedures for the detection of vaginal adenosis. Obstet Gynecol 47:268–271, 1976.

Gupta J, Pilotti S, Shah KV, et al. Human papillomavirus-associated early vulvar neoplasia investigated by in situ hybridization. Am J Surg Pathol 11:430–434, 1987.

Gupta RK, Belton JH, Bronowics M. Cytologic diagnosis of primary squamous cell carcinoma of Bartholin's gland. Acta Cytol 21:303–305, 1977.

Hansen K, Egholm M. Diffuse vaginal adenosis. Three cases combined with imperforate hymen and haematocolpos. Acta Obstet Gynecol Scand 54:287–292, 1975.

Hart WR. Vulvar intraepithelial neoplasia: Historical aspects and current status. Int J Gynecol Pathol 20:16–30, 2001.

Haye KR, Maiti H, Stanbridge CM. Cytological screening to detect subclinical anal human papillomavirus (HPV) infection in homosexual men attending genitourinary medicine clinic. Genitourin Med 64:378–382, 1988.

Hendrix RC, Behrman SJ. Adenocarcinoma arising in a supernumerary mammary gland in the vulva. Obstet Gynecol 8:238–241, 1956.

Herbst AL. Clear cell adenocarcinoma and the current status of DES-exposed females. Cancer 48:484–488, 1981.

Herbst AL, Bern HA (eds). Developmental Effects of Diethylstilbestrol (DES) in Pregnancy. New York, Thieme-Stratton, 1981.

Herbst AL, Green TH, Ulfelder H. Primary carcinoma of the vagina. Am J Obstet Gynecol 106:210–218, 1970.

Herbst AL, Kurman RJ, Scully RE, Poskanzer DC. Clear-cell adenocarcinoma of the genital tract in young females. N Engl J Med 287:1259–1264, 1972.

Herbst AL, Robboy SJ, Scully RE, Poskanzer DC. Clear-cell adenocarcinoma of the vagina and cervix in girls: analysis of 170 registry cases. Am J Obstet Gynecol 119:713–724, 1974.

Herbst AL, Ulfelder H, Poskanzer DC. Adenocarcinoma of the vagina. Association of maternal stilbestrol with tumor appearance in young women. N Engl J Med 284:878–881, 1971.

Hilgers RD, Malkasian GD, Soule EH. Embryonal rhabdomyosarcoma (botryoid type) of the vagina. Am J Obstet Gynecol 107:484–502, 1970.

Hill EC. Clear cell carcinoma of the cervix and vagina in young women. Am J Obstet Gynecol 116:470–484, 1973.

Hillemanns P, Ellerbrock TV, McPhillips S, et al. Prevalence of anal human papillomavirus infection and anal cytologic abnormalities in HIV-seropositive women. AIDS 10:1641–1647, 1996.

Holohan M, Coughlan M, O'Loughlin S, Dervan P. Crohn's disease of the vulva. Case report. Br J Obstet Gynaecol 95:943–945, 1988.

Hopkins MP, Kumar NB, Lichter AS, et al. Small cell carcinoma of the vagina with neuroendocrine features: a report of three cases. J Reprod Med 34:486–491, 1989.

Hummer WK, Mussey E, Decker DG, Dockerty MB. Carcinoma in situ of the vagina. Am J Obstet Gynecol 108:1109–1116, 1970.

Hunter CA Jr, Long KR. Study of microbiological flora of vagina. Am J Obstet Gynecol 75:865–871, 1958.

Husseinzadeh N, Newman NJ, Wesseler TA. Vulvar intraepithelial neoplasia: A clinicopathological study of carcinoma in situ of the vulva. Gynecol Oncol 33:157–163, 1989.

Ikenberg H, Gissmann L, Gross G, et al. Human papillomavirus type 16-related DNA in genital Bowen's disease and in Bowenoid papulosis. Int J Cancer 32:563–565, 1983.

Imbertson LM, Beaurline JM, Couture AM, et al. Cytokine induction in hairless mouse and rat skin after topical application of the immune response modifiers imiquimod and S-28463. J Invest Dermatol 110:734–739, 1998.

Jacobs E. Anal infections caused by herpes simplex virus. Dis Colon Rectum 19:151–157, 1976.

Jafari K, Cartnick EN. Microinvasive squamous-cell carcinoma of the vulva. Am J Obstet Gynecol 125:274, 1976.

Japaze H, Van Dinh T, Woodruff JD. Verrucous carcinoma of the vulva. Study of 24 cases. Obstet Gynecol 60:462–466, 1982.

Jee KJ, Kim YT, Kim KR, et al. Loss in 3p and 4p and gain of 3q are concomitant aberrations in squamous cell carcinoma of the vulva. Mod Pathol 14:377–381, 2001.

Johnson DE, Lo RK, Srigley J, Ayala AG. Verrucous carcinoma of the penis. J Urol 133:216–218, 1985.

Johnson LD, Palmer AE, King NW Jr, Hertig AT. Vaginal adenosis in cebus apella monkeys exposed to DES in utero. Obstet Gynecol 57:629–635, 1981.

Jones RW, Rowan DM. Vulvar intraepithelial neoplasia: III. A clinical study of the outcome in 113 cases with relation to the later development of invasive vulvar carcinoma. Obstet Gynecol 84:741–745, 1994.

Jorgensen EO. White lesions of the vulva. Med Clin North Am 58:755–758, 1974.

Joura EA, Lösch A, Haider-Angeler M-G, et al. Trends in vulvar neoplasia. Increasing incidence of vulvar intraepithelial neoplasia and squamous cell carcinoma of the vulva in young women. J Reprod Med 45:613–615, 2000.

Kanbour AI, Klionsky B, Murphy AI. Carcinoma of the vagina following cervical cancer. Cancer 34:1838–1841, 1974.

Kaplan AL, Kaufman RH, Birken RA, Simkin S. Intraepithelial carcinoma of the vulva with extension to the anal canal. Obstet Gynecol 58:368–371, 1981.

Karney MY, Cassidy MS, Zahn CM, Snyder RR. Melanosis of the vagina: A case report. J Reprod Med 46:389–391, 2001.

Kashimura M, Matsuura Y, Kawagoe T, et al. Cytology of vulvar squamous neoplasia. Acta Cytol 37:871–875, 1993.

Kaufman RH, Bornstein J, Adam E, et al. Human papillomavirus and herpes simplex virus in vulvar squamous cell carcinoma in situ. Am J Obstet Gynecol 158:862–871, 1988.

Kiviat NB, Critchlow CW, Holmes KK, et al. Association of anal dysplasia and human papillomavirus with immunosuppression and HIV infection among homosexual men. AIDS 7:43–49, 1993.

Koenig C, Tavassoli FA. Nodular hyperplasia, adenoma, and adenomyoma of Bartholin's gland. Int J Gynecol Pathol 17:289–294, 1998.

Koss LG. Tumors of the Urinary Bladder. Atlas of Tumor Pathology, Second Series, Fascicle 11). Washington DC, Armed Forces Institute of Pathology, 1975, 1985 (Supplement).

Koss LG, Brockunier AJ. Ultrastructural aspects of Paget's disease of the vulva. Arch Pathol 87:592–600, 1969.

Koss LG, Ladinsky S, Brockunier A. Paget's disease of the vulva. Report of 10 cases. Obstet Gynecol 31:513–525, 1968.

Koss LG, Melamed MR, Daniel WW. In situ epidermoid carcinoma of cervix and vagina following radiotherapy for cervical cancer. Cancer 14:353–360, 1961.

Kovi J, Tillman RL, Lee SM. Malignant transformation of condyloma acuminatum: A light microscopic and ultrastructural study. Am J Clin Pathol 61:702–710, 1974.

Kraus FT, Perez-Mesa C. Verrucous carcinoma: Clinical and pathologic study of 105 cases involving oral cavity larynx, and genitalia. Cancer 19:26–38, 1966.

Krebs HB. Treatment of vaginal intraepithelial neoplasia with laser and topical 5-fluorouracil. Obstet Gynecol 73:657–660, 1989.

Kurman RJ, Prabha AC. Thyroid and parathyroid glands in the vaginal wall: Report of a case. Am J Clin Pathol 59:503–507, 1973.

Kurman RJ, Scully RE. The incidence and histogenesis of vaginal adenosis: An autopsy study. Hum Pathol 5:265–276, 1974.

Lacey HB, Wilson GE, Tilston P, et al. A study of anal intraepithelial neoplasia in HIV positive homosexual men. Sex Transm Infect 75:172–177, 1999.

Lathrop JC, Ree HJ, McDuff HC Jr. Intraepithelial neoplasia of the neovagina. Obstet Gynecol 65:91S–94S, 1985.

Lavand'Homme P. Late carcinoma of the artificial vagina formed from the rectum. Brux Med 6:407–414, 1938.

Law CL, Thompson CH, Rose BR, Cossart YE. Anal intercourse: a risk factor for anal papillomavirus infection in women? Genitourin Med 67:464–468, 1991.

Lee RA, Symmonds RE. Recurrent carcinoma in situ of the vagina in patients previously treated for in situ carcinoma of the cervix. Obstet Gynecol 48:61–64, 1976.

Leiman G, Markowitz S, Veiga-Ferreira MM, Margolis KA. Renal adenocarcinoma presenting with bilateral metastases to Bartholin's glands: Primary diagnosis by aspiration cytology. Diagn Cytopathol 2:252–255, 1986.

Lin JI, Caracta PF, Ny CHG, et al. Malacoplakia of the vagina. South Med J 73:326–328, 1979.

Loening T, Riviere A, Henke RP, et al. Penile/anal condylomas and squamous cell cancer: A HPV DNA hybridization study. Virchows Arch [A] 413:491–498, 1988.

Logani S, Lu D, Quint WGV, et al. Low-grade vulvar and vaginal intraepithelial neoplasia: Correlation of histologic features with human papillomavirus DNA detection and MIB-1 immunostaining. Mod Pathol 16:735–741, 2003.

Lowhagen GB, Bergbrant IM, Bergstrom T, et al. PCR detection of Epstein-Barr virus, herpes simplex virus and human papillomavirus from the anal mucosa in HIV-seropositive and HIV-seronegative homosexual men. Int J STD AIDS 10:615–618, 1999.

Mabuchi K, Bross DS, Kessler II. Epidemiology of cancer of the vulva. A case-control study. Cancer 55:1843–1848, 1985.

Masukawa T, Friedrich EG Jr. Cytopathology of Paget's disease of the vulva: Diagnostic abrasive cytology. Acta Cytol 22:476–478, 1978.

May HC. Carcinoma in situ of vagina subsequent to hysterectomy for carcinoma in situ of cervix. Am J Obstet Gynecol 76:807–811, 1958.

Medak H, Burlakow P, McGrew EA, Tiecke R. The cytology of vesicular conditions affecting the oral mucosa: Pemphigus vulgaris. Acta Cytol 14:11–21, 1970.

Meisels A, Fortin R. Condylomatous lesions of the cervix and vagina. I. Cytologic patterns. Acta Cytol 20:505–509, 1976.

Melnick S, Cole P, Anderson D, Herbst A. Rates and risks of diethylstilbestrol-related clear-cell adenocarcinoma of the vagina and cervix. An update. N Engl J Med 316:514–516, 1987.

Merchant S, Murad TM, Dowling EA, Durant J. Diagnosis of vaginal carcinoma from cytologic material. Acta Cytol 18:494–503, 1974.

Mitsudo S, Nakanishi I, Koss LG. Paget's disease of the penis and adjacent skin. Its association with fatal sweat gland carcinoma. Arch Pathol Lab Med 105:518–520, 1981.

Montanari GD, Marconato A, Montanari GR, Grismondi GL. Granulation tissue on the vault of the vagina after hysterectomy for cancer: Diagnostic problems. Acta Cytol 12:25–29, 1968.

Moracci E, Berlingieri D. Hormonal evaluation of vaginal smears from artificial vagina. Acta Cytol 17:131–134, 1973.

Morley GW. Cancer of the vulva: A review. Cancer 48:597–601, 1981.

Moscicki AB, Hills NK, Shiboski S, et al. Risk factors for abnormal anal cytology in young heterosexual women. Cancer Epidemiol Biomarkers Prev 8:173–178, 1999.

Mossler JA, Woodard BH, Addison A, McCarty KS. Adenocarcinoma of Bartholin's gland. Arch Pathol Lab Med 104:523–526, 1980.

Mudhar HS, Smith JHF, Tidy J. Primary vaginal adenocarcinoma of intestinal type arising from an adenoma: Case report and review of the literature. Int J Gynecol Pathol 20:204–209, 2001.

Murad TM, Durant JR, Maddox WA, Dowling EA. The pathologic behavior of primary vaginal carcinoma and its relationship to cervical cancer. Cancer 35:787–794, 1975.

Nakao CY, Nolan JF, DiSaia PJ, et al. Microinvasive epidermoid carcinoma of the vulva with an unexpected natural history. Am J Obstet Gynecol 120:1122–1123, 1974.

Nauth HF. Vulva-Zytologie. Lehrbuch und Atlas. Stuttgart, Georg-Thieme Verlag, 1986.

Norris HJ, Bagley GP, Taylor HB. Carcinoma of the infant vagina. Arch Pathol 90:473–479, 1970.

Okagaki T, Clark BA, Zachow KR, et al. Presence of human papillomavirus in verrucous carcinoma (Ackerman) of the vagina. Arch Pathol Lab Med 108:567–570, 1984.

Oriel JD. Genital and anal papillomavirus infections in human males. In Syrjanen K, Gissmann L, Koss LG (eds). Papillomaviruses and Human Disease. Berlin-Heidelberg-New York, Springer Verlag, 1987, pp 182–196.

Orr JW Jr, Schingleton HM, Gore H, et al. Cervical intraepithelial neoplasia associated with exposure to diethylstilbestrol in utero: A clinical and pathologic study. Obstet Gynecol 58:75–82, 1981.

Palefsky JM. Anal squamous intraepithelial lesions: relation to HIV and human papillomavirus infection. J Acquir Immune Defic Syndr 21:S42–S48, 1999.

Palefsky JM, Gonzales J, Greenblatt RM, et al. Anal intraepithelial neoplasia and anal papillomavirus infection among homosexual males with group IV HIV disease. JAMA 263:2911–2916, 1990.

Palefsky JM, Holly EA, Hogeboom CJ, et al. Anal cytology as a screening tool for anal squamous intraepithelial lesions. J Acquir Immune Defic Syndr Hum Retrovirol 14:415–422, 1997.

Palefsky JM, Holly EA, Hogeboom CJ, et al. Virologic, immunologic, and clinical parameters in the incidence and progression of anal squamous intraepithelial lesions in HIV-positive and HIV-negative homosexual men. J Acquir Immune Defic Syndr Hum Retrovirol 17:314–319, 1998.

Palefsky JM, Holly EA, Ralston ML, et al. Anal cytological abnormalities and anal HPV infection in men with Centers for Disease Control group IV HIV disease. Genitourin Med 73:174–180, 1997.

Palefsky JM, Holly EA, Ralston ML, et al. Anal squamous intraepithelial lesions in HIV-positive and HIV-negative homosexual and bisexual men: prevalence and risk factors. J Acquir Immune Defic Syndr Hum Retrovirol 17:320–326, 1998.

Palefsky JM, Holly EA, Ralston ML, et al. High incidence of anal high-grade squamous intra-epithelial lesions among HIV-positive and HIV-negative homosexual and bisexual men. AIDS 12:495–503, 1998.

Palefsky JM, Shiboski S, Moss A. Risk factors for anal human papillomavirus infection and anal cytologic abnormalities in HIV-positive and HIV-negative homosexual men. J Acquir Immune Defic Syndr 7:599–606, 1994.

Paquin ML, Davis JR, Weiner S. Malacoplakia of Bartholin's gland. Arch Pathol Lab Med 110:757–758, 1986.

Parmley TH, Woodruff JD, Julian CG. Invasive vulvar Paget's disease. Obstet Gynecol 46:341–346, 1975.

Partridge EE, Murad T, Shingleton HM, et al. Verrucous lesions of the female genitalia. I. Giant condylomata. Am J Obstet Gynecol 137:412–418, 1980.

Partridge EE, Murad T, Shingleton HM, et al. Verrucous lesions of the female genitalia. II. Verrucous carcinoma. Am J Obstet Gynecol 137:419–424, 1980.

Penn I. Cancers of the anogenital region in renal transplant recipients: Analysis of 65 cases. Cancer 58:611–616, 1986.

Peters WA, Kumar NB, Morley GW. Microinvasive carcinoma of the vagina: A distinct clinical entity? Am J Obstet Gynecol 153:505–507, 1985.

Pilotti S, Della Torre G, Rilke F, et al. Immunohistochemical and ultrastructural evidence of papilloma virus infection associated with in situ and microinvasive squamous cell carcinoma of the vulva. Am J Surg Pathol 8:751–761, 1984.

Powell JL, Franklin EW III, Nickerson JF, Burell MO. Verrucous carcinoma of the female genital tract. Gynecol Oncol 6:565–573, 1978.

Prasad KR, Kumari GS, Arcuna CA, et al. Fibroadenoma of ectopic breast tissue in the vulva. A case report (published erratum appears in Acta Cytol 40:146, 1996). Acta Cytol 39:791–792, 1995.

Raju RR, Goldblum JR, Hart WR. Pagetoid squamous cell carcinoma in situ (Pagetoid Bowen's disease) of the external genitalia. Int J Gynecol Pathol 22:127–135, 2003.

Ramzy I, Smout MS, Collins JA. Verrucous carcinoma of the vagina. Am J Clin Pathol 65:644–653, 1976.

Ridley CM, Frankman O, Jones ISC, et al. New nomenclature for vulvar disease: International Society for Study of Vulvar Disease. Hum Pathol 20:495–496, 1989.

Ritchi RN. Primary carcinoma of the vagina following a Baldwin reconstruction for congenital absence of the vagina. Am J Obstet Gynecol 18:794–796, 1929.

Robboy SJ, Friedlander LM, Welch WR, et al. Cytology of 575 young women with prenatal exposure to diethylstilbestrol. Obstet Gynecol 48:511–515, 1976.

Robboy SJ, Herbst AL, Scully RE. Clear cell adenocarcinoma of the vagina and cervix in young females. Analysis of 37 tumors that persisted or recurred after primary therapy. Cancer 34:606–614, 1974.

Robboy SJ, Hill EC, Sandberg EC, Czernobilsky B. Vaginal adenosis in women born prior to the diethylstilbestrol era. Hum Pathol 17:488–492, 1986.

Robboy SJ, Noller KL, O'Brien P, et al. Increased incidence of cervical and vaginal dysplasia in 3,980 diethylstilbestrol-exposed young women. JAMA 252:2979–2983, 1984.

Robboy SJ, Welch WR, Young RH, et al. Topographic relation of cervical ectropion and vaginal adenosis to clear cell adenocarcinoma. Obstet Gynecol 60:546–551, 1982.

Robboy SJ, Young RH, Welch WR, et al. Atypical vaginal adenosis and cervical ectropion. Cancer 54:869–875, 1984.

Rose PG, Roman LD, Reale FR, et al. Primary adenocarcinoma of the breast arising in the vulva. Obstet Gynecol 76:537–539, 1990.

Rotmensch J, Rosenshein N, Dillon M, et al. Carcinoma arising in neovagina: case report and review of the literature. Obstet Gynecol 61:534–536, 1983.

Rutledge F. Cancer of the vagina. Am J Obstet Gynecol 97:635–655, 1967.

Ryan DP, Compton CC, Mayer RJ. Carcinoma of the anal canal. N Engl J Med 342:792–800, 2000.

Sagerman PM, Choi YJ, Hu Y, Niedt GW. Human papilloma virus, vulvar dystrophy, and vulvar carcinoma: differential expression of human papillomavirus and vulvar dystrophy in the presence and absence of squamous cell carcinoma of the vulva. Gynecol Oncol 61:328–332, 1996.

Schneider A, de Villiers E-M, Schneider V. Multifocal squamous neoplasia of the female genital tract: Significance of human papillomavirus infection of the vagina after hysterectomy. Obstet Gynecol 70:294–298, 1987.

Scholefield JH, Johnson J, Hitchcock A, et al. Guidelines for anal cytology: To make cytological diagnosis and follow up much more reliable. Cytopathol 9:15–22, 1998.

Sedlacek TV, Riva JM, Magen AB, et al. Vaginal and vulvar adenosis: an unexpected side effect of CO2 laser vaporisation. J Reprod Med 35:995–1001, 1990.

Serraino D, Carrieri P, Pradier C, et al. Risk of invasive cervical cancer among women with, or at risk for, HIV infection. Int J Cancer 82:334–337, 1999.

Sharkey FE, Clark RL, Gray GF. Perianal Paget's disease: Report of 2 cases. Dis Colon Rectum 18:245–248, 1975.

Sherman ME, Paull G. Vaginal intraepithelial neoplasia. Reproducibility of pathologic diagnosis and correlation of smears and biopsies. Acta Cytol 37: 699–704, 1993.

Sherman ME, Friedman HB, Busseniers AE, et al. Cytologic diagnosis of anal intraepithelial neoplasia using smears and Cytyc ThinPreps. Mod Pathol 8: 270–274, 1995.

Sillman FH, Sentovich S, Shaffer D. Ano-genital neoplasia in renal transplant patients. Ann Transplant 2:59–66, 1997.

Sonek M, Bibbo M, Wied GL. Colposcopic findings in offspring of DES-treated mothers as related to onset of therapy. J Reprod Med 16:65–71, 1976.

Sonnex C, Scholefield JH, Kocjan G, et al. Anal human papillomavirus infection: a comparative study of cytology, colposcopy and DNA hybridisation as methods of detection. Genitourin Med 67:21–25, 1991.

Spitzer M, Molho L, Seltzer VL, Lipper S. Vaginal glomus tumor: Case presentation and ultrastructural findings. Obstet Gynecol 66:86–88, 1985.

Stafl A, Mattingly RF, Roley DV, Fetherston WC. Clinical diagnosis of vaginal adenosis. Obstet Gynecol 43:118–128, 1974.

Strand CL, Windhager HA, Kim EH, Chiranand N. Prompt regression of cystic vaginal adenosis following cessation of oral contraceptive therapy. Am J Clin Pathol 64:483–487, 1975.

Sturgeon SR, Brinton LA, Devesa SS, et al. In situ and invasive vulvar cancer incidence trends (1973 to 1987). Am J Obstet Gynecol 166:1482–1485, 1992.

Surawicz CM, Crtichlow C, Sayer J, et al. High grade anal dysplasia in visually normal mucosa in homosexual men: seven cases. Am J Gastroenterol 90: 1776–1778, 1995.

Syrjänen KJ. Human papillomavirus (HPV) lesions of the vulva: Histopathology. In Patologia Benigna E Maligna Della Vulva, Edizioni Internazionali, pp 39–47, 1988.

Taft PD, Robboy SJ, Herbst AL, Scully RE. Cytology of clear-cell adenocarcinoma of genital tract in young females: Review of 95 cases from the Registry. Acta Cytol 18:279–290, 1974.

Tambouret R, Pitman MB, Bell DA. Benign glandular cells in posthysterectomy vaginal smears. Acta Cytol 42:1403–1408, 1998.

Toki T, Kurman RJ, Park JS, et al. Probable nonpapillomavirus etiology of squamous cell carcinoma of the vulva in older women: A clinicopathologic

study using in situ hybridization and polymerase chain reaction. Int J Gynecol Pathol 10:107–125, 1991.

Tsukada Y, Lopez RG, Pickren JW, et al. Paget's disease of the vulva: A clinicopathologic study of eight cases. Obstet Gynecol 45:73–78, 1975.

Tyring SK, Arany I, Stanley MA, et al. A randomized, controlled, molecular study of condylomata acuminata clearance during treatment with imiquimod. J Infect Dis 178:551–555, 1998.

Ulbright TM, Alexander RW, Kraus FT. Intramural papilloma of the vagina. Cancer 48:2260–2266, 1981.

Ulfelder H. Stilbestrol, adenosis, and adenocarcinoma. Am J Obstet Gynecol 117:794–800, 1973.

Underwood PB, Smith RT. Carcinoma of the vagina. JAMA 217:46–52, 1971.

Vallejos H, Del Mistro A, Kleinhaus S, et al. Characterization of human papillomavirus types in condylomata acuminata in children by in situ hybridization. Lab Invest 56:611–615, 1987.

Van Hoeven KH, Randleman GA, Artymyshyn RL. Cytologic findings in lichen sclerosus. Acta Cytol 41:474–480, 1997.

Van Nagell JR Jr, Tweeddale DN, Roddick JW Jr. Primary adenoacanthoma of the Bartholin gland: Report of a case. Obstet Gynecol 34:87–90, 1969.

Vandrie DM, Puri S, Upton RT, Demeester LJ. Adenosquamous carcinoma of the cervix in a woman exposed to diethylstilbestrol in utero. Obstet Gynecol 61:84S–87S, 1983.

Venuti A, Marcante ML. Presence of human papillomavirus type 18 in vulvar carcinomas and its integration into the cell genome. J Gen Virol 70: 1587–1592, 1989.

Veridiano NP, Weiner EA, Tancer ML. Squamous cell carcinoma of the vagina associated with vaginal adenosis. Obstet Gynecol 47:689–692, 1976.

Virgili A, Marzola A, Corazza M. Vulvar hidradenoma papilliferum. A review of 10.5 years' experience. J Reprod Med 45:616–618, 2000.

Wade TR, Kopf AW, Ackerman AB. Bowenoid papulosis of the penis. Cancer 42:1890–1903, 1978.

Wade TR, Kopf AW, Ackerman AB. Bowenoid papulosis of the genitalia. Arch Dermatol 115:306–308, 1979.

Ward KA, Houston JR, Lowry BE, et al. The role of early colposcopy in the management of females with first episode anogenital warts. Int J STD AIDS 5:343–345, 1994.

Webb JB, Lott M, O'Sullivan JC, Azzopardi JG. Combined adenoid cystic and squamous carcinoma of Bartholin's gland. Br J Obstet Gynaecol 91: 291–295, 1984.

Webb MJ, Symmonds RE, Weiland LH. Malignant fibrous histiocytoma of the vagina. Am J Obstet Gynecol 119:190–192, 1974.

Wharton JT, Gallager S, Rutledge FN. Microinvasive carcinoma of the vulva. Am J Obstet Gynecol 118:159–162, 1974.

Wied GL. Interpretation of inflammatory reactions in vagina, cervix, and endocervix by means of cytologic smears. Am Clin Pathol 28:233–242, 1957.

Wilbur DC, Maurer S, Smith NJ. Behçet's disease in a vaginal smear. Report of acase with cytologic features and their distinction from squamous cell carcinoma. Acta Cytol 37:525–530, 1993.

Wilkinson EJ, Brown HM. Vulvar Paget's disease of urothelial origin: A report of three cases and a proposed classification of vulvar Paget disease. Hum Pathol 33:549–554, 2002.

Williams SL, Rogers LW, Quan HQ. Perianal Paget's disease: Report of seven cases. Dis Colon Rectum 19:30–40, 1976.

Woodruff H, Dockerty MB, Wilson RB, Pratt JH. Papillary hidradenoma of the vulva: A clinicopathologic study of 69 cases. Am J Obstet Gynecol 110: 501–508, 1971.

Woodruff JD, Baens JS. Interpretation of atrophic and hypertrophic alterations in the vulva epithelium. Am J Obstet Gynecol 86:713–723, 1963.

Xi LF, Critchlow CW, Wheeler CM, et al. Risk of anal carcinoma in situ in relation to human papillomavirus type 16 variants. Cancer Res 58: 3839–3844, 1998.

Yoonessi M, Goodell T, Satchidanand S, et al. Microinvasive squamous carcinoma of the vulva. J Surg Oncol 24:315–321, 1983.

Young AW Jr, Herman EW, Tovell HMM. Syringoma of the vulva: Incidence, diagnosis, and cause of pruritus. Obstet Gynecol 55:515–518, 1980.

Zaleski S, Setum C, Benda J. Cytologic presentation of alveolar soft-part sarcoma of the vagina. Acta Cytol 30:665–670, 1986.

Tumors of the Ovary and Fallopian Tube

15

THE OVARY

HISTOLOGIC RECALL

The anatomy of the ovaries was discussed in Chapter 8. Because components of the normal ovary may be observed in cytologic preparations, a brief summary of the histology is provided (Fig. 15-1).

The central portion of the ovaries is formed by the **hilum,** the site of entry of the vascular supply and lymphatic drainage. The **hilum** also contains **clusters of large endocrine cells with eosinophilic, granular cytoplasm,** similar to **Leydig cells** of the testis, that may contain rod-like Reinke's crystalloids. The ovary is surrounded by a **surface or germinative epithelium.** The bulk of the ovary is formed by **ovarian stroma.**

The surface epithelium, which is closely related to the mesothelium, is composed of a single layer of cuboidal cells with scanty basophilic cytoplasm and spherical nuclei. The surface epithelium often forms invaginations into the cortex of the ovary or **small cysts.** It should be noted that cortical cysts may be mistaken for ovarian follicles on ultrasound examination and may be incidentally aspirated during the harvest of ova for in vitro fertilization.

The **ovarian stroma** is composed of small spindly cells, some of which are capable of endocrine function. The superficial part of the ovarian stroma, **the cortex,** contains **ova** in various stages of maturation. The **ova,** numerous at birth, are reduced in number in the mature ovary and reside in the cortical stroma, where each ovum is surrounded by a single layer of epithelial cells, forming a **primitive follicle.** The maturation of the ova begins at puberty. Under the impact of **pituitary follicle-stimulating hormone (FSH),** a few select follicles begin to enlarge. It is not known how and why the selection is taking place. The epithelial cells surrounding the ovum begin to multiply, become larger and multilayered, and are named **granulosa cells.** The ovum is separated from the granulosa cells by a homogeneous membrane, known as the **zona pellucida.** As the maturation of the ovum progresses, the number of cell layers of the granulosa increase. At the same time stromal cells surrounding the ovum become larger and, named **theca cells,** form a multilayered envelope around the follicle. The **granulosa and theca cells secrete estrogens** that induce the proliferative phase in the endometrium (see Chap. 13). As the follicle matures and enlarges, the granulosa cells form a cavity filled with a hormone-rich fluid. The ovum, still surrounded by granulosa cells, now protrudes into the follicular cavity;

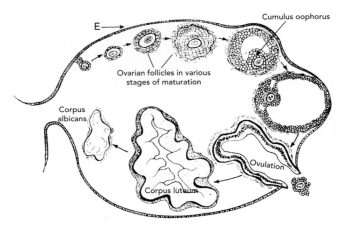

Figure 15-1 Schematic representation of events in ovulation (indicated in *arrows*) from a primitive follicle to formation of corpus albicans (see text). E, epithelium.

the protrusion is named **cumulus oophorus** (Fig. 15-2A). At this point, the follicle is named after the Dutch anatomist who first described it in the 17th century, a follicle of **De Graaf or Graafian follicle.** The graafian follicles are now visible on the surface of the ovary as small protrusions, but **normally only one of them will spontaneously rupture and discharge the mature ovum together with the follicular fluid into the peritoneal cavity,** followed by bleeding into the cavity of the follicle. Again, it is not known how and why the single follicle is selected. The ovulation takes place under the impact of **pituitary luteinizing hormone (LH),** that also causes enlargement of the granulosa cells that converts the collapsed follicle into a **large, grossly visible yellow structure, the corpus luteum, that secretes progesterone,** thus inducing the secretory phase of the endometrium (Fig. 15-2B). The yellow color of the corpus luteum is due to a high lipid content of the hormone-producing component cells. The discharged ovum is captured by the fimbria of the fallopian tube, pending fertilization by a spermatozoon in the lumen of the tube. Unless pregnancy intervenes, the corpus luteum undergoes atrophy and

fibrosis, resulting in a small **white scar [corpus albicans or (plural) corpora albicantia]** within the cortex of the ovary. If pregnancy occurs, the corpus luteum persists, becomes larger, and is known as **corpus luteum of pregnancy.**

METHODS OF INVESTIGATION

Cervicovaginal Preparations

In the study of the ovary, cervicovaginal preparations may serve two purposes:

- They may contribute to the **diagnosis of ovarian tumors that shed recognizable cancer cells.**
- They allow an assessment of the **hormonal status of women,** bearers of estrogen-producing tumors. **This method occasionally contributes to the recognition of primary or recurrent tumors, particularly of granulosa cell tumors.**

Endometrial Aspirations

Occasionally ovarian tumors may be recognized in material aspirated from the endometrium. The techniques were described in Chapter 13.

Transvaginal Aspiration for In Vitro Fertilization

In vitro fertilization requires harvesting ova that are exposed to spermatozoa in vitro and then re-implanted into the suitably primed uterus. The ovary is stimulated by hormonal treatment to achieve maturation of several ova at the same time. The viable ova are harvested by ultrasound-guided transvaginal needle aspirates of maturing Graafian follicles (Fig. 15-3). **Cytologic examination of the aspirated material is not warranted unless the aspirated fluid is discolored or the amount is larger than the normal 2 to 3 ml** (Greenebaum et al, 1992; Yee et al, 1994). When this occurs, it is assumed that either the aspirated follicle contained a blighted ovum or that a small cortical ovarian cyst has

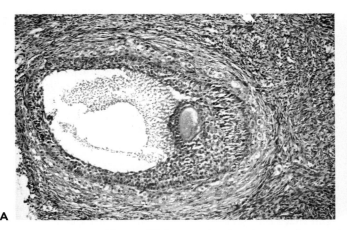

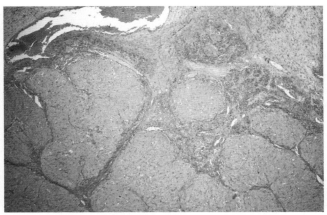

Figure 15-2 Graafian follicle (*A*) and corpus luteum (*B*). *A.* The follicle, lined by granulosa cells, contains fluid rich in estrogens. The ovum, still surrounded by a few layers of granulosa cells, protrudes into the follicle (**cumulus oophorus**). The granulosa cells are surrounded by layers of modified stromal cells, the **theca cells.** *B.* Corpus luteum composed of clusters of modified granulosa cells, secreting progesterone.

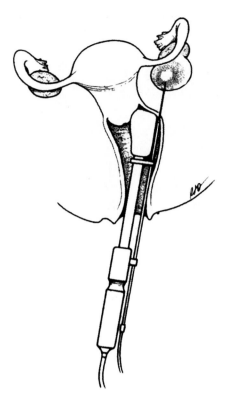

Figure 15-3 Ovarian puncture device. Automated, spring-loaded puncture device, with a 21-gauge needle attached, used to aspirate ovarian cysts under ultrasound guidance. (Drawing courtesy of Dr. Ellen Greenebaum, Columbia University College of Physicians and Surgeons, New York, NY.)

been aspirated. **The main purpose of the cytologic examination is to identify benign or malignant cells in cysts, masquerading as follicles. It should be stressed that malignant tumors diagnosed during harvesting of ova are vanishingly rare** (Greenebaum et al, 1992; Rubenchik et al, 1996).

Aspiration Biopsy (FNA)

The purpose of direct ovarian aspiration is identification of the nature of cystic and solid tumors. The procedure can be performed **transvaginally** under ultrasound guidance or during **peritoneoscopy.** The general principles of the fine needle-syringe aspiration technique, or FNA, are discussed in Chapter 28. Initially, ovarian aspirates were performed using equipment devised for aspiration of the prostate (see Chap. 33 and Fig. 33-1). Currently, a **spring-loaded puncture device** with a 21-gauge needle attached to a collection trap is used for transvaginal aspirations (Fig. 15-3). For aspirations performed during peritoneoscopy, a small caliber needle attached to a syringe may suffice. With the progress in imaging, it is now possible to determine in advance whether the ovarian lesion is cystic or solid, or a combination of both.

The use of the aspiration technique for the diagnosis of malignant tumors of the ovary is highly controversial because of the danger of rupturing the capsule of a cancer, whether cystic or solid, and consequent spillage of malig-

nant cells into the peritoneal cavity. The pros and contras of this technique have been well summarized by Greenebaum (1996). The advantages are a possible early diagnosis of ovarian tumors and avoidance of surgical procedures for benign cysts. De Crespigny et al (1989) and Greenebaum (1996) recommended that direct aspiration be limited to cystic lesions less than 10 cm in diameter without thick septa or solid areas on ultrasound imaging.

CYTOLOGY OF NORMAL OVARY

The normal cells that may be recognized in follicular aspirates obtained for purposes of in vitro fertilization are: **granulosa cells, theca cells, and ova.**

Granulosa Cells

Granulosa cells may be harvested from follicular cysts either before or after transformation into cells of corpus luteum **(luteinization).** The **nonluteinized granulosa cells** appear singly or in small, sometimes spherical (papillary) clusters, have a scanty eosinophilic cytoplasm and oval or bean-shaped nuclei that may show nuclear grooves (Fig. 15-4A). Mitoses may be observed. The nuclei are sometimes surprisingly large and hyperchromatic. There is usually a background of a few inflammatory cells, small macrophages, and debris. **Luteinized granulosa cells** are larger because of a more abundant, granular cytoplasm. The nuclei are sometimes in an eccentric position and are similar to nuclei of nonluteinized cells, except for the presence of visible chromocenters or small nucleoli (Fig. 15-4B) (Greenebaum, 1996; Selvaggi, 1996). **Smears with atypical granulosa cells may sometimes suggest a malignant tumor.** The nuclei of such cells may be enlarged and granular, with larger nucleoli and may present a difficult problem of differential diagnosis. Selvaggi (1991) also stressed that the granulosa cell lining of some of the follicular cysts may be atypical and difficult to interpret. **Knowledge of clinical and ultrasonographic data is important in preventing diagnostic errors. Caution is advised before the diagnosis of a malignant tumor is made in such samples.** In a few such follicles, excised for verification of atypical cytologic findings, only benign ovarian structures were observed (Dr. Ellen Greenebaum, personal communication, 2003).

Theca Cells

The theca cells have not been identified with certainty. Greenebaum et al (1992) assumed that some of the smaller granulosa cells may represent luteinized theca cells. Selvaggi (1996) does not mention their existence in routine aspirates.

See Chapter 8 for comments on, and illustrations of, ova.

OVARIAN TUMORS

In spite of their modest size, the ovaries are the site of benign proliferative processes and of malignant tumors of a bewildering variety of histologic patterns, clinical behavior, and

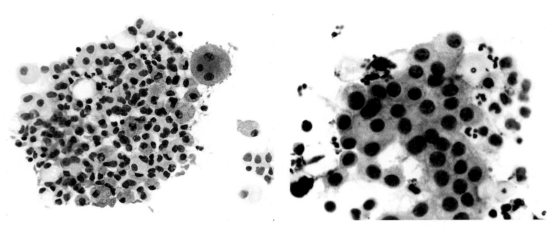

A   **B**

Figure 15-4 **Luteinized and nonluteinized granulosa cells.** *A.* Granulosa cells, one of which with three nuclei, are enlarged and luteinized. The cytoplasm contains pigment of unknown nature. *B.* A sheet of luteinized granulosa cells at high magnification. Note the abundant cytoplasm, dark nuclei, and general similarity to small hepatocytes. (Both photographs courtesy of Dr. Ellen Greenebaum, Columbia University College of Physicians and Surgeons, New York, NY.)

significance. A description and discussion of all of these is beyond the scope of this work, and readers are referred to the authoritative reviews of this subject (Cannistra, 1993; Scully et al, 1998). Only tumors and tumorous conditions that have a cytologic correlation will be discussed here.

Tumors of the ovary are classified, on the basis of their origin, into several groups, listed in Table 15-1. From the point of view of diagnostic cytology, the most important

are **cysts, malignant epithelial tumors** and **tumors with hormonal activity** (granulosa and theca cell tumors).

Benign Ovarian Cysts

Benign ovarian cysts are by far the most common tumors of the ovaries. Besides follicular cysts resulting from events in ovulation, described above, benign cystic lesions of the

TABLE 15-1

SIMPLIFIED CLASSIFICATION OF OVARIAN TUMORS

| Tissue of origin | Epithelial tumors | |
	Benign	Malignant
Germinative epithelium and its variants	Serous cysts (cystomas)	Serous carcinomas, Borderline (low malignant potential) serous tumors, Psammocarcinoma
	Mucous cysts (cystomas)	Mucous carcinomas, Borderline tumors
	Endometriosis Endometriotic cyst	Endometrioid carcinomas
	Brenner tumor	Malignant Brenner tumor, Clear cell (mesonephric) carcinomas Rare types of carcinomas
Granulosa-stroma cells		Granulosa cell tumor
Theca-stroma cells	Thecoma	Malignant variant extremely rare
Sertoli and Leydig cells (ovarian equivalent)	Hilar cell tumor	Sertoli-Leydig cell tumors (masculinizing)
Germ cells and embryonal structures	Benign teratoma (Dermoid cysts)	Malignant tumors derived from teratomas (carcinomas, carcinoid). Also dysgerminoma, Gonadoblastoma, Endodermal sinus tumor, Yolk sac tumor (Embryonal carcinoma)
Gestational trophoblasts		Choriocarcinoma
Very rare tumors	See Chapter 17	

ovary include **small cortical cysts,** caused by invagination of the surface epithelium, **corpus luteum cysts, cysts occurring in endometriosis, and serous or mucinous cysts (cystomas).** The serous and mucinous cystomas may be monolocular or multilocular and may vary in size from tiny cysts, measuring a few millimeters in diameter, to very large cysts up to 20 or even more centimeters in diameter. **Corpus luteum cysts** are formed because of bleeding into the center of the corpus luteum. The **cortical inclusion cysts, serous cysts, and paraovarian cysts** are lined by small cuboidal cells, similar to the cells of ovarian epithelium (Fig. 15-5B). The **mucinous cysts** are lined by tall, columnar, mucus-secreting cells, akin to those lining the endocervical canal. Occasionally, both types of epithelia may be found side by side. **Endometriotic cysts** are usually formed by bleeding occurring in foci of endometriosis and usually contain liquefied blood and hemosiderin-laden macrophages in their center. Endometrial glands, sometimes accompanied by scanty endometrial stroma and hemosiderin-laden macrophages, are found in the wall of the cyst.

Cytology

Most fluids aspirated from benign ovarian cysts are **acellular,** as confirmed by Mulvany (1996). The type of such cysts may be sometimes determined by biochemical studies of the aspirated fluid (see below). The cytologic evidence of cyst type is usually scanty and the precise type of cysts cannot always be determined. The description below is based on relatively few cases of benign cysts with diagnostic cellular features.

Cortical Inclusion Cysts and Ovarian or Paraovarian Serous Cysts

These cysts may shed sheets of small, cuboidal cells with scanty cytoplasm and spherical, granular nuclei (Fig. 15-5A–C). **Ciliated epithelial cells** and ciliated cell fragments **(ciliated bodies),** are sometimes observed. Rivasi et al (1993) observed such cells in nearly 10% of aspirates from 320 ovarian cysts. Calcified debris or psammoma bodies may be present. For an extensive discussion of psammoma bodies, see below.

Greenebaum (1994) reported a case of a benign serous cyst with isolated, markedly atypical lining cells with large nuclei and a nondiploid DNA histogram. Occasionally the cyst fluid contains numerous macrophages (Fig. 15-5D).

Corpus Luteum Cysts

The aspirates from **corpus luteum cysts** may contain old, liquefied blood and foam cells (macrophages) and may be

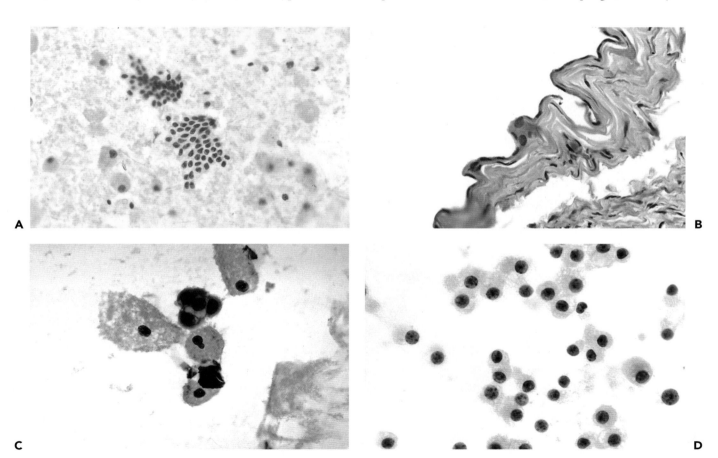

Figure 15-5 Ovarian cyst aspirates. A. aspirate from a simple serous cyst showing orderly clusters of small cuboidal cells in the background of squamous cells. B. Histologic section of the ovarian cyst represented in A. C. Aspirate of a paraovarian cyst in a 24-year-old woman. The smear shows squamous cells and small cuboidal cells assumed to be benign epithelial cyst lining. D. Aspirate of benign ovarian cyst in a young woman. The field shows monotonous macrophages. (A,B courtesy of Dr. Ellen Greenebaum, Columbia University College of Physicians and Surgeons, New York, NY; D courtesy of Dr. M. Zaman, New York Medical College, Valhalla, NY.)

difficult to distinguish from the contents of an endometriotic cyst (see below). The aspirates may also contain **large, luteinized granulosa cells**. As has been noted above, such cells may be quite atypical because of large nuclei and nucleoli and may be confused with cancer cells. In a case reported by Burke et al (1997), the corpus luteum cyst occurred in an **ovarian remnant** after total abdominal hysterectomy and oophorectomy; the luteinized cells were mistaken for cancer cells.

Cysts of Unknown Derivation

In a personally observed case, the fluid from a benign cyst in a 17-year-old patient contained cells and cell clusters closely **resembling normal urothelium,** particularly multinucleated large cells resembling the superficial urothelial umbrella cells (Fig. 15-6A,B). It is possible, although unproven, that this cyst was related to a Brenner tumor (see below). The cyst also contained crystalline structures of unknown significance (Fig. 15-6C).

Mucinous Cysts

These may be occasionally recognized because of the presence of columnar, mucus-containing cells with small, basally located nuclei, similar to endocervical cells. The differential diagnosis between a benign mucinous cyst and a mucinous carcinoma (see below) may be impossible on cytologic evidence alone.

Endometriosis of the Ovary

Endometriosis is characterized by the presence of old, liquefied blood, **hemosiderin-containing macrophages,** and clusters of poorly preserved cuboidal epithelial cells of endometrial type. Endometrial stromal cells are very rarely seen.

Biochemical Studies of Fluids From Ovarian Cysts

Biochemical studies of acellular or cellular fluids aspirated from ovarian cysts may sometimes provide additional information on the nature of the cysts. Thus, estradiol-17β is elevated in follicle cysts but not in other cysts (Geier and Strecker, 1981; Mulvany et al, 1995, 1996; Greenebaum,

1996). The antibody to the antigen CA125 may be elevated in a variety of benign and malignant lesions of the ovary. Carcinoembryonic antigen (CEA) may be elevated in mucinous ovarian tumors and in metastatic carcinomas of colonic origin (Pinto et al, 1990).

Endosalpingiosis

Strictly speaking, endosalpingiosis **is not an ovarian disease.** It is described here because of its **important role in the diagnosis and differential diagnosis of ovarian tumors.**

Endosalpingiosis, a term first suggested by Sampson (1930), is defined as the **presence of multiple glandular cystic inclusions on the surface of the ovary, fallopian tubes, uterine serosa, and elsewhere in the pelvic peritoneum, omentum and even in pelvic lymph nodes.** Clement and Young (1999) described a rare form of **endosalpingiosis with tumor-like masses,** involving the uterus and rectum.

The cysts are lined by cuboidal or columnar epithelial cells, some of which are ciliated. Contrary to endometriosis, the cysts show no evidence of bleeding. Endometrial stromal cells are absent. The most important aspect of endosalpingiosis is the presence within the cysts of **numerous,** concentrically calcified, approximately spherical structures, known as **psammoma bodies** (Fig. 15-7). **In the presence of pelvic endosalpingiosis, psammoma bodies may also be observed in the endometrium and the endocervix.** It is not clear whether this phenomenon represents a transfer of psammoma bodies from the pelvic peritoneum to the uterus or represents "burned-out" foci of endosalpingiosis in this location. **In such cases, psammoma bodies may be observed in cervicovaginal samples.**

In the absence of an ovarian tumor, endosalpingiosis is a benign disorder; in the presence of an ovarian tumor, the possibility of metastases must be ruled out. For example, in 16 cases of endosalpingiosis, described by Zinsser and Wheeler (1982), there were four ovarian tumors that could have been a source of metastases. The significance of psammoma bodies in cytologic material is discussed below in reference to ovarian cancer and, in Chapter 16, to peritoneal

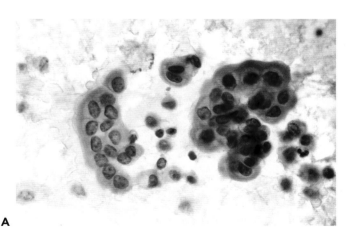

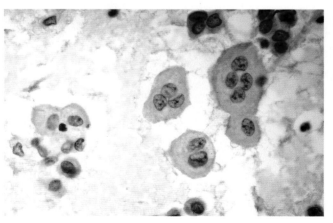

A

B

Figure 15-6 **Ovarian cyst in a 17-year-old woman with lining suggestive of urothelial origin.** *A.* Several clusters of fairly large epithelial cells with one flat surface. *B.* Multinucleated epithelial cells, closely resembling umbrella cells of urothelial origin (see Chapter 22).

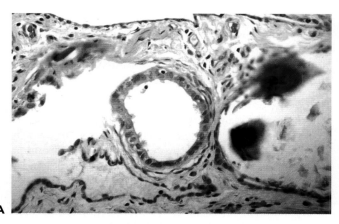
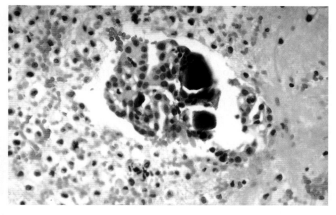

Figure 15-7   Endosalpingiosis. *A.* Cyst lined with ciliated cells and containing calcified psammoma bodies on the surface of the fallopian tube. *B.* Fragment of endometriotic cyst with psammoma bodies in peritoneal wash specimen.

lavage. It must be noted that **calcified deposits** resembling psammoma bodies may also occur as an isolated event in **fallopian tubes and the endometrium** (Fig. 15-8).

Primary Carcinomas

Epidemiology and Risk Factors

Cancer of the ovary is second only to carcinoma of the breast as cause of deaths among American women, with 23,100 new cases and 14,000 deaths projected for the year 2000 (Greenlee et al, 2000). The very high mortality from ovarian cancer reflects the dissemination of the tumor at the time of the diagnosis because of absence of symptoms in the early stages of the disease (Cannistra, 1993). The disease occurs mainly in women past the age of 40 with median age of 58 at the time of diagnosis. The overall 5-year survival rate is only 40% and is stage dependent. **Staging of ovarian carcinomas** is shown in Table 15-2. Stage I disease (confined to one ovary) offers a much higher survival rate than stage II to IV disease, the higher stages reflecting the degree of spread of cancer beyond the ovary of origin.

Various epidemiologic risk factors related to obstetrical, endocrine, and gynecologic events have been explored, none with conclusive results (Runnebaum and Stickeler, 2001). However, mutations in **breast cancer genes BRCA1 and BRCA2** constitute a **high risk factor** for familial ovarian carcinomas. The risk in women with BRCA1 mutations is the extraordinary 45% whereas for BRCA2 mutations, it is about 25% (summary in Runnebaum and Stickeler 2001). Ovarian cancers associated with BRCA1 mutation appear to have a more favorable clinical course when compared with sporadic cancers (Rubin et al, 1996). The presence of intratumoral T cells is apparently related to better survival (Zhang et al, 2003). It is of note that oral contraceptives may reduce the risk of ovarian cancer in these women (Narod et al, 1998).

Prophylactic salpingo-oophorectomy in women with BRCA1 or BRCA2 mutations repeatedly revealed small, occult ovarian cancers and other benign epithelial abnormalities (Salazar et al, 1996; Kauff et al, 2002; Stoler, 2002). Occult **carcinomas of the fallopian tubes and the peritoneum** also came to light in such studies. Agoff et al (2002) and Stoler (2002) emphasized the diagnostic value of peritoneal lavage in such patients (see Chap. 16).

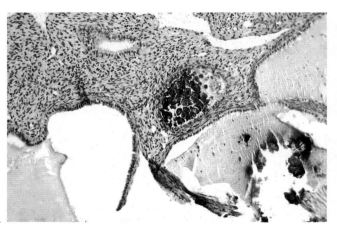
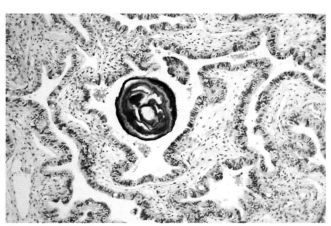

Figure 15-8   Psammoma bodies in normal organs of the female genital tract. *A.* In endometrium. *B.* In fallopian tube. The finding in *B* is sometimes described as salpingolith.

An added advantage of prophylactic salpingo-oophorectomy appears to be a reduction in breast cancer (Kauff et al, 2002).

Early detection of ovarian carcinoma may conceivably improve the prognostic outlook. The current status of efforts toward early detection of ovarian cancer are summarized at the end of this chapter.

Classification

As shown in Table 15-1, the principal groups of ovarian carcinomas are:

- Serous carcinomas
- Mucin-producing carcinomas
- Endometrioid carcinomas

All these tumors may be cystic, solid, or a combination of the two presentations. Not uncommonly, the tumors involve both ovaries simultaneously.

Histology

Serous Carcinomas

These tumors usually originate from ovarian cysts lined by markedly atypical cuboidal epithelium that often forms papillary projections. The gland-forming tumors may range from borderline types, of relatively low malignant potential, to highly malignant, nearly solid tumors capable of distant metastases (Figs. 15-9B,D and 15-10D). A characteristic feature of these tumors is the formation of **calcified psam-moma bodies** (calcospherites). Their diagnostic significance is discussed below. **Similar primary tumors may occur in the peritoneum** (see Chap. 26). A case of a peritoneal serous carcinoma in a patient with **BRCA1 gene mutation** was reported by Agoff et al (2002).

Borderline Serous Tumors

This is a well-differentiated variant of papillary serous adenocarcinoma, with orderly epithelium, resembling vaguely the histologic structure of the fallopian tube. Such tumors were previously classified as *endosalpingiomas* but today the preferred term is **"borderline serous tumors"** or serous tumors of **"low malignant potential"** (Fig. 15-11).

Separation of borderline serous tumors from serous carcinomas is the subject for a considerable debate (Scully et al, 1998; Prat, 1999). In general, the borderline tumors are composed of cysts and well-differentiated papillary structures lined by one or two layers of uniform cuboidal or columnar cells, that do not invade either the stroma of the tumor or the adjacent ovary. The prognosis of the tumor is usually very good with long-term survival of about 90%, although late recurrences may be observed.

A fairly common event in these tumors is the presence of **tumor deposits** or "implants" on the **serosal surfaces of adjacent organs,** the peritoneum and the omentum. The deposits are classified as either **invasive** or **noninvasive.** In the invasive deposits, there is obvious spread of the tumor cells to the adjacent fat or connective tissue. In the noninva-

---

TABLE 15-2

STAGING OF PRIMARY CARCINOMA OF THE OVARY (FIGO)*

Stage

I Growth limited to the ovaries
   Ia Growth limited to one ovary; no ascites; no tumor on the external surface; capsule intact
   Ib Growth limited to both ovaries; no ascites; no tumor on the external surfaces; capsules intact
   Ic† Tumor either stage Ia or Ib, but with (1) tumor on surface of one or both ovaries or (2) capsule(s) ruptured or (3) ascites present containing malignant cells or (4) positive peritoneal washings
II Growth involving one or both ovaries with pelvic extension
   IIa Extension and/or metastases to the uterus and/or tubes
   IIb Extension to other pelvic tissues
   IIc† Tumor either stage IIa or IIb, but with (1) tumor on surface of one or both ovaries or (2) capsule(s) ruptured or (3) ascites present containing malignant cells or (4) positive peritoneal washings
III Tumor involving one or both ovaries with peritoneal implants outside the pelvis and/or positive retroperitoneal or inguinal nodes (superficial liver metastasis equals stage III); tumor is limited to the true pelvis, but with histologically proven malignant extension to small bowel or omentum
   IIIa Tumor grossly limited to the true pelvis with negative nodes but with histologically confirmed microscopic seeding of abdominal peritoneal surfaces
   IIIb Tumor of one or both ovaries with histologically confirmed implants of abdominal peritoneal surfaces, none exceeding 2 cm in diameter; nodes are negative
   IIIc Abdominal implants > 2 cm in diameter and/or positive retroperitoneal or inguinal nodes
IV Growth involving one or both ovaries with distant metastases; if pleural effusion is present, there must be positive cytology to allot a case to stage IV (parenchymal liver metastasis equals stage IV)

* Based on findings at clinical examination and/or surgical exploration. The histology is to be considered in the staging, as is cytology as far as effusions are concerned. It is desirable that a biopsy be taken from suspicious areas outside of the pelvis.
† To evaluate the impact on prognosis of the different criteria for allotting cases to stage Ic or IIc, it would be of value to know: (1) if rupture of the capsule was (a) spontaneous or (b) caused by the surgeon, or (2) if the source of malignant cells detected was (a) peritoneal washings or (b) ascites. (From McGowan L. Peritoneal fluid washings [letter to editor]. Acta Cytol 33:414–415, 1989.)

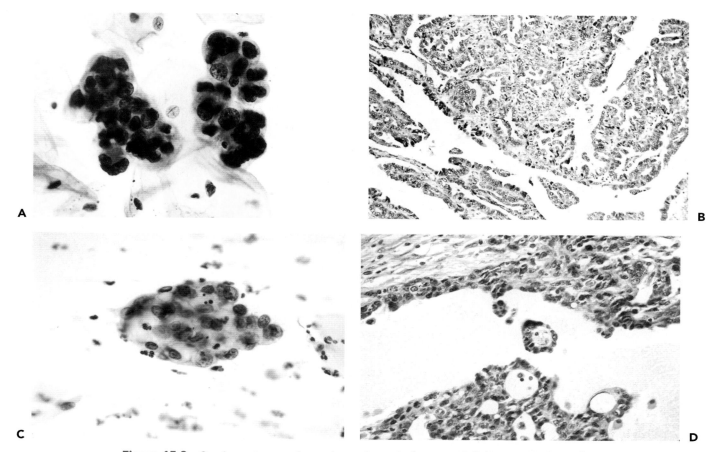

Figure 15-9   Ovarian serous carcinoma in cervicovaginal smears. *A,C.* large compact papillary clusters of tightly packed large malignant cells corresponding to the ovarian serous carcinomas shown in *B* and *D.*

sive deposits, the tumor nodules are circumscribed implants on serosal surfaces. The nature of the deposits is enigmatic and many of them may represent synchronous primary events in the serosal surfaces rather than true metastases. Seidman et al (2002) explored the possibility that the "implants" may be somehow related to chronic salpingitis with psammoma bodies, named salpingoliths. The deposits may contain **numerous psammoma bodies** that may be either sparse or absent in the primary tumor. In any event, the prognosis of borderline serous tumors is much less favorable if the serosal deposits are invasive (summary in Prat, 1999). The same observation pertains to **tumor deposits in regional, usually paraortic, lymph nodes.** Many of these deposits are probably benign glandular inclusions of no prognostic significance but some represent real metastases (Prade et al, 1995; Moore et al, 2000).

Psammocarcinomas

A group of serous carcinomas exceptionally rich in calcified psammoma bodies has been identified as tumors with better prognosis than the common serous cancer and named **psammocarcinomas** (Gilks et al, 1990). My old chief, Dr. Fred Stewart, believed that psammocarcinomas may be self-healing or "burnt out," serous carcinomas, leaving behind collections of psammoma bodies. The tumor may be related to **endosalpingiosis,** described above.

Peritoneal Mimickers of Ovarian Serous Carcinomas

It has also been observed that **tumors mimicking ovarian serous carcinomas may originate in the peritoneum.** Various names have been applied to this group of rare tumors: **peritoneal papillary serous carcinoma, multifocal extraovarian serous carcinoma, and serous surface papillary carcinoma** (review in Mills et al, 1988). **Borderline lesions** of this type may also occur (Bell and Scully, 1990). The survival of patients is very poor, probably because these rare tumors are disseminated at the time of diagnosis. The cytologic presentation of such tumors in fluids is similar to that of primary ovarian tumors (see Fig. 16-8).

Mucin-Producing (Mucinous) Carcinomas

These tumors usually originate in ovarian cysts and are usually multiloculated. The mucinous tumors may reach very large sizes and their surgical removal with intact capsule should be curative of the disease. Usually, the epithelial lining resembles **intestinal epithelium rich in goblet cells, occasionally containing Paneth cells.** In some tumors, the epithelial lining resembles the **endocervical epithelium** in the form of **tall, columnar, mucus-producing cells with relatively small, spherical, basally-placed nuclei. The number of cell layers and level of nuclear abnormalities are the criteria of separation between the benign, border-**

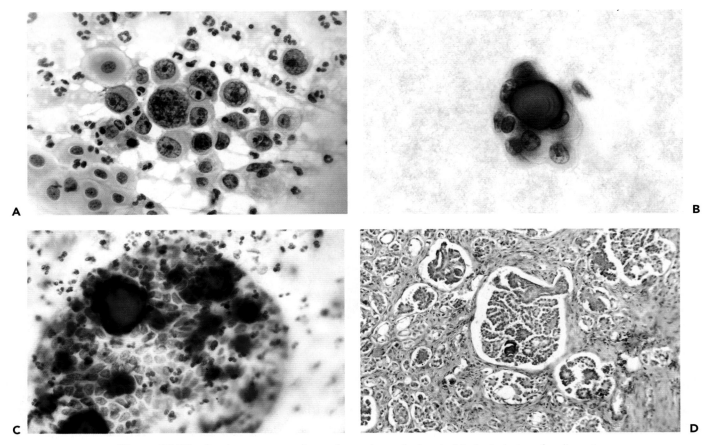

Figure 15-10   Ovarian serous carcinoma in cervicovaginal material. *A.* A cluster of malignant cells of variable sizes corresponding to a poorly differentiated serous carcinoma of the ovary. This presentation is unusual and not characteristic of ovarian tumors. *B,C.* Psammoma bodies in vaginal smears in the presence of serous carcinoma of the ovary shown in *D.* Note that the psammoma body shown in *B* is surrounded by large malignant cells. In *C,* the psammoma body occurred in a papillary cluster of malignant cells. *D.* Serous carcinoma of the ovary showing numerous psammoma bodies.

line or fully malignant tumors but are not always valid (Fig. 15-12).

The mucinous tumors, even with a low grade of nuclear abnormality, may spread to the abdominal cavity, particularly if inadvertently ruptured during removal or sampling. The characteristic pattern of spread of the tumors is on the surfaces of abdominal viscera, particularly the omentum and the intestinal serosa. The resulting lesion is accompanied by ascites, is **akin to pseudomyxoma peritonei,** described in Chapter 26, and does not respond to treatment. It has been shown that **similar tumors may synchronously occur in the appendix** and may be the source of peritoneal spread (Young et al, 1991). Molecular evidence suggests that most **pseudomyxomas are of appendiceal origin** (Szych et al, 1999). **Mural nodules,** that may have the configuration of poorly differentiated sarcomas, may be observed in the wall of mucinous tumors.

Borderline Mucinous Tumors

This is a poorly defined group of ovarian neoplasms characterized by focal nuclear abnormalities in the multilayered lining of multiloculated mucinous cystic tumors (Fig. 15-12C). Their behavior depends on the preservation of their capsule. Late recurrences have been observed (summary in

Prat, 1999). Peritoneal implants may also be observed in such tumors.

Endometrioid Carcinomas

These tumors are presumably derived from areas of endometriosis, although this origin is often difficult to prove. Histologically, the tumors **resemble endometrial carcinomas in all their various forms** (see Chap. 13). Squamous differentiation within the tumor is common, and it may range from small foci with squamoid features **(adenoacanthoma)** to tumors with a poorly differentiated squamous component **(adenosquamous carcinoma).** While glandular features are usually present, solidly growing tumors may occur. Synchronous occurrence of the ovarian tumors of this type with endometrial carcinomas has been repeatedly observed.

Rare Types of Ovarian Carcinoma

Tumors resembling the so-called **clear cell carcinomas** of the cervix and vagina (see Chaps. 11 and 14) are well known and are sometimes still referred to as **"mesonephric" tumors.**

Small cell carcinoma is a rare tumor resembling oat cell carcinoma of the lung (Dickersin et al, 1982; Eichhorn et al, 1992). In about two-thirds of the cases, there is an eleva-

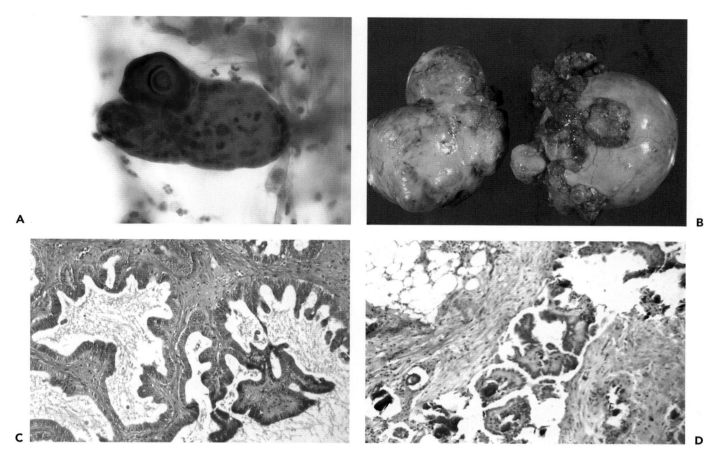

Figure 15-11 Borderline serous tumor of ovary in a 50-year-old woman. *A.* A tightly packed cluster of small malignant cells containing a large psammoma body. *B.* Gross appearance of the ovaries upon removal. Note tumor growth on the surface of the ovary. *C.* A very well differentiated borderline serous tumor of ovary. *D.* The tumor has spread to the adjacent omentum which shows numerous psammoma bodies. After removal of the ovaries and the omentum, the patient was free of disease for 10 subsequent years. (Case courtesy of Dr. Short, Chicago, IL.)

tion of serum calcium **(hypercalcemia).** Young et al (1994) stressed that the **differential diagnosis** of these tumors includes **granulosa cell tumor** and an ovarian involvement by **abdominal small round cell desmoplastic tumor,** discussed in Chapter 26.

Carcinomas originating in ovarian teratomas are predominantly of squamous type. Malignant carcinoids and thyroid carcinomas can also occur in teratomas (Baker et al, 2001). **Ovarian squamous cancers not occurring in teratomas are rare** (Pins et al, 1996). **Yolk sac (or endodermal sinus tumors) and embryonal carcinomas of the ovary** occur mainly in children and young adolescents. Malignant tumors with hormonal activity are described below.

Tumors of mesothelial lining of the ovary **(ovarian mesotheliomas)** are discussed in Chapter 26.

Cytology

Cervicovaginal Samples and Endometrial Aspirations

In about 20% to 30% of patients with **advanced** ovarian carcinoma, regardless of histologic type, **malignant cells**

may be observed in cervicovaginal preparations and occasionally in endocervical and endometrial aspirates (Jobo et al, 1999). Conversely, the presence of ovarian cancer cells in cervicovaginal smears usually, but not always, indicates advanced disease. The cancer cells may be derived from a primary tumor, via the fallopian tubes and the endometrial cavity, but may also reflect metastatic foci either within the endometrial cavity or in the vagina.

When seen in cervicovaginal smears or in endometrial aspirates, the tumor cells of nearly all ovarian cancers form **clusters, often of papillary configuration, made up of large malignant cells with prominent, large nuclei, containing multiple, often large, irregular nucleoli** (see Fig. 15-9). Single, usually large cancer cells with hyperchromatic nuclei containing large nucleoli may also be observed (see Fig. 15-10A). **Cytoplasmic vacuoles** are fairly common but may be the **dominant feature of cells derived from the relatively uncommon mucinous cystadenocarcinomas** (see Fig. 15-12A). The latter may also shed cells of **columnar configuration.** As a general rule, **cancer cells of ovarian origin are larger than cells of endometrial origin,** but there are exceptions. The exact identification of histologic type of carcinoma in cytologic material is not always easy.

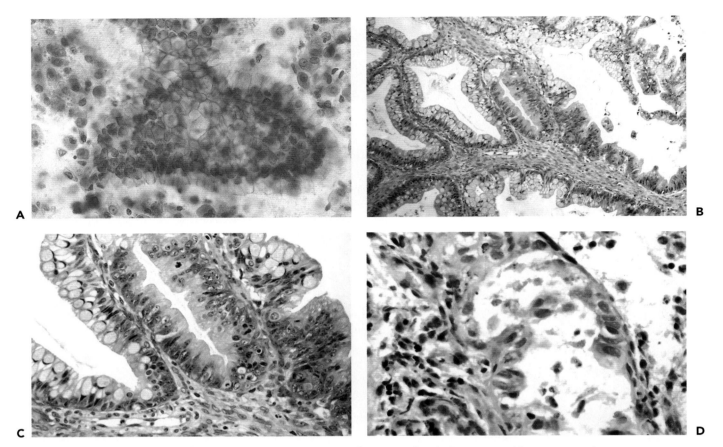

Figure 15-12 Mucinous adenocarcinoma and mucinous borderline tumor with recurrence. *A.* Direct aspirate of a mucinous cystadenocarcinoma of the ovary showing, at its periphery, tall, columnar, mucus-producing cells. *B.* The ovarian tumor corresponding to *A. C.* Borderline mucinous tumor of ovary in a 38-year-old woman observed in 1985. *D.* A cell block of an aspirated cul-de-sac nodule of the same patient in 1995. The nodule, with malignant features, retains some resemblance to the original mucinous tumor.

The most helpful hint is offered by **psammoma bodies,** concentrically calcified, spherical structures of various sizes.

Psammoma bodies are commonly found in **serous carcinoma of the ovary,** less commonly in the **borderline serous tumors,** very rarely in **endometrioid carcinomas,** and practically never in mucous tumors. It must be noted that **primary endometrial carcinomas may occasionally form psammoma bodies** (see Chap. 13).

When observed in cytologic preparations, psammoma bodies either are accompanied by cancer cells or are found isolated. In **high-grade serous carcinomas,** the psammoma bodies are usually accompanied by readily identifiable **large cancer cells,** as described above (see Fig. 15-10B,C). In such cases, there are usually no problems of cancer identification. In **borderline serous tumors, the cells accompanying the psammoma bodies are smaller and are arrayed in tightly packed papillary clusters** (see Fig. 15-11A). The number of cells in such clusters is very variable, ranging from a few to several hundred. The nuclear abnormalities are relatively inconspicuous, and the nucleoli are small. The finding of psammoma bodies accompanied by cancer cells is suggestive of tumor spread beyond the ovary, even in the absence of clinical symptoms.

Endosalpingiosis is the most important entity in the

differential diagnosis of serous ovarian carcinomas with which it shares the presence of numerous psammoma bodies in cervicovaginal smears and other cytologic preparations (see Fig. 15-7). In this condition, the psammoma bodies are either isolated or sometimes accompanied by a few small epithelial cells. These rare events may cause a great deal of diagnostic difficulty because they mandate a search for an ovarian carcinoma. Kern (1991), on review of nearly 10,000 cervicovaginal smears, noted that the presence of psammoma bodies was **more common in benign conditions (i.e., endosalpingiosis) than in ovarian carcinoma.** In a more recent study, Parkash and Chacho (2002) observed that over one half (11 of 20) of cervicovaginal smears containing psammoma bodies came from patients without cancer. **Also, calcified fragments of IUDs, some mimicking psammoma bodies, have been observed in patients wearing intrauterine contraceptive devices** (see Chap. 10), but the fragments are usually small and unstructured, lack the characteristic concentric lamination and are not accompanied by cancer cells. They may, however, be surrounded by macrophages.

Still, the presence of psammoma bodies in a cervicovaginal preparation or in an endocervical or endometrial aspiration, particularly in the absence of an intrauterine

contraceptive device, calls for a thorough investigation of the female genital tract to rule out a malignant tumor, most likely of ovarian origin. For a discussion of psammoma bodies and calcified debris in peritoneal washings, see Chapter 16.

Takashina et al (1988) compared the performance of **cervicovaginal smears** and **endometrial aspirates** in 114 patients with clinically documented **ovarian cancer** of various types and stages. The cervicovaginal smears were positive in 19% of the patients. Cancer cells were also found in 13 of 31 (42%) endometrial aspiration smears. The presence of ascitic fluid increased the rate of positive smears. Jobo et al (1999) confirmed that satisfactory **endometrial aspirations** provided diagnostic material in about 25% of 210 patients with ovarian cancer. The results were stage dependent: the smears were diagnostic of cancer in 3.9% for stage I tumors and over 50% in stage IV. It is of incidental interest that two occult ovarian serous adenocarcinomas were also observed by us during the search for occult endometrial cancer (see Chap. 13 and Fig. 15-10C,D). In both instances, the cancer cells were identified in vaginal pool smears and in direct endometrial samples.

Direct Needle Aspirates (FNA) of Ovaries

The methods of aspiration were discussed above. Direct aspirates from ovarian carcinomas are, as a rule, richer in cells than are aspirates from benign epithelial tumors. The cytologic recognition of a malignant tumor is usually not difficult. Even in well-differentiated types of carcinoma, the smeared aspirate contains approximately **spherical (papillary) groups of cancer cells, often with characteristic nuclear features, such as enlargement and hyperchromasia, large nucleoli, and thickening of the nuclear membrane** (Fig. 15-13). In **serous adenocarcinoma,** the cells may form a monolayer, but such a finding is insufficient for a reliable distinction between a serous and endometrioid carcinoma. Psammoma bodies are rarely seen in direct aspirates. **Mucinous ovarian carcinoma** may be recognized by the presence of **mucus-producing columnar cells embedded in masses of mucus** (see Fig. 15-11A). **Clear cell adenocarcinomas** may resemble clear cell adenocarcinoma of the kidney (see Chap. 40).

In serous lesions of **"borderline malignancy,"** the needle aspirates usually are more cellular than in benign cystomas, often forming **large flat clusters of well-adhering cells with only slight nuclear enlargement and minimal hyperchromasia.**

The accuracy of aspiration biopsy cytologic diagnosis in patients with ovarian enlargement or cancer was reported by Kjellgren and Ångström (1971, 1979), Geier et al (1975), Nadji et al (1979), and Geier and Strecker (1981). In these reports, ovarian cancer was accurately identified in

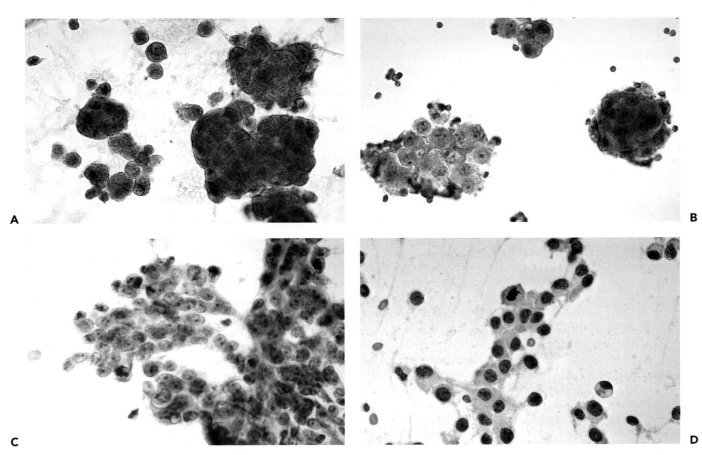

Figure 15-13 **Direct aspirates of ovarian serous carcinomas.** *A,B.* The sample was obtained by direct aspirate of an ovarian mass. It shows large clusters of malignant cells. *C,D.* Aspirate of a vaginal nodule in a patient with previously treated serous ovarian carcinoma. *C.* Clusters of malignant cells. In *D,* the malignant cells are dispersed and show fairly abundant cytoplasm and mitotic activity.

approximately 85% to 90% of cases. The proportion of false-positive cytologic reports in histologically benign lesions varied from 0% to about 5%. None of these authors reported on spread of tumor cells after the procedure. The caveats pertaining to this method of diagnosis of ovarian tumors were discussed above.

Tumors With Hormonal Activity

Theca and granulosa cell tumors, or a combination thereof, usually originate in cells forming ovarian follicles. It is quite likely that at least some of them originate in the ovarian stroma. These tumors may occur in all age groups, although they are uncommon in children. **Theca cell tumors** are grossly solid and hard and are made up of bundles of elongated, spindly cells resembling fibroblasts. The tumor is rich in cholesterol and other fats, which usually gives it a yellowish hue on section. Theca cell tumors are benign with very rare exceptions (Yang and Mesia, 1999). **Granulosa cell tumors,** which may be either benign or malignant, are generally soft and fleshy and have a number of different histologic patterns. These tumors are principally composed of small or medium-sized cells forming nests or sheets and sometimes **rosette-like clusters** resembling primitive follicles, known as the **Call-Exner bodies. Nuclear folds or "grooves"** are commonly observed in these tumors. Many uncommon histologic variants of this tumor have been recognized (Scully et al, 1998). Granulosa-theca cell tumors show a combination of both tumor types.

Most, although not all, of these tumors have marked **hormonal activity,** usually of estrogenic type. Occasional cases of masculinization have also been recorded with these tumors, hence a testosterone-like metabolic pathway may occur. The estrogenic function of the theca and granulosa cell tumors may be reflected in the morphology of the endometrium and in the squamous epithelium of the vagina and the cervix. **Endometrial hyperplasia and endometrial carcinoma** are known complications of these tumors, as discussed in Chapter 13.

Cytology

Cervicovaginal Smears

Hormonal Patterns. The cytologic identification of the hormonal effect on the squamous epithelium depends on the age of the patient. **In a woman of childbearing age,** it is extremely difficult to detect increased estrogenic effect on a single vaginal smear. However, if serial smears, as described in Chapter 9, show a consistent preovulatory (estrogenic) pattern, an abnormality of the estrogen output may be suspected. **In children and in postmenopausal women,** the presence of a very high level of maturation of squamous cells in a vaginal smear is suggestive of an **abnormal estrogen activity, which may be caused by an estrogen-producing ovarian tumor.**

Granulosa and granulosa-theca cell tumors have an unpredictable behavior and may recur and even metastasize, sometimes several years after the removal of the primary lesion. The **recurrent tumors** may also be estrogen producers and may be **heralded by an estrogenic smear pattern,** which is particularly evident in postmenopausal

women (Fig. 15-14A,C). On rare occasions, **other ovarian tumors** such as mucinous cystadenoma, may also show luteinization of ovarian stromal cells and have an **estrogenic effect** on smears. **Masculinizing tumors of the ovary** (Sertoli and Leydig cell tumors, hilar cell tumors, gonadoblastomas) have occasionally been recorded as **suppressing the maturation of squamous epithelium,** resulting in low estrogenic level in smears during the childbearing age (Rakoff, 1961).

Tumor Cells. In rare cases of **malignant granulosa cell tumors** with disseminated metastases, malignant cells of variable sizes with scanty cytoplasm and hyperchromatic nuclei with fairly large nucleoli have been observed in cervicovaginal smears. In the absence of history or clinical data, the precise classification of the tumor cannot be established.

Aspiration Biopsy (FNA)

Needle biopsy usually yields preponderantly granulosa cells. Granulosa cells appear in smears in **variable-sized clusters of medium-sized cells with granular cytoplasm and monomorphic, coffee-bean shaped oval nuclei, with inconspicuous nucleoli** (Fig. 15-15D). **Nuclear "grooves"** are common and have been repeatedly reported in metastatic granulosa cell tumors (Ehya, 1986; Ali, 1998; Thirumala et al, 1998). Zajicek observed that the presence of mitotic figures is suggestive of a malignant variant of the tumor.

Yang and Mesia (1999) reported a case of an extremely rare **malignant fibrothecoma** of ovary. The aspiration biopsy smears disclosed tightly packed small cells with uniform nuclei, diagnosed as "low-grade neoplasm."

Germ Cell Tumors

Benign Germ Cell Tumors

Benign Teratomas

Benign germ cell tumors are ovarian teratomas, also known as **dermoid cysts.** The tumors, usually observed in young women, are often bulky and composed of a **variety of tissues derived from two or three embryonal layers,** including skin and its appendages which are often the dominant component (hence the name dermoid cyst), brain tissue, gut, lung, thyroid etc. **So-called monomorphic teratomas** contain only one tissue type, such as the thyroid (**struma ovarii).**

Cells derived from benign teratomas have never been observed in routine cervicovaginal material. The diagnosis may be established or suspected in direct aspirates.

The aspirates of dermoid cysts usually contain **smelly amorphous matter (sebum) mixed with squamous epithelial cells and inflammatory cells, including foreign body giant cells.** Equally characteristic is the presence of **hairs,** provided that contamination of the smear by skin hair can be ruled out (Kjellgren and Ångström, 1979). The presence of columnar epithelial **cells of respiratory or intestinal type** is also indicative of a benign teratoma. Occasionally, unusual cells may be found in aspirates. Thus, Mulvany and Allan (1996) reported the presence of orderly clusters of **choroidal cells** in an aspirate from an **ependymal cyst** developing in a mature teratoma (Fig. 15-15). Canda

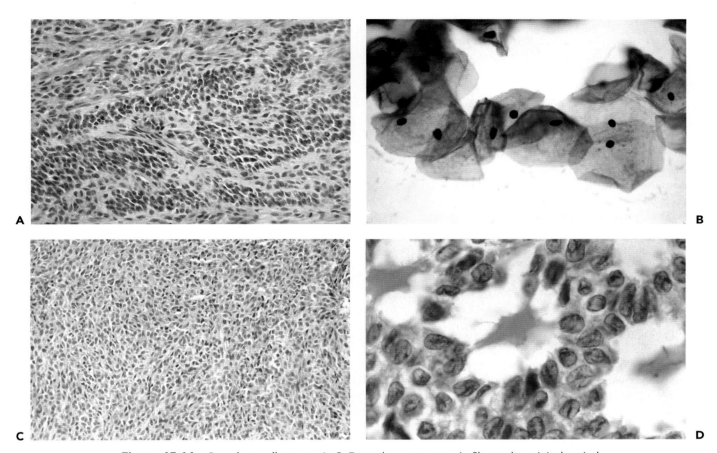

Figure 15-14 **Granulosa cell tumor.** *A–C.* From the same case. *A.* Shows the original typical granulosa cell tumor removed at the age of 50. *B.* Five years later, the patient showed a remarkably high level of squamous cell maturation (high estrogen level) in her vaginal smear. Active search for recurrent granulosa cell tumor led to the discovery of a small metastatic nodule shown in *C. D.* Direct aspirate of a metastatic granulosa cell tumor. In this photograph at high magnification, the cells form a gland-like structure corresponding to a Call-Exner body. The large nuclei of the tumor show nuclear folds or creases. (*D* courtesy of Dr. Hormoz Ehya, Fox Chase Cancer Center, Philadelphia, PA.)

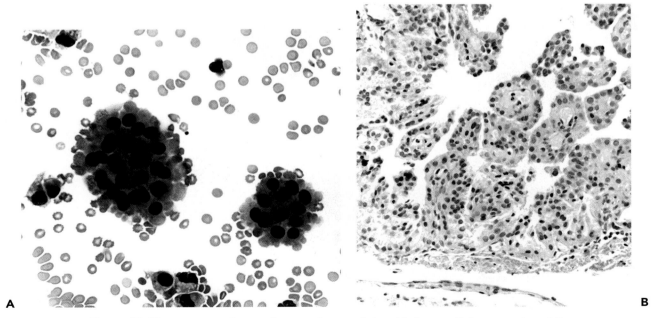

Figure 15-15 Teratoma of ovary showing clusters of choroid plexus cells in cyst aspirate (*A*). The corresponding tissue pattern in the resected teratomatous cyst is shown in *B*. (Photos courtesy of Dr. N. J. Mulvaney, Traralgon, Victoria, Australia.)

et al (2001) reported the presence of **Curshmann's spirals** in fluid aspirated from a dermoid cyst, lined by bronchial epithelium. For further comments on Curshmann's spirals, see Chapters 10, 19, and 25.

Sex Cord Tumor with Annular Tubules

Another benign ovarian tumor with cytologic implications is the rare ovarian sex cord tumor with annular tubules, observed in **Peutz-Jeghers syndrome.** The association of this tumor with **endocervical adenocarcinoma of the adenoma malignum type** has been noted (Young et al, 1982; Szyfelbein et al, 1984; see Chap. 12).

Hirschman et al (1998) described the cytologic features of this rare neoplasm in peritoneal washings in a most unusual case of ruptured tumor. The tumor was characterized by cellular tubular structures and absence of single tumor cells.

Malignant Germ Cell Tumors

Brenner Tumor

These tumors, composed of **nests of epithelial cells resembling the urothelium** (transitional epithelium) and **mucinous cysts,** may be benign or malignant. We have no experience with the cytologic patterns of these tumors. However, we observed cells suggestive of urothelial origin in an ovarian cyst, illustrated in Figure 15-6. Because the cyst was not excised, the exact derivation of these cells could not be established.

Dysgerminoma

The tumors resemble **seminomas of testis** and are composed of **sheets of large cancer cells in a background rich in lymphocytes.** The cells of this tumor are approximately spherical and are provided with pale nuclei with single large nucleoli. The cytologic presentation in needle aspirates corresponds to that of seminoma in the testis. Hees et al (1991) emphasized the presence of a **striated "tigroid" background in the air-dried MGG-stained smears,** representing cell debris, a feature also characteristic of germ cell tumors of testis (see Chap. 33 and Fig. 33-19).

Malignant Teratoma

Malignant teratomas of the ovary are exceedingly rare. The malignant component may be made up of undifferentiated small malignant cells, resembling neuroblastoma. In rare cases, a **carcinoid** or a **carcinoma,** most often of **squamous type,** rarely of **thyroid type,** may arise in a dermoid cyst. Baker et al (2001) reported the presence of **mucin-producing carcinoids** in teratomas. There is no record of such cases in the cytologic literature.

Embryonal Carcinoma

We observed one instance of the highly malignant **embryonal adenocarcinoma** in cervicovaginal smears from a 15-year-old girl. The tumor shed small malignant cells with prominent nucleoli, either singly or in papillary clusters. The

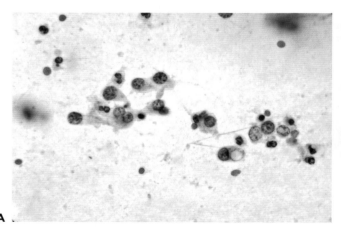

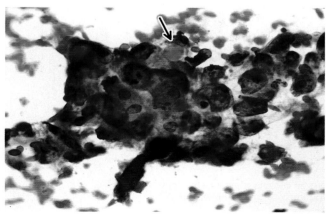

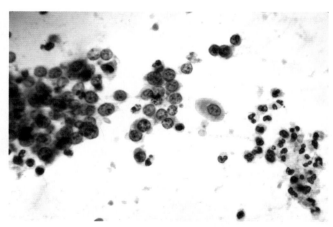

Figure 15-16 **Embryonal carcinoma of ovary.** *A,B.* The tumor in cervicovaginal smears was characterized by small cancer cells, singly and in papillary clusters, suggestive of an adenocarcinoma. *C.* Yolk sac tumor of ovary. High magnification to show hyaline body (*arrow*) adjacent to a cluster of tumor cells. (*C* courtesy of Dr. Hormoz Ehya, Fox Chase Cancer Center, Philadelphia, PA.)

smear pattern was suggestive of an adenocarcinoma (Fig. 15-16A,B). Other rare tumors are discussed in Chapter 17.

Yolk Sac Tumor (Endodermal Sinus Tumor)

This is an uncommon, highly malignant tumor of ovaries occurring in children and young people. The tumors may be primary in the **ovary, testis,** or the **sacrococcygeal region.** The tumor is histologically characterized by a loose network of cells wherein one finds solid nests of cells and the so-called **Schiller-Duval bodies,** papillary structures lined by columnar cells, centered around a fibrovascular core containing a single vessel (Yang, 2000). **Eosinophilic, periodic acid-Schiff (PAS) positive, spherical hyaline bodies** are commonly found in the cytoplasm of the tumor cells (Fig. 15-16C). Although the tumors produce **α-feto-protein,** the hyaline bodies are not immunoreactive with the specific antigen because they represent electron-dense granules of not further specified nature. Because, in most cases, the tumors are advanced at the time of diagnosis, they are recognized in ascitic fluid or in aspirates of metastases. **Clusters of epithelial cells containing the characteristic hyaline cytoplasmic inclusions** (which may also appear as isolated hyaline structures) allow the precise diagnosis of these tumors (Morimoto et al, 1981; Kapila et al, 1983; Roncalli et al, 1988; Domínguéz-Franjo et al, 1993; Mizrak and Elkinci, 1995).

DNA Analysis of Ovarian Tumors

It has been shown by several observers that common ovarian cancers have a better prognosis if their DNA content measured by flow cytometry is within the diploid range (Atkin, 1984; Friedlander et al, 1984; Iverson and Laerum, 1985; Kallioniemi et al, 1988). Greenebaum et al (1994) found the technique useful in separating benign (diploid) from suspicious or malignant (nondiploid) aspirates from ovarian cysts. For further comments, see Chapter 47.

DIAGNOSIS OF OCCULT OVARIAN CARCINOMA

The high frequency and poor outcome of ovarian carcinoma, with spread beyond the ovary at the time of diagnosis, has led to numerous efforts at early detection of these tumors. It is now known from the results of prophylactic salpingo-oophorectomy in high risk women with mutations of BRCA1 and 2 that small ovarian tumors and other possibly precancerous epithelial changes may be observed (Bell and Scully, 1994; Salazar et al, 1996; Kauff et al, 2002). Finding such tiny tumors before further spread has been a major challenge over many years.

Routine Cervicovaginal Smears

The finding of cancer cells suggestive of an adenocarcinoma in cervicovaginal smears or in an endocervical or endometrial aspiration in an **asymptomatic patient** presents a difficult clinical dilemma. A thorough clinical examination, an ultrasound examination, a CT scan, a peritoneoscopy, or even an exploratory laparotomy may reveal a clinically occult ovarian (see Fig. 15-9) or a tubal carcinoma (see below). Occasionally, this may lead to the diagnosis of a **carcinoma still confined to the ovary,** hence offering a good chance for a cure. In my experience, however, most ovarian carcinomas diagnosed by cervicovaginal cytology are usually advanced and have formed metastases, usually to the omentum or the lower genital tract. Thus, routine cytologic preparation offers limited hope for the diagnosis of ovarian cancer in early stages. Other tumors that must be considered in the differential diagnosis are endometrial carcinoma and metastatic carcinoma from a distant site.

Detection of Early Ovarian Carcinoma by Special Techniques

Because the results of treatment of fully developed ovarian carcinoma are not satisfactory, in 1962, Graham et al suggested the use of **cul-de-sac aspiration via the vaginal route (culdocentesis)** for the diagnosis of early, clinically occult ovarian cancers. The original study was based on examination of 576 volunteer patients and gave eight positive results. Seven patients were explored and the ovaries examined: one had metastatic breast cancer, one had no demonstrable lesion, four had papillary ovarian lesions of "borderline malignancy," and one had a "probable borderline lesion." Subsequently (1964 and 1967), these authors reported on an additional eight ovarian lesions showing abnormalities of surface epithelium. Because of current interest in early carcinomas of the ovary, especially **"early ovarian intraepithelial neoplasia or dysplasia"** of the surface epithelium (Plaxe et al, 1990), histologic sections of the original ovaries reported by Graham et al (1964), were re-examined by Werness and Eltabbakh (2000). On re-examination, the eight ovaries were considered to be within normal limits. Long-term follow-up of 7 of the 8 patients was noncontributory and none of them had any evidence of ovarian cancer. The experience with this method of ovarian cancer detection since the publication of the 1964 and 1967 reports by Graham et al has remained inconclusive. Several published papers (McGowan et al, 1966; Grillo et al, 1966; Zervakis et al, 1969; Funkhouser et al, 1975) gave equivocal results. Keettel et al (1974) gave a pessimistic appraisal of the value of the procedure.

Although early carcinomas may be occasionally observed on the surface of the ovaries (Bell and Scully, 1994), most ovarian cancers develop within ovarian cysts that remain intact, possibly for long periods of time. Therefore, there is significant doubt that the cul-de-sac aspiration will indeed significantly contribute to the salvage of lives.

As reported by Greenebaum et al (1992, 1996), it is occasionally possible to discover an early ovarian cancer while harvesting ova in in vitro fertilization patients. This event is exceedingly rare. The procedure has been described in the earlier part of this chapter.

Transvaginal sonographic screening (TVS) has been shown to be capable of uncovering ovarian lesions, although in some early studies (Goswamy et al, 1983), many false alarms were generated because of enlarged benign ovaries. Three per cent of screened women without evidence of malignant disease required laparoscopy or laparotomy. Recently, Van Nagell et al (2000) reported on the efficacy of TVS in 14,469 women, ages 50 or older (or younger women with family history of ovarian cancer), conducted from 1987 to 1999. The principal criteria for laparoscopy or exploratory laparotomy were: large ovarian volume or papillary or complex tissue projections in cysts, verified on a repeat examination 4 to 6 weeks after the original sonogram. In 180 women explored 17 ovarian cancers were detected, most in stages I and II of disease. In the remaining 163 women, numerous other benign ovarian lesions were observed. Eight additional women subsequently developed ovarian cancer in the absence of sonographic abnormalities. The conclusions of this paper suggested that **TVS in fortuitous cases leads to the detection of occult ovarian cancer with a low positive predictive value of only 9.4% but a high negative predictive value of 99.07%.** In other words, a negative TVS offers a high degree of assurance that the risk of ovarian cancer in a given patient is low. Unfortunately, the system fails in the detection of ovarian cancer in ovaries with normal volume. **The procedure may be of particular value in women who have germ-line mutations of breast cancer genes (BRCA1 and 2)** (Rubin et al, 1996).

There is no evidence that serologic studies, particularly measuring the serum levels of antibodies with a high degree of specificity for ovarian cancer, such as CA 125 or OV 632, are applicable as a screening test for ovarian cancer, although the determinations may be of value in recurrent cancer (Niloff et al, 1968; Koelma et al, 1988; Malkasian et al, 1988).

Proteomics

Most recently, protein patterns in blood plasma, characteristic of ovarian cancer, generated by **proteomic spectra,** obtained with mass spectroscopy, have been reported as a promising approach to early detection of ovarian cancer (Bicsel et al, 2001; Petricoin et al, 2002; Rai et al, 2002). Algorithms generated by proteomics have been effectively applied to the identification of patients with ovarian cancer with sensitivity of 100% and specificity of 95% (Petricoin et al, 2002). Excellent results were also claimed by combining proteomics with other markers, such as CA 125 (Rai et al, 2002). The value of the proteomics still needs testing on a large population.

FALLOPIAN TUBE

HISTOLOGIC RECALL

The epithelium of the fallopian tubes is composed of three types of cells. The dominant cell type is the **columnar ciliated cells** that closely resemble in size and configuration similar cells observed in the lining of the endocervical canal. The second cell type is the **secretory cells** that are interspersed among ciliated cells which they resemble, except for clear cytoplasm and the absence of cilia. The luminal aspect of the secretory cells often shows "snouts" of secretions on their surface. The third cell types are the least frequent **intercalary or peg cells,** narrow cells with thin, dark-staining nucleus. The epithelium is separated from the two muscular layers by a thin lamina propria of connective tissue.

Normal tubal epithelial cells are virtually never seen in normal cervicovaginal smears, except as the so-called tubal metaplasia, discussed in Chapter 10.

BENIGN DISORDERS

The fallopian tubes may be affected by a variety of benign disorders, some of which may have cytologic implications.

Inflammatory disorders, such as **tuberculosis** and **chlamydia** infection may cause tubal obstruction and dilatation **(hydrosalpinx)** that may lead to **tubal pregnancy.** These conditions may be sometimes mistaken for tumors. Seidman et al (2002) observed that **chronic salpingitis** with formation of psammoma bodies (named here **salpingoliths;** see Fig. 15-12B) may be related to serous carcinoma of ovary and peritoneal implants.

A variety of **cysts,** ranging from **simple serous paraovarian cysts** to **endometriosis** and **endosalpingiosis,** may be observed on the serosal surface of the tubes. Some of these cysts, if of significant sizes, may be aspirated. The cytologic presentation of these cysts is identical to ovarian cysts, discussed above. More importantly, perhaps, these cystic structures may be sometimes recognized in peritoneal washings, discussed below.

CARCINOMA OF FALLOPIAN TUBES

Histology and Clinical Features

Carcinoma of the fallopian tube resembles ovarian and endometrial adenocarcinomas and may occur in a **variety of histologic patterns, some papillary, some solid.** A stage of **carcinoma in situ** has been recognized.

Most lesions are usually discovered too late for effective treatment, although they often produce vaginal spotting or bleeding for which no obvious cause can be found (review in Nordin, 1994). Sedlis (1961), upon review of the literature, pointed out that those patients who had the benefit of routine cytologic examination had a surprisingly high percentage (40%) of positive diagnoses. Fidler and Lock (1954) go so far as to say: "The triad of vaginal spotting or hemorrhage, lower abdominal pain and pelvic mass, when accompanied by positive cytology and negative cervical and endometrial biopsy is practically diagnostic of tubal carcinoma." This is an extreme view, since many cancers of other origins may have a similar clinical and laboratory presentation. Heselmeyer et al (1998) observed high levels of genomic instability in 12 tubal carcinomas studied by comparative genomic hybridization. The tumors were free of human papillomavirus but most were strongly reactive with p53 antibody. These authors attributed the poor prognosis of these tumors to their genetic and molecular features.

In a recent communication, Agoff et al (2002) reported high frequency of tubal carcinoma in women with **proven or suspected BRCA1 or 2 mutations.** In four of the seven cases reported, the **tumors were occult** and two of them were discovered in pelvic washings in patients undergoing **prophylactic salpingo-oophorectomy.**

Tubal Carcinoma in Cervicovaginal Smears and Endometrial Samples

Tubal carcinoma may be recognized **in cervicovaginal smears** and in **direct endometrial samples.** The **cytologic presentation of tubal carcinoma cannot be distinguished from that of an ovarian adenocarcinoma. Large malignant cells,** sometimes with vacuolated cytoplasm, hyperchromatic large nuclei, and **prominent nucleoli,** are found in cervicovaginal smears singly and in papillary clusters (Figs. 15-17 and 15-18). If the lesion is small, **the problems of localization of tubal carcinoma** may prove to be difficult, not only clinically or at the time of surgery, but even at the time of examination of the specimen by the patholo-

gist. This sequence of events is illustrated in Figure 15-19. As in cases of occult carcinomas of the ovary, discussed above, if the results of the clinical and ultrasound examination of the vagina, cervix, and endometrium are normal, a laparotomy may be needed to clarify the origin of malignant cells. A case of a **tubal carcinoma in situ,** diagnosed in an endometrial sample, was reported by Luzzatto et al (1996). The smear pattern in this case was again identical to an ovarian carcinoma because of the presence of **psammoma bodies** and cells of adenocarcinoma.

Excellent results of cytologic examination in 128 patients with tubal cancer were reported by Takashina and Kudo (1985) on the basis of **cervicovaginal smears** (positive in 38% of 58 patients) and **direct endometrial samples** (positive in 80% of 15 patients). Hirai et al (1987) and Takeshima et al (1997) also reported good diagnostic results by **endometrial aspiration smears** in 6 of 20 patients with tubal cancer. We also observed a case of occult tubal carcinoma diagnosed in an endometrial aspiration from an asymptomatic patient during the search for occult endometrial cancer (see Fig. 15-18).

Rare tumors of the fallopian tube include **mesodermal mixed tumors** (Kinoshita et al, 1989), a **carcinosarcoma** (Axelrod et al, 1989), and a **glassy cell carcinoma** (Herbold et al, 1988).

For further discussion of rare tumors see Chapter 17.

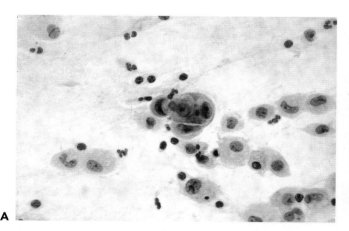

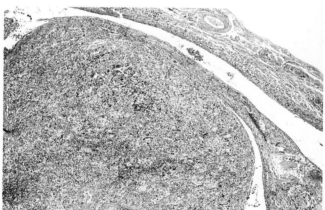

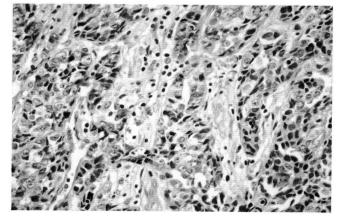

Figure 15-17   Carcinoma of a fallopian tube discovered on cervicovaginal smear. *A.* A cervicovaginal smear with a single cluster of cells suggestive of an adenocarcinoma. The tumor was clinically occult. *B,C.* Low and higher power views of the fallopian tube showing a poorly differentiated adenocarcinoma.

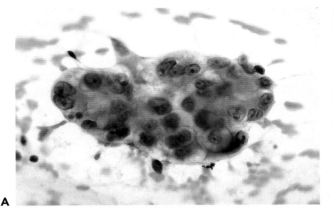

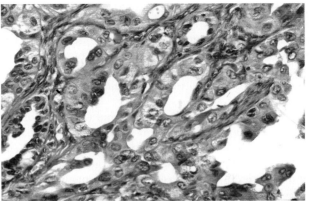

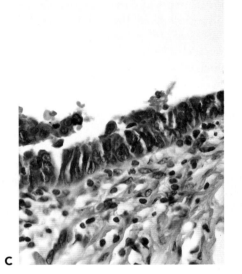

Figure 15-18 **Adenocarcinoma of fallopian tube detected on endometrial aspiration smear.** *A.* A large papillary cluster of cancer cells with very large nuclei and prominent nucleoli observed in an endometrial aspirated sample. This appearance is identical to that observed in serous carcinomas of ovary. *B,C.* Histologic appearance of fallopian tube. *B.* Adenocarcinoma composed of very large cells. *C.* An area of carcinoma in situ at the periphery of invasive tumor shown in *B.*

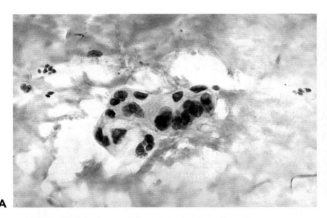

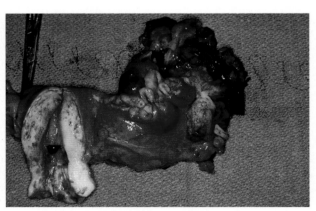

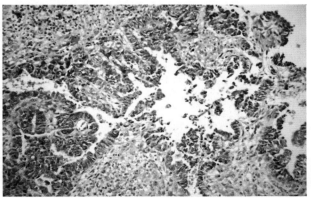

Figure 15-19 **Adenocarcinoma of fallopian tube.** The tumor was very difficult to localize in the surgical specimen. *A.* A papillary cluster of malignant cells in cervicovaginal smear. *B.* The gross appearance of the uterus and the fallopian tube. The fallopian tube was folded but not thickened. *C.* Adenocarcinoma of fallopian tube was identified and diagnosed only after numerous cross sections of the tube were examined.

BIBLIOGRAPHY

Agoff SN, Mendelin JE, Grieco VS, Garcia RL. Unexpected gynecologic neoplasms in patients with proven or suspected BRCA-1 or -2 mutations. Implications for gross examination, cytology, and clinical follow-up. Am J Surg Pathol 26:171–178, 2002.

Ali SZ. Metastatic granulosa-cell tumor in the liver. Cytopathologic findings and staining with Inhibin. Diagn Cytopathol 19:293–297, 1998.

Ångström T, Kjellgren O, Bergman F. The cytologic diagnosis of ovarian tumors by means of aspiration biopsy. Acta Cytol 16:336–341, 1972.

Asmussen M, Kaern J, Kjoerstad K, et al. Primary adenocarcinoma localized to the fallopian tubes: Report on 33 cases. Gynecol Oncol 30:183–186, 1988.

Atkin NB. Prognostic value of cytogenetic studies of tumors of the female genital tract. In Koss LG, Coleman DV (eds). Advances in Clinical Cytology, Vol 2. New York, Masson, 1984, pp 103–121.

Axelrod JH, Herbold DR, Freel JH. Carcinosarcoma of the fallopian tube. Gynecol Oncol 32:398–400, 1989.

Baker PM, Oliva E, Young RH, et al. Ovarian mucinous carcinoids including some with a carcinomatous component: A report of 17 cases. Am J Surg Pathol 25:557–568, 2001.

Barnhill D, Heller P, Brzozowski P, et al. Epithelial ovarian carcinoma of low malignant potential. Obstet Gynecol 65:53–59, 1985.

Bell DA, Scully RE. Serous borderline tumors of the peritoneum. Am J Surg Pathol 14:230–239, 1990.

Bell DA, Scully RE. Early de novo ovarian carcinoma: a study of 14 cases. Cancer 73:1859–1864, 1994.

Bell DA, Weinstock MA, Scully RE. Peritoneal implants of ovarian serous borderline tumors: Histologic features and prognosis. Cancer 62:2212–2222, 1988.

Benson PA. Cytologic diagnosis in primary carcinoma of fallopian tube: Case report and review. Acta Cytol 18:429–434, 1974.

Benson PA. Psammoma bodies found in cervicovaginal smears: Case report. Acta Cytol 17:64–66, 1973.

Beyer-Boon ME. Psammoma bodies in cervicovaginal smears: An indicator of the presence of ovarian carcinoma. Acta Cytol 18:41–44, 1974.

Bicsel VE, Liotta LA, Petricoin EF III. Cancer proteomics: from biomarker discovery to signal pathway profiling. Cancer J 7:69–78, 2001.

Bjersing L, Frankendal B, Angström T. Studies on feminizing ovarian mesenchymoma (granulosa cell tumor). I. Aspiration biopsy, cytology, histology, and ultrastructure. Cancer 32:1360–1369, 1973.

Bostwick DG, Tazelaar HD, Ballon SC, et al. Ovarian epithelial tumors of borderline malignancy. A clinical and pathologic study of 109 cases. Cancer 58:2052–2065, 1986.

Buchino JJ, Buchino JJ. Malignant mixed mullerian tumor of the fallopian tube. Arch Pathol Lab Med 111:386–387, 1987.

Burke M, Talerman A, Carlson JA, Bibbo M. Residual ovarian tissue mimicking malignancy in a patient with mucinous carcinoid tumor of the ovary: A case report. Acta Cytol 41:1377–1380, 1997.

Burmeister RE, Fechner RE, Franklin RR. Endosalpingiosis of the peritoneum. Obstet Gynecol 34:310–318, 1969.

Canda T, Ozkal S, Ozer E. Curschmann's spirals in cyst fluid associated with a teratoma of the ovary: A case report. Acta Cytol 45:441–444, 2001.

Cannistra SA. Cancer of the ovary. N Engl J Med 329:1550–1559, 1993.

Clement PB, Young RH, Scully RE. Malignant mesotheliomas presenting as ovarian masses. A report of nine cases, including two primary ovarian mesotheliomas. Am J Surg Pathol 20:1067–1080, 1996.

Clement PB, Young RH. Florid cystic endosalpingiosis with tumor-like manifestations. A report of four cases including the first reported cases of transmural endosalpingiosis of the uterus. Am J Surg Pathol 23:166–175, 1999.

Coffin CM, Adcock LL, Dehner LP. The second-look operation of ovarian neoplasms: A study of 85 cases emphasizing cytologic and histologic problems. Int J Gynecol Pathol 4:97–109, 1985.

Creasman WT, Lukeman J. Role of the fallopian tube in dissemination of malignant cells in corpus cancer. Cancer 29:456–457, 1972.

Dalrymple JC, Bannatyne P, Russell P, Solomon HJ, et al. Extraovarian peritoneal serous papillary carcinoma: A clinicopathologic study of 31 cases. Cancer 64:110–115, 1989.

Davila RM. Cytology of benign cystic uterine adnexal masses. Acta Cytol 37:385–390, 1993.

DeCrespigny LC, Robinson HP, Davoren RA, Fortune D. The "simple" ovarian cyst: Aspirate or operate? Br J Obstet Gynaecol 96:1035–1039, 1989.

Dekmezian R, Sneige N, Ordonez NG. Ovarian and omental ependymomas in peritoneal washings: Cytologic and immunocytologic features. Diagn Cytopathol 2:62–68, 1986.

Dharan M. Intraoperative cytology of small cell carcinoma of the ovary with hypercalcemia: A case report. Acta Cytol 37:61–66, 1993.

Dickersin GR, Kline IW, Scully RE. Small cell carcinoma of the ovary with hypercalcemia. A report of 11 cases. Cancer 49:188–197, 1982.

Dictor M. Malignant mixed mesodermal tumor of the ovary: A report of 22 cases. Obstet Gynecol 65:720–724, 1985.

Differding JT. Psammoma bodies in a vaginal smear. Acts Cytol 11:199–201, 1967.

Dockerty MB, Mussey E. Malignant lesions of uterus associated with estrogen-producing ovarian tumors. Am J Obstet Gynecol 61:147–153, 1951.

Dominguez-Franjo P, Vargas J, Rodriguez-Peralto JL, et al. Fine needle aspiration biopsy findings in endodermal sinus tumors: A report of four cases with cytologic, immunochemical and ultrastructural findings. Acta Cytol 37:209–215, 1993.

Ehrmann RL, Federschneider JM, Knapp RC. Distinguishing lymph node metastases from benign glandular inclusions in low-grade ovarian carcinoma. Am J Obstet Gynecol 136:737–746, 1980.

Ehya H, Lang WR. Cytology of granulosa cell tumor of the ovary. Am J Clin Pathol 85:402–405, 1986.

Eichhorn J, Bell DA, Young RH, et al. DNA content and proliferative activity in ovarian small cell carcinomas of the hypercalcemic type. Am J Clin Pathol 98:579–586, 1992.

Feichter GE, Kuhn W, Czernobilsky B, et al. DNA flow cytometry of ovarian tumors with correlation to histopathology. Int J Gynecol Pathol 4:336–345, 1985.

Fidler HK, Lock DR. Carcinoma of the fallopian tube detected by cervical smear. Am J Obstet Gynecol 67:1103–1111, 1954.

Freese VU. Ein Beitrag zur Zytologie des Tubenkarzinoms. Geburtshilfe Fraunheilk 17:173–180, 1957.

Friedlander ML, Hedley DW, Taylor IW, et al. Influence of cellular DNA content on survival in advanced ovarian cancer. Cancer Res 44:397–400, 1984.

Funkhouser JW, Hunter KK, Thompson NJ. The diagnostic value of cul-de-sac aspiration in the detection of ovarian carcinoma. Acta Cytol 19:538–541, 1975.

Gallion HH, van Nagell JR Jr, Donaldson ES, Powell DE. Ovarian dysgerminoma: Report of seven cases and review of the literature. Am J Obstet Gynecol 158:591–595, 1988.

Geier G, Kraus H, Schuhmann R. Fine needle aspiration biopsy in ovarian tumors. In DeWatteville H, et al (eds). Diagnosis and Treatment of Ovarian Neoplastic Alterations. Amsterdam, Excerpta Medica, 1975, pp 73–76.

Geier GR, Strecker JR. Aspiration cytology and E2 content in ovarian cytology. Acta Cytol 25:400–406, 1981.

Gilks CB, Bell DA, Scully RE. Serous psammocarcinoma of the ovary and peritoneum. Int J Gynecol Pathol 9:110–121, 1990.

Gonzalez-Crussi F. The human yolk sac and yolk sac (endodermal dermal sinus) tumors: A review. Perspect Pediatr Pathol 5:179–215, 1979.

Goswamy RK, Campbell S, Whitehead MI. Screening for ovarian cancer. Clin Obstet Gynaecol 10:621–643, 1983.

Graham JB, Graham RM. Cul-de-sac puncture in the diagnosis of early ovarian carcinoma. J Obstet Gynecol Br Commonw 74:371–378, 1967.

Graham JB, Graham RM, Schueller EF. Preclinical detection of ovarian cancer. Cancer 17:1414–1432, 1964.

Graham RM, Bartels JD, Graham JB. Screening for ovarian cancer by cul-de-sac aspiration. Acta Cytol 6:492–495, 1962.

Graham RM, Van Niekerk WA. Vaginal cytology in cancer of the ovary. Acta Cytol 6:496–499, 1962.

Greenebaum E. Aspirating malignant ovarian cysts. Lab Med 27:607–611, 1996.

Greenebaum E. Aspirating nonneoplastic ovarian cysts. Lab Med 27:462–467, 1996.

Greenebaum E, Mayer JR, Stangel JJ, Hughes P. Aspiration cytology of ovarian cysts in in vitro fertilization patients. Acta Cytol 36:11–18, 1992.

Greenebaum E, Yee HT, Liu J. DNA ploidy of ovarian and adnexal cyst fluid. A useful adjunct to cytology. Acta Cytol 38:201–208, 1994.

Greenebaum E. Aspirating benign and borderline ovarian cysts. Lab Med 27:538–541, 1996.

Greenlee RT, Murray T, Bolden S, Wingo PA. Cancer statistics 2000. CA Cancer J Clin 50:7–33, 2000.

Grillo D, Stienmier RH, Lowell DM. Early diagnosis of ovarian carcinoma by culdocentesis. Obstet Gynecol 28:346–350, 1966.

Gurley AM, Hidvegi DF, Cajulis RS, Bacus S. Morphologic and morphometric features of low grade serous tumours of the ovary. Diagn Cytopathol 11:220–225, 1994.

Guzman J, Hilgarth M, Bross KJ, et al. Malignant ascites of serous papillary ovarian adenocarcinoma: An immunocytochemical study of the tumor cells. Acta Cytol 32:519–522, 1988.

Hees K, de Jonge JP, von Kortzfleisch DH. Dysgerminoma of the ovary: Cytologic, histologic and electron microscopic study of a case. Acta Cytol 35:341–344, 1991.

Heine W, Buttner HH, Kuhne D, Richter I. Granulosazelltumor bei einem 3 jahrigen Mädchen. Pediatr Prax 13:561–565, 1974.

Herbold DR, Axelrod JH, Bobowski SJ. Glassy cell carcinoma of the fallopian tube: A case report. Int J Gynecol Pathol 7:384–390, 1988.

Heselmeyer K, Hellstrom AC, Blegen H, et al. Primary carcinoma of the fallopian tube: comparative genomic hybridization reveals high genetic instability and a specific, recurring pattern of chromosomal aberrations. Int J Gynecol Pathol 17:245–254, 1998.

Highman WJ. Calcified bodies and the intrauterine device. Acta Cytol 15:473–475, 1971.

Hirai Y, Chen J-T, Hamada T, et al. Clinical and cytologic aspects of primary fallopian tube carcinoma: A report of 10 cases. Acta Cytol 31:834–840, 1987.

Hirschman SA, Dottino P, Deligdisch L, Szporn A. Cytology of sex cord tumor with annular tubules: a case report. Diagn Cytopathol 18:362–364, 1998.

Hoffman MS, Cavanagh D, Walter TS, et al. Adenocarcinoma of the endometrium and endometrioid carcinoma of the ovary associated with pregnancy. Gynecol Oncol 32:82–85, 1989.

Honore LH, Nickerson KG. Papillary serous cystadenoma arising in a paramesonephric cyst of the parovarium. Am J Obstet Gynecol 125:870–871, 1976.

Hsu YK, Parmley TH, Rosenshein NB, Bhagavan BS, Woodruff JD. Neoplastic and non-neoplastic mesothelial proliferations in pelvic lymph nodes. Obstet Gynecol 55:83–88, 1980.

Iverson OE, Laerum OD. Ploidy disturbances in endometrial and ovarian carcinomas. A review. Anal Quant Cytol Histol 7:327–336, 1985.

Jensen RD, Norris HJ. Epithelial tumors of the ovary: Occurrence in children and adolescents less than 20 years of age. Arch Pathol 94:29–34, 1972.

Jobo T, Arai M, Iwaya H, Kato Y, et al. Usefulness of endometrial aspiration cytology for the preoperative diagnosis of ovarian carcinoma. Acta Cytol 43:104–109, 1999.

Johnson TL, Kumar NB, Hopkins M, Hughes JD. Cytologic features of ovarian tumors of low malignant potential in peritoneal fluids. Acta Cytol 32:513–518, 1988.

Johnston WW, Goldston WR, Montgomery MS. Clinicopathologic studies in feminizing tumors of the ovary. III. The role of genital cytology. Acta Cytol 15:334–338, 1971.

Jose B, Mendoza E, Chu AM, Sharma S. Dysgerminoma of the ovary. J Surg Oncol 26:202–204, 1984.

Julian CG, Woodruff D. The biologic behavior of low-grade papillary serous carcinoma of the ovary. Obstet Gynecol 40:860–867, 1972.

Kallioniemi OP, Mattila J, Punnonen R, Koivula T. DNA ploidy level and cell cycle distribution in ovarian cancer: Relation to histopathological features of the tumor. Int J Gynecol Pathol 7:1–11, 1988.

Kapila K, Hajdu S, Whitmore WF, et al. Cytologic diagnosis of metastatic germ cell tumors. Acta Cytol 27:245–251, 1983.

Karp LA, Czernobilsky B. Glandular inclusions in pelvic and abdominal para-aortic lymph nodes: A study of autopsy and surgical material in males and females. Am J Clin Pathol 52:212–218, 1969.

Kauff ND, Satagopan JM, Robson ME, et al. Risk-reducing salpingo-oophorectomy in women with a BRCA1 or BRCA2 mutation. N Engl J Med 346:1609–1615, 2002.

Keettel WC, Pixley EE, Buchsbaum HJ. Experience with peritoneal cytology in the management of gynecologic malignancies. Am J Obstet Gynecol 120:174–182, 1974.

Kennedy AW, Biscotti CV, Hart WR, Webster KD. Ovarian clear cell adenocarcinoma. Gynecol Oncol 32:342–349, 1989.

Kern SB. Prevalence of psammoma bodies in Papanicolaou-stained cervicovaginal smears. Acta Cytol 35:81–88, 1991.

Kern WH. Benign papillary structures with psammoma bodies in culdocentesis fluid. Acta Cytol 13:178–180, 1969.

Kinoshita M, Asano S, Yamashita M, Matsuda T. Mesodermal mixed tumor primary in the fallopian tube. Gynecol Oncol 32:313–315, 1989.

Kjellgren O, Ångström T, Bergman F, Wiklund D-E. Fine-needle aspiration biopsy in diagnosis and classification of ovarian carcinoma. Cancer 28:967–976, 1971.

Kjellgren O, Øngström T. Transvaginal and transrectal aspiration biopsy in diagnosis and classification of ovarian tumors. In Zajicek J (ed). Aspiration Biopsy Cytology, Part 2: Cytology of Infradiaphragmatic Organs. Basel, S Karger, 1979, pp 80–103.

Koelma IA, Nap M, van Steenis GJ, Gleuren GJ. Tumor markers for ovarian cancer. A comparative immunohistochemical and immunocytochemical study of two commercial monoclonal antibodies (OV632 and OC125). Am J Clin Pathol 90:391–396, 1988.

Koss LG. Early diagnosis of uterine and ovarian carcinoma. Oncology. Proceedings of the 10th International Cancer Congress 4:211–220, 1970.

Koss LG, Rothschild EO, Fleisher M, Francis JE Jr. Masculinizing tumor of the ovary apparently with adrenocortical activity: A histologic, ultrastructural and biochemical study. Cancer 23:1245–1258, 1969.

Kreuzer GF, Paradowski T, Wurche KD, Flenker H. Neoplastic or nonneoplastic ovarian cyst? The role of cytology. Acta Cytol 39:882–886, 1995.

Kurman RJ, Norris HJ. Endodermal sinus tumor of the ovary: A clinical and pathological analysis of 71 cases. Cancer 38:2404–2419, 1976.

Leo S, Rorat E, Parekh M. Primary malignant melanoma in a dermoid cyst of the ovary. Obstet Gynecol 41:205–210, 1973.

LiVolsi VA, Merino MJ, Schwartz PE. Coexistent endocervical adenocarcinoma and mucinous adenocarcinoma of ovary: A clinicopathologic study of four cases. Int J Gynecol Pathol 1:391–402, 1983.

Luzzatto R, Brucker N. Benign inclusion cysts of the ovary associated with psammoma bodies in vaginal smears. Acta Cytol 25:282–284, 1981.

Luzzatto R, Sisson G, Luzatto L, et al. Psammoma bodies and cells from in situ fallopian tube carcinoma in endometrial smears: a case report. Acta Cytol 40:295–298, 1996.

Malkasian GD Jr, Knapp RC, Lavin PT, et al. Preoperative evaluation of serum CA 125 levels in premenopausal and postmenopausal patients with pelvic masses: Discrimination of benign from malignant disease. Am J Obstet Gynecol 15:314–316, 1988.

McCaughey WTE, Schryer MJP, Lin X, Al-Jabi M. Extraovarian pelvic serous tumor with marked calcification. Arch Pathol Lab Med 110:78–80, 1986.

McGarvey RN. Cytologic diagnosis of ovarian cancer: Report of case, review of literature. Obstet Gynecol 5:257–261, 1955.

McGowan L, Stein DB, Miller W. Cul-de-sac aspiration for diagnostic cytologic study. Am J Obstet Gynecol 96:413–417, 1966.

McMurray EH, Jacobs AJ, Perez CA, et al. Carcinoma of the fallopian tube. Cancer 58:2070–2075, 1986.

Michael H, Roth LM. Invasive and noninvasive implants in ovarian serous tumors of low malignant potential. Cancer 57:1240–1247, 1986.

Mills SE, Andersen WA, Fechner RE, Austin MB. Serous surface papillary carcinoma. A clinicopathologic study of 10 cases and comparison with stage III–IV ovarian serous carcinoma. Am J Surg Pathol 12:827–834, 1988.

Mizrak B, Elkinci C. Cytologic diagnosis of yolk sac tumor. Acta Cytol 39:936–940, 1995.

Momtazee S, Kempson RL. Primary adenocarcinoma of the fallopian tube. Obstet Gynecol 32:649–656, 1968.

Moore WF, Bentley RC, Berchuck A, et al. Some müllerian inclusion cysts in lymph nodes may sometimes be metastases from serous borderline tumors of the ovary. Am J Surg Pathol 24:710–718, 2000.

Morimoto N, Ozawa M, Amano S. Diagnostic value of hyaline globules in endodermal sinus tumor: Report of two cases. Acta Cytol 25:417–420, 1981.

Mulvany N, Ostor A, Teng G. Evaluation of estradiol in aspirated ovarian cystic lesions. Acta Cytol 39:663–668, 1995.

Mulvany NJ. Aspiration cytology of ovarian cysts and cystic neoplasms. A study of 235 aspirates. Acta Cytol 40:911–920, 1996.

Mulvany NJ, Allan P. Choroidal cells in ovarian cyst fluid: a case report. Acta Cytol 40:302–306, 1996.

Nadji M, Greening SE, Sevin B-U, et al. Fine needle aspiration cytology in gynecologic oncology. II. Morphologic aspects. Acta Cytol 23:380–388, 1979.

Narod SA, Risch H, Moslehi R, et al. Oral contraceptives and the risk of hereditary ovarian cancer. N Engl J Med 339:424–428, 1998.

Nestler JE, Jakubowicz DJ, Evans WS, Pasquali R. Effects of metformin on spontaneous and clomiphene-induced ovulation in the polycystic ovary syndrome. N Engl J Med 338:1876–1880, 1998.

Nguyen HN, Averette HE, Janicek MSO. Ovarian carcinoma. A review of the significance of familial risk factors and the role of prophylactic oophorectomy in cancer prevention. Cancer 74:545–555, 1994.

Niloff JM, Knapp RC, Lavin PT, et al. Prognosis of granulosa-theca tumors of the ovary. Cancer 21:255–263, 1968.

Nordin AJ. Primary carcinoma of the fallopian tube: a 20-year literature review. Obstet Gynecol Surv 49:349–361, 1994.

Parkash V, Chacho MS. Psammoma bodies in cervicovaginal smears: Incidence and significance. Diagn Cytopathol 26:81–86, 2002.

Petricoin EF, Ardekani AM, Hitt BA, et al. Use of proteomic patterns in serum to identify ovarian cancer. Lancet 359:572–577, 2002.

Picoff RC, Meeker CI. Psammoma bodies in the cervicovaginal smear in association with benign papillary structures of the ovary. Acta Cytol 14:45–47, 1970.

Pins MR, Young RH, Daly WJ, Scully RE. Primary squamous cell carcinoma of the ovary: Report of 37 cases. Am J Surg Pathol 20:823–833, 1996.

Pinto MM, Bernstein LH, Parikh F, Lavy G. Measurement of CA 125, carcinoembryonic antigen, and alpha-fetoprotein in ovarian cyst fluid: diagnostic adjunct to cytology. Diagn Cytopathol 6:160–163, 1990.

Pinto MM, Greenebaum E, Simsir A, et al. CA-125 and carcinoembryonic antigen assay vs. cytodiagnostic experience in the classification of benign ovarian cysts. Acta Cytol 5:1456–1462, 1997.

Plaxe SC, Deligdisch L, Dottino PR, Cohen CJ. Ovarian intraepithelial neoplasia demonstrated in patients with stage I ovarian carcinoma. Gynecol Oncol 38:367–372, 1990.

Podratz KC, Podczaski ES, Gaffey TA, et al. Primary carcinoma of the fallopian tube. Am J Obstet Gynecol 154:1319–1326, 1986.

Prade M, Spatz A, Bentley R, et al. Borderline and malignant serous tumor arising in pelvic lymph nodes: Evidence of origin in benign glandular inclusions. Int J Gynecol Pathol 14:87–91, 1995.

Prat J. Ovarian tumors of borderline malignancy (tumors of low malignant potential): A critical appraisal. Adv Anat Pathol 6:247–274, 1999.

Qazi FM, Geisinger KR, Barrett RJ, et al. Cervicovaginal psammoma bodies. The initial presentation of the ovarian borderline tumor. Arch Pathol Lab Med 112:564–566, 1988.

Rai AJ, Zhang Z, Rosenzweig J, et al. Proteomic approaches to tumor marker discovery. Identification of biomarkers for ovarian cancer. Arch Pathol Lab Med 126:1518–1526, 2002.

Rakoff A. Vaginal cytology of endocrinopathies. Acta Cytol 5:153–167, 1961.

Resta L, Sabatini R, Restaino A. Ovarian dysgerminoma: A clinicopathologic study. Neoplasma 31:459–464, 1984.

Rivasi F, Gasser B, Morandi P, Philippe E. Ciliated bodies in ovarian cyst aspirates. Acta Cytol 37:489–493, 1993.

Robboy SJ, Scully RE. Ovarian teratoma with glial implants on the peritoneum. An analysis of 12 cases. Hum Pathol 1:643–653, 1970.

Roncalli M, Gribaudi G, Simoncelli D, Servida E. Cytology of yolk-sac tumor of the ovary in ascitic fluid. Acta Cytol 32:113–116, 1988.

Ronnett BM, Shmookler BM, Diener-West M, et al. Immunohistochemical evidence supporting the appendiceal origin of pseudomyxoma peritonei in women. Int J Gynecol Pathol 16:1–9, 1997A.

Ronnett BM, Shmookler BM, Sugarbaker PH, Kurman RJ. Pseudomyxoma peritonea: new concepts in diagnosis, origin, nomenclature, and relationship to mucinous borderline (low malignant potential) tumors of the ovary. Anat Pathol 2:197–226, 1997B.

Rosenblum NG, LiVolsi VA, Edmonds PR, Mikuta JJ. Malignant struma ovarii. Gynecol Oncol 32:224–227, 1989.

Rubenchik I, Auger M, Casper RF. Fine-needle aspiration cytology of ovarian cysts in in vitro fertilization patients: a study of 125 cases. Diagn Cytopathol 15:341–344, 1996.

Rubin DK, Frost JK. The cytologic detection of ovarian cancer. Acta Cytol 7:191–195, 1963.

Rubin SC, Benjamin I, Behbakht K, et al. Clinical and pathological features of ovarian cancer in women with germ-line mutations of BRCA1. N Engl J Med 335:1413–1416, 1996.

Runnebaum IB, Stickeler E. Epidemiological and molecular aspects of ovarian cancer risk. J Cancer Res Clin Oncol 127:73–79, 2001.

Salazar H, Godwin AK, Daly MB, et al. Microscopic benign and invasive malignant neoplasms and a cancer-prone phenotype in prophylactic oophorectomies. J Natl Cancer Inst 88:1810–1820, 1996.

Sampson JA. Postsalpingectomy endometriosis (endosalpingiosis). Am J Obstet Gynecol 20:443–480, 1930.

Schenck SB, Mackles A. Primary carcinoma of fallopian tubes with positive smears. Am J Obstet Gynecol 81:782–783, 1961.

Schuldenfrei R, Janovski NA. Disseminated endosalpingiosis associated with bilateral papillary serous cystadenocarcinoma of the ovaries: A case report. Am J Obstet Gynecol 84:382–389, 1962.

Schwinn CP, Bernstein GS, Willie S. Culdocentesis. *In* Wied GL, Koss LG, Reagan JW (eds). Compendium on Diagnostic Cytology, 6th ed. Chicago, Tutorials of Cytology, 1988.

Scully RE, Mark EJ, McNeely WF, et al. Case Records of the Massachusetts General Hospital: Case 39–1997. N Engl J Med 337:1829–1837, 1997.

Scully RE, Mark EJ, McNeely WF, et al. Case Records of the Massachusetts General Hospital: Case 3–1998. N Engl J Med 338:248–254, 1998.

Scully RE, Mark EJ, McNeely WF, et al. Case Records of the Massachusetts General Hospital: Case 14–1999. N Engl J Med 340:1491–1497, 1999.

Scully RE, Mark EJ, McNeely WF, McNeely BU. Case Records of the Massachusetts General Hospital: Case 13–1995. N Engl J Med 332:1153–1159, 1995.

Scully RE, Young RH, Clement PB. Tumors of the ovary, maldeveloped gonads, fallopian tube, and broad ligament. Atlas of Tumor Pathology. Third Series. Fascicle 23. Washington DC, AFIP, 1998, 51–168.

Sedlis A. Primary carcinoma of the fallopian tube. Obstet Gynecol Surv 16: 209–226, 1961.

Seidman JD, Sherman ME, Bell KA, et al. Salpingitis, salpingoliths, and serous tumors of the ovaries: Is there a connection? Int J Gynecol Pathol 21: 101–107, 2002.

Selvaggi SM (ed). Guides to Clinical Aspiration Biopsy. Female Pelvic Organs. Baltimore, Williams and Wilkins, 1996.

Selvaggi SM. Fine needle aspiration cytology of ovarian follicle cysts with cellular atypia from reproductive-age patients. Diagn Cytopathol 7:189–192, 1991.

Shingleton HM, Middleton FF, Gore H. Squamous cell carcinoma of the ovary. Am J Obstet Gynecol 120:556–560, 1974.

Silverberg SG. Ultrastructure and histogenesis of clear cell carcinoma of the ovary. Am J Obstet Gynecol 115:394–400, 1973.

Sneige N, Fernandez T, Copeland LJ, Katz RL. Muellerian inclusions in peritoneal washings. Potential source of error in peritoneal washings. Acta Cytol 30:271–276, 1986.

Sommers SC, Long ME. Ovarian carcinoma: Pathology, staging, grading and prognosis. Bull NY Acad Med 49:858–869, 1973.

Song YS. The cytological diagnosis of carcinoma of the fallopian tube. Am J Obstet Gynecol 70:29–33, 1955.

Spencer TR Jr, Marks RD Jr, Fenn JO, Jenrette JM, Lutz MH. Intraperitoneal P-32 after negative second-look laparotomy in ovarian carcinoma. Cancer 63:2434–2437, 1989.

Stanley MW, Horowitz CA, Frable WJ. Cellular follicular cyst of the ovary: Fluid cytology mimicking malignancy. Diagn Cytol 7:48–52, 1991.

Stoler MH. Prophylactic surgical pathology. Am J Surg Pathol 26:257–259, 2002.

Szych C, Staebler A, Connolly DC, et al. Molecular genetic evidence supporting the clonality and appendiceal origin of pseudomyxoma peritonei in women. Am J Pathol 6:1849–1855, 1999.

Szyfelbein WM, Young RH, Scully RE. Adenoma malignum of cervix. Cytologic findings. Acta Cytol 28:691–698, 1984.

Takashina T, Ito E, Kudo R. Cytologic diagnosis of primary tubal cancer. Acta Cytol 29:367–372, 1985.

Takashina T, Ona M, Kanda Y, et al. Cervicovaginal and endometrial cytology in ovarian cancer. Acta Cytol 32:159–162, 1988.

Takeshima N, Hirai Y, Yamauchi K, Hasumi K. Clinical usefulness of endometrial aspiration cytology and CA-125 in the detection of fallopian tube carcinoma. Acta Cytol 41:1445–1450, 1997.

Tan LK, Flynn SD, Carcangiu ML. Ovarian serous borderline tumors with lymph node involvement: Clinicopathologic and DNA content study of seven cases and review of the literature. Am J Surg Pathol 18:904–912, 1994.

Teilum G. Special Tumors of Ovary and Testis and Related Extragonadal Lesions. Copenhagen, Einar Munksgaard, 1971.

Thirumala SD, Putti TC, Medalie NS, Wasserman PG. Skeletal metastases from a granulosa-cell tumor of the ovary: report of a case diagnosed by fine-needle aspiration cytology. Diagn Cytopathol 19:375–377, 1998.

Valicenti JF, Priester SK. Psammoma bodies of benign endometrial origin in cervicovaginal cytology. Acta Cytol 21:550–552, 1977.

Van Nagell JR, DePriest PD, Reedy MB, et al. The efficacy of transvaginal sonographic screening in asymptomatic women at risk for ovarian cancer. Gynecol Oncol 77:350–356, 2000.

Wachtel E. The cytology of tumors of the ovary and fallopian tube. Clin Obstet Gynecol 4:1159–1171, 1961.

Webb MJ, Decker DG, Mussey E. Cancer metastatic to the ovary. Obstet Gynecol 45:391–396, 1975.

Weir MM, Bell DA, Young RH. Grade 1 peritoneal serous carcinomas: A report of 14 cases and comparison with 7 peritoneal serous psammocarcinomas and 19 peritoneal serous borderline tumors. Am J Surg Pathol 22:849–862, 1998.

Werness BA, Eltabbakh GH. Ovarian dysplasia identified by cul-de-sac aspiration: A reexamination of previously reported cases [Letter to the Editor]. Int J Gynecol Pathol 19:190–192, 2000.

Yang GCH. Fine-needle aspiration cytology of Schiller-Duval bodies of yolk-sac tumor. Diagn Cytopathol 23:228–232, 2000.

Yang GC, Mesia AF. Fine-needle aspiration cytology of malignant fibrothecoma of the ovary. Diagn Cytopathol 21:284–286, 1999.

Yee H, Greenebaum E, Lerner J, et al. Transvaginal sonographic characterization combined with cytologic evaluation in the diagnosis of ovarian and adnexal cysts. Diagn Cytopathol 10:107–112, 1994.

Young RH, Gilks CB, Scully RE. Mucinous tumors of the appendix associated with mucinous tumors of the ovary and pseudomyxoma peritonei: A clinicopathological analysis of 22 cases supporting an origin in the appendix. Am J Surg Pathol 15:415–429, 1991.

Young RH, Hart WR. Metastatic intestinal carcinomas simulating primary ovarian clear cell carcinoma and secretory endometrioid carcinoma. A clinicopathologic and immunohistochemical study of five cases. Am J Surg Pathol 22:805–815, 1998.

Young RH, Oliva E, Scully RE. Small cell carcinoma of the ovary, hypercalcemic type: A clinicopathologic analysis of 150 cases. Am J Surg Pathol 18: 1102–1116, 1994.

Young RH, Welch WR, Dickersin GR, Scully RE. Ovarian sex cord tumor with annular tubules. Review of 74 cases including 27 with Peutz-Jeghers syndrome and four with adenoma malignum of the cervix. Cancer 50:1384–1402, 1982.

Zervakis M, Howdon WM, Howdon A. Cul-de-sac needle aspiration: its normal and abnormal cytology and its value in the detection of ovarian cancer. Acta Cytol 13:507–514, 1969.

Zhang L, Conejo-Garcia JR, Katsaros D, et al. Intratumoral T cells, recurrence, and survival in epithelial ovarian cancer. N Engl J Med 348:203–213, 2003.

Zinsser KR, Wheeler JE. Endosalpingiosis in the omentum: A study of autopsy and surgical material. Am J Surg Pathol 6:109–117, 1982.

Peritoneal Washings or Lavage in Cancers of the Female Genital Tract

Cytologic sampling of **fluid from the peritoneal cavity** or, more specifically, from the pelvic cul-de-sac (pouch of Douglas), at the time of surgery was first proposed for ovarian tumors by Keettel and Pixley (1958). **The purpose of the procedure was to improve the staging of these tumors.** In 1958, Keettel and Pixley published preliminary results indicating that this procedure may provide **evidence of spread of ovarian cancer in the absence of visible lesions.** In 1986, this concept was incorporated into the official **staging of ovarian cancer** by the International Federation of Gynecology and Obstetrics (FIGO), shown in Table 15-2.

This staging system attributes an important diagnostic role to the cytologic examination of ascitic and peritoneal fluids: the presence of cancer cells modifies the staging of ovarian tumors from stages Ia or Ib to Ic and from IIa and IIb to IIc. The higher staging calls for a different approach to treatment with the recognition that surgery alone is not likely to be curative of the disease. In current practice the aspiration of pelvic fluid is often supplemented by washings of the cul-de-sac, the fluids being submitted for cytologic examination. Additional data on cytology of ascitic and pleural fluids in ovarian cancer are provided in Chapter 26.

The principal applications of pelvic peritoneal lavage are:

■ Staging of ovarian, and, somewhat less commonly, other gynecologic cancers
■ Securing evidence of persisting or recurring cancer during the second-look surgical procedures
■ Occasional discovery of occult cancer during exploratory laparotomies or laparoscopies for benign disease
■ Incidental discovery of metastatic cancer from nongynecologic sites

SECURING AND PROCESSING THE SPECIMEN

McGowen et al (1966) advocated the **aspiration of accumulated peritoneal fluid** as the first step upon surgical entry into the abdominal cavity, using a laryngeal cannula with a blunted end, attached to a syringe. A **washing or lavage** of the pelvic peritoneum can be performed using small amounts of normal saline solution or similar fluid that can be repeatedly instilled and reaspirated. If the fluid cannot be processed by the laboratory without delay, the addition of a fixative is recommended (see Chap. 44). **Cul-**

docentesis, an aspiration of pelvic peritoneal fluid across the vaginal wall, may be used for the same purposes. Aspirations may also be performed by skilled operators at the time of a **laparoscopy.** Luesley et al (1990) advocated the use of **direct scrapings or brushings** of the peritoneal surfaces as superior to lavage specimens. We do not have any experience with this technique.

The processing of peritoneal aspirates or lavage samples calls for centrifugation of the specimen and preparation of smears or cytospin preparations, as described in Chapter 44. In our experience the use of **cell blocks** supplementing smears is often diagnostically helpful. Poorly preserved specimens of peritoneal fluid, submitted without fixative after a substantial delay, or unfixed smears prepared by inexperienced personnel may be difficult to interpret. In this type of material, overstained and poorly preserved mesothelial cells may be mistaken for cancer cells. The risk of a false-positive diagnosis in such cases is substantial.

CYTOLOGY OF PERITONEAL LAVAGE

Benign Cells and Conditions

The principal benign cellular components of peritoneal fluids are mesothelial cells, macrophages, leukocytes, and epithelial cells or cell fragments derived from the peritoneal lining and various benign cysts and other structures. The fluids may also contain **"collagen balls,"** described by Wojcik and Naylor (1992), calcified debris and, occasionally, psammoma bodies.

Mesothelial Cells

The principal characteristics of mesothelial cells are described in great detail in Chapter 25. In the context of the peritoneal fluid, the mesothelial cells are fairly easy to recognize when well preserved: the cells are of medium size, comparable to small parabasal squamous cells, and have a generally basophilic, delicate cytoplasm, wherein the outer zone is often lighter than the inner, perinuclear zone (Fig. 16-1A). However, depending on the technique used in processing the material and speed of fixation, the mesothelial cells may **vary in size** and staining properties among specimens. When in **flat sheets,** the mesothelial cells are often separated from each other by narrow clear gaps or "windows" (Fig. 16-1B,C). Sometimes, **long strips of mesothelial cells,** forcibly removed from their setting, may be observed in cell blocks (Fig. 16-1D). The cells have **central, round, but sometimes slightly indented nuclei,** occasionally containing visible **small nucleoli** (Fig. 16-1A,B). The presence of nucleoli may be

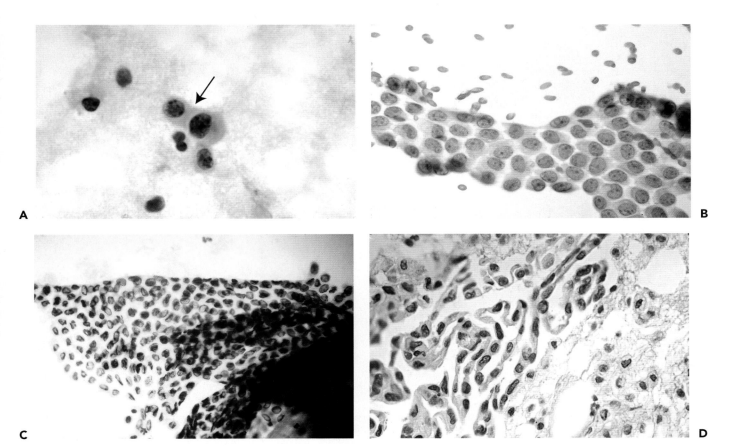

A

B

C

D

Figure 16-1 **Pelvic washings: mesothelial cells.** *A.* Isolated mesothelial cells with approximately spherical nuclei and tiny nucleoli. A gap or "window" (*arrow*) may be seen between the two cells in the center. *B.* Sheet of mesothelial cells in pelvic lavage. Note the uniform appearance of the nuclei, each containing a small nucleolus. The gaps or "windows" among the cells are well shown. *C.* A very large sheet of mesothelial cells in peritoneal lavage. *D.* A cell block of pelvic lavage corresponding to *C* showing strips of benign mesothelium.

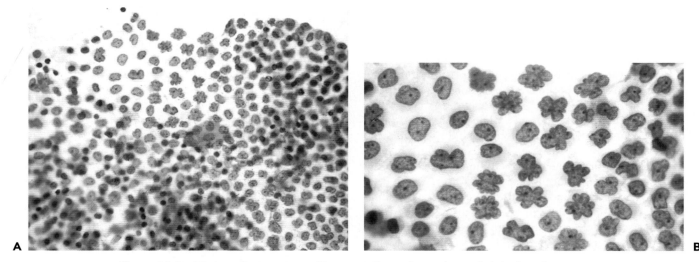

Figure 16-2   "Daisy cells" in peritoneal lavage. *A.* Sheet of normal mesothelial cells with transition to cells showing multiple nuclear indentations, rendering them similar to daisies. *B.* High-power view of daisy cells. (Courtesy of Dr. W.-K. Ng, Pamela Youde Nethesole Eastern Hospital, Hong Kong, China.)

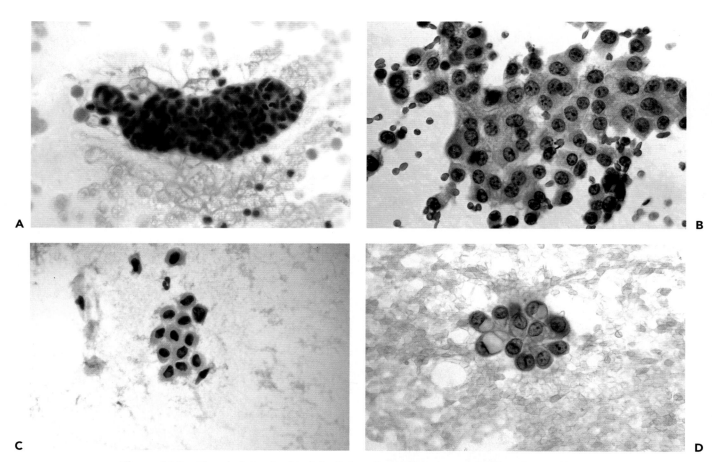

Figure 16-3   **Mesothelial and epithelial cells in peritoneal lavage.** *A.* A papillary cluster of benign mesothelial cells, mimicking adenocarcinoma. Note the monotonous makeup of the benign cluster. *B.* A sheet of mesothelial cells showing gaps or "windows" between the cells and the presence of small nucleoli. *C,D.* Sheets of benign epithelial cells in cul-de-sac lavage. In *C,* the cells are somewhat similar to mesothelial cells, except for angulated cytoplasm. *D.* Small papillary cluster of benign epithelial cells, some showing cytoplasmic vacuolization. The nuclei are small, each containing a tiny nucleolus.

troublesome to an inexperienced observer, who may confuse such cells with cancer cells; the fairly monotonous size of the mesothelial cells and their nuclei should prevent the erroneous diagnosis. Through the courtesy of Dr. Wai-Kuen Ng of the Pamela Youde Nethersole Eastern Hospital in Hong Kong, I was privileged to see a very unusual variant of mesothelial cells in peritoneal washings characterized by **lobulated nucleus.** The term **"daisy cells"** has been appended to these cells, which were apparently observed before in peritoneal washings. A transition between normal mesothelial cells and **"daisy cells"** is shown in Figure 16-2. Such cells have not been observed by us in any other fluid and, hence, appear to be a unique feature of peritoneal mesothelial cells.

It is not uncommon, however, to see mesothelial cells in large, densely packed sheets wherein the individual cells are difficult to study (Fig. 16-3A,B). As a rule, **the diagnosis of cancer should not be made unless the characteristics of cells and their nuclei can be studied in detail;** the thick sheets or dense clusters of mesothelial cells are no exception to this rule.

Benign Epithelial Cells

Benign epithelial cells of various types may be observed in peritoneal washings, especially after a vigorous irrigation. These may represent a variety of structures, from ruptured **benign inclusion cysts,** commonly found on the surfaces of tubes and ovaries, foci of **endosalpingiosis** and **endometriosis,** or benign **ciliated tubal epithelium.** The cells may be of **cuboidal or columnar configuration** (Figs. 16-3C,D and 16-4A,B) and may appear singly or may form sheets or even papillary clusters, composed of small cuboidal or columnar cells with **inconspicuous nuclei and nucleoli.** Some of the cells **may be ciliated.** Detached **ciliated tufts of tubal origin** may also be observed (Poropatich and Ehya, 1986). Sidawy et al (1987) correlated the presence of the ciliated tufts with stages of menstrual cycle and observed them only in the secretory stage (Fig. 16-4C,D).

Leukocytes and Macrophages

In **"first look"** specimens and in the absence of cancer, the leukocytes are usually few in number, **except in the presence of an inflammatory process.** In the latter condition, macrophages accompanied by leukocytes of various types, fibrin and necrotic material may be observed. Cancerous processes may also be accompanied by an inflammatory reaction. In **"second look"** procedures, a marked inflammatory reaction is often present (see below).

Macrophages may vary in size: most are mononucleated

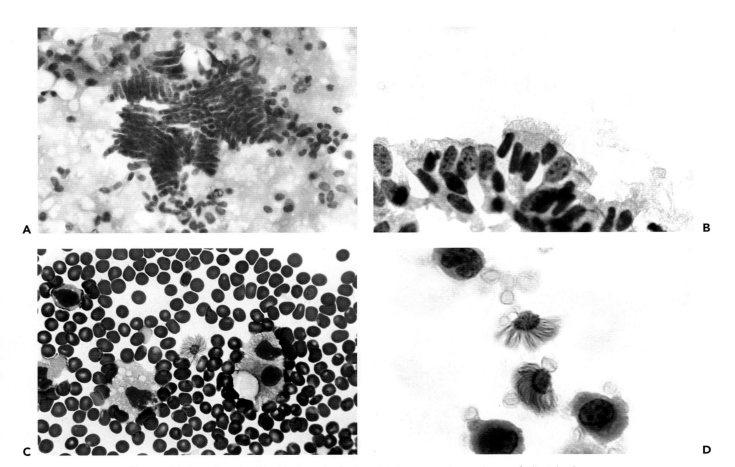

Figure 16-4   Ciliated cells and ciliated tufts in pelvic lavage. A. Large sheets of ciliated columnar cells representing epithelial lining of the fallopian tubes. B. High-power view of a cluster similar to that shown in A showing cilia on the surface of the cells. C,D. Isolated ciliated tufts in pelvic lavage. The details of the tufts are well shown at oil immersion magnification in D. (C,D photographs courtesy Dr. Mary Sidawy, George Washington University, Washington DC.)

cells, **comparable in size to mesothelial cells,** but having **finely vacuolated cytoplasm** and **peripheral, spherical or kidney-shaped nuclei** of similar size. **Large cytoplasmic vacuoles** may occur, pushing the nucleus to the periphery. Evidence of **phagocytosis** in the form of ingested particles of pigment, such as hemosiderin, helps in the identification of these cells, although sometimes cancer cells are also capable of phagocytosis. Macrophages may also form large, either **mono- or multinucleated giant cells;** the latter are commonly observed in patients with chronic inflammatory processes or as a reaction to foreign bodies, such as powder, usually observed after a surgical intervention. Macrophages are more common in "second look" procedures.

Collagen Balls

Under this term, Wojcik and Naylor (1992) analyzed the frequency and origin of peculiar **homogenous structures, lined by a single layer of cuboidal cells** that may be observed in about 5% of pelvic fluids and lavage specimens (Fig. 16-5A,B). In one such case, the structures could be traced to small collagenous excrescences on the surface of an ovary, hence, the conclusion that the small cuboidal cells represent ovarian epithelium. We have observed the collagen balls in **benign and malignant peritoneal lavage specimens** and, therefore, they have no diagnostic significance.

Foreign, Plant, and Ganglion Cells

During cul-de-sac aspirations performed with a needle-syringe system, a loop of bowel may be inadvertently penetrated. **Epithelial cells of intestinal origin or** bowel contents in the form of **plant cells** may be observed. The **enteric cells** are usually columnar and may occur in large clusters. The **plant cells** may be identified by a thick, transparent cellulose wall and fine, refractile cytoplasmic granules (see Chapters 8 and 19). Rare findings in aspirates include **large ganglion cells,** with abundant granular cytoplasm and peripheral nuclei, inadvertently removed from presacral ganglia (Fig. 16-5C,D).

Endometriosis

In abdominal endometriosis two types of cells may be seen side by side: **small cuboidal or columnar epithelial cells, usually in small sheets,** and, very rarely, very small, spindly stromal cells; these cells are usually accompanied by **hemosiderin-laden macrophages.** An iron stain may be occasionally helpful in establishing the diagnosis (see Chap. 34). Stowell et al (1997) examined the accuracy of cytologic examination of peritoneal fluids in the diagnosis of endometriosis and concluded that the identification of epithelial cells of endometrial origin is difficult but that the presence

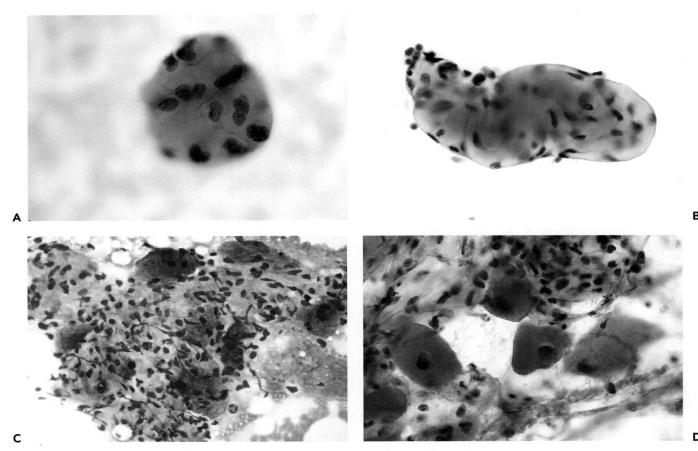

Figure 16-5 **Collagen balls and ganglion cells.** *A,B.* Collagen balls are sharply demarcated fragments of a homogeneous substance surrounded by a few small epithelial cells. *C,D.* Low- and high-power view of ganglion cells inadvertently aspirated in peritoneal lavage. *C.* DiffQuik.

of hemosiderin-laden macrophages should alert the pathologist to the possibility of this disorder.

Endosalpingiosis

In endosalpingiosis the fluids are characterized by the presence of **calcified debris and psammoma bodies that can be numerous,** and are sometimes surrounded by inconspicuous, small, benign epithelial cells (Fig. 16-6; see also Fig. 15-7). Psammoma bodies may also occur within fragments of glandular structures or surrounded by inflammatory exudate and cell debris (Fig. 16-6C).

In incidental biopsies, **small cystic structures,** lined by cuboidal, occasionally ciliated, epithelial cells and containing calcified debris or psammoma bodies, may be observed on the surface of the fallopian tubes, the ovaries, and elsewhere in the peritoneum (see Fig. 15-7). For a discussion on the possible relationship of endosalpingiosis to psammocarcinoma, see Chapter 15.

The presence of psammoma bodies in peritoneal lavage may be perplexing, particularly in the presence of ovarian abnormalities that may be unrelated to the cytologic findings (Sidawy and Silverberg, 1987). In general, **psammoma bodies or calcified debris observed in peritoneal washings, do not have the same diagnostic significance as in vaginal and cervical material** (see Chap. 15) or in effusions (see Chap. 26) **and, unless accompanied by cancer cells, should be interpreted with great caution.** Focal calcium deposits, not uncommon in the peritoneum, may be dislodged by vigorous lavage and may mimic psammoma bodies.

Diagnostic Problems in the Absence of Cancer

Ravinsky (1986), Zuna and Mitchell (1988), and Zuna et al (1989) presented comprehensive reviews of their experiences with peritoneal lavage. In the absence of cancer, **benign ovarian cysts and endometriosis** presented significant diagnostic dilemmas. Zuna and Mitchell (1988) recorded diagnostic difficulties in 12% of 149 benign peritoneal washings. In my experience, besides atypical mesothelial cells and, rarely, atypical epithelial cells, **endosalpingiosis is the most common source of diagnostic difficulty,** particularly if there is an association of psammoma bodies with sheets of epithelial cells. Selvaggi (2003) recommended the use of cell blocks and immunostains in difficult cases. Sams et al (1990) reported an exceedingly rare case of **ectopic pancreas** that shed cells mistaken for cancer cells.

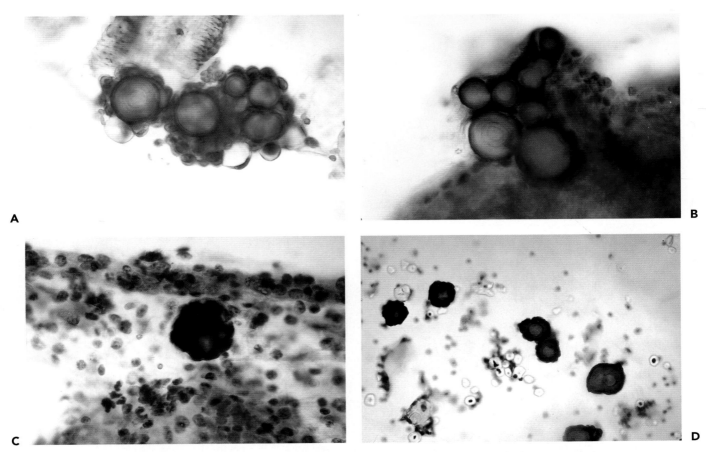

Figure 16-6   Endosalpingiosis in peritoneal lavage. *A.* A cluster of psammoma bodies surrounded by a layer of small epithelial cells. In *B,* the psammoma bodies are superimposed upon each other. *C.* Psammoma bodies surrounded and accompanied by sheets of epithelial cells. *D.* Isolated, calcified psammoma bodies from a case of endosalpingiosis. (*A,B* case courtesy of Dr. F. Bonetti, Verona, Italy.)

PERITONEAL LAVAGE IN OVARIAN CANCER

"First Look"

The most common indication for peritoneal washings is **staging or upstaging of ovarian carcinomas.** Usually, but not always, cancer cells stand out as a different population of cells, easily separated from benign cells.

Serous Adenocarcinomas

Malignant cells most often observed in peritoneal washings are derived from fully developed carcinomas of the serous type. Such cells occur **singly** and in **structured, approximately spherical clusters.** The cytoplasm is usually delicate and finely vacuolated. The dominant feature of these cells is **nuclear abnormalities, such as nuclear enlargement, irregular nuclear configuration and the presence of prominent, often multiple nucleoli** (Fig. 16-7). Such malignant cells may be occasionally confused with benign mesothelial or epithelial cells which, however, are usually much smaller. **Papillary clusters of cancer cells with nuclear hyperchromasia,** of the type commonly observed in cells of ovarian cancer in cervicovaginal material (see above),

are less common but may occur (Fig. 16-8A,B). **A central core of connective tissue may be sometimes observed in the papillary clusters,** a feature that is usually better seen in cell block preparations (Fig. 16-7B). **Psammoma bodies** may occur, but, unless accompanied by cancer cells, have limited diagnostic value, as discussed above (Fig. 16-7D).

Serous carcinomas of the peritoneum, some of which may be **occult,** shed large cohesive clusters of cancer cells (see Fig. 16-9C,D). For further discussion and examples of this entity, see Chapter 26.

The **low-grade (borderline) serous ovarian tumors** shed **atypical but not clearly cancerous epithelial cells, usually forming cohesive clusters** (see Fig. 15-11). The nuclear abnormalities are usually more modest than in high-grade carcinomas, specifically the **nucleoli are usually small and inconspicuous,** but in some cases the cells are similar to those of a well-differentiated serous carcinoma. Gurley et al (1994) compared by image analysis the nuclear features of borderline serous tumors with low-grade carcinomas. The borderline tumors displayed less nuclear pleomorphism and were diploid, whereas the carcinomas were aneuploid. This paper pointed out the difficulties of precise cytologic classification of the spectrum of well-differentiated

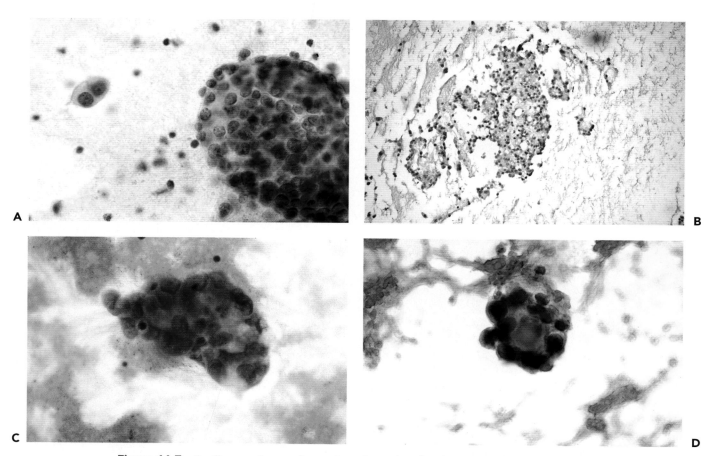

Figure 16-7 **Papillary carcinoma of ovary in peritoneal wash.** *A,B.* From the same case showing a large papillary cluster of malignant cells and dispersed malignant cells at the periphery of the cluster. *B.* Cell block showing the glandular structure of the tumor. *C.* Another example of serous carcinoma of ovary in cul-de-sac washings. The large cancer cells form a papillary cluster. Note the large nuclei and nucleoli. *D.* Psammoma body in a case of serous carcinoma in pelvic lavage. Note that the psammoma body is surrounded by large cancer cells with hyperchromatic nuclei.

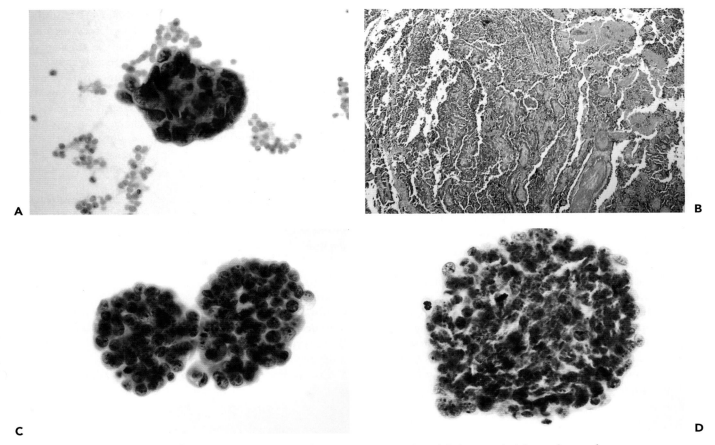

Figure 16-8 Ovarian and peritoneal serous carcinomas in pelvic lavage. *A.* A large cluster of cancer cells in pelvic lavage corresponding to the tumor shown in *B. C,D.* Large compact papillary clusters of cancer cells in a case of primary peritoneal serous carcinoma in pelvic lavage.

serous tumors in peritoneal lavage specimens, a point also stressed by Mulvany (1996).

Mucinous Carcinomas and Borderline Tumors

In the absence of obvious spread to the peritoneum, resulting in **pseudomyxoma peritonei** and accumulation of ascitic fluid (discussed in Chapter 26), these tumors are **practically never observed** in peritoneal lavage specimens. However, **late recurrences** of the tumors may occur and may be diagnosed in cytologic preparations. In such preparations, the malignant nature of the cells is unmistakable (see Fig. 15-12).

Endometrioid Carcinoma

The cytologic presentation of endometrioid ovarian carcinoma in peritoneal lavage **is identical to that of metastatic endometrial cancer,** discussed below.

Other ovarian tumor types may occasionally be encountered, and their identification depends on the make-up of the primary tumor. Ravinsky (1986) reported examples of **clear cell carcinoma of the ovary** (also observed by Mulvany, 1996), **malignant granulosa cell tumor** and a **malignant teratoma.**

Clinical Significance

Peritoneal samples showing evidence of **serous or endometrioid carcinoma** indicate either the **presence of the tumor on the surface of the ovary, or as a metastatic deposit on the peritoneal surfaces.** They may also indicate the existence of a **primary peritoneal tumor, a mimicker of serous carcinoma.** In Mulvany's experience (1996), approximately one half of 14 patients with serous carcinomas were **upgraded as a consequence of peritoneal lavage containing cancer cells.** However, this study was limited to lavages showing definite cancer cells and the author did not attempt to present the rate of false-negative lavages. In the experience of Mathew and Erozan (1997), upstaging of gynecologic cancer occurred in 12, or 3%, of 125 cancer cases.

In **borderline serous tumors,** the cytologic abnormalities in lavage specimens may indicate the presence of **peritoneal deposits that may be either invasive or noninvasive and this important prognostic difference cannot be determined in peritoneal lavage.** Cheng et al (1998) reviewed their experience with 90 patients with ovarian tumors of low malignant potential. In one third of these patients, cancer cells were observed in peritoneal lavage specimens, most often with tumors of serous type, less often with mucinous tumors. Positive cytology correlated well with the presence of peritoneal implants, regardless whether or not the implants were invasive. Gammon et al (1998) observed positive peritoneal washing results in four patients below the age of 25.

For further descriptive comments on ovarian cancer cells in fluids, see Chapter 26.

"Second Look"

Second-look procedures are performed in patients previously treated by surgery, radiotherapy, chemotherapy, or a combination thereof, to determine the presence of residual or recurrent ovarian cancers. **The purpose of the second-look procedure is to ascertain whether the disease has been eradicated, and hence whether or not the patient requires additional treatment.** At the time of the second-look procedure, it is customary to obtain multiple biopsies of any area of the peritoneum or mesentery that shows thickening or other changes suggestive of residual disease; the examination of the peritoneal fluid or washings is a part of this procedure.

If the cytologic examination of the peritoneal fluid in untreated patients is fraught with pitfalls, the difficulties are often increased in patients previously treated. The therapeutic regimens affect not only the residual cancer but also many of the benign structures, notably the mesothelium. Occasionally, acute or chronic inflammatory processes intervene, rendering the diagnostic process even more difficult.

To be sure, in some patients who failed to respond to therapy, **easily recognizable cancer cells may be observed** (Fig. 16-9A–C). Sagae et al (1988) suggested that in such cases quantitation of the malignant cells (comparing the initial sampling with the second sampling) may be of prognostic value.

In most patients, however, the **dominant cell population is benign mesothelial cells, showing effects of therapy.** Such cells may be **enlarged** and have a **thickened, often eosinophilic cytoplasm and proportionately enlarged nuclei, wherein prominent chromocenters or nucleoli may be present** (Fig. 16-9D). It is quite easy to confuse such cells with epithelial cancer cells. Sagae et al (1988) observed that mesothelial cell changes are more significant with the intraperitoneal use of alpha-2 interferon than with cisplatin. In my experience, however, any intensive radiotherapy or chemotherapeutic regimen can cause mesothelial cell abnormalities.

Another source of difficulty is the presence of **multinucleated and sometimes atypical macrophages.** With vigorous lavage, the **epithelial lining cells of ruptured benign peritoneal inclusion cysts** may contribute to the difficulty, especially if showing radiation changes (see Chapter 18).

Results

Coffin et al (1985) estimated that **diagnostic difficulties may occur in about one third of the second-look cases.** Biopsy evidence has shown that in many second-look procedures the residual cancer may be encased in foci of fibrosis, and hence not be accessible to peritoneal washings. Rubin and Frost (1963), on the basis of experience with 173 pa-

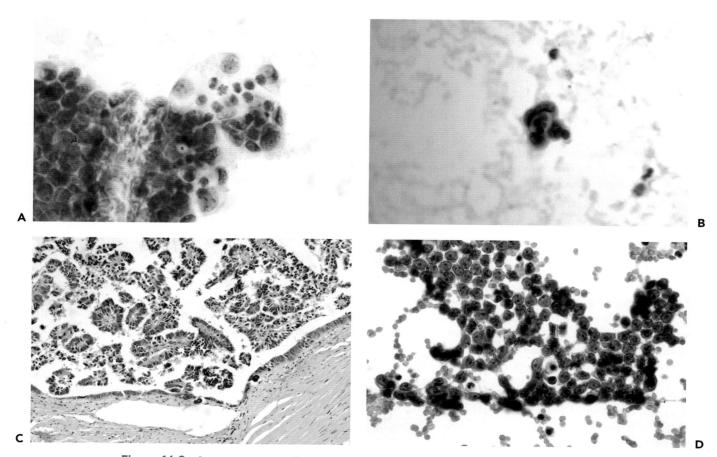

Figure 16-9   Serous carcinoma of ovary on "second look" pelvic lavage. *A,B.* Large cancer cells with hyperchromatic nuclei and large nucleoli corresponding to metastatic ovarian carcinoma in the jejunum shown in *C. D.* A fairly disorderly cluster of overstained mesothelial cells mimicking cells of serous carcinoma.

tients, reported failure of the cytologic procedure to diagnose residual carcinoma in 66% of patients with overt disease and in 78% of patients with microscopic foci of residual cancer. These results appear pessimistic. Zuna et al (1989) reported significantly better results, with a failure rate in only about 30% of patients with documented residual cancer. Kudo et al (1990) reported positive lavage results in 8 of 18 patients with documented residual disease and in 4 of 23 patients without residual disease. However, three of the four patients with allegedly "false-positive" results subsequently developed recurrent cancer and died of it. **It thus appears that the greatest value of the "second look" cytology is in an occasional detection of recurrences that escape the customary multi-biopsy evaluation.**

It is quite evident that the quality of the specimens, care in their preparation for cytologic study, and competence in the interpretation of the material may account for the variability of the results. Still, there is no evidence that the cytology of the peritoneal fluid in second-look surgical procedures can replace the standard multiple biopsies, though it may occasionally supplement them. To firmly establish the significance of pelvic lavage in these situations, a long-term follow-up study of patients after the "second look" procedure would be desirable.

PERITONEAL WASHINGS IN CANCERS OTHER THAN CANCER OF THE OVARY

Endometrial Carcinoma

The spread of endometrial cancers to the peritoneum of the cul-de-sac is probably more common than recognized so far. A particularly important culprit may be the relatively uncommon **serous papillary endometrial carcinoma** that may form metastases even if the primary tumor shows only superficial invasion of the myometrium. We have also observed several **adenoacanthomas** and **adenosquamous carcinomas** with relatively limited invasion of the myometrium and the presence of cancer cells in the peritoneal lavage.

Cytology

Endometrial **adenocarcinomas** can be recognized in lavage preparations as **clusters of malignant cells of various sizes, often of approximately spherical, papillary configuration,** very similar to serous ovarian cancer. The cytoplasm of these cells is usually delicate and sometimes vacuolated. The nuclei are usually large, hyperchromatic, of irregular contour, and provided with clearly visible but not particularly large nucleoli (Fig. 16-10). The **serous-papillary en-**

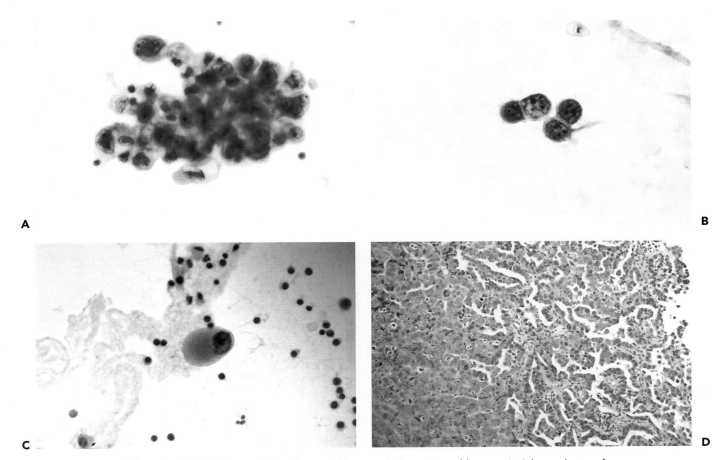

Figure 16-10 Endometrial carcinoma of low grade in peritoneal lavage. *A.* A large cluster of cancer cells with large, somewhat hyperchromatic nuclei and nucleoli. *B.* Doublets of cancer cells mimicking the arrangement of mesothelial cells. However, the nucleocytoplasmic ratio is modified in favor of the hyperchromatic, coarsely granular nuclei. *C.* A single cancer cell with an eccentrically located nucleus, containing nucleolus. *D.* Endometrial carcinoma, the source of cells seen in *A–C.*

dometrial carcinoma may shed cancer cells and cell clusters identical to those of serous ovarian carcinoma (Mesia et al, 1999). Single malignant cells have the same features as the cells in clusters. Sometimes, however, they are difficult to identify because of their similarity to atypical mesothelial cells and macrophages. **Similar cells are observed in ovarian endometrioid carcinomas.**

The **squamous component of adenoacanthomas and adenosquamous carcinomas** may have several different presentations. **Single squamous cancer cells** may be recognized within clusters of adenocarcinoma cells, or sometimes lying singly. As a general rule, these cells have **thick, sharply demarcated orange-staining cytoplasm** in a well-executed Papanicolaou stain. The **nuclei are sometimes large and hyperchromatic but more often are obliterated or seen as a pale nuclear outline ("ghost cells").** Occasionally irregularly contoured **sheets of keratin-forming cells** may occur (Fig. 16-11). In our experience, **the combination of cells of adenocarcinoma and squamous cells in peritoneal lavage occurs only in endometrial carcinomas.** So far, we have never seen this association in other tumors but one can think of several candidate tumors, such as ovarian adenoacanthomas and endocervical adenocarcinoma with a squamous component.

In a very large study of 298 women with endometrial carci-

noma, Gu et al (2000) compared positive peritoneal washings, observed in 32 patients with tumor type and stage. Ten percent of 262 patients with endometrioid carcinoma had positive washings, some with low stage and grade of disease. The frequency of positive washings for other tumor types (including serous carcinoma) was similar. The conclusions of the paper that positive peritoneal washing in endometrial cancer could not be correlated with stage, grade or histologic type of disease, is in keeping with several other studies cited in this paper and with personal experience.

Clinical Significance

Several publications on record suggest that the **presence of cancer cells in peritoneal lavage is of value in the prognosis of endometrial cancer, even of low stage and low grade** (Yazigi et al, 1983; Ide, 1984; Heath et al, 1988; Hirai et al, 1989; Mulvany, 1996; Zuna and Behrens, 1996). These authors reported increased mortality from endometrial cancer in the presence of cancer cells in the peritoneum. On the other hand, absence of cancer cells appears to be a favorable prognostic sign, although the rate of false negative examinations has not been established. Szpak et al (1981) correlated the number of malignant cells per 100 ml of washing fluid and documented a generally better response to therapy in patients with a low count of cancer

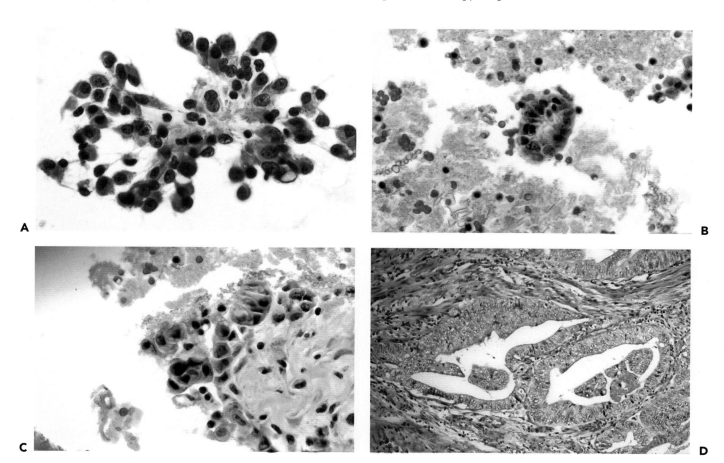

Figure 16-11 **Adenosquamous carcinoma of endometrium in peritoneal wash.** *A.* A large cluster of cancer cells with hyperchromatic nuclei. *B.* Cancer cells forming a glandular structure (cell block). *C.* Clusters of squamous cells in the same peritoneal wash. *D.* The adenoacanthoma in a 33-year-old woman, corresponding to cells shown in *A–C.* (Case courtesy of Dr. David Burstein, Mount Sinai Hospital, New York, NY.)

cells than in patients with a high count, although there were some exceptions.

However, several studies failed to attribute prognostic significance of positive peritoneal washings in stage I endometrial cancer (Lurain et al, 1989; Kadar et al, 1992; Gu et al, 2000). Still, there is little doubt that the procedure is desirable as part of a work-up of all patients with endometrial carcinoma. Still, a major follow-up study, taking into account response to therapy and long-term survival, may shed additional light on its clinical value.

Carcinomas of the Uterine Cervix

Peritoneal lavage in staging of squamous and adenocarcinomas of the uterine cervix has been the subject of several studies (Roberts et al, 1986; Morris et al, 1992; Patsner et al, 1992). A case of a small-cell, endocrine carcinoma was reported by Mulvany (1996). It is evident that **direct spread to the peritoneum occurs only in advanced, fully invasive carcinomas** and is not the preferred mode of spread of carcinoma of the cervix which tends to metastasize to lymph nodes.

Cytology
Cytologic findings depend on tumor type. **Well-differentiated squamous cancers of the cervix are virtually never observed in peritoneal lavage.** In **poorly differentiated squamous cancer,** the recognition of cancer cells is relatively easy. The cells occur singly and are characterized by **marked nuclear abnormalities and large nucleoli.** The presence of clusters of large, undifferentiated cancer cells usually corresponds to poorly differentiated squamous (epidermoid) carcinomas. In **adenocarcinomas,** clusters of **slender, columnar cancer cells** may be observed, sometimes forming **rosettes.** In the absence of clinical data it is virtually impossible to guess the origin of such cells that mimic any number of primary or metastatic tumors from various sites.

Results
Roberts et al (1986) studied peritoneal washings in 139 patients with invasive carcinoma of the uterine cervix. Positive cytologic findings generally reflected high-risk factors, such as high stage of disease. Morris et al (1992) and Patsner (1992) expressed significant reservations about the value of peritoneal lavage in cervical cancers, particularly of low stage.

Carcinoma of Fallopian Tubes

The significance of peritoneal washings in carcinoma of the fallopian tubes has been underestimated. We observed a case of **occult tubal carcinoma** first observed as brain metastasis,

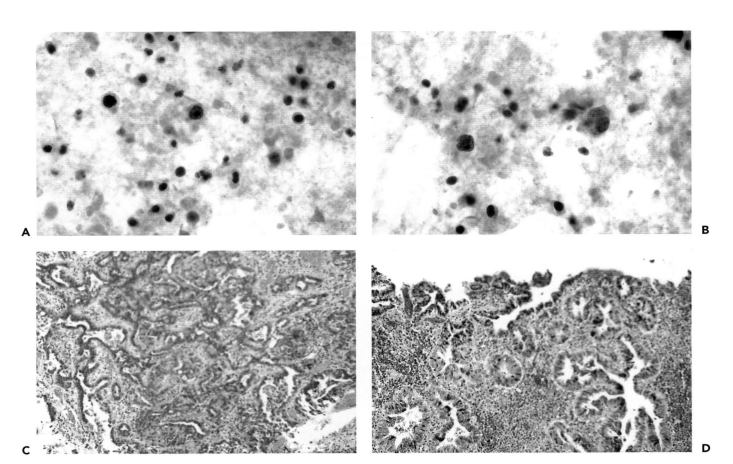

Figure 16-12 Tubal carcinoma with first clinical manifestation as a brain metastasis. *A,B.* Cancer cells of a fallopian tube carcinoma in peritoneal lavage obtained at the time of hysterectomy. *C.* Metastatic adenocarcinoma to the brain which was ultimately traced to the fallopian tube. *D.* Carcinoma in situ of the fallopian tube. The tumor was invasive elsewhere.

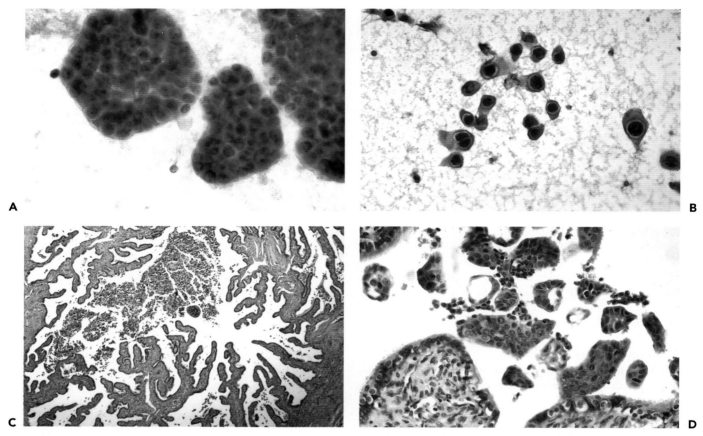

Figure 16-13 Metastatic mammary carcinoma in pelvic lavage 6 years after mastectomy. *A.* large papillary clusters of cancer cells. In *B*, the handful of cancer cells is dispersed. *C,D*. The presence of tumor cells within the lumen of the fallopian tube under low power in *C*, higher power in *D*. (Case courtesy of Dr. Belur Bhagavan, Baltimore, MD.)

with positive peritoneal washings prior to salpingo-oopho-rectomy (Fig. 16-12). Several such cases were described by Agoff et al (2002) in patients with BRCA1 and 2 gene mutations. Mulvany (1996) reported the presence of cancer cells in 5 cases of **tubal carcinoma,** two of them with **psammoma bodies.**

Other Primary Tumors

Geszler et al (1986) observed that the presence of cancer cells in stage I **mesodermal mixed tumors** (see Chap. 17) had a significant negative impact on prognosis. With growing experience other uncommon tumors of the female genital tract will be recognized in peritoneal lavage fluids.

Metastatic Cancers

Although uncommon, metastatic cancers from other sites may also be observed in peritoneal washings. In my experience, **mammary carcinoma is the most common offender,** although, other cancers are sometimes observed. Occasionally, the cancer cells reach the peritoneal cavity via the fallopian tubes and are discovered in peritoneal washings in the absence of visible metastases (Fig. 16-13). A case of metastatic melanoma of the vulva identified in peritoneal fluid was described by Izban et al (1999).

BIBLIOGRAPHY

Abu-Ghazaleh S, Johnston W, Creasman WT. The significance of peritoneal cytology in patients with carcinoma of the cervix. Gynecol Oncol 17: 139–148, 1984.

Agoff SN, Mendelin JE, Grieco VS, Garcia RL. Unexpected gynecologic neoplasms in patients with proven or suspected BRCA-1 or -2 mutations. Implications for gross examination, cytology, and clinical follow-up. Am J Surg Pathol 26:171–178, 2002.

Bell DA, Scully RE. Serous borderline tumors of the peritoneum. Am J Surg Pathol 14:230–239, 1990.

Bloch T, Davis TE Jr, Schwenk GR Jr. *Giardia lamblia* in peritoneal fluid. Acta Cytol 31:783–784, 1987.

Burmeister RE, Fechner RE, Franklin RR. Endosalpingiosis of the peritoneum. Obstet Gynecol 34:310–318, 1969.

Cheng L, Wolf NG, Rose PG, et al. Peritoneal washing cytology of ovarian tumors of low malignant potential: Correlation with surface ovarian involvement and peritoneal implants. Acta Cytol 42:1091–1094, 1998.

Chua KL, Hjerpe A. Human papillomavirus analysis as a prognostic marker following conization of the cervix uteri. Gynecol Oncol 66:108–113, 1997.

Coffin CM, Adcock LL, Dehner LP. The second-look operation of ovarian neoplasms: A study of 85 cases emphasizing cytologic and histologic problems. Int J Gynecol Pathol 4:97–109, 1985.

Covell JL, Carry JB, Feldman PS. Peritoneal washings in ovarian tumors. Potential sources of error in cytologic diagnosis. Acta Cytol 29:310–316, 1985.

Creasman WT, DiSaia PJ, Blessing J, et al. Prognostic significance of peritoneal cytology in patients with endometrial cancer and preliminary data concerning therapy with intraperitoneal radiopharmaceuticals. Am J Obstet Gynecol 141:921–929, 1981.

Creasman W, Rutledge F. The prognostic value of peritoneal cytology in gynecologic malignant disease. Am J Obstet Gynecol 110:773–781, 1971.

Dekmezian R, Sneige N, Ordonez NG. Ovarian and omental ependymomas in peritoneal washings: Cytologic and immunocytologic features. Diagn Cytopathol 2:62–68, 1986.

Gammon R, Hameed A, Keyhani-Rofagha S. Peritoneal washing in borderline epithelial ovarian tumors in women under 25: the use of cell block preparations. Diagn Cytopathol 18:212–214, 1998.

Geszler G, Szpak CA, Harris RE, et al. Prognostic value of peritoneal washings in patients with malignant mixed mullerian tumors of the uterus. Am J Obstet Gynecol 155:83–89, 1986.

Gu M, Shi W, Barakat RR, et al. Peritoneal washings in endometrial carcinoma. A study of 298 patients with histopathologic correlation. Acta Cytol 44: 783–789, 2000.

Gurley AM, Hidvegi DF, Cajulis RS, Bacus S. Morphologic and morphmetric features of low grade serous tumours of the ovary. Diagn Cythopathol 11: 220–225, 1994.

Heath R, Rosenman J, Varia M, Walton L. Peritoneal fluid cytology in endometrial cancer: Its significance and the role of chromic phosphate (32P) therapy. Int J Radiat Oncol Biol Phys 15:815–822, 1988.

Hirai Y, Fujimoto I, Yamauchi K, et al. Peritoneal fluid cytology and prognosis in patients with endometrial carcinoma. Obstet Gynecol 73:335–338, 1989.

Ide P. Prognostic value of peritoneal fluid cytology in patients with endometrial cancer stage I. Eur J Obstet Gynecol Reprod Biol 18:343–349, 1984.

Izban KF, Candel AG, Hsi ED, Salvaggi SM. Metastatic melanoma of the vulva identified by peritoneal fluid cytology. Diagn Cytopathol 20:152–155, 1999.

Johnson TL, Kumar NB, Hopkins M, Hughes JD. Cytologic features of ovarian tumors of low malignant potential in peritoneal fluids. Acta Cytol 32: 513–518, 1988.

Kadar N, Homesley HD, Malfetano JH. Positive peritoneal cytology is an adverse factor in endometrial carcinoma only if there is other evidence of extrauterine disease. Gynecol Oncol 46:145–149, 1992.

Keettel WC, Pixley E. Diagnostic value of peritoneal washings. Clin Obstet Gynecol 1:592–606, 1958.

Keettel WC, Pixley EE, Buchsbaum HJ. Experience with peritoneal cytology in the management of gynecologic malignancies. Am J Obstet Gynecol 120: 174–182, 1974.

Kern WH. Benign papillary structures with psammoma bodies in culdocentesis fluid. Acta Cytol 13:178–180, 1969.

Kudo R, Takashina T, Ito E, Mizuuchi H, et al. Peritoneal washing cytology at second-look laparotomy in cisplatin-treated ovarian cancer patients. Acta Cytol 34:545–548, 1990.

Kyle RA, Pierre RV, Bayrd ED. Multiple myeloma and acute leukemia associated with alkylating agents. Arch Int Med 135:185–192, 1975.

Luesley DM, Williams DR, Ward K, et al. Prospective comparative cytologic study of direct peritoneal smears and lavage fluids in patients with epithelial ovarian cancer and benign gynecologic disease. Acta Cytol 34:539–544, 1990.

Lurain JR, Rumsey NK, Schink JC, et al. Prognostic significance of positive peritoneal cytology in clinical stage I adenocarcinoma of the endometrium. Obstet Gynecol 74:175–179, 1989.

Mathew S, Erozan YS. Significance of peritoneal washings in gynecologic oncology. The experience with 901 intraoperative washings at an academic medical center. Arch Pathol Lab Med 121:604–606, 1997.

Mazurka JL, Krepart GV, Lotocki RJ. Prognostic significance of positive peritoneal cytology in endometrial carcinoma. Am J Obstet Gynecol 158:303–306, 1988.

McGowan L, Bunnag B. Morphology of mesothelial cells in peritoneal fluid from normal women. Acta Cytol 18:205–209, 1974.

McGowan L, Stein DB, Miller W. Cul-de-sac aspiration for diagnostic cytologic study. AM J Obstet Gynecol 96:413–417, 1966.

McLellan R, Dillon MB, Currie JL, Rosenshein NB. Peritoneal cytology in endometrial cancer: A review. Obstet Gynecol Surv 44:711–719, 1989.

Mesia AF, Tarafder D, Shanerman AI, Cohen JM. Peritoneal cytology in uterine papillary serous carcinoma. Acta Cytol 43:605–609, 1999.

Mills SE, Andersen WA, Fechner RE, Austin MB. Serous surface papillary carcinoma. A clinicopathologic study of 10 cases and comparison with stage III–IV ovarian serous carcinoma. Am J Surg Pathol 12:827–834, 1988.

Moore WF, Bentley RC, Berchuck A, Robboy SJ. Some Müllerian inclusion cysts in lymph nodes may sometimes be metastases from serous borderline tumors of the ovary. Am J Surg Pathol 24:710–718, 2000.

Morris PC, Haugen J, Anderson B, Buller R. The significance of peritoneal cytology in stage 1B cervical cancer. Obstet Gynecol 80:196–198, 1992.

Mulvany N. Cytohistologic correlation in malignant peritoneal washings. Analysis of 75 malignant fluids. Acta Cytol 40:1231–1239, 1996.

Patsner B. Peritoneal cytology in patients with stage 1B cervical cancer undergoing radical hysterectomy: limited value. Eur J Gynaecol Oncol 13:306–308, 1992.

Poropatich C, Eyha H. Detached ciliary tufts in pouch of Douglas fluid. Acta Cytol 30:442–444, 1986.

Pretorius RG, Lee KR, Papillo J, et al. False-negative peritoneal cytology in metastatic ovarian carcinoma. Obstet Gynecol 68:619–623, 1986.

Ravinsky E. Cytology of peritoneal washings in gynecologic patients: Diagnostic criteria and pitfalls. Acta Cytol 30:6–16, 1986.

Roberts WS, Bryson SC, Cavanagh D, et al. Peritoneal cytology and invasive carcinoma of the cervix. Gynecol Oncol 24:331–336, 1986.

Rubin DK, Frost JK. The cytologic detection of ovarian cancer. Acta Cytol 7: 191–195, 1963.

Sagae S, Berek JS, Fu YS, Chang N, et al. Peritoneal cytology of ovarian cancer patients receiving intraperitoneal therapy: Quantitation of malignant cells and response. Obstet Gynecol 72:782–788, 1988.

Sams VR, Benjamin E, Ward RH. Ectopic pancreas: A cause of false-positive peritoneal cytology. Acta Cytol 34:641–644, 1990.

Selvaggi SM. Diagnostic pitfalls of peritoneal washing cytology and the role of cell blocks in their diagnosis. Diagn Cytopathol 28:335–341, 2003.

Sidawy MK, Chandra P, Oertel YC. Detached ciliary tufts in peritoneal washings: A common finding. Acta Cytol 31:841–844, 1987.

Sidawy MK, Silverberg SG. Endosalpingiosis in female peritoneal washings: A diagnostic pitfall. Int. J Gynecol Pathol 6:340–346, 1987.

Sneige N, Fernandez T, Copeland LJ, Katz RL. Müllerian inclusions in peritoneal washings. Potential source of error in peritoneal washings. Acta Cytol 30:271–276, 1986.

Spencer TR Jr, Marks RD Jr, Fenn JO, et al. Intraperitoneal P-32 after negative second look laparotomy in ovarian carcinoma. Cancer 63:2434–2437, 1989.

Stewart CJ, Kennedy JH. Peritoneal fluid cytology in serous borderline tumours of the ovary. Cytopathol 9:38–45, 1998.

Stowell SB, Wiley CM, Perez-Reyes N, Powers CN. Cytologic diagnosis of peritoneal fluids. Applicability to the laparoscopic diagnosis of endometriosis. Acta Cytol 41:817–822, 1997.

Szpak CA, Creasman WT, Vollmer RT, Johnston WW. Prognostic value of cytologic examination of peritoneal washings in patients with endometrial carcinoma. Acta Cytol 25:640–646, 1981.

Uras C, Altinkaya E, Yardimci H, et al. Peritoneal cytology in the determination of free tumour cells within the abdomen in colon cancer. Surg Oncol 5: 259–263, 1996.

Walts AE. Optimization of the peritoneal lavage. Diagn Cytopathol 18: 265–269, 1998.

Wheeler DT, Bell KA, Kurman RJ, Sherman ME. Minimal uterine serous carcinoma. Diagnosis and clinicopathologic correlation. Am J Surg Pathol 24: 797–806, 2000.

Wojcik EM, Naylor B. Collagen balls in peritoneal washings: Prevalence, morphology, origin and significance. Acta Cytol 36:466–470, 1992.

Yazigi R, Piver MS, Blumenson L. Malignant peritoneal cytology as prognostic indicator in stage I endometrial cancer. Obstet Gynecol 62:359–362, 1983.

Zervakis M, Howdon WM, Howdon A. Cul-de-sac needle aspirations: Its normal and abnormal cytology and its value in the detection of ovarian cancer. Acta Cytol 13:507–514, 1969.

Ziselman EM, Harkavy SE, Hogan M, et al. Peritoneal washing cytology. Use and diagnostic criteria in gynecologic neoplasms. Acta Cytol 28:105–110, 1984.

Zuna RE, Behrens A. Peritoneal washing cytology in gynecologic cancers: Long-term follow-up of 355 patients. J Natl Cancer Inst 88:980–987, 1996.

Zuna RE, Mitchell ML. Cytologic findings in peritoneal washings associated with benign gynecologic disease. Acta Cytol 32:139–147, 1988.

Zuna RE, Mitchell ML, Mulick KA, Weijchert WM. Cytohistologic correlation of peritoneal washing: Cytology in gynecologic disease. Acta Cytol 33: 327–336, 1989.

Rare and Unusual Disorders of the Female Genital Tract

17

This chapter contains descriptions of uncommon benign and malignant lesions, that for the most part, may affect several component organs of the female genital tract.

RARE BENIGN DISORDERS

Deficiency of Folic Acid

Deficiency in folic acid (or vitamin B12) leads to impaired DNA synthesis during hematopoiesis, resulting in abnormal maturation of erythrocytes (and other blood cells) known as **megaloblastic anemia.** The disease is characterized mainly by a marked enlargement of erythrocytes and abnormalities of leukocytes. Folic acid deficiency may also impair DNA synthesis in other organs, such as the oral cavity and the gastrointestinal tract, where it can cause cellular enlargement (see Chaps. 21 and 24). In 1962 and 1966, Van Niekerk reported cell changes observed in **squamous cells in cervical smears** in patients with **megaloblastic anemia** and, hence, a folic acid deficiency, during the puerperium. The principal changes observed were generalized **enlargements of intermediate squamous cells** (diameter of 70 μm or larger), accompanied by an **enlargement of the nucleus** (diameter of 14 μm or more). Van Niekerk also observed **multinucleation** and **cytoplasmic vacuolization** in an average of 3.5% of cells. Other findings included phagocytosis, clumping, and folding of nuclear chromatin. The changes were apparently reversible after appropriate therapy. Van Niekerk's observations were generally confirmed by Klaus (1971), who considered **nuclear folding** as the most frequent event (6% of cells) and nuclear enlargement the second most frequent event (4% of cells). In Klaus' experience, the cytologic changes may be observed 8 to 10 weeks before clinical onset of megaloblastic anemia. Subsequently, Whitehead et al (1973) linked similar cell changes with contraceptive therapy but the conclusive proof of this association is lacking.

Changes apparently caused by folic acid deficiency are deceptively similar to early neoplastic changes in the uterine cervix such as the **dyskaryosis (dysplasia)** of the superficial and intermediate squamous cells, **consistent with a low-grade squamous intraepithelial lesion, and abnormalities caused by a human papillomavirus infection** (see Chap. 11). It is of interest in this regard that folic acid deficiency may apparently enhance the patient's susceptibility to infection with human papillomavirus (Harper et al, 1994; Butterworth et al, 1992). Somewhat similar cell abnormalities may be observed as an **early effect of radiotherapy** (see Chap. 18). Because the cytologic follow-up of such lesions may be unreliable, it is prudent to have the patient undergo an appropriate work-up that should include a colposcopic evaluation of the uterine cervix before accepting the diagnosis of folic acid deficiency as secure.

Pemphigus Vulgaris

Pemphigus vulgaris (from Greek, *pemphis* = blister) is a disorder usually affecting the skin and the mucous membranes of the oral cavity (see Chapter 21). It may sometimes involve the lower female genital tract. Several such cases were described in the gynecologic and dermatologic literature (see Krain et al, 1973). The disease is caused by **antibodies to desmoglein 3, a component protein of desmosomes** (Amagai et al, 1996) **causing a disruption of desmosomes in the lower layers of the squamous epithelium** leading to the formation of fluid-filled blisters, vesicles or bullae. The latter contain atypical squamous cells (**cells of Tznack et al, 1951,** who first described them) that can be observed in smears of broken vesicles. These are **squamous cells of bizarre shapes, sometimes with cytoplasmic protrusions, characterized by clear cytoplasm and nuclei and large nucleoli, occurring singly and in clusters. The antibodies coating these cells can be demonstrated by immunofluorescence,** as first shown by Beutner and Jordan in 1964. Libcke (1970) and Friedman et al (1971) each reported atypical squamous cells in cases of pemphigus vulgaris **involving the squamous epithelium of the cervix.** A number of additional cases of genital pemphigus, some also involving the vulva and vagina, were described (Kaufman et al, 1969). In a case described by Valente et al (1984), the atypical squamous cells were interpreted as suspicious, yet corresponded to clinically **occult pemphigus blisters** discovered in the hysterectomy specimen. In a case reported by Dvoretsky et al (1985), pemphigus was associated with a microinvasive carcinoma of the uterine cervix and, in a case reported by Krain et al (1973), with endometrial carcinoma. Because genital pemphigus can cause vaginal bleeding, it is obvious that a thorough examination of the female genital tract is required to rule out the possibility of a malignant tumor associated with this disease. For further discussion and illustrations of pemphigus, see Chapters 21 and 34.

Malakoplakia

This rare disorder of macrophages, unable to cope with colibacteria because of an enzymatic deficiency, is described in detail and illustrated in Chapter 22. The characteristic, **spherical cytoplasmic Michaelis-Guttmann bodies** (representing enlarged and often calcified lysosomes), **observed in medium size macrophages, are diagnostic of this disorder in smears.** The findings in cervicovaginal smears were described in several cases of malakoplakia involving the **vagina and uterine cervix** (Lin et al, 1979; Chalvardijan et al, 1980; Wahl, 1982; Valente et al, 1984; Falcon-Escobedo et al, 1986). In an electron microscopic study, Kapila and Verma (1989) identified the characteristic coliform bacteria within the Michaelis-Guttmann bodies in a case of cervical malakoplakia. Thomas et al (1978) described a case of this disorder involving the **endometrium** and causing abnormal bleeding.

Amyloidosis of the Cervix

A case of amyloidosis limited to the uterine cervix was reported by Yamada et al (1988). There are no known cytologic findings in this very rare disorder.

Eosinophilic Granuloma (Langerhans' Cell Granulomatosis)

This uncommon lesion, composed of Langerhans cells resembling macrophages and a mixture of eosinophilic polymorphonuclear leukocytes with other inflammatory cells, is known to involve the female genitals (Zinkham, 1976; Issa et al, 1980). There is no information on the cytologic presentation of this lesion in cervicovaginal smears. For discussion of this entity in other organs, see Chapters 19 and 35.

Ectopic Prostatic Tissue in the Uterine Cervix

Larraza-Hernandez et al (1997) and Nucci et al (2000) reported the presence of ectopic prostatic tissue in the uterine cervix, presenting in one case as a cervical mass (thought to be a fibroid) and in three cases as an incidental finding in tissue obtained for treatment of high-grade squamous intraepithelial lesions.

BENIGN TUMORS

Leiomyomas

These benign tumors of smooth muscle usually involve the myometrium of the body of the uterus and may reach substantial sizes. They are virtually always encapsulated and do not normally shed any cells in cytologic samples from the uterus. Occasionally, however, ulcerated leiomyomas of the uterus, particularly if located in the uterine cervix, may shed **benign smooth muscle cells** that can be recognized in cervicovaginal smears. These slender cells are **spindly, elongated, usually occur in parallel bundles, and show oval, finely granular nuclei,** often located in the approximate center of the cell. Similar cells may be sometimes observed following **abortion** and after a **mechanical injury to the** cervix (see Chap. 8). **Endometrial abnormalities** may occur in the presence of large leiomyomas (see Chap. 13).

Other Benign Tumors

Other benign tumors of the uterus, vulva or vagina, such as **rhabdomyoma** (Gad and Eusebi, 1975; Gold and Bossen, 1976), **syringoma** (Young et al, 1980), **glomus tumor** (Spitzer et al, 1985), and **granular cell tumor** (Coates and Hales, 1973), are exceedingly rare and they have not been observed in smears. Granular cell tumors of the breast, and sometimes of other organs, may be recognized in aspiration biopsies (see Chaps. 20 and 29).

RARE MALIGNANT TUMORS

Sarcomas

Sarcomas and other malignant tumors of mesenchymal origin constitute about 2% to 3% of all malignant tumors of the female genital tract. Their most common primary site is the uterine corpus, followed by the cervix and vagina. Most sarcomas are **homologous** (i.e., made up of a single tissue type, such as smooth or striated muscle or fat). However, a substantial number of malignant mesenchymal tumors of the uterus, known as the **mesodermal or Müllerian mixed tumors,** contain a **mixture of epithelial and sarcomatous** components. The histologic and cytologic aspects of these and other sarcomas are discussed below.

Most sarcomas originate within the depths of the affected organ and do not reach the exfoliating surface until they have grown to a substantial size and have produced surface ulceration. In the vast majority of such cases, the patients are symptomatic and have clinically obvious disease. Thus, **routine cytologic examination of the female genital tract rarely contributes to the primary diagnosis of these tumors, except for the mesodermal mixed tumor.** In most cases, the role of cytology is relegated to the **recognition of recurrent disease.** In many instances, even this exercise is fraught with considerable difficulty. Occasionally, however, cytologic evaluation may contribute to the diagnosis and clinical handling of the patient.

Tumors of Smooth Muscle (Leiomyosarcomas)
Histology
Leiomyosarcomas are the most common sarcomas of the female genital tract. Nearly all tumors originate in the smooth muscle of the uterine corpus, although they may be primary in the muscle of the uterine cervix and, exceedingly rarely, in other genital organs such as the fallopian tube or the wall of the vagina. The tumors are composed of **criss-crossing bundles of abnormal smooth muscle cells,** characterized by large, hyperchromatic nuclei. Several rare variants of these tumors are known to occur, chief among them the **epithelioid leiomyosarcoma,** a tumor composed of large, polygonal cells mimicking an epithelial tumor. The prognosis of uterine leiomyosarcomas depends on the size of the tumor, its relationship to adjacent organs, and its histologic differentiation or grade. Small tumors inciden-

tally found within the myometrium or arising within benign leiomyomas generally offer an excellent prognosis. However, tumors attached to adjacent viscera are often fatal, regardless of grade. **Well-differentiated tumors,** closely resembling benign leiomyomas, except for nuclear abnormalities and sometimes high mitotic count **(grade I),** usually have a much better prognosis than tumors composed of bundles of clearly malignant cells **(grade II).** Highly disorganized tumors made up of bizarre large or small cancer cells **(grades III and IV)** have a nearly uniformly fatal prognosis (Spiro and Koss, 1965; Bodner et al, 2003). Voluminous literature pertaining to the classification and recognition of leiomyosarcomas, particularly the differentiation between atypical leiomyomas and low-grade leiomyosarcomas (Bell et al, 1994), has very limited bearing on cytologic observations.

Cytology
Massoni and Hajdu (1984) stressed the very low rate of primary leiomyosarcomas recognized in cervicovaginal material. **Cells from the well-differentiated forms of leiomyosarcoma (grade I) have never been seen by us or identified in routine smears.** However, more anaplastic forms of this tumor (grades II through IV), once ulcerated or metastatic, may shed **highly abnormal, often grotesque cancer cells. If such cells are elongated, as is sometimes the case, a more specific diagnosis of tumor type may be attempted** (Fig. 17-1). Single or multiple abnormal nuclei of variable sizes may be noted. **Nuclear hyperchromasia is variable, and irregular, large nucleoli may be present.** The difference between cells of a high grade leiomyosarcoma and normal smooth muscle cells is obvious. Quite often, however, cancer cells shed from a leiomyosarcoma are **polygonal rather than elongated and may be mistaken for cells of a carcinoma.**

Elongated, spindly, or bizarre malignant cells are not unique to leiomyosarcomas and may occur in other sarcomas and in mesodermal mixed tumors. Similar cells may also occur in invasive epidermoid carcinomas, particularly of the spindle- and giant-cell variety (see below).

Klijanienko et al (2003) reported a large series of leiomyosarcomas of various types and primary extrauterine locations, diagnosed by direct thin needle aspiration. To my knowledge, no attempts have been made to apply this technique to uterine tumors.

Tumors of Striated Muscle (Rhabdomyosarcomas)
Although the female genital tract does not normally contain striated muscle, isolated cells of this type may occasionally be found in benign myometria. This, however, is not an essential prerequisite for the occurrence of rhabdomyosarcoma, which apparently may originate from any type of mesenchymal cell. **Pure embryonal-type sarcomas of striated muscle origin are most commonly observed in the vagina or the cervix of young children and young adults as botryoid sarcomas** (Daya and Scully, 1988). Occasional rhabdomyosarcomas of **alveolar type** have been observed in other organs of the female genital tract, for example, in the uterine corpus (Donkers et al, 1972) and the vulva (Ima-

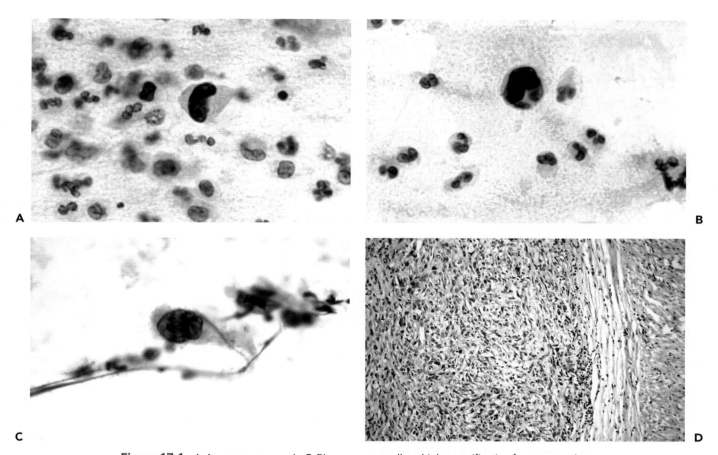

Figure 17-1 **Leiomyosarcomas.** *A–C.* Bizarre cancer cells at high magnification from two patients with recurrent tumor. *D.* The histologic appearance of the tumor corresponding to *A* and *B.* The diagnosis of a poorly differentiated malignant tumor could be easily made but the specific diagnosis of a leiomyosarcoma could not be established in the absence of past history.

chi et al, 1991). Rhabdomyosarcomas are a **common component of mesodermal mixed tumors** (see below).

Botryoid sarcoma (from the Greek, *botrys* = bunch of grapes) is a form of immature (embryonal) rhabdomyosarcoma that forms **grape-like, translucent tumor nodules** usually in the vagina, much less commonly in the uterine cervix of young girls, who are rarely older than five years of age, but sometimes also in young adults. Similar tumors may occur in the **urinary bladder of children of both sexes** and in the **prostate** of boys. The grape-like structures are surfaced by an intact squamous epithelium. The tumor cells form a **dense subepithelial layer** (cambium layer) composed of very small cancer cells, surrounding the loosely structured bulk of the tumor wherein larger **cancer cells, some with cytoplasmic cross-striations** or marked cytoplasmic eosinophilia, may be identified.

Previously considered nearly invariably fatal (Daniel et al, 1959), the tumors are now curable in a large proportion of cases with a combination of radiotherapy and chemotherapy (review in Brand et al, 1987). Daya and Scully (1988) stressed better prognosis of botryoid sarcoma of the uterine cervix in young adults than in children.

Cytology
The diagnosis of primary botryoid sarcomas is usually made by clinical inspection and biopsy. Cytologic diag-

nosis is superfluous in such instances. **Even if vaginal smears are obtained, the tumor cells may be absent because of the protective epithelial layer.** However, in recurrent and in metastatic tumors, **small, elongated, spindly tumor cells may be observed** in vaginal smears or in urinary sediment (see Chap. 26). In rare instances, **cytoplasmic cross-striations** may occur that allow a precise classification of the tumor.

Differentiated rhabdomyosarcomas are very rare in the female genital tract (Brand et al, 1989). One can then anticipate the finding of bizarre tumor cells with cytoplasmic cross-striations, characteristic of rhabdomyoblasts (see Fig. 17-6). The cytologic findings in two cases of alveolar rhabdomyosarcoma of the vulva were reported by Imachi et al (1991), who did not observe cytoplasmic striations in the tumor cells.

Endometrial Stromal Sarcomas
The endometrial stromal tumors originate either in the endometrium or in foci of uterine endometriosis (adenomyosis). There are two presentations of this tumor: a low-grade and a high-grade tumor.

Histology and Clinical Features
The **low-grade,** well-differentiated form of the tumor (previously named **the endolymphatic stromal myosis**) is com-

posed of orderly bundles of small cells similar to endometrial stroma, sometimes forming **ribbon-like organoid structures (so called "plexiform tumorlets") and occasionally small glands, mimicking primitive endometrial glands.** Clement and Scully (1989) **misinterpreted the "tumorlets" for sex cord-like elements,** seen in rare ovarian tumors, but the origin of these structures from endometrial stroma has been clearly documented by Larbig et al (1965). The tumor cells may occasionally **differentiate into smooth muscle cells, particularly in metastatic foci.** Oliva et al (2001) pointed out that cells with markedly **eosinophilic cytoplasm** may occur in such tumors. The tumor has several other interesting features: it has the tendency to **invade vessels of the uterus and adjacent pelvis,** sometimes forming **solid, spaghetti-like cylinders** that can be pulled from the affected vessels by a forceps. For this reason, the tumor **may be confused with intravenous leiomyomatosis,** as in a paper by Clement et al (1988). The tumor may have an erratic, protracted clinical course, stretching over a period of many years (Koss et al, 1965). **It may form local, retroperitoneal, or distant metastases, for example, to the bladder or lung, often many years after surgical removal of the primary tumor** (28 years in a personally observed case), and still be **consistent with long-term survival** following aggressive treatment of metastases. Late pulmonary metastases were also described by Abrams et al (1989). The tumor may also respond to **hormonal manipulation with progesterone,** not unlike an endometrial carcinoma. **Because of the unusual, often favorable behavior of this tumor, its diagnosis in metastatic foci may be life-saving.**

The **high grade endometrial stromal sarcomas are infrequent.** In a small series by Koss et al (1965), only 1 of 10 stromal sarcomas could be so classified. The tumor has a similar distribution to the low-grade variant but is composed of obviously malignant larger cells and has aggressive behavior.

Cytology

Several examples of this tumor were described in cervicovaginal smears (Hsiu and Stawicki, 1979; Becker and Wong, 1981) and in other cytologic samples such as effusions (Massoni and Hajdu, 1984; Hajdu and Hajdu, 1976). So far as one can tell, the reported cases represented the **high-grade variant of the disease.** In general, the authors stressed the **small size and the relatively monotonous appearance of the round or oval malignant cells,** accompanied by occasional elongated cells with tapering cytoplasm, named **comet cells** by Hsiu and Stawicki (1979). Except for hyperchromasia and variability in size, the nuclei had no distinguishing features. Mitotic figures were observed in two of three cases reported by Becker and Wong (1981). In all cases described, the tumor was far advanced and symptomatic; all patients, save one, died of disease shortly after diagnosis.

There are no reported cases of primary diagnosis of the **low-grade stromal sarcoma.** However, **metastases** of this tumor may be amenable to diagnosis by needle aspiration biopsy that may lead to aggressive treatment and long-term survival. As an example, the aspirate of one of many **large, cannon-ball pulmonary metastases** in a 38-year-old woman contained **small, spindly, rather benign-looking cells and scattered glands, resembling benign endometrial glands** (Fig. 17-2). The cytologic finding led to the review of hysterectomy material obtained 8 years previously, which was initially diagnosed as a benign abnormality (stromal nodule). The review disclosed a low-grade endometrial stromal sarcoma. After surgical removal of all but one of the pulmonary metastases, followed by progesterone therapy, the patient remained well for several years without any evidence of active disease. In another more recent case with only short follow-up, the aspirate of lung metastases yielded small cells resembling normal endometrial stroma (Fig. 17-3).

Other Sarcomas

Exceedingly uncommon sarcomas may be observed in the female genital tract.

Epithelioid sarcomas are very rare sarcomas of soft tissue that characteristically mimic epithelial tumors, hence their name. A few cases of this disease involving the vulva were reported in the cytologic literature (Ulbright et al, 1983; Hernandez-Ortiz et al, 1995). In aspirated material, the authors reported the presence of **polygonal malignant cells with eosinophilic cytoplasm,** large nuclei and prominent nucleoli, mimicking cells of a clear cell carcinoma. It is unlikely that an accurate cytologic diagnosis of these tumors can be established in the absence of clinical history.

A case of **malignant fibrous histiocytoma of the cervix,** with cytologic findings, was described by Fukuyama et al (1986). The cytologic features included **multinucleated and elongated (spindly) cancer cells.** Zaleski et al (1986) and Foschini et al (1989) each reported a case of **alveolar soft-part sarcoma of the vagina.** In keeping with the pseudoepithelial histologic appearance of this tumor, **large malignant cells, with eosinophilic granular cytoplasm, singly and in clusters,** were observed in the cervicovaginal smears. The nuclei were eccentric and provided with large nucleoli. Characteristic **intracytoplasmic crystalloids** were documented by periodic acid-Schiff (PAS)-stain and by electron microscopy.

An **osteosarcoma, a liposarcoma, and a Wilms' tumor of the uterine cervix** were described (Bloch et al, 1988; Bell et al, 1985; Brooks and LiVolsi, 1987) but there is no information on their cytologic presentation in this anatomic location. A **synovial sarcoma-like** tumor of the vagina was described by Okagaki et al (1976). For cytologic presentation of sarcomas of various types and organs in aspiration biopsies, see Chapter 35.

Malignant Mesodermal Mixed Tumors (Müllerian Mixed Tumors)

The highly malignant mesodermal mixed tumors are most often of **endometrial origin; similar tumors, however, may also occur in the uterine cervix, fallopian tube, the ovary, and organs of other than Müllerian origin, such as the urinary bladder** (Mortel et al, 1974; Dictor, 1985; Wu et al, 1973; see also Chapter 23). Hence, the commonly used term "Müllerian mixed tumors," is not accurate. In the female genital tract, the most common mesodermal mixed tumors of the endometrium occur chiefly in the menopausal

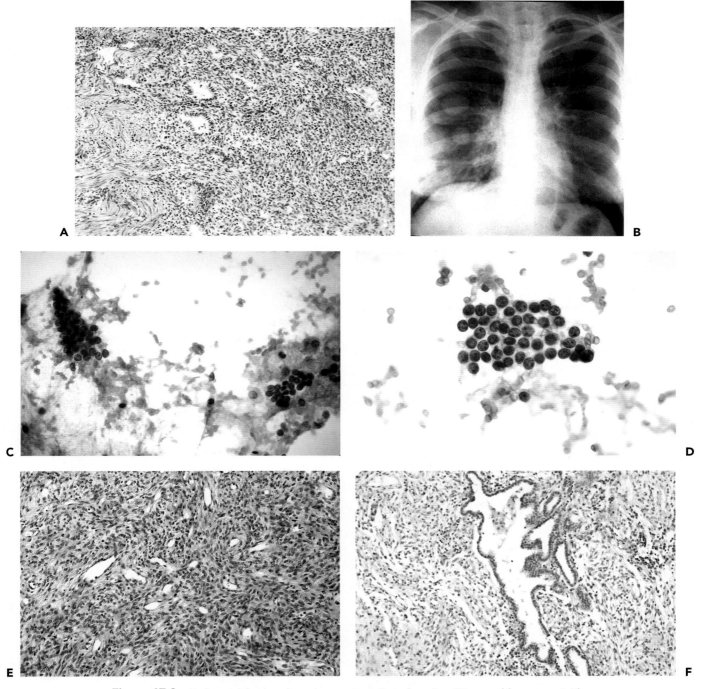

Figure 17-2   Endometrial stromal sarcoma metastatic to lung in a 38-year-old woman. *A.* The original uterine tumor observed in 1975. The tumor was composed of small, spindly cells and formed small glands. The diagnosis of ''stromatosis'' was established. *B.* The chest x-ray of this patient in 1983 showing multiple cannonball-type metastases. *C,D.* Aspiration smears of a pulmonary lesion. *C.* A low-power view of the aspiration smear showing clusters of epithelial cells and a few scattered spindly cells. *D.* Epithelial clusters resembling benign endometrial glands. *E.* Resected pulmonary nodule showing a histologic pattern somewhat similar to the original uterine tumor shown in *A.* Elsewhere the metastases differentiated into smooth muscle. *F.* The metastatic foci formed gland-like structures which were reflected in the aspiration biopsy shown in *C* and *D.* This patient is known to have survived 10 years after the resection of the pulmonary nodules.

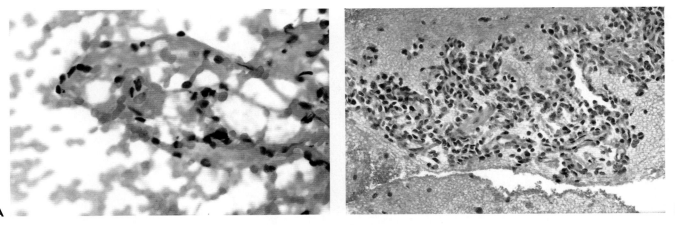

Figure 17-3 **Endometrial stromal sarcoma metastatic to lung.** *A.* The aspiration of the lung nodule. The smear is composed mainly of short spindly cells without conspicuous nuclear abnormalities. *B.* A biopsy of pulmonary nodule showing endometrial stromal sarcoma forming glands.

age group and often appear clinically as **polypoid lesions, sometimes protruding through the external os of the cervix.**

When these tumors show only elements of **carcinoma with spindle cell stroma,** they are usually classified as **carcinosarcomas or spindle cell carcinomas** (see below).

Histology

These tumors **are composed of a mixture of undifferentiated and differentiated sarcomas and carcinomas. The most common differentiated sarcoma is rhabdomyosarcoma** (see Fig. 17-4C,D). Other sarcomatous elements may resemble endometrial stromal sarcoma, leiomyosarcoma,

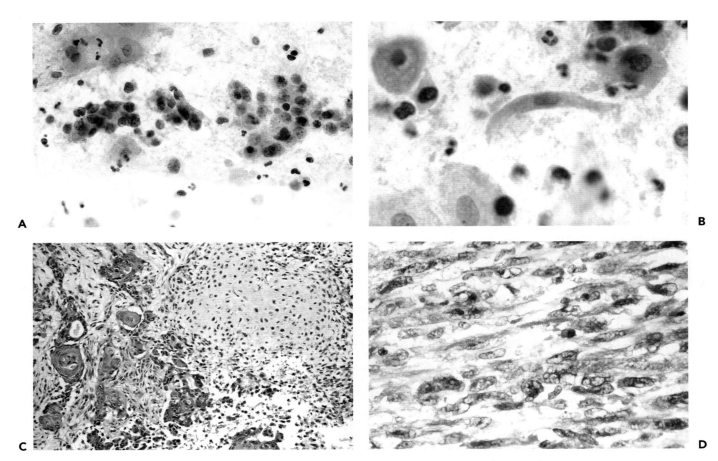

Figure 17-4 **Mesodermal (Müllerian) tumor of the uterus.** *A.* Clusters of epithelial cells resembling a poorly differentiated carcinoma. *B.* Spindly cells, some of which had cross striations in the cytoplasm. *C.* Histology of tumor shown in *A* and *B.* In this field, one can observe poorly differentiated carcinoma with focal squamous differentiation and a fragment of chondrosarcoma. In *D,* striated spindly cells brought out by trichrome stain reflect the presence of a rhabdomyosarcoma.

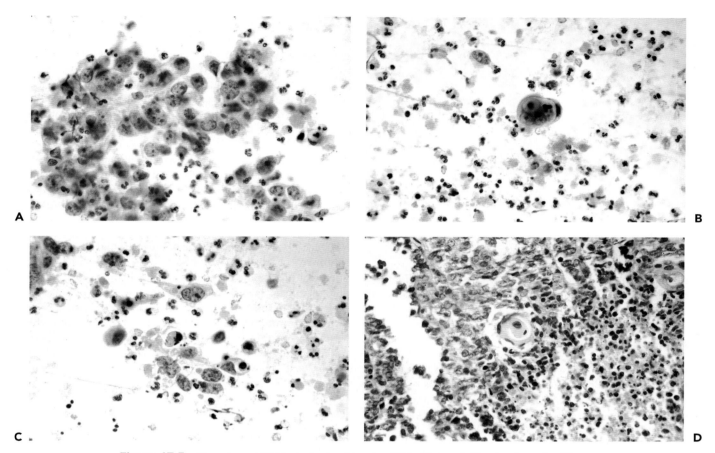

Figure 17-5   Mesodermal (Müllerian) mixed tumor of the uterus. *A.* Sheets of poorly differentiated malignant epithelial cells. *B.* A cluster of malignant cells suggestive of a squamous pearl. *C.* A few elongated cancer cells and a few cancer cells, most likely corresponding to the undifferentiated component of the tumor. *D.* The histology of one area of the tumor composed mainly of small, poorly differentiated cells and a poorly differentiated carcinoma forming a squamous pearl.

chondrosarcoma, or liposarcoma (see Fig. 17-5D). The carcinomatous components are in the form of adenocarcinoma, squamous carcinoma, or a mixture of both. Clement and Scully (1974) identified a subvariant of mesodermal mixed tumors in which the epithelial component was morphologically benign and named it **adenosarcoma.** However, the behavior of adenosarcoma was similar to that of malignant mesodermal mixed tumor. In 1989, the same authors described a very rare variant of mesodermal mixed tumor with **sex-cord–like elements.** An exceedingly rare, histologically benign variant of mesodermal mixed tumor has been described (Vellios et al, 1973; Demopoulos et al, 1973).

Cytology

The mesodermal mixed tumors may sometimes be recognized in cervicovaginal smears prior to clinical diagnosis. The **background of the smears** is usually filled with necrotic material and fresh and old blood. Fully developed mesodermal mixed tumors usually shed abundant cancer cells (Figs. 17-4 and 17-5). The **predominant malignant cells** are usually **small, of uneven size, round or elongated, with scanty cytoplasm and relatively large, hyperchromatic nuclei, wherein conspicuous nucleoli can often be seen.** Elongated, spindle-form small malignant cells may

also occur. These cells correspond to the sarcomatous component of these tumors, made up of small cells. Cells of **coexisting carcinomas resemble those of endometrial carcinoma, squamous carcinoma, or both. Sometimes, carcinoma cells are the only malignant component observed in smears.** More often, however, there is an association of elements of adeno- or squamous carcinoma with the small malignant cells described above, which is fairly characteristic of mesodermal mixed tumor. Cells of **rhabdomyosarcoma,** showing **cytoplasmic cross-striations** or at least markedly eosinophilic cytoplasm, are rarely seen. When they occur, however, they are diagnostic of **rhabdomyosarcoma** which, in most cases, is a component of a mesodermal mixed tumor (Fig. 17-6). Identifiable cells from other forms of sarcoma, such as **chondrosarcoma,** are exceedingly rare.

Mesodermal mixed tumor should be differentiated from **endometrial or cervical carcinomas with undifferentiated components,** which may be made up of spindly and giant tumor cells, thereby suggesting a co-existing sarcoma. Such tumors are often referred to as **carcinosarcomas,** but the name **spindle-cell or spindle- and giant cell carcinoma** appears more appropriate (see below). The prognosis of these tumors is better than that of mesodermal mixed tumors (Norris and Taylor, 1966; Mortel et al, 1974). The

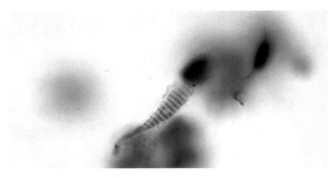

Figure 17-6 Ascitic fluid with metastatic mesodermal (Müllerian) mixed tumor of the uterus. Cytoplasmic cross striations are indicative of a rhabdosarcoma-like element in the tumor. Oil immersion magnification. (Case courtesy of Dr. Misao Takeda, Jefferson Medical College, Philadelphia, PA.)

separation of mesodermal mixed tumors from undifferentiated carcinomas in limited biopsy material may be very difficult.

Malignant Lymphomas

Current classification of malignant lymphomas is discussed in Chapter 31. **Primary malignant lymphomas** of the female genital tract are uncommon and only sporadic cases of such tumors occurring in the uterine cervix, vagina or

ovary were recorded prior to 1980 (Johnson and Soule, 1957; Vieaux and McGuire, 1964; Iliya et al, 1968; Buchler and Kline, 1972; Katayama et al, 1973; Stransky et al, 1973; Delgado et al, 1976; Carr et al, 1976; Whitaker, 1976; Krumermann and Chung, 1978; Tunca et al, 1979). Within recent years, additional cases of primary malignant lymphomas of the uterine cervix have been reported (Komaki et al, 1984; Harris and Scully, 1984; Taki et al, 1985; Mann et al, 1987; Strang et al, 1988; Andrews et al, 1988; Perren et al, 1992; Clement, 1993; Gabriele and Gaudiano, 2003). We have personally observed several examples of malignant lymphoma of the uterine cervix and vagina. **Vaginal bleeding** may be the first manifestation of this group of diseases.

Cytology

The cytologic recognition of **small-cell malignant lymphomas** (or chronic lymphocytic leukemias which have identical presentation) in cervicovaginal smears is difficult. The cytologic samples contain a monotonous population of small lymphocytes without distinguishing features, except for **granularity of the nuclei and irregularities of the nuclear contour.** Young et al (1985) cautioned that benign inflammatory lymphoid infiltrates of the cervix, endometrium, and vulva may mimic malignant lymphomas. Lymphocytic cervicitis (see Chap. 10) is a case in point. The presence of polyclonal plasma cells and lymphocytes or polymorphonuclear leukocytes within the lymphocytic

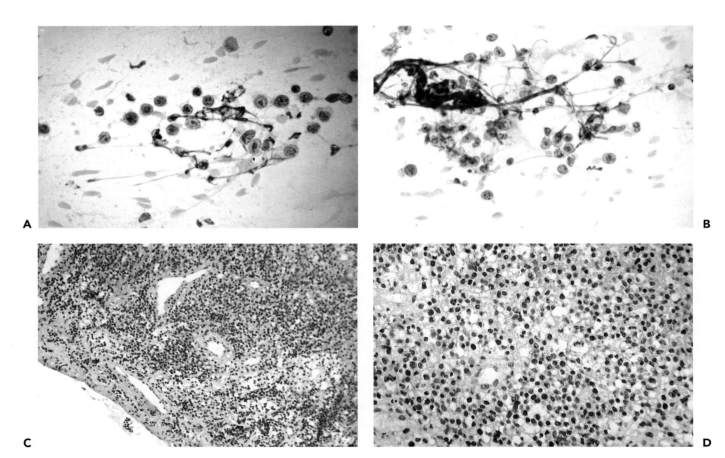

Figure 17-7 Large cell malignant lymphoma primary in the uterine cervix. *A,B.* Cervical smears showing dispersed cells of lymphocytic lineage with prominent large nucleoli. *C,D.* Aspects of the cervical lymphoma which was originally misinterpreted as a poorly differentiated carcinoma.

lesion should be construed as a warning that the lesion may be inflammatory.

The cytologic presentation of **primary large-cell lymphomas** is identical with that of secondary involvement (described in detail in Chaps. 26 and 31). The malignant cells, with nuclei rarely larger than 15 μm in diameter, **are dispersed and, as a rule, do not form clusters.** The cells **vary somewhat in size, have scanty cytoplasm and have stippled, occasionally folded, cleaved, or creased nuclei that are often provided with large nucleoli** (Fig. 17-7). Occasionally, the **nuclei may form small nipple-like protrusions** that should be distinguished from similar protrusions occurring in the much larger columnar endocervical cells (see Chap. 8). The most important **differential diagnosis** of large cell lymphomas is with **poorly differentiated carcinomas.** In the latter, clustering and molding of malignant cells is commonly seen and the nuclei are rarely cleaved or creased. Still, it is advisable to use **immunocytochemistry** to determine the nature of the tumor. This was described, with impressive results, in two more recent papers on this topic (Matsuyama et al, 1989; Dhimes et al, 1996).

The **difficulties in the differential diagnosis of large-cell lymphomas** of the cervix may **extend to the biopsy material.** Before the era of immunologic markers, large-cell lymphomas were repeatedly mistaken for anaplastic small cell carcinomas treated by surgery, occasionally with disastrous consequences for the patient. An abnormality of **decidual cells** in the cervix, **mimicking a large cell lymphoma** (reticulum cell sarcoma in the original article) has been reported by Armenia et al (1964).

Nasiell (1964) presented a well-documented case of **Hodgkin's disease,** apparently confined to the cervix, with a primary diagnosis by cervical smear. **Multinucleated tumor cells, similar to Reed-Sternberg cells,** were described (Fig. 17-8). A similar case was described by Uyeda et al (1969).

Granulocytic Sarcoma (Chloroma)

This tumor-like manifestation of chronic myelocytic leukemia may occur in the female genital tract. The tumor may appear greenish on gross presentation because of the presence of myeloperoxidase in tumor cells and, hence, were named **chloroma** (from Greek, *chloros* = green). Abeler et al (1983) described two cases of this disease affecting the uterine cervix. Oliva et al (1997) described 11 patients with this disorder, affecting the female genital tract, mainly the **ovaries** (7 cases), but also the **vagina** (3 cases) and, in one case, the **uterine cervix.** The diagnosis was confirmed by histochemistry, disclosing enzymes and products characteristic of myelogenous leukemia. Spahr et al (1982) were the first to describe the cytologic presentation of this condition in the cervix, diagnosed by **cervical smears prior to clinical evidence of chronic myelogenous leukemia.** The smear was characterized by the presence of highly **abnormal large cells, mimicking malignant lymphoma,** but with **eosinophilic cytoplasm that gave a positive reaction for Leder's esterase,** a characteristic histochemical reaction for myelogenous leukemia. At autopsy, the diagnosis of chloroma of the uterus and bowel was

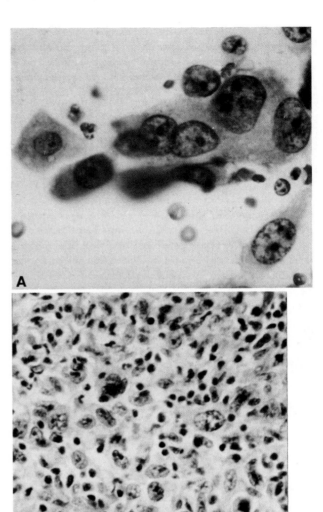

Figure 17-8   Primary Hodgkin's disease of the uterine cervix in a 39-year-old woman. Primary diagnosis by smear. *A.* Cervical smear showing a multinucleated cancer cell with large nucleoli and a few mononucleated cells showing similar nuclear features. *B.* Histologic presentation of cervix lesion. The patient was free of disease 3 years after hysterectomy. (From Nasiell M. Hodgkin's disease limited to the uterine cervix: A case report including cytological findings in the cervical and vaginal smears. Acta Cytol 8:16–18, 1964.)

established; the bone marrow showed pre-leukemic abnormalities. A similar case was described by Kapadia et al (1978) in an elderly patient with known acute myelocytic leukemia. An example of this entity is illustrated in Chapter 27.

Neuroendocrine Tumors

Histology

This group of tumors of the uterine cervix may have variable morphologic characteristics, ranging from the rare classical **carcinoid tumors** (Albores-Saavedra et al, 1976; Walker

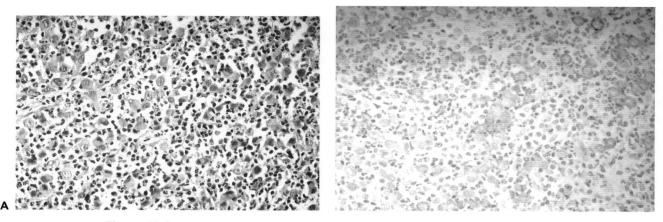

Figure 17-9 **Histologic presentation of a lymphoepithelioma-like tumor of the uterine cervix in a 33-year-old Chinese woman.** The keratin stain in *B* shows the epithelial component of the tumor which is obscured in *A* by the proliferation of lymphocytes. (Case courtesy of Prof. Shanmugaratnan, Singapore.)

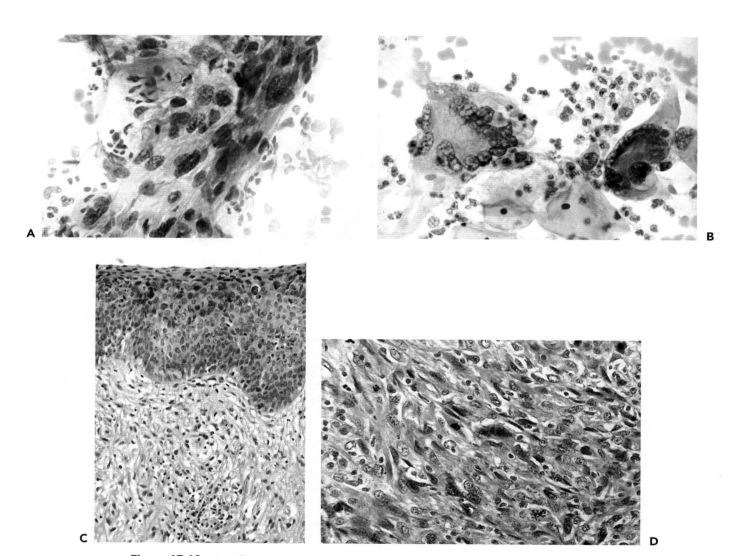

Figure 17-10 **Spindle and giant cell carcinoma of cervix.** *A.* Tumor cells in spindly configuration. *B.* Multinucleated giant cells observed in the same smear. *C.* The overall structure of the invasive tumor topped by a carcinoma in situ. *D.* Detail of tumor stroma composed of spindly cells with numerous giant cells.

and Mills, 1987; Seidel and Steinfeld, 1988), to **carcinomas resembling small cell squamous carcinomas,** to the highly malignant variant resembling **oat cell carcinoma** (Johannessen et al, 1980; Walker et al, 1988). The term **neuroendocrine carcinomas** has been applied to some of these tumors. The **common denominator** of these tumors is the presence of **cytoplasmic neurosecretory granules** in electron microscopy and immunochemical reactions documenting the presence of endocrine activity, such as **chromogranin, serotonin, and synaptophysin.** Such tumors may also occasionally occur in the endometrium and the ovary. The endocrine activity of the vast majority of these tumors has no clinical significance. As discussed in Chapter 11, in an exceptional case, the **endocrine function of these tumors may have systemic effects,** as in a case of **serotonin-producing cervical carcinoid** (Hirahatake et al, 1990) or an **insulin-producing cervical, small cell carcinoma,** causing hypoglycemia (Seckl et al, 1999). It must be added that metastatic carcinoma of the cervix to the pituitary may cause **diabetes insipidus** (Salpietro et al, 2000).

It has now been shown that **neuroendocrine features,** such as neuroendocrine granules and corresponding immunohistologic reactions, can be observed in about **one-third of invasive cervical carcinomas of various types,** but mainly of the small-cell type (Barrett et al, 1987; van Nagell et al, 1988). The endocrine features have no bearing on the diagnosis. In some of these tumors, squamous carcinoma in situ has been observed in adjacent epithelium (Johannessen et al, 1980), although this feature has not been stressed by other observers. Groben et al (1985), Seidel and Steinfeld (1988), and Stoler et al (1991) commented on the poor outcome of such tumors, even if diagnosed at low initial stage. Stoler et al (1991) observed the presence of **HPV type 18, and sometimes type 16,** in 18 of 20 endocrine carcinomas.

Cytology

In view of the diversity of morphologic types of cervical carcinomas with endocrine features, it is not surprising that their cytologic presentation is equally diverse. In general, these tumors **cannot be identified in smears as having neuroendocrine features.** In most cases, the cells in smears have the features of **high-grade carcinoma composed of small cells,** described in Chapter 11. In a case described by Miles et al (1985), the cancer cells in the cervical smear had the appearance of **cells of an epidermoid carcinoma and adenocarcinoma, next to undifferentiated cancer cells.** Although the presence of neuroendocrine granules was documented in the tumor and a positive reaction to serotonin was observed in the exfoliated cells, the morphologic appearance of the tumor was that of an adenosquamous carcinoma. Russin et al (1987) reported another case that had the cytologic presentation of an **adenocarcinoma with psammoma bodies.** In a case of **carcinoid of the uterine cervix,** Hirahatake et al (1990) described a population of small malignant cells with granular nuclei and prominent nucleoli and, hence, cytologic features not specific for carcinoid tumors (see Chaps. 11 and 20). Reich et al (1999), describing a case of malignant carcinoid in an 18-year-old woman, stressed **molding of tumor cells,** a feature commonly observed in oat cell carcinoma (see Chap. 20).

Lymphoepithelioma-Like Cervical Carcinoma

A rare tumor of the cervix in which **undifferentiated cancer cells were accompanied by a large population of lymphocytes** was observed by us in a young Chinese patient in the 1970s. The cytoplasm of the carcinoma cells was strongly positive with keratin antibodies. The tumor had a **striking similarity to a nasopharyngeal tumor,** known to occur with high frequency among Chinese, particularly from the southern provinces of China (see Chap. 21). Similar tumors of the uterine cervix were initially described by Mills et al (1985) and Hafiz et al (1985), and subsequently by several other observers (Halpin et al, 1989; Weinberg et al, 1993; Tseng et al, 1997; Reich et al, 1999) (Fig. 17-9). **Epstein-Barr virus (EBV),** which is often associated with nasopharyngeal tumors of this type, was observed by Tseng et al (1997) in 11 of 15 cases of cervical tumors, but also the presence of HPV in four of them. Noel et al (2001) were unable to identify EBV but confirmed the presence of HPV in two additional patients.

Reich et al (1999) described the **cytologic features** of one such tumor in cervicovaginal smears. The dominant feature was the presence of **large, pale cancer cells** with prominent nucleoli, **accompanied by numerous lymphocytes** and, hence, identical to the cytologic presentation of the nasopharyngeal tumors, described in Chapter 21. Proca et al (2000) described the cytologic findings in two patients with advanced tumors of this type. The findings were not specific.

Spindle and Giant Cell Carcinomas (Carcinosarcomas)

Histology

Rare cancers of the uterine cervix, vagina and endometrium may show unusual patterns, such as **spindle cell configuration, often accompanied by multinucleated giant cells (spindle and giant cell carcinoma sometimes referred to as "carcinosarcoma").** In the **cervix or vagina,** such tumors always contain a component of **squamous cancer,** either in the form of a high-grade precursor lesion on the surface of the tumor (HGSIL) or as nests of keratin-forming tumor cells within the invasive tumor and, therefore, must be considered as variants of squamous carcinoma. Grayson et al (2001) reported the presence of HPV type 16 in three of eight tumors. Of special interest was the presence of the virus in the sarcomatous component of the tumors, documenting still further that the spindly cells are merely a variant of squamous cancer. Spindly cell tumors with a glandular component are also observed in the endometrium (Mortel et al, 1974). It is generally thought that such tumors are variants of malignant mesodermal mixed tumors, described above.

Cytology

The cytologic appearance of these rare tumors is characteristic: **in cervicovaginal smears,** the tumors shed **spindly tumor cells and multinucleated giant cells, usually accompanied by scattered asquamous cancer cells** (Fig. 17-10). We have not observed any other tumors with these cytologic features.

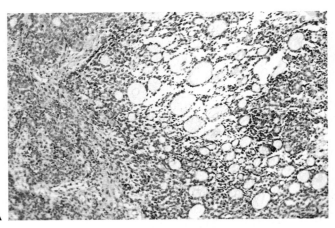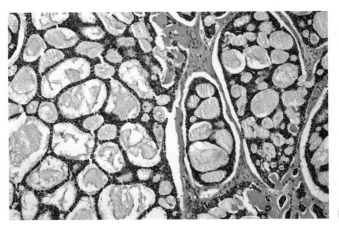

Figure 17-11   Adenoid-cystic carcinomas of cervix. *A.* Low-power view of the tumor which is associated with a squamous carcinoma. *B.* Details of another tumor in which the configuration of the cystic spaces is well shown. Cytologic presentation of this tumor is discussed at length in Chapter 32.

Merkel Cell Carcinoma of the Vulva

A case of this most unusual tumor, with extensive metastases, was reported by Bottles et al (1984). For description of histologic and cytologic features of Merkel cell carcinoma, see Chapter 34.

Adenoid Cystic Carcinomas

Clinical Data

These are rare but highly malignant tumors of the uterine cervix, occurring mainly in women past the age of 60. Prempree et al (1980) documented that even for tumors of clinical stage I, the five-year postsurgical survival was only 50% to 70%, even after radiotherapy. For tumors of higher stages, there were virtually no 5-year survivors in a compiled series of 43 patients. Ferry and Scully (1988) documented that these tumors have a more aggressive behavior pattern than their counterparts in the salivary glands (see Chap. 32). Thus, the **adenoid cystic carcinoma of the cervix must be considered a highly lethal tumor,** at par with the more common tumors of this type in the salivary glands (see Chap. 32). The tumor may occur in women of all ages but also in younger women (De La Maza et al, 1972; Ramzy et al, 1975; King et al, 1989). A case of metastatic adenoid cystic carcinoma of cervix to the lung, mimicking primary bronchial tumor, was reported by Ryden et al (1974).

Histology

The tumor is characterized by **densely packed, uniform small cancer cells, forming extracellular, cyst-like spaces, filled with eosinophilic homogeneous material** consisting of **reduplication of basement membrane.** The tumors also contain small glandular structures producing mucus (Fig. 17-11). Morphologically, the tumors are similar to a common **carcinoma of salivary gland origin** (Ferry and Scully, 1988). **Similar tumors** may be occasionally observed in **the breast, bronchus, prostate and other sites.** When first described by the surgeon Billroth in the 1880s, the tumors were thought to be relatively benign with emphasis on the

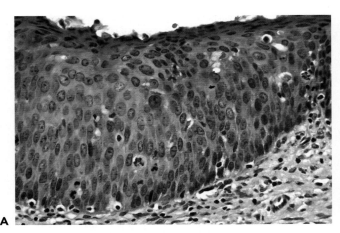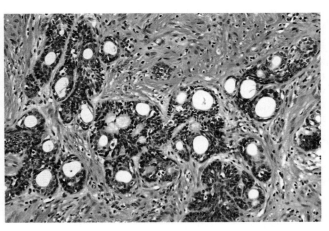

Figure 17-12   Basaloid cystic carcinoma of cervix. *A.* Carcinoma in situ on the surface of the cervix was the source of abnormal cells in smears. *B.* An area of basaloid-cystic carcinoma adjacent to carcinoma in situ. The tumor was infiltrating but showed no evidence of recurrence after removal. (Case courtesy of Dr. William Hart, The Cleveland Clinic, Cleveland, OH.)

cylindrically-shaped spaces within the tumor, hence the name *cylindroma.* In spite of slow evolution, the tumors are fully capable of metastases. In the **uterine cervix,** the adenoid cystic carcinomas are **commonly associated with squamous carcinoma in situ or invasive squamous cancer** and thus must be considered a rare variant of squamous carcinoma of the cervix (Ravinsky et al, 1996; Vuong et al, 1996).

Cytology

We have not seen an example of adenoid cystic carcinoma of the uterine cervix. Bittencourt et al (1979) from Brazil reported six such tumors and described the cytologic findings. Several additional case reports can be found in more recent literature (Dayton et al, 1990; Ravinsky et al, 1996; Vuong et al, 1996). The smears contained **sheets of small, fairly uniform cells.** In fortuitous cases, **central spaces with the characteristic hyaline deposits could be observed.** These cytologic findings are identical with tumors of the same histologic type observed in the salivary glands, trachea, or bronchus. In smears of cervix, **malignant cells of squamous type may accompany or even conceal the presence of adenoid cystic carcinoma,** which may be an incidental finding in biopsies.

Adenoid Basal Cell Carcinoma (Epithelioma)

This unusual low-grade tumor is usually discovered as an **incidental finding** in conization or hysterectomy specimens of **elderly women,** obtained because of cervical smears, usually showing a high grade squamous intraepithelial lesion or squamous carcinoma (Peterson and Neumann, 1995; Powers et al, 1996). The lesion was apparently first described by Baggish and Woodruff (1971) and by Daroca and Durandhar (1980). The lesion is composed of nests of **small basaloid cells surrounding small cystic spaces,** thus has some similarity to adenoid cystic carcinoma (Ferry and Scully, 1988; Grayson et al, 1999). However, the lesion is usually limited in size and does not spread through the cervix as observed in adenoid cystic carcinoma (Fig. 17-12). Brainard and Hart (1998) emphasized the essentially benign nature of the lesion and suggested that the term **"epithelioma"** be used to describe it, thus preventing unnecessary treatment.

Cviko et al (2000) hypothesized that the lesion is a peculiar form of basal cell differentiation of squamous carcinoma with good prognosis. HPV type 16 was observed in the squamous components in several cases (Jones et al, 1997; Grayson et al, 1997).

Cytology

The diagnosis of adenoid basal cell carcinoma is usually an incidental finding in patients with cytologic diagnosis of a squamous intraepithelial lesion (SIL). Powers et al (1996) observed clusters of small epithelial cells on **retrospective** review of abnormal smears in three such patients. These authors concluded that the cytologic diagnosis of adenoid basal carcinoma could not be established. The smear pattern in 11 of 12 patients studied by Brainard and Hart (1998) was that of a high-grade SIL that led to the discovery of the lesion. It may be concluded that it is **virtually impossible to recognize this tumor type in cervicovaginal smears.**

Primary Mammary Carcinoma of the Vulva

Primary mammary carcinomas may occur along the anlage of the mammary glands, **the linea lacta,** which stretches from the axilla to the vulva. On the rarest occasion, mammary carcinoma may be observed in the vulva (Cho et al, 1985). Such tumors may be diagnosed by aspiration biopsy. Metastatic mammary cancer must always be ruled out. Another point of differential diagnosis is **carcinoma of sweat glands** that may occur in the vulva and may mimic mammary carcinoma to perfection. For description of cytologic features of mammary carcinoma, see Chapter 29.

Transitional and Squamotransitional Carcinomas of the Cervix

These very uncommon and poorly defined tumors are most likely variants of squamous cancer that may occur within the cervix and the endometrium. Lininger et al (1998) reported the presence of HPV type 16 in some of these neoplasms. There are no reported cases of cytologic presentation of these tumors.

Malignant Melanoma

General Data and Histology

Primary malignant melanomas are most **common in the vulva** (Chung et al, 1975; Ariel, 1981; Bradgate et al, 1990), **less frequent in the vagina** (summary in Gupta et al, 2002), **and exceedingly rare in the uterine cervix** (summary in Deshpande et al, 2001). These highly malignant tumors are usually capable of **pigment formation,** although the nonpigment-producing variety may also be observed. The tumors originate in embryologically-derived neuroepithelial cells that are incorporated into the epidermis of the skin and other epithelia. The configuration of malignant melanomas is often similar to tumors of epithelial origin in the form of solid sheets of cancer cells. Hence, the **differential diagnosis between a melanoma and a carcinoma is, at times, very difficult in the absence of pigment.** A very rare, benign condition, **melanosis of vagina,** may clinically mimic a malignant melanoma (Karney et al, 2001).

Histologic variants of melanoma, such as balloon cell melanoma, spindle cell, or sarcomatoid melanoma, are discussed in Chapter 34. In histologic sections from the female genital tract, so-called **junctional changes** may sometimes be observed, although they are less common than in melanomas of the skin. When present, clear, large cells of melanoma are found singly and in clusters at the junction of the epithelium and subepithelial connective tissue (Fig. 17-13A). These findings are usually diagnostic of malignant melanoma in histologic material, but are rarely reflected in cytologic preparations.

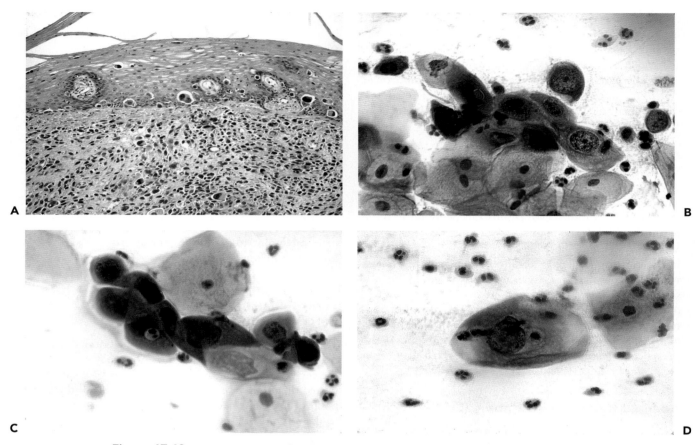

Figure 17-13 Various aspects of malignant melanoma of vagina. A. Histology of the tumor showing the so-called junctional change in the epithelium. B,C. Large tumor cells with pigmented cytoplasm from a 24-year-old woman. D. Giant squamous cell from the same smear as B and C.

Cytology

Cytologic presentation of primary malignant melanoma is similar for all organs of the female genital tract. The tumors can mimic almost any form and type of a malignant tumor. Most often, the tumors shed **large malignant cancer cells, with abundant cytoplasm, large hyperchromatic nuclei, and sometimes very large, prominent nucleoli** (Figs. 17-13 and 17-14). The presence of **intracytoplasmic granules of brown melanin pigment** usually clinches the diagnosis (see Fig. 17-13B,C). A frequent cytologic finding in melanomas of the vagina or cervix is the presence of **multinucleated cancer cells containing two or three, rarely more, peripherally placed large nuclei with large, often multiple nucleoli** (Fig. 17-14B). Occasionally, **intranuclear cytoplasmic inclusions (intranuclear vacuoles)** or "holes" may be noted (Hajdu and Hajdu, 1976). Intranuclear cytoplasmic inclusions and intracytoplasmic pigment deposits were observed in cancer cells in a cervical smear from a case of primary melanoma of the cervix reported by Fleming and Main (1994). For further discussion of intranuclear cytoplasmic inclusions in malignant melanomas, see Chapter 34. In the case shown in Figure 17-14, cells of an amelanotic malignant melanoma, and the original biopsy of the cervix, were interpreted initially as a poorly differentiated carcinoma. At autopsy, melanin pigment was documented in liver metastases.

It is of interest that, in the presence of melanoma, **abnormalities of squamous cells may be observed in vaginal smears. Most striking is the presence of very large squamous cells with abnormal nuclei** (Fig. 17-13D), or of pigment-bearing benign squamous cells. Such cells may signal the presence of disseminated melanoma elsewhere. The exact site of origin of such cells has not been determined, but their origin in the squamous epithelium of the vagina or cervix seems highly probable.

A few additional case reports of the cytologic presentation of primary malignant melanomas of the uterine cervix are on record (Mudge et al, 1981; Yu and Ketabchi, 1987; Holmquist and Torres, 1988). In the case of Holmquist and Torres, **spindle-shaped malignant cells were observed and initially interpreted as leiomyosarcoma;** the primary tumor involving the cervix and the vagina was a spindle-cell melanoma. A primary **malignant melanoma of the vulva** was diagnosed cytologically by Ehrmann et al (1962). Most lesions of this type are large and ulcerated when seen by the physician. The best hope for prophylaxis is a surgical excision of every pigmented lesion of the vulva.

Benign, melanin-containing **blue nevi,** which occasionally occur in the stroma of the uterine cervix (Goldman and Friedman, 1967; Jiji, 1971; Kudo et al, 1983), are not known to shed any abnormal cells in cervical smears.

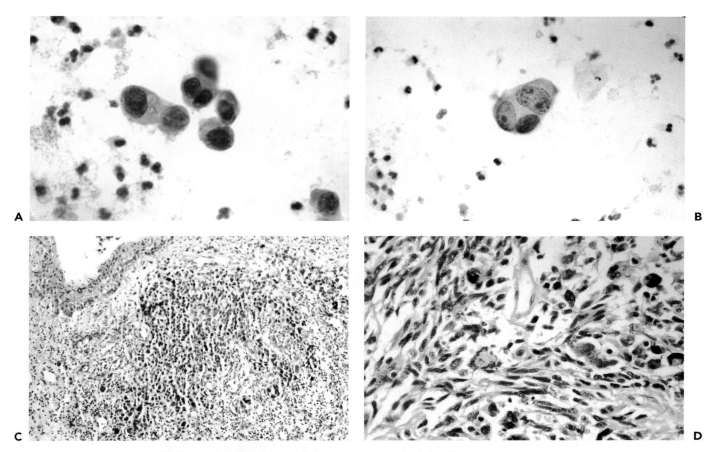

Figure 17-14   Primary melanoma of the uterine cervix, initially mistaken for an anaplastic carcinoma. *A.* A small cluster of large tumor cells with prominent hyperchromatic nuclei shown at high magnification. *B.* A multinucleated tumor cell showing the peripheral arrangement of the large nuclei, provided with large nucleoli. There was no evidence of pigment in this smear. *C.* Original biopsy of the cervix showing a subepithelial malignant tumor composed of small cells. There was no evidence of junctional changes or of melanin formation and the patient was treated for carcinoma. *D.* The patient died of her tumor 2 years after the original smear and biopsy and melanin formation was clearly evident in the liver metastasis.

UNUSUAL MALIGNANT TUMORS IN INFANTS AND CHILDREN

Endodermal Sinus Tumor

These rare tumors occur primarily in the ovary but also occasionally in the vagina or uterine cervix (Larry et al, 1985; Kohorn et al, 1985). Ishi et al (1998) described the cytologic features of one such tumor in a 10-year-old girl with high serum levels of alpha fetoprotein. **Cytoplasmic hyaline inclusions** were observed in the cytoplasm of tumor cells. For further discussion of this tumor, see Chapter 15.

Primitive Neuroectodermal Tumors

These very rare tumors have been described in the vagina and cervix (Horn et al, 1997; Pauwels et al, 2000; Karseladze et al, 2001). Ward et al (2000) described the cytologic findings in a vaginal tumor. Approximately **spherical monotonous tumor cells** with large nuclei and scanty rim of cytoplasm corresponded to rosettes characterizing this neoplasm.

CYTOLOGY OF CANCERS METASTATIC TO THE FEMALE GENITAL TRACT

A great many malignant tumors may produce metastases to the uterus or the vagina. Occasionally, the metastases may involve or reach the surface of these organs and the cancer cells may be found in the cervicovaginal preparations. Some of the cancer cells may also find their way to the vagina through the fallopian tubes, the endometrial cavity, and the endocervical canal, as has been shown by Bhagavan and Weinberg in 1969. It has been stated that, in **metastatic carcinoma, the background of cervicovaginal smears is often free of necrotic material and debris** ("tumor diathesis") when compared with primary carcinomas. **This is correct in some, but not all, cases.** Inflammation, necrosis and blood may be observed in smears, particularly if metastatic cancer has formed a large lesion with a necrotic surface. **Knowledge of clinical history** is usually helpful in assessing the cytologic findings. Still, the history of a treated or co-existing malignant tumor outside of the female genital tract does not rule out a second primary tumor within the genital tract. For example, the association of mammary carcinoma with syn-

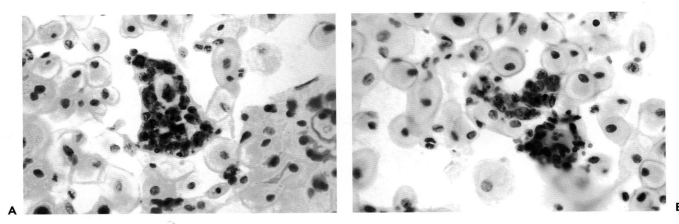

Figure 17-15 Metastatic endometrial carcinoma in the vagina of a 65-year-old woman. *A,B.* Two aspects of the same smear showing clusters of small malignant cells with somewhat enlarged hyperchromatic nuclei. In the absence of history of prior endometrial carcinoma, the precise diagnosis could not be established.

chronous or metachronous carcinomas of the uterine cervix, endometrium, and ovaries is not uncommon.

Even if accurate clinical history is available, the correct cytologic recognition of a metastatic tumor, and its organ of origin, is not necessarily easy, and it is based largely on experience. In many instances, the diagnosis of metastatic cancer may be suspected, because the exfoliated malignant cells do not quite resemble any of the known patterns of cancer of the female genital tract. This is, admittedly, an area in which cytologic diagnosis falls into the realm of art, rather than science, but this is occasionally true of the histologic diagnosis of cancer as well.

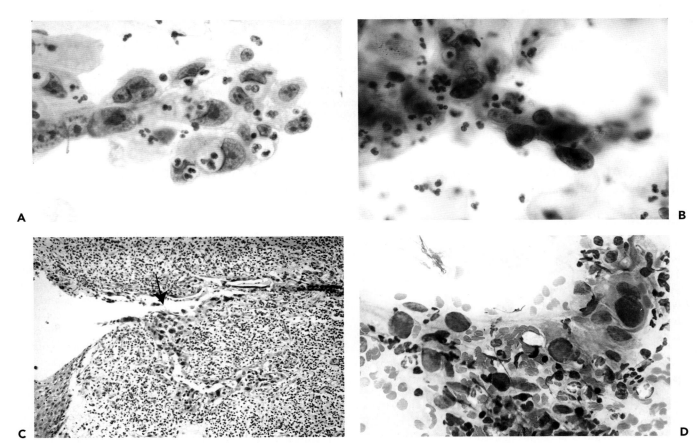

Figure 17-16 Choriocarcinoma metastatic to cervix in a 20-year-old woman. *A,B.* Two aspects of the cervical smear showing very large cancer cells with hyperchromatic nuclei. *C.* Cervical biopsy from the same case showing metastatic choriocarcinoma to the uterine cervix. *D.* Another case of choriocarcinoma with the cervical smear showing numerous, very large cancer cells. (*A–C* case courtesy Dr. John Lukeman, M.D. Anderson Cancer Center, Houston, TX.)

Metastases From Other Component Organs of the Female Genital Tract

Cancers primary in one organ of the female genital tract may metastasize to another organ. For example, metastases of ovarian or endometrial carcinoma to the vagina are not uncommon (Fig. 17-15). The cytologic presentation is often similar to that of the primary tumors (see Chaps. 13 and 14).

Choriocarcinoma

Choriocarcinoma, a tumor of **trophoblasts from the chorionic villi** of the placenta, must be mentioned briefly. The tumors may be a consequence of pregnancy (**gestational choriocarcinoma**) or may be derived from **germ cells of the ovary or testis** (review in Berkowitz and Goldstein, 1996). The gestational choriocarcinomas are relatively uncommon in the Western world, but are exceedingly frequent in Asia, parts of Africa, and Latin America. Many of the tumors are preceded by an important abnormality of placental villi, the **hydatidiform mole,** characterized by a grape-like swelling of the villi, visible to the naked eye. The hydatidiform moles can be **complete** (diploid) or **incomplete** (triploid). Only the complete moles are capable of progession to choriocarinoma. Follow-up of these tumors is based on serum levels of **human chorionic gonadotrophins (hCG).** Fully **malignant cho-** riocarcinoma may **metastasize extensively,** sometimes to the uterine cervix.

Cytology

In the rare cases of metastatic chroriocarcinoma to the lower genital tract, one can sometimes observe the component cells of choriocarcinoma that reflect **the two families of trophoblasts, the small cytotrophoblasts and the very large, multinucleated syncytiotrophoblasts.** The innocent-appearing, small cytotrophic cells may be overlooked but syncytiotrophic cells are striking. The similarity of the large, multinucleated syncytiotrophic tumor cells to benign syncytiophoblasts must be noted (see Chapter 8). In most cases, however, only large cancer cells with single nuclei may be observed (Fig. 17-16). Because of the excellent response of these tumors to chemotherapy, the accurate recognition of the cytologic pattern may be of vital importance to the patient. History of recent pregnancy and high levels of human chorionic gonadotropin are helpful in diagnosis.

The possibility of early diagnosis of these tumors by cytologic techniques should be considered in those geographic areas of the world where the tumor is frequent.

Metastases From Adjacent Organs

Carcinomas of the colon and rectum are relatively frequent invaders of the female genital tract. Young and Hart

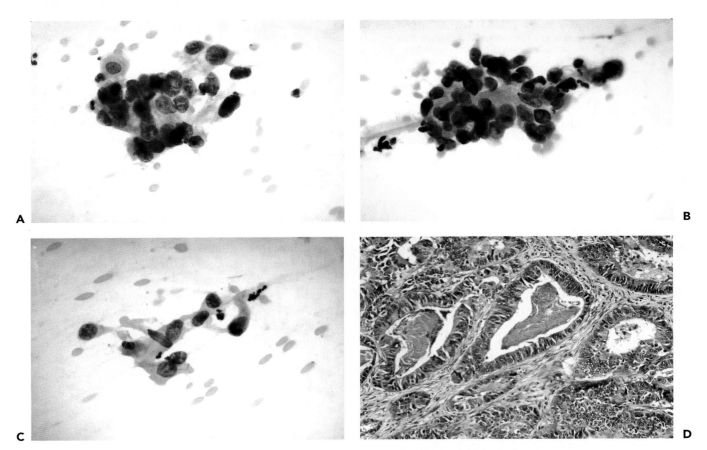

Figure 17-17   Various aspects of rectal adenocarcinoma metastatic to the uterine cervix. In A, the columnar shape of the cancer cells is evident. In B, the cancer cells form a gland-like structure. In C, the cells are columnar and dispersed. D. A histologic section of the original tumor.

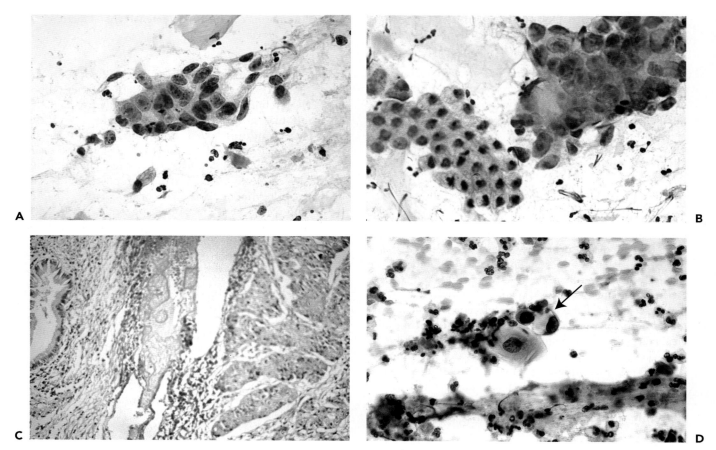

Figure 17-18   Colonic carcinoma, first diagnosed in cervical smears in a 68-year-old woman. *A.* A cluster of columnar cancer cells. *B.* A cluster of benign endocervical cells next to a cluster of tumor cells, some of which show cytoplasm distended with mucus. *C.* Histologic section of colonic carcinoma invading the uterine cervix. *D.* Another example of metastatic colonic carcinoma. The cancer cells in the center of the field have a "signet ring" configuration (*arrow*).

(1998) pointed out that metastatic cancers from the intestinal tract may mimic primary carcinomas of the ovary. A well-known manifestation of metastatic gastrointestinal cancer to the ovary is the **Krukenberg tumor** in which signet ring cancer cells are mixed with a spindle cell reaction in the ovarian stroma. Clinical complaints referable to the genital tract may be the first evidence of disease. In rare cases, the diagnosis of colonic cancer may be first established in cervicovaginal smears.

The most common cytologic presentation of colorectal carcinoma is **cancer cells, occurring singly or in thick clusters, composed of large, often columnar cells** with finely stippled or vacuolated cytoplasm, suggestive of mucus production (Figs. 17-17 and 17-18). The columnar cells are sometimes arranged in **parallel, palisade-like clusters** or form **rosettes.** The **nuclei are large,** usually but not always hyperchromatic, often provided with **large nucleoli.** Less often, the cancer cells are of the **signet-ring type,** i.e., approximately **spherical, with a large hyperchromatic nucleus pushed to the periphery by a large cytoplasmic mucus vacuole** (Fig.17-18D.)

The **differential diagnosis of colonic carcinoma** comprises primary **adenocarcinoma of the endocervix** and **vaginal adenocarcinoma,** the latter particularly in a young

woman with a history of maternal exposure to diethylstilbestrol (DES) (see Chap. 14). The presence of **normal endocervical cells in the smear is in favor of metastatic colonic carcinoma** (Fig. 17-18B). Rarely, benign endocervical or endometrial cells with large mucus vacuoles and normal nuclei may mimic signet ring cells of colonic carcinoma.

Urothelial (transitional cell) carcinoma of the bladder may form metastases to the female genital tract. In the absence of clinical history, the finding of **large, multinucleated tumor cells with one sharply delineated surface** (umbrella cells; see Chap. 22) may occasionally allow for a specific diagnosis. In most cases, however, there are no distinguishing cytologic features that may allow the exact identification of tumor type (Fig. 17-19). It is of note that **metastatic bladder cancer to the vagina or penis may result in changes similar to Paget's disease** (Koss, 1985) (Fig. 17-19D; see Chap. 23). For further comments on metastatic urothelial carcinoma in fluids, see Chapter 26.

Metastases From Distant Sites

Mammary carcinoma is by far the most common source of metastases to the female genital tract. The cytologic

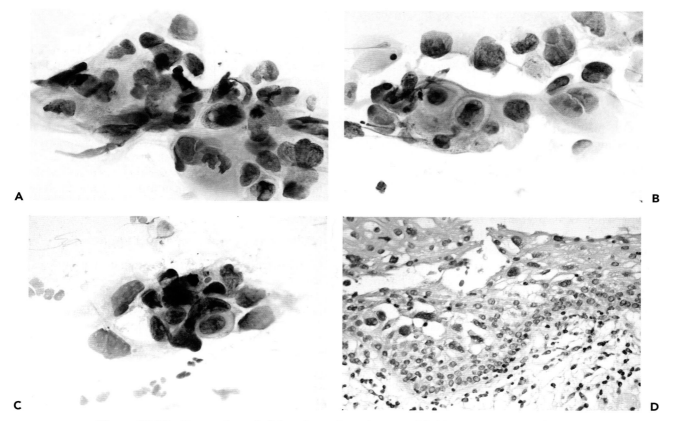

Figure 17-19 **Metastatic urothelial carcinoma from the urinary bladder to vagina.** *A–C.* Clusters of obvious malignant cells, some of which have columnar configuration. Note the sharply demarcated cytoplasm in some of the cells. *D.* Biopsy of vagina showing the pagetoid appearance of the epithelium.

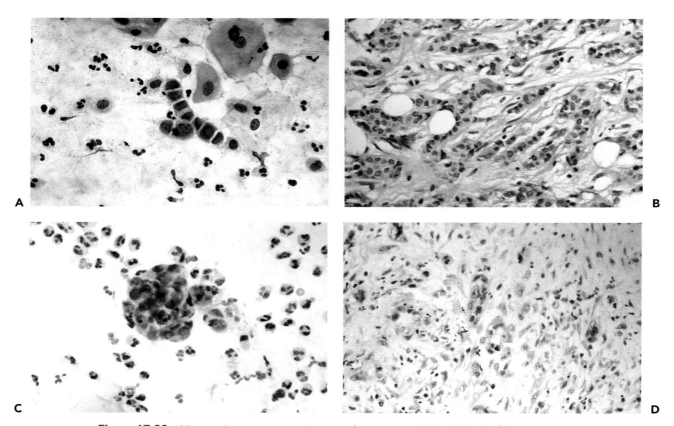

Figure 17-20 **Metastatic mammary carcinoma to the uterus.** *A.* A classical single-file arrangement of breast cancer cells consistent with lobular carcinoma, shown in *B. C.* Another aspect of metastatic mammary carcinoma in which the cells form a papillary cluster. *D.* Biopsy from same case as *C* showing metastatic mammary carcinoma to the cervix.

presentation is very variable. Occasionally, **cancer cells are arranged in "single file,"** suggestive of lobular carcinoma (Fig. 17-20A,B) but, more often, the smear contains clusters of malignant cells suggestive of adenocarcinoma without distinguishing features (Figs. 17-20C,D, 17-21). Metastatic mammary carcinoma, particularly of the **lobular type, may also have a signet ring cell pattern with a large vacuole occupying the center of the cell and the nucleus pushed to the periphery.** The **mammary signet ring cells are much smaller than the cells from tumors of the gastrointestinal tract** (see Chap. 29). As a further point of distinction, **a central condensation of mucus** may be observed **within the cytoplasmic vacuoles in mammary, but not the gastrointestinal cancer.** Tamoxifen therapy does not protect women from developing metastatic mammary cancer, as shown in Figure 17-21C,D. Metastatic mammary carcinoma to endometrial polyps caused by tamoxifen have been reported (Houghton et al, 2003). For further description of mammary cancer cells, see Chapter 29.

Cancers of a variety of other distant primary sites may occasionally form metastases to the female genital tract. We have observed **bronchogenic, pancreatic,** and **renal carcinomas,** to name only a few, although their exact identification is rarely possible in the absence of clinical history and prior histologic or cytologic material for purposes of comparison. Metastases from **gastric cancer** were described by Matsuura et al (1997), from a **salivary duct carcinoma** (Vinette-Leduc et al, 1999), and from a variety of sites by Gupta and Balsara (1999). **Metastatic melanoma** to the vagina, an extremely uncommon event, may also occur (Chung et al, 1980; Gupta et al, 2003). Undoubtedly, other metastases will be described in the future but their cytologic features are not likely to be specific.

Malignant Lymphomas and Leukemias

Generalized non-Hodgkin's malignant lymphomas may involve the female genital tract with a frequency that is perhaps not sufficiently appreciated. They may mimic primary cancer of the cervix, and also of the vagina, the uterus, and the ovaries. The alert pathologist, regardless of whether he or she is dealing with a histologic or a cytologic preparation, may be in a position to render the correct diagnosis **by merely considering malignant lymphoma in the differential diagnosis.**

Large-cell malignant lymphomas are the most com-

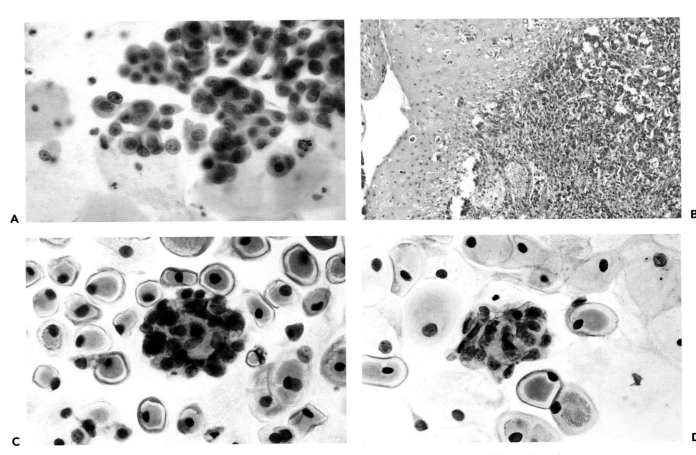

Figure 17-21 Metastatic mammary carcinoma in cervicovaginal smears. *A.* Large, loosely structured clusters of relatively small malignant cells. The precise diagnosis of tumor type could not be established on morphology alone. *B.* Biopsy of cervix in this case showing a large area of metastatic mammary carcinoma in the uterine cervix. *C,D.* Metastatic mammary carcinoma in a 65-year-old woman receiving Tamoxifen therapy. *C.* A classical papillary cluster in the background of an atrophic smear. *D.* A smaller cluster of malignant cells in the same smear as C.

mon form of malignant lymphoma to invade the female genital tract. **Small-cell lymphomas and acute leukemias** are cytologically identical. The cytologic presentation is identical to primary tumors of this type, described above. In leukemias, there is often evidence of bleeding, and numerous erythrocytes may obscure the pattern of the smear. Ceelan and Sakurai (1962) reported cytologic evidence of leukemia in 17 of 61 consecutive leukemic patients from whom cervical smears were obtained. It has also been recorded by Kanter and Mercer (1950) that ulcerative lesions of the vagina may occur in **monocytic leukemia.**

Metastatic **Hodgkin's disease** may occasionally be observed in cervical smears. Uyeda et al (1969) described classic Reed-Sternberg cells with two "mirror-image" large nuclei and prominent nucleoli in a patient with this disorder.

BIBLIOGRAPHY

Abeler V, Kjorstad KE, Langholm R, Marto, PF. Granulocytic sarcoma (chloroma) of the uterine cervix: Report of two cases. Int J Gynecol Pathol 2: 88–92, 1983.

Abell MR: Primary melanoblastoma of the uterine cervix. Am J Clin Pathol 36:248–255, 1961.

Abell MR, Ramirez JA. Sarcomas and carcinosarcomas of the uterine cervix. Cancer 31:1176–1192, 1973.

Abrams J, Talcott J, Corson JM. Pulmonary metastases in patients with low-grade endometrial stromal sarcoma. Clincopathologic findings with immunohistochemical characterization. Am J Surg Pathol 13:133–140, 1989.

Albores-Saavedra J, Larraza O, Poucell S, Rodriguez-Martinez HA. Carcinoid of the uterine cervix. Cancer 38:2328–2342, 1976.

Amagai M, Koch PJ, Nishikawa T, Stanley JR. Pemphigus vulgaris antigen (desmoglein 3) is localized in the lower epidermis, the site of blister formation in patients. J Invest Dermatopathol 106:76–78, 1996.

Andrews SJ, Hernandez E, Woods J, Cook B. Burkitt's-like lymphoma presenting as a gynecologic tumor. Gynecol Oncol 30:131–136, 1988.

Ariel IM. Malignant melanoma of the female genital system: A report of 48 patients and review of the literature. J Surg Oncol 16:371–383, 1981.

Armenia CS, Shaver DN, Melvin WM. Decidual transformation of the cervical stroma simulating reticulum cell sarcoma. Am J Obstet Gynecol 89: 808–816, 1964.

Baggish M, Woodruff JD. Adenoid basal lesions of the uterine cervix. Obstet Gynecol 37:807–819, 1971.

Barrett RJ, Davos I, Leuchter RS, Lagasse LD. Neuroendocrine features in poorly differentiated and undifferentiated carcinomas of the cervix. Cancer 60: 2325–2330, 1987.

Becker SN, Wong JI. Detection of endometrial stromal sarcoma in cervicovaginal smears. Report of three cases. Acta Cytol 25:272–276, 1981.

Bell DA, Shimm DS, Gang DL. Wilms' tumor of the endocervix. Arch Pathol Lab Med 109:371–373, 1985.

Bell SW, Kempson RL, Hendrickson MR. Problematic uterine smooth muscle neoplasms: A clinicopathologic study of 213 cases. Am J Surg Pathol 18: 535–558, 1994.

Benda JA, Platz CE, Anderson B. Malignant melanoma of the vulva: A clinical-pathologic review of 16 cases. Int J Gynecol Pathol 5:202–216, 1986.

Benitez E, Rodriguez HA, Rodriguez-Cuevas H, Chavez GB. Adenoid cystic carcinoma of the uterine cervix. Report of a case and review of 4 cases. Obstet Gynecol 33:757–762, 1969.

Berkowitz RS, Goldstein DP. Chorionic tumors. N Engl J Med 335:1740–1748, 1996.

Beutner EH, Jordon RE. Demonstration of skin antibodies in sera of pemphigus vulgaris patient by indirect immunofluorescent staining. Proc Soc Exp Biol Med 117:505–510, 1964.

Bhagavan BS, Weinberg T. Cytopathologic diagnosis of metastatic cancer by cervical and vaginal smears with report of a case. Acta Cytol 13:377–381, 1969.

Bittencourt AL, Guimaraes JP, Barbosa HS, et al. Adeno cystic carcinoma of the uterine cervix: Report of six cases and review of the literature. Acta Med Port 1:697–706, 1979.

Bloch T, Roth LM, Stehman FB, et al. Osteosarcoma of the uterine cervix associated with hyperplastic and atypical mesonephric rests. Cancer 62: 1594–1600, 1988.

Bodner K, Bodner-Adler B, Kimberger O, et al. Evaluating prognostic parameters in women with uterine leiomyosarcoma. A clinicopathologic study. J Reprod Med 48:95–100, 2003.

Bottles K, Lacey CG, Goldberg J, et al. Merkel cell carcinoma of the vulva. Obstet Gynecol 63:61S–65S, 1984.

Bradgate MG, Rollason TP, McConkey CC, Powell J. Malignant melanoma of

the vulva: a clinicopathological study of 50 women. Br J Obstet Gynaecol 97:124–133, 1990.

Brainard JA, Hart WR. Adenoid basal epitheliomas of the uterine cervix. A reevaluation of distinctive cervical basaloid lesions currently classified as adenoid basal carcinoma and adenoid basal hyperplasia. Am J Surg Pathol 22:965–975, 1998.

Brand E, Berek JS, Nieberg RK, Hacker NF. Rhabdomyosarcoma of the uterine cervix. Sarcoma botryoides. Cancer 60:1552–1560, 1987.

Brand E, Fu YS, Lagasse LD, Berek JS. Vulvovaginal melanoma: Report of seven cases and literature review. Gynecol Oncol 33:54–60, 1989.

Brooks JJ, LiVolsi VA. Liposarcoma of the vulva. Am J Obstet Gynecol 156: 73–75, 1987.

Buchler DA, Kline JC. Primary lymphoma of the vagina. Obstet Gynecol 40: 235–237, 1972.

Butterworth CE Jr, Hatch KD, Macaluso M, et al. Folate deficiency and cervical dysplasia. JAMA 267:528–533, 1992.

Carr I, Hill AS, Hancock B, Neal FE. Malignant lymphoma of the cervix uteri: Histology and ultrastructure. J Clin Pathol 29:680–686, 1976.

Ceelan GH, Sakurai M. Vaginal cytology in leukemia. Acta Cytol 6:370–372, 1962.

Ces-Blance JA. Sarcoma of the vagina. An unusual cytologic diagnosis. Acta Cytol 21:547–549, 1977.

Chalvardijan A, Picard L, Shaw R, Davey R, Cairns JD: Malacoplakia of the female genital tract. Am J Obstet Gynecol 138:391–394, 1980.

Chin JL, Wolf RM, Huben RP, Pontes JE. Vaginal recurrence after cystectomy for bladder cancer. J Urol 134:58–61, 1985.

Cho D, Buscema J, Rosenshein NB, Woodruff JD. Primary breast cancer of the vulva. Obstet Gynecol 66:79S–81S, 1985.

Chung A, Casey MJ, Flannery JT, et al. Malignant melanoma of the vagina: report of 19 cases. Obstet Gynecol 55:720–727, 1980.

Chung AF, Woodruff JM, Lewis JL Jr. Malignant melanoma of the vulva: Report of 44 cases. Obstet Gynecol 45:638–646, 1975.

Clement PB. Miscellaneous primary neoplasms and metastatic neoplasms. In Clement P, Young R, (eds). Contemporary Issues in Surgical Pathology, Vol 19. Tumors and Tumorlike Lesions of the Uterine Corpus and Cervix. New York, Churchill Livingstone, 1993, pp 395–404.

Clement PB, Scully RE. Müllerian adenosarcoma of the uterus. Cancer 34: 1138–1149, 1974.

Clement PB, Scully RE. Müllerian adenosarcomas of the uterus with sex cord-like elements. A clinicopathologic analysis of eight cases. Am J Clin Pathol 91:664–672, 1989.

Clement PB, Young RH, Scully RE. Intravenous leiomyomatosis of the uterus. A clinicopathological analysis of 16 cases with unusual histologic features. Am J Surg Pathol 12:932–945, 1988.

Coates JB III, Hales JS. Granular cell myoblastoma of the vulva. Obstet Gynecol 41:796–799, 1973.

Copeland LJ, Cleary K, Sneige N, Edwards CL. Neuroendocrine (Merkel cell) carcinoma of the vulva: A case report and review of the literature. Gynecol Oncol 22:367–378, 1985.

Cviko A, Briem B, Granter SR, et al. Adenoid basal carcinomas of the cervix: A unique morphological evolution with cell cycle correlates. Hum Pathol 31:740–744, 2000.

Dance EF, Fullmer CD. Extrauterine carcinoma cells observed in cervicovaginal smears. Acta Cytol 14:187–191, 1970.

Daniel WW, Koss LG, Brunschwig, A. Sarcoma botryoides of the vagina. Cancer 12:74–84, 1959.

Daroca PJ, Durandhar HN. Basaloid carcinoma of the uterine cervix. Am J Surg Pathol 4:235–239, 1980.

Daw E. Extragenital adenocarcinoma metastatic to the cervix uteri. Am J Obstet Gynecol 114:1104–1105, 1972.

Daya DA, Scully RE. Sarcoma botryoides of the uterine cervix in young women: A clinicopathological study of 13 cases. Gynecol Oncol 29:290–304, 1988.

Dayton V, Henry M, Stanley MW, et al. Adenoid cystic carcinoma of the uterine cervix. Cytologic features. Acta Cytol 34:125–128, 1990.

De La Maza LM, Thayer BA, Naeim F. Cylindroma of the uterine cervix with peritoneal metastases: Report of a case and review of the literature. Am J Obstet Gynecol 112:121–125, 1972.

Delgado G, Smith JP, Luis D, Gallagher S. Reticulum-cell sarcoma of the cervix. Am J Obstet Gynecol 125:691–694, 1976.

Dellenbach P, Hartmann JM, Methlin G. Rhabdomyosarcome du vagin chez la femme. A propos d'un cas. Rév Fr Gynécol 69:265–268, 1974.

Demopoulos RI, Denarvaez R, Kaji V. Benign mixed mesodermal tumors of the uterus: A histogenetic study. Am J Clin Pathol 60:377–383, 1973.

de Muelenaere GF. Vaginal metastases in endometrial carcinoma. Am J Obstet Gynecol 118:168–172, 1974.

Deshpande AH, Munshi MM. Primary malignant melanoma of the uterine cervix: Report of a case diagnosed by cervical scrape cytology and review of the literature. Diagn Cytopathol 25:108–111, 2001.

Dhimes P, Alberti N, DeAgustin P, Tubio J. Primary malignant lymphoma of the uterine cervix: report of a case with cytologic and immunohistochemical diagnosis. Cytopathol 7:204–210, 1996.

Dictor M. Malignant mixed mesodermal tumor of the ovary: A report of 22 cases. Obstet Gynecol 65:720–724, 1985.

Donkers B, Kazzaz BA, Meijering JH. Rhabdomyosarcoma of the corpus uteri. Am J Obstet Gynecol 114:1025–1030, 1972.

Dvoretsky PM, Bonfiglio TA, Patten SF Jr, Helmkamp BF. Pemphigus vulgaris and microinvasive squamous-cell carcinoma of the uterine cervix. Acta Cytol 29:403–410, 1985.

Ehrmann RL, Younge PA, Level VL. The exfoliative cytology and histogenesis of an early primary malignant melanoma of the vagina. Acta Cytol 6:245–254, 1962.

Falcon-Escobedo R, Mora-Tiscareno A, Pueblitz-Peredo S. Malacoplakia of the uterine cervix. Histologic, cytologic, and ultrastructural study. Acta Cytol 30: 281–284, 1986.

Favre Y, Genton CY, Ziogas V, Schreiner WE. Carcinomes non gynecologiques, occultes, diagnostiqués au travers de leurs métastases ovariennes. Schweiz Med Wochenschr 116:845–851, 1986.

Ferry JA, Scully RE. Adenoid cystic carcinoma and adenoid basal carcinoma of the uterine cervix. A study of 28 cases. Am J Surg Pathol 12:134–144, 1988.

Fleming H, Mein P. Primary melanoma of cervix. A case report. Acta Cytol 38: 65–69, 1994.

Foschini MP, Eusebi V, Tison V. Alveolar soft part sarcoma of the cervix uteri. A case report. Pathol Res Pract 184:354–358, 1989.

Fox H, Langley FA, Govan ADT, Hill AS, Bennett MH. Malignant lymphoma presenting as an ovarian tumour: A clinicopathological analysis of 34 cases. Br J Obstet Gynaecol 95:386–390, 1988.

Friedman D, Haim S, Paldi E. Refractory involvement of cervix uteri in a case of pemphigus vulgaris. Am J Obstet Gynecol 110:1023–1024, 1971.

Fukuyama M, Matsui T, Hozumi K, et al. Malignant fibrous histiocytoma of the vagina—a case report (Japanese). J Jpn Soc Clin Cytol 25:1086–1091, 1986.

Gabriele A, Gaudiano L. Primary malignant lymphoma of the cervix. A case report. J Reprod Med 48:899–901, 2003.

Gad A, Eusebi V. Rhabdomyoma of the vagina. J Pathol 115:179–181, 1975.

Gallager HS, Simpson CB, Ayala AG. Adenoid cystic carcinoma of the uterine cervix. Cancer 27:1398–1402, 1971.

Garcia-Valdecasas R, Rodriguez-Rico L, Linares J, Galera H, Salvatierra V. Malignant melanoma of the vagina. A case diagnosed cytologically. Acta Cytol 18:535–537, 1974.

Garret R. Extrauterine tumor cells in vaginal and cervical smears. Obstet Gynecol 14:21–27, 1959.

Genton CY, Kunz J, Schreiner WE. Primary malignant melanoma of the vagina and cervix uteri: Report of a case with ultrastructural study. Virchows Arch [A] 393:320–327, 1981.

Gersell DJ, Mazoujian G, Mutch DG, Rudloff MA. Small-cell undifferentiated carcinoma of the cervix. A clinicopathologic, ultrastructural, and immunocytochemical study of 15 cases. Am J Surg Pathol 12:648–698 1988.

Ghavimi F, Exelby PR, Lieberman PH, et al. Multidisciplinary treatment of embryonal rhabdomyosarcoma in children: A progress report. Natl Cancer Inst Monogr 56:111–120, 1981.

Gold JH, Bossen EH. Benign vaginal rhabdomyoma. A light and electron microscopic study. Cancer 37:2283–2294, 1976.

Goldman RL, Friedman NB. Blue nevus of the uterine cervix. Cancer 20: 210–214, 1967.

Gordon HW, et al. Adenoid cystic (cylindromatous) carcinoma of the uterine cervix: Report of two cases. Am J Clin Pathol 58:51–57, 1972.

Grafton WD, Kamm RC, Cowley LH. Cytologic characteristics of adenoid cystic carcinoma of the cervix uteri. Acta Cytol 20:164–166, 1976.

Grayson W, Taylor LF, Cooper K. Adenoid basal carcinoma of the uterine cervix: Detection of integrated human papillomavirus in a rare tumor of putative "reserve cell" origin. Int J Gynecol Pathol 16:307–312, 1997.

Grayson W, Taylor LF, Cooper K. Adenoid cystic and adenoid basal carcinoma of the uterine cervix: Comparative morphologic, mucin, and immunohistochemical profile of two rare neoplasms of putative "reserve cell" origin. Am J Surg Pathol 23:448–458, 1999.

Grayson W, Taylor LF, Cooper K, et al. Carcinosarcoma of the uterine cervix. A report of eight cases with immunohistochemical analysis and evaluation of human papillomavirus status. Am J Surg Pathol 25:338–347, 2001.

Grimalt MA, Arguells M, Ferenczy A. Papillary cystadenofibroma of endometrium: A histochemical and ultrastructural study. Cancer 36:137–144, 1975.

Groben P, Reddick R, Askin F. The pathologic spectrum of small cell carcinoma of the cervix. Int J Gynecol Pathol 4:42–57, 1985.

Gupta D, Balsara G. Extrauterine malignancies. Role of Pap smears in diagnosis and management. Acta Cytol 43:806–813, 1999.

Gupta D, Malpica A, Deavers MT, Silva EG. Vaginal melanoma. A clinicopathologic and immunohistochemical study of 26 cases. Am J Surg Pathol 26:1450–1457, 2002.

Gupta D, Neto AG, Deavers MT, et al. Metastatic melanoma to the vagina: Clinicopathologic and immunohistochemical study of three cases and literature review. Int J Gynecol Pathol 22:136–140, 2003.

Hafiz MA, Kragel PJ, Toker C. Carcinoma of the uterine cervix resembling lymphoepithelioma. Obstet Gynecol 66:829–831, 1985.

Hajdu SI, Hajdu EO. Cytopathology of Sarcomas and Other Nonepithelial Malignant Tumors. Philadelphia, W.B. Saunders, 1976.

Hajdu SI, Koss LG. Cytologic diagnosis of metastic myosarcoma. Acta Cytol 13:545–551, 1969.

Hall DJ, Schneider V, Goplerud DR. Primary malignant melanoma of the uterine cervix. Obstet Gynecol 56:525–529, 1980.

Halpin TF, Hunter RE, Cohen MB. Lymphoepithelioma of the uterine cervix. Gynecol Oncol 34:101–105, 1989.

Harper JM, Levine AJ, Rosenthal DL, et al. Erythrocyte folate level, oral contraceptive use and abnormal cervical cytology. Acta Cytol 38: 324–330, 1994.

Harris NL, Scully RE. Malignant lymphoma and granulocytic sarcoma of uterus and vagina. Cancer 53:2530–2545, 1985.

Havys DM, Shimada H, Raney RB, et al. Sarcoma of the vagina and uterus: The intergroup Rhabdomyosarcoma Study. J Pediatr Surg 20:718–724, 1985.

Hernandez-Ortiz MJ, Valenzuela-Ruiz P, Gonzalez-Estecha A, et al. Fine needle aspiration cytology of primary epithelioid sarcoma of the vulva. A case report. Acta Cytol 39:100–103, 1995.

Hilgers RD, Malkasian GD, Soule EH. Embryonal rhabdomyosarcoma (botryoid type) of the vagina. Am J Obstet Gynecol 107:484–502, 1970.

Hirahatake K, Hareyama H, Kure R, et al. Cytologic and hormonal findings in a carcinoid tumor of the uterine cervix. Acta Cytol 34:119–124, 1990.

Holmquist ND. The exfoliative cytology of mixed mesodermal tumors of the uterus. Acta Cytol 6:373–375, 1962.

Holmquist ND, Torres J. Malignant melanoma of the cervix: Report of a case. Acta Cytol 32:252–256, 1988.

Horn LC, Fischer U, Bliek K. Primitive neuroectodermal tumor of the cervix uteri: A case report. Gen Diagn Pathol 142:227–230, 1997.

Houghton JP, Ioffe OB, Silverberg SG, et al. Metastatic breast lobular carcinoma involving tamoxifen-associated endometrial polyps: Report of two cases and review of tamoxifen-associated polypoid uterine lesions. Mod Pathol 16: 395–398, 2003.

Hsiu J-G, Stawicki ME. The cytologic findings in two cases of stromal sarcoma of the uterus. Acta Cytol 23:487–489, 1979.

Iliya FA, Muggia FM, O'Leary JA, O'Leary TM. Gynecologic manifestations of reticulum cell sarcoma. Obstet Gynecol 31:266–269, 1968.

Imachi M, Tsukamoto N, Kamura T, et al. Alveolar rhabdomyosarcoma of the vulva. Report of two cases. Acta Cytol 35:345–349, 1991.

Ishi K, Suzuki F, Saito A, et al. Cytodiagnosis of vaginal endodermal sinus tumor. A case report. Acta Cytol 42:399–402, 1998.

Issa PY, Salem PA, Brihi E, Azoury RS. Eosinophilic granuloma with involvement of female genitalia. Am J Obstet Gynecol 137:608–612, 1980.

Jiji V. Blue nevus of the endocervix. Arch Pathol Lab Med 92:203–205, 1971.

Johannessen JV, Capella C, Solcia E, Davy M, Sobrinho-Simoes M. Endocrine cell carcinoma of the uterine cervix. Diagn Gynecol Obstet 2:127–134, 1980.

Johnson CE, Soule EH. Malignant lymphoma as a gynecologic problem. Obstet Gynecol 9:149–157, 1957.

Jones MW, Kkounelis S, Papadaki H, et al. The origin and molecular characterization of adenoid basal carcinoma of the uterine cervix. Int J Gynecol Pathol 16:301–306, 1997.

Kanter AF, Mercer TH. Ulcerative vaginitis in a case of acute monocytic leukemia. Am J Obstet Gynecol 60:455–456, 1950.

Kapadia SB, Krause JR, Kanbour AI, Hartsock RJ. Granulocytic sarcoma of the uterus. Cancer 41:687–691, 1978.

Kapila K, Verma K. Intracellular bacilli in vaginal smears in a case of malakoplakia. Acta Cytol 33:410–411, 1989.

Karney MY, Cassidy MS, Zahn CM, Snyder RR. Melanosis of the vagina. A case report. J Reprod Med 46:389–391, 2001.

Karseladze AI, Filipova NA, Navarro S, Llombart-Bosch A. Primitive neuroectodermal tumor of the uterus. A case report. J Reprod Med 46:845–848, 2001.

Katayama I, Hajian G, Evjy JT. Cytologic diagnosis of reticulum cell sarcoma of the uterine cervix. Acta Cytol 17:498–501, 1973.

Kaufman RH, Watts JM, Gardner HL. Pemphigus vulgaris genital involvement; report of 2 cases. Obstet Gynecol 33:264–266, 1969.

Kempson RL. Sarcomas and related neoplasms. In Norris HJ, Hertig AT, Abell MR (eds). The Uterus. Baltimore, Williams & Wilkins, 1973, pp 298–319.

King LA, Talledo OE, Gallup DG, et al. Adenoid cystic carcinoma of the cervix in women under age 40. Gynecol Oncol 32:26–30, 1989.

Kitay DZ, Wentz WB. Cervical cytology in folic acid deficiency of pregnancy. Am J Obstet Gynecol 104:931–938, 1969.

Klaus H. Quantitative criteria of folate deficiency in cervico-vaginal cytograms, with report of a new parameter. Acta Cytol 16:50–53, 1971.

Klijanienko J, Caillaud J-M, Lagace R, Vielh P. Fine-needle aspiration of leiomyosarcoma: A correlative cytohistopathological study of 96 tumors in 68 patients. Diagn Cytopathol 28:119–125, 2003.

Kohorn EI, McIntosh S, Lytton B, et al. Endodermal sinus tumor of the infant vagina. Gynecol Oncol 20:196–203, 1985.

Komaki R, Cox JD, Hansen RM, et al. Malignant lymphoma of the uterine cervix. Cancer 54:1699–1704, 1984.

Korhonen M, Stenback F. Adenocarcinoma metastatic to the uterine cervix. Gynecol Obstet Invest 17:57–65, 1984.

Koss LG. Tumors of the Urinary Bladder. Supplement. Atlas of Tumor Pathology, Fascicle II, Second Series. Washington, DC: Armed Forces Institute of Pathology, 1985.

Koss LG, Spiro RH, Brunschwig A. Endometrial stromal sarcoma. Surg Gynecol Obstet 121:431–537, 1965.

Krain LS, Rosenthal I, Newcomer VD. Pemphigus vulgaris involving the cervix associated with endometrial carcinoma of the uterus. A case report with immunofluorescent findings. Int J Dermatol 12:220–228, 1973.

Krumermann M, Chung A. Solitary reticulum cell sarcoma of the uterine cervix with initial cytodiagnosis. Acta Cytol 22:46–50, 1978.

Kudo R, Nagayama T, Miura M, Fukunaga N. Blue nevus of the uterine cervix. Arch Pathol Lab Med 107:87–90, 1983.

Larbig GG, Clemmer JJ, Koss LG, Foote FW Jr. Plexiform tumorlets of endometrial stromal origin. Am J Clin Pathol 44:32–35, 1965.

Larraza-Hernandez O, Molberg KH, Lindberg G, et al. Ectopic prostate tissue in the uterine cervix. Int J Gynecol Pathol 16:291–293, 1997.

Larry J, Copeland LJ, Sneige N, et al. Endodermal sinus tumor of the vagina and cervix. Cancer 38:2404–2419, 1985.

Levitan Z, Gordon AN, Kaplan AL, Kaufman RH. Primary malignant melanoma of the vagina: Report of four cases and review of the literature. Gynecol Oncol 33:85–90, 1989.

Libcke JH. The cytology of cervical pemphigus. Acta Cytol 14:42–44, 1970.

Lin JI, Caracta PF, Ny CHG, et al. Malacoplakia of the vagina. South Med J 73: 326–328, 1979.

Lininger RA, Wistuba I, Gazdar A, et al. Human papillomavirus type 16 is detected in transitional cell carcinomas and squamotransitional cell carcinomas of the cervix and endometrium. Cancer 83:521–527, 1998.

Linthicum CM. Primary malignant melanoma of the vagina. A case report. Acta Cytol 15:179–181, 1971.

Luksch F. Leukemia cells in vaginal smears [Letter]. Acta Cytol 8:95, 1964.

Mann R, Roberts WS, Gunasakeran S, Tralins A. Primary lymphoma of the uterine cervix. Gynecol Oncol 26:127–134, 1987.

Massoni EA, Hajdu SI. Cytology of primary and metastatic uterine sarcomas. Acta Cytol 28:93–100, 1984.

Masubuchi S, Nagai I, Hirata M, Kubo H, Masubuchi K. Cytologic studies of malignant melanoma of the vagina. Acta Cytol 19:527–532, 1975.

Matsuura Y, Saito R, Kawagoe T, et al. Cytologic analysis of primary stomach adenocarcinoma metastatic to the uterine cervix. Acta Cytol 41:291–294, 1997.

Matsuyama T, Tsukamoto N, Kaku T, et al. Primary malignant lymphoma of the uterine corpus and cervix. Acta Cytol 33:228–232, 1989.

McElin TW, Wagner AL Jr. Primary malignant vaginal lymphoma. Case report. Am J Obstet Gynecol 110:883–885, 1971.

Miles PA, Herrera GA, Mena H, Trujillo I. Cytologic findings in primary malignant carcinoid tumor of the cervix. Acta Cytol 29:1003–1008, 1985.

Mills SE, Austin MB, Randall ME. Lymphoepithelioma-like carcinoma of the uterine cervix. Am J Surg Pathol 9:883–889, 1985.

Mortel R, Koss LG, Lewis JL Jr, D'Urso JR. Mesodermal mixed tumors of the uterine corpus. Obstet Gynecol 43:248–252, 1974.

Mudge TJ, Johnson J, MacFarlane A. Primary malignant melanoma of the cervix. Br J Obstet Gynaecol 88:1257–1259, 1981.

Mullins JD, Hilliard GD. Cervical carcinoid (argyrophyl cell carcinoma) associated with an endocervical adenocarcinoma: A light and ultrastructural study. Cancer 47:785–790, 1981.

Nasiell M. Hodgkin's disease limited to the uterine cervix. A case report including cytological findings in the cervical and vaginal smears. Acta Cytol 8: 16–18, 1964.

Ng ABP, Teeple D, Lindner EA, Reagan JW. The cellular manifestations of extrauterine cancer. Acta Cytol 18:108–117, 1974.

Ng KH, Chan DPC, Prathap K. Primary melanoma of the vagina. Aust NZ J Obstet Gynaecol 12:65–67, 1972.

Noel J-C, Lespagnard L, Fayt I, et al. Evidence of human papilloma virus infection but lack of Epstein-Barr virus in lymphoepithelioma-like carcinoma of uterine cervix: Report of two cases and review of the literature. Hum Pathol 32:135–138, 2001.

Norris HJ, Taylor HB. Mesenchymal tumors of the uterus. III. A clinical and pathologic study of 31 carcinosarcomas. Cancer 19:1459–1465, 1966.

Nucci MR, Ferry JA, Young RH. Ectopic prostatic tissue in the uterine cervix. A report of four cases and review of ectopic prostatic tissue. Am J Surg Pathol 24:1224–1230, 2000.

Okagaki T, Ishida T, Hilgers RD. A malignant tumor of the vagina resembling synovial sarcoma. Cancer 37:2306–2320, 1976.

Oliva E, Clement PB, Young RH, Scully RE. Mixed endometrial stromal and smooth muscle tumors of the uterus. A clinicopathologic study of 15 cases. Am J Surg Pathol 22:997–1005, 1998.

Oliva E, Clement PB, Young, RH. Epithelioid endometrial and endometrioid stromal tumors: A report of four cases emphasizing their distinction from epithelioid smooth muscle tumors and other oxyphilic uterine and extrauterine tumors. Int J Gynecol Pathol 21:48–55, 2001.

Oliva E, Ferry JA, Young RH, et al. Granulocytic sarcoma of the female genital tract: a clinicopathologic study of 11 cases. Am J Surg Pathol 21:1156–1165, 1997.

Parker JE. Cytologic findings associated with primary uterine malignancies of mixed cell types (malignant mixed Müllerian tumor). Acta Cytol 8:316–320, 1964.

Pauwels P, Ambros P, Hattinger C, et al. Peripheral primitive neuroectodermal tumour of the cervix. Virchows Arch 436:68–73, 2000.

Perren T, Farrant M, McCarthy K, et al. Lymphomas of the cervix and upper vagina: A report of five cases and a review of the literature. Gynecol Oncol 44:87–95, 1992.

Peterson LS, Neumann AA. Cytologic features of adenoid basal carcinoma of the uterine cervix. A case report. Acta Cytol 39:563–568, 1995.

Powers CN, Stastny JF, Frable WJ. Adenoid basal carcinoma of the cervix: a potential pitfall in cervicovaginal cytology. Diagn Cytopathol 14:172–177, 1996.

Prasad KR, Kumari GS, Arcuna CA, et al. Fibroadenoma of ectopic breast tissue in the vulva. A case report [published erratum appears in Acta Cytol 40: 146, 1996]. Acta Cytol 39:791–792, 1995.

Prempree T, Villasanta U, Tang C-K. Management of adenoic cystic carcinoma of the uterine cervix (cylindroma). Cancer 46:1631–1635, 1980.

Proca DM, Hitchcock CL, Keyhani-Rofagha S. Exfoliative cytology of lymphoepithelioma-like carcinoma of the uterine cervix. Acta Cytol 44:410–414, 2000.

Qizilbash AH. Blue nevus of the uterine cervix: Report of a case. Am J Clin Pathol 59:803–806, 1973.

Ramzy I, Yuzpe AA, Hendelman J. Adenoid cystic carcinoma of the uterine cervix. Obstet Gynecol 45:679-683, 1975.

Ravinsky E, Safneck JR, Chantziantoniou N. Cytologic features of primary adenoid cystic carcinoma of the uterine cervix. A case report. Acta Cytol 40: 1304–1308, 1996.

Reich O, Pickel H, Purstner P. Exfoliative cytology of a lymphoepithelioma-like carcinoma in a cervical smear. A case report. Acta Cytol 43:285–288, 1999.

Rossi G, Bonacorsi G, Longo L, et al. Primary high-grade mucosa-associated lymphoid tissue-type lymphoma of the cervix presenting as a common endocervical polyp. Arch Pathol Lab Med 125:537–540, 2001.

Roszel JF. Canine metastatic mammary carcinoma cells in smears from genital epithelium. Vet Pathol 11:20–28, 1974.

Russin VL, Valente PT, Hanjani P. Psammoma bodies in neuroendocrine carcinoma of the uterine cervix. Acta Cytol 31:791–795, 1987.

Ryden SE, Silverman EM, Goldman RT. Adenoid cystic carcinoma of the cervix presenting as a primary bronchial neoplasm. Am J Obstet Gynecol 120: 846–847, 1974.

Salpietro FM, Romano A, Alafaci C, Tomasello F. Pituitary metastasis from uterine cervical carcinoma: a case presenting as diabetes insipidus. Br J Neurosurg 14:156–159, 2000.

Seckl MJ, Mulholland PJ, Bishop AE, et al. Hypoglycemia due to an insulin-secreting small-cell carcinoma of the cervix. N Engl J Med 341:733–736, 1999.

Seidel RJ Jr, Steinfeld A. Carcinoid of the cervix: Natural history and implications for therapy. Gynecol Oncol 30:114–119, 1988.

Silverberg SG. Leiomyosarcoma of the uterus. Obstet Gynecol 38:613–628, 1971.

Song YS. Significance of positive vaginal smears in extrauterine carcinomas. Am J Obstet Gynecol 73:341–348, 1957.

Spahr J, Behin FG, Schneider V. Preleukemic granulocytic sarcoma of cervix and vagina. Initial manifestation by cytology. Acta Cytol 26:56–60, 1982.

Spiro RH, Koss LG. Myosarcoma of the uterus. A clinicopathological study. Cancer 18:571–588, 1965.

Spitzer M, Molho L, Seltzer VL, Lipper S. Vaginal glomus tumor: Case presentation and ultrastructural findings. Obstet Gynecol 66:86–88, 1985.

Stoler MH, Mills SE, Gersell DJ, Walker AN. Small-cell neuroendocrine carcinoma of the cervix. A human papillomavirus type 18-associated cancer. Am J Surg Pathol 15:28–32, 1991.

Strang P, Sorbe B, Sundestrom C. Primary aneuploid lymphoma of the uterine cervix: A case report. Gynecol Oncol 30:302–305, 1988.

Stransky GC, Acosta AA, Kaplan AL, Friedman JA. Reticulum cell sarcoma of the cervix. Obstet Gynecol 41:183–187, 1973.

Taki I, Aozasa K, Kurokawa K. Malignant lymphoma of the uterine cervix. Cytologic diagnosis of a case with immunocytochemical corroboration. Acta Cytol 29:607–611, 1985.

Tang C-K, Toker C, Harriman B. Müllerian adenosarcoma of the uterine cervix. Hum Pathol 12:579–581, 1981.

Tateishi R, Wada A, Hayakawa K, et al. Argyrophil cell carcinomas (apudomas) of the uterine cervix: Light and electron microscopic observations of five cases. Virchows Arch [A] 366:257–274, 1975.

Taylor CW. Müllerian mixed tumour. Acta Pathol Microbiol Scand 80:48–55, 1972.

Thomas W, Sadeghhieh B, Fresco R, et al. Malacoplakia of the endometrium, a probable cause of postmenopausal bleeding. Am J Clin Pathol 69:637–641, 1978.

Tseng CJ, Pao CC, Tseng, LH, et al. Lymphoepithelioma-like carcinoma of the uterine cervix: association with Epstein-Barr virus and human papillomavirus. Cancer 80:91–97, 1997.

Tunca JC, Reddi PR, Shah SH, Slack ST. Malignant non-Hodgkin's-type lymphoma of the cervix uteri occurring during pregnancy. Gynecol Oncol 7: 385–393, 1979.

Tzanck A, Melki GR, Aron-Brunetiere R. Cytodiagnosis of pemphigus. Acta Unio Int Contra Cancrum 7:727–729, 1951.

Ulbright, TM, Brokaw SA, Stehman FB, Roth LM. Epithelioid sarcoma of the vulva. Evidence suggesting a more aggressive behavior than extra-genital epithelioid sarcoma. Cancer 52:1462–1469, 1983.

Uyeda CK, Stephens SR, Bridger WM. Cervical smear diagnosis of Hodgkin's disease. Report of a case. Acta Cytol 13:652–655, 1969.

Valente PT, Ernst CS, Atkinson BF. Pemphigus vulgaris with subclinical involvement of the uterine cervix. Report of a case with persistence of abnormal Papanicolaou smears posthysterectomy. Acta Cytol 28:681–683, 1984.

van Dinh T, Woodruff JD. Adenoid cystic and adenoid basal carcinomas of the cervix. Obstet Gynecol 65:705–709, 1985.

van Nagell JR Jr, Powell DE, Gallion HH, et al. Small cell carcinoma of the uterine cervix. Cancer 62:1586–1593, 1988.

Van Niekerk WA. Cervical cells in megaloblastic anaemia of the puerperium. Lancet 1:1277–1279, 1962.

Van Niekerk WA. Cervical cytological abnormalities caused by folic acid deficiency. Acta Cytol 10:67–73, 1966.

Van Velden DJJ, Chuang JT. Cylindromatous carcinoma of the uterine cervix. A case report. Obstet Gynecol 39:17–21, 1972.

Vang R, Medeiros LJ, Silva EG, et al. Non-Hodgkin's lymphoma of the vagina. A clinicopathologic analysis of 14 patients. Am J Surg Pathol 24:719–725, 2000.

Vellios F, Ng ABP, Reagan, JW. Papillary adenofibroma of the uterus: A benign mesodermal mixed tumor of Müllerian origin. Am J Clin Pathol 60: 543–551, 1973.

Vieaux JW, McGuire DE. Reticulum cell sarcoma of the cervix. Am J Obstet Gynecol 89:134–135, 1964.

Vinette-Leduc D, Yazdi HM, Payn G, Villeneuve N. Metastatic salivary duct carcinoma to the uterus: report of a case diagnosed by cervical smear. Diagn Cytopathol 21:271–275, 1999.

Vuong PN, Neveux Y, Schoonaert MF, et al. Adenoid cystic (cylindromatous) carcinoma associated with squamous cell carcinoma of the cervix uteri: cytologic presentation of a case with histologic and ultrastructural correlations. Acta Cytol 40:289–294, 1996.

Wahl RW. Malacoplakia of the uterine cervix. Acta Cytol 26:591–694, 1982.

Walker AN, Mills SE. Unusual variants of uterine cervical carcinoma. Pathol Ann 22:277–310, 1987.

Walker AN, Mills SE, Taylor PT. Cervical neuroendocrine carcinoma: A clinical and light microscopic study of 14 cases. Int J Gynecol Pathol 7:64–74, 1988.

Ward BS, Hitchcock CL, Keyhani S. Primitive neuroectodermal tumor of the uterus: A case report. Acta Cytol 44:667–672, 2000.

Waxman M, Vuletin JC. Endocervical blue nevus. Arch Pathol Lab Med 101:160, 1977.

Webb MJ, Symmonds RE, Weiland LH. Malignant fibrous histiocytoma of the vagina. Am J Obstet Gynecol 119:190–192, 1974.

Welch JW, Hellwig CA. Reticulum cell sarcoma of the uterine cervix: Report of a case. Obstet Gynecol 22:293–294, 1963.

Weinberg E, Hoisington S, Eastman AY, et al. Uterine cervical lymphoepithelial-like carcinoma. Absence of Epstein-Barr virus genomes. Am J Clin Pathol 99:195–199, 1993.

Whitaker D. The role of cytology in the detection of malignant lymphoma of the uterine cervix. Acta Cytol 20:510–513, 1976.

Whitehead N, Reyner F, Lindenbaum J. Megaloblastic changes in the cervical epithelium. Association with oral contraceptive therapy and reversal with folic acid. JAMA 226:1421–1424, 1973.

Wu JP, Tanner WS, Fardal PM. Malignant mixed Müllerian tumor of the uterine tube. Obstet Gynecol 41:707–712, 1973.

Yamada M, Hatakeyoma S, Yamamoto E, et al. Localized amyloidosis of the uterine cervix. Virchows Arch [A] 413:265–268, 1988.

Young AW Jr, Herman EW, Tovell HMM. Syringoma of the vulva: Incidence, diagnosis, and cause of pruritus. Obstet Gynecol 55:515–518, 1980.

Young EE, Gamble CN. Primary adenocarcinoma of the rectovaginal septum arising from endometriosis. Report of a case. Cancer 24:597–601, 1969.

Young RH, Hart WR. Metastatic intestinal carcinomas simulating primary ovarian clear cell carcinoma and secretory endometrioid carcinoma. A clinicopathologic and immunohistochemical study of five cases. Am J Surg Pathol 22:805–815, 1998.

Young RH, Harris NL, Scully RE. Lymphoma-like lesions of the lower female genital tract: A report of 16 cases. Int J Gynecol Pathol 4:289–299, 1985.

Yu HC, Ketabchi M. Detection of malignant melanoma of the uterine cervix from Papanicolaou smears: A case report. Acta Cytol 31:73–76, 1987.

Zaleski S, Setum C, Benda J. Cytologic presentation of alveolar soft-part sarcoma of the vagina. Acta Cytol 30:665–670, 1986.

Zaloudek CJ, Norris HJ. Adenofibroma and adenosarcoma of the uterus: A clinicopathologic study of 35 cases. Cancer 48:354–366, 1981.

Zinkham WH. Multifocal eosinophilic granuloma. Am J Med 60:457–463, 1976.

Effects of Therapeutic Procedures on the Epithelia of the Female Genital Tract

18

HEAT, COLD, AND LASER TREATMENT

Heat, in the form of cautery, is an ancient remedy for local treatment of various lesions. In its more modern form, as the **electrocautery,** it has enjoyed great popularity in the treatment of various benign disorders of the female genital tract, such as chronic cervicitis. Large loop electrosurgical excision procedure (**LEEP**) of precancerous lesions of the cervix is another application of electrocautery. Other forms of locally destructive therapy include: cold, in the form of **cryosurgery,** and energy, transmitted in the form of a **laser** beam, used in the treatment of intraepithelial neoplastic lesions of the uterine cervix and of the vagina (see Chaps. 11 and 14). Because cytology, and particularly the cervicovaginal preparations, are extensively used as a follow-up measure after treatment, it is important to distinguish cell changes caused by therapy from evidence of recurrent cancer.

All these forms of therapy have in common cell changes that are of two types:

■ **Initial changes,** caused by tissue and cell necrosis under the impact of treatment
■ **Secondary changes,** caused by epithelial regeneration following the injury

Initial Changes

In principle, cervicovaginal samples should not be obtained for about 6 weeks following treatment. However, ever so often, smears are obtained sooner and the cell changes seen in such material are described here. Immediately after, and for about 7 days following treatment, **tissue and cell necrosis are** the predominant features observed in cytologic and histologic material (Fig. 18-1A). The necrosis is of the coagulative type and, hence, the affected epithelia

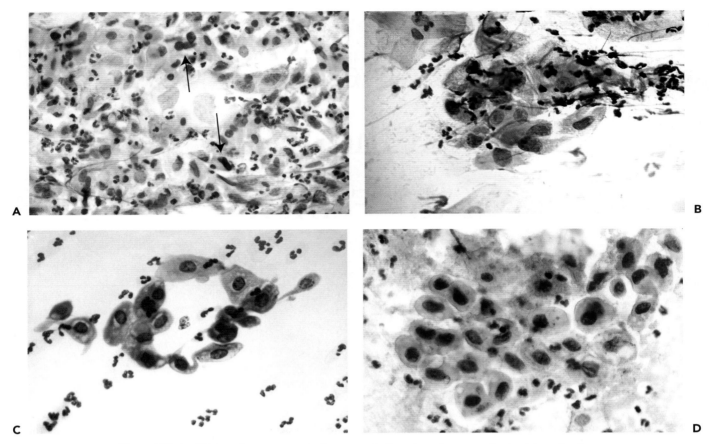

Figure 18-1   Effects of cryosurgery and cautery. *A.* Overview of a smear obtained 6 weeks after cryosurgery for carcinoma of the cervix. Marked inflammation, distortion of squamous cells, and a few suspicious cells with hyperchromatic nuclei (*arrows*) are seen. *B.* Nuclear and cellular enlargement and nuclear haziness one week after cautery. *C.* Parabasal cells with basophilic cytoplasm and somewhat enlarged nuclei showing "repair" 2 weeks after cautery. *D.* Smear obtained 4 weeks after cautery showing markedly atypical metaplastic squamous cells. It is impossible to determine from this smear pattern whether or not this patient has been cured. Further follow-up is essential.

may retain their overall structure, even though their component cells may be severely injured.

In **cervicovaginal smears,** the background usually contains cell debris and evidence of **acute inflammation in the form of polymorphonuclear leukocytes.** The resilient **squamous cells** may become **enlarged because of cytoplasmic vacuolization** but often **retain their cytoplasmic silhouette.** Their **nuclei are either "empty" or smudged,** without any internal structure, or show nuclear **pyknosis and karyorrhexis** (Fig. 18-1B). The more fragile **endocervical cells** may be **enlarged and vacuolated, sometimes misshapen,** with **opaque or fragmented nuclei.** For the most part, however, the endocervical cells rarely survive intact and usually are fragmented. Holmquist et al (1976) emphasized "distortion" or odd shapes of endocervical cells after carbon-dioxide laser treatment. Similar observations were reported after cryosurgery (Hasegawa et al, 1975).

Thomas (1997) described an unusual procedure in the form of **immediate post-LEEP endocervical brush to determine** the presence of residual disease or lesions located beyond the reach of the loop. The endocervical cells were often elongated and showed distortion of nuclear configuration with oddly shaped, often "smudgy" nuclei. Thomas

(1997) stressed the difficulties in the interpretation of such smears, compounded by the presence of blood and necrosis. The value of this procedure has not been ascertained.

Secondary Changes

The secondary changes are more common because they may persist for several weeks, when most of the follow-up smears are obtained. Starting on or about 8 days after treatment, the smear background usually shows evidence of inflammation and sometimes persisting necrosis. **Lymphocytes and macrophages, the latter sometimes multinucleated, are the dominant inflammatory cells.** In the epithelial cells, **cytoplasmic vacuolization** may persist for as long as 6 weeks after cautery and for several months after cryosurgery (Gondos et al, 1970). Another persisting change is **slight nuclear enlargement, hyperchromasia,** and the appearance of **nuclear "folds" or lines.** Within 1 week after treatment, **sheets of parabasal squamous cells** of various sizes, with well-preserved, dark nuclei with stippled chromatin granules and basophilic cytoplasm, may be observed, signaling the beginning of regeneration or "repair" of the squamous epithelium (Fig. 18-1C). Sheets of **smooth muscle** cells may be observed in **endocervical brush samples,** particularly if the sampling was obtained before epithelial regeneration has been completed or if the brushing was very vigorous.

In somewhat later stages of epithelial regeneration, cell changes of **florid squamous metaplasia or "repair,"** as described in detail in Chapter 10, may be noted. Sheets or clusters of **parabasal squamous cells with basophilic cytoplasm and relatively large, often granular nuclei** with **prominent, large nucleoli** may be observed. Nucleolar prominence has been emphasized by Hasegawa et al (1975) in patients after cryosurgery. **Mitotic figures** can occur in such epithelial fragments. These changes may persist for about six weeks after treatment.

The duration of the therapy-induced cell changes is variable and depends on the anatomic extent and mode of treatment. The procedures used are not standardized and, consequently, significant differences occur among practitioners and institutions. If the treatment is confined to a small area of the cervix, its effects will be less noticeable and of shorter duration than if much of the epithelium of the exo- and endocervix has been treated or removed together with the underlying connective tissue and muscle.

The most important practical point is the **determination of whether intraepithelial neoplasia has been destroyed by treatment. In our experience, the diagnosis of residual disease should not be made until at least six weeks have elapsed after treatment,** or until complete healing of the therapy-induced changes has taken place. **Prior to that time, cancer cells derived from the original, adequately treated lesion may still occur in smears, even in patients with a favorable response. Past the 6 week deadline,** the presence of cancer or dyskaryotic (dysplastic) cells may be interpreted in the customary fashion, described in previous chapters, and their presence indicates **persisting disease.** However, the post-treatment cytologic examination to detect persisting lesions is not fully reliable and has its difficulties and failures. An example of this problem is shown in Figure 18-1D wherein the differentiation between atypical repair and recurrent lesion proved to be difficult until further smears revealed a low-grade squamous intraepithelial lesion (LGSIL). Thus, it is advisable to combine the cytologic follow-up with colposcopy and testing for high-risk human papillomavirus (HPV). Chua and Hjerpe (1997) reported that the **presence of high risk human papillomavirus,** determined by PCR, was an important indicator of recurrent high-grade precancerous lesions. There is no information on the value of this procedure in patients treated by laser or cryotherapy.

TOPICAL ANTIBIOTICS

A topical application of broad-spectrum antibiotics may result in **massive desquamation of the squamous epithelium** of the cervix and the vagina, as discussed in Chapter 11. Sometimes cancer cells may be concealed by sheets of benign epithelial cells. In some cases of carcinoma in situ, we have observed sloughing of the cancerous epithelium,

with resulting disappearance of the lesion. Before pronouncing an in situ carcinoma as "cured" by this method, it is essential to follow the patient for at least 3 years, since cancer cells may reappear in smears at a time when least expected. It would not be wise to rely on this chance action of antibiotics for treatment of precancerous lesions. These observations are reported here as a matter of scientific interest only.

RADIOTHERAPY

Nearly all of the information on the effects of radiotherapy on the organs of the female genital tract, be it as **external irradiation, radium** or implanted **radioactive seeds,** pertains to treatment of **carcinoma of the uterine cervix or vagina.** Although the changes in the benign epithelia of the female genital tract are the same for all forms of radiotherapy and all tumors, regardless of location, the changes observed in cancer cells are limited to cervical carcinoma, because there is very little reliable information on cancers in other component organs of the female genital tract. The effects of radiotherapy may be described as acute and chronic.

Acute Effect on Benign Epithelia

Graham (1947) studied extensively the immediate effect of radiation on benign **squamous epithelium** of the cervix and the vagina. She noted and described the following cellular changes:

- Marked cellular enlargement accompanied by a proportional nuclear enlargement
- A peculiar "wrinkling" of the nuclei
- Vacuolization of the cytoplasm or, occasionally, of the nucleus
- Multinucleation
- Appearance of bizarre cell forms

The changes represent the damaging effect of radiation on individual cells and various stages of cell death (Fig. 18-2A). The most striking change in such smears is **generalized cellular enlargement,** usually affecting the cytoplasm and the nucleus, **without a change in the nucleocytoplasmic ratio. For the most part, the enlarged nuclei are homogeneous and pale, easily recognized as benign. The "wrinkling" of the nucleus,** described by Graham, **occurs rather rarely. Unfortunately, in squamous cells,** radiation may also produce **nuclear hyperchromasia, multinucleation,** and **bizarre forms** (Fig. 18-2C) and may render the differential diagnosis from cancer cells very difficult.

The endocervical cells are well preserved, but there is a **marked vacuolization and enlargement of both the cytoplasm and the nucleus** (Fig. 18-2B). Within the nucleus, **granules of chromatin** stand out against the pale background. Corresponding changes may be noted in histologic sections. **Bizarre nuclear abnormalities,** common in squamous cells, are **less frequent in endocervical cells.** Similar observations were reported by Little (1968), Boschann (1981), and Shield et al (1992).

The acute changes in the squamous and endocervical cells usually recede a few weeks after completion of ra-

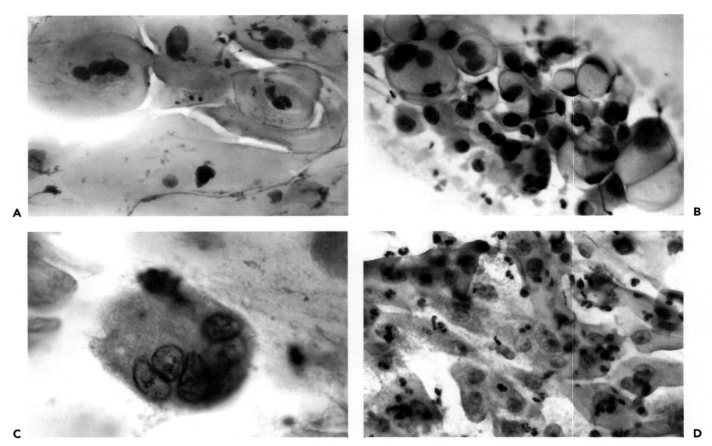

Figure 18-2 Radiation effect in cervical smears. *A.* Huge, multinucleated squamous cells after 60 Gy administered to the uterine cervix. *B.* Radiation effect on endocervical cells. The cells are markedly enlarged and contain huge cytoplasmic vacuoles. *C.* A huge multinucleated giant cell after 60 Gy. *D.* Persisting radiation effect 4 months after completion of treatment. Sheets of elongated squamous cells with hazy nuclei may be observed.

diotherapy in favor of the chronic changes, described below. In some patients, however, **these changes may persist for several months after completion of radiation therapy.**

Persistent Effect on Benign Epithelia

In some patients who have undergone radiation therapy to the pelvic area, there may be persistence of radiation effect upon the **benign squamous** and the **endocervical epithelia,** stretching over a **period of many years.** We have observed such changes 28 years after the completion of radiotherapy. The biologic phenomena that account for this effect are unknown. It may be speculated that, in susceptible patients, the genetic make-up of the irradiated epithelium has been altered. The occurrence of **post-radiation carcinoma in situ** (see below) and of **cancer in organs within the field of radiation** support this hypothesis. Neither the amount of radiation nor the manner of application appears to play a role; it is rather a matter of individual response to radiation injury.

The **cytologic manifestations of a late radiation effect** differ from the acute radiation effect. The phenomena of acute injury to the cell, such as nuclear and cytoplasmic vacuolization and nuclear necrosis are absent. Commonly,

there still is a persisting **slight enlargement of cells and their nuclei.** The **squamous cells often desquamate in cohesive sheets of elongated cells, sometimes mimicking smooth muscle cells, with elongation of the rather homogeneous nuclei** (Fig. 18-2D). Among the elongated nuclei, a few are often hyperchromatic. Multinucleation is less frequent than in the acute radiation response. The **nuclei of endocervical cells** may also show **persisting enlargement and some hyperchromasia** (Fig. 18-3A). The changes are sufficiently characteristic for an experienced and knowledgeable observer to diagnose late radiation effects in cervicovaginal smears.

Effect on Cancer Cells

During radiotherapy, the cancer cells, regardless of type, undergo essentially the same changes as the benign epithelial cells, that is, **cellular and nuclear ballooning and extensive vacuolization of both the cytoplasm and the nucleus.** Occasionally, extensive fragmentation of the nuclei may be observed, most likely a form of cell death or **apoptosis** (see Chap. 6). Squamous cancer cells usually retain some of their cytoplasmic characteristics and can be recognized; however, poorly differentiated cancer cells and cells of adenocarcinomas usually cannot be specifically classified. Marked radia-

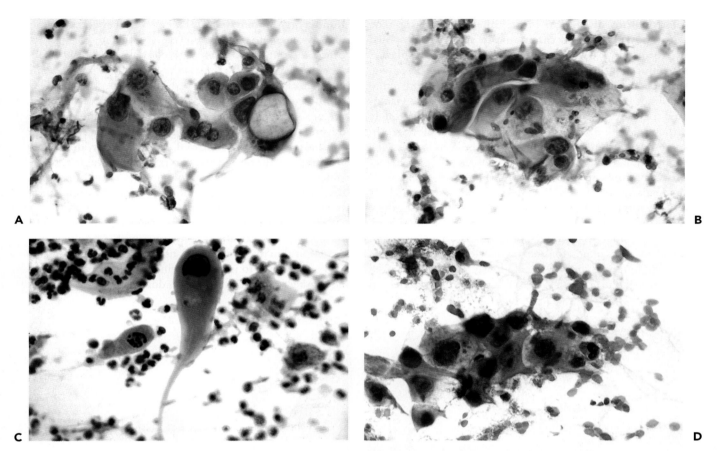

Figure 18-3   Persisting radiation effect. *A.* Endocervical and squamous cells 5 months after completion of radiotherapy. Persisting large cytoplasmic vacuoles and distortion of cell configuration may be noted. *B.* Same case as in *A.* There is a marked atypia of squamous cells with large nuclei and nucleoli. It is difficult to determine from this smear whether or not the patient had recurrent cancer. *C.* Obvious bizarre squamous cancer cells 6 months after completion of radiation treatment. In this case, the diagnosis of recurrent cancer was secure. *D.* Malignant cells 4 months after completion of radiotherapy for cervix cancer.

tion effect may enhance or obliterate some of the features of malignant cells, such as abnormal structure of the nuclear chromatin and the presence of large nucleoli (Fig. 18-3B). However, **some measure of hyperchromasia usually persists, as does an abnormal nucleocytoplasmic ratio.**

Differential Diagnosis Between Radiated Benign and Malignant Cells

The question of differentiation between irradiated benign and malignant cells is of academic interest only. **If the malignant cells display radiation effect** that obliterates their characteristic features, they are not capable of reproduction; therefore, they **provide no information on the presence or the absence of viable tumor. Only those cancer cells that are either unaffected or only slightly affected by radiation are of concern in the diagnosis of persistent or recurrent tumor.**

In reference to cancer of the uterine cervix, **persistence of unaffected cancer cells in smears during and after treatment suggests that a tumor is not responding to radiation.** However, as reported by Zimmer (1959), cancer

cells may persist for as long as 3 weeks after completion of treatment, and yet the patients appeared to be cured and did not show tumor recurrence for several years. Such cases are exceptional. It must be stressed that, in spite of apparent favorable cytologic response of the tumor to treatment, the tumor may persist within the subepithelial stroma or other areas not accessible to cytologic sampling. In such situations, the absence of cytologic evidence of persisting carcinoma is of no clinical value whatever.

Recurrent cancer of the uterine cervix, after successful initial treatment, may be recognized in cervicovaginal smears and its manifestations are identical to those of primary cancer, sometimes in the background of smears showing slight persisting radiation effect (Fig. 18-3C,D).

Postradiation Carcinoma In Situ in the Cervix and Vagina (Post-Irradiation Dysplasia)

In 1961, we reported on a group of patients who, after a disease-free time interval ranging from 1.5 to 17 years **following successful radiotherapy for invasive squamous cancer** of the cervix, developed **cytologic abnormalitiesconsistent with carcinoma in situ or closely** related forms of cervical intraepithelial neoplasia. The term **"post-irradiation carcinoma in situ"** was proposed by Koss et al (1961). The term **"postradiation dysplasia"** was subsequently used by Patten et al (1963) in describing this lesion. The abnormal epithelium, located on either the irradiated cervix or vagina, **often could not be visualized** on inspection or colposcopy and was exceedingly difficult to localize within the scarred genital tract. In some cases, numerous biopsies of the cervix and the vaginal mucosa were required to confirm the presence of **postradiation carcinoma in situ** (Fig. 18-4). In one of the patients of the original series who was treated by hysterectomy for the postradiation carcinoma in situ, there was associated residual metastatic carcinoma in an obturator lymph node that would not have been discovered and removed were it not for the vaginal lesion. It is of note that Fujimura et al (1991), Holloway et al (1991), and Longatto Filho et al (1997) observed the **presence of**

human papillomavirus (HPV) in cervicovaginal smears of 18 women after completion of radiotherapy for invasive cancer of the uterine cervix. Holloway et al (1991) observed HPV type 16 in cancer of the cervix recurring after therapy.

Subsequently, in a number of personally observed cases, the ominous significance of these lesions became apparent. **Several patients, with postradiation carcinoma in situ (or dysplasia) who were followed conservatively, developed invasive carcinomas of the cervix or of the vagina,** sometimes after many years of follow-up. In yet other patients, disseminated metastatic carcinoma developed within a short period of time (Figs. 18-5 and 18-6).

The cytologic presentation of these lesions failed as a means of prognostication. Some cases with a cytologic presentation akin to classic squamous carcinoma required many years to progress to invasive carcinoma (see Fig. 18-6); others, with a cytologic presentation dominated by dyskaryotic

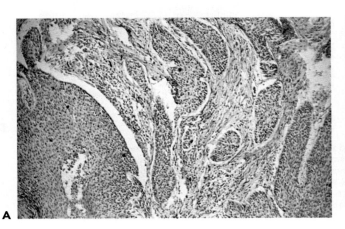

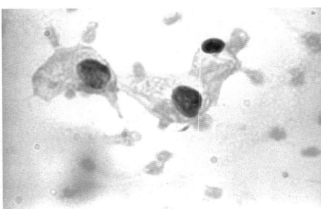

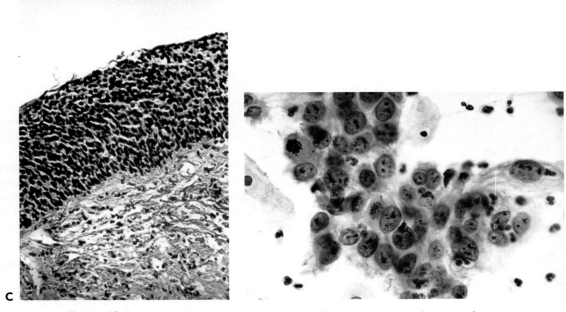

Figure 18-4   Postradiation carcinoma in situ (dysplasia). *A.* The original pattern of invasive squamous carcinoma treated by radiotherapy in 1946. *B.* Cervical smear obtained 13 years later (in 1959) showing large dyskaryotic (dysplastic) cells with markedly enlarged nuclei. *C.* Classical carcinoma in situ in a biopsy obtained in 1959. *D.* Another example of postradiation carcinoma in situ. The smear shows large granular nuclei with prominent nucleoli and mitoses.

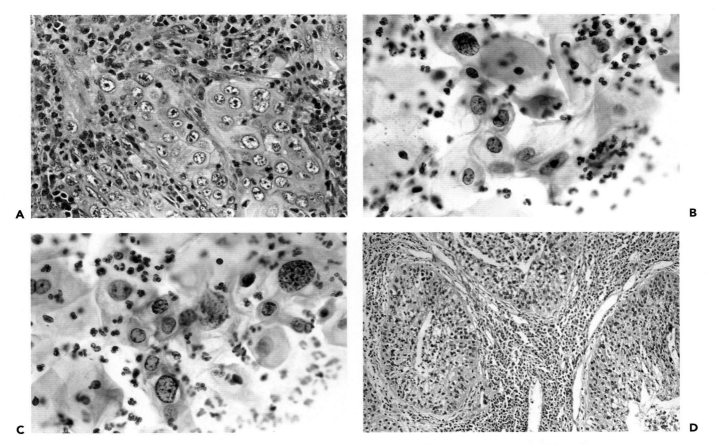

Figure 18-5 **Postradiation carcinoma of cervix.** *A.* The original squamous cancer treated by radiotherapy in 1958. *B.* Smear obtained in 1975 showing markedly abnormal cells corresponding to an intraepithelial neoplastic lesion. Several of the cells resemble koilocytes, suggestive of HPV infection. *C.* Another field of the smear shown in *B. D.* Squamous carcinoma in the left external iliac node observed in 1975, after the smear shown in *B* and *C.*

(dysplastic) superficial and intermediate squamous cells, hence resembling a low-grade lesion, were followed by rapid progression and dissemination of the tumor (Fig. 18-5).

Patten et al (1963) reported on a group of 28 patients with similar cytologic and histologic patterns, and elected to call the lesion **"post-irradiation dysplasia."** One of his patients developed invasive squamous carcinoma after 19 months of follow-up. Wentz and Reagan (1970) subsequently reported on 84 patients with "post-irradiation dysplasia." Seventy-one of these patients developed the lesion within 3 years or less after completion of radiotherapy for invasive carcinoma of the cervix, whereas 13 patients developed the lesion 3 to 12 years after completion of therapy. Forty-seven (56%) of the 84 patients developed recurrent carcinoma and the majority of them died of disease. **The probability of developing recurrent cancer was much higher for patients who developed the post-irradiation change within 3 years or less than for the patients with a delayed onset.** The overall 5-year survival rate for the 84 patients was only 44%, although most of them initially had carcinomas of stage I (30 patients) and stage II (44 patients), wherein a much better survival rate could be expected for these stages of disease. This study fully confirmed the **serious prognostic significance of the post-irradiation intraepithelial lesion, regardless of the name attached to it.**

Okagaki et al (1974) studied 60 patients who received radiotherapy for carcinoma of the cervix of various stages. Twenty-three patients (38.5%) showed evidence of post-irradiation lesions. The study of **DNA content of the abnormal cells** by destaining the slides and re-staining with Feulgen stain showed diploid, polypoid, or aneuploid patterns. Twenty-seven of the 60 patients died; 13 of these had "post-irradiation dysplasias," 6 of which were aneuploid. Two of the 33 surviving patients also had aneuploid dysplasia. The conclusions of this paper, suggesting that **DNA measurements are of prognostic value,** have been confirmed by Davey et al (1992, 1998).

Regardless of the controversy over the name of the cytologic and histologic lesions observed following completion of radiotherapy for invasive cancer of the uterine cervix, it may be unequivocally stated that the presence of **post-irradiation intraepithelial neoplasia** carries with it a **very serious prognostic connotation.** The majority of these patients will die of invasive and metastatic carcinoma, unless rapidly treated.

The use of periodic cytologic examinations is mandatory following irradiation treatment of cervical cancer to detect local recurrences promptly and to treat them without delay. The early identification of post-irradiation intraepithelial neoplasia should lead to vigorous treatment of patients at risk.

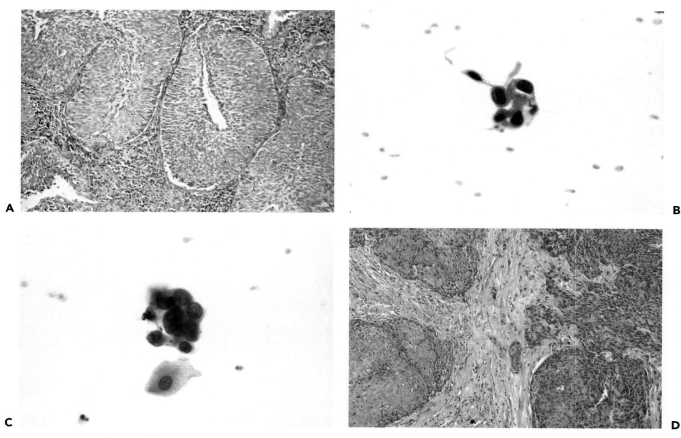

Figure 18-6 **Postradiation carcinoma of the cervix.** *A.* Original squamous cancer treated by radiotherapy in 1968. *B,C.* Cervical smears obtained in 1970 showing small clusters of cancer cells. *D.* Recurrent carcinoma of the cervix documented in 1971, hence 3 years after completion of radiation treatment.

Postradiation Cancers of Other Pelvic Organs

A successful radiotherapeutic eradication of a primary cancer of the cervix or endometrium puts the surviving patient at risk for the development of other cancers within the radiation field. An **excess of leiomyosarcomas and endometrial carcinomas** has been observed in such patients (Smith and Bowden, 1948; Meredith et al, 1986). Carcinomas of the bladder and rectum may also occur (Fehr and Prem, 1974; Kapp et al, 1982; Russo et al, 1997). **Soft tissues and pelvic bone are also at risk and sarcomas may develop in these organs.** It is empirically assumed that **at least 6 years must elapse** between the conclusion of radiotherapy and the development of the new cancers within the irradiated area **for the tumors to be classified as radiation related.** It is of note that some of the radiation-related cancers, notably of the uterus, may be diagnosed in cervicovaginal smears (Meredith, 1986). We have identified **several endometrial carcinomas in vaginal smears in patients previously irradiated for a variety of diseases, including endometrial hyperplasia** (see Chap. 13).

Other Complications of Therapy for Cancer of the Cervix

Chlamydia Trachomatis and Herpesvirus

Several observers reported the presence of *chlamydia trachomatis and herpesvirus* in patients treated for cancer of the

uterine cervix (Longatto Filho et al, 1990, 1991; Maeda et al, 1990). The cytologic findings were identical with those described in Chapter 10.

Vaginal and Sexuality Changes

Hartman and Diddle (1972) observed vaginal stenosis after radiotherapy for cervix cancer. Bergmark et al (1999) reported that significant abnormalities of the vagina (shortening and atrophy) occurred in about 25% of women treated for cancer of the, regardless of mode of therapy. These changes, which interfered with sexual function, have not been correlated with cytologic findings but it may be hypothesized that they correspond to women with postradiation changes in benign epithelium, described earlier.

THE SEARCH FOR PROGNOSTIC FACTORS IN RADIOTHERAPY OF CERVICAL CANCER

The treatment of cervical cancer has undergone an almost cyclic evolution since the turn of the 20th century. The surgical treatment devised by the great pioneers, such as Wertheim and Schauta during the last years of the 19th century, gave way to radiation therapy early in the 20th century, followed by a revival of the surgical approach in the 1960s. Currently, both the radiotherapy and surgical treatment have their advocates and their opponents.

It is obvious to all students of cervical cancer that the response of the tumor to adequate therapy is not always the same, in spite of apparently similar clinical presentation of the disease and similar manner of treatment. With the introduction of **molecular genetics,** it has been shown that the modification of certain genes governing control of the cell cycle, notably the retinoblastoma gene (Rb) and p53, or expression of the oncogene HER2-neu, may be associated with poor treatment results in some cancers (see Chap. 7). Very little is known about genetic factors influencing the results of treatment for invasive carcinoma of the uterine cervix (see Chap. 11). Attempts have been made in the years past to determine whether histologic, cytologic or cytogenetic observations, or ploidy of tumor DNA, may provide prognostic information. These efforts had only modest success in providing clinically relevant prognostic profiles.

Histology as a Prognostic Factor

Glücksmann and Cherry (1956) attempted to correlate the changes in consecutive biopsies of the tumor with the **response to radiation therapy.** These investigators observed that **the well-differentiated squamous carcinomas respond to radiotherapy better than the less well-differentiated varieties.** Wentz and Reagan (1959) also correlated the histologic type of invasive cervix cancer with response to radiotherapy. The results were somewhat different from Glücksmann's, inasmuch as the response to radiotherapy was best for the large-cell nonkeratinizing carcinoma, followed by keratinizing carcinoma. The response of the small cell cancer was poor.

Our own group (Sidhu et al, 1970) observed that the **results of surgical treatment of carcinoma, stage I, also depended on tumor type.** Keratinizing carcinomas did poorly, but the **survival of patients with small cell cancer was surprisingly satisfactory.** We also noted that the presence of a **lymphoid infiltrate in the cervical stroma of the resected tumors was a favorable prognostic factor,** suggestive of a good immune response. Also, **patients older than 45 years** of age at the time of diagnosis **fared much better than younger patients.**

Cytology as a Prognostic Factor

The late Ruth and John Graham (1951, 1953, 1954, 1960) attempted to define the **biologic response of the patients to radiotherapy by changes in benign cells in cervicovaginal smears.** Thus, the **radiation response (RR)** was the percentage of benign superficial squamous cells displaying radiation effect. Subsequently, the Grahams attributed significance to the presence of small squamous epithelial cells with finely vacuolated cytoplasm, staining lavender in Papanicolaou's stain **(sensitivity response or SR).** They reported that the presence of these cells correlated well with response to radiotherapy. Although the work of the Grahams initially found support, chiefly among Scandinavian workers, it has never received general acceptance.

The concept that there are differences in the individual response to radiotherapy found some initial support in studies by Davis et al (1960). These workers measured the patients' response to radiation by administering **1,500 rads to the mucosa of the cheek of patients with cervical cancer.** By counting **multinucleated squamous cells in smears from the buccal mucosa** as the index of radiation sensitivity, they initially found a surprisingly **good correlation between the response of the buccal epithelium and the radiocurability of cervical cancer.** However, in follow-up studies, the results of treatment were not convincingly favorable in patients with a "good" oral radiation response (Sugimori and Gusberg, 1969).

There is no doubt that the response of the benign squamous epithelium to radiotherapy is quite variable, with some patients showing a remarkable response and others hardly any. Work by Feiner and Garin (1963), from my laboratory, on patients with ovarian and endometrial cancer treated by radiation, disclosed that nearly all the patients had a good radiation response. The reasons for this response remain obscure. In our hands, the correlation of the radiation response to the clinical outcome was not satisfactory.

Cytogenetics and DNA Ploidy as a Prognostic Factor

Atkin and his co-workers (1962, 1964, 1984) and Cox et al (1969) used **cytogenetic techniques** to assess radiosensitivity of invasive carcinoma of the uterine cervix. Atkin's data, based initially on karyotype analysis, and subsequently on DNA measurements, strongly suggested that **patients with aneuploid cervical cancers respond better to radiotherapy and live longer than patients with diploid tumors. Conversely, the prognosis of endometrial and ovarian carcinomas with DNA content in the diploid range was superior to aneuploid cancer.** As discussed in Chapter 11, the issue of DNA measurements in cells derived from precancerous lesions or cancer of the cervix, is highly controversial and may depend a great deal on the techniques used. DNA measurements by image analysis are discussed in Chapter 46 and by flow cytometry in Chapter 47.

EFFECTS OF CANCER CHEMOTHERAPY AGENTS ON EPITHELIA OF THE UTERINE CERVIX

The prototype of chemotherapeutic anti-cancer agents is **mustard gas** [bis(β-chloroethyl)sulfide], a substance first used as a war gas with devastating effects in 1917 during the battle of Ypres. During World War II, it was discovered that a related derivative, the alkylating agent nitrogen mustard (HN$_2$), was capable of selectively damaging lymphoid tissue in experimental animals. The target of action of alkylating agents is cellular DNA. Cross-linking of the double helix has been documented in vitro (summary in Koss, 1967). This mechanism interferes with the mitotic apparatus of cells and thereby causes cell death and, as a sideline, the morphologic abnormalities. This property of alkylating agents has been subsequently utilized in treatment of certain malignant diseases of humans, such as leukemia and malignant lymphomas. Several other alkylating compounds were synthesized during the ensuing years for chemotherapy of cancer.

In the late 1950s, after the introduction of these compounds as therapeutic agents, significant cellular **abnormalities in the squamous epithelium of the uterine cervix were observed in the autopsy material of patients dying of leukemia** (Fig. 18-7). Subsequently, sporadic observations in cervical smears of patients undergoing chemotherapy for various forms of cancer, also disclosed abnormalities of squamous cells (Fig. 18-7B). In retrospect, these charges were **consistent with activation of human papillomavirus (HPV) infection.** In the case illustrated in Figure 18-7A, the patient was a **12-year-old virgin,** strongly suggesting that the viral infection was an activation of a pre-existing virus. Two other alkylating agents, **cyclophosphamide (Cytoxan, Endoxan) and busulfan (Myleran) had a major effect on a variety of benign tissues, resulting in significant cytologic abnormalities.**

Cyclophosphamide, an agent extensively used in the treatment of a broad variety of neoplastic diseases, has its effect **primarily on the epithelium of the urinary bladder** and is discussed in Chapter 22.

Busulfan, a drug previously used exclusively in the treatment of **chronic myelogenous leukemia,** was often administered in small doses (1 to 6 mg/day) over several years. Currently, it is also used as one component of chemotherapeutic regimens prior to **bone marrow transplants.**

Its therapeutic effect on neoplastic cells is beyond the scope of this chapter, but Busulfan also causes **notable changes in benign cells of normal organs.** Changes have been observed in the **lungs, the pancreas, the spleen, the urinary tract, the uterine cervix, the breast and other tissues.** Detailed descriptions of the changes in the respiratory and urinary tracts will be found in Chapters 19 and 22, respectively. Changes in the pancreas and the spleen are irrelevant to the topic at hand. A summary may be found in prior publications (Gureli et al, 1963; Nelson and Andrews, 1964; Koss et al, 1965; Feingold and Koss, 1969).

Busulfan Effect on Cervicovaginal Smears

The epithelial abnormalities were observed initially in the cervices of five patients receiving busulfan alone and in four patients receiving other forms of therapy in addition to busulfan. Busulfan frequently **induces artificial menopause** after variable periods of administration; the smears assume the **pattern of postmenopausal atrophy.** The abnormalities involving principally squamous cells, resemble those seen in spontaneously occurring low-grade lesions or carcinoma in situ. **Cell enlargement, nuclear enlargement and hyperchromasia, coarse granulation of chromatin, and variation in nuclear size and shape,** may be observed (Fig. 18-8). **Cytoplasmic vacuolization, such as that seen in koilocytes,** was also noted and may represent an infection with (HPV) in immunodeficient patients (see Chap. 11). Because of atrophy, the abnormal cells may show **distortion caused by dryness and, frequently, loss of cytoplasm** (Fig. 18-8C). The changes resemble somewhat late irradiation effect, but the nuclear changes are much more pronounced. In several instances when the patients could be followed, the abnormalities persisted or increased, although the drug was discontinued. The **histologic appearance** of the lesions of the cervix resembles that of spontaneously occurring **low-grade neoplastic lesions** or **flat condyloma** (see Fig. 18-8B,D). There are no studies of HPV in these lesions known to us, but the morphology is strongly **suggestive of a permissive HPV infection.** However, HPV is not likely to be a factor in nuclear abnormalities in the epithelia of lung, breast, or pancreas. The possibility that the alkylating agents are carcinogenic in humans was raised early on by Shimkin (1954) and by Boyland (1964). Interestingly, a patient re-

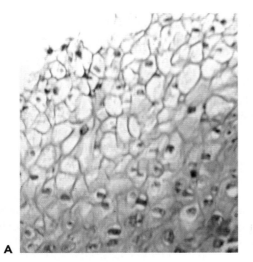

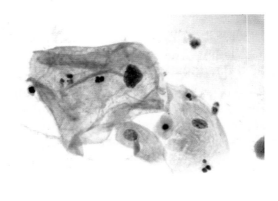

A

B

Figure 18-7 **Effect of chemotherapy on cervical smears.** *A.* Section of the uterine cervix obtained in 1957 at postmortem examination of a 12-year-old girl treated for acute leukemia with a variety of drugs. The tissue pattern closely resembles the warty changes observed in condylomas. Also note scattered nuclear abnormalities. *B.* Effect of Thiothepa administered for a malignant tumor. A large squamous cell resembling a koilocyte is shown in the cervical smear.

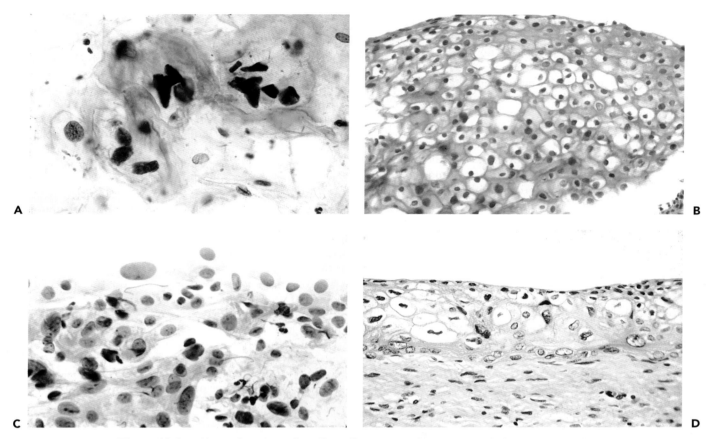

Figure 18-8   Effects of Myeleran (busulfan) effect in cervical smears. *A.* Cell changes very similar to spontaneously-occurring koilocytosis were observed several years after onset of busulfan treatment for chronic myelogenous leukemia. *B.* Biopsy of cervix corresponding to *A* showing a "warty lesion" with marked koilocytosis, suggestive of an active HPV infection. *C.* Nuclear enlargement and hyperchromasia in an atrophic smear of a woman treated with busulfan for chronic myelogenous leukemia. *D.* Postmortem changes in the squamous epithelium of the uterine cervix of the patient shown in *C.* The change is suggestive of human papillomavirus activation.

ported by Nelson and Andrews (1964) developed breast cancer while under treatment with busulfan. We have observed two patients, one who developed a carcinoma of the vulva under similar circumstances (Koss et al, 1965) and another who developed invasive carcinoma of the cervix after 5 years of busulfan therapy.

Other alkylating agents, such as **Thiotepa,** may occasionally induce similar abnormalities of squamous cells in cervical epithelium (see Fig. 18-7B). It is known that patients surviving an intensive course of chemotherapy for various cancers are at a high risk for future cancers and their benefit must be carefully assessed in view of the risk factors (Kyle et al, 1975; Leone et al, 1999; Oddou et al, 1998).

IMMUNE DEFICIENCY

Immunosuppressive Agents in Organ Transplantation

Suppression of the human immune system has been introduced into the medical armamentarium with the onset of the era of **organ transplantation.** To prevent rejection of the transplanted organ, it became important to suppress, at least

temporarily, the natural immune rejection mechanism. Immunosuppression may also be incidental to cancer chemotherapy (see above). Several of the alkylating and other chemotherapeutic agents are immunosuppressive by depressing one or more of the cell types active in immune response (see Chap. 5). Some of the most important immunosuppressive agents currently used are **cyclosporine, azathioprine (Imuran), human anti-lymphocytic serum, certain corticoids such as prednisolone, and certain alkylating agents such as cyclophosphamide (Cytoxan, Endoxan) and busulfan (Myeleran).** The mechanisms of action of these various agents are very different and the interested reader is referred to other sources for further information.

The introduction of immunosuppression on a large scale, while effective in preventing transplant rejection in many patients, has substantially increased the frequency of certain disorders that hitherto were extremely rare. This pertains to several bacterial, fungal, and viral diseases, which are discussed in Chapters 10 and 19 and to recognition that for the **immunosuppressed patient, there is a significantly increased risk of cancer** (Kyle et al, 1975; Oddou et al, 1998; Leone et al, 1999). The same applies to **patients with the acquired immunodeficiency syndrome (AIDS).** Although the most frequently observed malignant tumors are malignant lymphomas, a very wide spectrum of other types of malignant tumors have been observed.

The uterine cervix is among the high-risk organs. Gupta et al (1969) were the first to record a case of **cervical dysplasia associated with azathioprine therapy,** followed by a report by Kay et al (1970). Besides various levels of intra-epithelial neoplasia (dysplasia, carcinoma in situ), invasive carcinomas have also been observed (for summary, see Chassot et al, 1974; and Penn, 1969, 1980, 1981).

The **cervical cytologic abnormalities** in the immuno-suppressed patient are generally **similar to those observed in routine material from patients with precancerous lesions or cancer of the cervix** (Fig. 18-9A,B). Occasionally, however, **unusually large sizes and bizarre configuration of the abnormal cells may be observed** (Fig. 18-9C,D). These epithelial abnormalities are capricious and their significance is unpredictable: in some instances, a carcinoma in situ has been observed and treated (see Fig. 18-9A,B); in other instances, the cell changes disappeared after arrest of immunosuppressive therapy (see Fig. 18-9C,D). The experience to date strongly suggests that long-term follow-up of these patients, many of whom are very young, should be the rule, as is true with similar patients of the nonimmunosuppressed group. Again, the possibility that human papillomavirus may play a role in these changes cannot be ruled out.

Other Forms of Immunosuppression

In a study of cervical and vaginal lesions associated with human papillomavirus (HPV), Shokri-Tabibzadeh et al (1981) reported from this laboratory on four women, three with **treated Hodgkin's disease and one with a not-further-classified form of immune deficiency.** In the four women, **cytologic and histologic neoplastic changes** were observed, and the presence of **viral particles** could be documented by electron microscopy (see Fig. 11-6). In one of these women, an invasive carcinoma of the vulvar introitus was observed. The **immune deficiency** of patients with treated **Hodgkin's disease** is well known and such patients are at a very high **risk for development of other tumors** (Arseneau et al, 1977; Brody et al, 1977; Krikorian et al, 1979; Tucker et al, 1988). The **uterine cervix** appears to be a major target, probably because of **superinfection with HPV and its consequences.**

The confirmation of this relationship was obtained from a study of women with **AIDS.** As summarized in Chapter 11, women with AIDS have a statistically significant greater increase in HPV-associated cytologic abnormalities than that found for AIDS-free controls, matched for age, race, and sexual activity. Numerous other observations on the relationship have documented that AIDS is a major risk factor for cervical cancer precursors and invasive cancer.

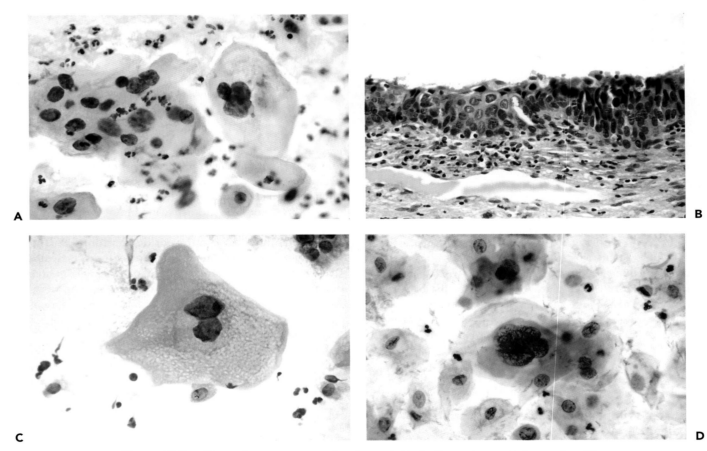

Figure 18-9 **Effects of immunosuppressive drugs.** *A.* Markedly atypical cervical smear in a 27-year-old woman who received a renal transplant 2 years prior. *B.* A classical carcinoma in situ (HGSIL) observed in the patient shown in *A. C,D.* Atypia of squamous cells observed in a 24-year-old renal transplant recipient. The change vanished after reduction in the dosage of immunosuppression drugs. (*C,D* case courtesy of Dr. Clifford Urban.)

ORAL CONTRACEPTIVE DRUGS

Oral Contraceptives and Cervical Intraepithelial Neoplasia

Widespread use of contraceptive hormonal agents has stimulated interest in the possible impact of these drugs on carcinogenesis of the uterine cervix. The studies were triggered by fortuitous observations that recipients of Planned Parenthood advice apparently had a high rate of precancerous lesions of the uterine cervix. Several such studies are now on record and they generally show a **trend toward higher rates of cervical epithelial neoplasia among women users of oral contraceptive drugs** than in the control groups who use barrier contraceptives (Melamed et al, 1969; see also Chap. 11). However, there is no agreement on whether the differences are attributable to the effect of the drugs, to a protective effect of barrier contraception, or to the social and behavioral characteristics of the women selecting oral contraceptives in preference to other modes of birth control. It is possible that **protection from human papillomavirus superinfection** is provided to women using barrier contraceptives. Regardless of these considerations, Planned Parenthood clinics now generally offer cytologic screening to women requesting and using contraceptives, undoubtedly with beneficial results for the recipients.

There are no known morphologic differences in the cytologic presentation of precancerous lesions and carcinoma of the uterine cervix in the users of any of the current methods of contraception.

Other Effects

Oral contraceptives that contain progesterone may cause nuclear enlargement in isolated endocervical cells, which can be quite substantial (Fig. 18-10A,C). The changes, when seen in histologic material, often are **combined with microglandular hyperplasia** (see Chap. 10), wherein **single endocervical cells have enlarged, hyperchromatic nuclei, akin to the Arias-Stella phenomenon in pregnancy** (Fig. 18-10D; also see Chap. 8). After discontinuation of

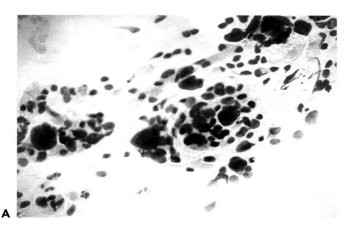

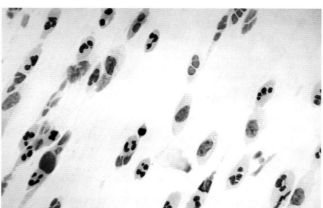

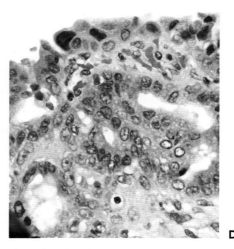

A

B

C

D

Figure 18-10 **Effect of contraceptive medication.** *A.* Enlarged nuclei of endocervical cells in a 27-year-old woman, a long-term user of contraceptive medication. *B.* The same patient 6 months after discontinuation of therapy. The endocervical cell pattern was completely normal. *C.* A multinucleated endocervical giant cell, strongly resembling the Arias-Stella phenomenon in a patient on contraceptive medication. *D.* Biopsy of endocervix corresponding to smear shown in *C.* The endocervical lining shows several large cells with hyperchromatic nuclei. The abnormality disappeared 6 months after discontinuation of medication.

the drugs, the changes usually disappear (Fig. 18-10B). Although the exact mechanism of this phenomenon is not known, it may be assumed that the large cells have polyploid nuclei, as has been shown for the Arias-Stella phenomenon. The differential diagnosis comprises dyskaryotic or malignant endocervical cells. The drug-induced changes are usually limited to a few endocervical cells, surrounded by a population of normal nuclei. In case of doubt, discontinuation of the drug and follow-up studies will usually solve the dilemma.

Liver Abnormalities in Users of Oral Contraceptives

Although this subject is of no consequence for gynecologic cytology, it must be mentioned that abnormalities of the liver in the form of **hamartomas, adenomas, and even hepatomas and angiosarcomas,** have been observed in women using oral hormonal contraceptives. The pertinent references are listed in the bibliography. For cytologic manifestations of liver lesions in aspirated samples, see Chapter 38.

BIBLIOGRAPHY

Antoniades K, Campbell WN, Hecksher RH, et al. Liver cell adenoma and oral contraceptives. Double tumor development. JAMA 234:628–629, 1975.

Arseneau JG, Canellos GP, Johnson R, DeVita VT Jr. Risk of new cancers in patients with Hodgkin's disease. Cancer 40:1912–1916, 1977.

Atkin NB. The chromosomal changes in malignancy; an assessment of their possible prognostic significance. Br J Radiol 37:213–218, 1964.

Atkin NB. Prognostic value of cytogenetic studies of tumors of the female genital tract. In Koss LG, Coleman DV (eds). Advances in Clinical Cytology, Vol 2. New York, Masson, 1984, pp 103–121.

Atkin NB, Richards BM. Clinical significance of ploidy in carcinoma of the cervix: Its relation to prognosis. Brit Med J 2:1445–1446, 1962.

Balachandran I, Galagan KS. Cervical carcinoma in situ associated with azathioprine therapy. A case report and review. Acta Cytol 28:699–702, 1984.

Bergmark K, Avall-Lundqvist E, Dickman PW, et al. Vaginal changes and sexuality in women with a history of cervical cancer. N Engl J Med 340:1383–1389, 1999.

Birkeland SA. Malignant tumors in renal transplant material. Cancer 51:1571–1575, 1983.

Boschann VHW. Zytologie und Histologie nach Strahlentherapie in der Gynäakologie. Fortschr Med 99:1840–1844, 1981.

Boyce JG, Lu T, Nelson JH Jr, Joyce D. Cervical carcinoma and oral contraception. Obstet Gynecol 40:139–146, 1972.

Boyland E. The carcinogenic activity of drugs employed in the treatment of cancer and leukemia. Bull. Union Int Cancer 2:6, 1964.

Brody RS, Schottenfeld D, Reid A. Multiple primary cancer risk after therapy for Hodgkin's disease. Cancer 40:1917–1926, 1977.

Campos J. Persistent tumor cells in the vaginal smears and prognosis of cancer of the radiated cervix. Acta Cytol 14:519–522, 1970.

Castro EB, Rosen PP, Quan SHQ. Carcinoma of large intestine in patients irradiated for carcinoma of cervix and uterus. Cancer 31:45–52, 1973.

Cerilli J, Hattan D. Immunosuppression and oncogenesis. Am J Clin Pathol 62:218–223, 1974.

Chassot PG, Guttmann RD, Beaudoin JG, et al. Cancer in renal allograft recipients. Immunol Cancer Prog Exp Tumor Res 19:91–101, 1974.

Christopherson WM, Mays ET, Barrows GH. Liver tumors in women on contraceptive steroids. Obstet Gynecol 46:221–223, 1975.

Chua KL, Hjerpe A. Human papillomavirus analysis as a prognostic marker following conization of the cervix uteri. Gynecol Oncol 66:108–113, 1997.

Cox LW, Stanley MA, Harvey NDM. Cytogenetic assessment of radiosensitivity of carcinoma of uterine cervix. Obstet Gynecol 33:82–91, 1969.

Dabancens A, Prado R, Larraguibel R, Zanartu J. Intraepithelial cervical neoplasia in women using intrauterine devices and long-acting injectable progestogens as contraceptives. Am J Obstet 119:1052–1056, 1974.

Davey DD, Gallion H, Jennings CD. DNA cytometry in postirradiation cervical-vaginal smears. Hum. Pathol 23:1027–1031, 1992.

Davey DD, Zaleski S, Sattich M, Gallion H. Prognostic significance of DNA cytometry of postirradiation cervicovaginal smears. Cancer Cytopathol 84:11–16, 1998.

Davis HJ, Jones HW Jr, Dickson RJ. Bioassay of host radiosensitivity; index of radiocurability applied to cervical carcinoma. Cancer 13:358–361, 1960.

Dougherty CM. Cervical cytology and sequential birth control pills. Obstet Gynecol 36:741–744, 1970.

Fehr PE, Prem KA. Malignancy of the uterine corpus following irradiation therapy for squamous cell carcinoma of the cervix. Am J Obstet Gynecol 119:685–692, 1974.

Feiner LL, Garin A. Cytological response to radiation in noncervical cancers of the female genital tract. Cancer 16:166–169, 1963.

Feingold ML, Koss LG. Effects of long-term administration of busulfan. Arch Intern Med 124:66–71, 1969.

Forni AM, Koss LG, Geller W. Cytologic study of the effect of cyclophosphamide on the epithelium of the urinary bladder in man. Cancer 17:1348–1355, 1964.

Fujimura M, Ostrow RS, Okagaki T. Implication of human papillomavirus in post-irradiation dysplasia. Cancer 68:2181–2185, 1991.

Glücksmann A, Cherry CP. Incidence, histology, and response to radiation of mixed carcinomas (adenoacanthomas) of uterine cervix. Cancer 9:971–979, 1956.

Gondos B, Smith LR, Townsend DE. Cytologic changes in cervical epithelium following cryosurgery. Acta Cytol 14:386–389, 1970.

Graham J, Graham R, Schultz M. Cancer of the uterine cervix. Harvard study, 1954 through 1956. Am J Obstet Gynecol 89:421–431, 1964.

Graham JB, Graham RM. Sensitization response in patients with cancer of the uterine cervix. Cancer 13:5–14, 1960.

Graham JB, Graham RM, Liu W. Prognosis in cancer of uterine cervix based on vaginal smear before treatment; SR-sensitization response. Surg Gynecol Obstet 99:555–562, 1954.

Graham RM. Effect of radiation on vaginal cells in cervical carcinoma. I. Description of cellular changes. II. Prognostic significance. Surg Gynecol Obstet 84:153–165; 166–173, 1947.

Graham RM. Prognosis of cancer of cervix by vaginal smear; correlation with 5 year results. Surg Gynecol Obstet 93:767–774, 1951.

Graham RM, Graham JB. Cellular index of sensitivity to ionizing radiation; sensitization response. Cancer 6:215–223, 1953.

Graham RM, Graham JB. Cytological prognosis in cancer of uterine cervix treated radiologically. Cancer 8:59–70, 1955.

Green TH Jr. Further trial of a cytologic method for selecting either radiation or radical operation in the primary treatment of cervical cancer. Am J Obstet Gynecol 112:545–555, 1972.

Gupta PK, Pinn VM, Taft PD. Cervical dysplasia associated with azathioprine (Imuran) therapy. Acta Cytol 13:373–376, 1969.

Gureli N, Denham SW, Root SW. Cytologic dysplasia related to busulfan (Myleran) therapy; report of case. Obstet Gynecol 21:466–470, 1963.

Hartman P, Diddle AW. Vaginal stenosis following irradiation therapy for carcinoma of the cervix uteri. Cancer 30:426–429, 1972.

Hasegawa T, Tsutsui F, Kurihara S. Cytomorphologic study on the atypical cells following cryosurgery for the treatment of chronic cervicitis. Acta Cytol 19:533–537, 1975.

Haselow RE, Nesbit M, Dehner LP, et al. Second neoplasms following mega-voltage radiation in a pediatric population. Cancer 42:1185–1191, 1978.

Holloway RW, Farrell MP, Castellano C, et al. Identification of human papillomavirus type 16 in primary and recurrent cervical cancer following radiation therapy. Gynecol Oncol 41:123–128, 1991.

Holmquist ND, Bellina JH, Danos ML. Vaginal and cervical cytologic changes following laser treatment. Acta Cytol 20:290–294, 1976.

Kapp DS, Fischer D, Grady KJ, Schwartz PE. Subsequent malignancies associated with carcinoma of the uterine cervix: Including analysis of the effect of patient and treatment parameters on incidence and site of metachronous malignancies. Int J Radiat Oncol Biol Phys 8:197–205, 1982.

Karnofsky DA, Clarkson BD. Cellular effects of anticancer drugs. Annu Rev Pharmacol 3:357–428, 1963.

Kay S, Frable WJ, Hume DM. Cervical dysplasia and cancer developing in women on immunosuppression therapy for renal homotransplantation. Cancer 26:1048–1052, 1970.

Kinlen LJ, Eastwood JB, Kerr DNS, et al. Cancer in patients receiving dialysis. Br J Med 280:1401–1403, 1980.

Kjellgren O. Radiation reaction in vaginal smear and its prognostic significance: studies on radiologically treated cases of cancer of uterine cervix. Acta Radiol 168(Suppl):1–170, 1958.

Koss LG. A light and electron microscopic study of the effects of a single dose of cyclophosphamide on various organs in the rat. I. The urinary bladder. Lab Invest 16:44–65, 1967.

Koss LG, Melamed MR, Daniel WW. In situ epidermoid carcinoma of cervix and vagina following radiotherapy for cervix cancer. Cancer 14:353–360, 1961.

Koss LG, Melamed MR, Mayer K. The effect of busulfan on human epithelia. Am J Clin Pathol 44:385–397, 1965.

Krikorian JG, Burke JS, Rosenberg SA, Kaplan HS. Occurrence of non-Hodgkin's lymphoma after therapy for Hodgkin's disease. N Engl J Med 300:452–458, 1979.

Kripke ML, Borsos T. Immunosuppression and carcinogenesis. Isr J Med Sci 10:888–903, 1974.

Kurohara SS, Vongtama VY, Webster JH, George FW. Post-irradiational recurrent epidermoid carcinoma of the uterine cervix. Am J Roentgenol Radium Ther Nucl Med 111:249–259, 1971. Kyle RA, Pierre RV, Bayrd ED. Multiple myeloma and acute leukemia associated with alkylating agents. Arch Intern Med 135:185–192, 1975.

Kyle RA, Pierre RV, Bayrd ED. Multiple myeloma and acute leukemia associated with alkylating agents. Arch Int Med 135:185–192, 1975.

Leone G, Mele L, Pulsoni A, et al. The incidence of secondary leukemias. Haematol 84:937–945, 1999.

Little JB. Cellular effects of ionizing radiation. N Engl J Med 278:369–376, 1968.

Longatto Filho A, Maeda MYS, Oyafuso MS, et al. Herpes simplex virus in post-radiation smears of uterine cervix: a morphologic and immunocytochemical study. Acta Cytol 34:652–656, 1990.

Longatto Filho A, Maeda MYS, Oyafuso MS. Identification of *Chlamydia trachomatis*, herpes simplex virus and human papillomavirus in irradiated uterine cervix: critical analysis of potential virus problems in Papanicolaou smears routine. Rev Inst Adolfo Lutz 51:93–99, 1991.

Longatto Filho A, Maeda MY, Oyafuso MS, et al. Cytomorphologic evidence of human papillomavirus infection in smears from the irradiated uterine cervix. Acta Cytol 41:1079–1084, 1997.

Maeda MYS, Longatto Filho A, Shih LWS, et al. Chlamydia trachomatis in cervical uterine-irradiated cancer patients. Diagn Cytopathol 6:86–88, 1990.

Matas AJ, Simmons RL, Kjellstrand CM, et al. Increased incidence of malignancy during chronic renal failure. Lancet 1:883–886, 1975.

McLennan MT, McLennan CE. Cytologic radiation response in cervical cancer. A critical appraisal, including the effect of supervoltage radiation. Obstet Gynecol 24:161–168, 1964.

McLennan MT, McLennan CE. Significance of cervicovaginal cytology after radiation therapy for cervical carcinoma. Am J Obstet Gynecol 121:96–100, 1975.

Melamed MR, Koss LG. Developments in cytological diagnosis of cancer. Med Clin North Am 50:651–666, 1966.

Melamed MR, Koss LG, Flehinger BJ, et al. Prevalence rates of uterine cervical carcinoma in situ for women using the diaphragm or contraceptive oral steroids. Br Med J 3:195–200, 1969.

Meredith RF, Eisert DR, Kaka Z, et al. An excess of uterine sarcomas after pelvic irradiation. Cancer 58:2003–2007, 1986.

Merrill JA. Radiosensitivity studies in treatment of cancer of the cervix. Cancer 19:143–148, 1966.

Morgenfeld MC, Goldberg V, Parisier H, et al. Ovarian lesions due to cytostatic agents during the treatment of Hodgkin's disease. Surg Gynecol Obstet 134:826–828, 1972.

Mullen DL, Silverberg SG, Penn I, Hammond WS. Squamous cell carcinoma of the skin and lip in renal homograft recipients. Cancer 37:729–734, 1976.

Nelson BM, Andrews GA. Breast cancer and cytologic dysplasia in many organs after busulfan (Myleran). Am J Clin Pathol 42:37–44, 1964.

Nissen ED, Kent DR. Liver tumors and oral contraceptives. Obstet Gynecol 46:460–467, 1975.

Oddou S, Vey N, Viens P, et al. Second neoplasms following high-dose chemotherapy and autologous stem cell transplantation for malignant lymphomas: a report of six cases in a cohort of 171 patients from a single institution. Leuk Lymphoma 31:187–194, 1998.

Okagaki T, Meyer AA, Sciarra JJ. Prognosis of irradiated carcinoma of cervix uteri and nuclear DNA in cytologic postirradiation dysplasia. Cancer 33:647–652, 1974.

Ory HW, Jenkins R, Byrd JY, et al. Cervical neoplasia in residents of a low-income housing project: An epidemiologic study. Am J Obstet Gynecol 123:275–277, 1975.

Patten SF Jr, Reagan JW, et al. Post-irradiation dysplasia of uterine cervix and vagina. An analytical study of the cells. Cancer 16:173–182, 1963.

Penn I. Some contributions of transplantation to our knowledge of cancer. Transplant Proc 12:676–680, 1980.

Penn I. Depressed immunity and the development of cancer. Clin Exp Immunol 46:459–474, 1981.

Penn I, Hammond W, Brettschneider L, Starzl TE. Malignant lymphomas in transplantation patients. Transplant Proc 1:106–112, 1969.

Penn I, Starzl TE. A summary of the status of de novo cancer in transplant recipients. Transplant Proc 4:719–732, 1972.

Porreco R, Penn I, Droegemueller W, et al. Gynecologic malignancies in immunosuppressed organ homograft recipients. Obstet Gynecol 45:359–364, 1975.

Russo F, Spina C, Coscarella G, et al. Radiotherapy of cancer of the uterine cervix and successive appearance of new malignant growth in the irradiated field. Minerva Ginecol 49:345–354, 1997.

Sandmire HF, Austin SD, Bechtel RC. Carcinoma of the cervix in oral contraceptive steroid and IUD users and nonusers. Am J Obstet Gynecol 125:339–345, 1976.

Schneider V, Kay S, Lee HM. Immunosuppression: High risk factor for the development of condyloma acuminata and squamous neoplasia of the cervix. Acta Cytol 27:220–224, 1983.

Schramm G. Development of severe cervical dysplasia under treatment with azathioprine (Imuran). Acta Cytol 14:507–509, 1970.

Sherlock S. Progress report. Hepatic adenomas and oral contraceptives. Gut 16:753–756, 1975.

Shield PW, Daunter B, Wright RG. Post-irradiation cytology of cervical cancer patients. Cytopathol 3:167–182, 1992.

Shimkin MB. Pulmonary-tumor induction in mice with chemical agents used in the clinical management of lymphomas. Cancer 7:410–413, 1954.

Shokri-Tabibzadeh S, Koss LG, et al. Association of human papillomavirus with neoplastic processes in genital tract of four women with impaired immunity. Gynecol Oncol 12:S129–S140, 1981.

Sidhu GS, Koss LG, Barber HRK. Relation of histologic factors to the response of stage I epidermoid carcinoma of the cervix to surgical treatment. Analysis of 115 patients. Obstet Gynecol 35:329–338, 1970.

Simmons RL, Kelly WD, Tallent MB, Najarian JS. Cure of dysgerminoma with widespread metastases appearing after renal transplantation. N Engl J Med 283:190–191, 1970.

Smith RF, Bowden L. Cancer of corpus uteri following radiation therapy for benign uterine lesions. Am J Roentgenol Radium Ther Nucl Med 59:796–804, 1948.

Stern E, Clark VA, Coffelt CF. Contraceptives and dysplasia: Higher rate for pill choosers. Science 169:497–498, 1970.

Sugimori H, Gusberg SB. Quantitative measurements of DNA content of cervical cancer cells before and after test dose radiation. Am J Obstet Gynecol 104:829–838, 1969.

Takamizawa H, Wong K. Effect of anticancer drugs on uterine carcinogenesis. Obstet Gynecol 41:701–706, 1973.

Thomas DB. Relationship of oral contraceptives to cervical carcinogenesis. Obstet Gynecol 40:508–518, 1972.

Thomas PA. Postprocedural Pap smears: a LEEP of faith? Diagn Cytopathol 17:440–446, 1997.

Tucker MA, Coleman CN, Varghese A, Rosenberg SA. Risk of second cancers after treatment for Hodgkin's disease. N Engl J Med 318:76–81, 1988.

Wagoner JK. Leukemia and other malignancies following radiation therapy for gynecological disorders. *In* Boice JD Jr, Fraumeni JF Jr (eds). Radiation Carcinogenesis: Epidemiology and Biological Significance. New York, Raven Press, 1984, pp 153–159.

Walker D, Gill TJ, Corson JM. Leiomyosarcoma in a renal allograft recipient treated with immunosuppressive drugs. JAMA 215:2084–2086, 1971.

Wegmann W, Largiader F, Binswanger U. Maligne Geschwülste nach Nierentransplantation. Schweiz Med Wochenschr 104:809–814, 1974.

Wentz WB, Reagan JW. Survival in cervical cancer with respect to cell type. Cancer 12:384–388, 1959.

Wentz WB, Reagan JW. Clinical significance of postirradiation dysplasia of the uterine cervix. Am J Obstet Gynecol 106:812–817, 1970.

Wilkinson E, Dufour DR. Pathogenesis of microglandular hyperplasia of the cervix uteri. Obstet Gynecol. 47:189–195, 1976.

Worth AJ, Boyes DA. A case control study into the possible effects of birth control pills on preclinical carcinoma of the cervix. J Obstet Gynaecol Br Commonw 79:673–679, 1972.

Zimmer TS. Late irradiation changes; cytological study of cervical and vaginal smears. Cancer 12:193–196, 1959.

Zippin C, Bailar JC, Kohn GI, et al. Radiation therapy for cervical cancer; late effects on life and on leukemia incidence. Cancer 28:937–942, 1971.

The Lower Respiratory Tract in the Absence of Cancer: Conventional and Aspiration Cytology

19

Revised by Myron R. Melamed

ANATOMY

The respiratory tract serves the dual purpose of supplying oxygen to and removing carbon dioxide from the circulating blood. This exchange takes place at the level of the pulmonary alveoli. Oxygen-rich air is inhaled, and carbon-dioxide rich air is exhaled through a complex series of conduits extending from the upper or cranial portions of the respiratory tract (e.g, the nasal cavity and the mouth*) to the thin-walled terminal alveoli of the lung via the larynx, trachea, and bronchi. The trachea and main bronchi are rigid, resisting collapse as pressures within the thorax change during respiratory movements. The musculature of the thorax and

---

* The mouth is often considered, anatomically, as a portion of the digestive rather than the respiratory tract. However, since material from the buccal cavity is frequently seen during the cytologic investigation of the respiratory tract, it was felt that the anatomic and histologic descriptions are properly placed here.

the diaphragm initiate inspiration by expanding the thoracic cage, thereby creating negative pressure within the pleural cavity that is transmitted to the elastic lungs. A very thin layer of fluid facilitates the movement of the pleural surfaces against each other (see anatomy of the serous cavities in Chap. 25).

The respiratory tract may be roughly divided into three portions. The cranial portion is supported by the bones of the skull and the cervical vertebrae; it comprises the nasal cavity and the paranasal sinuses, the buccal cavity, and the pharynx. The intermediate portion is composed of the larynx, trachea and the main bronchi; it stretches from the larynx to the hilus of each lung. The third portion is the lung proper, composed of lobar, segmental and smaller bronchi, and the alveolar system with its extraordinarily rich blood supply (Fig. 19-1A). A brief discussion of the various anatomic components follows.

Upper Airway

The **nasal cavity** functions principally as a conduit for inspired air, but also serves in warming and moistening the air, and trapping larger dust particles. It is subdivided by the turbinate bones into **three compartments,** of which the uppermost is partially lined by the **olfactory mucosa** containing receptors for the sense of smell. The middle and lower compartments are purely respiratory. All three nasal compartments communicate through small orifices directly into the **paranasal sinuses.** The nasal cavity opens posteriorly into the **pharynx,** a space demarcated posteriorly by the spine and its muscles, reaching upward to the base of the skull and downward to be in direct continuity with the esophagus and the larynx. Of importance within the pharynx is the presence of rich deposits of **lymphoid tissue,** especially the tonsils, located anterolaterally on each side of the pharynx, and the pharyngeal or third tonsil (adenoids) located posteriorly near the base of the skull. The **mouth** or **buccal cavity** also opens posteriorly into the pharynx; the **tongue** with its complex and exquisitely developed musculature occupies the central portion of the buccal cavity. The ducts of numerous **salivary glands** open into the buccal cavity, providing a constant flow of saliva.

Intermediate Airway

Inferiorly, the pharynx communicates with the **larynx** anteriorly and continues posteriorly as the **esophagus.** The **epiglottis** forms a lid capable of closing the larynx during the act of swallowing and thereby prevents entrance of food particles into the lower respiratory tract. The larynx is contained within a system of cartilages and is in direct continuity with the **trachea,** a semi-rigid tube kept open by C-shaped rings of cartilage that are incomplete posteriorly where the trachea is in contact with the esophagus. Within the thorax, approximately at the level of the fourth thoracic vertebra, the trachea divides into two main branches—the **left and right mainstem bronchi.**

Lower Airway

Each mainstem bronchus enters the corresponding lung accompanied by branches of the pulmonary artery and veins

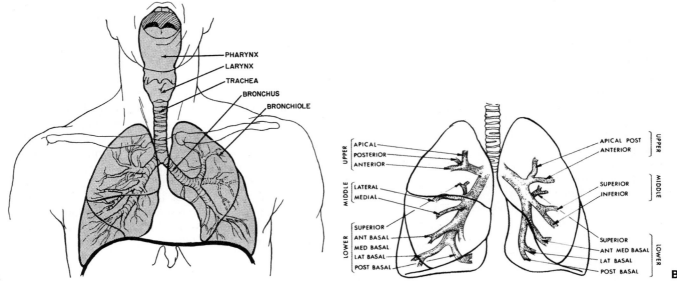

Figure 19-1   **Diagrams of the respiratory tract.** *A.* Upper respiratory tract. *B.* Lower respiratory tract, showing lobar and segmental branching of the bronchial tree.

in an area designated as **the hilus.** The **left lung** is partially separated by fissures into **two lobes; the right lung** has **three lobes.** Thus, the mainstem bronchi divide into **two lobar bronchi on the left and three on the right.** Subsequently, each lobar bronchus divides into **segmental bronchi** (10 on the right and 9 on the left; Fig. 19-1B), which undergo 18 dichotomous divisions into **subsegmental bronchi and bronchioles** that, in turn, form the thin-walled **respiratory bronchioles,** each of which opens into several alveoli. Although the lumina of individual bronchi become smaller with each bronchial division, the total air-carrying volume increases progressively to reach its greatest capacity at the level of the alveoli, which form the bulk of the pulmonary parenchyma.

Each **alveolus** is a small, thin-walled sac, described in detail below. Capillary branches of the **pulmonary artery** run in the alveolar walls or **alveolar septa,** bringing blood that is poor in oxygen from the right ventricle and carrying away oxygenated blood in interlobular venules to pulmonary veins to the left atrium. The exchange of gases takes place across the alveolar wall. The lung itself is nourished by branches of the **bronchial arteries** that come from the aorta and follow the branching bronchi into the lung along with the pulmonary vessels, returning blood through the pulmonary veins.

Except at the hilus, the lungs are entirely surrounded by the **visceral layer of the pleura.**

HISTOLOGY OF THE NORMAL RESPIRATORY TRACT

Epithelial Lining

Two principal types of epithelium are encountered within the upper respiratory tract and the bronchial tree: **nonkera-** tinizing, **stratified squamous epithelium,** which has no distinguishing features, and a characteristic **respiratory epithelium.** The **olfactory mucosa,** present in the uppermost portion of the nasal cavity, does not play a significant role in the cytology of the respiratory tract. The epithelia lining the respiratory alveoli and the alveolar macrophages will be described separately.

Squamous Epithelium

Stratified squamous epithelium lines the anterior portion of the **nasal cavity,** the **mouth, tonsils,** and central and lower portions of the **pharynx.** In general, the mucosa overlying and tightly adherent to bony structures, the hard palate, for example, and buccal mucosa that is subject to chronic irritation as in patients with poor dental hygiene, tends to form a superficial layer of keratin and therefore appears white; elsewhere throughout most of the mouth and oropharynx, it is nonkeratinizing (Fig, 19-2A). In the **larynx,** the upper or buccal aspect of the **epiglottis** is lined by nonkeratinizing stratified squamous epithelium, and the **vocal cords** are lined by a layer of thin, yet mechanically very resistant squamous epithelium (Fig. 19-2B). The remainder of the laryngeal mucosa may show islands of stratified squamous epithelium alternating with respiratory epithelium.

Respiratory Epithelium

Respiratory epithelium surfaces the major portion of the **nasal cavity,** the **paranasal sinuses,** the upper or nasal portion of the **pharynx and adenoids,** parts of the **larynx,** all of the **trachea,** and the **bronchial** tree (McDowell et al, 1978).

The respiratory epithelium is a **pseudostratified columnar epithelium,** characterized by the presence of **ciliated columnar cells** with interspersed **mucus-secreting goblet cells.** The term *pseudostratified* is used to describe epithelia

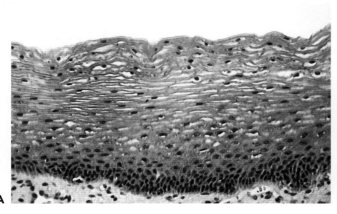
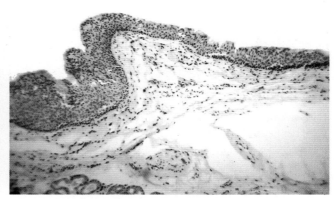

Figure 19-2   Stratified squamous epithelium. *A.* **Oral mucosa.** Note the similarity to squamous epithelium of the vagina, which is characteristically layered and matures toward the surface. There is no keratinization. *B.* **Vocal cord.** The epithelium is stratified squamous but composed of tightly coherent small cells.

with nuclei located at different levels, hence the stratified appearance, although most cells are attached to the basement membrane. **The cilia** are anchored to the luminal surface of the bronchial cells by a row of points of attachment, combining to form a readily visible dark line or **terminal plate** (see Chap. 2). At their opposite end, where the columnar cells attach to the basement membrane, they are tapered, leaving a triangular space between the cells within which are small, triangular **basal or reserve cells** that are the source of epithelial regeneration. The basic structure of the respiratory epithelium is illustrated in Figure 19-3A.

The **goblet cells** derive their name from an approximately triangular shape, resembling a wine goblet, with the nucleus placed at the narrow, basal end of the cell, while the clear supranuclear cytoplasm is distended by mucus-forming small vacuoles (Fig. 19-3B). The number of goblet cells is variable. They may be numerous under certain pathologic circumstances, such as chronic bronchitis and asthma. The fine structure of ciliated columnar and goblet cells is shown in an electron micrograph in Figure 19-3C. The goblet cells **produce a thin layer of mucus** that carpets the surface of the ciliated epithelium. This **mucus carpet** (also known as the **mucociliary escalator**) captures respired dust particles and is kept moving by the coordinated motion of the beating cilia in the direction of the larynx where it is removed by coughing. This function is lost in patients who suffer from genetic abnormalities of ciliary structure and function known as **immobile ciliary syndrome,** discussed below.

Within the trachea and the main bronchi, the epithelium is truly stratified with two, three, or more layers of columnar cells, not all of which reach the surface. The cells that do not reach the surface have no cilia, an example of cellular differentiation determined by spatial arrangement. Goblet cells and ciliated cells progressively decrease in number in the smaller bronchial branches, and give way to nonciliated columnar and cuboidal cells. The epithelium of the smaller bronchioles is single layered and epithelial cells are low, columnar, or cuboidal.

The terminal bronchiolar epithelium includes **Clara cells,** nonmucus-secreting cells that produce **surfactant** (see below). They are characterized by protruding apical cytoplasm containing PAS-positive, diastase-resistant secretory material (Fig. 19-3D) and characteristic electron-dense, apical cytoplasmic granules (Cutz and Conen, 1971). They can be identified also by immunocytochemical staining with antibody to human surfactant-associated glycoproteins (Balis et al, 1985).

A small number of basally placed **neuroepithelial cells** known as **Feyrter** or **Kulchitsky** cells also are present, primarily at airway bifurcations. They are most numerous in fetal lungs but relatively sparse in the adult and are characterized by dense core neurosecretory granules in electron micrographs. In some individuals living at high altitudes or with chronic lung disease, there may be multiple minute **hyperplastic nests of these neuroendocrine cells,** which have been termed **tumorlets.** They have been shown to secrete a number of polypeptide hormones (McDowell et al, 1976b), including corticotropin that in one reported case was the cause of **Cushing's syndrome** (Arioglu et al, 1998). The Kulchitsky cells are considered to be the parent cells of carcinoid tumors (see Chap. 20).

The terminal bronchioles open into a vestibule-like respiratory bronchiole with nearly flat epithelium from which respired air enters several communicating alveoli.

The Alveoli

The roughly spherical thin-walled alveolus is the functional unit of the lung, where exchange of oxygen and carbon dioxide takes place between air space and capillary. Ultrastructural studies have shown the wall of the alveolus to be surfaced by two types of epithelial cells, pneumocytes type I and pneumocytes type II, represented schematically in Figure 19-4A. **Pneumocytes type I** are flattened cells, few in number, with extremely attenuated cytoplasm that surfaces at least 90% of the alveolar wall. They have few cytoplasmic organelles, are metabolically inactive, cannot be visualized in conventional histologic sections, and are not capable of regeneration.

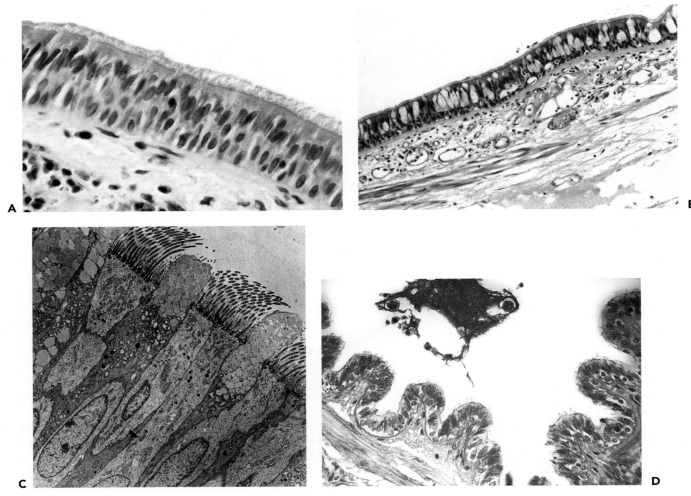

Figure 19-3 Respiratory epithelium of a medium-sized bronchus and terminal bronchiole. *A.* The characteristic pseudostratified appearance of this ciliated columnar epithelium is due to the midcellular location of nuclei of the columnar cells and the basal location of nuclei of the small basal or reserve cells that lie between tapered ends of the columnar cells at their attachment to the basement membrane. *B.* Mucus-secreting goblet cells are interspersed between the ciliated columnar cells in this section of bronchial mucosa. The goblet cells are increased in patients with asthma or chronic bronchitis. *C.* Electron micrograph showing the ciliated columnar epithelial cells and interspersed goblet cells. Mucus is being extruded from the goblet cells. *D.* The respiratory epithelium of the terminal bronchiole is single-layered, cuboidal and nonciliated. Interspersed surfactant-secreting Clara cells are PAS positive (stained red). (*C:* Courtesy of Dr. R. Erlandson, ×1,600.)

The remaining 10% of the alveolar surface is occupied by more plump, rounded, or cuboidal **pneumocytes type II.** Although they too are scarcely (if at all) visible in conventional histologic sections of normal lung, these cells are capable of proliferating and can become hyperplastic in a broad variety of chronic inflammatory lung diseases. They are the source of regenerating pneumocytes type I. They express epithelial cytokeratins (Fig. 19-4B), are metabolically very active and, like the Clara cells, they synthesize **alveolar surfactant, a detergent-like protein that lines the inner surface of the alveoli, lowering surface tension and preventing collapse of the air spaces** (Fig. 19-4C) (Groniowski and Byczyskowa, 1964; Askin and Kuhn, 1971). Surfactant accumulates in the cytoplasm of pneumocytes type II in the form of characteristic, large **osmiophilic lamellar inclusions** that can be demonstrated by electron microscopy (Fig.19-4D). **The precursor proteins of surfactant and the lamellar inclusions are markers of pneumocytes type**

II. As noted, these cells can regenerate if injured, and are also capable of differentiating into pneumocytes type I (Kasper and Haroske, 1996).

Pneumocytes are not likely to be recognized in specimens of sputum or bronchial brushing, but they can be identified in bronchoalveolar lavage (BAL) and fine-needle aspiration (FNA) specimens of lung from patients with chronic lung disease and may be mistaken for adenocarcinoma (see below).

Pulmonary Alveolar Macrophages

In histologic material that has been handled carefully and processed without excessive delay, large phagocytic cells containing particles of dust are observed within nearly all of the alveoli (Fig. 19-5). These cells are sometimes referred to as **dust cells** or **pneumocytes type III.** Exceedingly large numbers of macrophages may be observed in the alveoli of

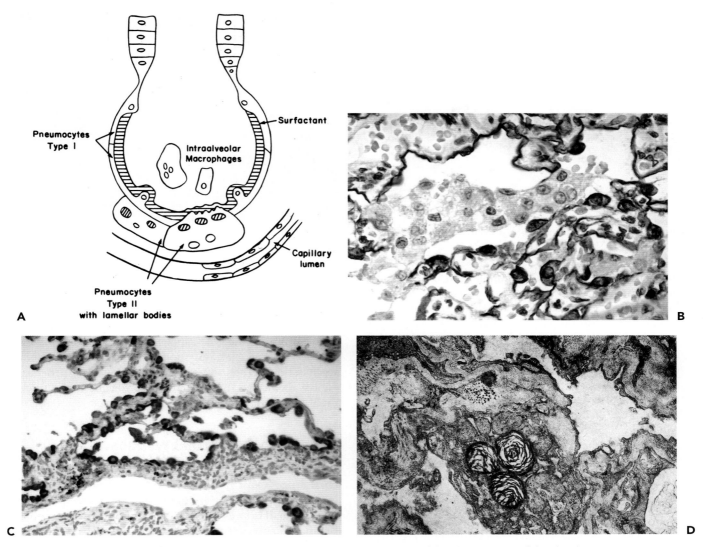

Figure 19-4   Pulmonary alveoli. *A.* Schematic representation of the ultrastructure of the alveolus showing pneumocytes type I and II, the latter with large nuclei and abundant cytoplasm within which are osmiophilic, dark inclusions. Overlying the pneumocytes is a layer of surfactant, and in the alveolar wall is a capillary separated from the alveolus by a basement membrane. *B.* The alveolus here is stained with anti-cytokeratin antibody (AE1/AE3) that demonstrates plump pneumocytes type II surfacing the alveolar wall, and the flat, greatly attenuated cytoplasm of type I pneumocytes. Pulmonary macrophages lie within the lumen of the alveolus. (Immunoperoxidase reaction with hematoxylin counterstain.) *C.* Immunoperoxidase reaction with anti-surfactant antibody, identifying the surfactant produced by pneumocytes type II. *D.* Electron micrograph of an alveolus showing the concentrically laminated cytoplasmic inclusions of surfactant precursor in the cytoplasm of a type II pneumocyte. (*C:* Courtesy of Dr. Allen Gown.) (*D:* ×1,600).

people who are heavy cigarette smokers or live in a dusty atmosphere. The ultrastructure of alveolar macrophages is consistent with a metabolically active cell provided with microvilli, lysosomes, and vacuolated inclusions. The **bone marrow origin** of alveolar macrophages was demonstrated in mice by Brunstetter et al (1971), and in humans by Thomas et al (1976) and Nakata et al (1999) who used the **FISH** (fluorescent in situ hybridization) technique (see Chaps. 3 and 4) to demonstrate a Y chromosome in the alveolar macrophages of a female recipient of bone marrow from a male donor. The **phagocytic function of alveolar macrophages** is called upon in terminal bronchioles and alveoli where the respiratory tract lacks cilia, thus providing

an additional defense against inspired foreign particles. In a series of ingenious experiments, Harmsen et al (1985) have shown that labeled particles instilled into the lung are not passively transported across the alveolar membrane but are phagocytized by alveolar macrophages that then migrate to lymph nodes.

CYTOLOGIC SAMPLING METHODS

Sputum

Spontaneously produced or artificially induced sputum is by far the simplest and most useful method of investigating

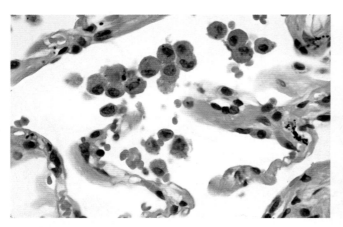

Figure 19-5 **Alveolar macrophages** within the alveoli.

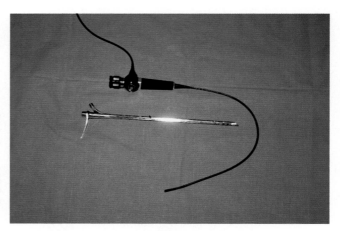

Figure 19-6 Flexible fiber bronchoscope and a rigid broncho-scope.

the respiratory tract. Multiple samples can be obtained at home or in the doctor's office or clinic without discomfort to the patient, and the diagnostic yield is excellent in many benign and nearly all malignant disorders. Patients should be instructed that the diagnostic material comes from deep portions of the lungs. They should be told to clear their nasal passages and rinse their mouth with water, discarding that material before collecting a specimen. **Ideal diagnostic material is obtained from a spontaneous deep cough,** which should be expelled directly into a wide-mouth container with fixative (vodka or whiskey will do, if necessary) and stored in the refrigerator where it can remain for as long as 2 to 3 weeks before processing in the laboratory. Often the best specimens are obtained on arising in the morning when a change in position will initiate a deep cough that expels bronchial secretions accumulated over-night.

Unfortunately, few patients are adequately instructed in how to produce a good deep cough specimen, and the material submitted may consist entirely of mouth contents or **saliva that is of no diagnostic value.** Even with good cough specimens, the presence of contaminating material from the mouth or nasopharynx can obscure diagnostic cells and make evaluation more difficult.

For patients with a nonproductive cough or no cough, it is possible to induce coughing by inhalation of a heated aerosol of 20% polypropylene glycol in hypertonic (10%) saline (or in water if the patient is salt restricted). One container may be used to collect three or four deep cough specimens. The composition of an adequate sputum sample is described below, and methods of processing are described in Chapter 44.

Bronchial Brushings

With the introduction of flexible bronchoscopes (Fig. 19-6) capable of reaching subsegmental bronchi, the cytologic diagnosis of lung cancer relies heavily on direct bronchial brushings. Cell samples are obtained with a small brush threaded through a separate channel in the fiberoptic bronchoscope, guided to a selected site under visual control. The method permits sampling of a visualized mucosal abnor-

mality or systematic sampling of all segmental bronchi to **confirm and localize occult in situ or early invasive carcinomas** detected by sputum cytology or suspected radiologically. Brushings may be supplemented by tissue biopsies or by transbronchial aspiration biopsy of lesions within reach of the fiberoptic bronchoscope, but in our experience, are less useful than BAL specimens for diagnosis of a more distal peripheral bronchoalveolar carcinoma.

Bronchial Aspirates and Washings

Although **brushings provide a better sample of the bronchial mucosa at a given site or sites, aspirates and washings provide information on the status of the respiratory tract in small bronchi beyond reach of the bronchoscopic brush.** Bronchial washing specimens are obtained under bronchoscopic guidance by first aspirating the accumulated contents of the bronchus (or bronchi) in an initial sample. Then, additional samples are obtained by repeatedly instilling and reaspirating (about 50 ml) normal saline from the selected bronchus or bronchi. The composition of samples is discussed below, and methods of processing it can be found in Chapter 44.

Bronchoalveolar Lavage (BAL)

BAL was introduced initially as a **therapeutic** procedure to clear the alveolar spaces of accumulated secretions blocking gaseous exchange, for example, in **alveolar proteinosis** (see below) and **bronchial asthma** (summary in Ramirez et al, 1965). Subsequently, the technique has been used for **diagnostic** purposes primarily in suspected *Pneumocystis carinii* **pneumonia,** replacing open lung biopsy (Stover et al, 1984; Fleury et al, 1985), and in the diagnosis of interstitial lung disease (Stoller et al, 1987). It has been used to identify various other **bacterial, fungal, parasitic, and sometimes viral** agents causing pulmonary infections, particularly in patients with **acquired immunodeficiency syndrome (AIDS)** (Broaddus et al, 1985; Kraft et al, 1998; Scaglia et al, 1998) and children with chronic granulomatous disease, an inherited defect of phagocytic oxidative enzymes (Abati et al, 1996). It has also been reported of value in investigating and monitoring other inflammatory reactions in the lung, for example **ozone injury** of the alveolar epithelium (Bhalla, 1999), **bronchiolitis obliterans organizing pneumonia (BOOP)** (Lamont et al, 1998) and chronic pulmonary diseases, mainly **sarcoidosis** and various forms of **pulmonary pneumoconioses.** In patients suspected radiologically of having pulmonary **alveolar microlithiasis,** a rare disease characterized by the presence of alveolar calcospherites, the calcospherites can be demonstrated in BAL fluid (see below) (Mariotta et al, 1997).

A recent and important application of BAL is in detecting rejection and/or infection in recipients of **lung transplants.** Rejection is heralded by an increasing percentage of polymorphonuclear leukocytes in the lavage specimen (Chan et al, 1996; Henke et al, 1999). BAL may sometimes disclose an unsuspected carcinoma, particularly **bronchoalveolar carcinoma,** which can mimic diffuse inflammatory lung disease radiologically and has been reported in patients monitored after lung transplantation (Garver et al, 1999).

Procedure

Under local anesthetic, the bronchoscope is passed to the lung segment of interest, usually a secondary or tertiary bronchus, and wedged to occlude the bronchial lumen. From 100 to 300 ml of normal saline is instilled in 20 to 50 ml aliquots, reaspirated, and the collected fluid is forwarded to the laboratory for processing. Evaluation of the lavage fluid is based on differential cell counts and immunophenotyping the cells present, as well as chemical analysis and bacteriologic study of the fluid retrieved from the alveolar spaces (Reynolds and Newball, 1974; summaries in Reynolds et al, 1977; Hunninghake et al, 1979; Crystal et al, 1984; Bitterman et al, 1986). If the lavage is properly performed, the cell content will be limited to the epithelium of the bronchioles beyond the point of occlusion and to the contents of the alveoli, mainly alveolar macrophages and inflammatory cells. Certain characteristics of the macrophages may be evaluated, for example, their ability to produce fibronectin or other factors stimulating the growth of fibroblasts leading to pulmonary fibrosis (Bitterman et al, 1983). The proportion and type of immunostimulated lymphocytes and the presence or absence of polymorphonuclear leukocytes also may be useful in evaluating the nature of the pulmonary disorder. The fluid may also be examined for the presence of surfactant. Recognition of microorganisms is described below.

Needle Aspiration Biopsy

The general principles of aspiration biopsy technique are discussed in Chapter 28. Special features of needle aspiration biopsy of the lung are described here and in Chapter 20.

There are two techniques of pulmonary aspiration biopsy: **percutaneous aspiration** of lung lesions and **transbronchial aspiration** via fiberoptic bronchoscopy. Percutaneous needle biopsy of the lung is most commonly performed to investigate peripheral lesions that are inaccessible to the bronchoscope and do not desquamate cells into the bronchial tree. Computed tomography (CT) or, less commonly, ultrasound is used to guide the direction and depth of insertion of the biopsy needle; fluoroscopy is no longer used. Transbronchial needle aspirates, first suggested by Wang et al (1981), serve to sample enlarged para-hilar or para-bronchial lymph nodes or other near-hilar masses that cannot easily be reached by percutaneous needle biopsy.

Contraindications to percutaneous needle biopsy include the following:

- Hemorrhagic diathesis
- Anticoagulant therapy (unless previously discontinued with restoration of normal clotting time)
- Severe pulmonary hypertension
- Advanced emphysema
- Suspected arteriovenous malformation or aneurysm
- Suspicion of hydatid cyst (see below)
- Uncooperative patient

Percutaneous Biopsy With Small-Caliber Needles (FNA)

When the lesion is close to the chest wall, it can be reached with a thin, relatively short needle (external diameter, 0.6 mm; length, 10 cm). For deeper lesions, a longer, flexible needle (14 to 20 cm) with the same diameter can be inserted though a thicker (17-gauge) needle that serves as a guide.

Local anesthesia is applied to the chest wall and pleura. The guide is introduced into the chest wall, care being taken not to let it penetrate into the pleural space. The finer needle is inserted through the guide, and when it reaches the target in the lung, the aspiration is performed, moving the needle to and fro as for palpable lesions. A **single-grip syringe** may be used to assist in the aspiration procedure (see Chap. 28).

Percutaneous Aspiration With Large-Caliber Needles

Thin needles may be unsuitable for small (2 cm or less) deep-lying lesions. Such needles may bend during passage through the pulmonary parenchyma, and the target may be missed. A wider bore, sturdy needle (0.9 to 1 mm external diameter) will not bend easily and may be more accurately guided to the lesion. A stylus inserted into the needle lends additional rigidity to the needle and also prevents tissues from the thoracic wall entering the lumen of the needle as it is inserted.

The technique of aspiration biopsy with a large-caliber needle is as follows. The patient is usually positioned horizontally on an adjustable table. An entry point, marked on the skin, is chosen so that the lesion can easily be reached. The skin, chest wall, and pleura are anesthetized. Premedication and general anesthesia are usually not necessary. With CT guidance, the needle is inserted at the designated entry point (close to the upper margin of a rib to avoid the intercostal artery) and introduced into the lesion. Care is taken to avoid large blood vessels and bronchi. The patient is instructed to breathe normally. When the needle has reached the lesion, a change in consistency usually will be noticed. With the tip of the needle in the lesion, the operator rotates it clockwise and counter-clockwise to loosen small tissue fragments around the tip. The stylus is then withdrawn, a 10- or 20-ml syringe is attached, and **the loosened tissue is aspirated into the needle while the patient holds his or her breath.** The aspirated material need not (should not) be drawn beyond the lumen of the needle. Negative pressure is released and the needle is withdrawn from the chest. The aspirated material is expressed onto glass slides; the number of slides depends on the amount of aspirate. Air-dried and wet-fixed smears are prepared. The needle may be washed with sterile normal saline and the contents are preserved for cell blocks or for bacteriologic examination.

Screw-Needle Biopsy

Now rarely used, this method is of historical interest as a technique designed to obtain diagnostic material from **fibrocalcific granulomas, hamartomas, and other lesions that are not easily penetrated or aspirated with a regular needle.** The intent is to avoid exploratory thoracotomy for diagnosis of a benign lesion. The procedure of inserting the needle is the same as for the large-caliber needle, described above. When the large-caliber needle reaches the lesion, **the stylus is removed and replaced by one with a sharp point on a screw tip that is rotated into the target mass.** The tumor, now fixed by the screw, can be penetrated by the needle. After some rotary movements, the instrument is withdrawn from the chest. The screw stylus is removed from the needle, and loose cellular material is deposited on a glass slide by rotating the screw. The material is smeared on one or more slides, except for sizeable tissue fragments that are embedded in paraffin for sectioning (Dahlgren and Nordenstrøm, 1966).

Complications of Percutaneous Aspiration Biopsy

Serious complications are rare. The three most common complications of immediate importance are **pneumothorax, hemorrhage, and air embolism.** Also important, but exceedingly rare and of less immediate concern, is the possibility of seeding cancer in the needle track.

Pneumothorax

The frequency of pneumothorax among patients in the Karolinska Hospital series, who underwent single or multiple aspiration biopsies to obtain a cytologic diagnosis, was about 27% (Dahlgren and Nordenstrøm, 1966). An approximately similar frequency of pneumothorax was recorded at Montefiore Medical Center. In most cases, the pneumothorax is asymptomatic and detected only by follow-up chest x-ray taken routinely after 6 to 12 hours; it resolves spontaneously, and no treatment is necessary. In about 3% of patients, the pneumothorax requires hospitalization and treatment (Kamholz et al, 1982). Factors influencing the frequency and severity of pneumothorax include the size and site of the lesion, the patient's age, presence of emphysematous blebs, and the operator's experience. Pneumothorax is more common in elderly patients and in patients with

small, deeply seated lesions. The risk of pneumothorax precludes aspiration biopsy of the lung as an office procedure. It should be performed only where emergency thoracic surgical assistance is available if needed.

Hemorrhage

Some bleeding into the lung can be expected with every needle aspiration biopsy. In most cases, the bleeding is of no consequence. An occasional patient will experience transient hemoptysis, but we have not encountered more severe or persistent hemoptysis. In one instance, cardiac tamponade was reported following FNA of a lesion near the mediastinum (Kucharczyk et al, 1982).

Air Embolism

Aberle et al (1987) reported the death of a patient with Wegener's granulomatosis due to air embolism following percutaneous FNA. This extremely rare complication was never encountered during a series of 3,799 aspiration biopsies of the lung on 2,726 patients from Karolinska Sjukhuset (Dahlgren and Nordenstrøm, 1966), nor has it been observed in many hundreds of patients at Montefiore Medical Center and Westchester Medical Center.

Spread of Cancer in the Needle Track

This complication is extremely rare. In the Karolinska Hospital series, more than 1,250 pulmonary carcinomas were diagnosed by aspiration biopsy, but implantation metastasis was reported in only one patient, a 73-year-old man with inoperable squamous cell carcinoma (Sinner and Zajicek, 1976). Sacchini et al (1989) reported implants of pulmonary adenocarcinoma in the chest wall of a 57-year-old woman 3 months following percutaneous FNA and resection of the lung cancer; a single additional case was reported by Moloo et al (1985). Similar complications were observed and illustrated by Koss et al (1992) and by Yoshikawa et al (2000). Considering that many thousands of such procedures are performed annually worldwide, this complication is still rare enough to be reportable.

Transbronchial Needle Aspiration

Transbronchial needle aspiration, first described in 1981 by Wang et al, is performed **during bronchoscopy** when an extrabronchial lesion is suspected. A thin, flexible needle is inserted through the bronchial wall into the suspected lesion via the bronchoscope, and the cellular material is aspirated and processed as for percutaneous biopsies.

CYTOLOGY OF THE NORMAL RESPIRATORY TRACT

Squamous Epithelium

The squamous epithelium of the buccal cavity is constantly washed by saliva; therefore, the changes induced by cellular dryness are exceedingly uncommon. The exfoliated **superficial squamous cells,** which predominate in specimens of saliva as they do in scrape smears of other squamous mucosal surfaces, are similar in all respects to the superficial and intermediate squamous cells of the female genital tract.

There may be karyomegaly of occasional cells without apparent significance (Fig. 19-7A). Occasionally also, smaller **squamous cells** with relatively large but uniform nuclei may be present, comparable to the parabasal cells of cervicovaginal cytology specimens (Fig. 19-7B). They may be present singly, but are often in plaques and encountered more commonly in **inflammatory disorders** of the oral cavity. They are presumed to represent incomplete maturation of regenerating epithelium. **Onion-like arrangements of benign squamous cells (i.e., squamous pearls)** (Fig. 19-7C) and occasionally small spindly squamous cells also may be observed. **Anucleated squamous cells** are few, if present at all, but may exfoliate from the normal mucosa overlying and fixed to bone (e.g., hard palate), or from sites of chronic irritation as occurs with poor dentition. The presence of large numbers or plaques of anucleated squames (Fig, 19-7D) is abnormal and is an indication of **oral leukoplakia** (see Chap. 21).

Respiratory Epithelium

Contrary to squamous epithelium, which desquamates easily and is well represented in all exfoliated samples, the **normal respiratory epithelium does not desquamate freely.** Consequently, cells derived from this epithelium are **uncommon in sputum** and are typically seen in **specimens obtained by bronchial brushing or aspiration,** or after other procedures that dislodge them from their epithelial setting, such as bronchoscopy. If they are present at all in a sputum specimen, it is an indication of prior instrumentation, trauma, or severe cough. However, respiratory epithelial cells may also originate in the **nasal cavity** or **nasopharynx;** therefore, their presence in a specimen is not absolute insurance of origin from the lower respiratory tract.

Ciliated Cells

Respiratory epithelium is readily recognized in cytologic material by the presence of **ciliated columnar cells** (Fig. 19-8A; see also Fig. 2-4).

Columnar cells may appear singly or in groups or clusters of cells, depending on how forcefully they have been dislodged. In brush specimens, **large numbers of bronchial cells** are commonly observed, sometimes forming clusters of considerable complexity (Fig. 19-8B), and sometimes also with **adherent reserve or basal epithelial cells** (Fig. 19-

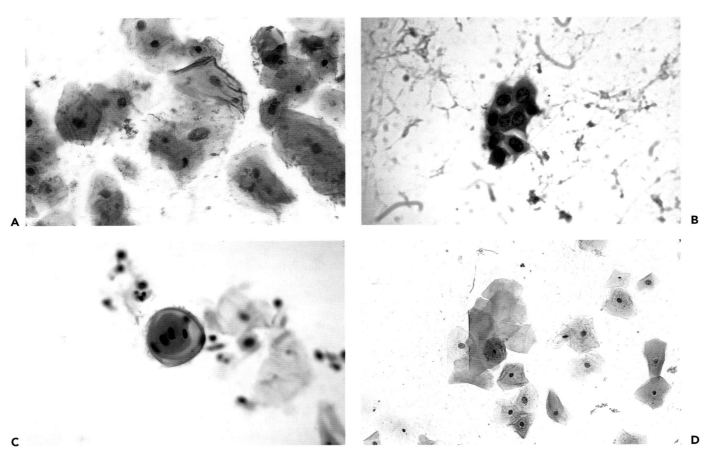

Figure 19-7 **Squamous cells in saliva.** *A.* Superficial squamous cells of oral mucosal origin similar to those of cervicovaginal specimens. Note the single cell exhibiting moderate karyomegaly, and the bacterial background typical of saliva. *B.* A cluster of small squamous cells from deep layers of the epithelium, resembling the parabasal cells of cervicovaginal specimens. They are derived from an inflamed or ulcerated mucosa. The cells retain "intercellular bridges" and exhibit some cytoplasmic and nuclear hyperchromasia. *C.* Benign squamous pearl. Nuclei are small and innocent in appearance, and usually more numerous than in a malignant pearl. *D.* A plaque of anucleated keratinized cells suggestive of leukoplakia.

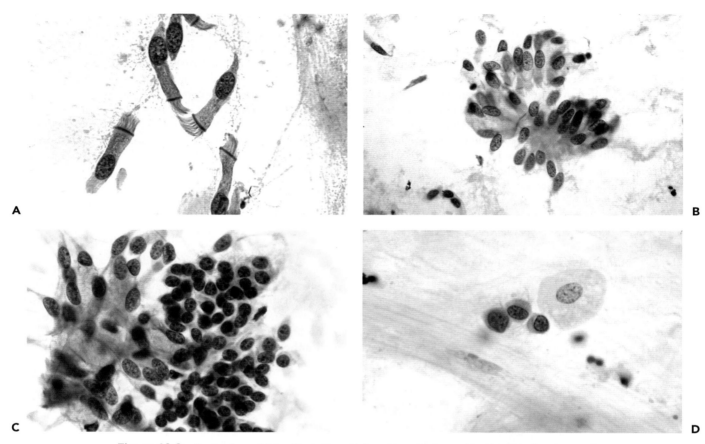

Figure 19-8   Benign bronchial cells. *A.* Bronchial washing specimen showing dissociated normal ciliated columnar bronchial cells. The terminal plates to which the cilia are attached are well demonstrated in these optimally fixed cells. Nuclei may be relatively large and bulge out the bronchial cell (oil immersion). *B.* Bronchial brushing specimen showing bronchial cells in a cluster with some cells projecting out of the cluster to give a "feathering" appearance. *C.* Another cluster of bronchial cells in a brush specimen with adherent basal or reserve cells. *D.* Cuboidal bronchial cells derived from a peripheral bronchiole. Note one flat cell border.

8C). At the periphery of such clusters, normal ciliated cells may appear at a right angle to the main axis of the cluster, giving the impression of **feathering,** clearly **an artefact** induced by brushing (Fig. 19-8B).

The individual cells, derived from larger bronchi, are typically **cilia bearing and columnar in configuration,** measuring about 30 to 50 μm in length and 10 to 15 μm in width. **Much smaller, approximately square bronchial cells** with scanty cytoplasm and a flat surface, with or without cilia, derived from terminal bronchioles, are occasionally observed (Fig. 19-8D).

There is a prominent **linear thickening** or **flat terminal plate** at the luminal end of the columnar cell, **anchoring the cilia** (Fig. 19-8A). On close inspection, under very high magnification by light microscopy, the terminal plate is composed **of a series of confluent dots representing roots of the cilia** or **basal corpuscles.** In a well-executed Papanicolaou stain, the **cilia stain a distinct pink color.** While cilia may be damaged or lost, **the terminal plate is usually preserved** (Dalhamn, 1970). The opposite or basal end of the cell tapers off to terminate in a whip-like process representing the former point of attachment to the basement membrane.

Clusters or sheets of dislodged respiratory cells lying flat on the slide and **viewed from the luminal surface** have a **honeycomb** appearance, formed by the cytoplasmic borders of adjacent cells, not unlike endocervical cells (Fig. 19-9A).

The **cytoplasm** of the ciliated epithelial cell seen in profile is **homogeneous** and lightly **basophilic** or less commonly eosinophilic. Rarely, small mucus vacuoles may be observed. In the supranuclear cytoplasm of some bronchial cells, there are **granules of brown lipochrome pigment,** more commonly found in older patients and considered a "wear and tear" pigment (Fig. 19-9B). Rarely, the entire cytoplasm may eventually be filled with this pigment.

The **nuclei are usually very finely textured and oval in shape,** with their long axis corresponding to the long axis of the cell. Sometimes, the nucleus appears to be larger than the transverse diameter of the slender cell, resulting in a slight bulge at the level of the nucleus (Figs. 19-8A and 19-10C). However, electron micrographs show that the nucleus is always surrounded by a rim of cytoplasm. Within most bronchial cell nuclei, there are usually one or two **small, but distinct, chromatin granules** and sometimes a **tiny nucleolus.** The **sex chromatin (Barr body)** may be readily recognized in females (see Fig. 2-4).

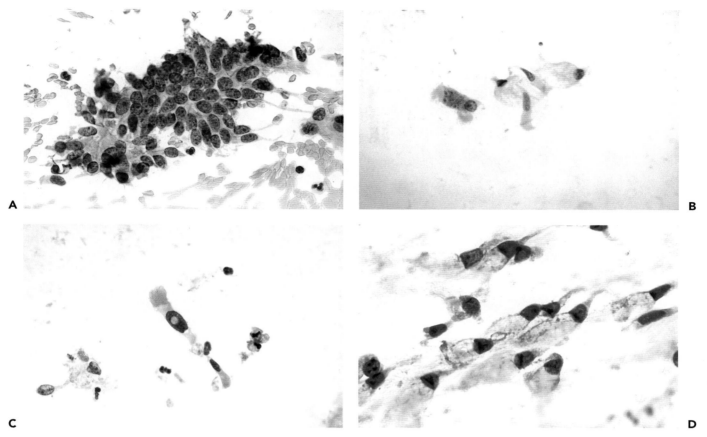

Figure 19-9   **Benign bronchial cells.** *A.* A plaque of bronchial cells seen on end has a honeycomb appearance much like endocervical cells. *B.* Lipochrome pigment in the cytoplasm of a bronchial cell. This is generally considered to be an aging phenomenon and has no diagnostic significance. *C.* Bronchial cell with a nuclear hole attributed to an artefact of preparation has no diagnostic significance. *D.* Dissociated single goblet cells in a bronchial brush specimen showing the supranuclear cytoplasm distended by multiple packets of mucin. (*D:* oil immersion.)

The **position of the nucleus** relative to the ciliated cell surface is variable, usually midway between the ciliated or luminal end of the cell and the tapered basal end. Chalon et al (1971) reported that in women of childbearing age, the position of the nucleus in the ciliated cells varies according to the time of the menstrual cycle, from a basal position in the proliferative phase of the cycle, to midposition after ovulation and to a position closer to the ciliated plate toward the end of the secretory phase. In men and postmenopausal women, he found that the position of the nucleus was always distant from the ciliated plate. Chalon et al attributed these variations to a changing mucopolysaccharide content of the cells during the cycle. To our knowledge, this has not been studied or confirmed by others.

The normal nuclei may also show **folds or creases** and sometimes, **intranuclear cytoplasmic inclusions,** or clear intranuclear "holes" (Fig. 19-9C). We find the latter to be more common in cancer cell nuclei. **Dense nuclear protrusions (nipples)** may also be observed in benign bronchial cells and are similar to those observed in endocervical cells at midcycle (see Chap. 8). Koizumi (1996) concluded that the "nipples" were a common nonspecific effect of mechanical forces during specimen collection or processing.

Goblet Cells

The mucus-producing **goblet cells** are less common than ciliated cells. They are approximately the same length but usually wider than the ciliated cells, with a **basally placed nucleus and distended supranuclear cytoplasm** that is tightly packed with faintly basophilic tiny **vacuoles** representing packages of mucus. The much wider cytoplasm of these cells toward their luminal surface accounts for the "goblet" shape (Fig. 19-9D). The nuclei, located near the narrow, basal end of the cell are similar to those of ciliated cells, described above. Cilia are absent but **faint streaks of mucus** topping the broad luminal end of the goblet cell, **may superficially resemble cilia,** and can easily be differentiated by the absence of a terminal plate. If there is goblet cell hyperplasia as a result of asthma or chronic irritation, goblet cells will be present in increased numbers in brush specimens, as in Figure 19-9D. This finding may be of clinical significance and should be recorded.

Basal or Germinative Cells

The **basal** or **germinative cells** of the respiratory epithelium are the source of epithelial regeneration and normally form a single layer of cells on the basement membrane. In response to inflammation or injury, these cells may proliferate

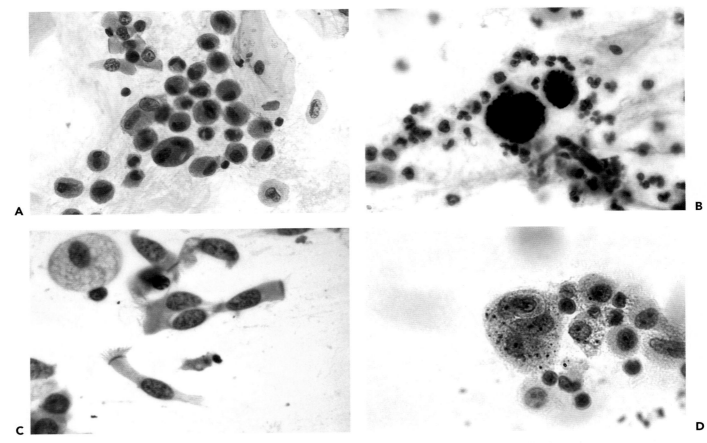

Figure 19-10 Pulmonary macrophages (dust cells). These cells come from the alveolar spaces, and are most abundant in BAL specimens. They are present in deep cough specimens of sputum, usually with a few leukocytes. There is variation in amount and staining of cytoplasm, which may have a yellowish color due to the presence of submicroscopic dust (A), or be densely crowded with phagocytized brown or black particles that obscure the nucleus (B). In the absence of phagocytosis, as illustrated in C, the cytoplasm may be finely vacuolated. Macrophages may be binucleated or multinucleated (D), and the reactive cells have multiple nuclei or prominent nucleoli. (C,D: oil immersion.)

and form several layers, resulting in **basal or reserve cell hyperplasia.** The significance of basal cell hyperplasia in the diagnosis of benign disease and neoplasia is addressed later in this chapter.

Other Epithelial Cells

Other components of the **normal respiratory tract epithelium** such as **Clara cells,** neuroendocrine **(Kulchitsky) cells,** or **pneumocytes types I and II** are difficult or impossible to identify in clinical specimens of cytologic material without use of special cytochemical techniques (see Figs. 19-3D and 19-4C). **Hyperplastic or atypical pneumocytes type II, which may be seen in certain benign lung disorders, can enter into the differential diagnosis of cancer** (see below).

Artefacts Induced by Delayed or Inadequate Fixation

If the fixation of the smears is delayed, there may be **drying artefact,** resulting in slight-to-moderate cellular and nuclear enlargement, loss of staining intensity and cellular detail, and often distortion of the bronchial cells with **loss of cilia,**

but usually preservation of the terminal plate. Artefacts of nuclear staining caused by drying are generally well recognized, and typically manifest as nuclear enlargement, hypochromasia, and loss of nuclear detail. Drying artefact is most marked at the periphery of cell clusters and in isolated single cells, yet the basic uniformity of nuclear size and structure and the preservation of the nucleocytoplasmic ratio is still appreciated, supporting a benign diagnosis. The drying artefact may enhance the vacuolated appearance of the goblet cells' cytoplasm.

Mesothelial Cells

Although limited to the serosal surface of the lung, these cells are commonly observed in needle aspirates of peripheral lung lesions. They form flat clusters of cells that are separated by clear spaces or "windows," but may contain large nucleoli and be mistaken for cancer cells. For further discussion, see Chapters 20 and 26.

Alveolar Macrophages

The alveolar macrophages are of great importance in evaluating cytologic material from the respiratory tract. **Their** presence confirms origin of the sample from pulmonary alveoli, hence the deeper portions of the respiratory tract, and sputum specimens are rarely of diagnostic value in their absence. Macrophages are most abundant in sputum specimens from cigarette smokers and in specimens from patients living in dusty environs, for example, from farmers. In BAL specimens, they are the predominant cell type, and present in abundance. The origin of these cells from bone marrow has been discussed above.

Macrophages appear most commonly as **spherical or oval cells** measuring from 10 to 25 μm or more in diameter. Their **cytoplasm,** usually amphophilic, may be abundant or limited in amount, basophilic or acidophilic, and usually contains a variable amount of phagocytized gray, brown, or black granular dust particles, hence the name **dust cells,** which is occasionally used. The dust particles may be below the resolving power of the microscope and simply lend a faint, usually yellowish color to the cytoplasm (Fig. 19-10A), or they may be numerous and dense, and completely obscure details of the cell structure (Fig. 19-10B). In smokers, as pointed out by Mellors (1957) and later by Roque and Pickren (1968), some of the granules fluoresce in ultraviolet light. In the absence of dust, the cytoplasm may contain fine vacuoles (Fig. 19-10C). As a rule, the periphery of the cells is sharply demarcated, but there may be one or several **cytoplasmic extensions or processes.** Walker and Fullmer (1971) described **nipple- or tail-shaped eosinophilic cytoplasmic extensions** of variable size, usually located at opposite ends of elongated macrophages. These cytoplasmic "tails" stain brilliantly eosinophilic, often in sharp contrast with the remainder of the cytoplasm. Such cells have been observed mainly in smokers and in people exposed to toxic inhalants (Frost et al, 1973), but their significance remains unknown.

The **nuclei of macrophages** vary in size and number but are generally round, oval, or kidney-shaped, about 5 to 10 μm in diameter, with fine, evenly dispersed chromatin and small nucleoli. Binucleation is common, as are **large multinucleated macrophages** (Fig. 19-10D), including an occasional giant macrophage resembling Langhans' or foreign body giant cells. Kern et al (2003) found multinucleated cells with 3 to 10 nuclei in the majority of their patients, and at least a few multinucleated giant cells with more than 10 nuclei in BAL specimens from 10% of their patients. The latter were most common in sarcoidosis, but also viral infections, asbestosis, and various interstitial lung diseases including hard metal pneumoconioses. Kinoshita et al (1999) described bizarre macrophages of possible diagnostic value in the BAL specimens of two hard-metal workers.

The pulmonary macrophages, which are best studied in BAL specimens, not only phagocytize and remove respired dust particles that are not eliminated by the ciliated bronchial cells, they are the **primary defense against invading organisms** and are responsible for **removing dead or damaged cells and any foreign matter.** They are metabolically active cells that also ingest and **process antigens for presentation to T lymphocytes** and thus mediate a great many immunologic reactions. Activated macrophages **produce cytokines that recruit other inflammatory cells and**

growth factors for fibroblasts and blood vessels (Abbas et al, 1991). Smoking adversely affects the pulmonary alveolar macrophages, as do a number of infectious and idiopathic disorders.

The functional activity of the alveolar macrophages can be estimated by a number of different techniques that include quantification of phagocytosis and immunocytochemical estimates of lysosomal enzyme activity—a marker of phagocytic cells. Like other monocytes, they express the **antigens CD-14 and CD-68,** and exhibit strong, diffuse, nonspecific esterase and acid phosphatase activity; 5'-nucleotidase is a marker of activated macrophages. Wehle and Pfitzer (1988) reported increased activity of nonspecific esterase in smokers and in persons with bronchial asthma.

Leukocytes

Polymorphonuclear leukocytes in small numbers are very common in cytologic specimens from the normal respiratory tract, especially in cigarette smokers. Kilburn and McKenzie (1975) pointed out that particulate matter in cigarette smoke recruits leukocytes to the bronchial tree. However, a finding of numerous polymorphonuclear leukocytes, particularly in the presence of necrotic material in an acutely ill patient, suggests a major inflammatory process such as **pneumonia** or **abscess** (Fig. 19-11A).

Eosinophils (Fig. 19-11B), or the elongated **Charcot-Leyden crystals** derived therefrom (Fig. 19-11C), suggest an **allergic process,** such as bronchial asthma.

Lymphocytes, singly or in pools, are a common finding in various inflammatory disorders; their presence in the appropriate clinical setting is consistent with **follicular bronchitis** (see below), but it must be remembered that they may be dislodged **from tonsillar tissue in subjects without disease.** In these benign conditions, there is typically a **mixture of mature small and medium lymphocytes** with scattered large reactive lymphoblasts and phagocytic macrophages (Fig. 19-11D). In lymphomas and leukemias, on the other hand, the lymphoid cells are more uniform. They present as small mature lymphocytes in the case of small-cell lymphocytic lymphoma or chronic lymphocytic leukemia, or as immature lymphoblasts or atypical mononuclear cells. Small-cell carcinoma is characterized by cells with irregular, hyperchromatic nuclei with coarse chromatin, nuclear molding, necrosis and streaks of DNA (see Chaps. 20 and 26). Tassoni (1963) stressed that pools of lymphocytes in small numbers may accompany lung cancer and that their presence warrants careful examination of the cytologic material. This has not been confirmed by others, and we have not found it useful. It should be noted that cigarette smokers have increased numbers of inflammatory cells in their airways and specifically, an **increased number of CD8+ (suppressor) T lymphocytes,** particularly in the presence of chronic obstructive pulmonary disease (Saetta et al, 1999).

Plasma cells are a frequent component of chronic inflammatory processes, particularly those involving the mouth and oropharynx.

Monocytes may be observed occasionally and are now known to be precursors of the larger alveolar macrophages.

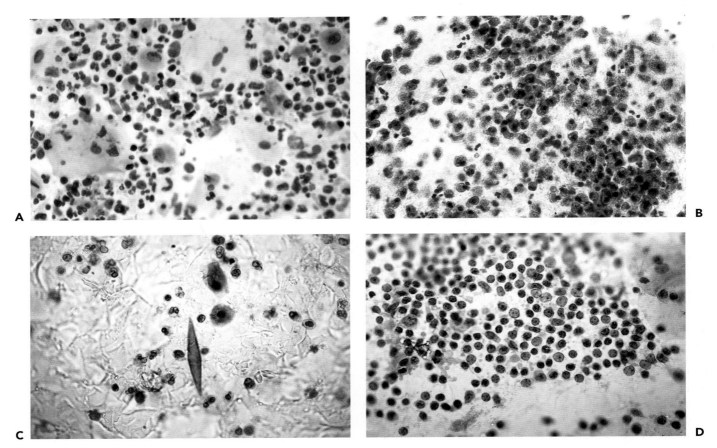

Figure 19-11 **Leukocytes.** *A.* Polymorphonuclear leukocytes (PMNs), when present as the predominant cell type in a cough specimen or bronchial aspirate, and particularly if associated with necrotic cellular debris, indicate an acute inflammatory process such as pneumonia, bronchiectasis, or lung abscess. *B.* Eosinophils, if present in at least moderate number, are an indicator of an allergic inflammatory process and most commonly associated with asthmatic bronchitis. *C.* Needle-shaped Charcot-Leyden crystals may accompany marked eosinophilia. (Bronchial wash, high magnification). *D.* Pools of lymphocytes may be dislodged by bronchoscopy or after vigorous coughing from tonsillar tissues or lymphoid aggregates in lymphocytic bronchitis (follicular bronchitis). Mature lymphocytes are mixed with follicular lymphoblasts and histiocytes. They should not be mistaken for lymphoma or for SSC (see Chap. 20) (High magnification).

Using fresh sputum, Chodosh (1970) found monocytes comprising 1% to 2% of the cells in specimens from patients with chronic bronchitis and chronic bronchial asthma.

Mast cells have also been observed in material obtained by bronchial brushing (Patterson et al, 1972).

Megakaryocytes released from the marrow in vertebral or pelvic bones enter the systemic venous system and **traverse, or are sometimes trapped in capillaries of the lung** (Fig. 19-12A). In passing through the **pulmonary capillary bed, the megakaryocytes become elongated and are stripped of cytoplasm that is broken into platelets** (Melamed et al, 1966). Inevitably, some find their way into the alveolar air space, and on rare occasions, **they may be found in sputum, bronchial brushings, or FNA specimens of the lung** (Fig. 19-12B). They may be relatively well-preserved, with **multilobate nuclei** and abundant cytoplasm, but more commonly are only **sausage-shaped nuclei.**

Other Nonepithelial Cells

Takeda and Burechailo (1969) reported the presence of **smooth muscle cells in sputum** of a patient who had the

pulmonary form of Wegener's granulomatosis with bronchial ulceration. They pointed out the difficulty in correctly identifying these cells. We have seen smooth muscle cells on occasion in bronchial brush specimens, presumably due to vigorous brushing (Fig. 19-12C).

Noncellular Endogenous Material

Curschmann's Spirals

Curschmann's spirals are **casts of inspissated mucus,** derived from and shaped by the lumens of small bronchi. The characteristic coiled appearance of the spirals, with a **dark central axis and a translucent periphery,** allows easy recognition (Fig. 19-13A).

The presence of Curschmann's spirals has long been considered diagnostic of **chronic bronchitis** or **asthma,** diseases in which there is an increased number of goblet cells and increased secretion of mucus. However, Curschmann's spirals are likely to be found in patients with goblet cell hyperplasia or metaplasia and increased mucus secretion of any cause. Walker and Fullmer (1970) documented that

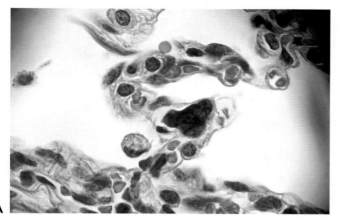

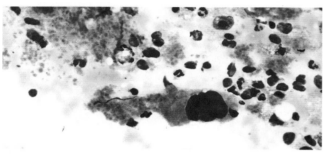

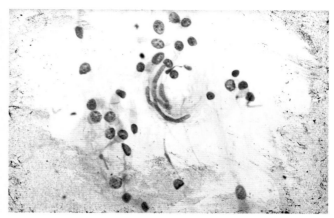

Figure 19-12 Uncommon cell types. *A.* Megakaryocyte trapped in alveolar capillary of lung. *B.* Megakaryocyte with multilobulated nucleus and abundant, ragged cytoplasm seen in an FNA of lung. Most megakaryocytic nuclei are stripped of cytoplasm as they pass through the alveolar capillaries. *C.* Bronchial brush specimen with a cluster of spindly **smooth muscle cells** that have elongated nuclei with rounded ends (*A:* Oil immersion).

over 90% of **asymptomatic cigarette smokers** have such spirals in their sputum. Plamenac et al (1972) found Curschmann's spirals in the sputum of former cigarette smokers for 6 years after cessation of smoking. There was no correlation found between the daily consumption of cigarettes and the number of spirals per specimen.

Inspissated Mucus

Inspissated, amorphous mucus may form **small, dark staining, structureless bodies (blobs)** that occasionally have the **size and shape of nuclei** (Fig. 19-13B,C). We have observed situations where they were **mistaken for nuclei of cancer cells,** particularly if they happened to overlay a cell. Close attention must be paid to the absence of any internal structure in the blobs of mucus.

Corpora Amylacea

Corpora amylacea are **spherical, translucent structures** that may be found in alveoli of people who have had previous episodes of pulmonary edema. Such structures, which in all likelihood represent a condensation of proteins, may be observed on occasion in sputum (Fig. 19-13D,E). Schmitz and Pfitzer (1984) described very similar "acellular bodies" in 1% of sputum specimens from 70 patients with a **variety of chronic pulmonary disorders,** including one with adenocarcinoma. They observed an association of the "acellular bodies" with Curshmann's spirals and correlated them with similar structures found at autopsy in alveolar spaces and dilated ducts of bronchial glands.

Amyloid

Amyloid was observed in irregular, amorphous fragments by Chen (1984) and by Neifer and Amy (1985) in the

bronchial brushings of patients who had documented tracheobronchial amyloidosis. The homogeneous, waxy appearance of the fragments should raise suspicion of amyloid, and their apple-green birefringence under polarized light after Congo red staining establishes the diagnosis (Fig. 19-14A,B). Neifer and Amy noted the **similarity of such fragments to corpora amylacea,** which may also stain with Congo red, but are spherical or oval structures that lack the apple-green birefringence of amyloid. Other cases of pulmonary amyloid nodules diagnosed by aspiration biopsy were reported by Tomashefski et al (1980) and Vera-Alvarez et al (1993). We have not seen such a case in cytologic material.

Pseudoamyloid

We observed a case of pseudoamyloid in a 73-year-old patient with an endobronchial lesion. Fragments of **faintly fibrillar, eosinophilic material indistinguishable from amyloid were observed in bronchial brushes** and in the cell block (Fig. 19-14C), which also contained a small fragment of bronchial epithelium. The material **failed to give the Congo red reaction** and was therefore classified as pseudoamyloid, a rare event in the lungs usually associated with light-chain deposits in the presence of multiple myeloma (Kijner et al, 1988; Stokes, et al, 1997).

Calcific Concretions

Small calcific concretions may be observed in sputum of people with **chronic pulmonary diseases, especially tuberculosis.** They also suggest the possibility of **alveolar microlithiasis,** a rare disorder of unknown etiology in which there are numerous calcific deposits within the alveoli that inter-

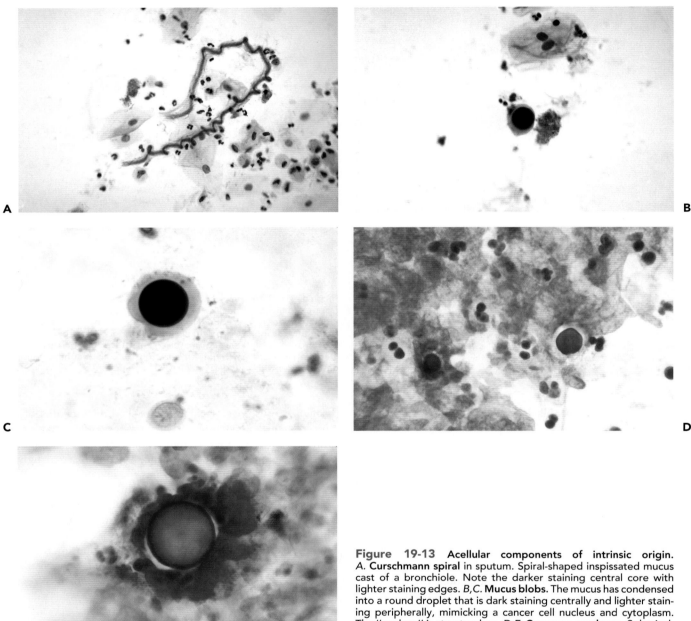

Figure 19-13 Acellular components of intrinsic origin. *A.* **Curschmann spiral** in sputum. Spiral-shaped inspissated mucus cast of a bronchiole. Note the darker staining central core with lighter staining edges. *B,C.* **Mucus blobs.** The mucus has condensed into a round droplet that is dark staining centrally and lighter staining peripherally, mimicking a cancer cell nucleus and cytoplasm. The "nucleus" is structureless. *D,E.* **Coropora amylacea.** Spherical, translucent, structureless condensates of protein, usually associated with pulmonary edema of some duration. (*C,E:* oil immersion.)

fere with respiratory exchange. The diagnosis may be suspected by radiologic findings that are often striking in patients with minimal symptoms (Brandenburg and Schubert, 2003) and can be confirmed by finding the calcospherites in sputum or bronchoalveolar washings (Fig. 19-15A,B). Unlike corpora amylacea, they are hard and crystalline and may fragment. They must be differentiated from **calcium oxalate crystals,** which are sometimes associated with and should suggest the possibility of fungal infection with aspergillus (see below).

Exogenous Foreign Material

Ferruginous Bodies (Asbestos Bodies)

Exposure to some forms of asbestos in respired air induces **pleural and pulmonary fibrosis,** risk of **malignant meso-**thelioma, and, in cigarette smokers, a five- to tenfold increased risk of **lung cancer** (see Chap. 26). The inhaled uncoated asbestos fibers, measuring less than 1 μm in diameter and about 50 μm or more in length, are translucent and scarcely visible (Fig. 19-16A). In the lung, they become coated with protein and iron (hence ferruginous), giving them a characteristic **golden-brown, segmented or beaded bamboo shape with knobbed or bulbous ends** (Fig. 19-16B). The fibers are sometimes partially enveloped by a macrophage, as was first described by Frost et al (1973). The coated ferruginous bodies of asbestos fibers measure from 5 to 200 μm in length and 3 to 5 μm in diameter. The larger fibers are removed by bronchial ciliary action. Asbestos exposure is most common among certain construction, shipbuilding, and

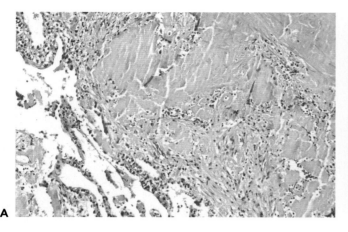

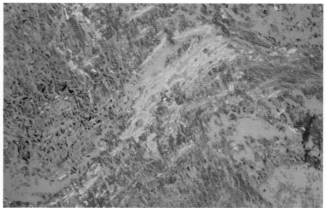

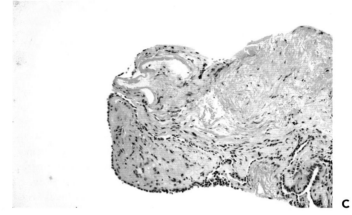

Figure 19-14   Amyloid. *A.* Amyloid involving lung, pale eosinophilic acellular material. *B.* **"Apple green" birefringence** of amyloid in polarized light after **Congo red stain.** *C.* Pseudoamyloid in a cell block section of tissue recovered by bronchial brush, resembling amyloid but not birefringent. Fragments of amyloid have been described in bronchial specimens (see text).

industrial workers, and in recent years, the workers involved in demolition of older buildings in which asbestos was used for insulation. **Routine sputum samples from individuals exposed to asbestos may contain the characteristic ferruginous bodies.** However, they are more abundant and **more easily demonstrated in BAL** specimens, and can be found in those specimens even in patients without known exposure to asbestos. There is a correlation between the number of ferruginous bodies in BAL samples and in lung tissue (Teschler et al, 1994),

and the presence of large numbers of ferruginous bodies in lavage specimens (>1 per 10^6 cells) is indicative of considerable asbestos exposure (Roggli et al, 1986).

Rosen et al (1972) examined digests of lung tissue in surgical and autopsy specimens and documented the presence of small numbers of typical asbestos ferruginous bodies in the lungs of virtually all people living in an urban area. They are most commonly present in the lower lobes. Using Smith and Naylor's method (1972), Bhagavan and Koss (1976) documented a dramatic in-

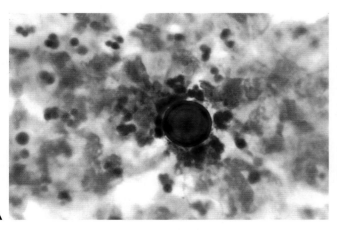

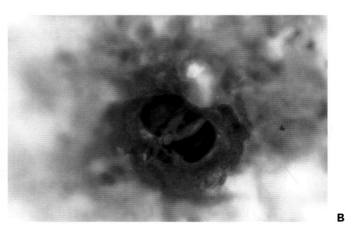

Figure 19-15   Pneumoliths in bronchial irrigation specimen from a 73-year-old woman with chronic lung disease. *A.* Pneumoliths are small, generally round laminated microcalcific bodies. *B.* Broken pneumolith (oil immersion).

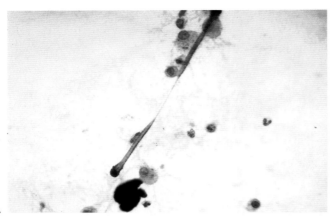
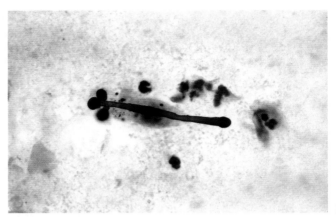

A

B

Figure 19-16 Acellular components of sputum or bronchial cytology of extrinsic origin. *A,B.* Ferruginous bodies. These are **asbestos bodies,** but mineral fibers of diverse origin can be similar in appearance. The fiber itself is thin and almost transparent (*A*), but has a golden-yellow coating of protein with iron (*B*), hence the name *ferruginous,* which is generic for all such fibers. Macrophages in a futile attempt to phagocytize and remove an asbestos fiber.

crease in the lung content of asbestos bodies over the three decades from 1940 to 1972. Surprisingly high counts of asbestos bodies were found without evidence of lung disease in digests of sputum and lung tissue from young children and juveniles as well as adults. Thus, the **presence of asbestos bodies in sputum does not necessarily imply asbestos-related disease,** and must be interpreted with appropriate caution after correlation with clinical and radiologic findings.

Asbestos bodies may be found in FNAs of lung lesions. In a series of 1,256 transthoracic FNAs, Leiman (1991) found them in 57 specimens from 55 patients. They were an incidental finding in all cases; in none was asbestos-induced fibrosis alone responsible for the lung mass aspirated, except for one patient with a mesothelioma.

Asbestos fibers are by far the most common substrate of ferruginous bodies, but **other mineral fibers may have a similar appearance** (Churg and Warnock, 1981; Mazzucchelli et al, 1996). Some of the nonasbestos ferruginous bodies are distinguished by a **fibrous core that is opaque or colored** rather than clear, and some **may be curved or branched** rather than straight. Rosen et al (1973) reported such "atypical" branching or segmentally thickened fibers in digests of lung and fibrous pleura.

Undigested Food Particles

Particles of food are commonly observed in sputum, particularly from patients with poor oral hygiene and must be recognized as contaminants.

Material of Plant Origin

Vegetable matter is one of the most common contaminants in sputum specimens. **The cells comprising fragments of plant tissue** have a characteristic **heavy cellulose cell wall** and are easily identified (Fig. 19-17A), but isolated plant cells that have lost the cellulose wall (Fig. 19-17B,C) may be confused with cancer because of their large dark nuclei. They are readily recognized after some experience, even in the absence of a heavy cellulose membrane, because of the

homogeneous staining of plant cell nuclei and the frequent presence of **refractile, pigment granules within the cytoplasm.** Weaver et al (1981) have provided a detailed study of plant cells in sputum.

Meat Fibers

Meat fibers composed of striated muscle are easily recognized by the presence of cytoplasmic cross-striations and peripherally placed nuclei. Smooth muscle cells are less commonly seen. They are elongated spindle cells with centrally placed ovoid nuclei and are without striations. Neither muscle cells, fat cells, cartilage cells, nor the occasional cells of epithelial origin that are found in undigested food have cellulose cell membranes.

Pollen

Sputum may contain pollen of plant origin, recognized as **spherical** or **oval, dark yellow or brown** structures of variable sizes, rarely smaller than 25 to 30 μm in diameter and provided with a characteristic thick, refractile cell wall (Fig. 19-17D). They are more commonly found in the spring and summer, and particularly if the processing laboratory is exposed to outside air (see Chap. 8).

Other Contaminants

The brown, septate, boat-shaped fungal organisms of **Alternaria species** (Fig. 19-18A) are present in earth and water and are a frequent contaminant. Radio et al (1987) pointed out that *Alternaria* has been found in bronchioalveolar lavage material and may rarely be a pathogen.

Small **nematodes** (Fig. 19-18B,C), also from tap water, may be found in sputum as in other cytologic specimens. They must be differentiated from **Strongyloides stercoralis** (see below). Usually, it is clear from the clinical setting that they are contaminants, but if there is doubt, repeat specimens should be obtained with care to prevent contamination.

Copepods, another contaminant of tap water (Fig.19-

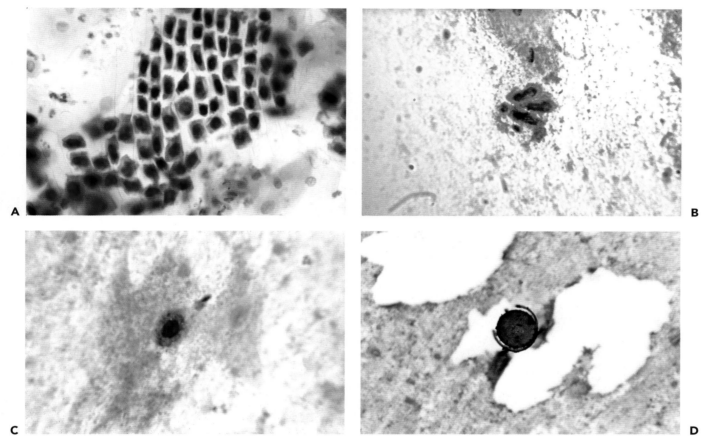

Figure 19-17   Vegetable (plant) cells. *A.* Plant cells in flat fragments with thick transparent cellulose walls. The **cellulose walls,** which do not stain with either Papanicolaou or hematoxylin/eosin stains specifically identify vegetable cells. *B,C.* Poorly preserved single vegetable cells may have lost their cellulose cell wall but are still identified by homogeneous staining nuclei and often by **pigmented granules in the cytoplasm.** *D.* **Pollen,** a common air contaminant. Their structure is variable depending on the flower or plant from which they come, but they are usually easily recognized.

18D), have been reported to cause disease on rare occasions (Van Horn et al, 1992).

Abundant bacterial or fungal growth in a poorly preserved specimen with minimal or no inflammatory infiltrate suggests that the specimen was left standing for many hours at room temperature without fixative, and the organisms present must be disregarded.

BENIGN CELLULAR ABNORMALITIES OF THE RESPIRATORY TRACT

Various noncancerous processes within the respiratory tract may affect the cytologic makeup of smears. **Many such disorders have common cytologic findings** and cannot be diagnosed with confidence on cytology grounds alone. **Knowledge of the roentgenologic and clinical findings is always desirable and often essential for specific classification of a pathologic process.** In cases of inflammation, bacteriologic studies are needed, as is a careful search for viral cytopathic changes and the presence of fungi or parasites. Even without specific classification, however, knowledge of the degenerative and reactive cytologic changes that

accompany inflammatory and other benign pathologic processes is essential if one is to avoid a false diagnosis of cancer.

Benign disorders of the respiratory epithelium may be manifested by abnormalities of:

- Respiratory bronchial epithelium
- Squamous epithelium
- Alveolar epithelium, particularly pneumocytes type II
- Pulmonary macrophages

Benign Abnormalities of Bronchial Epithelium

Abnormalities of Ciliated Cells
Cytologic techniques have been applied extensively to studies of the respiratory epithelium in various clinical settings. The information derived therefrom carries with it major diagnostic implications.

Acute Injury
The **loss of cilia and terminal plate** is a common response of the respiratory epithelium to acute injury. It was demonstrated experimentally in bovine lung exposed to cigarette smoke and viral infection (Sisson et al, 1994), and may be observed in thermally injured patients who have inhaled

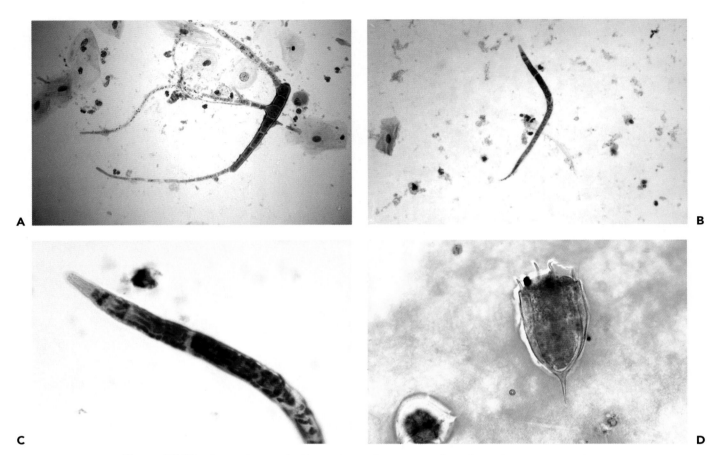

Figure 19-18 **Contaminants.** *A.* ***Alternaria* species,** a contaminant from air or tap water, is a genus of fungi and readily recognized by its shape and pigmented, segmented structure. *B,C.* **Nematodes,** also present in tap water, may be a contaminant and mistaken for pathogenic microfilaria. Compare with Figure 19-52B. Usually, it is clear from the clinical setting, that they are a contaminant. *D.* **Copepod,** a contaminant of tap water, rarely reported to cause infection. (*D:* High magnification; *C:* oil immersion.)

hot gases (Ambiavagar et al, 1974). In burn victims with great exposure to hot gases and smoke, there is extensive necrosis of respiratory epithelium followed by squamous metaplasia (see below), and severe degenerative changes including mitochondrial calcium deposits in surviving bronchial cells (Drut, 1998).

Chalon et al (1974) reported that in patients under anesthesia, after 3 hours inhalation of dry anesthetic gases, 40% of the respiratory epithelial cells showed loss of cilia, changes in cell configuration and staining, and some nuclear pyknosis. Such damage was preventable by humidification.

Nonspecific Abnormalities of Bronchial Cells

Multinucleation of Bronchial Cells

Multinucleation of bronchial lining cells may result from a failure of cell division after nuclear replication and division, and involve **single well-differentiated ciliated cells** (Fig. 19-19A); or it may be the result of cell fusion with formation of **true syncytia** (Fig. 19-19B). The number of nuclei in single cells may vary from 2 or 3 to about 20, whereas in syncytia, the number varies from few to over 100. The **nuclei** within the multinucleated cells are **small, regular, and equal in size.** Since it is known that certain viruses may

produce cell fusion, and thereby true syncytia, the **possibility of a viral infection** should be considered when syncytial multinucleation is observed. **However, in most cases, multinucleated bronchial cells are a nonspecific reaction to injury.** They have been observed within 48 to 72 hours after a variety of traumas, including bronchoscopy, x-ray therapy, and exposure to fumes. They should not be confused with tumor cells, with which they have no common traits.

Cell and Nuclear Enlargement

Occasional individual ciliated bronchial cells may be considerably larger than others **(cytomegaly),** sometimes **twice or more their normal size,** with **proportionally enlarged nucleus (karyomegaly), usually containing a single prominent nucleolus or multiple small nucleoli** (Fig. 19-19C). Here again, the cilia, or at least the terminal plates, are often well preserved. Such cells appear under a variety of circumstances, and like multinucleation and nucleolar enlargement (see below), they are a nonspecific response of the respiratory epithelium to various forms of injury. They may be observed after even **minor trauma** such as repeated bronchoscopies or **bouts of severe coughing,** and also **in inflammatory processes** such as **bronchitis, bacterial or viral pneumonia, or tuberculosis,** but also in cancer.

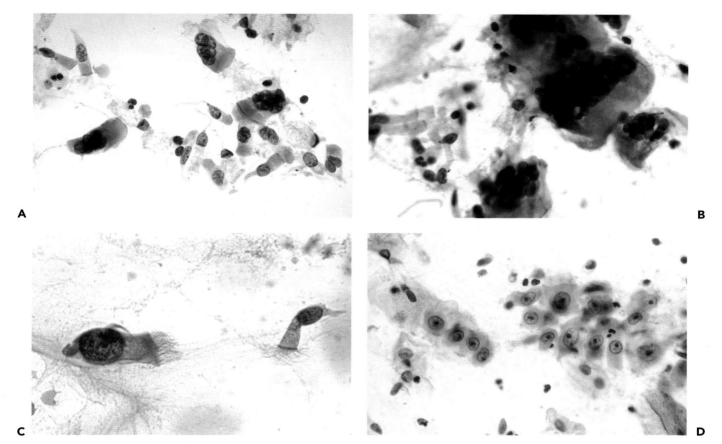

Figure 19-19   Nonspecific bronchial cell atypias. *A.* Multinucleation. *B.* Syncytia. *C.* Cytomegaly and karyomegaly. *D.* Nucleolar prominence in otherwise bland and uniform bronchial cells. The cells are cuboidal, with smoothly contoured round or oval nuclei and delicate chromatin. They are separate or in flat plaques, unlike the cells of adenocarcinoma, which cluster in groups of overlapping cells. (*C:* oil immersion.)

Cohen et al (1997) reported a 9-year-old boy with Ataxia-Telangiectasia (AT) who had aneuploid karyomegaly of bronchial cells obtained by bronchial brushings. They suggested that the finding of aneuploidy might be related to the known increased risk of cancer in this genetic disease. However, the child had had recurrent respiratory infections and was suffering from severe chronic obstructive lung disease; it is not clear whether the karyomegaly was due to the genetic defect of AT or simply reactive to injury and infection.

Nucleolar Enlargement

Under a broad variety of circumstances, **benign bronchial cells may display prominent single or multiple nucleoli.** The affected cells are either **normal** in size and shape or the cells are **more cuboidal and slightly enlarged.** Those that **retain their cilia or at least their terminal bar should not be mistaken for cells of adenocarcinoma** (see Chap. 20). Others having lost cilia and terminal bar are undergoing squamous metaplasia or repair (see below).

Ciliocytophthoria

Under this term, Papanicolaou (1956) reported a unique type of destruction of ciliated bronchial cells occurring in some inflammatory conditions of the lung, especially viral pneumonia. The distal ciliated portion of the cells is pinched off, resulting in the formation of **anucleated ciliated tufts** and **nucleated cytoplasmic remnants** (Fig. 19-20A,B). **Nuclear degeneration,** resembling apoptosis, and the presence of **cytoplasmic eosinophilic inclusions** of various sizes (Fig. 19-20C) complete the picture. Papanicolaou initially associated **ciliocytophthoria** (CCP) with bronchogenic carcinoma; he reported one case in which CCP preceded the appearance of tumor cells by 10 months. However, evidence has now shown that CCP is not a precancerous event, but a form of cellular degeneration often associated with viral infections and possibly due to adenovirus or other viral pneumonitis (see below).

Lipochrome Pigmentation

With aging, there is an accumulation of lipochrome pigment in bronchial epithelial cells, the so-called "wear and tear" pigment (see Fig. 19-9B). As already described it has no diagnostic significance. The pigment is brown, faintly granular and accumulates first in the supranuclear cytoplasm of intact, otherwise normal bronchial cells.

Immobile Cilia Syndrome

Abnormal cilia are common in bronchial epithelial cells of cigarette smokers and in patients with neoplastic and a number of chronic nonneoplastic diseases of lung (McDow-

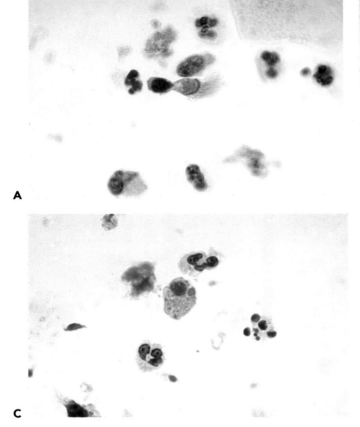

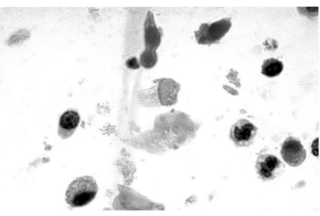

Figure 19-20   Ciliocytophthoria (CCP). Sputum specimen from a young woman on the second day of her illness with a viral pneumonia. *A.* The ciliated cytoplasmic end of a bronchial cell with pyknotic nucleus is pinched off. *B.* In the same specimen, there were detached anuclear ciliated cytoplasmic tufts and cell fragments with pyknotic nuclei. *C.* Degenerating cell with eosinophilic intracytoplasmic inclusion. (*A–C:* High magnification.)

ell et al, 1976a). However, the **immobile cilia syndrome** is a rare congenital **abnormality of cilia** caused by absence of dynein arms or defective radial spokes resulting in chaotic, uncoordinated beating of cilia. Young children with this disease suffer illnesses resulting from a **deficiency of mucociliary transport** (Afzelius, 1976, 1981). They typically present with recurrent respiratory infections and sinusitis. The classic form of this syndrome, described by Kartagener in 1933, and now known as the **Kartagener syndrome,** comprises **bronchiectasia, chronic sinusitis, and situs inversus.** Because spermatozoan flagella are also affected, sterility in males has been noted. The disorder can be diagnosed only by electron microscopy (see Chap. 2). Transposition of ciliary microtubules is another cause of impaired motility of cilia (Sturgess et al, 1980). Moreau et al (1985) reported that **cytologic samples from bronchial and nasal brushings** may be suitable for electron microscopic examination to determine if the ciliary structure is deformed; however, it should be noted that in some cases, ciliary abnormalities in respiratory epithelium may be a result rather than a cause of chronic or repeated respiratory infections.

Abnormalities of Goblet Cells

In chronic inflammatory processes, as for example in chronic bronchitis, bronchiectasis, and asthma, there may be hyperplasia of goblet cells in bronchial mucosa and increased mucus secretion. Sputum, bronchial aspirates, and washings from such patients contain an **increased number of goblet cells,** some of which may be significantly **larger than normal.** This finding has no other known significance.

Benign Proliferative Processes in Respiratory Epithelium

Benign proliferations of the respiratory epithelium may occur as a reaction to injury, usually an inflammatory process, and cause **papillary hyperplasia, basal (reserve) cell hyperplasia or squamous metaplasia of bronchial mucosa.** These processes can have a major impact on the cytology of the respiratory tract.

Papillary Hyperplasia of the Respiratory Epithelium (Creola Bodies)

Histology
Hyperplastic respiratory epithelium is most commonly observed in chronically inflamed, dilated bronchi, that is, **bronchiectasis,** but may be seen in other **chronic pulmonary disorders, in bronchial asthma, and in viral pneumonitis.** The mucosa **undergoes folding and formation of papillary projections** (Fig. 19-21A). The **epithelial surface** of these hyperplastic areas is composed of **normal ciliated and goblet cells,** with deeper layers of smaller intermediate or basal epithelial cells. The individual epithelial cells may have visible nucleoli but are generally uniform, coherent, and do not show the nuclear hyperchromasia,

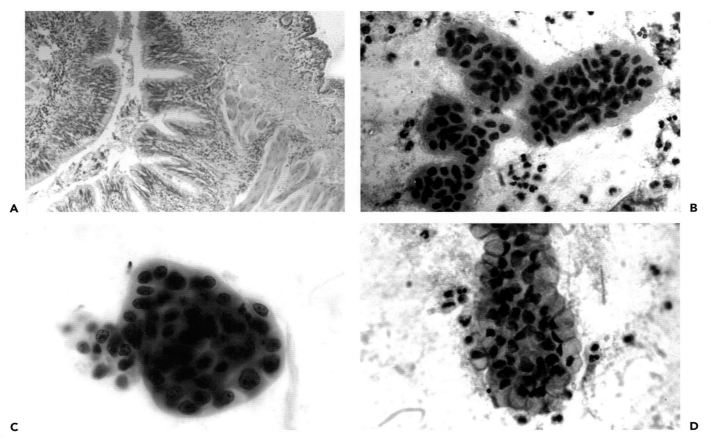

Figure 19-21   Creola bodies. *A.* Hyperplastic bronchial mucosa in bronchiectasis, a source of apillary fragments of bronchial epithelium in pulmonary cytology specimens. *B,C.* Fragments of hyperplastic reactive bronchial epithelium (Creola bodies) that in *C* are from a 28-year-old patient with AIDS who has had chronic lung infections. The most peripheral cells have a smooth surface configuration and are recognizable as bronchial cells; deeper in the cluster are intermediate or basal cells. *D.* Creola body surfaced by mucin-secreting cells. Creola bodies should not be mistaken for papillary carcinoma.

coarse chromatin, or very prominent nucleoli of adenocarcinoma (see Chap. 20).

Cytology

The hyperplastic bronchial mucosa sheds **spherical** or **ovoid papillary clusters of bronchial cells.** As in histologic sections, the **surface** is **formed of well-preserved respiratory epithelial cells with cilia or terminal plates,** whereas the core of these clusters is composed of uniform small cells (Fig. 19-21B,C). Cilia are not always well preserved. When the hyperplastic mucosa is rich in **goblet cells,** they will be displayed in the surface layers of the exfoliated clusters (Fig. 19-21D). Of some importance is the occasional presence of **tiny, usually single nucleoli** within the nuclei of cells lining the papillae. They should not be mistaken for the much larger nucleoli of adenocarcinoma (see Chap. 20). These cell clusters were first described as a possible diagnostic pitfall by Koss and Richardson in 1955. They were subsequently called **Creola bodies** by Naylor (1962), who named them for a patient with asthma who produced sputum specimens with numerous such clusters. Naylor warned against misinterpreting these papillary cell clusters as papillary adenocarcinoma. He and Railey (1964) identified the papillar-

yclusters in sputa of 42% of asthmatic patients, frequently present during the asthmatic attack. Folded fragments of mucosa dislodged by endoscopic procedures may be mistaken for Creola bodies.

A large number of such papillary clusters may be observed in cytologic specimens from adults with acute respiratory disorders of viral etiology, or from infants and children with viral pneumonitis or acute respiratory distress syndrome (ARDS) (see also Fig. 19-32). In those patients, there is usually a prompt return to normal after the acute illness has subsided. Sheets of bronchial cells originating in hyperplastic bronchial epithelium have been reported in **Wegener's granulomatosis** (Hector, 1976).

Of prime importance in differentiating these papillary clusters of cells from the somewhat similar cell clusters that may be observed in well-differentiated bronchioloalveolar adenocarcinoma are:

- The presence of cilia or a terminal plate on the free surface of the outermost cells
- The presence of normal goblet cells on the free surface of the cluster, indicating benign disease

■ Nuclei of normal size and configuration, whereas in adenocarcinomas they are larger and are provided with large nucleoli

Further points of differential diagnosis are discussed in Chapter 20.

Basal Cell Hyperplasia
Histology
The small basal or germinative cells situated next to the basement membrane in the respiratory epithelium are normally unobtrusive and may escape the attention of a casual observer (see the section on the Respiratory Epithelium above). Basal (or reserve cell) hyperplasia is the result of **abnormal multiplication of these basal cells,** which can form **many layers occupying a substantial portion of the thickened epithelium.** Usually, the surface of the altered epithelium is topped with a layer of ciliated respiratory epithelium and goblet cells, confirming that the process of epithelial maturation is preserved (Fig. 19-22A). Because

the basal cells are small and their nuclei occupy much of the total cell volume, the **epithelium may have a disturbing hyperchromatic appearance. Unlike small-cell carcinoma, however, the benign hyperplastic basal epithelium is composed of uniform cells in an orderly arrangement.** The problem of recognition occurs only if the maturing surface of the epithelium is lost.

Basal cell hyperplasia is a nonspecific response of the respiratory epithelium, usually induced by chronic inflammatory processes. Affected bronchi may be found in **chronic bronchitis** and **bronchiectases,** especially with **bronchiectatic cavities,** in **tuberculosis** and in other forms of chronic inflammation including **organizing pneumonia** and **mycotic infections,** particularly with mycetomas. However, such changes may also occur in bronchi adjacent to bronchogenic carcinoma.

Cytology
Normally, the basal cells are firmly adherent to the basement membrane and therefore exceedingly uncommon in spu-

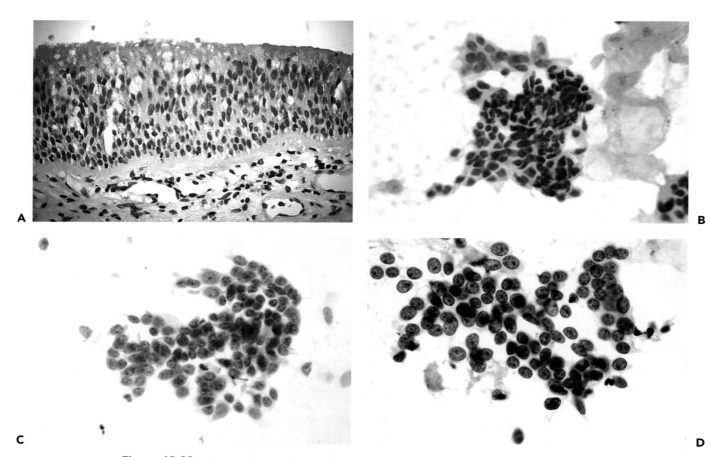

Figure 19-22   **Basal cell hyperplasia of bronchial epithelium.** *A.* Histologic section of bronchial mucosa showing basal cell (reserve cell) hyperplasia. Note that there are several layers of basal epithelium. *B,C.* Basal cell hyperplasia in bronchial brush specimens. The cells are small and generally uniform with scanty cytoplasm and relatively large hyperchromatic nuclei. They differ from small cell carcinoma in that the cells are coherent and nuclei are uniform and smoothly contoured without necrosis or molding, and without evidence of active proliferation. Often, there is either a straight edge to the cluster of cells, or some cells show evidence of maturation (see Chap. 20). *D.* Basal cells are best visualized when present in loose clusters of cells. At high magnification, they have scanty cytoplasm and uniform, smoothly contoured nuclei with dark staining but finely textured chromatin and a small nucleolus. They must be differentiated from large-cell lymphoma and SSC, discussed in Chapter 20. (*C,D:* oil immersion.)

tum. They are more commonly seen in specimens obtained by instrumentation in which there is forceful disruption of the epithelium, and they usually form coherent clusters of various sizes made up of small rounded or polygonal cells (Fig. 19-22B–D). Several such clusters of cells are often present in the same specimen, and sometimes in the company of ciliated cells that are also dislodged in the course of bronchial intubation or other manipulations. The latter may have been damaged in the process or destroyed by disease and atypical in appearance.

These **clusters of small basal cells with dark nuclei and scanty cytoplasm** are always disquieting, even to an experienced observer, as they **may suggest a small-cell malignant tumor.** Their interpretation becomes particularly difficult when the pathologist is pressured to make a diagnosis in cases suspected of carcinoma clinically or radiologically. Following are the characteristics of bronchial basal cells that allow their correct classification and diagnosis:

- The cells, as a rule, appear in **clusters that are tightly packed** and show little if any tendency to dissociate (see Fig. 19-22B). One edge of the cluster may be straight, presumably where detached from the basement membrane.
- The **cells are small,** somewhat larger than leukocytes, with relatively prominent but quite **uniform dark, round, or oval nuclei.** Nucleoli may be observed, but are tiny and inconspicuous (Fig. 19-22D). Cytoplasm is scanty and basophilic. At the periphery of at least some of the clusters, one usually finds larger cells with very similar nuclei but more cytoplasm, suggesting differentiation toward columnar or metaplastic squamous cells.
- Nuclear molding by adjacent cells, characteristic of small-cell (oat cell) carcinoma does not occur in the clusters of benign reserve cells. Other nuclear abnormalities observed in small-cell malignant tumors are absent (see Chap. 20).

The problem of diagnosis is compounded if the **clusters of small basal cells are loosely structured,** rather than compact, and may include cells with somewhat larger nuclei. (Fig. 19-22C–D). **Such instances of basal cell hyperplasia may be very difficult to differentiate from small-cell carcinoma,** and have been seen in association with carcinoma elsewhere in the bronchi. For other points of differential diagnosis, which includes carcinoid and malignant lymphoma, see Chapter 20.

Squamous Metaplasia

Squamous metaplasia is a common reaction to injury in the bronchus and is defined as the **replacement of respiratory mucosa by squamous epithelium.** It can be limited in extent or diffuse and implies the capability of germinative basal cells to form squamous epithelium under abnormal circumstances. Both basal cell hyperplasia and squamous metaplasia result from chronic irritation of the respiratory tract and may be considered a means of defense or adaptation of the mucosa to abnormal circumstances. Whether squamous metaplasia may or may not revert to normal ciliated epithelium is not known; possibly the process is revers-

ible in its early stages, but cytologic studies suggest that well-developed squamous metaplasia persists relatively unchanged for many years (Grunze, 1958).

The **mechanism of formation** of squamous metaplasia of the bronchus is uncertain. While it may fairly rapidly follow massive damage or loss of respiratory epithelium, for example, in bronchopulmonary dysplasia of newborns (see below), in most cases, it appears to be a more gradual process of progressive squamous differentiation.

Some histologic studies have implicated squamous metaplasia as **a step in the development of squamous lung cancer.** There is increased frequency of squamous metaplasia in cigarette smokers and with advancing age, paralleling an increased risk of lung cancer. Some observers also report increased atypia of squamous metaplasia in cigarette smokers with increasing number of cigarettes smoked (Kierszenbaum, 1965; Nasiell, 1966; Saccomanno et al, 1970). However, the relationship of squamous metaplasia to squamous lung cancer has been brought into question by the frequent finding of squamous metaplasia without lung cancer (see below), and by our own studies of cigarette smokers in whom orderly squamous metaplasia is found in mainstem and lobar bronchi, whereas early lung cancer most often begins more distally in segmental bronchi. In the very early lung cancers that we have studied, squamous carcinoma in situ of the bronchus has not necessarily been associated or in continuity with squamous metaplasia. On the other hand, *atypical* squamous metaplasia is a potential precursor of **bronchogenic squamous carcinoma** (see Chap. 20).

Squamous metaplasia is a common finding in patients free of cancer. For example, Spain et al (1970) found squamous metaplasia in the bronchial tree of 50% of 500 healthy adults of all ages who died accidentally. Cytologic evidence of metaplasia was reported by Plamenac et al in wind instrument players (1969), commonly in men past the age of 65 (1970), and in former cigarette smokers (1972). Good et al (1975) reported atypical metaplastic changes in the sputum of users of pressurized spray cans. These cytologic reports, not supported by histologic evidence, should be considered with some caution. **Histologically documented squamous metaplasia has been observed in a broad spectrum of benign inflammatory lung disorders,** including chronic bronchitis, bronchiectasis, lung abscesses, and granulomatous inflammations. Squamous metaplasia may also occur in areas of pulmonary infarcts and after radio- and chemotherapy. Therefore, **squamous metaplasia of the bronchial epithelium without atypia must not be regarded as a precancerous lesion.**

Squamous metaplasia has never been implicated in the development of bronchiolar or adenocarcinoma of the lung, or of small-cell (oat cell) carcinoma, both of which are also attributable to cigarette smoking.

Histology

As noted, squamous metaplasia is seen in mainstem and lobar bronchi. In the earliest evidence of squamous metaplasia, the respiratory columnar epithelium is replaced by a superficial layer of flattened cells in association with basal cell hyperplasia. This may involve only limited areas of bronchus, usually at bifurcation sites, or progress to extensive complete replacement of respiratory epithelium by nonkeratinizing squamous epithelium (Fig. 19-23A). Very often, the squamous epithelium lining the surface of the bronchus is not "pure" but includes scattered respiratory cells, or metaplastic squamous cells with intracellular mucin. Other cells that are only partially differentiated may retain their cuboidal or columnar shape and a flat free surface, but lack cilia and a terminal bar. These features of the metaplastic epithelium are important indications of their common origin with respiratory epithelium from undifferentiated reserve cells.

The frequent coexistence of basal cell hyperplasia with squamous metaplasia suggests that the former precedes the latter, but whether this is always the case is open to conjecture. The two processes can be seen side by side in cytologic material.

Cytology

Cells in **sputum** that originate from orderly squamous metaplasia of the bronchus may be difficult or impossible to differentiate from the normal squamous cells of the mouth, pharynx, or larynx. In **bronchial washings, aspirates, and brush specimens,** however, the presence of squamous cells can be explained only by squamous metaplasia (excluding the common occurrence of contamination from the upper respiratory tract). Squamous metaplasia is typically represented by **small squamous cells, often in clusters or sheets of cells with eosinophilic cytoplasm, resembling the parabasal cells of squamous epithelium or showing partial differentiation to respiratory epithelium.** The metaplastic cells **usually adhere well to each other and may have nuclei that are vesicular and open** (Fig. 19-23B,C) or hyperchromatic (Fig. 19-23D). As in histologic sections, the bronchial origin of metaplastic squamous epithelium is best demonstrated when the periphery of the cluster is composed of cuboidal or columnar cells with a straight edge or terminal plate (Fig. 19-23B). The cytologic features of squamous metaplasia of bronchial epithelium are not unlike squamous metaplasia of endocervical epithelium (see Chap. 10), in which the relatively small cuboidal cells have an angular configuration and hyperchromatic nuclei (Fig, 19-23D). Significant cytologic abnormalities resulting from squamous metaplasia of the trachea following intubation or laryngectomy are discussed below.

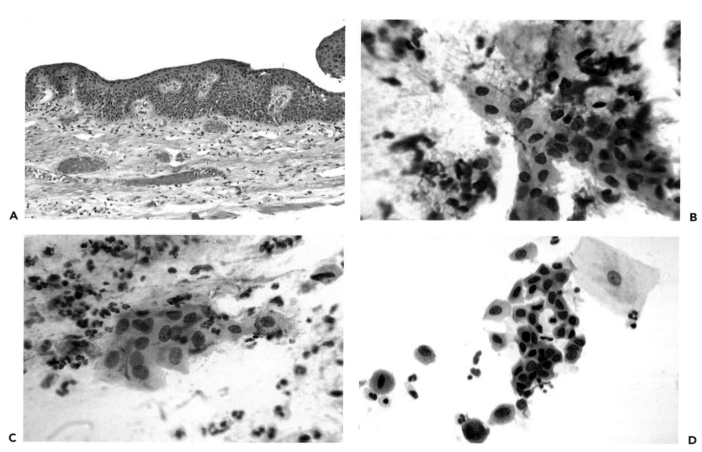

Figure 19-23 **Squamous metaplasia of bronchial epithelium.** *A.* Histologic section of bronchus showing squamous epithelium completely replacing the respiratory epithelium in an example of fully developed mature squamous metaplasia. *B,C.* Squamous metaplasia in a cough specimen of sputum. The cells are cuboidal, with moderately abundant eosinophilic or amphophilic cytoplasm. They form loosely coherent flat plaques, much like endocervical squamous metaplasia with usually one straight edge. *D.* Bronchial brush specimen showing squamous metaplasia. The cells form a loosely coherent flat plaque of cuboidal, relatively small cells with amphophilic or eosinophilic cytoplasm. Alveolar macrophages and a mature squamous cell are present for comparison.

Tracheitis Sicca

Squamous metaplasia is part of the repair process after injury to bronchopulmonary tissues, and in some circumstances, there may be significant atypia. Particularly severe atypias of squamous cells have been described in the trachea and tracheobronchial aspirates of patients with prolonged tracheal intubation and patients with **tracheitis sicca** (dry tracheitis) who have permanent tracheostomies following laryngectomy for carcinoma. They are at high risk of developing a new primary carcinoma of lung, and we have recommended monitoring them at regular intervals by tracheal aspiration cytology (see Chap. 20). The dry and constantly irritated mucosa of the upper trachea undergoes squamous metaplasia, sometimes with keratinization and marked nuclear atypia of superficial cells (Fig. 19-24A). **The desquamated squamous epithelial cells are of variable, abnormal shapes with abundant deeply eosinophilic cytoplasm and enlarged, hyperchromatic nuclei, usually accompanied by keratinized squamous cells with pyknotic or karyorrhectic nuclei.** The presence of these latter cells in a tracheobronchial specimen postlaryngectomy indicates cautious interpretation. Even so, cytologic abnormalities as have been extensively studied and described by Nunez et al (1966) may be indistinguishable from squamous carcinoma (Fig. 19-24B,C) and can lead to an erroneous diagnosis. It is essential to have the history of tracheostomy and to be aware that the epithelial abnormality is in the trachea, whereas squamous lung cancer arises more distally in lobar or segmental bronchi. If in doubt, additional specimens should be obtained from lobar bronchi, which will yield only benign bronchial epithelium in patients with tracheitis sicca.

"Repair"

In 1988, Rosenthal introduced the term *repair* to describe cytologic abnormalities in the bronchial tree that were reminiscent of those occurring in the uterine cervix (see Chap. 10). The principal feature of these abnormalities is the presence of prominent nucleoli in otherwise unremarkable bronchial epithelial cells (see Fig. 19-19D). To our knowledge, there is no diagnostic significance to this finding, so long as the bronchial epithelial cells retain intact structure. Enlarged nucleoli may also occur in metaplastic cells of **patients who have had prolonged tracheal intubation.** Such cells, usually observed in tracheal aspirates, have been described and illustrated in Chapter 21.

Prominent nucleoli may also be observed in bronchial cells from patients with **respiratory distress syndrome,** including infants receiving oxygen therapy (discussed in the closing pages of this chapter), in burn patients (Cooney et al, 1972), and after radiotherapy (see below). Pneumocytes type II with prominent nucleoli are also seen in atypical pneumonias (see discussion below and Figs. 19-27 and 19-28).

Benign Abnormalities of the Squamous Epithelium

Inflammatory Changes

Inflammatory changes within the **squamous mucosa of the upper respiratory tract** are of some importance in cytologic

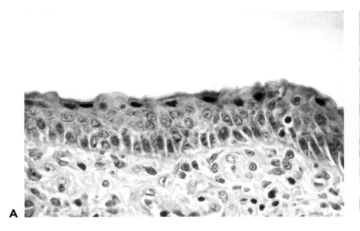

A

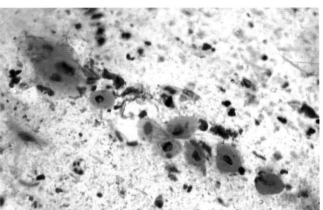

B

C

Figure 19-24 Tracheitis sicca. *A.* There is marked nuclear hyperchromasia in superficial cells of the dry, metaplastic tracheal epithelium. *B,C.* Tracheal aspirate cytology smear and cell block section from another patient with postlaryngectomy tracheitis sicca showing metaplastic squamous cells mimicking squamous carcinoma. (*B:* High magnification.)

interpretation since they can produce cellular abnormalities that may be confused with squamous cancer. In acute inflammatory processes involving the oral or oropharyngeal mucosa, there may be **necrosis of squamous cells,** manifested by nuclear pyknosis and apoptosis (karyorrhexis) with frayed cytoplasm. If there is **ulceration or erosions,** numerous **small squamous cells** originating from the deeper layers of the squamous epithelium make their appearance singly or in clusters (see Fig. 19-7B). The **nuclei** of such cells often have **coarse chromatin** and a **heavy nuclear membrane.** Any confusion with squamous cancer should be readily ruled out by the uniform appearance of these cells, their smooth nuclear configuration, and presentation in coherent cell clusters. These changes are also discussed in Chapter 21. Significant abnormalities of squamous cells may occur as a consequence of **radiotherapy** (see below).

"Pap" Cells

In sputum of patients with an **upper respiratory tract infection and laryngitis,** especially during cold weather, **small squamous cells with dark, round or oval, single nuclei** may be seen. (Fig.19-25A). They have been named **Pap cells.** Dr. Papanicolaou is alleged to have observed these cells in his own sputum, examined because of a cough, and was concerned about their appearance. Indeed, superficial observation may give rise to some concern because of the nuclear hyperchromasia. However, the small size and regular nuclear outline of these generally uniform squamous cells should readily identify them. Histologic section of inflamed laryngeal mucosa in at least some cases demonstrates reactive epithelium that appears to be the source of these cells (Fig. 19-25B). "Pap cells" are not a specific indicator of laryngitis and are probably derived from other sites of regenerative epithelium in the respiratory tract as well.

Abnormalities of Alveolar Lining Cells

Bronchial "Metaplasia" of Alveolar Epithelium

In a variety of chronic fibrosing and obstructive processes, **the pulmonary alveoli are lined by one or more layers**

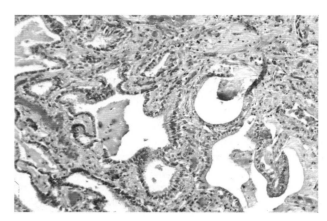

Figure 19-26   Bronchial metaplasia of alveoli. Histologic section of "honeycomb lung" in which alveolar epithelium is replaced by cuboidal or columnar bronchial epithelium.

of small cuboidal or columnar epithelial cells that are in continuity with and identical or similar to the adjoining bronchioles (Fig. 19-26). This process is observed in **chronic pneumonias of varying etiology,** in **pulmonary fibrosis,** in **areas adjacent to scars** or old infarcts, and in some disorders associated with cystic degeneration of the lungs, the **so-called honeycomb lung** (Meyer and Liebow, 1965). It is generally accepted that in most cases this is not true metaplasia of alveolar epithelium, but results from an extension of the distal bronchial epithelium.

Cytology

It may be possible to recognize bronchial metaplasia of air spaces in honeycomb lung by the presence of cuboidal or columnar epithelial cells accompanying the alveolar macrophages in a carefully performed BAL specimen. Such a specimen ordinarily contains few or no bronchial epithelial cells, and their presence would suggest alveolar bronchial metaplasia.

Abnormalities of Pneumocytes Type II

Pneumocytes type II are **highly reactive cells that respond to various pathologic processes by morphologic changes**

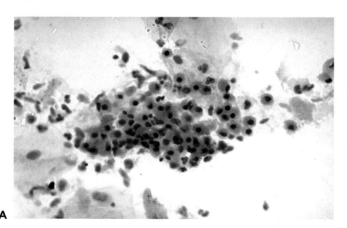

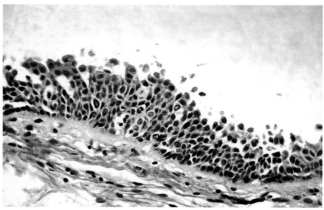

Figure 19-25   Pap cells. A. Small squamous cells found in sputum of some patients with laryngitis, thought to be shed from regenerating epithelium of the larynx. B. Histologic section of larynx showing hyperplasia of immature regenerating laryngeal epithelium in a patient with prolonged severe laryngitis.

that may perfectly mimic adenocarcinoma or its precursor lesions in cytologic samples.

Histology

In a great variety of pathologic conditions, the **pulmonary alveoli are lined by or contain large and prominent alveolar epithelial cells** (Fig. 19-27A). These cells are **pneumocytes type II, as evidenced by positive immunoreaction with antisurfactant antibody** (Fig. 19-27B), **positive cytokeratin expression, and by electron microscopy** (see Fig. 19-4C,D). The **cells are large, cuboidal or rounded, with large, vesicular or hyperchromatic nuclei and readily visible, often prominent nucleoli.** While this is a benign reactive process, it may closely mimic atypical alveolar hyperplasia, a putative precursor of adenocarcinoma (Nakayama et al, 1990) (see Chap. 20). The spectrum of pulmonary diseases with reactive hyperplasia of pneumocytes type II is vast and includes **viral pneumonitis, chronic pneumonias, pulmonary fibrosis of various etiologies, fibrosing alveolitis, infarcts, and effects of radio- and chemotherapy.** Pneumocytes type II may form small tumor nodules in **tuberous sclerosis** (Myers, 1999).

Cytology

In past studies of cytologic material from the respiratory tract, reactive hyperplastic pneumocytes were usually identified descriptively as atypical or abnormal "bronchoalveolar cells." Their identity as pneumocytes type II is relatively recent (Grotte, 1990). Although their benign nature is usually evident in histologic sections, when seen **in cytologic preparations, atypical pneumocytes type II are a potentially important source of false-positive diagnoses of adenocarcinoma** (Nakanishi, 1990; Nakayama et al, 1990; Kerr et al, 1994; Kitamura et al, 1999). They may be seen in sputum, bronchial aspirates, BAL or FNA specimens from patients with persisting pneumonic infiltrates. These pneumocytes appear singly, in flat plaques, or in rosette-like

groups of epithelial cells about the size of parabasal cells (Fig. 19-28A–C). They have finely textured cyanophilic cytoplasm and frequently fine or sometimes large cytoplasmic vacuoles (Fig. 19-28D). **Nuclei are large and may be smoothly configured with finely textured chromatin, or irregular with moderately coarse chromatin and single or multiple nucleoli.** In some cases, it may be difficult or impossible to differentiate from atypical alveolar hyperplasia or even adenocarcinoma.

The cells illustrated in Figure 19-28D were transiently present in the sputum of a patient following pulmonary infarction and raised suspicion of adenocarcinoma, but were ultimately interpreted as atypical type II pneumocytes. Scoggins et al (1977) described three patients with pulmonary infarction and false cytologic diagnoses of adenocarcinoma. Bewtra et al (1983) reported nine cases in which the most severe cytologic abnormalities were in the second and third week postinfarction. Johnston (1992) also stressed the misleading nature of cytologic atypias associated with pulmonary infarct. We have observed similar, marked cytologic abnormalities associated with pulmonary infarct, but their transient nature is an important diagnostic clue.

Viral pneumonias are another, more common source of reactive, hyperplastic pneumocytes. Figure 19-29A–C demonstrates cells observed in the sputum of a 60-year-old woman with a febrile illness diagnosed as viral pneumonia. Lung biopsies carried out because of suspected adenocarcinoma demonstrated interstitial fibrosis of usual interstitial pneumonia with obsolete alveoli lined by large cuboidal cells with large nuclei and nucleoli. Immunostaining by Dr. Allen Gown confirmed that alveolar lining cells bound pancytokeratin and surfactant (AT10) antibodies, confirming their identity as pneumocytes type II (Fig. 19-29D; see also Figs. 19-4C, 19-27B). The cells disappeared from her sputum 2 weeks later, and the patient has remained well for 10 years following this episode.

In a study of BAL cytology specimens from a series of 38 patients with **acute respiratory distress syndrome,**

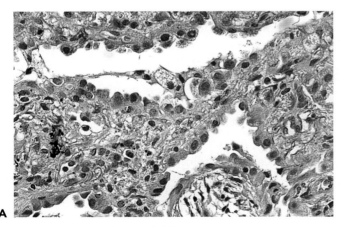
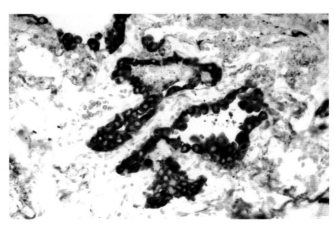

Figure 19-27 **Hyperplasia of pneumocytes, type II.** *A.* Histologic section of lung showing thickened alveolar septa surfaced by hyperplastic alveolar epithelium in a case of interstitial pneumonia. The cells are clearly different from bronchial epithelium and consistent with hyperplasia of type II pneumocytes. *B.* Same specimen of lung as in (*A*) above. The hyperplastic alveolar epithelial cells react with an antibody to surfactant in an immunoperoxidase reaction, confirming their identity as pneumocytes type II. (*B,* courtesy of Dr. Allen Gown, Seattle, Washington.)

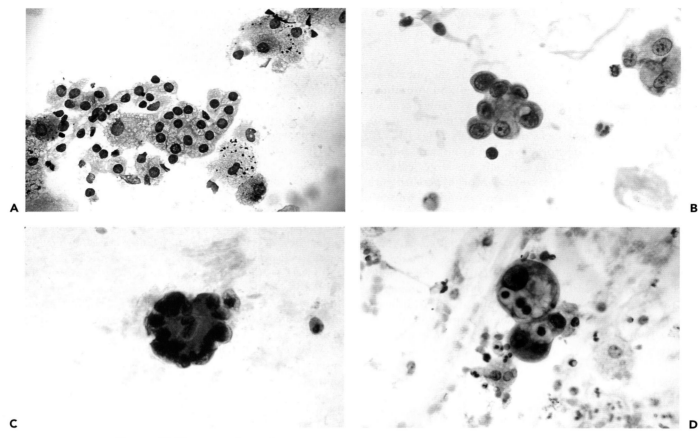

Figure 19-28 **Hyperplasia of pneumocytes type II.** *A.* FNA cytology specimen from the case illustrated in Figure 19-27. Flat plaques of cuboidal and rounded type II alveolar pneumocytes are seen among larger pulmonary macrophages (Diff-Quik). *B.* Alveolar pneumocytes in a bronchial lavage specimen of another patient. The cells are rounded with relatively large nuclei, delicate chromatin and prominent nucleoli. *C.* Rosette-like cluster of alveolar pneumocytes with hyperchromatic nuclei mimicking adenocarcinoma. *D.* Large, vacuolated cells with enlarged nuclei, coarse chromatin and prominent nucleoli. These cells mimicking adenocarcinoma were present transiently after pulmonary infarction and interpreted as reactive pneumocytes (Case courtesy of Dr. Eileen King, San Francisco, California).

Stanley et al (1992) noted that **type II pneumocytes were transiently present during the early and organizing (reparative) stages of the disease** but did not persist after day 32 following onset of illness. Chemotherapy for cancer also induces atypias that may mimic cancer, and in some cases probably represents drug-induced carcinogenesis. This is discussed in the closing pages of this chapter.

The important point is that **utmost caution is warranted in the interpretation of cytologic abnormalities from patients with known febrile illness, chronic lung disorder, unexplained diffuse opacity of the lung, and in patients receiving anticancer chemotherapy or radiotherapy.** Accurate and complete clinical information is essential to avoid diagnostic pitfalls.

Abnormalities of Pulmonary Macrophages (Dust Cells)

Alveolar macrophages may display morphologic abnormalities that require careful interpretation.

Nuclear Abnormalities

Multinucleation
Bi-, tri-, and multinucleated histiocytes or macrophages are often seen in sputum in the absence of any significant inflammatory process. Large giant cells with numerous peripheral nuclei, resembling the Langhans' cells of tuberculosis, may occur in nonspecific inflammatory processes (see below). Thus the **mere presence of multinucleated macrophages in cytologic material cannot be correlated with a specific disease state.**

Prominent Nucleoli
Prominent nucleoli are occasionally observed in macrophages. The concomitant presence of dust granules within the cytoplasm is helpful in identifying the cells correctly. This finding is of no diagnostic significance.

Degenerative Nuclear Changes
Degenerative nuclear changes that may be confused with cancer are rarely observed in alveolar macrophages. The **cells are typically large** and are provided with **correspondingly large, hyperchromatic, but homogeneous nuclei** that are

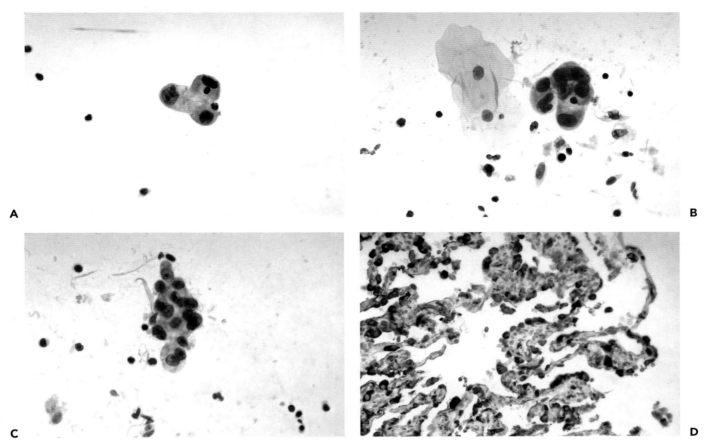

Figure 19-29   Atypical pneumocytes type II in viral pneumonia. *A–C.* Small clusters and single cells with large, hyperchromatic nuclei, some with visible nucleoli, in sputum of a 60-year-old woman with viral pneumonia. *D.* Lung biopsy revealed interstitial fibrosis consistent with usual interstitial pneumonia. The markedly prominent alveolar lining cells (pneumocytes) bind the anti-surfactant antibody A10 (*D,* courtesy of Dr. Allen Gown, PhenoPath Laboratories, Seattle, WA).

sometimes irregular and multiple. These cells are described and illustrated in Chapter 21.

Lipid Pneumonia

Lipid pneumonia may be exogenous or endogenous.

Exogenous Lipid Pneumonia

This disorder results from **aspiration of an oily substance into the lung.** Thus, habitual users of mineral oil or oily nose drops are subject to the disease. The **radiologic appearance** of exogenous lipid pneumonia is that of a localized **infiltrate or mass mimicking lung cancer,** usually in the lower lobes. Although this disorder is much less common today than a generation ago, it is still encountered from time to time, particularly among older persons, and differentiation from lung cancer is of paramount clinical importance.

Because oil aspirated into the lung cannot be absorbed or metabolized, it is **phagocytized by pulmonary macrophages** that carry some of the oil droplets to regional lymph nodes. However, much of the oil remains within the lung where the oil-containing macrophages generate a **granulomatous inflammatory reaction** in the pulmonary parenchyma. This so-called **golden pneumonia** gets its name from the gross appearance of the lipid-rich pneumonic tissues.

Cytology

Sputum is an excellent medium for diagnosis of lipid pneumonia. A deep cough specimen contains lipid-filled macrophages that are diagnostic of this disease. **The characteristic finding of large macrophages with large cytoplasmic vacuoles or abundant bubbly or lacy, vacuolated cytoplasm, representing lipid-filled vacuoles, is pathognomonic of this disease** (Fig. 19-30A). The **nuclei are single or multiple, but small and unremarkable** in appearance. The **differential diagnosis** is limited to **mucus-producing cancer cells,** which, as a rule, have less cytoplasm and display highly **abnormal nuclei.** Also, the cytoplasmic mucin in cancer cells is almost invariably limited to a single vacuole, unlike the bubbly, multiple vacuoles in the cytoplasm of lipid histiocytes. If in doubt, a fresh specimen of sputum can be stained for fat with Oil-red-O (Fig. 19-30B) or Sudan black.

Pulmonary macrophages in the presence of mucus-producing lung cancer may contain phagocytized mucin, but again, as a usually single, fairly large vacuole. Rarely will there be confusion with the cells of lipid pneumonia, and in those unusual cases, the issue can be settled by **staining for mucin** to determine the nature of the cytoplasmic droplets.

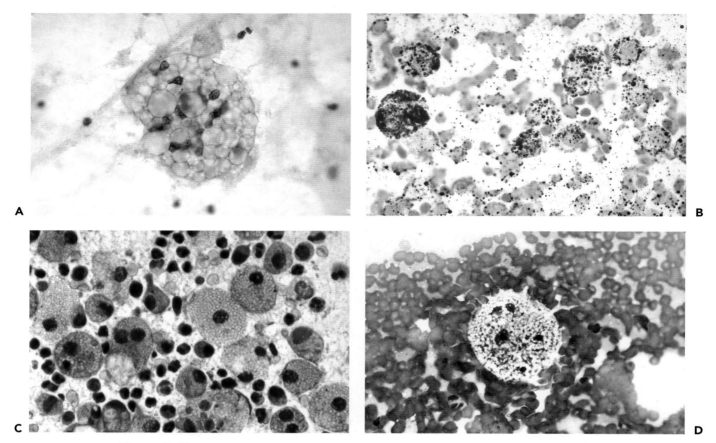

Figure 19-30 Lipid pneumonia. *A.* A large multinucleated macrophage with phagocytized lipid (lipophage) in sputum of a patient with lipid pneumonia. The **multiple cytoplasmic vacuoles or abundant lacy cytoplasm of mono- or multinucleated macrophages are pathognomonic.** *B.* **Oil-red-O stain** for lipid in an unfixed, air-dried specimen. *C.* Endogenous lipid pneumonia due to tissue destruction in association with organizing pneumonia. These lipid-filled histiocytes have very fine vacuoles, are usually mononuclear and not enlarged. *D.* Lipid histiocytes of endogenous lipid pneumonia in an FNA sample stained with Diff-Quik.

Endogenous Lipid Pneumonia

Endogenous lipid pneumonia is a complication of pulmonary disease in which there is tissue destruction and release of tissue lipids that are phagocytized by macrophages. The lipid-filled macrophages accumulate at these sites of tissue damage. This may involve lung parenchyma distal to an obstructing bronchial lesion such as **carcinoma,** or in association with **organizing pneumonia, necrotizing granulomatous inflammation,** or other chronic inflammatory and destructive processes including the effects of **radiotherapy.** Endogenous lipid pneumonia is more common today than exogenous lipid pneumonia. The **radiologic presentation is typically that of the primary lung disease, and endogenous lipid pneumonia is usually an incidental finding.**

Cytology

Macrophages with large, bubbly vacuoles, so characteristic of exogenous lipid pneumonia in sputum, are rarely observed in endogenous lipid pneumonia. **Small, finely vacuolated macrophages** are more characteristic (Fig. 19-30C,D), but they are seldom recognized in sputum and are not specific since they can also be found in sputum of smok-

ers (Roque and Pickren, 1968). The cytologic diagnosis of endogenous lipid pneumonia **is virtually always made by aspiration biopsy (FNA), obtained because of clinical suspicion of bronchogenic carcinoma.** The **characteristic lipid-filled macrophages** may be accompanied by cancer cells. In cases in which such macrophages are observed, the nature of the principal lesion must be urgently clarified by additional cytologic or histologic samples.

The differential diagnosis is primarily with mucinous adenocarcinoma, as discussed above. Among the **few other conditions that mimic endogenous lipid pneumonia** are **Gaucher's disease** involving the lungs, and side effects of **Amiodarone,** a cardiac anti-arrythmic drug that is associated with interstitial fibrosis and foamy macrophages in the lung. Both entities are described below.

Heart Failure Cells (Hemosiderin-Laden Macrophages, Siderocytes)

"Heart failure cells," so named because they may be found in sputum or BAL specimens of patients with chronic congestive heart failure, are **pulmonary macrophages containing a large amount of phagocytized hemosiderin,** which sometimes obscures the nuclei of the macrophages.

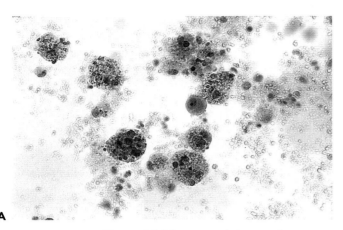

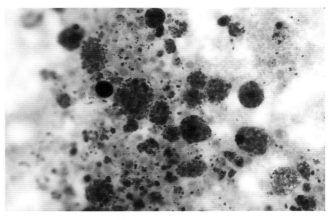

A   B

Figure 19-31 "Heart failure" cells. *A.* Hemosiderin blood pigment in the cytoplasm of macrophages has a characteristic crystalline brown or golden appearance. Hemosiderin may be so abundant in some histiocytes as to obscure the nucleus. *B.* If in doubt, hemosiderin can be identified by a deep blue color in the Prussian blue, ferroferricyanide stain for iron.

The **hemosiderin,** a product of hemoglobin breakdown, is a **golden-brown, iron-containing crystalline pigment** (Fig. 19-31A). Such cells are the sequelae of bleeding into the pulmonary parenchyma. In **heart failure,** bleeding into the air spaces of the lung is usually caused by microscopic oozing from congested alveolar septal capillaries. The hemoglobin breakdown products are phagocytized by macrophages. It should be emphasized that "heart failure cells" are not a specific indicator of heart disease, but may be seen, for example, **after pulmonary infarction** or bleeding of any cause into the lung. Friedman-Mor et al (1976) observed hemosiderin-laden macrophages (siderocytes) in specimens from patients in **shock,** and Naylor found them in patients with **Goodpasture's syndrome** (personal communication), a disease in which vascular damage results from autoantibodies to the basement membrane. In the very rare cases of **primary pulmonary hemosiderosis,** the sputum also can be expected to have an abundance of hemosiderin-containing macrophages.

Granules of hemosiderin should not be confused with other pigments that may be phagocytized by macrophages. **Common dust particles** are usually black and coarse, or so fine as to alter the coloration of the cytoplasm without visible particulates. **Brown melanin pigment** lacks the crystalline appearance of hemosiderin. The rare occurrence of **bile** in severely jaundiced patients, or in the cytoplasm of metastatic hepatocellular carcinoma, is a vaguely greenish, granular, but not crystalline pigment. If in doubt, **hemosiderin pigment can be easily identified by the characteristic blue color of iron in the Prussian blue ferroferricyanide staining reaction** (Fig. 19-31B).

CYTOLOGY OF INFLAMMATORY PROCESSES

Acute Bacterial Inflammation

Cytology

Acute bacterial inflammatory processes include **pneumonias** of various etiologies, lung **abscess** and **purulent bron-**chitis, and result in tissue breakdown. In these diseases, the **sputum** and **aspirated bronchial material** are partly or wholly made up of **purulent exudate,** a mixture of necrotic cellular material and intact and damaged polymorphonuclear leukocytes (see Fig. 19-11A). The Papanicolaou-stained smears appear predominantly **basophilic** (cyanophilic) because of the abundance of necrotic nuclear material forming **threads and amorphous masses of DNA** that stain blue with hematoxylin. Although one is often tempted to consider such smears to be of limited diagnostic value, careful study may reveal underlying (or complicating) causes of the inflammatory process, including various bacterial, fungal, viral, or parasitic infections. The identification of causative organisms is of special importance for effective treatment of patients with AIDS. Also, **because lung cancer, particularly squamous carcinomas, may occasionally be masked by coexisting inflammation, careful screening for cancer cells is mandatory.**

Identification of Specific Bacterial Organisms

The great majority of acute inflammatory processes in the lung are caused by bacteria, most commonly ***pneumococci, streptococci, staphylococci,*** and ***Klebsiella*** **species.** Even with special bacteriologic stains, there are few morphologic features that allow more than a presumptive identification of the bacterial agent or agents in cytologic preparations. Staphylococci, streptococci, and pneumococci may sometimes be tentatively identified by their configuration and growth patterns in chains (streptococci) or clusters (staphylococci). Gram-negative intracellular micrococci are typical of *Neisseria* species. The gram-positive organisms stain blue with hematoxylin. ***Legionella micdadei,*** a cause of Legionnaire's disease, was identified in bronchial washings and pleural fluid by Walker et al (1983) as either extracellular or intracellular small, delicate, gram-negative and acid-fast positive bacilli within the cytoplasm of neutrophils and macrophages. In most cases, bacteriologic culture is required for confirmation and specific classification of the causative organisms and to determine their antibiotic sensitivities. A growing list of **nucleic acid probes and monoclonal antibodies** provide new bacteriologic techniques to accelerate and enhance diagnostic results. Other less common agents that may occasionally cause acute inflammation are discussed below.

Atypical Pneumonias

Atypical pneumonias in adults are caused by *mycoplasma,* **by viruses** including adenovirus, rhinovirus and influenza virus, by **some fungi** including *Pneumocystis carinii* and occasionally bacterial agents. In children and some adults, **respiratory syncytial virus** may be at fault (see below for discussion of fungal and viral manifestations in cytologic material).

The patients usually have symptoms of an **acute febrile respiratory illness with a poorly defined segmental infiltrate on x-ray.** In most cases, the disease is transient, lasting from a few days to a few weeks, and ends by resolution of the pulmonary infiltrate. In some patients, however, the disease may become chronic with progressive interstitial fibrosis.

Cytology

During the **acute and subacute stages** of atypical pneumonias, cytologic samples of **sputum** may pose **significant problems in differential diagnosis.** Following a vigorous bout of coughing, there is often abundant desquamation of **ciliated bronchial cells,** some showing nonspecific atypias in the form of **cellular and nuclear enlargement and enlarged nucleoli.** Other nonspecific abnormalities may include occasional **papillary clusters of hyperplastic bron-**chial cells (Creola bodies) and **ciliocytophthoria** (see above), which can occur in any viral infection (Pierce and Hirsch, 1958), but is particularly likely in adenovirus pneumonia (Pierce and Knox, 1960). An extraordinary exfoliation of papillary groups of bronchial epithelium (Creola bodies) seen in the bronchial aspirate from a 1-year-old child with viral pneumonia is illustrated in Figure 19-32A–C.

Abnormalities of type II pneumocytes, previously discussed and illustrated in Figure 19-29, are another consequence of the pneumonic process.

Knowledge of the clinical setting is always important, but particularly in these difficult cases. Significant epithelial abnormalities in the smaller bronchioles and adjacent alveolar lining cells were noted in autopsy studies of viral pneumonias as long ago as the influenza pandemic of 1918 (Winternitz, 1920). **Thus, the history of an acute, febrile illness should act as a deterrent to the cytologic diagnosis of cancer.** The patient should be monitored with additional specimens until symptoms abate and radiologic abnormalities resolve, or until there is confirmed evidence of cancer on repeat specimens. The cytologic changes accompanying viral pneumonia can be expected to clear over a period of 4 to 6 weeks, and often sooner.

Chronic Inflammatory Processes

Chronic Bronchitis and Pneumonia

These disorders are usually the sequelae of acute bacterial infections or atypical pneumonias and are recognized clini-

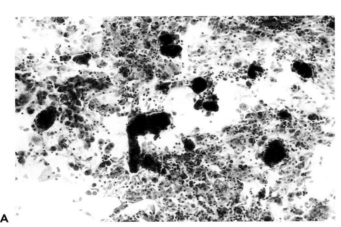

A

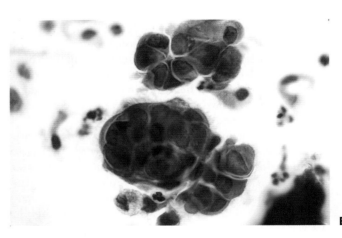

B

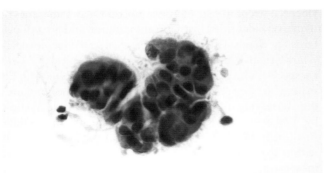

C

Figure 19-32 Bronchial cell atypia in viral pneumonia. A–C. Numerous groups of hyperplastic bronchial epithelial cells (Creola bodies) with hyperchromatic nuclei in the bronchial aspirate of a 1-year-old boy with atypical (viral) pneumonia. Note the persistence of cilia in some of the cells. (Case courtesy of Dr. Goodman.) (B,C: oil immersion.)

cally because of persisting cough, low-grade fever, and various roentgenologic images. The cytologic manifestations of chronic bronchitis and pneumonia in sputum and bronchial washings encompass a range of benign abnormalities. **Nonspecific atypias of bronchial lining cells** and **squamous metaplasia** are the most typical reactions to chronic inflammatory processes. **Reserve cell (basal cell) hyperplasia** and an **increase in mucin-secreting cells** are common.

Chodosh (1970), who followed patients with chronic bronchitis by total and differential cell counts of 24-hour sputum samples, observed that the total number of exfoliated epithelial cells rose and fell according to the stage and activity of their disease, yet the differential count of various epithelial cell types (e.g., ciliated, nonciliated, goblet cells) remained relatively constant. As expected, there was an increase in neutrophils and a drop in macrophages during acute exacerbations of disease, whereas the reverse sequence occurred during recovery.

Diffuse Alveolar Damage

Diffuse alveolar damage is the result of injury to distal alveoli resulting from a single injurious event, usually within the prior few days to weeks. The damage may be extensive, or it may be limited to a small region of the lung. There are a great variety of causes including inhalants, drugs, oxygen toxicity, irradiation, shock, and sepsis. Histologically, there is an early, acute phase characterized by pulmonary edema, a proteinaceous exudate, and **hyaline membrane formation.** This is followed in a few days or a week by hyperplasia of type II pneumocytes in what is apparently a reparative effort. The damage may resolve or may be followed by organization and fibrosis.

Cytologic samples obtained by BAL early in the course of the disease consist of amorphous proteinaceous material, alveolar macrophages, neutrophils, and atypical type II pneumocytes, described above (Beskow et al, 2000).

Interstitial Lung Diseases

Under this heading, there are a number of clinically divergent lung disorders grouped as **idiopathic interstitial pneumonias.** They have **common cytologic denominators** and cannot be specifically identified on the basis of cytologic findings, although various special techniques have been applied to specimens of BAL in an attempt to clarify the nature of some abnormalities. In this group of diseases, it is essential to have accurate knowledge of clinical history and roentgenologic findings to avoid errors of interpretation.

Idiopathic Interstitial Pneumonias
Pathology and Clinical Data
The interstitial pneumonias were first defined by Liebow (1975) and recently reclassified by Katzenstein (1997). Idiopathic interstitial pneumonias comprise a heterogeneous group of disorders of unknown etiology (hence "idiopathic"), having in common **inflammation and progressive fibrosis of alveolar spaces, resulting in obliteration of alveoli and synchronous dilatation of bronchioles,**

leading to formation of pseudoglandular spaces. Nogee et al (2001) described a mutated gene regulating the production of surfactant protein C in a case of familial interstitial disease in an adolescent girl. There is no evidence, so far, that this or similar mechanisms are operative in other sporadic cases. The final stage of the disease is the so-called **honeycomb lung (or end-stage lung)** characterized by grossly visible cysts surrounded by firm, fibrosed lung tissue. **Early histologic changes include hypertrophy of alveolar pneumocytes type II, gradually replacing alveolar epithelium by cuboidal cells with large nuclei,** and **hypertrophy of bronchiolar epithelium with bronchiolar metaplasia in alveoli.**

The common clinical denominator of these disorders is **progressive difficulty in breathing (dyspnea)** caused by the impaired exchange of oxygen and carbon dioxide across the alveolar septum (alveolar-capillary block). Roentgenologic studies show a diffuse and progressive opacification of both lung fields.

Although from a cytologic point of view, this entire group of diseases can be considered as a single entity, there are subtle clinical and histologic differences among the various entities, which have been subclassified as follows:

- Usual interstitial pneumonia (UIP)
- Nonspecific interstitial pneumonia (NSIP)
- Desquamative interstitial pneumonia (DIP)
- Acute interstitial pneumonia (AIP) or Hamman-Rich syndrome
- Respiratory bronchiolitis-interstitial lung disease (RB-ILD)
- Chronic "idiopathic" pulmonary fibrosis

In addition, several diseases of known or suspected cause may result in a similar clinical and pathologic picture and may be considered in this group of disorders. These are:

- **Farmer's lung** and various other types of **allergic pneumonitis (eosinophilic pneumonia)**
- **Pneumoconioses** (e.g., silicosis, asbestosis, anthracosis)
- **Sarcoidosis** (see below)
- **Drug-induced pneumonitis** (to be discussed separately later in this chapter)

Cytology
While the diagnosis often is apparent from clinical and radiologic findings, there may sometimes be **striking atypias of reactive bronchiolar epithelium or pneumocytes type II that can raise questions of adenocarcinoma.** These were discussed above.

Localized chronic interstitial inflammatory processes that mimic lung cancer are most likely to be investigated by FNA biopsy. In most cases, the aspirate is easily recognized as inflammatory and benign, but on occasion, there is **exuberant reactive hypertrophy and hyperplasia of bronchoalveolar epithelium derived from pseudoglandular spaces in the lung, lined by atypical cuboidal cells.** The aspirate may then yield **globoid or ovoid papillary clusters** of cuboidal bronchiolar or alveolar lining cells with small but visible nucleoli, usually arranged in a monolayer (Figs. 19-27 and 19-28). The small size of these cells, their uniform appearance, and regular small nuclei should help prevent a mistaken diagnosis of adenocarcinoma. Kern (1965) reported significant cell abnormalities in sputum of 11 patients with interstitial pneumonia, some with the **Hamman-Rich syndrome.** In two patients, the atypical cells led to an erroneous diagnosis of adenocarcinoma. In retrospect, Kern was dealing with atypical pneumocytes, type II.

Another important source of diagnostic error in aspiration biopsy of the lung, particularly in chronic inflammatory disease, is the presence of mesothelial cells, discussed in Chapters 20 and 26.

With the introduction of **BAL,** many attempts have been made to identify these inflammatory disease processes more specifically by differential cell counts and immunophenotyping the cells, and by chemical analysis of the supernatant. The fundamental cytologic observations are as follows: **In normal, nonsmoking persons, the total cell count in BAL specimens is lower than in smokers;** the difference is caused by an **increase in alveolar macrophages in smokers.** In various **interstitial lung diseases, there is an increase in macrophages, lymphocytes, and polymorpho-**nuclear **leukocytes.** A chronic process is favored when lymphocytes are predominant, and a more acute inflammatory pneumonitis is favored when polymorphonuclear leukocytes are increased. Further characterization of macrophages and lymphocyte subtypes has been possible for some time through immunophenotyping (Costabel et al, 1985), but is of little practical value at present, except perhaps in suspected lymphoproliferative disorders.

BAL has also been studied in **adult respiratory distress syndrome** (summary in Hyers and Fowler, 1986). This potentially lethal, but occasionally reversible disorder is a complication of prolonged exposure to high concentrations of oxygen. It is characterized by the presence of **polymorphonuclear leukocytes and high-molecular-weight plasma proteins** in the lavage specimen, reflecting the increased permeability of damaged alveolar capillaries and interstitial tissues in the alveolar septa.

Giant-Cell Interstitial Pneumonia

Hard-metal workers who are exposed to the dust of a number of metallic industrial pollutants such as tungsten, cobalt, diamond dust, titanium, beryllium, and others may develop a peculiar form of chronic interstitial lung disease characterized by the presence of **large multinucleated giant cells**

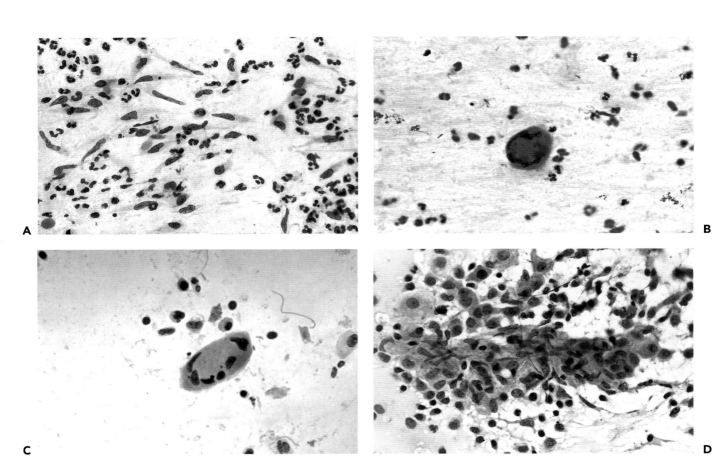

Figure 19-33 Tuberculosis. *A.* Slender, elongated epithelioid cells with elongated, sometimes carrot-shaped nuclei and (*B*) multinucleated Langhans' giant cell in the sputum of a patient with tuberculosis. (Case courtesy of the late Dr. Magnus Nasiell, Stockholm.) *C.* Multinucleated Langhans'-like cell in sputum of a patient with viral pneumonia. The finding of such a cell per se is nonspecific. *D.* FNA of tuberculosis in lung showing a cluster composed of epithelioid histiocytes and spindle cells suggestive of a granuloma.

and fibrosis of interalveolar septa. There are several reports of cytologic abnormalities in this disease (Valicenti et al, 1979; Davison et al, 1983; Tabatowski et al, 1988). The **sputum, bronchial washings, and BAL** fluid in such patients are reportedly characterized by the presence of **numerous giant cells with multiple nuclei.** Particles of phagocytosed material may be observed in the cytoplasm, and the metals can be characterized by analytical electron microscopy. Kinoshita et al (1999) reported two well-documented cases due to tungsten carbide and cobalt in which **bizarre macrophages** were found in BAL specimens. It now appears that the likelihood of disease, at least in the case of exposure to **beryllium,** is greatly increased in individuals with a genetic predisposition to develop sensitivity to this metal (Marshall, 1999). Tabatowski et al emphasized that the cytologic diagnosis of interstitial pneumonia must be supported by clinical and occupational data. The **presence of giant cells in cytologic samples is not specific,** per se, as such cells may occur in a broad variety of chronic inflammatory disorders, and sometimes without an obvious cause.

Giant-cell pneumonia of newborn infants and children is idiopathic or ascribed to a virus, most commonly to measles.

Aspiration Pneumonia

Individuals who have a suppressed cough reflex, for example, as the result of a stroke, alcohol or drug intoxication or postanesthesia, are at risk of aspiration pneumonia (Marik, 2001). Aspiration pneumonia may be acute or chronic. In **acute aspiration pneumonia,** foreign material inspired and then expelled in a sputum sample cannot be distinguished from contaminants of the oral cavity; the cytologic findings are nonspecific and reflect the degree of associated acute inflammation. **A finding of foreign material in bronchial aspirate or lavage specimens** excludes the possibility of oral cavity contamination and is **diagnostic of aspiration.**

In cases of **chronic aspiration pneumonia,** one may find foreign material within the inflammatory exudate in a cough specimen, either partially embraced by macrophages or phagocytized by foreign body giant cells. The exudate is pleomorphic, and includes many polymorphonuclear leukocytes as well as the lymphocytes and histiocytes that typically characterize chronic inflammation. The diagnosis of aspiration pneumonia, whether acute or chronic, may have important legal implications.

Quantitation of lipid-laden macrophages has been proposed as an index of aspiration pneumonitis (Corwin and Irwin, 1985) and applied to BAL in adult patients (Silverman et al, 1989; Langston and Pappin, 1996; Knauer-Fischer and Ratjen, 1999) and to various cytologic samples from infants and children (Colombo and Hallberg, 1987; Collins et al, 1995; Yang et al, 2001). The lipid-laden macrophages can be visualized in air-dried, unfixed smears by staining with the oil-soluble dye, Oil-red-O (see Fig. 19-30B), or after fixing in formalin or formalin vapor (Yang et al, 2001). We found that the stain can work adequately on conventionally prepared smears of bronchial irrigation or sputum specimens preserved in 50% alcohol but not

processed through xylol or other lipid solvents. The proportion of lipid-laden cells versus the total number of macrophages was proposed as a grade of risk by Corwin and Irwin (1985). The grading system later was simplified by Yang et al (2001) who concluded that an absolute or relative increase of lipid-laden macrophages was a sensitive but not particularly specific method for the diagnosis of aspiration pneumonitis in pediatric patients.

Specific Inflammatory Processes

Tuberculosis

Clinical Data

Tuberculosis, caused by the **acid-fast *mycobacterium tuberculosis,*** is a worldwide infectious disease still rampant in the developing countries. It has seen a recent resurgence in the US and other industrialized countries because of AIDS. The disease has two principal forms depending on the portal of entry of the highly infectious organisms. The common **pulmonary form** is caused by inhalation, whereas the rare **intestinal form** is caused by ingestion, usually in milk.

The disease is characterized by formation of minute granules (granulomas), composed of immobilized macrophages that resemble epithelial cells and are therefore called **epithelioid cells.** Fusion of the epithelioid cells leads to the formation of giant cells with a peripheral wreath of nuclei known as **Langhans' cells.** The center of these granulomas often is necrotic and the cheese-like necrotic tissue is known as **caseous necrosis.**

In pulmonary tuberculosis, the upper lobes are first involved, and as the disease progresses, large areas of confluent granulomas undergo caseous necrosis. Expulsion of the necrotic material through the bronchi leads to formation of **cavities** that are the hallmark of late stages of the disease. The sputum of patients with cavitating tuberculosis is rich in acid-fast bacteria and is the most important source of infection to others. Prevention of cavity formation by drugs is the main goal of public health measures.

Early diagnosis followed by treatment is curative of pulmonary tuberculosis. The customary mode of disease detection is by culture of the organism or by a specific polymerase chain reaction (PCR) (see Chap. 3). Still, there are many cases of the disease that are not recognized clinically and may be mistaken for other infectious or neoplastic diseases. Recognizing the possibility of tuberculosis in cytologic samples would be of paramount importance to the patient and to society.

Cytology

Nasiell et al (1972) were among the first to study the sputum and bronchial secretions of a large group of patients with pulmonary tuberculosis. They reported identifying the component cells of the tubercle, the **epithelioid cells,** and **Langhans' giant cells,** in sputum (Fig. 19-33A,B). The identifiable **epithelioid cells** usually appeared in loose clusters as **elongated or somewhat spindly slender cells, sometimes carrot-shaped with one end broader than the** other, and were a bit smaller than bronchial cells. They had eosinophilic cytoplasm with poorly defined cell borders, and pale nuclei that generally followed the elongated shape of the cells. It is likely that epithelioid cells with a more rounded configuration were present as well, but could not be distinguished from other mononuclear macrophages. The **multinucleated Langhans' giant cells** have **peripherally arranged nuclei, but multinucleated giant cells with centrally placed nuclei also may be present.**

The original study by Nasiell et al was reported to show a high degree of specificity for epithelioid cells and Langhans' giant cells, and the combination of the two was considered most specific. In a later report from the same group, however, their original observations could not be sustained (Roger et al, 1972). **In our own experience, the presence of multinucleated giant macrophages in cytologic material, even giant cells of Langhans' type, is of limited diagnostic value.** Such cells may be observed in a broad variety of other inflammatory disorders (Fig. 19-33C), and in occasional patients for unknown reasons.

Percutaneous FNAs usually yield only granular necrotic debris and a mixture of inflammatory cells, a dirty aspirate, including mono- and multinucleated macrophages with, perhaps, occasional comma-shaped epithelioid cells. The presence of a granuloma-like cluster of spindly (comma-shaped) epithelioid cells and histiocytes in an FNA should raise question of tuberculosis, but is not diagnostic (Fig. 19-33D).

In the BAL specimens of patients with active tuberculosis and sarcoidosis, Hoheisel et al (1994) reported an increased proportion of lymphocytes, predominantly activated T cells. The CD-4/CD-8 ratio of lymphocytes was increased in sarcoidosis (see below) but not in tuberculosis.

The frequently **similar radiologic presentation of tuberculosis and lung cancer, and their occasional coexistence,** must be borne in mind when the cytologic diagnosis of tuberculosis is contemplated. **Confirmation of tuberculosis by bacteriologic studies is essential, particularly in high-risk patients with AIDS** in whom the disease is severe and likely to disseminate. In such patients, the granulomas are less well formed, more often necrotic, and likely to contain a greater number of acid-fast organisms. Unfortunately, stains for acid-fast bacilli in sputum smears or cell block sections have been of very limited value in our hands.

Mycobacterium Avium Intracellulare

Pulmonary infections with the acid-fast bacterium, *Mycobacterium avium intracellulare* (MAI), have acquired new significance with the onset of AIDS, and brief discussion of this disease is warranted. Once an extremely rare cause of disease in the human, it is now one of the most common opportunistic infections in AIDS and other immunodeficient patients, in whom it is a potentially lethal infection. The organism is found worldwide in soil and water. Beginning in the lung or gastrointestinal tract, it disseminates throughout the reticuloendothelial system and to the central nervous system. The involved tissues are choked with numerous swollen, foamy macrophages that contain enormous numbers of acid-fast organisms. **Massive abdominal lymphadenopathy and splenomegally caused by an overwhelming MAI infection may mimic a malignant lymphoma.** We are unaware of any systematic cytologic study of pulmonary MAI infection. However, in FNA smears of lymph nodes from those patients, numerous bacterial rods are found within large foamy macrophages. In hematologic stains such as Diff-Quick, the organisms do not stain, but appear as clear or pale oblong structures within the cytoplasm of macrophages (see Chap. 31). In the immunocompetent patient with pre-existing chronic lung disease, MAI can sometimes cause a superimposed indolent granulomatous and cavitating infection that is clinically and pathologically similar to tuberculosis. Indolent infections with *M. avium* have been reported in elderly patients without a known predisposing immunologic defect (Prince et al, 1989).

Other Bacterial Infections

Material for culture can be secured in sputum, BAL, bronchial brush, or FNA specimens. On occasion, unusual bacterial organisms may be identified directly in such specimens. For example, Lachman (1995) identified *Rhodococcus equi* in BAL and bronchial brush specimens, and Hsu and Luh (1995) reported *Fusobacterium nucleatum* in an FNA.

Sarcoidosis

The granulomatous disease, sarcoidosis, **differs from tuberculosis in that there is no caseous necrosis within the granulomas.** The disease is most common in young African–Americans, and whereas the lung is frequently affected, **sarcoidosis is a systemic disease** of unknown cause. In most patients, the disease is chronic, involving lymphoid tissue and many other organs including the eye, bones, heart, etc.

Mycobacterium tuberculosis has long been suspected of having some role in the pathogenesis of sarcoid, perhaps associated with a defect of cellular immunology. Bacterial proteins of *M. tuberculosis* have been reportedly demonstrated in sarcoid tissue by PCR. Nasiell et al observed both epithelioid cells and multinucleated giant cells in sputum of some of their patients with sarcoidosis.

We have observed well-formed granulomas composed of epithelioid cells and Langhans' giant cells in FNA specimens of several cases of pulmonary sarcoidosis (Fig. 19-34A–C). A characteristic, though not invariable or fully specific feature is the presence of **laminated crystalline inclusions (Schaumann's bodies)** in multinucleated giant cells (Fig. 19-34D). Such cells are suggestive of sarcoidosis.

Zaman et al (1995) reported their findings in **BAL specimens** from a series of 26 patients with sarcoidosis and concluded that in an appropriate clinical setting, **a combination of the following would suggest pulmonary sarcoidosis: multinucleated giant cells** with highly reactive nuclear changes; **reactive alveolar macrophages** and **epithelioid cells;** lymphocytosis; and a clean background. As noted above, Hoheisel et al (1994) found an increased

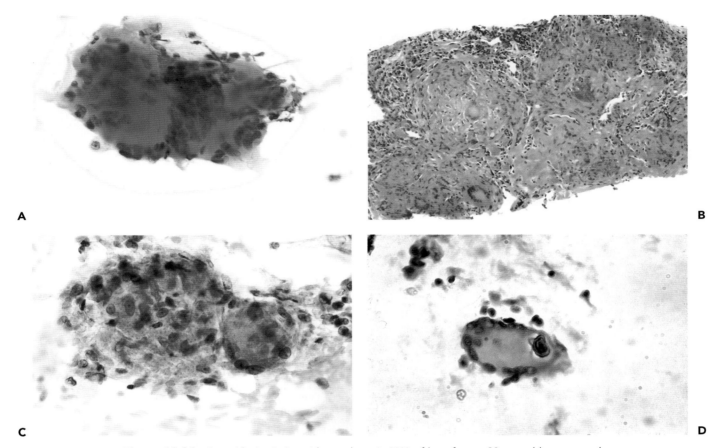

Figure 19-34   Sarcoidosis. *A.* Sarcoid granuloma in FNA of lung from a 38-year-old woman and (*B*) confluent noncaseating granulomas in a needle core biopsy of lung from the same patient. *C.* Sarcoid granuloma in bronchial cytology of another patient. Note the multinucleated Langhans' giant cell with adherent rounded and elongated epithelioid cells. *D.* Schaumann body, a laminated crystalline inclusion in a multinucleated Langhans' giant cell, considered very suggestive of sarcoidosis. This was in a sputum specimen from a woman later confirmed to have sarcoidosis on biopsy of a neck node (*D*, courtesy of Dr. Klaus Schreiber).

percentage of lymphocytes in BAL specimens with predominance of activated T cells and an increased CD-4/CD-8 ratio. It should be re-emphasized that the finding of multinucleated giant cells or lymphocytosis in itself is nonspecific, and can be observed in a variety of inflammatory processes or even in the absence of disease.

If sarcoid is suspected clinically, a transbronchial FNA of mediastinal lymph node may be more effective than percutaneous aspirate (Koerner et al 1975). In those cases, care must be taken not to confuse the epithelioid cells with cancer cells. Even with cytologic or histologic evidence of noncaseating granulomas, however, prudence requires that a final diagnosis of sarcoidosis be confirmed clinically and by negative bacteriologic study.

Actinomycosis and Nocardiosis

Actinomycosis and nocardiosis are suppurative infections caused by **gram-positive branching filamentous bacteria** once thought to be fungi because of their morphology. Both are saprophytic organisms, but may be pathogenic in patients with impaired cellular immunity. Actinomyces grow under conditions of reduced oxygen, and are common in-

habitants of the tonsillar crypts and gingival crevices. The organism does not invade healthy tissues and in order to cause disease it must be injected into the tissue under anaerobic conditions, thus usually in association with trauma, for example, in the oral cavity. **Consequently, they may be present in the sputum as contaminants of no clinical importance.** They are **readily identified** by their pattern of growth in colonies **made up of dense masses of hematoxylin-stained, tangled filaments** that radiate outward and tend to be eosinophilic at the periphery (Fig. 19-35A). In the female genital tract, actinomycotic colonies are usually associated with long-term use of an intrauterine device (see Chap. 10). **Pulmonary lesions caused by actinomyces** usually represent secondary or complicating infections of already-damaged or inflamed lung tissue. Actinomyces derived from tonsillar crypts may produce **lung abscesses** from which the organism can grow into the pleura and chest wall with resulting empyema and fistulous tracts. The actinomycotic colonies are visible grossly as small yellow particles **(sulfur granules). If the organism is observed in bronchial brush or bronchial aspirate from an infected segment of lung, or is found in a FNA of a pulmonary lesion, its role as a pathogen is secure** (Koss et al, 1992).

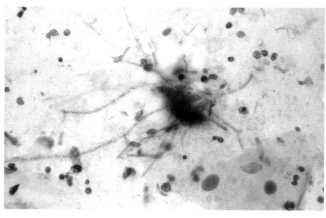

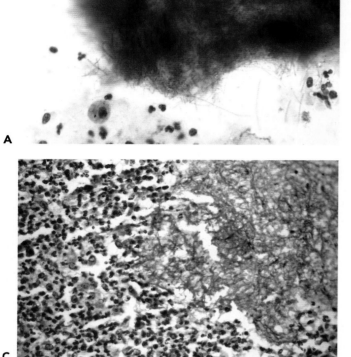

Figure 19-35   Actinomyces and nocardia. *A.* The long filamentous actinomyces are best visualized at the periphery of the colony and are a common contaminant in specimens of sputum. *B.* Nocardia in sputum, a loose cluster of long, thin, branching filamentous organisms. *C.* Nocardial lung abscess in the same patient.

The clinical presentation of **nocardiosis** is similar to actinomycosis, and usually also is an infection of immunocompromised individuals. It is caused by inhalation of the organism, which is widely present in the soil. **Nocardia is an aerobic branching filamentous bacterium that is gram-positive and resembles actinomyces** but is weakly acid-fast. The organism may cause pulmonary abscesses (Fig. 19-35B,C). It does not usually form colonies ("sulfur granules") characteristic of actinomyces. Culture is required for positive identification of the organism.

Wegener's Granulomatosis

Wegener's granulomatosis is a disease of unknown etiology, characterized by vasculitis of small and medium size vessels and necrotizing granulomatous inflammation involving the upper respiratory tract and lung, where it may sometimes mimic cavitating tuberculosis. Glomerulonephritis and generalized vasculitis are common. In the proper clinical setting, the diagnosis may be suggested by **FNA** of lung that yields **amorphous or filamentous necrotic tissue** (a "dirty" background) and an **inflammatory cellular infiltrate** containing mono- and multinucleated macrophages and, in some cases, epithelioid cells (Fekete et al, 1990; Pitman et al, 1992; Kaneishi et al, 1995). Five cases diagnosed by transbronchial biopsy were reported by Lombard et al (1990). Takeda and Burechailo (1969) observed **smooth muscle cells** in the sputum of a patient with Wegener's granulomatosis, and Hector (1976) described sputum cytology in two

cases of Wegener's granulomatosis, but the findings were nonspecific. There is no evidence that sputum is an effective diagnostic technique for this disease.

The diagnosis must be verified by biopsy and by **positive anti-neutrophil cytoplasmic antigen test (cANCA) confirmed by enzyme-linked immunosorbent assay (ELISA) for proteinase 3** (Savige et al, 1999; van der Geld, 2000).

Langerhans' Cell Histiocytosis (Langerhans' Cell Granulomatosis, Eosinophilic Granuloma)

Langerhans' cell histiocytosis in the lung is part of a spectrum of diseases characterized by monoclonal proliferation and infiltration of many organs by Langerhans' cells (Willman et al, 1994; Vassallo et al, 2000). The **Langerhans' cells** are dendritic, antigen-presenting cells, characterized by expression of the CD1a antigen and the presence (in electron micrographs) of penta-layered, rod-shaped intracytoplasmic structures known as **Birbeck granules** (Birbeck et al, 1961).

The Langerhans' cells are associated with eosinophils and, in its localized form, the disorder is called **eosinophilic granuloma.** In cases of multiorgan involvement, the disease was once thought to be a different entity and was called **histiocytosis X** or **Letterer-Siwe disease.** These terms are now obsolete. **The Hand-Schüller-Christian syndrome (a triad of exophthalmos, diabetes insipidus, and bone lesions involving primarily the skull)** is a disease of childhood most often caused by eosinophilic granuloma.

Langerhans' cell granulomatosis is now thought to represent a reactive rather than a neoplastic process (Lieberman et al, 1996; Vassallo et al, 2000; Yousem, et al, 2001), although clonality has been reported in extrapulmonary lesions (Willman, 1994). It accounts for an estimated 5% of adult patients with interstitial lung disease (Gaensler et al, 1980) who may present with cough and dyspnea. In chest x-rays, the upper and middle lobes of the lung are predominantly involved with interstitial infiltrates, sometimes accompanied by cystic changes. The disease can occur as a single, isolated nodule and mimic carcinoma of the lung (Fichtenbaum, 1990; Khoor et al, 2001).

Cytology

When suspected clinically, the diagnosis can be supported by **BAL in which more than 5% of large mononuclear cells are CD1a positive** (Chollet et al, 1984; Auerswald et al, 1991).

Occasionally, a transbronchial or percutaneous aspirate may yield Langerhans' cells measuring 10 to 12 μm and **resembling macrophages with long cytoplasmic processes. The round or oval nuclei are finely textured and typically have a cleaved or convoluted contour, resulting in an appearance of nuclear creases.** These cells **do not show any evidence of phagocytosis and are CD1a and S-100 positive.** In a classical case, the Langerhans' cells are accompanied by **numerous eosinophils** and lymphocytes; Charcot-Leyden crystals may occasionally be present (see Fig. 19-11C). However, this classic cytologic presentation is uncommon. Most patients have a good prognosis, although some may end with pulmonary insufficiency due to fibrosis and cystic change; thus the importance of an accurate diagnosis (Colby and Lombard, 1983). In most cases, confirmation of the diagnosis will require lung biopsy, which may be successfully performed as a transbronchial biopsy, in at least some instances. For additional discussion, see Chapters 31 and 36.

SPECIFIC VIRAL INFECTIONS

Over the years, specific cytopathic changes have been described for different viral infections of the respiratory tract. Credit for many of the initial observations goes to Naib et al (1963, 1968). The issue is particularly important for patients with AIDS, who are prone to viral infections that may be treated with antiviral pharmacologic agents. Infectious viruses are obligatory cellular parasites, often forming inclusion bodies as they multiply within cells. Table 19-1, modified from Naib et al (1968), summarizes the principal cytopathic changes attributed to several different, common viral infections identified by culture. Frable et al (1977) described their findings in 33 cases of upper respiratory tract viral infection diagnosed by cytology. A description of cell changes for each specific virus follows.

Herpes Simplex Virus

As discussed in Chapter 10, herpes simplex is a DNA virus related to herpes virus type II, varicella-zoster virus, and to cytomegalovirus. Until a few years ago, herpetic tracheobronchitis and pneumonia had been considered rare disorders affecting markedly debilitated patients. We now know it is not uncommon. Herpesvirus infection has been observed in burn patients (Foley et al, 1970) and in cancer patients (Rosen and Hajdu, 1971). It is a fairly **frequent cause of respiratory tract disease** that affects children as well as adults, although again, particularly patients with AIDS. At the Montefiore Hospital, 30

TABLE 19-1					
DIFFERENTIAL DIAGNOSIS OF MORPHOLOGIC MANIFESTATIONS OF VIRAL INFECTIONS IN THE RESPIRATORY TRACT OF MEN					
	Epithelial Target Cell	Cytoplasmic Inclusions	Nuclear Inclusions	Multinucleated Giant Cells	Cell De-generation
Herpes simplex	Respiratory squamous	No	Yes, ground-glass and eosinophilic	Yes	No
Cytomegalovirus	Respiratory	Yes, eosinophilic or basophilic with halo	Yes, basophilic or eosinophilic, large halo	Occasional	No
Parainfluenza	Respiratory	Yes, eosinophilic with halo	No	No	Yes
Adenovirus	Respiratory	No	Yes, multiple basophilic	No	No
Respiratory syncytial virus	Respiratory	Multiple basophilic with halos	No	100%	Slight
Measles	Respiratory	Multiple small eosinophilic	Rare	100%	Slight

(Modified from Naib ZM, et al. Cytological features of viral respiratory tract infection. Acta Cytol 12:162, 1968.)

documented cases of herpetic pneumonia were observed during a 2-year period from January 1975 to December 1976, and many more since that time. Yet, while several of the patients had cancer or were immunodeficient, about half had **no clinical evidence of immune incompetence.** Similar observations were recorded by Frable et al (1977). Lindgren et al (1968) observed that herpes virus may be recovered from respiratory secretions of adults without evidence of disease. Clinically, most patients present with **high fever** and **intractable cough,** with or without roentgenologic evidence of pneumonia. Vesicles and ulcerative lesions may be present in the mouth and the upper respiratory tract (Fig. 19-36A).

Cytologic examination of **sputum reveals multinucleated cells with moderately enlarged basophilic nuclei of ground-glass appearance** (Fig. 19-36B), **or nuclei with margination of chromatin and large intranuclear eosino-**philic inclusions (Fig. 19-36C,D). **The nuclei are molded by contact with each other.** There are **no cytoplasmic inclusions.** Herpes virus can be specifically identified in cells and tissues by immunocytochemistry with monoclonal antibody and by in situ hybridization with cDNA (see Chaps. 3 and 4). Most immunocompetent patients recover spontaneously without antiviral therapy.

It cannot be sufficiently emphasized how essential the cytologic or virologic identification of this disease is for the patient. **Patients with a history of treated cancer may develop herpetic pneumonia that mimics metastatic tumor. In those patients, a cytologic finding of herpes may prevent unnecessary or even harmful treatment.** It is worth emphasizing that in debilitated patients with advanced stages of cancer or AIDS, herpetic pneumonia may complicate diseases caused by other infectious agents, primarily fungi.

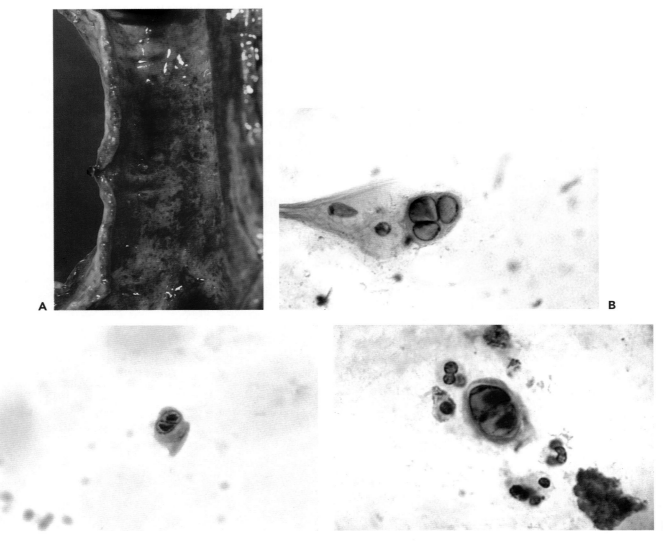

Figure 19-36 **Herpes simplex.** *A.* Herpetic tracheitis showing confluent shallow ulcers in the congested mucosa. *B.* A multinucleated cell with nuclear molding and ground-glass nuclei in suptum specimen. *C.* Binucleated bronchial cell with preserved terminal bar and cilia and a single well-formed, homogeneous nuclear inclusion in each nucleus. *D.* Binucleated bronchial cell with nuclear molding, a homogeneous central inclusion within each nucleus, and nuclear clearing about the inclusion with margination of chromatin. (*B,C:* High magnification; *D:* oil immersion.)

Varicella-Zoster Virus

Varicella-zoster virus is closely related to the herpes virus. Skin lesions such as varicella (chicken pox) and herpes zoster are caused by this virus. In children, and in patients with AIDS, the virus can cause pneumonia. **Herpes virus-type inclusions** may be observed in epithelial cells of the bronchioles and within the desquamated cells in the alveoli.

Cytomegalovirus

Cytomegalovirus (CMV) is a DNA virus related to herpes. In debilitated infants and immunocompromised patients, the virus may cause a fatal illness.

CMV is characterized in **histologic sections and cytologic specimens** by the presence of **markedly enlarged cells (hence the name)** with **large, basophilic intranuclear inclusions surrounded by a clear halo, and sometimes, tiny satellite basophilic inclusions in the cytoplasm** (Fig. 19-37A,B). They may be demonstrated in sputum (Fig. 19-37C,D), as first shown by Naib (1963) and Warner et al (1964). While most affected cells are mononuclear, Naib (1963) also noted that the inclusions may be seen in multinucleated giant cells. Epithelial and endothelial cells are involved widely throughout the body, including **bronchiolar** and alveolar epithelial cells and macrophages. In infants, the characteristic inclusions are best demonstrated in exfoliated renal tubular cells in the urinary sediment (see Chap. 22). In patients with AIDS, CMV infection may be associated with multiple other viral and fungal agents. In questionable cases, the virus can be documented by immunocytology with a specific antibody, by in-situ hybridization, or by PCR.

Adenovirus

Koprowska (1961) described **eosinophilic intranuclear inclusions** attributed to adenovirus in respiratory epithelial cells within smears of respiratory secretions. Naib et al (1968) pointed out that **the affected respiratory cells and their nuclei are usually enlarged but retain their cilia. The enlarged nuclei contain multiple spherical eosinophilic inclusions with halos** (Fig.19-38). The **inclusions in some cells merge into a single basophilic mass.** The term **smudge cell** was used to describe them. Pierce and Knox (1960) observed **massive ciliocytophthoria** in adenovirus infection (see above).

Parainfluenza Virus

In children with this viral infection, Naib et al (1968) described **uniform epithelial cell degeneration** with

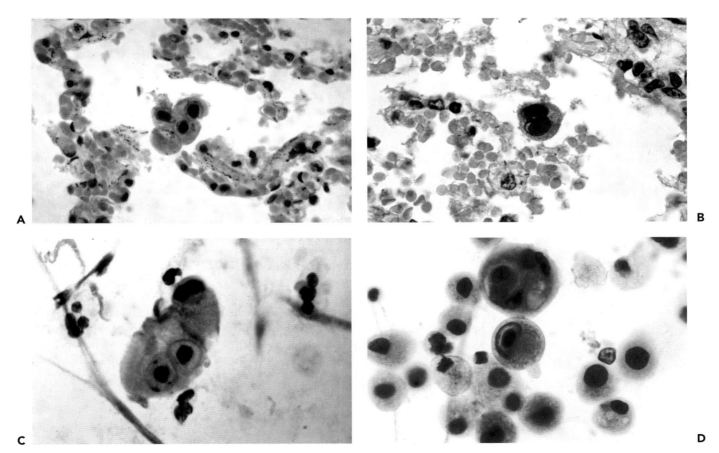

A   B

C   D

Figure 19-37   Cytomegalovirus (CMV) targets epithelial and endothelial cells, which are enlarged with large nuclei that contain a homogeneous basophilic inclusion with surrounding halo. There may be one or more tiny cytoplasmic inclusions. *A,B.* Histologic sections of lung showing cytomegalovirus inclusions in desquamated cells within alveoli. *C,D.* Sputum with cytomegalovirus inclusions in exfoliated cells. (*C,D:* oil immersion.)

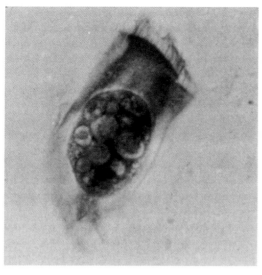

Figure 19-38 Adenoviral infection: enlarged bronchial cells with preservation of cilia. In the nucleus are multiple round, in reality, eosinophilic inclusions with halos (oil immersion). (Courtesy of Dr. Zuher Naib, Atlanta, GA.)

ciliocytophthoria of respiratory epithelial cells. There are **multiple eosinophilic cytoplasmic inclusions, but no intranuclear inclusions.**

Respiratory Syncytial Virus

This infection, which can be fatal, **occurs principally in infants or children with primary immunodeficiency.** It may be seen in immunocompromised patients following bone marrow or organ transplant, or after chemotherapy for neoplastic disease. It may occur in normal individuals.

The classical cytologic finding in infections with respiratory syncytial virus (RSV) is the formation of **very large syncytial cell aggregates,** measuring 100 μm or more in diameter (Fig. 19-39). Naib et al (1968) described **multiple, deeply basophilic inclusion bodies with clear halos** within the degenerated cytoplasm of the multinucleated

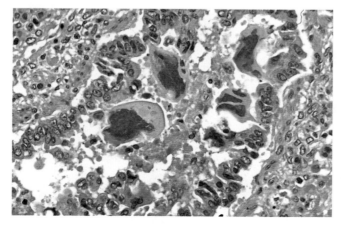

Figure 19-39 **Respiratory syncytial virus (RSV).** Histologic section of lung from autopsy of an infant who died with RSV bronchitis, showing the large multinucleated syncytial cells in a bronchiole destroyed by inflammation.

syncytial giant cells. Immunocompromised children with fatal RSV infection typically have a giant cell pneumonia (Hall et al, 1986).

In what may have been an earlier stage or more subtle form of the disease, Zaman et al (1996) described one or more discrete **eosinophilic cytoplasmic inclusions in mononuclear pneumocytes** of a BAL specimen from a 45-year-old man who was immunocompromised after stem cell transplantation for multiple myeloma. Multinucleated giant cells were rare. There were no nuclear inclusions and no nuclear molding. Parham et al (1993) also described **pink intracytoplasmic inclusions** in a May-Grunwald–Giemsa–stained BAL specimen of a child with RSV following bone marrow transplantation, confirmed by immunofluorescence and electron microscopy.

Measles (Rubella)

This common infection of childhood is caused by an RNA virus of the paramyxoma family. The infection is usually of a transient nature, but may be fatal in debilitated children in developing countries or in immunocompromised patients regardless of age. The disease is characterized by formation of **multinucleated giant cells (Warthin-Finkelday cells)** that may occur throughout the reticuloendothelial system, mainly in lymphoid tissue and lymph nodes. **Measles pneumonia** is one of the potentially fatal manifestations of the disease.

As early as 1955, Tompkins and Macauly reported finding **Warthin-Finkelday giant cells in nasal secretions before** the appearance of other clinical signs of measles such as Koplik's spots and skin rash, an observation later confirmed by Beals and Campbell (1959) and by Mottet and Szanton (1961). It was proposed as a means of early cytologic diagnosis of measles.

The Warthin-Finkelday cells **have up to 100 nuclei and contain spherical eosinophilic intracytoplasmic and intranuclear inclusions.** Similar cells were observed by Naib et al (1968) in material from the respiratory tract and by Abreo and Bagby (1991) in sputum. Harboldt et al (1994) described **two types of giant cells** in an immunosuppressed patient with measles pneumonia: **Warthin-Finkelday giant cells** and **syncytial epithelial giant cells.** The latter are formed by coalescence of hyperplastic alveolar epithelial cells, probably pneumocytes type II, and contain no more than 35 nuclei, whereas Warthin-Finkelday giant cells, which are found throughout the reticuloendothelial system, contain up to 100 nuclei. Both types of giant cells have **intranuclear and intracytoplasmic, sharply demarcated eosinophilic inclusions.**

Polyomavirus

The **homogeneous basophilic nuclear inclusions of polyomavirus,** affecting mainly the urinary tract and the central nervous system, may occur in bronchial cells (Fig. 19-40). The virus may also cause a **fishnet chromatin structure** identical with that seen in urothelial cells (see Chap. 22).

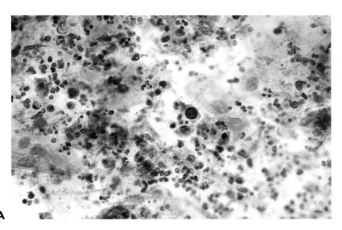

A

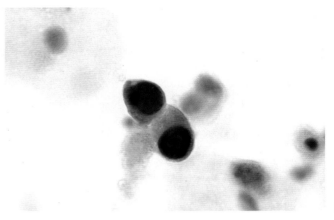

B

Figure 19-40   Polyoma virus. *A.* Sputum specimen with viral inclusion in bronchial cell. *B.* At higher magnification, the nuclei of affected cells have lost chromatin structure and appear homogeneously basophilic and slightly enlarged. In a later stage of degeneration, the chromatin takes on a coarse "fishnet" structure (*B:* oil immersion).

The pulmonary infection appears to be incidental and has no known clinical significance.

Human Papillomavirus

Koilocytes, cells that are pathognomonic of a permissive human papillomavirus infection, have been observed in cytologic material derived from **solitary papillomas of the bronchus.** The possible role of the virus in the pathogenesis of solitary bronchial papillomas and in bronchogenic squamous cancer is discussed in Chapter 20. Human papillomavirus in **laryngeal and tracheobronchial papillomatosis** is discussed in Chapter 21.

NONSPECIFIC INTRACYTOPLASMIC INCLUSIONS

Small eosinophilic intracytoplasmic inclusions are not infrequently observed in desquamated bronchial cells of patients with or without cancer. Similar inclusions are commonly seen in cells of the urinary sediment (see Chap. 22 for further discussion of their nature). The **eosinophilic cytoplasmic inclusions seen in ciliocytophthoria** (see above) are morphologically similar. These inclusions represent degenerative cytoplasmic aggregates of intermediate filaments and have no diagnostic significance. They should not be confused with viral inclusions. It has been suggested that such inclusions are more numerous in the presence of metastatic urothelial cancer. This has not been our experience.

PULMONARY MYCOSES

Although lung diseases caused by fungi have been known for many years in endemic areas, the movements of populations, treatment of patients with immunosuppressive agents, and mainly the onset of AIDS have significantly increased the prevalence of this group of diseases in the US and other countries. **Many of the organisms can be identified in routinely Papanicolaou-stained cytologic material from the respiratory tract,** although some require culture or special staining procedures for identification. Sputum or BAL specimens are commonly used for diagnosis, and fiberoptic bronchoscopy with BAL cytology is reported to approach 90% sensitivity; together with transbronchial biopsy, diagnostic yield has been as high as 98% (Broaddus, 1985). With the availability of new drugs, the proper identification of these organisms has become an urgent, potentially life-saving task.

Pathogenic Fungi

This group of fungi is primary pathogens (i.e., they are capable of causing disease in otherwise normal, healthy persons). Only a few of the most common and most important organisms seen in cytologic preparations will be discussed here. The reader is referred to other sources for more extensive description.

Cryptococcus neoformans (hominis)

Once uncommon, cryptococcal infections are now **frequently observed in AIDS, and occasionally in immunosuppressed leukemic patients.** The diagnosis is of considerable clinical importance. While the disease typically presents as a **meningitis** (see Chap. 27), the lung is believed to be the site of entry for the fungus (see below); hence, its **early detection and treatment may prevent dissemination.**

Histology

Lung involvement may be **diffuse or localized.** In the **diffuse form,** as the organism extends throughout the alveolar space, its thick mucoid capsular material **can suggest pulmonary alveolar proteinosis.** In its **localized granulomatous form, the fungal lesions can mimic bronchogenic carcinoma** (Fig. 19-41A). The cryptococcal infection in

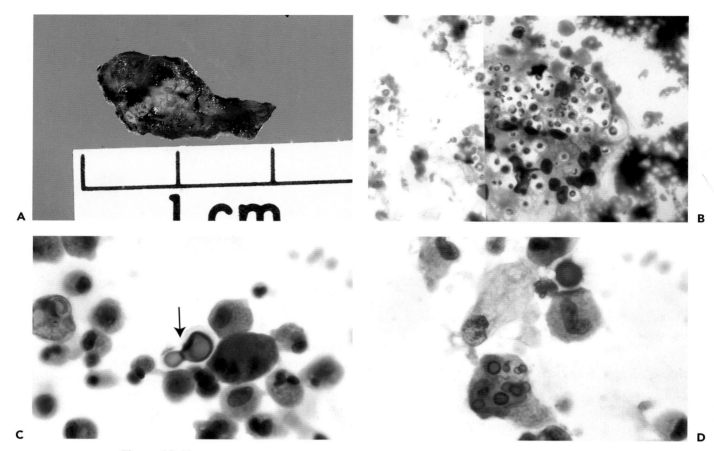

Figure 19-41 *Cryptococcus. A.* Gross photograph of cryptococcal pneumonia, which has a grey-white mucoid appearance and may mimic a mucinous lung cancer. *B.* A cluster of cryptococcal spores in sputum under high magnification. Note that the thick capsule is only faintly stained by the Papanicolaou stain. *C.* Narrow-based budding of *Cryptococcus (arrow). D.* Cryptococcal yeast varies in size; some are phagocytized by macrophages, others lie free. The capsules stain red with mucicarmine. (*B–D:* Oil immersion.)

lung and particularly in meninges has a characteristic sticky mucoid appearance that should suggest the proper diagnosis on gross examination.

Cytology

The **spherical yeast form of the organism,** as it is seen in the sputum, varies greatly in size from 5 to 25 μm in diameter, and has a thick, sharply demarcated **transparent capsule** (Fig. 19-41B). It produces a single, **teardrop-shaped bud (spore) attached to the mother cell by a narrow pedicle** (Fig. 19-41C). The organisms are faintly stained in both Papanicolaou and Diff-Quick stains. They may be found free or phagocytized within mononuclear alveolar macrophages or multinucleated giant phagocytes (Fig. 19-41D). **The thick mucoid capsule stains with mucicarmine** (Fig. 19-41D), **periodic acid-Schiff (PAS), and Gomori methenamine silver stains, facilitating identification in sputum as in spinal fluid** (see Chap. 27). In fresh sputum specimens, the organisms can be stained supravitally with 1% cresyl blue in distilled water and counterstained with Sudan IV in 70% alcohol (Beemer et al, 1972).

Blastomyces dermatitidis

Pulmonary blastomycosis caused by ***Blastomyces dermatitidis*** was described in detail by Johnston and Amatulli

(1970). The disease, observed mainly in young people, produces **granulomatous lesions and abscesses** in the skin. The fungus may also **involve the lungs wherein it causes pneumonias that can mimic bronchogenic carcinoma.** It may be fatal if untreated. **Primary diagnosis of this disease by cytologic examination of sputum** should be the rule.

In sputum, the **yeast forms of the organism are spherical, about the same size or larger than *Cryptococcus,* from which they differ by absence of the thick, mucoid capsule** (Fig. 19-42A). **The organism has a refractile, thick wall, stained by methenamine silver** (Fig. 19-42B). It **produces single buds, which are often rounded and are attached to the mother cell by a broad, flat surface.** The form of the bud and its attachment differ from the teardrop-shaped bud of *Cryptococcus.* The organisms may be phagocytized by macrophages or found free. Other forms of blastomycosis have not been reported in cytologic material.

Coccidioides immitis

Coccidiomycosis, previously endemic to the San Joaquin Valley in California, the western and southwestern regions of the US, and Central and South America, now has a worldwide distribution. In New York State, there have been approximately 30 cases a year for the last 5 to 10 years,

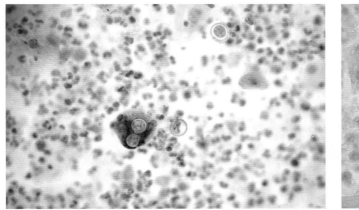
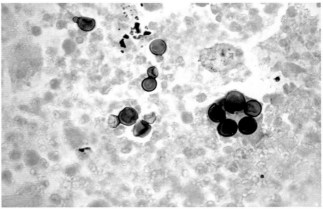

Figure 19-42 Blastomycosis. *A.* Sputum with two blastomyces yeast in a macrophage. *B.* Blastomyces are stained by Grocott silver stain. Note the cluster of organisms, which were engulfed by a phagocytic giant cell, not well shown. There are other extracellular organisms, including one with broad-based budding.

almost all in immunodepressed individuals who have traveled to endemic areas (Chaturvedi et al, 2000). The **pulmonary form of the disease** produces **infiltrates that may be pneumonic, may mimic tuberculosis because of cavitary lesions,** or may present as a **lung mass that can simulate a neoplasm.** In most cases, primary infections are asymptomatic and the disease is self-limiting; but in a small percentage of patients, progressive generalized forms of the disease may occur.

The organism in sputum has been described by Naib (1962), Guglietti and Reingold (1968), and Johnston (1992) as **large spherules with thick walls, measuring from 20 to 100 μm in diameter. Minute endospores may be observed within the spherule in sputum** (Fig. 19-43A), often more readily than in histologic sections. The endospores stain reddish in Papanicolaou stain (Guglietti and Reingold, 1968). Rosenthal (1988) observed the organisms in **FNA** of cavitary lesions; and Raab et al (1993) described and illustrated the cytologic findings in 73 patients diagnosed by FNA. They noted large amounts of granular, eosinophilic debris in the smears, with a paucity of inflamma-

tory cells. Many of the spherules had a crushed or fractured appearance, and some were calcified.

Paracoccidioides brasiliensis

Paracoccidiomycosis is endemic to Brazil and other parts of South America. The fungus ***Paracoccidioides brasiliensis*** is characterized by large spores surrounded by multiple peripheral buds, sometimes described as a ship's wheel (Fig. 19-44). Tani and Franco (1984) examined sputum and bronchial cytology specimens from **45 patients with lung involvement** and were able to identify the organism in Grocott-stained specimens from 43 of the 45 patients, primarily in cell block sections. Most of the specimens were purulent or hemorrhagic and contained epithelioid cells and multinucleated giant cells within inflammatory exudate. They concluded that cytology was an effective diagnostic technique for this infection.

Histoplasma capsulatum

Histoplasmosis is seen predominantly in the southern states and the Ohio and Tennessee valleys. Many organs of

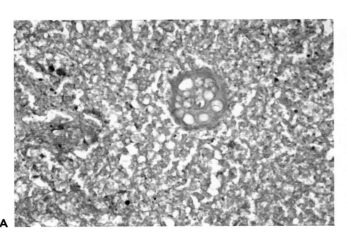
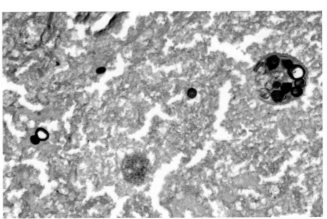

Figure 19-43 Coccidiomycosis. *A.* Large thick-walled spherule in sputum, almost as large as an intermediate squamous cell, containing endospores. *B.* Methenamine silver stain of same specimen. (Case courtesy of Ms. Carol Bales and Ms. Gretchen Torres.)

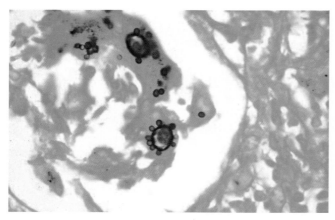

Figure 19-44   Paracoccidiomycosis: Thick-walled spherules with peripheral buds resembling the spokes on a ship's wheel (high magnification).

the body may be affected. The **pulmonary forms** of the infection **can mimic tuberculosis** and may be a cause of **sclerosing mediastinitis.**

The **tiny organisms** (2 to 4 μm in diameter) are best recognized when seen within the **cytoplasm of a macrophage,** which they may fill with **tiny dot-like structures with clear halos** (Fig. 19-45). Johnston (1992) reported great difficulty in identifying this organism in sputum, and without special stains such as the Grocott methenamine silver stain, it is virtually impossible. The disease is not uncommon in AIDS patients (Salzman et al, 1988; Tomita and Chiga, 1988) and when suspected, the organisms are best demonstrated by silver staining of BAL specimens. (Blumenfeld and Gan, 1991).

Sporothrix schenkii

Pulmonary **sporotrichosis** is uncommon. Clinically, it may mimic tuberculosis, but there are no specific signs or symptoms.

Farley et al (1991) described finding **multiple, small** (2–4 μm) **ovoid, eosinophilic intracytoplasmic yeast in**

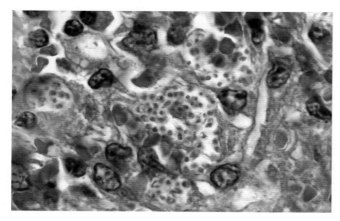

Figure 19-45   Histoplasmosis: Numerous tiny dot-like yeast with clear halos are seen here engulfed by histiocytes in the spleen. They measure about 2 μm (oil immersion).

macrophages of Papanicolaou-stained sputum from two patients with culture-confirmed sporotrichosis. Gori et al (1997) reported making this diagnosis by sputum cytology in an HIV-infected patient.

The yeast has a nonstaining cell wall, giving the appearance of a thin halo. They closely resemble *Histoplasma capsulatum,* from which they may be differentiated by their tendency to form **elongated, budding cigar bodies 2 to 3 μm thick and up to 10 μm in length.** Hyphae formation at body temperature is unusual. This fungus should not be confused with *Candida albicans,* which is extracellular and often forms pseudohyphae (see below).

Rhinosporidium seeberi

Rhinosporidiosis is primarily an infection of the nasal mucosa and upper respiratory tract, endemic in parts of India, Central, and South America. In tissues, the **fungus is in the form of a large sphere or sporangium measuring 25 to 300 μm in diameter. The sporangium has a thick homogeneous wall and clear cytoplasm containing many small endospores.** The fungus cannot be cultured, and diagnosis requires direct examination of tissue or cell samples. Gori and Scasso (1994) reported cytologic findings in two cases.

Opportunistic Fungi

The opportunistic fungi that are normally found as saprophytes may become pathogenic in debilitated or immunocompromised patients. Masses of such fungi may inhabit bronchi as **fungus balls (mycetomas)** for prolonged periods, and may cause significant atypias of the bronchial lining that can lead to an erroneous diagnosis of cancer, as illustrated below. The error may be compounded by the radiologic presentation of a single pulmonary lesion mimicking cancer.

Fungi of the class ***Phycomycetes,*** which include ***Aspergillus*** and ***Mucor*** species, are widely distributed in nature and can produce an alarming and often **deadly form of pneumonia** in susceptible individuals. They have a propensity to invade pulmonary vessels, thereby causing infarction, necrosis, and abscess formation **(phycomycosis).** Organs such as the **orbit** and **brain** can be infected as well. This dramatic clinical picture with its ominous prognosis, has now been recognized as a **fairly frequent complication of intensive multiagent chemotherapy** of cancer and **in AIDS** patients. Chest x-rays may show pneumonic consolidation, solitary or multiple nodules or masses, and cavitation with or without intracavitary masses (mycetomas) (McAdams et al, 1997).

Candida albicans (Monilia or Thrush)

Budding yeast and/or **pseudohyphae** of Candida may be observed in specimens taken from the **oral cavity** or **vagina** where the warm, moist environment provides ideal growth conditions (see Chaps. 10, 15, and 21). In well patients, it is usually considered an innocuous tenant. In immunosuppressed or debilitated patients, and not infrequently in terminal cancer patients, **it may become invasive and dissem-**

inated, causing urinary tract and pulmonary infections (Fig. 19-46), and sometimes septicemia with endocarditis. Its presentation in sputum and other pulmonary specimens is as described in other sites (see the chapters cited above).

Pseudohyphae of monilia must be differentiated from hyphae of *Trichoderma* sp, a common contaminant (Fig. 19-46B).

Aspergillus Species (Aspergillosis)

Aspergillus may produce a **diffuse pulmonary infection or solitary lung lesions (so-called solitary aspergilloma),** observed mainly in debilitated and AIDS patients. It has a strong tendency to invade blood vessels with infarction and necrosis of tissues, and cavitation harboring a fungus ball (mycetoma). Early cytologic diagnosis of aspergillosis leading to effective treatment may be life-saving.

Microscopic Features

The **rigid, thick, brown, septate hyphae of the fungus** are readily identified when present in sputum or bronchial wash specimens (Fig. 19-47A). The **hyphae branch at an angle of approximately 45°,** one of the features that differentiates this fungus from the *Mucor* species (see below). Under proper aerobic conditions, **fruiting heads or conidiospores** will be formed (Fig. 19-47B).

A characteristic feature of aspergillosis, mainly with the species *Aspergillus niger,* is the formation of calcium oxalate crystals, first reported in cytologic material by Reyes et al (1979). The crystals, which may be observed in sputum, bronchial washings, BAL, and pleural fluid are colorless, sheaf-shaped structures that are strongly birefringent under polarized light. Presence of the crystals alone, even if the organism cannot be identified, is highly suggestive of aspergillosis. The **differential diagnosis** includes the **rhomboid, birefringent crystals of barium sulfate,** once used as a roentgenographic contrast medium (Shahar et al, 1994), and the very rare **intracellular calcium crystals** observed by Vigorita et al (1979) in a patient with tuberculosis.

Thick-walled bronchiectatic or abscess cavities containing fungus balls (mycetomas) (Fig. 19-47C) may be surfaced by atypical metaplastic squamous epithelium (Fig. 19-47D) or ragged reactive hyperplastic basal epithelium (Fig. 19-47E,F).

Mucor Species (Mucormycosis)

This family of fungi, like aspergillus, is **capable of invading blood vessel walls and causing vascular thromboses and infarcts** (mucormycosis). Its principal representative is *Mucor,* but several other related fungi may cause disease (Johnston, 1992). Infection with *Mucor* occurs in diabetics and in debilitated or immunocompromised patients.

The fungi are recognized by **broad, ribbon-like, non-septate hyphae of variable diameter** that branch at 90° (Fig. 19-48). Unlike *Aspergillus,* the hyphae are wavy and folded. The organism has been identified in sputum, bronchial brushings, and BAL.

Pneumocystis carinii

Pneumocystis carinii, a ubiquitous organism, has assumed a major role in pulmonary pathology and cytology since the onset of AIDS. Because of its microscopic appearance, the organism was long considered to be a protozoan parasite, although its molecular biologic features now indicate that it is a fungus (Edman et al, 1988). The mature organism forms **small cysts,** measuring 4 to 6 μm in diameter, **containing tiny trophozoites** that, upon rupture of the cyst, are released, and in turn, mature to form new cysts. Before the onset of AIDS, **pneumonia caused by *P. carinii*** was only occasionally observed in **debilitated infants and immunocompromised adults.** Today, it is often the **first and dominant major complication of AIDS.** The clinical presentation of *P. carinii* pneumonia is highly variable, ranging from minimal pulmonary infiltrate to rapidly progressive and extensive pneumonia. Because recovery depends on prompt treatment, rapid diagnosis is essential.

Once the disease is suspected in an immunodeficient patient, either because of respiratory symptoms or clinical signs, BAL specimens are generally recommended for diagnosis (Stover et al, 1984; Broaddus et al, 1985). Bronchial

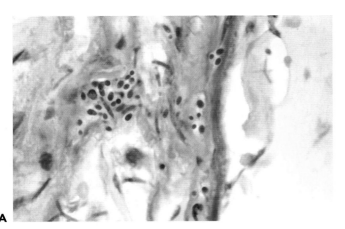
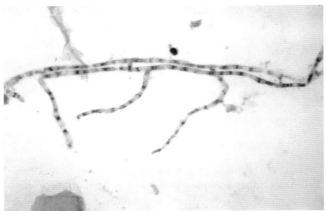

A **B**

Figure 19-46 *A. Candida.* Spores and pseudohyphae growing in the bronchial mucosa. See other chapters for additional illustrations. *B. Trichophyton* sp, a common cause of dermatophycomycosis and a contaminant in saliva resembling candida pseudohyphae (*A,B*: High magnification).

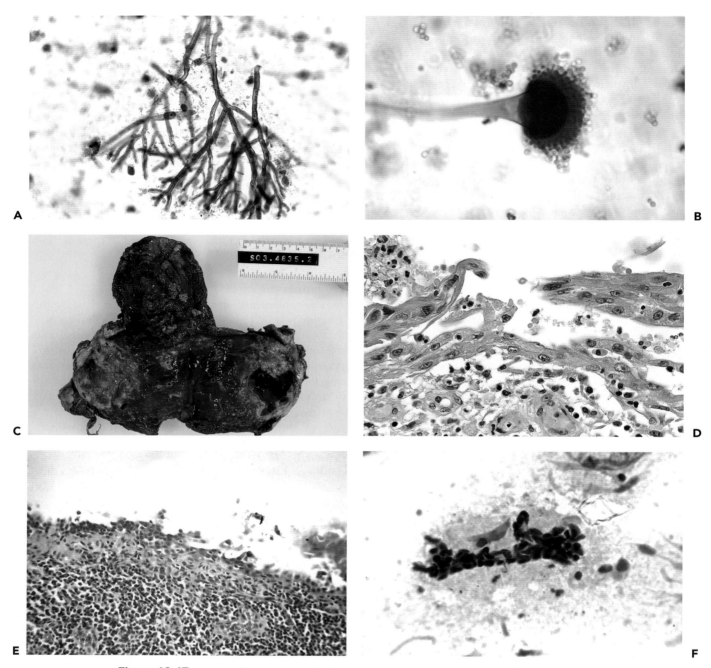

Figure 19-47 Aspergillus. A. Aspergillus in sputum showing septate, rather rigid hyphae branching at an acute angle. B. Fruiting head of aspergillus identified at autopsy, a response to aerobic conditions. (Case courtesy of Dr. M. B. Zaman.) C. Thick-walled abscess cavity with aspergilloma. Both halves of the cavity are shown. D. Atypical squamous metaplasia of the cavity wall shown in C. E. Markedly inflamed wall of another bronchiectatic cavity containing an aspergillus fungus ball (aspergilloma). The lumen is lined by irregular reactive basal epithelial cells. Elsewhere, there was marked basal cell hyperplasia. F. A cluster of small, dark, tightly packed basal epithelial cells in bronchial washings from the same patient prior to surgery. The cells are consistent with origin from the lining epithelium illustrated in E. (B: High magnification.) (E and F from Koss and Richardson, 1955.)

brushing is of limited additional value (Djamin et al, 1998). **BAL has almost completely replaced open lung biopsy, which was previously considered necessary for diagnosis.** While the organisms also may be found in spontaneous or induced sputum (Bigby et al, 1986), and in bronchial washings, they are generally few and difficult to identify.

Cytology

The **P. carinii organisms themselves are not easily identified in conventional smears** with the Papanicolaou or Diff-Quick stain, though their very likely presence is signaled by the finding of **finely vacuolated or foamy proteinaceous alveolar casts** in bronchial wash specimens (Naimey and

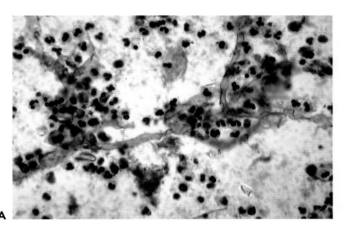

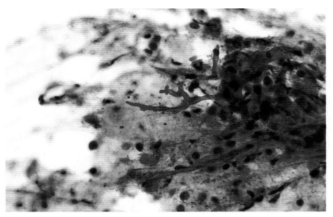

A B

Figure 19-48 **Mucormycosis.** *A.* Bronchial aspirate with mucormycosis in a patient with malignant lymphoma. *B.* Mucormycosis in brushing cytology of upper respiratory tract from an immunosuppressed patient with kidney transplant. The hyphae are folded and wavy, flat and broad compared with aspergillus, and nonseptate. They branch at right angles compared to the rigid, acute angle branching of aspergillus. (*A,B:* High magnification.)

Wuerker, 1995). In the proper clinical setting, these casts are essentially diagnostic of *Pneumocystis* infection (Fig. 19-49A). The cysts, which are unstained by conventional cytology stains, account for the vacuoles found in the casts. They are **spherical, oval, or cup-shaped structures with one flat surface, measuring 4 to 6 μm in diameter. Within the cysts, one or two tiny dot-like trophozoites or sporozoites, measuring 0.5 to 1 μm in diameter, may be seen** (Sun and Chess, 1986). The trophozoites that are released

from a cyst appear as numerous small dots. **The walls of the cysts and the trophozoites** are stained and readily identified by the Grocott methenamine silver (GMS) or Gram-Weigert stain (Fig. 19-49B,C).

P. carinii also can be visualized in unstained or Papanicolaou-stained slides by their **bright yellow fluorescence** under the fluorescence microscope (Ghali et al, 1984; Chandra et al, 1988), but this diagnostic technique is seldom used. It should be noted that **the walls of cryptococci also**

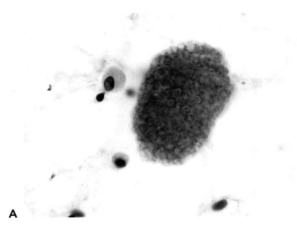

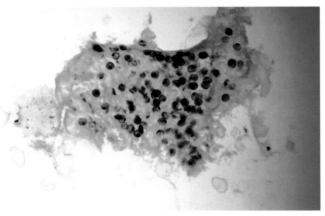

A B

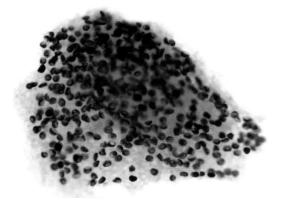

Figure 19-49 *Pneumocystis carinii.* *A.* Bronchial wash specimen showing a proteinaceous cast of an alveolus containing many tiny vacuoles. The vacuoles are due to the presence of unstained Pneumocystis cysts. The Grocott methenamine silver stain (*B*) or Gram-Weigert stain (*C*) may be used to stain the cysts.

C

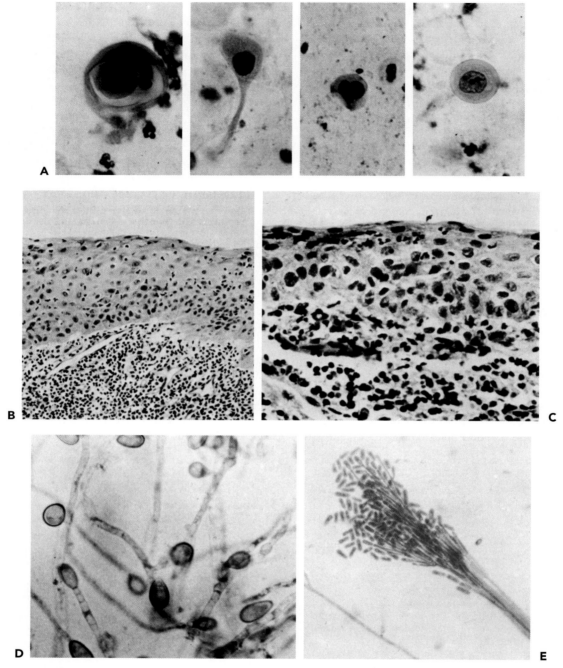

Figure 19-50 *Allescheria boydii.* Pulmonary mycetoma caused by *Allescheria boydii.* A. Composite photograph of cell abnormalities found in the patient's sputum. These were thought to represent squamous cancer. Cyst lining, partly well differentiated (*B*) and partly atypical squamous epithelium (*C*). The causative organism: conidia on conidiophores (*D*) and a tuft of conidiophores (*E*). (From Louria DB, et al. Pulmonary mycetoma due to *Allescheria boydii.* Arch Intern Med 117:748-751, 1966.) (*D*: oil immersion.)

are fluorescent (Sun and Chess, 1986), but the size and configuration of the *P. carinii* organisms are quite different. A number of **monoclonal antibodies to *P. carinii*** are now available for immunocytologic identification of the organisms (Kovacs et al, 1986; Blumenfeld and Kovacs, 1988; Elvin et al, 1988). Kovacs et al (1988) reported over 90% sensitivity and 100% specificity in the immunocytologic diagnosis of *P. carinii* in induced sputum samples. The more sensitive **PCR** technique has been described recently by the same group (Olsson, 1996); but it may be too sensitive, picking up cases in which these ubiquitous organisms are present without infection. In a comparison of immunofluorescence and PCR with direct staining techniques, Armbruster et al (1995) favored a combination of the **Diff-Quick stain and the fluorescent dye, Fungifluor.** For the present, we find the **methenamine silver staining technique** on **BAL** specimens to be our diagnostic method of choice.

***P. carinii* trophozoites must be differentiated from**

histoplasma, which does not form cysts, has a more uniformly round configuration, and does not present in clusters. Because histoplasma elicits a granulomatous reaction, it is very rarely seen in sputum or BAL specimens. The differential diagnosis is more important in histologic sections than in cytologic samples.

Alternaria

This species was discussed as a contaminant (see above). It may be a cause of hypersensitivity pneumonitis in wood-pulp workers (Schleuter et al, 1972) and can rarely cause pulmonary granuloma (Lobritz et al, 1979).

Cytology of Mycetomas

Mycetomas are fungus balls lodged in a bronchiectatic cavity. The markedly inflamed, thick wall of an aspergilloma cavity (see Fig. 19-47C) can simulate a cavitating carcinoma on x-ray. The **epithelial lining of such a cavity** may undergo reactive basal cell hyperplasia and squamous metaplasia with **marked atypia that may lead to a diagnostic error in cytologic samples.** Figures 19-47E and F illustrate an early case in which cells shed from the reactive basal cell hyperplasia surfacing an aspergilloma cavity were mistakenly interpreted as small-cell carcinoma (SSC).

In our experience, the most striking cytologic abnormalities were seen in a case of pulmonary mycetoma caused by **Allescheria boydii,** reported by Louria et al (1966). This patient with an unusual, clinically suspect solitary lesion of the right upper lobe of the lung had **markedly abnormal squamous cells in specimens of sputum** on several occasions, resulting in an erroneous diagnosis of squamous cancer (Fig. 19-50). The fungus ball lay within a solitary cyst that was lined in part by well-differentiated squamous epithelium and in part by highly atypical epithelium from which the abnormal cells undoubtedly originated. There are few safeguards to prevent such errors occurring from time to time.

Opportunistic Organisms as Contaminants

Opportunistic fungi and certain other organisms are common contaminants in specimens of sputum, some because they are saprophytic inhabitants of the mouth and orophar-

ynx and others derived from air or water during collection and processing. How very common they are was demonstrated by my colleague, Dr. M. B. Zaman, in an unpublished study of the sputum specimens obtained from men enrolled in the Early Lung Cancer study described in Chapter 20. Zaman examined the sputum specimens from 4,968 male cigarette smokers who were followed for 5 to 8 years with examinations of sputum cytology scheduled every 4 months. Ninety percent of the men had five or more sputum specimens examined. The most common organisms of interest were *Actinomyces, Candida,* and *Aspergillus* (Table 19-2); less commonly found organisms are listed in Table 19-3. Obviously, the mere presence of these organisms in sputum of a patient with or without symptoms of pulmonary disease is no guarantee that the organism is causative of infection.

PARASITES

Amoebiasis

Entamoeba histolytica was identified in sputum by Kenney et al (1975) in a case of amoebiasis involving the lung. The parasite was identified by its characteristic nucleus and

---

TABLE 19-3

FUNGI AND OTHER ORGANISMS UNCOMMONLY FOUND IN SPUTUM SPECIMENS OF 4,968 CLINICALLY WELL CIGARETTE-SMOKING MEN

Organism	No. men with organism in sputum
Aspergillus	73
Mucor	5
Sporotrich	1
Geotrich	2
Alternaria	11
Algae	8
Unclassified	11
Total	111

TABLE 19-2

OPPORTUNISTIC ORGANISMS COMMONLY FOUND IN SPUTUM SPECIMENS OF CIGARETTE-SMOKING MEN

Organism in sputum	No. men with opportunistic organisms	
	With lung cancer (154)	No lung cancer (4814)
Actinomyces	145 (94%)	4586 (95%)
Candida	61 (40%)	1605 (33%)
Aspergillus	5 (3%)	68 (1.4%)

phagocytized erythrocytes (Fig. 19-51). Other usually saprophytic amoebae have been recovered in sputum and in BAL specimens from immunocompromised patients (Newsome et al, 1992).

Trichomoniasis

Trichomonas buccalis (T. elongatus) is a common inhabitant of the oral cavity in conditions of poor hygiene. Walton and Bacharach (1963) reported finding trichomonads in three specimens from the respiratory tract, but did not classify them further. It is not known whether the organisms were an oral contaminant. (See also a report by Osbome et al, 1984.) Trichomonads are described in detail in Chapter 10.

Strongyloidiasis

The larval form of the small nematode *Strongyloides stercoralis* (threadworm) penetrates the victim's skin and achieves wide circulation through the bloodstream before maturing and settling in the small intestine. **Autoinfection by larvae produced in the intestine is common and accounts for the hyperinfective forms of this disease,** usually under poor hygienic conditions and in the immunodeficient patient. The case described by Kenney and Webber (1974) occurred in an immunocompetent person, but the 32 fatal cases described by Purtilo et al (1974) were in patients with a wide variety of disorders including malignant tumors, burns, radiation exposure, and other debilitating diseases in which the common denominator was reduced cell-mediated immunity. It must be emphasized that only two people in this group of patients had blood eosinophilia.

Cytology

There are several reports of cytologic diagnosis of strongyloidiasis in sputum, summarized by Johnston (1992). Examination of **sputum** may lead to early diagnosis and treatment of this potentially fatal disorder. In one striking example that we observed, the **fresh sputum specimen was quivering** due to movement of the **filariform larvae** in the case of a patient with hyperinfective disease (Fig. 19-52A,B). The larvae have a worm-like configuration, with a thick, rounded forward end and a characteristic **V-shaped notch at the sharply pointed tail end of the filiform.** The noninfective **rhabditiform larvae** with cross striations of the body may also be recognized (Fig. 19-52C) (Humphreys and Hieger, 1979).

Ancylostoma Duodenale (Hookworm)

Acute superinfection with hookworm is uncommon, and hookworm larvae in sputum have not been reported to date. A variety of filariform organisms not further identified but commonly present in drinking water may closely resemble them (see Fig. 19-18B,C). With knowledge of the clinical setting, there should be no difficulty in recognizing these as contaminants.

Echinococcus

Lung cysts caused by the larval form of the **tapeworm *Echinococcus granulosus* or *E. multilocularis* (hydatid cysts)** are endemic in Europe and Asia. Oztek et al (1997) found scolices of the tapeworm in Papanicolaou-stained sputum or bronchial washings/brushings from 11 of 111 patients in Turkey with histologically proven hydatid cysts, and hooklets in specimens from 26 patients. The disease is being seen with increased frequency in the US. Allen and Fulmer (1972) reported identifying the **scolex of the parasite with its characteristic hooklets in the sputum** of a patient with the disease and two cases were reported by Tomb and Matossian (1976) (Fig. 19-53A). A case diagnosed by FNA biopsy of lung was reported by Koss et al (1992).

Giardia lamblia

The presence of this gastrointestinal parasite in **BAL** fluid was reported by Stevens and Vermeire (1981). It is commonly found in biopsies of duodenum, and may be seen in cytologic specimens (see Chap. 24).

Lung Flukes

Paragonimus westermani is a common invader of the lung in parts of East Asia, namely in Korea, parts of China, Thailand, and Indonesia. The infection is acquired by eating uncooked, infected shellfish. The **pulmonary lesions clinically resemble chronic tuberculosis** and may form **cavities** that communicate with the bronchus. Generalized spread of the infection to other organs, including the brain, may occur and can be fatal. The parasite is identified by **finding ova in the sputum,** which is typically blood-tinged and contains many leukocytes, including **eosinophils,** and **Charcot-Leyden crystals. The ova measure about 100** μm in their long axis, and have a thick, yellowish-brown,

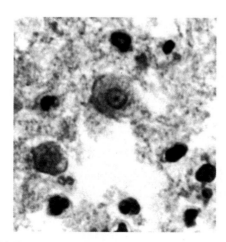

Figure 19-51 *Entamoeba histolytica.* Cell block of sputum in a patient with intestinal amoebiasis and lung abscess. The organism may be identified by the characteristic round eccentric nucleus, with a central karyosome and finely granular nuclear material. (From Kenney M, et al. Amebiasis. Unusual location in lung. NY State J Med 75:1542-1543, 1975. © Medical School of the State of New York.)

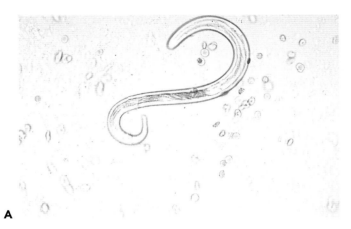

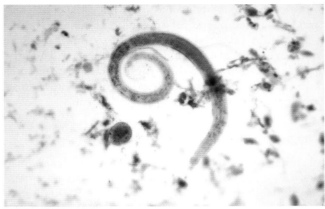

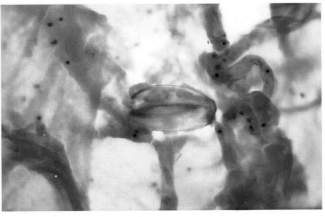

Figure 19-52 **Strongyloides stercoralis.** *A.* Unstained sputum specimen from a 69-year-old man with hyperinfection complicating lung cancer. The microfilaria were readily visualized in sputum that was literally quivering on the slide due to their vigorous movement. *B.* Stained specimen. One can just make out the blunt, rounded, forward end and bifid sharp tail. *C.* In another patient, the rhabditiform larvae were found in sputum (and in spinal fluid). Note the cross-striations. (*B,C:* H&E Stain.)

oval shell with a more thickened, distinctly flattened end or operculum (Fig. 19-53B).

Willie and Snyder (1977) reported finding the ova in bronchial washings, and McCallum (1975) in fluid from a lung cyst. Rangdaeng et al (1992) identified the ova in a **FNA of a lung abscess** from a 19-year-old Nigerian woman with a history of prior treatment for lymphoma of the breast.

Microfilariae

Filariasis is a common disease in developing countries, but rare in the US and Europe. Avasthi et al (1991) reported

a patient from India in whom the diagnosis of Bancroftian microfilariasis was made by FNA of the lung from a 25-year-old man who had coexisting pulmonary tuberculosis. See also reports by Anupindi et al (1993) and Walter et al (1983) describing various species of filariae in pulmonary material.

Dirofilariasis

Dirofilaria immitis, the dog heartworm, may be transmitted to humans by mosquitoes. The microfilaria are carried

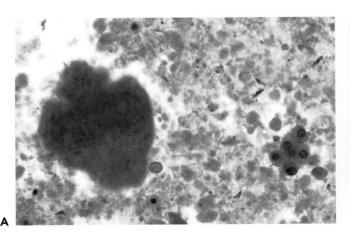

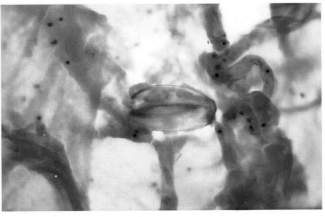

Figure 19-53 *A.* **Echinococcus granulosus.** Scolex with hooklets in an FNA specimen that penetrated the right lower lobe of lung and entered a hydatid cyst of the liver. *B.* ***Paragonimus westermani* ovum.** (Case courtesy of Nancy Morse.) (*A:* H&E stain; *A,B:* High magnification.)

through the venous circulation to the lung where they die, causing small **peripheral infarcts** and **granulomas.** Akaogi et al (1993) reported a case of pulmonary dirofilariasis in which transbronchial brushing cytology yielded **papillary bronchiolar epithelium with high nuclear/cytoplasmic ratio, macronucleoli and nuclear irregularity mimicking carcinoma.** The organism was not identified.

Microsporidia

Intestinal microsporidiosis caused by tiny intracellular parasites of the **Microsporidians** family is an important cause of **debilitating diarrhea** and weight loss in immunodeficient **AIDS patients (Weber et al, 1994).** The organism rarely involves the lung and only a small number of such cases have been reported in patients with disseminated disease (Lanzafame et al, 1997; Scaglia et al, 1998; Schwartz et al, 1993). Remadi et al (1995) identified **microsporidian spores, measuring about 1.5 μm, within macrophages in BAL specimens from an AIDS patient.** The tiny spores are not easily seen in Papanicolaou-stained preparations, but may be visualized with a fluorescent mycology stain or by immunofluorescence antibody staining.

OTHER BENIGN DISEASES AND CONDITIONS OF THE RESPIRATORY TRACT

There are a few other conditions of the respiratory tract in which cytologic techniques may contribute to the diagnosis and treatment.

Alveolar Proteinosis

Pulmonary alveolar proteinosis, first described by Rosen et al in 1958, is now understood to be a disease of impaired macrophage function. The disease may be primary and idiopathic or secondary to infections, hematologic disorders, inhaled fumes, or inorganic dusts. In its most common acquired form, it is an autoimmune disorder caused by antibodies targeting cell surface receptors for granulocyte-macrophage colony stimulating factor, which is expressed on alveolar macrophages. Most patients present with insidious onset of progressive exertional dyspnea and cough; the 5-year survival rate is about 75% with deaths due to respiratory failure or uncontrolled infection. **Biopsies of the lung show preserved alveolar architecture with alveoli filled by phospholipid-rich proteinaceous material** that ultimately blocks respiratory exchange and may lead to the death of the patient (Fig. 19-54A).

There is good evidence that the material filling the alveoli is surfactant, probably due to defective removal by alveolar macrophages (Golde et al, 1976) rather than excess production by type II pneumocytes (see Trapnell et al, 2003, for a recent review). BAL has been the treatment of choice, and it provides symptomatic relief, improved physiologic and radiologic findings, and increased survival.

Sputum of patients with pulmonary alveolar proteinosis

has been studied by Carlson and Mason (1960), Burkhalter et al (1996), Mermolja et al (1994), and by the late Dr. M. Wilson Toll in our laboratories (unpublished data). The presence of **chunks or globules of amorphous or fibrillar PAS-positive proteinaceous casts** containing or associated with cellular debris, macrophages and inflammatory cells is **suggestive of this disease in the proper clinical setting.** It is not diagnostic, and Toll has pointed out that **very similar material may be observed in sputum of patients with other chronic lung disorders** (Fig. 19-54B).

The diagnosis considered clinically can be confirmed by BAL (Martin et al, 1980). BAL specimens are opaque, muddy or milky in appearance. Smears and cell block sections contain granular, lipoproteinaceous, eosinophilic material that may be mistaken for mucus or casts of *P. carinii.* It is **brightly stained in the PAS reaction,** with or without diastase digestion, and contains **large, foamy alveolar macrophages with PAS-positive cytoplasmic inclusions** and a few inflammatory cells of other types. Surfactant proteins have been demonstrated by immunohistochemical stains (Wang et al, 1997; Schoch et al, 2002); and multilamellar osmiophilic bodies and tubular myelin, similar to condensed surfactant, have been demonstrated in the alveolar material by electron microscopy (Sosolik et al, 1998).

Malakoplakia

Malakoplakia is a rare enzymatic disorder of **macrophages that have an impaired ability to process and digest coliform bacteria, which accumulate in lysosomes.** The peculiar granulomas that characterize the disease are composed of epithelioid histiocytes with abundant cytoplasm that contains **concentrically laminated bodies (Michaelis-Guttmann bodies),** rich in calcium and iron, formed on enlarged lysosomes containing residual bacteria. The granulomas are located in the bronchial wall subjacent to the epithelium and may be identified in **bronchial brushings that disrupt the epithelium, releasing characteristic epithelioid macrophages with Michaelis-Guttmann bodies** (Fig. 19-55C). Malakoplakia was first observed in the urinary bladder as umbilicated soft yellow plaques (from Greek, *malakos* = soft, hence, soft plaque). It is described in detail in Chapter 22. Two cases of bronchial malakoplakia that we encountered are illustrated in Figure 19-55. Schwartz et al (1990) and Shin et al (1999) reported cases diagnosed by transbronchial biopsy; and Sughayer et al (1997) and Lambert et al (1997) reported cases diagnosed by percutaneous FNA. The causative organism in all these cases was ***Rhodococcus equi.***

Rheumatoid Granuloma

Rheumatoid granulomas may occur in the lung and pleura. Although there is a classic cytologic presentation of rheumatoid pleurisy in effusions (see Chap. 25), only very limited information is available on the cytologic findings in sputum or bronchoalveolar specimens. Johnston and Frable (1979) described one patient in whom bronchial washings disclosed necrotic material and cells of uncertain derivation, possibly

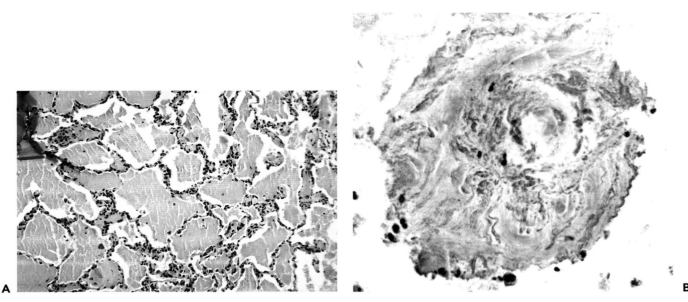

Figure 19-54 **Pulmonary alveolar proteinosis.** *A.* Histologic section showing structurally intact alveoli filled with dense protein precipitate. There is very little cellular reaction. *B.* Protein cast, mimicking proteinosis. Proteinaceous material observed in a cell block of sputum (high magnification). There was no evidence of pulmonary proteinosis, which is a frequent finding.

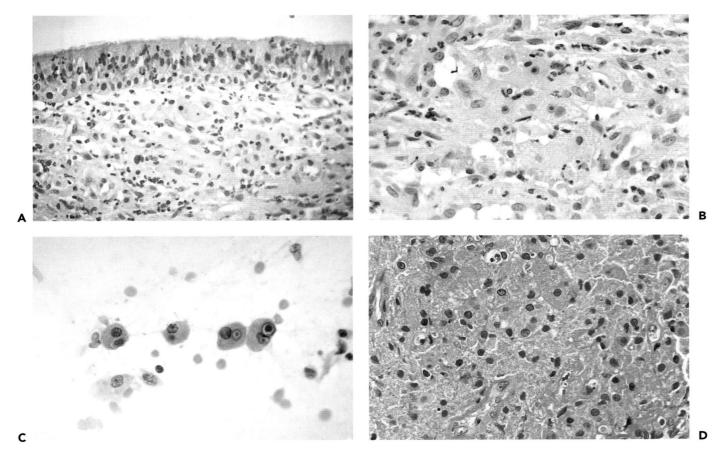

Figure 19-55 **Malakoplakia.** *A.* Subepithelial bronchial nodule composed of large epithelioid histiocytes with abundant eosinophilic cytoplasm. *B.* Careful inspection at higher magnification reveals Michaelis-Guttmann bodies within the cytoplasm of some epithelioid cells. *C.* Bronchial brush cytology specimen showing epithelioid cells with intracytoplasmic Michaelis-Guttmann bodies. *D.* Bronchial malakoplakia in a 15-year-old girl with congenital AIDS. A Gram stain showed the bacteria *Rhodococcus equi* within the epithelioid histiocytes. (*A–C:* Courtesy of Dr. Timothy Greaves, Los Angeles, CA.)

epithelioid macrophages. Kolarz et al (1993) reported that patients with rheumatoid arthritis had an increased number of activated (HLA-DR+) helper (CD4) lymphocytes in BAL specimens, which was most marked in patients with lung involvement.

Gaucher's Disease

Gaucher's disease is a **familial disorder of lipid metabolism,** caused by a defective enzyme, glucocerebrosidase, resulting in an accumulation of faulty glucocerebrosides in various organs, mainly the liver, spleen, and bone marrow. The disease may be observed in infants, juveniles, or adults and is diagnosed by recognition of the characteristic large macrophages that store the cerebrocide.

Gaucher's disease involving the lung was described by Schneider et al (1977) and diagnosed by aspiration biopsy of a pulmonary infiltrate by Johnston and Frable (1979). Carson et al (1994) identified Gaucher cells in a BAL specimen from a child. **The characteristic Gaucher cells in this type of specimen resemble mononuclear pulmonary macrophages with small eccentric nuclei and abundant striated and finely vacuolated cytoplasm.** An example of Gaucher cells is illustrated in Chapter 38. They may be superficially similar to the foam cells of lipid pneumonia but have **striated and strongly PAS-positive cytoplasm** (due to accumulated cerebroside), and numerous irregular lysosomes by electron microscopy.

Inflammatory Pseudotumor (Sclerosing Hemangioma)

These uncommon benign lesions form a well-delineated pulmonary mass that can mimic lung cancer on x-ray. They occur mainly in adolescents and young adults. There are several histologic variants: some of the lesions are composed predominantly of proliferating fibroblasts **(benign fibrous histiocytoma type),** and some predominantly of inflammatory cells, often with a dominant plasma cell component **(plasmacytoma type).** This diversity of histologic patterns

resulted in a number of different names attached to these lesions, among which are **sclerosing hemangioma, benign fibrous histiocytoma, plasmacytoma, and granulomatous inflammatory lesions.**

We have observed several examples of this lesion diagnosed by percutaneous lung aspiration (Koss et al, 1992). Smears of the aspirates from the **benign fibrous histiocytoma type** disclosed **loosely structured bundles of slender fibroblasts and single, slender fusiform cells,** accompanied by scattered inflammatory cells (Fig. 19-56A,B). In the **plasmacellular type,** the smears disclosed mainly **plasma cells in company of macrophages and scattered fibroblasts.** Somewhat similar observations were reported in a needle aspirate by Bakhos et al (1998), and in bronchial brushing cytology by Usuda et al (1990). In the bronchial wash specimen from a case presenting as an endobronchial polyp, Devouassoux-Shisheboran et al (2004) reported numerous clusters and sheets of small to medium, mononuclear cells with round or oval nuclei, dispersed chromatin, inconspicuous nucleoli, and scanty cyanophilic cytoplasm. Numerous foamy macrophages were also present.

Follicular (Lymphocytic) Bronchitis

Follicular bronchitis is uncommon and of unknown etiology, but presumably reflects a chronic inflammatory process. It is characterized by **lymphoid deposits in the submucosa of the bronchi,** similar to follicular cervicitis.

Bronchial brushing may remove fragments of lymphoid tissue, and the resulting smear shows **dense aggregates of lymphocytes of varying degrees of maturity** (see Fig. 19-11D). Mitotic figures may be observed among follicle center cells. Similar clusters of lymphocytes may be dislodged from tonsillar tissue, and it may be difficult to exclude this possibility. The cytologic presentation is essentially that of follicular cervicitis (see Chap. 10). The **differential diagnosis comprises small (oat) cell carcinoma, lymphoma and leukemia,** none of which forms equally dense aggregates of lymphoid cells in a mixed pattern of immature and mature lymphocytic cells.

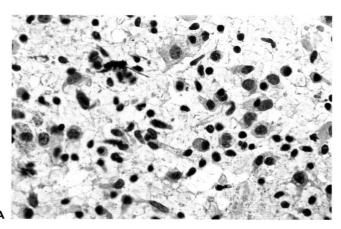
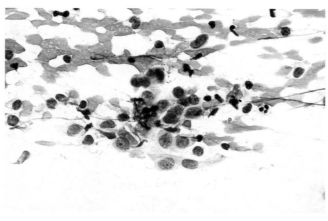

A
B

Figure 19-56 Inflammatory pseudotumor. *A,B.* An FNA of a pseudotumor of lung in a 40-year-old man demonstrates a mixed pattern of spindly fibroblasts, histiocytes, and variable numbers of plasma cells. The appearance is that of a chronic inflammatory process (high magnification).

THERMAL INJURY

Acute Thermal Injury

The effects of inhaling hot gases and smoke have been studied by Ambiavagar et al (1974) in burn victims. In severely burned patients, there was extensive necrosis ("burning") of cells. The **mucus** aspirated from the respiratory tract of such patients was **thick.** There was **marked destruction of ciliated cells.** In less severely burned patients, the abnormalities were less marked, and normal ciliated cells were present next to injured cells. **The degree of cytologic damage correlated well with prognosis;** patients with severe cellular damage either died or survived only with the greatest difficulty. Patients with relatively slight damage recovered. **Mitochondrial calcification** was noted in ciliated cells of burn patients by electron microscopy (Drut, 1998).

Cooney et al (1972) reported abnormal squamous cells in the sputum of 36 burn patients admitted to a burn center. The cells were enlarged, polygonal, oval, or spindly, often multinucleated and provided with hyperchromatic nuclei. They probably represented atypical squamous metaplasia of bronchial lining. Evidence of **viral pneumonitis** (herpes and cytomegalovirus) and **moniliasis** were seen in five of those patients.

Chronic Thermal Injury

Ambiavagar et al (1974) followed a few burn patients by repeated cytologic sampling from the respiratory tract and reported an increase of squamous cells in specimens aspirated from the trachea and bronchi as the patients recovered. They suggested that **squamous metaplasia was taking place** in the injured tracheobronchial tree. We observed **atypical squamous metaplasia of bronchial mucosa in sputum and bronchial brush specimens from firemen exposed to smoke inhalation;** the lesion was reversible.

TREATMENT EFFECTS

Certain forms of therapy, especially radiation and cancer chemotherapy, may cause significant changes within the respiratory tract as in tissues of other organs, notably in the uterine cervix and urinary bladder (see Chaps. 18 and 22). The abnormalities of bronchial cells and pneumocytes type II observed after radiotherapy are similar to irradiation-induced atypias in other cell types. Both the squamous and respiratory epithelia may be greatly affected, and they may produce cells so abnormal as to suggest the presence of a malignant tumor.

Radiation Therapy

Squamous Epithelium

Acute radiation changes may be observed in squamous cells in sputum for several weeks or months after completion of irradiation and care must be taken that they not be mistaken for residual squamous carcinoma. Much of this is due to the effect of irradiation on oropharyngeal epithelium, but metaplastic squamous mucosa of the tracheobronchial tree also may be affected. Radiation atypia has been observed not only as a result of direct irradiation, but also when the target of therapy is in the neck or thorax. The mechanism is unknown but likely due to scattering of the radiant energy from nearby target tissues (abscopal effect). Minimal cellular changes may persist for months or years after the acute effects regress.

Cytology

The radiation changes induced in squamous epithelium are not unlike those seen in the female genital tract (see Chap. 18). Of these, **marked cellular enlargement** associated with proportionate enlargement of the nucleus is of prime interest, because it may be mistaken for cancer. **The enlarged nuclei of huge irradiated squamous cells are often wrinkled or wavy, and have a peculiar "empty" look with very finely granular chromatin** (Fig. 19-57A). Other changes include **multinucleation, prominent nucleoli** (Fig. 19-57B), and **nuclear or cytoplasmic vacuolization. Nuclear hyperchromasia with cytoplasmic keratinization may be indistinguishable from squamous carcinoma.** Figure 19-57C shows irradiation atypia simulating a squamous cancer pearl in sputum of a 20-year-old man following irradiation to the chest for metastatic choriocarcinoma.

Chronic radiation effects may be seen for many months after completion of treatment. The squamous cells show slight irregularity and mild hyperchromasia of nuclei, and cytoplasmic eosinophilia (Fig. 19-57D). The diagnosis is made only with knowledge of the history of prior irradiation.

Respiratory Epithelium

The acute effects of irradiation on respiratory epithelium may occasionally result in **nonspecific multinucleation of ciliated bronchial cells** described earlier (see Fig. 19-19A,B). **However, the most characteristic effect, strongly suggestive of irradiation, is marked enlargement of all cellular components with preservation of the nucleocytoplasmic ratio. These otherwise well-formed large bronchial cells have prominent nuclei, and either enlarged nucleoli or several large chromatin granules** (Fig. 19-58A). Multinucleation and intranuclear cytoplasmic inclusions or nuclear holes in the enlarged cells are very suggestive of irradiation effect (Fig. 19-58B). In extreme cases, **bizarre cellular forms** with cellular and nuclear enlargement may far exceed what is usually seen with carcinoma, and one should exercise great diagnostic caution even in the absence of a history of irradiation. In fact, **the finding of very bizarre giant cells is more commonly caused by radiation than by the uncommon giant cell carcinoma.** The history of irradiation warrants very careful search for remnants of the terminal bar or cilia, which may prevent an unwarranted diagnosis of cancer.

Chronic Radiation Injury

Radiation-induced changes in the lung parenchyma progress with time following completion of treatment, and

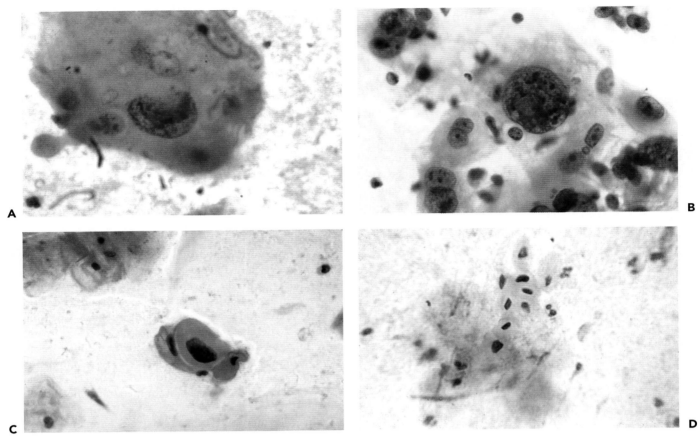

Figure 19-57 Acute irradiation effect on squamous epithelium. *A.* Sputum specimen from a young woman with Hodgkin's disease following irradiation to the neck and mediastinum. There is marked cellular and nuclear enlargement with loss of nuclear chromatin texture. This degree of cellular and nuclear enlargement is virtually pathognomonic of acute irradiation effect. The cell may be of oral mucosal origin and presumably was irradiated by scattering of the radiation beam. *B.* Cellular enlargement, multinucleation, nuclear vacuolization, and prominent chromocenters or nucleoli. *C.* Sputum specimen from a 20-year-old patient after irradiation to the lung for metastatic choriocarcinoma. This keratinized squamous pearl is indistinguishable from squamous carcinoma. *D.* **Late irradiation effect on squamous epithelium:** The cytologic pattern is nonspecific, and interpretation is based on clinical correlation with the known history of prior irradiation. There is cytoplasmic eosinophilia and slight nuclear enlargement with hyperchromasia. Note the strong similarity to radiation-induced atrophy and atypia in cervicovaginal smears. (*C:* oil immersion.)

often appear clinically and histologically out of proportion to the irradiation administered. In histologic sections, the initial marked enlargement of bronchial epithelial cells is accompanied by bronchial metaplasia of alveoli and/or hyperplasia of pneumocytes type II with proliferation of interstitial fibroblasts and progressive interstitial fibrosis (Fig. 19-58C). The presence of a few irradiated bronchial cells may be the only evidence of pulmonary parenchymal irradiation in such cases (Fig. 19-58D).

With the passage of time, there is **progressive diffuse interstitial pulmonary fibrosis** associated with metaplastic changes within the alveolar and bronchial lining epithelia. Enlargement of **pneumocytes type II** and **squamous metaplasia** are the dominant epithelial abnormalities.

Cytology

The late irradiation effects in sputum and bronchial brush specimens vary from minimal nonspecific atypias and squamous metaplasia, as is often seen in the absence of irradia-

tion (see Fig. 19-23), to **less common extreme degrees of atypical squamous metaplasia.** In this latter instance, **the cells of bronchial origin may show marked cytoplasmic eosinophilia, distortion of cell shapes, and nuclear hyperchromasia or pyknosis, combining to create a cytologic image mimicking epidermoid cancer.** The exfoliated cells are sometimes arranged in strips, consistent with origin in the bronchial epithelium.

Carcinoma Versus Radiation Effect

From time to time, the cytopathologist may be called upon to **determine whether or not there is residual viable carcinoma in patients undergoing irradiation for lung cancer. Acute radiation pneumonitis** is accompanied by pulmonary edema, desquamation of a great many **degenerated bronchoalveolar epithelial cells,** much necrosis, strands of smeared nuclear material, and an accumulation of leukocytes. In this material, it is nearly impossible to exclude the

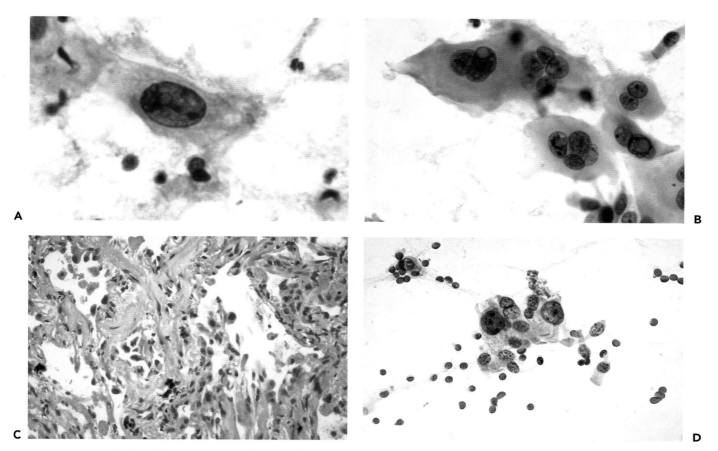

Figure 19-58   Acute irradiation effect on bronchial epithelium. *A.* Marked enlargement of bronchial cell with proportional enlargement of nucleus after 6,000 rad irradiation. *B.* Cellular enlargement, multinucleation, nuclear vacuolization and loss of chromatin structure. Cilia may be retained (oil immersion). **Late irradiation effect on lung.** *C.* Interstitial fibrosis is a late effect of irradiation, with hypertrophic alveolar epithelium and prominent nuclei in alveolar and stromal cells. *D.* Marked nuclear enlargement and hyperchromatic in a patient treated for lung cancer.

presence of rare cancer cells. Equally difficult in some cases, as noted above, is the differential diagnosis between marked radiation-induced atypical metaplasia and cancer, particularly when recurrence of irradiated squamous carcinoma is anticipated. **A good rule is to not make the diagnosis of cancer unless cancer cells not affected by irradiation are clearly identified at least 6 weeks after completing treatment.** That is usually the case if there is viable residual or recurrent carcinoma. The history of radiation should caution against the cytologic diagnosis of cancer on less-than-certain evidence.

Chemotherapy

Chemotherapy-induced histologic abnormalities of the bronchial epithelium were first reported by Weston and Guin in 1955, in children undergoing leukemia treatment. They observed nuclear abnormalities such as enlargement and hyperchromasia in normal epithelia. Similar histologic abnormalities have been noted in adult patients receiving chemotherapy, especially alkylating agents.

Busulfan

Busulfan (Myleran), an alkylating agent used for treating chronic myelogenous leukemia, is discussed in Chapter 18.

It is capable of inducing severe alterations in bronchial and alveolar epithelium, and in interstitial tissues of the lung (for summary of pertinent early literature, see Koss et al, 1965; Feingold and Koss, 1969). The pulmonary abnormalities received the name of **busulfan lung** (Heard and Cooke, 1968). Clinically, these patients are dyspneic because of **interstitial pulmonary fibrosis** that radiologically may mimic diffuse, lymphangitic spread of carcinoma.

Very large cells with correspondingly large, hyperchromatic or sometimes vesicular nuclei are seen in histologic sections of the bronchial epithelium (Fig. 19-59A), **bronchioles and alveoli** (Fig. 19-59B), and **are found in sputum** (Figs. 19-59C) and bronchial brush (Fig. 19-59D) specimens. The most severely damaged, abnormal cells are pneumocytes type II.

In the case of busulfan-induced atypias of the respiratory tract, as with drug-induced changes in the uterine cervix, the differential diagnosis with cancer may present a significant challenge. There is increasing evidence, as discussed in Chapter 18, that the changes induced by some of the alkylating agents are carcinogenic.

A case is on record of bronchogenic adenocarcinoma occurring in a patient receiving long-term busulfan therapy (Min and Gyorkey, 1968). Another such case seen by one

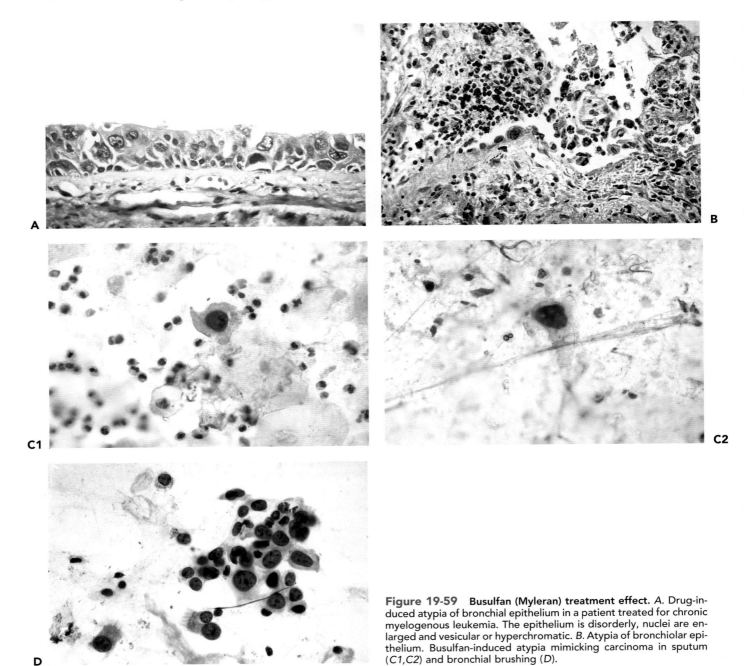

Figure 19-59   Busulfan (Myleran) treatment effect. *A.* Drug-induced atypia of bronchial epithelium in a patient treated for chronic myelogenous leukemia. The epithelium is disorderly, nuclei are enlarged and vesicular or hyperchromatic. *B.* Atypia of bronchiolar epithelium. Busulfan-induced atypia mimicking carcinoma in sputum (*C1,C2*) and bronchial brushing (*D*).

of us (LGK) was that of a 69-year-old man with chronic myelogenous leukemia who had been receiving busulfan therapy (4 mg/day) for 2½ years. He developed severe dyspnea, suggestive of acute busulfan lung. His sputum contained a moderate number of abnormal squamous cells suggestive of busulfan effect and other cells that were highly suggestive of carcinoma. This patient's chest radiograph showed only diffuse fibrosis with no localizing lesion, and he was not treated. At autopsy, a small, poorly differentiated squamous carcinoma was found in a busulfan lung. It should be noted that **busulfan is often administered to patients prior to bone marrow transplant** and may account for cellular abnormalities seen in some of those patients. Other changes caused by busulfan are described in Chapters 18 and 22.

Bleomycin

Bleomycin, an antibiotic with antineoplastic properties, has been used for several years in treating testicular tumors and squamous carcinomas of various organs. The drug induces **keratinization and death of squamous cancer cells,** which in turn, induces formation of **multinucleated macrophages that phagocytize keratin** (Burkhardt et al, 1976). The principal effect of the drug on the lung is the development of an interstitial pneumonia and interstitial fibrosis (Luna et al, 1972) that is **similar to busulfan lung except that cellular abnormalities are minimal** (Fig. 19-60A). Extensive squamous metaplasia of the bronchial lining is observed on occasion, and significant cytologic atypia has been observed when bleomycin is used in conjunction with other drugs in combination chemotherapy (Fig. 10-60B).

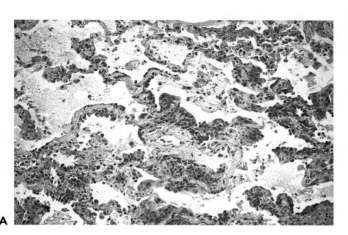

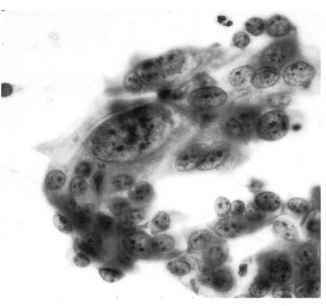

Figure 19-60   Bleomycin effect. *A.* Bleomycin treatment of lymphoma resulted in interstitial pulmonary fibrosis with only minimal alveolar epithelial hyperplasia. *B.* In combination with Chloromycetin, Bleomycin caused marked atypia of bronchial epithelium in a brush specimen.

Of interest, the interstitial fibrosis of Hamman-Rich syndrome also was associated with epithelial atypias in a report by Kern (1965) who classified cells as "suspicious" in 2 of 11 such patients.

Cyclophosphamide

Cyclophosphamide (Cytoxan), an alkylating agent widely used in treatment of neoplastic disease, is noted primarily for its effect on urothelium of the bladder (see Chap. 22). It may cause significant atypias of bronchial and alveolar epithelium as well. Figure 19-61A shows metaplasia and atypia of bronchoalveolar epithelium attributed to cyclophosphamide treatment in a woman with breast cancer. Bronchial cell atypia in a bronchial brush specimen of another patient receiving Cytoxan is shown in Figure 19-61B,C.

We observed diffuse pulmonary fibrosis in a patient receiving **cyclophosphamide** in large doses for 3 years. Several additional cases of this type have been recorded, summarized in early reports by Patel et al (1976) and Mark et al (1978).

A case report of pulmonary fibrosis and busulfan-like syndrome caused by **chlorambucil** (Leukeran) was described by Rose (1975). Cole et al (1978) reported alveolar lining cell dysplasia as well as interstitial pulmonary fibrosis in a patient who was treated with chlorambucil for polycythemia vera. Wada et al (1968) observed a statistically **significant increase in lung cancer among workers engaged in the manufacture of mustard gas,** which is closely related to nitrogen mustard, the prototype of all chemotherapeutic alkylating agents including cyclophosphamide and chlorambucil.

Methotrexate

This drug acts by inhibition of the enzyme folic acid reductase and is extensively used in the treatment of various

neoplastic diseases including **choriocarcinoma** and **certain leukemias.** It has also been used in the treatment of patients with **psoriasis, rheumatoid arthritis,** and other benign disorders. The drug causes liver abnormalities and occasionally pulmonary complications (Clarysse et al, 1969) in the form of **interstitial pneumonias** and apparently **granulomas** (Filip et al, 1971). Van der Veen et al (1995) described two **fatal cases of pulmonary fibrosis** in aged patients after low-dose methotrexate therapy for rheumatoid arthritis. Postmortem examination disclosed extensive pulmonary fibrosis, obliterative bronchiolitis and hyperplasia of type II pneumocytes. There are no known cytologic studies of these patients.

Carmustine (bis-Chloroethylnitrosourea [BCNU])

Nitrosoureas are a group of anticancer chemotherapeutic agents used extensively in the therapy of many malignant tumors including leukemias, lymphomas, melanomas, Ewing's tumor, various carcinomas, and brain tumors. Fatal interstitial pulmonary fibrosis has been reported by Holoye et al (1976).

One of our patients who died apparently as a **consequence of chemotherapy for a brain tumor had cytologic abnormalities in what we now believe to be reactive type II pneumocytes that were a perfect mimic of adenocarcinoma** (Fig. 19-62 A,B), **including cells in mitosis** (Fig.19-62C). The patient, whose death was attributed to viral pneumonia, had been treated with the chemotherapeutic drug, carmustine (BCNU). At autopsy, there was no evidence of tumor in the lung. There was interstitial pulmonary fibrosis and cell gigantism (Fig. 19-62D) that was first thought to represent drug effect but later attributed to viral pneumonia. It was probably due to the combined effect of the chemotherapeutic drug and viral infection. Additional

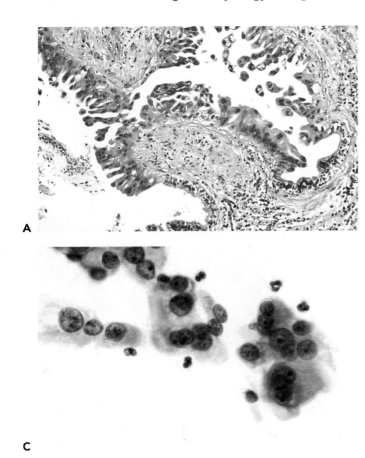

A

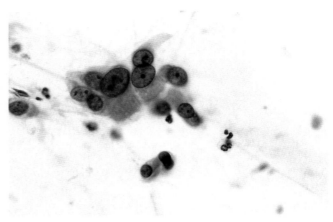

B

C

Figure 19-61 Cyclophosphamide (Cytoxan) effect. *A.* Histologic section of lung from a woman who had been receiving cyclophosphamide treatment for breast cancer and developed respiratory symptoms. There was atypical bronchial metaplasia of terminal bronchioles and alveolar epithelium. She did not have lung metastases. *B,C.* Bronchial brush cytology specimens from another patient on long-term cyclophosphamide treatment showing nuclear enlargement with prominent chromocenters and small nucleoli in bronchial cells.

experience is still required to ascertain the precise effects of this drug on the cytology of the lung.

Combination Chemotherapy

Single-drug chemotherapy is now the exception rather than the rule, increasing the likelihood of drug-induced cytologic atypias. Examples of bronchial cell abnormalities in a BAL specimen from a 22-year-old man on multidrug therapy for acute lymphocytic leukemia is illustrated in Figure 19-63A,B, and in squamous cells in sputum from another patient with Hodgkin's disease in Figure 19-63C. Bronchial epithelial atypia in a child on multidrug therapy for leukemia is shown in Figure 19-63 D. Complete and accurate clinical information is increasingly important in the interpretation of cytologic specimens.

Amiodarone

Amiodarone is representative of a new class of very potent antiarrhythmic drugs used to treat cardiac arrhythmias. The drug, taken over a number of years in large doses, may cause a **variety of toxic effects** involving a number of organs such as the skin, thyroid, liver, bone marrow, and others. In a certain proportion of patients, **lung lesions** may develop. The frequency of lung disease has been significantly reduced with lower doses of the drug, averaging 200 mg daily.

The **clinical manifestations** of pulmonary toxicity include **progressive dyspnea and cough.** A pleural effusion may occasionally be observed (Stein et al, 1987). Roentgenologic findings are **bilateral pulmonary infiltrates,** initially affecting mainly the lower lung lobes. **The basic injury from the drug appears to be an accumulation of phospholipids in the cytoplasm of macrophages.** The appearance has suggested a **drug-induced storage disease. Large mono- and multinucleated macrophages with finely vacuolated, foamy cytoplasm are characteristic of this disorder and have been described in BAL or in pleural fluid** (Martin et al, 1985; Stein et al, 1987; Mermolja et al, 1994; Bedrossian et al, 1997) (Fig.19-64). Stein et al (1987) stressed the **similarity of the foamy macrophages to cells in lipid pneumonia.** Osmiophilic lamellar inclusion bodies were observed in lysosomes by electron microscopy (Colgan et al, 1984; Dake et al, 1985), corresponding to foamy inclusions in alveolar macrophages by light microscopy (Israel-Biet et al, 1987; Myers et al, 1987; Bedrossian et al, 1997). **Reactive hyperplasia and damage to type II pneumocytes, a massive accumulation of large alveolar macrophages,** and **interstitial fibrosis** have been reported (Colgan et al, 1984).

Amiodarone lung must be differentiated from other disorders with similar clinical and roentgenologic presentation; the diagnosis requires correlation of clinical and roentgenologic data. Because **BAL** is safer than open lung biopsy for seriously ill patients, it is the **preferred diagnostic proce-**

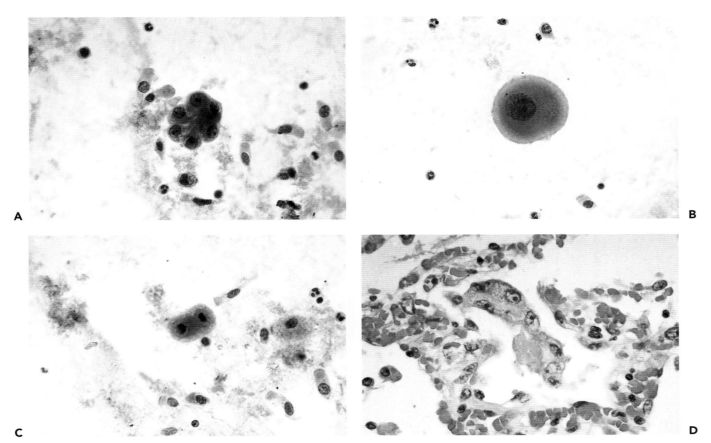

Figure 19-62   BCNU. Probable effects of carmustine (bis-chloroethylnitrosourea, BCNU) and viral pneumonia. Bronchopulmonary cytology and lung tissue at autopsy of a 29-year-old man with an astrocytoma treated by irradiation to the brain and systemic chemotherapy with BCNU. The patient died of respiratory failure after a febrile illness of 2 weeks' duration. *A.* Round papillary cluster of cells with prominent nucleoli. *B.* A single, very large cell with prominent nucleolus. *C.* Cell in telophase of miosis. *D.* Autopsy sections of lung showed interstitial fibrosis and scattered cells with giant nuclei, probably a drug effect. Alveoli were lined by prominent type II pneumocytes, and in this illustration, a syncytium of desquamated atypical pneumocytes with prominent nucleoli are seen within an alveolus.

dure to identify abnormal macrophages. Whether induced sputum may be equally effective has not been tested.

Organ Transplantation

Bone Marrow Transplantation

Autologous and allogeneic bone marrow transplants are used to **protect the hematopoietic system of the patient from the effects of high-dose chemotherapy and sometimes total body irradiation.** This approach is used in the treatment of **patients with systemic cancer,** most commonly patients with lymphoma, leukemia and, until recently, for metastatic breast cancer. The transplant recipients are **severely immunosuppressed** by their drug treatment and are **susceptible to opportunistic infections.** Lobenthal and Hajdu (1990) described their findings in various cytologic specimens that included cerebrospinal fluid and respiratory tract samples from 328 patients receiving bone marrow transplants, mainly for treatment of leukemias. Sputum, bronchial washing and **BAL** specimens of 92 patients were examined. Their principal observations were **marked enlargement and nuclear hyperchromasia** of epi-

thelial cells, presumably pneumocytes type II, attributed to total body irradiation. In several patients, ***P. carinii*** and **cytomegalovirus infections** were observed. The investigators were not successful in predicting recurrent leukemia in these patients based on cytologic changes.

Abu-Farsakh et al (1995) studied the **BAL specimens** from 77 recipients of bone marrow transplants who developed pulmonary symptoms or lung infiltrates on chest x-ray. The purpose of the study was to determine whether cytologic findings in BAL were of prognostic value. Bizarre epithelial cell changes were observed in specimens from 14 patients, some of which affected pneumocytes type II. These cells had markedly enlarged, hyperchromatic nuclei that were similar to the nuclear changes observed in atypical pneumonias, interstitial pulmonary fibrosis, or busulfan lung (see above). Also of note was the presence of 36 nonbacterial infections, 14 caused by fungi, mainly *Aspergillus,* and 19 that were viral (14 with **cytomegalovirus** and 5 with **herpes simplex**). In this series, there were three statistically significant **indicators of a poor prognosis:** (1) low lymphocyte counts (<5/hpf); (2) presence of hemosiderin laden macrophages; and (3) opportunistic viral or fungal infections.

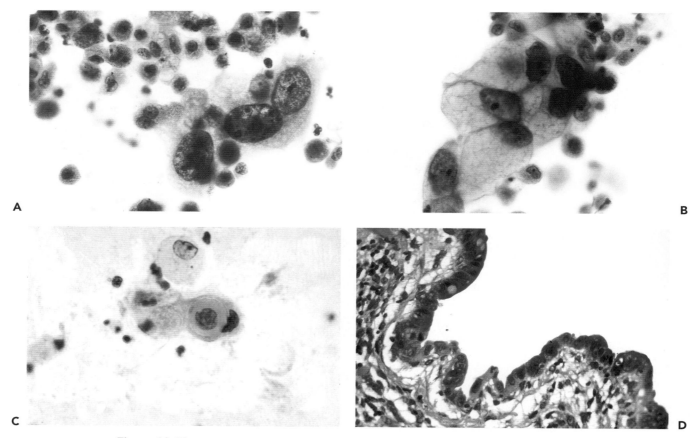

Figure 19-63   Atypia induced by combination chemotherapy. *A,B.* BAL cytology from a 22-year-old man under treatment for acute lymphocytic leukemia, showing enlarged and atypical columnar cells (*A*) and goblet cells (*B*). *C.* Squamous pearl perfectly mimicking squamous carcinoma in bronchial irrigation cytology of a young woman with Hodgkin's disease. She was treated with Velban, Leukeran, and radiotherapy. *D.* Chemotherapy- induced bronchial epithelial atypia in a child with acute leukemia. (*A–C:* High magnification.)

Lung Transplantation

Selvaggi (1992) reported her observations on six patients receiving lung transplantation. **BAL specimens** were used to **monitor the rejection of the transplanted organs.** The principal cytologic findings included **hyperplasia of pneumocytes type II** and the presence of inflammatory cells. **Cytomegalovirus** and **candida species** infections were each observed in one patient. When compared with concurrent lung biopsies, cytologic studies were a poor predictor of organ rejection.

NEONATAL LUNG DISEASE

Bronchopulmonary Dysplasia of Newborns

Northway and Rosan (1969) define **bronchopulmonary dysplasia** as a disorder of the respiratory tract occurring in neonates with respiratory distress syndrome, treated with intermittent positive-pressure respirators and high oxygen concentration for more than 6 days. The high oxygen pressure induces pulmonary injury, which can be monitored by radiographic and cytologic examination of pulmonary secretions. Northway and Rosan identified four stages of

bronchopulmonary dysplasia that can be described as follows:

- **Stage I** of oxygen toxicity (1 to 3 days of age) is characterized by **bronchial epithelial necrosis.** The chest radiograph shows fine granular densities, and the **cytologic examination of aspirated secretions shows excessive shedding of normal bronchial cells.**

- **Stage II** (4 to 10 days of age) is characterized by **nearly complete opacification of both lungs. Cytologic examination** shows **loss of ciliated respiratory cells. Abnormal, bizarre cell forms** appear toward the end of this stage, indicating progressive necrosis and the beginning of epithelial regeneration. This stage of disease still responds favorably to withdrawn or reduced oxygen therapy.

- **Stage III** (10 to 20 days of age) is a period of **cellular atypia and transition** to chronic disease. Radiographic examination shows areas of radiolucency in the previously completely opacified lungs. **Cytologic specimens** show **squamous metaplasia** and **mitotic activity** suggestive of healing of the denuded epithelial areas (D'Ablang et al, 1975). There is an increase in thick and viscid mucus secretions.

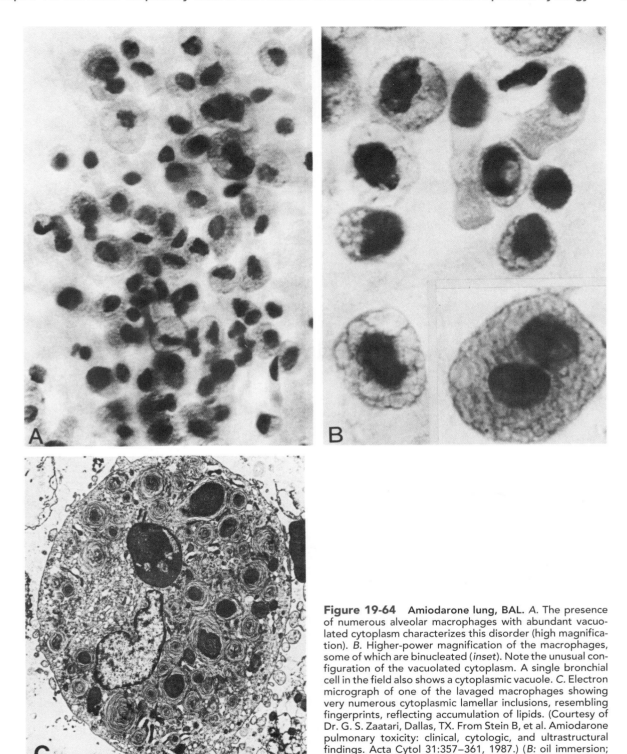

Figure 19-64 Amiodarone lung, BAL. *A.* The presence of numerous alveolar macrophages with abundant vacuolated cytoplasm characterizes this disorder (high magnification). *B.* Higher-power magnification of the macrophages, some of which are binucleated (*inset*). Note the unusual configuration of the vacuolated cytoplasm. A single bronchial cell in the field also shows a cytoplasmic vacuole. *C.* Electron micrograph of one of the lavaged macrophages showing very numerous cytoplasmic lamellar inclusions, resembling fingerprints, reflecting accumulation of lipids. (Courtesy of Dr. G. S. Zaatari, Dallas, TX. From Stein B, et al. Amiodarone pulmonary toxicity: clinical, cytologic, and ultrastructural findings. Acta Cytol 31:357–361, 1987.) (*B*: oil immersion; *C*: ×11,000.)

■ **Stage IV** represents **irreparable, chronic lung disease.** The **cytologic findings** in this stage of the disease show **progressive squamous metaplasia** and atypia, probably of pneumocytes type II. At autopsy, the lungs show squamous metaplasia of bronchial lining, marked interstitial fibrosis, and emphysema. D'Ablang et al confirmed the above findings in a major study, and suggested that care-

ful monitoring by x-ray examination and **cytology could identify the high-risk infants** (Fig. 19-65).

Other Pulmonary Disorders in Neonates

Doshi et al (1982) reported on the value of tracheal aspiration cytology in a number of pulmonary disorders other

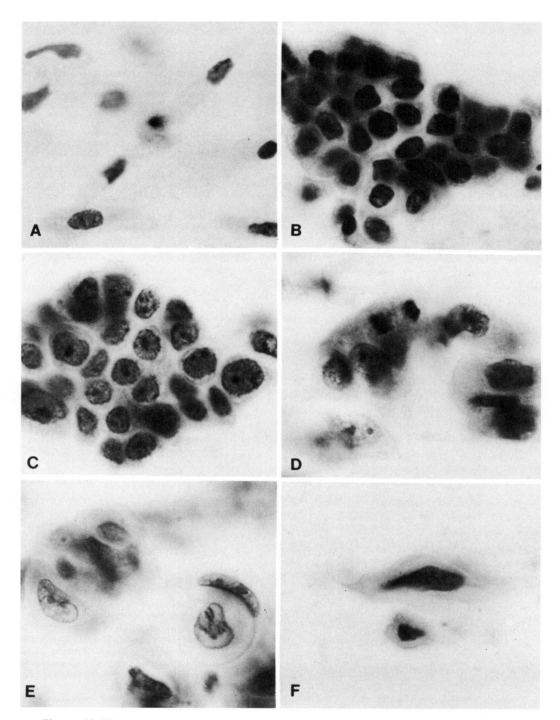

Figure 19-65 Cytologic manifestations of bronchopulmonary dysplasia of newborns in aspirated bronchial secretions. *A,B.* Stage II: respiratory columnar cells with loss of cilia (*A*); cohesive clusters of deep bronchial epithelial cells (*B*). *C,D.* Stage III: atypical cells of bronchial epithelial origin (*C*); some cells with mitotic activity (*D*). The findings correspond to regeneration of bronchial epithelial lining. *E,F.* Stages III and IV: squamous metaplasia of bronchial lining (*E*); bizarre squamous cells (*F*). These findings correspond to replacement of bronchial epithelium by atypical squamous metaplasia, evidence of irreversible pulmonary damage. (*A–F:* High magnification.) (From D'Ablaing G, et al. Neonatal pulmonary cytology and bronchopulmonary dysplasia. Acta Cytol 19:21–27, 1975.)

than bronchopulmonary dysplasia. Thus, **hyaline membrane disease, pneumonia, amniotic fluid, meconium aspiration,** and **pulmonary hemorrhage** were described. Of note was the finding of **massive desquamation of bronchial cells, ciliocytophthoria** and fragments of hyaline membranes in hyaline membrane disease. **Meconium aspiration** was characterized by the presence of **fragmented squames** and **coarse cellular debris. Anucleated squames** were the dominant cytologic finding in **amniotic fluid aspiration** (see Chap. 27).

ACKNOWLEDGMENT

Thanks are due to my colleagues Dr. L. G. Koss and Dr. M. B. Zaman who provided many of the illustrations for this chapter.

BIBLIOGRAPHY

Abati A, Cajigas A, Holland SM, Solomon D. Chronic granulomatous disease of childhood: Respiratory cytology. Diagn Cytopathol 15:98–102, 1996.

Abbas AK, Lichtman AH, Pober JS. Cellular and molecular immunology. Philadelphia, WB Saunders, 1991, p 417.

Aberle DR, Gamsu G, Golden JA. Fatal systemic arterial air embolism following lung needle aspiration. Radiology 165:351–353, 1987.

Abreo F, Bagby J. Sputum cytology in measles infection. A case report. Acta Cytol 35:719–721, 1991.

Abu-Farsakh HA, Katz RL, Atkinson N, Champlin RE. Prognostic factors in bronchoalveolar lavage in 77 patients with bone marrow transplants. Acta Cytol 39:1081–1088, 1995.

Afzelius BA. "Immotile cilia syndrome" and ciliary abnormalities induced by infection and injury. Am Rev Respir Dis 124:107–109, 1981.

Afzelius BA. A human syndrome caused by immotile cilia. Science 193:317–319, 1976.

Aisner SC, Gupta PK, Frost JK. Sputum cytology in pulmonary sarcoidosis. Acta Cytol 21:394–398, 1977.

Akaogi E, Ishibashi O, Mitsui K, et al. Pulmonary dirofilariasis cytologically mimicking lung cancer. A case report. Acta Cytol 37:531–534,1993.

Allen AR, Fulmer CD. Primary diagnosis of pulmonary echinococcosis by the cytologic technique. Acta Cytol 16:212–216, 1972.

Ambiavagar M, Chalon J, Zargham I. Tracheobronchial cytologic changes following lower airway thermal injury. J Trauma 14:280–289, 1974.

Anupindi L, Sahoo R, Rao RV, et al. Microfilariae in bronchial brushing cytology of symptomatic pulmonary lesions. A report of two cases. Acta Cytol 37:397–399, 1993.

Arioglu E, Doppman J, Gomes M, et al. Cushing's syndrome caused by corticotropin secretion by pulmonary tumorlets. N Engl J Med 339:883–886, 1998.

Armbruster C, Pokieser L, Hassl A. Diagnosis of *Pneumocystis carinii* pneumonia by bronchoalveolar lavage in AIDS patients: Comparison of Diff-Quik Fungifluor stain, direct immunofluorescence test and polymerase chain reaction. Acta Cytol 39:1089–1093, 1995.

Askin FB, Kuhn C. The cellular origin of pulmonary surfactant. Lab Invest 25:260–268, 1971.

Auerswald U, Barth J, Magnussen H. Value of CD-1 positive cells in bronchoalveolar lavage fluid for the diagnosis of pulmonary histiocytosis X. Lung 169:305–309, 1991.

Avasthi R, Jain AP, Swaroop K, Samal N. Bancroftian microfilariasis in association with pulmonary tuberculosis. Acta Cytol 35:717–718, 1991.

Bakhos R, Wojcik EM, Olson MC. Transthoracic fine-needle aspiration cytology of inflammatory pseudotumor, fibrohistiocytic type: A case report with immunohistochemical studies. Diagn Cytopathol 19:216–220, 1998.

Balis JU, Paterson JF, Pacija JE, et al. Distribution and subcellular location of surfactant associated glycoprotein in the lung. Lab Invest 52:657–669, 1985.

Beals AJ, Campbell WA. Rapid cytologic method for the diagnosis of measles. J Clin Pathol 12:335–337, 1959.

Bedrossian CWM, Luna MA, Mackay B, Lichtiger B. Ultrastructure of pulmonary bleomycin toxicity. Cancer 32:44–51, 1973.

Bedrossian CW, Warren CJ, Ohar J, Bhan R. Amiodarone pulmonary toxicity: cytopathology, ultrastructure, and immunocytochemistry. Ann Diagn Pathol 1:47–56, 1997.

Beemer AM, Kuttin ES, Pinkenson M. Cytology for early diagnosis of cryptococcal tracheo-bronchitis. Mykosen 15:359–365, 1972.

Berkheiser SW. Epithelial proliferation of the lung associated with cortisone administration. A pathological and experimental study. Cancer 16:1354–1364, 1963.

Berkheiser SW. Bronchiolar proliferation and metaplasia associated with bronchiectasis, pulmonary infarcts, and anthracosis. Cancer 12:499–508, 1959.

Beskow CO, Drachenberg CB, Bourquin PM, et al. Diffuse alveolar damage: Morphologic features in bronchoalveolar fluid. Acta Cytol 44:640–646, 2000.

Bewtra C, Dewan N, O'Donahue WJ Jr. Exfoliative sputum cytology in pulmonary embolism. Acta Cytol 27:489–496, 1983.

Bhagavan BS, Koss LG. Secular trends in prevalence and concentration of pulmonary asbestos bodies—1940 to 1972. A necropsy study. Arch Pathol Lab Med 100:539–541, 1976.

Bhalla DK. Ozone-induced lung inflammation and mucosal barrier disruption: Toxicology, mechanisms and implications. J Toxicol Environ Health B Crit Rev 2(1):31–86, 1999.

Bhatt ON, Miller MSR, LeRiche J, King EG. Aspiration biopsy in pulmonary opportunistic infections. Acta Cytol 21:206–209, 1977.

Bigby TD, Margolskee D, Curtis JL, et al. The usefulness of induced sputum in the diagnosis of *Pneumocystis carinii* pneumonia in patients with the acquired immunodeficiency syndrome. Am Rev Resp Dis 133:515–518, 1986.

Birbeck MS, Breathnach AS, Everall JD. An electron microscopic study of basal melanocytes and high-level clear cells (Langerhans cells) in vitiligo. J Invest Dermatol 37:51–64, 1961.

Bitterman PB, Rennard SI, Keogh BA, et al. Familial idiopathic pulmonary fibrosis: Evidence of lung inflammation in unaffected family members. N Engl J Med 314:1343–1347, 1986.

Bitterman PB, Adelberg S, Crystal RG. Mechanisms of pulmonary fibrosis: Spontaneous release of the alveolar macrophage-derived growth factor in the interstitial lung disorders. J Clin Invest 72:1801–1813, 1983.

Blanc PL, Guibaud S, Bedock B, Robert D. Diagnostic de l'embolie amniotique par lavage broncho-alveolaire. Presse Med 16:479–480, 1987.

Bleiweiss IJ, Jagirdar JS, Klein MJ, et al. Granulomatous *Pneumocystis carinii* pneumonia in three patients with the acquired immune deficiency syndrome. Chest 94:580–583, 1988.

Blumenfeld W, Gan GL. Diagnosis of histoplasmosis in bronchoalveolar lavage fluid by intracytoplasmic localization of silver-positive yeast. Acta Cytol 35:710–712, 1991.

Blumenfeld W, Kovacs JA. Use of monoclonal antibody to detect *Pneumocystis carinii* in induced sputum and bronchoalveolar lavage fluid by immunoperoxidase staining. Arch Pathol Lab Med 112:1223–1236, 1988.

Bonfiglio TA. Fine needle aspiration biopsy of the lung. Pathol Annu 16:159–180, 1981.

Brandenburg VM, Schubert H. Images in clinical medicine. Pulmonary alveolar microlithiasis. N Engl J Med 348:1555, 2003.

Broaddus C, Dake MD, Stulbarg MS, et al. Bronchoalveolar lavage and transbronchial biopsy for the diagnosis of pulmonary infections in the acquired immunodeficiency syndrome. Ann Intern Med 102:747–752, 1985.

Brody RS, Schottenfeld D, Reid A. Multiple primary cancer risk after therapy for Hodgkin's disease. Cancer 40:1917–1926, 1977.

Brunstetter M-A, Hardie JA, Schiff R, et al. The origin of pulmonary alveolar macrophages. Arch Intern Med 127:1064–1068, 1971.

Bryan WTK, Bryan MP. Structural changes in the ciliated epithelial cells during the common cold. Trans Am Acad Ophthalmol Otolaryngol 57:297–303, 1953.

Burkhalter A, Silverman JF, Hopkins MB, Geisinger KR. Bronchoalveolar lavage cytology in pulmonary alveolar proteinosis. Am J Clin Pathol 106:504–510, 1996.

Burkhardt A, Bommer G, Gebbers J-D, Holtje W-J. Riesezellenbildung bei Bleomycintherapie oraler Plattenzellenarcinome. Virchows Arch [A] 369:197–214, 1976.

Burns WA, McFarland W, Matthews MJ. Busulfan induced pulmonary disease. Am Rev Respir Dis 101:408, 1970.

Cahan W, Melamed MR, Frazell EL. Tracheobronchial cytology after laryngectomy for carcinoma. Surg Gynecol Obstet 123:15–21, 1966.

Caldwell JE, Porter DD. Herpetic pneumonia in alcoholic hepatitis. JAMA 217:1703, 1971.

Capers TH, Lee D. Pulmonary cytomegalic inclusion disease in an adult. Am J Clin Pathol 33:238–242, 1960.

Carey FA, Wallace WA, Fergusson RJ, et al. Alveolar atypical adenomatous hyperplasia in association with primary pulmonary adenocarcinoma: A clinicopathologic study of ten cases. Thorax 47:1041–1043, 1992.

Carlson DJ, Mason EW. Pulmonary alveolar proteinosis: Diagnosis of probable case by examination of sputum. Am J Clin Pathol 33:48–54, 1960.

Carson KF, Williams CA, Rosenthal DL, et al. Bronchoalveolar lavage in a girl with Gaucher's disease: A case report. Acta Cytol 38:597–600, 1994.

Chalon J, Katz JS, Gorstein F, Tumdorf H. Malignant disease and tracheobronchial epithelial multinucleation. Cancer 37:1874–1881, 1976.

Chalon J, Tayyab MA, Ramanathan S. Cytology of respiratory epithelium as a predictor of respirator complications after operation. Chest 67:32–35, 1975.

Chalon J, Katz JS, Ramanathan S, et al. Tracheobronchial epithelial multinucleation in malignant disease. Science 183:525–526, 1974.

Chalon J. Changes in tracheobronchial cytology noted during anesthesia. NY State J Med 74:2185–2189, 1974.

Chalon J, Loew DAY, Orkin LR. Tracheobronchial cytologic changes during the menstrual cycle. JAMA 218:1928–1931, 1971.

Chamberlain DW, Braude AC, Rebuck AS. A critical evaluation of bronchoalveolar lavage. Criteria for identifying unsatisfactory specimens. Acta Cytol 31:599–605, 1987.

Chan CC, Abi-Saleh WJ, Arroliga AC, et al. Diagnostic yield and therapeutic impact of flexible bronchoscopy in lung transplant recipients. J Heart Lung Transplant 15: 196–205, 1996.

Chandra P, Delaney MD, Tuazon CU. Role of special stains in the diagnosis of *Pneumocystis carinii* infection from bronchial washing specimens in patients with the acquired immune deficiency syndrome. Acta Cytol 32:105–108, 1988.

Chaturvedi V, Ramani R, Gromadzki S, et al. Coccidiomycosis in New York State. Emerging Infectious Diseases 6:25–29, 2000.

Cheever AW, Valsamis MP, Rabson AS. Necrotizing toxoplasmic encephalitis and herpetic pneumonia complicating treated Hodgkin's disease. N Engl J Med 272:2629, 1965.

Chen KTK. Cytology of tracheobronchial amyloidosis. Acta Cytol 28:133–135, 1984.

Chodosh S. Examination of sputum cells. N Engl J Med 282:854–857, 1970.

Chollet S, Soler P, Dournovo P, et al. Diagnosis of pulmonary histiocytosis X by immunodetection of Langerhans cells in bronchoalveolar lavage fluid. Am J Pathol 115:225–232, 1984.

Churg AM, Warnock ML. Asbestos and other ferruginous bodies: Their formation and clinical significance. Am J Pathol 102:447–456, 1981.

Clarysse AM, Cathey WJ, Cartwright GE, et al. Pulmonary disease complicating intermittent therapy with methotrexate. JAMA 209:1861–1864, 1969.

Cohen MC, Sanchez-Marull R, Drut R. Aneuploid nucleomegaly of bronchial cells in Ataxia-Telangiectasia Diag Cytopathol 17: 484–486, 1997.

Colby TV, Lombard C. Histiocytosis X in the lung. Hum Pathol 14:847-856, 1983.

Cole SR, Myers, TJ, Klatsky AU. Pulmonary disease with chlorambucil therapy. Cancer 41:455–459, 1978.

Colgan T, Simon GT, Kay JM, et al. Amiodarone pulmonary toxicity. Ultrastruct Pathol 6:199–207, 1984.

Collins KA, Geisinger KR, Wagner PH, et al. The cytologic evaluation of lipid-laden alveolar macrophages as an indicator of aspiration pneumonia in young children. Arch Pathol Lab Med 119:229–231, 1995.

Colombo JL, Hallberg TK. Recurrent aspiration in children: Lipid laden alveolar macrophages quantitation. Pediatr Pulmonol 3:86–89, 1987.

Cooney W, Dzuira B, Harper R, Nash G. The cytology of sputum from thermally injured patients. Acta Cytol 16:433–437, 1972.

Corwin RW, Irwin RS. The lipid laden alveolar macrophage as a marker of aspiration in parenchymal lung disease. Am Rev Resp Dis 132:576–581, 1985.

Costabel U, Teschler H, Guzman J, Kroegel C. Bronchoalveolar lavage: Interim evaluation following 10 years clinical use. Med Klin 85:376–387, 1990.

Costabel U, Bross KJ, Ruble KH, et al. La-like Antigens on T-cells and their subpopulations in pulmonary sarcoidosis and in hypersensitivity pneumonitis. Am Rev Respir Dis 131:337–342, 1985.

Costabel U, Matthys H, Gusman J, Freidenberg N. Multinucleated cells in bronchoalveolar lavage. Acta Cytol 29:189–190, 1985.

Costabel U, Bross KJ, Matthys H. Augmentation of natural killer cells in the bronchoalveolar lavage fluid of hypersensitivity pneumonitis compared to pulmonary saxcoidosis. Am Rev Respir Dis 127(Suppl):68, 1983.

Crystal RG, Bitterman PB, Rennard SI, et al. Interstitial lung disease of unknown cause: Disorders characterized by chronic inflammation of the lower respiratory tract. N Engl J Med 310:154–166; 235–244, 1984.

Crystal RG, Gadek JE, Ferrans VJ, et al. Interstitial lung disease: Current concepts of pathogenesis, staging, and therapy. Am J Med 70:542–568, 1981.

Crystal RG, Fulmer JD, Roberts WC, et al. Idiopathic pulmonary fibrosis: Clinical, histologic, radiographic, physiologic, scintigraphic, cytologic, and biochemical aspects. Ann Intern Med 85:769–788, 1976.

Cutz E, Conen PE. Ultrastructure and cytochemistry of Clara cells. Am J Pathol 62:127–141, 1971.

D'Ablaing G, Bernard B, Zaharov L, et al. Neonatal pulmonary cytology and bronchopulmonary dysplasia. Acta Cytol 19:21–27, 1975.

Dahlgren SE, Ekstrom P. Aspiration cytology in the diagnosis of pulmonary tuberculosis. Scand J Respir Dis 53:196–201, 1972.

Dahlgren S, Nordenstrom B. Transthoracic Needle Biopsy. Stockholm: Almqvist & Wiksell, 1966.

Dahlgren SE. Needle biopsy of intrapulmonary hamartoma. Scand J Respir Dis 47:187–194, 1966.

Dake MD, Madison JM, Montgomery CK, et al. Electron microscopic demonstration of lysosomal inclusion bodies in lung, liver, lymph nodes, and blood leukocytes of patients with amiodarone pulmonary toxicity. Am J Med 78:506–512,1985.

Dalhamn T: In vivo and in vitro ciliotoxic effects of tobacco smoke. Arch Environ Health 21:633–734, 1970.

Daniele RP, Elias JA, Epstein PE, Rossman MD. Bronchoalveolar lavage: Role in pathogenesis, diagnosis, and management of interstitial lung disease. Ann Intern Med 102:93–108, 1985.

Daniele RP, Altose MD, Rowland DR Jr. Immunocompetent cells from the lower respiratory tract of normal human lungs. J Clin Invest 59:986–996, 1975.

Dauzier G, Willis T, Barnett RX. Pneumocystis carinii pneumonia in an infant. Am J Clin Pathol 26:787–793, 1956.

Davison AG, Haslam PL, Corrin B, et al. Interstitial lung disease and asthma in hard metal workers. Bronchoalveolar lavage, ultrastructural and analytical findings and results of bronchial provocation tests. Thorax 38:119–128, 1983.

De Fine LA, Saleba KP, Gobson BB, et al. Cytologic evaluation of bronchoalveolar lavage specimens in immunosuppressed patients with suspected opportunistic infections. Acta Cytol 31:235–242, 1987.

De Mattos MC, De Oliveira ML. Respiratory cytopathology: Paracoccidiomycosis associated either with tuberculosis or bronchogenic carcinoma. Diagn Cytopath 8:198–199, 1992.

DeGroodt M, Sebruyns M. Cytodiagnosis of generalized cytomegalic inclusion made in patients during life. JAMA 173:116, 1960.

del Rio C, Guarner J, Honing EG, Slade BA. Sputum examination in the diagnosis of Pneumocystis carinii pneumonia in the acquired immunodeficiency syndrome. Arch Pathol Lab Med 12:1229–1232, 1988.

DeMay RM. The Art and Science of Cytopathology. Chicago ASCP Press, 1996.

Demedts M, Gheysens B, Nagels J, et al. Cobalt lung in diamond polishers. Am Rev Respir Dis 130:130–135, 1984.

Devouassoux-Shisheboran M, de la Fouchardière A, Thivolet-Bèjuié F, et al. Endobronchial variant of sclerosing hemangioma of lung: Histological and cytological features on endobronchial material. Mod Pathol 17; 252–257, 2004.

Djamin RS, Drent SM, et al. Diagnosis of Pneumocystis carinii pneumonia in HIV-positive patients: Bronchoalveolar lavage vs. bronchial brushing. Acta Cytol 42:993–998, 1998.

Doshi N, Kanbour A, Fujikura T, Klionski B. Tracheal aspiration cytology of neonates with respiratory distress. Histopathologic correlation. Acta Cytol 26:15–21, 1982.

Douglas RG, Anderson MS, Weg JG, et al. Herpes simplex virus pneumonia. Occurrence in an allotransplanted lung. JAMA 210:902–904, 1969.

Drut R. Calcified mitochondria in epithelial cells of the respiratory tract in upper respiratory thermal injury. Diagn Cytopathol 19;288–289, 1998.

Edman JC, Kovacs JA, Masur HE, et al. Ribosomal RNA sequence shows Pneumocystis carinii to be a member of fungi. Nature 334:519–522, 1988.

Elvin KM, Bjorkman A, Linder E, et al. Pneumocystis carinii pneumonia: Detection of parasites in sputum and bronchoalveolar lavage fluid by monoclonal antibodies. Br J Med 297:381–384, 1988.

Farber L. Sputum cytology in patients following enzyme aerosol therapy. Dis Chest 31:169–179, 1957.

Farber SM, Pharr SL, Traut HF, et al. Metaplasia and dyskeratosis of bronchial epithelial cells following inhalation of trypsin and desoxyribonuclease. Lab Invest 3:33–38, 1954.

Farber SM, Wood DA, Pharr SL, Pierson B. Significant cytologic findings in non-malignant pulmonary disease. Dis Chest 31:1–13, 1957.

Farley ML, Fagan MF, Mabry LC, Wallace RJ Jr. Presentation of Sporothrix schenkii in pulmonary cytology specimens. Acta Cytol 35:389–395, 1991.

Farley ML, Mabry L, Munoz LA, Discrens HW. Crystals occurring in pulmonary cytology specimens. Association with Aspergillus infection. Acta Cytol 29: 737–744, 1985.

Feingold ML, Koss LG. Effects of long term administration of busulfan. Arch Intern Med 124:66–71, 1969.

Fekete P S, Campbell WG, et al. Transthoracic needle aspiration biopsy in Wegener's granulomatosis. Morphologic findings in five cases. Acta Cytol 34:155–160, 1990.

Fichtenbaum CJ, Kleinman GM, Haddad RG. Eosinophilic granuloma of the lung presenting as a solitary pulmonary nodule. Thorax 45: 905–916, 1990.

Filip DJ, Logue GL, Harle TS, Farrar WH. Pulmonary and hepatic complications of methotrexate therapy of psoriasis. JAMA 216:881–882, 1971.

Fisher ER, Davis E. Cytomegalic inclusion disease in the adult. N Engl J Med 258:1036–1040, 1958.

Fleury J, Escudier E, Pocholle MJ, et al. Cell populations obtained by bronchoalveolar lavage in Pneumocystis carinii pneumonitis. Acta Cytol 29: 721–726, 1985.

Foley FD, Greenawald KA, Nash G, Pruitt BA Jr. Herpes virus infection in burned patients. N Engl J Med 282:652–656, 1970.

Foraker SHA, Haesaert S. Cytomegalic virus inclusion body in bronchial brushing material. Acta Cytol 21:181–182, 1977.

Frable WJ, Frable MA, Seney FD Jr. Virus infections of the respiratory tract, cytopathologic and clinical analysis. Acta Cytol 21:32–36, 1977.

Frable WJ, Kay S. Herpes virus infection of the respiratory tract. Electron microscopic observation of the virus in cells obtained from a sputum cytology. Acta Cytol 21:391–393, 1977.

Freedman SI, Ang EP, Haley RS. Identification of coccidioidomycosis of the lung by fine needle aspiration biopsy. Acta Cytol 30:420–424, 1986.

Friedman-Mor Z, Chalon J, Katz JS, et al. Tracheobronchial and pulmonary cytologic changes in shock. J Trauma 16:58–62, 1976.

Frost JK, Gupta PK, Erozan YS, et al. Pulmonary cytologic alterations in toxic environmental inhalation. Hum Pathol 4:521–536, 1973.

Gaensler EA, Carrington CB. Open biopsy for chronic diffuse infiltrative lung disease: Clinical, roentgenographic, and physiologic correlations in 502 patients. Ann Thorac Surg 30:411–426, 1980.

Garver RI Jr, Zorn GL, Wu X, et al. Recurrence of bronchioloalveolar carcinoma in transplanted lungs. N Engl J Med 340:1071–1074, 1999.

George RB, Mogabgab WJ. Atypical pneumonia in young men with rhinovirus infections. Ann Intern Med 71:1073–1078, 1969.

Ghali VS, Garcia RL, Skolom J. Fluorescence of P carinii in Papanicolaou smears. Hum Pathol 15:907–909, 1984.

Gigliotti F, Stokes DC, Cheatham AB, et al. Development of murine monoclonal antibodies to Pneumocystis carinii. J Immunol Method 154:315–322, 1986.

Glezen WP, Fernald GW, Lohr JA. Acute respiratory disease of university students with special reference to the etiologic role of herpesvirus hominis. Am J Epidemiol 101:111–121, 1975.

Golde DW, Territo M, Finley MJ. Defective lung macrophages in pulmonary alveolar proteinosis. Ann Intern Med 85:304–309, 1976.

Good WO, Ellison C, Archer VE. Sputum cytology among frequent users of pressurized spray cans. Cancer Res 35:316–321, 1975.

Gori S, Lupetti A, Moscato G, et al. Pulmonary sporotrichosis with hyphae in a human immunodeficiency virus infected patient. A case report. Acta Cytol 41:519–521, 1997.

Gori S, Scasso A. Cytologic and differential diagnosis of rhinosporidiosis. Acta Cytol 38:361–366, 1994.

Greaves TS, Strigle SM. The recognition of Pneumocystis carinii in routine Papanicolaou-stained smears. Acta Cytol 29:714–720, 1985.

Greenwood MF, Holland P. The mammalian respiratory tract surface. A scanning electron microscopic study. Lab Invest 27:296–304, 1972.

Gronbeck C II. Pneumocystis carinii pneumonia presenting as cavitary lung disease. Milit Med 153:314–316, 1988.

Groniowski J, Biczvskowa W. Structure of the alveolar lining film of the lungs. Nature 204:745–747, 1964.

Grotte D, Stanley MW, Swanson PE, et al. Reactive type II pneumocytes in bronchoalveolar lavage fluid from adult respiratory distress syndrome can be mistaken for cells of adenocarcinoma. Diagn Cytopathol 6:317–322, 1990.

Grunze H. Long term cytology study of squamous metaplasia of bronchial mucosa. Transactions of the Sixth Annual Meeting of the inter-Society Cytology Council. 1958, pp 153–156.

Guglietti LC, Reingold IM. The detection of Coccidioides immitis in pulmonary cytology. Acta Cytol 12:332–334, 1968.

Hall CB, Powell KR, MacDonald NE, et al. Respiratory syncytial viral infection in children with compromised immune function. N Engl J Med 315:77–81, 1986.

Haque A, Plattner SB, Cook RT, Hart MN. *Pneumocystis carinii:* Taxonomy as viewed by electron microscopy. Am J Clin Pathol 87:504–510, 1987.

Harboldt SL, Dugan JM, Tronic BS. Cytologic diagnosis of measles pneumonia in a bronchoalveolar lavage specimen. A case report. Acta Cytol 38:403–406, 1994.

Harmsen AG, Muggenburg BA, Snipes MB, Bice DE. The role of macrophages in particle translocation from lungs to lymph nodes. Science 230:1277–1280, 1985.

Hartz JW, Geisinger KR, Scharyj M, Muss HB. Granulomatous pneumocystosis presenting as a solitary pulmonary nodule. Arch Pathol Lab Med 109:466–469, 1985.

Haslam PL, Turton CWG, Heard B, et al. Bronchoalveolar lavage in pulmonary fibrosis: Comparison of cells obtained with lung biopsy and clinical features. Thorax 35:9–18, 1980.

Hawkins CC, Gold JWM, Whimbey E, et al. Mycobacterium avium complex infections in patients with the acquired immunodeficiency syndrome. Ann Intern Med 105:184–188, 1986.

Heard BE, Cooke RA. Busulphan lung. Thorax 23:187–193, 1968.

Hector MF. Sputum cytology in two cases of Wegener's granulomatosis. J Clin Pathol 29:259–263, 1976.

Henke JA, Golden JA, et al. Persistent increases of BAL neutrophiles as a predictor of mortality following lung transplant. Chest 115:403–409, 1999.

Herout V, Vortel V, Vondrackova A. Herpes simplex involvement of the lower respiratory tract. Am J Clin Pathol 46:411–416, 1966.

Hers JFP, Mulder J. Rapid tentative postmortem diagnosis of influenza with the aid of cytological smears of the tracheal epithelium. J Pathol Bacteriol 63:329–332, 1951.

Hoheisel JB, Tabak I, Teschler H, et al. Bronchoalveolar lavage cytology and immunocytology in pulmonary tuberculosis. Am J Respir Crit Care Med 149:460–483, 1994.

Holoye PY, Jenkins DE, Greenberg SD. Pulmonary toxicity in long-term administration of BCNU. Cancer Treat Rep 60:1691–1694, 1976.

Hopewell PC, Luce JM. Pulmonary involvement in the acquired immunodeficiency syndrome. Chest 87:104–112, 1985.

Hsu CY, Luh KT. Cytology of pulmonary *Fusobacterium nucleatum* infection. A case report. Acta Cytol 39:114–117, 1995.

Humphreys K, Hieger LB. *Strongyloides stercoralis* in routine Papanicolaou-stained sputum smears. Acta Cytol 23:471–475, 1979.

Hunninghake G, Gadek J, Weinberger S, et al. Comparison of the alveolitis of sarcoidosis and idiopathic pulmonary fibrosis. Chest 75:266–267, 1979.

Hunninghake GW, Gadek JE, Kawanami O, et al. Inflammatory and immune processes in the human lung in health and disease: Evaluation by bronchoalveolar lavage. Am J Pathol 97:149–206, 1979.

Hunninghake GW, Kawanami O, Ferrans VJ, et al. Characterization of the inflammatory and immune effector cells in lung parenchyma of patients with interstitial lung disease. Am Rev Respir Dis 123:407–412, 1981.

Hyers TM, Fowler AA. Adult respiratory distress syndrome: Causes, morbidity, and mortality. Fed Proc 45:25–29, 1986.

Israel-Biet D, Venet A, Caubarrere L, et al. Bronchoalveolar lavage in amiodarone pneumonitis. Cellular abnormalities and their relevance to pathogenesis. Chest 91:214–221, 1987.

Jain U, Mani K, Frable J. Cytomegalic inclusion disease: Cytologic diagnosis from bronchial brushing material. Acta Cytol 17:467–468, 1973.

Jampolis RW, McDonald J, Clagett OT. Mineral oil granuloma of the lungs: An evaluation of methods for identification of mineral oil in tissue. Surg Gynecol Obstet 97:105–119, 1953.

Johnston WW. Role of cytopathology in the diagnosis of opportunistic infections of the respiratory tract and other nongynecologic sites. *In* Wied et al (eds). Compendium on Diagnostic Cytology, ed 7. Chicago, Tutorials of Cytology, 1992, pp 194–204.

Johnston WW. Type II pneumocytes in cytologic specimens. A diagnostic dilemma. Am J Clin Pathol 97:608–609, 1992.

Johnston WW, Frable WJ. Diagnostic Respiratory Cytopathology. New York, Masson Publishing, 1979.

Johnston WW, Frable WJ. The cytopathology of the respiratory tract. Am J Pathol 84:372–424, 1976.

Johnston WW, Amatulli J. The role of cytology in the primary diagnosis of North American blastomycosis. Acta Cytol 14:200–204, 1970.

Johnston WW, Schlein B, Amatulli J. Cytopathologic diagnosis of fungus infection. Acta Cytol 13:488–495, 1969.

Jordan SW, McLaren LC, Crosby JH. Herpetic tracheobronchitis. Cytologic and virologic detection. Arch Intern Med 135:784–788, 1975.

Kamholz SL, Pinsker KL, Johnson J, Schreiber K. Fine needle aspiration biopsy of intrathoracic lesion. NY State J Med 82:736–739, 1982.

Kaneishi NK, Howell LP, Russell LA, et al. Fine needle aspiration cytology of pulmonary Wegner's granulomatosis with biopsy correlation. Acta Cytol 39:1094–1100, 1995.

Kartagener M. Zur Pathogenese der Bronchiectasien: Bronchiectasien bei situs viscerum inversus. Beitr Klin Tuberk 83:489–501, 1933.

Kasper M, Haroske G. Alterations in the alveolar epithelium after injury leading to pulmonary fibrosis. Histol Histopathol 11:463–483, 1996.

Katzenstein A-LA. Katzenstein and Askin's Pathology of Non-Neoplastic Lung Disease. vol 13. *In* Livolsi VA (ed). Major Problems in Pathology 3rd ed. Philadelphia, WB Saunders, 1997.

Kenney M, Eveland LK, Yermakov V. Amebiasis. Unusual location in lung. NY State J Med 75:1542–1543, 1975.

Kenney M, Webber CA. Diagnosis of strongyloidiasis in Papanicolaou-stained sputum smears. Acta Cytol 18:270–273, 1974.

Kern I, Keclj P, Kosnik M, Mermolja M. Multinucleated giant cells in bronchoalveolar lavage. Acta Cytol 47: 426–430, 2003.

Kern WH, Dermer GB, Tiemann RM. Comparative morphology of histiocytes from various organ systems. Quantitative cytologic and ultrastructural studies. Acta Cytol 14:205–215, 1970.

Kern WH. Cytology of hyperplastic and neoplastic lesions of terminal bronchioles and alveoli. Acta Cytol 9:372–380, 1965.

Kerr KM, Carey FA, King G, Lamb D. Atypical alveolar hyperplasia Relationship with pulmonary adenocarcinoma, p53 and c-erb B-2 expression. J Pathol 174:249–256, 1994.

Khoor A, Myers JL Tazelaar HD, Swensen SJ. Pulmonary Langerhans cell histiocytosis presenting as a solitary nodule. Mayo Clin Proc 76: 209–211, 2001.

Kierszenbaum AL. Bronchial metaplasia. Observations on its histology and cytology. Acta Cytol 9:365–371, 1965.

Kijner CH, Yousem SA. Systemic light chain deposition disease presenting as multiple pulmonary nodules. A case report and review of the literature. Am J Surg Pathol 12:405–413, 1988.

Kilburn KH, McKenzie WM. Leukocyte recruitment to airways by cigarette smoke and particle phase in contrast to cytotoxicity of vapor. Science 189: 634–637, 1975.

Kim CJ, Ko L, Bukantz SC. Ciliocytophthoria (CCP) in asthmatic children with reference to viral and respiratory infection and exacerbation of asthma. J Allergy 35:159–168, 1964.

Kinoshita M, Sueyasu Y, Watanabe H, et al. Giant cell interstitial pneumonia in two hard metal workers: The role of bronchoalveolar lavage in diagnosis. Respirology 4:263–266, 1999.

Kinsella DL Jr. Bronchial cell atypias: Report of preliminary study correlating cytology with histology. Cancer 12:463–472, 1959.

Kirschner RH, Esterly JR. Pulmonary lesions associated with busulfan therapy of chronic myelogenous leukemia. Cancer 27:1074–1080, 1971.

Kitamura H, Kameda Y, Ito T, Hayashi H. Atypical adenomatous hyperplasia of the lung. Implications for the pathogenesis of peripheral lung adenocarcinoma. Am J Clin Pathol 111:610–622, 1999.

Knauer-Fischer S, Ratjen F. Lipid-laden macrophages in bronchoalveolar lavage fluid as a marker for pulmonary aspiration. Pediatr Pulmonol 27:419–422, 1999.

Koerner SK, Sakowitz AJ, Appelman RI, et al. Transbronchial lung biopsy for the diagnosis of sarcoidosis. N Engl J Med 293:268–270, 1975.

Koizumi JH. Nipplelike protrusions in endocervical and other cells. Acta Cytol 40:519–528, 1996.

Koizumi JH, Sommers HM. *Afyobacterium yenopi* and pulmonary disease. Am J Clin Pathol 73:826–830, 1980.

Kolarz G, Scherak O, Popp W, et al. Bronchoalveolar lavage in rheumatoid arthritis. Br J Rheumatol 32: 556–561, 1993.

Koprowska I. Intranuclear inclusion bodies in smears of respiratory secretions. Acta Cytol 5:219–228, 1961.

Koss LG, Melamed MR, Mayer K. The effect of busulfan on human epithelia. Am J Clin Pathol 44:385–397, 1965.

Koss LG, Richardson HL. Some pitfalls of cytological diagnosis of lung cancer. Cancer 8:937–947, 1955.

Koss LG, Woyke S, Olszewski W. Aspiration Biopsy. Cytologic Interpretation and Histologic Bases, 2nd ed. New York, Igaku Shoin, 1992.

Kovacs JA, Ng VL, Masur H, et al. Diagnosis of *Pneumocystis carinii* pneumonia: Improved detection in sputum with use of monoclonal antibodies. N Engl J Med 318:589–593, 1988.

Kovacs JA, Gill V, Swan JC, et al. Prospective evaluation of a monoclonal antibody in diagnosis of *Pneumocystis carinii* pneumonia. Lancet 2:1–4, 1986.

Kraft M, Cassell GH, Henson JE, et al. Detection of mycoplasma pneumoniae in the airways of adults with chronic asthma. Am J Respir Crit Care Med 158: 998–1001, 1998.

Kucharczyk W, Weisbrod GL, et al. Cardiac tamponade as a complication of thin-needle aspiration lung biopsy. Chest 82:120–121, 1982.

Lachman MF. Cytologic appearance of *Rhodococcus equi* in bronchoalveolar lavage specimens. A case report. Acta Cytol 39:111–113, 1995.

Lambert C, Gansler T, Mansour KA, et al. Pulmonary malakoplakia diagnosed by fine needle aspiration. A case report. Acta Cytol 41:1833–1838, 1997.

Lamont J, Verbeken E, Verschakelen J, et al. Bronchiolitis obliterans organising pneumonia. A report of 11 cases and a review of the literature. Acta Clin Belg 53:328–336, 1998.

Langston C, Pappin A. Lipid-laden alveolar macrophages as an indicator of aspiration pneumonia. Arch Pathol Lab Med 120:326–327, 1996.

Lanzafame M, Bonora S, Di Perri G, et al. *Microsporidium* species in pulmonary cavitary lesions of AIDS patients infected with Rhodococcus equi. Clin Infect Dis 25:926–927, 1997.

Leiman G. Asbestos bodies in fine needle aspirates of lung masses. Acta Cytol 35:171–174, 1991.

Leung AN, Brauner MW, Caillat-Vigneron N, et al. Sarcoidosis activity: Correlation of HRCT findings with those of 67 Ga scanning, bronchoalveolar lavage and serum angiotensin converting enzyme assay. J Comput Assist Tomogr 22:229–234, 1998.

Lieberman PH, Jones CR, Steinman RM, et al. Langerhans cell (eosinophilic) granulomatosis. Am J Surg Pathol 20:519–552, 1996.

Liebow AA. Definition and classification of interstitial pneumonias in human pathology. Prog Resp Res 8:1, 1975.

Lindgren KM, Douglas RG Jr, Couch RB. Significance of herpes virus hominis in respiratory secretions of man. N Engl J Med 278:517–523, 1968.

Liu W. An Introduction to Respiratory Cytology. Springfield IL, Charles C. Thomas, 1964.

Lobenthal SW, Hajdu SI. The cytopathology of bone marrow transplantation. Acta Cytol 34:559–566, 1990.

Lobritz RW, Roberts TH, Marraro RV, et al. Granulomatous pulmonary disease secondary to Alternaria. JAMA 241:596–597, 1979.

Lombard CM, Duncan SR, Rizk NW, Colby TV. The diagnosis of Wegener's granulomatosis from transbronchial biopsy specimens. Hum Pathol 21: 838–842, 1990.

Louria DB, Lieberman PH, Collins HS, Blevins A. Pulmonary mycetoma due to Allescheria boydii. Arch Intern Med 117:748–751, 1966.

Ludwig ME, Otis RD, Cole SR, Westcott JL. Fine needle aspiration cytology of pulmonary hamartomas. Acta Cytol 26: 671–677, 1982.

Luna MA, Bedrossian CWM, Lichtiger B, Salem PA. Interstitial pneumonitis associated with bleomycin therapy. Am J Clin Pathol 58:501–510, 1972.

Mahmoud AAF. Parasitic protozoa and helminths: Biological and immunological challenges. Science 246:1015–1022, 1989.

Marik PE. Aspiration pneumonitis and aspiration pneumonia. N Engl J Med 344:665–671, 2001.

Mariotta S, Guidi L, et al. Pulmonary alveolar microlithiasis; Review of Italian reports. Eur J Epidemiol 13:587–590, 1997.

Mark GJ, Lehimgar-Zadeh A, Ragsdale BD. Cyclophosphamide pneumonitis. Thorax 33:89–93, 1978.

Marshall E. Beryllium screening raises ethical issues. Science 285:178–179, 1999.

Martin RJ, Coalson JJ, Rogers RM, et al. Pulmonary alveolar proteinosis: The diagnosis by segmental lavage. Am Rev Respir Dis 121:819–825, 1980.

Martin WJ, Osborn MJ, Douglas WW. Amiodarone pulmonary toxicity: Assessment by bronchial lavage. Chest 88:630–631, 1985.

Mazzucchelli L, Radelfinger H, Kraft R. Nonasbestos ferruginous bodies in sputum from a patient with graphite pneumoconiosis. Acta Cytol 40: 552–554, 1996.

McAdams HP, Rosado de Christenson M, Strollo DC, Patz EF Jr. Pulmonary mucormycosis: Radiologic findings in 32 cases. Am J Roentgenol 168: 1541–1548, 1997.

McCallum SM. Ova of the lung fluke Paragonimus kellicotti in fluid from a cyst. Acta Cytol 19:279–280, 1975.

McDowell EM, Barrett LA, et al. The respiratory epithelium. I Human bronchus. J Natl Cancer Inst 61:539–549, 1978.

McDowell EM, Barrett LA, Trump BF. Observations on small granule cells in adult human bronchial epithelium and in carcinoid and oat cell tumors. Lab Invest 34:202–206, 1976b.

McDowell EM, Barrett LA, et al. Abnormal cilia in human bronchial epithelium. Arch Pathol Lab Med 100:429–436, 1976a.

McKee G, Parums DV. False-Positive cytodiagnosis in fibrosing alveolitis. Acta Cytol 34:105–107, 1990.

Medici TC, Chodosh S. Qualitative und quantitative Exfoliativzytologie bei chronischer Bronchitis. Schweiz Med Wochenschr 104:859–864, 1974.

Melamed MR, Cliffton EE, Mercer C, Koss LG. The megakaryocyte blood count. Am J Med Sci 252:301–309, 1966.

Mellors RC. Cellular localization of fluorescent products derived from cigarette smoke: Studies in experimental animals and in man by fluorescent microscopy. Am J Pathol 33(Abstr):611, 1971.

Mermolja M, Rott T, Debeljak A. Cytology of bronchoalveolar lavage in some rare pulmonary disorders: Pulmonary alveolar proteinosis and amiodarone pulmonary toxicity. Cytopathol 5:9–16, 1994.

Metzger JB, Garagusi VF, Kerwin DM. Pulmonary oxalosis caused by Aspergillus niger. Am Rev Respir Dis 129:501–502, 1984.

Meyer EC, Liebow AA. Relationship of interstitial pneumonia, honeycombing and atypical epithelial proliferation to cancer of the lung. Cancer 18: 322–351, 1965.

Min KW, Gyorkey F. Interstitial pulmonary fibrosis, atypical epithelial changes and bronchiolar cell carcinoma following busulfan therapy. Cancer 22: 1027–1032, 1968.

Mitchell ML, King DE, Bonfiglio TA, Patten SF. Pulmonary fine needle aspiration cytopathology. A five-year correlation study. Acta Cytol 28:72–76, 1984.

Moloo Z, Finley RJ, Lefcoe MS, et al. Possible spread of bronchogenic carcinoma to the chest wall after a transthoracic fine needle aspiration biopsy. A case report. Acta Cytol 29:167–169, 1985.

Moreau MF, Chretien MF, Dubin J, et al. Transposed ciliary microtubules in Kartagener's syndrome. A case report with electron microscopy of bronchial and nasal brushings. Acta Cytol 29:248–253, 1985.

Mottet NK, Szanton V. Exfoliated measles giant cells in nasal secretions. Arch Pathol 72:434–437, 1961.

Myers JL. Micronodular pneumocyte hyperplasia: The versatile type 2 pneumocyte all dressed up in yet another brand new suit. Adv Anat Pathol 6:49–55, 1999.

Myers JL, Kennedy JI, Plumb VJ. Amiodarone lung: Pathologic findings in clinically toxic patients. Hum Pathol 18:340–354, 1987.

Mylius EA, Gullvag B. Alveolar macrophage count as an indicator of lung reaction to industrial air pollution. Acta Cytol 30:157–165, 1986.

Naib ZM, Stewart JA, Dowdle WR, et al. Cytological features of viral respiratory tract infection. Acta Cytol 12:162–171, 1968.

Naib ZM. Cytologic diagnosis of cytomegalic inclusion-body disease. Am J Dis Child 105:153–159, 1963.

Naib ZM. Exfoliative cytology of fungus diseases of the lung. Acta Cytol 6: 413–416, 1962.

Naimey GL, Wuerker RB; Comparison of histologic stains in the diagnosis of Pneumocystis carinii. Acta Cytol 39:1124–1127, 1995.

Nakanishi K. Alveolar epithelial hyperplasia and adenocarcinoma of the lung. Arch Pathol Lab Med 114:363–368, 1990.

Nakata K, Gotoh H, Watanabe J, et al. Augmented proliferation of human alveolar macrophages after allogeneic bone marrow transplantation. Blood 93:667–673, 1999.

Nakayama H, Noguchi M, Tsuchiya R, et al. Clonal growth of atypical adenomatous hyperplasia of the lung: Cytofluorimetric analysis of nuclear DNA content. Mod Pathol 3:314–320, 1990.

Nash G. Necrotizing tracheobronchitis and bronchopneumonia consistent with herpetic infection. Hum Pathol 3:283–291, 1972.

Nash G, Major O, Foley FD. Herpetic infection of the middle and lower respiratory tract. Am J Clin Pathol 54:857–863, 1970.

Nasiell M. Sputum-cytologic changes in smokers and nonsmokers in relation to chronic inflammatory lung diseases. Acta Pathol Microbiol Scand 74: 205–213, 1968.

Nasiell M. Abnormal columnar cell findings in bronchial epithelium. A cytologic and histologic study of lung cancer and non-cancer. Acta Cytol 11: 397–402, 1967.

Nasiell M. Metaplasia and atypical metaplasia in the bronchial epithelium. A histopathologic and cytopathologic study. Acta Cytol 10:421–427, 1966.

Nasiell M, Roger V, Naisell K, et al. Cytologic findings indicating pulmonary tuberculosis. 1. The diagnostic significance of epithelioid cells and Langhans' giant cells found in sputum or bronchial secretions. Acta Cytol 16:146–151, 1972.

Naylor B, Railey C. A pitfall in the cytodiagnosis of sputum of asthmatics. J Clin Pathol 17:84–89, 1964.

Naylor B. The shedding of the mucosa of the bronchial tree in asthma. Thorax 17:69–72, 1962.

Neifer RA, Amy RWM. Cytology of tracheobronchial amyloidosis (Letter). Acta Cytol 29:187–188, 1985.

Newsome AL, Curtis FT, Culbertson CG, Allen SD. Identification of Acanthamoeba in bronchoalveolar lavage specimens. Diagn Cytopath 8:231–234, 1992.

Nogee LM, Dunbar AE, Wert SE, et al. A mutation in the surfactant protein C gene with familial interstitial lung disease. N Engl J Med 344:573–579, 2001.

Northway WH Jr, Rosan RC. Oxygen therapy hazards in the neonate. Hosp Pract 4:59–67, 1969.

Nowakovsky S, McGrew EA, Medak H, et al. Manifestations of viral infections in exfoliated cells. Acta Cytol 12:227–236, 1968.

Nunez V, Melamed MR, Cahan W. Tracheobronchial cytology after laryngectomy for carcinoma of larynx. 11. Benign atypias. Acta Cytol 10:38–48, 1966.

O'Driscoll BR, Hasleton PS, Taylor PM, et al. Active lung fibrosis up to 17 years after therapy with carmustine (BCNU) in childhood. N Engl J Med 323:378–382, 1990.

Ognibene FP, Shelhamer J, Gill V, et al. The diagnosis of Pneumocystis carinii pneumonia in patients with the acquired immunodeficiency syndrome using segmental bronchoalveolar lavage. Am Rev Respir Dis 129:929–932, 1984.

Olsson M, Elvin K, Lidman C, et al. A rapid and simple nested PCR assay for the detection of Pneumocystis carinii in sputum samples. Scand J Infect Dis 28:547–600, 1996.

Orenstein M, Webber CA, Heunch AE. Cytologic diagnosis of Pneumocystis carinii infection by bronchoalveolar lavage in acquired immune deficiency syndrome. Acta Cytol 29:727–731, 1985.

Osborne PT, Gillman LJ, Uthman EO. Trichomonads in the respiratory tract. A case report and literature review. Acta Cytol 28:136–138, 1984.

Oztek I, Baloglu H, Demirel D, et al. Cytologic diagnosis of complicated pulmonary unilocular cystic hydatidosis. A study of 131 cases. Acta Cytol 41: 1150–1166, 1997.

Papanicolaou GN. Degenerative changes in ciliated cells exfoliating from bronchial epithelium as cytologic criterion in diagnosis of diseases of lung. NY State J Med 56:2647–2650, 1956.

Paradis IL, Ross C, Dekker A, Dauber J. A comparison of modified methenamine silver and toluidine blue stains for the detection of Pneumocystis carinii in bronchoalveolar lavage specimens from immunosuppressed patients. Acta Cytol 34:511–516, 1990.

Parham DM, Bozeman P, Killian C, et al. Cytologic diagnosis of respiratory syncytial virus infection in a bronchoalveolar lavage specimen from a bone marrow transplant recipient. Am J Clin Pathol 99:588–592, 1993.

Patchefsky AS, Israel HL. Pulmonary Wegener's granulomatosis. Ann Clin Lab Sci 3:249–258, 1973.

Patel AR, Shah PC, Rhee HL, et al. Cyclophosphamide therapy and interstitial pulmonary fibrosis. Cancer 38:1542–1549, 1976.

Patterson R, Head LR, Suszko IM, Zeiss CR, Jr. Mast cells from human respiratory tissue and their in vitro reactivity. Science 175:1012–1014, 1972.

Pfitzer P. Zytodiagnostik der Lungenerkrankungen. GBK Mitteilungsdienst. 15(52):11–14, 1987.

Pfitzer P, Wehle K, Blanke M, Burrig K-F. Fluorescence microscopy of Papanicolaou-stained bronchoalveolar lavage specimens in the diagnosis of Pneumocystis carinii. Acta Cytol 33:557–559, 1989.

Pickren JW. Identification of oil-red-O stained granules in sputum macrophages. JAMA 215:1985, 1971.

Pierce CH, Hirsch JG. Ciliocytophthoria: Relationship to viral respiratory infections of humans. Proc Soc Exp Biol Med 98:489–492, 1958.

Pierce CH, Knox AW. Ciliocytophthoria in sputum from patients with adenovirus infections. Proc Soc Exp Biol Med 104:492–495, 1960.

Pilotti S, Rilke F, Gribaudi G, et al. Transthoracic fine needle aspiration biopsy in pulmonary lesions: Updated results. Acta Cytol 28:225–232, 1984.

Pitman MB, Szytelbein WM, Niles J, Fienberg R. Clinical utility of fine needle aspiration biopsy in the diagnosis of Wegener's granulomatosis. A report of two cases. Acta Cytol 36:222–229, 1992.

Plamenac P, Nikulin A, Pikula B. Cytologic changes of the respiratory epithelium in iron foundry workers. Acta Cytol 18:34–40, 1974.

Plamenac P, Nikulin A, Pikula B. Cytology of the respiratory tract in former smokers. Acta Cytol 16:256–260, 1972.

Plamenac P, Nikulin A, Kahvic M. Cytology of the respiratory tract in advanced age. Acta Cytol 14:526–530, 1970.

Plamenac P, Nikulin A. Atypia of the bronchial epithelium in wind instrument players and in singers: A cytopathologic study. Acta Cytol 13:274–278, 1969.

Prince DS, Peterson DD, Steiner RM, et al. Infection with Mycobacterium avium complex in patients without predisposing conditions. N Engl J Med 321:863–868, 1989.

Prior C, Klima G, Gattringer C, et al. Cell profiles in serial bronchoalveolar laveage after human heart-lung transplantation. Acta Cytol 36:19–25, 1992.

Purtilo DT, Meyers WM, Connor DH. Fatal strongyloidiasis in immunosuppressed patients. Am J Med 56:488–493, 1974.

Raab SS, Silverman JF, Zimmerman KG. Fine needle aspiration biopsy of coccidiomycosis. Spectrum of cytologic findings in 73 patients. Am J Clin Pathol 99: 582–587, 1993.

Radio SJ, Rennard SI, Ghafouri MA, Linder J. Cytomorphology of *Alternaria* in bronchoalveolar lavage specimens. Acta Cytol 31:243–248, 1987.

Ramirez RJ, Kieffer RF Jr, Ball WC Jr. Bronchopulmonary lavage in man. Ann Intern Med 63:819–828, 1965.

Rangdaeng S, Alpert LC, Khiyami A, et al. Pulmonary paragonimiasis. Report of a case with diagnsis by fine needle aspiration cytology. Acta Cytol 36: 31–36, 1992.

Reddy PA, Gorelick DF, Christianson CF. Giant cell interstitial pneumonia (GIP). Chest 58:319–325, 1970.

Remadi S, Dumais J, Wafa K, MacGee W. Pulmonary microsporidiosis in a patient with the acquired immunodeficiency syndrome. A case report. Acta Cytol 39:1112–1116, 1995.

Rennard SI, Hunninghake GW, Bitterman PB, Crystal RG. Production of fibronectin by the human alveolar macrophage: Mechanism for the recruitment of fibroblasts to sites of tissue injury in interstitial lung diseases. Proc Natl Acad Sci USA 78:7147–7151, 1981.

Repsher LH, Schroter G, Hammond WS. Diagnosis of *Pneumocystis carinii* pneumonitis by means of endobronchial brush biopsy. N Engl J Med 287: 340–341, 1972.

Reyes CV, Kathuria S, MacGlashan A. Diagnostic value of calcium oxalate crystals in respiratory and pleural fluid cytology. Acta Cytol 23:65–68, 1979.

Reynolds HY, Fulmer JD, Kazmierowski JA, et al. Analysis of cellular and protein content of broncho-alveolar lavage fluid from patients with idiopathic pulmonary fibrosis and chronic hypersensitivity pneumonitis. J Clin Invest 59:165–175, 1977.

Reynolds HY, Newball HH. Analysis of proteins and respiratory cells obtained from human lungs by bronchial lavage. J Lab Clin Med 84:559–573, 1974.

Rhodin JAG. Ultrastructure and function of the human tracheal mucosa. Am Rev Respir Dis 93(Suppl):1–15, 1966.

Roger V, Nasiell M, Nasiell K, et al. Cytologic findings indicating pulmonary tuberculosis. II. The occurrence in sputum of epithelioid cells and multinucleated giant cells in pulmonary tuberculosis, chronic non-tuberculosis inflammatory lung disease and bronchogenic carcinoma. Acta Cytol 16: 538–541, 1972.

Roggli VL, Piantadosi CA, Bell DY. Asbestos bodies in bronchoalveolar lavage fluid. A study of 20 asbestos exposed individuals and comparison to patients with other chronic interstitial lung diseases. Acta Cytol 30:470–476, 1986.

Roque AL, Pickren JW. Enzymatic changes in fluorescent alveolar macrophages of the lungs of cigarette smokers. Acta Cytol 12:420–429, 1968.

Rose MS. Busulphan toxicity syndrome caused by chlorambucil. Br Med J 2: 123, 1975.

Rosemond GP, Burnett WE, Hall JH. Value and limitations of aspiration biopsy for lung lesions. Radiology 52:506–510, 1949.

Rosen P, Gordon P, Savino A, Melamed M. Ferruginous bodies in benign fibrous pleural plaques. Am J Clin Pathol 60:608–612, 1973.

Rosen P, Hajdu SI. Visceral herpesvirus infections in patients with cancer. Am J Clin Pathol 56:459–465, 1971.

Rosen P, Melamed MR, Savino A. The "ferruginous body" content of lung tissue: A quantitative study of 86 patients. Acta Cytol 16:207–211, 1972.

Rosen PP, Martini N, Armstrong D. *Pneumocystis carinii* pneumonia diagnosis by lung biopsy. Am. J Med 58:794–802, 1975.

Rosen SH, Castleman B, Liebow AA. Pulmonary alveolar proteinosis. N Engl J Med 258:1123–1142, 1958.

Rosenthal DL. Cytopathology of Pulmonary Disease (Monographs in Clinical Cytology). Basel, Karger, 1988.

Rosenthal DL, Wallace JM. Fine needle aspiration of pulmonary lesion via fiberoptic bronchoscopy. Acta Cytol 28:203–210, 1984.

Russell HT, Nelson BM. Pneumocystis in American infants. Am J Clin Pathol 26:1334–1340, 1956.

Sacchini V, Galimberti V, Marchini S, Luini A. Percutaneous transthoracic needle aspiration biopsy: A case report of implantation metastasis. Eur J Surg Oncol 15:179–183, 1989.

Saccomanno G, Saunders RP, Klein MG, et al. Cytology of the lung in reference to irritant, individual sensitivity and healing. Acta Cytol 14:377–381, 1970.

Saetta S, Baraldo S, Corbino L, et al. CD 8+ cells in the lungs of smokers with chronic obstructive pulmonary disease. Am J Respir Crit Care Med 160: 711–717, 1999.

Saito Y, Imai T, Sato M, et al. Cytologic study of tissue repair in bronchial epithelium. Acta Cytol 32:622–628, 1988.

Saltini C, Hance AJ, Ferrans VJ, et al. Accurate quantification of cells recovered by bronchoalveolar lavage. Am Rev Respir Dis 130:650–658, 1984.

Salzman SH, Smith RL, Aranda CP. Histoplasmosis in patients at risk for the acquired immunodeficiency syndrome in a nonacademic setting. Chest 93: 916–921, 1988.

Sandritter W, Meuller D, Schaefer H, Schienter HG. Histochemie von Sputumzellan. II. Quantitative ultraviolettmikrospektrophotometrische Nucleinsaeurebestimmungen. Zeitschr Pathol Frankf 68:710–727, 1958.

Sanerkin NG, Evans DMD. The sputum in bronchial asthma: Pathognomonic patterns. J Pathol Bacteriol 89:535–541, 1965.

Sargent EN, Turner AF, Gordonson J, et al. Percutaneous pulmonary needle biopsy. Report of 350 patients. Am J Roentgenol Radium Ther Nucl Med 122:758–768, 1974.

Savige J, Gillis D, Benson E, et al. International consensus statement on testing and reporting of antineutrophil cytoplasmic antibodies (ANCA). Am J Clin Pathol F111:507–513, 1999.

Scaglia M, Gatti S, Sacchi L, et al. Asymptomatic respiratory tract microsporidiosis due to *Encephalitozoon hellem* in three patients with AIDS. Clin Infect Dis 26:174–176, 1998.

Schleuter DP, Fink JN, Hensley GT. A hypersensitivity pneumonitis caused by *Alternaria*. Ann Intern Med 77: 907–914, 1972.

Schmitz B, Pfitzer P. Acellular bodies in sputum. Acta Cytol 28:118–125, 1984.

Schneider EL, Epstein CJ, Kabak M, Brandes D. Severe pulmonary involvement in adult Gaucher's disease. Report of three cases and review of the literature. Am J Med 63:475–480, 1977.

Schober R, Bensch KG, Kosek JC, Northway WH. Origin of membranous intra-alveolar material in pulmonary alveolar proteinosis. Exp Mol Pathol 21: 246–258, 1974.

Schoch OD, Schanz U, Koller M, et al. BAL findings in a patient with pulmonary alveolar proteinosis successfully treated with GM-CSF. Thorax 57:277–280, 2002.

Schumann GB, Roby TJ, Swan GE, Sorensen KW. Quantitative sputum cytologic findings in 109 nonsmokers. Am Rev Respir Dis 139:601–603, 1989.

Schwartz DA, Ogden PO, Blumberg HM, Honig E. Pulmonary malakoplakia in a patient with the acquired immunodeficiency syndrome. Differential diagnostic considerations. Arch Pathol Lab Med 114:1267–1272, 1990.

Schwartz DA, Visvesvara GS, Leitch GJ, et al. Pathology of symptomatic microsporidial (*Encephalitozoon hellem*) bronchiolitis in the acquired immunodeficiency syndrome: A new respiratory pathogen diagnosed from lung biopsy, bronchoalveolar lavage, sputum, and tissue culture. Hum Pathol 24: 937–943, 1993.

Scoggins WG, Smith RH, Frable WJ, O'Donohue WJ Jr. False positive diagnosis of lung carcinoma in patients with pulmonary infarcts. Ann Thorac Surg 24:474–480, 1977.

Selvaggi SM. Bronchoalveolar lavage in lung transplant patients. Acta Cytol 36: 674–679, 1992.

Shahar J, Mailman D, Meitzen G. Crystals in pulmonary cytologic preparations in association with aspiration of barium. A case report. Acta Cytol 38: 415–416, 1994.

Shin MS, Cooper JA Jr, Ho KJ. Pulmonary malacoplakia associated with Rhodococcus equi infection in a patient with AIDS. Chest 115:889–892, 1999.

Silverman JF, Turner RC, West RL, Dillard TA. Bronchoalveolar lavage in the diagnosis of lipoid pneumonia. Diagn Cytopathol 5:3–8, 1989.

Sinner WN, Zajicek J. Implantation metastasis after percutaneous transthoracic needle aspiration biopsy. Acta Radiol Diagn (Stockh) 17:473–480, 1976.

Sisson JH, Papi A, Beckmann JD, et al. Smoke and viral infection cause cilia loss detectable by bronchoalveolar lavage cytology and dynein ELISA. Am J Respir Crit Care Med 149:205–213, 1994.

Smith MJ, Naylor B. A method for extracting ferruginous bodies from sputum and pulmonary tissue. Am J Clin Pathol 58:250–254, 1972.

Smith P, Heath D, Moosair H. The Clara cell. Thorax 29:147–163, 1974.

Sosolik RC, Gammon RR, Julius CJ, Ayers LW. Pulmonary alveolar proteinosis. Acta Cytol 42:377–383, 1998.

Spain DM, Bradess VA, Tarter R, Matero A. Metaplasia of bronchial epithelium. Effect of age, sex, and smoking. JAMA 211:1331–1334, 1970.

Spencer H. Pathology of the Lung. New York, Macmillan, 1962.

Stanley MW, Henry-Stanley MJ, Gajl-Peczalska KJ, Bitterman PB. Hyperplasia of type II pneumocytes in acute lung injury. Am J Clin Pathol 97: 669–677, 1992.

Stein B, Zaatari GS, Pine JR. Amiodarone pulmonary toxicity. Clinical, cytologic, and ultrastructural findings. Acta Cytol 31:357–361, 1987.

Stevens WJ, Vermeire PA. *Giardia lamblia* in bronchoalveolar lavage fluid. Thorax 36:875, 1981.

Stokes MB, Jagirder J, Burchstin O, et al. Nodular pulmonary immunoglobulin light chain deposits with coexistent amyloid and non-amyloid features in an HIV-infected patient. Mod Pathol 10:1059–1065, 1997.

Stoller JK, Rankin JA, Reynolds HY. The impact of bronchoalveolar lavage cell analysis on clinicians' diagnostic reasoning about interstitial lung disease. Chest 92:839–843, 1987.

Stover DE, Zaman MB, Hajdu SI, et al. Bronchoalveolar lavage in the diagnosis of diffuse pulmonary infiltrates in the immunosuppressed host. Ann Intern Med 101:1–7, 1984.

Studdy PR, Rudd RM, Gellert AR, et al. Bronchoalveolar lavage in the diagnosis of diffuse pulmonary shadowing. Br J Dis Chest 78:46–54, 1984.

Sturgess JM, Chao J, Turner JA. Transposition of ciliary microtubules: Another cause of impaired ciliary motility. N Engl J Med 303:318–322, 1980.

Sughayer M, Ali SZ, Erozan YS, et al. Pulmonary malacoplakia associated with Rhodococcus Equi infection in an AIDS patient. Report of a case with diagnosis by fine needle aspiration. Acta Cytol 41:507–512, 1997.

Sun T, Chess Q. Fluorescence not specific for Pneumocystis carinii. Acta Cytol 30:549–552, 1986.

Sun T, Chess Q, Tanenbaum B. Morphologic criteria for the identification of Pneumocystis carinii in Papanicolaou-stained preparations (letter). Acta Cytol 30:80–82, 1986.

Tabatowski K, Roggli VL, Fulkerson WJ, et al. Giant cell interstitial pneumonia in a hard-metal worker. Cytologic, histologic and analytical electron microscopic investigation. Acta Cytol 32:240–246, 1988.

Takahashi M, Hayata Y. Cytology of the Lung: Techniques and Interpretation. Tokyo, New York, Igaku-Shoin, 1983.

Takeda M, Burechailo FA. Smooth muscle cells in sputum. Acta Cytol 13:696–699, 1969.

Tani EM, Franco M. Pulmonary cytology in paracoccidioidomycosis. Acta Cytol 28:571–575, 1984.

Tao LC. Guides to Clinical Aspiration Biopsy. Lung Pleura and Mediastinum. New York, Igaku-Shoin, 1988.

Tassoni EM. Pools of lymphocytes: Significance in pulmonary secretions. Acta Cytol 7:168–173, 1963.

Taxay EP, Montgomery RD, Wildish DM. Studies of pulmonary alveolar microlithiasis and pulmonary alveolar proteinosis. Am J Clin Pathol 34:532–545, 1960.

Teschler H, Friedrichs KH, Hoheisel GB, et al. Asbestos fibers in bronchoalveolar lavage and lung tissue of former asbestos workers. Am J Respir Crit Care Med 149:641–645, 1994.

Thomas ED, Ramberg RE, Sale GE, et al. Direct evidence for a bone marrow origin of the alveolar macrophage in man. Science 192:1016–1018, 1976.

Tomashefski JF Jr, Cramer SF, Abramowsky C, et al. Needle biopsy diagnosis of solitary amyloid nodule of the lung. Acta Cytol 24:224–227, 1980.

Tomb JA, Matossian RM. Diagnosis of pulmonary hydatidosis by sputum cytology. Johns Hopkins Med J 139 Suppl:38–40, 1976.

Tomita T, Chiga M. Disseminated histoplasmosis in acquired immunodeficiency syndrome: Light and electron microscopic observations. Hum Pathol 19:438–441, 1988.

Tompkins V, Macaulay JC. A characteristic cell in nasal secretions during prodromal measles. JAMA 157:711, 1955.

Trapnell BC, Whitsett JA, Nakata K. Pulmonary alveolar proteinosis. N Engl J Med 239: 2527–2539, 2003.

Trump GF, McDowell EM, et al. The respiratory epithelium. III. Histogenesis of epidermal metaplasia and carcinoma in situ in the human. J Natl Cancer Inst 61:563–575, 1978.

Usuda K, Saito Y, Imai T, et al. Inflammatory pseudotumor of the lung diagnosed as granulomatous lesion by preoperative brushing cytology. A case report. Acta Cytol 34:685–689, 1990.

Valicenti JF Jr, McMaster KR, Daniell CJ. Sputum cytology of giant cell interstitial pneumonia. Acta Cytol 23:217–221, 1979.

Valicenti JV, Daniell C, Gobien RP. Thin needle aspiration cytology of benign intrathoracic lesions. Acta Cytol 25:659–664, 1981.

van der Geld YM, Huitema MG, Franssen CF, et al. In vitro T lymphocyte responses to proteinase 3 (PR3) and linear peptides of PR3 in patients with Wegener's granulomatosis (WG). Clin Exp Immunol 122:504–513, 2000.

Van der Veen MJ, Dekker JJ, Dinant HJ, et al. Fatal pulmonary fibrosis complicating low dose methotrexate therapy for rheumatoid arthritis. J Rheumatol 22:1766–1768, 1995.

Van Horn KG, Tatz JS, Li KI, Newman L. Copepods associated with a perirectal abscess and copepod pseudo-outbreaks in stools for ova and parasite examinations. Diagn Microbiol Infect Dis 15:561–565, 1992.

Vassallo R, Ryu JR, Colby TV, et al. Pulmonary Langerhans' cell histiocytosis. N Eng J Med 342:1969–1978, 2000.

Vera-Alvarez J, Marigil-Gomez M, Abascal-Agorreta M, Pons-Bosque J. Local-

ized pulmonary amyloidosis diagnosed by fine needle aspiration cytology. Acta Cytol 37:846–848, 1993.

Vernon SE. Nodular pulmonary sarcoidosis. Diagnosis with fine needle aspiration biopsy. Acta Cytol 29:473–476, 1985.

Vigorita VJ, Gupta PK, Bargeron CB, Frost JK. Occurrence and identification of intracellular calcium crystals in pulmonary specimens. Acta Cytol 23:49–52, 1979.

Wada S, Miyanishi M, Nishimoto Y, et al. Mustard gas as a cause of respiratory neoplasia in man. Lancet 1:1161–1163, 1968.

Walker AN, Walker GK, Feldman PS. Diagnosis of Legionella micdadei pneumonia from cytologic specimens. Acta Cytol 27:252–254, 1983.

Walker KR, Fullmer CD. Observations of eosinophilic extracytoplasmic processes in pulmonary macrophages. Progress report. Acta Cytol 15:363–364, 1971.

Walker KR, Fullmer CD. Progress report on study of respiratory spirals. Acta Cytol 14:396–398, 1970.

Walter A, Krishnaswami H Cariappa A. Microfilariae of Wuchereria bancrofti in cytologic smears. Acta Cytol 27:432–436, 1983.

Walton BC, Bacharach T. Occurrence of trichomonads in the respiratory tract: Report of three cases. J Parasitol 49:35–38, 1963.

Wang FBM, Stern EJ, Schmidt RA, Pierson DJ. Diagnosing pulmonary alveolar proteinosis. A review and an update. Chest 111: 460–466, 1997.

Wang KP, Marsh BR, Summer WR, et al. Transbronchial needle aspiration for diagnosis of lung cancer. Chest 80:48–50, 1981.

Wang SE, Nieberg RK. Fine needle aspiration cytology of sclerosing hemangioma of the lung: A mimicker of bronchioloalveolar carcinoma. Acta Cytol 30:51–54, 1986.

Warner NE, McGrew EA, Nanos S. Cytologic study of the sputum in cytomegalic inclusion disease. Acta Cytol 8:311–315, 1964.

Weaver KM, Novak PM, Naylor B. Vegetable cell contaminants in cytologic specimens. Their resemblance to cells associated with various normal and pathologic states. Acta Cytol 25:210–214, 1981.

Weber R, Bryan RT, Schwartz DA, Owen RL. Human microsporidial infections. Clin Microbiol Rev 7:426–461, 1994.

Wehle K, Pfitzer P. Nonspecific esterase activity of human alveolar macrophages in routine cytology. Acta Cytol 32:153–158, 1988.

Weinberger SE, Kelman JA, Elson NA, et al. Bronchoalveolar lavage in interstitial lung disease. Ann Intern Med 89:459–466, 1978.

Weston JT, Guin GH. Epithelial atypias with chemotherapy in 100 acute childhood leukemias. Cancer 8:179–186, 1955.

Willie SM, Snyder RX. The identification of Paragonimus westermani in bronchial washings. Case report. Acta Cytol 21:101–102, 1977.

Willman CL, Busque L, Griffith BB, et al. Langerhans' cell histiocytosis (histiocytosis X)—a clonal proliferative disease. N Engl J Med 331:154–160, 1994.

Winternitz MC, Wasun LM, McNamara FP. The pathology of influenza. New Haven, Yale University Press, 1920.

Yang YJ, Steele CT, Anbar RD, et al. Quantitation of lipid-laden macrophages in evaluation of lower airway cytology specimens from pediatric patients. Diagn Cytopathol 24:98–103, 2001.

Yeager HJ, Zimmet SM, Schwartz SL. Pinocytosis by human alveolar macrophages. Comparison of smokers and nonsmokers. J Clin Invest 54:247–251, 1974.

Yoshikawa T, Yoshida J, Nishimura M, et al. Lung cancer implantation in the chest wall following percutaneous fine needle aspiration biopsy. Jpn J Clin Oncol 30:450–452, 2000.

Yousem SA, Colby TV, Chen YY, et al. Pulmonary Langerhans' cell histiocytosis: Molecular analysis of clonality. Am J Surg Pathol 25:630–636, 2001.

Zaharopoulos P, Wong JY. Cytologic diagnosis of rhinoscleroma. Acta Cytol 28:139–142, 1984.

Zakowski P, Fligiel S, Berlin GW, Johnston BL Jr. Disseminated Mycobacterium avium-intracellulare infection in homosexual men dying of acquired immunodeficiency. JAMA 248:2980–2982, 1982.

Zaman SS, Elshami A, Gupta PK. Bronchoalveolar lavage cytology in pulmonary sarcoidosis. Acta Cytol 39:1117–1123, 1995.

Zaman SS, Seykora JT, Hodinka RL, et al. Cytologic manifestations of respiratory syncytial virus pneumonia in bronchoalveolar lavage fluid. Acta Cytol 40:546–551, 1996.

Zavala DC, Schoell JE. Ultrathin needle aspiration of the lung in infections and malignant disease. Am Rev Respir Dis 123:125–131, 1981.

Tumors of the Lung: Conventional Cytology and Aspiration Biopsy

20

Revised by Myron R. Melamed

At the onset of the 21st century, cancer of the lung remains the most common cause of cancer deaths in men and women alike, as it has been for many years (Landis et al, 1999). The link between lung cancer and cigarette smoking was emphasized half a century ago by Wynder and Graham (1950) and became officially recognized in 1957 when the Surgeon General of the United States, Leroy E. Burney, issued a statement declaring, "Excessive smoking is one of the causative factors in lung cancer." This was followed by a Public Health Service Monograph, "Smoking and Health" published in 1964 (PHS monograph 1103) that exhaustively reviewed the health effects of cigarette smoking and clearly established the relationship between cigarette smoking and lung cancer. It may be assumed that a subsequent decrease in cigarette smoking accounts for the recent modest drop in the incidence and deaths from this disease in the US. The relationship between cigarette smoking and lung cancer is complex, however, and individuals differ in their susceptibility to the carcinogenic effects of cigarette smoking and probably other environmental agents (Spitz, 1999); the challenge of the future will be to identify those who are constitutionally at risk.

Lung cancer is also an occupational disease. The earliest recorded cases of occupational lung cancer, first recognized in 1879, were among the Schneeberg and Joachimstal miners of Czechoslovakia who were exposed to radon gas in material known as *Pitchblende,* from which Pierre and Marie Curie extracted and isolated radium. In the US, lung cancer in Colorado uranium miners has been attributed to radiation (Archer et al, 1974; Saccomanno et al, 1988). Arsenic, long known to produce cutaneous hyperkeratoses, is now also recognized as a cause of lung cancer. At least 12 substances found in the workplace are considered to be lung carcinogens in humans, and 5% of lung cancers in the US have been attributed to occupational exposure (Doll and Peto, 1981). The industrial agents reported to cause lung cancer include chloromethyl ether, mustard gas, polycyclic aromatic hydrocarbons, crystalline silica, nickel, chromium, beryllium, cadmium, and asbestos, the last in association with cigarette smoking (Braun and Truant, 1958; Cordova et al, 1962; Talcott et al, 1989; Rosenman and Stanbury, 1996; Steenland et al, 1996; Beckett, 2000). Of these, asbestos is of particular interest to the cytopathologist because these fibers can be identified in specimens of sputum (see Chap. 19). Asbestos fibers may be observed in sputum simultaneously with cancer cells, as was first demonstrated by An and Koprowska in 1962. For a comprehensive review of the pathology of asbestos associated diseases, see Roggli et al, 1992.

Finally, human papillomavirus (HPV) has been implicated in the pathogenesis of squamous lung cancer. Syrjänen et al (1989) reported finding HPV types 6 and 16 in 9 of 131 squamous lung cancers. On the other hand, Stremlau et al (1985) hybridized tissue from 24 lung tumor biopsies with 10 different HPV types and found only 1 carcinoma with HPV (type 16). The latter occurred in a woman with a history of treated cervical carcinoma and the lung tumor may have represented metastatic cancer. Thus, the evidence that **HPV has a role in carcinogenesis of the lung is unconfirmed.** See also comments on the role of HPV in cervical cancer (Chap. 11), lesions of the oral cavity and larynx (Chap. 21), and the esophagus (Chap. 24).

The relative frequency of the histologic subtypes of lung cancer in the US has changed dramatically over the last several decades (Vincent et al, 1977; Johnston, 1988; Devesa et al, 1991; Sobue et al, 1999). Squamous cancers, which were predominant in the 1950s and 1960s, now account for no more than 30% of cases. At the same time, **peripheral adenocarcinomas of the lung have increased in frequency and are now the most common type of lung cancer in the US.** The reason for this is unknown but has been attributed to changes in the manufacture of cigarettes, the use of filter tips, or the possible effects of other environmental cofactors. As a result, **sputum cytology, which best detects early squamous carcinomas, is less useful as a screening tool now than in prior years.** On the other hand, **percutaneous aspiration of peripheral lung lesions has become increasingly important in early diagnosis of small peripheral carcinomas,** even as tiny as 2 to 5 mm, and may prove of value in assessing lesions found by high-resolution spiral or helical computed tomography (CT) (Henschke et al, 1999).

Surgery remains the treatment of choice for all but small-cell lung cancer; even with recent advances in chemotherapy and radiotherapy, the **best opportunity for long-term survival and cure of lung cancer lies in early diagnosis and surgical resection.** A major feasibility study of early lung cancer detection, encompassing over 30,000 cigarette-smoking men who were followed for 5 to 8 years (Berlin et al, 1984; Flehinger et al, 1984; Fontana et al, 1984; Frost et al, 1984) has now been concluded (Melamed et al, 1984; Melamed and Flehinger, 1987; Flehinger et al, 1988; Melamed, 2000) and is summarized below. The results of this study failed to show a decrease in death rates from lung cancer, leading the **American Cancer Society and other influential agencies to recommend against screening for lung cancer. Chest x-rays and sputum cytology were considered to be diagnostic tools for symptomatic patients only. Because symptomatic lung cancer is usually advanced lung cancer, however, the opportunity for early diagnosis and cure is lost.** In a recent evaluation of the statistical basis for this recommendation, Dempster (1998) concluded that **the study data "strongly support a finding**

of benefit from routine screening of high-risk populations." Flehinger and Kimmel (1987) have estimated that
annual radiographic screening alone would decrease mortality from adenocarcinoma of the lung by up to 18%. The
results of extensive Japanese lung cancer studies also suggest
that surgical removal of very small adenocarcinomas, discovered by the new methods of CT, can improve the cure rate
significantly (Noguchi et al, 1995).

Ongoing studies of lung cancer detection, using **spiral
CT** (spiral or helical CT), known as the Early Lung Cancer
Action Project **(ELCAP),** summarized later in this chapter,
may yet modify future recommendations regarding screening for lung cancer (Henschke, 2000). This project, if successful, is likely to pose new challenges for interpretation
of cytology of sputum, bronchial brushes, bronchoalveolar
lavage, and particularly transbronchial and percutaneous
needle aspirates.

It must be emphasized that **cytology is a method of
choice in the diagnosis of radiologically detected lung
lesions suspected of being malignant.** Thus, it is appropriate to analyze briefly the existing methods of diagnosis of
lung cancer with attention to the role of cytology.

METHODS OF DIAGNOSIS OF LUNG CANCER

Asymptomatic Population

The original approach to the detection and diagnosis of
early lung cancer in asymptomatic, high-risk individuals was
based on an examination of conventional chest roentgenograms and sputum cytology. At present, spontaneously produced or artificially induced sputum only rarely leads to the
discovery of an occult lung cancer (see below). Most early
(small) lung cancers in asymptomatic individuals are incidental findings on routine chest roentgenograms, and increasingly sophisticated imaging techniques such as spiral
CT are now proposed to screen for the very earliest, potentially curable cancers. Whether these techniques will lead
to earlier diagnosis and more successful treatment of lung
cancer is the subject of ongoing studies.

Symptomatic Population

Roentgenologic Techniques

For patients with symptoms of cough, hemoptysis or chest
pain and radiologic abnormalities, whether or not suggestive
of lung cancer, there are several avenues of further investigation. Conventional and high-resolution CT may help clarify
the nature of a suspicious lesion or narrow the diagnostic
possibilities. More specific diagnosis requires morphologic
examination and analysis by cytologic techniques or by biopsy.

Cytologic Techniques

Cytologic examination of sputum, bronchial secretions, and
aspirates has a dual purpose:

- To determine the presence of tumor
- To classify the tumor as accurately as possible according to predominant histologic type. This task is of considerable importance, since it may influence the mode
  of treatment in individual cases. The **identification of
  small-cell carcinoma (SSC) versus all other (non-SSC)
  types is of primary importance.**

In competent hands and with experience, cytologic procedures serve to render the diagnosis of lung cancer with
precision, speed, and accuracy equal to or even superior
to other techniques. The benefits of cytologic methods are
substantial, as they often offer the option of treatment planning without the need for an open biopsy. It should be
emphasized, however, that **the interpretation of cytologic
findings must always be made in the context of clinical
findings,** since certain benign processes can induce cellular
changes that mimic a malignant neoplasm (see Chap. 19).

Sputum

Sputum cytology is the oldest and simplest of these diagnostic procedures and is readily available to every medical practitioner (summary in Wandall, 1944). **It can provide a
diagnosis in about 80% of primary lung carcinomas,**
depending on tumor type and stage. As already noted, cytology of sputum is most effective in the diagnosis of squamous
carcinomas of the lung, although other types of cancer can
be recognized and diagnosed as well. Sputum cytology also
may provide a substrate to **search for diagnostic molecular
markers of lung cancer** (Tockman et al, 1997; Ahrendt et
al, 1999).

Bronchial Brushings and Washings

Samples obtained by the fiberoptic bronchoscope also are
very effective in the diagnosis and differential diagnosis of
cancer. Brush specimens, obtained directly from the suspect
lesion, often provide an **excellent sample and exact information on the location of the disease.** The rigid bronchoscope, now seldom used, limits examination to the
mainstem, lobar, and lower lobe segmental bronchi.

Bronchoalveolar Lavage (BAL)

This technique was discussed in detail in Chapter 19. With
increasing incidence of peripheral adenocarcinomas, **BAL
has begun to play a more important role in the diagnosis
of lung cancer.** Initial reports of lung cancer diagnosed by
BAL (Springmeyer et al, 1983; Lindner et al, 1987) were
supported by a recent study in which BAL was positive for
malignant cells in 14 of 30 patients with endoscopically
invisible tumors, whereas transbronchial biopsy was positive
in only 5 of those patients (Wongsurakiat et al, 1998). **The
technique was also very effective in the diagnosis of
lymphangitic carcinomatosis caused by metastatic cancer (Levy et al, 1988),** but not as useful for other metastatic
cancer. As ever-smaller lesions of the lung are detected by
spiral CT, whether used as a diagnostic or screening tool,
BAL will come under further evaluation (Sone et al, 1998;
Henschke et al, 1999). **BAL specimens may also be used
for molecular analyses in the search for diagnostic or
prognostic markers** (Tockman, 2000).

Percutaneous Fine-Needle Aspiration Biopsy (FNA)

This method, performed under radiologic guidance, was described in Chapter 19, with a discussion of potential complications. It has been recognized since the 1970s as a critically important diagnostic technique (Koss et al, 1992), and is particularly valuable in the diagnosis of space-occupying lesions located in the periphery of the lung and in the mediastinum. The technique is used with increasing frequency to investigate pulmonary infiltrates as well as more discrete masses in the lung.

Transbronchial FNA Biopsy

Transbronchial FNA biopsy (TBFNA) is performed during fiberoptic bronchoscopy for diagnosis of tumor masses located outside the bronchial lumen. In early reviews of this procedure (Schenk et al, 1987; Gay et al, 1989), the method was found to be useful in selected cases of primary and metastatic cancer. It is also of potential value in the recognition and diagnosis of inflammatory disease and certain benign mediastinal or parabronchial masses.

Cell Block Technique

Given an adequate specimen, a selected portion of the sputum, bronchial brush specimen or needle aspirate may be fixed, embedded in paraffin and processed by histologic techniques to supplement the cytologic examination. **Cell block sections provide the advantage of a microbiopsy, and are highly recommended for examination of any specimen in which tiny tissue fragments are present or if there is residual material after the smears have been prepared. It is not recommended as a substitute for the cytologic technique.** Cell block sections are particularly useful if immunostains or other special stains are required.

CT-Guided Core Biopsies

This method utilizes an automatic gun provided with an 18- or 20-gauge cutting needle to obtain core biopsies of lung lesions. The method has been applied with a success rate which depends on the size of the lesions (Haramati, 1995; Arakawa et al, 1996; Laurent et al, 2000). Thus, Tsukada et al (2000) recorded a diagnostic accuracy of about 66% for lesions 6 to 10 mm in diameter, 79% for lesions 11 to 20 mm in diameter, 87% for lesions 21 to 30 mm in diameter, and 93% for larger lesions. Connor et al (2000) reported on a comparison of fluoroscopic or CT-guided core biopsies with FNA on 103 patients. These investigators concluded that **the core biopsy was superior to FNA for the diagnosis of benign lesions and superior to FNA in establishing tumor type in cancer.** The reported rate of complications, mainly pneumothorax (about 30%) and hemoptysis (1% to 2%), was comparable for both methods, with about 3% of patients requiring treatment for pneumothorax.

Haramati (personal communication, July 11, 2001) now utilizes the guided core biopsies for presumed benign lesions and FNA for presumed malignant lesions, with excellent results. It is likely that core biopsies of lung lesions will be carried out more frequently in the future, as interventional radiologists become increasingly skilled with this technique.

The cytopathologist will be called upon to evaluate these specimens.

CLASSIFICATION OF LUNG CANCER

Most lung cancers are derived from the epithelium of the bronchi and bronchioles, although some tumors may originate in epithelial cells lining the alveoli. The term **bronchogenic carcinomas** is commonly used to describe these tumors. They may be classified into the following **main groups:**

- Carcinomas exhibiting predominantly squamous differentiation, classified as **squamous** or **epidermoid carcinomas.**
- Carcinomas forming glandular patterns, **mimicking bronchi or alveoli, classified as bronchogenic adenocarcinomas of various types or as bronchioloalveolar carcinomas.**
- Carcinomas composed of undifferentiated small cells, resembling the **basal or reserve cells of the bronchial epithelium,** forming the group of **small cell carcinomas** or SSCs.
- Carcinomas **composed of undifferentiated or poorly differentiated large cells, some of which may exhibit glandular or squamous differentiation, or even endocrine features.**
- Rare types of carcinomas, including tumors with endocrine features.

Carcinomas of lung may have **mixed histologic patterns,** in which case minor components are disregarded and the carcinoma is classified by the predominant pattern; if there are two different major components, the tumor is classified as a mixed-pattern carcinoma.

Most important from the clinical point of view is an accurate cytologic diagnosis of SCC and its differentiation from all other (non–small-cell) carcinomas. SCC is highly responsive to irradiation and chemotherapy, which is the treatment of choice, whereas all other malignant lung tumors (except for malignant lymphomas) are best treated by surgery.

Malignant lymphomas, soft-part sarcomas, metastatic tumors and other less-common pulmonary neoplasms will be described separately. **Benign tumors** and **tumors of low malignant potential,** will be discussed in the closing pages of this chapter.

As a basis for the discussion of cytologic findings, the classification of bronchogenic carcinomas shown in Table 20-1 has been adopted here. It should be emphasized that this classification is not rigid and that transitions between and among the various types of bronchogenic carcinoma may be observed. In a thorough analysis of histologic types of 234 cases of lung cancer, Reid and Carr (1961) emphasized that only 37% of these tumors were homogeneous and the remainder were mixed, although they often showed a single dominant pattern. Roggli et al (1985) also found variations in the histologic pattern in two thirds of lung cancers, and in 45% there was more than one major histologic classification. This has been our experience also, and

TABLE 20-1

CLASSIFICATION OF PRIMARY LUNG CARCINOMAS AND RELATED TUMORS

Squamous carcinoma
    Keratinizing (well-differentiated)
    Poorly differentiated (epidermoid)
Large-cell undifferentiated carcinoma*
Small-cell undifferentiated carcinoma (SCC)
    Oat cell carcinoma
    Intermediate cell type
Adenocarcinoma
    Adenocarcinoma of central bronchial origin
      "Acinar" carcinoma
      Solid carcinoma with mucin formation
      Papillary carcinoma
    Bronchioloalveolar carcinoma
Adenosquamous carcinoma
Mucoepidermoid carcinoma
Spindle and giant-cell carcinoma
Neuroendocrine tumors
    Carcinoid
    Atypical carcinoid (well-differentiated
      neuroendocrine carcinoma)
    Large-cell carcinoma with endocrine
      differentiation
Rare carcinomas

Although a more detailed classification was recently proposed for the World Health Organization by an expert pathology panel of the International Association for the study of Lung Cancer (Travis et al, 1999), the simple classification shown here is adequate for our purpose.
*Most of these are undifferentiated large-cell adenocarcinomas, undifferentiated squamous carcinomas, or a mixture of both.

it has considerable bearing on the cytologic diagnosis of tumor types in sputum and bronchial material.

STAGING OF PRIMARY LUNG CANCER

The *TNM* system, which is based on characteristics of the primary *t*umor, lymph *n*odes, and presence of *m*etastases, was devised by the American Joint Committee on Cancer (AJCC, 1997). It is widely used to classify invasive lung carcinomas into five stages, and is of value for prognosis and as a guide to therapy.

- **Occult carcinoma:** Tumor proven by cytologic diagnosis but not visualized by radiologic imaging or bronchoscopy, and location not found
- **Stage 0:** Squamous carcinoma in situ, and microinvasive carcinoma
- **Stage IA:** Carcinoma confined to the lung, no more than 3 cm in diameter
- **Stage IB:** Carcinoma confined to the lung, greater than 3 cm in diameter

- **Stage II:** Carcinoma with metastases to peribronchial or hilar lymph nodes or invading tissue adjacent to lung
- **Stage III:** Carcinoma with metastases to mediastinal lymph nodes
- **Stage IV:** Carcinoma with distant metastases

Surgically resectable stage IA carcinomas have a 5-year survival rate of about 70% (Melamed and Flehinger, 1987; Melamed et al, 1981; Flehinger et al, 1992; Melamed, 2000). Stage II carcinomas have a 5-year survival rate of about 30% (Beahrs, 1992). In stage III tumors, the survival rate is 10% at 5 years, and in stage IV tumors, it is almost anecdotal (Beahrs, 1992; AJCC, 1997). All SSCs are stage IV by definition.

The **optimal goal of cytology is to detect lung cancer in the earliest possible stage, ideally at stage T0, which defines initially occult carcinomas diagnosed by cytology in the absence of roentgenologic abnormalities, or stage 1A, which comprises localized carcinomas smaller than 3 cm in diameter without evidence of metastases.** As already noted, these two groups of early-stage carcinomas offer significantly better prognosis than the more advanced tumors in stages II through IV. The role of pulmonary cytology in the diagnosis of low-stage lung cancer is considered in more detail later in this chapter.

In daily practice, however, cytology has very limited application as a screening technique for detecting lung cancer in asymptomatic populations and serves mainly to clarify the nature of lesions in the lung or mediastinum discovered by radiologic examination.

CYTOLOGIC DIAGNOSIS OF BRONCHOGENIC CARCINOMA

Effect of Specimen Collection Method

Sputum and Bronchial Specimens
Cancer cells found in sputum or bronchial secretions originate from loosely bound and often necrotic peripheral cells of the tumor, facing the lumen of the bronchus. They differ significantly from the tumor cells obtained in brush specimens or needle aspirates of more viable tumor. **Thus, the desquamated cells of squamous or SSCs often occur singly, are poorly preserved, and show nuclear condensation or pyknosis.** The cytologic diagnosis of cancer in these specimens depends in large part on the interpretation of these poorly preserved tumor cells with the understanding that they are often not representative of the tumor as a whole. These sampling artifacts are consistent and diagnostically very useful, however, and with practice, such cells can be recognized and correctly classified with a high degree of accuracy.

Adenocarcinomas of central bronchial origin shed characteristic tumor cells in clusters. However, the more commonly peripherally located tumors are unlikely to shed more than a few tumor cells into the bronchus.

In Saccomanno's technique of sputum processing (Saccomanno et al, 1963), described in detail in Chapter 44, the specimen is collected in 50% ethanol with 2% carbowax and blended briefly to homogeneity in a Waring blender before preparation of smears from the centrifuged sediment. The morphology of Papanicolaou-stained cancer cells is the same as in direct smears of sputum. There is some evidence, however, that **the diagnosis of SSC based on the distribution of widely separated single cells in Saccomanno's preparations may be more difficult than in conventional smears.**

Bronchial wash and brush specimens collect cells from the surface and the deeper layers of the tumor. Consequently, they exhibit a mixture of viable and poorly preserved or necrotic tumor cells. Squamous and SSCs comprise most of the carcinomas within reach of the bronchial brush. **Nuclear structure in the viable cells is more transparent and nuclear hyperchromasia is less marked than in desquamated tumor cells found in sputum.** These differences are shown diagrammatically in Figure 20-1.

BAL specimens are designed to sample the distal bronchoalveolar tree (see Chap. 19). In peripheral adenocarcinomas, the lavage specimens may yield well-preserved **single cells and small papillary or flat clusters of large tumor cells.**

Needle Aspirates

In percutaneous and transbronchial needle aspirates, the samples are taken directly from the tumor, and usually from its viable portion. A technically good aspirate should contain an abundance of tumor cells, often with small fragments of tumor tissue. The tumor cells in needle aspirates can usually be classified according to tumor type as described below.

Differences in Smear Preparation and Staining Methods

Optimal assessment of cytology of various types of lung cancer is obtained by examining fixed smears stained by the Papanicolaou method. However, air-dried, methanol-fixed smears, stained with Diff-Quik or another hematologic stain are widely used, particularly for percutaneous aspiration cytology. In this type of material, the diagnosis of cancer is usually readily established but **differences among**

tumor types are less obvious. The brilliant qualities of cytoplasmic keratin staining, so obvious in Papanicolaou stain, are replaced by a bluish color that may be intense enough to obscure the nuclear structure of the cells. **The description of features that distinguish the types of cancer cells in bronchogenic carcinomas that follows is based on the Papanicolaou stain.** The results with other stains will be briefly noted when needed.

SQUAMOUS CARCINOMA

Clinical Data

Squamous carcinoma is a common form of primary lung cancer. Afflicting primarily cigarette-smoking men and women older than 50 years of age, these neoplasms originate mainly in the epithelium of secondary or tertiary bronchi (Melamed et al, 1977), and may cause bronchial obstruction. They are twice as frequent in upper lobes as middle or lower lobes; those that arise in the lower lobes are almost always in an upper segment. As they grow, the carcinomas extend proximally from segmental to lobar and eventually the mainstem bronchus (Fig. 20-2A). Cough, with or without hemoptysis, is by far the most common clinical symptom. **In the earliest stages of the disease, radiographic examination of the chest may fail to reveal any significant abnormality. Later, the radiographic abnormalities are of a tumor mass and/or atelectasis or pneumonitis secondary to obstruction of the bronchial lumen.**

Histology

The **well-differentiated,** keratinizing squamous cancers are composed of sheets of cells attempting to form squamous epithelium (Fig. 20-2B), often with abundant keratin formation and keratin pearls. **Central keratinization and necrosis is characteristic, particularly in larger tumors, and may lead to cavity formation within the tumor** (Fig. 20-2C,D).

In poorly differentiated, that is, nonkeratinizing

CHANGES OF CHROMATIN PATTERNS CAUSED BY NUCLEAR DEGENERATION

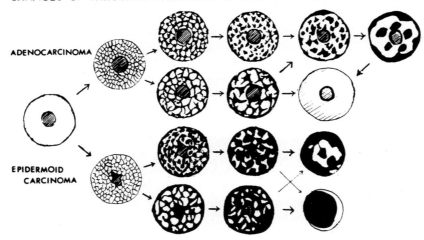

ADENOCARCINOMA

EPIDERMOID CARCINOMA

Figure 20-1 Diagrammatic presentation of effects of cell degeneration in bronchogenic carcinoma. Cancer cells removed by bronchial brush from the growing tumor (*left*) cannot be differentiated as to tumor type. The degenerative changes allow a differentiation between epidermoid carcinoma (nuclear pyknosis) and adenocarcinoma (nucleolar prominence). The cell types shown in the three rows of cells on the *left* are observed in brush specimens. The cell types seen in the three rows on the *right* are seen in sputum. (Courtesy of Dr. Shoji Hattori, Osaka, Japan.)

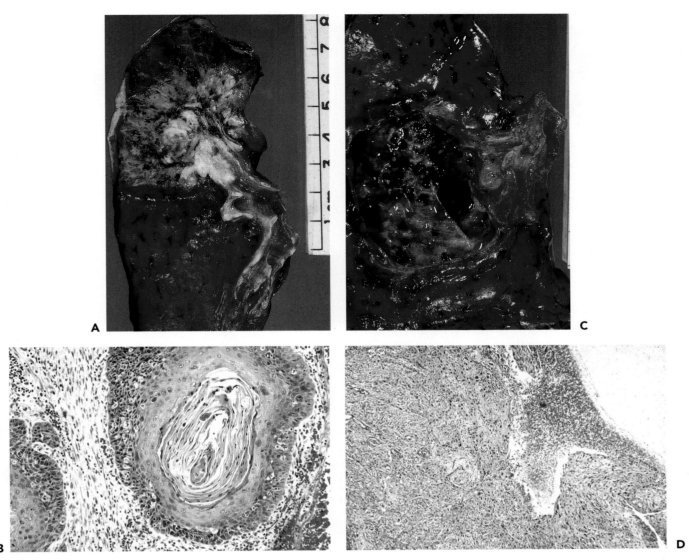

Figure 20-2 **Squamous carcinoma.** *A.* Gross appearance of squamous carcinoma, which originated in a segmental branch of the upper lobe bronchus and extended proximally into the lobar bronchus. *B.* Histologic section of well-differentiated keratinizing squamous carcinoma. The cancer cells grow in sheets mimicking squamous epithelium, with keratinization and necrosis in the poorly vascularized center of the tumor. *C.* Gross photograph of a cavitating squamous carcinoma. The cavity communicates with a large bronchus. *D.* Histologic section of the cavity wall shown in C. The tumor is composed of poorly differentiated squamous cancer cells.

squamous carcinomas (also known as epidermoid carcinomas), the cancer cells are usually smaller and keratin formation is less conspicuous, limited to individual cells or focal areas of the tumor. The arrangement of cancer cells in sheets is characteristic of these tumors as well (Figs. 20-2D and 20-5C).

Precursor lesions of squamous carcinoma (e.g., bronchogenic carcinomas in situ), are discussed below in the section on lung cancer detection.

Cytology

Sputum and Bronchial Secretions

Cytologic examination of sputum and/or aspirated bronchial secretions can yield a rapid and accurate diagnosis of squamous lung cancer, regardless whether the tumor is visu-

alized bronchoscopically or not. **Squamous cancer cells** are reminiscent of normal squamous epithelial cells, but differ from normal in several important features.

Abnormalities in Shapes and Sizes

Cells of squamous carcinoma **vary considerably in shape and size,** are typically found in a background of inflammation and necrosis, and often assume a most bizarre appearance (Fig. 20-3A,B). **Spindly cancer cells and tadpole** cells are quite common and their presence is characteristic of these neoplasms (Fig. 20-3B,C). **Very large squamous cells may appear next to very small cells.**

Cytoplasmic Abnormalities

The cytoplasm produces keratin and assumes **a brilliant orange or yellow color in Papanicolaou stain,** with a cer-

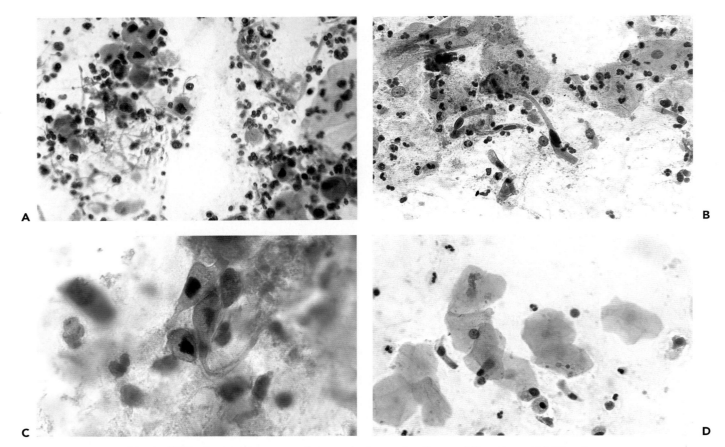

Figure 20-3 Squamous cancer cells in cytologic samples. Sputum (*A*) and bronchial (*B*) aspirate showing squamous cancer cells in an inflammatory background. The cells vary in shape and size, have deeply eosinophilic cytoplasm and relatively large, hyperchromatic nuclei without discernible internal structure ("ink spot" nuclei). An elongated, spindly squamous cancer cell is seen in *B*, and a "tadpole" cell in *C*. *D*. "Ghost" cells in a bronchial wash specimen, strongly suggestive of squamous cancer.

tain quality of **thickness and refractility** that may be brought out when the condenser of the microscope is lowered. The keratin also confers a **very sharp cell outline** (Fig. 20-3A,C). In some degenerating highly keratinized cancer cells, the densely yellow or orange cytoplasm **drowns out a fading nucleus** that is undergoing karyolysis. The resulting abnormally shaped **yellow or orange ghost cells** have only faint outlines of a nucleus, or no nucleus at all (Figs. 20-3D). **In the absence of nucleated cancer cells, the ghost cells in sputum or bronchial specimens are strongly suggestive, although not fully diagnostic of squamous carcinoma. Only in tracheitis sicca associated with tracheostomy are there likely to be benign squamous ghost cells with nuclear atypia that mimics malignant cells; otherwise the ghost cell nuclei are bland, if at all visible** (see Chap. 19).

Nuclear Abnormalities

Although **nuclear hyperchromasia is characteristic and typical,** it does not apply to all squamous cancer cells. As noted, **the nuclei of some cancer cells may be relatively pale,** especially the keratinized or necrotic cells that

are undergoing karyolysis ("ghost" cells; Fig. 20-3D). Peculiar **staining characteristics** of the nuclei are evident in tumor cells that are undergoing degeneration. They may sometimes have a **smudgy** or remarkably **homogeneous water color appearance. More often, the nuclei are deeply and evenly hyperchromatic, resembling India ink** (Fig. 20-3A–C). This is caused by pyknosis. On closer examination, chromatin structure is generally visible in such nuclei.

Significant aberrations of nuclear shape are common. Many nuclei are **angular or irregular in configuration** (Fig. 20-3A,C) and commonly variable in size as well as shape. Some have a **bizarre shape** (Fig. 20-3C).

The **nuclear/cytoplasmic ratio** varies considerably in this type of tumor and, although nuclei are on the whole quite large for cell size, there may be some very small pyknotic nuclei as well. **Reversal of the nuclear/cytoplasmic ratio in favor of the nucleus, so characteristic of cancer in general, is not of paramount importance in diagnosing the well-differentiated keratinizing form of squamous carcinoma.**

Uncommonly, **abnormal nucleoli** may be noted usually in poorly differentiated epidermoid cancer cells.

Phagocytosis of Cancer Cells by Cancer Cells

Multinucleated squamous cancer cells are not unusual (Fig. 20-4A) but on occasion, a **complete small cancer cell may be found within the cytoplasm of a larger cell (Fig. 20-4B).** While cancer cells are sometimes capable of phagocytosis of small particles, carbon or hemosiderin for example, the "cell in cell" phenomenon most likely is the **result of an abnormal mitotic division** with improper separation of the two daughter cells. Phagocytosis should not be confused with **emperipolesis,** the active infiltration of a cell (in this example, tumor cells) by leukocytes (Fig. 20-4C).

Incomplete separation of squamous daughter cells may result in the formation of a **squamous pearl,** that is, a concentrically arranged cluster of cancer cells (Fig. 20-4D). These must be distinguished from similar structures (benign pearls) occurring in the absence of cancer (see Fig. 19-7C). The **difference** lies in the **configuration and staining of the nuclei,** which in the malignant squamous pearls are hyperchromatic and of irregular shape, in keeping with squamous cancer. **The malignant pearl is usually smaller, with fewer cells and greater cytoplasmic keratinization.** Most importantly, in case of doubt, a search for single, clearly identifiable cancer cells in other fields of the specimen usually settles the problem.

Breakdown of Clusters

Squamous cancer **has a marked tendency to exfoliate as single cells** (see Fig. 20-3A). In fact, one should follow **the general rule that a diagnosis of this tumor type should not be made unless single cancer cells are found.** A dozen or so of the characteristic single tumor cells scattered over one or two smears may be sufficient to establish the diagnosis.

Mitotic Activity

Mitoses are very rare in keratinizing squamous carcinoma. In general, however, mitotic cells in a specimen of pulmonary origin, **although not diagnostic of cancer, call for careful investigation to rule out a malignant neoplasm.**

Cytology of Nonkeratinizing Squamous (Epidermoid) Carcinoma

The **nonkeratinizing carcinomas differ primarily in cytoplasmic staining, which in most cancer cells is basophilic**

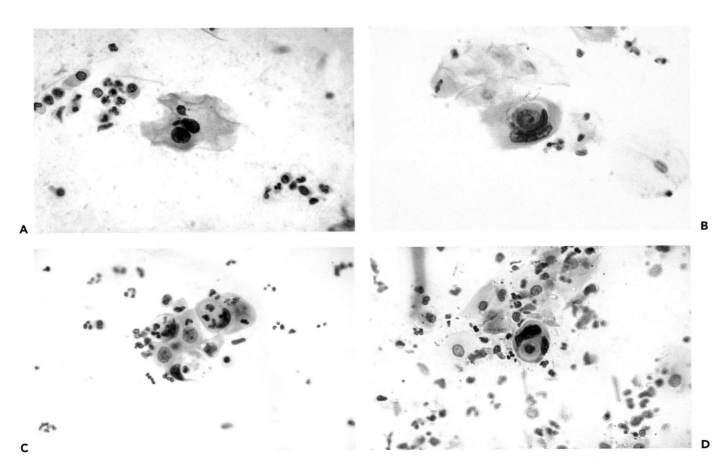

Figure 20-4 **Squamous cancer cells in cytology samples.** *A.* Multinucleated squamous cancer cell. *B.* "Cell in cell" formation of cancer cells, suggesting (incorrectly) phagocytosis. *C.* Emperipolesis, the active entry of lymphocytes or polymorphonuclear leukocytes into the cytoplasm of another cell, often a cancer cell. *D.* Malignant squamous pearl, formed by concentrically layered squamous cancer cells.

or **amphophilic** (Fig. 20-5A,B) **and more transparent** with less abundant cytoplasm **than in keratinizing carcinoma.** The nuclei are hyperchromatic with coarsely textured chromatin but usually not pyknotic. Less commonly, nuclear chromatin is more delicate and nucleoli may be visible. It is not unusual in such specimens to find a few keratinizing cancer cells, and these are of value in correctly classifying the tumor (Fig. 20-5B). They are derived from the more ischemic surface (Fig. 20-5C).

Bronchial Brush Specimens and Transbronchial Needle Aspirates

Several of the **key features that identify squamous carcinoma in sputum and bronchial secretions,** such as squamous pearls, keratinization, nuclear pyknosis, and the presence of single cancer cells **may have only scant representation in bronchial brush specimens and transbronchial needle aspirates.** This is particularly evident in poorly differentiated squamous (epidermoid) carcinomas. Cancer cells removed from actively growing peripheral portions of a squamous carcinoma do not exhibit nuclear pyknosis or cytoplasmic keratinization as found in the center of the tumor or at the bronchial surface (see Figs. 20-2B and 20-5C). **The viable, replicating tumor cells in an FNA occur in sheets or loose clusters wherein the cell outline may be ill-defined and the cytoplasm is cyanophilic (basophilic) rather than eosinophilic. The nuclei are large, coarsely granular, and may be hyperchromatic,**

but are rarely pyknotic. There may be visible or even prominent nucleoli. On occasion, thick cell clusters can assume a pseudopapillary configuration. Thus, bronchial brush and particularly FNA specimens of keratinizing and non-keratinizing squamous cancers may be very much the same.

In the absence of keratinization and nuclear pyknosis, as may be the case in poorly differentiated squamous (epidermoid) carcinoma, or if direct bronchial brushings or needle aspirates sample nonkeratinized areas of tumor, the distinction between a poorly differentiated squamous carcinoma and adenocarcinoma may be difficult. **In such cases, it is best to report the cytologic diagnosis as "positive for malignant cells, undifferentiated large-cell carcinoma," or as "non-SSC."** The principal differences between the cytologic presentation of exfoliated cells of squamous carcinoma in sputum and direct samples of tumor in bronchial brush specimens and transbronchial aspirates are summarized in Table 20-2.

Percutaneous Needle Aspirates

Squamous lung cancers usually arise in the secondary or tertiary bronchi. Most are centrally located and are accessible to bronchoscopic study. In our experience, peripheral squamous cancers are quite uncommon and the majority are nonkeratinizing. Percutaneous aspiration biopsy may be needed for those few cases. The aspirate yields cells with large nuclei and variably stained cytoplasm that is

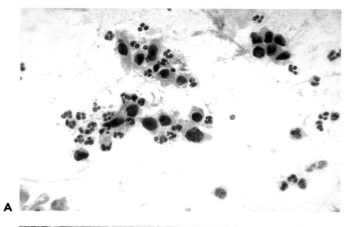
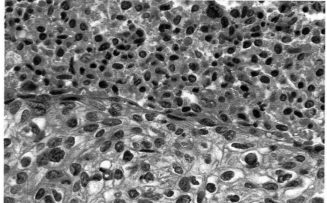
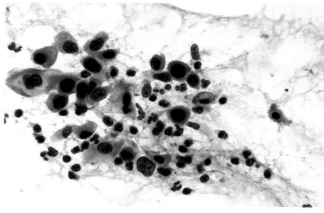

Figure 20-5 **Poorly differentiated (nonkeratinizing) squamous carcinoma** in sputum (*A*) and bronchial brush (*B*) specimens. The nuclei are hyperchromatic, coarsely textured and irregular. The tumor cells in sputum have scanty, pale eosinophilic cytoplasm, while in the bronchial brush specimen, they have amphophilic or sometimes basophilic cytoplasm. *C.* Junction of viable (*lower*) and nonviable (*upper*) tumor, the latter at the surface of the bronchus of origin. The condensed and hyperchromatic pyknotic nuclei are present in the necrotic portion of the tumor.

TABLE 20-2

SQUAMOUS CARCINOMA: PRINCIPAL DIFFERENCES IN THE CYTOLOGY OF CANCER CELLS IN SPUTUM VERSUS BRONCHIAL BRUSH SPECIMENS AND TRANSBRONCHIAL NEEDLE ASPIRATES

Cytologic Presentation	Sputum	Bronchial Brush and Transbronchial Needle Aspirates
Presence of cancer cells	Variable, may be few	Usually many
Cytoplasmic keratinization	Marked	Confined to a few cells; often absent
Abnormal N/C ratio	Variable	More commonly increased
Nuclear pyknosis	Marked	Not marked; often absent
Single cancer cells	Frequent	Infrequent
Cancer cells in clusters	Infrequent	Predominant
Nuclear structure detail	Difficult to see	Readily visible
Nucleoli	Inconspicuous or absent	Commonly visible and may be prominent

only moderate or sometimes scanty in amount. Nuclear chromatin may be coarse and hyperchromatic or more delicate with visible or even prominent nucleoli. Differentiation from large-cell carcinoma or adenocarcinoma is frequently difficult or impossible. Except for the extremely uncommon **keratinizing peripheral squamous cancers, which yield classic keratinized cancer cells, most of the nonglandular peripheral cancers are best classified as poorly differentiated large-cell carcinoma** (discussed later).

Correlation of Cytology With Histology in Keratinizing Squamous Lung Cancer

Because of selective sampling from the exposed surface of the tumors in sputum and bronchial washings, or if the periphery of the tumor is sampled in an FNA, **a dominant cell population of keratinized cancer cells in the former case, or their absence in the latter, may not accurately reflect the histology of the tumor.** Bronchial brushings or needle aspirates from the core of the tumor are generally more representative.

Squamous Lung Carcinoma Following Laryngectomy for Carcinoma

Cahan and Montemayor (1962) have shown that the incidence of squamous lung cancer is greatly increased in patients who have had prior cancers of the upper air passages, mainly the larynx. To secure cytologic material from patients who have had a laryngectomy for carcinoma and are left with a permanent tracheostomy, they obtained **tracheobronchial washings via the tracheal stoma.** In a survey of 308 such patients, there were 12 with positive cytology: 6 had metastatic carcinoma, but 6 had new

primary cancers of the lung, and in 4 of those patients, cytologic evidence preceded radiographic suspicion (Cahan et al, 1966). However, one must be warned that cells derived from the metaplastic squamous epithelium of tracheitis sicca (dry tracheitis) in patients with a permanent tracheostomy can sometimes mimic squamous carcinoma (see Chap. 19).

Determining the Site of Origin of Squamous Carcinoma

The histologic and cytologic presentation of bronchogenic squamous carcinoma is not unique. Tumors of identical morphology arise in the oral cavity, esophagus, and upper respiratory tract, not uncommonly as multiple, separate, simultaneous or sequential cancers of squamous origin. Metastatic carcinomas from more distant sites may also mimic primary bronchogenic squamous carcinoma, including, for example, carcinomas of bladder, uterine cervix, and the exceedingly rare squamous cancers of endometrium or breast. Thus, **cytologic evidence of squamous carcinoma in sputum, and even in samples taken directly from the lower respiratory tract, does not automatically indicate bronchogenic origin.** Clinical correlation is essential. Localization procedures in patients with occult bronchogenic carcinoma and carcinoma in situ are discussed below.

Differential Diagnosis of Bronchogenic Squamous Carcinoma

Diagnostic difficulties may be encountered in differentiating **nonneoplastic atypias of squamous cells of buccal, laryngeal, or tracheal origin** from bronchogenic squamous carcinoma (see Chap. 19). These difficulties can be minimized by attention to clinical data and a careful evaluation of cellular detail. **A history of prior or concurrent radiation treatment or prior laryngectomy should caution against the diagnosis of squamous carcinoma on limited evidence.** Other sources of possible error include vegetable (plant) cells, droplets of condensed mucus, and **epithelial atypias** associated with nonneoplastic disorders such as **pulmonary mycetomas** or **pemphigus,** all discussed in Chapters 19 and 21.

Tumor cells of other types that sometimes exhibit cytoplasmic eosinophilia in the Papanicolaou stain may mimic squamous or epidermoid carcinoma. This can occur with other forms of lung cancer and with metastatic cancers to the lung.

Large-Cell Undifferentiated Carcinoma

Histology

The large-cell undifferentiated bronchogenic carcinomas are composed of broad, diffusely infiltrating **sheets of usually moderate size tumor cells with moderate- to abundant-cytoplasm** (Fig. 20-6A). Many of these tumors are peripheral in origin and/or unrelated to major bronchi, and we believe they most likely represent undifferentiated adenocarcinomas. **By definition, they are without substantial squamous or glandular differentiation,** although they may exhibit focal features of squamous cancer or adenocarcinoma, sometimes side by side. They are derived from the same basal epithelial cells (reserve cells) that give rise to squamous and adenocarcinomas. Tateishi and Hattori (1982) considered these tumors to be undifferentiated carcinomas that lacked either light microscopic or ultrastructural evidence of maturation to other cell types, but Kodama et al (1985) found ultrastructural evidence of both glandular and, less commonly, squamous differentiation. As a practical point, more specific classification is irrelevant at this time, since all non–small-cell lung cancers have the same prognosis and are treated in the same way.

Cytology

The tumor cells, although frequently single, have a marked tendency to form loosely structured clusters composed of

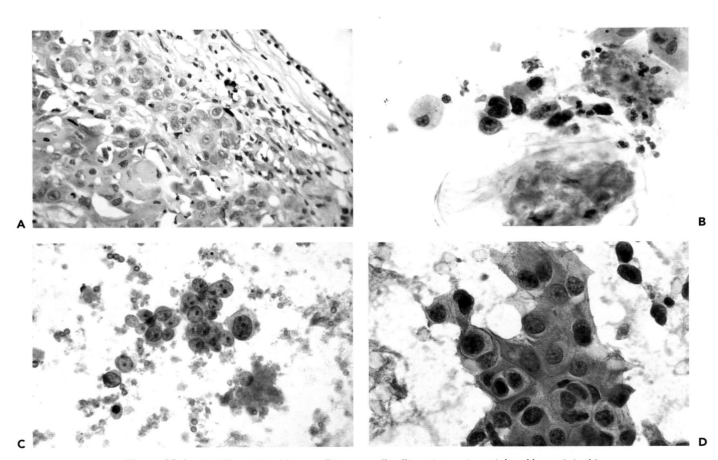

Figure 20-6 **Undifferentiated large-cell (non–small-cell) carcinoma in peripheral lung.** A. In this histologic section, the cancer cells are growing in sheets and have abundant, pale eosinophilic cytoplasm. Sputum (B) and bronchial brush (C) with cells from an undifferentiated large-cell carcinoma showing variations in staining pattern. The nuclei are either hyperchromatic with coarsely textured chromatin within the pale-staining cytoplasm (B), or have a more delicate chromatin structure with prominent nucleoli, resembling adenocarcinoma (C). A percutaneous FNA (D) shows sheets of large tumor cells with abundant cytoplasm corresponding to the histologic section shown in A.

cells of unequal sizes. Cells within the clusters are seldom superimposed; commonly, they lie flat next to each other (Fig. 20-6B,C). While some have little cytoplasm, most of the tumor cells are characterized by ample cytoplasm and they are comparable in size either to the cells of squamous carcinoma or adenocarcinoma. The cytoplasm is usually pale staining and delicate in appearance, and may be eosinophilic or basophilic. On rare occasions, **small red intracytoplasmic inclusions** are noted; they are wholly **comparable to those observed in urinary sediment** (see Chap. 22) and have no diagnostic significance. **The nuclei are large, sometimes of irregular contour, and sharply outlined.** They are characterized by **coarse hyperchromatic chromatin** (Fig. 20-6B), **or frequently by fine chromatin and single or multiple prominent nucleoli** (Fig. 20-6C), and rarely are pyknotic. Thus, the nuclear structure is more reminiscent of an adenocarcinoma (see below) than squamous carcinoma. Occasional **papillary cell clusters and cytoplasmic vacuoles may suggest differentiation toward adenocarcinoma.**

Sputum and Bronchial Brush Specimens

In this tumor type, the differences in cytologic presentation between sputum and bronchial brush specimens are not as marked as in keratinizing carcinoma. **The main features of the tumor cells, as described above, are observed in sputum and brush specimens.** The tumor cells more often form groups and clusters in brush specimens than in sputum. **Nuclear structure** is usually well preserved. The nuclear envelope often shows indentations and protrusions, resulting in **irregular nuclear contours.** The nuclei show **one or more large nucleoli** (Fig. 20-6C). **In the absence of keratinization, the differential diagnosis lies between undifferentiated large-cell carcinoma and adenocarcinoma and may be difficult to establish.** Fragments of tissue embedded in paraffin and processed as a cell block may facilitate the identification of tumor type.

Percutaneous and Transbronchial FNAs

Undifferentiated large-cell carcinomas are among the **easiest to identify as malignant because of the size of the cancer cells and their often-striking nuclear abnormalities,** which include **abnormal shapes and either coarse granulation of chromatin or more delicate chromatin with prominent nucleoli.** In needle aspirates, the tumor cells may be in sheets (Fig. 20-6D) or dispersed. **In air-dried, methanol-fixed smears stained with Diff-Quik or similar stains,** the nuclei of the tumor cells are large, but nuclear features are poorly visualized and the cytoplasm, which stains pale blue, has no definable structure. The differential diagnosis of non-SSC **should include primary and metastatic adenocarcinoma and attention should be directed to any history of previously treated cancer.**

Sources of Diagnostic Error

Except for markedly atypical squamous metaplasia ("repair"), radiation effect and drug effect (see Chap. 19), **there are virtually no benign cell abnormalities that could lead to a mistaken diagnosis of undifferentiated large-cell bronchogenic carcinoma.**

SMALL CELL CARCINOMA (SCC)

Clinical Features

In prior classification schemes, these highly aggressive malignant tumors were divided into two subgroups: **classical oat cell carcinoma,** and an **intermediate cell type of SSC.** Because these two subtypes do not differ clinically, the latest **World Health Organization (WHO) classification combines both subtypes as SCC** (Travis et al, 1999). The term **combined SSC** is used for the not uncommon occurrence of SCC with any non–small-cell component, for example, squamous, adenocarcinoma, or large-cell carcinoma.

However, there are **distinct cytologic differences between the small and intermediate cell types of SSC,** based on cell size and other morphologic characteristics, that are of importance in cytologic diagnosis. Though not recognized in the 1999 WHO classification, the distinction is important for our diagnostic purposes and the two subtypes will be described separately.

SSCs, as a group, share some important characteristics. These tumors, even when of very small size, **may induce endocrine paraneoplastic syndromes** because of active production of a broad variety of polypeptide hormones, including adrenocorticotropin (ACTH), antidiuretic hormone, parathormone, calcitonin, and gonadotropins. The clinical syndromes include **Cushing's syndrome, water retention, hypo- or hypercalcemia** (hypercalcemia is more commonly associated with squamous lung cancer), **gynecomastia, and antibody-induced central nervous system (CNS) disturbances with bulbar and cerebellar degeneration.** The CNS syndrome is induced by a polyclonal IgG (anti-Hu) antibody that binds to nuclei of SSC and of the affected neurons (Anderson et al, 1988; Rosenblum, 1993; Gultekin et al, 2000). The neurologic disorder may precede first clinical evidence of carcinoma. Thus, although hormone production has been demonstrated by immunohistochemistry in nearly one third of all lung carcinomas (Dirnhofer et al, 2000), the **paraneoplastic syndromes are most common in SSC.** It is essential that patients presenting with suspicion of a paraneoplastic syndrome undergo careful evaluation for a possible malignant tumor (Mizutani, 1988; Nathanson and Hall, 1997), and cytology may play an important role in the workup of these patients.

Because of the frequency of associated endocrine syndromes, it has been widely **assumed that SSCs are part of the spectrum of neuroendocrine tumors** (Colby et al,

1995), related to carcinoid tumors, and derived from the Kulchitsky cells, that is, the endocrine bronchial cells (Bensch, 1965). **Neuroendocrine cytoplasmic granules can be observed by electron microscopy** in both the carcinoids and SSCs (Bensch et al, 1968; Nomori et al, 1986); however, they are **numerous in carcinoid tumors and few in oat cell carcinomas.** It is not unusual to find a few neuroendocrine granules in other lung cancers that are not considered to be of neuroendocrine origin, and their presence in oat cell carcinoma may simply represent aberrant differentiation. Although immunohistologic stains for neuroendocrine markers such as synaptophysin may be positive, we have found the **stains for chromogranin are typically negative in oat cell carcinoma and consistently positive in carcinoid tumors** (Zaman, unpublished data). For other studies of oat cell carcinomas and carcinoids, see Fisher et al (1978).

The **epidemiology of oat cell carcinoma and carcinoid are markedly different** (Godwin and Brown, 1977). SSCs are highly aggressive, rapidly growing, and widely metastasizing malignant tumors that rarely are cured by surgery, unlike the very slowly growing carcinoids that typically evolve over a period of many years with high rates of cure by surgical excision. They differ also in **gene expression profiles recently studied with cDNA arrays that clearly indicate small-cell (oat cell) carcinomas are related to and are most likely derived from bronchial epithelial cells, whereas the bronchial carcinoids are neural-crest derived** (Anbazhagan et al, 1999). In a long-term study of uranium miners and others at risk of lung cancer Saccomanno et al (1974) described several patients with **cytologic evidence of squamous carcinoma in situ preceding the development of oat cell carcinoma.** It is therefore **quite likely that SSCs of the lung are epithelial tumors derived from the epithelium of the bronchi and not from endocrine cells.** It must be assumed that the paraneoplastic syndromes occurring in SSCs (and occasionally in squamous and other lung cancers) reflect the ability of epithelial bronchial cells to produce polypeptide hormones, accounting for the clinical manifestations.

Until about 1975, the prognosis of SSC, whether treated or untreated, was nearly hopeless, with rapid dissemination and death from disease occurring within a few months of diagnosis. Aggressive irradiation and multidrug therapy introduced and improved over the last quarter of a century may eradicate the primary tumor and some metastases, significantly extending survival (Perry et al, 1987), but remission is temporary and widespread seeding to distant organs including the CNS is common. **Carcinomatous meningitis is a fairly common complication in patients treated for SSC** (Balducci et al, 1984; Strady et al, 2000), **and may superficially resemble meningeal involvement by leukemia or lymphoma; cytologic examination of cerebrospinal fluid is of paramount importance in establishing the diagnosis** (see Chap. 27). Prophylactic radiotherapy of the CNS in patients with remission has decreased the risk of brain metastases and further increased 3-year survival (Auperin et al, 1999). Because the treatment of **small-cell lung cancer is different from that of non-SSCs, an accurate diagnosis of this tumor is essential and represents a major challenge in cytopathology.**

Oat Cell Type

Histology

SSCs arise from lobar or major segmental bronchi, similar in origin to squamous carcinomas. In contrast to the more slowly growing squamous carcinomas, SCC metastasizes early to hilar and mediastinal lymph nodes, and disseminates widely via the blood stream.

For many years, this rapidly fatal malignant tumor was considered by some to be a small cell sarcoma. James Ewing (1922) classified it as a "peribronchial sarcoma," a testimony to its anaplastic appearance. Even today, the correct diagnosis is not always easy, especially in biopsies of metastatic sites or when tissue or cytologic samples are scanty.

Histologically, small-cell (oat cell) carcinoma is composed of **sheets of small, round, ovoid, or spindly cells that characteristically seem separated from each other, and have been compared to grains of oats;** hence, the widely accepted name. The "oat cell" appearance of these tumor cells is exaggerated by tumor **necrosis, which is extremely common** (Fig. 20-7A). There may be **"crushing artifact" in biopsies, or streaks of hematoxylin-stained nuclear material (Azzopardi effect),** which is extremely characteristic of this tumor. In **well-fixed tumor tissue,** the sheets of tumor cells take on an **epithelial configuration,** often with **poorly formed glandular or tubular structures, rosettes, or islands of larger cells.** In some cases, SSC may assume a **lobular growth pattern with peripheral palisading of tumor cells, resembling and sometimes referred to as basaloid carcinoma** (Brambilla, 1992; Dugan, 1995). All variants of SSC have the same aggressive clinical course, and it is doubtful whether they deserve separate classification.

In keeping with their origin in the reserve cells of the bronchial epithelium, oat cell carcinomas may exhibit foci of glandular or squamous differentiation, and conversely the anaplastic squamous and adenocarcinomas of lung may mimic oat cell carcinoma. The term **combined SSC is** reserved for those tumors that have a **dominant pattern of SSC with a substantial component of other tumor types.**

Frequent genetic abnormalities observed in SSCs include a loss of the short arm of chromosome 3. Rarely, this abnormality may also occur in non–small-cell cancers (Brauch et al, 1987; Dennis and Stock, 1999).

Cytology

Sputum and Bronchial Secretions or Washings

Oat cell carcinoma may be difficult to diagnose because, at low (scanning) magnification, **the small cancer cells can**

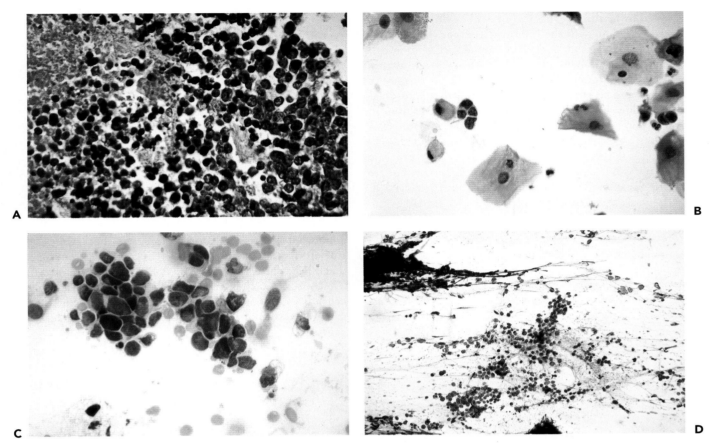

Figure 20-7   Small-cell (oat cell) carcinoma. *A.* Histology of SSC. The tumor is composed of small cells about twice the size of lymphocytes. Necrosis is common. *B.* The small, loosely clustered or single cells with irregular hyperchromatic nuclei and scanty cytoplasm may easily be misinterpreted as lymphocytes, or entirely overlooked. Note the molding of adjacent nuclei, a feature that is highly characteristic of SSC and is not seen with lymphocytes. *C.* A cluster of loosely coherent cells of SSC in a bronchial brush specimen. There is marked variation in cell configuration with molding of adjacent hyperchromatic nuclei. *D.* At low magnification, the loose clusters of small cells can easily be mistaken for lymphocytes. Note the streaks of hematoxylin-stained DNA from broken tumor cell nuclei, suggestive of SSC.

be misinterpreted as lymphocytes or may entirely escape the attention of an inexperienced observer (Fig. 20-7B). However, the cytologic presentation of this tumor is very characteristic and, once the hurdle of initial recognition has been overcome, the diagnosis is quite easy and accurate. This is of considerable importance to the clinician for reasons discussed above.

Sputum processed by the "pick-and-smear" technique is superior to Saccomanno's technique in the diagnosis of this tumor type (see Chap. 44). **Oat cell carcinomas shed loosely arranged clusters of small cells of variable sizes, somewhat larger than lymphocytes,** with molding of adjacent or superpositioned nuclei that are pressed together (Fig. 20-7B,C). In bronchial washings and aspirates, the tumor cell clusters are usually more cohesive than in sputum, and overlapping nuclei and flattening or "molding" of adjacent cells are more common.

Although the tumor cells are small, they have **relatively large nuclei, larger than lymphocytes, and a very scanty rim of cytoplasm.** The **cytoplasm is usually basophilic,** but on occasion may exhibit eosinophilia, suggesting keratin

formation. Often, the tumor cells are present as **bare nuclei,** or with only a small amount of adherent cytoplasm. Tumor cell necrosis is common.

Bauer and Erozan (1982) reported **psammoma bodies** in a case of SSC.

Bronchial Brush Specimens

There is better sampling of viable tumor in bronchial brush specimens than in sputum or bronchial washing, and a **greater proportion of well-preserved, viable tumor cells.** The tumor cells are variable in size, although they are generally small with very scanty cytoplasm. **The molding of adjacent nuclei in clusters of tumor cells** (Fig. 20-7C) **is very common. Two types of nuclei may be observed:** hyperchromatic or pyknotic nuclei and nuclei that are open or vesicular. The **best-preserved tumor cells have a coarsely granular nuclear pattern,** and some may have **small, discernible nucleoli. The cells with pyknotic nuclei are derived from necrotic parts of the tumor,** whereas tumor cells with vesicular nuclei are from nonnecrotic tumor

sampled by brushing. This feature will be illustrated and discussed below with the intermediate type of SSC. The nuclei are fragile and, regardless of the care with which the specimen has been obtained, **nuclear breakdown is extremely common. This "crush artifact" results in smudges and streaks of nuclear material that is of diagnostic value since this type of necrosis is uncommon in other tumors** (Azzopardi effect) (Fig. 20-7D). Sturgis et al (2000) ranked cell size, scanty cytoplasm, and nuclear molding as the most useful diagnostic features. Hyperplastic basal cells can be confused with oat cell carcinoma, but are smaller, more uniform without necrosis, and typically in coherent clusters (see Chap. 19).

Percutaneous Fine-Needle Aspirates

Although most oat cell carcinomas are located in major bronchi and can be diagnosed by sputum or bronchial brush, a small number of the tumors are peripheral and are best sampled by percutaneous biopsy. The cellular features described above for bronchial brush specimens are usually observed in needle aspiration biopsy smears as well. Groups of tumor cells are more common and cell detail is obscured, except in the loosely coherent single cells at the periphery of such clusters. Of special note, **there may be short chains of cancer cells in needle aspirates of oat cell carcinoma** (Fig. 20-8B), **often with flattening (molding) of adjacent cells. Visible nucleoli are uncommon.** In some aspirates, **the well-preserved cells dominate and differentiation of oat cell carcinoma from intermediate-type SSC is not possible** (see below).

Intermediate Type

Histology

These tumors resemble oat cell carcinomas except for their **somewhat larger size, more cytoplasm, more vesicular nucleus, and considerably less necrosis** (Fig. 20-8A). Their behavior is the same as that of oat cell carcinoma. In some cases, this tumor type may be mistaken for a small-cell adenocarcinoma or poorly differentiated epidermoid carcinoma, both of which have very different clinical significance.

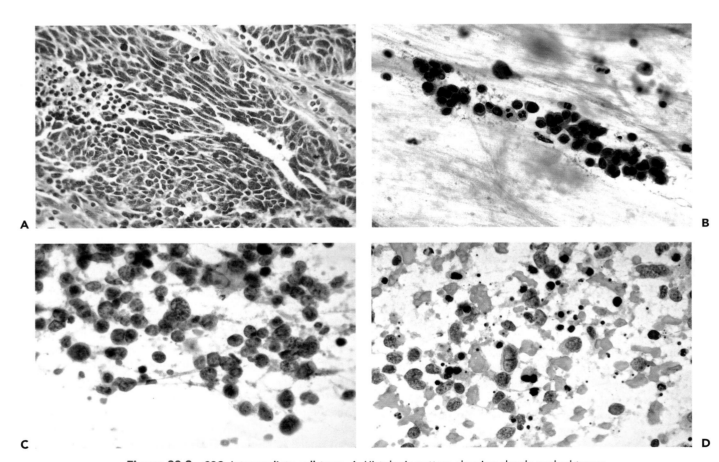

Figure 20-8 **SSC, intermediate cell type.** *A.* Histologic pattern showing closely packed tumor cells, somewhat larger than oat cell carcinomas but smaller than epidermoid and adenocarcinoma. The cells have more vesicular nuclei and more abundant cytoplasm than oat cell carcinoma, and may be polygonal or spindle-shaped; pyknotic nuclei are few. *B.* Bronchial aspirate showing a streak of nuclei with only wisps of cytoplasm. The hyperchromatic, coarsely textured nuclei, usually provided with one or more chromocenters or a small nucleolus, vary in size but are two to three times larger than a lymphocyte. *C.* Dispersed and loosely aggregated nuclei in a bronchial brush specimen. Nuclei have a vesicular chromatin pattern and clearly evident nucleoli. *D.* Single-cell necrosis and apoptosis are characteristic of SSC.

Cytology

Sputum and Bronchial Secretions or Washings

The cells desquamating from intermediate type SSC are similar to those of oat cell carcinoma, but are **somewhat larger, with more cytoplasm, and larger nuclei with finer chromatin structure. There are fewer pyknotic nuclei and less necrosis of tumor cells than in classical oat cell carcinoma. They may form cohesive sheets or structures** suggesting adenocarcinoma; in the Papanicolaou stain, the eosinophilic cytoplasm of some cells may be retained, suggesting kinship to epidermoid carcinoma (Fig. 20-8B).

Bronchial Brushings and Fine-Needle Aspirates

In these specimens, the cancer cells of intermediate type SSC present with a **fairly monotonous population of small, spherical, ovoid or elongated cancer cells, singly or in short groups, with vesicular or hyperchromatic, coarsely granular nuclei** (Fig. 20-8C). Small nucleoli may be present. The synchronous presence of both open and pyknotic nuclei is characteristic of this tumor type (Fig. 20-8D). Other characteristics that apply to both types of nuclei include **markedly irregular configuration and marked anisonucleosis. Karyorrhexis (apoptosis) and necrosis is not uncommon** (Fig. 20-8D), **but usually not with the streaks of nuclear material seen in oat cell carcinoma.**

These tumor cells may have a **clearly visible rim of pale cytoplasm and, as noted above, they may have features suggesting epidermoid or adenocarcinoma.** Focal glandular or epidermoid differentiation, as is sometimes found in these tumors, does not affect treatment.

The subclassification of intermediate type SSC into polygonal or fusiform variants proposed by Zaharopoulos et al (1982) and sometimes seen in histologic sections (Fig. 20-8A) is no longer used.

Sources of Diagnostic Error

- **Basal cell hyperplasia:** Clusters of small cells originating in areas of basal cell hyperplasia of the bronchial mucosa (see Chap. 19) may be mistaken for SSC. However, these compact clusters of uniform cells, in some cases with peripheral columnar differentiation, are readily distinguished from SSC.
- **Atypical basal cell hyperplasia** may occasionally present a diagnostic problem since it can include reactive cells with variable size nuclei and small nucleoli. However, **the cells are usually dislodged in tight clusters or fragments of epithelium, unlike SSCs.** The absence of single cancer cells strongly suggests a benign abnormality.
- **Lymphocytes: Clusters of lymphocytes seen in follicular bronchitis** also may suggest oat cell carcinoma, but they do not form coherent groups and are easily distinguished from epithelial cells. They consist of a usually mixed population of mature lymphocytes and lymphoblasts, smaller than the cells of oat cell carci-

noma, without nuclear pyknosis or necrosis (see Chap. 19).

- **Lymphoma:** Differentiation of intermediate type SSC from **large-cell lymphoma** may present some difficulty. **The cells of lymphoma are generally well preserved and distinctly separate without molding. They are more uniform than cells of SSC, and have nuclei with invaginations and protrusions, often with prominent nucleoli** (see below). The viable cells of carcinoma have nuclei that are more smoothly configured.
- **Carcinoid tumors: The cells of carcinoid tumors are found in sputum only after bronchoscopy or other trauma. In bronchial brushings and percutaneous aspirates, the tumor cells** are larger than the cells of SSC and form tightly coherent clusters with abundant well-preserved cytoplasm. Tumor cell necrosis is absent (see below).
- **Small-cell malignant tumors** that are morphologically identical with bronchogenic oat cell carcinoma occur in other organs (Gerald et al, 1991; Parkash et al, 1995) and are capable of metastases to the lung. Their cytologic presentation may be identical with that of oat cell carcinoma.

Tumor cells closely resembling oat cell carcinoma may be observed in pulmonary cytology from children with lung metastases of neuroblastoma, embryonal rhabdomyosarcoma, Ewing's tumor, and Wilms' tumor. Because SSC of lung is not seen in childhood, the diagnosis of metastatic cancer is virtually ensured.

ADENOCARCINOMA

Clinical Presentation

Adenocarcinoma of the lung is clearly associated with cigarette smoking, and has been increasing in frequency both in male and female cigarette smokers. Two forms of pulmonary adenocarcinoma may be differentiated on histologic and clinical grounds: **adenocarcinomas of so-called central bronchial origin and peripheral bronchioloalveolar or terminal bronchiolar carcinomas.** Both types begin within the lung parenchyma.

For didactic purposes, **the different histologic patterns of pulmonary adenocarcinoma and their cytologic presentation are described separately. In practice, except for some bronchioloalveolar carcinomas, cytologic separation of the two subtypes is seldom possible.**

Many, perhaps most, of these patients are asymptomatic at the time of diagnosis. The carcinomas are discovered by chest x-ray taken as part of a routine physical examination or at the time of hospitalization for other disease. The patients who are symptomatic with chest pain, dyspnea, or hemoptysis usually have advanced disease.

The diagnosis of adenocarcinoma calls for an evaluation of tumor location, size and extent, and metastatic status to determine surgical resectability. So far, the response of these tumors to chemotherapeutic agents has been modest at best, and the best hope of cure is through early detection and surgical resection.

Adenocarcinomas of Central Bronchial Origin

Histology

In the 1999 WHO classification of lung tumors, adenocarcinomas of central bronchial origin were subclassified into **acinar, papillary, and solid subtypes** (Travis et al, 1999). Although the exact site of origin of these tumors is still not certain, most are peripheral (Fig. 20-9A) and probably arise in **epithelium of sub-segmental bronchial branches or bronchioles.** A small number are of **mucus-gland origin.** There is no difference in management or prognosis of the different subtypes of adenocarcinoma. The **localized tumors** are commonly associated with areas of pulmonary fibrosis or scar. They either arise in the **vicinity of old scars or develop areas of scarring within ischemic parts of the tumor;** present evidence supports the latter view in most cases. The histology and growth patterns of localized adenocarcinoma are similar to those of adenocar-

cinomas else where in the body, and may be difficult to distinguish from metastatic tumor. The issue of precursor lesions for bronchogenic adenocarcinoma is discussed below.

The tumors may be **glandular (acinar)** in configuration (Fig. 20-9B), **papillary** (Fig. 20-9C), or composed of **solid nests or sheets of clear cells with intracellular mucin, usually in a few of the cells** (Fig. 20-9D). Solid sheets of tumor may show central (comedo) necrosis. Very often, there is a **combination of patterns.** Uncommonly, the tumors are exuberantly productive of mucin and are grossly gelatinous (Fig. 20-10A,B).

Adenocarcinomas with solid growth pattern are distinguished from large-cell carcinoma by the presence of mucus within at least some tumor cells. The distinction is of little practical importance because prognosis and treatment are not affected. It may be that many, if not most, undifferentiated large-cell carcinomas are adenocarcinomas of solid growth pattern. Regardless of histologic pattern, **the tumor cells vary in shape from polygonal to cuboidal to columnar.**

In 1976, Harwood et al described **a rare form of peripheral pulmonary adenocarcinoma, imitating mesothelioma.**

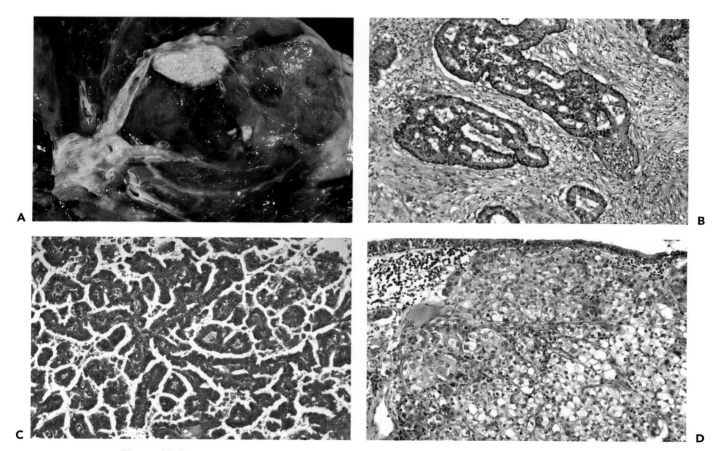

Figure 20-9 **Adenocarcinoma of lung.** *A.* Adenocarcinoma, arising in peripheral lung parenchyma adjacent to and invading a major segmental bronchus. *B.* Acinar adenocarcinoma of lung, associated with a desmoplastic reaction, is histologically indistinguishable from adenocarcinomas of other organs. *C.* Papillary adenocarcinoma of lung. *D.* Solid growth pattern of a clear cell adenocarcinoma of lung. An occasional tumor cell is mucicarminophilic (not shown).

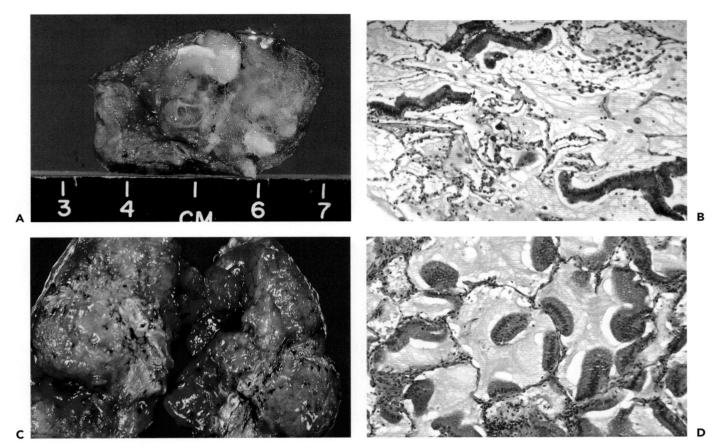

Figure 20-10 Adenocarcinoma of lung. *A.* Gross appearance of **mucinous (gelatinous) adenocarcinoma.** *B.* Histology: strips and scattered mucin-secreting cells within a lake of mucus. *C.* **Bronchioloalveolar carcinoma** spreading diffusely throughout both lungs (autopsy specimen). *D.* Histologic section of the type I tumor shown in *C.* The tumor cells are columnar with basal nuclei, growing upon the intact alveolar framework. There is no destruction of lung tissue.

Cytology

Sputum and Bronchial Secretions

There are no consistent differences in the cytologic presentation of the subtypes of central adenocarcinoma. The exfoliated **cancer cells** in sputum and bronchial secretions are **large, usually round or polygonal, occasionally columnar,** and are found in **clusters** or **singly** in sputum and bronchial wash specimens. The cell clusters have a three-dimensional **papillary** or approximately **spherical configuration** with tumor cells superimposed upon each other (Fig. 20-11A,B). **Cytoplasm of the cancer cells may be scanty or stripped away, but in well-preserved cells, it is moderate in amount, often finely vacuolated and faintly staining, usually basophilic. Single vacuolated tumor cells** may be mistaken for macrophages, **and on rare occasions are phagocytic,** but they have the nuclear features of cancer cells (Fig. 20-11C). Such cells are seen in the lumens of adenocarcinoma in histologic sections and represent desquamated, degenerating, mucin-secreting tumor cells. The larger mucin vacuoles often seem to displace the nucleus to one side, sometimes causing it to bulge out of the cell (Fig. 20-11C and 20-12C). This does not happen with histiocytes. We have occasionally observed **lipid-containing vacuolated mac-**

rophages accompanying the tumor cells of adenocarcinoma, consistent with an endogenous lipid pneumonia (see Chap. 19). Macrophages may also contain phagocytized mucin, but this is unusual and a positive mucicarmine stain can be of help in confirming the identity of mucin-secreting cancer cells.

In a phenomenon known as **emperipolesis,** tumor cells may be infiltrated by leukocytes (Fig. 20-11D).

The nuclei of pulmonary adenocarcinomas are best studied in single cancer cells. They are large for the size of the cells, with finely granular chromatin and usually slight to moderate hyperchromasia, **often with prominent, single or multiple nucleoli.** There may be **indentation of the nuclear membrane and sometimes an investigation of cytoplasm into the nucleus, forming the so-called nuclear holes** (Fig. 20-12A). **Multinucleation** is common. Nuclear pyknosis is rare.

Primary adenocarcinoma of the lung may be difficult to differentiate from anaplastic carcinoma of large-cell type, particularly if the tumor is represented by single cells without cell clusters. The presence of papillary clusters or columnar cancer cells clearly favors the diagnosis of adenocarcinoma.

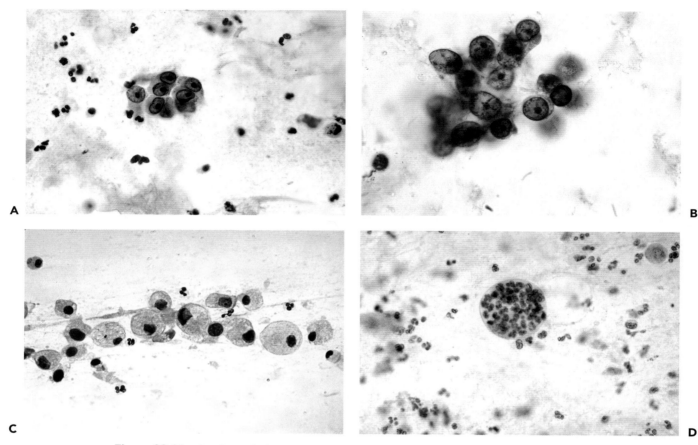

Figure 20-11 **Cytology of adenocarcinoma of lung.** *A,B.* Clusters of overlapping tumor cells with scanty, pale cytoplasm, relatively large nuclei, finely textured chromatin and prominent nucleoli. *C.* Single cancer cells with abundant finely vacuolated cytoplasm may mimic histiocytes, but are distinguished by nuclear abnormalities, including prominent nucleoli. *D.* Emperipolesis. Leukocytes have entered the cytoplasm of a cancer cell. (*A–D:* High magnification.)

Bronchial Brush Specimens

Bronchial brushing is of particular value in sampling small adenocarcinomas of the lung (Hattori et al, 1971). In well-sampled specimens, the tumor cells are more abundant than in a bronchial aspirate or wash. The cells often appear in **papillary clusters** (Fig. 20-12A), **or in sheets of large rounded or polygonal cells** (Fig. 20-12B). The latter may be mistaken for mesothelial cells but usually form glandular patterns and lack the intercellular "windows" of mesothelium. Suspect tumor cells in sheets are best studied by comparing their nuclei with those of clearly benign bronchial cells in the same smear. The brush specimens of **mucus-producing adenocarcinomas may yield tumor cells with large mucus vacuoles that displace the nucleus, superficially resembling goblet cells** (Fig. 20-12C). Some of the papillary adenocarcinomas of lung may have psammoma bodies, and on rare occasions, one may find **psammoma bodies** surrounded by tumor cells in a cytology specimen (Fig. 20-12D). Depending on fixation, the nuclei may be clear and vesicular or air-dried and pale staining, but they are provided with **readily visible and often prominent nucleoli.** In the uncommon small-cell variant of adenocarcinoma, the nuclei are about twice the size of nuclei of hyperplastic basal cells and must be differentiated from them and from the tumor cells of SSC (Fig. 20-13A).

Some **tumor cells may resemble normal ciliated bronchial cells,** but differ by their generally **larger size, greater nuclear/cytoplasmic ratio, the presence of prominent and sometimes multiple nucleoli,** and (most important) **the absence of cilia.** Ciliated cancer cells are very rare.

It was previously pointed out in reference to sputum cytology that the diagnosis of bronchogenic squamous carcinoma should *not* be made in the absence of single cancer cells. A contrary situation applies in the interpretation of **brush specimens of bronchogenic adenocarcinoma,** wherein the identification of **cancer cell clusters is of major diagnostic importance.**

Percutaneous needle aspiration cytology is the same for all types of pulmonary adenocarcinoma and is discussed below.

Bronchioloalveolar Carcinoma (Terminal Bronchiolar Carcinoma)

The recognition and classification of bronchioloalveolar carcinoma (BAC) as a specific subtype of non–small-cell lung cancer has taken on new importance following recent advances in targeted, molecular-based chemotherapy. Muta-

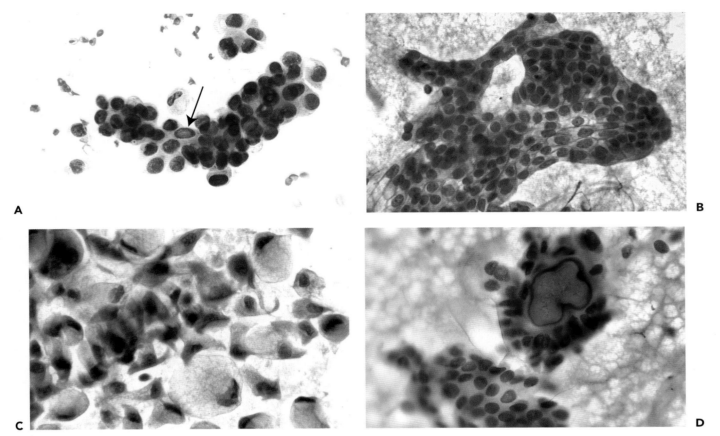

Figure 20-12   Cytology of adenocarcinoma of lung. *A.* Elongated or sometimes spherical papillary clusters of adenocarcinoma may superficially resemble the "Creola bodies" (see Chap. 19). The tumor cells have coarsely granular, hyperchromatic nuclei with "nuclear holes" or nuclear cytoplasmic inclusions (*arrow*). Nucleoli are scarcely visible in these cells. *B.* Well-differentiated adenocarcinoma of lung composed of uniform glandular cells mimicking mesothelioma in an FNA cytology specimen. Note the glandular formations within the cell cluster. *C.* Single cells of mucus-secreting adenocarcinoma with large cytoplasmic vacuoles, superficially resembling goblet cells. Note that the nucleus is displaced to the periphery by the mucus vacuole in some cells. *D.* A psammoma body surrounded by cells of adenocarcinoma of lung in an FNA. (C: mucicarmine stain, high magnification.)

tions in the tyrosine kinase domain of the epidermal growth factor receptor (EGFR) are believed to initiate a series of intracellular signaling reactions that promote cell survival and contribute to carcinogenesis. Two drugs designed to interface with tyrosine kinase signaling (Iressa and Tarceva) have had a dramatic response in patients with BAC, particularly nonsmokers. The drugs are ineffectual in other non–small-cell lung cancers (Ebright, 2002; Lynch, 2004; Zakowski, personal communication, Nov. 19, 2004).

Histology

These tumors arise in bronchiolar or alveolar epithelium of peripheral lung tissue and may present as a **localized mass or masses** in lung parenchyma similar to central adenocarcinoma (see Fig. 20-9A) or as a **diffuse pneumonic type** of infiltrating carcinoma that represents intrapulmonary spread (see Fig. 20-10C). In the **diffuse type** of lung cancer, there is **extensive replacement of large portions of the pulmonary parenchyma by adenocarcinoma.** The proliferating tumor cells are uniform and orderly in appearance and **utilize the alveolar framework for support so that at least initially, the basic architec-**

ture of the lung remains well preserved, so-called lepidic spread (see Fig. 20-10D). Tumor cells often form papillary projections into the alveolar space. These diffusely spreading bronchioloalveolar carcinomas may be divided into two types (Manning et al, 1984): **type I, characterized by tall, mucus-producing cells with basal nuclei lining the tumor septa** (see Fig. 20-10D); and **type II, wherein the septa are lined by smaller, cuboidal cancer cells with more centrally located nuclei** (see below). The 1999 WHO classification of these tumors retained this division as **mucus-producing** and **non–mucus-producing** bronchioloalveolar carcinomas. Surfactant apoproteins can be demonstrated in the latter, consistent with origin in Clara cells and type II pneumocytes (Mizutani et al, 1988). A mixed form of these tumors has also been recognized. As the tumor progresses, there is invasion and destruction of lung parenchyma, and the proliferating tumor cells become more malignant in appearance and form solid tumor masses. As with the other non–small-cell lung cancers, survival depends on successful surgical resection and results are best for the small, localized tumors.

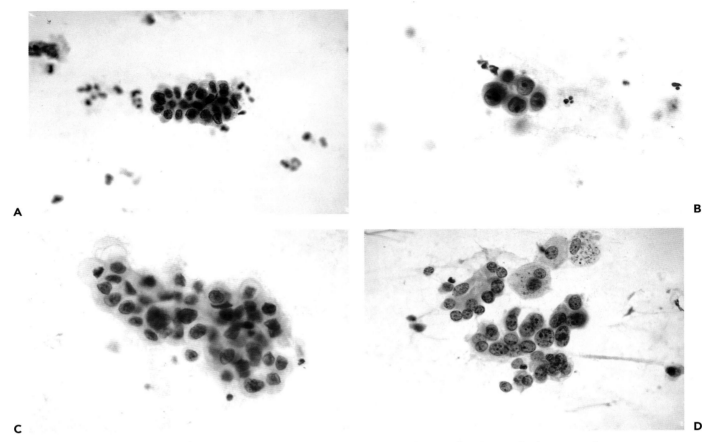

Figure 20-13   Bronchioloalveolar carcinoma, type II. *A.* Sputum showing a cohesive group of small tumor cells with scanty cytoplasm and uniform hyperchromatic nuclei. The nuclei are only 1.5 to 2.5 times the size of bronchial basal cell nuclei and may be mistaken for small-cell (oat cell) carcinoma (SCC), but do not have the other features of SCC (see Fig. 20-7). *B.* Sputum with a cluster of glandular cancer cells that have delicate chromatin, prominent nucleoli and scanty, pale-staining cytoplasm. *C.* Sputum: a cluster of disarranged, overlapping glandular cancer cells with variably sized nuclei and a moderate amount of pale, eosinophilic cytoplasm. *D.* Bronchial brush specimen with loosely coherent cells of adenocarcinoma with uniform, round nuclei that are only slightly larger than the nuclei in the nearby benign bronchial cells. The tumor cells show delicate nuclear chromatin, prominent nucleoli, and very scanty, lightly stained cytoplasm.

Years ago, the well-differentiated (type I) tumors, made up of uniform, columnar, mucus-secreting cells growing along alveolar septa, were classified as **pulmonary adenomatosis.** Many of these patients died of respiratory failure without evidence of metastases, and there was a question about whether the tumors were malignant. This form of adenocarcinoma has striking morphologic similarity to a communicable viral disease of **sheep,** first observed in South Africa under the name *jaagsiekte* (the "driving disease" in Afrikaans, so called because the frantic, oxygen-deprived sheep break into a gallop just before death). The concept of "pulmonary adenomatosis" is now obsolete, as **all types of bronchioloalveolar carcinomas are capable of metastasis.**

Cytology

Sputum and Bronchial Secretions

Sputum is by far the best diagnostic medium for this group of tumors. **In nonmucus-producing type II tumors, the sputum contains variable numbers of well-demarcated, rounded, or papillary clusters of tumor cells.** Such clusters are composed of overlapping small, **round, or roughly cuboidal cancer cells with scanty clear or lightly stained cytoplasm and moderately hyperchromatic nuclei with one or two small nucleoli** (Fig. 20-13A-C). Small-cell adenocarcinoma (see Fig. 20-13A) may have to be differentiated from small-cell (oat cell) carcinoma, but cell groups of adenocarcinoma are tightly clustered, and the component cells lack the molding and necrosis so characteristic of SSC. As already noted, some of the papillary clusters of cancer cells may resemble and **must be distinguished from the so-called Creola bodies** (see below and Chap. 19). Other, loosely coherent cell clusters may be flat, composed of relatively uniform cells with usually distinct cell borders and finely textured nuclei with small nucleoli (Fig. 20-13D). **Isolated single cancer cells are few, and may be difficult to identify** in this tumor type. Thus, the diagnosis rests on identifying tumor cell clusters.

In the mucus-producing type I bronchioloalveolar carcinoma, characterized by tall columnar mucus-secreting cells (see Fig. 20-10D), the cytologic presentation is different. The sputum contains single recognizable malignant cells as well as cell clusters. The tumor cells are larger than those of type II carcinoma and have abundant mucus-producing clear cytoplasm (Fig. 20-14A). They have one or two finely textured nuclei with sharply defined nuclear membranes and visible or sometimes prominent nucleoli (Fig. 20-14B). Tumor cell clusters may be composed of overlapping cells or of flat coherent groups of cells with a glandular or acinar configuration (Fig. 20-14C). Columnar cancer cells are uncommon. Some may have a flat free cell border and mimic benign bronchial cells, but they do not have cilia or a terminal bar. We have seen only a single case of pulmonary adenocarcinoma with cilia on the surface of tumor cells (which were accompanied by conventional cancer cells), and it was clearly an exception to the very good rule that ciliated cells should not be considered malignant.

Bronchial Brush Specimens

The tumor cells in bronchial brush specimens are similar to those described above, except that the collection procedure results in formation of flat groups and strips. Figure 20-15A illustrates an example of bronchial brush cytology in type II bronchioloalveolar carcinoma. The cancer cells have relatively large nuclei, easily visible nucleoli, and a moderate amount of pale-staining cytoplasm. Some may

have a columnar or cuboidal configuration. The smaller nuclei of benign bronchial cells that are present are useful for comparison. Figure 20-15B is an example of bronchioloalveolar carcinoma, type I. The cells are large with abundant transparent cytoplasm and spherical nuclei, some with nucleoli. The differential diagnosis must include metastatic mucin-secreting adenocarcinoma, including colonic carcinoma (see below). The tumor cells **in bronchial brush specimens** of bronchioloalveolar carcinoma **may mimic normal bronchial cells, but their presence in sheets of cells, absence of cilia and terminal bar, and their nuclear features identify them as adenocarcinoma.**

Percutaneous Fine Needle Aspirates

Bronchogenic adenocarcinoma is the most frequently seen primary tumor in percutaneous needle aspirates of the lung. **If the aspirate is performed well, there should be an abundance of tumor cells,** similar to the tumor cells illustrated above in bronchial brush specimens. One should be cautious of making a diagnosis based on a few isolated cells in a milieu of otherwise benign epithelial and inflammatory cells. As in other specimens, cytologic criteria for identification of the tumor type depend on the degree of differentiation: **gland-forming cancers are characterized by papillary, glandular, or rosette-like cell clusters and usually few single cuboidal or columnar cancer cells.** In some cases, the delicate cytoplasm of these glandular cancer cells may be damaged or lost, and the smear then contains **sheets or clusters of stripped**

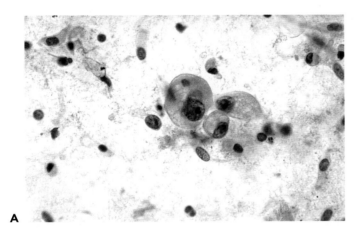

A

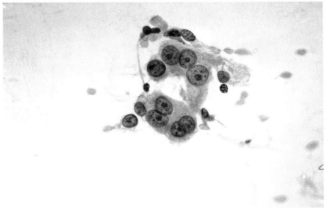

B

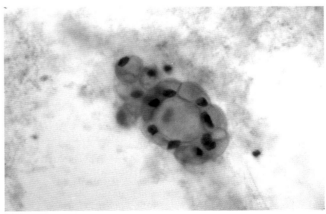

C

Figure 20-14 **Bronchioloalveolar carcinoma, type I,** showing large mucus-secreting, single cancer cells with abundant clear or vacuolated cytoplasm, and large round or ovoid nuclei with delicate chromatin, distinct nuclear membrane and prominent nucleoli. The cluster of cells in *C* mimics an acinus.

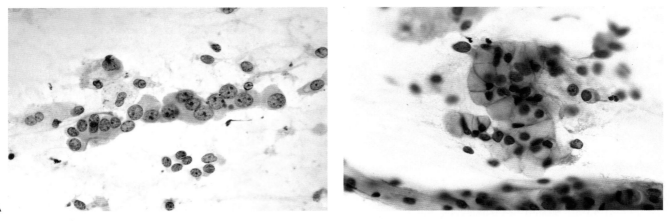

Figure 20-15 Brush cytology of bronchioloalveolar carcinoma, type II (*A*) compared with type I (*B*). Note the larger, mucus-producing cancer cells in *B*.

nuclei with prominent nucleoli (Fig. 20-16A). Well-preserved cells may retain their columnar or cuboidal shape and form chains of cells (Fig. 20-16B) or gland-like patterns, not usually seen in undifferentiated large-cell carcinoma. The latter have denser staining, sharply defined polygonal or irregularly configured cytoplasm. In many instances, these two sometimes arbitrarily divided types of cancer cannot be differentiated.

In the mucus-producing type I tumors, the cancer cells in FNA specimens tend to be larger and often of cuboidal or columnar configuration with abundant pale-staining amphophilic cytoplasm that may be solid or

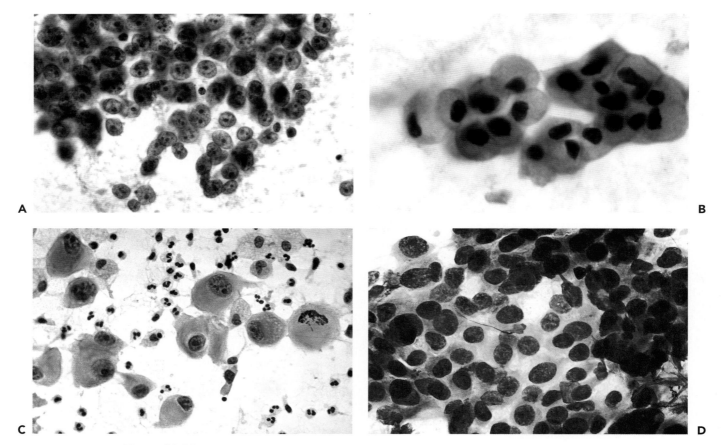

Figure 20-16 FNAs of bronchioloalveolar carcinoma are similar to bronchial brush specimens but more cellular. *A.* Nuclei may be stripped of cytoplasm but retain their fine chromatin structure and prominent nucleoli. *B.* Cuboidal and columnar mucin-secreting cells of type I bronchioloalveolar carcinoma in linear and pseudoglandular arrangement. *C.* Single large cells of adenocarcinoma. Note the abnormal mitotic figure. *D.* Diff-Quik stain of a wet-fixed smear.

finely vacuolated (Fig. 20-16C,D), or may contain large mucus vacuoles. On occasion, single cancer cells **resembling macrophages** are found in aspirates of usually well-differentiated tumors. They are approximately oval or rounded large cells with abundant cytoplasm and large nuclei with coarse chromatin and visible or prominent nucleoli. They differ by their nuclear features from the macrophages that are invariably present, with which they can be compared, and they are almost always accompanied by other more obvious cancer cells. In methyl green pyronin, or Diff-Quik stain, cytoplasmic features may not be well demonstrated.

It must be stressed that it is not always possible to distinguish bronchioloalveolar carcinoma from other forms of bronchogenic adenocarcinoma, or from some metastatic tumors. Zakowski emphasizes the presentation in flat sheets of cells in imprint cytology, with irregular nuclei, nuclear grooves, and intranuclear cytoplasmic inclusions (personal communication). The tumor location and growth pattern as observed in the chest x-ray may be of help in distinguishing these tumor subtypes.

An unusual case of adenocarcinoma in which the needle aspiration cytology mimics mesothelium is illustrated in Figure 20-12B. This pseudomesotheliomatous lesion is of importance in the differential diagnosis of mesothelioma and is discussed in Chapter 26.

Sources of Diagnostic Error

The cytologic presentation of bronchioloalveolar and bronchogenic adenocarcinoma is similar, as noted above, and pitfalls in diagnosis of both tumor types may be discussed together.

In specimens of sputum, perhaps **the most difficult diagnostic problems** occur with the spherical **clusters of bronchial cells desquamated from hyperplastic bronchial mucosa in bronchiectasis, asthma, and other chronic respiratory disorders (Creola bodies)** (see Chap. 19). Such clusters differ from papillary clusters of cancer cells in that they are composed of generally uniform cells **without significant nuclear abnormalities** and particularly **without the prominent nucleoli** that characterize the cells of adenocarcinoma. Furthermore, in clusters from adenocarcinoma, the cells are often superimposed upon one another, whereas the benign cells from hyperplastic mucosal lesions are usually arranged in an orderly "flat" fashion. **Peripheral palisading of columnar cells, the presence of ciliated cells in the cluster, and the presence of identifiable goblet cells speak in favor of a benign condition.** Ultimately, the presence of clearly malignant cells is of critical diagnostic importance, whether they are found singly or in the clusters that characterize most specimens from adenocarcinomas.

Chemotherapeutic drugs, particularly **busulfan (Myleran),** may induce bronchial cell abnormalities reminiscent of adenocarcinoma (see Chap. 19).

Also important in the differential diagnosis of adenocarcinoma is **hyperplasia of pneumocytes type II,** which occurs under various circumstances discussed at length in Chapter 19. The reactive pneumocytes are **large cells with prominent nucleoli** occurring singly and in small clusters. They may be seen in cytologic specimens from patients with a broad variety of benign lung disorders, including viral pneumonitis, adult respiratory distress syndrome (Stanley et al, 1992), chronic obstructive bronchiolitis, pulmonary infarction, and as an effect of treatment. Although atypical pneumocytes in those specimens may mimic the cells of adenocarcinoma, they are usually few in number. In cases of viral pneumonia or other febrile illnesses, the cytologic abnormalities are transient and usually persist no longer than 2 or 3 weeks. Thus, repeat follow up examination may clarify the issue. Diffuse opacity of lung fields in the absence of a discrete tumor should serve as a warning that one may be dealing with a benign process.

Another potential source of cytologic error is the not uncommon presence of a few large bronchial cells with large nuclei (see Chap. 19). Such cells retain their columnar or cuboidal shape and, if they are ciliated or at least provided with a terminal plate, it is an indicator of benign atypia rather than cancer. Variations of nuclear size and abnormal nucleolar features that are diagnostic of adenocarcinoma are usually absent in an inflammatory or reactive atypia.

Objective and measurable cytomorphologic differences between reactive and neoplastic cells have been reported, but they are not entirely consistent (Zaman et al, 1997; Fiorella et al, 1998). A good rule to follow **when cytologic evidence of cancer is scanty is to take a conservative approach to the diagnosis.**

Differentiation of primary from metastatic adenocarcinoma of similar histologic type is clinically important but may prove impossible on cytologic grounds alone. If the past history of the patient or radiologic findings suggest the possibility of metastatic tumor, the burden of proof lies with the diagnosis of a new primary carcinoma of lung. Cytologic features that characterize the most common types of metastatic carcinomas in the lung are described later on in this chapter.

Precursor Lesions of Bronchogenic Adenocarcinoma

Histologic Observations

Friedrich (1939), Rössle (1943), and later Spencer (1985) pointed out the **association of peripheral lung cancers, mainly adenocarcinomas, with subpleural scars.** Alveolar interstitial fibrosis is almost always present at the margins of scarring in the lung, regardless of cause, and is associated with **reparative hyperplasia of bronchiolar and alveolar epithelial cells, a change that was thought to precede neoplasia in some cases.** The occurrence of bronchioloalveolar carcinoma in patients with scarring due to tuberculosis, cystic lung disease, or long-standing scleroderma (progressive systemic sclerosis) of the lung are cited as examples of neoplasia arising in the epithelial hyperplasia that accompanies alveolar septal fibrosis (Meyer and Liebow, 1965; Talbott and Barrocas, 1980; Bielefeld, 1991; Paksoy et al, 1995). However, Shimosato et al (1982) have made a persuasive argument that **most scars associated with lung cancer are formed after the tumor develops,** and are caused by fibrosis of areas of tumor necrosis. Our own experience in the early lung cancer program at Memorial Sloan-Kettering Cancer Center, described below, is consistent with this view, since the vast majority of new lung cancers had no evidence of prior lung scar.

Meyer and Liebow (1965) described "atypical acinar proliferation" in lungs with honeycombing and interstitial fibrosis, and considered it to be a precursor of peripheral lung cancer. Later, Shimosato (1982) suggested that **atypical adenomatous hyperplasia (AAH) of bronchoalveolar epithelium may arise** in otherwise unremarkable lung tissue as a precursor of **peripheral adenocarcinomas of the lung.** The atypical is characterized by a layer of prominent cuboidal or columnar cells lining the terminal bronchioles and adjacent alveoli (Fig. 20-17), with or without slight interstitial fibrosis. The nuclei of these cells are often enlarged and somewhat hyperchromatic and may contain visible nucleoli, but rarely reach the level of abnormality observed in adenocarcinoma. At the time of this writing (2004), there is consensus that the origin of most bronchioloalveolar carcinomas is from the **epithelium of terminal bronchioles and the lining of adjacent alveoli, and that AAH is the likely precursor lesion of at least some peripheral adenocarcinomas** (Shimosato et al, 1982; Noguchi et al, 1995).

The original suggestions by Montes et al (1977), Sidhu and Forrester (1977), and Jacques and Currie (1977) that **pneumocytes type II as well as Clara cells may participate in the pathogenesis of bronchioloalveolar carcinoma** have been amply confirmed by histochemistry, electron microscopy, and immunopathology (Bolen and Thorning, 1982; Espinoza et al, 1984; Linnoila et al, 1992). Both cell types have been demonstrated in the nonmucinous variant of bronchioloalveolar carcinomas (Singh et al, 1981; Dermer, 1982; Espinoza et al, 1984), although some tumors are preferentially composed of pneumocytes or of Clara cells (summary in Axiotis and Jennings, 1988). Ogata and Endo (1984) observed Clara-type cells in other forms of bronchogenic carcinoma.

It must be pointed out that **atypical adenomatous hyperplasia is similar to the hyperplasia of alveolar lining epithelium observed in certain inflammatory and chronic obstructive pulmonary diseases,** discussed in Chapter 19. In the examples of the benign reactive processes described, the **sputum contained abnormal pneumocytes type II with large nuclei and nucleoli, mimicking cells of adenocarcinoma, without evidence of progression to cancer.** Thus, the entity of AAH may be difficult, and in some cases impossible, to differentiate from atypical reactive hyperplasia and, like other precancerous lesions, it may not always progress to carcinoma.

Cytology

Once in a while, abnormal ciliated bronchial cells may be observed in bronchial washings or brushings from patients with lung cancer. **The affected ciliated cells have enlarged and hyperchromatic nuclei** and sometimes show an abnormally coarse nuclear chromatin pattern or prominent nucleoli. In an unpublished study, Koss found marked nuclear atypia of bronchial cells in bronchial washings and aspirates from 4 of 100 consecutive patients with lung cancer, and moderate atypia in 19 others. **Similar abnormalities of ciliated cells may be observed in isolated instances of cancer metastatic to the lung, but also in obstructive pulmonary disease, acute radiation reaction, and chemotherapy effect** (see Chap. 19). However, **in a patient who has no other evidence of lung disease, a finding of marked bronchial cell atypia, although not diagnostic of cancer, should alert one to the possibility of an early occult adenocarcinoma.**

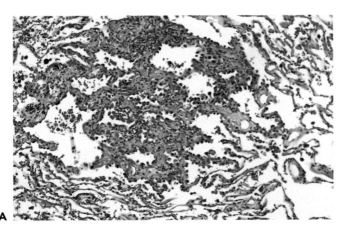
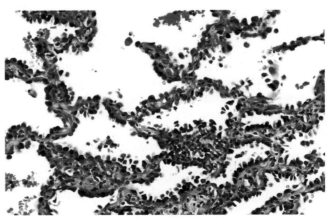

A **B**

Figure 20-17 Atypical adenomatous hyperplasia of alveolar epithelium, a putative precursor of bronchioloalveolar carcinoma.

ADENOSQUAMOUS CARCINOMA

The term **adenosquamous carcinoma** is used to define bronchogenic carcinomas combining features of both epidermoid carcinoma and adenocarcinoma. While many undifferentiated large-cell carcinomas exhibit minor areas of glandular or squamous differentiation, the adenosquamous diagnosis is reserved for those **tumors composed predominantly of the two cell types.** Most show evidence of mucin secretion by special stains in addition to frank keratinization, and some have **minor components of undifferentiated large-cell or even SSC. Their cytologic presentation varies depending on the histologic pattern.**

Mucoepidermoid Carcinoma

The true mucoepidermoid carcinomas of lung are rare tumors, accounting for less than 0.2% of primary lung cancers (Colby et al, 1995). They arise in major bronchi or their branches, either from mucus glands in the bronchial wall or from the mucus-secreting surface epithelium, and form polypoid masses in the bronchial lumen.

Histology

As is suggested by their name, the mucoepidermoid carcinomas mimic similar tumors of salivary gland origin (see Chap. 32), and are composed of a **mixture of differentiated and undifferentiated (intermediate) squamous cancer cells with interspersed mucinous glands or mucin-secreting single cells** (Fig. 20-18A). The **low-grade tumors** are localized, predominantly mucin-secreting, and have a generally good prognosis following resection. **High-grade tumors, usually characterized by a poorly differentiated squamous component with interspersed mucicarminophilic cells** are invasive, capable of metastasis, and resemble adenosquamous carcinomas of the lung, differing primarily in their **gross presentation as a polypoid intrabronchial mass.**

Cytology

We have seen brush cytology from a 61-year-old woman with this diagnosis. The dominant cancer cells were of a mucus-producing adenocarcinoma (Fig. 20-18B,C). There were only a few isolated, keratinized cancer cells (Fig. 20-18D). The patient was treated by surgery, but the tumor rapidly recurred with a pleural effusion. The diagnosis of

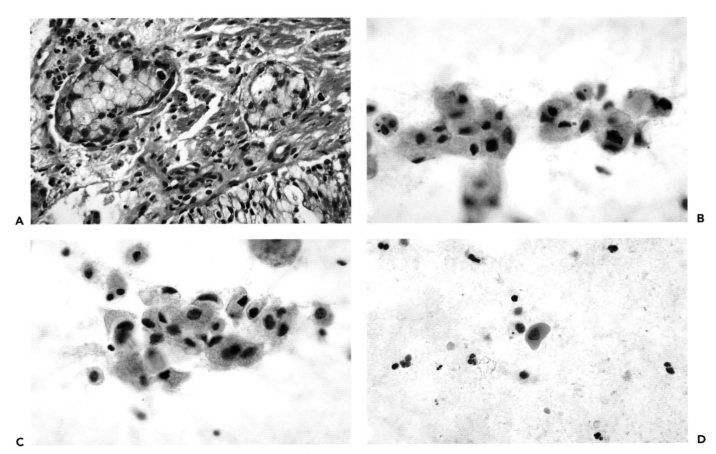

Figure 20-18   Mucoepidermoid carcinoma of lung in a 61-year-old woman. A. A tumor of bronchial mucus glands similar to the corresponding tumor of salivary gland origin composed of mucin-secreting glandular and epidermoid tumor cells. In bronchial brush specimens, the presence of both mucin-secreting (B,C) and epidermoid or squamous (D) cells may be observed.

these uncommon tumors depends on **finding within the same specimen cells of squamous and adenocarcinoma.**

GIANT-CELL CARCINOMA (SPINDLE AND GIANT-CELL CARCINOMA)

These uncommon malignant tumors of lung constitute not more than 2% of all lung cancers. They may be considered a **subset of undifferentiated large-cell carcinomas,** and are characterized by the presence of **very large, often multi-nucleated, bizarre tumor giant cells** with equally **bizarre nuclei** and frequently **very large nucleoli** (Fig. 20-19). In the spindle and giant-cell variant, there is a sarcomatoid component of **spindly, elongated cancer cells resembling sarcoma** (Fig. 20-19C). Ozzello and Stout (1961) first documented the epithelial origin of these tumors, which was later confirmed by immunochemical expression of epithelial antigens (Fishback et al, 1994). Although the tumors have a bizarre appearance, common to all spindle and giant-cell tumors of various organs, their **prognosis appears to be about the same as that of other non–small-cell lung carcinomas** (Hellstrom and Fisher, 1963; Herman et al, 1966; Ginsberg et al, 1992).

In sputum, bronchial aspirates, bronchial brush specimens, or needle aspiration cytology, the presence of isolated **very large, single or multinucleated tumor cells with huge bizarre nuclei is virtually diagnostic of this neoplasm** (Fig. 20-20B,D). **Smaller, undifferentiated malignant cells are almost always present as well.** Spindly tumor cells are rare. Although it has been suggested that these tumors may represent a bizarre variant of adenocarcinoma, we have not found cytologic evidence to support this in our material, nor have Broderick et al (1975) or Naib (1961). In one of our cases, the tumor was accompanied by a **squamous carcinoma in situ,** strongly suggesting that the tumor was of squamous derivation.

Differential Diagnosis

Spindle and giant-cell carcinomas of other organs (e.g., the thyroid, esophagus, uterine cervix) may metastasize to the lung, as do many **sarcomas,** any of which may shed cells identical with those described above. These are rare tumors, however, and it is usually obvious clinically that the lung lesion is a metastasis. Perhaps the most important differential diagnosis is the **effect of radiotherapy** on more common types of primary lung cancer. **Irradiation and sometimes chemotherapy** may produce huge distorted

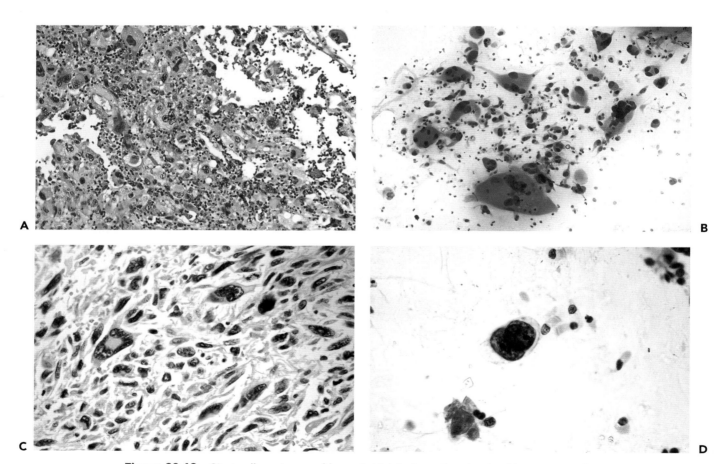

Figure 20-19 Giant-cell carcinoma of lung. *A.* Histologic section showing bizarre tumor giant cells with large nuclei. *B.* Bronchial brush specimen in same case. *C,D.* Histologic section and bronchial brush cytology of a sarcomatoid giant-cell carcinoma. Compare the huge size of cancer cells with normal bronchial cells.

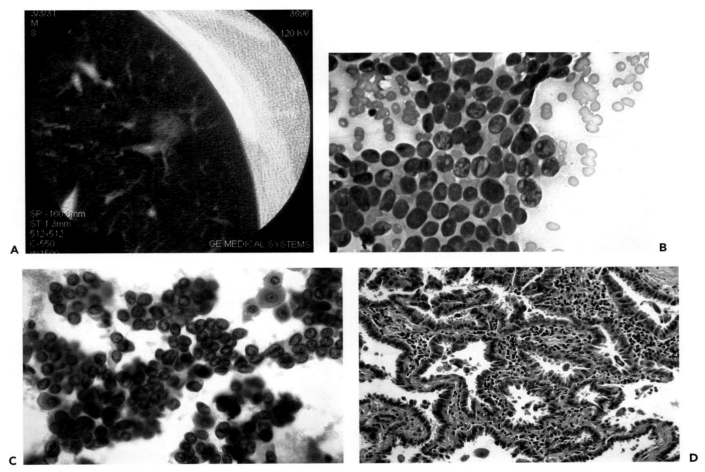

Figure 20-20   Early lung cancer detected in the ELCAP program. *A.* Spiral CT radiograph showing a well-delineated "ground glass" density (less than 1 cm in diameter). *B.* FNA showing monolayered clusters of uniform epithelial tumor cells with nucleoli and intranuclear cytoplasmic inclusions. *C.* FNA showing clusters of uniform tumor cells with well-defined nuclear membrane, and some with pinpoint nucleoli. *D.* Histologic section of the resected tumor revealed a well-differentiated bronchioloalveolar carcinoma. (*B:* Diff-Quik stain; *C:* H&E.) (Case courtesy of Dr. Madeline Vazquez, New York Hospital, New York, NY.)

tumor giant cells that in the absence of clinical data cannot be differentiated from giant-cell carcinoma.

SECOND PRIMARY LUNG CANCERS

Individuals who have had non–small-cell lung cancer and survived following resection are at increased risk of another lung cancer, which was estimated at about 2% per year by Pairolero et al (1984). Martini and Melamed (1975) reported a series of 50 patients with multiple primary lung cancers, 18 synchronous and 32 metachronous. In 31 patients, the second carcinoma was of the same histologic type, mostly squamous. In the remaining 19 patients, the histology was different. Similar observations were made by Broghamer et al (1985) who reported cytologic studies on 17 of 23 patients with second primary lung cancers. In 10 cases, cytologic diagnosis preceded histologic verification. Cytology is mandatory in monitoring patients after curative resection of lung cancer. It can present diagnostic difficulties in patients treated by adjuvant or postoperative irradiation.

PRECURSOR STAGES OF BRONCHOGENIC SQUAMOUS CARCINOMA

It is logical to assume that bronchogenic carcinomas, in common with other malignant epithelial tumors, are **preceded by a sequence of epithelial changes during malignant transformation before invasion.** Little is known about the histologic abnormalities occurring in the formative stages of **adenocarcinoma, although atypical adenomatous hyperplasia is a presumed precursor lesion (see above).** Virtually nothing is known about the precursor stages of **SSC.** The best information is available for **squamous carcinoma** and the precursor lesion known as **squamous carcinoma in situ.**

Historical Overview

In 1935, a Finnish investigator, Lindberg, observed that squamous metaplasia is a frequent finding in the bronchi of patients with lung cancer. Subsequent histologic studies, notably by Auerbach et al (1957) and by Nasiell (1966), supported this observation and squamous metaplasia was considered to be an important step in the genesis of bronchogenic squamous carcinoma. The possible mechanism of formation and frequency of occurrence of squamous metaplasia were discussed in Chapter 19.

Auerbach et al (1957, 1961) systematically mapped epithelial changes in the bronchial tree of cigarette smokers at autopsy, and found varying degrees of cytologic abnormality in patchy areas of the bronchial epithelium. However, even in the most severely affected bronchi, large areas of normal or nearly normal respiratory epithelium were present. There was no good explanation for the patchy distribution of epithelial abnormalities but, because the sites of bronchial division (bronchial spurs) were most frequently affected, it was thought that local variation in airflow might play a role in this phenomenon. The epithelial abnormalities were most frequent and most severe in patients who had invasive squamous carcinoma. Auerbach's work suggested that histologically identifiable bronchial epithelial abnormalities precede the development of epidermoid carcinoma. **It was generally assumed that the initial carcinogenic event was squamous metaplasia that progressed to atypical metaplasia. In the most severe of these epithelial changes, the entire thickness of the epithelium was occupied by abnormal cells resembling the cells of invasive carcinoma, and this lesion was termed carcinoma in situ.** A somewhat similar sequence of events was observed in experimental carcinogenesis of the trachea in hamsters (Schreiber et al, 1974; McDowell and Trump, 1983).

Saccomanno et al (1974) described their experience with long-term cytologic studies of a large population of uranium miners in comparison with cigarette smokers and nonsmokers. They proposed a sequence of epithelial events in the development of bronchogenic epidermoid carcinoma, which is summarized in Table 20-3.

On the basis of cytologic data, Saccomanno et al (1974) recorded the time of transition from moderate cytologic atypia to invasive epidermoid carcinoma at 4.8 years (ranging from 0.3 to 9 years) and from carcinoma in situ to invasive epidermoid carcinoma at 2.5 years (ranging from 0.5 to 6.2 years). Updated figures, based on cytologic and clinical observation of a larger group of patients and kindly provided by Dr. Saccomanno in 1977, suggest somewhat longer average times of transition: 9.4 years for transition from moderate atypia to invasive carcinoma and 3.2 years for transition from carcinoma in situ to invasive carcinoma. A similar sequence had been suggested previously by Koprowska et al (1965) and by Nasiell (1966).

The concept of squamous metaplasia as a precursor lesion of bronchogenic carcinoma was subsequently challenged by Melamed et al (1977). In a detailed histologic study of the resected lobectomy specimens from patients with in situ or incipient invasive epidermoid carcinoma of lung, they found **no transition from squamous metaplasia or basal hyperplasia to carcinoma.** On the contrary, **the carcinomas seemed to arise de novo from transformed basal (reserve) cells of the bronchial epithelium.** Further, squamous metaplasia, which is a common finding in the absence of carcinoma, was seen predominantly in the mainstem and lobar bronchi, whereas the earliest in situ and focally invasive carcinomas were found to arise in more distal segmental and subsegmental bronchi. Melamed et al concluded that **neoplastic transformation of bronchial epithelium induced by respired carcinogens** (such as tobacco smoke) **proceeds independently of squamous metaplasia and basal hyperplasia.** The latter were believed to be a nonspecific reaction to the irritating smoke. These views received support from the observations of an **abrupt transition between normal respiratory epithelium and carcinoma in situ without intervening squamous metaplasia, and from the location of squamous metaplasia commonly in mainstem and lobar bronchi, whereas in situ carcinoma was most commonly found more distally in subsegmental bronchi** (Fig. 20-21). It is also known from Auerbach's work that the frequency of atypical metaplasias in the bronchial tree of smokers vastly exceeds the expected number of invasive bronchogenic cancers. Hence, it is reasonable to assume that few of these lesions progress to carcinoma and the outcome in any given case is unpredictable. The readers should be cautioned, however, that many pathologists still regard squamous metaplasia to be an essential precursor of squamous lung cancer.

Despite differing views on the pathogenesis of lung cancer, most pathologists are in agreement on the criteria for diagnosis of **in situ carcinoma** of the bronchus, which may be well or poorly differentiated. Some pathologists prefer the term **dysplasia** for the well-differentiated carcinomas in situ. The cytology of these lesions is discussed below.

The natural history of bronchogenic squamous carcinoma in situ, the probability of progression, and the time required for progression to invasive cancer are not yet known. Certainly, not all atypical squamous metaplasias will progress to in situ or invasive cancer, and there are only a very few patients with biopsy-confirmed carcinoma in situ who have been followed without treatment (because of med-

TABLE 20-3

SEQUENCE OF EPITHELIAL EVENTS IN THE DEVELOPMENT OF BRONCHOGENIC EPIDERMOID CARCINOMA

Squamous metaplasia
↓
Squamous metaplasia with mild atypia
↓
Squamous metaplasia with moderate atypia
↓
Squamous metaplasia with marked atypia
↓
Squamous carcinoma in situ
↓
Invasive squamous carcinoma

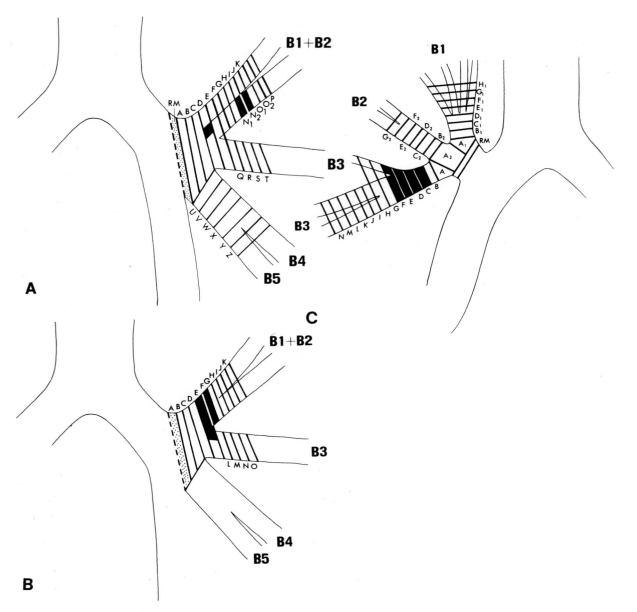

Figure 20-21   *A–C.* Diagrammatic presentation of three cases of occult bronchogenic carcinoma in situ discovered by sputum cytology. The lesions, shown in black, are surrounded by normal bronchial epithelium. Areas of squamous metaplasia (gray area) seen in *A* and *B* are separated from carcinoma in situ by a zone of normal bronchial epithelium. B1, B2, B3, etc, refer to segmental bronchi. Small capital letters in the drawings refer to sequential tissue blocks. (Modified from Melamed et al. Radiologically occult in situ and invasive epidermoid lung cancer: Detection by sputum cytology in a survey of asymptomatic cigarette smokers. Am J Surg Pathol 1:5–16, 1977.)

ical contraindications or refusal of surgery). In one well-documented case seen by one of us (M.R.M.), and in another seen by Woolner at the Mayo Clinic (personal communication), the time of progression from in situ to invasive carcinoma was at least 5 years. In two other cases seen by one of us (LGK), time intervals of 4 to 6 years elapsed from cytologic diagnosis of bronchogenic carcinoma until clinical cancer developed. Nasiell et al (1977) reported time intervals of 8 to 9 years from *cytologic* diagnosis of bronchogenic carcinoma in situ to the clinical diagnosis of cancer. One of his patients with documented bronchogenic carcinoma in situ was followed for 13 years without clinical evidence

of invasive cancer. These anecdotal experiences suggested a **transit time of 5 to 10 years for progression of in situ to invasive squamous carcinoma.** In a mathematical model based on data from the Memorial Sloan-Kettering early lung cancer study, Flehinger and Kimmel (1987) and Flehinger et al (1988) estimated a **minimum of 4 years duration for the early stage of lung cancer.** Thus, there appears to be ample opportunity for early detection and treatment of at least some lung cancers (see below). There is still very limited experience with treatment of carcinoma in situ by locally ablative photodynamic therapies (Cortese and Edell, 1993). With few exceptions, even very limited foci of in

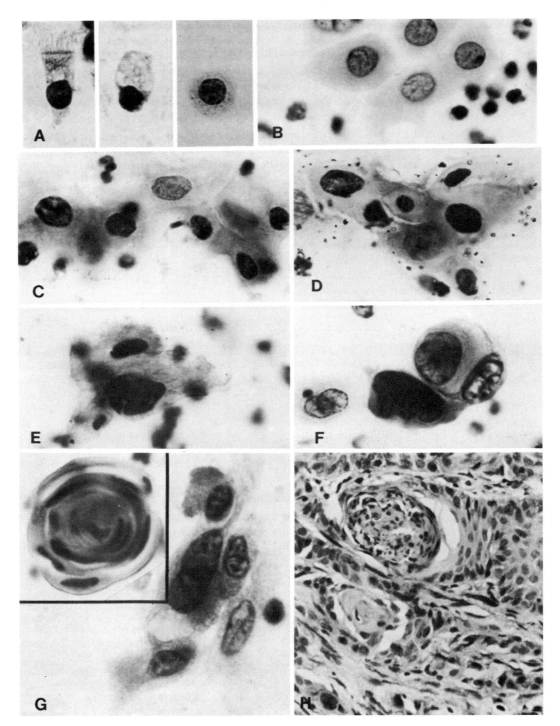

Figure 20-22 Sequential cytologic abnormalities observed in experimental carcinogenesis of the respiratory tract in Syrian golden hamsters, induced by intratracheal injections of benzo[a]pyrene and ferric oxide. The tumors closely resemble human lung cancers. *A.* Normal ciliated respiratory cell, a goblet cell, and a macrophage. *B,C.* Cells from areas of squamous metaplasia of the trachea after 7 weeks of carcinogen application; the cells in *C* show considerable nuclear abnormalities. *D–F.* Increasing cell abnormalities after 12, 15, and 18 weeks of carcinogen application. *G.* Cells and (*H*) tissue of squamous carcinoma located at carina of the trachea. (*A–F:* Oil immersion; *H:* high magnification.) (Modified from Schreiber H, Nettlesheim, P. A new method for pulmonary cytology in rats and hamsters. Cancer Res 32:737–745, 1972. Courtesy of Dr. H. Schreiber, Oak Ridge, Tenn.)

situ or microinvasive carcinoma require lobectomy. Further, **eradication of in situ or invasive carcinoma in one bronchus does not exclude the possibility of additional carcinomas occurring in other areas of the bronchial tree** (see above, second primary lung cancers). Thus, the management of bronchogenic squamous carcinoma in situ is still a dilemma, and likely to remain so for many years.

Cytology of Sputum

As noted, Saccomanno proposed some of the most detailed diagnostic criteria for cytologic identification of the presumed precursors of bronchogenic epidermoid carcinoma and described their progression to invasive carcinoma. His work was primarily with uranium miners in western Colorado who were exposed to naturally occurring radon gas, but were also cigarette smokers. Saccomanno's views received support from cytologic studies of experimental carcinoma of the respiratory tract in hamsters, conducted by Schreiber et al (1974) (Fig. 20-22). He considered squamous metaplasia of the bronchial epithelium to be an important link in the chain of events.

Simple Squamous Metaplasia

In the absence of nuclear atypia, squamous metaplasia cannot be considered a precancerous lesion. As discussed in Chapter 19, it is a common finding, particularly among individuals exposed to irritating dusts or gases, or subject to recurrent respiratory tract infections. The cytologic presentation of simple squamous metaplasia without atypia was described and illustrated in Chapter 19.

Squamous Metaplasia With Atypia

In contrast to simple squamous metaplasia, a finding of squamous metaplasia with nuclear abnormalities should raise the possibility of a precancerous lesion. Atypical squamous metaplasia may accompany squamous carcinoma

in situ (see below), or in some cases of apparent progression to invasive carcinoma, **it may already represent carcinoma in situ.** In other instances, there is regression of atypical squamous metaplasia, or at least no apparent progression of the lesion. Risse et al (1988) followed a group of 46 patients with a diagnosis of "severe dysplasia" by sputum cytology, and 21 eventually developed lung cancer while 25 did not.

Cytology

Squamous metaplasia is manifested in sputum and bronchial specimens by **loosely structured clusters of small squamous cells with variably sized atypical nuclei** (Fig. 20-23). **The clusters have a mosaic pattern and one straight edge, a configuration suggesting origin from the surface of the bronchial mucosa** (see Chap. 19). **The distinction between markedly atypical squamous metaplasia and carcinoma in situ often is subtle, and a matter of judgment. The presence of single, well-differentiated abnormal cells (with or without similar cells in clusters) points toward the diagnosis of squamous carcinoma in situ; the cells derived from atypical squamous metaplasia are less well differentiated and more likely to remain in coherent groups.**

As a practical matter, **all patients with atypical squamous cells in sputum or bronchial samples should be carefully followed.** Repeat examinations of additional cytology specimens will be necessary to ensure that sampling is adequate, and they must be diligently searched for single cancer cells. In some instances, **a very few single malignant cells have been identified in specimens several years before bronchogenic carcinoma was diagnosed.** It is not known whether the exfoliated cells came from a precursor lesion or an occult and indolent invasive carcinoma. Several examples of markedly atypical squamous cells interpreted as atypical metaplasia preceding carcinoma in situ were reported from the Cooperative Early Lung Cancer study. In our own experience in that same study, however, **the cancer cells appeared abruptly in the sputum of patients without prior significant atypia.**

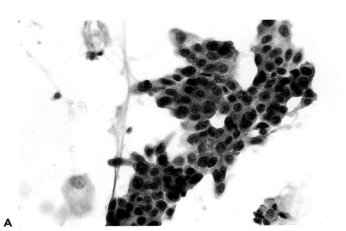

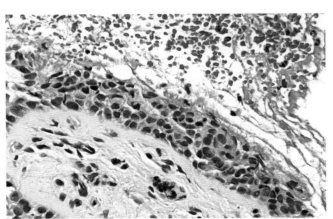

Figure 20-23 **Atypical squamous metaplasia.** *A.* Bronchial brushing of RUL segmental bronchus from a 53-year-old man who subsequently was diagnosed with SSC of the left upper lobe. The cells are coherent, but small and disorderly with relatively large, coarsely textured, hyperchromatic nuclei and amphophilic cytoplasm. *B.* Histologic section of the same site. The lesion could be classified either as atypical metaplasia or early carcinoma in situ.

Differential Diagnosis

There are many conditions that may mimic **atypical squamous metaplasia.** These include small squamous cells from the deep layers of buccal epithelium and larynx, frequently present in inflammatory or ulcerative processes (see Chap. 21), "Pap cells" from the larynx (see Chap. 19), tracheitis sicca associated with tracheostomy (see Chap. 19), and non-specific inflammatory changes occurring in metaplastic bronchial cells. Atypical metaplastic cells may also be confused with the **atypical squamous cells of pemphigus** involving the upper respiratory tract (see Chap. 21); with non-specific cell abnormalities observed in **viral pneumonia;** with specific viral infections, mainly **herpes simplex;** and with **drug-induced changes** (see Chap. 19).

Potential Markers of Progression of Atypical Metaplasia to Cancer

There are still too few follow-up studies of atypical metaplastic lesions to predict their behavior or even to define them reliably from one laboratory to another. This presents a practical problem in management of the individual patient and also in evaluating studies of drugs intended to prevent progression or reverse presumed precancerous lesions (Mel-

amed and Flehinger, 1993). DNA aneuploidy has been reported in some cases of atypical squamous metaplasia (Nasiell et al, 1978; Hirano et al, 1994), and may be a marker of progression.

Tockman et al (1997) reported **overexpression of the heterogeneous nuclear riboprotein (hnRNP) A2/B1** in archival sputum specimens of patients with atypical squamous metaplasia progressing to squamous carcinoma in situ. This finding was supported by a prospective study of Chinese miners at high risk of lung cancer (Qiao et al, 1997), and by a study of bronchial lavage specimens (Fielding et al, 1999). Expression of **p53 and K-ras point mutations** in sputum cells also may precede morphologic diagnosis of lung cancer by some months and perhaps even years (Mao et al, 1994). However, the sensitivity of these tests is low, and their applicability to the detection of small peripheral lung cancers has yet to be documented (Gazdar and Minna, 1999).

Cytology of Squamous Carcinoma In Situ

In sputum specimens from many of our own cases of squamous carcinoma in situ, and from specimens graciously

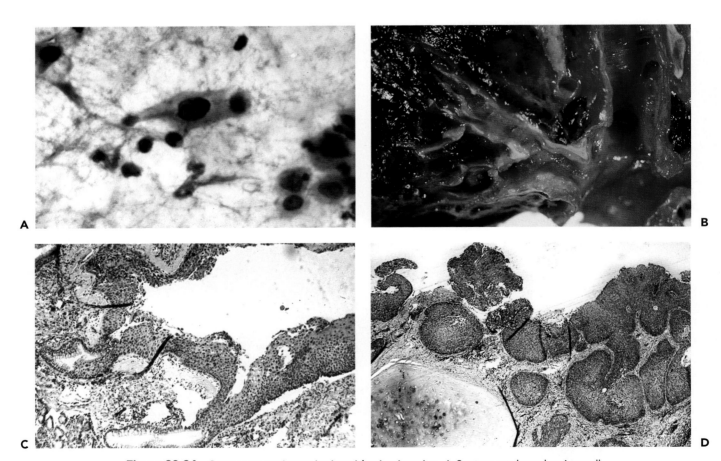

Figure 20-24   Squamous carcinoma in situ with microinvasion. *A.* Sputum cytology showing well-differentiated, single squamous cancer cell with opaque eosinophilic cytoplasm and hyperchromatic, irregular enlarged nucleus. *B.* Gross appearance of the resected lobe of lung showing thickened mucosa with loss of rugal folds in the segmental bronchus with carcinoma in situ. *C,D.* Histologic sections showing carcinoma in situ. *D.* Microinvasive carcinoma. (From Melamed MR, Koss LG, Cliffton EE. Roentgenologically occult lung cancer, diagnosed by cytology. Report of 12 cases. Cancer 16: 1537–1551, 1963.)

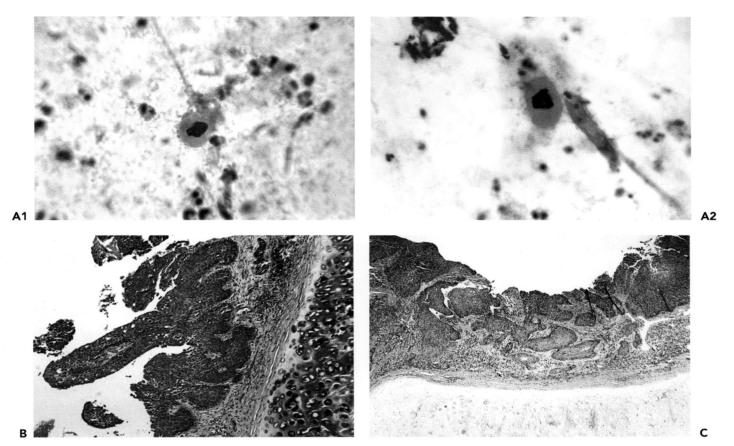

Figure 20-25   Carcinoma in situ with microinvasive carcinoma. *A1,A2.* Sputum with single well-differentiated squamous cancer cells. Same patient with papillary carcinoma in situ at the bifurcation of a segmental bronchus (*B*) and adjacent flat carcinoma in situ with microinvasion (*C*). (From Melamed MR, Zaman MB, Flehinger BJ, Martini N. Radiologically occult in situ and incipient invasive epidermoid lung cancer. Detection by sputum cytology in a survey of asymptomatic cigarette smokers. Am J Surg Pathol 1:5–16, 1977.)

loaned to us by others,[*] **the most consistent finding has been the presence of well-differentiated squamous cells with the nuclear abnormalities of cancer occurring usually singly or, uncommonly, in small clusters** (Figs. 20-24 to 20-26). They are similar to the **dyskaryotic squamous cells of keratinizing squamous carcinoma in situ of uterine cervix** (see Chap. 11). Similar cells may be seen in squamous carcinomas in situ of other organs, such as the esophagus and larynx (see Chaps. 21 and 24).

The characteristic cells are typically large, superficial squamous cells with moderately abundant predominantly eosinophilic, but occasionally basophilic cytoplasm. They are smoothly contoured; the bizarre cell forms sometimes seen in invasive squamous carcinoma are uncommon. **Nuclei are hyperchromatic, irregular, and enlarged in proportion to the surrounding cytoplasm,** resulting in a higher-than-normal nucleocytoplasmic ratio. As discussed above, the differential diagnosis between markedly atypical squamous metaplasia ("grave" atypia of Dr. John Frost)

and epidermoid carcinoma in situ is a matter of judgment. In case of doubt, further cytologic and clinical studies are indicated.

In **bronchial brush specimens, the abnormal squamous cells often form clusters and groups as well as single cells.** The cell groups are made up primarily of **superficial squamous cells, as in sputum, with cytoplasm that is often eosinophilic and sometimes frankly keratinized. Nuclei are significantly enlarged and usually coarsely textured, hyperchromatic, and irregular.** The break-up of the clusters and the presence of single cells, if any, speak in favor of fully developed carcinoma in situ. Detached fragments of epidermoid carcinoma in situ may occasionally be dislodged in a bronchial brush or wash specimen, and recognized in cell block preparations (Fig. 20-26C). Such rare events suggest that carcinoma in situ is more readily detached from the surface of the bronchus than is normal bronchial epithelium. Similar observations have been made for carcinomas in situ of the uterine cervix and the bladder (see Chaps. 11 and 23).

One of the features of carcinoma in situ is the failure to differentiate normally, as is seen, for example, in the lack

---

[*] The late Dr. G. N. Papanicolaou, Dr. L. Woolner, Rochester, MN, and the late Dr. M. Nasiell, Stockholm, Sweden.

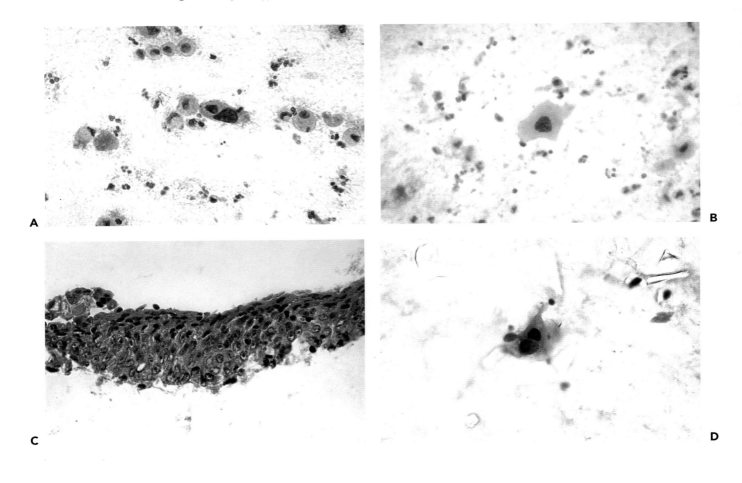

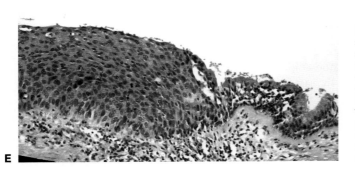

Figure 20-26 **Squamous carcinomas in situ.** *A,B.* Sputum with single well-differentiated squamous cancer cells. *C.* Carcinoma in situ in a mucosal strip from the right bronchial wash specimen of a patient who had had left pneumonectomy for lung cancer 2 years earlier (cell block section). *D,E.* Similar well-differentiated squamous cancer cell from another patient with carcinoma in situ, and histologic section of segmental bronchus with carcinoma in situ showing the abrupt transition from normal bronchial mucosa without squamous metaplasia. (From Melamed MR, Zaman MB, Flehinger BJ, Martini N. Radiologically occult in situ and incipient invasive epidermoid lung cancer: Detection by sputum cytology in a survey of asymptomatic cigarette smokers. Am J Surg Pathol 1:5–16, 1977.)

of cilia (Fig. 20-27). In more advanced invasive carcinomas, the cellular and nuclear abnormalities are generally more marked, an observation confirmed by us and others (Tao et al, 1982), but **whether cells derived from squamous carcinoma in situ can be distinguished from cells of early invasive squamous carcinoma is still a matter of debate.** Erozan et al (1979) reported measurable differences between the cells of carcinoma in situ versus microinvasive and fully invasive cancer. Greenberg et al (1987), using sophisticated image analysis methods, also concluded that there were measurable differences between cells from reversible atypias, carcinoma in situ, and invasive cancer. In our view, the number of cases of in situ and microfocally invasive squamous lung cancer is still too low to draw firm conclusions.

Clinical Approach to Patients With Cancer Cells in Sputum in the Absence of Radiologic Abnormalities

A diagnosis of carcinoma by sputum cytology in the absence of localizing radiologic findings must be confirmed on at least two separate specimens on two different days to rule out laboratory error. The diagnosis and treatment of such cases should then be governed by the following principles:

Once the cytologic diagnosis of cancer has been established, **a thorough examination of the buccal cavity, nasopharynx, larynx, etc., must be undertaken to rule out a possible source of cancer cells from the upper respiratory tract.**

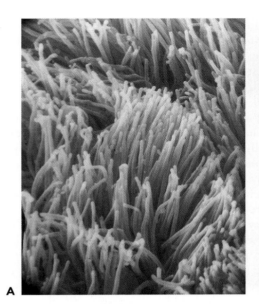
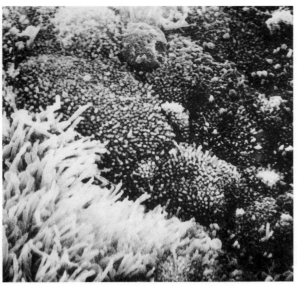

Figure 20-27   Scanning electron micrograph of squamous carcinoma in situ of bronchus. *A.* Normal bronchus showing surface cilia. *B.* Carcinoma in situ at the margin with adjacent bronchial mucosa showing short microvilli replacing cilia. (Courtesy of Dr. Patricia Saigo.)

If the above procedures are negative, a thorough investigation of the bronchial tree is indicated. Fiberoptic bronchoscopy, preferably with videotape recording, is mandatory, and may have to be repeated if the source of the cancer cells is not found. Localized roughening and redness of the bronchial mucosa, and loss of the normal rugal folds, especially at a bronchial bifurcation or spur, may be the only visible evidence of squamous carcinoma in situ or microinvasive squamous carcinomas.

Even in the presence of a suspicious mucosal lesion, but particularly in the absence of a visible abnormality, **systematic bronchial brushing should be carried out,** and separately labeled specimens must be obtained from each lobar, segmental, and subsegmental bronchus. Bronchial brushing samples and biopsies from tertiary and sometimes quaternary bronchi are technically feasible, and have been successful in confirming and localizing occult carcinomas. **We have never seen a case of confirmed positive sputum cytology in which fiberoptic bronchoscopy in skilled hands failed to localize the malignant lesion.**

Under no circumstances should the patient be explored surgically before the source of the cancer cells has been localized and the surgical procedure defined in advance. Carcinoma in situ and related lesions of the bronchus cannot be visualized or palpated at thoracotomy, and surgery will fail if it is undertaken before establishing the exact site of the lesion. In such a case, a renewed attempt at localization in the future will be made more difficult by the operative procedure, which will only delay definitive treatment, as happened to two of the first patients we encountered.

A patient with positive sputum cytology may have a radiographically visible lesion that is benign and unrelated to an early, occult cancer located elsewhere in the bronchial tree. This was observed in two of our early patients, one with bronchiectases, and another with a Ghon tubercle. In the latter case, thoracotomy and resection of the radiologically visible lesion delayed definitive treatment and was followed by invasive carcinoma with a fatal outcome. If thoracotomy is undertaken on the assumption that a radiologic lesion is the source of the cancer cells in sputum, frozen section confirmation should be obtained for confirmation at the time of surgery.

PROGRAMS FOR DETECTION OF OCCULT BRONCHOGENIC CARCINOMA

History

The concept that early detection of lung cancer might lower mortality from that disease was first tested in the Philadelphia Pulmonary Neoplasm Research Project (Boucot et al, 1970; Weiss et al, 1982), the North West London study (Brett, 1969) and the South London Cancer Study (Nash et al, 1968). These surveys were based on photofluorogram chest x-rays used in mass surveys to detect tuberculosis and were not suited for detection of early lung cancer. Although they were successful in finding some unsuspected advanced cancer cases, the surveys failed to show that they could lower the mortality of lung cancer. **Cytology has played a key role in all subsequent efforts to detect early occult lung cancer.**

In 1951, Papanicolaou and Koprowska reported the **first documented case of radiographically occult carcinoma in situ of the bronchus diagnosed by cytology,** thus offering promise of a new technique for detection of preinvasive, potentially curable lung cancer. The first application of this procedure in a cancer detection survey of cigarette smokers was between 1959 and 1961 in New York City. Of 643 cigarette-smoking men aged 40 and over, two were found with occult carcinoma (see Fig. 20-24).

A number of reports of single and small groups of patients with radiologically occult carcinoma detected by sputum cytology were subsequently published (Lerner et al, 1961; Melamed et al, 1963; Holman and Okinaka, 1964; Pearson and Thompson, 1966; Lilienfeld et al, 1966; Woolner et al, 1966; Grzybowski and Coy, 1970; Woolner et al, 1970; Marsh et al, 1972; Martini et al, 1974). These reports, and the introduction of fiberoptic bronchoscopy to localize occult carcinomas discovered by sputum cytology, led to a large multicenter evaluation of sputum cytology as a lung cancer detection technique.

Early Lung Cancer Detection Studies Sponsored by the National Cancer Institute

Between 1972 and 1974, three major screening programs were initiated, sponsored by the National Cancer Institute under the direction of Dr. Nathaniel Berlin. They were designed to evaluate sputum cytology as an adjunct to the chest x-ray for lung cancer detection. The goal was to determine whether systematic, periodic examinations of sputum cytology, supplementing the chest x-ray, could lead to a significant reduction in the death rate from lung cancer in a selected population at high risk. The Johns Hopkins Medical Institutions, the Mayo Clinic, and the Memorial Hospital for Cancer were the participating institutions. A total of 31,360 asymptomatic male cigarette smokers, aged 45 or older, were recruited by the three groups into a study that continued for 5 to 8 years, until November, 1982, with up to 2 years of additional follow-up. Details of the study design have been published in a *Manual of Procedures* available from the National Cancer Institute (NIH publication no. 79-1972).

There were some differences among the three institutions. The men in the Hopkins and Memorial studies were recruited from the general populations of Baltimore and New York City, respectively, and randomly divided into a study group, offered annual chest x-rays (full size PA and lateral) and sputum cytology every 4 months, or into a control group that was offered the annual chest x-ray only. The Mayo population was recruited from their outpatient clinic, and excluded men with any suspicion of lung cancer on initial examination. All had chest x-rays and sputum cytology on entry and those without evidence of lung cancer were assigned to a "close surveillance" group that was offered x-ray and sputum cytology every 4 months, or to a "control" group that was advised initially but not reminded to seek periodic chest x-rays.

Prevalence Data
The lung cancer cases that have accumulated in the study population and are discovered in the initial screening examination are defined as prevalence cases. They include indolent cancers that may have been present for months or years.

In the initial (prevalence) screening, there were 160 patients with lung cancer detected among the 21,127 men who had dual screening with both sputum cytology and chest x-ray (0.75%); 93 cancers were detected by x-ray only, 37 by cytology only, and 30 by both techniques (Fontana et al, 1984; Frost et al, 1984; Flehinger et al, 1984; summary in Berlin et al, 1984). **Sputum cytology was useful almost exclusively for detection of squamous carcinomas, especially those located in subsegmental and larger central bronchi.** Most of the 93 lung cancers detected by x-ray only were adenocarcinomas or undifferentiated large-cell carcinomas; almost all of the peripheral adenocarcinomas were found by x-ray. Nearly half of the cancers detected by x-ray alone were stage I, and more than 80% of the cancers detected by cytology alone were stage I, that is, localized and potentially curable by resection. The 5-year survival rate for the patients with resected stage I lung cancer was 75% to 80%; and the 10-year survival in this study was 65%, which should be compared with the expected 12% 5-year survival rate for lung cancer nationally. These data emphasize the importance of screening asymptomatic individuals at high risk of lung cancer if one is to identify the disease in an early and curable stage.

Incidence Data
New lung cancers that developed after the initial screening are referred to as incident cases. They were observed during the year following the initial or subsequent negative annual examination and provide information on the rate of development of lung cancer. The most detailed incidence data come from the Memorial Hospital study in New York (Melamed et al, 1984; Melamed and Flehinger, 1987; Melamed, 2000), but are not significantly different from the other two institutions.

Of the 10,040 men recruited into the program in New York City, a total of 354 developed lung cancer, of which 293 were diagnosed during the screening period of 5 to 8 years and 61 during the postscreening follow-up period. Fifty-three men had lung cancer detected on the initial screening examination (prevalence = 0.5%), and 137 were detected by subsequent repeat screenings. Thus, 190 of 293 lung cancers diagnosed during the screening period (65%) were detected by screening. The remaining 103 patients had lung cancer detected clinically because of symptoms or radiologic findings between scheduled screening examinations (interval cases). Not surprisingly, **over half of the rapidly growing small-cell (oat cell) carcinomas (12 of 21) were interval cases, diagnosed clinically because of symptoms.** As in the prevalence study, most of the lung cancers found by cytology were squamous carcinomas, and most of those found by x-ray were adenocarcinomas (Tables 20-4 to 20-6). **Sixty-one additional cases were diagnosed clinically during the 2 years of follow-up after screening was discontinued, mostly in symptomatic patients who had advanced disease.**

The patients in this study with lung cancer diagnosed as a result of symptoms had an estimated 13% survival at 7 years, which is comparable to the estimated overall survival of 13% at 5 years for lung cancer throughout the US. Thus,

TABLE 20-4

HISTOLOGY OF LUNG CANCER IN 10,040 PARTICIPANTS IN NEW YORK LUNG CANCER DETECTION PROGRAM

Cell Type	Detected by Screening	Interval Cases	Postscreening	Total
Epidermoid	61	29	21	111
Adenocarcinoma	105	37	22	164
Undifferentiated large cell	9	8	6	23
Oat cell	15	28	12	55
Carcinoid	0	1	0	1
Total	190	103	61	354

From Melamed and Flehinger (1987).

TABLE 20-5

STAGE OF LUNG CANCERS IN NEW YORK LUNG CANCER DETECTION STUDY

	According to Mode of Detection			
	Detected by Screening	Interval Cases	Postscreening	Total
Stage 1	100	20	12	132
Stage 2	15	3	5	23
Stage 3	75	80	44	199
Total	190	103	63	354

From Melamed and Flehinger (1987).

TABLE 20-6

LUNG CANCER CELL TYPE ACCORDING TO METHOD OF DETECTION IN 4,968 MEN SCREENED BY CYTOLOGY AND X-RAY

	Method of Detection				
Cell Type	Cytology	X-Ray	Both	Interval	Total
Epidermoid	20	8	8	10	46
Adenocarcinoma	5	44	3	21	73
Undiff. large cell	1	3	0	2	6
Oat cell	1	5	3	12	21
Carcinoid	0	0	0	1	1
Total	27	60	14	46	147

From Melamed and Flehinger (1987).

for all practical purposes, **symptomatic lung cancer is late lung cancer, and the cure rates are dismal.**

Conclusions From the Early Lung Cancer Study

As mentioned in the opening pages of this chapter, there is good evidence that some early stage lung cancers detected by screening have high resectability and survival rates but, so far, there is no convincing statistical proof that screening lowers death rates from lung cancer (Fontana, 2000; Kubik, 2000). If this seems paradoxical, it has been suggested that some lung cancers discovered by screening are indolent and would never have progressed to cause illness and death (Black, 2000; Parkin and Moss, 2000). However, there is no persuasive evidence that this theory is correct. Thus, Flehinger et al (1992) reported 5-year survival of only 0% to 8% for untreated stage I lung cancer patients with adeno- and large-cell carcinoma, whereas 5-year survival ranged from 52% to 62% for men with the same tumor types and the same stage who were treated by surgery. Similarly, the higher death rates from lung cancer in black, compared to white, patients can be explained by lower rates of surgical treatment (Bach et al, 1999).

It is now virtually impossible to do a randomized study of lung cancer screening that denies chest x-rays to high-risk individuals. In the absence of such a study, it has become impossible to demonstrate that screening lowers the death rate from lung cancer (recently reviewed by Patz et al, 2000). In a mathematical model of the progression kinetics of lung cancer developed by Flehinger and Kimmel (1987, 1988) from data collected in the NCI study of lung cancer screening described above, it was concluded that annual screening could reduce lung cancer deaths by up to 18%.

Pending future developments in the new lung cancer screening programs based on spiral CT and summarized below, **the American Cancer Society recommends that physicians should decide for each individual patient whether the risk of lung cancer is sufficient to warrant periodic radiologic examination of the chest and cytologic investigation of any suspect lesion. The following categories of patients should receive special attention:**

- **Long-term cigarette smokers** over 55 years of age
- **Any adult with a history of persistent cough,** with or without hemoptysis
- **Any patient with recurrent pneumonia,** obstructive lung disease, or a localized pathologic process in the lung
- **Any patient with persisting or unexplained radiographic abnormalities,** whether or not considered benign
- **Industrial workers or others exposed to pulmonary carcinogens,** and particularly asbestos or radioisotopes (uranium mining)

Lung Cancer Screening Based on Spiral (Helical) Computed Tomography

Recent technical advances in CT (helical or spiral CT) have greatly shortened exposure times and significantly reduced irradiation to patients. Screening examinations of the chest now take 20 seconds or less and require no contrast medium (Kaneko et al, 1996; Sone et al, 1998; Nitta et al, 1999). This technique is now being applied to lung cancer detection in a number of programs, one of which is the "Early Lung Cancer Action Project" (ELCAP).

The ELCAP project, which now encompasses several institutions in the US and abroad, has undertaken a program of annual screening of asymptomatic patients at various degrees of risk for lung cancer (Henschke et al, 1999, 2000). Small pulmonary nodules, observed on the initial scan, are investigated further by high-resolution CT and classified as to their appearance. Nodules with evidence of calcification are presumed to be granulomas and are followed clinically. Nodules with homogeneous, opaque appearance ("ground-glass opacities") and irregular margins are investigated further.

Most of the nodules discovered by spiral CT are smaller than 1 cm, and most are benign, so that identifying the few that are very small carcinomas can be a challenge. With contemporary technology, **detailed three-dimensional images of the nodules are available for precise measurements and study of their configuration, which can then be followed to detect possible progression on repeat scans** (Yankelevitz et al, 2000). It is assumed that nodules of irregular configuration or those that change shape or grow in size are more likely to be malignant than smoothly configured nodules of constant shape and volume.

The institutions participating in these studies use different approaches to investigate the nature of suspicious nodules: some use large-caliber (18-gauge) needles to perform a "mini-biopsy" of the nodule; others **rely on cytologic evaluation of the nodules by percutaneous thin-needle aspirations** (Henschke et al, 1999, Yankelevitz et al, 2000). Most of the malignant lesions discovered by this approach are peripheral adenocarcinomas, a smaller number are squamous carcinomas (see Fig. 20-20). Unfortunately, the percutaneous aspirations are not without complications, as discussed in detail in Chapter 19. **Approximately 30% of the patients develop pneumothorax, although almost all are minor and resolve spontaneously without intervention.** Of concern has been the possibility of **tumor cell implantation** in the needle track. Sinner and Zajicek (1976) reported only one such instance in more than 1,250 lung cancer cases, and single, additional cases were reported by Moloo et al (1985) and Sacchini et al (1989). **This very rare complication is even more unlikely if fine-bore needles are used (< 0.6 mm diameter, 21-gauge).**

Results

Several groups of investigators have reported preliminary results of their studies, which include an early report from the US (Henschke et al, 1999), and a larger experience from Japan (Kaneko et al, 1996; Sone et al, 1998). It is clear that selection of the population at risk will impact results. Thus, the Henschke study admits men age 60 and higher with 10 or more years of smoking history. The **prevalence** of lung cancer on the first screen of 1,000 patients was 2.7% (27 cases), whereas on the next 1,184 examinations, which includes a second screening of the same group and gives an **approximation of incidence,** there were only 7 new cases (0.6%). More than 80% of the cancers discovered were in surgically resectable stage I (see Fig. 20-20).

In other studies dealing with lesser risk populations, the prevalence of lung cancer was much lower. In the study by Sone et al (1998), which accepted smokers and nonsmokers of both sexes, age 40 and higher, lung cancer was detected in 40 of 7,847 patients (0.5%), and was the same for smokers and nonsmokers. Miettinen (2000) discussed the cost-effectiveness of the screening programs. At the time of this writing (2004), none of the health agencies of the US government or the American Cancer Society have formally endorsed these screening programs. In describing a statistical model of expected true and false-positive findings with helical CT for lung cancer detection, Mahadevia et al (2003) considered estimates of the uncertainty of benefits, the potential harm of false-positive invasive tests and high costs, and concluded that these screening examinations were not cost-effective.

UNCOMMMON PRIMARY MALIGNANT TUMORS OF LUNG

Neuroendocrine Tumors

The neuroendocrine tumors as a group have been separated from other pulmonary neoplasms by histology and their presumed common origin in the endocrine bronchial cells (Kulchitsky's cells). They are characterized by the presence of **membrane-bound, dense-core neuroendocrine cytoplasmic inclusions in electron micrographs,** and **positive immunocytochemical reactions with specific monoclonal antibodies for chromogranin, synaptophysin,** or for **polypeptide hormones such as serotonin, ACTH, gastrin, etc.** (see also Chap. 45). **Endocrine activity may be evident clinically in the form of various polypeptide-related syndromes, such as the carcinoid syndrome** (see below). The prototypical neuroendocrine tumor of lung is the carcinoid and its variants. Small-cell (oat cell) carcinoma and its relationship to endocrine tumors was discussed above.

Carcinoid Tumors

Histology and Clinical Data

Carcinoid tumors of the lung occur in adults of any age and are unrelated to cigarette smoking. The tumors are generally circumscribed and grow under and lift the sometimes-ulcerated overlying bronchial epithelium. They present most frequently as a nodular tumor projecting into and partially obstructing a major bronchus (Fig. 20-28A). Like their counterpart in the bowel, carcinoids of the lung are **composed of nests, rosettes, or ribbons of tightly packed, quite regular, small, polyhedral cells** (Fig. 20-28B). **Variants may be composed of spindle cells** (Fig. 20-28C) **or contain an admixture of large, eosinophilic oncocytic cells with granular cytoplasm**. They typically produce serotonin and sometimes other polypeptide hormones, and stain for chromogranin, a neurosecretory marker (Fig. 20-

28D). Carcinoid tumors commonly arise in the bowel and their products are detoxified in liver. The **carcinoid syndrome (i.e.,** flushing of skin, diarrhea, bronchospasm, and sometimes endocardial and valvular fibrosis of the right side of the heart) results from **serotonin secretion** by metastatic carcinoid in the liver, bypassing detoxification (see Chap. 24). Interestingly, the carcinoid syndrome has been described, not only with pulmonary carcinoid, but also in bronchogenic carcinoma (Majcher et al, 1966).

The majority of carcinoids arise in and partially obstructs larger bronchi, and cause symptoms at an early, still-localized stage. They are diagnosed by conventional radiographic studies and bronchoscopic biopsy or brushing cytology. The uncommon peripheral carcinoids are diagnosed by needle-aspiration cytology or a needle core biopsy. If detected early, they can be cured by surgery. If untreated, carcinoids will gradually enlarge and most eventually metastasize.

Cytology

As the tumors are covered entirely or almost entirely by intact bronchial epithelium, and since the tumor cells are quite coherent and do not exfoliate easily, an initial **diagnosis of pulmonary carcinoid by cytologic examination of sputum or bronchial secretions is highly unlikely.** However, the diagnosis has been made on postbronchoscopy sputum specimens from patients suspected of bronchogenic carcinoma, as a consequence of mucosal disruption during the diagnostic procedure. We have also observed tumor cells in **sputum specimens of patients with metastatic carcinoid of intestinal origin,** and in patients with the related pancreatic islet cell tumors (see below).

The diagnosis is usually established on **bronchial brush specimens or by percutaneous needle aspiration.** In **postbronchoscopy sputum or bronchial brush specimens,** the cells of bronchial carcinoid are 15 to 20 μm in diameter. They are typically dispersed (Fig. 20-29A,B) or in small groups, sometimes forming **flat, loosely structured glandlike clusters** (Fig. 20-29C) (Lozowski et al, 1979). Carcinoid tumor cells are generally uniform and have a characteristic appearance: variably cuboidal or rectangular with faintly basophilic transparent cytoplasm in Papanicolaou stain, and eccentric nuclei. The position of the nucleus gives a vaguely plasmacytoid appearance (Fig. 20-29B). The nuclear chromatin is finely granular, often described as "salt and pepper." There may be tiny nucleoli.

In the **uncommon variant of carcinoid with oncocytic cells** (Matsumoto, 1993), the smears may show the classical features of carcinoid with an admixture of **variable numbers of oncocytes, singly and in clusters** (Fig. 20-29D). The oncocytes are readily recognized as **larger cells about the size of macrophages, with abundant, granular, eosinophilic cytoplasm and small vesicular nuclei.** There have been reports in which the cytologic pattern is dominated by the presence of oncocytes (Ogino, 2000). Because primary oncocytomas of lung are exceedingly rare, **the finding of oncocytes in bronchial brush specimens or aspirates from a lung tumor should immediately raise the possibility of a carcinoid or, more remotely, a granular cell tumor.**

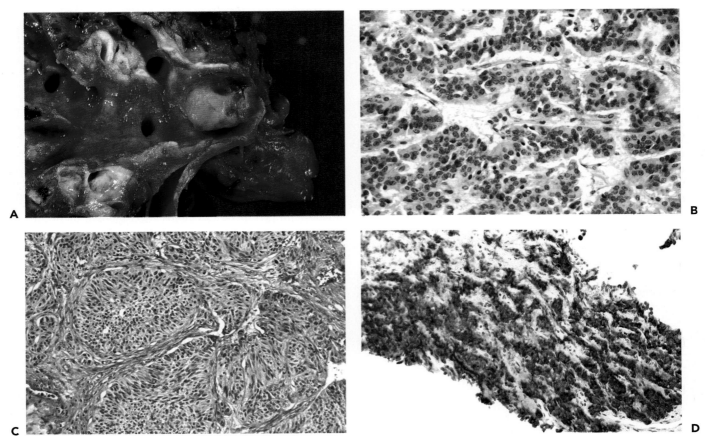

Figure 20-28   Carcinoid of lung. *A.* Gross appearance of a carcinoid tumor of lobar bronchus in an adult female. The smooth-surfaced polypoid tumor obstructs the lumen of the bronchus. *B.* Histologic section showing cuboidal tumor cells in trabecular pattern or nests. *C.* Carcinoid tumor with an organoid spindle cell pattern. *D.* Immunoperoxidase reaction for chromogranin is strongly positive for neurosecretory granules in this needle core biopsy.

With increasing use of **percutaneous needle aspiration biopsy,** cytologic samples of bronchial carcinoids are now being seen more frequently (Nguyen, 1995). The cytologic presentation in needle aspirates is similar to bronchial brushing specimens but usually more cellular (Collins and Cramer, 1996). **Occasional large, sometimes multinucleated giant cells may be observed, not an uncommon finding in endocrine tumors of all origins.** In an occasional case, the nuclei may be more darkly stained, but we have not observed the markedly hyperchromatic nuclei described by Kyriakos and Rockoff (1972) in brush specimens.

Peripheral carcinoids are often composed of spindle cells (see Fig. 20-28C) **and may yield fusiform or polygonal cells** (Jordan et al, 1987) **with spindle-shaped nuclei and scant cytoplasm in percutaneous needle aspirates.** Generally, the **cytologic diagnosis of carcinoid is suggested by monotony of nuclear size, delicate "salt and pepper" chromatin structure,** and **absence of necrosis.** As noted, carcinoids may have a rosette pattern in histologic section, and Pilotti et al (1983) described two carcinoids with **glandular features in needle aspirates.** In such very unusual cases, the differentiation of carcinoid from adenocarcinoma and sometimes from SSC may cause diagnostic problems. Strong staining for chromogranin (see Fig. 20-28D) supports the diagnosis of carcinoid.

Atypical Carcinoid Tumors

Synonyms: well-differentiated neuroendocrine carcinomas, peripheral SSCs resembling carcinoid tumors.

Histology

The uncommon atypical carcinoid tumors were defined by Arrigoni et al (1972) as circumscribed **tumors with the basic histologic pattern of carcinoid but characterized by tumor cell pleomorphism; variably sized and atypical nuclei, a high mitotic rate; prominent nucleoli and focal necrosis.** They have a more aggressive clinical course than conventional carcinoids, and in 1983, Gould et al introduced the term **well-differentiated neuroendocrine carcinoma** to describe these tumors. Because even the conventional carcinoid may be malignant, however, there seems little rationale for this designation. Mark and Ramirez (1985) preferred to call them peripheral SSCs resembling carcinoid tumors. Craig and Finley (1982) described a spindle cell variant of these tumors, which is more likely to arise in peripheral lung, and more likely to be seen in percutaneous needle aspirates. The current WHO nomenclature is simply "atypical carcinoid."

All of these designations pertain to the same group of uncommon lung tumors that combine the basic histologic features of carcinoid tumors with focal areas of anaplastic

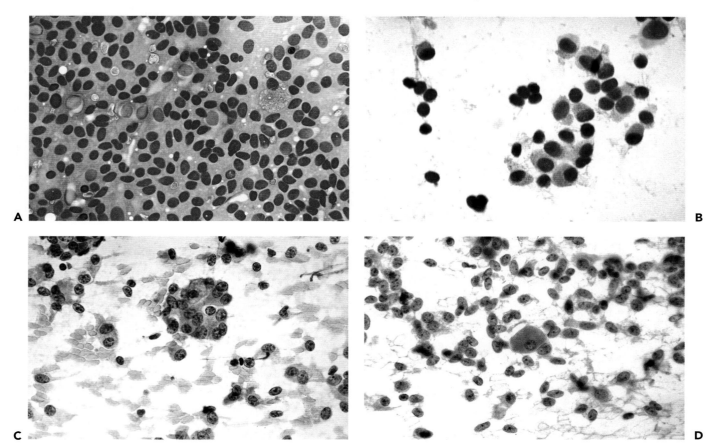

Figure 20-29   Cytologic patterns of carcinoid tumor of lung in FNA and bronchial brushings. *A.* Pulmonary carcinoid tumor in a 34-year-old woman. In the aspiration smear, the cells are evenly spread with uniform, ovoid or round nuclei, delicate chromatin and tiny nucleoli. There are few clusters of overlapping cells and no molding or necrosis. *B.* Aspirate of carcinoid tumor in which there are flat plaques or clusters of cells with deeper-staining cytoplasm and peripheral nuclei of plasmacytoid appearance. *C.* Bronchial brush specimen with flat clusters and single tumor cells with a moderate amount of pale-staining cytoplasm, uniform, round or slightly ovoid nuclei with delicate "salt and pepper" chromatin and small nucleoli. *D.* Oncocytic cell type of carcinoid in aspiration smear. The tumor cells have abundant eosinophilic cytoplasm.

cell growth, mimicking SSC of intermediate type. By high-resolution image analysis, the nuclei of anaplastic carcinoids are intermediate between conventional carcinoid and SSC (Larsimont et al, 1990). **Whereas atypical carcinoids have a more aggressive clinical course than the conventional carcinoids, they offer a significantly greater chance of surgical cure than SSC** (Ferguson et al, 2000).

Cytology

Experience with the cytology of these tumors is limited. Frierson et al (1987) describe eight such tumors in samples obtained by percutaneous needle aspiration. The cells differed from those of typical carcinoid by more likely formation of cell clusters, more **variability in nuclear size,** and the presence of some cells with **increased nuclear hyperchromasia or prominent nucleoli. Atypical carcinoid was distinguished from SSC, intermediate type, by tumor cells often arranged in organoid pattern with more abundant cytoplasm, open, nonpyknotic nuclei, a** lower level of nuclear abnormalities, and absence of nuclear molding or necrosis (Fig. 20-30).

In one cytologic study of 22 cases, Jordan et al (1987) described small sheets and cohesive **clusters of polygonal or fusiform cells with clear cytoplasm, medium-sized ovoid nuclei with single or multiple nucleoli, and rosette-like acinar clusters with palisading. Molding of nuclei was absent.** There were 13 long-term survivors among the 22 patients.

Although these features may be evident on retrospective review of histologically documented cases, in practice, the **prospective cytologic diagnosis of this group of tumors is extremely difficult.** In several cases from the Massachusetts General Hospital, seen courtesy of Dr. Wanda Szyfelbein, and personally reviewed (LGK), the diagnosis rendered was **carcinoid with atypical features. In practice, regardless of cytologic classification, resectable lung neoplasms should be excised and examined histologically so long as the diagnosis is not that of an oat cell carcinoma or SSC, intermediate type.**

Large-Cell Neuroendocrine Carcinomas

Some **non–small-cell undifferentiated carcinomas of lung are distinguished from other non–small-cell tu-**

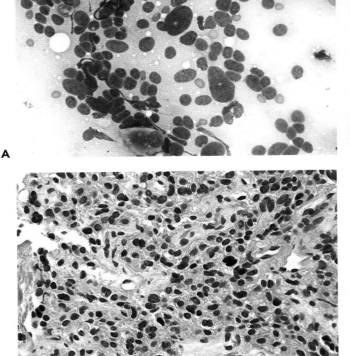

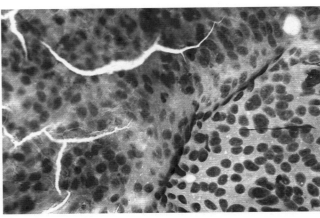

Figure 20-30 Atypical carcinoid of lung. *A.* FNA of an atypical peripheral carcinoid of lung in a 73-year-old woman. There are occasional cells with large nuclei among an otherwise generally uniform but unevenly distributed population of cells. The aspirate could be mistaken for adenocarcinoma. *B.* A thick part of the same smear in which the trabecular and nesting patterns of carcinoid tumor are evident side by side. *C.* Histologic section. Chromogranin stain was strongly positive. (*A,B*: Diff-Quik stain.)

mors only **by expression of neuroendocrine markers in immunocytochemical stains for chromogranin, synaptophysin, etc.** They constitute an estimated 3% of lung cancers (Jiang et al, 1998), and **cannot be differentiated from the morphologically similar tumors by conventional cytology alone.**

Minute Pulmonary Chemodectomas (Tumorlets)

The chemodectomas, first described by Whitwell (1955), are minute neuroendocrine tumors, often multiple, derived from Kulchitsky cells and believed to be related if not identical with carcinoids. Arioglu et al (1998) reported a case of **Cushing's syndrome** caused by corticotropin-secreting pulmonary tumorlets. We know of no case diagnosed by cytology, however, one should be aware that high-resolution spiral CT examinations may lead to the discovery and needle biopsy of a tumorlet.

Adenoid Cystic Carcinoma

Histology

These are highly malignant tumors of slow evolution, corresponding to the adenoid cystic carcinoma of salivary gland origin (Conlan, 1978). They are derived from **bronchial mucous glands,** and are therefore tumors of trachea and large bronchi. They have a very characteristic appearance, composed of **sheets of small, quite uniform cells, forming cystic spaces filled with homogeneous hyaline material that is derived from reduplicated basement membrane**

material (Fig. 20-31A). While they are common in the salivary glands, adenoid cystic carcinomas are uncommon in the lower respiratory tract. For comments on such tumors in the trachea, see Chapter 21, and in the salivary glands, see Chapter 32.

Cytology

Adenoid cystic carcinomas do not easily exfoliate, and the diagnostic cells are more likely to be found in bronchial brushing specimens than in sputum, and more often in recurrent than in primary tumors. The cytologic presentation is quite characteristic: **clusters of uniform, small cells with scanty cytoplasm and monotonous, dark nuclei, arranged around a core of homogeneous basement membrane material, which is faintly stained either cyanophilic or eosinophilic with the Papanicolaou stain** (Fig. 20-31B). The material stains purple with Diff-Quik and other metachromatic stains. In **percutaneous aspirates,** we have observed tumor cells forming large **overlapping spherical structures** composed of uniform small cells. Hyaline cores were not visible within the tumor globes, but could be seen as isolated extruded bodies in the smear background. In the absence of the hyaline cores, one may make a descriptive diagnosis of a tumor composed of small cells, and suggest adenoid cystic carcinoma as one possibility, but a more specific diagnosis may not be possible. The cytology of metastases from salivary gland tumors is identical.

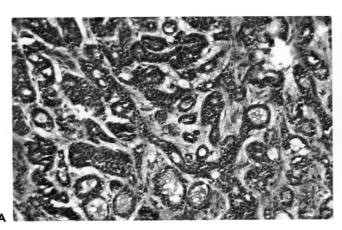 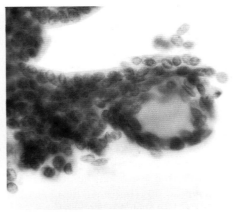

A   **B**

Figure 20-31   Adenoid cystic carcinoma of lung. *A.* Histologic section of adenoid cystic carcinoma of bronchus, showing a tumor composed of uniform small cells surrounding cystic spaces filled with hyaline basement membrane material. *B.* Bronchial brush cytology in which the small tumor cells form the characteristic cystic spaces. See also Chapter 32.

Mixed Malignant Tumors (Carcinosarcomas)

There are very uncommon malignant tumors in which a **malignant epithelial component is associated with a sarcomatous component such as rhabdomyosarcoma** (Davis et al, 1984; Takeda et al, 1994; Berho et al, 1995; M. Koss et al, 1999). Ishizuka et al (1988) and Parafiniuk et al (1994) reported the cytologic findings in sputum of patients with such a tumor. **Cells of ordinary squamous carcinoma were associated with tumor cells of variable configuration with cytoplasmic cross-striations, classified as rhabdomyoblasts.** Finley et al (1988) reported the immunocytochemistry and electron microscopy studies of a needle aspirate of pulmonary carcinosarcoma. The histology and cytology of these tumors in the uterus are described in Chapter 17.

Pulmonary and Pleuropulmonary Blastomas

Pulmonary blastomas are exceedingly uncommon **and highly malignant tumors of embryonal type** that may be compared to Wilms' tumor of the kidney (see Chap. 40). The tissues comprising the tumor resemble fetal lung. They are composed of **malignant embryonal connective tissue within which are tubular structures lined by cuboidal or columnar cells mimicking primitive bronchioles** (Barnard, 1952; Spencer, 1961; Souza et al, 1965). Variants may be entirely epithelial or mesenchymal. Although pulmonary blastomas are often considered tumors of children and young adults, they may occur at any age, and the median age is reported to be in the fourth decade (M. Koss et al, 1991).

Non et al (1976) described the cytologic presentation of one such case in the **sputum** of a 73-year-old patient. He observed numerous clusters of **large cancer cells derived from adenocarcinoma** together with **clusters of smaller cells derived from the undifferentiated sarcomatous component.** Spahr et al (1979) also reported a single case of blastoma in which cells of carcinoma were accompanied by small stromal cells. Jacobsen and Francis (1979) described 10 cases of pulmonary blastoma in elderly patients

of both sexes, studied by several cytologic techniques. **Most specimens were diagnosed as carcinomas of various types by sputum and bronchial washings.** The diagnoses of **sarcoma and of a "mixed tumor" were each rendered only once in percutaneous aspiration biopsy material.** It is evident from their report that cytologic sampling by routine techniques may be biased in favor of carcinoma; the sarcomatous component of a mixed tumor is best recognized by direct FNA sampling.

Pleuropulmonary blastoma, an embryonal malignant tumor of children, arises in lung in association with pleura. Unlike the pulmonary blastoma of adults, it is composed of **embryonal mesenchymal elements without a malignant epithelial component** (Manivel et al, 1988). Nicol and Geisinger (2000) described a case in which a percutaneous needle aspirate yielded a **mixture of primitive blastemal cells and spindle-shaped cells,** presenting as dispersed single cells and cohesive aggregates. In reports by Gelven et al (1997) and Drut and Pollono (1998), **myxoid matrix was present as well.** The differential diagnosis includes all the small, round cell malignant tumors of childhood.

Sarcomas

For an in-depth discussion of soft part sarcomas, see Chapter 35. Primary pulmonary sarcomas are very uncommon and few are intrabronchial in origin. Those that arise in the lung seldom erode the bronchial wall (except for malignant lymphomas) (see below), and they do not exfoliate easily. Thus, finding tumor cells of sarcoma in sputum is an exceptional event. On the other hand, aggressive investigation of lung masses by **percutaneous or transbronchial needle aspiration biopsy** may lead to at least a presumptive diagnosis of sarcoma. The most common are leiomyosarcoma, malignant fibrous histiocytoma and fibrosarcoma, but precise classification of tumor type by cytology is difficult (Guccion and Rosen, 1972; Nascimento et al, 1982; Suster, 1995; Keel et al, 1999).

Leiomyosarcoma

These uncommon tumors, composed of bundles of malignant smooth muscle cells, may form an intrabronchial polypoid mass, as in a case described by Krummerman (1977) (Fig. 20-32A), but more often appear as parenchymal tumors. There are a few cases on record in which the **spindly malignant cells** were observed in **sputum** (Fleming and Jove, 1975), **bronchial brushings** (Sawada et al, 1977), or in **a bronchial aspirate** (Krummerman, 1977). In most cases, the diagnosis is obtained by **percutaneous FNA.**

In the reported cases, **spindly, but fairly plump** malignant cells were observed (Fig. 20-32B), some with bifurcated ends. We observed one such case in a 17-year-old male with a very large intrapulmonary tumor mass who shed some of the relatively inconspicuous spindly tumor cells in sputum. The diagnosis was confirmed by a percutaneous needle aspirate that disclosed densely clustered and dispersed elongated tumor cells with moderately enlarged, finely granular nuclei and conspicuous, irregular, but not very large nucleoli (Fig. 20-32C). The tumor was resected, and the diagnosis of leiomyosarcoma was confirmed in histologic material.

Malignant Fibrous Histiocytoma

These tumors, cytologically similar to fibrosarcoma and leiomyosarcoma, have been reported by Barbas et al (1997) to yield **spindle-shaped cancer cells with "comet" configuration** in a bronchial brush specimen. Sampling is scanty at best in bronchial specimens, and much better in percutaneous needle aspirates. Hsiu et al (1987) and Kawahara et al (1988) diagnosed malignant fibrous histiocytoma by needle aspirate. The smears showed a mixture of malig-

nant spindle and polygonal cells with a few giant cells. In addition to the cytologic patterns described above, we have seen aspirates of a small number of these tumors that also contained cells with ample cytoplasm mimicking an epithelial tumor.

The diagnosis of **Kaposi's sarcoma** must be considered in AIDS patients and others who are immunosuppressed and present with space-occupying lesions of the lung. One of us (LGK) has seen the percutaneous FNA cytology slide from a case of Kaposi's sarcoma reported by Haramati (1995). In this and a few other cases, the smears contained thick bundles and dispersed spindly cells with enlarged oval, hyperchromatic nuclei in a background of blood. In the proper clinical setting, it is possible to make a diagnosis of spindle cell tumor consistent with Kaposi's sarcoma (Fig. 20-33) and in doubtful cases demonstrating expression of herpes virus 8 in tumor cells.

Synovial sarcoma, a malignant soft-tissue tumor commonly found in the extremities in association with synovial or bursal tissues, may rarely arise in other sites including lung and/or pleura (Essary et al, 2002). The tumor may be biphasic with spindle sarcomatous and epithelial components or a monophasic spindle-cell sarcoma. We have encountered one such case, presenting as a solitary intraparenchymal monophasic spindle-cell sarcoma, but have no experience with FNA cytology. Costa (1997) reported the FNA cytology of a metastatic, monophasic synovial sarcoma in the lung. The tumor was characterized by the presence of groups of spindle cells with ovoid nuclei and scant cyto-

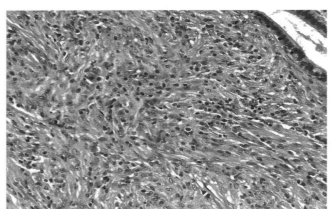

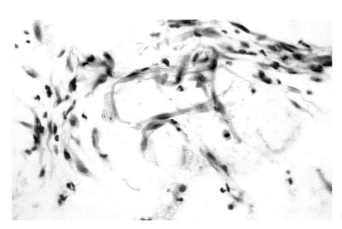

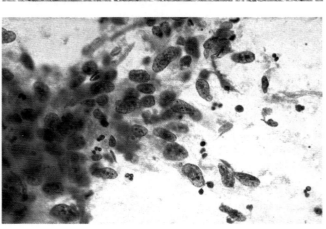

Figure 20-32 **Leiomyosarcoma of lung.** *A,B.* Case of Dr. Krummerman showing a polypoid spindly leiomyosarcoma that projected into the bronchus (*A*), and yielded spindly, smooth muscle tumor cells in a bronchial aspirate (*B*). *C.* Aspiration biopsy of lung in another patient, a 17-year-old boy. Note elongated cancer cells.

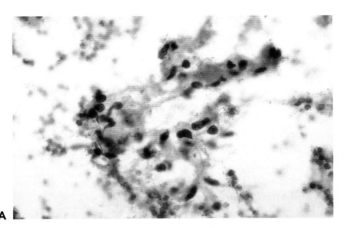
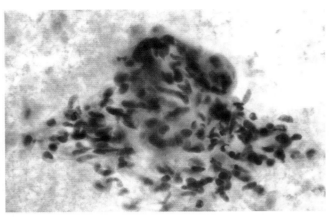

Figure 20-33 Kaposi's sarcoma involving lung in a patient with AIDS. An FNA of lung tumor showing spindly tumor cells singly and in small clusters. The cytologic findings were consistent with diagnosis of Kaposi's, which was subsequently confirmed.

plasm (for further discussion of these tumors, see Chap. 35).

Other Sarcomas

Medalie et al (1998) reported a patient with **pulmonary artery sarcoma diagnosed by FNA.** The diagnosis was made by a finding of pleomorphic and spindly malignant cells in an FNA of a lung nodule from a patient with an intraluminal filling defect of the left main pulmonary artery.

Differential Diagnosis of Spindle-Cell Sarcomas

The **differential diagnosis of primary pulmonary spindle-cell sarcomas** should include the **solitary fibrous tumor of pleura (fibrous mesothelioma: pleural fibroma). It is a benign, often pedunculated, spindle-cell fibroblastic pleural tumor** that is typically rich in collagen, does not exfoliate, and is often sparsely cellular in percutaneous needle aspirates. The **spindle cells obtained by needle aspirate show varying degrees of nuclear atypia, and are immunoreactive with CD-34.** The smears frequently contain **thick collagen and sometimes-recognizable capillaries** as well as **clusters of mesothelial cells** (Ali et al, 1997; Apple et al, 1997; Drachenberg et al, 1998). Sarcomatous malignant mesothelioma must also be included in the differential diagnosis. Primary tumors of the pleura are discussed in Chapter 26.

Lymphangiomyomatosis is an uncommon, cytologically "benign," but locally aggressive vascular tumor that is rich in smooth muscle and can mimic low-grade spindle-cell sarcoma in a FNA. Buhl et al (1988) drew attention to the **organoid configuration of tumor cells as a possibly useful diagnostic feature in the needle aspirate.** These tumors are not likely to exfoliate into sputum or bronchial specimens. Ackley et al (1998) reported a case with lymph node metastases diagnosed by needle aspiration cytology.

In general, the cytologic presentation of all sarcomas of lung is similar, and classification of tumor type on cytologic material alone is virtually impossible. A specific classification requires histologic material and often a battery of immunostains.

Further, it should be emphasized that **malignant spindle cells in sputum or a bronchial aspirate are much more likely to be derived from a spindle cell or sarcomatoid carcinoma than a sarcoma.** Thus, it is quite possible for a sarcoma of lung to be misinterpreted as spindle-cell carcinoma. Conversely, a **mistaken diagnosis of sarcoma** may be due to exfoliated cells of a primary or metastatic spindle-cell carcinoma in lung (Nakajima, 1999).

A very unusual example of **exfoliated, degenerating smooth muscle cells** resembling the cells of a spindle-cell sarcoma was reported by Takeda and Burechailo (1969) in a patient with **Wegener's granulomatosis and ulcerative tracheobronchitis.** Thus, **knowledge of clinical data is indispensable** before cytologic diagnosis of rare entities can be rendered. With the present increasing use of percutaneous needle aspiration biopsy, additional examples of these exceedingly rare primary pulmonary sarcomas certainly will be reported.

Primary Pulmonary Lymphomas

Lymphomas originating primarily within the lower respiratory tract are rare. It must be assumed that they **arise within intrapulmonary lymph nodes or in deposits of lymphoid tissue.** The current classification of malignant lymphomas is complex, based on cytology, antigen expression by immunocytochemistry and flow cytometry, and cytogenetics. An overview is provided in Chapter 31. In this description of the cytologic presentation of malignant lymphomas in the lung, it is sufficient to group them into categories of **small-cell and large-cell lymphomas and Hodgkin's disease.** The cytologic presentation of lymphomas secondarily involving lung is identical (see below).

In an authoritative review of primary pulmonary lymphomas, 36 cases were reported from a major cancer center by L'Hoste et al (1984). Twenty-one patients had a small-cell plasmacytoid lymphoma; most of the others had a large-cell lymphoma. Many of the small-cell lymphomas were originally diagnosed as pseudolymphoma, based on their slow clinical evolution. Most have been reclassified as mucosa-associated lymphomas (MALT lymphomas), and the term *pseudolymphoma* must now be considered obsolete.

In our experience, **primary small-cell lymphoma of lung cannot be diagnosed with confidence from exfoliative cytology in sputum, bronchial washings, or brushings.** An abundance of uniform, morphologically normal lymphocytes or plasmacytoid cells, with or without intermixed lymphoblasts, may very well represent an inflammatory lesion or reactive hyperplasia of lymphoid tissue (see Chap. 19). Even in patients with known lymphocytic lymphoma and a pulmonary tumor, the presence of a uniform population of small lymphocytes, while consistent with lymphoma, cannot be considered diagnostic. In principle, it is possible to make the diagnosis if a monoclonal population of lymphoid cells is demonstrated, either by flow cytometry or by immunocytochemical staining of the cells on a slide, or if the diagnosis is confirmed by chromosomal karyotyping on a portion of the specimen (see Chap. 4). This is rarely possible in specimens of sputum, bronchial aspirates, or wash specimens.

Similarly, percutaneous needle aspiration biopsy of lung has been of little help in the diagnosis of primary pulmonary lymphocytic lymphoma, although the cytology of these tumors is better demonstrated in needle aspirates than in sputum or bronchial brushings. Needle aspirates do have the potential advantage of providing more material for immunocytochemistry and flow cytometry to confirm and classify suspected lymphoma.

On the other hand, **large-cell lymphomas can be recognized in conventional cytologic specimens,** and particularly in FNAs. Bardales et al (1996) reported several such cases diagnosed by sputum cytology.

Cytology of Large-Cell Malignant Lymphoma

The exfoliated cells of large-cell lymphoma are comparable in size to SSC of the lung, and to metastatic small-cell malignant tumors from which they must be distinguished. The lymphoma cells have **round or oval, sometimes folded or indented nuclei with finely textured or vesicular chromatin and often-prominent nucleoli** (Fig. 20-34). **Like SSC of lung, they may have a narrow rim of cytoplasm. However, the bizarre cell forms, variations in cell size and necrosis that are common in SSC are not seen in lymphoma. Most importantly, the lymphoma cells lie singly, only touching each other in crowded cell specimens, unlike the loosely coherent clusters of superimposed cells of SSC; cell molding, which is so common in SSC, is not seen in lymphoma. The degree of nuclear pyknosis and hyperchromasia is much greater in SSC than in lymphoma, whereas nucleolar prominence is significantly greater in large-cell lymphoma.**

A case of the very rare "signet ring cell" lymphoma of the lung was described by Vernon (1981). The tumor mim-

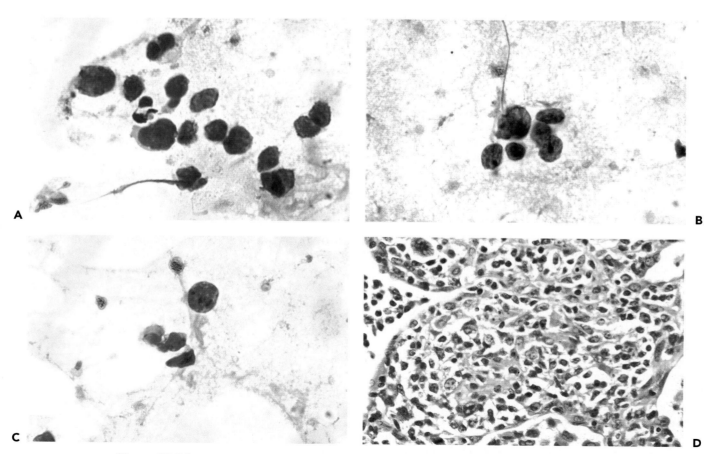

Figure 20-34 **Primary large-cell lymphoma of lung.** *A–C.* FNA of lung showing variably sized nuclei of lymphoid cells with irregular nuclear configuration, finely granular chromatin, and prominent nucleoli. Cytoplasm is scanty or absent. *D.* Histologic section of lung from the same case showing large-cell lymphoma. (*A–C:* Oil immersion.)

ics small-cell adenocarcinoma. For further discussion of this and other common and uncommon types of malignant lymphoma, see Chapter 31.

When lymphoma is suspected and the cytologic diagnosis is uncertain, one can gain considerable help from the ancillary diagnostic techniques of cytogenetics, immunocytochemistry and flow cytometry (see Chaps. 4, 45, and 47). **Primary Hodgkin's disease of the lung** is exceedingly rare (Kern et al, 1961). To date, we have not encountered a single case diagnosed initially by cytology. The lung is commonly involved secondarily, however, particularly in cases of **mediastinal Hodgkin's disease,** and there are several examples of such cases diagnosed by cytology, as discussed below.

Langerhans' cell tumors and their variants are discussed in Chapter 19.

PRIMARY BENIGN TUMORS AND TUMORS OF LOW MALIGNANT POTENTIAL

As a group, the primary benign tumors of lung do not exfoliate well and, when present, the exfoliated cells may not be recognized as tumor cells. Cytology plays a role here when specimens are obtained by bronchial brushing or by needle aspirates.

Squamous Papillomas of Bronchi

These uncommon lesions are usually observed in children and young adolescents as multiple papillary squamous tumors involving the larynx, trachea, and bronchi **(juvenile papillomatosis),** and are discussed in Chapter 21. HPV has been detected in mucosal swabs of these lesions (Sun et al, 2000). Their growth may subside after puberty, and without other predisposing factors, they progress to carcinoma only on rare occasions (Guillou et al, 1991).

In contrast, the very rare histologically similar **squamous papillomas of bronchus** of older adults (Fig. 20-35) have a high risk of progression to squamous carcinoma (DiMarco et al, 1978). The tumors resemble condylomata acuminata of the genital tract (see Chap. 11), and HPV has been demonstrated in koilocytes of this lesion by means of anti-HPV antibody and electron microscopy (Trillo and Guha, 1988); the subtype of virus was not determined. Rubel and Reynolds (1979) described **marked dyskaryosis and koilocytosis of squamous cells in bronchial brushings, similar to the HPV-induced changes in the uterine cervix. Hyperkeratotic atypia of squamous cells** (Fig. 20-35C) was

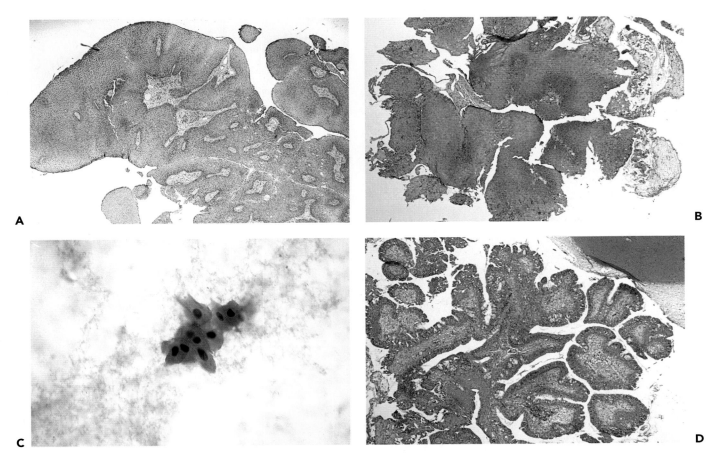

Figure 20-35 Bronchial papillomas. *A,B.* Squamous papillomas. The tumors are composed of uniform, cytologically benign squamous epithelium. *C.* Hyperkeratotic squamous cell atypia in bronchial wash specimen. *D.* Bronchial epithelial papilloma. *B,C,* and *D* are from papillomas in the left upper lobe bronchus of the same patient.

noted in a bronchial wash specimen from the patient illustrated in Figure 20-35B who also had a **bronchial papilloma** surfaced by benign bronchial epithelium (Fig. 20-35D). The only other case of which we are aware in which a solitary bronchial papilloma presented with cellular abnormalities in a cytologic specimen was described by Roglic et al (1975). Although the investigators failed to diagnose the lesion prospectively, a review of the photographic illustrations in their report strongly suggests that **atypical squamous cells resembling koilocytes were present in the bronchial brushings. Nonspecific atypias of squamous cells were observed in sputum** of two patients seen in consultation by one of us (LGK). In another very recent case that we saw, there was sufficient cytologic atypia in the intraoperative imprint cytology of a squamous papilloma from the upper respiratory tract to raise suspicion of squamous carcinoma.

The **differential diagnosis of benign squamous papilloma includes well-differentiated exophytic squamous carcinoma.** The two entities may have identical gross and superficially similar microscopic appearances, but even very orderly squamous carcinomas have significant atypia of squamous cells and usually demonstrable invasion of the underlying tracheobronchial wall. Such tumors shed squamous cancer cells, some of which may resemble koilocytes. The possibility of HPV infection has been raised in these cases (Syrjäanen et al, 1989). There are reports of HPV type 16 identified in a verrucous carcinoma of the larynx (Brandsma et al, 1986), and HPV type 11 in specimens from a patient with malignant laryngotracheobronchial papillomatosis of the lung metastatic to the liver (Byrne et al, 1987).

Granular Cell Tumor

Benign granular cell tumors have been observed in many different organs including the tongue, skin and breast, as well as the larynx and bronchus (Majmudar et al, 1981) and uncommonly in peripheral lung (Schulster et al, 1975). While extremely unusual, there are examples of malignant granular cell tumors in the bronchus (Steffelaar et al, 1982; Klima and Peters, 1987; Parayno and August, 1996). The tumors are of uncertain origin, although probably derived from the neural Schwann cell (Alvarez-Fernandez and Carretero-Albinana, 1987). In the bronchus, they are **subepithelial in location and composed of sheets of large cells with small nuclei and abundant, granular eosinophilic cytoplasm** that contains numerous lysosomes (Fig. 20-36A,B). Granular cell tumors may grow to substantial

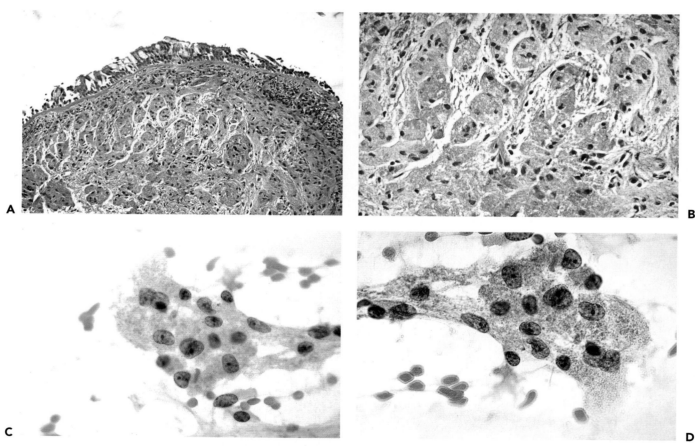

Figure 20-36 Granular cell tumor of bronchus. *A,B.* Histologic section of a granular cell tumor of bronchus. The tumor lies under the epithelium and is composed of large cells with abundant, granular, eosinophilic cytoplasm. Nuclei are relatively small and round. *C,D.* Bronchial brush specimen shows coherent groups of large cells with abundant, delicate, finely granular cytoplasm and vesicular nuclei with smooth nuclear border and small nucleoli. Cell boundaries are indistinct at high magnification.

size and cause bronchial obstruction, thereby clinically mimicking bronchogenic cancer. Naib and Goldstein (1962) were the first to describe the cytologic presentation of this tumor, followed later by Glant et al (1979).

Cytology

Granular cell tumors do not exfoliate easily, and we are unaware of any cases diagnosed by sputum cytology. In **bronchial brushings and aspirates, the tumor presents in cohesive sheets of large cells with slightly hyperchromatic but round or oval nuclei, visible nucleoli and abundant, granular, faintly basophilic cytoplasm. Cell borders are ill-defined** (Fig. 20-36C,D). **Single tumor cells are usually poorly preserved, and their cytoplasm is often frayed** (Thomas et al, 1984; Fuzesi et al, 1989; Chen, 1991; Guillou et al, 1991). Smith et al (1998) described a granular cell tumor in the **posterior superior mediastinum,** diagnosed by percutaneous needle aspiration. As in bronchial brush specimens, the tumor cells were large, polygonal or spindly, with granular cytoplasm and indistinct cell borders. In agreement with Glant et al (1979), we found that the **most important feature distinguishing cells of granular cell tumor from macrophages is the coherent clustering of the tumor cells, virtually never seen with macrophages.** The distinction between benign and malignant granular cell tumors is based on conventional cytologic criteria, and on clinical presentation; however, the malignant granular cell tumors are so rare that the reader is cautioned not to make the diagnosis without very strong evidence.

Oncocytoma

These benign tumors are fairly common in the salivary glands and in the thyroid, less common in other organs such as the kidney, but are **extremely rare in the lung where they may be related to carcinoid tumors** (see above). Pulmonary oncocytomas, like those at other sites, are composed of **sheets of large, eosinophilic cells with large, sometimes multiple, often hyperchromatic nuclei. Characteristically, the cytoplasm of the tumor cells is filled with mitochondria** (Black, 1969; Fernandez and Nyssen, 1982; Alverez-Fernandez and Carretero-Albinana, 1987; Santoz-Briz et al, 1977).

The cytology of bronchogenic oncocytoma was described in a case report by Cwierzyk et al (1985). **They observed large cells with granular cytoplasm, dark nuclei, and prominent nucleoli in bronchial brushings, similar to the cells of oncocytomas of other organs.** Laforga and Aranda (1999) recently described a case of multicentric oncocytomas of the lung studied by FNA in which cell aggregates and fragments of tissue were made up of rounded tumor cells with granular cytoplasm that reacted immunocytochemically with anti-mitochondrial antibodies.

Clear Cell (Sugar) Tumor

These are very rare, sharply demarcated benign lung tumors of unknown histogenesis, so named by Liebow and Castleman (1971) because of a strongly positive periodic acid-Schiff (PAS) reaction for glycogen content in the clear cytoplasm of the tumor cells. The tumors do not shed cells into sputum or bronchial secretions. In a percutaneous aspirate, Nguyen (1989) described **large irregular clusters of polygonal and spindle-shaped, benign-appearing cells with finely vacuolated, granular, PAS-positive cytoplasm and small nuclei.** Large cells with granules radiating out from the nucleus were referred to as "spider" cells. The tumor cells may contain **finely granular brown lipochrome pigment** and, since the cells **react with HMB-45 antibody** to pre-melanosomes, the diagnosis of melanoma has to be excluded. The differential diagnosis must include other clear-cell tumors, including the rare clear-cell bronchogenic carcinoma and metastatic tumors with clear cytoplasm, such as renal cell carcinoma and clear-cell sarcoma.

Hamartomas

These are relatively common intrapulmonary **malformations** that may present as **coin lesions or may mimic lung cancer in roentgenologic images.** They are well-circumscribed tumors that shell out easily from lung parenchyma and have a chondroid or fibrous texture on a cut surface. Histologically, they are composed of **cartilage, fibrous or loosely structured fibromyxoid connective tissue associated with bronchial epithelium and rudimentary bronchial structures lined by epithelial cells of respiratory type** (Fig. 20-37A). Hamartomas do not communicate with bronchi and cannot be diagnosed on sputum or bronchial material. Percutaneous needle aspiration is the only diagnostic method short of thoracotomy. Still, the aspirates are often unsatisfactory because the tumor is too firm for the needle to penetrate and is pushed away by it; the "screw needle" described in Chapter 19 was devised to overcome this. If an adequate sample is obtained, **fragments of loosely structured connective tissue, fibromyxoid stromal components** (which are S-100 positive), **and benign epithelium occasionally with bits of cartilage may be observed** (Fig. 20-37B–D) (Dahlgren, 1966; Ramzy, 1976; Sinner, 1982; Wiatrowska et al, 1995). The **epithelial cells, which are derived from the rudimentary bronchi, may show some atypia, including intranuclear cytoplasmic inclusions or nuclear holes** as described in Chapter 19.

Primary Pulmonary Meningioma

Meningiomas, whether primary or metastatic, are exceedingly rare in the lung, but have been described and may be multiple (see Lockett et al, 1997, for a review of reported cases). Ueno et al (1998) were able to make an intraoperative diagnosis on cytology imprints of a thoracoscopically resected tumor by the presence **of whorled nests of cells accompanied by psammoma bodies.** Minute meningotheliomatous tumors (Travis et al, 1999) or chemodectomas are a different entity, and like tumorlets, they are not likely to be sampled. For further description of the cytology of meningiomas, see Chapter 42.

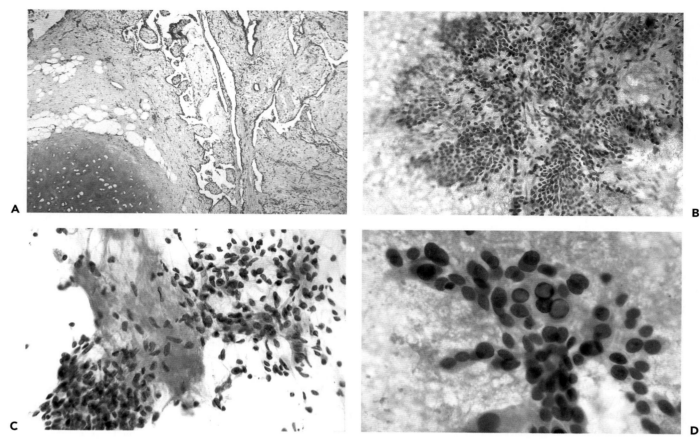

Figure 20-37   **Hamartoma of lung.** *A.* Hamartomas are circumscribed tumors composed of fibrous tissue, bronchial epithelium, usually with cartilage or other connective tissue elements. *B–D.* FNA showing the unique mixture of epithelial and stromal components that characterize this tumor. Cartilage, if present, is virtually diagnostic. Note the nuclear holes in *D.*

Inflammatory pseudotumor (plasma cell granuloma; inflammatory myofibroblastic tumor) was discussed in Chapter 19.

CYTOLOGY OF TUMORS METASTATIC TO THE LUNG (OTHER THAN LYMPHOMAS)

Patients with a past history of cancer at another site who develop a lung lesion must be thoroughly investigated with the following options to be considered:

■ The lesion is a metastasis
■ The lesion is benign with special consideration of:
  (a) Bacterial, viral, or mycotic infection
  (b) Effect of treatment by radio- or chemotherapy
■ The lesion is a primary lung cancer

The benign lesions and complications of therapy have been discussed in Chapter 19. Here we consider **recognition of metastatic tumors by cytologic techniques.** The dominant thought in these investigations should be that the lesion is **not a metastasis until documented. It is important to emphasize that knowledge of the clinical findings** and **review of prior histologic and cytologic material are important safeguards** to ensure maximal accuracy of a di-

agnosis that often carries with it major therapeutic and prognostic consequences for the patient.

Metastatic tumors in the lung may be identified by cytologic techniques (although not necessarily classified) in about half of the cases, including a great variety of tumors from many different primary sites (Koss et al, 1964). The probability of a positive diagnosis in any particular case is a function of tumor type, size and location in the lung, and the type of cytologic sample. Kern and Schweizer (1976) found **sputum cytology** to be as effective a diagnostic technique for metastatic cancer as for primary carcinoma of the lung. However, many metastatic tumors do not communicate with a bronchus, at least until they are relatively large. In our experience, the yield in sputum or bronchial aspirates is somewhat less for metastatic than for primary lung cancers (Koss et al, 1964). The yield from transbronchial or percutaneous needle aspirates is not affected by presence or absence of bronchial communication, but is more successful for larger metastases in easier reach of the aspirating needle.

Burke and Melamed (1968) reported on 92 consecutive patients (two-thirds males and one-third females) with (exfoliative) cytologic evidence of metastatic cancer to the lung, confirmed by histologic or clinical evidence. Their study antedated the common use of needle aspiration cytology. The most **frequent primary source of metastases was carcinoma of the esophagus, followed in order of frequency by colon, breast, lymphoma and leukemia, prostate, stomach, malignant melanoma, and a group of miscellaneous tumors of other sites.** Eighty-six patients had radiographic evidence of metastatic disease, but **in 6 patients, sputum cytology revealed metastatic carcinoma in the absence of roentgenologic abnormalities,** possibly due to lymphangitic spread; in four of these six patients, an autopsy was performed and confirmed metastatic tumor. **In a more recent report from the same institution that included FNA cytology but excluded the esophagus, the most common primary sites of metastases to lung, in decreasing frequency, were breast, colon, kidney, bladder, and melanoma** (Zaman et al, 1986). It should be noted that these observations were from a cancer hospital with many referrals of problem cases and may not be representative of other institutions. However, it is clear that a broad spectrum of primary tumors metastatic to the lung is amenable to cytologic diagnosis.

Identification of Site of Origin of Metastatic Cancer

In the absence of clinical history, the cytologic diagnosis of primary versus metastatic cancer may be very difficult. With knowledge of age and gender, however, there are cytologic patterns in which preference for the primary site of origin of a metastatic carcinoma may be expressed.

Colon

Metastatic colonic carcinomas typically shed **cuboidal or columnar cells in clusters with one straight border, superficially resembling bronchial epithelial cells. The cells are not ciliated and they do not have a terminal bar. Nuclei are relatively large, larger than most bronchial cells, and ovoid, usually with coarsely textured chromatin** (Fig. 20-38A). **There is almost always tumor necrosis and the cytology smears have a dirty background with much necrotic and inflammatory cellular debris** (Fig. 20-38B). **An FNA may yield tall columnar cells aligned in a linear strip with a picket fence appearance, usually with some single cells,** resembling bronchial cells (Fig. 20-38C), but it should be remembered that few if any columnar bronchial cells are found in aspirates of peripheral lung, and columnar cells are rarely shed from primary adenocarcinomas of lung. Thus, the presence of **a linear strip of columnar cells in sputum, or in a bronchial or needle aspirate, whether obviously malignant or not, should arouse suspicion of metastatic colonic carcinoma, particularly if**

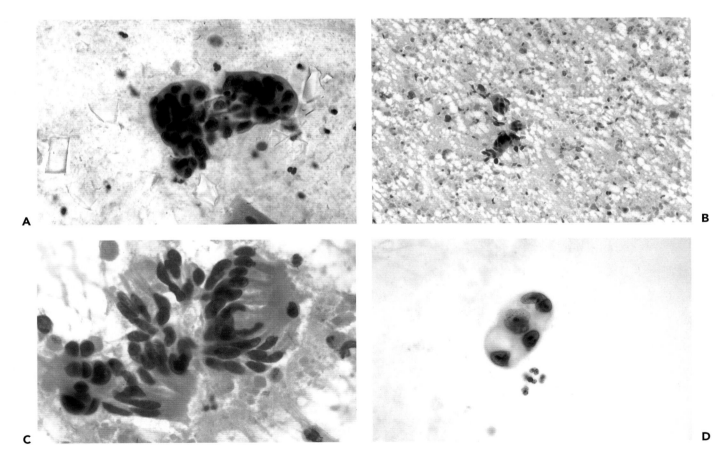

Figure 20-38 **Metastatic colonic carcinoma in lung.** *A.* Of greatest differential diagnostic value is the presence of a linear group of columnar cells with one straight border. *B.* Also of diagnostic value is necrotic cellular debris in the background. *C.* The presence of clusters of columnar cells, or a strip of columnar cells with a straight edge, even if benign appearing, is highly suspicious of metastatic colonic carcinoma. *D.* Evidence of mucin secretion is consistent with, but not specific for, colonic carcinoma.

associated with necrotic cellular debris. Metastatic colonic carcinomas also shed mucin-secreting cancer cells (Fig. 20-38D), including so-called "signet ring cells." The late Dr. John Frost emphasized that the nuclei of signet ring cancer cells "pushed the cell membrane out," something one does not see with benign vacuolated cells. Necrosis is a frequent finding and colonic carcinoma must be considered if cells of adenocarcinoma with no specific features lie in a background of necrotic cellular debris.

Koizumi and Schon (1997) emphasized that **nuclear hyperchromasia may be absent** in some metastatic colonic cancers, and that the cancer cells may have **pale nuclei** with **distinct nuclear membranes and prominent nucleoli** (Fig. 20-38D). These investigators also found that the metastatic tumors sometimes shed smaller cancer cells than the corresponding primary tumor, perhaps due to differences in needle aspirate versus brush cytology techniques.

Breast

Metastatic mammary carcinoma is by far the most common source of metastatic lung cancer in women. The tumors shed a great variety of **tumor cells that vary in size and configuration but generally match the histologic pattern of the tumor** (Fig. 20-39A,B). **Most often, they present in groups and clusters, sometimes in papillary configuration, but also as single malignant cells that may be large, moderate in size, or small.** Regardless of cell size, the **nuclei are relatively large and may be vesicular with nucleoli** (Fig. 20-39A), **or they may be hyperchromatic and irregular or angular in configuration with nucleoli that are less conspicuous** (Fig. 20-39C). The cytology in bronchial secretions is similar to sputum and typically diagnostic of adenocarcinoma, although not usually organ specific (Fig. 20-39D). **A feature of small-cell mammary carcinoma, usually lobular carcinoma, is the arrangement of tumor cells in single file** (Indian file) (Fig. 20-39C). In some cases of metastatic lobular carcinoma, the cancer cells are miniature signet ring cells, with a mucus vacuole in the center of the cell pushing the nucleus to one side. Other small-cell cancers can mimic this pattern, notably SSC of lung (see Chap. 29).

The cells from rare cases of metastatic carcinoma of male breast are identical to those derived from duct carcinomas of female breast.

Clinical history is paramount in the diagnosis of metastatic mammary carcinoma. If confirmatory evidence is desired, it may be of help to stain for cytoplasmic mucin and to demonstrate estrogen receptor expression by immunocy-

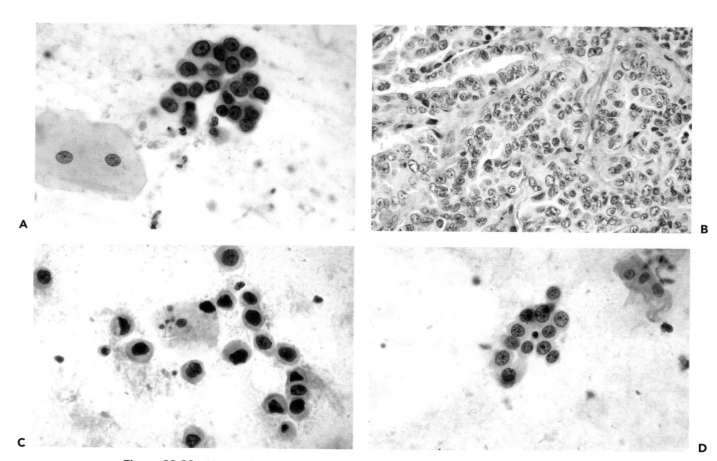

Figure 20-39 **Metastatic mammary carcinoma.** *A.* This is the most common presentation in sputum as clusters and single small cancer cells, some with vesicular nuclei and small nucleoli, others with hyperchromatic nuclei. *B.* Histologic section of the primary infiltrating duct carcinoma from the same case. *C.* Sputum cytology from another case showing small tumor cells with hyperchromatic nuclei in "single file." *D.* Bronchial wash specimen showing a cluster of small cells with vesicular nuclei and small nucleoli, similar to the sputum specimen in *A.*

tochemistry, although neither is specific whether present or absent. For further discussion of metastatic mammary carcinoma, see Chapter 26.

Kidney

Metastatic renal carcinoma may be observed in patients with an occult primary tumor. Until the recent almost routine use of CT and ultrasound examinations of patients with vague abdominal symptoms small, asymptomatic renal carcinomas escaped detection and as many as **one-third of renal cortical carcinomas were first diagnosed in a metastatic site.** Many still are. **The tumor cells contain abundant cytoplasmic lipid, accounting for the classical clear cell appearance of the tumor** (Fig. 20-40A). **The cytologic diagnosis is suggested by cancer cells with large vesicular nuclei and prominent nucleoli, with abundant clear or faintly staining delicate cytoplasm.** Often, the fragile cytoplasm is lost as the tumor cells are aspirated or exfoliated, and the cells present as bare nuclei or with only wisps of cytoplasm. They may be single or in small clusters (Fig. 20-40B).

Although this classical presentation is commonly observed, renal cancer may exhibit diverse other cytologic patterns, including cells with granular eosinophilic cytoplasm, or elongated or **spindly cancer cells mimicking sarcoma** (Fig. 20-40C). In such cases, positive **immunostaining** for **keratins** and **vimentin** is often helpful, as this combination of staining is observed in few other tumors.

Urothelial Carcinoma

Metastatic urothelial carcinomas can rarely be identified as to site of origin. We have seen cases in which the needle aspirate yielded **tumor cells similar to umbrella cells,** for example, **large, flat, mononuclear or multinuclear crescent-shaped cells,** with a thick, refractile cell border corresponding to the asymmetric unit membrane (see Chap. 22) (Fig. 20-41A). We have not observed such cells in other metastatic tumors. More commonly, however, the aspirate contains nondescript epithelial tumor cells, or spindly, columnar or cuboidal cells (Fig. 20-41B). In exceptional cases, the FNA of a lung metastasis may have a remarkable resemblance to fragments of low-grade papillary urothelial tumors of the bladder (see Chap. 23).

Some observers report **cercariform cells** to be diagnostic of metastatic urothelial cancer in aspirates (FNA). The cells are described as cancer cells with exceptionally long cytoplasmic processes that have a bulbous or flattened end (Powers and Elbadawi, 1995; Renshaw and Madge, 1997; Hida and Gupta, 1999). Although we have observed elongated cancer cells in aspirates of well-differentiated metastatic urothelial carcinomas (Fig. 20-41), we do not consider them to be specific. **Antibody to uroplakin** has been shown to specifically recognize metastatic urothelial cancer in tissues and in circulating blood (Moll et al, 1995; Wu et al, 1998; Li et al, 1999).

Renshaw et al (1997) investigated the frequency of small cells with **eosinophilic cytoplasmic inclusions** in pulmo-

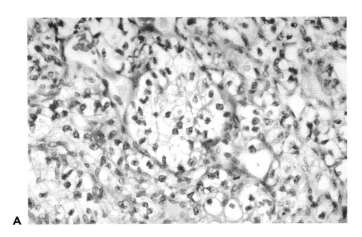

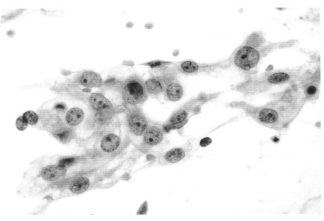

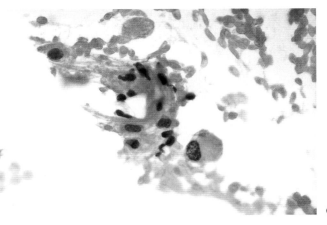

Figure 20-40 **Metastatic renal cortical carcinoma.** *A.* Primary renal carcinoma showing the typical highly vascularized tumor composed of large cells with clear cytoplasm. *B.* FNA of tumor metastatic to the lung, yielding cells with large, round or oval vesicular nuclei with small nucleoli. The delicate cytoplasm is stripped away, leaving only a few adherent wisps of cytoplasmic material. *C.* Not uncommonly, the cells of renal cortical carcinoma have granular, eosinophilic cytoplasm, and may be spindly or sarcomatoid.

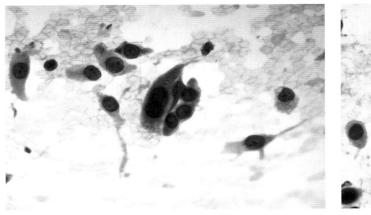

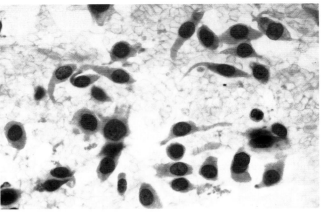

Figure 20-41   Metastatic urothelial carcinoma. *A.* A finding of umbrella cells shown here is unusual but strongly suggestive of urothelial carcinoma. *B.* More commonly, the aspirate will contain spindly and columnar or cuboidal epithelial cancer cells.

nary effusions and concluded that **such cells are more common in the presence of metastatic urothelial carcinoma than in lung cancer.** As discussed in Chapter 22, the inclusions are composed of cytoplasmic filaments in cells undergoing degeneration, and are very common in benign urothelial cells in the urinary sediment. Their alleged association with metastatic urothelial cancer is puzzling and awaits confirmation and evaluation.

Malignant Melanoma

Metastatic melanomas may mimic all types of malignant tumors and present considerable difficulties in diagnosis, particularly in patients whose primary tumor is either unknown or was treated many years before as a "benign nevus." Metastatic melanoma in the lung **usually sheds nonpigmented cancer cells** and in the absence of clinical history, they are seldom specifically identified. The diagnosis of metastatic malignant melanoma may be suspected, however, if the **cells have very large nucleoli and/or intranuclear inclusions of invaginated cytoplasm (nuclear holes). If the cancer cells are large and contain the fine, dusty brown pigment of melanin,** a definitive diagnosis of melanoma can be established (Fig. 20-42). It is important

to remember, however, that in patients with **disseminated melanoma and sometimes in heavily suntanned individuals, the alveolar macrophages may contain phagocytized melanin,** usually seen as a **very fine yellowish brown coloration of the cytoplasm;** and the sputum may contain **macrophages with engulfed pigment that must not be confused with pigmented melanoma cells.** The differential diagnosis of pigments commonly present in macrophages is discussed in Chapter 19. If the nucleus is obscured by what is believed to be melanin, the pigment should be removed by bleaching and the slide restained to permit evaluation of the suspect cells. The **cells of melanoma are usually larger than pigment-containing macrophages, and they exhibit the nuclear abnormalities of cancer cells. If material is available for a cell block, immunostaining with the antibody to pre-melanosomes (HMB-45 or Melan-A) will be positive in most melanoma cells and negative in macrophages. The antibody to S-100 protein is more sensitive but less specific, and is most useful if negative. Metastatic melanoma should always be included in the differential diagnosis of metastatic malignant tumors of unknown primary site.**

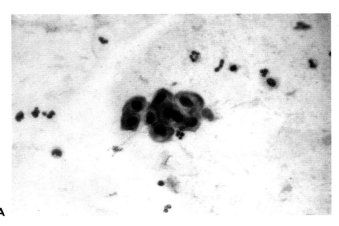

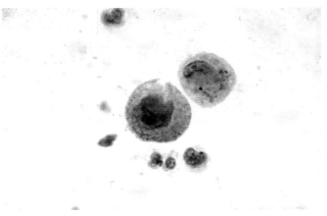

Figure 20-42   Metastatic malignant melanoma in sputum. Large nucleoli and fine cytoplasmic pigment are strongly suggestive, if not diagnostic of melanoma. (*B:* oil immersion.)

Pancreatic Islet Cell Tumor

We have encountered one case of metastatic pancreatic islet cell tumor in an FNA of lung from a 75-year-old man. The tumor cells formed loosely cohesive, flat clusters of uniform cells with eccentrically placed nuclei, occasional giant nuclei, and a moderate amount of cytoplasm (Fig. 20-43). Not surprisingly, the cytology was indistinguishable from that of a carcinoid tumor (see Chap. 39).

Tumors with Psammoma Bodies

Concentrically laminated, calcified psammoma bodies may be observed in specimens of sputum, bronchial aspirates, or FNA cytology. Their interpretation depends on the company they keep. If the calcified bodies are not accompanied by cancer cells, the **possibility of a primary calcific process in the lung** (pulmonary alveolar microlithiasis, pneumoliths) must be considered (see Chap. 19). Once this has been ruled out by the presence of suspicious or frankly malignant cells accompanying the psammomas, the relationship of the cells to the calcific deposits is of diagnostic importance.

■ The most common source of cancer cells with psammomas in sputum is **papillary bronchioloalveolar or adenocarcinoma** of lung. The psammomas may be separate or **only loosely related to moderate-size cancer cells** (see Fig. 20-12D).

■ If the psammomas lie **within clusters of obvious, large cancer cells,** metastatic **ovarian** or, much less likely, endometrial or tubal carcinomas must be considered. In most such cases, before there are lung metastases, there is clinical evidence of a pelvic mass or intra-abdominal metastases with ascites.

■ If the psammomas are integrated within clusters of smaller, generally uniform and innocuous-appearing cancer cells, metastatic **thyroid carcinoma** is a strong possibility. One should search for tumor cells with nuclear creases or intranuclear cytoplasmic inclusions (see Chap. 30).

Rare examples of other tumors associated with psammoma bodies have been reported, including **metastatic breast cancer with giant cells** (Ludwig and Gero, 1987), and **metastatic ameloblastoma** (Levine et al, 1981). We have also observed **psammoma bodies in mesothelioma,** usually in effusions or needle aspirates of tumor (see Chap. 26).

Metastatic Carcinomas, Not Further Specified

Most metastatic carcinomas occur as single cells or in clusters with no specific cytologic features for assigning tumor type or organ of origin. One can only make an educated guess based on clinical and radiologic findings, age, gender, etc. Papillary groups of tumor cells with vacuolated cytoplasm that are readily identified as adenocarcinoma may originate from metastatic carcinomas of the breast, prostate, pancreas, bowel, stomach or endometrium, and often cannot be differentiated from primary bronchogenic adenocarcinomas.

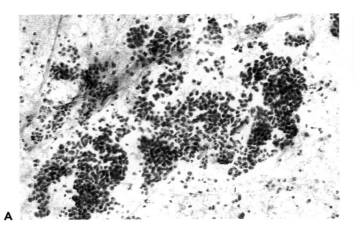

A

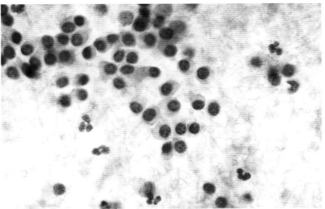

B

C

Figure 20-43 **Metastatic pancreatic islet cell tumor.** FNA of the pulmonary metastasis yielded flat clusters of uniform cells of "plasmocytoid" configuration indistinguishable from carcinoid tumor. The presence of an occasional cell with a larger nucleus is not unusual.

The problem of metastatic squamous carcinoma in the lung is even more vexing because it is much less common than metastatic adenocarcinoma, and the tumor cells cannot be differentiated from those of a primary squamous lung cancer. Thus, cells from **metastatic squamous carcinomas of the esophagus, the buccal cavity or larynx, and even the uterine cervix may all look alike,** and in the absence of accurate clinical information, one may erroneously assume that they are derived from a primary bronchogenic carcinoma. On the other hand, the history of a treated carcinoma of another organ does not rule out the possibility of a second primary bronchogenic carcinoma.

The cytologic diagnosis of a new primary lung cancer should be favored in patients with a past history of carcinoma of different histologic and cytologic type. For example, the diagnosis of lung cancer would be favored in a patient with a history of adenocarcinoma who now has squamous cancer cells in a cytologic specimen, or vice versa. A word of caution is indicated here: **cells originating from metastatic cancers of any type may appear eosinophilic in exfoliated material because of poor preservation. Thus, cytoplasmic eosinophilia of a few poorly preserved cells is not a sufficient criterion to label cancer cells as squamous.**

Special stains are sometimes of help in classification of a metastatic tumor. Examples are the immunocytochemical demonstration of **thyroglobulin in thyroid carcinoma;** calretinin for mesothelioma; cytokeratin and vimentin to distinguish epithelial from nonepithelial tumors (except that renal carcinoma and mesothelioma may contain both); prostate-specific antigen or prostatic acid phosphatase in prostatic cancer; HMB-45, Melan-A, and S-100 in malignant melanoma; alkaline phosphatase in the case of osteogenic sarcoma; estrogen or progesterone receptor expression in breast cancer; and lymphocyte common antigen (CD-45) for lymphoid cells.** None of these are entirely specific, and must be interpreted with consideration of cytologic morphology and clinical context. Among the more useful conventional special stains **is mucicarmine staining for identification of mucin-secreting adenocarcinoma.** Unfortunately, there is rarely enough material in difficult cases to carry out the battery of special stains and immunocytochemical reactions that are possible with histologic specimens. In fortuitous cases, a cell block may be available for such studies.

Metastatic Sarcomas

Metastatic sarcomas are much less common than metastatic carcinomas, but more common than primary sarcomas of lung. Ali et al (1998) reported making the diagnosis of metastatic leiomyosarcoma by cytologic examination of sputum but, except for such rare examples (see below), the **sarcomas are best sampled by percutaneous needle aspiration** (Kim et al, 1986). Even with adequate sampling, **specific classification of a metastatic sarcoma, or differentiation from sarcomatoid carcinoma (Fig. 20-44A–C) may not be possible without the primary tumor for comparison.** Hajdu and Koss (1969) and Hajdu and Hajdu

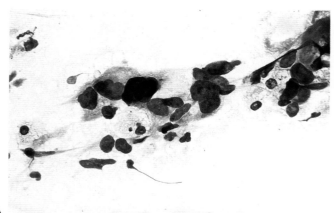

A

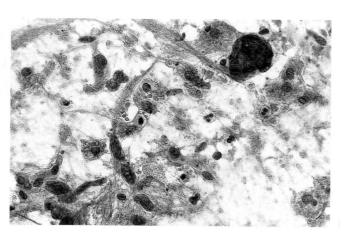

B

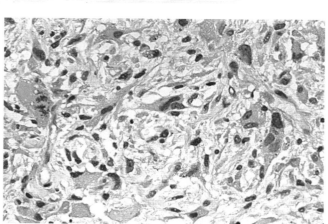

C

Figure 20-44 Metastatic sarcomatoid squamous carcinoma. *A,B.* FNA of pulmonary metastasis from sarcomatoid squamous carcinoma of the esophagus in a 48-year-old man. *C.* Biopsy of sarcomatoid carcinoma of esophagus in the same case. (*A:* Diff-Quik stain; *B:* Papanicolaou stain.)

(1975) pointed out that spindly tumor cells are shed by some metastatic sarcomas, whereas others, and particularly embryonal rhabdomyosarcomas, may be remarkably pleomorphic. We have not always been able to classify the pulmonary metastases of solid small-cell malignant tumors of childhood. Nor have we often been successful, for example, in the search for striations in known cases of metastatic rhabdomyosarcoma. However, **it is possible to make an educated guess of tumor type based on cytologic pattern with knowledge of the patient's age and clinical and radiologic findings (see below).**

Publications within the last several years have included reports of needle aspirates of metastatic **epithelioid sarcoma** (Niemann and Bottles, 1993), **chondrosarcoma** (Abdul-Karim et al, 1993), **synovial sarcoma** (Costa et al, 1997; Silverman et al, 2000), **Ewing's sarcoma** (Collins et al, 1998), **osteosarcoma** (Nicol et al, 1998) and **alveolar soft part sarcoma** (Logrono et al, 1999). We have observed metastatic Ewing's sarcoma (Fig. 20-45A) and metastatic testicular embryonal carcinoma (Fig. 20-45B) in sputum cytology specimens. Koss previously illustrated a multinucleated tumor cell of metastatic testicular choriocarcinoma in sputum (1992).

Criteria for the cytologic diagnosis and classification of metastatic sarcoma are not different from those of primary sarcoma. In most cases, the primary site and type of tumor are already known when needle aspiration of a clinically suspected metastasis is performed, usually to confirm the clinical diagnosis and exclude an incidental benign neoplasm, or to rule out an inflammatory process that may be a consequence of therapy. Caution is indicated before making a diagnosis on very scanty evidence, or if cytologic morphology is not consistent with the clinical setting. **In the final analysis, knowledge of the clinical history and review and comparison of the cytologic findings with histologic sections of a previously removed or biopsied cancer is key to the identification and classification of many metastatic tumors.**

Malignant Lymphomas Secondarily Involving Lung

Non-Hodgkin's Lymphoma

Lymphomas of all types may make their appearance in sputum or bronchial aspirates. As already noted, **well-differentiated small-cell lymphoma/chronic lymphocytic leukemia (SCL/CLL) presents as single or loosely aggregated small lymphocytes that differ little from normal lymphocytes** (Fig. 20-46A). They may exhibit slight variability in size, minimal granularity of nuclei, and sometimes slight hyperchromasia or visible nucleoli, but these are subtle differences. **Also subtle, but of diagnostic value, the cells of SCL/CLL are much more uniform than those of nonneoplastic lymphoid tissue; they do not show the variability and variety of cell types that constitute the pattern of cells from inflammatory processes or hyperplastic lymphoid tissue that may be dislodged from tonsillar tissue or lymphoid nodules in the bronchial wall.**

Large-cell lymphomas shed cells that are more easily recognized as lymphoma. They are most readily diagnosed in FNA specimens in which they comprise a single population of cells that contrasts with the mixed population of reactive lymphoid tissue. **The cells are twice the size of mature lymphocytes, or larger, and in the case of large-cell anaplastic (K1) lymphomas, they may be as large as small-cell (oat cell) carcinoma or some soft tissue sarcomas, or even larger.** On occasion, they may be mistaken for anaplastic carcinoma, even in histologic section. As in effusions, they have nuclei that are irregularly round or ovoid with nuclear protrusions, indentations and folds, and finely textured or vesicular nuclei, many with prominent nucleoli (Fig. 20-46B,C). The cells are often stripped of their delicate cytoplasm, and it is useful to search for cytoplasmic fragments (**lymphoglandular bodies**) in the background of the smear (Fig. 20-46C). Since primary carcinomas of the lung may occur in patients with a past history of lymphoma, the differential diagnosis with small-cell (oat

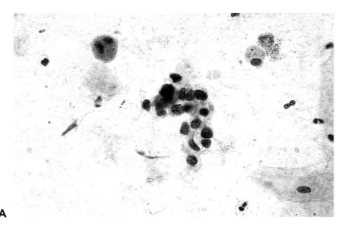

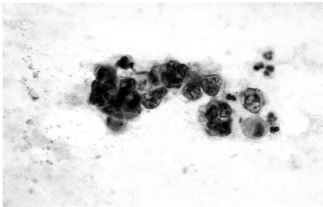

A
B

Figure 20-45 **Metastatic small-cell tumors.** *A.* Metastatic malignant tumor cells in the sputum of a 21-year-old man with known bone tumor. In this setting, the cluster of small, coherent malignant cells can confidently be reported as consistent with **Ewing's sarcoma.** *B.* **Metastatic embryonal carcinoma** in a specimen of sputum. The tumor cells are clearly malignant, with visible nucleoli. In a young man with known testicular tumor, the differential diagnosis includes embryonal carcinoma and seminoma. The variation in nuclear configuration and chromatin texture, variable nucleoli, and abundant cytoplasm all favor embryonal carcinoma.

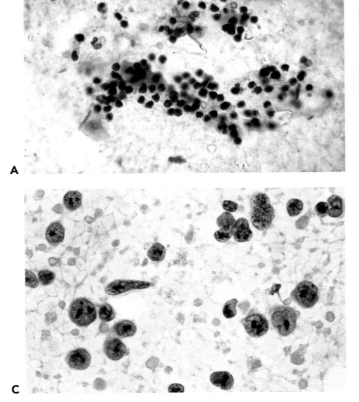

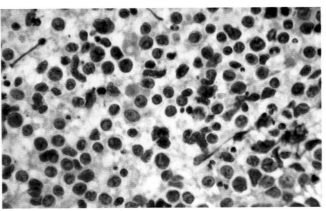

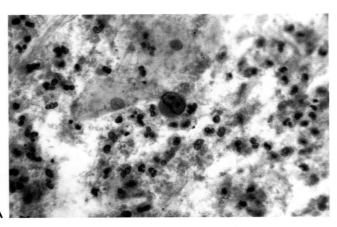

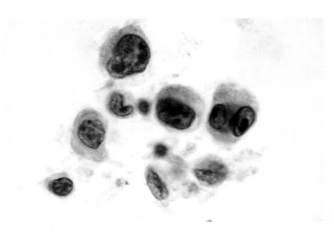

Figure 20-46 Malignant lymphoma/leukemia. *A.* Sputum specimen with a loose aggregate of uniform small lymphocytes from a patient with chronic lymphocytic leukemia involving lung. *B,C.* Large-cell lymphoma in a bronchial brush (*B*) and FNA (*C*) specimen from two different patients. The tumor cells are much larger than mature lymphocytes, approaching the size of SSC, but loosely arranged without forming coherent clusters. Nuclei are irregularly rounded or ovoid with indentations, protrusions and creases, finely textured chromatin, and prominent chromocenters or nucleoli. Note the "lymphoglandular bodies," best seen in *C.* (*C:* oil immersion.)

cell) carcinoma is of particular importance, especially if sampling is scanty (see above for a discussion of the distinguishing features of SSC versus lymphoma).

Hodgkin's Disease

In a review of the cytology of sputum and bronchial lavage specimens from patients with Hodgkin's disease involving the lung (Suprun and Koss, 1964), **mono- and binucleated cells were observed that had prominent nuclei and large eosinophilic nucleoli.** The resemblance to classic binucleated Reed-Sternberg cells was striking (Fig. 20-47A,B). Yet

even in those cases, **in the absence of a clinical history, differentiation from other types of cancer was tentative at best.** The difficulty was compounded in patients with a history of prior radiotherapy to the mediastinum, in whom the resulting cellular atypia with marked nuclear pyknosis and often striking cytoplasmic eosinophilia made cell classification very difficult.

In most cases, only rare single tumor cells are found in sputum of patients with Hodgkin's disease but, on rare occasions, we have seen Reed-Sternberg cells within groups of tumor cells resembling those of large-cell lymphoma (Fig.

Figure 20-47 Hodgkin's disease. *A.* Binucleated Reed-Sternberg cell with prominent nucleoli in sputum. *B.* Reed-Sternberg cells together with less specific tumor cells identical to those of large-cell lymphoma in sputum of a patient with pulmonary involvement by Hodgkin's disease. (*B:* oil immersion.)

20-47B). Others who have described tumor cells of Hodgkin's disease in cytology specimens include Reale et al (1983) who reported six cases and Fullmer and Morris (1972) who were able to establish the diagnosis of mediastinal Hodgkin's disease by sputum cytology. Levij (1972) described a patient with **cavitary** Hodgkin's disease in the lung diagnosed by cytology. More recently, Sharma et al (1986), Bardales et al (1996) and Stanley et al (1993) reported additional cases of Hodgkin's disease with lung involvement.

Mycosis Fungoides

In **disseminated mycosis fungoides, a T-cell lymphoma of skin, pulmonary involvement** is common and the cytologic diagnosis of malignant lymphoma has been made in bronchial brushings (Ludwig and Balachandran, 1983) and in sputum (Rosen et al, 1984; Shaheen and Oertel, 1984). The diagnosis of lung involvement by mycosis fungoides can be made only in patients with known cutaneous disease, in whom **small or large mononuclear lymphoid cells with cerebriform nuclei** are found in company of atypical lymphocytic cells (see also Chap. 34).

Primary Pulmonary Thymoma

These rare intrapulmonary tumors have been observed in percutaneous aspiration biopsies, and the aspirates may be confused with large-cell lymphoma (Fig. 20-48). They are similar to primary thymomas of mediastinum, described in Chapter 37.

Plasmacytoma (Plasma Cell Myeloma, Multiple Myeloma)

Plasma cell tumors have been described in needle aspirates of various organs and in effusions, but rarely in sputum or bronchial aspirates. Geisinger et al (1986) reported one such case among 126 patients studied. The diagnosis is made on finding an increased number of **plasma cells with atypical and immature forms in sputum or bronchial specimens of** patients known to have disseminated plasmacytoma and

suspected of lung involvement clinically or radiologically. In some cases, the aspirate may contain lymphoid blast cells that suggest lymphoma but not necessarily plasmacytoma. Before making the diagnosis of plasma cell myeloma on a needle aspirate of an infiltrate in the lung that is rich in plasma cells, one would have to consider plasma cell granuloma (a pseudotumor with plasma cells) and other chronic inflammatory processes in the differential diagnosis (see Chap. 19).

Leukemia

Leukemic cells in blastic phase may occasionally be identified in sputum. This finding can be of assistance in evaluating the clinical status of the patient and in planning therapy. The cytology is not unlike that of non-Hodgkin's lymphoma (see also Chap. 26).

Microvascular Cytology

An interesting technique for sampling and identifying the cancer cells in cases of lymphangitic spread of metastatic cancer was proposed by Masson et al (1989). They reported finding cancer cells in blood samples obtained by wedged pulmonary artery catheter and examined by cytologic techniques. Success was claimed in seven of eight patients (see also Chap. 30 for comments on cancer cells in the blood).

Accuracy of Pulmonary Cytology

Principal Sources of Error in the Diagnosis of Bronchogenic Carcinoma

Careful collection and processing of cytology specimens and close correlation with clinicoradiologic imaging is absolutely necessary if one is to achieve optimum diagnostic results. In general, a false-positive diagnosis is more serious an error than a false-negative diagnosis, and Tables 20-7, 20-8, and 20-9 list the principal sources of such errors. Above all,

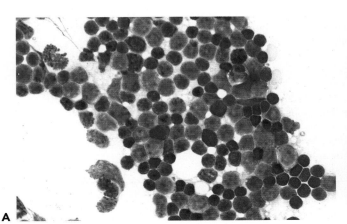
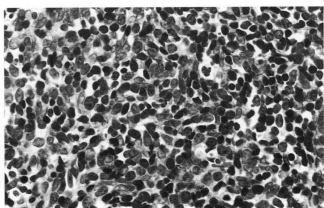

A   B

Figure 20-48 **Subpleural pulmonary thymoma.** *A.* FNA. *B.* Histologic section. Differentiation from lymphoma by cytologic features alone may not be possible. (Diff-Quik.)

TABLE 20-7

PRINCIPAL SOURCES OF ERROR IN THE CYTOLOGIC DIAGNOSIS OF PRIMARY SQUAMOUS LUNG CANCER

Sources of Error	Helpful Diagnostic Features
Irradiation effect on benign squamous cells	History of radiation; bizarre enlarged cells, smudgy nuclei, vacuoles, multinucleation
Tracheitis sicca	Permanent tracheostomy; abnormal squamous cells from near stoma in cough specimen or aspirate; not in bronchial specimen
Atypical squamous metaplasia	Atypical cells in clusters, no single cells. Often after mechanically assisted respiration (ARDS)
Cancer chemotherapy (particularly Myleran)	History of chemotherapy, primarily for leukemia or organ transplant. Cellular changes often bizarre. May be seen in children on chemotherapy.
Mycetoma with atypical squamous metaplasia	Presence of fungus. X-ray shows cavity with "fungus ball."
Vegetable cells; pollen	Thick refractile cell wall, characteristic morphology, yellow pigment
Mucoepidermoid carcinoma	A rare tumor arising in major bronchi; abnormal squamous cells accompanied by mucus-secreting glandular cells
Metastatic squamous carcinoma	History of cancer, radiologic findings
Upper respiratory tract carcinoma	Cancer cells in sputum, not in bronchial specimens; negative chest x-ray; origin located by careful exam of upper respiratory mucosa and scrape cytology or biopsy of suspicious lesions

TABLE 20-8

PRINCIPAL SOURCES OF ERROR IN THE CYTOLOGIC DIAGNOSIS OF ADENOCARCINOMA OF LUNG

Sources of Error	Helpful Diagnostic Features
Papillary fragments of hyperplastic bronchial epithelium ("Creola" bodies)	Presence of goblet cells within the papillary fragments of bronchial epithelium. Cilia or terminal plates of surface epithelium. History of asthma, bronchiectasis.
Atypical bronchial cells; cytomegaly, karyomegaly	Presence of cilia or terminal plates; cells often retain columnar or cuboidal shape
Numerous goblet cells misinterpreted as mucinous adenocarcinoma	Retained columnar shape, small basal nuclei. History of asthma, chronic bronchitis.
Post-bronchoscopy bronchial cell atypia	Bronchial cells with hyperchromatic nuclei; columnar shape, terminal bar (cilia lost). History of recent bronchoscopy.
Atypical pneumocytes, type II	History of acute febrile respiratory illness, with persisting symptoms. May occur in pulmonary infarct and some chronic pulmonary disorders. Atypia is usually transitory.
Viral cytopathic changes	Familiarity with cytopathic effects of cytomegalovirus, herpesvirus, respiratory syncytial virus, adenovirus.
Reactive mesothelium	Present only in percutaneous needle aspirates. Flat sheets of epithelial cells with prominent nucleoli; intercellular "windows."
Pemphigus	Correlate with clinical history of painful mucosal and cutaneous blisters.
Mucoepidermoid carcinoma	A rare tumor, arising from major bronchi. Presence of mucus-secreting glandular cells accompanied by atypical squamous cells.
Metastatic adenocarcinoma	History. Radiologic evidence of multiple tumors.

TABLE 20-9

PRINCIPAL SOURCES OF ERROR IN THE CYTOLOGIC DIAGNOSIS OF SMALL CELL CARCINOMA OF LUNG

Sources of Error	Helpful Diagnostic Features
Reserve (basal) cell hyperplasia	Compact clusters of uniform small cells. No single cells, no molding. No nuclear smudging or necrosis. Often a straight edge to the cluster.
Pools of lymphocytes	Small mature lymphocytes singly and in loose aggregates, mixed with monocytes and reactive or immature lymphocytes that have nucleoli. No coherent groups of cells. No molding, nuclear smudging or necrosis.
Small-cell adenocarcinoma	Overlapping groups and single cancer cells with smoothly configured round or ovoid vesicular nuclei and nucleoli. No molding. No nuclear smudging. May have mucin vacuoles.
Lymphoma	Single cells and loose clusters of noncoherent cells. Nuclei show protrusions and invaginations. Visible and often prominent nucleoli. Lymphoglandular bodies and micronuclei (apoptotic bodies).
Carcinoid	Uniform cells in coherent flat groups with uniform, regular nuclei. "Salt and pepper" chromatin. No necrosis. Present only in bronchial brush or FNA specimens.
Small "blue cell" tumors: Ewing's tumor; Wilms tumor; neuroblastoma; embryonal rhabdomyosarcoma; pleuropulmonary blastoma	Tumors primarily of children and adolescents. May be mistaken for lymphoma but form coherent clusters.
Droplets of condensed mucus	Smooth, round, "ink drop" appearance with no chromatin structure. Usually single.

inconsistencies between clinical findings and cytologic diagnosis must not be allowed to go unresolved.

Sputum

In data from early studies still valid today, positive identification of lung cancer in good sputum samples from an unselected series of patients with the disease was in the range of 60% to 70% (Koss et al, 1964; Johnston, 1982; Pilotti et al, 1982; Ng and Horak, 1983; Rosenthal, 1988). Cancer cells exfoliate intermittently, and the number of positive diagnoses achieved in a single sample may be increased by as much as 10% with three or more samples over a period of several days. As was discussed earlier, the highest diagnostic yield is with squamous carcinomas arising in lobar or segmental bronchi, whereas relatively few peripheral adenocarcinomas shed cells into the sputum until they grow large enough to break into a sizable bronchus.

Bronchial Secretions

Atay and Brandt (1975) studied this in great detail. Of the 885 patients with bronchogenic carcinoma that they examined, 79% of the patients with centrally located tumors and 45% with peripheral tumors had positive cytology in bronchial secretions. Using the TNM clinical classification system (see p 647), these investigators documented increasing efficiency of cytologic diagnosis with increasing tumor size: from 30% for smaller, localized tumors to a maximum of 62% to 65% for larger, more extensive tumors (T3, T4). There was also increased diagnostic yield from tumors with more extensive metastases, ranging from 49% for N0 tumors (no lymph node metastases) to 72% for tumors with

extensive nodal and other metastases (N3, M1). Biopsy diagnoses, as well, are generally easier to obtain from the more advanced tumors.

Fiberoptic Bronchoscopy and Brushing

The rigid bronchoscope has now been superseded by fiberoptic bronchoscopy, permitting visualization and cytologic sampling of third and fourth order bronchial branches. Solomon et al (1974) obtained positive cytologic diagnoses by fiberoptic bronchoscopic brushing in 41 of 46 patients with bronchogenic carcinoma. In a study of 224 patients, Bibbo et al (1973) reported positive diagnoses in 60% of primary peripheral adenocarcinomas and 81% of peripheral squamous carcinomas of lung by fiberoptic bronchial brushing, compared with fewer than 20% by sputum. Interestingly, an additional 12% of patients had positive sputum after the bronchial brushing. Thus, the superiority of fiberoptic bronchial brushing for cytologic diagnosis of peripheral lung cancers, as originally described by Hattori et al (1964, 1971), was firmly established soon after its introduction. In a further advantage, the brushings provide bronchopulmonary samples for microbiologic studies that may contribute to the diagnosis of inflammatory disease in distal portions of the lung.

Needle Aspirates

Beginning with major reviews of results by Dahlgren and Nordenstrøm (1966) and Dahlgren and Lind (1972), percutaneous needle aspiration cytology of primary lung cancers has been widely accepted as an accurate diagnostic method, and this technique greatly increased the number of small peripheral lung tumors that could be diagnosed by cytology. The cell sample must be technically adequate, representative of the disease, and properly identified as to its source and clinical setting. Under these conditions, a positive diagnosis based on adequate sampling and reported by an experienced examiner should be comparable to a biopsy. Still, erroneous positive cytologic diagnoses of lung cancer (false-positive cases) do occur, even under the best of circumstances. In a College of American Pathologists (CAP) report of data from 436 institutions in North America, there were 0.8% false-positive diagnoses, that is, 8 per 1,000; the false-negative rate was ten times higher, 8% (Zarbo and Fenoglio-Preiser, 1992). Some of the principal causes of diagnostic error, discussed in this chapter, include chronic lung disease with proliferation of bronchioloalveolar lining epithelium and reactive proliferation of mesothelium that may be observed in needle aspirates. Errors can be minimized, and the effect on patient care lessened by close communication between pathologist, radiologist and surgeon or pulmonologist, and by confirming the cytologic diagnosis with biopsy or frozen section at the time of thoracotomy. Confirmation is especially important when the diagnosis is based on scanty evidence or if cytologic findings are inconsistent with the clinical or radiologic diagnosis.

Many benign lesions can be identified in adequately sampled cases, including some of the benign tumors described above, inflammatory lesions discussed in this chapter and Chapter 19, and especially certain infectious processes. Still, a report of "negative for malignant cells," with or without some specific diagnosis, does not necessarily exclude a coexisting cancer that may be present in an adjacent, unsampled area. Zakowski et al (1992) attributed the relatively poor negative predictive value of needle aspirates (53%) to inaccurate or inadequate sampling of many cases. They recommended that scanty or insufficient specimens be reported as such, and not as negative. We agree with this recommendation. On the other hand, a positive diagnosis based on adequate sampling and reported by a competent observer should have the same accuracy as a tissue biopsy.

In summary, it should be emphasized that only by combined judicious use of all three methods of diagnosis (i.e., radiography, bronchoscopy, and cytology) can optimal diagnostic results be achieved.

ACKNOWLEDGMENTS

Thanks are due to my colleagues Dr. L. G. Koss and Dr. M. B. Zaman, who provided many of the illustrations for this chapter and Chapter 19.

BIBLIOGRAPHY

Abdul-Karim FW, Wasman JK, Pitlik D. Needle aspiration cytology of chondrosarcomas. Acta Cytol 37:655–660, 1993.

Aberle DR, Gamsu G, Golden JA. Fatal systemic arterial air embolism following lung needle aspiration. Radiology 165:351–353, 1987.

Ackley CD, Heineman L, Dodd LG. Utility of fine needle aspiration in the diagnosis of recurrent pulmonary lymphangioleiomyomatosis: A case report. Diagn Cytopathol 19:458–461, 1998.

Ahrendt SA, Chow JT, Xu LH, et al. Molecular detection of tumor cells in bronchoalveolar lavage fluid from patients with early stage lung cancer. J Natl Cancer Inst 91:332–339, 1999.

AJCC Cancer Staging Manual, 5th ed. Philadelphia, Lippincott Williams & Wilkins, 1997.

Ali SZ, Hoon V, Hoda S, et al. Solitary fibrous tumor. A cytologic-histologic study with clinical, radiologic and immunohistochemical correlations. Cancer 81:116–121, 1997.

Ali SZ, Kronz JD, Plowden KM, Erozan YS. Metastatic pulmonary leiomyosarcoma: Cytopathologic diagnosis on sputum examination. Diagn Cytopathol 18:280–283, 1998.

Alvarez-Fernandez E, Carretero-Albinana L. Bronchial granular cell tumor. Presentation of three cases with tissue culture and ultrastructural study. Arch Pathol Lab Med 111:1065–1069, 1987.

An SH, Koprowska I. Primary cytologic diagnosis of asbestosis associated with bronchogenic carcinoma. Acta Cytol 6:391–398, 1962.

Anbazhagan R, Tihan T, Bornman DM, et al. Classification of small cell lung cancer and pulmonary carcinoid by gene expression profiles. Ca Res 59: 5119–5122, 1999.

Anderson C, Ludwig ME, O'Donnell M, Garcia N. Fine needle aspiration cytology of pulmonary carcinoid tumors. Acta Cytol 34:505–510, 1990.

Anderson NE, Rosenblum MK, Graus F, et al. Autoantibodies in paraneoplastic syndromes associated with small-cell lung cancer. Neurology 38: 1391–1398, 1988.

Apple SK, Nieberg RK, Hirschowitz SL. Fine needle aspiration biopsy of solitary fibrous tumor of the pleura. A report of two cases with a discussion of diagnostic pitfalls. Acta Cytol 42:1528–1533, 1997.

Arakawa H, Nakajima Y, Kurihara Y, et al. CT-guided transthoracic needle biopsy: A comparison between automated biopsy gun and fine needle aspiration. Clin Radiol 51:503–506, 1996.

Aranda C, Sidhu G, Sasso LA, Adams FV. Transbronchial lung biopsy in the diagnosis of lymphangitic carcinomatosis. Cancer 42:1995–1998, 1978.

Archer VE, Saccomanno G, Jones JH. Frequency of different histologic types of bronchogenic carcinoma as related to radiation exposure. Cancer 34: 2056–2060, 1974.

Arioglu E, Doppman J, Gomes M, et al. Cushing's syndrome caused by corticotropin secretion by pulmonary tumorlets. N Engl J Med 339:883–886, 1998.

Arrigoni MG, Woolner LB, Bernatz PE. Atypical carcinoid tumor of lung. J Thorac Cardiovasc Surg 64:413–421, 1972.

Atay A, Brandt HJ. Ergebnisse zytologischer Untersuchungen des Bronchialsekrets bei Lungentumoren in Verhaltnis zum Tumorstadium (TNM System). Dtsch Med Wochenschr 100:1269–1274, 1975.

Auerbach O, Garfinkel L, Parks VR. Histologic type of lung cancer in relation to smoking habits, year of diagnosis and sites of metastases. Chest 67:382–387, 1975.

Auerbach O, Gere JB, Forman JB, et al. Changes in bronchial epithelium in relation to smoking and cancer of lung: Report of progress. N Engl J Med 256:97–104, 1957.

Auerbach O, Stout AP, Hammond EC, Garfinkel L. Changes in bronchial epithelium in relation to cigarette smoking and in relation to lung cancer. N Engl J Med 265:253–267, 1961.

Auerswald U, Barth J, Magnussen H. Value of CD-1 positive cells in bronchoalveolar lavage fluid for the diagnosis of pulmonary histiocytosis X. Lung 169: 305–309, 1991.

Auperin A, Amagada R, Pignon JP, et al. Prophylactic cranial irradiation for patients with small-cell lung cancer in complete remission. Prophylactic Cranial Irradiation Overview Collaborative Group. N Engl J Med 341: 476–484, 1999.

Axiotis CA, Jennings TA. Observations on bronchioloalveolar carcinomas with special emphasis on localized lesions. A clinicopathological, ultrastructural, and immunohistochemical study of 11 cases. Am J Surg Pathol 12:918–931, 1988.

Bach PB, Cramer LD, Warren JL, Begg C. Racial differences in the treatment of early stage lung cancer. N Eng J Med 341:1198–1205, 1999.

Bakhos R, Wojcik EM, Olson MC. Transthoracic fine-needle aspiration cytology of inflammatory pseudotumor, fibrohistiocytic type: A case report with immunohistochemical studies. Diagn Cytopathol 19:216–220, 1998.

Balducci L, Little DD, Khansur T, Steinberg MH. Carcinomatous meningitis in small cell lung cancer. Am J Med Sci 287:31–33, 1984.

Barbas CSV, Caperozzi VL, Takagaki TY, et al. Primary malignant fibrous histiocytoma of lung. Report of a case with bronchial brushing cytology features. Acta Cytol 41:919–923, 1997.

Bardales RH, Powers CN, Frierson HF Jr, et al. Exfoliative respiratory cytology in the diagnosis of leukemias and lymphomas in the lung. Diagn Cytopathol 14:108–113, 1996.

Barkan GA, Caraway NP, Jiang F, et al. Comparison of molecular abnormalities in bronchial brushings and tumor touch preparations. Cancer 105:35–43, 2005.

Barnard WG. Embryoma of the lung. Thorax 7:299–301, 1952.

Bauer TW, Erozan YS. Psammoma bodies in small cell carcinoma of the lung: A case report. Acta Cytol 26:327–330, 1982.

Beahrs OH. Manual for staging of cancer, 4th ed. American Joint Commision on Cancer (AJCC). Philadelphia, JB Lippincott, 1992.

Bean WJ, Graham WL, Jordan RB, Evenson LW. Diagnosis of lung cancer by the transbronchial brush biopsy technique. JAMA 206:1070–1072, 1968.

Beck WC, Reganis JC. Primary lymphoma of lung: Review of literature report of case and addition of 8 other cases. J Thorac Surg 22:323–328, 1951.

Beckett WS. Occupational respiratory diseases. N Engl J Med 342:406–413, 2000.

Bedrossian CW, Warren CJ, Ohar J, Bhan R. Amiodarone pulmonary toxicity: Cytopathology, ultrastructure and immunocytochemistry. Ann Diagn Pathol 1:47–56, 1997.

Bensch KG, Corrin B, Pariente R, Spence H. Oat-cell carcinoma of the lung. Its origin and relationship to bronchial carcinoid. Cancer 22:1163–1172, 1968.

Bensch KG, Gordon GB, Miller LR. Studies of the bronchial counterpart of the

Kulchitsky (argentaffin) cell and innervation of bronchial glands. J Ultrastruct Res 12:668–686, 1965.

Berho M, Moran CA, Suster S. Malignant mixed epithelial/mesenchymal neoplasms of the lung. Semin Diagn Pathol 12:123–139, 1995.

Berlin NI, Buncher CR, Fontana RS, et al. The National Cancer Institute Cooperative Early Lung Cancer Detection Program: Results of the initial screen (Prevalence). Am Rev Resp Dis 130:545–549 (Introduction), 565–570 (Summary and Conclusions), 1984.

Bernhardt H, Killian JJ, Eastridge C. Gastric washings as a source of malignant cells from bronchial secretions. JAMA 183:189, 1963.

Berquist TH, Bailey PB, Cortese DA, Miller WE. Transthoracic needle biopsy: Accuracy and complications in relation to location and type of lesion. Mayo Clin Proc 55:474–481, 1980.

Bhatt ON, Miller MSR, LeRiche J, King EG. Aspiration biopsy in pulmonary opportunistic infections. Acta Cytol 21:206–209, 1977.

Bibbo M, Fennessy JJ, Lu C-T, et al. Bronchial brushing technique for the cytologic diagnosis of peripheral lung lesions. A review of 693 cases. Acta Cytol 17:245–251, 1973.

Bielefeld P. Systemic scleroderma and malignant diseases. A review of literature. Rev Med Intern 12:350–354, 1991.

Black H, Ackerman LV. Importance of epidermoid carcinoma in situ in histogenesis of carcinoma of lung. Ann Surg 136:44–55, 1952.

Black WC. Overdiagnosis: An underrecognized cause of confusion and harm in cancer screening. J Natl Cancer Inst 92:1280–1282, 2000.

Black WC III. Pulmonary oncocytoma. Cancer 23:1347–1357, 1969.

Bolen JW, Thorning D. Histogenetic classification of pulmonary carcinomas. Peripheral adenocarcinomas studied by light microscopy, histochemistry, and electron microscopy. Pathol Annu 17:77–100, 1982.

Bonfiglio TA. Fine needle aspiration biopsy of the lung. Pathol Ann 16:159–180, 1981.

Boucot KR, Cooper DA, Weiss W. The Philadelphia Pulmonary Neoplasm Research Project. Med Clin North Am 54:549–553, 1970.

Brambilla E, Moro D, Veale D, et al. Basal cell (basaloid) carcinoma of the lung. Hum Pathol 23:993–1003, 1992.

Brandsma JL, Steinberg BM, Abramson AL, Winkler B. Presence of human papillomavirus type 16 related sequences in verrucous carcinoma of the larynx. Cancer Res 46:2185–2188, 1986.

Brauch H, Johnson B, Hovis J, et al. Molecular analysis of the short arm of chromosome 3 in small-cell and non-small-cell carcinoma of the lung. N Engl J Med 317:1109–1113, 1987.

Braun DC, Truant TD. Epidemiological study of lung cancer in asbestos miners. Arch Ind Health 17:634–653, 1958.

Brett GZ. Earlier diagnosis and survival in lung cancer. Br Med J 4:260–262, 1969.

Broderick PA, Corvese NL, LaChance T, Allard J. Giant cell carcinoma of lung: A cytologic evaluation. Acta Cytol 19:225–230, 1975.

Broghamer WL, Richards ME, Biscopink RJ, Faurest SH. Pulmonary cytologic examination in the identification of the second primary carcinoma of the lung. Cancer 56:2664–2668, 1985.

Buhl L, Larsen KE, Bjorn-Hansen, L. Lymphangiomatosis. Is fine needle aspiration cytodiagnosis possible? Acta Cytol 32:559–562, 1988.

Bull JC, Grimes OF. Pulmonary carcinosarcoma. Chest 65:9–12, 1974

Burke MD, Melamed MR. Exfoliative cytology of metastatic cancer in lung. Acta Cytol 12:61–74, 1968.

Byrne JC, Tsao, M-S, Fraser RS, Howley PM. Human papillomavirus-11 DNA in a patient with chronic laryngotracheobronchial papillomatosis and metastatic squamous cell carcinoma of the lung. N Engl J Med 317:873–878, 1987.

Cafer D, Bonfiglio TA, Patten SF. Fine needle aspiration cytopathology of bronchial carcinoid tumors. An analytic study of the cells. Acta Cytol 24:67, 1980.

Cahan WG, Melamed MR, Frazell EL. Tracheobronchial cytology after laryngectomy for carcinoma. Surg Gynecol Obstet 123:15–21, 1966.

Cahan WG, Montemayor PB. Cancer of larynx and lung in the same patient: A report of 60 cases. J Thorac Cardiovasc Surg 44:309–320, 1962.

Calhoun P, Fledman PS, Armstrong P, et al. The clinical outcome of needle aspirations of the lung when cancer is not diagnosed. Ann Thorac Surg 41:592–596, 1986.

Cardozo PL, DeGraaf S, DeBoer MJ, et al. The results of cytology in 1000 patients with pulmonary malignancy. Acta Cytol 11:120–131, 1967.

Carey JM, Geer AE. Bronchogenic carcinoma complicating pulmonary tuberculosis: Report of 8 cases and review of 140 cases since 1932. Ann Intern Med 49:161–180, 1958.

Carter D, Marsh BR, Baker RR, et al. Relationships of morphology to clinical presentation in ten cases of early squamous cell carcinoma of the lung. Cancer 37:1389–1396, 1976.

Chamberlain DW, Braude AC, Rebuck AS. A critical evaluation of bronchoalveolar lavage. Criteria for identifying unsatisfactory specimens. Acta Cytol 31:599–605, 1987.

Chen KT. Cytology of bronchial benign granular-cell tumor. Acta Cytol 35:381–384, 1991.

Chopra SK, Genovesi MG, Simmons DH, Gothe B. Fiberoptic bronchoscopy in the diagnosis of lung cancer. Comparison of pre- and post-bronchoscopy sputa, washings, brushings and biopsies. Acta Cytol 21:524–527, 1977.

Chow LT, Chan SK, Chow WH, Tsui MS. Pulmonary sclerosing hemangioma. Report of a case with diagnosis by fine needle aspiration. Acta Cytol 36:287–292, 1992.

Colby TV, Koss MN, Travis WD. Tumors of the Lower Respiratory Tract in Atlas of Tumor Pathology. Washington, DC, AFIP, 1995.

Collins BT, Cramer HM. Fine needle aspiration cytology of carcinoid tumors. Acta Cytol 40:695–707, 1996.

Collins BT, Cramer HM, Frain BE, Davis MM. Fine needle aspiration biopsy of metastatic Ewing's sarcoma with MIC2 (CD 99) immunocytochemistry. Diagn Cyopathol 19:382–384, 1998.

Conlan AA, Payne WS, Woolner LB, Sanderson DR. Adenoid cystic carcinoma (cylindroma) and mucoepidermoid carcinoma of the bronchus: Factors affecting survival. J Thorac Cardiovasc Surg 76:369–377, 1978.

Connor S, Dyer J, Guest P. Image-guided automated needle biopsy of 106 thoracic lesions: A retrospective review of diagnostic accuracy and complication rates. Eur Radiol 10:490–494, 2000.

Cordova JF, Tesluk H, Knudtson KP. Asbestosis and carcinoma of the lung. Cancer 15:1181–1187, 1962.

Cortese DA, Edell ES. Role of phototherapy, laser therapy, brachytherapy, and prosthetic stents in the management of lung cancer. Clin Chest Med 14:149–159, 1993.

Costa I, Lerma E, Esteve E, et al. Aspiration cytology of lung metastasis of monophasic synovial sarcoma: Report of a case. Acta Cytol 41:1289–1292, 1997.

Craig JD, Finley RJ. Spindle cell carcinoid of lung. Cytologic, histopathologic and ultrastructural features. Acta Cytol 26:495–498, 1982.

Craver LF. Diagnosis of malignant lung tumors by aspiration biopsy and by sputum examination. Surgery 8:947–960, 1940.

Cwierzyk TA, Glasberg SS, Virshup MA, Cranmer JC. Pulmonary oncocytoma. Report of a case with cytologic, histologic, and electron microscopic study. Acta Cytol 29:620–623, 1985.

Dahlgren S, Nordenstrom B. Transthoracic Needle Biopsy. Stockholm, Almqvist & Wiksells, 1966.

Dahlgren SE. Aspiration biopsy of intrathoramic tumors. Acta Pathol Microbiol Scand [B]. 70:566–576, 1967.

Dahlgren SE. Needle biopsy of intrapulmonary hamartoma. Scand J Res Dis 4:187–194, 1966.

Dahlgren SE, Lind B. Comparison between diagnostic results obtained by transthoracic needle biopsy and by sputum examination. Acta Cytol 16:53–58, 1972.

Davis MP, Eagan RT, Weiland LH, Pairolera PC. Carcinosarcoma of the lung: Mayo Clinic experience and response to chemotherapy. Mayo Clin Proc 59:598–603, 1984.

Dempster AP. Logicist statistics I. Models and modeling. Statistical Science 13:248–276, 1998.

Dennis TR, Stock AD. A molecular cytogenetic study of chromosome 3 rearrangements in small cell lung cancer: Consistent involvement of chromosome band 3q13.2. Cancer Genet Cytogenet 113:134–140, 1999.

Dermer GB. Origin of bronchioloalveolar carcinoma and peripheral bronchial adenocarcinoma. Cancer 49:881–887, 1982.

Devesa SS, Shaw GL, Blot WJ. Changing patterns of lung cancer incidence by histological type. Cancer Epidemiol Biomarkers Prev 1:29–34, 1991.

DiMarco AF, Montenegro H, Payne CB Jr, Kwon KH. Papillomas of the tracheobronchial tree with malignant degeneration. Chest 74:464–465, 1978.

Dirnhofer S, Freund M, Rogatsch H, et al. Selective expression of trophoblastic hormones by lung carcinoma: Neuroendocrine tumors exclusively produce human chorionic gonadotropin alpha-subunit (hCGalpha). Hum Pathol 31:966–972, 2000.

Doll R, Peto R. The causes of cancer: Quantitative estimates of avoidable risks of cancer in the United States today. J Natl Cancer Inst 66:1191–1308, 1981.

Drachenberg CB, Bourquin PM, Cochran LM, et al. Fine needle aspiration biopsy of solitary fibrous tumor. Report of two cases with histologic immunohistochemistry and ultrastructural correlation. Acta Cytol 42:1003–1010, 1998.

Drut R, Pollono D. Pleuropulmonary blastoma: Diagnosis by fine-needle aspiration cytology: A case report. Diagn Cytopathol 19:303–305, 1998.

Dudgeon LS, Wrigley CH. On demonstration of particles of malignant growth in sputum by means of wet-film method. J Laryngol 50:752–762, 1935.

Dugan JM. Cytologic diagnosis of basal cell (basaloid) carcinoma of the lung: A report of two cases. Acta Cytol 39:539–542, 1995.

Ebright MI, Zakowski MF, Martin J, et al. Clinical pattern and pathologic stage but not histologic features predict outcome for bronchioloalveolar carcinoma. Ann Thorac Surg 74:1640–1646, 2002.

Ellis FH Jr, Woolner LB, Schmidt HW. Metastatic pulmonary malignancy; Study of factors involved in exfoliation of malignant cells. J Thorac Surg 20:125–135, 1950.

Erozan YS, Pressman NJ, Donovan PA, et al. A comparative cytopathologic study of noninvasive squamous cell carcinoma of the lung. Anal Quant Cytol 1:50–56, 1979.

Espinoza CG, Balis JU, Saba SR, et al. Ultrastructural and immunohistochemical studies of bronchioloalveolar carcinoma. Cancer 54:2182–2189, 1984.

Essary LR, Vargas SO, Fletcher CD. Primary pleuropulmonary synovial sarcoma: Reappraisal of a recently described anatomic subset. Cancer 94:459–469, 2002.

Ewing J. Neoplastic Diseases. 2nd ed. Philadelphia, WB Saunders, 1922.

Fabian E, Nagy M, Mesozaros G. Experiences with bronchial brushing method. Acta Cytol 19:320–321, 1975.

Fekette PS, Cohen C, DeRose PB. Pulmonary spindle cell carcinoid: Needle aspiration biopsy, histologic and immunohistochemical findings. Acta Cytol 34:50–56, 1990.

Fennessy JJ, Fry WA, Manalo-Estrella P, Frias Hidvegi DVS. The bronchial brushing technique for obtaining cytologic specimens from peripheral lung lesions. Acta Cytol 14:25–30, 1970.

Ferguson MK, Landreneau RJ, Hazelrigg SR, et al. Long-term outcome after resection for bronchial carcinoid tumors. Eur J Cardiothorac Surg 18: 156–161, 2000.

Fernandez MA, Nyssen J. Oncocytoma of the lung. Can J Surg 25:332–333, 1982.

Fielding P, Turnbull L, Prime W, et al. Heterogeneous nuclear ribonucleoprotein A2/B1 up-regulation in bronchial lavage specimens: A clinical marker of early lung cancer detection. Clin Cancer Res 5:4048–4052, 1999.

Finley JL, Silverman JF, Dabbs DJ. Fine-needle aspiration cytology of pulmonary carcinosarcoma with immunocytochemical and ultrastructural observations. Diagn Cytopathol 4:239–243, 1988.

Fiorella RM, Gurley SD, Dubey C. Cytologic distinction between bronchioalveolar carcinoma and reactive/reparative respiratory epithelium: A cytomorphometric analysis. Diagn Cytopathol 19:270–273, 1998.

Fishback N, Travis W, Moran C, et al. Pleomorphic (spindle/giant cell) carcinoma of the lung: A clinicopathologic study of 78 cases. Cancer 73: 2936–2945, 1994.

Fisher ER, Palekar A, Paulson JD. Comparative histopathologic, histochemical, electron microscopic and tissue culture studies of bronchial carcinoids and oat cell carcinomas of lung. Am J Clin Pathol 169:165–172, 1978.

Flanagan P, Roeckel IE. Giant cell carcinoma of the lung: Anatomic and clinical correlation. Am J Med 36:214–221, 1964.

Flehinger BJ, Kimmel M. The natural history of lung cancer in a periodically screened population. Biometrics 43:127–144, 1987.

Flehinger BJ, Melamed MR. Current status of screening for lung cancer. Curr Perspect Thoracic Oncol 4:1–15, 1994.

Flehinger BJ, Kimmel M, Melamed MR. Natural history of adenocarcinoma–large cell carcinoma of the lung: Conclusions from screening programs in New York and Baltimore. J Natl Cancer Inst 80:337–344, 1988.

Flehinger BJ, Kimmel M, Melamed MR. The effect of surgical treatment on survival from early lung cancer. Implications for screening. Chest 101: 1013–1018, 1992.

Flehinger BJ, Melamed MR, Zaman MB, et al. Early lung cancer detection: Results of the initial (prevalence) radiologic and cytologic screening in the Memorial Sloan Kettering study. Am Rev Respir Dis 130:555–560, 1984.

Fleming WH, Jove DF. Primary leiomyosarcoma of the lung with positive sputum cytology. Acta Cytol 19:14–20, 1975.

Fontana RS, Sanderson DR, Taylor WF, et al. Early lung cancer detection: Results of the initial (prevalence) radiologic screening in the Mayo Clinic study. Am Rev Respir Dis 130:561–565, 1984.

Fontana RS. The Mayo lung project. Cancer 89(Suppl):2352–2355, 2000.

Foot NC. Identification of types of pulmonary cancer in cytologic smears. Am J Pathol 28:963–983, 1952.

Francis D, Jacobsen M. Pulmonary blastoma: Preoperative cytologic and histologic findings. Acta Cytol 23:437–442, 1979.

Friedberg EC. Giant cell carcinoma of the lung. Cancer 18:259–264, 1965.

Friedrich G. Periphere lungenkrebse auf dem boden pleuranaher narben. Virchows Arch 304:230, 1939.

Frierson HF Jr, Covell JL, Mills S. Needle aspiration cytology of atypical carcinoid of the lung. Acta Cytol 31:471–475, 1987.

Frost JK, Ball WC Jr, Levin M, et al. Early lung cancer detection: Results of the initial (prevalence) radiologic and cytologic screening in the Johns Hopkins study. Am Rev Respir Dis 130:549–554, 1984.

Fullmer CD, Morris RP. Primary cytodiagnosis of unsuspected mediastinal Hodgkin's disease (report of a case). Acta Cytol 16:77–81, 1972.

Fullmer CD, Parrish CM. Pulmonary cytology. A diagnostic method for occult carcinoma. Acta Cytol 13:645–651, 1969.

Fuzesi L, Hoer PW, Schmidt W. Exfoliative cytology of multiple endobronchial granular cell tumor. Acta Cytol 33:516–518, 1989.

Gay PC, Brutinel WM. Transbronchial needle aspiration in the practice of bronchoscopy. Mayo Clin Proc 64:158–162, 1989.

Gazdar AF, Minna JD. Molecular detection of early lung cancer (editorial comment). J Natl Cancer Inst 91:299–301, 1999.

Geisinger KR, Buss DH, Kawamoto EH, Ahl ET Jr. Multiple myeloma. The diagnostic role and prognostic significance of exfoliative cytology. Acta Cytol 30:334–340, 1986.

Gelven PL, Hopkins MA, Green CA, et al. Fine-needle aspiration cytology of pleuropulmonary blastoma: Case report and review of the literature. Diagn Cytopathol 16:336–340, 1997.

Gephardt GN, Belovich DM. Cytology of pulmonary carcinoid tumors. Acta Cytol 26:434–438, 1982.

Gerald WL, Miller HK, Battifora H, et al. Intra-abdominal desmoplastic small round-cell tumor. Report of 19 cases of a distinctive type of high grade polyphenotypic malignancy affecting young individuals. Am J Surg Pathol 15:499–513, 1991.

Ginsberg SS, Buzard AC, Stern H, Carter D. Giant cell carcinoma of the lung. Cancer 70:606–610, 1992.

Givens CD Jr, Marini JJ. Transbronchial needle aspiration of a bronchial carcinoid tumor. Chest 88:152–153, 1985.

Gladhill EY, Spriggs JB, Binford CH. Needle aspiration in the diagnosis of lung carcinoma. Am J Clin Pathol 19:235–242, 1949.

Glant MD, Wall RW, Ransburg R. Endobronchial granular cell tumor: Cytology of a new case and review of the literature. Acta Cytol 23:477–482, 1979.

Godwin JD, Brown CC. Comparative epidemiology of carcinoid and oat-cell tumors of the lung. Cancer 40:1671–1673, 1977.

Gould VE, Linnoila RI, Memoli VA, Warren WH. Neuroendocrine cells and neuroendocrine neoplasms of the lung. Pathol Annu 18:287–330, 1983.

Granberg I, Willems JS. Endometriosis of lung and pleura diagnosed by aspiration biopsy. Acta Cytol 21:295–297, 1977.

Greenberg SD, Spjut HJ, Estrada RG, et al. Morphometric markers for the evaluation of preneoplastic lesions of the lung. Diagnostic evaluation by high-resolution image analysis of atypical cells in sputum specimens. Anal Quant Cytol Histol 9:49–54, 1987.

Grunze H. A critical review and evaluation of cytodiagnosis in chest diseases. Acta Cytol 4:175–198, 1960.

Grzybowski S, Coy P. Early diagnosis of carcinoma of the lung: Simultaneous screening with chest x-ray and sputum cytology. Cancer 25:113–120, 1970.

Guccion JG, Rosen SH. Bronchopulmonary leiomyosarcoma and fibrosarcoma: A study of 32 cases and review of the literature. Cancer 30:836–847, 1972.

Guillou L, Gloor E, Anani PA, Kaelin R. Bronchial granular-cell tumor: Report of a case with preoperative cytologic diagnosis on bronchial brushings and immunohistochemical studies. Acta Cytol 35:375–380, 1991.

Guillou L, Sahli R, Chaubert P, et al. Squamous cell carcinoma of the lung in a nonsmoking, nonirradiated patient with juvenile laryngotracheal papillomatosis: Evidence of human papillomavirus-11 DNA in both carcinoma and papillomas. Am J Surg Pathol 15:891–898, 1991.

Gultekin SH, Rosai J, Demopoulos A, et al. Hu Immunolabeling as a Marker of Neural and Neuroendocrine Differentiation in Normal and Neoplastic Human Tissues: Assessment Using a Recombinant Anti-Hu Fab Fragment. Intl J Surg Pathol 8:109–117, 2000.

Gupta PK, Verma K. Calcified (psammoma) bodies in alveolar cell carcinoma of the lung. Acta Cytol 16:59–63, 1972.

Gupta RK. Value of sputum cytology in the differential diagnosis of alveolar cell carcinoma from bronchogenic adenocarcinoma. Acta Cytol 25: 225–258, 1981.

Hajdu SI, Hajdu EO. Cytopathology of Sarcomas and Other Nonepithelial Malignant Tumors. Philadelphia, WB Saunders, 1975.

Hajdu SI, Koss LG. Cytologic diagnosis of metastatic myosarcomas. Acta Cytol 13:545–551, 1969.

Haramati LB. CT-guided automated needle biopsy of the chest. Am J Roentgenol 165:53–55, 1995.

Harwood TR, Gracey DR, Yokoo H. Pseudomesotheliomatous carcinoma of the lung: A variant of peripheral lung cancer. Am J Clin Pathol 65:159–167, 1976.

Hattori S, Matsuda M, Nishihara H, Horai T. Early diagnosis of small peripheral lung cancer: Cytologic diagnosis of very fresh cancer cells obtained by the TV-brushing technique. Acta Cytol 15:460–467, 1971.

Hattori S, Matsuda M, Sugiyama T, Matsuda H. Cytologic diagnosis of early lung cancer: Brushing method under x-ray television fluoroscopy. Dis Chest 45:129–142, 1964.

Healy TM. Cytology of the sputum in carcinoma of the lung: 515 cases. Isr J Med Sci 140:523–528, 1971.

Heitmiller RF, Mathisen DJ, Ferry JA, et al. Mucoepidermoid lung tumors. Ann Thorac Surg 47:394–399, 1989.

Hellstrom HR, Fisher ER. Giant cell carcinoma of lung. Cancer 16:1080–1088, 1963.

Henschke CI. Early lung cancer action project. Cancer 89(Suppl):2472–2482, 2000.

Henschke CI, McCauley DI, Yankelevitz DF, et al. Early lung cancer action project: Overall design and findings from baseline screening. Lancet 354: 99–105, 1999.

Herbut PA, Clerf LH. Bronchogenic carcinoma: Diagnosis by cytologic study of bronchoscopically removed secretions. JAMA 130:1006–1012, 1946.

Herman BL, Bullock WK, Waken JK. Giant cell adenocarcinoma of the lung. Cancer 19:1337–1346, 1966.

Hida CA, Gupta PK. Cercariform cells: Are they specific for transitional cell carcinoma? Cancer 87:69–74, 1999.

Hirano T, Franzen B, Kato H, et al. Genesis of squamous cell lung carcinoma: Sequential changes of proliferation, DNA ploidy, and p53 expression. Am J Pathol 144:296–302, 1994.

Holman CW, Okinaka A. Occult carcinoma of the lung. J Thor Cardiovasc Surg 47:466–471, 1964.

Hsiu JG, Kreuger JK, D'Amato NA, Morris JR. Primary malignant fibrous histiocytoma of the lung: Fine needle aspiration cytologic features. Acta Cytol 31: 345–350, 1987.

Ishizuka T, Yoshitake J, Yamada T, et al. Diagnosis of a case of pulmonary carcinosarcoma by detection of rhabdomyosarcoma cells in sputum. Acta Cytol 32:658–662, 1988.

Jacobsen M, Francis D. Pulmonary blastoma: Preoperative cytologic and histologic findings. Acta Cytol 23:437–442, 1979.

Jacques J, Currie W. Broncho-alveolar carcinoma: A Clara cell tumor? Cancer 40:2171–2180, 1977.

Jiang SX, Kameya T, Shoji M, et al. Large cell neuroendocrine carcinoma of the lung: A histologic and immunohistochemical study of 22 cases. Am J Surg Pathol 22:526–537, 1998.

Johnston WW. Cytologic diagnosis of lung cancer. Principles and problems. Pathol Res Pract 181:1–36, 1981.

Johnston WW. Fine needle aspiration biopsy versus sputum and bronchial material in the diagnosis of lung cancer: A comparative study of 168 patients. Acta Cytol 32:641–646, 1988.

Johnston WW. Histologic and cytologic patterns of lung cancer in 2,580 men and women over a 15-year period. Acta Cytol 32:163–168, 1988.

Johnston WW. Ten years of respiratory cytopathology at Duke University Medical Center. III. The significance of inconclusive cytopathologic diagnoses during the years 1970–1974. Acta Cytol 26:759–766, 1982.

Johnston WW, Frable WJ. Diagnostic Respiratory Cytopathology. New York, Masson Publishing, 1979.

Johnston WW, Frable WJ. The cytopathology of the respiratory tract. Am J Pathol 84:372–414, 1976.

Jordan AG, Predmore L, Sullivan MM, Memoli VA. The cytodiagnosis of well-differentiated neuroendocrine carcinoma. Acta Cytol 31:464–470, 1987.

Kamholz SL, Pinsker KL, Johnson J, Schreiber K. Fine needle aspiration biopsy of intrathoracic lesion. NY State J Med 82:736–739, 1982.

Kaneko M, Eguchi K, Ohmatsu H, et al. Peripheral lung cancer screening and detection with low-dose spiral CT versus radiography. Radiology 201:798–802, 1996.

Kanhouwa SB, Matthews MJ. Reliability of cytologic typing of lung cancer. Acta Cytol 20:229–232, 1976.

Karcioglu ZA, Someren AD. Pulmonary blastoma: A case report and review of literature. Am J Clin Pathol 6:287–297, 1974.

Katzenstein, A-LA, Gmelich JT, Carrington CB. Sclerosing hemangioma of the lung: A clinicopathologic study of 51 cases. Am J Surg Pathol 4:343–356, 1980.

Kaw YT, Nayak RN. Fine needle aspiration biopsy cytology of sclerosing hemangioma of the lung: A case report. Acta Cytol 37:933–937, 1993.

Kawahara E, Nakanishi I, Kuroda Y, Morishita T. Fine needle aspiration biopsy of primary malignant fibrous histiocytoma of the lung. Acta Cytol 32:226–230, 1988.

Keel SB, Bacha E, Mark EJ, et al. Primary pulmonary sarcoma: A clinicopathologic study of 26 cases. Mod Pathol 12;1124–1131, 1999.

Kern WH. Cytology of hyperplastic and neoplastic lesions of terminal bronchioles and alveoli. Acta Cytol 9:372–380, 1965.

Kern WH, Schweizer CW. Sputum cytology of metastatic carcinoma of the lung. Acta Cytol 20:514–520, 1976.

Kern WH, Crepean AG, Jones JC. Primary Hodgkin's disease of the lung: Report of 4 cases and review of the literature. Cancer 14:1151–1165, 1961.

Kerr KM, Carey FA, King G, Lamb D. Atypical alveolar hyperplasia: Relationship with pulmonary adenocarcinoma, p53 and c-erb B-2 expression. J Pathol 174:249–256, 1994.

Kim K, Naylor B, Han IH. Fine needle aspiration cytology of sarcomas metastatic to the lung. Acta Cytol 30:688–694, 1986.

Kitamura H, Kameda Y, Ito T, Hayashi H. Atypical adenomatous hyperplasia of the lung. Implications for the pathogenesis of peripheral lung adenocarcinoma. Am J Clin Pathol 111:610–622, 1999.

Kleinert R, Popper H. Giant fibroma of the lung: A morphological study. Virchows Arch 410:363–367, 1987.

Klima M, Peters J. Malignant granular cell tumor. Arch Pathol Lab Med 111:1070–1073, 1987.

Knudtson KP. Method of study of squamous metaplasia, atypical change, and early bronchogenic carcinoma of bronchial mucosa in smokers and nonsmokers. Cancer 9:84–85, 1956.

Kodama T, Shimosato Y, Koide T, et al. Large cell carcinoma of the lung: Ultrastructural and immunohistochemical studies. Jpn J Clin Oncol 15:431–441, 1985.

Koizumi JH, Schon DS. Cytologic features of colonic adenocarcinoma: Differences between primary and metastatic neoplasms. Acta Cytol 41:419–426, 1997.

Koprowska I, An SH, Corsey D, et al. Cytologic patterns of developing bronchogenic carcinoma. Acta Cytol 9:424–430, 1965.

Koss LG. Cytologic diagnosis of lung cancer. Acta Pathol Jpn 8:99–111, 1958.

Koss LG, Melamed MR, Goodner JT. Pulmonary cytology: A brief survey of diagnostic results from July 1st 1952 until December 31st 1960. Acta Cytol 40:104–113, 1964.

Koss LG, Woyke S, Olszewski W. Aspiration Biopsy. Cytologic Interpretation and Histologic Bases. New York, Igaku-Shoin, 1984.

Koss LG, Woyke S, Olszewski W. Aspiration Biopsy. Cytologic Interpretation and Histologic Bases. 2nd ed. New York, Igaku-Shoin, 1992.

Koss MN, Hochholzer, L, O'Leary T. Pulmonary blastomas. Cancer 67:2368–2381, 1991.

Koss MN, Hochholzer L, Frommelt RA. Carcinosarcoma of the lung: A clinicopathologic study of 66 patients. Am J Surg Pathol 23:1514–1526, 1999.

Krumerman MS. Leiomyosarcoma of the lung: Primary cytodiagnosis on two consecutive cases. Acta Cytol 21:103–108, 1977.

Kubik AK, Parkin DM, Zatloukal P. Czech study on lung cancer screening: Posttrial follow-up of lung cancer deaths up to year 15 since enrollment. Cancer 89(Suppl):2363–2368, 2000.

Kuschner M, Beckler PA. Cancer of the lung: The cytology of sputum prior to the development of carcinoma. Acta Cytol 9:413–421, 1965.

Kyriakos M, Rockoff SD. Brush biopsy of bronchial carcinoid: A source of cytologic error. Acta Cytol 16:261–268, 1972.

L'Hoste RH Jr, Filippa DA, Lieberman PH, Bretsky S. Primary pulmonary lymphomas: A clinicopathologic analysis of 36 cases. Cancer 54:1397–1406, 1984.

Laforga JB, Aranda FI. Multicentric oncocytoma of the lung diagnosed by fine-needle aspiration. Diagn Cytopathol 21:51–54, 1999.

Landis SH, Murray T, Bolden S, Wingo PA. Cancer statistics, 1999. Cancer 49:8–31, 1999.

Lange E, Hoeg K. Cytologic typing of lung cancer. Acta Cytol 16:327–330, 1972.

Larsimont D, Kiss R, de Lanoit Y, Melamed MR. Characterization of the morphonuclear features and DNA ploidy of typical and atypical carcinoids and small cell carcinomas of the lung. Am J Clin Pathol 94:378–383, 1990.

Laurent F, Latrabe V, Vergier B, et al. CT-guided transthoracic needle biopsy of pulmonary nodules smaller than 20 mm: Results with an automated 20 gauge coaxial cutting needle. Clin Radiol 55:281–287, 2000.

Lavoie RR, McDonald JR, Kling GA. Cavitation in squamous carcinoma of the lung. Acta Cytol 21:210–214, 1977.

Lerner MA, Rosbach H, Frank HA, Fleischner FG. Radiologic localization and management of cytologically discovered bronchial carcinoma. N Engl J Med 264:480–485, 1961.

Levij IS. A case of primary cavitary Hodgkin's disease of the lungs, diagnosed cytologically. Acta Cytol 16:546–549, 1972.

Levine SE, Mossler JA, Johnston WW. The cytologic appearance of metastatic ameloblastoma. Acta Cytol 25:295–298, 1981.

Levy H, Horak DA, Lewis MI. The value of bronchial washings and bronchoalveolar lavage in the diagnosis of lymphangitic carcinomatosis. Chest 94:1028–1030, 1988.

Li SM, Zhang ZT, Chan S, et al. Detection of circulating uroplakin-positive cells in patients with transitional cell carcinoma of the bladder. J Urol 162:931–935, 1999.

Liang XM. Accuracy of cytologic diagnosis and cytotyping of sputum in primary lung cancer: Analysis of 161 cases. J Surg Oncol 40:107–111, 1989.

Liebow AA. Tumors of the Lower Respiratory Tract. Atlas of Tumor Pathology, section 5: fascicle 17. Washington, DC, Armed Forces Institute of Pathology, 1952.

Liebow AA, Castleman B. Benign clear cell (sugar) tumors of the lung. Yale J Biol Med 43:213–222, 1971.

Lilienfeld A. An evaluation of radiologic and cytologic screening for the early detection of lung cancer: A cooperative pilot study of the American Cancer Society and the Veterans Administration. Cancer Res 26:2083–2121, 1966.

Lindberg K. Uber die Formale Genese des Lungerkrebses. Helsingfors Mercator Trycken Aktiebolaget, 1935.

Lindner J, Radio SJ, Robbins RA, et al. Bronchoalveolar lavage in the cytologic diagnosis of carcinoma of the lung. Acta Cytol 31:796–801, 1987.

Linnoila TI, Jensen SM, Steinberg SM, et al. Peripheral airway cell marker expression in non–small cell lung carcinoma. Am J Clin Pathol 97:233–243, 1992.

Lockett L, Chiang V, Scully N. Primary pulmonary meningiomas: Report of a case and review of the literature. Am J Surg Pathol 21:453–560, 1997.

Logrono R, Filipowicz EA, Eyzaguirre EJ, Sawh RN. Diagnosis of primary fibrosarcoma of the lung by fine-needle aspiration and core biopsy. Arch Pathol Lab Med 123:731–735, 1999.

Logrono R, Wojtowycz MM, Wunderlich DW, et al. Fine needle aspiration cytology and core biopsy in the diagnosis of alveolar soft part sarcoma presenting with lung metastases: A case report. Acta Cytol 43:464–470, 1999.

Lozowski W, Hajdu SI, Melamed MR. Cytomorphology of carcinoid tumors. Acta Cytol 23:360–365, 1979.

Ludwig ME, Otis RD, Cole SR, Westcott JL. Fine needle aspiration cytology of pulmonary hamartomas. Acta Cytol 26:671–677, 1982.

Ludwig RA, Balachandran I. Mycosis fungoides. The importance of pulmonary cytology in the diagnosis of a case with systemic involvement. Acta Cytol 27:198–201, 1983.

Ludwig RA, Gero M. Bronchoscopic cytology of metastatic breast carcinoma with osteoclastic giant cells. Acta Cytol 31:305–308, 1987.

Lynth TJ, Bell DW, Sordella R, et al. Activating mutations in the epidermal growth factor receptor underlying responsiveness of non–small-cell lung cancer to gefitinib. N Engl J Med 350:2129–2139, 2004.

Mahadevia PJ, Fleisher LA, Frick KD, et al. Lung cancer screening with helical computed tomography in older adult smokers: A decision and cost-effectiveness analysis. JAMA 289:313–322, 2003.

Majcher SJ, Lee ER, Reingold IM, et al. Carcinoid syndrome in bronchogenic carcinoma. Arch Intern Med 117:57–63, 1966.

Majmudar B, Thomas J, Gorelkin L, Symbas PN. Respiratory obstruction caused by a multicentric granular cell tumor of the laryngotracheobronchial tree. Hum Pathol 12:283–286, 1981.

Manivel JC, Priest JR, Watterson J, et al. Pleuropulmonary blastoma: The so-called pulmonary blastoma of childhood. Cancer 62:1516–1526, 1988.

Manning JT, Spjut HJ, Tschen JA. Bronchoalveolar carcinoma: The significance of two histopathologic types. Cancer 54:525–534, 1984.

Mao L, Hruban RH, Boyle JO, et al. Detection of oncogene mutations in sputum precedes diagnosis of lung cancer. Cancer Res 54:1634–1637, 1994.

Mark EJ, Ramirez JE. Peripheral small-cell carcinoma of the lung resembling carcinoid tumor. Arch Pathol Lab Med 109:263–269, 1985.

Marsh BR, Frost JK, Erozan YS, Carter D. Occult bronchogenic carcinoma: Endoscopic localization and television documentation. Cancer 30:1348–1352, 1972.

Martini N, Melamed M. Multiple primary lung cancers. J Thorac Cardiovasc Surg 70:606–612, 1975.

Martini N, Beattie EJ, Cliffton EE, Melamed MR. Radiologically occult lung cancer: Report of 26 cases. Surg Clin North Am 54:811–823, 1974.

Masson RG, Krikorian J, Lukl P, et al. Pulmonary microvascular cytology in the diagnosis of lymphangitic carcinomatosis. N Engl J Med 321:71–76, 1989.

Matsumoto S, Muranaka T, Hanada K, Takeo S. Oncocytic carcinoid of the lung. Radiat Med 11:63–65, 1993.

McCaughey WTE, Wade OL, Elmes PC. Exposure to asbestos dust and diffuse pleural mesotheliomas. Br Med J 2:1397, 1962.

McDowell EM, Trump BF. Histogenesis of preneoplastic and neoplastic lesions in tracheobronchial epithelium. Surv Synth Pathol Res 2:235–279, 1983.

McGrath AK Jr. Cytologic Diagnosis of Lung Cancer. Springfield, IL, Charles C Thomas, 1950.

Medalie NS, Vallejo CE, Wasserman P. Metastatic pulmonary sarcoma: Report of a case with diagnosis by fine needle aspiration. Acta Cytol 42:968–972, 1998.

Melamed MR. Lung cancer screening results in the National Cancer Institute New York study. Cancer 89(Suppl):2356–2362, 2000.

Melamed MR, Flehinger BJ. Early lung cancer as a target for chemoprevention. J Cell Biochem 17F(Suppl):57–65, 1993.

Melamed MR, Flehinger BJ. Detection of lung cancer: Highlights of the Memorial Sloan-Kettering Study in New York City. Schweiz Med Wochenschr 117:1457–1463, 1987.

Melamed MR, Flehinger B, Miller D, et al. Preliminary report of the lung cancer detection program in New York. Cancer 39:369–382, 1977.

Melamed MR, Flehinger BJ, Zaman MB. Impact of early detection on the clinical course of lung cancer. Surg Clin North Am 67:909–924, 1987.

Melamed MR, Flehinger BJ, Zaman MB, et al. Screening for early lung cancer: Results of the Memorial Sloan-Kettering study in New York. Chest 86:44–53, 1984.

Melamed MR, Flehinger BJ, Zaman M, et al. Detection of true pathologic stage l lung cancer in a screening program and effect on survival. Cancer 47:1182–1187, 1981.

Melamed MR, Koss LG, Cliffton EE. Roentgenologically occult lung cancer, diagnosed by cytology: Report of 12 cases. Cancer 16:1537–1551, 1963.

Melamed MR, Zaman MB, Flehinger BJ, Martini N. Radiologically occult in situ and incipient invasive epidermoid lung cancer: Detection by sputum cytology in a survey of asymptomatic cigarette smokers. Am J Surg Pathol 1:5–16, 1977.

Meyer EC, Liebow AA. Relationship of interstitial pneumonia, honeycombing and atypical epithelial proliferation to cancer of the lung. Cancer 18:322–351, 1965.

Miettinen OS. Screening for lung cancer: Can it be cost-effective? CMAJ 162:1431–1436, 2000.

Mills SE, Cooper PH, Walker AN, Kron IL. Atypical carcinoid tumor of the lung: A clinicopathological study of 17 cases. Am J Clin Pathol 6:643–654, 1982

Mitchell ML, King DE, Bonfiglio TA, Patten SF. Pulmonary fine needle aspiration cytopathology: A five-year correlation study. Acta Cytol 28:72–76, 1984.

Mizutani T, Maeda S, Hayakawa K, et al. Paraneoplastic cortical cerebellar degeneration: A neuropathological study of an autopsy case in comparison with cortical cerebellar degeneration in alcoholics. Acta Neuropathol (Berl) 77:206–212, 1988.

Mizutani Y, Nakajima T, Morinaga S, et al. Immunohistochemical localization of pulmonary surfactant apoproteins in various lung tumors: Special reference to nonmucus producing lung adenocarcinomas. Cancer 61:532–537, 1988.

Moll R, Wu XR, Lin JH, Sun TT. Uroplakins, specific membrane proteins of urothelial umbrella cells, as histological markers of metastatic transitional cell carcinomas. Am J Pathol 147:1383–1397, 1995.

Moloo Z, Finley RJ, Lefcoe MS, et al. Possible spread of bronchogenic carcinoma to the chest wall after a transthoracic fine needle aspiration biopsy: A case report. Acta Cytol 29:167–169, 1985.

Montes M, Binette JP, Chaudhry AP, et al. Clara cell adenocarcinoma: Light and electron microscope studies. Am J Surg Pathol 1:245–253, 1977.

Naib ZM. Giant cell carcinoma of the lung: Cytological study of the exfoliated cells in sputum and bronchial washings. Dis Chest 40:69–73, 1961.

Naib ZM, Goldstein AA. Exfoliative cytology of a case of bronchial granular cell myoblastoma. Dis Chest 42:645–647, 1962.

Nakajima M, Kasai T, Hashimoto H, et al. Sarcomatoid carcinoma of the lung: A clinicopathologic study of 37 cases. Cancer 86:608–616, 1999.

Nascimento AG, Unni KK, Bernatz PE. Sarcomas of the lung. Mayo Clin Proc 57:355–359, 1982.

Nash FA, Morgan JM, Tomkins JG. South London Cancer Study. Br Med J 2:715–721, 1968.

Nasiell M. Abnormal columnar cells in sputum and bronchial epithelium: A study of lung cancer and non-cancer cases. Acta Cytol 11:397–402, 1967.

Nasiell M. Metaplasia and atypical metaplasia in the bronchial epithelium: A histopathologic and cytopathologic study. Acta Cytol 10:421–427, 1966.

Nasiell M, Kato H, Auer G, Zetterberg A, et al. Cytomorphological grading and Feulgen DNA analysis of metaplastic and neoplastic bronchial cells. Cancer 41:1512–1521, 1978.

Nasiell M, Sinner W, Tornvall G, et al. Clinically occult lung cancer with positive sputum cytology and primary negative radiological findings. Scand J Respir Dis 58:1–11, 1977.

Nathanson L, Hall TC. Introduction: Paraneoplastic syndromes. Semin Oncol 24:265–268, 1997.

Ng ABP, Horak GC. Factors significant in the diagnostic accuracy of lung cytology in bronchial washings and sputum. I. Bronchial washings. II. Sputum samples. Acta Cytol 27391–27402, 1983.

Nguyen G-K. Cytopathology of pulmonary carcinoid tumors in sputum and bronchial brushings. Acta Cytol 39:1152–1160, 1995.

Nguyen G-K. Aspiration biopsy cytology of benign clear cell ("sugar") tumor of the lung. Acta Cytol 33:511–515, 1989.

Nicol KK, Geisinger KR. The cytomorphology of pleuropulmonary blastoma. Arch Pathol Lab Med 124:416–418, 2000.

Nicol KK, Ward WG, Savage PD, Kilpatrick SE. Fine-needle aspiration biopsy of skeletal versus extraskeletal osteosarcoma. Cancer 84:176–185. 1998.

Niemann TH, Bottles K. Cytologic diagnosis of metastatic epithelioid sarcoma: A cytologic mimic of squamous cell carcinoma. Am J Clin Pathol 100:171–173, 1993.

Nitta N, Takahashi M, Murata K, Morita R. Ultra low-dose helical CT of the chest: Evaluation in clinical cases. Radiat Med 17:1–7, 1999

Noguchi M, Morikawa A, Kawasaki M, et al. Small adenocarcinoma of the lung: Histologic characteristics and prognosis. Cancer 75:2844–2852, 1995.

Nomori H, Shimosato Y, Kodama T, et al. Subtypes of small cell carcinoma of the lung: Morphometric, ultrastructural, and immunohistochemical analyses. Hum Pathol 17:604–613, 1986.

Non DP Jr, Lang WR, Patchefsky A, Takeda M. Pulmonary blastoma: Cytopathologic and histopathologic findings. Acta Cytol 20:381–386, 1976.

O'Donnell RH, Mann RH, Grosh JL. Asbestos, an extrinsic factor in the pathogenesis of bronchogenic carcinoma and mesothelioma. Cancer 19:1143–1148, 1966.

Ogata T, Endo K. Clara cell granules of peripheral lung carcinoma. Cancer 54:1634–1644, 1984.

Ogino S, al-Kaisi N, Abdul-Karim FW. Cytopathology of oncocytic carcinoid tumor of the lung mimicking granular cell tumor: A case report. Acta Cytol 44:247–250, 2000.

Ozzello L, Stout AP. The epithelial origin of giant cell carcinoma of the lung confirmed by tissue culture: Report of a case. Cancer 14:1052–1056, 1961.

Pairolero PC, Williams DE, Bergstralh EJ, et al. Postsurgical stage 1 bronchogenic carcinoma: Morbid implications of recurrent disease. Ann Thorac Surg 38:331–338, 1984.

Paksoy N, Elpek O, Ozbilim G, et al. Bronchioloalveolar carcinoma in progressive systemic sclerosis. Acta Cytol 39:1182–1186, 1995.

Paladugu R, Benfield J, Pak H, et al. Bronchopulmonary Kulchitsky cell carcinomas: A new classification scheme for typical and atypical carcinoids. Cancer 55:1303–1311, 1985.

Papanicolaou GN, Koprowska I. Carcinoma in situ of right lower bronchus: Case report. Cancer 4:141–146, 1951.

Parafiniuk M, Pankowski J, Janowski H, Wojcik J. Cause of rare pulmonary tumors. Two cases of pulmonary carcinosarcoma. Pneumonol Alergol Pol 62:513–519, 1994.

Parayno PP, August CZ. Malignant granular cell tumor. Report of a case with DNA ploidy analysis. Arch Pathol Lab Med 120:296–300, 1996.

Parkash V, Gerald W, Parma A, et al. Desmoplastic small round cell tumor of the pleura. Am J Surg Pathol 19:659–665, 1995.

Parkin DM, Moss SM. Lung cancer screening. Improved survival but no reduction in deaths—the role of "overdiagnosis." Cancer 89(Suppl):2369–2376, 2000.

Patz EF Jr, Goodman PC, Bepler G. Screening for lung cancer. N Engl J Med 343:1627–1633, 2000.

Patz EF Jr, Rossi S, Harpole DH Jr, et al. Correlation of tumor size and survival in patients with stage 1A non-small cell lung cancer. Chest 117:1568–1571, 2000.

Pearson FG, Thompson DW. Occult carcinoma of the bronchus. Can Med Assoc J 94:825–833, 1966.

Perry MC, Eaton WL, Propert KJ, et al. Chemotherapy with or without radiation therapy in limited small-cell carcinoma of the lung. N Engl J Med 316:912–918, 1987.

Pfitzer P, Knoblich PG. Giant carcinoma cells of bronchogenic origin. Acta Cytol 12:256–261, 1968.

Pilotti S, Rilke F, Lombardi L. Pulmonary carcinoid with glandular features. Report of 2 cases with positive fine needle aspiration cytology. Acta Cytol 27:511–514, 1983.

Pilotti S, Rilke F, Gribaudi G, Ravasi GL. Sputum cytology for the diagnosis of carcinoma of the lung. Acta Cytol 26:649–654, 1982.

Pilotti S, Rilke F, Gribaudi G, et al. Transthoracic fine needle aspiration biopsy in pulmonary lesions: Updated results. Acta Cytol 28:225–232, 1984.

Pilotti S, Rilke F, Gribaudi G, Spinelli P. Cytologic diagnosis of pulmonary carcinoma on bronchoscopic brushing material. Acta Cytol 26:655–660, 1982.

Powers CN, Elbadawi AC. "Cercariform" cells: A clue to the cytodiagnosis of transitional cell origin of metastatic neoplasms? Diagn Cytopathol 13:15–21, 1995.

Qiao,YL, Tockman MS, Li I, et al. A case-cohort study of an early biomarker of lung cancer in a screening cohort of Yunnan tin miners in China. Cancer Epidemiol Biomarkers Prev 6:893–900, 1997.

Raeburn C, Spencer H. A study of the origin and development of lung cancer. Thorax 8:1, 1953.

Ramzy J. Pulmonary hamartomas. Cytologic appearance of fine needle aspiration biopsy. Acta Cytol 2015–2019, 1976.

Ranchod RM, Levine GD. Spindle-cell carcinoid tumors of the lung: A clinicopathologic study of 35 cases. Am J Surg Pathol 4:315–331, 1980.

Reale FR, Variakojis D, Compton J, Bibbo M. Cytodiagnosis of Hodgkin's disease in sputum specimens. Acta Cytol 27:258–261, 1983.

Reid JD, Carr AH. The validity and value of histological and cytological classifications of lung cancer. Cancer 14:673–698, 1961.

Renshaw AA, Madge R. Cercariform cells for helping distinguish transitional cell carcinoma from non-small cell lung carcinoma in fine needle aspirates. Acta Cytol 41:999–1007, 1997.

Renshaw AA, Madge R, Granter SR. Intracytoplasmic eosinophilic inclusions (Melamed-Wolinska bodies). Association with metastatic transitional cell carcinoma in pleural fluid. Acta Cytol 41:995–998, 1997.

Risse EKJ, Vooijs GP, van't Hof M. The quality and diagnostic outcome of postbronchoscopy sputum. Acta Cytol 31:166–169, 1988.

Risse EKJ, Vooijs GP, van't Hof MA. Diagnostic significance of "severe dysplasis" in sputum cytology. Acta Cytol 32:630–634, 1988.

Robbins E, Silverman G. Coexistent bronchogenic carcinoma and active pulmonary tuberculosis. Cancer 2:65–97, 1949.

Roger V, Nasiell M, Linden M, Enstad I. Cytologic differential diagnosis of bronchioloalveolar carcinoma and bronchogenic adenocarcinoma. Acta Cytol 20:303–307, 1976.

Roggli VL, Greenberg SD, eds. Pathology of asbestos associated diseases. Boston, Little Brown and Company, 1992.

Roggli VL, Vollmer RT, Greenberg SD, et al. Lung cancer heterogeneity: A blinded and randomized study of 100 consecutive cases. Hum Pathol 16:569–579, 1985.

Roglic M, Jukic S, Damjanoc I. Cytology of the solitary papilloma of the bronchus. Acta Cytol 19:11–13, 1975.

Rohwedder JJ, Weatherbee L. Multiple primary bronchogenic carcinoma with a review of the literature. Am Rev Respir Dis 109:435–445, 1974.

Rosen SE, Vonderheid EC, Koprowska I. Mycosis fungoides with pulmonary involvement. Cytopathologic findings. Acta Cytol 28:51–57, 1984.

Rosenblum MK. Paraneoplastic and autoimmunologic injury of the nervous system: The anti-Hu syndrome. Brain Pathol 3:199–212, 1993.

Rosenman KD, Stanbury M. Risk of lung cancer among former chromium smelter workers. Am J Ind Med 29:491–500, 1996.

Rosenthal DL. Cytopathology of Pulmonary Disease (Monographs in Clinical Cytology). Basel, S Karger, 1988.

Rosenthal DL, Wallace JM. Fine needle aspiration of pulmonary lesion via fiberoptic bronchoscopy. Acta Cytol 28:203–210, 1984.

Rossle R. Die Narbenkrebse der lungen. Schweiz Med Wschr 39:1200, 1943.

Rubel LR, Reynolds RE. Cytologic description of squamous cell papilloma of the respiratory tract. Acta Cytol 23:227–230, 1979.

Russell WO, Neidhardt HW, Mountain CF, et al. Cytodiagnosis of lung cancer: A report of a four-year laboratory clinical, and statistical study with a review of the literature on lung cancer and pulmonary cytology. Acta Cytol 7:1–44, 1963.

Sacchini V, Galimberti V, Marchini S, Luini A. Percutaneous transthoracic needle aspiration biopsy: A case report of implantation metastasis. Eur J Surg Oncol 15:179–183, 1989.

Saccomanno G, Archer VE, Auerbach O, et al. Development of carcinoma of the lung as reflected in exfoliated cells. Cancer 33:256–270, 1974.

Saccomanno G, Ruth GC, Auerbach O, Kuschner M. Relationship of radioactive radon daughters and cigarette smoking in the genesis of lung cancer in uranium miners. Cancer 62:1402–1408, 1988.

Saccomanno G, Saunders RP, Archer VE, et al. Cancer of the lung: The cytology of sputum prior to the development of carcinoma. Acta Cytol 9:413–423, 1965.

Saccomanno G, Saunders RP, Archer VE, et al. Possibilities of early diagnosis of bronchogenic carcinoma. Acta Cytol 10:351–357, 1975.

Saccomanno G, Saunders RP, Ellis H, et al. Concentrations of carcinoma or atypical cells in sputum. Acta Cytol 7:305–310, 1963.

Sanderson DR, Fontana RS, Woolner LB, et al. Bronchoscopic localization of radiographically occult lung cancer. Chest 65:608–612, 1974.

Santos-Briz A, Terron J, Sastre R, et al. Oncocytoma of the lung. Cancer 40:1330–1336, 1977.

Sargent EN, Turner AF, Gordonson J, Schwinn CP, Pashky O. Percutaneous pulmonary needle biopsy. Report of 350 patients. Am J Roentgenol Radium Ther Nucl Med 122:758–768, 1974.

Sawada K, Fukuma S, Seki Y, et al. Cytological features of primary leiomyosarcoma of the lung; Report of a case diagnosed by bronchial brushing procedure. Acta Cytol 21:770–773, 1977.

Schenk DA, Bryan CL, Bower JH, Myers DL. Transbronchial needle aspiration in the diagnosis of bronchogenic carcinoma. Chest 87:83–85, 1987.

Schreiber H, Saccomanno G, Martin DH, Brennan L. Sequential cytologic changes during development of respiratory tract tumors induced in hamsters by benzo[a]pyrene ferric oxide. Cancer Res 34:689–698, 1974.

Schreiber H, Schreiber K, Martin DH. Experimental tumor induction in a circumscribed region of the hamster trachea: Correlation of histology and exfoliative cytology. JNCI 54:187–197, 1975.

Schulster PL, Khan FA, Azueta V. Asymptomatic pulmonary granular cell tumor presenting as a coin lesion. Chest 68:256–258, 1975.

Selikoff IJ, Churg J, Hammond EC. Asbestos exposure and neoplasia. JAMA 188:22–46, 1964.

Seo IS, Azzarelli B, Warner TF, et al. Multiple visceral and cutaneous granular cell tumors: Ultrastructural and immunocytochemical evidence of Schwann cell origin. Cancer 53:2104–2110, 1984.

Shaheen K, Oertel YC. Mycosis fungoides cells in sputum: A case report. Acta Cytol 28:483–486, 1984.

Sharma SK, Panda JN, Dawar R, Gullena JS. Hodgkin's disease with pulmonary involvement. Jpn J Med 25:73–74, 1986.

Shimosato Y, Kodamo T, Kameya T. Morphogenesis of peripheral type adenocarcinoma of the lung. Chapt. 3. *In* Shimosato Y, Melamed M, Nettesheim P (eds). Morphogenesis of Lung Cancer. Boca Raton, CRC Press, 1982.

Sidhu GS, Forrester EM. Glycogen-rich Clara cell-type bronchioloalveolar carcinoma. Cancer 40:2209–2215, 1977.

Silverman JF, Landreneau RJ, Sturgis CD, et al. Small cell variant of synovial sarcoma: Fine-needle aspiration with ancillary features and potential diagnostic pitfalls. Diagn Cytopathol 23:118–123, 2000.

Singh G, Katyal SL, Torikata C. Carcinoma of type II pneumocytes. Am J Pathol 102:195–208, 1981.

Sinner WN. Fine needle biopsy of Hamartomas of the lung. AJR 138:65–69, 1982.

Sinner WN, Zajicek J. Implantation metastasis after percutaneous transthoracic needle aspiration biopsy. Acta Radiol Diag 17:473–480, 1976.

Sklar JL, Chung A, Bensch KG. Oncocytic carcinoid tumor of the lung. Am J Surg Pathol 4:287–292, 1980.

Smith AR, Gilbert CF, Strausbach P, Silverman JF. Fine needle aspiration cytology of a mediastinal granular cell tumor with histologic confirmation and ancillary studies: A case report. Acta Cytol 42:1011–1016, 1998.

Smith JH, Frable WJ. Adenocarcinoma of the lung. Cytologic correlation with histologic types. Acta Cytol 18:316–320, 1974.

Smoking and Health. Report of the Advisory Committee to the Surgeon General of the Public Health Service. Public Health Service Publication No 1103: US Government Printing Office, Washington DC, 1964.

Sobue T, Ajiki W, Tsukuma H, et al. Trends of lung cancer incidence by histologic type: A population-based study in Osaka, Japan. Jpn J Cancer Res 90:6–15, 1999.

Solomon DA, Solliday NH, Gracey DR. Cytology in fiberoptic bronchoscopy. Comparison of bronchial brushing, washing and postbronchoscopy sputum. Chest 65:616–619, 1974.

Sone S, Takashima S, Li F, et al. Mass screening for lung cancer with mobile spiral computed tomography scanner. Lancet 351:1242–1245, 1998.

Souza RC, Peasley ED, Takaro T. Pulmonary blastomas: A distinctive group of carcinosarcoma of lung. Ann Thorac Surg 1:259–267, 1965.

Spahr J, Draffin RM, Johnston WW. Cytopathologic findings in pulmonary blastoma. Acta Cytol 23:454–459, 1979.

Spencer H. Pathology of the Lung. 4th ed. New York, Pergamon Press, 1985.

Spencer H. Pulmonary blastomas. J Pathol Bacteriol 85:161–165, 1961.

Spitz MR, Wei Q, Guojun L, Wu X. Genetic susceptibility to tobacco carcinogenesis. Cancer Invest 17:645–659, 1999.

Spjut HJ, Fier DJ, Ackerman LV. Exfoliative cytology and pulmonary cancer: A histopathological and cytologic correlation. J Thorac Surg 30:90–107, 1955.

Springmeyer SC, Hackman R, Carlson JJ, McClellan JE. Bronchioloalveolar cell carcinoma diagnosed by bronchoalveolar lavage. Chest 83:278–279, 1983.

Stanley C, Wolf P, Haghighi P. Reed-Sternberg cells in sputum from a patient with Hodgkin's disease: A case report. Acta Cytol 37:90–92, 1993.

Stanley MW, Henry-Stanley MJ, Gajl-Peczalska DJ, Bitterman PB. Hyperplasia of type II pneumocytes in acute lung injury. Cytologic findings of sequential bronchoalveolar lavage. Am J Clin Pathol 97:669–677, 1992.

Steenland K, Loomis D, Shy C, Simonsen N. Review of occupational lung carcinogens. Am J Ind Med 29:474–490, 1996.

Steffelaar JW, Nap M, von Haelst UJ. Malignant granular cell tumor. Report of a case with special reference to carcinoembryonic antigen. Am J Surg Pathol 6:665–672, 1982.

Sternberg WH, Sidransky H, Ochsner S. Primary malignant lymphomas of lung. Cancer 12:806–819, 1959.

Strady C, Ricciarelli A, Nasca S, et al. Carcinomatous meningitis and solid tumors. Oncol Rep 7:203–207, 2000.

Stremlau A, Gissmann L, Ikenberg H, et al. Human papillomavirus type 16 related DNA in an anaplastic carcinoma of the lung. Cancer 55:1737–1740, 1985.

Sturgis CD, Nassar DL, D'Antonio JA, Raab SS. Cytologic features useful for distinguishing small cell from non-small cell carcinoma in bronchial brush and wash specimens. Am J Clin Pathol 114:197–202, 2000.

Sun JD, Weatherly RA, Koopmann CF Jr, Carey TE. Mucosal swabs detect HPV in laryngeal papillomatosis patients but not family members. Int J Pediatr Ortorhinolaryngol 53:95–103, 2000.

Suprun H, Koss LG. The cytological study of sputum and bronchial washings in Hodgkin's disease with pulmonary involvement. Cancer 17:674–680, 1964.

Suster S. Primary sarcomas of the lung. Semin Diagn Pathol 12:140–157, 1995.

Syrjäanen K, Syrjäanen S, Kellokoski J, et al. Human papillomavirus (HPV) type 6 and 16 DNA sequences in bronchial squamous cell carcinomas demonstrated by in situ DNA hybridization. Lung 167:33–42, 1989.

Szyfelbein WM, Ross JS. Carcinoids, atypical carcinoids and small-cell carcinomas of the lung. Differential diagnosis of fine-needle aspiration biopsy specimen. Diagn Cytopathol 4:1–8, 1988.

Tabei SZ, Abdollahi MD, Nili F. Diagnosis of metastatic adamantinoma of the tibia by pulmonary brushing cytology. Acta Cytol 32:579–581, 1988.

Takeda M, Burechailo FA. Smooth muscle cells in sputum. Acta Cytol 13:696–699, 1969.

Takeda S, Nanjo S, Nakamoto K, et al. Carcinosarcoma of the lung. Report of a case and review of the literature. Respiration 61:113–116, 1994.

Talbott JH, Barrocas M. Carcinoma of the lung in progressive systemic sclerosis: A tabular review of the literature and a detailed report of the roentgenographic changes in two cases. Semin Arthritis Rheum 9:191–217, 1980.

Talcott JA, Thurber WA, Kantor AF, et al. Asbestos-associated diseases in cohort of cigarette-filter workers. N Engl J Med 321:1220–1223, 1989.

Tao LC, Chamberlain DW, Delarue NC, et al. Cytologic diagnosis of radiographically occult squamous cell carcinoma of the lung. Cancer 50:1580, 1982.

Tao L-C, Weisbrod GL, Pearson FG, et al. Cytologic diagnosis of bronchioalveolar carcinoma by fine-needle aspiration biopsy. Cancer 57:1564–1570, 1986.

Tassoni EM. Pools of lymphocytes: Significance in pulmonary secretions. Acta Cytol 7:168–173, 1963.

Tateishi R, Hattori S. Ultrastructure of large cell and giant cell carcinomas in the lung in relation to histogenesis. Chapt. 3. *In* Shimosato Y, Melamed MR, Nettesheim P (eds). Morphogenesis of Lung Cancer. Boca Raton, CRC Press, 1982.

Thomas L, Risbaud M, Gabriel JB, et al. Cytomorphology of granular-cell tumor of the bronchus: A case report. Acta Cytol 28:129–132, 1984.

Thunnissen FBJM, Arends JW, Buchholtz RTF, ten Velde G. Fine needle aspiration cytology of inflammatory pseudotumor of the lung (plasma cell granuloma). Report of four cases. Acta Cytol 33:917–921, 1989.

Tockman MS, Mulshine JL, Piantadosi S, et al. Prospective detection of preclinical lung cancer: Results from two studies of heterogeneous nuclear ribonucleoprotein A2/B1 overexpression. Clin Cancer Res 3:2237–2246, 1997.

Tockman MS. Advances in sputum analysis for screening and early detection of lung cancer. Cancer Control 7:19–24, 2000.

Travis WD, Colby TV, Corrin B, et al. Histological typing of lung and pleural tumours. World Health Organization International Histological Classification of Tumours, 3rd ed. Berlin, Springer, 1999.

Trillo A, Guha, A. Solitary condylomatous papilloma of the bronchus. Arch Pathol Lab Med 112:731–733, 1988

Tsukada H, Satou T, Iwashima A, Souma T. Diagnostic accuracy of CT-guided automated needle biopsy of lung nodules. Am J Roentgenol 175:239–243, 2000.

Turnbull AD, Huvos AG, Goodner JT, Foote FW Jr. Mucoepidermoid tumors of bronchial glands. Cancer 28:539–544, 1971.

Ueno M, Fujiyama J, Yamazaki I, et al. Cytology of primary pulmonary meningioma: Report of the first multiple case. Acta Cytol 42:1424–1430, 1998.

Umiker W, Storey C. Bronchogenic carcinoma in situ: Report of case with positive biopsy, cytological examination, and lobectomy. Cancer 5:369–374, 1952.

Unterman DH, Reingold IM. The occurrence of psammoma bodies in papillary adenocarcinoma of the lung. Am J Clin Pathol 57:297–302, 1972.

Usuda K, Saito Y, Imai T, et al. Inflammatory pseudotumor of the lung diagnosed as granulomatous lesion by preoperative brushing cytology: A case report. Acta Cytol 34:685–689, 1990.

Valaitis J, McGrew EA, Chomet B, et al. Bronchogenic carcinoma in situ in asymptomatic high risk population of smokers. J Thorac Cardiovasc Surg 57:325–332, 1969.

Valicenti JV, Daniell C, Gobien RP. Thin needle aspiration cytology of benign intrathoracic lesions. Acta Cytol 25:659–664, 1981.

Vernon SE. Cytodiagnosis of "signet-ring" cell lymphoma. Acta Cytol 25:291–294, 1981.

Vincent RG, Pickren JW, Lane WW, et al. The changing histopathology of lung cancer: A review of 1682 cases. Cancer 39:1647–1655, 1977.

Wandall HH. Study on neoplastic cells in sputum: As contribution to diagnosis of primary lung cancer. Acta Chir Scand 93(Suppl):1–143, 1944.

Wang KP, Marsh BR, Summer WR, et al. Transbronchial needle aspiration for diagnosis of lung cancer. Chest 80:48–50, 1981.

Wang SE, Nieberg RK. Fine needle aspiration cytology of sclerosing hemangioma of the lung: A mimicker of bronchioloalveolar carcinoma. Acta Cytol 30:51–54, 1986.

Weiss W, Boucot KR, Seidman H. The Philadelphia Pulmonary Neoplasm Research Project. Clin Chest Med 3:243–256, 1982.

Whitwell F. Tumourlets of the lung. J Pathol Bact 70:529–541, 1955.

Wiatrowska BA, Yazdi HM, Matzinger FR, MacDonald LL. Fine needle aspiration biopsy of pulmonary hamartomas. Radiologic, cytologic and immunocytochemical study of 15 cases. Acta Cytol 39:1167–1174, 1995.

Wierman WH, McDonald JR, Clagett OT. Occult carcinoma of major bronchi. Surgery 35:335–345, 1954.

Wongsurakiat P, Wongbunnate S, Dejsomritrutai W, et al. Diagnostic value of bronchoalveolar lavage and postbronchoscopic sputum cytology in peripheral lung cancer. Respirology 3:131–137, 1998.

Woolner LB, McDonald JR. Diagnosis of carcinoma of lung; Value of cytologic study of sputum and bronchial secretions. JAMA 139:497–502, 1949.

Woolner LB, Andersen HA, Bernatz PE. "Occult" carcinoma of bronchus: Study of 15 cases of in situ or early invasive bronchogenic carcinoma. Dis Chest 37:278–288, 1966.

Woolner LB, David E, Fontana RS, et al. In situ and early invasive bronchogenic carcinoma. Report of 28 cases with postoperative survival data. J Thorac Cardiovasc Surg 60:275–290, 1970.

Woolner LB, Fontana RS, Bernatz PE. Early bronchogenic carcinoma. Problems in detection, localization, and treatment. Surg Clin N Am 53:761–768, 1973.

Woolner LB, Fontana RS, Cortese DA, et al. Roentgenologically occult lung cancer: Pathologic findings and frequency of multicentricity during a 10 year period. Mayo Clin Proc 59:453–466, 1984.

Wu RL, Osman I, Wu XR, et al. Uroplakin II gene is expressed in transitional cell carcinoma but not in bilharzial bladder squamous cell carcinoma: Alternative pathways of bladder epithelial differentiation and tumor formation. Cancer Res 58:1291–1297, 1998.

Wynder EL, Graham EA. Tobacco smoking as a possible etiologic factor in bronchiogenic carcinoma: A study of six hundred and eighty-four proved cases. JAMA 143:329–336, 1950.

Yankelevitz DF, Reeves AP, Kostis WJ, et al. Small pulmonary nodules: Volumetrically determined growth rates based on CT evaluation. Radiology 217:251–256, 2000.

Zaharopoulos P, Wong JY, Lamke CR. Endometrial stromal sarcoma. Cytology of pulmonary metastasis including ultrastructural study. Acta Cytol 26:49–54, 1982.

Zaharopoulos P, Wong JY, Stewart GD. Cytomorphology of the variants of small cell carcinoma of the lung. Acta Cytol 26:800–808, 1982.

Zakowski MF, Gatscha RM, Zaman MB. Negative predictive value of pulmonary fine needle aspiration cytology. Acta Cytol 36:283–286, 1992.

Zaman MB, Hajdu SI, Melamed MR, Watson RC. Transthoracic aspiration cytology of pulmonary lesions. Semin Diagn Pathol 3:176–187, 1986.

Zaman SS, van Hoeven KH, Slott S, Gupta PK. Distinction between bronchioloalveolar carcinoma and hyperplastic pulmonary proliferations: A cytologic and morphometric analysis. Diagn Cytopathol 16:396–401, 1997.

Zarbo RJ, Fenoglio-Preiser CM. Interinstitutional database for comparison of performance in lung fine-needle aspiration cytology: A College of American Pathologists Q-Probe Study of 5264 cases with histologic correlation. Arch Pathol Lab Med 116:463–470, 1992.

Zavala DC, Schoell JE. Ultrathin needle aspiration of the lung in infections and malignant disease. Am Rev Respir Dis 123:125–131, 1981.

Epithelial Lesions of the Oral Cavity, Larynx, Trachea, Nasopharynx, and Paranasal Sinuses

HISTOLOGIC RECALL

As briefly described in Chapter 19, the **oral cavity** (including the palate, tongue, pharynx, and floor of the mouth) is lined by **squamous epithelium with varying degrees of** surface keratinization. The **surface of the larynx,** facing the oral cavity, is also lined by **squamous epithelium.** The **inner aspects of the larynx** (including the vocal cords) are lined by a **nonkeratinizing epithelium composed of five to six layers of parabasal and intermediate squamous cells. Lower aspects of the larynx** and the adjacent **trachea** are, in part, lined by similar **nonkeratinizing epithelium** and, in part, **by ciliated epithelium, identical to bronchial epithelium,** described in Chapter 19. The **paranasal sinuses and the nasopharynx** are principally lined by an epithelium composed of cuboidal and columnar ciliated cells. **All ciliated epithelia contain mucus-producing goblet cells and may undergo squamous metaplasia,** as described in Chapter 19.

Minor salivary glands are dispersed throughout the oral cavity and adjacent organs. The tumors of these glands can be sampled only by aspiration biopsy. Aspiration biopsy may also be used for the study of deeply seated tumors of the various component organs and bony structures (Castelli et al, 1993; Das et al, 1993; Gunhan et al, 1993; Mondal and Raychoudhuri, 1993; Mathew et al, 1997; Domanski and Akerman, 1998; Shah et al, 2000). These issues are discussed in Chapters 32 and 36.

ORAL CAVITY

SAMPLING TECHNIQUES

Lesions of the oral cavity **can be sampled by smears obtained by scraping.** In most cases, the scrape smears may be obtained with a simple tongue depressor or a small curette. For oral lesions covered with **thick layers of keratin,** a more vigorous scraping with a **sharp metallic instrument may be advisable. A brush specifically designed to sample oral lesions** was described by Sciubba (1999).

INDICATIONS FOR CYTOLOGIC EXAMINATION

The principal application of cytologic techniques to epithelial lesions of the oral cavity is the diagnosis of occult carcinomas, not identified or not suspected on clinical inspection. As will be set forth in this chapter, cytologic methods are particularly valuable in screening for occult oral cancer, but may occasionally contribute to the diagnosis of early or unsuspected cancers of adjacent organs. King (1962) briefly summarized the early history of the application of cytologic techniques to lesions of the oral cavity.

CYTOLOGY OF ORAL SQUAMOUS EPITHELIUM IN THE ABSENCE OF DISEASE

Squamous Epithelial Cells

Normal squamous epithelium of the oral cavity sheds **superficial and intermediate squamous cells,** identical to squamous cells of the vagina and cervix, except that nuclear pyknosis is not observed. Such cells occur either singly or in clusters and are identical with squamous cells that are found in specimens of sputum and of saliva (see Chap. 19).

A **longitudinal condensation of the nuclear chromatin in the form of a nuclear bar with lateral extensions,** similar to that observed in **Anitschkow cells in the myocardium** in rheumatic heart disease, has been recorded in superficial squamous cells by Wood et al (1975). A similar cell change was also illustrated in the *Atlas of Oral Cytology* by Medak et al (1970). Such cells are commonly seen in smears of the **mucosal surface of the lower lip and the adjacent floor of the mouth** in perfectly healthy people (Fig. 21-1A). The change is probably related to "nuclear creases" but its significance is unknown. Similar cells may be observed in mesothelial cells in the pericardium surface of the conjunctiva and in other organs.

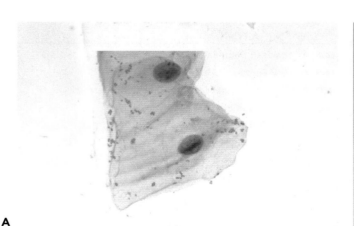

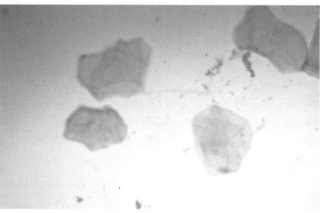

A

B

Figure 21-1   Normal cells in oral scrapings. A. Scrape smear of labial fold of lower lip. The squamous cell shows a nuclear bar with lateral extensions (caterpillar nuclei) similar to Anitschkow cells. B. Anucleated squamous cell from the palate. (A: High magnification.)

Fully keratinized squamous superficial cells without visible nuclei (keratinized squames) are a common component of oral smears, especially from the palate, and do not necessarily reflect a significant abnormality (Fig. 21-1B). All stages of transition between nonkeratinized and keratinized cells may be observed. Smaller **parabasal squamous cells** may be observed if the surface of the epithelium is vigorously scraped, or if an epithelial defect, such as an ulceration, is present.

In general, the cytology of the oral cavity in the absence of disease is simple and monotonous.

Squamous oral cells carry on their membranes **blood group antigens** (for review, see Dabelsteen et al, 1974).

Other Cells

Mucus-producing columnar cells originating in the **nasopharynx or the salivary gland ducts** may occasionally be observed. A vigorous scrape of the **tonsillar area** or the **base of the tongue** may result in **shedding of lymphocytes,** singly or in clusters.

Oral Flora

Oral flora, especially in patients with poor oral hygiene, is rich in a variety of saprophytic fungi and bacteria. A protozoon, *Entamoeba gingivalis,* is fairly common (Fig. 21-2A). It is a multinucleated organism larger than *Amoeba histolytica,* from which it differs because it does not phagocytize

red blood cells (see Chaps. 10 and 24). The presence of these organisms does not necessarily indicate an inflammatory process in the oral cavity. An unusual organism, *Simonsiella* species, was described in smears of oropharynx, sputum, and gastric aspirates by Greenebaum et al (1988). The large bacteria form caterpillar-like chains, each composed of 10 to 12 individual bacteria. The bacterial chains are readily observed overlying squamous cells (Fig. 21-2B). The organism is nonpathogenic, most likely to be observed in mouths of people with rich dietary intake, particularly fat and proteins.

Buccal Squamous Cells in Genetic Counseling and as a Source of DNA

Buccal smears are the cheapest and easiest-to-use laboratory test **to determine genetic sex,** by observing and counting **sex chromatin (Barr bodies) in squamous oral cells.** The Barr bodies can be recognized as a **half-moon shaped chromatin condensation at the nuclear membrane** (see Chaps. 4, 7, 8, 11, and 29). Although, theoretically, in genetic females all squamous cells with nonpyknotic, open vesicular nuclei should contain a Barr body, in practice, it can be identified in fewer than half of these cells by light microscopy of oral smears stained with Papanicolaou's stain. Further, peripherally placed **chromocenters** and **focal thickening of the nuclear membrane may mimic Barr bodies.** There is some controversy about whether the frequency of

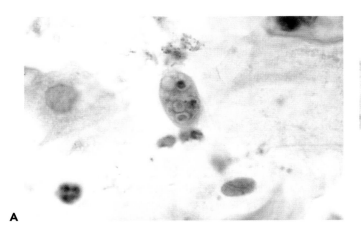

A

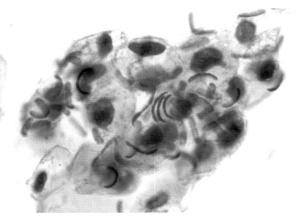

B

C

Figure 21-2   Microorganisms in oral smears. A. *Entamoeba gingivalis,* a common inhabitant of the buccal cavity. B,C. *Simonsiella* organism. Note the caterpillar-like appearance of the bacterium in C. (*A,B:* Pap stain; *C:* Methylene blue; *A,C:* Oil immersion.)

visible sex chromatin varies during the menstrual cycle (Chu et al, 1969; Ashkenazi et al, 1975).

For all practical intents and purposes, the finding of **about half a dozen or more cells** with a clear-cut single sex chromatin body is **diagnostic of the XX female chromosomal constitution** (see Chap. 4). An **excess of Barr bodies** (very rarely more than two in a cell) indicates an excess of X chromosomes (**"superfemale,"** with cells containing 47 chromosomes with XXX). Occasionally, **malignant cells may contain two or more Barr bodies,** reflecting aneuploidy.

The presence of **Barr bodies in cells in a phenotypic male strongly suggests Klinefelter's syndrome** (47 chromosomes, YXX). **The absence of Barr bodies in a phenotypic female** suggests **Turner's syndrome** or another form of gonadal dysgenesis (see Chap. 9).

Buccal cells collected in mouthwash or by other techniques may be valuable as **a source of DNA** for various tests, including person identification (Heath et al, 2001).

INFLAMMATORY DISORDERS

Acute and Chronic Inflammatory Processes

Superficial **erosion or ulceration** of the squamous epithelium occurs frequently in the course of diffuse or localized inflammatory processes or poor oral hygiene. As a result, the normal population of superficial and intermediate squamous cells in smears is partially or completely replaced by **parabasal squamous cells** from the deeper epithelial layers. Such cells **may vary in size and shape;** their principal feature is relatively **large, occasionally multiple, round or oval vesicular nuclei** of monotonous sizes. As is common in nuclei of younger cells, **chromocenters** may be readily observed against a pale nuclear background; occasionally, **small nucleoli** may be noted. The cytoplasm is often poorly preserved (Fig. 21-3). In the presence of a **diffuse stomatitis or gingivitis,** the preponderance of the irregularly shaped parabasal cells may result in an initial impression of a significant epithelial abnormality; close attention to nuclear detail will prevent an erroneous diagnosis of cancer.

In chronic ulcerative processes, **mono- and multinucleated macrophages** may also occur. Purulent exudate or **leukocytes** of various types are a common component of smears in these situations. **Plasma cells** are frequently observed, particularly in smears from the posterior oral cavity or pharynx.

Specific Inflammatory Disorders

Actinomycosis

As discussed in Chapter 19, bacteria of the *Actinomyces* species are **common saprophytes** of the oral cavity, usually found within tonsillar crypts. They may be acquired by chewing on bacterium-carrying plants, and are usually of no clinical significance. However, they may invade the traumatized or ulcerated mucosa and form an abscess or sinus

tract. As discussed in Chapters 10 and 19, the organism can be recognized in Papanicolaou-stained oral smears as masses of matted bacterial filaments. The identity of the organism should be confirmed by culture if there is clinical evidence of an inflammatory process. **The presence of *Actinomyces* in oral smears must always be correlated with clinical findings to distinguish between saprophytic and pathogenic organisms.**

Oral Herpes

This common disorder, characterized by blisters and painful ulcerations, is caused by Herpesvirus type 1 that can be identified by the **characteristic nuclear changes** described and illustrated in Chapters 10 and 19. Kobayashi et al (1998) observed the pathognomonic cell changes in smears of only 4 of 11 patients in whom the diagnosis could be confirmed by culture and, in some cases, by in situ hybridization.

Moniliasis (Thrush)

Clinically, moniliasis forms a characteristic white coating of the oral cavity. This organism may be identified with ease by finding the characteristic fungal spores and pseudohyphae (see Chap. 10). This harmless infection, previously occurring mainly in debilitated patients and diabetics, has been recognized as **one of the first manifestations of the acquired immunodeficiency syndrome (AIDS).**

Blastomycosis

Sivieri de Araujo et al (2001) described the application of oral smears for diagnosis of **Paracoccidiomycosis (South American blastomycosis),** a common and serious disorder in Latin American countries. The yeast form is described in Chapter 19.

CHANGES IN ORAL SQUAMOUS CELLS IN DEFICIENCY DISEASES

In diseases associated with **deficiencies in vitamin B_{12} and in folic acid, such as pernicious anemia,** the squamous cells of the oral mucosa may show significant **enlargement of both the nucleus and the cytoplasm** (Graham and Rheault, 1954; Massey and Rubin, 1954; Boen, 1957). Similar changes may be observed in the related disorder, **megaloblastic anemia** (Boddington and Spriggs, 1959), and in **tropical sprue** (Staats et al, 1965). The findings were documented by comparison with normal cell populations and are statistically impressive. Vitamin B_{12} and folic acid are essential for DNA synthesis. If there is an insufficient supply of either factor, the DNA synthesis becomes disturbed, with resulting cell enlargement (Beck, 1964). There is evidence that this change is not confined to the oral epithelium but may affect many tissues (Foroozan and Trier, 1967). In reference to the uterine cervix, the changes were discussed in Chapter 17. For changes in the gastrointestinal tract, see Chapter 24.

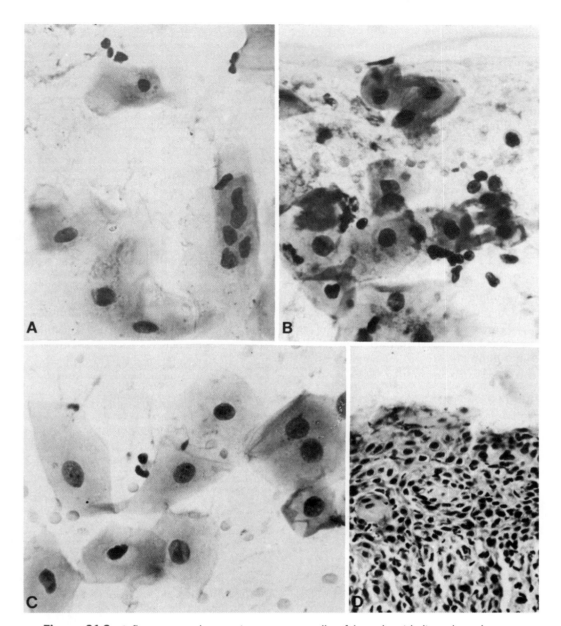

Figure 21-3 Inflammatory changes in squamous cells of buccal epithelium; buccal scrape smears. *A.* The cytoplasm is poorly preserved. A multinucleated cell may be noted. *B,C.* There is considerable variation in cell sizes, but the nuclei are, on the whole, uniform, an important diagnostic feature. Note chromocenters. Some of the dark-staining nuclei are showing early pyknosis. *D.* Histologic section of ulcerative gingivitis. Inflammatory changes in buccal epithelium. (Case courtesy of Dr. Sigmund Stahl, New York, NY.)

In my own experience, the oral smears from **patients with a variety of disorders,** probably having **malnutrition as a common denominator,** may occasionally have a population of large squamous cells with vesicular nuclei and numerous chromocenters. The finding should lead to a hematologic work-up of the patients. A marked enlargement of squamous cells may also be caused by **radiotherapy** (see below).

Nieburgs described nuclear enlargement and "discontinuous nuclear membrane" in buccal squamous cells in 72% of patients with cancer. He considered this **malignancy associated change (MAC)** as reflecting "an altered mitotic function of cells." Some of Nieburgs' material was air-dried

and the observations may be an artifact. The specific association of the buccal cell changes with cancer remains unproven. For further comments on MAC, see Chapter 7.

OTHER BENIGN DISORDERS

Benign Leukoplakia

Heavy keratin formation on the surface of oral epithelium is a common phenomenon occurring at the line of teeth occlusion, the palate, parts of gingiva, and occasionally elsewhere. The **milky white appearance** of such areas is best classified clinically as leukoplakia and appears histologically as a benign squamous epithelium, topped with layers of keratin. This **benign disorder** must be differentiated from **precancerous leukoplakia, which may have a similar clinical appearance. The differences are based on cytologic and histologic features,** discussed in detail below.

Cytology of benign leukoplakia is very simple, with **fully keratinized, yellow or yellow-orange stained cells without nuclei (anucleated squames)** being characteristic of this disorder (see Fig. 21-1B). However, **such cells may also be seen in normal oral smears;** therefore, the cytologic diagnosis should always be correlated with clinical findings.

"Hairy" Oral Leukoplakia

This is a benign lesion characteristically located on the **lateral aspect of the tongue** that was first observed in **AIDS patients.** The lesion shows vacuolization (ballooning) of squamous cells and intranuclear inclusions. The lesion was shown to be associated with **Epstein-Barr virus** (EBV) (Greenspan et al, 1986). There is no information on the cytologic presentation of this uncommon lesion.

Darier-White's Disease (Keratosis Follicularis)

Darier-White's disease is primarily a **chronic, benign, hereditary skin disease** presenting as small pink papules that may become confluent. The **oral mucosa may be involved** and show a rough pebbly surface or verrucous plaques. **Histologically,** the disease is characterized by the formation of slits or spaces within the epidermis and by **disturbances of keratinization** referred to as "corps ronds" (round bodies) and "grains." The corps ronds are miniature epithelial pearls, often containing a single large cell with a degenerated nucleus in the center. The grains are elongated, prematurely keratinized cells.

According to Witkop et al (1961), **smears from oral lesions of Darier's disease** show **parabasal squamous cells with numerous chromocenters,** corresponding to the cells lining the intraepithelial slits. Cells containing **round cytoplasmic eosinophilic inclusions,** probably corresponding to premature keratinization, may be observed. The **corps ronds** appear in smears as **epithelial pearls**—a simple one consists of a single keratinized cell within a cell; in more elaborate arrangements several keratinized cells may be found in the center of the pearl (Fig. 21-4A). **The grains** correspond to single, heavily keratinized, elongated cells.

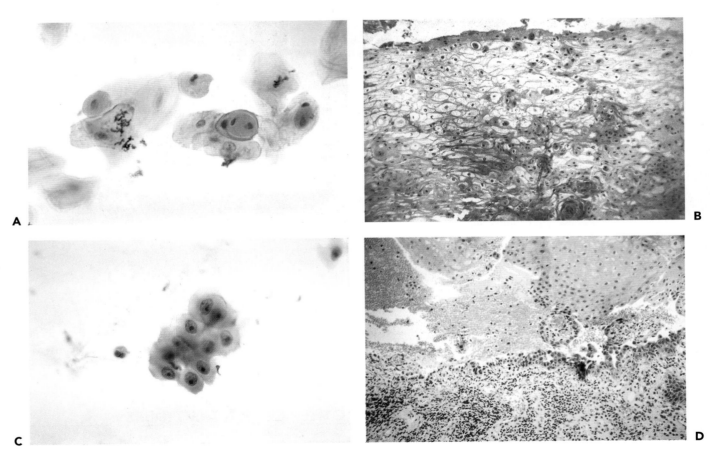

Figure 21-4   Benign abnormalities of oral epithelium. *A,B.* Hereditary intraepithelial dyskeratosis (Witkop). *A.* Typical squamous cells forming pearls (corps ronds or round bodies). Note normal size nuclei. Such cells may also be observed in Darier-White disease (see text). *B.* Tissue sections corresponding to *A* showing formation of squamous pearls (see text). *C,D.* Pemphigus vulgaris. *C* shows typical cluster of Tzanck's cells with pale nuclei containing very large nucleoli. *D.* Tissue sections corresponding to *C* showing the formation of a bulla in the oral epithelium.

Burlakow et al (1969) also pointed out that squamous cells scraped from the oral lesions may remain attached to each other by one end, not unlike leaves attached to the branch of a tree. The **"leafing out" pattern** associated with "corps ronds" and "grains" was considered by these authors as **diagnostic of this disorder.**

Hereditary Benign Intraepithelial Dyskeratosis (Witkop)

In this rare hereditary disorder, there is formation of **white spongy folds and plaques** of thickened mucosa within the oral cavity. The bulbar conjunctiva and the cornea may also be involved. The **histologic findings** in the oral epithelium disclose a marked **epithelial hyperplasia** accompanied by a **disorder of keratinization** in the form of pearl formation, which is not unlike the corps ronds of Darier's disease (Fig. 21-4B). In smears from such lesions, one sees **keratinized squamous cells** with elongated, dense nuclei and **"pearls"** composed of a large, orange-staining central degenerated cell, surrounded by a halo and an outer elongated cell with a preserved sickle-shaped nucleus (Fig. 21-4A). **Scrapings from the eye** in these patients showed identical cells. Witkop et al (1960, 1961) suggested that this cytologic presentation is diagnostic of this uncommon disorder.

White Sponge Nevus of Cannon

In this exceedingly uncommon hereditary disorder, there is a **spongy hypertrophy of squamous epithelium involving the oral, vaginal, and anal mucosa.** Abnormal keratinization may be noted. In cytologic preparations, **intracytoplasmic eosinophilic inclusions** may be observed (Witkop et al, 1960). A case of this rare entity was reported by Morris et al (1988). Electron microscopic investigation of the cytoplasmic "inclusions" disclosed bundles of "tonofilaments" of unspecified diameter, most likely representing keratin filaments, in keeping with Witkop's suggestion.

VESICLE- OR BULLAE-FORMING CONDITIONS

In a number of pathologic conditions, most of which can be diagnosed clinically, **liquid-filled blisters (vesicles) or large bullae may occur within the oral cavity.** As a general rule, the vesicles or bullae break down, and **the resulting ulcerations may become the subject of a cytologic scrutiny. One such condition is herpes simplex** of the oral cavity, which was discussed above.

With rare exceptions, the vesicle-forming disorders are manifestations of dermatologic disease and the involvement of the oral cavity is usually secondary. The most important such disorders are **erythema multiforme** and **various forms of pemphigus** (Wu et al, 2000). Specialized sources should be consulted for a detailed description and classification of these diseases.

Although **erythema multiforme** can affect the mucosa of the mouth, the diagnosis is usually based on clinical examination. There is no information on cytologic features of this transient disease, which is characterized by red plaques and small vesicles involving the skin. On the other hand, the nearly uniformly fatal **pemphigus vulgaris may have its primary manifestations in the oral cavity.**

Pemphigus Vulgaris

As has been discussed in Chapter 17, the disease is caused by **antibodies to desmoglein 3, a component protein of desmosomes, causing a disruption of desmosomes in the lower layers of the squamous epithelium,** leading to the formation of fluid-filled blisters, vesicles or bullae (Fig. 21-4D). The latter contain the atypical **cells of Tzanck,** which can be observed in smears of broken vesicles. The Tzanck cells are **squamous cells with frayed cytoplasm,** approximately of the size of large parabasal cells, occurring singly and in clusters. Occasionally, these cells show **cytoplasmic extensions. The most important feature of these cells is the presence of large, clear nuclei containing conspicuous large nucleoli that are usually single but may be multiple** (Fig. 21-4C). **These cells may be readily mistaken for cells of an adenocarcinoma.** "Cell-in-cell" arrangements, similar to those in epithelial "pearls" may be occasionally observed. **Multinucleated macrophages** may be observed in smears of treated pemphigus (Medak et al, 1970).

As a consequence of the autoimmune events, the **cells shed from pemphigus are coated with immunoglobulins.** Decker et al (1972), Lascaris (1981), and several other observers have documented, by **immunofluorescence,** the presence of coating immunoglobulins in smears from pemphigus. Faravelli et al (1984) used IgG peroxidase–antiperoxidase reaction to provide a permanent record of the immunoglobulin coat on the surfaces of acantholytic cells in smears of oral pemphigus. Harris and Mihm (1979) provided a summary of the immunologic differential diagnoses between pemphigus and other bullous lesions of the oral cavity. A current summary of the immunologic events leading to pemphigus vulgaris and related disorders may be found in an editorial by Bhattacharya and Templeton (2000). Takahashi et al (1998) reported a case wherein there was **simultaneous presence of herpes simplex and of pemphigus** in the oral cavity, both reflected in the oral smear.

Other skin diseases, too numerous to describe within the frame of this work, may involve the oral mucosa. Because the dermatologic features overshadow the oral presentation, there is no information on cytologic abnormalities in these disorders.

CHANGES CAUSED BY THERAPY

Changes in oral epithelial cells caused by **radiation therapy** were studied by Zimmer in my laboratory (unpublished) and by Umiker (1965). The changes are similar to those observed and described for the uterine cervix and consist of **marked enlargement** of squamous cells and their nuclei (see Chap. 18). They may occur either as a result of administration of the radiated beam **directly to the oral cavity or to adjacent organs, such as the neck.**

Bhattathiri et al (1998) studied the **response of cells of squamous carcinoma** of the oral cavity to radiation and reported that the **nuclear abnormalities are radiation-dose related.** As has been described in Chapter 18, the response of oral squamous epithelium to small doses of radiation was used as an index to gauge the response of squamous cancer of the uterine cervix to radiotherapy.

Changes caused by **chemotherapy** were observed by Witkop (1962). He noted nuclear degeneration and "cell-within-cell" structures following treatment with **methotrexate** and other anticancer chemotherapeutic agents. **Severe stomatitis,** caused by excessive shedding and ulceration of the buccal epithelium, is a common complication of treatment with various chemotherapeutic agents.

MALIGNANT LESIONS

Invasive Squamous Carcinoma and Its Precursors

Risk Factors

Abuse of **tobacco and alcohol** are the key epidemiologic factors in patients developing cancer of the oral cavity and the larynx. Tobacco in any form, such as pipe-, cigar-, or cigarette smoking, reverse smokers (people holding the burning end of a cigarette in their mouth), betel-nut chewers (tobacco powder is often wrapped inside the betel leaf) represent high-risk populations. The latter two forms of tobacco use are seen mainly in India and other parts of Southeast Asia. It is not known why alcohol abuse contributes to oral carcinogenesis. In the United States, African-Americans appear to have a higher risk of oral squamous cancer than people of other ethnic backgrounds (Skarsgard et al, 2000).

The presence **of human papillomavirus (HPV)** in oral cancer has been suspected for some years (Syrjänen, 1987) and has now been documented in benign and malignant lesions of the oral cavity. Garelick and Taichman (1991) observed HPV types 2, 4, 6, 11, 13, and 32 in the benign lesions, including leukoplakia, and HPV types 16 and 18 in oral carcinomas. Paz et al (1997) observed HPV sequences in only 15% of squamous cancers of the esophagus and the head and neck area. HPV was mainly observed in tumors of the tonsillar area and in some metastases. The presence of HPV had no prognostic significance. Mork et al (2001) considered infection with HPV type 16 as a risk factor in squamous cancer of the head and neck. These authors suggested oral sex as a possible source of virus. El-Mofty and Lu (2003) reported the presence of HPV type 16 only in **squamous carcinoma of the palatine tonsil** and considered this disease to be a distinct entity in patients age 40 or younger.

Clinical Aspects and Histology

Invasive squamous carcinoma is the most common malignant lesion of the oral cavity. The disease may occur in the epithelium of the **mouth, tongue, cheek, palate, tonsils, and pharynx.** Most patients with invasive squamous carcinomas show **ulcerative lesions with indurated borders** that are easily identified as cancer on clinical inspection. Rarely, inflammatory processes may imitate ulcerative oral cancer. However, some oral carcinomas, when first observed, **are not ulcerated.** Some of these lesions may have **wart-like configurations (verrucous carcinomas)** and others may present as **areas of redness (erythroplakia) or as white patches with irregular borders,** somewhat similar in appearance to benign **leukoplakia.** A biopsy confirmation of the nature of the disease is always recommended.

The invasive squamous cancers can be **graded,** with **well-differentiated, keratin-producing cancers, including verrucous lesions, classified as grade I, poorly differentiated carcinomas composed of small cells as grade III. The intermediate grade II, characterized by medium-size cells showing squamous differentiation, is by far the most common.** Except for verrucous carcinomas, which usually have a fairly good prognosis, grading has limited prognostic value. The **size and the depth of invasion of the primary tumor (stage)** is a more important prognostic factor. Stage I lesions are limited in size and depth of invasion. Stage IV lesions are cancers with distant metastases, usually to lymph nodes of the neck, which must be evaluated prior to therapy. Surgical treatment of oral cancers is often disfiguring and debilitating, whereas radiotherapy and chemotherapy are not always effective. **The 5-year survival of about 60% for stage I disease and less than 20% for stage IV, is not satisfactory** (Shah, 1992; Skarsgard et al, 2000; Charabi et al, 2000).

Forastiere et al (2001) summarized the sequence of molecular events leading to the occurrence and progression of squamous cancer of the head and neck area. The most common molecular event is a **mutation of p53 gene** that may occur even in relatively minor epithelial changes, classified as "dysplasia" (see below).

Cytology

In most cases, the diagnosis of invasive squamous cancer of the oral cavity is established by biopsy of clinically suspicious lesions. It has become apparent, however, during a large study of oral cancer detection (see below) that many dentists who are in the best position to see the abnormalities, often do not recognize the malignant nature of very early carcinomas. If given an opportunity to sample such questionable lesions by a painless and bloodless cytologic procedure, they may choose to do so, whereas they may be reluctant to recommend a biopsy.

The cytologic diagnosis of ulcerated invasive lesions is relatively simple **if care has been taken to remove the layer of necrotic surface material prior to cytologic sampling.** Regardless of the type of tumor, the smear background nearly always shows necrotic material, blood, and numerous leukocytes.

Cytologic preparations closely reflect the degree of keratinization of the lesion. In **heavily keratinized squamous cancer,** the cancer cells are characterized by **orange- and yellow-staining cytoplasm** and **large, sometimes pyknotic, dark-staining irregular nuclei** (Fig. 21-5A,B). **"Ghost" cells,** with heavily keratinized cytoplasm and virtually no residual nuclear material, are frequent, as are **keratinized "pearls" of malignant cells.** In **nonulcerated, invasive, keratinizing carcinomas,** particularly the **verrucous type,** the cytologic diagnosis of cancer may be **obscured by abundant, fully keratinized "ghost" cells, without perceptible nuclear abnormalities.** Reddy and Kameswari (1974) studied 165 patients with keratinizing carcinoma of the hard palate in reverse smokers in India and were able to reach the diagnosis in only 60% of the patients. Similar results were reported by Bànóczy and Rigó (1976). **In such cases, close attention must be paid to relatively minor nuclear abnormalities, which may occur in only a few cells; nuclear enlargement and irregularity of outline, with or without nuclear hyperchromasia, are of diagnostic significance.** In case of doubt, a biopsy should be recommended.

In **poorly differentiated squamous carcinomas,** the cytoplasmic keratinization is not prominent, but the **nuclear abnormalities, such as large nucleoli and a coarse pattern of chromatin distribution,** are evident (Fig. 21-5C,D). In the latter form of oral cancer, **the nucleocytoplasmic ratio is usually modified in favor of the nucleus, a feature not always observed in the cells of the keratinizing variety.** To anyone familiar with the principles of cytologic diagnosis of cancer, the diagnosis of invasive squamous carcinoma of the oral cavity will cause little difficulty if the potential pitfalls discussed above are considered.

PRECURSOR LESIONS OF SQUAMOUS CANCER

Because of poor results of treatment of invasive squamous carcinoma, the discovery of precursor lesions may prove to be lifesaving. **Precancerous lesions of the squamous epithelium of origin** must invariably precede invasive cancer.

Clinical Presentation and Histology

On clinical inspection, there are two types of precancerous lesions in the oral cavity:

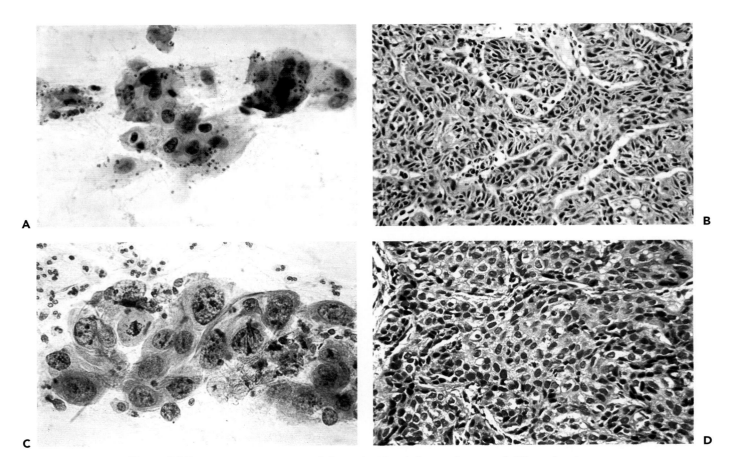

Figure 21-5   Squamous carcinoma of the oral cavity. *A.* Smears from a well-differentiated squamous cancer containing squamous cancer cells with enlarged, hyperchromatic nuclei. *B.* An infiltrating squamous carcinoma, corresponding to *A. C.* Smear from a poorly differentiated squamous carcinoma showing classical cancer cells with enlarged nuclei containing numerous large nucleoli. *D.* The tissue section of a poorly differentiated squamous carcinoma corresponding to *C.*

- **The common white lesions** with irregular, jagged borders, usually referred to as precancerous leukoplakias, are clinically similar to the benign leukoplakias, and correspond to precancerous lesions with a heavily keratinized surface and nuclear abnormalities in well-differentiated squamous cells (Fig. 21-6). The white color of the lesion is caused by the opaque surface layer of keratinized epithelium. The term mild or moderate dysplasia is often attached to such lesions.
- **The less common red lesions (erythroplakia)**, corresponding to the nonkeratinizing precursor epithelial lesions, are usually composed of smaller cancer cells with minimal or absent keratinization of surface (carcinomas in situ or severe dysplasia) (Fig. 21-7). The red color is due to the vascularized stroma underlying the often thin epithelium. The lesion is a definitive precursor of invasive squamous cancer and has been so recognized in the studies by Sandler (1962, 1963), Shafer et al (1975), and Mashberg et al (1977). Niebel and Chomet (1964) proposed in vivo staining of the oral mucosa with toluidine blue to demarcate the territories of these lesions.
- **In some fortuitous cases,** incidentally discovered, there are no visible oral lesions. Acetowhite areas, after application of 3% acetic acid solutions, may be observed in such patients (Fig. 21-8).

Subdø et al (2001) studied the **DNA content** of oral biopsies as a **prognostic marker in oral keratinizing lesions (leukoplakia)** that were either **histologically benign or atypical ("dysplasia").** Of the 45 patients with histolog-ically benign leukoplakia, 5 (11%) developed squamous carcinoma after a follow-up period of 5 years or more. Four of the 5 patients had an abnormal (aneuploid) DNA pattern. Only 1 patient with normal (diploid) DNA pattern developed oral cancer. Of the 150 patients with histologic atypia or dysplasia, 36 (24%) developed invasive cancer after a follow-up ranging from 4 to 57 months, mean 35 months. With only 3 exceptions, all cancers developed in patients with abnormal (tetraploid or aneuploid) DNA patterns. Lippman and Hong (2001) enthusiastically supported the conclusions of this work, which suggests that detectable and measurable nuclear abnormalities, as previously reported by Califano et al (2000), may be of practical use in assessing the behavior of oral leukoplakia.

Subdø et al (2002) also followed 37 patients with **"erythroplakia"** for a median observation time of 53 months. There were 12 patients with normal (diploid) DNA distribution and none of them developed invasive cancer after a median follow-up period of 98 months. On the other hand, 23 of 25 patients with aberrant DNA content developed invasive squamous cancer. The histologic grade of the lesion, sex of patients, and use of tobacco were not significant as prognostic factors.

Although the red oral lesions progress to cancer with a much higher frequency than white lesions, this study strongly suggests that a stratification of these lesions is possible by relatively simple image analysis of the DNA content. For further comments on DNA measurement techniques, see Chapters 46 and 47.

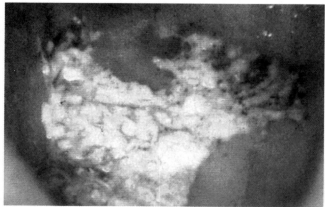

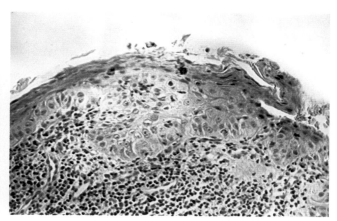

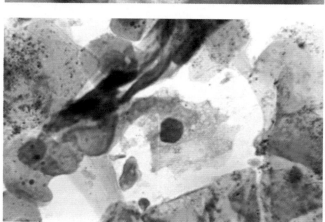

Figure 21-6 **Atypical leukoplakia (moderate dysplasia) of oral cavity.** *A.* Clinical appearance of the white lesion with jagged edges. *B.* The keratinizing lesion of the oral epithelium with scattered nuclear abnormalities. Note marked inflammatory infiltrate in the stroma. *C.* Atypical squamous cells with an enlarged hyperchromatic nucleus in oral smear.

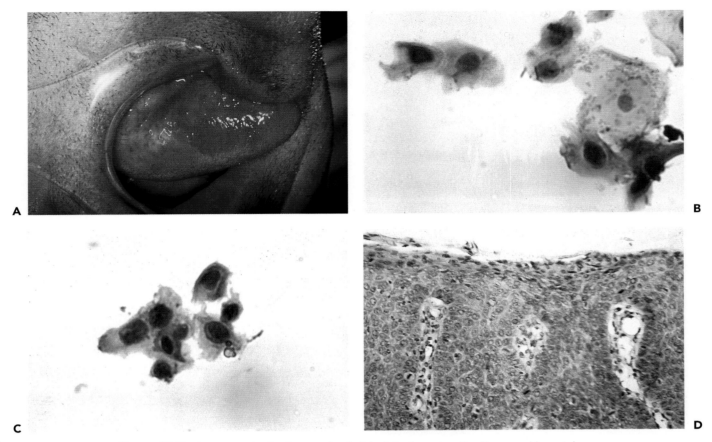

Figure 21-7   **Carcinoma in situ (severe dysplasia) of the buccal cavity discovered by cytology.**
A. Shows the reddened area of tongue (erythroplakia), the site of the lesion. *B,C.* Scrape smear of oral epithelium showing squamous cancer cells with abundant cytoplasm. *D.* Histology of carcinoma in situ corresponding to *A–C.*

Cytology

Keratinizing Lesions (Precancerous Leukoplakia, Mild or Moderate Dysplasia)

The accurate cytologic diagnosis of **keratinizing carcinoma in situ or of precancerous leukoplakia** may prove difficult, particularly if abnormal cells in smears are overshadowed by keratinized benign cells or anucleated squames. However, after **thorough screening** of cytologic material, it is rare not to find at least a **few cells suggesting** either a **borderline squamous lesion** or **a well-differentiated squamous cancer with keratinized cytoplasm and nuclear enlargement** (see Fig. 21-6C). In these situations, knowledge of the clinical presentation of the lesion is invaluable and should lead to a **confirmatory biopsy,** even though the cytologic evidence may be very scanty.

Hong et al (1986) reported that oral administration of 13-*cis*-retinoic acid had a beneficial effect on the size and degree of cellular abnormalities in oral precancerous leukoplakias of some patients, but had fairly severe toxic effects.

Nonkeratinizing Lesions (Carcinoma In Situ, Severe Dysplasia)

The terms **oral carcinoma in situ or severe dysplasia,** as distinct from precancerous leukoplakia, refers to malignant epithelial lesions without significant keratin formation on

their surfaces. As mentioned above, nearly all of these lesions present **clinically as areas of redness (erythroplakia)** but may be **clinically occult.**

Scrape smears from such lesions are characterized by a mixture of malignant **well-differentiated parabasal or intermediate squamous cells,** with translucent cytoplasm and **significant nuclear enlargement and hyperchromasia** (see Figs. 21-7 and 21-8). The term **dyskaryosis,** or "**dysplastic cells,**" used in the discussion of precursor lesions of carcinoma of the uterine cervix is applicable here (see Chap. 11). It is not uncommon to observe in such smears a few **squamous cancer cells with markedly keratinized cytoplasm and marked nuclear abnormality.** On the whole, the smear pattern in oral carcinoma in situ is remarkably similar to that of a high-grade squamous precursor lesion of carcinoma of the uterine cervix of well-differentiated type. These observations were confirmed in the study of carcinoma in situ recurring after treatment of invasive oral cancer (see below).

Stahl et al (1964), in discussing the implications of dyskaryosis in oral mucosal lesions, pointed out the necessity of long-term follow-up of patients showing such cells in their smears. The same authors noted that experimentally induced cancer of the cheek pouch of the hamster is also heralded by the appearance of dyskaryotic cells.

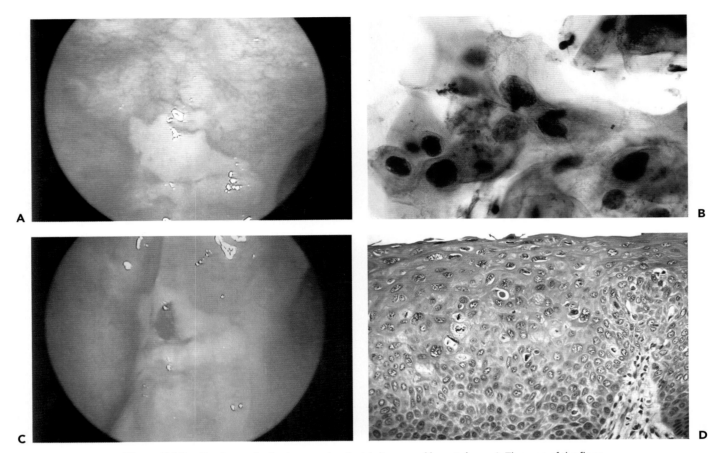

Figure 21-8 **Carcinoma in situ (severe dysplasia) diagnosed by cytology.** *A.* The area of the floor of the mouth without visible lesions. *B.* Cytologic presentation of an incidentally discovered lesion. *C.* Acetowhite biopsied area in the floor of the mouth after application of 3% acetic acid solution. *D.* Biopsy of a very high-grade intraepithelial lesion with marked mitotic activity. There was no invasion.

RESULTS OF CYTOLOGIC SCREENING FOR OCCULT CARCINOMA AND PRECURSOR LESIONS

The difficulty of clinical identification of precancerous leukoplakia and carcinoma in situ, both easily curable precursor stages of oral cancer, was not fully appreciated until an extensive cytologic study of mouth lesions was conducted by the Veterans Administration, guided by the late Dr. H. Sandler (Sandler, 1962; Sandler et al, 1963). As a consultant, I (LGK) was privileged to review a major portion of the material resulting from this study. There were 2,758 patients with visible mouth lesions screened by cytology, and there were 287 histologically documented cases of invasive carcinoma. Many of these lesions were very small (26 were less than 1 cm in diameter, and 69 were less than 2 cm in diameter); many were not ulcerated, not indurated, and not fixed to the underlying tissue. **Eighty three of these lesions (approximately 29%) were not recognized clinically as cancers** by the examining dentists.

There were also 28 patients with squamous carcinoma in situ. Only 11 of the lesions were suspected of being cancer by the examining dentists, whereas 17 **(about two-thirds) were considered benign.** Thirteen lesions were **reddish in color,** 6 were white, and the rest were of various colors; only 6 were ulcerated and only 5 indurated. **Thus, redness**

of circumscribed areas of oral epithelium erythroplakia is frequently characteristic of carcinoma in situ (see Fig. 21-7A).

The comparison of Sandler's data with observations on a nonscreened population surveyed by Shafer (1975) is enlightening. Shafer reviewed the clinical and histologic data on 82 oral carcinomas in situ (including 16 lesions of the lip), diagnosed by biopsy only. While in Sandler's survey, 28 carcinomas in situ were found in 2,758 patients with visible mouth lesions (1%), in Shafer's survey, there were 66 oral carcinomas in situ in 45,702 histologic accessions (0.0014%). It may be argued that the two populations of patients were unequal. Sandler's patients were men, mainly older than 50 years of age, many among them drinkers and smokers, who were much more prone to oral cancer than Shafer's unselected population. Nevertheless, Sandler's rate of discovery of carcinoma in situ was 10 times higher than in Shafer's population. The comparison of clinical findings is also enlightening; roughly one-half of Sandler's lesions were red, whereas there were only 16% of such lesions in Shafer's survey, strongly suggesting that **even the most competent observers consider red oral lesions as benign and do not perform biopsies. Such lesions should be the prime target for cytologic screening.**

A survey by Stahl et al (1967) confirmed that cytologic screening for oral cancer is feasible. Practicing dentists in the area of New York City were instructed to obtain **smears from all *visible* abnormalities of the oral cavity.** Although only a small proportion of the invited dentists responded, 47 oral cancers were found in 2,297 patients examined. Eleven of the 47 cancers (24%) were clinically unsuspected, thus confirming the results of the Veterans Administration study quoted above. It does not appear feasible or reasonable to cytologically screen all dental patients. However, a **scrape smear of an oral lesion may well permit more conservative surgery for earlier lesions and may be lifesaving.** Shiboski et al (2000) recently emphasized a major deficiency in the professional and public education regarding early diagnosis of oral cancer.

Sandler's, Shafer's, and Mashberg and Meyer's studies pointed out that the **floor of the mouth was the most frequently affected site of oral squamous cancer,** followed by lateral surface of **tongue** and **soft palate.** These should be the areas of the oral cavity that deserve a careful inspection during routine dental examination.

Within recent years, there has been a revival of interest in cytologic detection of oral cancers in the United States, based on evaluation of oral smears by a semiautomated cell analysis system **OralCDx** (Sciubba, 1999). A specially designed brush was used to secure cell samples from the visible lesions of the oral cavity. Of the 945 lesions sampled by cytology, 131 (about 14%) were biopsy-confirmed "dysplastic" lesions or carcinomas. In these cases, the smears were judged to be either "positive" or "atypical." In 29 patients (22% of the biopsy-documented lesions), **the malignant nature of the lesion was not suspected clinically,** a result remarkably similar to the Stahl (1967) study cited above. The histologic findings in these patients have not been reviewed by independent observers and, thus, it is not possible to determine how many of the "dysplasias" were truly precancerous lesions.

In situations in which an exceptionally high risk of oral cancer exists, more extensive surveys may be justified. Wahi, from Agra, India, demonstrated the value of cytologic techniques among **betel-nut chewers,** who have a very high incidence of oral carcinoma. His results (personal communication, 1966) are summarized in Table 21-1. The data strongly suggest that high-risk candidates for oral cancer, such as tobacco chewers and heavy cigar- and pipe smokers, represent a primary target for screening for oral cancer by cytologic techniques.

CYTOLOGIC DIAGNOSIS OF RECURRENT ORAL CANCER AFTER TREATMENT

Local recurrences of oral cancer after treatment by surgery, radiation, or a combination of these two techniques are sufficiently common to warrant a close follow-up of all patients. The **possibility of a residual or second primary cancer within the same anatomic area** is also very high in treated patients. **There is excellent evidence that the addition of cytologic techniques to the follow-up examination may result in the diagnosis of a recurrent or new cancer before it is suspected clinically.**

TABLE 21-1	
CYTOLOGIC DIAGNOSIS OF ORAL CARCINOMA AMONG BETEL-NUT CHEWERS	
Total cases of oral cancer studied	812
Clinically unsuspected	69
(66 squamous carcinoma, 2 reticulum cell sarcoma, 1 adenocarcinoma)	
Clinical diagnoses on 69 unsuspected cases	
Leukoplakia	26
Ulceration	27
Trismus	9
Dysphagia	4
Tonsillar enlargement	3
Cytologic diagnoses on the same cases	
Malignant cells	39
Cells suggestive of cancer	21
Dyskaryotic cells, possibly malignant	9

(Prof. P.N. Wahi, Agra, India, personal communication.)

Umiker (1965) reported on four such cases following radiation treatment. Hutter and Gerold (1966) applied cytologic techniques in the follow-up of patients previously treated by surgery. In limiting the application of cytology to the patients *without* visible lesions, they uncovered clinically unsuspected recurrent cancer in 10 of 177 patients investigated (6%). These authors were using material scraped from the general area of prior surgery by an endometrial curette. The results are summarized in Table 21-2.

An interesting aspect of Hutter and Gerold's work concerns the time that elapsed between the cytologic evidence of recurrent carcinoma and the appearance of a clinical abnormality, however slight, amenable to a biopsy. In several of the cases, 4 to 6 months of follow-up by a very experienced observer were required to see a lesion, usually an area of redness or a whitish patch. In six of the eight patients with cytologic diagnosis of recurrent carcinoma, the major histologic component of the lesion was a carcinoma in situ, either with or without superficial infiltration. In this work, the degree of accuracy of cytologic identification of carcinoma in situ was extremely high and is summarized in Table 21-3.

This work, as well as the results of cancer detection surveys described above, strongly suggest that the **silent stage of carcinoma in situ, whether primary or recurrent, is not readily identifiable clinically and precedes invasive squamous carcinoma of the oral cavity.** This stage of cancer may last for several months, and possibly much longer, before producing a visible lesion. Carcinoma in situ may be accurately identifiable by cytology, as is the case with many other organs discussed in this book.

OTHER TUMORS

Besides squamous carcinoma, other benign or malignant tumors involving the oral cavity may occasionally be diag-

---

TABLE 21-2

RESULTS OF CYTOLOGIC FOLLOW-UP ON PATIENTS WITH TREATED CANCER OF THE OROPHARYNX WITHOUT VISIBLE LESIONS AT THE SITE OF PRIOR SURGERY

Total patients examined		177	(100%)
Positive smears	12		
Suspicious smears	2		
		14	(9%)
Carcinoma confirmed	8		
Died	3	(2 with evidence of cancer)	
Still being followed without clinical evidence of lesion (smears still positive)	<u> 3</u>		
	14		

(Hutter RVP, Gerold FP. Cytodiagnosis of clinically inapparent oral cancer in patients considered to be high risks. A preliminary report. Am J Surg 112:541–546, 1966.)

---

nosed by smear. We have observed cases of a **benign mixed tumor** of salivary glands and of **adenoid cystic carcinoma,** located in the palate, and diagnosed on scrape smears. For description of these tumors, see Chapter 32. We have also seen a case of **primary malignant melanoma** of the oral mucosa. The smears were characterized by the presence of obvious malignant cells and macrophages containing melanin pigment (Fig. 21-9). King (1962) reported several examples of cytologic findings in a few uncommon tumors, such as an ulcerating **osteosarcoma of the jaw,** two **malignant lymphomas** (one of palate and one of mandible), and a case of **ulcerating adenoid cystic carcinoma.** A number of observers used aspiration biopsies (FNAs) to investigate the nature of palpable tumors of the oral cavity (Castelli et al, 1993; Das et al, 1993; Gunhan et al, 1993; Mondan and Raychoudhuri, 1993; Mathew et al, 1997; Damanski and Åkerman, 1998; Shah et al, 1999). Most lesions examined were **tumors of the salivary glands, dental anlage tu**

mors, and tumors of the jaws, topics that are discussed in Chapters 32 and 36. Of note were several cases of **malignant lymphomas,** involving the base of the tongue and the tonsils and several **metastatic carcinomas.** We have also observed a case of **lymphoblastic leukemia** in a child recognized on a scrape smear of an oral lesion. For discussion of cytologic presentation of malignant lymphoma, see Chapter 31.

THE LARYNX

METHODS OF INVESTIGATION

It is evident that cytologic examination of the larynx is possible only if an otorhinolaryngologist interested in this nonin-

---

TABLE 21-3

COMPARISON OF CYTOLOGIC DIAGNOSIS WITH HISTOLOGIC FINDINGS IN EIGHT CASES OF RECURRENT ORAL EPIDERMOID CARCINOMA

Number of Patients	Cytologic Diagnosis	Histologic Findings
4	Epidermoid carcinoma}	2 {Invasive carcinoma
		2 {In situ and infiltrating carcinoma
		1 {Carcinoma in situ
3	Carcinoma in situ	3 [Carcinoma in situ with foci of
1	Suspect carcinoma in situ}	very superficial invasion

(Modified from Hutter RVP, Gerold FP. Cytodiagnosis of clinically inapparent oral cancer in patients considered to be high risks. A preliminary report. Am J Surg 112:541–546, 1966.)

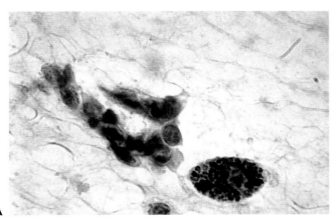
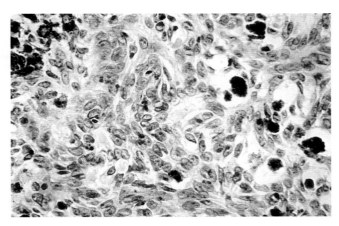

Figure 21-9 **Primary malignant melanoma of oral cavity.** *A.* The smear contained small cancer cells and a large macrophage with phagocytosis of melanin pigment. *B.* Tissue biopsy of the same lesion, showing accumulation of melanin.

vasive method of diagnosis is willing to obtain a cytologic sample during a **direct or indirect laryngoscopy.** Most papers describing the cytology of the larynx were written by interested clinicians, usually in association with a cytopathologist. A variety of methods were described to obtain the cell samples, ranging from a **simple cotton swab to sophisticated scrapers or brushes.** Carcinoma of the larynx may also be discovered in **samples of sputum** (see Chap. 20).

BENIGN LESIONS

Reaction to Intubation

The common practice of insertion of tubes into the larynx may lead to a necrosis and ulceration of the epithelium, followed by repair. It is not uncommon to have samples of the material aspirated for toilette purposes submitted for cytologic examination.

Sheets of small squamous cells with **marked nuclear abnormalities** are commonly observed in such patients (Fig. 21-10). Of particular interest is the presence of large nucleoli, a feature commonly seen in "repair." These cells may be mistaken for poorly differentiated squamous- or adenocarcinoma, unless the clinical history of intubation is available. As a general rule, **the diagnosis of cancer should not be made in samples obtained from intubated patients or patients on respirators.**

Another form of reaction to long-term intubation is **tracheitis sicca,** mimicking squamous cancer, described in Chapter 19.

Rhinoscleroma

A cytologic diagnosis of **rhinoscleroma of the larynx** was reported by Zaharopoulos and Wong (1984). **Large macrophages with phagocytized encapsulated bacilli (Mikulicz cells)** were illustrated. The bacterium causing the disease is

the gram-negative *Klebsiella rhinoscleromatis,* which usually causes obstructive nasal lesions, responding to antibiotics.

TUMORS

Papillomatosis

Laryngeal papillomatosis was briefly mentioned in reference to papillomatosis of the bronchus (see Chap. 20). The interest in this disease has grown exponentially since its association with **human papillomavirus (HPV) type 11** was documented (Gissmann et al, 1982; Mounts et al, 1982; Mounts and Shah, 1984). Laryngeal papillomas are **squamous papillomas,** histologically very **similar to condylomata acuminata** (see Chaps. 11 and 14). As a rule, the lesions are multiple, may grow rapidly, and may cause obstruction of the larynx. It has been reported that the number of immunoactive intraepithelial cells (Langerhans' cells) is markedly reduced in these lesions (Chardonet et al, 1986).

The disease occurs in two forms: a **juvenile form** affecting children, with the onset usually under the age of 5, and an uncommon **adult form** that usually manifests itself after the age of 20. It is postulated that in the juvenile form, HPV type 11 is **transmitted from the mother to the offspring during birth.** In fact, many of the mothers give a history of genital condylomata acuminata. Both forms are characterized by a chronic course and recurrences after treatment. Persistence of HPV in the laryngeal epithelium after removal of the lesions has been documented (Steinberg et al, 1983). A spread of the lesions into the trachea and the bronchi is common. Obstruction of the airway is an ever-existing danger. **Malignant transformation of laryngeal papillomas into squamous carcinoma, although rare, does occur.** In a case reported by Byrne et al (1987), the presence of HPV type 11 in the primary tumor and in the metastases was observed.

There has been no attempt known to this writer to use cytologic techniques for the diagnosis of primary or recur-

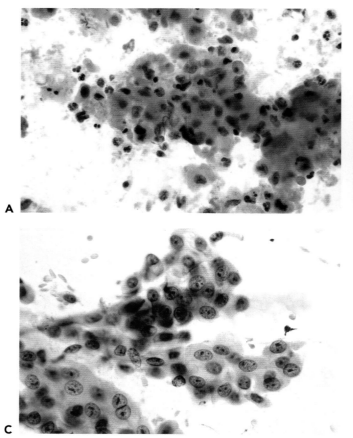

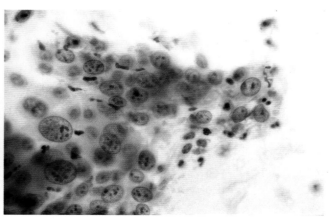

Figure 21-10 "Repair" reaction in laryngeal and tracheal aspirates. *A.* A sheet of small squamous cells with sporadic nuclear enlargement and hyperchromasia in a 30-year-old man on a respirator for 2 weeks. *B.* A sheet of small squamous cells with prominent nucleoli aspirated through a laryngectomy opening. *C.* Sheets of columnar cells of respiratory type with prominent nucleoli, aspirated through a laryngeal tube.

rent laryngeal papillomatosis. However, the cytologic findings in the **bronchial manifestations are consistent with HPV infection** (see Chap. 20).

Carcinoma

The vast majority of the malignant tumors of the larynx are **squamous carcinomas,** many of which are keratin-producing. Brandsma et al (1986) reported the presence of **HPV type 16** in one such cancer. Invasive cancers of the larynx are nearly always symptomatic, with persisting hoarseness as the presenting symptom. The grading and staging of laryngeal carcinomas is similar to that of the oral cavity. A stage of **carcinoma in situ,** often classified as **"dysplasia,"** preceding invasive cancer, is well known.

Cytology

Although biopsy is the method of choice in the diagnosis of these tumors, Frable and Frable (1968), Beham et al (1997), and Malamou-Mitsi et al (2000) reported high levels of cytologic accuracy in smears obtained at the time of direct laryngoscopy, prior to biopsy. The cytologic findings are **identical to those described for similar cancers of the oral cavity.**

There is ample evidence that **invasive carcinoma of the larynx is preceded by carcinoma in situ.** The latter lesion may either be **keratinized, hence, white on inspection**

(leukoplakia), or **nonkeratinized, which produces an area of redness.** It must be stressed that not all areas of leukoplakia harbor carcinoma. **Hyperkeratosis may also occur in the absence of cancer.**

In one of the early attempts at cytologic diagnosis of laryngeal lesions, a cotton swab smear of the larynx led to diagnosis of **squamous carcinoma in situ** in a man age 50 with mere redness of the vocal cords. **Dyskaryotic (dysplastic) squamous cells with abundant cytoplasm and enlarged, hyperchromatic nuclei were characteristic of this lesion** (Fig. 21-11).

Lundgren et al (1981) used a small wooden pin and a small brush to obtain cell samples from the larynx of 350 patients during direct laryngoscopies. The technical quality of the smears and the accuracy of the procedure were judged to be good. **Several cases of carcinoma in situ and "severe" and "moderate" dysplasia** were recorded. It is evident that the term **"dysplasia"** was used to describe a precancerous lesion because 46 of the 120 patients with this cytologic diagnosis proved to have invasive cancer, and 37 had carcinomas in situ. There were 26 lesions judged benign on biopsy, 25 of them with the diagnosis of "moderate dysplasia" and some of them possibly occult carcinomas, as documented by the authors in one case with adequate follow-up. There were also 33 malignant lesions missed by cytology for various reasons. The sensitivity of the procedure was estimated at 83% and the specificity at 84%. In a recent

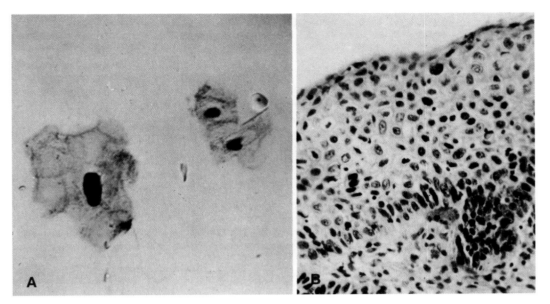

Figure 21-11   Carcinoma in situ of larynx. Primary diagnosis by smear. *A.* Swab smear of a slightly reddened larynx in a 54-year-old man. Note the excellent differentiation of abnormal cells resembling "dyskaryosis." *B.* The lesion proved to be a carcinoma in situ as shown here.

publication based on a small number of patients, Malamou-Mitsi et al (2000) reported a specificity of 100% and sensitivity of more than 90%.

A relatively large number of occult carcinomas of the larynx were discovered in **sputum** during the search for occult bronchogenic carcinomas (see Chap. 20). The cancer cells in sputum do not differ from those of a bronchogenic squamous carcinoma. It must be stressed that **identical cytologic presentation may also be observed in similar carcinomas of the oral cavity, the nasopharynx, and the trachea. These areas must be investigated if the sputum is positive and if there is no clinical evidence of oral or lung cancer.**

There are very few benign cytologic abnormalities of the larynx that can mimic squamous carcinoma. The **small squamous cells found in sputum in cases of laryngitis, known as Pap cells,** are perhaps the only finding of note (see Chap. 19). Frable and Frable (1968) and Lundgren et al (1981) pointed out that **radiation changes,** similar to those observed in the uterine cervix or the lung, may occur in larynges that have been irradiated for invasive carcinoma (see Chaps. 18 and 19). The importance of careful follow-up of patients after laryngectomy for carcinoma has been stressed elsewhere (see Chap. 20).

Other malignant tumors of the larynx are uncommon. These include **carcinomas of minor salivary glands** (Spiro et al, 1973) and the rare **small-cell endocrine tumor** of the same origin (Koss et al, 1972). An exceedingly rare form of **squamous carcinoma of the larynx with a spindle cell component** (pseudosarcoma) has been reviewed by Goellner et al (1973). The prognosis of this tumor is surprisingly favorable, as is the case with similar tumors of the esophagus (see Chap. 24). The cytologic presentation of these rare tumors has not been described.

THE TRACHEA

REPAIR REACTION

As described above, an injury to the trachea during intubation or tracheostomy may result in florid squamous metaplasia or "repair" reaction. **Sheets of immature squamous cells** with monotonous, but somewhat enlarged, clear nuclei containing large nucleoli may be seen (see Fig. 21-10).

CARCINOMAS

Primary carcinomas of the trachea are uncommon. The symptomatology of tracheal carcinoma is the same as for bronchogenic carcinoma—cough and hemoptysis. Rarely, such lesions may cause asthmatic attacks (Baydur and Gottlieb, 1975).

Carcinomas of the trachea are primarily of two types: squamous carcinoma, which **may be synchronous or metachronous with bronchogenic carcinoma** and is often keratinizing; and **adenoid cystic carcinoma of minor salivary (mucous) glands.** The latter lesion is identical with adenoid cystic carcinoma of major salivary or bronchial glands and is described in the appropriate chapters.

Hajdu and Koss (1969) reported the cytologic findings in 14 patients with tracheal carcinoma, of which 10 were squamous and 4 were adenoid cystic. The **squamous cancer** was recognized either in **sputum** or in **tracheobronchial aspirates** in 9 of 10 patients. All 4 **adenoid cystic carcinomas** were recognized in **direct tracheal aspirates.**

The **cytologic presentation of squamous carcinoma** of

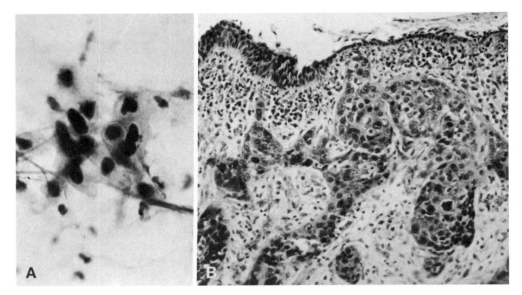

Figure 21-12 **Epidermoid carcinoma of trachea.** *A.* Cluster of cells of epidermoid carcinoma in sputum. Note the enlarged, hyperchromatic nuclei. *B.* Histologic appearance of tumor. (From Hajdu SI, Koss LG. Cytology of carcinoma of the trachea. Acta Cytol 13:256–259, 1969.)

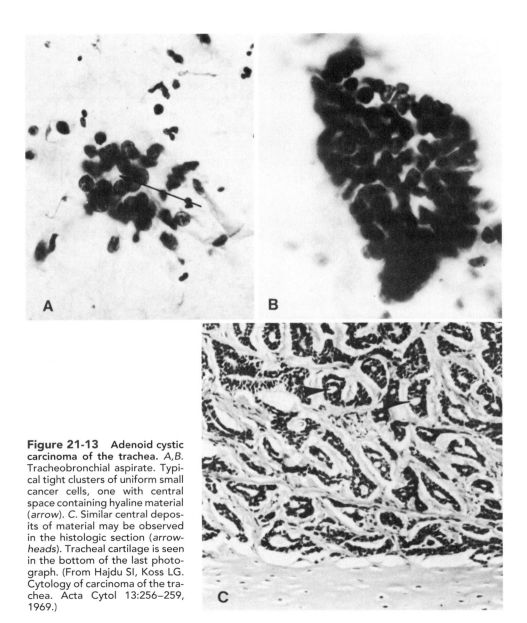

Figure 21-13 **Adenoid cystic carcinoma of the trachea.** *A,B.* Tracheobronchial aspirate. Typical tight clusters of uniform small cancer cells, one with central space containing hyaline material (*arrow*). *C.* Similar central deposits of material may be observed in the histologic section (*arrowheads*). Tracheal cartilage is seen in the bottom of the last photograph. (From Hajdu SI, Koss LG. Cytology of carcinoma of the trachea. Acta Cytol 13:256–259, 1969.)

the trachea was in every way similar to squamous carcinoma of the bronchus (see Chap. 20) or the larynx (Fig. 21-12). As is the case in other organs, the **adenoid cystic carcinoma was characterized by tightly packed clusters of small cancer cells** with scanty cytoplasm, often surrounding a **central core** of transparent hyaline material composed of layers of reduplicating basement membranes and forming the "cystic" component of the tumor (Fig. 21-13).

THE NASOPHARYNX

METHODS OF SAMPLING AND INDICATIONS

Cytologic examination of the nasopharynx requires direct scraping, which is best performed under visual control with a fiberoptic instrument.

The diagnostic sampling has several applications including to confirm an allergic disorder, such as asthma, or the detection of nasopharyngeal neoplasms, as narrated below.

NORMAL SMEARS

Scrape smears from nasopharyngeal epithelium contain **squamous cells, ciliated respiratory type cells, and goblet cells;** hence, their makeup is similar to that of bronchial smears (Fig. 21-14).

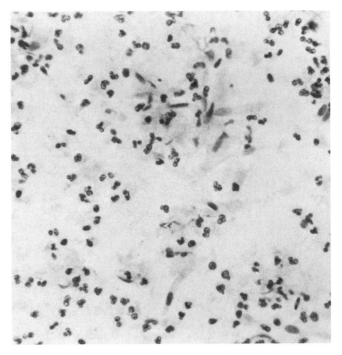

Figure 21-14 Nasopharynx: inflammation. Note a mixture of ciliated columnar cells against a background of polymorphonuclear leukocytes.

INFLAMMATORY DISORDERS AND BENIGN TUMORS

Cytology of the nasopharynx has been extensively studied in patients with **common colds or upper respiratory tract viral infections.** In smears, there is **partial or total necrosis of the exfoliated respiratory epithelium and changes similar to ciliocytophthoria, described** in Chapter 19. In **asthma,** a marked increase of **eosinophilic leukocytes** may be noted.

In an aspirate of the nasopharynx, we observed **markedly atypical degenerated macrophages** with markedly enlarged and hyperchromatic, yet homogeneous single or multiple nuclei, shown in Figure 21-15. The cells were mistaken for cancer cells but long-term follow-up of the patient failed to reveal a primary or metastatic tumor.

Fortin and Meisels (1974) reported a case of **rhinosporidiosis** of the nasal cavity, a disease caused by a fungus *Rhinosporidium seeberi*. The disorder causes polyp-like lesions. Large numbers of ovoid spores are characteristic of this infection. An incidental finding of **amyloidosis** in a smear from a nasopharyngeal carcinoma was reported by Chan et al (1988).

A number of disorders on the border of inflammation and neoplasia may affect the nasopharynx. Among them are **Wegener's granulomatosis (lethal midline granuloma),** which may culminate in a malignant lymphoma. There is limited information on the cytologic presentation of these disorders. The presence of **smooth muscle cells** in sputum in a case of Wegener's granulomatosis with ulceration of bronchial lining was reported by Takeda and Burechailo (1969; see Chap. 20).

Jones et al (2000) described a rare disorder known as **pyogenic granuloma** or **pregnancy tumor** of the nasal cavity of pregnant women. The disorder, also known as **hemangiomatous granuloma,** is a red, rapidly growing tumor of unknown etiology (reviews in Smulian et al, 1994; Sills et al, 1996). The tumor may be mistaken for other neoplasms with a rich capillary component, such as malignant hemangioma or Kaposi's sarcoma. There are no reports on cytologic presentation of pyogenic granuloma but the technique should prove useful in the differential diagnosis.

MALIGNANT TUMORS

Nasopharyngeal Carcinoma

For unknown reasons, the incidence of carcinoma of the nasopharynx is very high among **ethnic Chinese** (Chien et al, 2001). In Norway, nasopharyngeal epidermoid carcinoma was observed in **nickel workers** (Torjussen et al, 1979) in whom various stages of precancerous abnormalities ranging from loss of cilia to squamous metaplasia, to carcinoma in situ, could be observed.

The association of nasopharyngeal carcinomas with **Epstein-Barr (EB) virus** is well documented (summaries in Purtilo and Sakamoto, 1981; Cohen, 2000; Chien et al, 2001). It is not known what role, if any, the virus plays in

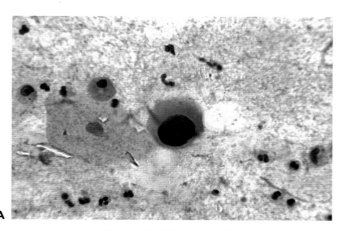
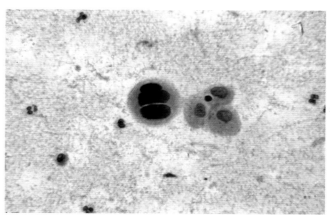

A

B

Figure 21-15   Atypical benign macrophages in nasopharyngeal aspirate. *A* and *B* show cells with markedly enlarged, hyperchromatic nuclei, mistaken for cancer cells. In *B*, the abnormal nuclei are multiple. In *B*, the huge size of the abnormal cells may be compared with that of three normal macrophages in the same field. A careful work-up of the patient and many years of follow-up failed to reveal any evidence of cancer. Hence, it may be assumed that the cells are degenerated, markedly atypical, but benign macrophages.

the genesis of the tumors. However, **the presence of the EB virus, documented by molecular techniques in aspirated cell samples from metastatic tumors in neck lymph nodes, supports the presumption of origin from a primary nasopharyngeal carcinoma** (Feinmesser et al, 1992). The presence in serum of serologic markers for EB virus was predictive of nasopharyngeal carcinoma (Chien et al, 2001).

Histology

Muir and Shanmugaratnam (1967) studied 994 cases of carcinoma of the nasopharynx and subdivided the tumors into **three main groups of tumors,** namely, **squamous carcinoma, nonkeratinizing carcinoma, and undifferentiated carcinoma,** the latter including **nonkeratinizing carcinomas** and the tumors known as **lymphoepitheliomas** (also known as Schmincke's or Regaud's tumors). Only 1% of the tumors were found to be of other types and included **mucus-producing carcinomas** of colonic type and **olfactory neuroblastomas (esthesioneuroblastomas),** discussed below. The significance of this tumor classification in reference to response to radiation treatment and survival showed that undifferentiated carcinoma offered the best prognosis (Shanmugaratham et al, 1979).

The **lymphoepitheliomas are characteristically composed of large, undifferentiated tumor cells with pale nuclei and large nucleoli, embedded in a stroma rich in lymphocytes.** Primary lymphoepitheliomas may be asymptomatic but tend to **metastasize early to the lymph nodes of the neck** and **the metastasis may be the first manifestation of the tumor, a fact also emphasized by** Dr. MY Ali, at the University of Singapore.

Pathmanathan et al (1995) reported that clonal proliferation of cells infected with EB virus, obtained from the nasopharynx, was diagnostic of **precancerous lesions** such as **dysplasia and carcinoma in situ.** The authors speculated that the presence of **EB virus transforming gene** LMP-1 was essential for neoplastic proliferation to take place.

Cytology

Ali (1965) adopted cytologic techniques to the diagnosis of nasopharyngeal carcinoma, using swab smears, obtained with cotton-tipped applicators. **Squamous or epidermoid carcinomas of the nasopharynx do not significantly differ from squamous cancers in other locations. Undifferentiated carcinomas** (including lymphoepitheliomas) were characterized by **large cancer cells with scanty cytoplasm and prominent irregular nuclei, often with large multiple nucleoli** (Fig. 21-16). The **lymphoepitheliomas** also contained a **population of lymphocytes** in the smear. Because these tumors often metastasize to lymph nodes of the neck (as noted, sometimes as the first manifestation of disease), **aspiration biopsy of the lymph node metastases is of significant diagnostic value** (Fig. 21-17). In most instances, the tumors cannot be specifically identified, except that they are epithelial in nature. As has been discussed above, the presence of EB virus in the material aspirated from lymph nodes supports the nasopharyngeal origin of the tumor (Feinmesser et al, 1992).

Results

Ali's results are summarized in Table 21-4. The results pertain largely to fully developed malignant tumors from symptomatic patients and are generally less satisfactory than results from other sites within the head and neck area. The difficulty of obtaining adequate samples from ulcerated and bulky tumors may account for these results. Ali's results compare favorably with those obtained by others and quoted by Ali from sources largely inaccessible to this author. With the exception of two small studies in the United States (Morrison et al, 1949; Hopp, 1958), the accuracy is below 50% of all cancers investigated. In view of the very high incidence of cancers of the nasopharynx among the Chinese, a cancer detection project, having for its purpose developing more effective cytology sampling with improved diagnosis of these lesions in preclinical stages, would seem

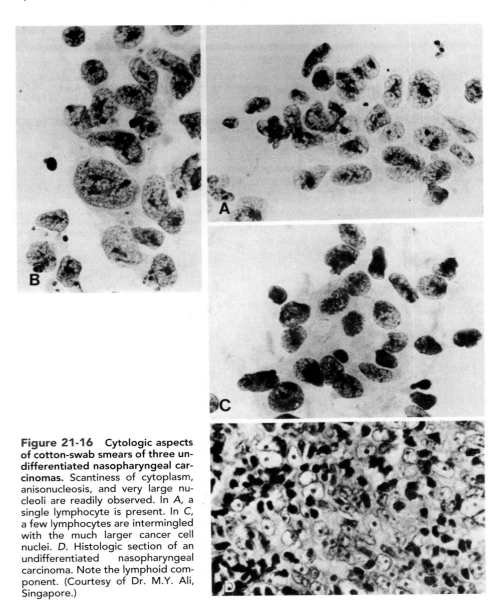

Figure 21-16 Cytologic aspects of cotton-swab smears of three undifferentiated nasopharyngeal carcinomas. Scantiness of cytoplasm, anisonucleosis, and very large nucleoli are readily observed. In *A*, a single lymphocyte is present. In *C*, a few lymphocytes are intermingled with the much larger cancer cell nuclei. *D*. Histologic section of an undifferentiated nasopharyngeal carcinoma. Note the lymphoid component. (Courtesy of Dr. M.Y. Ali, Singapore.)

worthwhile. The observation of Pathmanathan et al (1995), cited above, may conceivably serve this purpose.

OTHER TUMORS

The rare **adenocarcinomas of colonic type** were not studied cytologically. **Olfactory neuroblastoma or esthesioneuroblastoma** is a rare tumor of the nasopharynx of adults, derived from olfactory neural elements. The tumor structurally mimics a neuroblastoma, although it has a much better prognosis. **Rosette formation by small tumor cells,** with an accumulation of **neurofibrils** in the center is characteristic of this tumor. A case of this rare tumor diagnosed cytologically from a scrape smear of the nasal vault was reported by Ferris et al (1988). Another such case, diagnosed by thin-needle aspiration of the tumor, was reported by Jelen et al (1988). The cytologic features of neuroblastoma in aspiration biopsy are discussed in Chapter 40.

Other rare tumors of the nasopharynx such as **chordoma, craniopharyngioma,** and **plasmocytoma** will be briefly described and illustrated in appropriate chapters (also see article by Scher et al, 1988).

PARANASAL SINUSES

Malignant tumors of the paranasal sinuses comprise **squamous or epidermoid carcinomas, adenocarcinomas,** mainly of minor salivary (mucous) gland origin, the so-called **schneiderian carcinomas,** resembling urothelial carcinomas, and an occasional rarity such as a primary **melanoma or sarcoma.** In debatable clinical situations, washings from the paranasal sinuses may be submitted for cytologic evaluation. In most instances, the cytologic material shows evidence of acute or chronic inflammation, reflecting sinusitis. Occasionally, however, evidence of cancer may be ob-

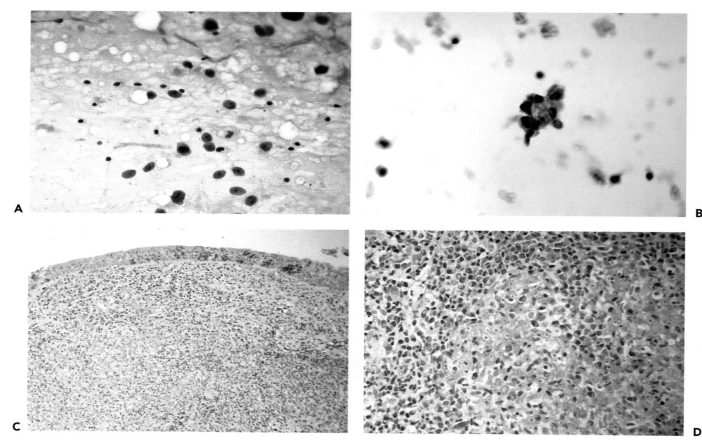

Figure 21-17 **Metastatic nasopharyngeal carcinoma to lymph nodes as the first manifestation of disease.** *A,B.* Scattered, small malignant cells, singly and in clusters, and lymphocytes in an aspirated sample from the enlarged neck nodes in a 23-year-old Chinese patient. *C,D.* Biopsy of the polypoid tumor of the nasopharynx. *C* shows the surface of the lesion, lined by benign epithelium. *D* shows the tumor composed of sheets of large epithelial cells surrounded by lymphocytes (lymphoepithelioma).

TABLE 21-4

THE ACCURACY OF DETECTION OF MALIGNANT CELLS IN NASOPHARYNGEAL SMEARS

| | Total Number Examined | Histologically Confirmed Malignancy | | | Histologically Negative for Cancer | | Overall Accuracy |
		Total	Positive Cytology	%	Total	Negative Cytology	%
Normal controls	25	–	–	–	25	25	100
Cases clinically suspected for cancer	138	79	35	44.3	59	59	68.1

[Ali MY. Cytodiagnosis of Nasopharyngeal Carcinoma (Its Histological and Cytological Bases). Thesis, Department of Pathology, University of Singapore, 1965.]

served, thereby clarifying the clinical situation. The cytologic presentation of these malignant tumors is identical with tumors of similar histological pattern arising in the oral cavity, larynx, trachea, and nasopharynx.

BIBLIOGRAPHY

Ali MY. Cytodiagnosis of Nasopharyngeal Carcinoma (Its Histological and Cytological Bases). Thesis, Department of Pathology, University of Singapore, 1965.

Altmann F, Ginsberg I, Stout AP. Intraepithelial carcinoma (cancer in situ) of larynx. Arch Otolaryngol 56:121–133, 1952.

Ashkenazi YE, Goldman B, Dotan A. Rhythmic variation of sex chromatin and glucose-6-phosphate dehydrogenase activity in human oral mucosa during the menstrual cycle. Acta Cytol 19:62–66, 1975.

Bánoczy J, Rigó O. Comparative cytologic and histologic studies on oral leukoplakia. Acta Cytol 20:308–312, 1976.

Baydur A, Gottlieb LS. Adenoid cystic carcinoma (cylindroma) of the trachea masquerading as asthma. JAMA 234:829–831, 1975.

Beck WS. Metabolic basis of megaloblastic erythropoiesis. Medicine 43:715–726, 1964.

Beham A, Regauer S, Friedrich G, Beham-Schmid CH. Value of exfoliative cytology in differential diagnosis of epithelial hyperplastic lesions of the larynx. Acta Otolaryngol 527:92–94, 1997.

Benisch BM, Tawfik B, Breitenbach EE. Primary oat cell carcinoma of the larynx; and ultrastructural study. Cancer 36:145–148, 1975.

Bhattacharya S, Templeton A. Pemphigus: Decoding the cellular language of cutaneous autoimmunity [editorial]. N Engl J Med 343:60–61, 2000.

Bhattathiri NV, Bindu L, Remani P, et al. Radiation-induced acute immediate nuclear abnormalities in oral cancer cells: serial cytologic evaluation. Acta Cytol 42:1084–1090, 1998.

Boddington MM, Spriggs AI. The epithelial cells in megaloblastic anaemias. J Clin Pathol 12:228–234, 1959.

Boen ST. Changes in nuclei of squamous epithelial cells in pernicious anaemia. Acta Med Scand 159:425–431, 1957.

Brandsma JL, Steinberg BM, Abramson AL, Winkler B. Presence of human papillomavirus type 16 related sequences in verrucous carcinoma of the larynx. Cancer Res 46:2185–2188, 1986.

Bridger GP, Nassar VH. Carcinoma in situ involving the laryngeal mucous glands. Arch Otolaryngol 94:389–400, 1971.

Bryan MP, Bryan WTK. Cytologic and cytochemical aspects of ciliated epithelium in the differentiation of nasal inflammatory diseases. Acta Cytol 13:515–522, 1969.

Bryan WTK, Bryan MP. Cytologic diagnosis in otolaryngology. Trans Am Acad Ophthalmol Otolaryngol 63:597–615, 1959.

Burlakow P, Medak H, McGrew EA, Tiecke R. The cytology of vesicular conditions affecting the oral mucosa: Part 2. Keratosis follicularis. Acta Cytol 13:407–415, 1969.

Byrne JC, Tsao M-S, Fraser RS, Howley PM. Human papilomavirus-11 DNA in a patient with chronic laryngotracheobronchial papillomatosis and metastatic squamous-cell carcinoma of the lung. N Engl J Med 317:873–878, 1987.

Cahan WG, Montemayor PB. Cancer of larynx and lung in the same patient; a report of 60 cases. J Thorac Cardiovasc Surg 44:309–320, 1962.

Califano J, Westra WH, Meininger G, et al. Genetic progression and clonal relationship of recurrent premalignant head and neck lesions. Clin Cancer Res 6:347–352, 2000.

Castelli M, Gattuso P, Reyes C, Solans EP. Fine needle aspiration biopsy of intraoral and pharyngeal lesions. Acta Cytol 37:448–450, 1993.

Chan MKM, McGuire LJ, Lee JCK. Cytology of amyloidosis in smears of nasopharyngeal carcinoma. Acta Cytol 32:429–430, 1988.

Charabi B, Torring H, Kirkegaard J, Hansen HS. Oral cancer—results of treatment in the Copenhagen University Hospital. Acta Otolaryngol Suppl 543:246–247, 2000.

Chardonnet Y, Viac J, Leval J, et al. Laryngeal papillomas: Local cellular immune response, keratinization and viral antigen. Virchows Arch [B] 51:421–428, 1986.

Chien Y-C, Chen J-Y, Liu M-Y, et al. Serologic markers of Epstein-Barr virus infection and nasopharyngeal carcinoma in Taiwanese men. N Engl J Med 345:1877–1882, 2001.

Chu EW, Malmgren RA, Kazam E. Variability of sex chromatin counts. Acta Cytol 13:72–75, 1969.

Cohen JI. Epstein-Barr virus infection. N Engl J Med 343:481–492, 2000.

Costa J. Nasopharyngeal carcinoma. Hum Pathol 12:386, 1981.

Crissman JD, Zarbo RJ. Dysplasia, in situ carcinoma, and progression to invasive squamous cell carcinoma of the upper aerodigestive tract. Am J Surg Pathol 13(Suppl 1):5–16, 1989.

Dabelsteen E, Fejerskov O, Francois D. Ultrastructural localization of blood group antigen A and cell coat on human buccal epithelial cells. Acta Pathol Microbiol Scand [B] 82:113–121, 1974.

Das DK, Gulati A, Bhatt NC, et al. Fine needle aspiration cytology of oral and pharyngeal lesions. A study of 45 cases. Acta Cytol 37:333–342, 1993.

Decker JW, Rubin MB, Goldschmidt H, Heiss HB. Immunofluorescence of Tsanck smears in pemphigus vulgaris. Acta Derm Venereol 52:116–118, 1972.

Djalilian M, Zuijko RD, Weiland LH, Devine KD. Olfactory neuroblastoma. Surg Clin North Am 57:751–762, 1977.

Domanski HA, Akerman M. Fine-needle aspiration cytology of tongue swellings: A study of 75 cases. Diagn Cytopathol 18:387–392, 1998 (corrected and republished in Diagn Cytopathol 19:229–234, 1998).

El-Mofty SK, Lu DW. Prevalence of human papillomavirus type 16 DNA in squamous cell carcinoma of the palatine tonsil, and not the oral cavity, in young patients. A distinct clinicopathologic and molecular disease entity. Am J Surg Pathol 27:1463–1470, 2003.

Faravelli A, Sironi M, Villa E, Radice F. Immunoperoxidase study of cytologic smears in oral pemphigus. Acta Cytol 28:414–418, 1984.

Feinmesser R, Miyazaki I, Cheung R, et al. Diagnosis of nasopharyngeal carcinoma by DNA amplification of tissues obtained by fine-needle aspiration. N Engl J Med 326:17–21, 1992.

Ferris CA, Schnadig VJ, Quinn FB, Jardins LD. Olfactory neuroblastoma: Cytodiagnostic features in a case with ultrastructural and immunohistochemical correlation. Acta Cytol 32:381–385, 1988.

Fisher HR, Miller AH. Carcinoma in situ of larynx: 10 year study of its histopathological classification, prognosis and treatment. Ann Otol Rhinol Laryngol 67:695–702, 1958.

Forastiere A, Koch W, Trotti A, Sidransky D. Head and neck cancer. N Engl J Med 345:1890–1900, 2001.

Foroozan P, Trier JS. Mucosa of the small intestine in pernicious anemia. N Engl J Med 227:553–559, 1967.

Fortin R, Meisels A. Rhinosporidiosis. Acta Cytol 8:170–173, 1974.

Frable WJ, Frable MA. Cytologic diagnosis of carcinoma of the larynx by direct smear. Acta Cytol 12:318–324, 1968.

Garelick JA, Taichman LB. Human papillomavirus infection of the oral mucosa. Am J Dermatopathol 13:386–395, 1991.

Gissmann L, Wolnik L, Ikenberg H, et al. Papillomavirus types of 6 and 11 sequences in genital and laryngeal papillomas and in some cervical cancers. Proc Natl Acad Sci USA 80:560–563, 1983.

Goellner JR, Devine KD, Weiland LH. Pseudosarcoma of the larynx. Am J Clin Pathol 59:312, 1973.

Goldsby JW, Staats OJ. Nuclear changes of intra-oral exfoliated cells of six patients with sickle cell disease. Oral Surg 16:1042–1048, 1963.

Graham RM, Rheault MH. Characteristic cellular changes in epithelial cells in pernicious anemia. J Lab Clin Med 43:235–254, 1954.

Greenebaum E, Levi MH, McKitrick JC. Cytologic manifestation of an unusual bacterial form, Simonsiella species. Acta Cytol 32:465–470, 1988.

Greenspan J, Greenspan D, Lannette ET. Replication of Epstein-Barr virus within the epithelial cells of oral "hairy" leukoplakia, and AIDS-associated lesion. N Engl J Med 313:1456–1471, 1986.

Gunhan O, Dogan N, Celasun B, et al. Fine needle aspiration cytology of oral cavity and jaw bone lesions. A report of 102 cases. Acta Cytol 37:135–141, 1993.

Hajdu SI, Koss LG. Cytology of carcinoma of the trachea. Acta Cytol 13:225–259, 1969.

Harris TJ, Mihm MC. Cutaneous immunopathology: The diagnostic use of direct and indirect immunofluorescence techniques in dermatologic disease. Hum Pathol 10:625–653, 1979.

Healy GB, Gelber RD, Trowbridge AL, et al. Treatment of recurrent respiratory papillomatosis with human leukocyte interferon. N Engl J Med 319:401–407, 1988.

Heath EM, Morken NW, Campbell KA, et al. Use of buccal cells collected in mouthwash as a source of DNA for clinical testing. Arch Pathol Lab Med 125:127–133, 2001.

Hilding AC. Summary of some known facts concerning the common cold. Trans Am Laryngol Assoc 66:87–108, 1944.

Hong WK, Endicott J, Itri LM, et al. 13-cis-Retinoic acid in the treatment of oral leukoplakia. N Engl J Med 315:1501–1505, 1986.

Hopp ES. Cytologic diagnosis and prognosis in carcinoma of mouth, pharynx, and nasopharynx. Laryngoscope 68:1281–1287, 1958.

Hutter RVP, Gerold FP. Cytodiagnosis of clinically inapparent oral cancer in patients considered to be high risks. A preliminary report. Am J Surg 112:541–546, 1966.

Jelen M, Wozniak, Rak J. Cytologic appearance of esthesion euroblastoma in a fine needle aspirate. Acta Cytol 32:377–380, 1988.

Jones JE, Nguyen A, Tabaee A. Pyogenic granuloma (pregnancy tumor) of the nasal cavity. A case report. J Reprod Med 45:749–753, 2000.

Kashima HH, Mounts P. Tumors of the head and neck, larynx, lung, and esophagus and their possible relation to HPV. In Syrjänen K, Gissmann L, Koss LG (eds). Papillomaviruses and Human Disease. Berlin, Springer-Verlag, 1987, pp 138–157.

King OH. The cytology of common and uncommon oral malignancies. Acta Cytol 6:348–354, 1962.

Kishi K, Nishijima K, Medak H, Burlakow P. Cytochemical study of exfoliated cells of oral mucosa. I. The glycogen deposition and keratinization. Acta Med Okayama 29:103–109, 1975.

Kobayashi TK, Ueda M, Nishino T, et al. Brush cytology of herpes simplex virus infection in oral mucosa: Use of the ThinPrep processor. Diagn Cytopathol 18:71–75, 1998.

Korman NJ, Eyre RW, Klaus-Kovtun V, Stanley JR. Demonstration of an adhering-junction molecule (plakoglobin) in the autoantigens of pemphigus foliaceus and pemphigus vulgaris. N Engl J Med 321:621–635, 1989.

Koss LG, Spiro RH, Hajdu S. Small cell (oat cell) carcinoma of minor salivary gland origin. Cancer 20:737–741, 1972.

Kraus FT, Perez-Mesa C. Verrucous carcinoma. Clinical and pathologic study of 105 cases involving oral cavity, larynx, and genitalia. Cancer 19:26–38, 1966.

Lascaris G. Oral pemphigus vulgaris: An immunofluorescent study of fifty-eight cases. Oral Surg 51:531–534, 1981.

Levin ES, Lunin M. The oral exfoliative cytology of pemphigus. A report of two cases. Acta Cytol 13:108–110, 1969.

Lind P, Syrjänen S, Syrjäanen K, et al. Immunoreactivity and human papillomavirus (HPV) in oral precancer and cancer lesions. Scand J Dent Res 94: 419–426, 1986.

Lindeberg H, Syrjänen S, Karja J, Syrjäanen K. Human papillomavirus type 11 DNA in squamous cell carcinomas and pre-existing multiple laryngeal papillomas. Acta Otolaryngol (Stockh.) 107:141–149, 1989.

Lippman SM, Hong WK. Molecular markers of the risk of oral cancer [editorial]. N Engl J Med 344:1323–1325, 2001.

Longmore RB, Cowpe J. Nuclear area and Feulgen DNA content of normal oral squames. Anal Quant Cytol 4:33–38, 1982.

Lundgren J, Olofsson J, Hellquist HB, Strandh AJ. Exfoliative cytology in laryngology: Comparison of cytologic and histologic diagnoses in 350 microlaryngoscopic examination: A prospective study. Cancer 47:1336–1343: 1981.

Makowska W, Zawisza EE. Cytologic evaluation of the nasal epithelium in patients with hay fever. Acta Cytol 19:564–567, 1975.

Malamou-Mitsi VD, Assimakopoulos DA, Goussia A, et al. Contribution of exfoliative cytology to the diagnosis of laryngeal lesions. Acta Cytol 44: 993–999, 2000.

Mashberg A. Erythroplasia vs. leukoplakia in the diagnosis of early asymptomatic oral squamous carcinoma (editorial). N Engl J Med 297:109–110, 1977.

Mashberg A, Meyers H. Anatomical site and size of 222 early asymptomatic oral squamous cell carcinomas. A continuing prospective study of oral cancer. II. Cancer 37:2149–2157, 1976.

Massey BW, Rubin CE. Stomach in pernicious anemia: Cytologic study. Am J Med Sci 227:481–492, 1954.

Mathew S, Rappaport K, Ali SZ, et al. Ameloblastoma. Cytologic findings and literature review. Acta Cytol 41:955–960, 1997.

Medak H, Burlakow P, McGrew EA, Tiecke R. The cytology of vesicular conditions affecting the oral mucosa: Pemphigus vulgaris. Acta Cytol 14:11–21, 1970.

Medak H, McGrew EA, Burlakow P, Tiecke RW. Atlas of Oral Cytology. US Department of Health, Education, and Welfare, Publication No. 1949 (1970).

Medak H, McGrew EA, Burlakow P, Tiecke RW. Correlation of cell populations in smears and biopsies from the oral cavity. Acta Cytol 11:279–288, 1967.

Mondal A, Raychoudhuri BK. Peroral fine needle aspiration cytology of parapharyngeal lesions. Acta Cytol 37:694–698, 1993.

Montgomery PW, von Haam E. Study of exfoliative cytology in patients with carcinoma of oral mucosa. J Dent Res 30:308–313, 1951.

Montgomery PW, von Haam E. Study of exfoliative cytology of oral leucoplakia. J Dent Res 30:260–264, 1951.

Mork J, Lie AK, Glattre E, et al. Human papillomavirus infection as a risk factor for squamous cell carcinoma of the head and neck. N Engl J Med 344: 1125–1131, 2001.

Morris R, Gansler TS, Rudisill MT, Neville B. White sponge nevus: Diagnosis by light microscopic and ultrastructural cytology. Acta Cytol 32:357–361, 1988.

Morrison LF, Hoop ES, Wu R. Diagnosis of malignancy of the nasopharynx. Cytological studies by the smear technique. Ann Otol 58:18–32, 1949.

Mounts P, Shah KV. Respiratory papillomatosis: Etiological relation to genital tract papillomaviruses. Prog Med Virol 29:90–114, 1984.

Mounts P, Shah KV, Kashima H. Viral etiology of juvenile and adult onset squamous papilloma of the larynx. Proc Natl Acad Sci USA 79:5425–5429 1982.

Muir CS, Shanmugaratnam K. The incidence of nasopharyngeal carcinoma in Singapore. In UICC Symposium on Cancers of the Nasopharynx and Accessory Sinuses. Flushing, NY, Medical Examination Publishing, 1967, pp 47–53.

Neiburgs HE, Herman BE, Reisman H. Buccal cell changes in patients with malignant tumors. Lab Invest 11:89–99, 1962.

Niebel HH, Chomet B. In vivo staining test for delineation of oral intraepithelial neoplastic change; preliminary report. J Am Dent Assoc 68:801–806, 1964.

Nunez V, Melamed MR, Cahan W. Tracheobronchial cytology after laryngectomy for carcinoma of larynx. II. Benign atypias. Acta Cytol 10:38–48, 1966.

Oberman HA, Rice DH. Olfactory neuroblastomas: A clinicopathologic study. Cancer 38:2494–2502, 1976.

Pathmanathan R, Prasad U, Sadler R, et al. Clonal proliferations of cells infected with Epstein-Barr virus in preinvasive lesions related to nasopharyngeal carcinoma. N Engl J Med 333:693–698, 1995.

Paz IB, Cook N, Odom-Maryon T, et al. Human papillomavirus (HPV) in head and neck cancer. An association of HPV 16 with squamous cell carcinoma of Waldeyer's tonsillar ring. Cancer 79:595–604, 1997.

Pizzetti F. Le precancerosi e il carcinoma in situ della laringe: Aspetti anatomopatologici. Tumori 60:467–470, 1974.

Purtilo DT, Sakamoto K. Epstein–Barr virus and human disease. Immune response determine the clinical and pathologic expression. Hum Pathol 12: 677–679, 1981.

Reddy CRRM, Kameswari VR. Oral exfoliative cytology in reverse smokers having carcinoma of hard palate. Acta Cytol 18:201–204, 1974.

Sandler HC (ed). Errors of oral cytodiagnosis. Report of follow-up of 1,801 patients. J Am Dent Assoc 72:851–854, 1966.

Sandler HC (ed). Oral Exfoliative Cytology. Veterans Administration Cooperative Study, 1962, Washington DC, Veterans Administration, 1963.

Sandler HC. Cytological screening for early mouth cancer. Interim report of the Veterans Administration Cooperative Study of Oral Exfoliative Cytology. Cancer 15:1119–1124, 1962.

Sandler HE, Freund HR, Stahl SS. Exfoliative cytology applied to detection and treatment of head and neck cancer. Surgery 46:479–485, 1959.

Scheman P. Mass survey for oral cancer by means of exfoliative cytological techniques. Oral Surg 16:61–67, 1963.

Scher RL, Oostinght PE, Levine PA, et al. Role of fine needle aspiration in the diagnosis of lesions of the oral cavity, oropharynx and nasopharynx. Cancer 62:2602–2606, 1988.

Sciubba JJ. Improving detection of precancerous and cancerous oral lesions. Computer-assisted analysis of the oral brush biopsy. J Am Dent Assoc 130: 1445–1457, 1999.

Shafer WG. Oral carcinoma in situ. Oral Surg Oral Med Oral Pathol 39: 227–238, 1975.

Shafer WG, Waldron CA. Erythroplakia of the oral cavity. Cancer 36: 1021–1028, 1975.

Shah SB, Singer MI, Liberman E, Ljung B-M. Transmucosal fine-needle aspiration diagnosis of intraoral and intrapharyngeal lesions. Laryngoscope 109: 1232–1237, 1999.

Shanmugaratnam K, Chan SH, De-Thé G, et al. Histopathology of nasopharyngeal carcinoma. Correlations with epidemiology, survival rates and other biological characteristics. Cancer 44:1029–1044, 1979.

Sharp GS, Bullock WK, Helsper JT. Multiple oral carcinoma. Cancer 14: 512–516, 1961.

Shedd DP, Hukill PB, Bahn S. In vivo staining properties of oral cancer. Am J Surg 110:631–634, 1965.

Shiboski CH, Shiboski SC, Silverman S Jr. Trends in oral cancer rates in the United States, 1973–1996. Community Dent Oral Epidemiol 28:249–256, 2000.

Sills ES, Zegarelli DJ, Hoschander MM, et al. Clinical diagnosis and management of hormonally responsive oral pregnancy tumor (pyogenic granuloma). J Reprod Med 41:467–470, 1996.

Silverman S. The cytology of benign oral lesions. Acta Cytol 9:287–295, 1965.

Silverman S, Becks H, Farber SM. Diagnostic value of intraoral cytology. J Dent Res 37:195–205, 1958.

Silverman S, Sheline GE. Effects of radiation on exfoliated normal and malignant oral cells. A preliminary study. Cancer 14:587–596, 1961.

Silverman SJ, Bhargava K, Mani NJ, Smith LW. Malignant transformation and natural history of oral leukoplakia in 57,518 industrial workers of Gujarat, India. Cancer 38:1790–1795, 1976.

Silverman SJ, Bilimoria KF, Bhargava K, et al. Cytologic, histologic and clinical correlations of precancerous and cancerous oral lesions in 57,518 industrial workers of Gujarat, India. Acta Cytol 21:196–198, 1977.

Sivieri de Araujo M, Mesquita RA, Correa L, et al. Oral exfoliative cytology in the diagnosis of paracoccidioidomycosis. Acta Cytol 45:360–364, 2001.

Skarsgard DP, Groome PA, Mackillop WJ, et al. Cancers of the upper aerodigestive tract in Ontario, Canada and the United States. Cancer 88:1728–1738, 2000.

Smulian JC, Rodis JF, Campbell WA, et al. Non-oral pyogenic granuloma in pregnancy. A report of two cases. Obstet Gynecol 84:672–674, 1994.

Spiro RH, Koss LG, Hajdu SI, Strong EW. Tumors of minor salivary glands. A clinicopathologic study of 492 cases. Cancer 31:117–129, 1973.

Staats OJ, Goldsby JW. Graphic composition of intraoral exfoliative cytology technics. Acta Cytol 7:107–110, 1963.

Staats OJ, Goldsby JW, Butterworth CE. The oral exfoliative cytology of tropical sprue. Acta Cytol 9:228–233, 1965.

Staats OJ, Robinson LH, Butterworth CE. The effect of systemic therapy on nuclear size of oral epithelial cells in folate related anemias. Acta Cytol 13: 84–88, 1969.

Stahl SS. Evaluation of oral cytology in large scale cancer screening studies. Annual Report on USPH Contract No. 86-63-149, May, 20, 1965 to May, 19, 1966.

Stahl SS, Koss LG, Brown RC Jr, Murray D. Oral cytologic screening in a large metropolitan area. J Am Dent Assoc 75:1385–1388, 1967.

Stahl SS, Sandler HC, Cahn LR. The significance of dyskaryotic cell in oral exfoliative cytology. Acta Cytol 8:73–79, 1964.

Steinberg BM, Topp WC, Schneider PS, Abramson AL. Laryngeal papillomavirus infection during clinical remission. N Engl J Med 308:1261–1264, 1983.

Sudbø J, Kildal W, Johannessen AC, et al. Gross genomic aberrations in precancers: Clinical implications of a long-term follow-up study in oral erythroplakias. J Clin Oncol 20:456–462, 2002.

Sudbø J, Kildal W, Risberg B, et al. DNA content as a prognostic marker in patients with oral leukoplakia. N Engl J Med 344:1270–1278, 2001.

Sudbø J, Ried T, Bryne M, et al. Abnormal DNA content predicts the occurrence of carcinomas in non-dysplastic oral white patches. Oral Oncol 37:558–565, 2001A.

Syrjänen SM. Human papillomavirus infections in the oral cavity. In Syrjäanen K, Gissmann L, Koss LG (eds). Papillomaviruses and Human Disease. Berlin, Springer-Verlag, 1987, pp 104–137.

Takahashi I, Kobayashi TK, Suzuki H, et al. Coexistence of Pemphigus vulgaris and herpes simplex virus infection in oral mucosa diagnosed by cytology, immuno-histochemistry, and polymerase chain reaction. Diagn Cytopathol 19:446–450, 1998.

Takeda M, Burechailo FA. Smooth muscle cells in sputum. Acta Cytol 13: 696–699, 1969.

Torjussen W, Solberg LA, Hogetveit AC. Histopathologic changes of nasal mucosa in nickel workers. Cancer 44:963–974, 1979.

Umiker W. Cytology in the radiotherapy of carcinoma of the oral cavity. Acta Cytol 9:296–297, 1965.

Umiker WO, Lampe I, Rapp R, Hiniker JJ. Oral smears in the diagnosis of carcinoma and premalignant lesions. Oral Surg 13:897–907, 1960.

von Haam E. Historical background of oral cytology. Acta Cytol 9:270–272, 1965.

Witkop CJ Jr. Epithelial intracellular bodies associated with hereditary dyskeratoses and cancer therapy. *In* Wied GL (ed). Proceedings of the First International Congress of Exfoliative Cytology. Philadelphia J. B. Lippincott, 1962, pp 259–268.

Witkop CJ Jr, Gorlin RJ. Four hereditary mucosal syndromes. Arch Dermatol 84:762–771, 1961.

Witkop CJ Jr, Shankle CH, Graham JB, et al. Hereditary benign intraepithelial dyskeratosis. II. Oral manifestations and hereditary transmission. Arch Pathol 70:696–711, 1960.

Wood TA Jr, DeWitt SH, Chu EW, et al. Anitschkow nuclear changes observed in oral smears. Acta Cytol 19:434–437, 1975.

Wu H, Wang ZH, Yan A, et al. Protection against pemphigus foliaceus by desmoglein 3 in neonates. N Engl J Med 343:31–35, 2000.

Zaharopoulos P, Wong JY. Cytologic diagnosis of rhinoscleroma. Acta Cytol 28:139–142, 1984.

The Lower Urinary Tract in the Absence of Cancer

22

URINARY TRACT CYTOLOGY: ITS ACCOMPLISHMENTS AND FAILURES IN HISTORICAL PERSPECTIVE

Examination of urine belongs among the oldest medical procedures in the history of mankind. Ancient Egyptians were aware of the importance of bloody urine in the diagnosis of bladder disorders that were later identified as cancer caused by the parasite *Schistosoma haematobium*. As noted in an important historical contribution by Badr (1981), the papyrus of Kahun, dated 1900 years B.C., contains a hieroglyphic describing hematuria (Fig. 22-1). The gross inspection of urine (often collected in special containers) or "uroscopy" was an important diagnostic procedure for many centuries. Fisman (1993) presented an amusing account of the role played by uroscopy in 17th century England and pointed out that this practice persisted until the early years of the 20th century. In 1856, Wilhelm Duschan Lambl, a

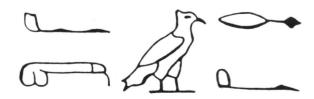

Figure 22-1 Hematuria, as recorded in the papyrus of Kahun (1900 B.C.), with reference to schistosomiasis. (From Badr M. Schistosomiasis in ancient Egypt. *In* El-Bolkainy M, Chu EW (eds). Detection of Bladder Cancer Associated with Schistosomiasis. Cairo, Egypt, The National Cancer Institute, 1981.)

Czech physician, published a remarkable paper on the use of the microscope for the examination of the urinary sediment at the bedside. Lambl described and illustrated a number of bladder conditions, including cancer (Fig. 22-2). This was the beginning of contemporary cytology of the urinary sediment. The reader is referred to other sources for a detailed description of these early events (Koss, 1995).

Nearly 150 years after the publication of Lambl's contribution on the cytology of the urinary sediment, the benefits and limitations of this method of diagnosis are still poorly understood by urologists and pathologists. It would be a safe bet that the opinions of individual urologists may vary from total indifference to the method as worthless in clinical practice, to the rare enthusiastic endorsement, with the majority expressing a moderate degree of interest in a method of occasional value.

The problem with cytology of the urinary tract is the lack of **basic understanding of the accomplishments and limitations of the method** and of the pathologic processes accounting for it. As will be set forth in this and the next chapter, it is **unrealistic to expect that the cytologic method will serve to recognize the presence or recurrence of low-grade papillary tumors.** It is equally **unrealistic** to expect that cytology of urine, or of the various ancillary sampling procedures, will help in **differentiating low-grade papillary tumors from other space-occupying lesions of the renal pelvis or ureter.** This accounts for the introduction of numerous noncytologic methods of diagnosis by commercial companies, discussed in the next chapter.

On the other hand, cytologic techniques are highly effective in detection and diagnosis **of high-grade malignant tumors,** particularly **flat carcinomas in situ,** which are the principal precursor lesions of invasive urothelial cancer. Cytology of urine is also valuable in the recognition of various **viral infections,** particularly **human polyomavirus, and the effects of various therapeutic procedures.** In our judg-ment, cytology of the urinary tract is **one of the most important diagnostic methods in urologic oncology,** provided:

- It is used properly by the urologist under well-defined circumstances and for well-defined reasons.
- It is performed by a laboratory competent in processing and interpretation of such specimens.
- The urologist and the pathologist understand the limitations of the method and are familiar with sources of error.

Application of Cytology in Forensic Sciences

An unusual application of cytology is the **identification of female cells in postcoital swab smears of the penis.** Fluorescence in situ hybridization techniques were used to record female cells with two X chromosome signals (Collins et al, 2000). The technique may be helpful in proving sexual contact in cases of presumed rape.

ANATOMY

The urinary tract is composed of the **kidneys, ureters, urinary bladder, and urethra.** The position of these organs in the abdominal cavity and the methods of cytologic sampling are shown in Figure 22-3.

The **two kidneys are fist-sized, encapsulated organs** located laterally in the retroperitoneal space. The principal function of the kidney is to **filter** blood and eliminate harmful products of metabolism and other impurities that are excreted in **urine.** The bulk of the kidney is constituted by the filtering apparatus or **nephrons,** each composed of the principal filtering device, or the **glomerulus,** connected to a series of **tubules.** The filtrate generated by the glomeruli

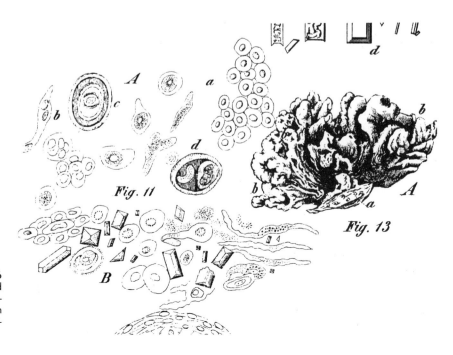

Figure 22-2 Figures from Lambl's 1856 paper. Figure 11 illustrates various cells and crystals observed in the urinary sediment. Figure 13 shows a "Papillary pseudoplasma from the urethra of a girl"—undoubtedly a condyloma acuminatum.

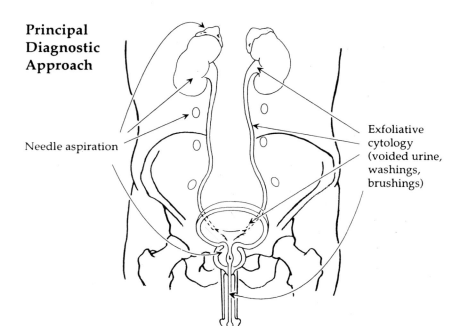

Principal Diagnostic Approach

Needle aspiration

Exfoliative cytology (voided urine, washings, brushings)

Figure 22-3 Diagram of the principal organs of the urinary tract and the methods of investigation by either exfoliative or aspiration cytology. (Diagram by Dr. Diane Hamele-Bena, College of Physicians and Surgeons of Columbia University, New York, NY.)

undergoes many modifications in the tubulus until the final product of the filtration process, or the **urine,** is excreted into the **renal pelvis,** whence it travels through the **ureters** to the **bladder.**

The kidney is essential to the maintenance of osmotic equilibrium in the blood. It also contributes to the regulation of blood pressure and has several other ancillary functions. It is beyond the scope of this book to provide details on the complex structure and function of the kidneys and interested readers are referred to specialized sources for further information.

The **ureters** are firm cylindrical structures, about 20 to 25 cm in length and about 0.5 cm in diameter. In their course toward the bladder, the ureters cross the pelvic brim and enter the bony pelvis, and thence the **urinary bladder.** In the **female,** the **ureters pass near the lowest segment of the uterus** to reach the bladder. This relationship is important in patients with **invasive cancer of the uterine cervix** that can surround and obstruct the ureters.

The bladder is a balloon-shaped organ composed from inside out of an **epithelium,** a connective tissue layer known as **lamina propria,** and an elastic **muscular wall (muscularis propria).** These component tissues work in unison to allow expansion of bladder volume while accumulating urine and collapse with voiding. Under pathologic circumstances, the bladder is capable of accommodating up to several liters of urine without rupture.

Lamina propria is a thin layer of connective tissue supporting the urothelium. It is rich in vessels and in most individuals, but not all, contains an **interrupted thin layer of smooth muscle cells (muscularis mucosae). The nests of Brunn and the cysts of cystitis cystica** are located within the lamina propria. **Muscularis propria, or the principal muscle of the bladder,** is composed of two thick concentric layers of smooth muscle, in continuity with the **muscular wall of the ureters.**

The **embryologic derivation** of the bladder is in part from the **cloaca,** or the **terminal portion of the embryonal intestinal tract.** A vestigial organ, the **urachus,** a remnant of the embryonal omphaloenteric duct, connects the bladder dome with the umbilicus. Other parts of the bladder are derived from the **genital tubercle.** This dual embryonal origin accounts for the **variety of epithelial types** that may occur in the bladder (see below). The basal portion of the urinary bladder contains the **trigone,** a triangular area with the apex directed forward to the urethra. The two **ureters enter the bladder** at the posterior angles of the trigone. The urine passes from the bladder into the **urethra,** which begins at the apex of the trigone. The important anatomic relationships of the trigone differ between females and males. In the **female,** the trigone **overlies the vesicovaginal septum and the vagina,** whereas in the **male,** the immediately underlying organs are the **prostate and seminal vesicles.** It is evident that cancers of these various organs may extend to the trigone and vice-versa.

The **female urethra** has only a very short course and opens into the upper portion of the **vaginal vestibule,** somewhat behind and below the clitoris (see Chap. 8). In the **male,** the urethra runs **across and through the prostate** and enters the **penis.** The anatomy of the prostate is discussed in Chapter 33.

THE UROTHELIUM

Histology

Urine is a toxic substance and, hence, the **renal pelves, ureters, bladder, and urethra must be capable of preventing the seepage of urine into the capillary bed in the wall of these organs** or, in other words, **protecting the urine-blood barrier.** This protective function is, at least in part, vested in the **highly specialized type of epithelium** lining these organs. Because of its **unique structure and ultrastructure,** this epithelium should be referred to as the **urothelium,** but is often called by the **improper traditional term—transitional epithelium.** The urothelium is **uniquely flexible** and **adapts to the changing volume of urine in the bladder, without breaching the urine-blood barrier.**

In tissue sections, **the normal urothelium** is composed on **the average of seven layers of cells,** although **the number of cell layers may appear greater in contracted bladders and smaller in dilated bladders. The superficial cells of the urothelium, also known as the umbrella cells, are very large and are often multinucleated.** The term **umbrella cells** indicates that each superficial cell covers several smaller cells of the underlying deeper layer in an umbrella-like fashion. In **histologic sections** of the **bladder,** the umbrella cells vary in shape, according to the state of dilatation of the bladder. **In the dilated bladder, they appear flat;**

in the contracted bladder, they are more rounded or cuboidal (Fig. 22-4C,D). In the renal pelvis, the ureters, and the urethra, the umbrella cells are usually cuboidal in configuration. The structure of umbrella cells is much better seen in cytologic material than in tissue sections (see below). The **deeper cell layers** are made up of cuboidal cells with a single nucleus. The schematic representation of the dilated and contracted mammalian urothelium is shown in Figure 22-4A,B. Cordon-Cardo et al (1984) and Fradet et al (1987) documented immunologic differences between deeper and superficial cells of the urothelium by means of various monoclonal antibodies. It should be added that Petry and Amon (1966) believed that cells in all layers of the urothelium were attached to basement membrane by means of cytoplasmic extensions. We were unable to confirm this observation.

Ultrastructural observations disclosed that the umbrella cells in all mammals, including humans, are lined on their surface (facing the bladder lumen) by a **unique**

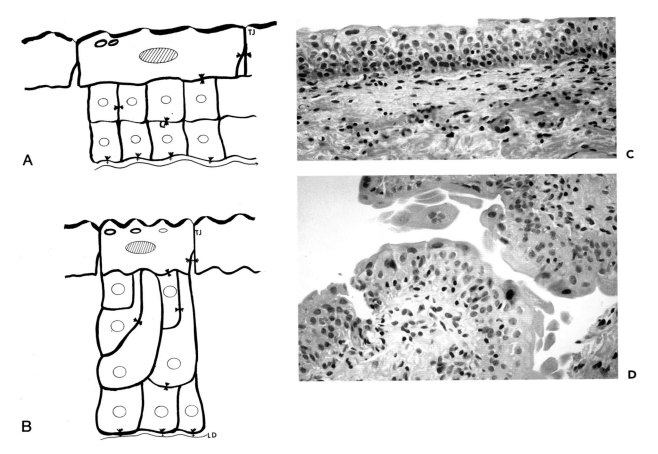

Figure 22-4 Diagrammatic representation of a dilated (*A*) and contracted (*B*) bladder urothelium to show the changes in cell configuration and the mechanism of cell movement. The superficial cells (umbrella cells) are shown lined by thick plaques of the asymmetric unit membrane, with intercalated segments of thin, symmetric membrane. The structure of the membrane can be compared with medieval armor in which flexible links between metal plates provided mobility for the bearer. Near the surface, the umbrella cells are linked by tight junctions (TJ). Abundant desmosomes bind the epithelial cells. Hemidesmosomes bind the epithelium to the lamina densa (LD). Note the difference in the configuration of the superficial cells in the dilated and contracted bladder. *C.* Histologic section of a dilated bladder, corresponding to *A. D.* Histologic section of a contracted bladder, corresponding to *B.* Note differences in the configuration of umbrella cells. (*A,B:* Modified from Koss LG. Some ultrastructural aspects of experimental and human carcinoma of the bladder. Cancer Res 37: 2824–2835, 1977.)

membrane known as the **asymmetric unit membrane (AUM)** (Hicks, 1966; Koss, 1969, 1977). The membrane has **two components—rigid, thick plaques** and **intervening segments of thin plasma membrane** or **hinges** (Fig. 22-5). The plaques, measuring about 13 nm in thickness, are composed of **three layers; the two outer layers are electron opaque and of unequal thickness,** the central layer is electron lucent. The term **asymmetric unit membrane** is descriptive of the difference in thickness of the electron-opaque components. It is assumed that the plaques may play a role in the urine-blood barrier, whereas the **intervening segments of plasma membrane act like hinges, providing flexibility to the plaques, thereby ensuring that the umbrella cells can adapt to changing urinary volume requirements** (Fig. 22-4C,D). There is some experimental evidence that the destruction of the superficial cells increases the permeability of the bladder to lithium ions (Hicks, 1966). Still, the urine-blood barrier remains in place, even in the absence of umbrella cells or of the asymmetric plaques, as is common in older persons (Jacob et al, 1978). Hu et al (2000) suggested that this function is vested in one of the membrane proteins, uroplakins (see below). Ablation of the uroplakin III gene in mice resulted in formation of smaller epithelial plaques and urothelial leakage. Still, it is likely that the urine-blood barrier function is also vested in other components of the bladder wall, such as the basement lamina and the muscle. For discussion of uroplakins, see below.

The AUM is produced in the Golgi complex of the superficial cells and travels to the surface packaged into oblong vesicles (Fig. 22-5), as was documented many years ago (Hicks, 1966; Koss, 1969, 1977). The **chemical structure** of the AUM has been unraveled. Its protein components, known as **uroplakins Ia, Ib, II, III,** have been analyzed and sequenced and their role as marker molecules will be discussed in the next chapter (Yu et al, 1990; Wu et al, 1990, 1994; 1996). The particles of the uroplakins form well-ordered hexagonal lattices (Walz et al, 1995). Liang et

al (1999) studied the **chemical make-up of the "hinges,"** located between the plaques in bovine urothelium. They reported that these segments of the urothelial surface membrane have a specialized chemical make-up, differing from the plaques.

The **deeper epithelial cells** are of approximately cuboidal shape and are attached to each other by numerous **desmosomes.** These cells have no specific ultrastructural features.

Of signal interest is a series of studies suggesting that the urothelium may have highly specialized **active functions,** such as regulating protein secretions in urine (Deng et al, 2001) and secretion of growth hormone (Kerr et al, 1998).

It is of note that human urothelial cells can be successfully cultured from the sediment of voided urine (Herz et al, 1979). The AUM may persist in several generations of these cells (Shokri-Tabibzadeh et al, 1982).

Epithelial Variants in the Lower Urinary Tract

Because of its diverse embryonal origin, the lower urinary tract may be partially lined by epithelia other than the urothelium. These are:

- Squamous epithelium of vaginal type
- Intestinal type glandular epithelium
- Brunn's nests and cystitis cystica

The location and distribution of these epithelial variants was documented by mapping studies of normal bladders (Morse, 1928; Wiener et al, 1979; Ito, 1981). The frequency of these epithelial variants is summarized in Table 22-1.

Squamous Epithelium of the Vaginal Type

The **trigone of the bladder in approximately 50% of normal adult women** and in a small proportion of men contains areas of **nonkeratinizing squamous epithelium of the vaginal type** (Fig. 22-6A). In cystoscopy, this area may appear as a gray membrane. Although this is merely an anatomic variant of bladder epithelium and evidence of in-

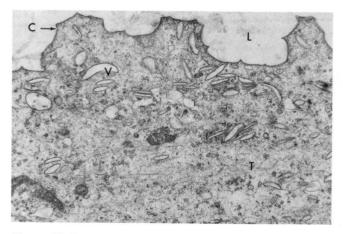

Figure 22-5 Electron micrograph of a superficial cell of moderately dilated rat bladder. Note the characteristic oblong vesicle (V) lined by a rigid, asymmetric unit membrane, morphologically identical with segments of the cell membrane (C). L, lumen of bladder. Fine tonofilaments (T) are evident as well as a few round vesicles and mitochondria. (×20, 400.)

TABLE 22-1

FREQUENCY OF EPITHELIAL VARIANTS IN 100 CONSECUTIVE NORMAL BLADDERS (61 MALE, 39 FEMALE; 8 CHILDREN AND 92 ADULTS)

Total bladders with one or more lesions: 93		
	Male	**Female**
Brunn's nests	53	36
Cystitis cystica	32	28
Vaginal metaplasia	3	19
None	6*	1*

* Two newborns: 1 male, 1 female. 5 males: 4 adults, 1, age 13. From Weiner et al, 1979.

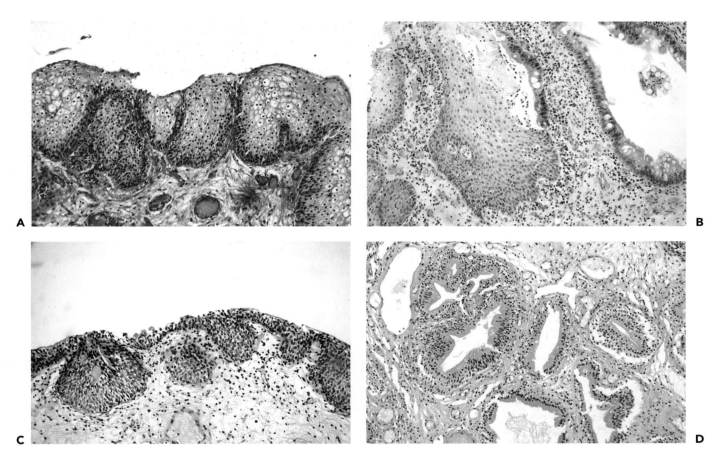

Figure 22-6   Variants of urothelium. *A.* Squamous epithelium of the vaginal type from the trigone of an adult woman. *B.* Glandular epithelium of intestinal type, adjacent to plugs of squamous epithelium from an exstrophic bladder in a 7-year-old child. *C.* Nests of Brunn. *D.* Cystitis cystica.

flammation is usually absent, this condition has been recorded clinically as **"urethrotrigonitis," "epidermidization,"** or **"membranous trigonitis."** In women, **this epithelium appears to be under hormonal control** and is the most likely source of squamous cells in **urocytograms,** described in Chapter 9.

Intestinal-Type Epithelium

Because the embryonal intestinal tract (the cloaca) participates in the formation of the lower urinary tract, areas of **mucus-producing intestinal-type epithelium with goblet cells may occur in the bladder, the ureters, and even the renal pelves.** In most patients, these areas are small, but **occasionally the bladder (sometimes also the ureters and the renal pelves) may be fully or partially lined by this type of the epithelium** (Fig. 22-6B). This is particularly evident in **exstrophy,** a congenital abnormality in which at birth, the bladder is located outside of the abdominal wall, but may also occur in anatomically normal organs (Koss, 1975). The intestinal type epithelium may contain **endocrine Paneth cells.** When the surface lined by intestinal epithelium is large, it presents a **high risk for adenocarcinoma.**

Brunn's Nests and Cystitis Cystica

The urothelium of the bladder may form small, usually round **buds, known as** the nests of von Brunn **(Brunn's**

nests) that extend into the lamina propria, occasionally to the level of the muscularis. Brunn's nests occur in approximately 80% of normal bladders. Occasionally, a florid proliferation of Brunn's nests may occur within the lamina propria (Volmar et al, 2003). Within the **center of Brunn's nests, there is often formation of cysts, which may be lined by mucus-producing columnar epithelium** (Fig. 22-6C). The cysts may become quite large and distended with mucus, giving rise to so-called **cystitis cystica or glandularis** (Fig. 22-6D). Gland-like cystic structures may also arise directly from the urothelium without going through the stage of Brunn's nests. Some of these structures **may express prostate-specific antigen** (Nowels et al, 1988). It is traditional to consider Brunn's nests and cystitis cystica as an expression of abnormal urothelial proliferation, either caused by an inflammatory process or as an expression of a neoplastic potential. This most **emphatically is not true.** The mapping studies of normal urinary bladders disclosed that such findings are common in normal bladders and must be considered as mere anatomic variants of the urothelium (Morse, 1928; Wiener et al, 1979; Ito, 1981).

Nephrogenic adenoma or adenosis is an uncommon benign lesion of the urinary bladder, composed of cystic spaces of various sizes lined by cuboidal epithelial cells (Koss, 1985). The lesion may contain elements of renal tubules. The lesion is of no diagnostic significance in urinary tract cytology, unless it becomes a site of an adenocarcinoma.

CYTOLOGY OF THE LOWER URINARY TRACT

As indicated in the anatomic diagram (see Fig. 22-3), there are two principal methods of cytologic sampling of the urinary tract: **exfoliative cytology** based on voided urine, washings or brushings of the epithelial surfaces, and **needle aspiration techniques** of solid organs, the kidneys, adrenals, retroperitoneum, and prostate. In this chapter, only the exfoliative cytology of the epithelial surfaces of the lower urinary tract is described. Aspiration biopsy of the solid organs is described in Chapters 33 and 40.

Methods of Specimen Collection

The principal methods of specimen collections are:

- Voided urine
- Catheterized urine
- Direct sampling techniques
    Bladder washings or barbotage
    Cell collection by retrograde catheterization of ureters
    Direct brushings

The selection of the method of specimen collection and processing depends on clinical circumstances and the goal of the examination. The advantages and disadvantages of the various methods are summarized in Table 22-2.

Voided Urine

This is by far the easiest and least expensive method of cytologic investigation of the urinary tract. The technique is valuable **as a preliminary assessment of a broad spectrum of abnormalities of the urethra, bladder, ureters and renal pelves** and, under special circumstances, of the kidney and prostate.

Urine is an acellular liquid product of renal excretory function. As the liquid passes through the renal tubules, renal pelvis, ureter, bladder, and urethra, it picks up desquamating cells derived from the epithelia of these organs. Inflammatory cells, erythrocytes, and macrophages are frequently seen. Voided urine normally has an acid pH and a high content of urea and other organic components; therefore, it is not isotonic. Consequently, **the urine is not a hospitable medium for desquamated cells, which are often poorly preserved and sometimes difficult to assess on microscopic examination.**

Collection

Morning urine specimens have the advantage of highest cellularity, but also the disadvantage of marked cell degeneration. **A specimen from the morning's second voiding is usually best. Three samples obtained on 3 consecutive days are diagnostically optimal** (Koss et al, 1985). Naib (1976) recommended hydration of patients to increase the yield of desquamated cells (1 glass of water every 30 minutes during a 3-hour period).

Processing

Unless the urine is processed without delay, the addition of a **fixative** is recommended. In our hands, the **best fixative is 2% polyethylene glycol (Carbowax) solution in 50% to 70% ethanol** (Bales, 1981). To achieve best results, the patient should be provided with a 250 to 300 ml widemouth glass or plastic container one-third filled with fixative. This makes it convenient for **home collection** of samples.

The urinary sediment can be processed in a variety of ways. The specimen can be centrifuged for 10 minutes at moderate speed and a **direct smear of the sediment** made on adhesive-coated slides. The urine **can be filtered** using one of the commercially available filtering devices, either for **direct viewing** of cells on the surface of the filter, or after transferring the filtered cells to a glass slide by imprinting them **(reverse filtration).** Alternatively, the cellular sediment can be placed on an adhesive-coated slide by use of a **cytocentrifuge,** preferably using the **method developed by Bales** (1981) in our laboratory. Several commercial methods of preparation of the urinary sediment have been developed within recent years. Urine sediment preparation by ThinPrep has been reported by Luthra et al (1999) as giving satisfactory results. Both ThinPrep and SurePath gave satisfactory results to Wright and Halford (2001). Still, these methods **may modify the appearance of urothelial cells, particularly their nuclei.** For further details on sample processing, see Chapter 44. The use of **phase microscopy** (de Voogt et al, 1975) and of **supravital stains** (Sternheimer, 1975) in the assessment of urine cytology has been suggested. Neither method received wide acceptance.

Catheterized Urine

The specimens are collected via a catheter and processed as described above for voided urine.

Direct Sampling Techniques

Bladder Washings or Barbotage

This procedure may be used to obtain **cellular specimens of well-preserved epithelium from patients at high risk for development of new or recurrent bladder tumors.** It is the specimen of choice for **DNA ploidy analysis** of the urinary epithelium, discussed in Chapters 23 and 47. The bladder should first be emptied by catheter. Bladder barbotage is then best performed **during or prior to cystoscopy** by instilling and recovering 3 to 4 times 50 to 100 ml of normal saline or Ringer's solution. The procedure can also be performed through **a catheter** but it is uncomfortable, particularly for male patients, and the results are less satisfactory.

Retrograde Catheterization of Ureters or Renal Pelves

This procedure is used **to establish the nature of a space-occupying lesion** of ureter or renal pelvis, observed by radiologic techniques. The most common application of the procedure is in the **differential diagnosis between a stone, a blood clot, or a tumor.** Other rare, space-occupying lesions of the **renal pelves** are **inflammatory masses, angi-**

TABLE 22-2

PRINCIPAL ADVANTAGES AND DISADVANTAGES OF VARIOUS CYTOLOGIC METHODS OF INVESTIGATION OF THE LOWER URINARY TRACT

Method	Advantages	Disadvantages	Remarks
Voided urine	Efficient method for **diagnosis of high grade tumors** (including carcinoma in situ) of bladder, ureters, and renal pelves. Unique method for the diagnosis of **human polyomavirus infection.** The method is of value in **monitoring** patients with locally treated tumors and patients with renal transplants. Examination can be repeated without harming the patient.	The findings are not consistent, and three or more specimens should be examined for optimal results. Sources of error must be known.	All methods fail in consistent identification of low-grade tumors. For exceptions, see text.
Catheterized urine	**Same** as voided urine. Less contamination with cells of female genital tract.	Same as voided urine.	
Bladder washings	**Same** as voided urine, but results confined to bladder. The diagnosis of high-grade tumors is sometimes easier. **Ideal medium for DNA measurements.**	The method is poorly tolerated by ambulatory patients, particularly males. Optimal results may require cystoscopy.	Fragments of low-grade tumors may sometimes be recognized, but beware of errors. See text. Useful to confirm occult carcinoma or CIS in bladder when cancer cells are found in voided urine.
Retrograde brushing	Occasionally useful in the identification and localization of high grade tumors of **ureters and renal pelves.**	A major source of diagnostic errors (see below and Chap. 23). The value of the procedure in the differential diagnosis of space-occupying lesions of ureters or renal pelves is very low.	
Drip urine collected from ureters	Efficient method of localization of high grade tumors of ureters and renal pelves.	A time-consuming procedure.	Separate catheters must be used for each side to avoid contamination.
Ileal bladder urine	Efficient in the diagnosis of metachronous **high grade tumors of ureters and renal pelves after cystectomy** for bladder cancer. Occasional primary lesions of ileal conduit may be observed.	Same as voided urine. Knowledge of cytologic presentation is essential.	A mandatory follow-up procedure after cystectomy for bladder cancer.

Modified from: Koss LG. Diagnostic Cytology of Urinary Tract. Philadelphia, Lippincott-Raven, 1996.

omas, and congenital aberrations of the vascular bed. In the **ureter,** there may be lesions caused by a **tumor, a stricture, or extraneous pressure.**

Another important application of this technique **is the localization of an occult malignant tumor diagnosed in voided urine sediment but not found in the bladder.** The purpose is to determine whether the tumor can be **localized in the left or right** kidney or ureter. For urine collection, **separate catheters must be used for each side** to avoid cross-contamination. The best results are obtained by **inserting the catheter to a depth of 3 to 4 cm into the ureters and by placing the other tip of the catheter in a container with fixative.** From 10 to 30 minutes may be needed to collect 5 to 10 ml of urine necessary for diagnosis. Although the procedure may be tedious to the patient, it is quite efficient in localizing the lesion.

The Direct Brushing Procedure

This procedure is used in the **investigation of space-occupying lesions in the ureters or renal pelves.** Brushing is performed through a ureteral catheter. The indications are the same as listed for retrograde catheterization.

Processing of Direct Samples

Bladder washings or barbotage specimens may be processed in a manner similar to voided urine, discussed above. **Retrograde catheterization specimens,** if liquid, are processed in a similar manner. **Direct brush specimens** are usually prepared in the cystoscopy suite by the urologist and submitted as **smears.** For **optimal preservation, the smears** should be immediately fixed in 50% ethanol for at least 10 minutes. Alternatively, the **brushes can be placed in a 50% alcohol fixative** and forwarded to the laboratory for further processing. See Chapter 44 for further comments on processing of this material.

Cellular Components of the Urinary Sediment

An **understanding of the complexities of the normal cell population** of the urinary sediment under various clinical circumstances is an **important first step for proper diag-** nostic utilization of cytology of the urinary tract. **Methods of sample collection and processing have a major impact on the interpretation of the cytologic images.** As always, information on **clinical circumstances** and **clinical procedures** leading to the collection of the cytologic samples may prevent major errors of interpretation, particularly in low-grade urothelial tumors.

The urinary sediment contains:

- Cells derived from the urothelium and its variants
- Cells derived from renal tubules
- Cells derived from adjacent organs
- Cells extraneous to the urinary tract, such as macrophages and blood cells

Normal Urothelial Cells

Normal urothelial cells have several features that set them apart from other epithelial cells. The **cells vary greatly in size:** the superficial umbrella cells are often very large and may contain multiple nuclei, whereas epithelial cells from the deeper layers of the urothelium are much smaller and usually have a single nucleus. Another important general feature of urothelial cells is their tendency to desquamate in **large, complex clusters, particularly after instrumenta-**

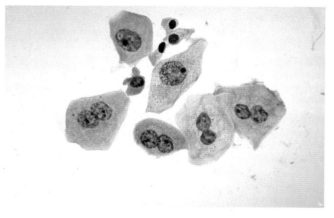
A

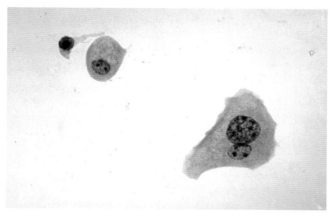
B

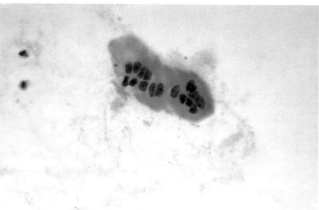
C

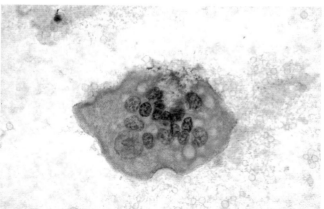
D

Figure 22-7   Umbrella cells and their variants. *A.* Umbrella cells from a bladder washing. Mononucleated and binucleated cells are seen side by side. Note that the nuclei of the binucleated cells are smaller than those of mononucleated cells. Also note one sharply demarcated rigid surface of these cells, corresponding to the asymmetric membrane. *B.* Two umbrella cells of different size, one with two nuclei of unequal size. *C.* A multinucleated umbrella cell with very small nuclei. *D.* A very large multinucleated umbrella cell with small nuclei.

tion. It must be stressed, once again, that **the appearance of the sediment varies according to the method of collection.**

Superficial Umbrella Cells

The **size of the umbrella cells is variable** and depends to some extent on the number of nuclei. The average **mononucleated umbrella cells** measure from **20 to 30 μm in diameter** and, hence, are much larger than the cells from deeper epithelial layers (see below). **Multinucleated** umbrella cells may be **substantially larger** (Fig. 22-7). These cells are usually **flat and polygonal** and usually have one **sharply demarcated, and sometimes angulated, surface.** The **abundant cytoplasm is thin and transparent, some-times faintly vacuolated,** and may contain **fat** (Masin and Masin, 1976) or **mucus-containing vacuoles** (Dorfman and Monis, 1964). Sometimes, the nature of the vacuoles cannot be ascertained (Fig. 22-8A).

The nuclei also vary in size. In **mononucleated cells,** the **spherical or oval nuclei** may measure from **8 to 20 μm in diameter,** depending on the size of the cell. The large nuclei reflect a tendency of urothelial cells to form **tetraploid** or even **octaploid nuclei** (Levi et al, 1969; Far-sund, 1974). This tendency to polyploidy appears to be part

and parcel of the pattern of normal urothelial differentiation but its mechanism is unknown. These features of normal umbrella cells are important in DNA measurements (Woj-cik et al, 2000). In well-preserved umbrella cells, the nuclei are **faintly granular but may contain prominent baso-philic chromocenters** that should not be **confused with large nucleoli.** Using some of the **newer methods of semi-automated processing the chromocenters may be eosino-philic,** accounting for additional difficulties in the inter-pretation of the samples (Fig. 22-8B). **In some samples processed by commercial methods, we have observed peculiar condensation of nuclear chromatin, mimicking mitotic figures** (Fig. 22-8C).

Multinucleated umbrella cells also vary in size. Most cells are binucleated and contain either nuclei of normal size and configuration or smaller. Other cells have **multiple nuclei of variable sizes** (see Fig. 22-7C). **Large and small nuclei often** occur side by side within the same cell. Still other umbrella cells may contain **10 or more small nuclei** and appear as multinucleated giant cells (see Fig. 22-8C,D). Umbrella cells derived directly from **the ureters** are often much larger with many more nuclei than in cells derived from the bladder. Occasionally, the nuclei in the large super-ficial cells are **clumped and degenerated and may be mis-**

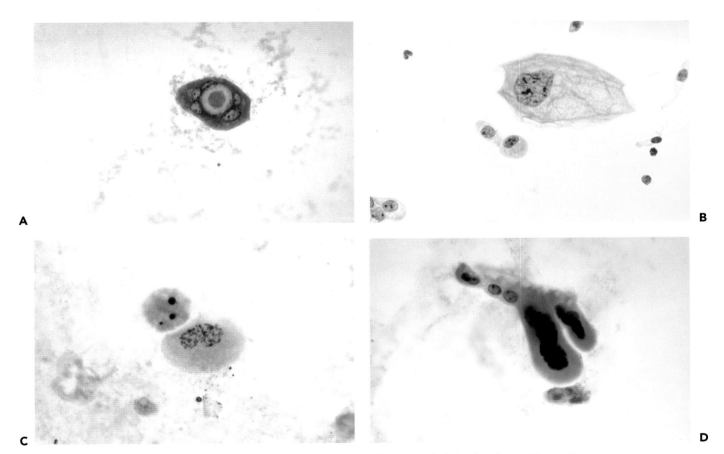

Figure 22-8 **Variants of superficial urothelial cells.** *A.* Urothelial cell with multiple small cyto-plasmic vacuoles and nuclear modification of unknown significance. *B.* An umbrella cell with an excep-tionally large nucleus containing multiple eosinophilic chromocenters that should not be mistaken for nucleoli. *C.* High magnification of urothelial cells with peculiar condensation of chromatin, which in the larger cell mimics a mitotic figure, probably a processing artifact (ThinPrep). *D.* Multinucleated umbrella cells with pyknotic, degenerated nuclei.

taken for nuclei of cancer cells, **an important source of diagnostic error** (see Fig. 22-8D).

Cells from the Deeper Layers of the Urothelium

Urothelial cells originating in the deeper layers of the urothelium, are rarely seen in voided urine, but are common in specimens obtained by or collected after instrumentation. These cells are much smaller than umbrella cells and are **comparable in size to small parabasal cervical squamous cells** and unlike the superficial cells, **show little variation in size.** When fresh and well preserved, these cells have **sharply demarcated transparent cytoplasm** that is often **elongated and whip-shaped** when the cells are removed by instruments. The cytoplasm is stretched at points of desmosomal attachments to neighboring cells, a phenomenon also observed in metaplastic cervical cells (see Chap. 8). The **finely granular nuclei may contain single chromocenters, mimicking nucleoli** (Fig. 22-9A,B). **Occasionally, the nuclei may be pyknotic, particularly in brushings** (Fig. 22-9C). **Similar cells in voided urine may have pale, transparent nuclei. Occasionally, mitotic figures may be**

noted, particularly in **urinary sediment obtained after a diagnostic or therapeutic surgical procedure** (Fig. 22-9D).

Clusters of Urothelial Cells

A very important feature of normal urothelium is its propensity to desquamate in fragments or clusters that are sometimes very complex. Although this feature is markedly enhanced in urine samples obtained by bladder catheterization, lavage, or any type of instrumentation, urothelial cell clusters may also occur in spontaneously voided urine. It appears that even abdominal palpation, the slightest trauma, or inflammatory injury to the bladder may enhance the shedding of clusters. **The clusters may be small and flat, composed of only a relatively few clearly benign cells** (Fig. 22-10A), or much larger and composed of **several hundred superimposed cells.** The clusters may round up and **appear to be spherical, oval, or "papillary" in configuration** (Fig. 22-10B). Occasionally, they are more **complex** (Fig. 22-10C) and sometimes **distorted** during smear preparation. The distor-

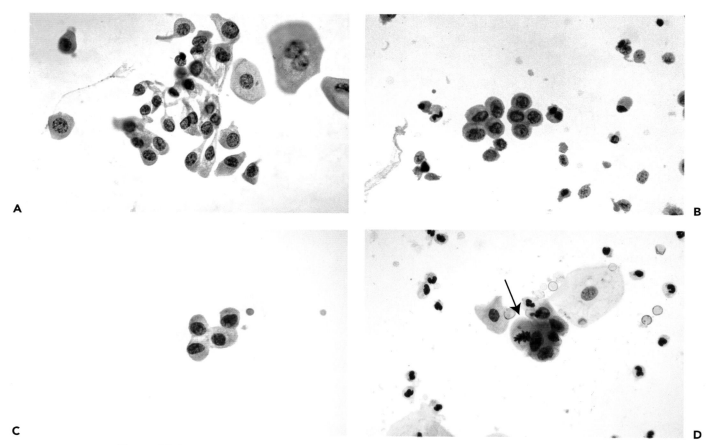

Figure 22-9 **Cells from deeper layers of the urothelium.** *A.* Specimen obtained by lavage of the bladder showing a large cluster of urothelial cells from deeper epithelial layers. Note that the cytoplasm of many of these cells is elongated because of desmosomal adherence. Peripheral to the cluster of small cells are several larger umbrella cells. *B.* Small urothelial cells from deeper layers in a bladder barbotage specimen. Note the faintly granular nuclei and abundance of peripheral cytoplasm. *C.* Small urothelial cells from deep epithelial layers in a specimen of retrograde brushings of the ureter. *D.* Small urothelial cells showing mitotic activity (*arrow*). This specimen was obtained 3 days after transurethral resection of the prostate.

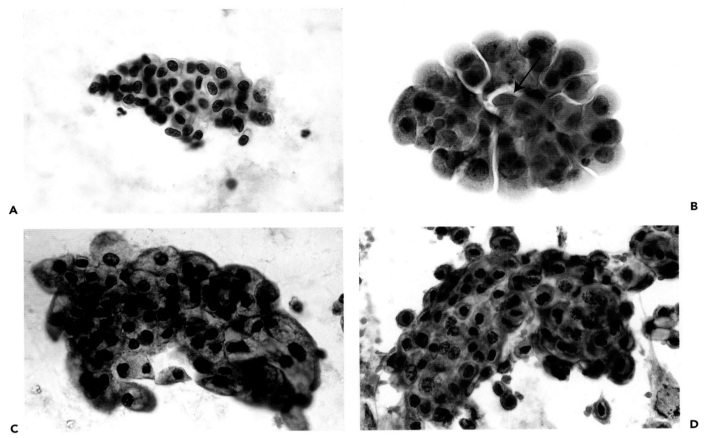

Figure 22-10   Clusters of benign urothelial cells. *A.* A cluster of approximately papillary configuration composed of small epithelial cells from the deeper epithelial layers. *B.* A cluster of large urothelial cells with umbrella cells at the periphery (high power). Note the spherical "papillary" structure of the cluster, a formation caused by contraction of muscularis mucosae, which may be seen as an eosinophilic structure in the center of that cluster (*arrow*). *C.* A large cluster of superficial and deep urothelial cells seen in a retrograde catheterization specimen. *D.* A large cluster of large and small urothelial cells in a lavage specimen of left kidney.

tion may be increased if frosted slides are used. The periphery of such clusters should be carefully examined under high magnification of the microscope. **On close inspection, the edge of the clusters is sharply demarcated, and the normal component cells of the urothelium may be readily observed** (Fig. 22-10D). It must be noted that in urine sediment prepared by the **ThinPrep method,** nuclear chromocenters sometimes stain pink or red and thus may be considered to be "atypical" or even malignant. **It is paramount in urinary cytology to avoid making the diagnosis of a papillary tumor based on the presence of clusters.** For further discussion of cytology of bladder tumors, see Chapter 23.

Cytologic Expressions of Epithelial Variants

It has been pointed out above that several epithelial variants may occur in bladder epithelium. **Intestinal-type epithelium may be the source of columnar, sometimes mucus-producing cells that are found in bladder washings and catheterized specimens but are uncommon in voided urine** (Fig. 22-11A). These cells have a generally clear cytoplasm and spherical, finely granular small nuclei. Harris et

al (1971) first described **ciliated columnar cells** in bladder washings (Fig. 22-11B).

There are no specific cytologic findings corresponding to Brunn's nests and cystitis cystica. Dabbs (1992) published his observations in renal pelvic washings in a case of **pyelitis cystica** but the findings, as illustrated, showed only clusters of normal urothelial cells.

Squamous epithelium sheds squamous cells of various degrees of maturity (Fig. 22-11C). The finding **is exceedingly common** and normal in adult women but is somewhat less frequent in men. In women, the urinary sediment may be used to assess their hormonal status (**"urocytogram"**), as discussed in Chapter 9. In both sexes, the harmless **squamous epithelium may become fully keratinized (leukoplakia),** presumably as a consequence of chronic irritation. The cytologic findings and significance of leukoplakia of the bladder are discussed below.

Renal Tubular Cells

Renal tubules are **lined by a single layer of epithelial cells** that vary somewhat in configuration according to the segment of the tubule. Of special interest in urine cytology is the terminal part of the tubular apparatus or the **collecting**

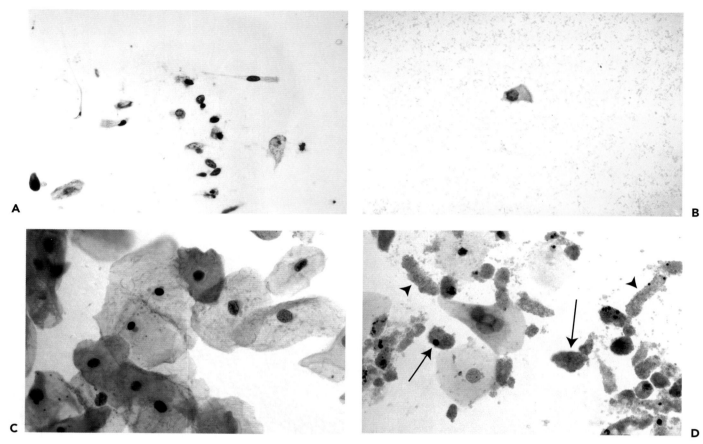

Figure 22-11 Variants of urothelial cells. *A.* Columnar urothelial cells in a bladder lavage. *B.* Small columnar cell with ciliated surface. *C.* Intermediate squamous cells. *D.* Renal tubular cells surrounding an umbrella cell. Note the small size, pyknotic nuclei, and granular cytoplasm of the tubular cells (*arrows*). Also present in this same field are a few granular casts (*arrowheads*).

ducts, lined by a single layer of cuboidal to columnar epithelial cells with clear cytoplasm and small spherical nuclei. These cells may be observed in the urinary sediment under various circumstances.

Renal tubular cells may be numerous whenever there is some **insult to the renal parenchyma,** for example, after an **intravenous pyelogram.** They may be found after an episode of **hematuria or hemoglobinuria.** The small cells are **poorly preserved, cuboidal or columnar in shape,** and are characterized by **small pyknotic nuclei and granular cytoplasm** (Fig. 22-11D). The presence of numerous, well-preserved tubular cells is of importance in monitoring renal transplant patients (see below). The renal tubular cells have **phagocytic properties** and may store the **dyes** used in intravenous pyelography, which are visualized as a yellow pigment in the cytoplasm. Khalil et al (1999) described **large, vacuolated renal tubular cells** with some similarity to macrophages, in the voided urine sediment of a patient with a rare disorder, **osmotic nephrosis.** The patient was treated with intravenous immunoglobulins stored in the cytoplasm. The identity of the cells was confirmed by immunochemistry and electron microscopy. **The presence of renal tubular cells in the urinary sediment must be correlated with clinical circumstances and does not necessarily indicate the presence of a renal disorder.**

Renal Casts

Accumulation of various proteins, erythrocytes, leukocytes, necrotic cells, and cellular debris **molded into longitudinal cylindrical structures** are known as **renal casts.** It is often assumed that the presence of casts indicates a severe renal disorder. However, carefully collected and fixed urinary sediment samples often reveal renal casts in the absence of disease.

In voided urine specimens collected in a 2% polyethylene glycol (Carbowax) solution in 70% ethanol (Bales, 1981; see Chap. 44), **renal tubular cells and casts are well preserved and observed with unexpected frequency, even in patients without overt evidence of renal pathology.**

The renal tubular casts are either **hyaline or granular.** The **hyaline casts** are composed of **homogeneous eosinophilic protein material,** sometimes with a few renal tubular cells attached at the periphery (Fig. 22-12A). The **granular casts** are composed of **cell debris mixed with degenerating renal tubular cells** with granular cytoplasm (Fig. 22-12B; see also Fig. 22-11D). Such casts are very common in renal transplant patients during episodes of rejection (see below) but may also be observed after urography during the period of elimination of the dye (Fischer et al, 1982). The presence of casts must be correlated with clinical data as it may indicate the presence of a renal parenchymal disorder.

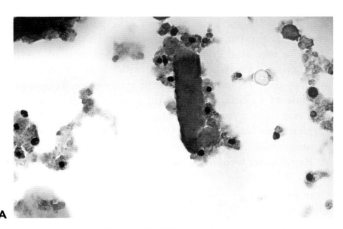
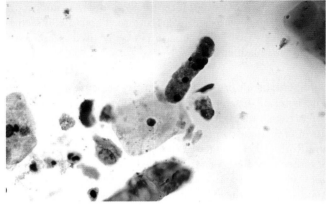

A   B

Figure 22-12   Renal casts. *A.* Hyaline cast. *B.* Tubular, granular cast (compare with Fig. 22-11D).

Cells Originating in Adjacent Organs

Cells from the Prostate, Seminal Vesicles, and Testis

These cells may be observed in the sediment of voided urine **after a vigorous prostatic palpation or massage.** The dominant component of such specimens are usually **spermatozoa** and their precursor cells, including **spermatogonia,** characterized by larger dark nuclei. The **normal prostatic glandular cells are difficult to recognize** as they are small and have few distinguishing characteristics. By far, the most important cells in such sediments are **cells derived from seminal vesicles,** which are **large and may have large, irregular, hyperchromatic but homogeneous nuclei, mimicking cancer cells.** They are almost invariably degenerated when expelled and are recognized by the presence of **yellow cytoplasmic lipochrome granular pigment.** For further description of these cells in health and disease, see Chapter 33.

Cells From the Female Genital Tract

The urinary stream may pick up cells from the vagina and the vulva. The most common are **normal squamous cells** (see above), **but abnormal cells reflecting neoplastic processes in the female genital tract may also occur** (see Chap. 23).

Other Cells

Blood Cells

Besides the urothelial and squamous cells, the normal urinary sediment may contain a few **leukocytes.** It is generally assumed that normal urinary sediment does not contain any red blood cells. Yet Freni (1977), using a careful collection technique, documented that **a few erythrocytes may be observed in virtually all healthy adults.** In 8.8% of this healthy population, there were 10 erythrocytes per single, high-power field. These observations were important because the presence of microscopic blood in urine has been suggested as a means of detecting bladder tumors.

Microhematuria

Microhematuria is by definition, the presence of erythrocytes in urine. Because normal people may show up to 10 erythrocytes per high-power field, the diagnosis should not be rendered unless the number of erythrocytes is higher. Cohen and Brown (2003) proposed a much lower threshold for the diagnosis of microhematuria, namely two erythrocytes per high-power field or a positive dipstick evaluation for hemoglobin. Microhematuria in asymptomatic persons has been the subject of several studies. Unfortunately, the populations studied were different and therefore no simple conclusion can be drawn. In an earlier study by Greene et al (1956), 500 Mayo Clinic patients with microhematuria were investigated and 11 of them were found to have cancer (7 of bladder and 2 of kidney). Most other patients had trivial and incidental disorders. In a study by Carson et al (1979) of 200 Mayo Clinic patients referred for a urologic workup, 22 (11%) had a tumor of the bladder and 2 had carcinoma of the prostate. It is of note in the Carson study, that **synchronous cytologic examination of urine was positive in 9 patients with occult carcinoma in situ and negative in 5 patients with low-grade papillary tumors** (see Chap. 23). On the other hand, in a study of **1,000 asymptomatic male** Air Force personnel, Froom et al (1984) found **microhematuria in 38.7%.** In only one subject, a "transitional cell carcinoma," not further specified, was observed. In a randomized 1986 study, Mohr et al observed microhematuria in 13% of asymptomatic adult men and women, with neoplasms of the bladder in 0.1% and of the kidney in 0.4% of the population studied. Bard (1988) observed no significant disease in 177 women with microhematuria, followed for more than 10 years.

The initial views on the significance of microhematuria suggested an aggressive investigation of all patients with this disorder. More recent opinions, notably by Mohr et al, Messing et al (1987), Bard (1988), and Grossfeld et al (2001) suggest that a **conservative follow-up of most asymptomatic patients is appropriate,** with cystoscopic work-up reserved for the patients with persisting significant hematuria or other evidence or suspicion of an important urologic disorder. Carson's study suggests that a **cytologic follow-up** may be helpful in some patients. Similar guidelines were more recently proposed by the American Urological Association (Grossfeld et al, 2001).

As Messing et al (1987) noted, microhematuria is a sporadic event that may occur intermittently and may not occur at all in patients with significant disease. Therefore, it seems quite unlikely that microhematuria may be used as a screening test for bladder tumors.

Renal versus Nonrenal Origin of Erythrocytes

The issue of differentiation of microhematuria caused by parenchymal renal disease, such as glomerulonephritis, versus microhematuria of other origin is controversial. Rathert and Roth (1991) suggested that a microscopic examination of either very fresh or rapidly fixed voided urine sediment does allow the separation of the two cell types. In phase microscopy, erythrocytes of renal origin were characterized by a **dense periphery in the form of a double ring, and an "empty" center.** Another manifestation of renal hematuria may be **partial breakdown of erythrocytes with the appearance of small, irregular, oddly shaped cells.** Other extrarenal erythrocytes acquire features akin to poikilocytosis, with the **periphery of the erythrocytes covered with spike-like excrescences or spherical protrusions.**

Mohammed et al (1993) and Van der Snoek et al (1994) (among others) suggested that the presence of **"dysmorphic" erythrocytes,** that is erythrocytes with abnormalities of shapes, was suggestive of a renal parenchymal disorder, whereas **"isomorphic erythrocytes** (i.e., red blood cells of normal shape) were representative of nonrenal origin of hematuria. Mohammed, using phase microscopy, indicated that the cut-off point of 20% of dysmorphic erythrocytes had a sensitivity of 90% and specificity of 100%. Van der Snoek used a cut-off point of 40%, achieving a sensitivity of 66.7%. The specificity of these observations was debated, among others, by Pollock et al (1989), Favaro et al (1997), Zaman and Proesmans (2000). Most recently, Nguyen (2003) examined the urinary sediments in 174 patients with various forms of glomerular disease and observed doughnut-shaped, target- or bleb-forming erythrocytes (collectively named **G1 or GIDE cells**) in a substantial proportion of cases. Nguyen proposed that the presence of GIDE cells above 10% of the erythrocyte population was a "specific diagnostic marker for glomerular disease." Unfortunately, the study did not include control patients with other possible causes of microhematuria and, thus, its specificity must still be proved.

Eosinophiluria

The presence of **bilobate eosinophils** in urine may be an indication of a drug-induced or spontaneous eosinophilic cystitis (see below). Nolan et al (1986) suggested the use of **Hansel's stain** (methylene blue and eosin-Y in methanol) to facilitate the recognition of eosinophils.

Acellular Components

Crystals

Urate crystals are commonly seen in poorly fixed urine specimens. The precipitation of urates occurs with a change in the pH of the urine, usually occurring after collection. The **crystals are usually semi-transparent, of odd shapes, and have no diagnostic significance,** except that they may

completely obscure cells present in the specimen. **Triple phosphate** crystals are transparent, often rectangular. **The star-like uric acid crystals** derived from stones, are rarely seen. From time to time, other crystals may be observed, such as the needle-like crystals of tyrosine or **hexagonal crystals of cystine.** Certain drugs, notably sulfonamides, may also form crystals of specific configuration. The reader is referred to Naib's book (1985) for a detailed description of uncommon crystals observed in the urinary sediment.

Renal casts were discussed above.

Contaminants

Urinary samples may sometimes contain **surgical powder** in the form of crystalline precipitates. Cotton threads may also occur. Occasionally, the **brown, septated fungus of the species *Alternaria,*** a contaminant from the water supply, may be observed. For a description and illustrations of this fungus, see Chapter 19.

COMPOSITION OF NORMAL SEDIMENT OF URINE SAMPLES ACCORDING TO THE MODE OF COLLECTION

Voided Urine

In **normal, spontaneously voided urine,** the **background is clean,** with only an occasional erythrocyte or leukocyte. (Table 22-3) There are usually **few urothelial cells, occurring singly and in small clusters.** An occasional large umbrella cell may be noted but most urothelial cells are small. The **nuclear structure** of these cells is **rarely well preserved** and most nuclei appear **spherical, pale and bland,** although an occasional **pyknotic or apoptotic nucleus** may be noted.

Squamous cells, usually of superficial type, are commonly present and **are usually more numerous in females than in males. In males,** the squamous cells are of **urethral origin.** In the **female,** some of the cells represent **vaginal contamination** and some are derived from **the vaginal-type epithelium in the area of the trigone commonly observed in normal women** (see above). The value of urinary sediment in estimating the **hormonal status** of the woman **(urocytograms)** is discussed in Chapter 9.

In **newborn children, regardless of sex,** the urinary sediment may contain a fairly **large proportion of mature squamous cells, reflecting the effect of maternal hormones.**

Catheterized Bladder Urine

Because catheters can damage the epithelium, catheterized bladder urine is usually much **richer in urothelial cells than voided urine.** The **single cells, which may vary enormously in size and configuration,** reflect the entire spectrum of urothelial cells ranging from the large umbrella to smaller cells from the deeper layers of the urothelium. Variants of the urothelium, particularly columnar cells are commonly present. Of special significance are **clusters of urothelial cells** that may be "papillary" or complex, as shown in Figure 22-10, in the absence of tumors.

TABLE 22-3

PRINCIPAL CYTOLOGIC FEATURES OF URINARY SEDIMENT ACCORDING TO METHODS OF COLLECTION

	Voided Urine	Catheterized Urine	Bladder Washings	Retrograde Catheterization	Brushings
Urothelial cells	sparse, poorly preserved	more numerous, sometimes in clusters	broad variety of urothelial cells, singly and in clusters*	as in bladder washings: complex clusters and umbrella cells*	numerous umbrella cells and complex clusters*
Squamous cells	common in adults and newborns of both sexes	rare	rare	absent	absent
Renal tubular cells and casts	common	rare	absent	absent	absent
Contaminants	common	rare	absent	absent	absent

* Important source of diagnostic error.

Bladder Washings (Barbotage)

These specimens offer an excellent panorama of the component cells of the urothelium, as discussed above. A broad variety of superficial umbrella cells and deeper urothelial cells and their variants may be seen. Cell clusters of various configurations are common and may be numerous.

Retrograde Ureteral Catheterization

Retrograde catheterization requires **threading a small catheter through the narrow lumens of the ureters.** Inevitably, the tip of the catheter dislodges urothelial cells from their setting, resulting in **specimens characterized by a large number of cell clusters next to single urothelial cells of a large variety of types.** It has been mentioned above that umbrella cells with a very large number of nuclei are particularly common in such specimens.

The cell **clusters** may be **numerous** and sometimes several dozen of them may be observed in a single specimen. **The multilayered, complex configuration of some of the clusters and their role as a source of false-positive reports has been stressed above.** An example of such an error seen by us in consultation is shown in Figure 22-13. In this case, the clusters were **misinterpreted as a "papillary tumor"** and the diagnosis was followed by a nephroureterectomy 4 days later. There was no evidence of a tumor. In the histologic sections of the ureter, the origin of the clusters could be traced to the large segments of the denuded urothelium scraped by the tip of the catheter. On review of the cytologic sample, the component cells of normal urothelium could be readily observed.

Brushings of Ureters and Renal Pelves

The samples, when prepared as **direct smears** by the urologist, are often **of limited diagnostic value** because of drying artifacts. The interpretation of numerous, **thick clusters of urothelial cells** is very difficult. We have seen several cases wherein the clusters were mistaken for evidence of a papillary tumor (see Fig. 22-13). Otherwise, the cytologic find-

ings are very similar to those described for retrograde catheterization.

It is a safe rule in diagnostic cytology of the urinary tract that in the absence of clear-cut criteria of cancer, such as a markedly altered nucleocytoplasmic ratio and changed nuclear configuration and texture (described in detail in Chapter 23), one should not attempt the diagnosis of a malignant tumor. This is particularly important with specimens obtained by brushing, retrograde ureteral catheterization or immediately thereafter, after instrumentation such as cystoscopy, or in bladder washings obtained under cystoscopic control. It is essential to be familiar with the enormous morphologic variability of the normal urothelial cells, which may exhibit chromocenters mimicking large nucleoli.

INFLAMMATORY PROCESSES WITHIN THE LOWER URINARY TRACT

Bacterial Infections

Bacterial infections involving the lower urinary tract may be **primary or secondary, acute or chronic.** The most common are **cystitis and pyelonephritis,** which are usually caused by a **bacterial infection.** Both disorders may cause high fever and **severe pain** in the lower abdomen, radiating to the groin. The histologic changes may include ulceration of the epithelium and infiltration of the wall of the organ by granulocytes in the acute phase and lymphocytes in the chronic phase. A variety of **pyogenic bacteria,** especially **cocci** but also *Escherichia coli* and *Pseudomonas aeruginosa (Bacillus pyocyaneus),* may be the predominant organisms. Wu et al (1996) documented that adhesion of *E. coli* to the urothelial surface is mediated by uroplakins.

In most cases, the bacterial infections are acute but may become chronic. **Of special significance are infections with gram-negative organisms occurring in debilitated patients who may develop septicemia, followed by irre-**

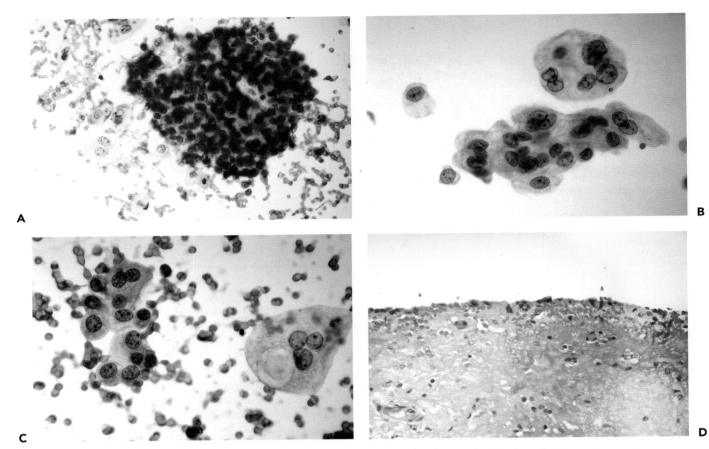

Figure 22-13 Benign urothelial cells in retrograde urine brushings, mistaken for cells of a papillary tumor. *A–C.* All three fields show large clusters of benign urothelial cells (*A* is overview). *D.* Surface of the ureter removed 3 days after the diagnosis of a "papillary tumor." The surface of the ureter was denuded by the brush.

versible shock leading to death. Occasionally, the offending organism may be observed in the urinary sediment and classified as bacillary or coccoid, but its exact identification must depend on bacteriologic data.

Contributory Factors

Obstructive processes, such as **strictures, compression, calculi, diverticula, or prostatic enlargement** that interfere with the free flow of urine, are common factors contributing to infection. **Cancers, intrinsic or extrinsic** to the lower urinary tract, may also create a favorable terrain for infection or may produce obstruction with the same effect. In **women, infections of the lower genital tract** may spread to the urethra and bladder. **Therapeutic procedures, such as in-dwelling catheters, particularly with inadequate toilette, may lead to severe infections, including the feared gram-negative septicemia.**

Some of the long-standing infectious processes are secondary to generalized infections. For instance, **tuberculosis of the bladder is usually secondary to pulmonary and renal tuberculosis.** Still, changes **mimicking tuberculosis** can be induced by treatment with Bacillus Calmette-Guérin (BCG), as described below.

Cytology

The background of the urinary sediment in acute inflammation shows **red blood cells and purulent material.** The latter shows **necrotic debris** and numerous **polymorphonuclear leukocytes** or, in more chronic forms of infection, numerous **lymphocytes.** The epithelial cells, singly and in clusters, typically are increased in number in the urine but the cells are often concealed by a heavy inflammatory exudate. **Degeneration and necrosis are the characteristic cellular changes in epithelial cells** (Fig. 22-14A,B). The degenerated cells are of variable size and configuration and are often **enlarged** because of markedly **vacuolated cytoplasm** that may be infiltrated with polymorphonuclear leukocytes (Fig. 22-14C). Of special diagnostic interest are the **nuclei** of the urothelial cells. They may be of somewhat **variable sizes and of irregular outline, but usually show an opaque or clear, transparent center surrounded by a rim of chromatin. This is an important point of differential diagnosis between inflammatory atypias and urothelial cancer. In the latter, the nuclear texture is quite different** (see Chap. 23). Occasionally, the nuclei of urothelial cells may show **chromatin condensation (pyknosis) and apoptosis,** that is, fragments of chromatin contained within the nuclear membrane. Contrary to cancer cells, the **nucleocytoplasmic ratio** in such cells is usually normal.

Other Cells Seen in Inflammation

Macrophages may make their appearance in the urine in varying numbers, indicating a more chronic inflammatory

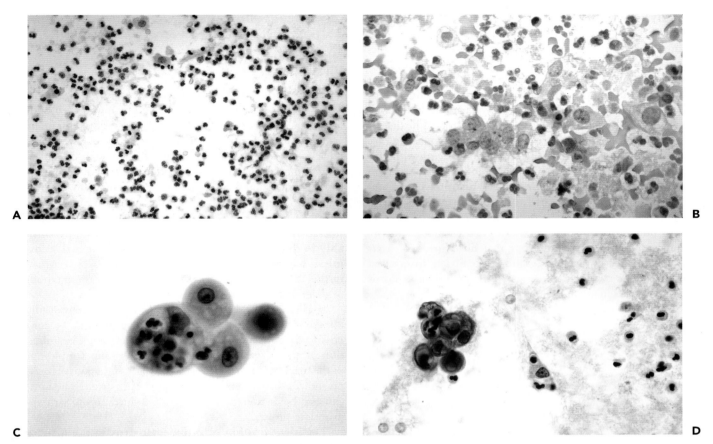

Figure 22-14   **Urine sediment in inflammation.** *A.* A low-power view of urine sediment containing numerous leukocytes. *B.* Poorly preserved urothelial cells surrounded by leukocytes and macrophages. Note the presence of nucleoli, possibly indicating a "repair" reaction. *C.* A cluster of urothelial cells with the cytoplasm infiltrated by polymorphonuclear leukocytes. *D.* Poorly preserved urothelial cells in the presence of an inflammatory exudate.

process. They include **mononucleated or multinucleated varieties, with faintly stippled spherical or kidney-shaped (remiform) nuclei, and characteristic faintly vacuolated basophilic cytoplasm, often showing evidence of phagocytosis.** They may be confused with vacuolated urothelial cells. Occasionally, **plasma cells** may be noted. In eosinophilic cystitis (see below), eosinophils may appear in the urinary sediment.

Specific Forms of Inflammation

Granulomatous Inflammation

Tuberculosis
Kapila and Verma (1984) described the presence of **comma-shaped epithelioid cells** in the urinary sediment of a patient with tuberculosis of the bladder. The slender, carrot-shaped cells forming a tubercle are characteristic, if present. Piscioli et al (1985) described the cytologic findings in the urinary sediment of 11 patients with tuberculosis. In 5 of them, he reported finding epithelioid cells, although the illustration provided was not convincing. In all 11 patients, **multinucleated cells of Langerhans' type** were observed. In my experience, this type of giant cell is extremely rare in urinary sediment and its presence has yet to be proven to be of

diagnostic value. Piscioli et al also described in 2 patients the presence of markedly atypical urothelial cells resembling cancer cells, which they traced to atypical hyperplastic urothelium that was similar to flat carcinoma in situ.

Granulomas after Bladder Surgery
Spagnolo et al (1986) described the presence of granulomas in the bladder walls of patients with two or more surgical procedures for bladder tumors. There were **two types of granulomas;** one type with **necrosis and palisading of peripheral cells resembling rheumatoid nodules,** and the other type was composed of **foreign body giant cells.** There is no known cytologic presentation of these granulomas and the entity is cited as a potential source of confusion with tuberculosis.

Inflammatory Pseudopolyp
A chronic inflammatory process in the bladder may result in a **protrusion of bladder epithelium around an inflamed stroma, mimicking a neoplastic lesion** on cystoscopy. Similar lesions were recently described in renal pelvis (Leroy et al, 2000). The urothelial cells in the urinary sediment show minor changes consistent with inflammation.

Interstitial Cystitis (Hunner's Ulcer)

This is a rare form of chronic ulcerative cystitis of unknown cause, first described by Hunner (1915) and extensively discussed by Smith and Denner (1972) and by Sant (1997). In an elaborate discussion, Elbadawi (1997) reported that ultrastructural studies of artificially distended bladders supported the hypothesis that altered nerve supply in the wall of the bladder may be the cause of this disorder. The disease causes painful cramping and high frequency of voiding. We studied the urinary sediment in several patients with this disorder, but except for evidence of inflammation, found **no specific cytologic abnormalities of note.** Dodd and Tello (1998) confirmed the absence of specific cytologic changes in this disorder, noting only acute inflammation with polymorphonuclear leukocytes and eosinophiles. Utz and Zincke (1973) pointed out that **nonpapillary carcinoma in situ may masquerade clinically as interstitial cystitis.** The cytologic presentation of carcinoma in situ is discussed in Chapter 23.

Eosinophilic Cystitis

Infiltration of the bladder wall with numerous eosinophils is most commonly observed **after cautery treatment** and may also occur in **patients with asthma or other allergic disorders. Spontaneous forms of eosinophilic cystitis may also occur** (Brown, 1960; Palubinskas, 1960; Hellstrom et al, 1979). The disease may produce **thickening of the wall of the bladder, mimicking an invasive carcinoma** (Hansen and Kristensen, 1993) or **cause obstruction of the urinary outlet** (Case record of the Massachusetts General Hospital, case 27-1998). In all such cases, the **urinary sediment may contain numerous bilobate eosinophils.** For discussion of eosinophiluria, see above. A true **eosinophilic granuloma (Langerhans' cell granulomatosis),** with simultaneous proliferation of eosinophils and macrophages, may also occur (Koss, 1975). For discussion of the cytologic presentation of eosinophilic granuloma, see Chapter 31.

Fungal Infections

The most common fungus observed in the urinary sediment is *Candida albicans.* The organism is observed mainly as **fungal spores** (yeast form), but pseudohyphae may occasionally be observed (see Fig. 10-10). This infection is **particularly serious in renal transplant recipients and other immunosuppressed patients.** It may lead to generalized fungal infection and septicemia or, in a rare case, to obstruction of the ureters by a fungal ball. The presence of casts of candida indicates upper urinary tract (renal) infection with an ominous prognosis.

Other fungi are uncommon. Eickenberg et al (1975) pointed out that the urinary tract may be affected in patients with systemic *North American blastomycosis* and that the organism can be identified in urine (see Fig. 19-42). We have also observed *Aspergillosis* in the urinary sediment of a patient with AIDS (see Fig. 19-47). Mukunyadzi et al (2002) reported a case of *histoplasmosis* diagnosed in urinary sediment. *Alternaria* species, a brown, septated fungus, is a common contaminant (see above and Fig. 19-18A).

Viral Infections

Cytomegalovirus (Cytomegalic Inclusion Disease)

This sometimes fatal, but fortunately uncommon, viral infection has been recognized in infants and children for many years. More recently, the frequency of cytolmegalovirus (CMV) has increased in adults as a consequence of the acquired immunodeficiency syndrome (AIDS) and immunosuppression, notably in recipients of bone marrow or renal transplants, and patients with various forms of cancer. This virus has been identified in patients with **infectious mononucleosis and may survive in the seminal fluid, presumably in the spermatozoa** (Lang et al, 1974). **Sexual transmission of the virus to a young woman** has been recorded in this case. Urinary sediment remains one of the methods of diagnosis of this serious disorder.

As discussed at length in Chapter 19, this often deadly disease is due to a virus of the herpesvirus group. The **conclusive diagnosis** intra vitam is made by cytologic examination of gastric washings, sputum or other lung samples, or of the urinary sediment. Precise methods of diagnosis, based on molecular markers, are now available as well. The virus can also be demonstrated by in situ hybridization with appropriate probes.

The **identification of cytomegalovirus in the urinary sediment of infants and children, and now in high-risk adults, has been a recognized diagnostic procedure for many years.** Urothelial cells may show all stages of infection. In the **early stages, multiple, small, basophilic viral inclusions are distributed throughout the nucleus and the cytoplasm and are surrounded by individual halos.** In **more advanced, classic forms** of the disease, **the epithelial cells are markedly enlarged and carry within their nuclei very large, basophilic inclusions, surrounded by a conspicuous clear halo. The residual chromatin is condensed at the nuclear periphery** (Fig. 22-15A). In the advanced stage of the disease, **cytoplasmic inclusions are somewhat less frequent.** Cellular inclusions of cytomegalovirus have been observed in the urinary sediment of **renal transplant recipients** (Bossen et al, 1969; Johnston et al, 1969), in young **patients with leukemia** (Chang, 1970) and in immunosuppressed patients.

The **differential diagnosis of cytomegalovirus is with human polyomavirus,** as discussed below. Cytomegalovirus infection is now treatable with antiviral agents.

It is of particular interest that the **incidental identification of cytomegalovirus in otherwise healthy adults does not carry with it the ominous prognosis** of this disease as seen in infancy and early childhood or in immunoincompetent patients. Apparently, many of the patients are carriers of the virus without suffering any direct ill effect.

Herpes Simplex Virus

Herpetic infection of the urinary tract was a rarity in the past. The recognition of the **typical multinucleated epithelial cells with molded, ground-glass nuclei and, on rare**

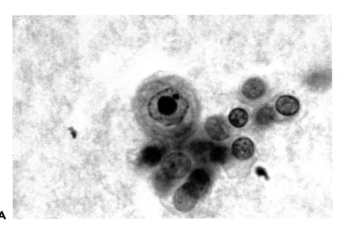
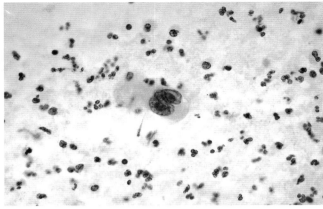

A   B

Figure 22-15 Viral manifestations in urinary sediment. *A.* Cytomegalovirus. Note very large intranuclear inclusion with a small satellite inclusion surrounded by a large perinuclear halo. *B.* Urothelial cell with eosinophilic nuclear inclusions characteristic of herpesvirus. (*B:* Oil immersion.)

occasions, of typical **eosinophilic intranuclear inclusions** has not posed any diagnostic dilemmas (Fig. 22-15B; also see Chaps. 10 and 19). This virus has been recognized in urinary sediment of **recipients of renal allografts** (Bossen and Johnston, 1975) and in a **patient with squamous cancer of the urinary bladder** (Murphy, 1976). Several such cases were personally observed by us in patients with and without cancer.

Human Polyomavirus (Decoy Cells)

Cytopathic changes induced by this virus in urothelial cells may be confused with cancer. This was first recognized in the 1950s, by the late Mr. Andrew Ricci, senior cytotechnologist at Memorial Hospital for Cancer in New York. He observed in the urinary sediment **cells with large, homogeneous, hyperchromatic nuclei, mimicking cancer cells, but not associated with bladder cancer** (Figs. 22-16A,B and 22-17A). Mr. Ricci named these cells **decoy cells.** The nature of the decoy cells remained unknown for many years. In the 1968 edition of this book, it was speculated that the change was due to an unidentified virus. This virus has been identified as **human polyomavirus** by Gardner et al (1971) and has been extensively studied by Coleman and her coworkers (1973, 1975, 1980, 1984). The virus belongs to the **Papovaviridae family** and is **related to the human papillomavirus.** Polyomaviruses have a somewhat smaller genome than the papillomaviruses and are somewhat differently organized (Frisque et al, 1984). **Electron microscopy** of nuclei containing polyomavirus inclusions shows many similarities to the human papillomavirus (HPV) infection (Fig. 22-18). Both viruses form **crystalline arrays of viral particles.** The polyomavirus particles are somewhat smaller than the papillomavirus particles.

Two strains of the human polyomavirus, both named after the initials of the patients, have been identified: the **JC strain,** isolated from a patient with the previously rare disease, **progressive multifocal leukoencephalopathy** (Padgett et al, 1971), and the **BK strain,** isolated from a **patient with a renal transplant** (Gardner et al, 1971). The two

strains differ from each other by the size of the virus particles and by serologic characteristics. It was thought for many years that the **two viral types are limited to specific anatomic territories, that is, the JC virus to the brain and the BK virus to the urinary tract. This is no longer the case, as JC viruses have been documented in the urinary tract** by polymerase chain reaction (PCR) (Itoh et al, 1998).

It has been documented by serologic studies that the **human infection with polyomaviruses is acquired in childhood and is nearly universal** (Padgett and Walker, 1976). **Thus, the cytologic manifestations of this infection reflect a reactivation of, or a superinfection with, the virus,** a sequence of events also proposed for the human papillomavirus (Koss, 1989; see Chap. 11). There is, however, a major difference between these two viruses: the **human papillomavirus is implicated in neoplastic events** in the skin, female genital tract, larynx, the esophagus, and perhaps even the bronchus (see appropriate chapters), but **there is no evidence that the polyomavirus is carcinogenic in humans,** although it plays a role in tumor formation in experimental animals.

The **activation** of polyomaviruses occurs in **immunosuppressed individuals,** patients receiving chemotherapy, such as cyclophosphamide (Cytoxan, see below), in **diabetics, in organ transplant recipients** (O'Reilly et al, 1981; Apperly et al, 1987), and in patients with **AIDS** (Filie et al, 2002). **Most importantly, however, virus activation may occur without any obvious cause** (Kahan et al, 1980; Minassian et al, 1994) and **last for a few weeks or even months without any ill effects** (Table 22-4). In such cases, shedding of the affected epithelial cells may be **intermittent.**

The polyomavirus plays an important role in the previously very rare **progressive multifocal encephalopathy,** currently on the rise in AIDS patients. Viral inclusions occur in nuclei of oligodendrocytes (summary in Berger and Major, 1994). Houff et al (1988) documented that the **JC type polyomavirus may proliferate in bone marrow cells and in mononuclear cells,** which may carry the virus to the brain, causing this disease.

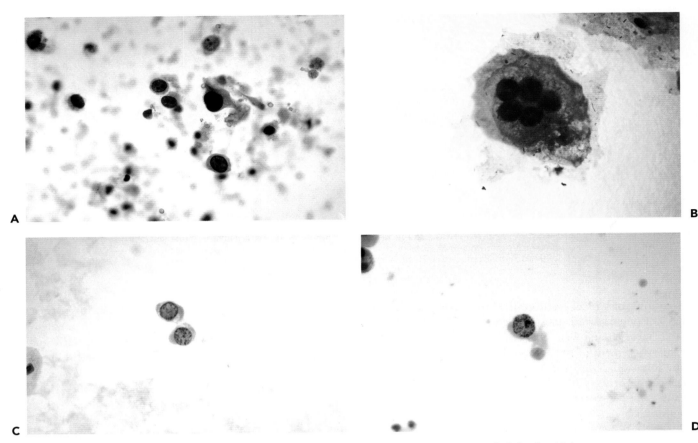

Figure 22-16   Human polyomavirus in urinary sediment. *A.* Numerous urothelial cells with large hyperchromatic homogeneous nuclear inclusions in a young person. *B.* A large multinucleated umbrella cell with each nucleus occupied by a large viral inclusion. *C.* Post-inclusion stage. The inclusions are very pale. *D.* Last stage of viral infection. The nucleus is filled with thin strands of chromatin within a thickened nuclear membrane. No viral particles are seen but the presence of the residual virus can be documented by immunochemistry.

Perhaps the most significant new development in reference to human polyomavirus is its role in **interstitial nephritis** in **AIDS and in renal transplant patients** (Rosen et al, 1983; Gardner et al, 1984; Drachenberg et al, 1999). It has been documented that **activation of the BK virus is a cause of renal dysfunction in patients with AIDS** (Nebuloni et al, 1999). **The same virus causes severe renal-allograft dysfunction** that may result in graft rejection unless treated (Pappo et al, 1996; Drachenberg et al, 1999; Nickeleit et al, 2000). Petrogiannis-Haliotis et al (2001) reported a case of **polyomavirus vasculopathy** in a patient after renal transplant. In all these situations, **classical evidence of polyomavirus activation may be observed in the sediment of voided urine,** as described below (Fig. 22-19). Drachenberg et al (1999) considered the **examination of voided urine sediment as the most effective diagnostic test for polyomavirus in renal transplant patients.**

A case of **polyomavirus infection with ureteral obstruction** in a renal allograph recipient was reported by Coleman et al (1973) and the possibility that the virus contributed to the obstruction of the cystic duct in a liver transplant recipient has been raised. It is not known whether these events were actually related to human polyomavirus infection.

The suggestion by Arthur et al (1986) and Apperley et al (1987) that the virus is the cause of **hemorrhagic cystitis** in bone marrow transplant recipients, has been disproved. In a series of 17 bone marrow transplant patients monitored by urinary cytology, the **presence of the virus-induced changes in urinary sediment could not be correlated with hemorrhagic cystitis** (Cottler-Fox et al, 1989). These conclusions have been confirmed by Drachenberg et al (1999).

The effects of human polyomavirus activation may be observed occasionally in **endocervical cells in smears of pregnant women** (Coleman et al, 1980) and in **bronchial cells** (see Chap. 19) but for reasons unknown, the most important and common manifestations are observed in urothelial cells in urinary sediment.

Cytology

There are **two types of polyomavirus manifestations** in the urinary sediment:

■ **A massive presence of infected cells,** observed mainly but not exclusively in children and young adults and in people of all ages with impaired immunity (see Fig. 22-16A). Ito et al (1998) attributed this type of infection to BK virus.

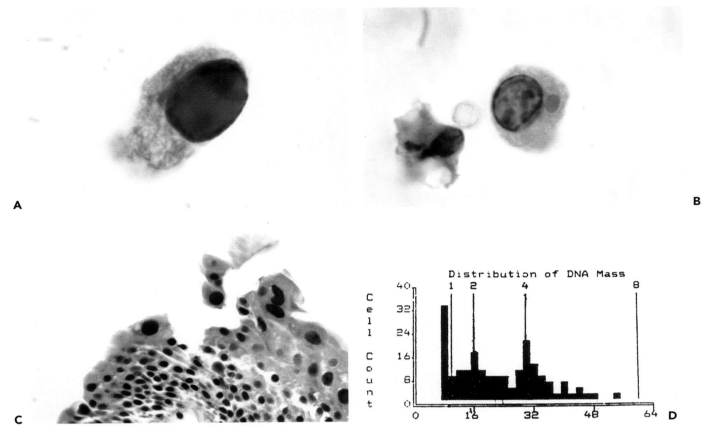

Figure 22-17   Polyomavirus infection. *A.* An oil immersion image of an infected cell showing the very large homogeneous nuclear inclusions surrounded by a thick nuclear membrane. *B.* Oil immersion view of a pale nuclear inclusion. In the cytoplasm, a nonspecific eosinophilic inclusion may be noted. *C.* Bladder biopsy in a case of polyomavirus infection. Several of the superficial umbrella cells show large viral inclusions. *D.* A histogram of DNA values in human polyomavirus infection. The nondiploid pattern of DNA distribution is readily seen.

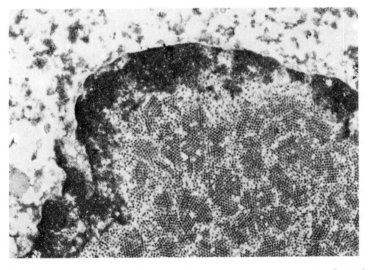

Figure 22-18   Electron micrograph of a cell in the human urinary sediment infected with human polyomavirus. The crystalline arrays of virus particles, measuring about 45 nm in diameter, are clearly shown.

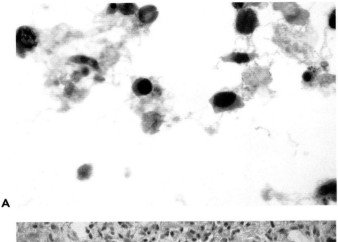

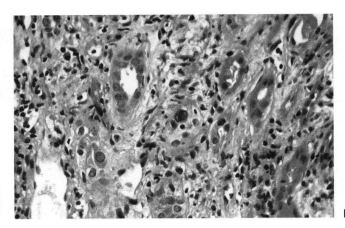

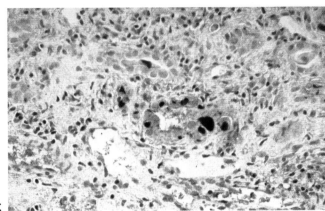

Figure 22-19 Polyomavirus nephropathy in a patient with AIDS. *A.* Urinary sediment showing numerous cells with viral inclusions. *B.* Kidney biopsy showing distortion of the tubules, many of which contain epithelial cells with large viral inclusions. *C.* Immunostain with antibody to SV40 virus showing positive staining reaction in cells of tubular lining.

- **Occasional, rare urothelial cells** with viral cytopathic changes, observed mainly in patients with no immunologic impairment (Fig. 22-17A). Ito et al (1998) attributed this type of infection to JC virus.

Regardless of viral type, two stages of the infection may be recognized in the urinary sediment and both are diagnostic of the disorder. These are the **inclusion stage** and the **postinclusion stage.**

Inclusion Stage
- **Classical basophilic inclusions:** The infected cells vary in size and many are markedly enlarged. In its classical presentation, the virus forms single, dense basophilic homogeneous intranuclear inclusions that blend with the thick nuclear membrane (see Figs. 22-16A,B, 22-17A, and 22-19A). A narrow, clear halo may sometimes be seen between the edge of the inclusion and the marginal rim of nuclear chromatin. In multinucleated umbrella cells, each nucleus may contain an inclusion (see Fig. 22-16B). Similar inclusions may be observed in the superficial layers of the urothelium in fortuitous bladder biopsies from an infected person (see Fig. 22-17C) and in cytologic preparations from progressive multifocal encephalopathy (Suhrland et al, 1987).
- **Pale inclusions:** In a proportion of infected cells, the nuclear inclusions become pale and transparent, forming a homogeneous clear space within the infected nucleus (see Figs. 22-16C and 22-17B). The pallor is usually best seen in the central portion of the inclusion and

it is nicely contrasted with the rim of the thick nuclear membrane. It is assumed, but it has not been proven, that this appearance of the inclusions is caused by leaching of the virus. Nonetheless, the pale inclusions are fully diagnostic of polyomavirus infection, as shown by immunochemistry (see below).

Postinclusion Stage. Presumably because of the leaching-out of the virus particles, **the nuclei of the infected cells that lost their viral content acquire a new appearance that, in my judgment, is just as characteristic of this infection as the inclusions.** The **enlarged nuclei** have an **"empty" appearance with a distinct network of chromatin filaments wherein scattered chromocenters may be observed** (see Fig. 22-16D). This has been described as a "fishnet-stocking" pattern. Transition forms between the inclusion-bearing cells and the "empty" cells may be observed. The presence of residual viral particles in such cells has been confirmed by **immunocytochemistry with an antigen to SV40 virus, which shares the antigenic properties with polyomaviruses,** obtained through the courtesy of Dr. Kertie Shah, Johns Hopkins School of Public Health, Baltimore, MD.

The scanty **cytoplasm of these dying or dead cells often contains small, irregular nonspecific eosinophilic inclusions which are not viral in nature** (see below).

Differential Diagnosis of Polyomavirus Infection
Although the similarities between the **basophilic polyomavirus inclusions and cytomegalovirus (CMV) inclu-**

sions are slight (see Figs. 22-15 with 22-16), inasmuch as the **polyomavirus inclusions have no halo and are not accompanied by satellite inclusions,** nonetheless, sometimes the differentiation cannot be securely made. In these cases, **the identity of the virus can be established** by immunologic, virologic, or serologic methods. Molecular techniques such as PCR (Ito et al, 1998) and in situ hybridization techniques with specific viral probes are also available. Electron microscopy may prove decisive because the CMV particles are very large (about 150 nm in diameter) and encapsulated, as are all the particles of the herpesvirus family, and do not form crystalline arrays. De LasCasas observed two cases of **adenovirus,** with intranuclear inclusions similar to those in polyomavirus and diagnosed by electron microscopy.

Diagnostic Significance of Polyomavirus Infection

The principal significance of the urothelial cell changes caused by polyomavirus activation is in an **erroneous diagnosis of urothelial cancer.** The so-aptly named **decoy cells** have been mistaken for cancer cells on many occasions and frequently resulted in a very extensive and unnecessary clinical work-up, which included biopsies of the bladder, and cost vast sums of money.

In AIDS patients with renal dysfunction and in renal transplant patients, a simple examination of the urinary sediment may lead to the diagnosis and treatment of interstitial nephritis (Fig. 22-19).

Unfortunately, **polyomavirus infection may also occur in patients with urothelial cancer, particularly if treated with cytotoxic drugs.** In these infrequent cases, the inclusion-bearing and the "empty" cells may appear side by side with cancer cells. As is discussed in Chapter 23, the characteristic features of urothelial **cancer cells *do not* include smooth, homogeneous appearance of the nucleus or the characteristic filamentous chromatin pattern of the empty nuclei.**

Human Papillomavirus (HPV)

Infection of the lower urinary tract with HPV occurs with fair frequency. Because the infection is **related to condylo-mata acuminata and possibly cancer of the urethra and bladder,** the topic is discussed in Chapter 23. However, it may be noted that **koilocytes in the urinary sediment in women may occur as a consequence of a "pick-up" of cells from the genital tract.** In such cases, further investigation of the genital organs is suggested before the much more complex investigation of the urinary tract is undertaken.

Cellular Inclusions in Urinary Sediment Not Caused by Viral Infection

Several types of cell inclusions that may be observed in the urinary sediment must be differentiated from viral inclusions.

Intracytoplasmic Eosinophilic Inclusions

On frequent occasions, **red, eosinophilic, opaque cytoplasmic inclusions, single or multiple,** may be noted within the benign or malignant epithelial cells in the urinary sediment. The inclusions vary in size and shape but most are **approximately spherical,** resembling droplets of red ink or red blood cells. Most of the inclusions appear in cells with a degenerated nucleus, as described for human polyomavirus infected cells. However, in some instances, the nucleus may still be well preserved (Figs. 22-20 and 23-15F). We have also observed **very large, homogeneous, eosinophilic cytoplasmic inclusions in poorly preserved urothelial** cells with vacuolated cytoplasm. Similar inclusions are frequently observed in degenerating intestinal **cells derived from ileal bladders** (see below). Dorfman and Monis (1964) documented that the inclusions contained mucopolysaccharides. Kobayashi et al (1984) reported a case of the rare **Kawasaki disease** with identical inclusions. Melamed and Wolinska (1961) studied these inclusions in a large number of cases. In this study, there was **no evidence of a specific association of the cytoplasmic inclusions with any known disease state.** Bolande's suggestion that these inclusions correlate with specific viral diseases of childhood was surely in error. Naib (personal communication) failed to identify any viral organisms in these inclusions and considers them as **products of cell degeneration,** possibly the result of prior viral infection. **Similar inclusions** may

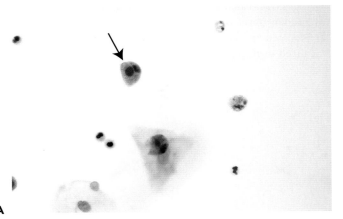
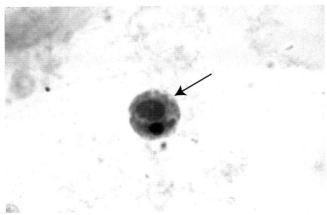

A   B

Figure 22-20 Nonspecific eosinophilic cytoplasmic inclusions (*arrows*). These single or multiple inclusions may vary in size from very small to rather large and vary in configuration (*B*: High magnification).

be observed in degenerating cells of the respiratory tract in **ciliocytophthoria** (see Chap. 19) and occasionally in cells from other organs. Most patients with intracytoplasmic eosinophilic inclusions in urinary sediment have some form of urinary tract disease or injury.

Inclusions Caused by Lead

Lead poisoning is not uncommonly observed in children and results in the formation of **intranuclear acid-fast inclusion bodies in renal tubular cells** (Fig. 22-21). Landing and Nakai (1959), who were the first to describe these inclusions, proposed that examination of the urinary sediment may lead to the correct diagnosis of the disease. This was confirmed by Schumann et al (1980) in industrial workers.

Eosinophilic Nuclear Inclusions

Such inclusions occurring in urinary sediment of women were described by Rouse et al (1986). Extensive investigations failed to uncover the nature of these inclusions. Electron microscopy was not performed.

Parasites

Trichomonas vaginalis

The parasite may be observed in the urinary sediment of both **female and male patients.** The presence of **Trichomonas vaginalis** in the male may be evident in urinary sediment **after prostatic massage** (for description of the parasite, see Chap. 10). A case of trichomonas infestation in a male patient with sterile pyuria was described by Niewiadomski et al (1998).

In female patients the parasites are usually of vaginal origin.

Schistosoma hematobium (Bilharzia) infestation

Infestation with the trematode or fluke **S. hematobium** is extremely widespread in certain parts of Africa, particularly along the Nile river (recent summary in Ross et al, 2002). The disease is transmitted from man to man through an intermediate host, a fresh-water snail. The mobile form of the parasite, the **cercariae,** penetrates the skin of people wading in the water, causing "**swimmers' itch.**" The cercariae travel to the veins of the pelvis, particularly the veins of the bladder, where they mature and copulate. The **ova,**

provided with a terminal spine (see Figs. 10-35 and 23-27D), are deposited mainly in the submucosa of the distal ureter and the urinary bladder, although the rectum and the uterus may also be involved. The involvement of the **female genital tract** with this infestation is discussed in Chapter 10.

The major importance of this infestation is its **frequent association with carcinoma of the bladder, mainly squamous carcinoma** (see Chap. 23). The reasons for this association are unclear; it may somehow be related to the severe inflammatory reaction and fibrosis of the bladder wall caused by the ova. **Keratin-forming squamous metaplasia of the urothelium is frequently observed and is thought to be a precursor of carcinoma.** The urinary sediment reflects such changes very closely: marked inflammatory epithelial changes, often associated with purulent exudate, are the rule in advanced schistosomiasis. In a study performed in our laboratories, numerous anucleated squames and squamous cells corresponding to squamous metaplasia were observed in 18 of 51 urine sediments from patients from Zimbabwe with schistosomiasis (Houston et al, 1966). Ova were not seen in this material. Somewhat similar observations were reported by Dimmette et al (1955).

Because of air travel and movement of infected people, the finding of *S. haematobium* is no longer confined to endemic areas. Clements and Oko (1983) reported such a case from New York City, and more such cases may be expected to occur in the Western world.

Filariasis

Filariasis, previously confined to endemic areas, may now be observed in other geographic settings. Webber and Eveland (1982) observed **Wuchereria bancrofti** filariae in urinary sediment of a patient in New York City. The presence of this worm is also discussed in reference to several other organs (see appropriate chapters).

URINARY CALCULI (LITHIASIS, STONES)

Urinary tract calculi (stones) cause **clinical symptoms** such as sudden onset of pain and hematuria. When the stones are located in the uretero-pelvic area, the pain is usually localized to the corresponding flank and may radiate to the

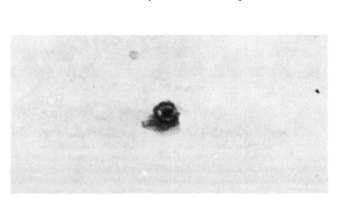

Figure 22-21   Lead poisoning. An intranuclear inclusion in an epithelial in urinary sediment (Hematoxylin-eosin; ×560. Courtesy of Dr. Benjamin Landing, Cincinnati, Ohio.)

groin. Radiologic examination usually reveals a **space-occupying lesion. The differential diagnosis includes lithiasis, tumor, or a blood clot.** The urologist may resort to cytologic techniques to clarify the nature of the lesion. Cytologic investigation of the urinary sediment is rarely of help in solving the dilemma. Urinary calculi have two major effects on the urinary specimen:

- They may cause a significant **desquamation of urothelial cells because of their abrasive effect.** On a rare occasion, **smooth muscle cells,** presumably derived from the wall of the ureter, may be observed.
- They may cause **atypias of urothelial cells,** which are for the most part nonspecific.

Abrasive Effect in Voided Urine

A stone or stones, particularly when lodged in the renal pelvis or ureter, or when being actively expelled through the narrow lumen of the ureter, **may act like an abrasive instrument. Significant and sometimes massive exfoliation of urothelial cells, singly and in clusters,** may occur and may be observed in the urinary sediment (Fig. 22-22A). Among the single cells, numerous large **multinucleated**

umbrella cells are sometimes quite striking. Because of the customary variation in the sizes of the nuclei, such cells have been **mistaken for cancer cells** by inexperienced observers.

More importantly, **cell clusters,** often numerous, may form **compact three-dimensional balls or "papillary" clusters** (Fig. 22-23A–C) that may be **mistaken for fragments of a papillary urothelial tumor.** Highman and Wilson (1982) observed papillary clusters of urothelial cells in voided urine in slightly more than 40% of 154 patients with calculi. They proposed that such clusters are predictive of calculi. They tested this hypothesis on more than 6,000 routine urine specimens and found similar clusters in 48 patients, of whom 30 were subsequently shown to harbor calculi. **In my experience, however, the presence of papillary clusters in voided urine is nonspecific, especially after palpation or catheterization of the bladder, and occurs in about 10% to 15% of all specimens from patients in whom no stones can be found.**

Stone-Induced Atypias of Urothelial Cells

In voided urine, urinary calculi may rarely cause alterations in the **shapes and sizes of urothelial cells, sometimes** with a **degree of nuclear hyperchromasia** that, in the absence

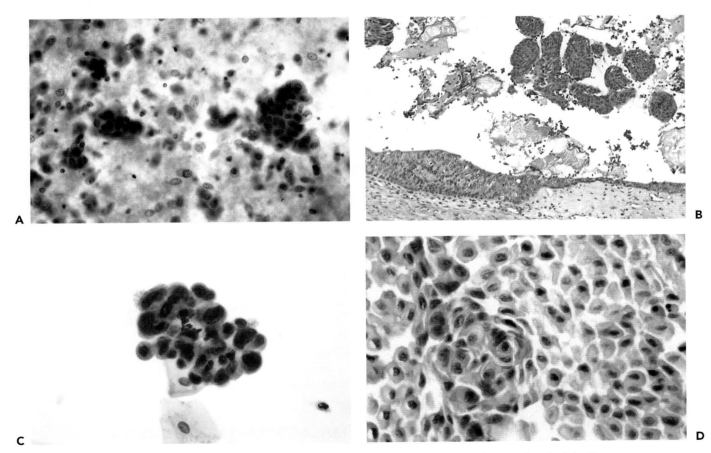

Figure 22-22 Cytologic manifestations of renal lithiasis. *A.* Numerous clusters of urothelial cells in a brush specimen. *B.* Lithiasis of renal pelves. There is some urothelial hyperplasia surrounding the remnants of a stone. Note numerous detached fragments of urothelium *C.* A papillary cluster in voided urine of a 51-year-old woman with lithiasis in a brush specimen. Note enlarged, somewhat hyperchromatic nuclei. *D.* Nuclear atypia in a case of lithiasis in a brush specimen. Note the pearl formation by urothelial cells with somewhat atypical and large nuclei.

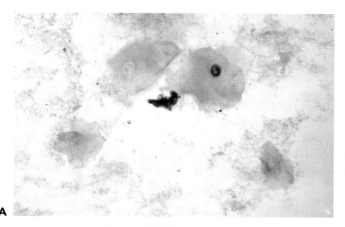
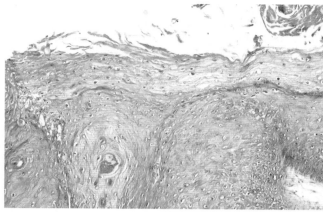

Figure 22-23 Leukoplakia in urinary sediment. *A.* Nucleated and anucleated squames in voided urine sediment. *B.* Biopsy of bladder wall showing a thick layer of keratin on the surface of the epithelium.

of any other nuclear changes, should be interpreted with caution (see Fig. 22-22D). **Crystalline deposits may be observed in the cytoplasm of such cells.**

The Dutch investigator, Beyer-Boon (1977), has recorded 11 cases of lithiasis that resulted in sufficiently abnormal cytologic patterns to warrant the diagnosis of bladder cancer, occasionally of high grade. Highman and Wilson (1982) observed markedly atypical urothelial cells in 10 of 154 patients with calculi. In 1 of the patients, a major abnormality of the urothelium was observed on biopsy. None of the patients developed bladder cancer after a follow-up of 1 to 3 years. Personal experience does not support these views. In the past 30 years, I am aware of only 2 patients for whom a presumably erroneous diagnosis of urothelial cancer was made in the presence of lithiasis. One must keep in mind that **cancer of the urothelium and lithiasis may co-exist** and, in the presence of highly abnormal urothelial cells, cancer should be suspected (see Chap. 23). In fact, Wynder (1963), considered lithiasis as an important epidemiologic factor in bladder cancer. Hence, in the presence of **cytologic findings suggestive of cancer, further investigation of patients is necessary, whether or not there is associated lithiasis.**

Retrograde Sampling of Renal Pelves and Ureters in Lithiasis

It is not unusual for the urologist confronted with a space-occupying lesion of renal pelvis or ureter to resort to **retrograde catheterization or direct brushing** under the assumption that the cell sample will solve the diagnostic dilemma. Although these procedures are **sometimes useful in high-grade tumors** (see Chap. 23), they generally fail in distinguishing a stone from a low-grade papillary tumor.

Regardless of the medium of diagnosis, whether voided urine or samples obtained by instruments, the **differentiation of lithiasis from low-grade tumors cannot be accomplished by cytology** and must be based on clinical and radiologic data.

LEUKOPLAKIA OF BLADDER EPITHELIUM

Chronic inflammatory processes in the urinary bladder often associated with **lithiasis,** or in Africa with **schistosomiasis,** may result in the formation of **squamous metaplasia,** which may occur anywhere in the bladder or the renal pelvis and should be differentiated from the squamous epithelium often observed in the trigone of the normal female. Squamous epithelium with a **thick layer of keratin on the surface** appears white on cystoscopy and is known as **leukoplakia** (Fig. 22-23B). **Keratinizing squamous cancer of the bladder may develop from this disorder** (see Chap. 23).

Cytology

Leukoplakia of the bladder sheds mature squamous cells and anucleated squames that are found in the urinary sediment. The **anucleated squames have a yellow cytoplasm in Papanicolaou stain** (Fig. 22-23A). The diagnostic significance of such findings varies. In **voided urine** from either a female or a male patient, the presence of mature nucleated squamous cells is of **no diagnostic value.** If a **catheterized specimen contains anucleated squames, the presence of leukoplakia in the urinary tract is probable and cystoscopy should be recommended.** Leukoplakia of the lower urinary tract must be considered a potentially dangerous lesion that may be associated with squamous carcinoma with which it may share similar cytologic presentation (see Chap. 23).

MALACOPLAKIA OF BLADDER

Clinical Data and Histology

Malacoplakia (from Greek: *malako* = soft and *plax* = plaque) is a rare disorder first described in the urinary bladder and subsequently observed in many other organs, such

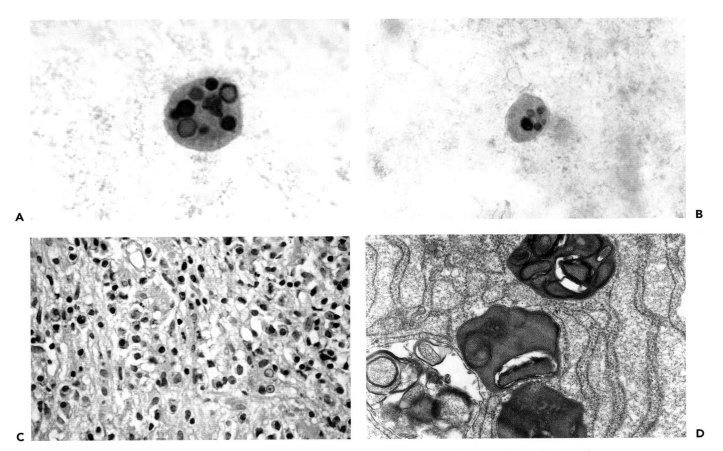

Figure 22-24 Malacoplakia of urinary bladder. *A,B.* Large macrophages with cytoplasmic inclusions or Michaelis-Gutmann bodies. Note the spherical appearance of the inclusions. *C.* Bladder biopsy corresponding to *A,* showing numerous macrophages containing Michaelis-Gutmann bodies. *D.* An electron micrograph of malacoplakia of the urinary bladder showing numerous very large lysosomes containing undigested remnants of bacteria. (*C:* PAS stain; *D:* approx. × 7,000.)

as the bronchus (see Chap. 19). The bladder lesion is characterized grossly by formation of **yellow soft plaques involving the urothelium and bladder wall.**

The lesions are located in the lamina propria and are separated from the lumen of the bladder by normal urothelium. The lesions are composed of **sheets of large, polygonal mononucleated macrophages.** The cytoplasm of these cells contains **spheroid, laminated, sometimes calcified concretions (Michaelis-Gutmann bodies)** (Fig. 22-24C). It has been shown that malacoplakia represents an **enzymatic deficiency of macrophages** that are unable to digest bacteria, are usually coliform. Electron microscopy has shown that the **Michaelis-Gutmann bodies represent giant cytoplasmic lysosomes containing phagocytosed bacteria that later become calcified in a concentric fashion and may contain iron** (Fig. 22-24D).

Cytology

Because malacoplakia is a subepithelial process, it is generally not accessible to cytologic sampling. However, if the epithelium is damaged, for example after a biopsy, the characteristic cytologic features of the disease may be recognized in the urinary sediment. In a case reported by Melamed (1962) and in other cases subsequently observed by us and others, **numerous cells in the urinary sediment of patients with malacoplakia contained one or more spherical Michaelis-Gutmann bodies. Concentric calcific laminations were readily identifiable in some, but not all, of the bodies** (Fig. 22-24A,B). Although urothelial cells may occasionally contain specks of calcium in the presence of lithiasis, the Michaelis-Gutmann bodies have a sufficiently unique appearance to be considered diagnostic of malacoplakia.

URINE OBTAINED THROUGH AN ILEAL BLADDER

An **ileal bladder or ileal conduit is a container constructed surgically from a segment of small bowel to function as a substitute bladder, usually after cystectomy for cancer** (Bricker, 1950). The ureters are transplanted and open into the lumen of the ileal bladder, which is usually anchored to the abdominal wall. The urine from the conduit is collected in a container. Another artificial bladder is the **Indiana pouch** built from cecum, ascending colon and the ileum that allows the patient to have some control of voiding (Rowland et al, 1987). For reasons that are discussed in detail in Chapter 23, cytologic follow-up of patients treated for bladder cancer is of considerable importance and requires familiarity with the make-up of the urinary sediment derived from the ileal conduit.

Cytology

Urinary sediments obtained from an ileal bladder are always **rich in small epithelial cells of small bowel origin,** which occur singly and in large clusters. **Rarely, the original columnar configuration of such cells is well preserved.** Typically, these **cells are spherical, oval, or somewhat irregular,** resembling macrophages (Fig. 22-25A). Their **cytoplasm is often frayed and may show vacuolization** and the **spherical nuclei, although of monotonous size, may appear hyperchromatic.** Most of these cells are very poorly preserved and show **nuclear pyknosis and apoptosis (karyorrhexis)** and **numerous nonspecific eosinophilic cytoplasmic inclusions** (Fig. 22-25B–D). There is no known clinical significance to these findings, which are present in most patients with an ileal bladder. The ileal bladder cells must be differentiated from cancer cells, derived from the ileal bladder, ureter, or renal pelvis, described in Chapter 23. Watari et al (2000) studied the urinary sediment on patients with Indiana pouch and failed to observe any intestinal-type cells.

CYTOLOGIC CHANGES CAUSED BY THERAPY

Urinary Sediment After Surgical Procedures

Urine samples, obtained shortly after transurethral resection of the prostate or other surgical procedures, usually show marked **acute inflammatory changes, sometimes with an admixture of eosinophils. Electrocautery,** used for biopsies, may cause **homogeneous nuclear enlargement and pyknosis in urothelial cells,** occasionally mimicking nuclear changes observed in bladder cancer. These changes may persist for 2 or even 3 weeks following the procedure. Errors in interpretation are avoided by knowledge of clinical history and cytologic follow-up 4 to 6 weeks after the surgical procedure. Fanning et al (1993) described a **spindly artifact** of urothelial cells after laser treatment caused by coagulation of epithelial surface. These authors cautioned against misinterpretation of such changes.

Epithelial regeneration that follows a biopsy or a surgical procedure may also result in some **atypia of urothelial cells and mitotic activity** that may be observed in urinary sediment. The **nuclei of the urothelial cells may show some granularity and sometimes contain visible nucleoli** and may show mitotic activity (Fig. 22-26A). As a rule,

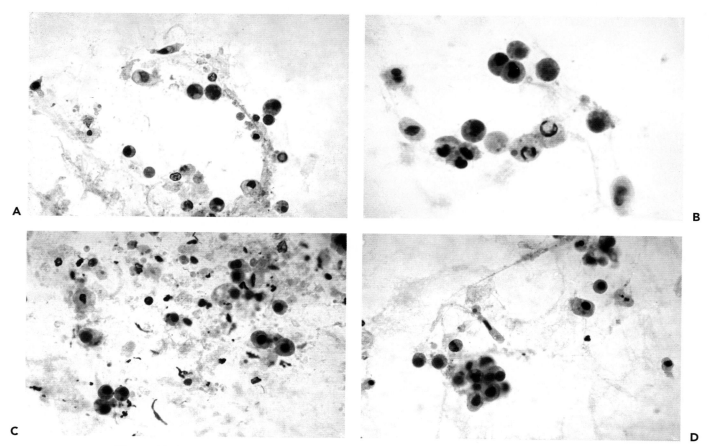

Figure 22-25   Cells derived from ileal bladders. The dominant cell in normal ileal bladder urine is a rounded, macrophage-like epithelial cell, undoubtedly derived from the intestinal lining. In Figures A, C, and D, scattered columnar intestinal epithelial cells may be observed. Note that the cytoplasm of most cells is degenerated and that many of them contain the nonspecific eosinophilic cytoplasmic inclusions or show nuclear disintegration. (B: High magnification).

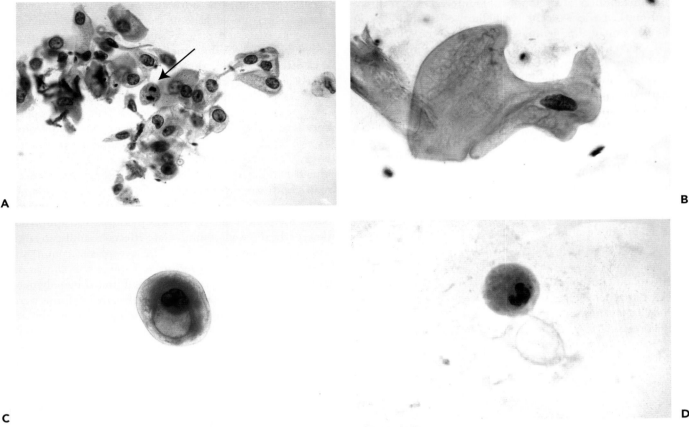

Figure 22-26 **Effect of treatment on urothelial cells.** *A.* Bladder brush a few days after transure-thral reaction for prostatic hypertrophy. Note the cluster of deeper urothelial cells, some showing mitotic activity (*arrow*). *B–D.* Effects of radiotherapy. *B.* A markedly distorted large urothelial cell after 35 GY. *C.* Same case as *B.* Note the large cytoplasmic vacuole. *D.* Radiation effect in a 20-year-old man with retroperitoneal Hodgkin's disease. The enlargement of the urothelial cell and nuclear break-down are shown.

these changes do not last more than **2 to 3 weeks after the procedure.** If significant cell abnormalities persist beyond that period, the possibility of a residual or recurrent malignant tumor cannot be ruled out.

Radiotherapy

Irradiation of the pelvic organs produces marked changes in the urinary bladder. Edema of the bladder wall is usually marked and there are also changes in blood vessels and the stroma. The **epithelial cells** share the fate of irradiated cells in other organs (see Chaps. 18 and 19) and **become enlarged.** The cytoplasm becomes **vacuolated and at times eosinophilic.** Their **nuclei** are also **enlarged,** occasionally showing **vacuolization, pyknosis and apoptosis (karyorrhexis)** (Fig. 22-26B–D). The value of cytologic assessment of radiotherapy for primary carcinoma of the bladder is discussed in Chapter 23.

Radiation changes in the **bladder** following **radiation treatment of carcinoma of the cervix** have resulted in serious diagnostic problems. Evaluating the **presence or absence of metastatic carcinoma of the cervix within the bladder** on the basis of the urinary sediment is at times **difficult** and, on at least one occasion, it was erroneous

because irradiated urothelial cells were mistaken for cells of epidermoid carcinoma. As elsewhere in similar situations, it appears wise to **withhold diagnostic judgment in the presence of radiation changes** until clear-cut evidence of cancer has been obtained.

Chemotherapy

Certain alkylating drugs, particularly **cyclophosphamide,** administered as an **immunosuppressive and therapeutic agent,** exercise a marked effect on the epithelium of the urinary bladder.

Cyclophosphamide

Cyclophosphamide (Cytoxan, Endoxan) is related to nitrogen mustard but is, per se, inactive until metabolized in the liver. In patients, the products of metabolism of the drug are rapidly excreted in the urine and have a marked cytotoxic effect, causing **hemorrhagic cystitis** that may lead to intractable hemorrhage necessitating surgical treatment (Berkson et al, 1973). This effect of cyclophosphamide may be attenuated or eliminated by hydration of the patient and by certain drugs.

Experimental evidence (Koss, 1967) **supports the view**

that metabolites of cyclophosphamide exercise a direct and marked effect on the epithelium of the bladder: in the rat, a single intraperitoneal injection of the drug in the dose of 200 or 400 mg/kg produced **rapid necrosis of the bladder epithelium, followed by marked atypical hyperplasia.** Cells from the hyperplastic epithelium showed **marked atypia, comparable to abnormalities observed in human material.** It has also been shown experimentally that by diverting the urine from the bladder, the drug effect could be prevented (Bellin et al, 1974).

Cyclophosphamide-induced abnormalities are not confined to the epithelium. There is experimental evidence that **subepithelial blood vessels and smooth muscle of the bladder may be severely damaged** (Bonikos and Koss, 1974). It has also been recorded that in children, fibrosis of the bladder wall may occur after exposure to this potent drug (Johnson and Meadows, 1971).

Effects on Urothelial Cells

The cytologic changes in patients receiving cyclophosphamide for a variety of malignant diseases were first described by Forni et al (1964). The changes observed were somewhat similar to those following radiation treatment. The most striking feature was **marked but variable cell enlargement,** usually pertaining to both the nucleus and the cytoplasm. The study of patients from the very beginning of treatment suggested that the **nuclear enlargement preceded cytoplasmic abnormalities.** The **enlarged nucleus was often eccentric, slightly irregular in outline, and nearly always markedly hyperchromatic.** The **chromatin granules** were at times **coarse** but their distribution was usually fairly even, giving the nucleus a **"salt-and-pepper" appearance** (Fig. 22-27). A **chromocenter or a nucleolus or two** were often well in evidence and **sometimes very large.** The large nucleoli were frequently distorted, with irregular and sharp edges. In **female patients, the sex chromatin body was often visibly enlarged.** Occasionally, multinucleated cells were noted with some variability in the sizes of the component nuclei. **Nuclear pyknosis and apoptosis (karyorrhexis)** were common **late effects,** resulting in large and hyperchromatic nuclei. The **cytoplasm** commonly showed **marked vacuolization** and sometimes contained particles of foreign material or was infiltrated by polymorphonuclear leukocytes. Occasionally, bizarre cell forms were observed. In some instances, the cytologic changes due to cyclophosphamide therapy may be extremely severe and **imitate urothelial carcinoma to perfection.** In cases showing such marked cell changes as those just described, the **smear**

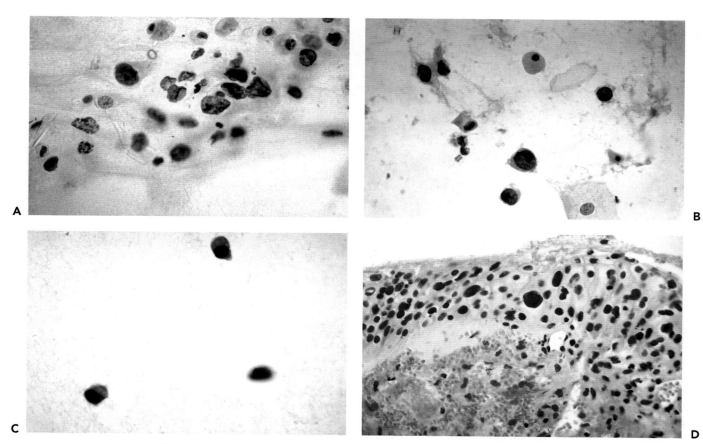

Figure 22-27   Effect of cyclophosphamide on urinary bladder epithelium. *A.* Smear pattern in voided urine showing numerous cells with large hyperchromatic nuclei. *B.* Similar nuclear abnormalities in a patient treated for large cell lymphoma. *C.* Nuclear enlargement and hyperchromasia in a patient treated for leukemia. *D.* Biopsy of bladder in the same patient as *C,* showing nuclear enlargement in the epithelium surmounting a hemorrhagic stroma, the latter is characteristic of cyclophosphamide effect.

background often contained numerous erythrocytes, cellular debris, and leukocytes.

It must be noted that there was no direct correlation between the degree of cytologic atypia and the dosage of the drug, as shown by Forni et al (1964). Histologic changes in biopsies of the bladder show very marked epithelial abnormalities which, at the height of the cyclophosphamide effect, are akin to carcinoma in situ (Fig. 22-27D), but can regress after cessation of therapy. It has been shown by Jayalakshmamma and Pinkel (1976) that **simultaneous radiotherapy enhances the effects of cyclophosphamide** on the bladder.

The cytologic changes caused by cyclophosphamide should **not be confused with synchronous urothelial cell abnormalities due to human polyomavirus activation,** which are quite common in such patients and were described above. The drug has an immunosuppressive effect and, thus, it may contribute to reactivation of the virus. As discussed above, there is no evidence that the polyomavirus activation has any bearing on the occurrence of **hemorrhagic cystitis** in patients with bone marrow transplants (Cottler-Fox et al, 1989). In fact, it is likely that the hemorrhagic cystitis may have been caused in these patients by cyclophosphamide.

The most significant complication of cyclophosphamide therapy has been the occurrence of cancer of the lower urinary tract, recorded in several patients **after long-term administration of large doses of the drug** for unrelated malignant disease, usually a lymphoma, but sometimes for a benign disorder (Schiff et al, 1982). **Bladder carcinomas** were reported by Worth (1971), Dale and Smith (1974), and by Wall and Clausen (1975). A squamous carcinoma of the bladder was personally observed in a 19-year-old girl with a history of 24 months of cyclophosphamide therapy (Fig. 22-28A) and an adenocarcinoma in a 77-year-old woman who received the drug for many years for Waldenstrom's macroglobulinemia (Siddiqui et al, 1996). **Carcinomas of the renal pelvis** (Fuchs et al, 1981, McDougall et al, 1981) and of **the ureter** (Schiff et al, 1982) were also recorded under similar circumstances. Several cases of

leiomyosarcoma of the bladder have been observed, usually several years after completion of treatment for a malignant lymphoma with large doses of cyclophosphamide (Rowland and Eble, 1983; Seo et al, 1985; Kawamura et al, 1993). Thrasher et al (1990) described a leiomyosarcoma of bladder after treatment for lupus nephritis. An example of a leiomyosarcoma of the bladder after cyclophosphamide therapy is shown in Figure 22-28B, courtesy of Dr. Lawrence Roth of Indianapolis, Indiana. Sigal et al (1991) described a **synchronous leiomyosarcoma and an invasive carcinoma** in a patient treated for lymphoma. An **excess of bladder cancer** was observed in patients treated with cyclophosphamide for **Hodgkin's disease** (Pedersen-Bjergaard, 1988) and **non-Hodgkin's lymphomas** (Travis et al, 1989). Although in some of the older patients, the bladder cancer may have been an incidental, new primary tumor, some of the observed patients were sufficiently young to suggest that the drug acted as a carcinogenic agent. This possibility is not unique to cyclophosphamide, and it has also been suggested for other alkylating agents (see Chap. 18). These observations strongly suggest that clinical and cytologic follow-up of patients receiving cyclophosphamide therapy is prudent. In patients in whom cell abnormalities develop and persist during and after cyclophosphamide therapy, clinical investigation of the bladder is warranted.

Busulfan

The marked effects of busulfan (Myeleran) on the epithelia of the cervix and the lung were described in Chapters 18 and 19. It is not surprising, therefore, that the drug also has a marked effect on the epithelium of the urinary tract. **Large cells with atypical large nuclei may be observed in renal tubules and the epithelium of the renal pelves. The urinary bladder** may even show **abnormalities resembling carcinoma in situ.** The **urinary sediment** of patients receiving busulfan may contain **abnormal epithelial cells,** difficult to differentiate from cancer cells. Examples of cell abnormalities caused by busulfan are shown in Chapter 18. The role of busulfan as a possible carcinogenic agent is ex-

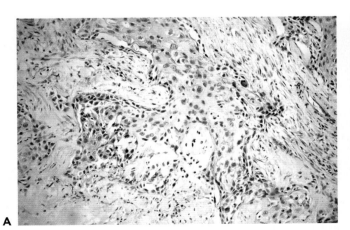
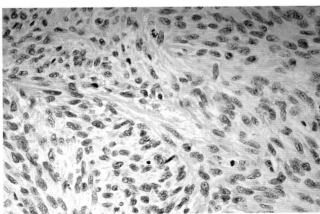

Figure 22-28 **Malignant tumors in patients treated with cyclophosphamide.** *A.* Urothelial carcinoma in a 47-year-old male with multiple myeloma. *B.* Leiomyosarcoma of bladder in a 17-year-old man treated for malignant lymphoma. (*B:* Courtesy of Dr. Lawrence Roth, Indianapolis, IN.)

tensively discussed in Chapter 19, to which the reader is referred for further information.

Intravesical Drug Therapy

A number of drugs such as **triethylenethiophosphoramide (Thiotepa), doxorubicin hydrochloride (Adriamycin), and mitomycin,** are being used intravesically for treatment of some bladder cancers, mainly carcinoma in situ, and for prevention of recurrences of papillary tumors. In my experience, **urothelial cell changes observed with these drugs are relatively trivial and consist of a radiomimetic effect** (cell and nuclear enlargement). I have not seen any drug-induced nuclear abnormalities that mimic carcinoma (except for an **occasional polyomavirus activation**). Thus, **the presence of identifiable cancer cells in the urinary sediment during the monitoring of such patients usually indicates a lack of tumor response to treatment.** In experimental dogs treated with intravesical doxorubicin and Thiotepa, similar observations were recorded: cell and nuclear enlargement, multinucleation, and karyorrhexis were the principal transient abnormalities noted (Rasmussen et al, 1980).

Immunotherapy with Bacillus Calmette-Guérin (BCG)

Immunotherapy with the attenuated *Mycobacterium bovis* strain, bacillus Calmette-Guérin (BCG) is now extensively used for treatment of flat carcinoma in situ of the bladder. The **monitoring of these patients by cytologic examinations of urinary sediment** is mandatory and the results are described in Chapter 23. The agent may produce **tubercle-like granulomas in the bladder wall, indistinguishable from tuberculosis. In a fortuitous case, clusters of epithelioid cells, forming a granuloma, may be observed in the urinary sediment** (Fig. 22-29). For further discussion of effects of treatment on bladder cancer, see Chapter 23.

Aspirin and Phenacetin

Prescott (1964) pointed out that the nephrotoxic effect of these drugs may be assessed in urinary sediment by performing **counts of renal tubular cells.** This is best accomplished by staining the sediment by the method described by Prescott and Brodie (see Chap. 44), which stains leukocytes deep blue, renal tubular cells pink, and erythrocytes red. This method was used by Prescott to demonstrate a marked increase in the desquamation of renal tubular cells in patients receiving aspirin, phenacetin, and related drugs. The significance of these drugs in the causation of carcinoma of the renal pelvis is discussed in Chapter 23.

URINARY SEDIMENT IN ORGAN TRANSPLANTATION

One of the greatest medical advances of our era has been the ability to substitute a diseased organ of a patient with a transplanted organ (allograft) obtained either from a living or deceased donor. Although knowledge of human immunology has made great strides and much more is known about the mechanisms of tissue matching and prevention of rejection than a few years ago, nevertheless, in spite of effective therapy, the rejection of the transplanted organ by the recipient remains a serious risk in every case. It is beyond the scope of this work to discuss all the manifestations of organ rejection. Only some of the effects on the urinary sediment will be discussed here in reference to bone marrow and renal transplantation.

Bone Marrow Transplantation

The procedure is used in **patients with treatment-resistant leukemias and lymphomas and in the treatment of some solid tumors and some patients with nonmalignant blood disorders** (summary in Stella et al, 1987). The preparation of the patients for a transplant involves **ablation of**

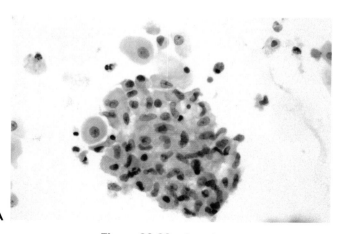
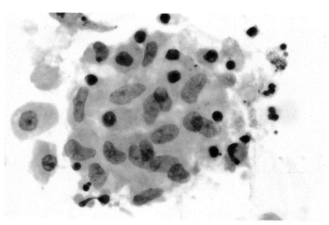

A   **B**

Figure 22-29   Granulomas in voided urine sediment of a patient treated with BCG for carcinoma cite A & B in situ of the bladder. Both photographs show plump epithelioid cells in a tight cluster. No giant cells were observed in this case; *B:* high power. (Case courtesy of Dr. Ruth Kreitzer, Mount Sinai Hospital, New York, NY.)

the marrow by total body irradiation and large doses of drugs, such as cyclophosphamide and busulfan (summary in Cottler-Fox et al, 1989). Perhaps the most common event in the bone marrow transplant patients is the **activation of polyomavirus infection, with resulting nuclear inclusions,** described and illustrated above.

Both radiation and drugs may affect the urothelial cells when applied singly, as discussed above. The combination of these procedures may be very difficult to interpret. As an example, the urinary sediment and bladder biopsies in a 43-year-old man with bone marrow transplant for leukemia are shown in Figure 22-30. The **urinary sediment** showed **radiomimetic effect** but also contained **bizarre malignant-looking cells with huge, hyperchromatic nuclei. The biopsy** of the bladder showed epithelial changes **mimicking urothelial carcinoma in situ.** The patient died and similar abnormalities were found in the epithelium of the bladder at postmortem examination. Because of multiple modes of treatment in this case, no single cause of the epithelial abnormalities can be ascertained. It is important, however, to recognize that cyclophosphamide may be the cause of bladder cancer (see above). In an excellent study, Stella et al (1992) compared change caused by conditioning therapy in bone marrow transplant recipients with cells har-

vested in urinary sediment from patients with bladder cancer. Although significant differences were observed in patients with low-grade tumors, the separation of therapy-induced changes from cells of high-grade carcinomas was very difficult.

Changes caused by radiotherapy and by cyclophosphamide may also occur simultaneously (Fig. 22-30A). Cell changes mimicking (or perhaps representing) cancer may be observed. On the other hand, it is known that organ transplant patients are prone to develop various forms of cancer, including carcinomas and malignant lymphomas (see discussion of this topic in Chap. 18). Hence, it remains a possibility that carcinomas in situ of the urinary bladder may occur in transplant patients.

Renal Transplantation

Renal transplantation in patients in uremia caused by renal failure is the oldest and one of the most successful procedures of its kind. Following the transplantation, the patients are immunosuppressed by a variety of drugs. The greatest danger to these patients is transplant rejection, which may be prevented by adjusting the dosage of the immunosuppressing agents.

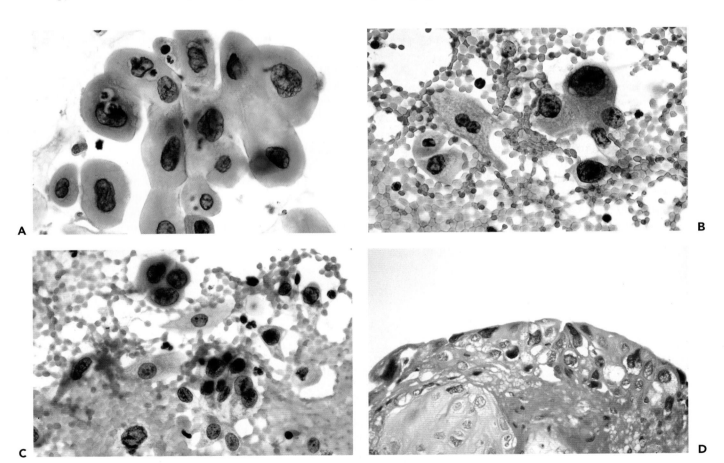

Figure 22-30   Urine sediment in a 45-year-old male treated with a bone marrow transplant for malignant lymphoma. *A.* Shows markedly enlarged urothelial cells, consistent with radiation effect. *B,C.* Show a variety of abnormal cells with large homogeneous nuclei next to urothelial cells of normal size and configuration. *D.* Shows a bladder biopsy with remarkable nuclear abnormalities in the epithelium consistent with a carcinoma in situ. (Case courtesy of Dr. Denise Hidvegi, Northwestern University, Chicago, IL.)

Monitoring of renal rejection by urinary sediment analysis was proposed in the late 1960s. Bossen et al (1970) studied a profile of urinary sediment that was composed of seven features observed before and during episodes of renal allograft rejection. These features were:

- Necrotic material forming the background of smears ("dirty background")
- Nuclear degeneration
- Tubular casts
- Erythrocytes
- Mixed cell clusters (epithelial and leukocytes)
- Lymphocytes
- Tubular cells

At least five of these features were observed in every patient prior to episodes of rejection. The **two most constant features were the presence of lymphocytes and of tubular cells.** The mere increase in cellularity of the smears was a hint of impending rejection. In the absence of rejection, the urinary sediment had low cellularity and a clean background. If the rejection episode was controlled by therapy, there was an improvement in the profile of features discussed above. Bossen et al recommend an evaluation of the **urinary sediment profile** for monitoring renal transplants **as more reliable than any single feature,** such as the presence of lymphocytes or tubular cells, as previously advocated by Kauffman et al (1964) and by Taft and Flax (1966). Schumann et al (1977) advocated use of the cytocentrifuge for the study of urinary sediment and confirmed that the presence of tubular cells, singly or in casts, was of great prognostic value of impending rejection (see Figs. 22-11D and 22-12). In a subsequent communication, Schumann et al (1981) discussed at length the criteria for **recognition of renal fragments and tubular cells** in the urinary sediment. These authors stressed the close relationship of tubular cells with casts and the cylindric fragments corresponding to tubular cells. With the use of Bales' method of urine fixation and processing, the recognition of casts in the sediment is significantly enhanced.

Spencer and Anderson (1979) stressed that numerous **viruses,** such as **cytomegalovirus, herpesvirus (including herpes zoster), and human papillomavirus** may become activated in the immunosuppressed renal allograft recipients. These authors reported that the infection with **cytomegalovirus was particularly serious. Human polyomavirus activation,** easily detected in voided urine, is also of major prognostic significance as narrated above (Drachenberg et al, 1999).

Since the publication of these early papers, considerable progress has been made in the **recognition of molecules that participate in organ rejection** (summary in Corey et al, 1997b). In a series of elaborate studies on serial urine samples in ten pediatric patients, processed by the method of Bales (see Chap. 44), these authors compared the predictive value of urine cytology with renal biopsies (Corey et al, 1997a) and conventional cytology with immunostaining for **receptors of adhesion molecules ICAM-1 and interferon gamma** and **TNF-α receptors,** two molecules that regulate the expression of ICAM-1 (Corey et al, 1997b). In conventional cytology, **organ rejection was anticipated when the urine sample contained less than 55% neutrophiles and more than 20% lymphocytes. The reading of the cytology specimens was more reproducible than the reading of biopsies.** In immunostudy of nonrejecting patients, the tubular cells expressed only the interferon gamma receptor. In the graft-rejecting patients, the tubular cells expressed ICAM-1 and TNFα receptors but not the interferon gamma receptor (Fig. 22-31). This study, in which each step was carefully controlled and each morphologic observation was confirmed by two observers, opened new possibilities in monitoring renal transplant patients.

Aspiration Biopsy

Häyry and von Willebrand (1981a) used percutaneous fine-needle aspiration technique (FNA) for monitoring of renal transplants. The technique, described in detail by the same authors (1981b, 1984), samples the cortical area of the graft. **Three types of cells are evaluated in smears** stained with

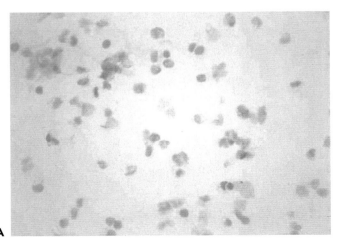
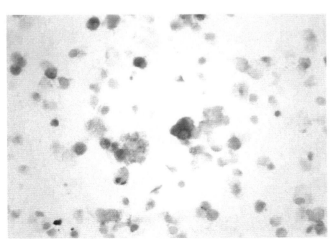

A

B

Figure 22-31 **Monitoring renal transplant rejection with ICAM.** *A.* Shows a negative control. *B.* Shows a renal cell with positive staining. For description of test, see text. (Courtesy of Dr. Flores Alfonso, Morristown Memorial Hospital, Morristown, NJ.)

May-Grünwald-Giemsa (MGG): the **large distal tubular cells,** either granulated or nongranulated, **small proximal tubular cells,** often forming clumps, and **endothelial cells.** The viability of these cells was evaluated on a scale from one to four, one indicating normal cells and four necrotic cells. The **extent of inflammation in the smear** was based on a **differential count** of leukocytes, **compared with the differential count in a simultaneously obtained sample of peripheral blood.** The results were compared with biopsy material and found to be accurate. Several **types of leukocytes** were recognized and classified in these samples. **Lymphocytes and monocytes** were the first inflammatory cells seen in the transplant. The appearance of **blast cells indicated that the function of the transplant deteriorated.** Granulocytes did not appear in the samples until late in rejection. **Platelets** were also studied with specific antibodies and have been shown to be **increased during rejection episodes.** Still, the finding of a **large number of tissue macrophages was the most secure evidence of acute transplant rejection.** Häyry, in a summary paper (1989), discusses the clinical value of the FNA technique and several ancillary laboratory procedures, as a most accurate method of monitoring renal transplants, leading to appropriate adjustments in antirejection therapy and salvage of allografts. The technique has been successfully used by Bishop et al (1989). It requires a dedicated team and a specialized laboratory for successful execution and has not achieved widespread acceptance.

Cyclosporine Effect

Cyclosporine is an immunomodulatory drug extensively used in organ transplant recipients to prevent rejection. The drug affects renal function in about 30% of the patients. Winkelmann et al (1985) and Stella et al (1987) described **necrosis of renal tubular epithelial cells** and the presence of **"tissue fragments" in the urine of bone marrow transplant patients** as evidence of cyclosporine toxicity. Similar conclusions were reached by Stilmont et al (1987). So far as one could judge from the photographs, the changes were not specific. Most unfortunately, many people knowledgeable about organ transplants who write about the cytologic findings in the urinary sediment are not familiar with the scope of urinary cytology. A number of published articles confuse common findings with transplant-specific findings. As an example, a paper by Stella et al (1992) shows cells with typical polyomavirus inclusions as evidence of "urothelial toxicity" following bone marrow transplantation. The **reader should be skeptical of much of the published work on this subject written by people with limited experience in urinary cytology.**

Because the allograft recipients routinely receive immunosuppressive drugs, they are subject to infections by agents that are uncommonly observed in nonsuppressed patients. These are mainly viral agents, which have been discussed in detail above. Such patients also run a substantial risk of developing malignant tumors, such as malignant lymphomas or other cancers, as discussed in Chapter 18.

BIBLIOGRAPHY

Alm P, Colleen S. A histochemical and ultrastructural study of human urethral uroepithelium. Acta Pathol Microbiol Immunol Scand 90:103–111, 1982.

Alroy J, Pauli BU, Weinstein RS, Merk FB. Association of asymmetric unit membrane plaque formation in the urinary bladder of adult humans with therapeutic radiation. Experientia 33:1645–1647, 1977.

Apperley JF, Rice SJ, Bishop JA, et al. Late-onset hemorrhagic cystis associated with urinary excretion of polyomaviruses after bone marrow transplantation. Transplantation 43:108–112, 1987.

Arthur RR, Shah KV, Baust ST, et al. Association of BK viruria with hemorrhagic cystis in recipients of bone marrow transplants. N Engl J Med 315:230–234, 1986.

Ashton PR, Lambird PA. Cytodiagnosis of malacoplakia. Report of case. Acta Cytol 14:92–94, 1970.

Bales CE. A semi-automated method for preparation of urine sediment for cytologic evaluation. Acta Cytol 25:323–326, 1981.

Bancroft J, Seybolt JF, Windhager HA. Cytologic diagnosis of cytomegalic inclusion disease. Acta Cytol 5:182–186, 1961.

Bard RH. The significance of asymptomatic hematuria in women and its economic implications—a ten year study. Arch Intern Med 148:2629–2632, 1988.

Bellin HJ, Cherry JM, Koss LG. Effects of a single dose of cyclophosphamide. V. Protective effect of diversion of the urinary stream on dog bladder. Lab Invest 30:43–47, 1974.

Berger JR, Kaszovitz B, Post MJ, Dickinson G. Progressive multifocal leukoencephalopathy associated with human immunodeficiency virus infection: A review of the literature with a report of sixteen cases. Ann Intern Med 107:78–87, 1987.

Berger JR, Major EO. Progressive multifocal leukoencephalopathy. In Broder S, Merigan TC Jr, Bolognesi E (eds). Textbook of AIDS Medicine. Baltimore, Williams & Wilkins, 1994, pp 385–400.

Berkson BM, Lome LG, Shapiro I. Severe cystitis induced by cyclophosphamide. Role of surgical management. JAMA 225:605–606, 1973.

Beyer-Boon ME. The Efficacy of Urinary Cytology. Doctor's thesis. University Medical Center, Leiden, 1977.

Bishop GA, Hall BM, Waugh J, et al. Diagnosis of renal allograft rejection by analysis of fine-needle aspiration biopsy specimens with immunostains and simple cytology. Lancet 2:645–649, 1986.

Blanc WA. Cytologic diagnosis of cytomegalic inclusion disease in gastric washings. Am J Clin Pathol 28:46–49, 1957.

Bolande RP. Inclusion-bearing cells in urine in certain viral infections. Pediatrics 24:7–12, 1959.

Bonikos DS, Koss LG. Acute effects of cyclophosphamide on rat urinary bladder muscle. Arch Pathol 97:242–245, 1974.

Bossen EH, Johnston WW. Exfoliative cytopathologic studies in organ transplantation. V. The diagnosis of rejection in the immediate postoperative period. Acta Cytol 21:502–507, 1977.

Bossen EH, Johnston WW. Exfoliative cytopathologic studies in organ transplantation. IV. The cytologic diagnosis of herpesvirus in the urine of renal allograft recipients. Acta Cytol 19:415–419, 1975.

Bossen EH, Johnston WW, Amatulli J, Rowlands DT. Exfoliative cytopathologic studies in organ transplantation. III. The cytologic profile of urine during acute renal allograft rejection. Acta Cytol 14:176–181, 1970.

Bossen EH, Johnston WW, Amatulli J, Rowlands DT. Exfoliative cytopathologic studies in organ transplantation. I. The cytologic diagnosis of cytomegalic inclusions disease in the urine of renal allograft recipients. Am J Clin Pathol 52:340–344, 1969.

Bricker EM. Bladder substitution after pelvic evisceration. Surg Clin North Am 30:1511–1521, 1950.

Brown EW. Eosinophilic granuloma of the bladder. J Urol 83:665–668, 1960.

Buckner CD, Rudolph RH, Fefer A, et al. High dose cyclophosphamide therapy for malignant disease. Toxicity, tumor response, and the effects of stored autologous marrow. Cancer 29:357–365, 1972.

Carson ICC, Segura JW, Greene LF. Clinical importance of microhematuria. JAMA 241:149–50, 1979.

Chang SC. Urinary cytologic diagnosis of cytomegalic inclusion disease in childhood leukemia. Acta Cytol 14:338–343, 1970.

Chappell LH, Lundin L. A pitfall in urine cytology. A case report. Acta Cytol 20:162–163, 1976.

Clark BG, Gherardi GJ. Urethrotrigonitis or epidermidization of the trigone of the bladder. J Urol 87:545–548, 1962.

Clements MS, Oko T. Cytologic diagnosis of schistosomiasis in routine urinary sediment. Acta Cytol 27:277–280, 1983.

Cohen RA, Brown RS. Microscopic hematuria. N Engl J Med 348:2330–2338, 2003.

Coleman DV. The cytological diagnosis of human polyomavirus infection and its value in clinical practice. In Koss LG, Coleman DV (eds). Advances in Clinical Cytology, vol 1. London, Butterworths, 1981, pp 136–159.

Coleman DV. The cytodiagnosis of human polyomavirus infection. Acta Cytol 19:93–96, 1975.

Coleman DV, Field AM, Gardner SD, et al. Virus-induced obstruction of the ureteric and cystic duct in allograft recipients. Transplant Proc 5:95–98, 1973.

Coleman DV, Gardner SD, Field AM. Human polyomavirus infection in renal allograft recipients. Br Med J 3:371–375, 1973.

Coleman DV, Wolfendale MR, Daniel RA, et al. A prospective study of human polyomavirus infection in pregnancy. J Infect Dis 142:1–8, 1980.

Colin AL, Howard RS. Asymptomatic microscopic hematuria. J Urol 124:389–391, 1980.

Collins KA, Cina MS, Pettenati MJ, Fitts M. Identification of femal cells in postcoital penile swabs using fluorescence in situ hybridization. Arch Pathol Lab Med 124:1080–1082, 2000.

Connery DB. Leukoplakia of the urinary bladder and its association with carcinoma. J Urol 69:121–127, 1953.

Cordon-Cardo C, Bander NH, et al. Immunoanatomic dissection of the human urinary tract by monoclonal antibodies. J Histochem Cytochem 32:1035–1040, 1984.

Corey HE, Alfonso F, Hamele-Bena D, et al. Urine cytology and the diagnosis of renal allograft rejection. I. Studies using conventional staining. Acta Cytol 41:1732–1741, 1997a.

Corey HE, Alfonso F, Hamele-Bena D, et al. Urine cytology and the diagnosis of renal allograft rejection. II. Studies using immunostaining. Acta Cytol 41:1742–1746, 1997b.

Cornish J, Lecamwasam JP, Harrison G, et al. Host defense mechanisms in the bladder. II. Disruption of the layer of mucus. Br J Exp Pathol 69:759–770, 1988.

Cottler-Fox M, Lynch M, Deeg HJ, Koss LG. Human polyomavirus: Lack of relationship of viruria to prolonged or severe hemorrhagic cystitis after bone marrow transplant. Bone Marrow Transplant 4:279–282, 1989.

Cowen PN. False cytodiagnosis of bladder malignancy due to previous radiotherapy. Br J Urol 47:405–412, 1975.

Crabbe JGS. "Comet" or "decoy" cells found in urinary sediment smears. Acta Cytol 15:303–305, 1971.

Crabtree WN, Murphy WM. The value of ethanol as a fixative in urinary cytology. Acta Cytol 24:452–455, 1980.

Csapo Z, Kuthy E, Lantos J, Ormos J. Experimentally induced malacoplakia. Am J Pathol 79:453–462, 1975.

Dabbs DJ. Cytology of pyelitis glandularis cystica. A case report. Acta Cytol 36:943–945, 1992.

Dale GA, Smith RB. Transitional cell carcinoma of the bladder associated with cyclophosphamide. J Urol 112:603–604, 1974.

De LasCasas LE, Hoerl HD, Bardales RH, et al. Utility of urinary cytology for diagnosing human polyoma virus infection in transplant recipients: A study of 37 cases with electron microscopic analysis. Diagn Cytopathol 25:376–381, 2001.

Deng F-M, Ding M, Lavker RM, Sun T-T. Urothelial function reconsidered: A role in urinary protein secretion. Proc Natl Acad Sci USA 98:154–159, 2001.

deVoogt HJ, Beyer-Boon ME, Brussec JAM. The value of phase contrast microscopy for urinary cytology. Reliability and pitfalls. Acta Cytol 19:542–546, 1975.

deVoogt HJ, Rathert P, Beyer-Boon ME. Urinary Cytology. New York, Springer-Verlag, 1977.

Dimette RM, Sproat HF, Kilimt CR. Examination of smears of urinary sediment for detection of neoplasms of bladder; survey of an Egyptian village infested with *Schistosoma haematobium*. Am J Clin Pathol 25:1032–1042, 1955.

Dodd LG, Tello J. Cytologic examination of urine from patients with interstitial cystitis. Acta Cytol 42:923–927, 1998.

Dolman CL, McLeod PM, Chang EC. Lymphocytes and urine in ceroid lipofuscinosis. Arch Pathol Lab Med 104:487–490, 1980.

Dorfman HD, Monis B. Mucin-containing inclusions in multinucleated giant cells and transitional epithelial cells of urine: Cytochemical observations on exfoliated cells. Acta Cytol 8:293–301, 1964.

Drachenberg CB, Beskow CO, Cangro CB, et al. Human polyomavirus in renal allograft biopsies: Morphological findings and correlation with urine cytology. Hum Pathol 30:970–977, 1999.

Eggensperger DL, King C, Gaudette LE, et al. Cytodiagnostic urinalysis. Three years' experience with a new laboratory test. Am J Clin Pathol 91:202–206, 1989.

Eickenberg H-U, Amin M, Lich RJ. Blastomycosis of the genitourinary tract. J Urol 113:650–652, 1975.

Elbadawi A. Interstitial cystitis: A critique of current concepts with a new proposal for pathologic diagnosis and pathogenesis. Urology 49(Suppl 5A):14–40, 1997.

Failde M, Eckert WG, Patterson JN. A comparison of a simple centrifuge method and the Millipore filter technic in urinary cytology. Acta Cytol 7:199–206, 1963.

Fanning CV, Staerkel GA, Sneige N, et al. Spindling artifact of urothelial cells in post-laser treatment urinary cytology. Diagn Cytopathol 9:279–281, 1993.

Favaro S, Bonfante L, et al. Is the red cell morphology really useful to detect the source of hematuria? Am J Nephrol 17:172–175, 1997.

Fetterman GH. New laboratory aid in clinical diagnosis of inclusion disease of infancy. Am J Clin Pathol 22:424–425, 1952.

Filie AC, Wilder AM, Brosky K, et al. Urinary cytology associated with human polyomavirus and indinavir therapy in HIV-infected patients. Am J Clin Pathol 117:922–926, 2002.

Fischer S, Nielson ML, Clausen S, et al. Increased abnormal urothelial cells in voided urine following excretory urography. Acta Cytol 26:153–158, 1982.

Fisher ER, Davis E. Cytomegalic-inclusion disease in adult. N Engl J Med 258:1036–1040, 1958.

Fisman D. Pisse-prophets and puritans: Thomas Brian, uroscopy, and seventeenth-century English medicine. Pharos 56:6–11, 1993.

Foot NC. Glandular metaplasia of the epithelium of the urinary tract. South Med J 37:137–142, 1944.

Forni AM, Koss LG, Geller W. Cytological study of the effect of cyclophosphamide on the epithelium of the urinary bladder in man. Cancer 17:1348–1355, 1964.

Fradet Y, Islam N, Boucher L, et al. Polymorphic expression of a human superficial bladder tumor antigen defined by mouse monoclonal antibodies. Proc Natl Acad Sci USA 84:7227–7231, 1987.

Freni SC, Freni-Titulaer LWJ. Microhematuria found by mass screening of apparently healthy males. Acta Cytol 21:421–423, 1977.

Froom P, Ribak J, Benbassat J. Significance of micro-haematuria in young adults. Br Med J 288:20–22, 1984.

Fuchs EF, Kay R, Poole R, et al. Uroepithelial carcinoma in association with cyclophosphamide ingestion. J Urol 126:544–545, 1981.

Gardner SD, Field AM, Coleman DV, Hulme B. New human papovavirus (BK) isolated from urine after renal transplantation. Lancet 1:1253–1257, 1971.

Gardner SD, MacKenzie EFD, Smith C, Porter AA. Prospective study of the human polyomaviruses BK and JC and cytomegalovirus in renal transplant recipients. J Clin Pathol 37:578–586, 1984.

Glucksman MD. Bladder cancer after cyclophosphamide therapy. Urology 16:553, 1980.

Goldstein ML, Whitman T, Renshaw AA. Significance of cell groups in voided urine. Acta Cytol 42:290–294, 1998.

Goudsmit J, Wertheim-van Dillen P, van Strein A, van der Noordaa J. The role of BK virus in acute respiratory tract disease and the presence of BKV DNA in tonsils. J Med Virol 10:91–99, 1982.

Greene LF, O'Shaughnessy EJ Jr, Hendricks ED. Study of five hundred patients with asymptomatic microhematuria. JAMA 161:610–613, 1956.

Grossfeld GD, Litwin MS, Wolf JS, et al. Evaluation of asymptomatic microscopic hematuria in adults: The American Urological Association best practice policy—Part I. Definition, detection, prevalence, and etiology. Part II. Patient evaluation, cytology, voided markers, imaging, cystoscopy, nephrology evaluation and follow-up. Urology 57:599–603, 604–610, 2001.

Gupta RJ, Schuster RA, Christian WD. Autopsy findings in a unique case of malacoplakia. Arch Pathol 93:42–48, 1972.

Hansen MV, Kristensen PB. Eosinophilic cystitis simulating invasive bladder carcinoma. Scand J Urol Nephrol 27:275–277, 1993.

Harris MJ, Schwinn CP, Morrow JW, et al. Exfoliative cytology of the urinary bladder irrigation specimen. Acta Cytol 15:385–399, 1971.

Häyry PJ. Fine-needle aspiration biopsy in renal transplantation. Kidney Intl 36:130–141, 1989.

Häyry PJ, von Willebrand E. Transplant aspiration cytology. Transplantation 38:7–12, 1984.

Häyry PJ, von Willebrand E. Monitoring of human renal allograft rejection with fine-needle aspiration cytology. Scand J Immunol 13:87–97, 1981a.

Häyry PJ, von Willebrand E. Practical guidelines for fine needle aspiration biopsy of human renal allografts. Ann Clin Res (Helsinki) 13:288–306, 1981b.

Hellstrom HR, Davis BK, Shonnard JW. Eosinophilic cystitis. A study of 16 cases. Am J Clin Pathol 72:777–784, 1979.

Henry L, Fox M. Histological findings in pseudomembranous trigonitis. J Clin Pathol 24:605–608, 1971.

Heritage J, Chesters PM, McCance DJ. The persistence of papovavirus BK DNA sequences in normal human renal tissue. J Med Virol 81:143–150, 1981.

Herz F, Gazivoda P, Papenhausen PR, et al. Normal human urothelial cells in culture. Subculture procedure, flow cytometric and chromosomal analyses. Lab Invest 53:571–574, 1985.

Herz F, Schermer HF, Koss LG. Short term culture of epithelial cells from urine of adults. Proc Soc Exp Biol Med 161:153–157, 1979.

Hicks RM. The mammalian urinary bladder: An accommodating organ. Biol Rev 50:215–246, 1975.

Hicks RM. The function of the Golgi complex in transitional epithelium. Synthesis of the thick cell membrane. J Cell Biol 30:623–643, 1966.

Hicks RM. The permeability of rat transitional epithelium. Keratinization and the barrier to water. J Cell Biol 28:21–31, 1966.

Hicks RM, Newman J. Scanning electron microscopy of urinary sediment. *In* Koss LG, Coleman DV (eds). Advances in Clinical Cytology, vol 2. New York, Masson Publishing, 1984, pp 135–161.

Hicks RM, Wakefield JSJ, Chowaniec J. Evaluation of a new model to detect bladder carcinogens or co-carcinogens: Results obtained with saccharin, cyclamate and cyclophosphamide. Chem Biol Interact 11:225–233, 1975.

Highman W, Wilson E. Urine cytology in patients with calculi. J Clin Pathol 35:350–356, 1982.

Hogan TF, Borden EC, McBain JA, et al. Human polyomavirus infection with JC and BK virus in renal transplant patients. Ann Intern Med 82:373–378, 1985.

Houff SA, Major EO, Katz DA, et al. Involvement of JC virus-infected mononuclear cells from the bone marrow and spleen in the pathogenesis of progressive multifocal leukoencephalopathy. N Engl J Med 318:301–305, 1988.

Houston W, Koss LG, Melamed MR, with technical assistance of M. Montague. Bladder cancer and schistosomiasis. A preliminary cytologic study. Trans Roy Soc Trop Med Hyg 60:89–91, 1966.

Hu P, Deng F-M, Liang F-X, et al. Ablation of uroplakin III gene results in small urothelial plaques, urothelial leakage, and vesicoureteral reflux. J Cell Biol 151:961–971, 2000.

Hunner GL. A rare type of bladder ulcer in women: Report of cases. Boston Med Surg 172:660–664, 1915.

Ito N, Hirose M, Shirai T, et al. Lesions of the urinary bladder epithelium in 125 autopsy cases. Acta Pathol Jpn 31:545–557, 1981.

Itoh S, Irie K, Nakamura Y, et al. Cytologic and genetic study of polyomavirus-infected or polyomavirus-activated cells in human urine. Arch Pathol Lab Med 122:333–337, 1998.

Jacob J, Ludgate CM, Forde J, Tulloch WS. Recent observations on the ultrastructure of human urothelium. 1. Normal bladder of elderly subjects. Cell Tissue Res 543:543–560, 1978.

Jayalakshmamma B, Pinkel D. Urinary-bladder toxicity following pelvic irradiation and simultaneous cyclophosphamide therapy. Cancer 38:701–707, 1976.

Johnston WW, Bossen EH, Amatulli J, Rowlands DT. Exfoliative cytopathologic studies in organ transplantation. II. Factors in the diagnosis of cytomegalic inclusion disease in urine of renal allograft recipients. Acta Cytol 13: 605–610, 1969.

Johnson WW, Meadows DC. Urinary bladder fibrosis and telangiectasia associated with long term cyclophosphamide therapy. N Engl J Med 284:290–294, 1971.

Kahan AV, Coleman DV, Koss LG. Activation of human polyomavirus infection—detection by cytologic technics. Am J Clin Pathol 74:326–332, 1980.

Kapila K, Verma K. Cytologic detection of tuberculosis of the urinary bladder. Acta Cytol 28:90–91, 1984.

Kauffman HM, Clark RF, Magee JH, et al. Lymphocytes in urine as an aid in the early detection of renal homograft rejection. Surg Gynecol Obstet 119: 25–36, 1964.

Kawamure J, Sakurai M, Tsukamoto K, Tochigi H. Leiomyosarcoma of the bladder eighteen years after cyclophosphamide therapy for retinoblastoma. Urol Int 51:49–53, 1993.

Kaye WA, Adri MNS, Soeldner JS, et al. Acquired effect in interleukin-2 production in patients with type I diabetes mellitus. N Engl J Med 315:920–924, 1986.

Kerr DE, Liang F, Bondioli KR, et al. The bladder as a bioreactor: Urothelium production and secretion of growth hormone into urine. Nature Biotech 16:75–79, 1998.

Khalil M, Shin HJC, Tan A, et al. Macrophagelike vacuolated renal tubular cells in the urine of a male with osmotic nephrosis associated with intravenous immunoglobulin therapy. A case report. Acta Cytol 44:86–90, 2000.

Kittredge WE, Brannan W. Cystitis glandularis. J Urol 81:419–440, 1959.

Kobayashi TK, Sugimoto T, Nishida K, Sawaragi I. Intracytoplasmic inclusions in urinary sediment cells from a patient with mucocutaneous lymph node syndrome (Kawasaki Disease). A case report. Acta Cytol 28:687–690, 1984.

Koss LG. Diagnostic Cytology of the Urinary Tract with Histopathologic and Clinical Correlations. Philadelphia: Lippincott-Raven, 1995.

Koss LG. From koilocytosis to molecular biology: The impact of cytology on concepts of early human cancer. Mod Pathol 2:526–535, 1989.

Koss LG. BK viruria and hemorrhagic cystitis (letter). N Engl J Med 316: 108–109, 1987.

Koss LG. Tumors of the Urinary Bladder. Atlas of Tumor Pathology, and series, Fascicle 11. Armed Forces Institute of Pathology 1975 (Supplement), 1985.

Koss LG. Urinary tract cytology. In Connolly JC (ed). Carcinoma of the Bladder. New York, Raven Press, 1981, pp 159–163.

Koss LG. Formal discussion of "clinical observations on 69 cases of in situ carcinoma of the urinary bladder." Cancer Res 37:2799, 1977.

Koss LG. Some ultrastructural aspects of experimental and human carcinoma of the bladder. Cancer Res 37:2824–2835, 1977.

Koss LG. The asymmetric unit membrane of the epithelium of the urinary bladder of the rat. An electron microscopic study of a mechanism of epithelium maturation and function. Lab Invest 21:154–168, 1969.

Koss LG. A light and electron microscopic study of the effects of a single dose of cyclophosphamide on various organs in the rat. I. The urinary bladder. Lab Invest 16:44–65, 1967.

Koss LG, Bartels PH, Sychra JJ, Wied GL. Computer analysis of atypical urothelial cells. II. Classification by unsupervised learning algorithms. Acta Cytol 21:261–265, 1977.

Koss LG, Melamed MR, Mayer K. The effect of busulfan on human epithelia. Am J Clin Pathol 44:385–397, 1965.

Koss LG, Sherman AB. Image analysis of cells in the sediment of voided urine. In Greenberg SD (ed). Computer Assisted Image Analysis Cytology. Basel, Karger, 1984, pp 148–162.

Koss LG, Sherman AB, Eppich E. Image analysis and DNA content of urothelial cells infected with human polyomavirus. Anal Quant Cytol 6:89–94, 1984.

Landing BH, Nakai H. Histochemical properties of renal lead-inclusions and demonstration in urinary sediment. Am J Clin Pathol 31:499–503, 1959.

Lang DJ, Kummer JF, Hartley DP. Cytomegalovirus in semen: persistence and demonstration in extracellular fluids. N Engl J Med 291:121–123, 1974.

Lawrence HJ, Simone J, Aur RJA. Cyclophosphamide-induced hemorrhagic cystitis in children with leukemia. Cancer 36:1572–1576, 1975.

Leroy X, Copin M-C, Graziana JP, et al. Inflammatory pseudotumor of the renal pelvis. A report of 2 cases with clinicopathologic and immunohistochemical study. Arch Pathol Lab Med 124:1209–1212, 2000.

Lewin KJ, Harell GS, Lee AS, Crowley LG. Malacoplakia. An electron-microscopic study: Demonstration of bacilliform organisms in malacoplakic macrophages. Gastroenterology 66:28–45, 1974.

Li SM, Zhang Z-T, Chan S, et al. Detection of circulating uroplakin-positive cells in patients with transitional cell carcinoma of the bladder. J Urol 162: 931–935, 1999.

Liang F, Kachar B, Ding M, et al. Urothelial hinge as a highly specialized membrane: Detergent-insolubility, urohingin association, and in vitro formation. Different 65:59–69, 1999.

Limas C, Lange P. T-antigen in normal and neoplastic urothelium. Cancer 58: 1236–124, 1986.

Loveless KJ. The effects of radiation upon the cytology of benign and malignant bladder epithelia. Acta Cytol 17: 355–360, 1973.

Luthra UK, Dey P, George J, et al. (Letter to the Editor) Comparison of ThinPrep

and conventional preparations: Urine cytology evaluation. Diagn Cytopathol 21:364–366, 1999.

Madersbacher H, Bartsch G. Eosinophile der Harnblase. Urol Int 27:149–159, 1972.

Martin BF. Cell replacement and differentiation in transitional epithelium; a histological and autoradiographic study of the guinea-pig bladder and ureter. J Anat 112:433–455, 1972.

Masin F, Masin M. Sudanophilia in exfoliated urothelial cells. Acta Cytol 20: 573–576, 1976.

Masukawa T, Garancis JC, Rytel MW, Mattingly RF. Herpes genitalis virus isolation from human bladder Acta Cytol 16:416–428, 1972.

McDougal WS, Cramer SF, Miller R. Invasive carcinoma of the renal pelvis following cyclophosphamide therapy for nonmalignant disease. Cancer 48: 691–695, 1981.

Melamed MR. The urinary sediment cytology in a case of malacoplakia. Acta Cytol 6:471–474, 1962.

Melamed MR, Koss LG, Ricci A, Whitmore WF. Cytohistological observations on developing carcinoma of the urinary bladder. Cancer 13:67–74, 1960.

Melamed MR, Wolinska WH. On the significance of intracytoplasmic inclusions in the urinary sediment. Am J Pathol 38:711–718, 1961.

Messing EM, Young TB, Hunt VB, et al. The significance of asymptomatic microhematuria in men 50 or more years old: Findings of a home screening study using urinary dipsticks. J Urol 137:919–922, 1987.

Minassian H, Schinella R, Reilly JC. Polyomavirus in the urine: Follow-up study. Diagn Cytopathol 10:209–211, 1994.

Mohammad KS, Bdesha AS, Snell ME, et al. Phase contrast microscopic examination of urinary erythrocytes to localize source of bleeding: An overlooked technique? J Clin Path 46:642–645, 1993.

Mohr DN, Offord KP, Owen RA, Melton ILJ. Asymptomatic microhematuria and urologic disease. JAMA 256:224–229, 1986.

Morse HD. The etiology and pathology of pyelitis cystica, ureteritis cystica, and cystitis cystica. Am J Pathol 4:33–50, 1928.

Mukunyadzi P, Johnson M, Wyble JG, Scott M. Diagnosis of histoplasmosis in urine cytology: Reactive urothelial changes, a diagnostic pitfall. Case report and literature review of urinary tract infections. Diagn Cytopathol 26: 243–246, 2002.

Murphy WM. Herpesvirus in bladder cancer. Acta Cytol 20:207–210, 1976.

Myerson D, Hackman RC, Nelson JA, et al. Widespread presence of histologically occult cytomegalovirus. Hum Pathol 15:430–439, 1984.

Naib ZM. Exfoliative cytology of renal pelvic lesions. Cancer 14:1085–1087, 1961.

Naib ZM. Exfoliative Cytology, 2nd ed. Boston: Little Brown, 1976; 3rd ed, 1985.

Nasuti JF, Fleisher SR, Gupta PK. Significance of tissue fragments in voided urine specimens. Acta Cytol 45:147–152, 2001.

Nebuloni M, Tosoni A, Boldorini R, et al. BK virus renal infection in a patient with the acquired immunodeficiency syndrome. Arch Pathol Lab Med 123: 807–811, 1999.

Newman J, Hicks RM. Surface ultrastructure of the epithelia lining the normal human lower urinary tract. Br J Exp Pathol 62:232–251, 1981.

Nguyen G-K. Urine cytology in renal glomerular disease and value of G1 cells in the diagnosis of glomerular bleeding. Diagn Cytopathol 29:67–73, 2003.

Nickeleit V, Klimkait T, Binet IF, et al. Testing for polyomavirus type BK DNA in plasma to identify renal-allograft recipients with viral nephropathy. N Engl J Med 342:1309–1315, 2000.

Niewiadomski S, Florentine BD, Cobb CJ. Cytologic identification of trichomonas vaginalis in urine from a male with long-standing sterile pyuria (letter). Acta Cytol 42:1060–1061, 1998.

Nolan ICR, Anger MS, Kelleher SP. Eosinophiluria—a new method of detection and definition of the clinical spectrum. N Engl J Med 315:1516–1519, 1986.

Norkin LC. Papovaviral persistent infections. Microbiol Rev 46:384–425, 1982.

Nowels K, Kent E, Rinsho K, Oyasu R. Prostate specific antigen and acid phosphatase-reactive cells in cytisis cystica and glandularis. Arch Pathol Lab Med 112:734–737, 1988.

O'Connor VJ, Greenhill JP. Endometriosis of the bladder and ureter. Surg Gynecol Obstet 80:113–119, 1945.

O'Flynn JD, Mullaney J. Leukoplakia of the bladder. Br J Urol 39:461–471, 1967.

O'Morchoe PJ, Riad W, Cowles LT, et al. Urinary cytological changes after radiotherapy of renal transplants. Acta Cytol 20:132–136, 1976.

Oravisto KJ. Epidemiology of interstitial cystitis. Ann Chir Gynaecol Fenn 64: 75–77, 1975.

O'Reilly RJ, Lee FK, Grossbard E, et al. Papovavirus excretion following marrow transplantation: Incidence and association with hepatic dysfunction. Transplant Proc 13:262–266, 1981.

Padgett BL, Walker DL. New human papillomaviruses. Prog Med Virol 21: 1–135, 1976.

Padgett BL, Walker DL, Zu Rhein GM, et al. Cultivation of papova-like virus from human brain with progressive multifocal encephalopathy. Lancet 1: 1257–1260, 1971.

Palubinskas AJ. Eosinophilic cystitis: case report of eosinophilic infiltration of the urinary bladder. Radiology 75:589–591, 1960.

Pedersen-Bjergaard J, Ersboli J, Hansen VL, et al. Carcinoma of the urinary bladder after treatment with cyclophosphamide for non-Hodgkin's lymphoma. N Engl J Med 318:1028–1032, 1988.

Petrogiannis-Haliotis T, Sakoulas G, Kirby J, et al. BK-related polyomavirus vasculopathy in a renal-transplant recipient. N Engl J Med 345:1250–1255, 2001.

Petry G, Amon H. The functional structure of the epithelium of the urinary bladder and its significance in urological cytodiagnosis. Klin Wochenschr 44:1371–1379, 1966.

Piscioli F, Pusiol T, Polla E, et al. Urinary cytology of tuberculosis of the bladder. Acta Cytol 29:125–131, 1985.

Pollock C, Pei-Ling L, Györy AZ, et al. Dysmorphism of urinary red blood cells—value in diagnosis. Kidney Int 36:1045–1049, 1989.

Prescott LF. Effects of acetylsalicylic acid, phenacetin, paracetamol, and caffeine on renal tubular epithelium. Lancet 1:91–96, 1965.

Prescott LF, Brodie DE. A simple differential stain for urinary sediment. Lancet 2:940, 1964.

Pund ER, Yount HA, Blumberg JM. Variations in morphology of urinary bladder epithelium. Special reference to cystitis glandularis and carcinomas. J Urol 68:242–251, 1952.

Rasmussen K, Petersen BL, Jacobo E, et al. Cytologic effects of thiotepa and Adriamycin on normal canine urothelium. Acta Cytol 24:237–243, 1980.

Rathert P, Roth SE. Urinzytologie. Praxis und Atlas, 2nd ed. Berlin, Springer-Verlag, 1991.

Reeves DS, Thomas AL, Wise R, et al. Lack of homogeneity of bladder urine. Lancet 1:1258–1259, 1974.

Rosen SH, Harmon W, Krensky AM, et al. Tubulointerstitial nephritis associated with polyomavirus (BK type) infection. N Engl J Med 308:1192–1196, 1983.

Ross AGP, Bartley PB, Sleigh AC, et al. Schistosomiasis. N Engl J Med 346: 1212–1220, 2002.

Rouse BA, Donaldson LD, Goellner JR. Intranuclear inclusions in urinary cytology. Acta Cytol 30:105–109, 1986.

Rowland RG, Eble JN. Bladder leiomyosarcoma and pelvic fibroblastic tumor following cyclophosphamide therapy. J Urol 130:344–346, 1983.

Rowland RG, Mitchell ME, Bihrle R, et al. Indiana continent urinary reservoir. J Urol 137:1136–1139, 1987.

Sant GR. Interstitial cystitis. Curr Opin Obstet Gynecol 9:332–336, 1997.

Schaeffer AJ. Interstitial cystitis. N Engl J Med 339:1253, 1998.

Schiff HI, Finkel M, Schapira HE. Transitional cell carcinoma of the ureter associated with cyclophosphamide therapy for benign disease: a case report. J Urol 128:1023–1024, 1982.

Schmid GH, Hornstein OP, Munstermann M, Potyka J. Periodical epithelial exfoliation of the urinary ducts in the male. Acta Cytol 16:352–362, 1972.

Schneider V, Smith MJV, Frable WJ. Urinary cytology in endometriosis of the bladder. Acta Cytol 24:30–33, 1980.

Schumann GB, Berring S, Hill RB. Use of the cytocentrifuge for the detection of cytomegalovirus inclusions in the urine of renal allograft patients. A case report. Acta Cytol 21:167–172, 1977.

Schumann GB, Burleson RL, Henry JB, Jones DB. Urinary cytodiagnosis of acute renal allograft rejection using the cytocentrifuge. Am J Clin Pathol 67: 134–140, 1977.

Schumann GB, Johnston JL, Weiss MA. Renal epithelial fragments in urine sediment. Acta Cytol 25:147–153, 1981.

Schumann GB, Lerner SI, Weiss MA, et al. Inclusion bearing cells in industrial workers exposed to lead. Am J Clin Pathol 74:192–196, 1980.

Scully RE, Mark EJ, McNeely WF, Ebeling SH. Case Records (#27-1998) of the Massachusetts General Hospital. N Engl J Med 339:616–622, 1998.

Seo IS, Clark SA, McGovern FD, et al. Leiomyosarcoma of the urinary bladder. 13 years after cyclophosphamide therapy for Hodgkin's disease. Cancer 55: 1597–1603, 1985.

Shokri-Tabibzadeh S, Herz F, Koss LG. Fine structure of cultured epithelial cells derived from voided urine of normal adults. Virchows Arch [B] 39: 41–48, 1982.

Siddiqui A, Melamed MR, Abbi R, Ahmed T. Mucinous (colloid) carcinoma of urinary bladder following long-term cyclophosphamide therapy for Waldenström's macroglobulinemia. Am J Surg Pathol 20:500–504, 1996.

Sigal SH, Tomaszewski JE, Brooks JJ, et al. Carcinosarcoma of bladder following long-term cyclophosphamide therapy. Arch Pathol Lab Med 115: 1049–1051, 1991.

Sinclair-Smith C, Kahn LB, Cywes S. Malacoplakia in childhood. Case report with ultrastructural observations and review of the literature. Arch Pathol 99:198–203, 1975.

Slavin RE, Millan JC, Mullins GM. Pathology of high dose intermittent cyclophosphamide therapy. Hum Pathol 6:693–709, 1975.

Smith BH, Dehner LP. Chronic ulcerating interstitial cystitis (Hunner's ulcer). A study of 28 cases. Arch Pathol 93:76–81, 1972.

Smith MG, Vellios F. Inclusion disease or generalized salivary gland virus infection. Arch Pathol 50:862–884, 1950.

Spagnolo DV, Waring PM. Bladder granulomata after bladder surgery. Am J Clin Pathol 86:430–437, 1986.

Spencer ES, Andersen HK. Viral infections in renal allograft recipients treated with long-term immunosuppression. Br Med J 2:829–830, 1979.

Stella F, Battistelli S, Marcheggiani F, et al. Urothelial toxicity following conditioning therapy in bone marrow transplantation and bladder cancer: Morphologic and morphometric comparison by exfoliative urinary cytology. Diagn Cytopathol 8:216–221, 1992.

Stella F, Troccoli R, Stella C, et al. Urinary cytologic abnormalities in bone marrow transplant recipients of cyclosporin. Acta Cytol 31:615–619, 1987.

Sternheimer R. A supravital cytodiagnostic stain for urinary sediments. JAMA 231:826–832, 1975.

Stilmant MM, Freelund MC, Schmitt GW. Cytologic evaluation of urine after kidney transplantation. Acta Cytol 31:625–630, 1987.

Streitz JM. Squamous epithelium in the female trigone. J Urol 90:62–66, 1963.

Suhrland MJ, Koslow M, Perchick A, et al. Cytologic findings in progressive multifocal leukoencephalopathy. Report of two cases. Acta Cytol 31: 505–511, 1987.

Sun T-T, Liang F-X, Wu X-R. Uroplakins as markers of urothelial differentiation. Adv Bladder Res 1:7–18, 1999.

Taft PD, Flax MH. Urinary cytology in renal transplantation; association of renal tubular cells and graft rejection. Transplantation 4:194–204, 1966.

Thrasher JB, Miller GJ, Wettlaufer JN. Bladder leiomyosarcoma following cyclophosphamide therapy for lupus nephritis. J Urol 143:119–121, 1990.

Travis LB, Curtis RE, Boice JD Jr, Fraumeni JF Jr. Bladder cancer after chemotherapy for non-Hodgkin's lymphoma. N Engl J Med 321:544–545, 1989.

Tyler DE. Stratified squamous epithelium in the vesical trigone and urethra: Findings correlated with the menstrual cycle and age. Am J Anat 111: 319–325, 1962.

Utz DC, Zinke H. The masquerade of bladder cancer in situ as interstitial cystitis. Trans Am Assoc Genitourin Surg 75:64–65, 1973.

Valente PT, Atkinson BF, Guerry D. Melanuria. Acta Cytol 29:1026–1028, 1985.

Van der Snoek BF, Hoitsma AJ, Van Weel C, Koene RA. Dysmorphic erythrocytes in urinary sediment in differentiating urological from nephrological causes of hematuria (in Dutch). Nederlands Tijdschrift voor Geneeskunde 138:721–726, 1994.

Volmar KE, Chan TY, De Marzo AM, Epstein JI. Florid von Brunn nests mimicking urothelial carcinoma. A morphologic and immunohistochemical comparison to the nested variant of urothelial carcinoma. Am J Surg Pathol 27: 1243–1252, 2003.

Wall RL, Clausen KP. Carcinoma of the urinary bladder in patients receiving cyclophosphamide. N Engl J Med,293:271–273, 1975.

Walz T, Häner M, Wu X-R, et al. Towards the molecular architecture of the asymmetric unit membrane of the mammalian urinary bladder epithelium: A closed "twisted ribbon" structure. J Mol Biol 248:887–900, 1995.

Watari Y, Satoh H, Matubara M, et al. Comparison of urine cytology between the ileal conduit and Indiana pouch. Acta Cytol 44:748–751, 2000.

Webber CA, Eveland LK. Cytologic detection of Wuchereria bancrofti microfilariae in urine collected during a routine work-up for hematuria. Acta Cytol 26:837–840, 1982.

Wenzel JE, Greene LF, Harris LE. Eosinophilic cystitis. J Pediatr 64:746–749, 1964.

Widran J, Sanchez R, Gruhn J. Squamous metaplasia of the bladder: A study of 450 patients. J Urol 112:479–482, 1974.

Wiener DP, Koss LG, Sablay B, Freed SZ. The prevalence and significance of Brunn's nests, cystitis cystica and squamous metaplasia in normal bladders. J Urol 122:317–321, 1979.

Winkelman M, Burrig KF, Koldovsky U, et al. Cyclosporin A altered renal tubular cells in urinary cytology. Lancet 2:667, 1985.

Wojcik EM, Brownlee RJ, Bassler TJ, Miller MC. Superficial urothelial cells (umbrella cells)—a potential cause of abnormal DNA ploidy results in urine specimens. Acta Cytol (In print), 2000.

Worth PHL. Cyclophosphamide and the bladder. Br Med J 3:182, 1971.

Wright RG, Halford JA. Evaluation of thin-layer methods in urine cytology. CytoPathol 12:306–313, 2001.

Wu X-R, Lin J-H, Walz T, et al. Mammalian uroplakins, a group of highly conserved urothelial differentiation-related integral membrane proteins. J Biol Chem 269:13716–13724, 1994.

Wu XR, Manabe M, Yu J, Sun TT. Large scale purification and immunolocalization of bovine uroplakins I, II, and III. Molecular markers of urothelial differentiation. J Biol Chem 265:19170–19179, 1990.

Wu X-R, Sun T-T, Medina JJ. In vitro binding of type 1-fimbriated Escherichia coli to uroplakins Ia and Ib: Relation to urinary tract infections. Proc Natl Acad Sci USA 93:9630–9635, 1996.

Wynder EL, Onderdonk J, Mantel N. An epidemiological investigation of cancer of the bladder. Cancer 16:1388–1407, 1963.

Yu J, Manabe M, Wu XR, et al. Uroplakin I. A 27-kD protein associated with the asymmetric unit membrane of mammalian urothelium. J Cell Biol 111: 1207–1216, 1990.

Zaman Z, Proesmans W. Dysmorphic erythrocytes and G1 cells as markers of glomerular hematuria. Pediatr Nephrol 14:980–984, 2000.

Tumors of the Urinary Tract in Urine and Brushings*

23

TUMORS OF THE UROTHELIUM (TRANSITIONAL EPITHELIUM) OF THE BLADDER

Epidemiology

In the United States, tumors of the bladder are the **fourth leading type of cancer in men** but are less common in women (Messing and Catalona, 1998). During the second half of the 20th century, a statistically significant increase in the rate of urothelial tumors, mainly tumors of the urinary bladder, has been observed in most industrialized countries

---

* Aspiration biopsy (FNA) of the prostate is discussed in Chapter 33 and of the kidney in Chapter 40.

(Cole et al, 1971, 1972; Wynder et al, 1977; Silverman et al, 1992). For the year 2001, the American Cancer Society projected more than 54,000 new cases and 12,400 deaths from tumors of the bladder (Greenlee et al, 2001).

The impact of **environmental factors** on the genesis of tumors of the bladder has been known since the publications by the German surgeon Rehn (1895 and 1896), who observed that workers in factories producing **aniline dyes** were at a high risk for this disease. It was subsequently shown that the carcinogenic compounds to which these workers were exposed were **aromatic amines,** such as 2-naphthylamine, para-aminodiphenyl (xenylamine), and 4-4'-diaminobiphenyl (benzidine) (Bonser et al, 1952; Boyland et al, 1954). Another compound known as MBOCA [4,4' methylenobis (2-chloroaniline)], an analogue of benzidine, has been shown to induce low-grade papillary tumors in the bladder (Ward et al, 1988). The drug **chlornaphazine,** related to the aromatic compounds, was shown to be carcinogenic for the bladder (Videbaek, 1964; Laursen, 1970). The effects of the alkylating agent **cyclophosphamide** as a carcinogen in the lower urinary tract were extensively discussed in Chapter 22. Women working in factories producing **phenacetin,** a common analgesic, and heavy users of the drug are also at increased risk for urothelial tumors that may involve the bladder but also the ureters and the renal pelves (Johansson et al, 1974; Mihatsch, 1979; Lomax-Smith, 1980; Piper et al, 1985). There also is evidence that workers in **rubber and cable, leather, and shoe repair industries** are at a high risk for bladder cancer, although the specific carcinogenic substances have not been clearly identified. Nortier et al (2000) reported that the use of a **Chinese herb (*aristolochia fangchi*)** may also be a risk for bladder tumors. Along similar lines, bladder tumors in cattle have been linked with consumption of another plant, bracken fern (***pteris aquilina***) (Pamukcu et al, 1964; Hirono et al, 1972). Experimental data suggested that bladder tumors in cattle fed bracken fern may also be associated with **bovine papillomavirus type 2** (Campo et al, 1992). A high level of **inorganic arsenic** in drinking water is another cause of bladder cancer (Cohen et al, 2000; Steinmaus, et al, 2000). Bladder cancer is by far the most common tumor in the population at risk, although organs such as the lungs may also be affected. Bladder tumors observed in Taiwan in areas of high arsenic concentration, are commonly associated with arteriosclerotic changes in lower extremities known as the "black foot" disease (Chiang et al, 1993; Chiou et al, 1995, 2001). The association has also been observed in Chile (Smith et al, 1998) and Argentina (Hopenhayn et al, 1996). The mechanisms of arsenic carcinogenicity are unknown (Simeonova and Luster, 2000).

Besides the environmental factors, there are other risk factors for tumors of the bladder. For example, **paraplegic and quadriplegic patients** are at risk, presumably because of inadequate voiding, and therefore exposure of the bladder to small doses of unknown carcinogenic agents contained in the urine (Kaufman et al, 1977; Bejany et al, 1987; Bickel et al, 1991). **Similar mechanisms may be responsible for bladder tumors in** otherwise normal men with **low intake of fluids** (Michaud et al, 1999) and enlargement of the prostate.

Work from this laboratory has shown that **prostatic enlargement, whether caused by hyperplasia or carcinoma, is another risk factor for cancer of the bladder.** Between January 1974 and August 1977, we observed 19 patients, seen primarily because of prostatic enlargement, whose urinary sediment disclosed an **occult urothelial carcinoma,** subsequently confirmed by biopsies of bladder. Further review of the files at Montefiore Medical Center, compiled by Dr. Allayne Kahan, disclosed 13 patients with coexisting carcinomas of the prostate and of the bladder and an additional 28 patients with benign prostatic hypertrophy and bladder cancer (unpublished data). Barlebo and Sørensen (1972) observed 2 patients with carcinoma in situ of the bladder, initially seen because of prostatic hypertrophy. A further association of bladder cancer with prostatic disease was reported by Mahadevia et al (1986), also from this laboratory. Mapping of 20 cystoprostatectomy specimens removed because of invasive high-grade bladder cancers or carcinoma in situ, or both, disclosed that occult carcinoma of the prostate was present in 14 of the 20 patients, **but only one of these lesions was suspected before cystectomy. These observations strongly suggest that in all patients with prostatic enlargement, whether benign or malignant, bladder cancer should be ruled out.** In fact, Nickel et al (2002) reported that three urothelial carcinomas in situ were observed among 150 patients with chronic prostatitis evaluated by urine cytology. Conversely, male patients with known tumors of the bladder should be investigated for coexisting prostatitic carcinoma. The urologists are generally unaware of this association.

Tumors of the bladder are observed with high frequency in some geographic areas. In the United States, these tumors are often observed in the state of New Jersey and in New Orleans, presumably because of a high level of exposure to **industrial waste.** In Egypt and many other African countries, an infection with the parasite ***Schistosoma haematobium (Bilharzia)*** is an important cause of bladder cancer, as discussed in Chapter 22 and in this chapter. Still, many patients with bladder tumors have no known risk factors. It is speculated that industrial pollution, cigarette smoking, or a combination of these and other yet unknown factors contribute to cancers of the lower urinary tract.

Terminology

The **unique features of the epithelium lining the lower urinary tract** were discussed at length in Chapter 22 and need not be repeated here. Many of these features, such as the **presence of the asymmetric unit membrane and umbrella cells,** are observed in tumors derived from this epithelium. Further, the presence of **uroplakins, proteins uniquely characterizing this epithelium** (summaries in Wu et al, 1994 and Sun et al, 1999), have been shown to be an important diagnostic and experimental tool, as discussed elsewhere in this chapter. For all these reasons, the term **urothelial tumors or carcinomas has been used in the previous additions of this book and in other writing, replacing the old term transitional cell tumors or**

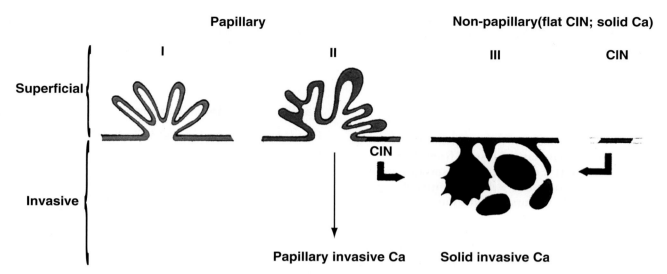

Figure 23-1   Schematic representation of two families of bladder tumors and the sequence of events in the development of tumors of the bladder. The drawing assumes that carcinoma in situ and related lesions are the cardinal step in the development of invasive cancer. (Diagram by Dr. Bogdan Czerniak.)

carcinomas (Koss, 1974, 1985, 1995). The term **urothelial tumors** has now been accepted by consensus of urologic pathologists (Epstein et al, 1998).

Classification and Natural History

The accomplishments and limitations of cytology in the diagnosis and follow-up of tumors of the bladder can only be understood against a background of histologic and clinical observations. It is of interest that cytologic observations on urinary sediment played a key role in establishing the current concepts of classification and natural history of these neoplasms (summary in Koss, 1995).

Two Pathways of Bladder Tumors

For many years, most urothelial tumors of the bladder, the ureter, and the renal pelves were thought to be malignant and were classified as "carcinomas," regardless of their morphology. Within the last half a century, evidence has been provided that there are significant differences in the behavior and prognosis among these tumors based on **their morphology and clinical presentation** (Fig. 23-1 and Table 23-1).

TABLE 23-1

CHARACTERISTICS OF TWO GROUPS OF UROTHELIAL TUMORS

Feature	Low-Grade Papillary Tumors	High-Grade Papillary Tumors and Invasive Carcinomas
Epithelial abnormality of origin	Hyperplasia	Flat carcinoma in situ and related abnormalities: atypical hyperplasia (or dysplasia)
Invasive potential	Low	High
Recognition in urine cytology	Poor	Good to outstanding, depending on grade and DNA ploidy
DNA ploidy pattern	Predominantly diploid	Predominantly aneuploid
Density of nuclear pores	Normal	Increased
Expression of Ca antigen (epitectin)	As in normal urothelium	Increased
Blood group isoantigen expression	Usually present	Usually absent
Mutation of p53 gene	Usually absent	Usually present

The urothelial tumors of the bladder may be classified into **two fundamental, although to some extent overlapping, groups with different patterns of behavior, different prognoses** and **different cytologic presentation.** These are:

- Papillary tumors
- Nonpapillary tumors

The papillary tumors of the urothelium have for the most part, a different natural history from the nonpapillary, flat tumors. It is of particular importance to recognize that many common, well-differentiated papillary tumors (low-grade tumors) should not be classified as "carcinomas" because they do not, or very rarely, progress to invasive cancer. On the other hand, **nonpapillary or flat urothelial lesions (carcinoma in situ and related abnormalities) are the principal precursor lesions of invasive urothelial cancer.** It is only recently that the community of urologic pathologists incorporated some of these concepts into the classification of tumors of the urothelium (Epstein et al, 1998), even though they have been advocated for many years in previous editions of this book and other writings (Koss, 1975, 1985, 1995).

Although this simple classification of urothelial tumors is based primarily on their morphologic characteristics, it is also supported by differences in **biologic and behavioral features** that will be briefly mentioned here and are discussed in detail below.

There are significant **differences in DNA content** among the different categories of urothelial tumors with **all, or nearly all, low-grade papillary tumors having a DNA content in the normal range (diploid) and all, or nearly all, high-grade lesions, whether papillary or nonpapillary, having an abnormal DNA content (aneuploid).** Several studies support further the concept of two pathways of bladder tumors. Thus, a study of the **density distribution of nuclear pores** (see Fig. 2-22 for description) was shown to correlate with DNA ploidy. The number and density of nuclear pores was significantly higher in aneuploid than in diploid tumors (Czerniak et al, 1984). The **expression of a monoclonal antibody Ca1 (epitectine),** a presumed marker of surfaces of cancer cells (Ashall et al, 1982), was also shown to be higher in all but one of 12 aneuploid tumors when compared with diploid tumors and normal urothelium (Czerniak and Koss, 1985). Molecular biology of these tumors is discussed further on in this chapter.

Very strong support for the concept of two pathways of bladder tumors has been recently offered based on experimental evidence in transgenic mice. Uroplakin II gene promoter was used to introduce two different oncogenes into the ova. **The mice bearing the Ha-ras oncogene developed superficial, noninvasive papillary tumors,** whereas mice bearing the **T antigen of the SV40 virus developed flat carcinomas in situ and invasive bladder cancers** (Zhang et al, 1999, 2001). Recent molecular studies of fibroblast growth factor receptors (FGRFR3), expressed in low-grade tumors, and p53 overexpression in high-grade tumors, also confirmed the concept of two pathways of bladder carcinogenesis (van Rhijn et al, 2004). It must be noted that in several recent studies, **genetic abnormalities were observed in morphologically normal urothelium adjacent to tumors** (Czerniak et al, 1995, 1999, 2000; Cianciulli et al, 2003).

Papillary Urothelial Tumors

Fundamental Structure and Clinical Presentation

Papillary urothelial tumors are **by far, the most common form of urothelial tumors** seen in the practice of urology. They occur in all age groups, even in children and adolescents, although they are more common in older patients. When first observed, they may be **single or multiple.** The **fundamental structure** of all papillary tumors is the same. The tumors form a **fern-like, cauliflower, or sea anemone–like protrusion** into the lumen of the organ, be it urinary bladder, renal pelvis, or the ureter. The papillary tumors may have a narrow base and a **single stalk** or may be **sessile, that is, having a broader base** with **multiple, branching stalks. Each stalk** is composed of a **central core of connective tissue and vessels, supporting epithelial folds of varying degrees of thickness and cytologic abnormality** (Fig. 23-2A,B). The make-up of the epithelium is used to classify these tumors further (see below).

It has been proposed, based on molecular analysis (Sidransky et al, 1991; Steiner et al, 1997) and comparative genomic hybridization (Simon et al, 2001), that multifocal papillary tumors of the bladder are of **monoclonal origin, that is, the result of proliferation of a single cell.** This theory assumes that multiple or recurrent tumors are the result of **intraepithelial migration of cells of the same clone.** In spite of molecular evidence, this **theory cannot be sustained.** There is no evidence whatever that urothelial cells, bound to each other by desmosomes, would undertake a perilous journey across long distances to settle in a different portion of the bladder epithelium and produce another papillary tumor. It is more likely that identical molecular abnormalities may affect cells in various segments of the bladder at different times as a result of a **"field change"** induced by carcinogens. For further discussion of molecular biology of urothelial tumors, see below.

Symptoms

The thin and delicate branches of the papillary tumor break easily, leading to the principal symptom of papillary tumors, **hematuria.** The bleeding is often intermittent, with episodes of hematuria occurring sporadically at the time of voiding. Hematuria may be significant, resulting in grossly bloody urine, or it may be relatively minor, resulting in microhematuria (for discussion of the significance of microhematuria, see Chap. 22). Hematuria may be associated with other symptoms such as dysuria and frequency of urination.

Precursor Lesions: Urothelial Hyperplasia

Papillary tumors are derived from **thickened urothelium, composed of more than the normal seven layers of cells**

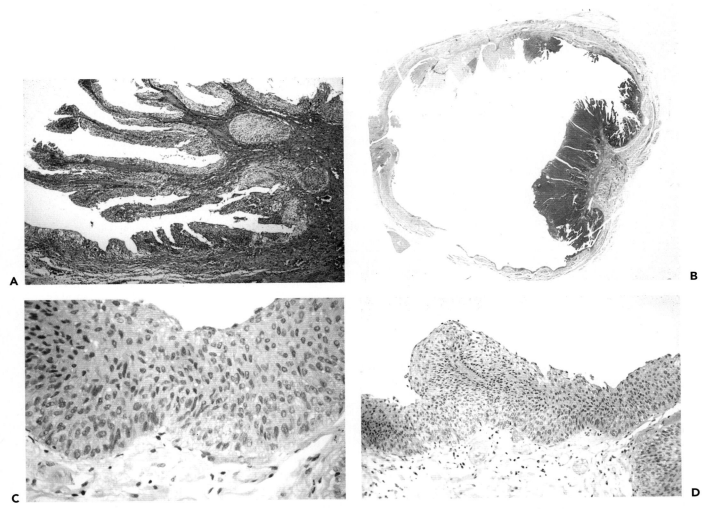

Figure 23-2   Papillary tumors of bladder. *A.* A typical papillary tumor with thin branches carrying capillary vessels. *B.* Sessile papillary tumor in whole bladder mount. *C.* Hyperplasia of urothelium. Note the increased number of epithelial layers and absence of nuclear abnormalities. *D.* Incipient papillary tumor. The presence of a capillary vessel within the hyperplastic epithelium is the cardinal event. (*B:* Case courtesy of Dr. Rolf Schade, Birmingham, UK.)

without nuclear abnormalities, a condition known as hyperplasia. The thickness of the urothelium may be quite **variable, ranging from a slight increase to 20 layers of cells or more.** The hyperplastic epithelium is well differentiated and its surface is usually formed by umbrella cells (Fig. 23-2C). **There are two morphologically identical types of hyperplasia:**

- Reactive hyperplasia
- Neoplastic hyperplasia

Reactive hyperplasia may occur in **inflammatory or reactive processes** or as a consequence of an **underlying space-occupying lesion.** Neoplastic hyperplasia may be the **source of well-differentiated, low-grade papillary tumors** and was shown in experimental systems by Koss and Lavin (1971), Koss (1977) and more recently in transgenic mice by Zhang et al (2001). **Because the two types of hyperplasia cannot be distinguished from each other morphologically,** the diagnosis depends on the environment in which

this change occurs. **Neoplastic hyperplasia** often contains **branches of submucosal vessels** that provide the blood supply and stalk of the growing tumor (Fig. 23-2D). This **interplay between mucosal thickening and vascular proliferation is an essential sequence of events in papillary tumors.** There are no molecular-biologic data explaining this phenomenon, but it may be speculated that a **combination of angiogenesis and a defect in the epithelial adhesion molecules must combine to form these tumors.** Taylor et al (1996) also considered urothelial hyperplasia as a precursor lesion of papillary tumors. **Urothelial hyperplasia cannot be identified cytologically.**

Histologic Grading of Papillary Tumors

In 1922, Broders, of the Mayo Clinic, observed that the behavior of papillary tumors of the bladder depended significantly on the **morphologic make-up of their epithelium and introduced the concept of tumor grading.** The current prevailing system of histologic grading is summarized

CLASSIFICATION AND GRADING OF PAPILLARY TUMORS OF THE BLADDER*

	Number of Epithelial Cell Layers	Superficial Cells	Nuclear Enlargement	Abnormalities Hyperchromasia
Papilloma	No more than 7	Present, albeit small	Not significant	Absent
Papillary tumors grade I (papillary neoplasm of low malignant potential)	More than 7	Usually present, albeit small	Slight to moderate	Slight in occasional cell
Papillary carcinoma grade II (papillary carcinoma, low grade)	More than 7, usually marked increase	Variable	Moderate to marked	Slight to moderate in 25–50% of cells
Papillary carcinoma grade III	More than 7, often marked increase	Usually absent	Marked; extreme variability of sizes	Marked in 50% or more of cells

* Note: In practice, it may prove difficult to fit any given case into this classification. Intermediate classifications such as I-II or II-III have been used. For all intents and purposes, a separation of tumors grade III from tumors grade IV is not warranted biologically and both groups can be considered as one.
Modified from Koss LG. Tumors of the Urinary Bladder. Atlas of Tumor Pathology, 2nd series, Fascicle 11. Washington, D.C., Armed Forces Institute of Pathology, 1975, WHO recommended terminology (1998).

in Table 23-2 (Koss, 1975, 1995, Epstein et al, 1998). **The grading is based on the degree of epithelial abnormality.**

Low-Grade Tumors

Papillomas and low-grade papillary tumors (papillary tumors of low malignant potential or **grade I papillary tumors)** share in common an **orderly epithelium** of variable thickness that shows **either no deviation or only minor deviation from normal urothelium. The size of the cells increases toward the surface, which is usually composed of umbrella cells** (Fig. 23-3A,B). The difference between these two entities are relatively trivial: in **papillomas, the thickness of the epithelium is within the normal seven-layer limit and there are no nuclear abnormalities.** In the **papillary tumors of "low malignant potential," the epithelial lining is somewhat thicker and less orderly, but umbrella cells are usually present on the surface. Although most nuclei are within normal limits, occasional enlarged and hyperchromatic nuclei may be present, particularly in grade I tumors.** Mitoses are infrequent.

Because of rarity of progression to invasive cancer, the term "carcinoma" should not be used in reference to this group of papillary tumors. Pich et al (2001) reported that papillary tumors of low malignant potential have a lower proliferation rate, lower expression of p53, and lower recurrence rate than tumors classified as low-grade papillary carcinomas. These differences are not reflected in the morphology of these tumors.

Papillary tumors may contain mucus-producing goblet cells in their lining. Papillomas of squamoid type may contain squamous "pearls" (see below).

High-Grade Tumors (Grades II and III)

Papillary tumors of higher grades show **significant cytologic abnormalities of the epithelial lining. Many of** these tumors are **broad-based or sessile** and are lined by an **epithelium that is usually composed of an increased number of layers of medium-sized cells that are arranged in a less orderly fashion and show a limited tendency to surface maturation (formation of umbrella cells) than the urothelium of low-grade tumors (Fig. 23-3C). Such tumors always show nuclear abnormalities in the form of hyperchromasia, variability in nuclear sizes, and mitotic activity. These tumors are usually referred to as** *papillary carcinomas,* subdivided into grades II and III.

Papillary carcinomas of high grade (grade III) are characterized by an **epithelium composed of highly abnormal cells of variable sizes with major nuclear abnormalities, readily recognized as cancer cells. Mitoses, often abnormal, are frequently observed** (Fig. 23-3D). In some of these tumors, the make-up of the epithelium may be **identical to flat carcinomas in situ,** described below.

The common **papillary carcinomas grade II** are intermediate between the tumors grade I and tumors grade III. Although **retaining the fundamental structure of the urothelium, they show varying degrees of epithelial maturation and nuclear abnormalities that may be distributed throughout the epithelium or limited to patchy areas.**

In practice, it is not unusual to observe **tumors with a mixture of patterns side by side.** Thus, combined grades of classification may have to be used, such as **grade I-II, II-III, etc.,** often combined with a descriptive comment. The problems of precise grading and, accordingly, behavior and prognosis of papillary tumors, particularly of the intermediate grade II, have led to several methods of objective analysis. There is evidence that the **grade II tumors may be separated into two prognostic groups according to their DNA content,** which may be within **normal or diploid range,** or **abnormal (aneuploid),** a feature that may play a major role in clinical behavior and cytologic recognition of these tumors (see below).

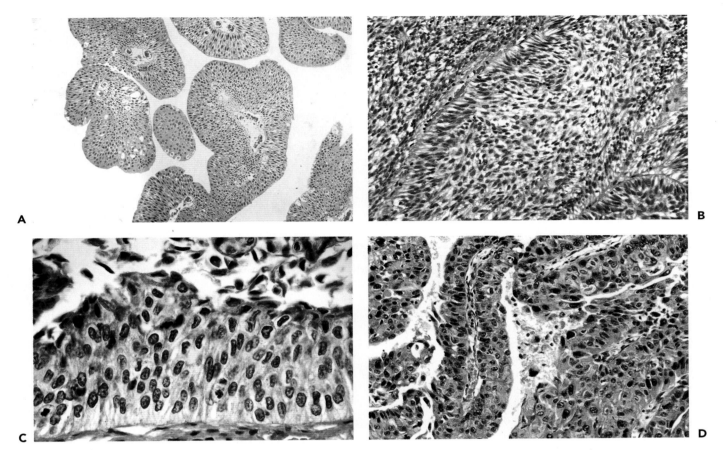

Figure 23-3 **Papillary tumors of bladder, various grades.** *A.* Papilloma, low power view. The somewhat thickened epithelium shows no nuclear abnormalities whatever. *B.* Papillary tumor, grade I (tumor of low malignant potential). The epithelium, although orderly, shows slight nuclear enlargement. *C.* Papillary carcinoma, grade II. The surface epithelium of this tumor shows significant nuclear enlargement, hyperchromasia, and mitotic activity. *D.* Papillary tumor, grade III or IV. The epithelium lining the tumor is composed of cancerous cells.

Papillary Tumors and Pseudoinvasion of Bladder Wall

Many papillary tumors, regardless of grade, may **have roots extending into the lamina propria** of the urothelium in the form of broad-based bands of cells in continuity with surface of urothelium. In my judgment and experience, **this extension should not be considered as evidence of invasion,** so long as there is **no splintering** of the tumor tissue into individual cells (Fig. 23-4).

Behavior Patterns

Papillary tumors when first seen by a urologist are either **single or multiple** and are **usually noninvasive** (i.e., they are confined to the urothelium or, at most, extending to the lamina propria) and therefore can be treated by simple excision. The **term "non-invasive papillary tumor" is much more accurate** than the term **"superficial bladder tumors,"** which has been extensively used and abused in the literature. For further discussion of this issue, see below "tumor staging."

Recurrence or New Tumors

After surgical removal of the primary papillary tumors, new such tumors may be observed in **the same or other areas** of the bladder and much less often, in **the ureters or the renal pelves.** The term, **recurrence,** which is in common use to describe these events, is **inaccurate,** inasmuch as the original tumors, if carefully removed, do not recur. The **new tumors** may be single or multiple and may be identical to the original tumor or show greater degree of epithelial abnormality (see Fig. 23-5). **The probability of "recurrence"** varies with the grade of the tumor: **low-grade tumors, such as papillomas or grade I tumors, are less likely to be followed by new tumors than are tumors of grade II or III.** Recurrent tumors are much more common in older patients than in children or adolescents. **Abnormal expression of cytokeratin, 20 (CK20),** normally confined to the superficial cell layers, was proposed **as a marker for recurrence of papillary tumors** (Harnden et al, 1995). However, Alsheikh et al (2001) found that the **CK20 staining differences** between the recurrent and nonrecurrent low-grade papillary tumors were **statistically not significant.**

Progression of Bladder Tumors to Invasive Cancer

The progression rate of urothelial papillomas to invasive cancer is extremely low. Cheng et al (1999C) confirmed this observation on 52 patients with a very long-term follow-

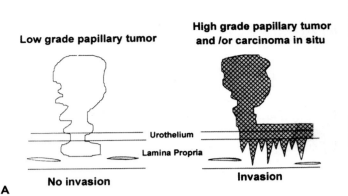

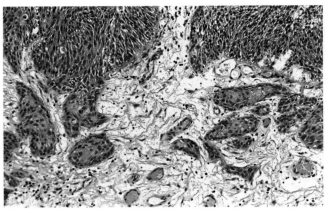

A

B

Figure 23-4 *A.* Schematic representation of pattern of invasion of papillary tumors. On the left, the roots of the tumor are located in the lamina propria. The roots have smooth borders and do not indicate invasion. On the right, the pattern of true invasion shows spike-like extensions of the tumor into the lamina propria. *B.* An illustration of an early invasion of the lamina propria of the bladder.

up. **The progression rate of the papillary tumors grade I (tumors of low malignant potential) is of the order of 3% or less.** Cheng et al (1999D) observed only four invasive carcinomas in a group of 112 patients with long-term follow up, although 29 patients had recurrent noninvasive papillary tumors. Similar observations were reported by McKenney et al (2003). In our experience, the invasive tumors in such patients are usually derived from occult carcinomas in situ (see below). Richter et al (1997) reported genetic differences between noninvasive and superficially invasive grade I tumors. These observations are of theoretical interest only and are discussed below.

The behavior of grade II papillary carcinomas depends on their DNA ploidy: papillary carcinomas grade II with a diploid DNA content have a similar behavior pattern to grade I papillary tumors. **High-grade papillary tumors, including carcinomas grade II, mainly those with abnormal (aneuploid) DNA content, and all carci-**

nomas grade III, progress to invasive carcinoma in a substantial proportion of cases, probably not less than 25%. Invasive carcinoma may **develop directly from sessile higher-grade papillary tumors, but it more commonly develops from adjacent areas of cystoscopically invisible urothelial abnormality, such as carcinoma in situ and related lesions** (see Fig. 23-1 and comments below on the derivation of invasive cancer of the bladder). In fact, the **prognosis of papillary tumors depends not only on the grade of the tumor but also on the level of histologic abnormality of the flat urothelium peripheral to the visible lesion (intraepithelial urothelial neoplasia),** discussed below. It must be stressed that the most invasive and metastatic bladder cancers **are not derived from papillary lesions but from flat carcinoma in situ and related lesions,** discussed below.

Nonpapillary Urothelial Tumors

Nonpapillary urothelial tumors occur in **two forms: invasive carcinoma and its precursor lesions, and flat carcinoma in situ and related abnormalities (intraurothelial neoplasia, or IUN).**

Invasive Urothelial Carcinomas

Clinical Presentation and Natural History
Most invasive cancers of the bladder are discovered **"de novo" in patients** seen because of hematuria, frequency, and other common nonspecific symptoms referable to a dysfunction of the bladder. On cystoscopy, either a protruding or an ulcerated lesion is observed. It has now been documented that in about **80% of the cases, primary invasive carcinomas of the bladder are *not* preceded by papillary tumors** (Brawn, 1982; Kaye and Lange, 1982); hence, the conclusion is that **most invasive bladder cancers are derived from cystoscopically invisible and usually asymptomatic flat lesions, namely carcinoma in situ and related abnormalities, discussed below.** In approximately 20% of cases of **invasive carcinoma preceded by papillary tu-**

Figure 23-5 Multiple recurrent low-grade papillary tumors in a whole bladder mount. Case courtesy of Dr. Rolf Schade, Birmingham, UK.

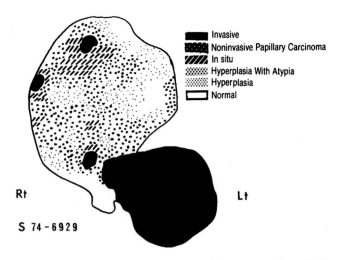

Invasive
Noninvasive Papillary Carcinoma
In situ
Hyperplasia With Atypia
Hyperplasia
Normal

Rt

Lt

S 74-6929

Figure 23-6 Mapping of urinary bladder, removed surgically because of a very large papillary tumor with extension into the lamina propria. Three peripheral foci of invasion are surrounded by carcinoma in situ and related abnormalities (dysplasia).

mors, it has been documented, by **mapping the urinary bladders,** that invasive cancer is usually **derived not from the papillary tumors but from adjacent epithelial segments showing carcinoma in situ or related lesions** (Koss et al, 1974, 1977; Koss, 1979) (Fig. 23-6).

Histologic Patterns

Urothelial carcinomas may show a **broad variety of histologic patterns** ranging from **urothelial carcinomas, solid or mimicking papillary tumors, to tumors composed of spindle and giant cells, mimicking sarcomas, to highly anaplastic large- and small-cell cancers, the latter akin to oat cell carcinoma** (Fig. 23-7A,B). Other variants of bladder cancer, such as **squamous carcinomas and adenocarcinomas,** may either occur as a **focal change in urothelial tumors or as a primary tumor type** (Fig. 23-7C,D). These variants may be recognized in cytologic material and will be discussed separately. Mahadevia et al (1989) pointed out that primary and metastatic bladder tumors may induce a **pseudosarcomatous stromal reaction,** mimicking a spindle-cell carcinoma or a sarcoma (Fig. 23-7C). Other rare variants of urothelial cancer are discussed below.

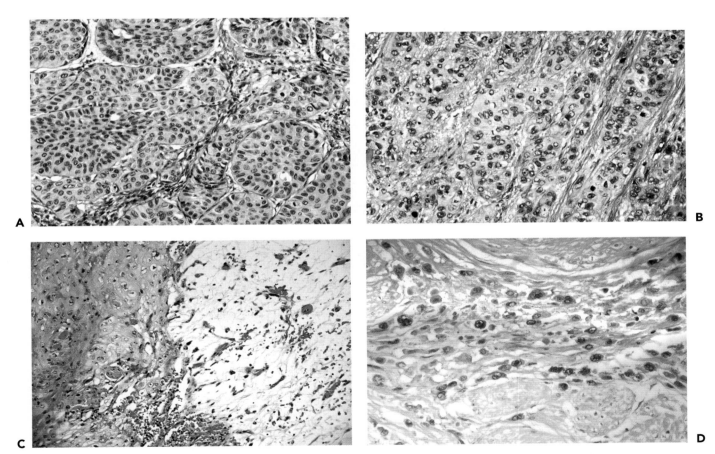

Figure 23-7 Patterns of invasive cancer of the urinary bladder. *A.* Urothelial carcinoma, grade II. The pattern mimics a papillary tumor. *B.* Urothelial carcinoma, grade III. The tumor is composed of sheets of poorly differentiated cancer cells. *C.* Squamous carcinoma with a pseudosarcomatous reaction. The presence of cancer cells in the loosely structured part of the tumor was documented by keratin staining. *D.* Leather bottle bladder showing the presence of signet ring cancer cells in the wall of the bladder. (*D*: Mucicarmine staining.)

Grading

Invasive carcinomas of the bladder composed of orderly sheets of cells resembling normal urothelium (grade I tumors) are very rare. Virtually all invasive tumors are **grade II, III,** or sometimes **IV,** depending on the **level of architectural and cytologic abnormality. Grade II tumors** mimic papillary tumors of higher grades and are composed of sheets of relatively uniform cancer cells separated from each other by bands of connective tissue. **Grade III tumors** are usually solid and are characterized by variability in the size of cancer cells and marked nuclear abnormalities. **Grade IV tumors** are either composed of large cancer cells, spindle and giant cells, or of small cancer cells (small-cell carcinomas).

Staging

Assuming competent treatment, the prognosis of invasive cancer of the bladder depends mainly on the stage of the disease at discovery and the presence or absence of metastases. The diagram in Figure 23-8 shows the principles of staging of bladder tumors. The staging is also applicable to tumors of the renal pelvis and ureters, although in these organs, therapeutic options are more limited. **Tumors with invasion limited to the lamina propria (Stage T_{IA}) fare better than tumors with invasion of the principal bladder muscle (muscularis propria). In the assessment of invasion,** the muscularis propria should **not be confused with the thin and incomplete layer of muscle observed in some patients in the lamina propria (muscularis mucosae).** In practice, tumors invading the main bladder muscle to various depth (stages T3 and T4) have a poor prognosis and do not

respond well to therapy, although there are some exceptions to this rule.

The left side of the diagram in Figure 23-8 pertains to **noninvasive tumors.** After many years, the staging system finally recognized the **major behavioral and prognostic differences between noninvasive papillary tumors, now designated as T_a, and flat carcinoma in situ, now designated as T_{IS}.** Still, even today (in 2004), many urologists (and some pathologists) speak of **"superficial carcinomas,"** without recognizing the major prognostic differences between the two entities. The difference is particularly significant from the cytologic point of view, as will be set forth below.

Precursor Lesions of Invasive Urothelial Carcinoma (IUN)

By far, the most important precursor lesion of invasive urothelial carcinoma is flat carcinoma in situ (Schade and Swinney, 1968). **However,** there are **lesser degrees of urothelial abnormalities** (urothelial atypia, dysplasia) that have been shown to be **precursor lesions of invasive urothelial tumors.** It was proposed (Koss et al, 1985; Koss, 1995) that **all these flat lesions, including carcinoma in situ, may be conveniently included under the term intraurothelial neoplasia (IUN), and subject to grading** in a manner similar to precancerous epithelial abnormalities of the uterine cervix (CIN) (see Chap. 12). The **term has been accepted as an alternate to carcinoma in situ and dysplasia in the new WHO nomenclature** (Epstein et al, 1998; Cina et al, 2001). Three grades of abnormality of the urothelium may be distinguished:

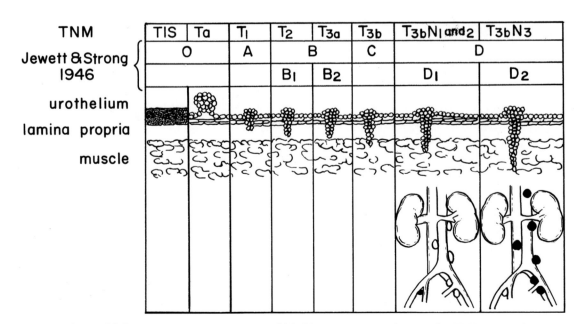

Figure 23-8 Modified clinical staging of bladder cancer according to the TNM system (top line). It was recognized that there are two types of noninvasive tumors: flat carcinoma in situ (TIS) and papillary tumors (Ta). The two entities have unequal prognosis inasmuch as most invasive cancers (T$_2$ and T$_3$) are derived from TIS (see text). N indicates lymph node metastases to pelvic nodes (N$_2$) and aortic nodes (N$_4$). The prognosis of invasive tumors depends on stage.

- Atypical urothelium (mild dysplasia) or atypical urothelial hyperplasia (UIN I or low-grade IUN)
- Markedly atypical urothelium (moderate or severe dysplasia) (IUN-II)
- Flat carcinoma in situ (UIN-III)
- IUN II and III can be combined as high-grade IUN.

Flat Carcinoma In Situ (IUN III)

Carcinoma in situ of the bladder was first described as **"Bowen's disease" of bladder epithelium** by Melicow and Hollowell (1952) as a microscopic abnormality of bladder epithelium, accompanying visible papillary tumors (Fig. 23-9). For several years, the significance of the lesion was not recognized until a major follow-up study of workers exposed to a potent carcinogen, *p*-aminodiphenyl (Melamed et al, 1960; Koss et al, 1965; Koss et al, 1969). This study documented that **clinically occult primary carcinoma in situ, identified in the sediment of voided urine because of the presence of cancer cells, is the principal precursor lesion of invasive cancer,** as confirmed by subsequent studies on the origins of primary invasive cancer of the bladder (Brawn, 1982; Kay and Lange, 1982).

Two forms of carcinoma in situ can be identified:

- **A primary form,** occurring as the initial lesion
- **A secondary form,** accompanying papillary lesions of the bladder (see Figs. 23-9).

Clinical Presentation

Carcinoma in situ of the bladder may be **completely asymptomatic** or may cause **nonspecific symptoms** commonly associated with cystitis or prostatic disease. Carcinoma in situ of the urinary bladder **cannot be recognized as a tumor on cystoscopic examination.** The most common visible alteration is **redness of the epithelial surface, sometimes described as "velvety redness,"** caused by inflammatory changes and vascular dilatation in the underlying stroma (Fig. 23-10). Other changes may mimic inflammation, **cobblestone mucosa, interstitial cystitis,** etc. However, **many carcinomas in situ do not form any visible abnormalities at all.** The **diagnosis** of the lesion **depends,** therefore, on **either recognition of cancer cells in the urinary sediment or a fortuitous biopsy of the urothelium.**

Histology

In its classical form, flat carcinoma in situ is recognized histologically as an abnormality of the urothelium composed of **cancer cells throughout its thickness.** The **thickness** of the cancerous epithelium **is variable:** some carcinomas in situ are composed of **only three or four layers of cells,** whereas others may be composed of **15 or even more layers of cells.** The cancer cells may vary in **size from large to very small,** corresponding to cell sizes observed in various forms of invasive urothelial carcinoma and the size of the cancer cells in the urinary sediment (Fig. 23-11A; see also Figs. 23-9D and 23-10C). The epithelium may sometimes show **differentiation in the superficial layers and the presence of umbrella cells on the surface.** Such lesions were sometimes referred to as "dysplasia" but in our experi-

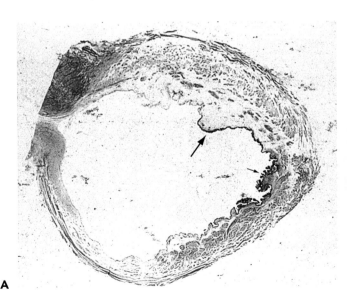

A

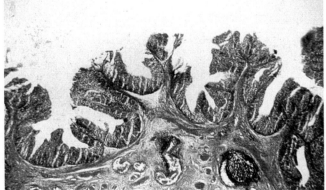

B

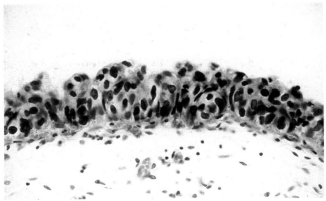

C

Figure 23-9 Cross-section of human bladder (*A*) with two types of tumors side-by-side: a papillary tumor (small arrow, *B*) and grossly invisible carcinoma in situ (large arrow, *C*). (Case courtesy Dr. Rolf Schade, Birmingham, UK.)

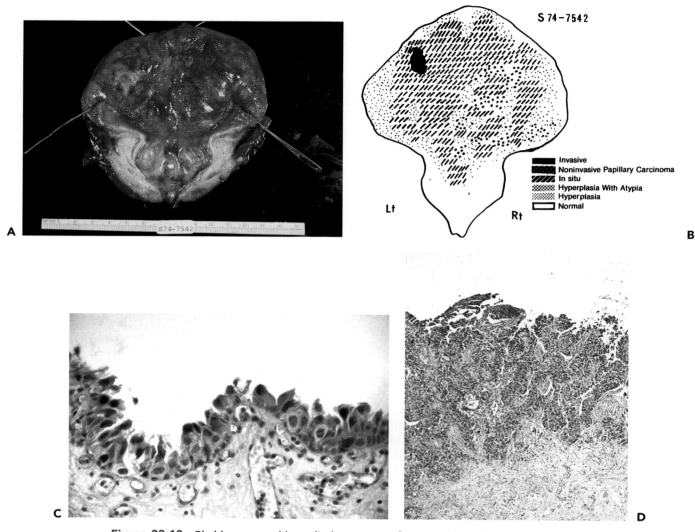

Figure 23-10 Bladder removed by radical cystectomy for extensive carcinoma in situ. *A.* The gross appearance of the bladder with markedly reddened epithelium. *B.* Mapping of the bladder showing one focus of occult invasive carcinoma. *C.* Histologic appearance of carcinoma in situ lining much of the bladder surface. *D.* The focus of unexpected superficial invasive carcinoma. The patient remained free of disease for 10 years after cystectomy.

ence, the diagnosis of carcinoma in situ can be established even **if the malignant cells are confined to three or four basal layers of the epithelium.** We also observed a case of carcinoma in situ of the bladder composed of large cancer cells with **eosinophilic cytoplasm,** resembling oncocytes. **Extension of carcinoma in situ into the nests of von Brunn should not be considered as evidence of invasion** (Fig. 23-11A).

Another form of **carcinoma in situ may mimic Paget's disease** (Fig. 23-11D) and is characterized by the presence of **large cancer cells with clear cytoplasm** within a relatively unremarkable epithelium (Koss, 1975; Yamada et al, 1984). It is of note that the **pattern of Paget's** disease **is repeated in the epithelia of the vulva, vagina, and penis** in **metastatic urothelial carcinoma** to these organs. Dr. Melamed observed a case of **carcinoma in situ of the blad-**

der infiltrated by large macrophages, mimicking Paget's disease.

Because the cancerous epithelium is fragile, sometimes only the **frayed remains of bottom layers may be observed in the biopsy** (Fig. 23-11C). The term **"denuding cystitis"** (Elliot et al, 1973) or, more recently, **"clinging variant of carcinoma in situ"** has been proposed to describe this phenomenon (Epstein et al, 1998). McKenney et al (2003) provided a comprehensive review of histologic patterns of urothelial carcinoma in situ.

Carcinoma in situ may be **multicentric** and involve several areas of the urothelium. As documented by biopsies of workers exposed to carcinogens, these lesions were **most often observed in the floor of the bladder** (the trigone area), including the periureteral areas, **followed by bladder neck.** The posterior and lateral walls of the

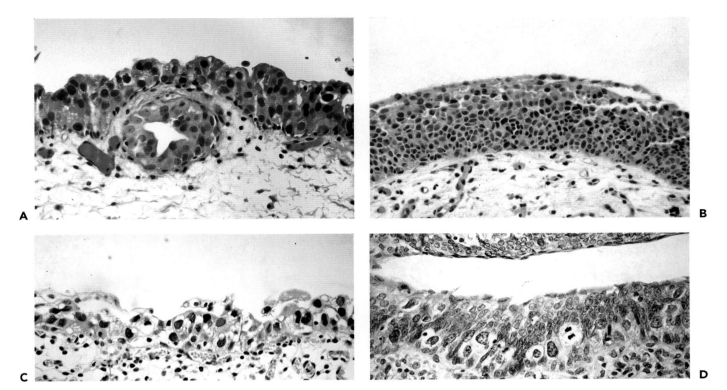

Figure 23-11 **Various forms of carcinoma in situ.** *A.* Lesion composed of large cells extending to nests of Brunn. *B.* Lesion composed of medium-sized cells. *C.* Lesion showing residual small cancer cells attached to the surface of the bladder ("clinging type"). *D.* Pagetoid type of carcinoma in situ with numerous clear cells in the epithelium.

bladder were next in frequency of involvement. The anterior wall or the dome were rarely involved. Cheng et al (2000A) confirmed that the trigone of the bladder was most often affected.

Carcinoma in situ **may extend to the distal ureters and the urethra in both female and male** patients (De Paepe et al, 1990; see Fig. 23-22). An **extension of carcinoma in situ of the bladder into the prostatic ducts is an important complication of this disease** (see Fig. 23-24). **This was observed in 9 of 20 cystectomy specimens with high-grade urothelial cancer** studied by complete mapping by Mahadevia et al (1986). **This observation has a major impact on treatment options because the tumor in the prostatic ducts is not accessible to and does not respond to immunotherapy with bacillus Calmette-Guérin (BCG).**

Behavior

The most important property of flat carcinoma in situ is its **progression to invasive carcinoma.** The invasion into lamina propria usually occurs in the form of **broad bands, sharp tongues, or single cancer cells** (see Fig. 23-10). Because invasion occurs from the deeper portions of the cancerous epithelium, it may completely escape the attention of the urologist, even in patients under close surveillance. The **rate of progression of untreated carcinoma in situ to invasive cancer is about 60% in 5 years** (summary in

Koss, 1975). Similar observations were reported by Utz et al (1970), Schade and Swinney (1973), and Farrow et al (1977). In a recent paper from the Mayo Clinic, **15-year survival** of 138 patients with this disease was reported to be **below 50%,** even though 41 patients received immediate and 34 delayed cystectomy (Cheng et al, 1999A). Most patients died of invasive and metastatic urothelial carcinoma.

Transit Time of Flat Carcinoma In Situ to Invasive Cancer

Follow-up data obtained on industrial workers and narrated below suggested that **progression of carcinoma in situ to invasive cancer can be rapid in some patients and occur within 2 years** after discovery. In other patients, however, the progression took up to 12 years (Table 23-3). These data were similar to those reported by Melamed et al (1964), which pertained to patients without carcinogen exposure seen at the Memorial and James Ewing Hospitals (Fig. 23-12). Additional data on several personally observed patients with sessile carcinoma in situ of the bladder, occurring ab initio, support the view that **from 2 to 7 years elapse from the time of initial cytologic observation until the development of invasive urothelial carcinoma.** Cheng et al (1999A) reported that the mean time interval for progression from carcinoma in situ to invasive cancer was 5 years. **These data confirm that urothelial carcinoma in situ of**

TABLE 23-3

DURATION OF SUSPICIOUS OR POSITIVE CYTOLOGY UNTIL HISTOLOGIC PROOF OF CARCINOMA – COMPARISON OF DATA FROM 1969 AND 1965

| | 1969 | | 1965 | |
| | Prior carcinoma | No prior carcinoma | Prior carcinoma | No prior carcinoma |
Duration				
<1 yr	1	6	0	0
12–20 mo	0	2	2*	1
21–32 mo	1	2	1	2
33–38 mo	1	1	2	1
50 mo	0	0	1	0
60 mo	0	1	0	0
77 mo	0	0	0	1
Total (26 patients)	3	12	6	5

(Koss LG, et al. Further cytologic and histologic studies of bladder lesions in workers exposed to para-aminodiphenyl: progress report. JNCI 43:233–243, 1969.)
* One patient with papilloma only.

the bladder is a life-threatening disease capable of progression to invasive cancer within a relatively short period of time.

Prout et al (1983, 1987) suggested that there were **differences in behavior of primary carcinoma in situ when compared with the secondary lesions of this type, preceded by or accompanying papillary tumors.** These authors claimed that the progression of the "secondary" carcinoma in situ to invasive cancer is less likely to occur. However, in our experience, the difference, if any, is not significant, as documented in Figure 23-12.

The principal features of carcinoma in situ of the urinary bladder are summarized in Table 23-4. The therapy of these lesions is discussed in the closing pages of this chapter.

Urothelial Atypia or Atypical Urothelial Hyperplasia (UIN-I or Low-Grade IUN)

As shown in Figure 23-13A, the **nuclei of urothelial cells show moderate nuclear enlargement, but no significant hyperchromasia.** This epithelial abnormality is often associated with, and may be, a **precursor lesion of papillary**

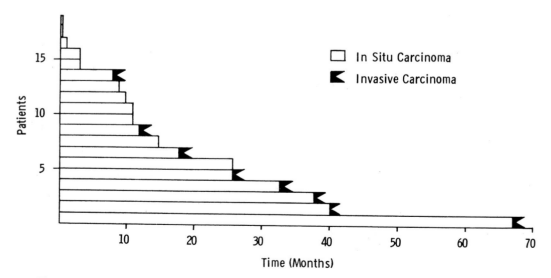

Figure 23-12   Follow-up study of a group of patients with secondary flat carcinoma in situ, conservatively treated. There was no history of carcinogen exposure in any of these patients. The black arrows indicate the time of diagnosis of invasive carcinoma. (From Melamed MR, et al. Natural history and clinical behavior of in situ carcinoma of the human urinary bladder. Cancer 17:1533–1545, 1964.)

TABLE 23-4

CHARACTERISTICS OF NONPAPILLARY CARCINOMA IN SITU OF THE BLADDER

- The lesion cannot be recognized cystoscopically as a tumor.
- Cystoscopic abnormalities may mimic inflammation; "velvety redness," "cobblestone epithelium," or "interstitial cystitis" were recorded. In other cases there are no cystoscopic abnormalities whatever.
- The lesion may extend into the ureters.
- In males, the lesion often extends into the prostatic ducts and the penile urethra.
- Because the lesion produces only nonspecific symptoms or may be asymptomatic, its diagnosis is based either on cytology of voided urine or on incidental biopsies of bladder epithelium.
- If untreated, carcinoma in situ will progress to invasive carcinoma in at least 60% of all patients within 5 years.

tumors, but its exact prospective significance is not fully known. I have not seen an invasive cancer derived from this level of urothelial abnormality. **In cytologic samples, slight atypia of urothelial cells, rarely of diagnostic significance, may be observed in the presence of this lesion.**

Markedly Atypical Urothelial Hyperplasia (Dysplasia, IUN-II, High-Grade IUN)

As shown in Figure 23-13B, the urothelium shows **markedly abnormal, enlarged and hyperchromatic nuclei.** Although **the degree of abnormality is perhaps somewhat less than in classic carcinoma in situ** (see Fig. 23-11), **the morphologic separation of the two lesions is highly subjective.** This type of lesion has been designated as **"dysplasia"** (Murphy and Soloway, 1982) or **"carcinoma in situ, grade II"** (Mostofi, 1979). The lesion was recently shown to have similar proliferative index and expression of p53 gene as classical carcinoma in situ (Cina et al, 2001).

In my experience, **this lesion is equivalent in its biologic behavior to carcinoma in situ** (Fig. 23-13C,D) in that it has a high potential for progression to invasive cancer, an observation confirmed by others (Wolf and Hjogaard, 1983; Harving et al, 1988; Rosenkielde et al, 1988). In a more recent study, the **progression of primary dysplasia, either to classical carcinoma in situ or to invasive cancer,** occurred in 7 of 36 patients (Cheng et al, 1999B). **These lesions cannot be differentiated cytologically from carcinoma in situ.**

Clinical Significance of Intraurothelial Neoplasia

In 1960, Eisenberg et al noted that the **prognosis of papillary tumors of the bladder was related to abnormalities** in peripheral urothelium adjacent to tumors. In patients with atypical peripheral epithelium, the probability of recurrent tumor or invasive cancer was significantly greater than in patients with normal urothelium. This casual observation was repeatedly confirmed in retrospective studies of bladder tumors by mapping (Koss et al, 1974, 1977; Koss, 1979) and in a prospective study by Althausen et al (1976), shown in Table 23-5. It may be noted that **the probability of occurrence of invasive cancer in patients with urothelial abnormalities increases with the level of atypia** and is very high for patients with peripheral carcinoma in situ.

CYTOLOGY OF TUMORS OF THE BLADDER

Lessons From Long-Term Follow-Up Study of Industrial Workers Exposed to Carcinogens

The **value and the efficacy of urinary tract cytology** could be documented during a 12-year follow-up of a group of about 500 workers exposed to a **potent bladder carcinogen, p-aminodiphenyl.** Following the example of Crabbe, who initiated cytologic screening of high-risk industrial workers in the United Kingdom (summary in Crabbe, 1961), the study was based on analysis of **cytologic findings in the sediment of voided urine and biopsy documentation of urothelial tumors** (Melamed et al, 1960; Koss et al, 1965, 1969). In this cohort, invasive carcinoma of the bladder developed in about 10% of the workers during the follow-up period.

p-aminodiphenyl is inhaled and the products of its metabolism are excreted in the urine within 48 to 72 hours after exposure. The initial exposure is usually accompanied by an episode of transient hematuria, with a prompt return to normalcy. There is no evidence that either p-aminodiphenyl or its metabolites are stored in the body. Hence, it has to be assumed that the genetic damage to the cells of the bladder epithelium, of as yet unknown nature, occurs during the few hours following exposure, even though it may not manifest itself clinically for many years. There appears to be **no direct correlation between the amount and length of exposure to carcinogens and the development of cancer of the bladder** (Koss et al, 1965). Persons with a casual contact with the carcinogen may develop carcinoma of the bladder, whereas numerous others with prolonged contact may remain free of disease for many years. Thus, a process of natural selection of an unknown nature protects some people from cancer of the bladder, even under most unfavorable conditions.

Following the initial effects of exposure to carcinogens, there was a period of clinical normalcy of unpredictable duration, often lasting as long as 10 to 15 years or more. During this period, the **cytologic findings** in the urinary sediment were normal. **Low-grade papillary tumors that occurred in some workers as the initial lesion could not be identified in the urinary sediment.**

Subsequently, in some of the exposed workers, slight and poorly defined cytologic abnormalities were observed in the

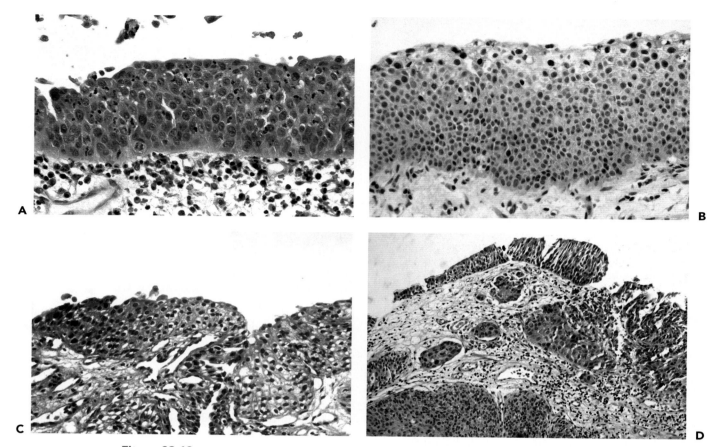

Figure 23-13 Intraurothelial neoplasia. Various aspects of precancerous lesions in the bladder, commonly referred to as "dysplasia." *A.* The hyperplastic epithelium is composed of cells with enlarged nuclei arranged in a relatively orderly pattern. *B.* Atypical hyperplasia. Scattered nuclear abnormalities are clearly evident within this epithelium. This lesion could be equally well diagnosed as carcinoma in situ. *C.* Atypical epithelium, classified as "dysplasia," which within 24 months led to invasive carcinoma shown in Figure 23-13D.

TABLE 23-5

DEVELOPMENT OF INVASIVE BLADDER CANCER IN PATIENTS WITH GRADE I OR II PAPILLARY TUMORS WITHIN 5 YEARS, ACCORDING TO STATUS OF PERIPHERAL EPITHELIUM

Status of Peripheral Epithelium	No. Patients	Development of Invasive Cancer No. Patients (%)	
Normal	41	3	7
Atypia	25	9	36
Carcinoma in situ	12	10	83
TOTAL	78	22	

(Althausen AF, et al. Non-invasive papillary carcinoma of the bladder associated with carcinoma in situ. J Urol 116:575–580, 1976, with permission.)

urinary sediment. The most conspicuous change, **limited to a very few cells,** was a **slight enlargement of the nuclei** of the urothelial cells, which in an occasional patient was **associated with slight hyperchromasia,** somewhat comparable to the "dyskaryosis" (or dysplasia) of squamous cells, observed during the formative stages of cervix cancer (see Chap. 11). The "dyskaryotic" cells, diagnosed as "atypia," appeared in the urine intermittently, sometimes over a period of several years. The cystoscopic findings in patients during this stage of the disease were essentially negative although, occasionally, an area of redness or "cystitis" was observed, which on biopsy, disclosed urothelial hyperplasia with slight nuclear abnormalities (see Fig. 23-17). In general, the cytologic findings during this period were not predictive of subsequent malignant events.

The Stage of Positive Cytology

After an unpredictably long period of either negative cytologic findings or slight cytologic abnormalities, there followed a period of clearly **positive cytologic findings,** associated with **papillary or nonpapillary high-grade bladder cancer or with flat carcinoma in situ.** In most patients, the **appearance of the cancer cells was sudden,** suggesting that the **development of high-grade malignant lesions in** the bladder is not necessarily preceded by diagnosable precursor stages. During this study, which was conducted many years ago with a group of general urologists, it proved difficult to obtain the biopsy confirmation of carcinoma in situ, particularly because many patients harboring this deadly disease were asymptomatic and their bladders showed no evidence of tumor on cystoscopy. Still, in many patients, biopsies were obtained and confirmed the presence of carcinoma in situ. This study documented that **cytology of voided urine is most useful in the discovery of high-grade urothelial tumors and notably flat carcinoma in situ of the bladder** (Melamed et al, 1960). Schulte et al (1986) and Crosby et al (1991) made fundamentally similar observations on a cohort of workers exposed to *β*-naphthylamine and benzidine.

Progression to Invasive Carcinoma

The follow-up studies on workers exposed to *p*-aminodiphenyl permitted the accumulation of data pertaining to the **duration of the stage of carcinoma in situ, as diagnosed cytologically.** In this group of patients, treatment was usually not instituted before the appearance of a clinically identifiable tumor. This experience is summarized in Table 23-3. At the conclusion of this study in 1970, there were 13 histologically documented instances of primary nonpapillary carcinoma in situ. In 7 of these patients, **invasive carcinoma developed within 1 or 2 years** after the initial cytologic diagnosis. The longest time interval observed was 12 years (Koss et al, 1969). **These data confirmed that urinary cytology is most useful in the discovery of precursor lesions of invasive cancer, notably flat carcinoma in situ, but has limited value in the diagnosis of urothelial abnormalities preceding this lesion.**

Comparison of Precancerous Events in the Bladder with the Uterine Cervix

The genesis of human bladder cancer may be compared with the processes within the human cervix, the only organ that has had the benefit of similar sustained investigative attention. In the cervix, there is usually clear cut-evidence of cytologic abnormalities prior to the development of high-grade lesions (see Chap. 11). In the urinary bladder, cytologic abnormalities preceding carcinoma in situ were either absent, or at best, not well defined and intermittent. Thus, **the option of early cancer prevention, which is paramount in cytologic screening for cancer of the uterine cervix is, at best, slight for the urinary bladder and limited to the discovery of carcinoma in situ and related lesions that are dangerous to the patient.** Although progression or regressions of high-grade cervical lesions may occur, the regression of untreated carcinoma in situ of the bladder appears to be extremely rare. Another **major difference between the cervix and the bladder is the time lapse between the occurrence of carcinoma in situ and its progression to invasive carcinoma: this appears to be considerably shorter for the urinary bladder.**

Urothelial Tumors

Targets of Cytologic Investigation

The success or failure of cytologic investigations of the urothelial tumors of the bladder, ureters, or the renal pelves depends on **morphology of the lesion. Thus, simple hyperplasias and low-grade papillary urothelial tumors** that are characterized by either **normal urothelium or by a urothelium with only slight and focal nuclear abnormalities, cannot be identified in cytologic material with any degree of certainty unless one is willing to assume responsibility for a large number of false-positive alarms. Cytology of the urinary tract is useful only in the identification of tumors or conditions that are associated with perceptible morphologic abnormalities of cells, hence, tumors of high-grade, with emphasis on flat carcinoma in situ and related lesions.**

Thus, the primary areas of application of cytologic techniques to the urinary tract are:

- **Detection and diagnosis of high-grade urothelial tumors**
- **Monitoring of patients after treatment for neoplastic lesions of the lower urinary tract, regardless of type or grade, because of risk for development of new high-grade lesions**
- **Under special circumstances, monitoring of high-risk, asymptomatic industrial workers exposed to known carcinogens. The benefits of this approach are discussed further in this chapter.**

Some caveats.

The cytologic diagnosis of neoplastic urothelial lesions is difficult. Some of the reasons for the diagnostic problems, already discussed in Chapter 22, are repeated here:

- The recognition of limitations of cytology of the urinary tract in the diagnosis of low-grade papillary tumors, by avoiding mistakes in the interpretation of benign cell changes, particularly those induced by inflammation, instrumentation, or lithiasis (stones)
- Mistakes in the interpretation of polyomavirus-infected cells for cancer cells
- Mistakes in the interpretation of cell abnormalities induced by or associated with therapy

Because the accuracy of the diagnosis relies often on subtle cytologic abnormalities, **impeccable technical processing of samples** is essential, as discussed in Chapters 22 and 44.

Urothelial Cancer Cells

The appearance of urothelial cancer cells **differs somewhat according to the medium of diagnosis, voided urine or bladder barbotage.**

Voided Urine

Depending on tumor type and grade, the **urothelial cancer cells vary in size** and may be equal to, **smaller, or larger than normal urothelial cells.** In voided urine, the cancer cells occur **singly** or in **small, loosely structured clusters.** Large aggregates of cancer cells are very uncommon, although they occur in specimens processed by the ThinPrep method.

The **configuration of cancer cells is variable.** Most of them are **approximately spherical or oval** with an irregular outline, but elongated or bizarre cell shapes have been observed, particularly in high-grade tumors. **Columnar cancer cells** and **large multinucleated cells mimicking umbrella cells** may be observed. The **cytoplasm is usually basophilic** and in well-preserved cells, **has sharp borders;** however, cells in voided urine are often **poorly preserved and the cytoplasm is frayed.** Cells with **eosinophilic cytoplasm** may occur, particularly if there is **a squamous component to the tumor. Cytoplasmic vacuoles** and nonspecific red inclusions are sometimes observed (Fig. 23-14).

The **nuclei of cancer cells are, as a rule, large for cell size and therefore there is a conspicuous change in the nucleocytoplasmic ratio in favor of the nuclei.** The nuclei are typically of **irregular, abnormal shape,** although some are approximately spherical or oval, sometimes showing small peripheral protrusions on close inspection. The most **important nuclear abnormality in urothelial cancer is hyperchromasia caused by abnormal** *nuclear texture:* **the chromatin is arranged in large, coarse, tightly packed or superimposed granules, rendering the nucleus dark and nontransparent** (Fig. 23-15). This is in marked **contrast**

with benign cells, which have a **finely textured "salt-and-pepper" appearance due to small chromatin granules, separated from each other by areas of translucent nucleoplasms** (Fig. 23-15A–G). Practically speaking, one can "see through" a normal nucleus but not through the nucleus of a cancer cell. **In high-grade tumors, abnormal mitotic figures are fairly common in the sediment** (Fig. 23-15H). **Multiple and large nucleoli may occasionally be present, particularly in flat carcinoma in situ and in invasive cancer, but they are much more difficult to see in voided urine** than in barbotage specimens, because of the marked nuclear hyperchromasia (Fig. 23-15G).

Except for the cells mimicking umbrella cells, we have not observed any cancer cell types that could be considered typical or unique of urothelial carcinoma. Although bizarre cell forms may occur in high-grade tumors, we have not observed **in voided urine, the elongated cells with long cytoplasmic processes with either bulbous or flattened ends ("fish tail" or "cercariform cells")** that were described as characteristic of metastatic urothelial cancer in aspirated samples (Johnson and Kini, 1993; Powers and Elbadawi, 1995; Renshaw and Madge, 1997; Hida and Gupta, 1999). It is possible that these authors classified the common columnar-shaped cancer cells, such as shown in Figure 23-15D, as "cercariform cells."

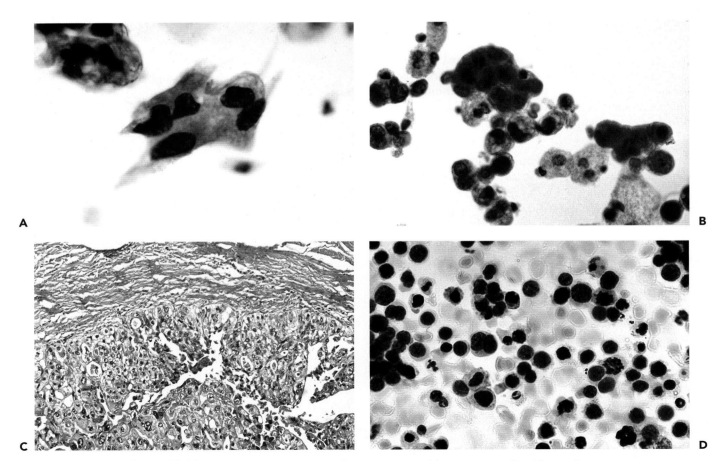

A   B

C   D

Figure 23-14 Cancer cells in urinary sediment. *A.* Several large cancer cells with very large, coarsely granulated, irregularly shaped nuclei. *B.* Cancer cells, appearing singly and in clusters, in voided urine sediment (ThinPrep). *C.* Invasive carcinoma corresponding to the smear shown in *B. D.* Small cell urothelial carcinoma in urinary sediment. (*A:* oil immersion.)

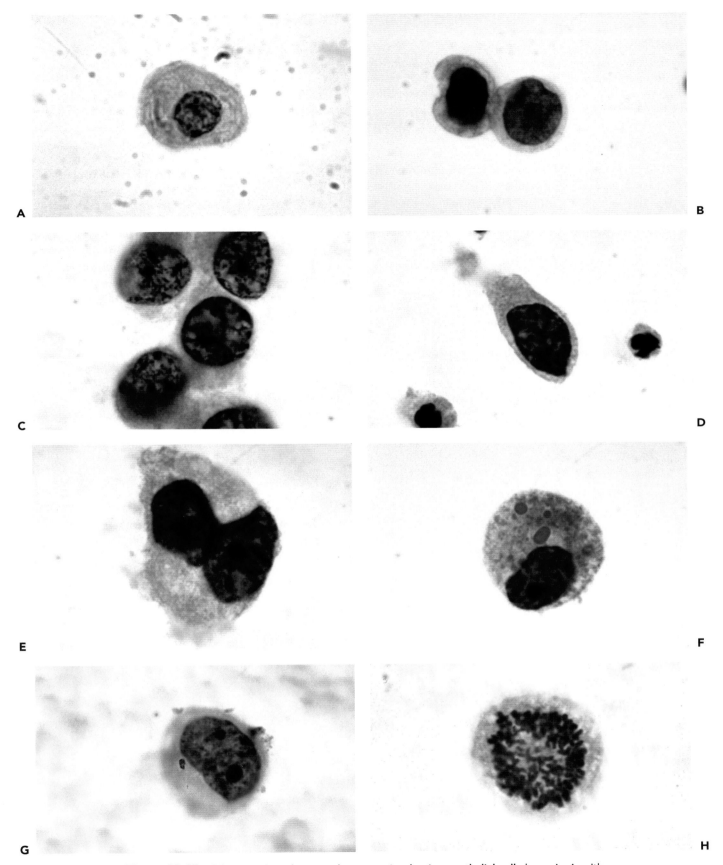

Figure 23-15 Oil immersion photographs comparing benign urothelial cell shown in *A*, with cancer cells shown in *B–H*. The differences in the nuclear structure are evident: the nuclei of cancer cells are significantly larger, coarsely granular, and show slight irregularities of contour. The cell in *D* has a columnar configuration. This is a common finding in bladder cancer. *E*. Shows a binucleated cancer cell. *F*. Shows a cancer cell with eosinophilic cytoplasmic inclusions. *G*. Cancer cell with prominent nucleoli. *H*. An abnormal mitotic figure.

Differential Diagnosis

Perhaps the most important points of **differential diagnosis** of urothelial cancer are urothelial cells infected with **polyomaviruses that show large, homogeneous, basophilic nuclear inclusions.** As discussed at length in Chapter 22, such cells are readily confused with cancer cells. We observed that in some specimens **processed by reverse filtration (ThinPrep),** the inclusions can be fractured. Other potential sources of error include the uncommon **pyknosis of normal nuclei, nuclear changes in lithiasis,** and in nuclear abnormalities **induced by treatment,** all discussed in Chapter 22. Errors can be avoided if the **high nucleocytoplasmic ratio** and the **granularity of the hyperchromatic nuclei,** such as shown in Figure 23-15, are considered essential criteria of diagnosis of urothelial cancer in well-preserved **single cells.**

Based on the degree of cell abnormalities and cell size in voided urine sediment, Bergkvist et al (1965) performed **grading of urothelial bladder tumors** and claimed high level of prognostic accuracy. Tumors with smaller cancer cells were considered to be of a higher grade than tumors with larger cells. This concept has received support from Esposti and Zajicek (1972) and Suprun and Bitterman (1975) but was not universally accepted and was replaced by image analysis and flow cytometry (see below).

Bladder Barbotage (Washings)

For description of technique of bladder barbotage, see Chapter 22. In this type of material, all cells, including cancer cells, are usually better preserved than in voided urine and their cytoplasm is more likely to be intact. The general features of cancer cells described above, that is, **variability in size and configuration and altered nucleocytoplasmic ratio,** are evident. The **nuclear texture** is also altered but the **degree of nuclear hyperchromasia is usually less** than in voided urine and the **nuclei are more transparent. Conspicuous, large, irregular, and sometimes multiple nucleoli** are much more common in cancer cells in bladder barbotage than in voided urine (Fig. 23-15G). A **word of caution** is necessary: in specimens processed by a proprietary procedure known as **ThinPrep, the chromocenters in normal urothelial cells, particularly the umbrella cells, may stain pink and may mimic nucleoli.** Experience with this technique is necessary to avoid errors of interpretation.

Scanning Electron Microscopy of Urothelial Cancer Cells

Jacobs et al reported in 1976, the results of scanning electron microscopy of cell surfaces in experimental bladder cancer. The presence of **irregular surface microvilli** may be ob-

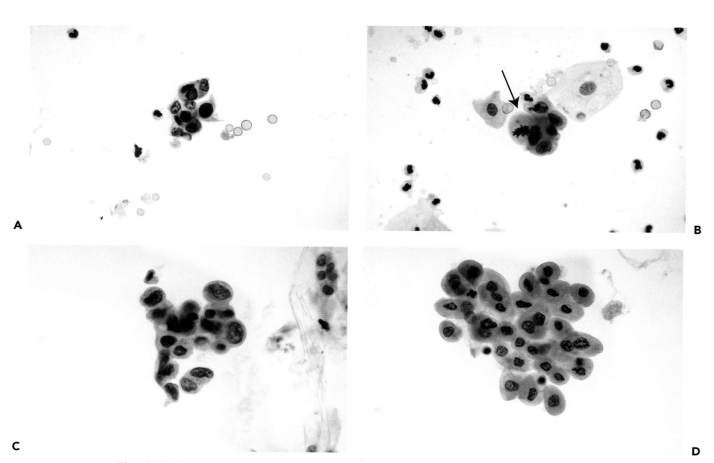

Figure 23-16 Various forms of atypia of urothelial cells in voided urine sediment, not diagnostic of cancer. *A,B.* Small clusters of urothelial cells with slight nuclear enlargement and hyperchromasia observed in the presence of lithiasis. *C,D.* Bladder lavage showing clusters of urothelial cells with slightly enlarged hyperchromatic nuclei. The bladder biopsies disclosed focal hyperplasia but no evidence of tumor in this patient.

served during the early stages of carcinogenesis. The applicability of this method to the human urinary sediment was tested in our laboratories (Domagala et al, 1979). The studies disclosed poor preservation of many urothelial cancer cells with loss of surface structure. Some, but not all, of the **better-preserved cancer cells had numerous surface microvilli of uneven length and configuration,** similar to those observed in cancer cells in effusion (see Chap. 26). By contrast, the surfaces of benign urothelial and some squamous cells showed only sparse microvilli of fairly regular configuration. This method is theoretically of diagnostic value but it is too costly and time consuming to be applicable to the practice of cytopathology.

Atypical Urothelial Cells

Atypical urothelial cells are a **common finding, particularly in voided urine and bladder barbotage, in inflammatory conditions, lithiasis, systemic therapy with alkylating drugs,** or **intravesical therapy,** and may also occur in **urothelial tumors of all grades.** The atypical cells are usually small, show **nuclear enlargement with a slight change in the nucleocytoplasmic ratio and a slight to moderate increase in nuclear hyperchromasia,** usually below the level of hyperchromasia and granularity of chromatin associated with obvious cancer (Fig. 23-16). Mitotic figures may be present (Fig. 23-16B, arrow). The term **"dys-**

plastic cells," proposed by Murphy (2000) in reference to small urothelial cells with enlarged nuclei, **is not justified,** as it implies a neoplastic event, whereas such cells may occur in a variety of benign situations and their origin in a specific epithelial abnormality is impossible to prove, even in the presence of a tumor.

The "atypical" urothelial cells may also occur in low-grade tumors, discussed below. In some cases, **the separation of "atypical" from "suspicious" or outright malignant cells** may become a matter for a debate that is not easily settled (Fig. 23-17). In such cases, it is important to secure a patient's history and cystoscopic findings before formulating a clinical recommendation. Usually, the significance of the "atypical" cells will be fairly easily determined. Still, in some cases, long-term follow-up and multiple bladder biopsies may be required to rule out a neoplastic process.

In a **computerized image analysis study** of atypical cells, an attempt was made to determine whether the atypical cells originating in benign conditions could be separated from those associated with urothelial tumors. Statistical analysis of several computer-generated features suggested that the atypical urothelial cells could be divided into two groups, one sharing cell features with benign cells and the other with malignant cells (Koss et al, 1977). On subsequent microscopic review, the urothelial cells with nuclei of round or oval configuration and only slight to moderate increase

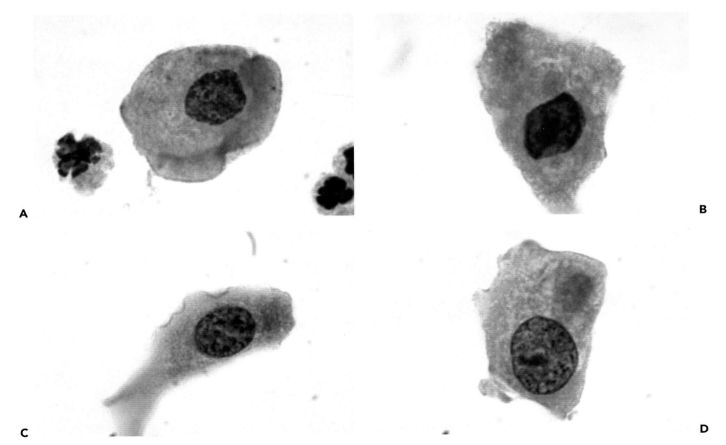

Figure 23-17 Oil immersion images of cells classified as markedly atypical or suspicious. The cells show no significant change in the nucleocytoplasmic ratio. The nuclei are generally spherical, although somewhat hyperchromatic and granular. In the presence of such cells, a search for a bladder tumor is mandatory.

in hyperchromasia belonged to the first group (ATY-I) whereas cells with irregular configuration of cytoplasm and nuclei and greater nuclear hyperchromasia, classed as atypical II (ATY-II) (Fig. 23-17), were commonly associated with bladder cancer (Koss et al, 1978). Unfortunately, the data obtained by a complex computer analysis of cell features were of little value in routine microscopic studies of the urinary sediment.

There is good evidence that the **DNA of nuclei of urothelial cells goes hand-in-hand with the level of cytologic abnormalities** (Koss et al, 1985). Thus, **atypical cells with abnormal (aneuploid) DNA content may belong to the "possibly malignant" group. The application of DNA measurements and other ancillary procedures to the analysis of atypical cells is discussed below, but in our view, does not replace morphologic assessment.**

Recognition of Specific Types of Urothelial Tumors in Urinary Sediment

Papillary Tumors of Low Grade (Papillomas and Grade I Papillary Tumors of Low Malignant Potential)

In the presence of these tumors, the **background of the cytologic preparations is usually clean** and there is rarely any evidence of inflammation or necrosis. Erythrocytes in varying numbers are usually present. By definition, these tumors are **lined by normal or only slightly abnormal, though sometimes thickened, urothelium** (see above). Hence, **cells derived therefrom cannot be identified as malignant.** The changes in **individual urothelial cells are nonspecific** and the feature of **slight nuclear enlargement,** proposed by Murphy (2000) as a characteristic of these tumors, **is not reliable because such changes may occur under a variety of benign circumstances.** Further, such atypical cells are more likely to occur in papillary carcinomas of low grade (see below).

It has been suggested that there are some **differences in the configuration of cell clusters** between low-grade papillary tumors and normal urothelium (Kannan and Bose, 1993). It is true that the surface of the clusters of normal urothelium is often composed of semilunar umbrella cells with smooth surface, as discussed in Chapter 22 and shown in Figure 22-10. However, clusters with "ragged borders" may also occur in a variety of benign conditions, such as instrumentation, inflammation, or stones (lithiasis) (Fig. 23-18A,B). The latter condition, named **"calculus artifact,"** was discussed at length in a study by Kannan and Gupta (1999), who documented the presence of cell clusters

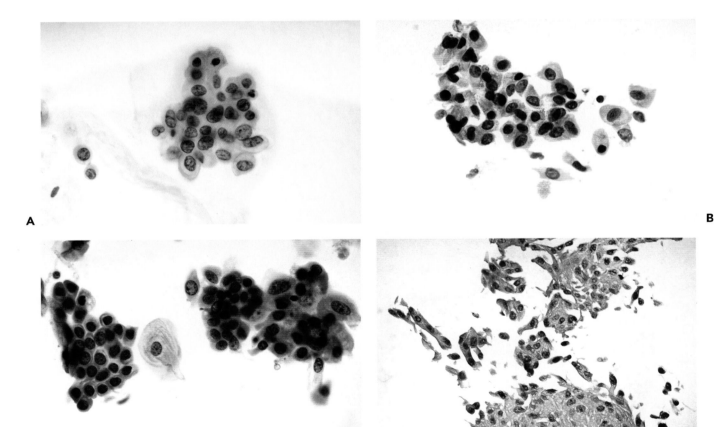

Figure 23-18 **Various aspects of low-grade papillary tumors (tumors with low malignant potential) in voided urine sediment.** *A,B.* A loosely structured cluster of urothelial cells with minimal nuclear enlargement and hyperchromasia. *C.* Comparison between two clusters of urothelial cells, one showing normal configuration (left) and one showing slight nuclear enlargement and hyperchromasia (right). *C.* Corresponds to a low-grade papillary tumor with slight nuclear enlargement shown in *D.* (*A–C:* High magnification.)

with irregular borders and slight level of nuclear atypia in 46 of 65 patients with lithiasis (also see discussion of lithiasis in Chap. 22).

Nasuti et al (2001) studied the frequency of **tissue fragments** captured on the surfaces of **filters** in 2,553 voided urine sediments. There were 174 patients with bladder biopsies. These authors concluded that **tissue fragments, particularly of tri-dimensional configuration, were more common in patients with urothelial tumors of various grades than in negative controls.** This has not been our experience. In a similar study of 5,001 urine specimens processed by **cytocentrifugation,** Goldstein et al (1998) failed to observe this relationship. Neither paper addressed the issue of instrumentation, such as cystoscopy, that may have been the cause of the tissue fragments, particularly in patients suspect of harboring a bladder tumor.

Wolinska et al (1985) systematically compared the findings in **voided urine sediment** from 51 patients known to have low-grade papillary tumors and 30 controls. The material was obtained from patients without prior cystoscopy. Except for somewhat increased cellularity and occasional presence of atypical cell shapes, such as elongated cells, there were no diagnostic findings of note, **confirming that the cytologic diagnosis of low-grade papillary tumors cannot be reliably established.** Similar conclusions have been reached by the Swedish investigators, Esposti and Zajicek (1972). Kern (1975), using planimetric studies, confirmed the essentially normal configuration of cells derived from such tumors. These observations, and our experience, strongly contradict Murphy et al (1984), who claimed that low-grade papillary tumors could be identified in 62% of patients, a view that was moderated in Murphy's subsequent publication (2000).

Direct washings or brushings of the urinary bladder contribute little to the diagnosis of low-grade papillary tumors. Harris et al (1971) were able to **diagnose such lesions only in cell blocks of the urinary sediment,** wherein biopsy-sized fragments of such tumors were observed. However, fragments of urothelium **may also occur in spontaneously voided urine in the absence of a tumor,** particularly after instrumentation (see Fig. 22-10). Within recent years, several attempts have been made to revive the matter of cytologic diagnosis of low-grade papillary tumors, predictably with conflicting results. Thus, Raab et al (1994), using logistic regression analysis of numerous parameters, suggested that **irregular nuclear borders, increased nucleocytoplasmic ratio, and cytoplasmic homogeneity** of urothelial cells in bladder washings were highly specific for low-grade tumors. The same group of investigators confirmed that the three criteria are valid in ThinPrep preparations with a sensitivity of 59% and specificity of 100% (Xin et al, 2003). Although the first two criteria may have some value, the "cytoplasmic homogeneity" is puzzling as it is clearly not related to the nature of these tumors. Renshaw et al (1996) failed to confirm these observations. Bastacky et al (1999) also were unable to recognize cell features characteristic of low-grade lesions. Sack et al (1995), in a cohort of 208 patients, recognized low-grade papillary tumors in 11 of 33 such patients but also committed an equal number of false-positive errors. **Thus, cytol-**

ogy of the urinary sediment does not lend itself to the diagnosis of papillary tumors of low grade.

There are **rare exceptions to this rule:** the finding of a **papillary cluster of urothelial cells with a central capillary** strongly suggests that the **cell cluster represents a broken fragment of a papillary tumor** (Fig. 23-19A). Also, **in the rare papillary tumors with a dominant squamous component, the cytologic findings can be suggestive of this diagnosis** (Fig. 23-19B,C).

On the other hand, if the urinary sediment shows obvious cancer cells and the biopsy discloses only a low-grade papillary lesion, the cytologic finding is of great clinical importance: it strongly suggests that a high-grade malignant lesion is present in the urinary tract. This may be another papillary lesion of high grade or, more often, nonpapillary carcinoma, in situ or invasive, located in the bladder, ureters, renal pelvis, or even within the prostatic ducts and the urethra. **Every effort must be made to localize and evaluate this lesion or lesions, because of their ominous prognosis.**

Papillary Tumors of High Grade (Papillary Carcinomas, Grades II and III)

In the urinary sediment, most of these lesions are characterized by the presence of **markedly atypical urothelial cells and recognizable cancer cells, occurring singly or in loosely structured clusters.** The number of single cancer cells increases with tumor grade. There are some important differences between the cytologic presentation of papillary tumors grade II and tumors grade III.

Papillary Tumors Grade II (Papillary Carcinomas, Low Grade)

Not all grade II tumors can be recognized cytologically. In 20 of 68 such tumors studied by Koss et al (1985), **only benign or somewhat atypical urothelial cells were observed, and the diagnosis could not be established** (Fig. 23-20). These were most likely grade II tumors with a DNA content in the diploid range. In aneuploid papillary tumors, grade II, **markedly atypical or frankly malignant cells can be recognized, either singly or in small clusters.** The cancer cells are **usually of medium size and rarely show marked abnormalities of configuration,** as in tumors of higher grade. The performance of cytology in debatable cases with "atypical," but not definitely malignant, cells can be improved by **analysis of DNA pattern.** Abnormal (aneuploid) DNA values are strongly suggestive of a neoplastic event. A number of new technological developments are also designed to recognize papillary tumors with negative or questionable cytologic presentation, with **fluorescent in situ hybridization (FISH)** being the most secure. These diagnostic options are discussed further on in this chapter.

Papillary Tumors Grade III (Papillary Carcinomas, High Grade)

All or nearly all papillary tumors grade III can be identified by cytology. These tumors shed **cancer cells that are of variable size and configuration** (Fig. 23-21). The papillary tumors, even highly anaplastic, may shed **cancer cells in**

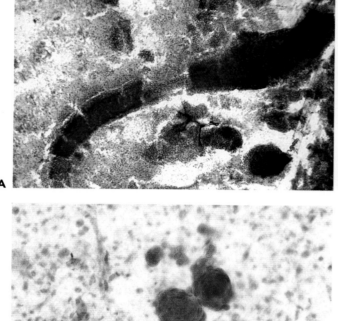

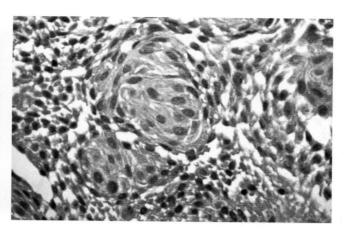

Figure 23-19 Papillary tumor. *A.* A remarkable example of fragments of papillary tumor with a capillary vessel in voided urine sediment. This appearance is diagnostic of a papillary tumor. *B,C.* Histologic and cytologic aspects of a low-grade papillary tumor of the bladder with formation of squamous pearls, which were seen in the urinary sediment, shown in *C.* (*A–C:* High magnification; *A:* courtesy of Dr. June Koizumi, New York Hospital, NY.)

large clusters, sometimes reminiscent of papillary arrangement of cells. However, **single cancer cells are always present and are usually numerous.** The **background** of smears often, but not always, shows evidence of **inflammation and necrosis.** Under these circumstances, it is impossible to determine whether or not a tumor is invasive and the variability in size and configuration of cancer cells is not helpful. It must be stressed that **in the presence of papillary tumors, particularly of high grades, the adjacent or remote peripheral urothelium of the bladder may show intraurothelial neoplasia of high grade (IUN III, equivalent of atypical hyperplasia or nonpapillary carcinoma in situ) whence occult invasion may take place** (see Fig. 23-4B).

Work-Up of Patients with Papillary Tumors
Because patients with papillary tumors may also harbor flat neoplastic lesions, which are more likely to progress to invasion than papillary lesions, a complete evaluation of patients with papillary bladder tumors requires **not only a biopsy of the visible lesion, but also an evaluation of the remaining urothelium by cytologic examination of voided urine sediment and by multiple superficial biopsies of the bladder to rule out the presence of a nonpapillary lesion. This recommendation is particularly important if the urinary sediment remains positive after resection of visible papillary lesion(s).** The recommended minimum work-up of such patients calls for cytologic analysis of **three**

voided urine samples on three consecutive days for optimization of results. The optimal approach to bladder biopsies is described below in reference to flat carcinoma in situ.

Nonpapillary Urothelial Carcinoma

Virtually all nonpapillary urothelial cancers, whether invasive or in situ, are made up of clearly identifiable cancer cells that can be readily recognized in the urinary sediment. **These lesions, particularly the nonpapillary carcinoma in situ and related lesions (IUN of high grade), are the principal target of cytologic studies of the urinary tract.**

Nonpapillary (Flat) Carcinoma In Situ
Voided urine sediment is the ideal diagnostic medium for the primary diagnosis of nonpapillary carcinoma in situ, whether located in the bladder, the renal pelvis, the ureters, or the urethra. Regardless of the method of preparation, the urinary sediment usually yields **persuasive evidence of cancer, reflecting the poor adhesiveness of cancer cells in the epithelial lesion** (Figs. 23-22 through 23-25). Because the shedding of cancer cells is sometimes intermittent, **three specimens of voided urine obtained on consecutive days are a secure means of diagnosis** (Koss et al, 1985, 1995).

The most common cytologic presentation of flat carcino-

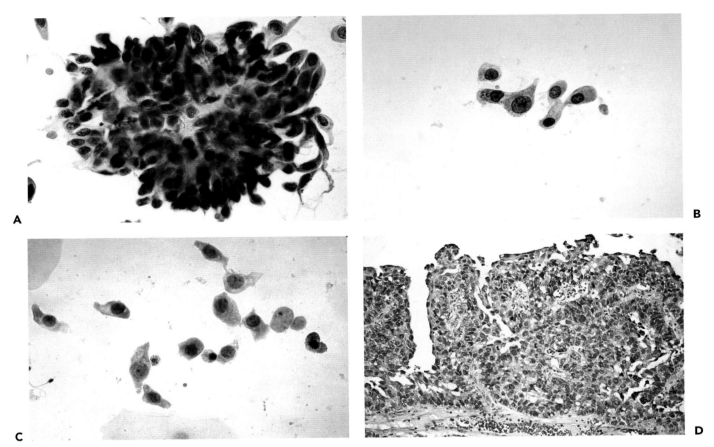

Figure 23-20 **Various aspects of cytologic presentation of a low-grade papillary tumor.** A. Brush specimen showing a cluster of urothelial cells with somewhat enlarged and hyperchromatic nuclei that appear to center around a core, possibly muscularis mucosae. *B,C.* Voided urine. The cells show slight enlargement of the nuclei but no significant hyperchromasia or change in the nucleocytoplasmic ratio. The papillary tumor corresponding to *B* and *C* is shown in *D*. The cytologic diagnosis of tumor in such cases is extremely difficult and unreliable.

mas in situ is a fairly **monotonous population of medium-sized or small urothelial cancer cells, comparable in size to benign urothelial cells from deeper layers of the urothelium.** The **cancer cells** usually appear **singly,** but occasionally form **small clusters. Occasionally, a few larger or bizarre cells may occur. Regardless of size, the cells have an irregular configuration and relatively scanty, usually basophilic cytoplasm, although cells with eosinophilic cytoplasms may occur.** The **nuclei** are relatively **large, hyperchromatic,** have an **irregular contour and show** an **abnormal chromatin texture. A coarse, filamentous arrangement of the chromatin is especially frequent. Enlarged nucleoli** are infrequent but may occasionally be noted. Condensation of nuclear chromatin or **pyknosis** is fairly common and, in such nuclei, the arrangement of chromatin cannot be studied.

In the sediment of about one-third of the patients with flat carcinoma in situ, the population of cancer cells is pleomorphic (see Fig. 23-21C,D). **The cancer cells vary in size and configuration although their nuclear characteristics are the same. Such smear patterns can be separated from patterns of invasive carcinoma only** by **smear background.** In the presence of

carcinoma in situ, the urine rarely contains more than a **few inflammatory cells or erythrocytes,** and there is usually **little evidence of necrosis, whereas marked inflammation and necrosis are commonly observed in invasive cancer.** Rarely, the cellular aberrations in carcinoma in situ may be so inconspicuous that they are interpreted as inflammatory changes, a verdict that is usually contradicted by nuclear abnormalities. However, in most patients the diagnosis is obvious, provided that the sources of error in the recognition of cancer cells, discussed above, are eliminated. Extension of carcinoma in situ to the ureters (Fig. 23-22) or prostatic ducts (Fig. 23-24) does not change the smear pattern.

From our laboratory, Voutsa and Melamed (1963) reported a systematic cytologic study of 20 patients with urothelial carcinoma in situ of the bladder. This study generally confirmed the observations reported above. **The cell pattern did not differ whether the lesion was primary or secondary to a previously treated tumor of the bladder.** These authors pointed out that **following a biopsy or fulguration, there may be a marked alteration of the smear pattern,** usually appearing within 24 hours after the procedure and lasting up to 4 weeks. A general **increase in the**

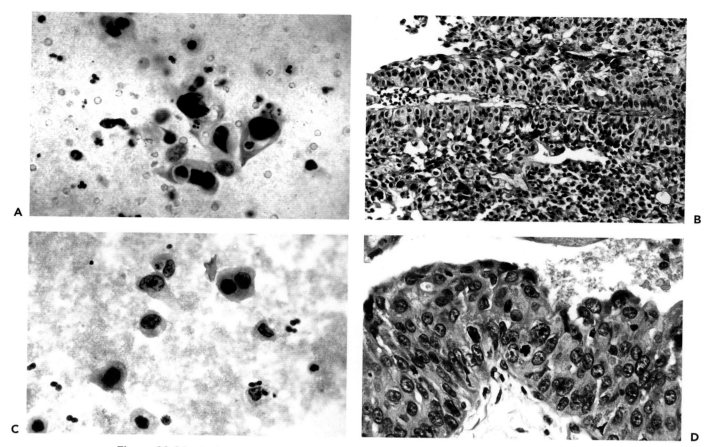

Figure 23-21 High-grade invasive urothelial cancer of the bladder. *A.* Irregularly shaped bizarre cancer cells, corresponding to the high-grade tumor, shown in *B. C.* Another aspect of urinary sediment in a high-grade carcinoma in situ, shown in *D.* This tumor was invasive elsewhere.

number of both benign and malignant cells, and occasionally **bizarre cell changes mimicking radiation changes,** were observed following such procedures.

Boon et al (1986), who studied 13 patients with primary carcinoma in situ and 10 patients with secondary carcinoma in situ of the bladder, did not fully agree with the observations recorded above. She found preponderantly pleomorphic cancer cells in 21 patients and clusters of cancer cells in 19 of the 23 patients. The observed differences may be caused by a different patient population and a different technical approach to the study of the urinary sediment.

Clinical Handling and Confirmatory Biopsy of Carcinoma In Situ

An **unequivocal cytologic diagnosis of urothelial carcinoma in the absence of cystoscopic evidence of a bladder tumor is usually diagnostic of a flat carcinoma in situ.** This diagnosis is often perplexing to the unsuspecting urologist who must be persuaded to obtain **biopsies** of the bladder, even in the total absence of cystoscopic abnormalities. Although on rare occasions the **cancer cells may reflect a high-grade cancer located in the renal pelvis or ureter,** it is still necessary in such cases **to rule out a bladder lesion first.** This can be fairly efficiently performed by bladder barbotage that provides a good sampling of bladder epithe-

lium with minimal contamination from the upper urinary tract.

Complete mapping of bladders with carcinoma in situ, as shown in Figure 23-22D, gives an excellent idea **of the spread of the lesion and often reveals foci of occult invasion. For obvious reasons, such mapping is not possible in patients whose bladders have not been removed. The closest approximation to mapping is multiple mucosal biopsies of the bladder epithelium** to localize the disease and define its extent. **The biopsies should be obtained with a cutting instrument that does not necessitate cauterization of the biopsy site.**

Besides biopsies of any visible, however trivial, abnormalities, multiple areas of the bladder must be sampled, at least:

- The trigone
- The anterior, posterior and lateral walls
- The dome
- In male patients, deep biopsies of the prostatic bed must be obtained to rule out extension of urothelial cancer into the prostatic ducts. This is of great clinical significance because such patients cannot be effectively treated by immunotherapy, unless the prostatic focus of disease is eradicated first.

Each biopsy should be submitted in a **separate, appro-**

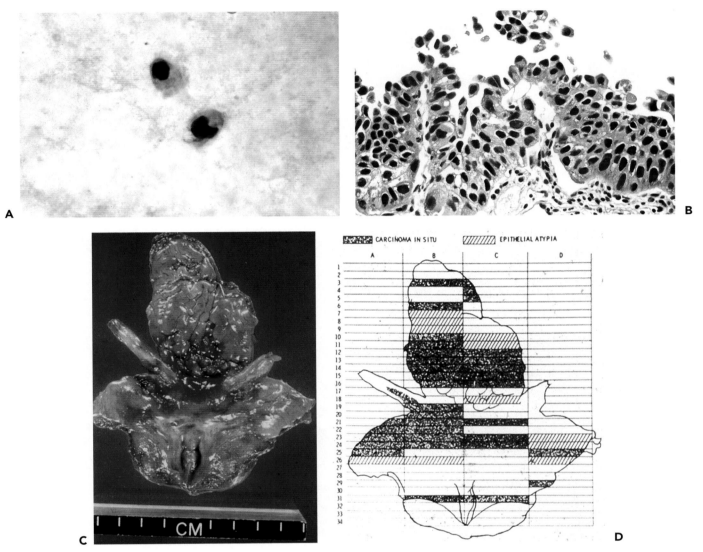

Figure 23-22   Urothelial carcinoma in situ. *A.* Voided urine. Small cancer cells with hyperchromatic nuclei and clean smear background are characteristic of this lesion (high magnification). *B.* Shows the histologic aspect of the extensive carcinoma in situ. In *C,* the gross appearance of the bladder shows areas of redness. *D.* The bladder was mapped showing several areas of carcinoma in situ extending beyond the area of redness, and also an extension of the tumor into the adjacent ureter. (Case courtesy of Dr. Myron R. Melamed, New York Medical College, Valhalla, NY.)

priately labeled bottle with fixative, in order to determine the distribution of the lesion and the location of occult invasion.

Laboratory Handling of Biopsies From Patients Suspected of Harboring Flat Carcinoma In Situ

Because the urothelium with a **carcinoma in situ is often fragile** and readily detached from the underlying stroma, it is important to ascertain **that all biopsy fragments are processed and examined.** DeBellis and Schumann (1986) proposed that **the liquid fixative** in which such biopsies are placed should be **processed by filtration (or cytocentrifuge),** as it may often contain small fragments of cancerous epithelium or detached cancer cells. **The mere absence of the epithelium in a bladder biopsy should raise a suspicion of a carcinoma in situ.** A search must be initiated in multiple cuts of the biopsies for a few **residual attached cancer cells,** now recognized as the **"clinging form of carcinoma in situ."**

As has been discussed in reference to the natural history of carcinoma of the bladder in industrial workers (see above), **the cytologic diagnosis of carcinoma in situ may remain unconfirmed for many years in the absence of an aggressive approach to bladder biopsies.** This has been repeatedly observed **in patients whose primary clinical problem is prostatic disease** and whose bladders did not receive the necessary attention. For further comments on the relationship of prostatic enlargement to bladder cancer, see comments on epidemiology of bladder cancer.

Invasive Nonpapillary Urothelial Carcinoma

In the cytologic preparation, there is usually evidence of **marked inflammation, bleeding, and necrosis.** In fully developed cancer, the predominant **cancer cells are of vari-**

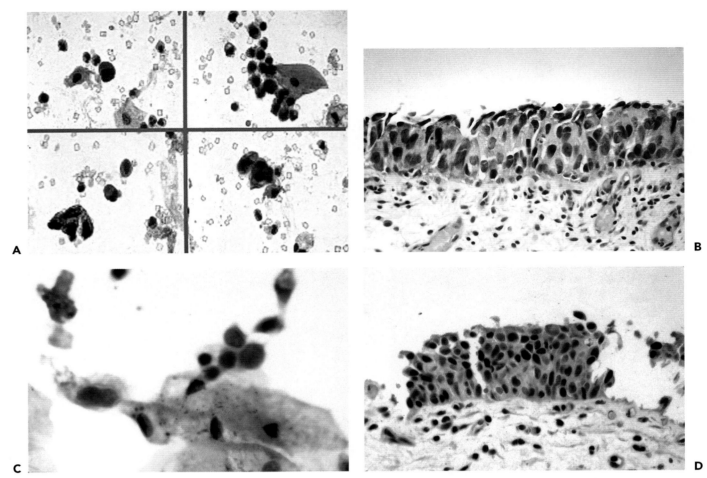

Figure 23-23 Urothelial carcinomas in situ. *A.* Various aspects of small cancer cells in the urinary sediment corresponding to the lesion shown in *B.* The images in *A* were generated by the Papnet device (with permission of TriPath Imaging, Burlington, NC). *C.* Another example of small cancer cells at high magnification in voided urine from a woman older than 30 years with multiple sclerosis and neurogenic bladder, corresponding to the lesion shown in *D.*

able sizes, of irregular configuration, with scanty cytoplasm and prominent, obviously abnormal, hyperchromatic nuclei, similar to cancer cells observed in high-grade papillary tumors (see Figs. 23-14 and 23-21). Although most cancer cells have a basophilic cytoplasm, the presence of **single keratinized cancer cells with eosinophilic cytoplasm is not rare.** Sometimes, early invasive carcinoma may give a smear pattern **identical with carcinoma in situ.** In some advanced cancers with necrotic surface, the yield of cancer cells may be very low.

Histologic Variants of Urothelial Carcinoma

Squamous (Keratinizing) Carcinoma

Histology and Natural History

The presence of a focal squamous component in urothelial carcinoma is a common finding. **Rarely, low-grade papillary tumors may have a squamous component** (see Fig. 23-19B,C). Also, **condylomata acuminata** may be mistaken for squamous carcinoma in situ (see below).

Bladder cancers made up predominantly or exclusively of squamous (keratinizing) cell types are less fre-

quent in the Western world than urothelial carcinomas, although they are **common among patients with *Schistosoma hematobium* infestation** (see Chap. 22 and introductory remarks to this chapter). **It is generally assumed that such tumors originate from areas of squamous metaplasia or leukoplakia,** although this cannot always be conclusively documented. Squamous carcinomas, like urothelial carcinomas, may be **graded** according to the degree of differentiation (Koss, 1975). The very **well-differentiated grade I** variety, which may mimic **verrucous carcinomas** of other organs, is notorious for **local growth and late occurrence of metastases.** Patients with this type of bladder cancer, particularly common in the presence of *Schistosoma,* may **die of uremia** because of obstruction of the urinary tract by tumor.

Squamous cancers of higher grades are fully capable of metastases and may occur not only in the **bladder** but also in the **ureters** and the **renal pelves.**

Cytology

In most cases, the cytologic presentation of squamous carcinoma of the urothelium closely resembles similar lesions of

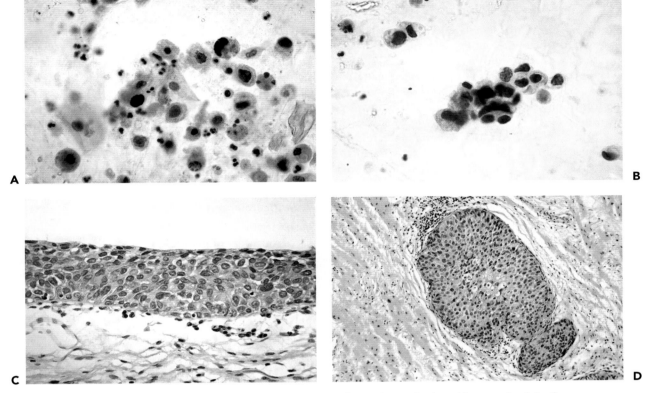

Figure 23-24 **Cytologic and histologic aspects of a carcinoma in situ with extension into the prostatic ducts.** *A,B.* Show scattered small cancer cells with hyperchromatic nuclei. *C.* A representative section of the lesion of the bladder, which was shown by mapping to extend into the prostatic ducts, as shown in *D.*

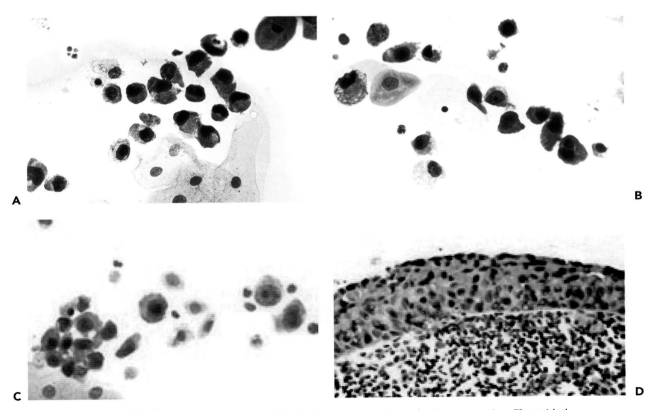

Figure 23-25 **Carcinoma in situ of bladder in characteristic cytologic presentation.** The voided urine sediment smears shown in *A–C* contained a fairly monotonous population of small cancer cells against a clean background. The histology of the lesion is shown in *D.*

the uterine cervix and bronchus (see Chaps. 12 and 20). The tumors shed **squamous cancer cells, some of bizarre configuration, with eosinophilic, often markedly keratinized cytoplasm. The nuclei are pyknotic** and occasionally may be totally submerged by keratin formation, with resulting formation of **"ghost" cells,** not unlike those observed in squamous carcinoma of the lung, described in Chapter 20 (Fig. 23-26). Clusters of cancer cells are common in bladder washings. Similar cells and tumor fragments may be observed in cell block preparations of urinary sediment.

In the **very rare squamous papillary urothelial tumors of low grade, concentrically arranged squamous cells or "squamous pearls"** may occasionally appear in urinary sediment (see Fig. 23-26B). **Condylomata acuminata of the bladder** may mimic the cytologic finding in squamous carcinoma (see below).

In cytologic material from **patients with S. haematobium infestation,** the presence of blood, pus, and necrotic debris may render the diagnosis of squamous bladder cancer very difficult. In fortuitous cases, **fragments of keratinized epithelium next to exceedingly well-differentiated squamous cancer cells** may be observed in the urinary sediment (Fig. 23-27). In a study performed at Memorial Hospital in New York City on urine sediments mailed in plastic bags from Bulawayo, Zimbabwe, the cytologic diagnosis of cancer could be rendered in only 15 of 29 patients with schistosomiasis and proved cancer of the bladder (Houston et al, 1966). Similar observations were made by Dimette (1955) and El-Bolkainy and Chu (1981).

In women, the presence of squamous cancer cells in the sediment of voided urine may indicate the presence of a neoplastic lesion in the female genital tract. The uterine cervix, vagina, or vulva may be the source of such cells.

Adenocarcinoma

Histology and Natural History

Occasional **foci of glandular differentiation in urothelial carcinoma are common.** These focal changes cannot be recognized in cytologic samples. **Primary adenocarcinomas** may occur anywhere in the lower urinary tract, most commonly in the **bladder, but occasionally in the renal pelvis or the ureter. Risk factors** for adenocarcinoma of the lower urinary tract are: **extensive intestinal metaplasia, extrophic bladders** and the benign **villous adenoma, a polypoid lesion lined by intestinal epithelium, similar to lesions observed in the colon** (Koss, 1975; Grignon et al, 1991; Cheng et al, 1999; Oliva et al, 2002). Such tumors

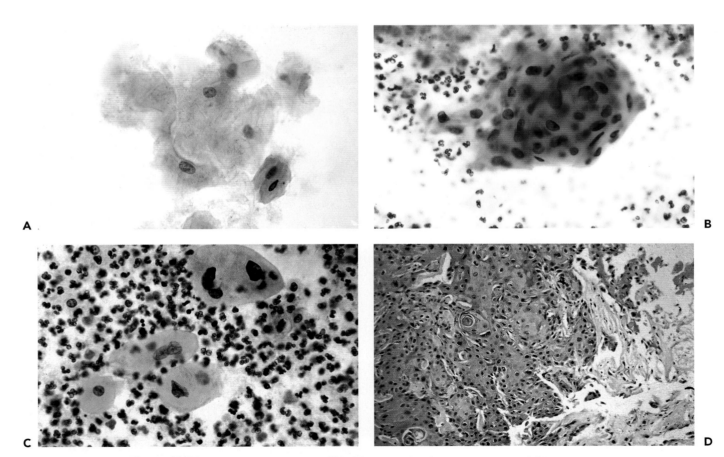

Figure 23-26 **Squamous carcinoma of bladder.** *A–C.* Cytologic presentation of this tumor type in the urinary sediment. In *A*, the sediment shows mainly anucleated squames accompanied by a few squamous cells with essentially normal nuclear features. *B.* A "pearl" of squamous cancer cells. *C.* Dispersed squamous cancer cells in a background of massive inflammation. *D.* A squamous carcinoma of the urinary bladder, corresponding to *A–C.*

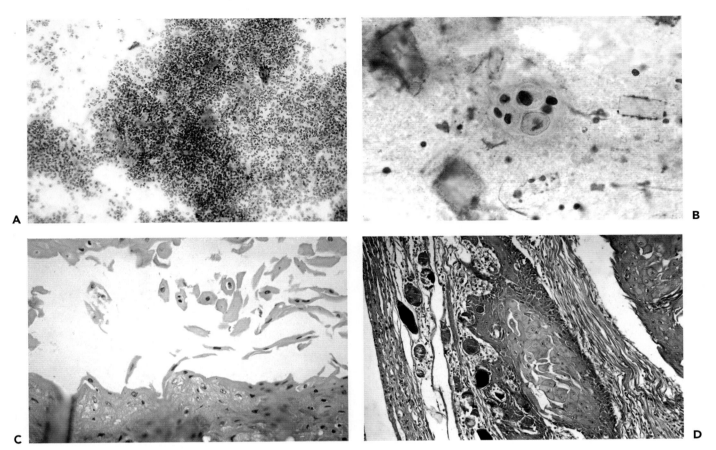

Figure 23-27 Squamous carcinoma of bladder in a patient with schistosomiasis. *A.* Massive inflammatory infiltrate is commonly seen in such patients. *B.* A "pearl" composed of squamous cells with nuclear atypia. *C.* Surface of a tumor composed mainly of anucleated squames. *D.* Wall of the bladder with invasive squamous carcinoma and ova of *Schistosoma hematobium.*

may also arise in **cystitis glandularis** and **nephrogenic adenomas** (see Chap. 22 and below).

Adenocarcinomas of the urothelium are predominantly **of enteric type.** Most such **tumors closely resemble carcinomas of the colon and may be made up of columnar, mucus-producing cells or signet-ring type cancer cells. The signet-ring cell type** typically diffusely infiltrates the wall of the bladder, **resulting in a markedly thickened, rigid bladder wall, or leather-bottle bladder** (see Fig. 23-7D). Rarely, adenocarcinomas may present with **mucinuria, characterized by a viscous appearance of the urine. Adenocarcinoma in situ of the bladder has been observed** (see Fig. 23-29A,B) (Koss, 1975). The rarity of primary, uncomplicated adenocarcinoma in situ was recently emphasized by Chan and Epstein (2001).

Nazeer et al (1996) described an **adenocarcinoma in situ of endocervical type** developing in a case of a woman harboring endocervical type glands in the wall of the bladder.

Bladder adenocarcinomas of **clear cell type,** resembling vaginal lesions occurring in daughters of DES-exposed women (see Chap. 13), may occasionally be observed (Oliva et al, 2002) (see Fig. 23-29C, D). Amin et al (1994) described an exceedingly uncommon type of adenocarcinoma, **resembling ovarian serous carcinoma,** and named it mi-

cropapillary variant of urothelial carcinoma. The prognosis of urothelial adenocarcinoma is stage related but generally poor because metastases may occur early in the course of the disease.

Adenocarcinomas derived from the urachus (remnants of the embryonal omphaloenteric duct) arise in the **dome of the bladder and along the course of the urachus,** terminating at the umbilicus. These tumors have no specific histologic features that would permit their separation from other adenocarcinomas of the lower urinary tract. A patient reported by Hom et al (1990) had an adenocarcinoma with endocrine component.

Cytology

In fortuitous cases, adenocarcinomas can be recognized in the urinary sediment because they shed **cells resembling those of colonic carcinoma.** These are often **columnar in configuration and have large, hyperchromatic nuclei and vacuolated cytoplasm** (Fig. 23-28A,B). Such cells may form **clusters** that may show a **spherical or rosette-like arrangement** (Fig. 23-28C,D). We were fortunate to have observed a rare case of **enteric adenocarcinoma in situ of the bladder. Numerous elongated or columnar cancer cells have been observed in the smear of the urinary sediment** (Fig. 23-29A,B). The cells were very similar to those

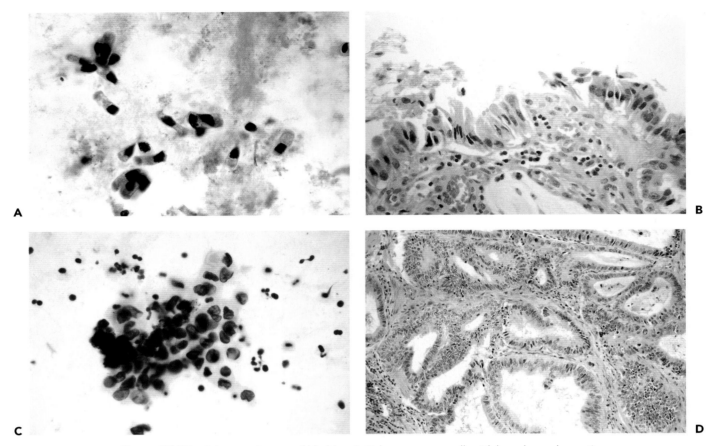

Figure 23-28 Adenocarcinomas of bladder. *A.* Columnar cancer cells with large hyperchromatic nuclei are representative of an adenocarcinoma, shown in *B. C.* A cluster of cancer cells, some of which at the periphery, have columnar configuration. *D.* The well differentiated adenocarcinoma corresponding to *C.*

of a fully developed adenocarcinoma, shown in Figure 23-28.

Occasionally, **somewhat smaller and more spherical cancer cells, with large, peripheral nuclei and vacuolated, mucin-containing cytoplasm, resembling signet-ring type cells of intestinal cancer,** may be observed. The presence of **very small signet ring cells in a woman may also indicate a metastatic mammary lobular carcinoma** (see below). Neither cell type can be differentiated from the cells of metastatic rectal or colonic adenocarcinoma discussed below (see Fig. 23-48). In many cases, however, **the sediment contains undifferentiated cancer cells and adenocarcinoma cannot be identified.** Occasionally, the **presence of mucin** may be observed in the background of the smears in the form of streaks of thick, eosinophilic precipitates. Reports of primary adenocarcinomas of the bladder by Trillo et al (1981) and DeMay and Grathwohl (1985) added no new information. Bardales et al (1998) reported a patient with **urachal adenocarcinoma** whose urinary sediment showed **bland columnar cells** and mucin.

In the rare cases of **clear-cell-type adenocarcinoma, papillary clusters of malignant cells with large nuclei, prominent nucleoli, and clear cytoplasm may be observed** (Fig. 23-29C,D). Similar cases were reported by Peven and Hidvegi (1985) and Doria et al (1996).

Diagnosis of Urothelial Tumors in Special Situations

Lithiasis

As was described in Chapter 22, the urinary sediment in lithiasis may contain numerous papillary clusters of urothelial cells that may be mistaken for a low-grade papillary tumor. Occasionally, lithiasis may also cause some nuclear atypia of urothelial cells. However, **lithiasis is a risk factor and may conceal the presence of a high-grade urothelialcarcinoma.** In the presence of lithiasis, the urinary sediment must be very carefully evaluated. In the presence of significant cellular abnormalities, a coexisting carcinoma must be ruled out.

Urothelial Carcinoma in Diverticula of the Bladder

Several cases of **urothelial carcinoma originating in outpouchings or diverticula of the bladder** have been observed in this laboratory (Fig. 23-30). The **cytologic presentation** of these lesions was identical to other urothelial cancers. However, the clinical localization of the lesions to a diverticulum proved to be difficult. It must be kept in mind that diverticula may have a very inconspicuous opening into the bladder, readily overlooked on cystoscopy.

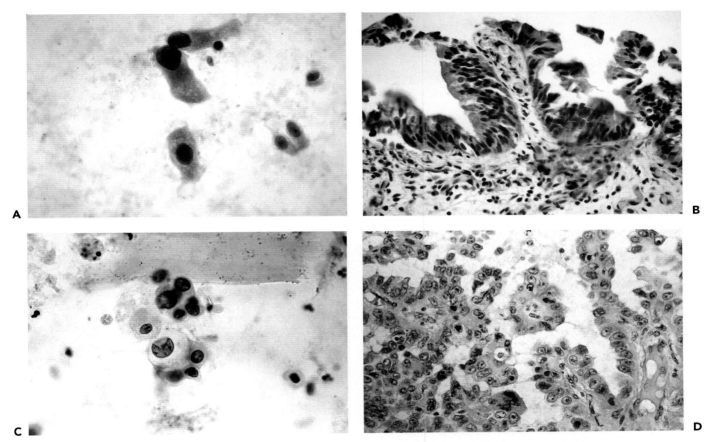

Figure 23-29   **Adenocarcinoma in situ.** *A.* Tall, columnar cells with nuclear enlargement and hyperchromasia correspond to the tumor on the surface of the bladder shown in *B. C,D.* Clear cell adenocarcinoma. *C* shows clusters of small cancer cells with clear cytoplasm, corresponding to the tumor shown in *D.*

Carcinoma of the Bladder and Prostatic Disease
In situ and invasive carcinomas of the bladder may occur in patients with prostatic enlargement, caused either by prostatic carcinoma or hyperplasia (Barlebo and Sorensen, 1972; Mahadevia et al, 1986). In such cases, the cancer cells are those of urothelial carcinomas, described above. The issue is discussed in the opening pages of this chapter.

UNCOMMON TUMOROUS CONDITIONS AND TUMORS OF THE BLADDER

Tumorous Conditions

Papillomatosis of Bladder
This is a rare disorder in which the entire surface of the bladder is covered with innumerable papillary fronds lined by essentially normal or minimally atypical urothelium. The condition is extremely difficult to treat conservatively and may require mucosal stripping or cystectomy (Lund, 1969). Little is known about the natural history of untreated papillomatosis (Koss, 1975). The lesion cannot be recognized cytologically.

Nephrogenic Adenoma (Adenosis of Bladder)
This uncommon lesion is composed of ducts and tubules, possibly of enteric origin (Koss, 1985, 1995). There are

two reports suggesting that nephrogenic adenomas may be recognized in urinary sediment. Stilmant et al (1986) reported the presence of markedly abnormal cells in four patients. Three of the patients, however, had documented bladder cancer with carcinoma in situ. The cells shown in the illustrations could well have originated from the malignant epithelium. Troster et al (1986) observed papillary urothelial clusters in the urine of one patient. The clusters had no specific features. It is **doubtful that nephrogenic adenoma can be recognized in urinary sediment.** However, **adenocarcinomas may develop in such lesions** and may shed cancer cells (see above).

Endometriosis
Endometriosis of the lower urinary tract, particularly of the bladder, is a rare condition in young women that may cause symptoms similar to those caused by a tumor. Schneider et al (1980) reported clusters of **endometrial cells in voided urine** in a case of endometriosis of the bladder (Fig. 23-31A,B). There were some similarities between cells from endometriosis and metastatic endometrial carcinoma (Fig. 23-31C). Bohlmeyer and Schroyer (1996), in reporting another case, pointed out that the endometrial cells in clusters in voided urine may be mistaken for cells of a urothelial carcinoma.

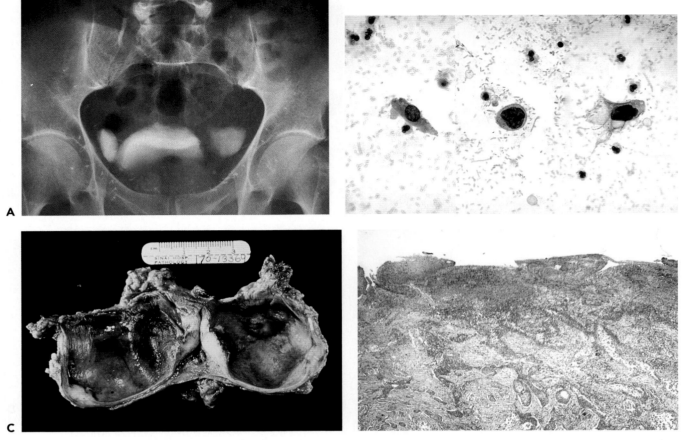

Figure 23-30   Carcinoma originating in bladder diverticulum. *A.* X-ray of bladder showing two diverticula, one of which contained a malignant tumor, shown in *C. B.* Composite picture of cancer cells from the voided urine sediment. *D.* Shows invasive carcinoma of bladder observed in the resected diverticulum shown in *C.*

Eosinophilic Granuloma

The disorder is discussed in Chapter 19. The rare eosinophilic granuloma may occur in the bladder or ureter. Because the lesion is subepithelial, there are no known specific cytologic findings.

Amyloidosis

Large deposits of amyloid in the wall of the bladder may elicit a granulomatous reaction with foreign body giant cells mimicking a tumor (Koss, 1975). There is no record of this diagnosis in either urine sediment or in direct aspirates of bladder wall.

Benign Tumors

Condylomata Acuminata

Condylomata acuminata may occasionally be observed in the urinary bladder (Koss, 1975). Petterson et al (1976) observed two such tumors in immunosuppressed patients following a renal transplant. With the passage of time, additional tumors of this type have been observed (summary in Del Mistro et al, 1988). **Condylomas of the bladder are often associated with condylomas of external genitalia, but may also occur as discrete tumors.** De Paepe et al

(1990) observed several such incidental lesions **in women with urothelial cancer of the bladder.**

In a report from this laboratory, three patients with bladder condylomas were studied in depth (Del Mistro et al, 1988). By in situ hybridization, the **presence of HPV types 6 and 11** was documented. The tumors are very difficult to treat and have a marked tendency to recur. Follow-up information on one of the patients studied by Del Mistro et al, strongly suggested that the lesion progressed to an invasive and metastatic squamous carcinoma of the bladder. **Progression of condylomata acuminata of the bladder to the verrucous variant of squamous carcinoma** has been reported by several other observers (Walther et al, 1986; Tenti et al, 1996; Bruske et al, 1997; Botella et al, 2000). In the case described by Botella, HPV type 11 was documented in the condyloma and the subsequent carcinoma.

It is of note that the **DNA content of the bladder condylomas is aneuploid,** an observation confirmed by Cheng et al (2000).

Histology

The tumors, composed of folds of squamous epithelium, resemble genital condylomata acuminata, characterized by the presence of **koilocytes in the superficial epithelial lay-**

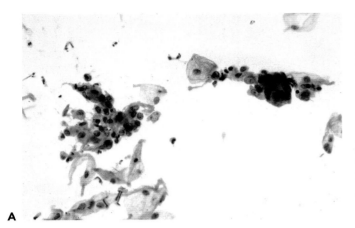

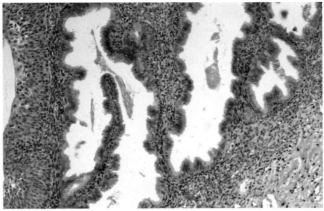

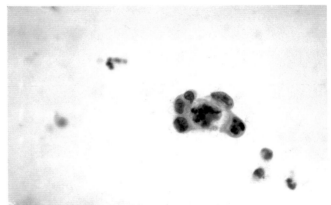

Figure 23-31   Endometriosis of bladder and metastatic endometrial carcinoma in bladder. *A.* Two clusters of small endometrial cells. *B.* Histologic section of bladder corresponding to *A* with an area of endometriosis. *C.* A small cluster of cells with vacuolated cytoplasm from an endometrial carcinoma, metastatic to bladder. (*A,B*: Courtesy of Dr. Volker Schneider, Freiburg I/B, Germany.)

ers. For a description of condylomas, see Chapter 11. In some tumors, marked **nuclear abnormalities** may be observed in epithelial cells (see Fig. 23-32D).

Cytology

In voided urine, **koilocyte-like cells can be observed** (Fig. 23-32A). For a definition and description of koilocytes, see Chapter 11. **In a female patient, the possibility of origin of these cells in the uterine cervix must be ruled out. In male patients, such cells may originate in penile urethra** (see below). Hartveit et al (1992) reported the presence of koilocytes in the urinary sediment of numerous patients with a variety of bladder lesions but we were unable to duplicate this experience.

More importantly, perhaps, in two of our three patients, the urinary sediment contained **large, highly abnormal squamous cells with keratinized cytoplasm and large, hyperchromatic and pyknotic nuclei** (Fig. 23-32B,C). "Cell-in-cell" arrangement was observed. Although in some of the cells perinuclear halos suggested a similarity to koilocytes, such cells were very **difficult to distinguish from cells of squamous carcinoma** (see Figs. 23-26 and 23-27). In the 3rd edition of this book, a lesion of the bladder with similar cytologic presentation was classified as **"squamous carcinoma in situ."** The question of whether this lesion represented a flat condyloma of the bladder or, in fact, a squamous carcinoma cannot be resolved in the absence of HPV hybridization and follow-up information. Clearly,

condylomata acuminata of the urinary bladder straddle the border between benign and malignant tumors, not unlike similar precancerous lesions of the uterine cervix (see Chap. 11 for further discussion of cervical lesions).

Squamous Papilloma of Bladder

Cheng et al (2000) described five squamous papillomas of the bladder and two of the urethra. The lesions failed to hybridize with HPV DNA and were diploid. These benign lesions are extremely rare and there is no information on their cytologic presentation.

Inverted Papilloma

An uncommon tumor of the urinary bladder, somewhat similar to a papilloma with a flat surface, was first described by Potts and Hirst in 1963. An uninterrupted layer of normal urothelium lines the surface of the tumor, which is made up of anastomosing strands of urothelium (Koss, 1975). The tumor is benign and there are **no known cytologic abnormalities associated with it.** An exceptional case of a malignant transformation of this tumor has been reported (Koss, 1985).

Villous Adenoma

Villous adenoma is a rare tumor of bladder of enteric origin that resembles similar tumors of the colon and rectum (Koss, 1975). There are **no known cell abnormalities in the urinary tract associated with this disorder.** Cheng et

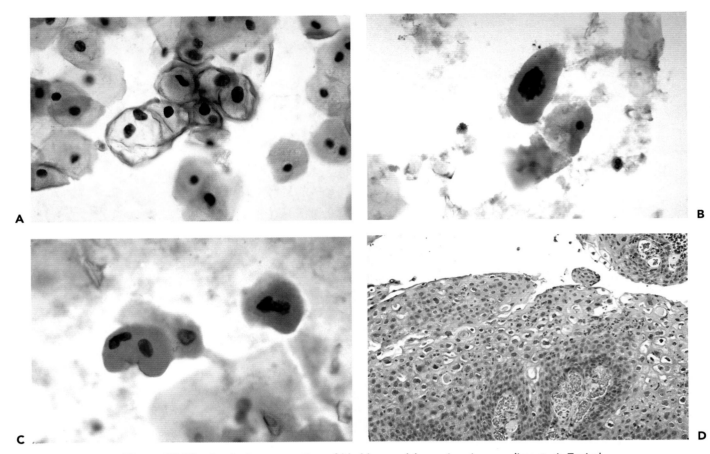

Figure 23-32 Cytologic presentation of bladder condylomas in urinary sediment. *A.* Typical koilocytes, a rather unusual finding. *B,C.* Various aspects of markedly atypical squamous cells derived from condyloma shown in *D.* The cells seen in *B* and *C* could be readily interpreted as squamous cancer cells.

al (1999) observed these uncommon tumors in the urachus, the dome, and the trigone of the bladder, and pointed out their **association with adenocarcinoma of the bladder** in 8 of 23 patients. Similar observations were reported by Seibel et al (2002). For discussion of cytologic findings in adenocarcinoma, see above.

Tumors With Malignant Potential

Pheochromocytoma (Paraganglioma)

Histology and Clinical Presentation

These endocrine tumors, classically composed of **nests or cords of large, eosinophilic epithelial calls** (Zellballen), separated from each other by thin mantles of richly vascularized connective tissue, produce hormones, the **catecholamines,** that may cause episodes of paroxysmal hypertension on voiding. The serum levels of metabolites of catecholamines, such as vanilmandelic acid (VMA), are usually elevated and, combined with a history of "fainting in the bathroom," a consequence of episodes of paroxysmal hypertension, will lead to the diagnosis. Most of these tumors are benign but malignant variants are known to occur (summary in Koss, 1975).

Cytology

Because these tumors are located within the wall of the bladder, there are no recorded cases of tumor cells in voided urine. Through the courtesy of Dr. Miguel Sanchez, we examined an aspiration smear in a case of malignant pheochromocytoma of bladder, mimicking a retroperitoneal tumor. Clusters of **large cells with abundant eosinophilic, granular cytoplasm** and inconspicuous **spherical nuclei** were observed. As is common in endocrine tumors, **much larger cells with single or multiple hyperchromatic nuclei** were scattered among the mononucleated cells (Fig. 23-33).

Carcinoids

Carcinoids of the bladder are morphologically identical to similar tumors occurring in the gastrointestinal tract and the lung and are composed of **sheets and ribbons of small cells, sometimes forming glands** (see Chaps. 20 and 24). Although usually benign, these tumors may display **malignant behavior,** as in the example cited by Koss (1985). There is no record of cytologic findings in bladder carcinoids but it may be assumed that the cytologic presentation would be similar to that of carcinoids in other organs, described in Chapters 20 and 24.

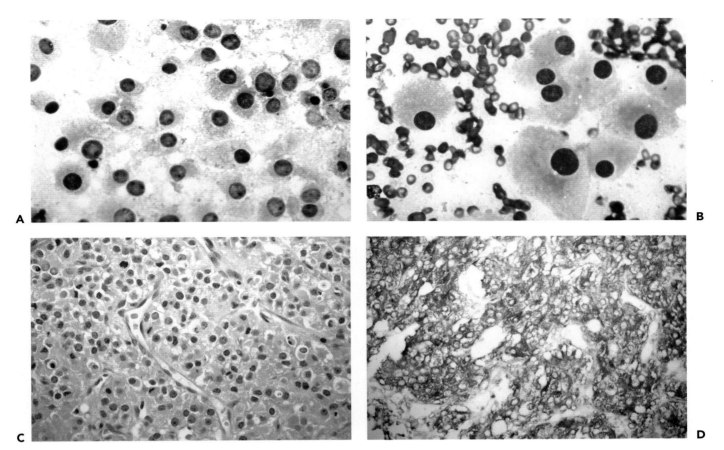

Figure 23-33   **Pheochromocytoma of bladder, metastatic to the retroperitoneum.** *A.* An aspiration smear of the retroperitoneal mass was composed of tumor cells of moderate size with granular cytoplasm. *B.* Tumor cells in air-dried smear stained with Giemsa, which enhances the granularity of the cytoplasm. *C.* The make-up of the tumor composed of "Zellballen." *D.* Positive stain with synaptophysin. Case courtesy of Dr. Miguel Sanchez, Englewood, NJ.

Malignant Tumors

Synchronous Carcinoma of the Bladder and Prostate (Uroprostatic Carcinoma)

Such tumors were recognized mainly in the European literature as **"transitional cell carcinomas of the prostate"** (Algaba et al, 1985), **"urothelial carcinomas in or of the prostate"** (Dhom and Mohr, 1977; Schujman et al, 1983; Goebbels et al, 1985). Dhom and Mohr, who reviewed the largest number of these cases, pointed out that when these tumors synchronously involved the bladder and the prostate, their prognosis was poor.

We observed three patients with this uncommon malignant tumor **that combined the features of primary bladder and prostate cancers.** In one of the patients, age 52, the disease was **first diagnosed on urinary sediment that indicated a high-grade urothelial cancer, which was confirmed by biopsy as a carcinoma in situ.** Subsequent biopsies of the enlarged prostate disclosed a **poorly differentiated malignant tumor** that combined with a **high level of prostate-specific antigen** in the serum, was considered to be a prostatic carcinoma and was treated with testosterone antagonists (Fig. 23-34). The patient died 2 years later with disseminated metastases. The outcome in the other two patients is not known as yet at the time of this writing. Genega

et al (2000) described an elaborate system of immunotyping to separate high-grade urothelial carcinomas from similar carcinomas of prostatic origin. It may well be that some of these tumors studied by Genega belong to the category of uroprostatic carcinomas.

Small-Cell (Oat Cell) Carcinomas

Small-cell carcinomas are either **pure,** composed of sheets and ribbons of small malignant cells akin to the oat cell carcinoma of the lung (see Chap. 20), or **mixed,** with either solid urothelial carcinomas or adenocarcinomas. The **endocrine features** of these tumors can be demonstrated either by immunomarkers or by electron microscopy (Cramer et al, 1981; Mills et al, 1987; Grignon et al, 1992). In some of these tumors, a **urothelial carcinoma in situ** can be documented, strongly suggesting that the tumors are variants of urothelial cancer (Koss, 1985). Some of these tumors may have ectopic hormonal activity (Partanen and Asikainen, 1985). These tumors have poor prognosis.

Cytology

Although **small-cell carcinomas** are uncommon, their cytology has been repeatedly described in recent years (van Hoeven

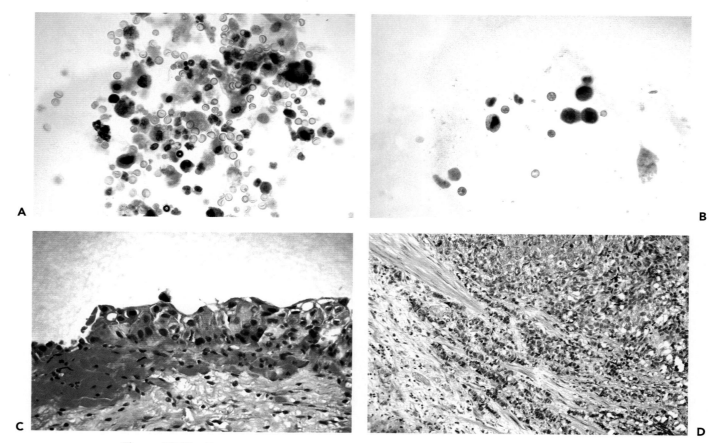

Figure 23-34   Uroprostatic carcinoma. *A,B.* Urinary sediment contained a large number of small cancer cells, corresponding to carcinoma in situ shown in *C. D.* Shows a synchronous, poorly differentiated prostatic carcinoma that resulted in the patient's death within two years.

and Artymyshyn, 1996; Ali et al, 1997; Acs et al, 2000). The **tumor cells are small, about two or three times larger than normal lymphocytes, are usually of approximately equal sizes and appear singly or in small chains and clusters,** wherein **molding** of adjacent cells can be observed. The **cytoplasm is very scanty,** often not visible. The relatively large **nuclei** show **fine granularity. Nucleoli are absent or very small** (see Fig. 23-14D). In some cases, **larger cancer cells corresponding to urothelial carcinoma** can be present next to the small cancer cells. The differential diagnosis includes other malignant tumors composed of small cells, such as malignant lymphomas, which, however, rarely form organized clusters or show molding of adjacent cells. For further discussion of malignant lymphoma, see below.

Spindle and Giant Cell Carcinomas

These tumors are uncommon and there are few reported cases in the literature (Holtz et al, 1972). We observed one such tumor in the wall of a bladder diverticulum. Although the diagnosis of a malignant tumor can be easily established in the urinary sediment, the exact identification of such exceedingly rare tumors is rarely, if ever, possible. **Pseudosarcomatous spindly pattern** observed in urothelial cancer was illustrated in Figure 23-7C. A case of **carcinosarcoma,** arising in a bladder diverticulum, was reported by Omeroglu et al (2002).

Urothelial Carcinomas Mimicking Plasmocytomas

Sahin et al (1991) described an unusual **malignant urothelial tumor of the bladder mimicking multiple myeloma, wherein the tumor cells, aspirated from a skull metastasis, were similar to plasma cells.** A similar case was reported by Zhang et al (2002).

Mesodermal Mixed Tumors (Heterologous Carcinosarcomas)

These exceedingly rare variants of urothelial carcinomas of the urinary bladder closely **resemble similar tumors observed in the female genital tract** (see Chap. 17). In a case observed by us, the **urinary sediment contained a mixture of malignant cells,** some of which had **features of urothelial carcinoma** and others had features suggesting a chondrosarcoma (Fig. 23-35).

Lymphoepithelioma-Like Carcinoma

These exceedingly uncommon tumors of the bladder are similar to nasopharyngeal tumors, described in Chapter 21 (Dinney, 1993; Amin et al, 1994). There is no information on the cytologic presentation of these tumors.

Nested Variant of Urothelial Carcinoma

This is an uncommon type of urothelial cancer with insidious onset. The tumor is difficult to recognize in biopsies

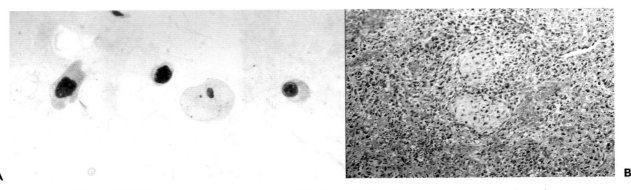

Figure 23-35   **Mesodermal mixed tumor of bladder.** *A.* The urinary sediment contained poorly differentiated cancer cells, corresponding to the mesodermal mixed tumor shown in *B.* In this area, the tumor was composed of poorly differentiated stroma and areas of cartilage. Elsewhere, the tumor contained elements of urothelial carcinoma that was in situ and invasive.

because of its **deceptively benign presentation:** it is composed of nests and gland-like formations of urothelial cells that are approximately cuboidal and have only moderately enlarged, hyperchromatic nuclei (Talbert and Young, 1989; Murphy and Deana, 1992; Billerey et al, 1999). When recognized, the tumor is often deeply invasive and this most likely accounts for its poor prognosis. Volmar et al (2003) pointed out the similarity of these tumors to florid proliferation of Brunn's nests, discussed in Chapter 22. The nested carcinoma apparently is derived from surface epithelium that is only minimally atypical and does not show any evidence of carcinoma in situ or related lesions (Young and Oliva, 1966; recently confirmed by Dr. Victor Reuter, MSKCC, personal communication). It is therefore not surprising that **cytology** of these tumors is **nondiagnostic.** Cardillo et al (2003) examined 13 urine sediments from 7 patients and reported that in nearly all cases, the tumor cells could not be differentiated from normal urothelial cells. The observed changes consisted of only trivial nuclear abnormalities such as slight nuclear enlargement, irregular nuclear contour and slight hyperchromasia. Enlarged nucleoli were occasionally observed. The authors concluded that one should not attempt to diagnose this tumor in cytologic preparations.

Sarcomas of the Bladder

These are mainly **rhabdomyosarcomas and leiomyosarcomas** (Koss, 1975) that occasionally shed cancer cells in urine. Krumerman and Katatikaru (1976) described a case of a **rhabdomyosarcoma** with intraepithelial spread in an adult. Generally, cells of sarcomas in the urinary sediment have malignant features, but usually cannot be accurately identified in the absence of prior histologic diagnosis or clinical history, including the age of the patient.

In children, **embryonal rhabdomyosarcomas (botryoid sarcomas)** of the vulva, vagina, prostate, and urinary bladder may occur. For an extensive discussion of these tumors, see Chapter 17. In Figure 23-36A,B, the cytologic findings in voided urine in a case of **botryoid embryonal rhabdomyosarcoma of bladder in a child** are illustrated. The small cancer cells have no distinguishing features and could not be further classified, except by comparison with

histology. By contrast, spindly cancer cells of adult forms of rhabdomyosarcoma may show cytoplasmic striations (Fig. 23-36C,D).

A case of **primary angiosarcoma** of the bladder was reported by Schindler et al (1999) in an aspirated sample.

Malignant Lymphomas

Cells of the very rare primary malignant lymphoma of the urinary bladder cannot be differentiated from the cells of systemic tumors of the same type, involving the lower urinary tract (see below). A case of **synchronous lymphoma and adenocarcinoma** of bladder was described by Stitt and Colapinto (1966).

Primary Melanomas

Primary melanomas of the bladder are exceedingly rare. Khalbuss et al (2001) described such a case in an 82-year-old woman and summarized prior literature. In a personally observed case, the sediment of voided urine contained rare malignant cells with large nuclei and prominent nucleoli, some containing brown melanin pigment in the cytoplasm. Phagocytized pigment was also observed in macrophages (Fig. 23-37).

Multiple Myeloma

Unusual primary carcinomas of bladder with cells mimicking plasma cells were mentioned above (Sahin et al, 1991; Zhang et al, 2002). We have not observed cells of a plasma cell myeloma in urinary sediment, although such cases were described by Auvigne et al (1956) and by Pringle et al (1974). However, **bizarre, multinucleated cells of renal tubular origin, a result of a so-called myeloma kidney,** may occur in the urinary sediment and are discussed below, in reference to voided urine cytology of the kidney.

Choriocarcinoma

Sporadic cases of primary choriocarcinoma of bladder in males have been reported (Weinberg, 1939). Such a case

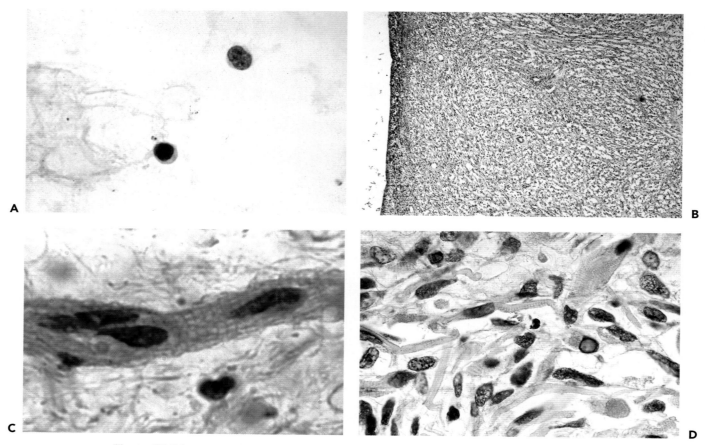

Figure 23-36 **Myosarcomas of bladder.** *A.* Small cancer cells observed at high magnification in urinary sediment from a child with botryoid sarcoma of bladder shown in *B. C,D.* Another example of botryoid sarcoma in a 9-year-old boy. The large cancer cells show cytoplasmic cross-striations in a smear (*C*) and tissue (*D*). (Oil immersion.)

was reported from this laboratory (Obe et al, 1983). The sediment of voided urine contained numerous malignant cells, most of which resembled cells of **urothelial carcinoma** but some that were **large and multinucleated, with large nuclei and nucleoli, consistent with syncytiotrophoblasts** (Fig. 23-38). The tumor and its cells gave a strongly positive reaction for human **chorionic gonadotro-**

pin. Because the tumor was accompanied by a **flat urothelial carcinoma in situ,** it most probably represented an **unusual transformation of a urothelial carcinoma.** Yokoyama et al (1992) reported one case of primary and one case of metastatic choriocarcinoma in the bladder with similar findings. The primary tumor was also accompanied by a carcinoma in situ.

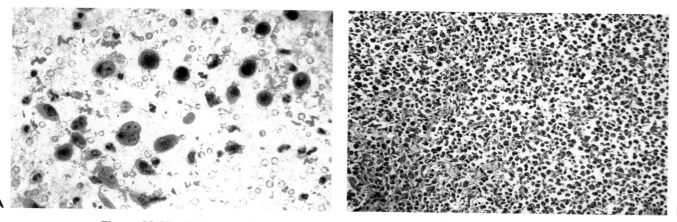

Figure 23-37 **Malignant melanoma primary in the bladder.** *A.* The urinary sediment contained scattered cancer cells and large macrophages filled with melanin pigment. *B.* Histologic section of the primary tumor.

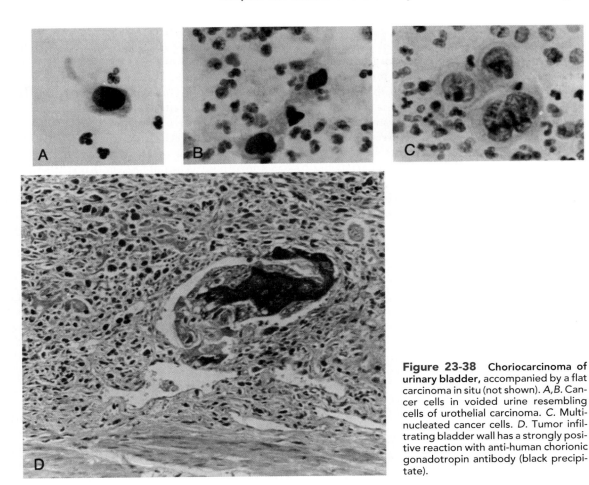

Figure 23-38 **Choriocarcinoma of urinary bladder**, accompanied by a flat carcinoma in situ (not shown). *A,B.* Cancer cells in voided urine resembling cells of urothelial carcinoma. *C.* Multinucleated cancer cells. *D.* Tumor infiltrating bladder wall has a strongly positive reaction with anti-human chorionic gonadotropin antibody (black precipitate).

Tumors Most Likely Induced by Chemotherapy

Rare tumors of the urinary tract apparently induced by **cyclophosphamide** were discussed in Chapter 22.

TUMORS OF THE RENAL PELVES AND THE URETERS

Natural History and Pathology of Urothelial Tumors

Primary urothelial tumors of the renal pelves and ureters encompass the full scale of urothelial tumors described in the bladder and can be either **papillary or nonpapillary in type.** The most frequent clinical symptom is hematuria, sometimes associated with evidence of renal failure. These tumors may be unilateral or bilateral. The bilateral tumors may occur simultaneously or in sequence and create a major diagnostic and therapeutic dilemma. Four patients with bilateral renal pelvic carcinomas were observed by us over a period of 2 years.

In most patients, **carcinomas of the renal pelves or ureters are synchronous or metachronous with urothelial tumors of the bladder.** In a series of 41 patients with carcinoma of the renal pelvis and ureters, 50% of the patients developed bladder tumors (Kakizoe et al, 1980). Herr et al (1996) reported upper urinary tract tumors in 18 of 86 patients (21%) with primary bladder tumors followed for

15 years (median 7.3 years). In 5 patients, the tumors occurred 10 to 15 years after treatment of the primary bladder neoplasm. **The sequence of events cannot be anticipated** and the presence of tumors in one of these locations must automatically trigger the search for other tumors. These patients require long-term follow-up in which cytology of urinary sediment plays a major role (Smart, 1964; Sherwood, 1971; Koss, 1979, Herr et al, 1996). **Urothelial carcinoma in situ of distal ureters is a common finding in extensive, high-grade urothelial carcinomas of the bladder** (summary in Koss, 1975; Koss et al, 1977).

Primary urothelial carcinomas of the renal pelves and ureters have also been observed **in association with use and abuse of analgesic drugs containing phenacetin.** Although most of the reported cases originated in Scandinavian countries, sporadic observations on this association have been recorded in other countries as well (Johansson et al, 1974; Mihatsch, 1979; Lomax-Smith and Seymour, 1980). An important **corollary of phenacetin toxicity is papillary necrosis of renal cortex,** which occurs in more than half of the patients. Carcinomas of the renal pelvis and ureters in patients receiving **cyclophosphamide** therapy have been recorded (see Chap. 22). It must be pointed out that the drug **busulfan** is capable of inducing major changes in renal pelvic epithelium that may mimic a carcinoma in situ (see Chap. 22 and Burry, 1974).

Mahadevia et al (1983) mapped seven high-grade urothelial carcinomas of the renal pelvis and two of the ureters and observed **peripheral atypical urothelium (dysplasia) in five patients and flat carcinoma in situ in four patients** (Fig. 23-39). Hence, it may be assumed that the sequence of events in renal pelvic and ureteral tumors is exactly the same as in the bladder. The findings were similar to the observations by Chasko et al (1981). **Extensive urothelial carcinoma in situ and related abnormalities were also observed in analgesic users** (Lomax-Smith and Seymour, 1980).

A few cases of **primary nonpapillary carcinoma in situ of the renal pelvis** diagnosed by cytology were recorded

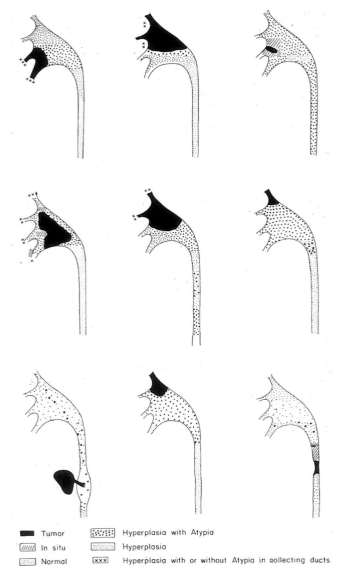

■ Tumor   ▦ Hyperplasia with Atypia
▨ In situ   ▨ Hyperplasia
▨ Normal   xxx Hyperplasia with or without Atypia in collecting ducts

Figure 23-39 **Mapping of seven carcinomas of the renal pelvis and two of the ureter.** The distribution of the various levels of epithelial abnormalities is shown. It may be noted that the areas of carcinoma in situ and epithelial atypia (UIN II) accompany every tumor. Tumor extension into the renal collecting tubules was observed in six of the seven carcinomas of renal pelves. (From Mahadevia PS, Karwa GL, Koss LG. Mapping of urothelium in carcinomas of the renal pelvis and ureter: A report of nine cases. Cancer 51: 890–897, 1983.)

(Papanicolaou and Foote, 1949; Murphy et al, 1974; Stagier et al, 1980; Dodd et al, 1997). I have also observed one such case by courtesy of Dr. Harold Block of El Paso, Texas (see below).

Fromowitz et al (1981) reported from this laboratory on two cases of **inverted papillomas** of the ureter. **The report was in error** because one of the tumors recurred with features of urothelial carcinoma, grade II. The second patient developed an adenocarcinoma of bladder. As was stated in a subsequent publication (Koss, 1985), **papillary urothelial tumors of the ureter** may develop a flat surface, probably for anatomic reasons, and **mimic an inverted papilloma.** Such tumors may be the source of the occasional reports of positive cytologic findings in benign inverted papilloma.

Grading and Prognosis

The **grading** is identical with that of urothelial cancers of the bladder (see above). Large, high-grade tumors have a poor prognosis. Although renal pelvic carcinomas are theoretically fully curable by surgery if diagnosed early, the mortality in the Johansson's series of 62 patients (1974) was in excess of 50%. The results were not significantly improved in a more recent series of cases (Guinan et al, 1992; Herr et al, 1996). A major factor complicating cure by surgery is the occurrence of tumors elsewhere in the urinary tract.

The prognosis of urothelial tumors of renal pelves or ureters depends primarily on **stage** of the disease, although tumor size and grade may play a role (Grabstald et al, 1971; Herr et al, 1996). Tumors invading through the wall of the renal pelvis or ureter have an ominous prognosis (Grabstald et al, 1971). The presence of carcinoma in situ in Mahadevia's study was of prognostic significance, inasmuch as two of four such patients developed metachronous carcinoma of the bladder, and one died of disseminated cancer. One of five patients with peripheral atypical urothelium also developed a tumor of the bladder. Weaver et al (2001) attempted to differentiate invasive from noninvasive urothelial carcinomas of the upper urinary tract by staining the cytologic samples with antibodies to CD 20 and CD 44 with uncertain results.

Adenocarcinoma and Carcinoid

Adenocarcinoma of the renal pelvis has been observed by us in a young woman with extensive **intestinal metaplasia of the renal pelvis and ureter. Mucinuria** may accompany such tumors. Sporadic cases of this tumor type have been reported in the literature (Bardales et al, 1998). A **carcinoid tumor** of renal pelvis was reported by Rudrick et al (1995).

Squamous Carcinoma

Sporadic cases of keratinizing squamous carcinoma of the renal pelves have been recorded, sometimes in association with lithiasis of long-standing, causing **squamous metaplasia.** Several such cases have been reported in Japanese literature.

Cytology

As discussed at length in Chapter 22, **the principal purpose of cytologic examination of the upper urinary tract is to determine whether the space-occupying lesion is a tumor or a benign abnormality.** Most patients are symptomatic, often with gross **hematuria.** Radiologic examination, either as intravenous or retrograde pyelograms or computed tomography may disclose the location and the size of the lesion though, occasionally, no definite lesion can be identified. The **principal lesions that must be considered in the differential diagnosis are:**

- Tumors
- Stones
- Blood clots
- Very rarely, anatomic or vascular abnormalities

Heedless of the limitations of the method in low-grade papillary urothelial neoplasms, the urologists not familiar with the benefits of voided urine will often attempt to secure samples by direct approach, either by brushings or by retrograde washings, barbotage, or by material obtained during ureteroscopy. Unless they are very skilled, many of the attempts at direct sampling will give unsatisfactory results. **Therefore, we strongly recommend that the first approach to the cytologic examination of the upper urinary tract should be by voided urine samples.** The meth-ods were discussed in Chapter 22, where an analysis of cytologic findings is discussed according to the method of collection.

Voided Urine

Cytologic presentation of **primary renal pelvic and ureteral urothelial tumors** is identical to tumors of the bladder (see above). Except for unusual conditions, discussed above, the **well-differentiated papillary urothelial tumors cannot be securely identified.** In high-grade urothelial carcinomas, the **population of malignant cells is sometimes surprisingly abundant** and readily identified (Fig. 23-40). The presence of a few **malignant cells of squamous type is common** in urothelial tumors. Such cells predominate in the rare **keratinizing carcinomas.**

In Mahadevia's study of **carcinomas of the renal pelves,** cited above, the urinary sediment disclosed **cancer cells in four of nine patients,** all with grade II or higher cancers. The sediment was considered **suspicious in three additional patients, atypical in one,** and was not examined in one.

Cytologic findings in a case of **adenocarcinoma of the renal pelvis** occurring in the **background of intestinal metaplasia,** were reported by Kobayashi et al (1985) and Yonekawa et al (2000). The findings suggested an adenocarcinoma because of the presence of clusters of cancer cells with **cytoplasmic vacuoles,** giving a positive stain for

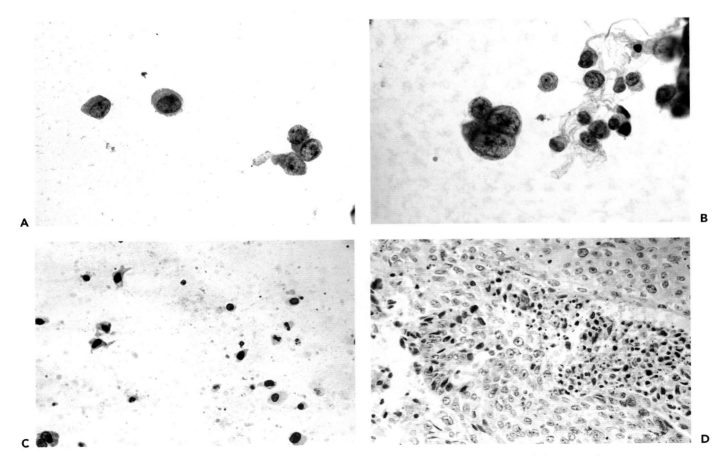

Figure 23-40   Renal pelvic carcinoma. *A,B.* The urinary sediment contained urothelial cancer cells of variable sizes corresponding to the pelvic tumor. *C.* Voided urine sediment (scanning power) containing small cancer cells corresponding to the tumor of renal pelvis shown in *D.*

mucin. **Mucinuria** may occur and may be recognized in smears of urinary sediment by thick, fibrillar eosinophilic background (Bardales et al, 1998).

In a malignant **carcinoid tumor** of renal pelvis, polygonal malignant cells with large nuclei and occasional nucleoli were observed in urine by Rudrick et al (1995).

Other rare tumors of the renal pelves, such as a **leiomyosarcoma** (Chow et al, 1994), were identified in fine-needle aspiration biopsies (FNA). See Chapter 40 for further comments on FNA of renal tumors.

Retrograde Catheterization

Cytologic examination of urine obtained by retrograde catheterization of ureters should be used for the purpose of localization of a high-grade tumor to either the left or right urether or renal pelvis. Such events **are rare** and occur under the following conditions:

- The patient's voided urinary sediment contains unequivocal cancer cells, consistent with a high-grade tumor, and there is no evidence of a bladder lesion.
- The roentgenologic examination of the urinary tract is either negative or inconclusive.
- It is not clear whether the tumor is located in the left or right renal pelvis or ureter.

As an example, **a selective catheterization procedure** was applied to the diagnosis of an **occult carcinoma in situ of the right renal pelvis** in an 80-year-old woman with hematuria, absence of roentgenologic abnormalities, a negative cystoscopy, and with abundant evidence of a high-grade carcinoma in voided urine (Fig. 23-41B–D).

As described in Chapter 22, **the urine specimens must be collected separately for each side** and great care must be exercised to avoid cross-contamination of the samples.

The cytologic findings are usually **complex because an abundant population of benign urothelial cells, occurring singly and in clusters, may obscure the presence of malignant cells** (see Chap. 22). Furthermore, perhaps as a result of multiple prior diagnostic procedures in some retrograde washings, the dispersed urothelial cells may show single cells with moderate nuclear hyperchromasia in the absence of tumor (Fig. 23-41A). Under these circumstances, great diagnostic caution is advised: the diagnosis of carcinoma should not be made unless the cytologic evidence is unequivocal.

Retrograde Brushing

Retrograde brushing is a method of direct sampling of the ureters, renal pelves, and renal calices that may be

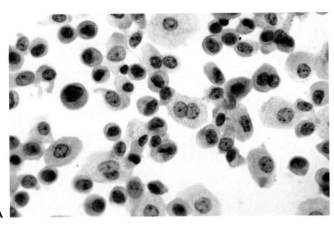

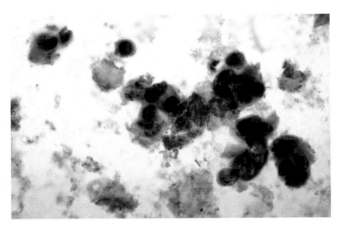

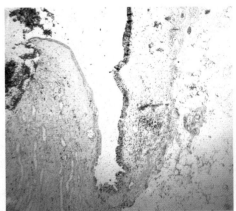

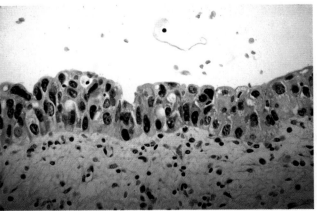

Figure 23-41   Carcinoma in situ of the renal pelvis and a potential source of error. *A.* The voided urine sediment after retrograde pyelogram, contained dispersed somewhat atypical benign urothelial cells, some of which show nuclear hyperchromasia and were thought to represent renal pelvic carcinoma. Nephrectomy failed to reveal any tumor. *B.* Left ureter sediment containing cancer cells corresponding to an asymptomatic and roentgenologically occult carcinoma in situ of the renal pelvis, shown in *C* and *D*. (*B,C,D*: Courtesy of Dr. Harold Block, El Paso, TX.)

performed under **radiologic control** or during **ureteroscopy** (endoscopic brushing). As is the case with retrograde irrigation material, **the samples are usually heavily contaminated with benign urothelial cells, occurring singly and in large clusters or clumps** that may cause significant problems of interpretation. In fact, in our consultation practice we have observed **more false-positive diagnoses of papillary tumors with this method of sampling than with other techniques. The diagnostic difficulties are increased if the sample contains somewhat atypical benign urothelial cells with enlarged nuclei, often the consequence of prior diagnostic procedures such as intravenous or retrograde pyelography** (see Fig. 23-41A). **The diagnosis of cancer can be rendered only in high-grade tumors and should be based on unequivocal evidence.**

Still, in skilled hands, the method offers the option of obtaining direct cytologic and tissue biopsy material for diagnosis (Gill et al, 1973). Bibbo et al (1974) reported excellent results with this method based on a small series of cases. Bian et al (1995) recognized in endoscopic brush specimens all high-grade malignant neoplasms of the renal pelves and suggested that the **smears are more informative than tiny tissue biopsies that can be obtained by this method.** Dodd et al (1997) compared endoscopic brush specimens with cytology of irrigation specimens and voided urine. Although these authors claimed that the brush cytology was a more specific and more sensitive sampling method, they **predictably failed to recognize seven low-grade papillary tumors. More importantly, however, Dodd et al failed to recognize four cases of flat carcinoma in situ that were diagnosed either in irrigation samples or in voided urine.** Zaman et al (1996) reported satisfactory diagnostic results with the brushing technique, which included **three renal carcinomas** (see below).

Personal experience confirms that cytologic samples obtained by retrograde brushing under fluoroscopic control may sometimes be informative and contribute in a major way to the diagnosis and localization of radiographically occult high-grade renal pelvic carcinoma (Fig. 23-42). **However, low-grade papillary tumors cannot reliably be detected by this technique.**

Ureteroscopic Biopsies

The technique of ureteroscopic biopsies of tumors of renal pelvis has been described (Tawfiek et al, 1997). At the time of this writing (2004), the procedure is not widely used and it is not likely to replace cytology in the near future.

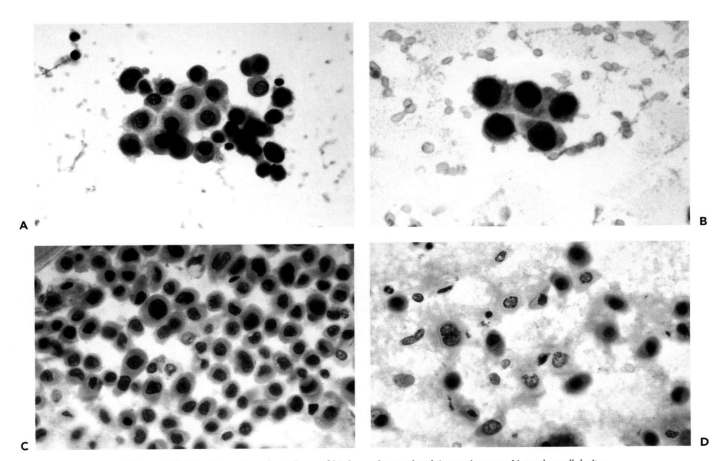

Figure 23-42 Examples of cytology of high grade renal pelvic carcinomas. Note the cellularity of the renal pelvic wash samples in *A* and *B* and renal pelvic brush specimen in *C* and *D*. Note the presence of mitoses in *D*. (*B*: High magnification.) *A* and *B*, same patient. *C* and *D*, each a different patient.

URINE FROM THE ILEAL CONDUIT (ILEAL BLADDER) OR OTHER ARTIFICIAL BLADDERS

Examination of urine from ileal bladders or other artificial bladders is a **mandatory follow-up procedure after radical cystectomy for urothelial tumors.** Cytologic findings in ileal bladder urine in the absence of cancer were discussed in Chapter 22. The recognition of cancer cells is not difficult because the cells are usually **larger than the cells from the ileal bladder and stand out because of large, hyperchromatic nuclei** (Fig. 22-43). **New primary cancers of the renal pelves or of the ureters following cancer of the bladder may occasionally be diagnosed in this fashion** before there is clinical evidence of disease. Since hydronephrosis is a common complication in patients with ileal bladder, a radiographic examination may show only slight changes in the renal pelvis that could be readily overlooked, were it not for the cytologic report.

In one of our early patients, **sequential bilateral primary high-grade urothelial carcinomas** of the renal pelves were observed following radical cystectomy for cancer of the bladder. Both kidneys were removed, and the patient was maintained on dialysis for several months pending renal transplant. Several additional patients with carcinomas of renal pelves or ureters following cystectomy for bladder cancer have been observed (Koss et al, 1977). Similar observations were reported by Malmgren et al (1971) and by Wolinska and Melamed (1973).

On rare occasions, **primary cancers of urothelial type** may develop in the ileal bladder epithelium, adjacent to the stoma (Grabstald, 1974). The tumors may be in situ or invasive. Although the pathogenesis of this event is not clear, it may be hypothesized that the intestinal epithelium undergoes some type of metaplasia that may become malignant. We have observed two such cases.

TUMORS OF THE URETHRA

Benign Tumors

Condylomata Acuminata

The most common benign tumors of the urethra in both sexes are condylomata acuminata. As was repeatedly dis-

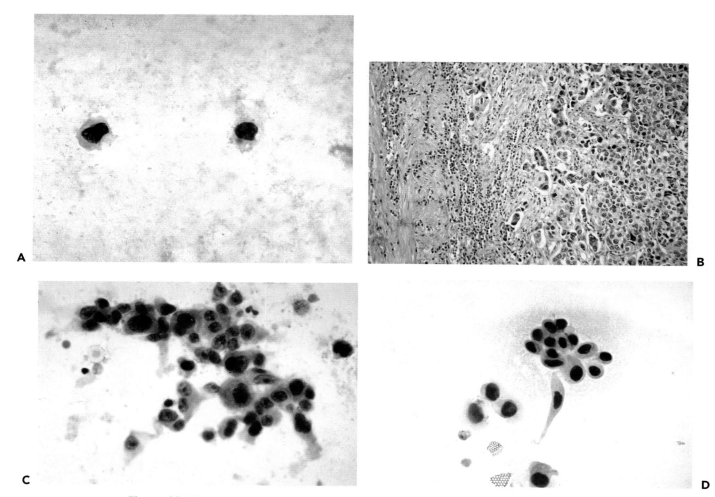

Figure 23-43 **Ileal bladder washings in a patient with carcinoma of the renal pelvis, following cystectomy for cancer of the urinary bladder.** *A.* Small cancer cells in urine from ileal bladder. *B.* Carcinoma of the renal pelvis following bladder cancer treated by surgical removal a few months earlier. *C,D.* Examples of ileal bladder urine in two patients with renal pelvic cancers following radical cystectomy for cancer of the urinary bladder.

cussed in the preceding pages, the tumors are associated with **human papillomavirus (HPV),** most commonly the **types 6 and 11,** but occasionally also 16 and 18. In a series of urethral condylomas in young male patients studied in this laboratory, Del Mistro et al (1987) observed the lesion in 16 young adult patients and in one boy, aged 9, who had an occult lesion. By in situ hybridization, **HPV types 6 and 11** were observed in 13 lesions, and **types 6 and 18** in one. In two lesions, only **type 11** was observed. One lesion and a recurrence thereof were negative with all probes. Four other recurrent lesions expressed the same type of viral DNA as the original lesion. Similar observations were reported in children (Vallejos et al, 1987).

In the female, condylomas of the urethra are usually visible lesions, associated with condylomas of external genitalia, a risk factor in cervical neoplastic events (see Chap. 11).

In the male, condylomas of the urethra occur in **two forms:** the **clinically evident lesions,** occupying the tip of the penile urethra at the meatus; and the **clinically occult lesions, located within the penile urethra.** The clinically obvious lesions are usually, but not always, associated with other genital condylomas. The frequency of occult lesions in the penile urethra is unknown, but there is concern that they may be the **source of infection of female partners** with HPV. They may also be **precursor lesions of squamous carcinomas of the male urethra,** which may also be associated with HPV infection (Malek et al, 1993). Giant penile condyloma of Buschke-Löwenthal, discussed in Chapter 11, is a closely related entity.

Histology

The visible papillary lesions are **identical with condylomas of the external female genitalia** (see Fig. 14-11A). The **condylomas of the penile urethra are generally flat lesions, mimicking cervical epithelial neoplasia (CIN) of low grade** and characterized by the presence of koilocytes in upper epithelial layers. Because of nuclear abnormalities, such as enlargement and hyperchromasia, which may be considerable, such lesions are readily **mistaken for a carcinoma in situ,** as became evident from several consultations. The association of condylomas with cancer of the bladder extending to the urethra was described by De Paepe et al (1990). Although the flat condylomas are benign by definition, and extremely unlikely to invade, all condylomas are difficult to treat because of a high rate of recurrence. See comments in Chapter 11 on new modes of treatment of condylomas.

Cytology

As in condylomas of the bladder, discussed above, **koilocytes** and **atypical squamous cells with enlarged, sometimes hyperchromatic nuclei** may be observed in voided urine sediments (see Fig. 23-32). In women, the cells may reflect a cervical or a vaginal lesion, but in the male, they usually indicate a lesion of the penile urethra or bladder. Cecchini et al (1988) performed **brushings of penile urethra** in 53 male partners of women with evidence of HPV infection (including CIN). Koilocytes were observed in smears of 26 (49%) of the men and none in the controls. Cecchini et al also performed colposcopy on the penile skin (**"penoscopy"**) on the male partners. In 5 of them, subclinical lesions were observed. Giacomini et al (1989) also studied the penile urethra, using a specially designed swab.

Subclinical infection of the penile skin has been considered by some as a source of infection with HPV for women (Sedlacek et al, 1986; Barrasso et al, 1987). The penile skin lesions are generally inconspicuous, histologically unimpressive, and not amenable to cytologic examination. For further discussion of the possible clinical significance of these lesions in transmission of human papillomavirus between sexes, see Chapter 11.

Adenomatous Polyps of Prostatic Urethra

Uncommon benign exophytic **papillary tumors** of the male urethra, with **histologic and immunologic features of prostatic epithelium,** may be the cause of hematuria or dysuria (Remick and Kumar, 1984; Chan et al, 1987). Schnadig et al (2000) described the cytologic findings in catheterized urine of several patients with this disorder. In some of these patients, **bland columnar cells** were observed.

Other Benign Tumors

Young et al (1996) described **urethral caruncles,** with markedly **atypical stroma, mimicking sarcomas or malignant lymphomas.** To our knowledge, these lesions have not been identified cytologically.

Malignant Tumors of the Female Urethra

De Paepe et al (1990) reported from our laboratories that the female **urethra was involved in 10 of 22 cases of bladder cancer.** The urethra may contain **urothelial carcinoma in situ, carcinoma in situ with extension to periurethral glands, or invasive cancer.** As an incidental finding in this study, 5 of 22 patients showed **condylomata of the urethra.**

Primary carcinomas of the female urethra are uncommon. Occasionally, the lesions occur in urethral diverticula. More than 80% of the lesions are **urothelial or squamous,** usually occurring in the anterior part of the urethra, whereas 20% are **adenocarcinomas of various types,** some originating in the glands of Littré (Grabstald, 1973; Sacks et al, 1975). Occasionally, **malignant melanomas** have been reported. There have been no known attempts to obtain routine smears of the urethra for purposes of early diagnosis of cancer. In fully developed cancer, the **voided urine** sediment may occasionally contain **cancer cells that reflect the type of the tumor.** Two examples of adenocarcinoma of the urethra are shown in Figure 23-44. One of them (Fig. 23-44C,D) originated in a diverticulum. Doria et al (1996) reported a similar case. In a case of **malignant melanoma of the urethra,** we observed, in a direct smear, **highly abnormal, but not diagnostic squamous cells, similar to cells observed in primary vaginal melanomas** (see Chap. 14).

Several personally observed patients with **treated squamous carcinoma of the distal (anterior) urethra** were followed by direct smears of the treated area. **Recurrent**

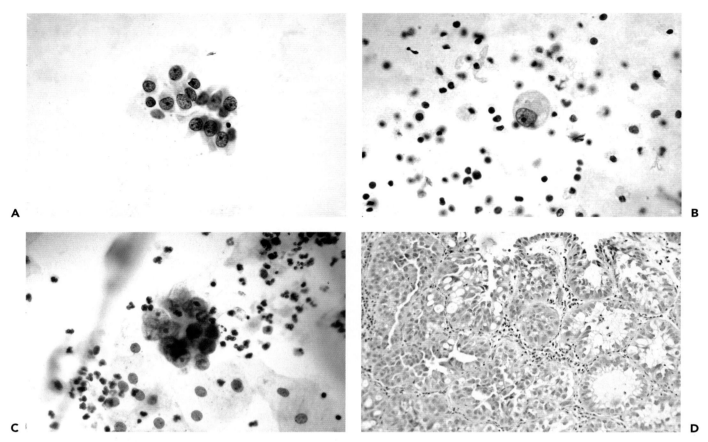

Figure 23-44 **Adenocarcinoma of female urethra in urinary sediment.** *A,B.* Cancer cells, singly and in clusters, showing vacuolated cytoplasm and nucleoli. *C.* A papillary cluster of cancer cells typical of an adenocarcinoma. *D.* Adenocarcinoma of the urethra that developed in a diverticulum corresponding to *C.*

disease could be diagnosed in some of them while still in the stage of carcinoma in situ. **The cytologic presentation was similar to that of carcinoma in situ of the cervix or the vagina, rather than of the urinary bladder.** This is in keeping with the epithelium of origin, which in the distal urethra is of the stratified squamous and not the urothelial type.

Malignant Tumors of the Male Urethra

Primary carcinomas of the male urethra not preceded by carcinoma of the bladder are exceedingly uncommon (Grabstald, 1973). However, **urothelial or squamous carcinomas of the prostatic portion of the male urethra may occur in about 10% of all patients after local treatment or radical cystectomy for carcinoma of the bladder** and, rarely, as a sequence of carcinoma of the prostatic ducts (Ritchie and Skinner, 1978). Penile discharge—mucoid, purulent, or hemorrhagic—may be observed on these occasions, and voided urine or washings of the urethra yield small cancer cells, singly or in clusters. Some of the observed lesions were carcinomas in situ or carcinomas in situ with superficial invasion (Fig. 23-45).

Primary malignant tumors of the anterior part of the male urethra are very rare. We observed several cases of

Paget's disease of the mucosa of the penile urethra and of the penile skin in patients with metastatic urothelial carcinoma of the bladder (Koss, 1985). There is no known cytologic counterpart of these rare events.

Carcinoid

Sylora et al (1975) described a case of **malignant carcinoid** of the urethra with extensive metastases and carcinoid syndrome. There is no information on the cytologic presentation of this tumor. For comments on carcinoids of the bladder, see above.

Adenocarcinoma of Endometrial Type of Prostatic Utricle

These tumors, originating in **prostatic utricle** (uterus masculinus), although very rare, may have the clinical presentation of a urethral tumor (Melicow and Tannenbaum, 1971; Epstein and Woodruff, 1985). In one such personally observed case, there were **malignant cells in the urinary sediment and in the washings of the urethra** (Fig. 23-46). The tumor proved fatal to the patient. Schnadig et al (2000) reported two such histologically confirmed cases, mimicking urethral polyps, with columnar cancer cells in catheterized urine. Masood et al (1991)

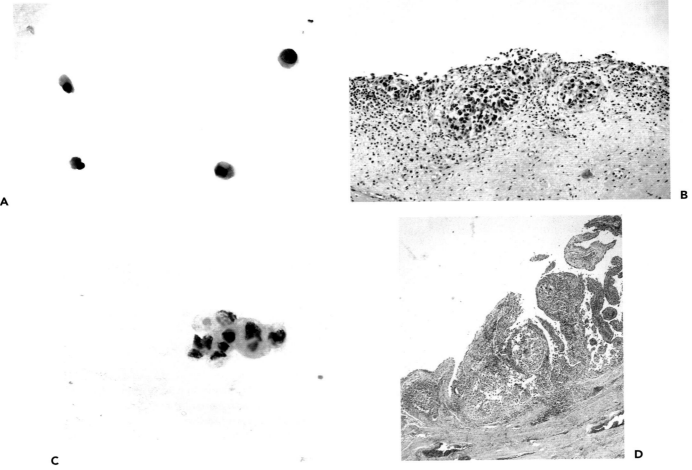

Figure 23-45 **Two examples of carcinoma of the male urethra after treatment for bladder cancer.** *A.* Small cancer cells correspond to the carcinoma in situ shown in *B. C.* Another patient showing a cluster of cancer cells corresponding to the high-grade noninvasive papillary tumor shown in *D.*

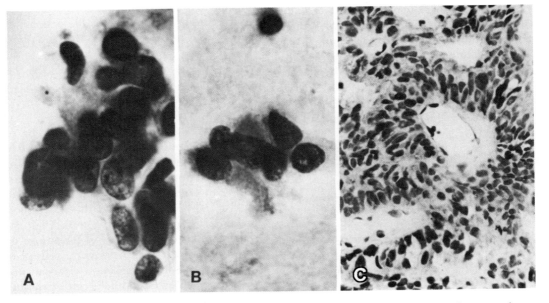

Figure 23-46 **Adenocarcinoma of prostatic utricle in a man, aged 57: urinary sediment and biopsy section.** *A,B.* Clusters of malignant cells that because of columnar configuration, are suggestive of adenocarcinoma. *C.* Histologic appearance of the tumor. (*A,B:* Oil immmersion; *C:* High magnification.)

reported a similar case, based on aspiration biopsy of the tumor. The presence of **grooved nuclei** was reported in the cancer cells.

METASTATIC TUMORS TO THE BLADDER AND OTHER ORGANS OF THE LOWER URINARY TRACT

Malignant tumors originating in adjacent organs, and less often in distant sites, may metastasize to the bladder wall and rarely other organs of the lower urinary tract. Many of these metastatic tumors may be detected cytologically and their discovery may be of value to the attending physician in evaluation of the patient. **The presence of a metastatic cancer does not rule out the possibility of a simultaneous primary tumor in the lower urinary tract.**

Metastases From Cancers of Adjacent Organs

Uterine Cervix

Cells of squamous carcinomas of the uterine cervix may be observed in the urinary sediment, either as a consequence of **direct extension of the cervical tumor to the trigone of the bladder or because of metastases.** These cells are **identical to those observed in primary squamous cancer of the bladder** (see Fig 23-26). In a female patient, the possibility of cervix cancer must always be investigated. The same rule applies to the finding of **koilocytes or dyskaryotic (dysplastic) squamous cells,** as mentioned above. So far, we have not observed cells of metastatic endocervical adenocarcinoma in urinary sediment.

Endometrium

Metastatic endometrial carcinoma should be considered in the differential diagnosis of adenocarcinoma, if the urinary sediment in a **postmenopausal female patient** contains **small- or medium-sized, approximately spherical, cancer cells with glandular features,** particularly if forming spherical (papillary) clusters or rosettes. In most such cases, the adenocarcinoma is of primary origin, either in the bladder or in another organ of the lower urinary tract, and the endometrial origin of such cells is exceedingly rare. We have observed very few cases of endometrial carcinoma in the urinary sediment over the past 50 years (see Fig. 23-31C). Bardales et al (1998) reported one such case. On the rarest occasion, **synchronous bladder tumors and endometrial carcinoma** may be recognized in urinary sediment (see Chap. 17).

Ovary

We observed two instances of metastatic ovarian carcinoma to the urinary bladder. In one of the two cases, the cancer cells were remarkably large with huge nuclei and nucleoli (Fig. 23-47).

Colon

Cells of colorectal carcinoma are a relatively frequent finding in urinary sediment and may be the result of either direct extension of rectal cancer to the urinary tract or metastases from a more distant portion of the bowel. In most such instances, the cytologic diagnosis is possible, or at least should be considered. Rarely, the **large cancer cells may be of signet-ring type.** More often, they are of **columnar configuration, sometimes forming rosettes or parallel bundles (palisades)** (Fig. 23-48A,B). The columnar cells of metastatic colonic carcinoma may be similar to cells of primary adenocarcinoma of the bladder (see Fig. 23-28). Koizumi and Schron (1997) pointed out that the **nuclei of metastatic colonic carcinoma may be pale and provided with large nucleoli, but this is very rarely seen in urinary sediment.** Occasionally, the finding of fecal material (plant cells) may lead to the diagnosis of a **vesicorectal fistula** that may be caused by rectal cancer.

Prostate

Cells of adenocarcinoma of the prostate may be occasionally observed in voided urine or in material obtained by prostatic massage. They are rather inconspicuous, usually small and difficult to identify in the absence of clinical data. Depending on the degree of differentiation of prostatic cancer, they are either **columnar, cuboidal, spherical, or oddly shaped.** The cells sometimes form papillary clusters but more often occur singly. The principal feature of these cells is the presence of **delicate cytoplasm and visible nucleoli.** Examples of cells of prostatic carcinoma in voided urine and other diagnostic media are shown in Chapter 33. A case of **prostatic duct carcinoma** diagnosed in urinary sediment was reported by Vandersteen et al (1997).

Metastatic Cancer From Distant Sites

Occasionally, carcinomas from more distant primary sites may be seen in the urinary sediment. An example of metastatic bronchogenic carcinoma is shown in Figure 23-48C,D. It is usually **not possible to determine on cytologic grounds, the origin of the primary tumor or for that matter, to determine whether the tumor is primary or metastatic.** There are two exceptions to this rule: **metastatic melanoma and tumors of the hematopoietic system.**

Metastatic Melanoma

Metastatic malignant melanoma may be recognized in the urinary sediment by the presence of pigment-containing malignant cells (Fig. 23-49A,B). In the **absence of pigment or pertinent clinical history, the specific diagnosis can rarely be established.** However, as pointed out by Piva and Koss (1964), even **the diagnosis of pigmented melanoma is not without its pitfalls. Pigment-containing renal tubular cells in cases of melanuria or pigmented macrophages** may be mistaken for cells of the metastatic tumor (Fig. 23-49C,D). Unless **clear-cut nuclear abnormalities, such as large nuclei with prominent nucleoli, are observed, the diagnosis of metastatic melanoma should not be made.** A case of metastatic melanoma with pigmented casts in the urinary sediment was described by Valente et al (1985).

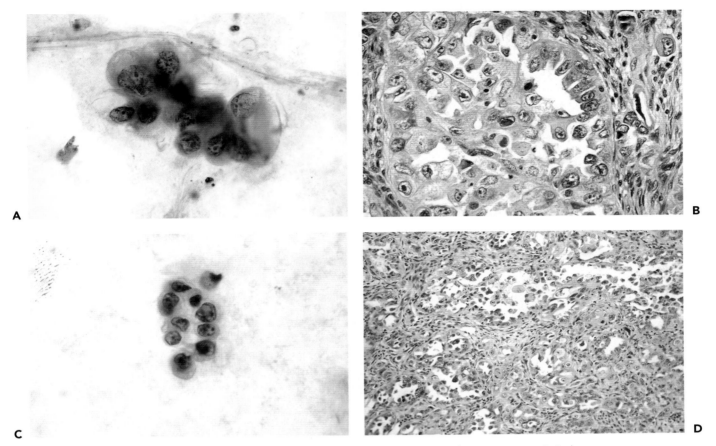

Figure 23-47 Two examples of metastatic ovarian carcinoma to the urinary tract. *A.* A cluster of very large cancer cells with clear cytoplasm, corresponding to the ovarian tumor shown in *B. C.* Clusters of much smaller cancer cells corresponding to metastatic ovarian carcinoma in the ureter, shown in *D.*

Lymphomas and Leukemias

Malignant lymphomas may involve the urinary bladder and malignant cells may be identified in the urine sediment. As is usual in lymphoma, **the tumor cells lie singly,** are **approximately spherical, have usually scanty cytoplasm and show nuclear abnormalities such as grooves or clefts and the peculiar nuclear protrusions** (nipples) observed in effusions (see Chap. 26). Tanaka et al (1993) described a case of **Ki-1 malignant lymphoma** in urinary sediment. The **tumor cells in such rare cases may be very large and show abundant cytoplasm.** The differential diagnosis of Ki-1 lymphoma from metastatic carcinoma requires knowledge of clinical history and immunostaining.

    Acute leukemias may sometimes begin with **hematuria. Blast cells may be identified in the urinary sediment** (Fig. 23-50A,B).

Multiple Myeloma

We have not observed cells of plasma cell myeloma in the urinary sediment. However, through the courtesy of Mr. Arthur Garutti, we observed a patient with renal impairment caused by multiple myeloma **(myeloma kidney)** who was shedding **bizarre multinucleated cells in his urinary sediment.** Undoubtedly, these cells **represented reactive renal tubular cells surrounding tubular casts of Bence-**

Jones protein, commonly observed in this disease (Fig. 23-50C,D).

ACCURACY OF CYTOLOGIC DIAGNOSIS OF TUMORS OF THE LOWER URINARY TRACT

Bladder

The evaluation of the accuracy of urinary cytology **depends on the expectations of the observer.** As was discussed above, it is totally unrealistic to expect that well-differentiated papillary urothelial tumors without obvious nuclear abnormalities (papillomas and low-grade papillary tumors) will yield diagnostic cells, either in voided urine or in specimens obtained by direct sampling (bladder washing or brushing). The rare exceptions to this rule were discussed above.

    On the other hand, the **finding of clearly malignant cells in the urinary sediment or bladder washings calls for a major investigative effort, even in the absence of cystoscopic or radiographic abnormalities. Nonpapillary carcinoma in situ may be present in the bladder, ureter, or renal pelvis in the absence of localizing evidence,** as documented in the preceding pages.

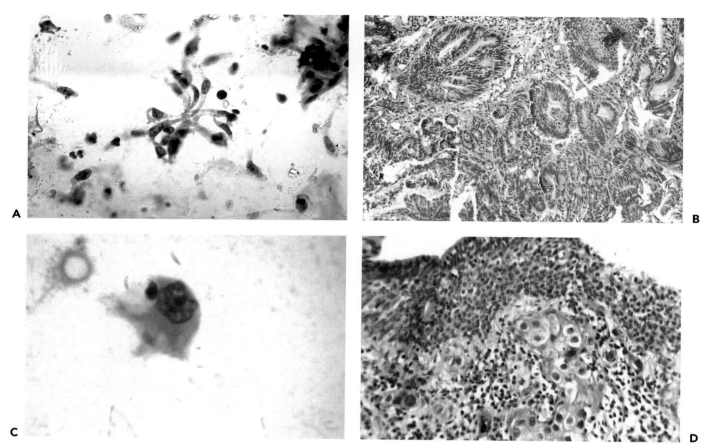

Figure 23-48 **Metastatic rectal and bronchogenic cancers to the bladder.** *A.* Urinary sediment with clusters of columnar cancer cells that are characteristic of colonic type of carcinoma. *B.* Histology of rectal adenocarcinoma corresponding to *A. C,D.* Metastatic bronchogenic carcinoma to bladder. *C* shows very large malignant cells with ample cytoplasm, corresponding to the metastatic bronchogenic carcinoma in the bladder shown in *D.*

The statistical evaluation of performance of urinary cytology published from various sources rarely reflect these elementary observations and thus result in **major confusion as to what urinary cytology can and cannot accomplish.** In experienced hands (Esposti and Zajicek, 1972), carcinoma of the bladder, grade II or above, was accurately identified in 78% of all cases. For high-grade tumors, the diagnostic accuracy reached 91%. None of the 52 cases diagnosed as papillomas and papillary carcinoma, grade I, could be identified cytologically. Morse and Melamed (1974) pointed out that the shedding of cancer cells in the voided urine is variable. Therefore, **three or more specimens must be examined for each patient.**

The results of a survey of the diagnostic efficacy of cytology of voided urine based on **three samples of voided urine** (Koss et al, 1985) is shown in Table 23-6. It may be noted that a **positive sediment observed in a single case of a papillary tumor grade I was subsequently shown to reflect a flat carcinoma in situ.** The results in papillary **tumors grade II closely reflected the distribution of the DNA values** in this group of tumors with positive findings limited to aneuploid tumors (Tribukait, 1984; see below). Nearly all high-grade tumors were identified in the urinary sediment as malignant or suspicious.

Shenoy et al (1985) and Murphy (1990) claimed a high rate of cytologic diagnoses for grade I tumors although, subsequently, Murphy has reduced the expectations (Murphy, 2000). Several other recent analyses of performance of urinary cytology in reference to urothelial tumors were discussed above (Raab et al, 1994; Renshaw et al, 1996; Bastacky et al, 1999). In spite of elaborate methods of analysis, only high-grade tumors could be reliably identified in cytologic samples. These results were confirmed by Curry and Wojcik (2002).

Tumors of Renal Pelves and Ureters

Similar comments apply to **tumors of the renal pelves and ureters.** Eriksson and Johansson (1976), who studied 43 such patients, obtained positive cytologic results in 19 patients, all with tumors grade II or higher. In a subsequent group of poorly differentiated tumors, an accuracy of 71% was recorded. These observations were confirmed by Mahadevia et al (1983) who reported that urinary sediment cytology is an excellent diagnostic tool in the diagnosis of high-grade carcinomas of the renal pelves and ureters.

Several **important sources of cytologic error,** discussed

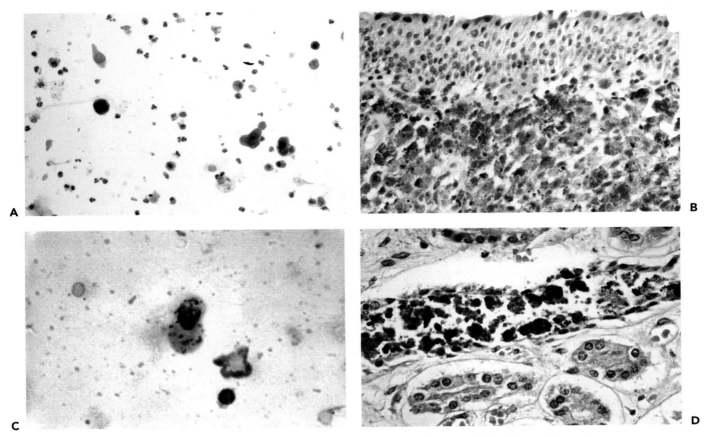

Figure 23-49   Metastatic melanoma to bladder. *A.* Pigmented cancer cells in urinary sediment. *B.* Pigment-producing cancer in wall of bladder, corresponding to *A*. *C,D.* Another case of disseminated melanoma with extensive phagocytosis of the pigment in renal tubules. *C* shows one of the pigment-containing macrophages in urinary sediment. *D* shows section of the kidney obtained at autopsy, corresponding to *C*.

in Chapter 22 and the preceding pages, must be emphasized: **instrumentation, lithiasis, inflammation, infection with human polyomavirus, effects of drugs, and radiotherapy.**

Is Cytologic Screening for Cancer of the Bladder Justified?

The most important accomplishment of cytology of the urinary tract is the diagnosis of clinically unsuspected cases of carcinoma, particularly carcinoma in situ. It has been documented above that this is indeed possible in screened industrial workers. There is considerable evidence that the salvage of such patients is potentially better than that of patients with advanced cancer, provided that treatment is applied before deep invasion or metastases occur.

The ultimate measure of success in a cancer detection endeavor is the extension of a good quality life for the patients. Unfortunately, as discussed above, the **survival rate of high-risk workers** who developed bladder cancer after exposure to *p*-aminodiphenyl was low. Because the study was conducted before contemporary methods of recognition and treatment of flat carcinoma in situ were available, most of these patients died with, or of the disease after a survival period of from 5 to 8 years. Although the follow-up of high-

risk industrial workers has been a highly rewarding scientific exercise that clarified many points of natural history of bladder cancer, the direct benefit of these studies to the workers was not satisfactory. Similar doubts were expressed in the United Kingdom (Fox and White, 1976).

With the spread of understanding of the role played by carcinoma in situ and related lesions in the development of invasive cancer of the urinary tract, the issue of cancer detection may deserve another look. In this regard, it is important to note that Farrow et al (1977), by performing routine cytologic examination of voided urine on 3,500 patients (without cystoscopically visible lesions) who attended the urologic clinic at the Mayo Clinic, observed 69 documented cases (1.9%) of **carcinoma in situ of the bladder.** Holmquist (1988) observed **12 unsuspected bladder cancers in a survey of urinary sediments in 9,870 routine urinalysis samples** (1.2 per 1,000). In the Holmquist study, the initial wet preparations were followed by two routine cytologic procedures whenever there was some suspicion of abnormality. Thus, this is a hitherto unexplored source of case findings that is deserving of further study. In the absence of a large population survey, the actual benefits of bladder cancer detection to the society cannot be ascertained. More recently, Nickel et al (2002) observed three

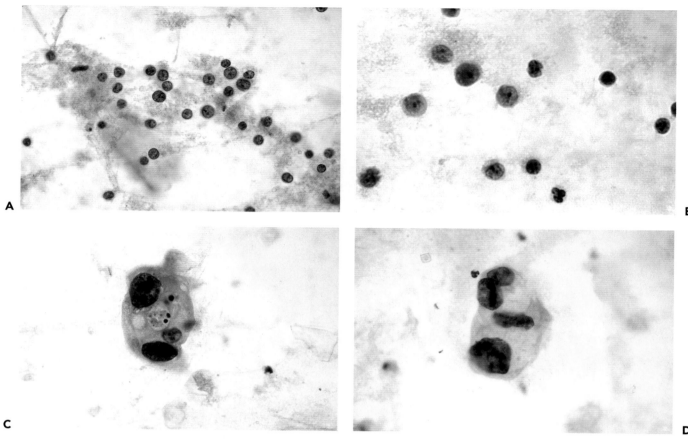

Figure 23-50   Hematologic disorders in urinary sediment. *A,B.* Urinary sediment containing blast cells in a child with hematuria, in acute blastic leukemia; the primary diagnosis was established in urinary sediment. *C,D.* Giant cells observed in the urinary sediment of a patient with multiple myeloma and evidence of renal damage. It is assumed that these cells represent renal tubular reaction to protein casts, which are common in this disease. (*B*: High magnification.) (*C,D*: Courtesy of Mr. Arthur Garutti, Port Jefferson, NY.)

cases of carcinoma in situ of bladder among 150 patients with "prostatitis" studied by voided urine cytology.

CYTOLOGIC MONITORING OF PATIENTS TREATED FOR TUMORS OF THE LOWER URINARY TRACT

The purpose of monitoring patients treated for tumors of the lower urinary tract is to detect tumor recurrence or formation of new tumors in a timely fashion. The **success of cytologic monitoring depends greatly on the type of tumor and the mode of therapy.**

Treatment Options and Their Impact

Surgical excision followed by cautery is still the therapeutic method of choice for primary and recurrent **superficial papillary bladder tumors. Tumors located in the renal pelvis may require nephrectomy. This mode of treatment does not impede cytologic follow-up. Radical**

cystectomy with the creation of an ileal- or other type of artificial bladder, is curative of nearly all flat carcinomas in situ and some invasive tumors. Such patients should be monitored by **examination of urine from the artificial bladder** for the possible occurrence of a carcinoma of upper urinary tract.

Radiotherapy, either as a primary treatment mode or as an adjunct to surgical treatment of invasive tumors, poses a **special challenge** to cytologic follow-up because of radiation-induced cell changes in benign and malignant cells, discussed below.

Immunotherapy, with intravesical instillation of the **attenuated bovine tuberculosis bacillus (bacillus Calmette-Guérin; BCG),** has become the treatment of choice for flat carcinoma in situ and related lesions of the **bladder** and has also been applied to urothelial tumors of the **renal pelvis.** Although the precise mechanism of effective treatment is still unknown, it is hypothesized that the inflammatory reaction attracts cytotoxic lymphocytes, which, in a manner not clearly understood, helps in replacing diseased epithelium by normal mucosa.

A substantial number of papers based on randomized

TABLE 23-6

COMPARISON OF HIGHEST CYTOLOGIC DIAGNOSIS IN THREE SPECIMENS OF VOIDED URINE WITH THE HIGHEST GRADE OF PRIMARY TUMOR IN THE NEAREST BIOPSY IN 203 EPISODES

Highest Histologic Diagnosis of Primary Tumor	No. of Cases	Highest Cytologic Diagnosis in 3 Specimens of Voided Urine	
		Negative or Atypical	Suspicious or Positive
Noninvasive papillary tumors	136	29 (22%)	107 (78%)
Grade I	6	5	1
Grade II	68	20	48
Grade III	62	4	58
Nonpapillary carcinoma *in situ*	14	0	14 (100%)
Invasive carcinoma (all grades)	27	2	25 (92%)
Carcinoma of ureter	4	0	4
Other cancers	2	1	1
No evidence of cancer	20	20	0
Total	203	52	151

(Koss LG, et al. Diagnostic value of cytology of voided urine. Acta Cytol 29:810–816, 1985, with permission)

trials have documented that, in some patients, long-term remissions and possibly cures of bladder lesions, can be achieved (Brosman, 1985; DeKernion et al, 1985; Pinsky et al, 1985; Herr et al, 1986; Guinan et al, 1987; Herr et al, 1989), but late recurrences of the tumors may occur (Herr et al, 1995). Although encouraging results for carcinoma in situ with prostatic extension were reported, still 10 of 23 such patients required cystectomy (Bretton et al, 1989). Similar data were reported by Cheng et al (2000). As described in Chapter 22, the treatment results in formation of **microscopic granulomas composed of epithelioid and giant cells of the Langhans' type in the wall of the bladder and in the adjacent prostate,** accompanied by a marked inflammatory reaction.

Intravesical chemotherapy with instillation of cytotoxic drugs, mainly the alkylating agent thiotepa and the antibiotic mitomycin, have been used after resection of papillary tumors to reduce the frequency of recurrences, and also in the treatment of carcinoma in situ and resected high-grade tumors to prevent the occurrence of invasive carcinoma (summary in Soloway, 1983, 1985). Therapeutic successes have been reported (Soloway, 1985) but persuasive evidence that these treatment modes are equal or superior to BCG is not available.

Photodynamic therapy of carcinoma in situ and small papillary tumors after priming with hematoporphyrin derivatives has been reported (Hisazumi et al, 1984; Prout et al, 1987). The parenterally injected compound localizes in rapidly growing tissues, such as carcinomas, and renders them susceptible to phototherapy by laser. Similar attempts at treatment of carcinoma in situ of the bronchus, esophagus, and oral cavity have been attempted.

Cytologic Monitoring

Cytologic monitoring of patients treated for tumors of the lower urinary tract is effective only in early detection of new or recurrent high-grade tumors. Urinary tract cytology has so far not replaced cystoscopy in the follow-up and identification of new low-grade papillary bladder tumors. In the experience of this writer, the best **method of monitoring bladder tumors is by cytologic analysis of voided urine specimens. After radical cystectomy, the patients must be monitored by periodic cytologic examination of urine from the ileal bladder** (see above). As pointed out by Herr et al (1996), the monitoring may be required for **many years after treatment.** Patients **treated for carcinoma of the renal relvis and ureter,** who are also prone to the development of new carcinomas elsewhere in the urinary tract, should also be monitored by urinary cytology.

Each monitoring sequence should be based on **three urine samples obtained on consecutive days** (see Chap. 22). **The presence of cancer cells, as described in the preceding pages, is always indicative of a recurrence or progression of urothelial carcinoma, regardless of the mode of treatment or presumed clinical status.** In fact, in several personally observed cases, urinary sediment that was positive for cancer cells, **in the presence of an apparently good clinical response to treatment,** anticipated an invasive or metastatic cancer that killed the patient. Harving et al (1988) documented that **cytologic analysis is more sensitive than multiple biopsies** in predicting tumor recurrence or progression. The need for cytologic monitoring was also emphasized by Hopkins et al (1983), who pointed out that **patients with seemingly innocuous low-grade**

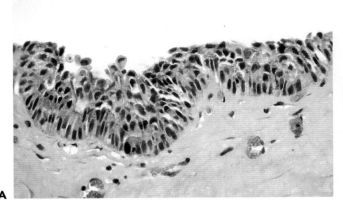 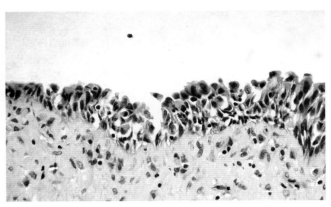

A B

Figure 23-51 **Radiation failure.** Two examples of residual carcinoma in situ in patients whose invasive tumor was eradicated by radiotherapy.

tumors may develop an unexpected invasive cancer of the bladder, presumably derived from adjacent carcinoma in situ and related lesions.

None of the cytotoxic drugs or BCG causes epithelial cell changes that could be confused with cancer. Although minor atypias in the form of cellular and nuclear enlargement may be observed with thiotepa, neither mitomycin nor BCG causes any significant cytologic abnormalities, except for granulomatous inflammation in BCG. The granulomas may be observed in the urinary sediment, as described in Chapter 22.

Monitoring of **patients undergoing radiotherapy** is difficult because of radiation changes affecting **benign epithelial cells,** as discussed in Chapter 22. Radiotherapy of carcinomas of the bladder may cause **nuclear pyknosis and ballooning of the tumor cells,** a change often reflected in smears of urinary sediment. The degree of nuclear abnormality in the cancer cells usually, but not always, allows a differentiation between the irradiated benign and the irradiated malignant cells. However, when the nuclei of irradiated benign cells show nuclear hyperchromasia, the differential diagnosis becomes difficult. In such situations, it is advisable to **withhold judgment until clear-cut evidence of cancer is obtained on subsequent samples of urine. The cells of bladder cancer recurring after radiotherapy are in no way different from the cells of the primary tumor.** Numerous biopsies or cystotomy often may be required to obtain histologic confirmation of a tumor, especially if there is considerable scarring of the bladder wall.

Cytologic studies of urinary sediment proved to be quite useful in following a group of patients with bladder cancer treated by radiation before undergoing surgery. If preliminary radiotherapy was successful, it resulted in rapid diminution in the numbers of cancer cells, and in four cases, in complete disappearance of cancer cells. In these latter cases, histologic studies of totally removed bladders failed to reveal the presence of cancer. However, **in several cases of carcinoma of the bladder, the urinary sediment remained positive in spite of a very favorable clinical response of the invasive tumor to radiotherapy. Subsequent surgical removal of the bladder revealed *residual carcinoma in situ***

that apparently did not respond to radiation treatment, **whereas the invasive tumor was obliterated** (Fig. 23-51). Similar observations were made with carcinoma of the cervix (see Chap. 18) and in carcinoma of the esophagus (see Chap. 24).

As emphasized above, the cytologic approach to monitoring of treated patients will fail in discovering new or recurrent low-grade papillary tumors. This fundamental fact has led to the development of a substantial number of new methods of monitoring of bladder tumors.

Monitoring of Tumors of the Lower Urinary Tract by Methods Other Than Cytology

DNA Ploidy Analysis

It has been known since the publications by Falor (1971), Falor and Ward (1973, 1976) and Granberg-Ohman et al (1984), that most **low-grade noninvasive bladder tumors had a chromosomal component in the normal diploid range and that high-grade tumors had grossly aneuploid karyotypes.** With the development of methods of **DNA quantification** by cytophotometry, image cytophotometry, and flow cytometry, enumeration of chromosomes could be replaced, to some degree, by measurements of DNA in cell populations. The methods, their accomplishments, and limitations, are described in Chapters 46 and 47.

The initial studies of **DNA content of bladder tumor cells,** conducted by **cytophotometry,** confirmed that low-grade papillary tumors are, for the most part, in the diploid range (i.e., have a DNA content identical or similar to normal tissues). With increasing grade, there was an increasing degree of abnormalities, reaching high aneuploid values for high-grade tumors (Lederer et al, 1972). With the developments in **flow cytometry,** rapid DNA measurements could be performed in a large number of bladder tumors (Fig. 23-52A). As was shown by Wijkstrøm et al (1984), the DNA values obtained by flow cytometry compared favorably with cytogenetic analysis.

Notable contributions to flow cytometric DNA studies of **bladder tumors** were made, among others, by Tribu-

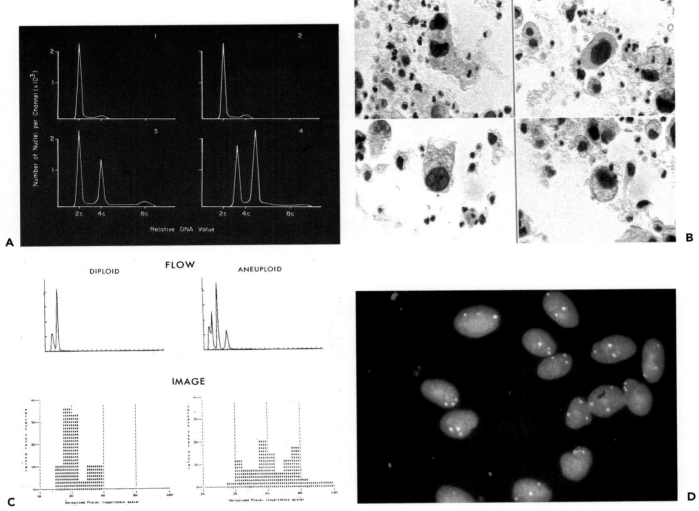

Figure 23-52   **DNA ploidy patterns of bladder tumors.** *A.* Flow cytometry. The two top diagrams (1,2) show diploid pattern of normal urothelium and a papillary tumor. The two bottom diagrams show marked aneuploidy of urothelial carcinoma. *B.* Shows Feulgen stained urine sediment to determine DNA ploidy by image analysis. *C.* Shows comparison of DNA analysis by flow cytometry (top) and image analysis (bottom). The diagrams on the right show an aneuploid pattern of bladder tumor. *D.* Fluorescent in situ hybridization (FISH) in bladder cells using probe to the centromere of chromosome 1. Many of the tumor cells showed triploidy of chromosome 1, even though the tumor was diploid by image analysis. (*D:* Courtesy of Drs. Hopman and Vooijs, Nijmegen, The Netherlands.)

kait, whose large experience is summarized in Table 23-7. It may be noted that DNA analysis confirms cytogenetic findings, inasmuch as **most noninvasive low-grade tumors have a DNA content in the diploid range. Tumors grade II are almost equally divided into diploid and aneuploid categories,** reflecting cytologic findings shown in Table 23-6. **Tumors grade III and all cases of flat carcinoma in situ (Tis) are aneuploid, confirming the clinical and pathologic observations on the origin of most high-grade invasive cancers of the urinary bladder from carcinomas in situ.** The analysis by stage also confirmed that most **deeply invasive bladder tumors were aneuploid.**

DNA Content of Bladder Washings (Barbotage)

Given the premise that the **DNA content of the epithelium of the bladder may be predictive of future behavior and,** **thereby, the prognosis of bladder tumors,** DNA measurements on bladder washings were initiated by Melamed et al (1976). A large number of papers from the Memorial-Sloan Kettering Cancer Center suggested that aneuploid DNA content of the cells in suspension, obtained either at the time of cytoscopy or by catheter (barbotage), was predictive of tumor persistence, recurrence, or impending invasion (Klein et al, 1982; Badalament et al, 1986, 1987, 1988). The method was shown to be particularly **effective in monitoring patients with carcinomas in situ undergoing treatment.**

Unfortunately, as is discussed in Chapter 47, although histograms that are clearly normal or abnormal are easy to interpret, many of the histograms obtained from bladder washings, particularly from patients with low-grade tumors, are not clear-cut, difficult to interpret, and require artificial classification schemes (Koss et al, 1989). Synchronous stud-

TABLE 23-7			
DISTRIBUTION OF DNA VALUES IN 277 UNTREATED BLADDER TUMORS			
Grade	No. in Group	Diploid	Aneuploid*
Distribution by Grade			
0	2	2	0
I	30 (100%)	24 (80%)	6 (20%)
II	107 (100%)	56 (52%)	51 (48%)
III	130 (100%)	6 (5%)	124 (95%)
Adenocarcinoma	8	1	7
Total	277	89	188
Distribution by Stage			
T_0	42 (100%)	32 (76%)	10 (24%)
T_1	118 (100%)	50 (42%)	68 (58%)
$T_{2,3,4}$	93 (100%)	7 (7.5%)	86 (92.5%)
Tis†	24 (100%)	0	24 (100%)
TOTAL	277	89	188

* Includes tetraploid–aneuploid tumors.
† Tis, flat carcinoma in situ.
(Modified from Tribukait B. Flow cytometry in surgical pathology and cytology of the genito-urinary tract. Koss LG, Coleman DV (eds.) Advances in Clinical Cytology. New York, Masson Publishing, 1984: pp 163–189.)

ies of the DNA content by image analysis and flow cytometry disclosed that some samples, which were considered normal (diploid) by flow cytometry, could contain small aneuploid cell populations that were revealed by image analysis and were of predictive value for tumor recurrence or progression (Koss et al, 1989). The method proved **unsatisfactory in attempting to predict recurrences of low-grade papillary tumors,** as is the case with conventional cytology. Attempts to replace bladder washings or barbotage with **samples of voided urine for flow cytometric analysis of DNA,** as suggested by deVere White et al (1988), **were not successful** in our hands.

Image Analysis

The principles of image analysis of cells are discussed in Chapter 46. For a number of years, our group has attempted to develop a system of objective, computer-based analysis of urothelial cells in voided urine sediments processed by the method of Bales, described in Chapter 44. The initial results indicated that several subgroups of urothelial cells could be identified with accuracy surpassing that of the human observer (Sherman et al, 1986). Furthermore, as discussed above, the "atypical" urothelial cells could be classified into two groups of diagnostic value. Automated processing of 119 specimens of voided urine yielded promising results (Sherman et al, 1984). However, subsequent studies revealed errors in the evaluation system that could not be corrected without a major improvement in the image capture and computer systems.

Work with an apparatus known as Papnet System, based on capture and selection of cell images by a neural network,

proved to be interesting. The apparatus was capable of identifying cancer cells in smears of the urinary sediment, whether prepared by conventional methods or processed as a liquid sample (Hoda et al, 1995). An example of the Papnet display of the urinary sediment in bladder cancer is shown in Figure 23-23A.

An interesting approach to the laboratory **processing of "atypical" or "suspicious" smears** of urinary sediment wasproposed by Dr. Jay Amberson (Dianon Systems, Inc., Stratford, CT). In such cases, a duplicate smear is stained with **Feulgen stain** and the **DNA profile** is established by rapid image analysis. In Feulgen-stained smears, cancer cells are easily recognized (Fig. 23-52B). If the DNA profile shows abnormal distribution of DNA (Fig. 23-52C), the urologist is informed of the possibility of a malignant lesion. Unfortunately, a full evaluation of the clinical benefits of this technique is not available at the time of this writing (2004). Wojcik et al (2001) adopted **laser scanning cytometry** for evaluation of DNA ploidy in urinary sediment and reported excellent results in recognition of malignant tumors. The same author pointed out that superficial umbrella cells may be a **source of abnormal ploidy** and, thus, should be excluded from measurements.

It is not likely that in the near future, quantitative image analysis will replace visual examination of cells in the urinary sediment, although the Feulgen technique is interesting and clearly deserving of further investigations.

Morphometry

A number of investigators, particularly a Dutch group headed by Baak, have advocated morphometric measurements of cellular and nuclear features **in histologic sections of bladder tumors** as a predictor of prognosis (Blomjous et al, 1989). The method is based on subjective selection of the microscopic field to be measured. To our knowledge, the method has not been applied to cytology of the urinary sediment.

New Technological Developments

Monoclonal Antibodies

Numerous monoclonal antibodies have been tested or are being developed as specific markers for the identification of bladder tumors with invasive potential (Cordon-Cardo et al, 1990; Fradet et al, 1984, 1986, 1987). Some of these monoclonal antibodies may be used in conjunction with flow cytometry to identify subpopulations of cells with particular characteristics and measure their DNA content. Other markers used for these purposes are monoclonal antibodies to keratin filaments, which facilitate the selection of epithelial cells from all other cells in bladder washings. In such studies, the DNA can be measured in epithelial cells only (Ramaekers et al, 1984, 1986). A commercially available test ImmunoCyt (Diagnocure, Saint-Foy, Quebec, Canada) has been reported to have better specificity and sensitivity for **detection of low-grade, low-stage tumors of the bladder** than conventional cytology (Fradet et al, 1997; Mian et al, 1999).

Nuclear Matrix Proteins

Keesee et al (1996) explored the possibility that the nuclear matrix proteins may show sufficient differences between normal and cancer cells to apply this system to bladder cancer detection and diagnosis. A test kit NMP22 (Matritech Corp., Newton, MA) was tested by a number of investigators (Soloway et al, 1996; Stampfer et al, 1998; Zippe et al, 1999) with interesting results, particularly in reference to low-grade papillary tumors. Del Nero et al (1999) reported a high sensitivity but also a high rate of false-positive results with this method.

Bladder Tumor Antigen

Bard bladder tumor antigen test, BTA stat, (Bard Diagnostics, Redmond, WA) is a latex agglutination assay for qualitative detection of basement membrane antigen in urine. Several investigators reported good specificity and sensitivity of this test when compared with urine cytology (Sarosdy et al, 1995; Leyh et al, 1997; Murphy et al, 1997; Sharma et al, 1999). Ramakumar et al (1999) observed that the test had high sensitivity, when compared with several other objective laboratory tests, particularly **telomerase activity** (Lin et al, 1996; Kyo et al, 1997).

Telomerase Activity

Telomerase, an enzyme that is essential for maintenance of chromosomal integrity, can be measured in urine by polymerase chain reaction (PCR) with appropriate primers. It has been reported that the method is more specific than any of the other methods of diagnosis of bladder tumors (Landman et al, 1998; Ramakumar et al, 1999).

Proteomics

The recently developed method of identification of proteins as markers of tumors has been applied to urinary sediment of patients with tumors of the urinary bladder (Vlahou et al, 2001). The method is experimental and is based on complex technology, using protein chips and mass spectrophotometry. Vlahou identified several **proteins that may be unique to tumors of the bladder.** The results of this study, while not spectacular, were interesting inasmuch as the authors claim 78% sensitivity in the detection of low-grade papillary tumors.

Induced Autofluorescence

Another approach to evaluation of the status of the bladder and therapy is based on direct **instillation of a compound 5-aminolevulinic acid (ALA),** which is absorbed by mucosal lesions such as flat carcinomas in situ, and induces the accumulation of endogenous **fluorescent protoporphyrins.** The lesions can then be visualized with Krypton ion laser and effectively resected (Kriegmair et al, 1994). Using this system, a reduction in the recurrence rate of such lesions was reported (Riede et al, 2001).

Blood Group Antigens

Kovarik et al (1968) suggested that the expression of blood group antigens in bladder tumors may be correlated with prognosis. The fundamental assumption of these studies was that those epithelial tumors that have retained the ability of normal epithelium to express the blood group antigen specific for the blood group of the patient were less likely to recur or progress than tumors that have lost the blood group antigen expression. In the initial studies, erythrocytes of known blood groups were used as markers (Kovarik et al, 1968; Weinstein et al, 1981; Yamase et al, 1981; Limas and Lange, 1982; Flanigan et al, 1983; Cordon-Cardo et al, 1988). Subsequently, serologic methods were developed, and the results were documented by the peroxidase-antiperoxidase system (Coon and Weinstein, 1981). Ultrastructural localization of antisera labeled with colloidal gold has also been documented (De Harven et al, 1987).

The concept, although theoretically valid, has been shown to be of limited practical value. The performance of the test, particularly on small bladder biopsies, was fraught with technical difficulties. The application of the method to cytologic samples has not been fully explored, although several successful attempts have been reported (Borgstrøm et al, 1985; Borgstrøm and Wahren, 1986). At the time of this writing (2004), the method has been abandoned and is reported here for its historical value.

Molecular Genetics in the Diagnosis and Prognosis of Urothelial Tumors

Progress in molecular biology has resulted in a number of observations pertaining to urothelial tumors, some of which may prove to be of clinical value.

In Situ Hybridization of Chromosomes (FISH)

Using **molecular probes** for identification of individual chromosomes (or their centromeres) by **fluorescent in situ hybridization (FISH),** Hopman et al (1988, 1989, 1991) could document, in tissue sections, that even the **diploid urothelial tumors have numerical abnormalities of individual chromosomes** (Fig. 23-52D). As summarized by Czerniak and Herz (1995), low-grade papillary tumors show fewer chromosomal abnormalities than high-grade tumors. An increase in the number of **chromosomes 1 and 7 (trisomy) and abnormalities of chromosome 9** were most commonly observed in **low-grade tumors.** Abnormalities in **chromosomes 3, 4, 8, 11, 17, and 18** were most commonly observed in **high-grade tumors.** This information has been applied to **recognition of cancer cells in urinary sediment** by Cajulis et al (1994) using the FISH technique with probes to centromeres of chromosomes 8 and 12. Cajulis documented the presence of **numerical chromosomal abnormalities** in cells in the urinary sediment in a substantial proportion of bladder tumors, some of which were diploid. The FISH technique has found a commercial application with a multicolor probe targeting **synchronously several chromosomes affected in tumors of the bladder and performed on sediment of voided urine** (UroVision, Vysis, Inc., Downers Grove, IL). The probe mixture targets chromosomes 3, 7, 17 and the 9p21 region (Fig. 23-53). The initial study of the probe claimed that the method was **more efficient than cytology in the diagnosis of low- and** **high-grade tumors and even carcinoma in situ of the bladder** (Sokolova et al, 2000; Halling et al, 2000).

Other Chromosomal Abnormalities

Further studies of chromosomal abnormalities in bladder tumors were performed by the techniques of **comparative genomic hybridization** (Kallioniemi et al, 1995) or by **molecular cloning with multiple marker probes to individual genes** (Czerniak et al, 2000). These studies documented that frequency of chromosomal abnormalities in bladder tumors is much higher than previously documented by cytogenetic techniques. For example, in chromosomes 4, 8, 9, 11, and 17, Czerniak et al identified **losses in 72 genetic loci, of which 47 were related in a statistical fashion to urothelial neoplasia.** Further, many of these chromosomal abnormalities were **also present in normal and minimally abnormal epithelia adjacent to tumors.** It is postulated that these damaged chromosomal loci represent the location of suppressor genes, most of which are unknown at this time (2004). Most recently, **the microarrays technique** has been used to identify genes that may be characteristic or unique for tumors of the bladder (Brown and Botstein, 1999).

Oncogenes and Tumor Suppressor Genes in Bladder Tumors

Although it is evident from the brief summary above that the issue of genetic abnormalities in bladder cancer has

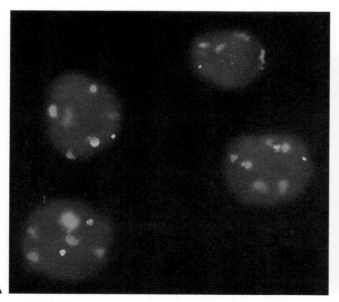

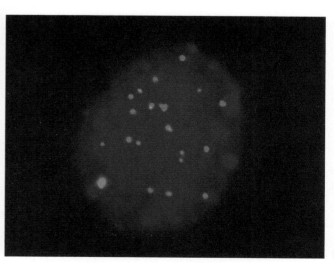

A   B

Figure 23-53 Bladder cells from urine hybridized with the UroVysion probe set. *A.* Composite image from a normal bladder. The UroVysion probe set contains SpectrumAqua CEP 17 (blue-green signals), SpectrumGreen CEP 7 (green signals), SpectrumGold LSI 9p21 (yellow signals), Spectrum Red CEP 3 (red signals). Nuclear DNA is stained with diamidinophenylindole (DAPI). Each nucleus contains two signals of each of the four probe colors as expected for diploid chromosomes. *B.* A composite image from a patient diagnosed with transitional cell carcinoma hybridized with UroVysion probe set. Greater than two signals are seen for CEP 17 (aqua), CEP 7 (green), and CEP 3 (red), indicating abnormally high chromosome copy numbers. In addition, both LSI 9p21 signals (yellow) are absent, indicating homozygous deletion of the chromosome 9p21 region (the 9p21 locus includes the tumor suppressor gene p16). (Photographs from Vysis, Inc.)

not been solved, some of the chromosomal abnormalities correspond to known loci for tumor suppressor genes and oncogenes. As early as 1990, Czerniak et al documented that **ploidy of bladder tumors could be correlated with a mutation of the *ras* oncogene.** The expression of the *ras* gene was **normal in diploid tumors** but was markedly **increased in aneuploid and invasive bladder carcinomas, particularly** when the mutation of the exon in position 12 was synchronous with an intron mutation. **The mutation could also be demonstrated in cells in voided urine sediment and in normal urothelium several years before the occurrence of invasive cancer** (Czerniak et al, 1992).

Sidransky et al (1991) also observed mutations of the **p53 inhibitory gene** in bladder tumors. It is known that this gene is involved in protecting the normal cell cycle, as discussed in Chapter 3. Several observers reported that the **mutation of the p53 gene is associated with rapid progression and poor prognosis in high-grade tumors of the bladder** (Sarkis et al, 1993; Esrig et al, 1994; Cordon-Cardo et al, 1994). This test is applicable to urinary sediment as reported by Hruban et al (1994) in reference to the bladder cancer of the late Vice President Hubert Humphrey. It is interesting to note, though, that Mr. Humphrey's **diagnosis of carcinoma in situ was established many years earlier by this writer and others by simple microscopic analysis of his urinary sediment and biopsies of bladder** (Koss, 1998, unpublished). Burton et al (2000) quantitated the expression of **p27,** a cyclin dependent inhibitor of cell cycle progression and of **caspase 3,** an important component of the apoptotic sequence, in attempting to establish the prognosis of urothelial carcinoma in situ. In a retrospective study, these authors documented that loss of p27 expression and increased expression of caspase 3 predicted progression of carcinoma in situ to invasive cancer with specificity of 85%.

Another tumor suppressor gene that controls the events of cell cycle is the **retinoblastoma (Rb) gene** (see Chap. 3). Abnormalities of this gene have been observed in **high-grade urothelial tumors with poor prognosis** (Cairns et al, 1991; Ishikawa et al, 1991; Cordon-Cardo et al, 1992).

There is no doubt that, with the passage of time, many additional genes will be identified that participate in carcinogenesis and will perhaps shed light on the genetic sequence of events in urothelial tumors. It remains to be seen, however, whether these labor intensive, costly techniques will soon replace cytology of the urinary tract as means of cancer detection and diagnosis.

The Urologist and Cytology of the Lower Urinary Tract

This brief summary of recent technologic developments in monitoring patients with tumors of the lower urinary tract reflects the **unhappiness of urologists with poor performance of urinary cytology in reference to low-grade, low-stage papillary urothelial tumors, which still**

require cystoscopic monitoring. It should be pointed out though that **these tumors are rarely, if ever, threatening the life of the patients** and that they can be easily diagnosed by cystoscopy during follow-up studies. Whether the expense of the new testing methods is ever going to provide lasting benefits to the patients, such as a reduced number of follow-up cystoscopies, is not clear, particularly in view of the high rate of false-positive results, reported by some of the investigators. **The most important benefit of urinary tract cytology is the recognition of high-grade tumors, either as a primary or a secondary event, with specificity unmatched by any of the new systems proposed.**

MALIGNANT TUMORS OF RENAL PARENCHYMA IN URINARY SEDIMENT

The technique of choice in the cytologic investigation of renal parenchymal lesions is the percutaneous needle biopsy, discussed at length in Chapter 40. However, **voided urine sediment, and occasionally retrograde brush technology,** may sometimes contribute to the **diagnosis of renal parenchymal tumors, if they extend to the renal pelvis and shed cancer cells in urine.** Tumors of renal parenchyma, remote from the renal pelvis, cannot be recognized in the urinary sediment.

Renal Adenocarcinoma

Most adenocarcinomas of the kidney usually originate in the renal cortex. The most common varieties are the **clear cell and granular cell** types. In **histologic material, the** large tumor cells have **large nuclei with prominent nucleoli,** surrounded by abundant, distinctly **granular or clear cytoplasm** that contains both glycogen and lipids. Renal carcinomas have a tendency to invade the renal pelvis and the renal vessels, with resulting **hematuria,** which is not infrequently the first evidence of the existence of the tumor (see Chap. 10).

Cytology

Cytologic detection of renal carcinoma in voided urine cannot occur unless the cancer cells desquamate into the urinary stream. Concomitant hematuria, which occurs often, may render the diagnosis exceedingly difficult. Moreover, the fragile renal cancer cells readily undergo degenerative changes so that even in the absence of hematuria, it is rare to see cells sufficiently well preserved for an unequivocal diagnosis.

Despite these problems, it is sometimes possible to recognize well-preserved cells of renal carcinomas in the urinary sediment. The cancer cells are fairly large, with a delicate, faintly vacuolated or finely granular cytoplasm, that is either eosinophilic or basophilic, and harbors distinctly abnormal, hyperchromatic large

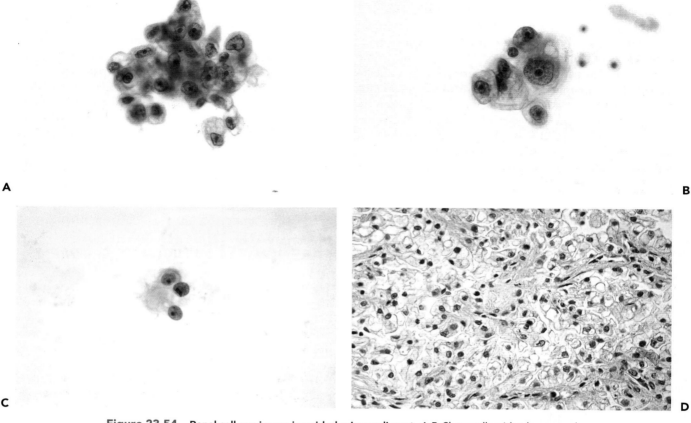

Figure 23-54 **Renal cell carcinoma in voided urine sediment.** *A,B.* Show cells with a large, markedly vacuolated cytoplasm, large pale nuclei with prominent nucleoli. *C.* Three small cancer cells with prominent nucleoli, corresponding to the clear cell renal carcinoma shown in *D.*

nuclei with large, often multiple nucleoli (Fig. 23-54). **Spindly cancer cells may also occur.** In diagnosing renal carcinoma, **one must be certain that the nuclear abnormalities are clearly evident,** since cytoplasmic granularity and vacuolization may be observed in macrophages and in benign cells of urothelial origin, the latter observed in specimens obtained by retrograde catheterization (see Chap. 22). In our experience, the urinary sediment is of questionable value in the diagnosis of primary renal parenchymal cancers, and an unequivocal cytologic diagnosis of renal carcinoma is a rare event.

These personal results are in contradistinction to the experience of other authors who reported a fair measure of success in the diagnosis of renal carcinoma. Umiker (1964) and Meisels (1963) reported between 25% and 50% of renal cancers as diagnosable by cytology. Piscioli et al (1983) claimed cytologic recognition of renal cancer in 19 of 44 cases. These results could not be duplicated by us.

Hajdu et al (1971) suggested the use of **fat stain (oil red-O) on cells of the unfixed urinary sediment.** The fat stain was positive in the form of distinct intracytoplasmic granules in 14 of 17 patients with renal cancer. The results could not be confirmed by Mount et al (1973) and the method has not received wide acceptance.

Other Types of Renal Carcinomas

Kennedy et al (1990), Mauri et al (1994), and Fallick et al (1997) each reported a case of **the rare carcinoma of the collecting ducts** diagnosed by urine cytology. Contrary to the common form of renal carcinoma, these tumors originate in the tubules of the renal medulla (ducts of Bellini) that open into the renal pelvis (Rumpelt et al, 1991). This may explain the success in the cytologic identification of this tumor.

Larson et al (1998) reported a case of **medullary carcinoma** of the kidney diagnosed in a retrograde brush specimen. The latter tumor is very rare as it occurs in young patients with sickle cell anemia and has a dismal prognosis. So far as one could judge from the illustrations, none of these uncommon tumors had sufficiently characteristic cytologic features for determination of tumor type.

Nephroblastoma (Wilms' Tumor)

This highly malignant tumor of childhood, discussed in Chapter 40, **may shed recognizable cancer cells in the urinary sediment. The cancer cells are small, spherical or elongated, and characteristically form clusters,** an appearance that does not occur with other cells of comparable size, whether inflammatory cells, leukemias, or lymphomas. These cells represent the epithelial component of the complex tumor. **When such cells are found in the urinary sediment of a child, the diagnosis of Wilms' tumor may**

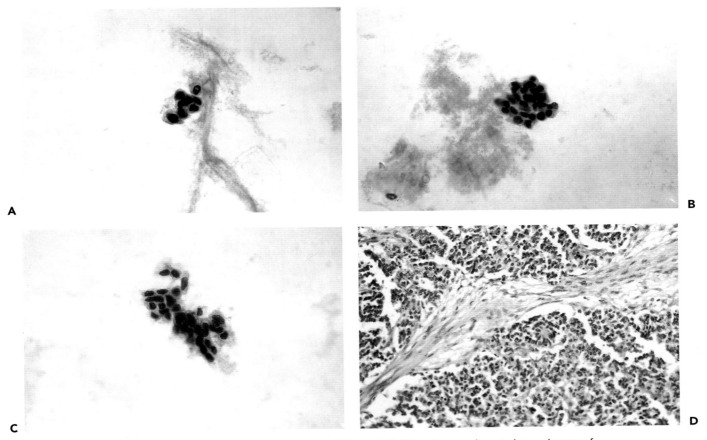

Figure 23-55 **Wilms' tumor in a 9-year-old boy.** *A–C.* The urinary sediment shows clusters of small cancer cells. *D.* Histology of the tumor.

be entertained (Fig. 23-55). The differential diagnosis includes all other "small blue cell tumors" of childhood and requires clinical data for confirmation.

Malignant Lymphoma

Sano and Koprowska (1965) reported an exceedingly rare case of **primary malignant lymphoma** of the kidney diagnosed on urinary sediment. Cheson et al (1984) reported a case of disseminated lymphoma with renal involvement. The cytologic presentation was comparable to other lymphomas in urinary sediment (see above).

BIBLIOGRAPHY

Acs G, Gupta PK, Baloch ZW. Cytomorphology of high-grade neuroendocrine carcinoma of the urinary tract. Diagn Cytopathol 23:92–96, 2000.

Ainsworth AM, Clark WH Jr, Mastrangelo M, Conger KB. Primary malignant melanoma of the urinary bladder. Cancer 37:1928–1936, 1976.

Algaba F, Santaularia JM, Lamas M, Ayala G. Transitional cell carcinoma of the prostate. Eur Urol 11:87–90, 1985.

Ali SZ, Reuter VE, Zakowski MF. Small cell neuroendocrine carcinoma of the urinary bladder. A clinicopathologic study with emphasis on cytologic features. Cancer 79:356–361, 1997.

Allegra SR, Broderick PA, Corvese NL. Cytologic and histogenetic observations in well differentiated transitional cell carcinoma of bladder. J Urol 107:777–782, 1972.

Alroy J, Pauli BU, Weinstein RS. Correlation between numbers of desmosomes and the aggressiveness of transitional cell carcinomas in human urinary bladder. Cancer 47:104–112, 1981.

Alsheikh MD, Mohamedali Z, Jones E, et al. Comparison of the WHO/ISUP classification and cytokeratin 20 expression in predicting the behavior of low-grade papillary urothelial tumors. Mod Pathol 14:267–272, 2001.

Althausen AF, Prout GR Jr, Daly JJ. Noninvasive papillary carcinoma of bladder associated with carcinoma in situ. J Urol 116:575–580, 1976.

Amin MB, Ro JY, Lee KM, et al. Lymphoepithelioma-like carcinoma of the urinary bladder. Am J Surg Pathol 18:466–473, 1994.

Amin MB, Ro JY, Troncoso P, et al. Micropapillary (ovarian serous carcinoma-like) variant of transitional cell carcinoma of the urinary bladder. Am J Surg Pathol 18:1224–1232, 1994.

Ashall F, Bramwell ME, Harris H. A new marker for human cancer cells: The Ca antigen and the Ca1 antibody. Lancet 2:1–7, 1982.

Atkin NB, Baker MC. Cytogenetic study of ten carcinomas of the bladder: Involvement of chromosomes 1 and 11. Cancer Genet Cytogenet 15:253–268, 1985.

Auvert J, Boureau M, Weisberger G. Embryonal sarcoma of the lower urinary tract in children: 5-year survival in two cases after radical treatment. J Urol 112:396–401, 1974.

Auvigne R, Auvigne J, Kerneis J Un cas de plasmocytome de la vessie. J Urol 62:85–90, 1956.

Badalament RA, Fair WR, Whitmore WF Jr, Melamed MR. The relative value of cytometry and cytology in the management of bladder cancer: The Memorial Sloan-Kettering Cancer Center experience. Semin Urol 6:22–30, 1988.

Badalament RA, Gay H, Whitmore WF Jr, et al. Monitoring intravesical bacillus Calmette-Guerin treatment of superficial bladder carcinoma by serial flow cytometry. Cancer 58:2751–2757, 1986.

Badalament RA, Hermansen DK, Kimmel M, et al. The sensitivity of bladder wash flow cytometry, bladder wash cytology, and voided cytology in the detection of bladder carcinoma. Cancer 60:1423–1427, 1987.

Baird SS, Bush L, Livingstone AG. Urethrectomy subsequent to total cystectomy for papillary carcinoma of the bladder. Case reports. J Urol 74:621–625, 1955.

Bales CE. A semi-automated method for preparation of urine sediment for cytologic evaluation. Acta Cytol 25:323–326, 1981.

Banigo OG, Waisman J, Kaufman JJ. Papillary (transitional) carcinoma in an ileal conduit. J Urol 114:626–627, 1975.

Bardales RH, Pitman MB, Stanley MW, et al. Urine cytology of primary and secondary urinary bladder adenocarcinoma. Cancer 84:335–343, 1998.

Barlebo H, Sorensen BL. Flat epithelial changes in the urinary bladder in patients with prostatic hypertrophy. Scand. J Urol Nephrol 6 (Suppl 15): 121–128, 1972.

Barlebo H, Sorensen BL, Soeberg Ohlsen A. Carcinoma in situ of the urinary bladder. Flat intraepithelial neoplasia. Scand J Urol Nephrol 6:213–223, 1972.

Barrasso R, De Brux J, Croissant O, Orth G. High prevalence of papillomavirus-associated penile intraepithelial neoplasia in sexual partners of women with cervical intraepithelial neoplasia. N Engl J Med 317:916–923, 1987.

Baschinsky DY, Chen JH, Vadmal MS, et al. Carcinosarcoma of the urinary bladder: An aggressive tumor with diverse histogenesis. A clinicopathologic study of 4 cases and review of the literature. Arch Pathol Lab Med 124:1172–1178, 2000.

Bastacky S, Ibrahim S, Wilczynski SP, Murphy WM. The accuracy of urinary cytology in daily practice. Cancer 87:118–128, 1999.

Bejany DE, Lockhart JL, Rhamy RK. Malignant vesical tumors following spinal cord injury. J Urol 138:1390–1392, 1987.

Bergkvist A, Ljunggvist A, Moberger G. Classification of bladder tumors based on the cellular pattern. Preliminary report of a clinical-pathological study of 300 cases with a minimum follow-up of eight years. Acta Chir Scand 130:371–378, 1965.

Bhansali SK, Cameron KM. Primary malignant lymphoma of the bladder. Br J Urol 32:440–454, 1960.

Bian Y, Ehya H, Bagley DH. Cytologic diagnosis of upper urinary tract neoplasms by ureteroscopic sampling. Acta Cytol 39:733–740, 1995.

Bibbo M, Gill WB, Harris MJ, et al. Retrograde brushing as a diagnostic procedure of ureteral, renal pelvic and renal calyceal lesions. A preliminary report. Acta Cytol 18:137–141, 1974.

Bickel A, Culkin DJ, Wheeler JS Jr. Bladder cancer in spinal cord injury patients. J Urol 146:1240–1242, 1991.

Billerey C, Marin L, Bittard H, et al. The nested variant of urothelial carcinoma of the urinary bladder: Report of five cases and review of literature. J Urol Pathol 1:89–100, 1999.

Blomjous EC, Schipper NW, Baak JP, et al. The value of morphometry and DNA flow cytometry in addition to classic prognosticators in superficial urinary bladder carcinoma. Am J Clin Pathol 91:243–248, 1989.

Bohlmeyer TJ, Shroyer KR. Endometriosis of the bladder: Cytologic findings and differentiation from transitional cell carcinoma (letter). Acta Cytol 40:382–383, 1996.

Bonser GM, Clayson DB, Jull JW, Pyrah LN. Carcinogenic properties of 2-amino-1-naphthol hydrochloride and its parent amine 2-naphthylamine. Br J Cancer 6:412–424, 1952.

Boon ME, Blomjous CE, Zwartendijk J, et al. Carcinoma in situ of the urinary bladder. Clinical presentation, cytologic pattern, and stromal changes. Acta Cytol 30:360–366, 1986.

Borgstrom E, Wahren B. Clinical significance of A, B, H isoantigen deletion of urothelial cells in bladder carcinoma. Cancer 58:2428–2434, 1986.

Botella E, Burgués O, Navarro S, et al. Warty carcinoma arising in condyloma acuminatum of urinary bladder. Int J Surg Pathol 8:253–259, 2000.

Boyland E, Harris J, Horning ES. Induction of carcinoma of bladder in rats with acetamindofluorene. Br J Cancer 8:647–654, 1954.

Brawn PN. The origin of invasive carcinoma of the bladder. Cancer 50:515–519, 1982.

Bretton PR, Herr HW, Whitmore WF Jr, et al. Intravesical bacillus Calmette-Guérin therapy for in situ transitional cell carcinoma involving the prostatic urethra. J Urol 141:853–856, 1989.

Brinton JA, Ito Y, Olsen BS. Carcinosarcoma of the urinary bladder. Cancer 25:1183–1186, 1970.

Broders AC. Epithelioma of the genitourinary organs, Ann Surg 75:574–604, 1922.

Brosman SA. The use of bacillus Calmette-Guérin in the therapy of bladder carcinoma in situ. J Urol 134:36–39, 1985.

Brown PO, Botstein D. Exploring the new world of the genome with DNA microarrays. Nat Genet 21:33–37, 1999.

Bruske T, Loch T, Thiemann O, et al. Pan-urothelial condyloma acuminatum with development of squamous cell carcinoma of the bladder and renal pelvis. J Urol 157:620–621, 1997.

Burton PBJ, Anderson CJ, Corbishly CM. Caspase 3 and p27 as predictors of invasive bladder cancer (Letter). N Engl J Med 343:1418–1420, 2000.

Cairns P, Proctor AJ, Knowles MA. Loss of heterozygosity at the RB locus is frequent and correlates with muscle invasion in bladder carcinoma. Oncogene 6:2305–2359, 1991.

Cajulis RS, Haines GK, et al. Cytology, flow cytometry, image analysis, and interphase cytogenetics by fluorescence in situ hybridization in the diagnosis of transitional cell carcinoma in bladder washes: A comparative study. Diagn Cytopathol 13:214–223, 1995.

Cajulis RS, Haines GK, Frias-Hidvegi D, et al. Cytology, flow cytometry, image analysis, and interphase cytogenetics by fluorescence in situ hybridization in the diagnosis of transitional cell carcinoma in bladder washes: A comparative study. Diagn Cytopathol 13:214–224, 1995.

Cajulis RS, Haines GK, Frias-Hidvegi D, McVary K. Interphase cytogenetics as an adjunct in the cytodiagnosis of urinary bladder carcinoma. A comparative study of cytology, flow cytometry and interphase cytogenetics in bladder washes. Anal Quant Cytol Histol 16:1–10, 1994.

Campo AM, Jarret WF, et al. Association of bovine papillomavirus type 2 and bracken fern with bladder cancer in cattle. Cancer Res 52:6898–6904, 1992.

Cardillo M, Reuter VE, Lin O. Cytologic features of the nested variant of urothelial carcinoma. A study of seven cases. Cancer Cytopathol 99:23–27, 2003.

Cecchini S, Cipparrone I, Confortini M, Scuden A. Urethral cytology of Cytobrush specimens. A new technique for detecting subclinical papillomavirus infection in men. Acta Cytol 32:314–317, 1988.

Chan JKC, Chow TC, Tsui MS. Prostatic-type polyps of the lower urinary tract: Three histogenic types? Histopathology 11:789–801, 1987.

Chan TY, Epstein JI. In situ adenocarcinoma of the bladder. Am J Surg Pathol 25:892–899, 2001.

Chasko SB, Gray GF, McCarron JP. Urothelial neoplasia of the upper urinary tract. In: Sommers SC, Rose PP, eds. Pathology Annual, Part 2. New York: Appleton-Century-Crofts, 1981:127–153.

Chaturvedi V, Hodges S, Johnston D, et al. Superimposed histologic and genetic mapping of chromosome 17 alterations in human urinary bladder neoplasia. Oncogene 14:2059–2070, 1997.

Cheng L, Cheville JC, Neumann RM, et al. Survival of patients with carcinoma in situ of the urinary bladder. Cancer 85:2469–2474, 1999A.

Cheng L, Cheville JC, Neumann RM, Bostwick DG. Natural history of urothelial dysplasia of the bladder. Am J Surg Pathol 23:443–447, 1999B.

Cheng L, Cheville JC, Neumann RM, Bostwick DG. Flat intraepithelial lesions of the urinary bladder. Cancer 88:625–631, 2000.

Cheng L, Darson M, Cheville JC, et al. Urothelial papilloma of the bladder. Clinical and biologic implications. Cancer 86:2098–2101, 1999C.

Cheng L, Leibovich BC, Cheville JC, et al. Paraganglioma of the urinary bladder: can biologic potential be predicted? Cancer 88:844–852, 2000.

Cheng L, Leibovich BC, Cheville JC, et al. Squamous papilloma of the urinary tract is unrelated to condyloma acuminata. Cancer 88:1679–1686, 2000.

Cheng L, Montironi R, Bostwick DG. Villous adenoma of the urinary tract: a report of 23 cases, including 8 with coexistent adenocarcinoma. Am J Surg Pathol 23:764–771, 1999.

Cheng L, Neumann RM, Bostwick DG. Papillary urothelial neoplasms of low malignant potential. Clinical and biologic implications. Cancer 86:2102–2108, 1999D.

Cheson BD, Schumann GB, Johnston JL. Urinary cytodiagnosis of renal involvement in disseminated histiocytic lymphoma. Acta Cytol 28:148–152, 1984.

Chiang HS, Guo HR, Hong CL, et al. The incidence of bladder cancer in the black foot disease endemic area in Taiwan. Br J Urol 71:274–278, 1993.

Chiou HY, Chiou ST, Hsu YH, et al. Incidence of transitional cell carcinoma and arsenic in drinking water: A follow-up study of 8,102 residents in an arseniasis-endemic area in northeastern Taiwan. Am J Epidemiol 153:411–418, 2001.

Chiou HY, Hsueh YM, Liaw KF, et al. Incidence of internal cancers and ingested inorganic arsenic: A seven-year follow-up study in Taiwan. Cancer Res 15:1296–1300, 1995.

Chow LT, Chan SK, Chow WH. Fine needle aspiration cytodiagnosis of leiomyosarcoma of the renal pelvis. A case report with immunohistochemical study. Acta Cytol 38:759–763, 1994.

Cianciulli AM, Leonardo C, Guadagni F, et al. Genetic instability in superficial bladder cancer and adjacent mucosa: An interphase cytogenetic study. Hum Pathol 34:214–221, 2003.

Cifuentes Delatte L, Oliva H, Navarro V. Intraepithelial carcinoma of the bladder. Urol Int 25:169–186, 1970.

Cina SJ, Lancaster-Weiss KJ, Lecksell K, Epsten JI. Correlation of Ki-67 and p53 with the new World Health Organization/International Society of Urological Pathology Classification System for Urothelial Neoplasia. Arch Pathol Lab Med 125:646–651, 2001.

Cohen SM, Shirai T, Steineck G. Epidemiology and etiology of premalignant and malignant urothelial changes. Scand J Urol Nephrol Suppl 205:105–115, 2000.

Cole P, Hoover R, Friedell GH. Occupation and cancer of the lower urinary tract. Cancer 29:1250–1260, 1972.

Collste LG, Devonec M, Darzynkiewicz. Z, et al. Bladder cancer diagnosis by flow cytometry. Correlation between cell samples from biopsy and bladder irrigation fluid. Cancer 45:2389–2394, 1980.

Coon JS, Weinstein RS. Detection of A, B, H tissue isoantigens by immunoperoxidase methods in normal and neoplastic urothelium. Comparison with the erythrocyte adherence method. Am J Clin Pathol 76:163–171, 1981.

Cooper PH, Waisman J, Johnston WH, Skinner DG. Severe atypia of transitional epithelium and carcinoma of the urinary bladder. Cancer 31:1055–1060, 1973.

Cordon-Cardo C, Dalbagni G, Saez GT, et al. p53 mutations in human bladder cancer: Genotypic versus phenotypic patterns. Int J Cancer 56:347–353, 1994.

Cordon-Cardo C, O'Brien JP, Boccia J, et al. Expression of the multidrug resistance gene product (P-glycoprotein) in human normal and tumor tissues. J Histochem Cytochem 38:1277–1287, 1990.

Cordon-Cardo C, Reuter VE, Lloyd KO, et al. Blood group-related antigens in human urothelium: enhanced expression of precuros LeX and LeY determinanys in urothelial carcinoma. Cancer Res 48:4113–4120, 1988.

Cordon-Cardo C, Sun TT. Uroplakin II gene is expressed in transitional cell carcinoma but not in bilharzial bladder squamous cell carcinoma: alternative pathways of bladder epithelial differentiation and tumor formation (published erratum appears in Cancer Res 58:2904, 1998). Cancer Res 58:1291–1297, 1998.

Cordon-Cardo C, Wartinger D, Petrylak D, et al. Altered expressions of the retinoblastoma gene product: prognostic indicator in bladder cancer. J Natl Cancer Inst 84:1251–1256, 1992.

Cordonnier JJ, Spjut HJ. Urethral occurrence of bladder carcinoma following cystectomy. J Urol 87:398–403, 1962.

Crabbe JGS. Cytology of voided urine and special reference to "benign" papilloma and some of the problems encountered in the preparation of the smears. Acta Cytol 5:233–240, 1961.

Cramer SF, Aikawa M, Cebelin M. Neurosecretory granules in small cell invasive carcinoma of the urinary bladder. Cancer 47:724–730, 1981.

Crane AR, Tremblay RG. Primary osteogenic sarcoma of the bladder. Ann Surg 118:887–908, 1943.

Crosby JH, Allsbrook WC Jr, Koss LG, et al. Cytologic detection of urothelial cancer and other abnormalities in a cohort of workers exposed to aromatic amines. Acta Cytol 35:263–268, 1991.

Cullen TH, Popham RR, Voss HJ. Urine cytology and primary carcinoma of the renal pelvis and ureter. Aust N Z J Surg 41:230–236, 1972.

Culp OS, Utz DC, Harrison EG Jr. Experiences with ureteral carcinoma in situ detected during operations for vesical neoplasms. J Urol 97:679–682, 1967.

Curry JL, Wojcik EM. The effects of the current World Health Organization/International Society of Urologic Pathologists bladder neoplasm classification system on urine cytology results. Cancer 96:140–145, 2002.

Czerniak B, Chaturvedi V, Hodges S, et al. Superimposed histologic and genetic mapping of chromosome 9 in progression of human urinary bladder neoplasia: implications for a genetic model of multistep urothelial carcinogenesis and early detection of urinary bladder cancer. Oncogene 18:1185–1196, 1999.

Czerniak B, Cohen GL, Etkind P, et al. Concurrent mutations of coding and regulatory sequences of the Ha-ras gene in urinary bladder carcinomas. Human Path 23:1199–1204, 1992.

Czerniak B, Deitch D, Simmons H, et al. Ha-ras gene codon 12 mutation and DNA ploidy in bladder carcinoma. Br J Cancer 62:762–763, 1990.

Czerniak B, Herz F. Molecular biology of common tumors of the urinary tract. Chapter 11. In Koss LG (ed). Diagnostic Cytology of the Urinary Tract. Philadelphia, New York, Lippincott-Raven, 1995.

Czerniak B, Koss LG. Expression of Ca antigen on human urinary bladder tumors. Cancer 55:2380–2383, 1985.

Czerniak B, Koss LG, Sherman A. Nuclear pores and DNA ploidy in human bladder carcinomas. Cancer Res 44:3752–3756, 1984.

Czerniak B, Li L, Chaturvedi V, et al. Genetic modeling of human urinary bladder carcinogenesis. Genes Chromosomes Cancer 27:392–402, 2000.

De Paepe ME, Andre R, Mahadevia P. Urethral involvement in female patients with bladder cancer. A study of 22 cystectomy specimens. Cancer 65:1237–1241, 1990.

Del Mistro A, Koss LG, Braunstein J, et al. Condylomata acuminata of the urinary bladder. Am J Surg Pathol 12:205–215, 1988.

Del Nero A, Esposito N, Curro A, et al. Evaluation of urinary level of NMP22 as a diagnostic marker for stage pTa-pT1 bladder cancer: comparison with urinary cytology and BTA test. Eur Urol 35:93–97, 1999.

DeBellis CC, Schumann GB. Cystoscopic biopsy supernate. A new cytologic approach for diagnosing urothelial carcinoma in situ. Acta Cytol 30:356–359, 1986.

DeHarven E, He S, Hanna W, et al. Phenotypically heterogeneous deletion of the A, B, H antigen from the transformed bladder urothelium. A scanning electron microscope study. J Submicrosc Cytol 19:639–649, 1987.

DeKernion JB, Haung M-Y, Linder A, et al. The management of superficial bladder tumors and carcinoma in situ with intravesical bacillus Calmette-Guérin. J Urol 133:598–601, 1985.

Del Mistro A, Braunstein JD, Halwer M, Koss LG. Identification of human papillomavirus types in male urethral condylomata acuminate by in situ hybridization. Human Path 18:936–940, 1987.

DeMay RM, Grathwohl MA. Signet-ring-cell (colloid) carcinoma of the urinary bladder. Acta Cytol 29:132–136, 1985.

deVere White RW, Deitch AD, Baker WC Jr, Strand MA. Urine: A suitable sample for deoxyribonucleic acid flow cytometry studies in patients with bladder cancer. J Urol 139:926–928, 1988.

deVere White RW, Olsson CA, Deitch AD. Flow cytometry: Role in monitoring transitional cell carcinoma of bladder. Urology 28:15–20, 1986.

Devonec M, Darzynkiewicz Z, Whitmore WF, Melamed MR. Flow cytometry for follow-up examinations of conservatively treated low stage bladder tumors. J Urol 126:166–170, 1981.

deVoogt HJ, Rathert P, Beyer-Boon ME. Urinary Cytology. New York, Springer-Verlag, 1977.

Dhom G, Mohr G. Urothelial carcinoma in the prostate. Urologe 16:70–72, 1977.

Dimmette RM, Sproat HF, Klimt CR. Examination of smears of urinary sediment for detection of neoplasms of bladder; survey of an Egyptian village infested with Schistosoma hematobium. Am J Clin Pathol 25:1032–1042, 1955.

Dinney CP, Ro JY, Babaian RJ, Johnson DE. Lymphoepithelioma of the bladder: a clinicopathological study of 3 cases. J Urol 149:840–841, 1993.

Dodd LG, Johnston WW, Robertson CN, Layfield LJ. Endoscopic brush cytology of the upper urinary tract. Evaluation of its efficacy and potential limitations in diagnosis. Acta Cytol 41:377–384, 1997.

Domagala W, Kahan AV, Koss LG. The ultrastructure of surfaces of positively identified cells in the human urinary sediment: A correlative light and scanning electron microscopic study. Acta Cytol 23:147–155, 1979.

Doria MI Jr, Saint Martin G, Wang HH, et al. Cytologic features of clear cell carcinoma of the urethra and urinary bladder. Diagn Cytopathol 14:150–154, 1996.

Droller MJ, Walsh PC. Intensive intravesical chemotherapy in the treatment of flat carcinoma in situ: Is it safe? J Urol 134:1115–1117, 1985.

Eisenberg RB, Roth RB, Schweinsberg MH. Bladder tumors and associated proliferative mucosal lesions. J Urol 84:544–550, 1960.

El-Bolkainy M, Chu EW (eds). Detection of bladder cancer associated with schistosomiasis. Cairo, Egypt: National Cancer Institute, Cairo University, Al Ahram Press, 1981.

Elliot JA, Moloney PL, Anderson GH. "Denuding cystitis" and in situ urothelial carcinoma. Arch. Pathol 96:91–94, 1973.

Epstein JI, Amin MB, Reuter VR, Mostofi FK. The World Health Organization/International Society of Urological Pathology consensus classification of urothelial (transitional cell) neoplasms of the urinary bladder. Am J Surg Pathol 22:1435–1448, 1998.

Epstein JI, Woodruff JM. Adenocarcinoma of the prostate with endometrioid features: A light microscopic and immunohistochemical study of ten cases. Cancer 57:111–119, 1985.

Eriksson O, Johansson S. Urothelial neoplasms of the upper urinary tract. A correlation between cytologic and histologic findings in 43 patients with urothelial neoplasma of the renal pelvis or ureter. Acta Cytol 20:20–25, 1976.

Esposti PL, Moberger G, Zajicek J. The cytologic diagnosis of transitional cell tumors of the urinary bladder and its histologic basis. A study of 567 cases of urinary-tract disorder including 170 untreated and 182 irradiated bladder tumors. Acta Cytol 14:145–155, 1970.

Esposti PL, Zajicek J. Grading of transitional cell neoplasms of the urinary bladder from smears of bladder washings. A critical review of 326 tumors. Acta Cytol 16:529–537, 1972.

Esrig D, Elmajian D, Groshen S, et al. Accumulation of nuclear p53 and tumor progression in bladder cancer. New Engl J Med 331:1259–1264, 1994.

Fadl-Elmula I, Gorunova L, Mandahl N, et al. Cytogenetic monoclonality in multifocal uroepithelial carcinomas: evidence of intraluminal tumour seeding. Br J Cancer 81:6–12, 1999.

Fallick ML, Hutchinson M, Alroy J, Long JP. Collecting-duct carcinoma presenting as upper tract lesion with abnormal urine cytology. Diagn Cytopathol 16:258–261, 1997.

Falor WH. Chromosomes in noninvasive papillary carcinoma of the bladder. JAMA 216:791–794, 1971.

Falor WH, Ward RM. Cytogenetic analysis: A potent index for recurrence of early carcinoma of the bladder. J Urol 115:49–52, 1976.

Farrow GM, Utz DC, Rife CC. Morphological and clinical observations in patients with early bladder cancer treated with total cystectomy. Cancer Res 36:2495–2501, 1976.

Farrow GM, Utz DC, Rife CC, Greene LF. Clinical observations on 69 cases of in situ carcinoma of the urinary bladder. Cancer Res 37:2794–2798, 1977.

Farsund T. Selective sampling of cells for morphological and quantitative cytology of bladder epithelium. J Urol 128:267–271, 1982.

Flanigan RC, King CT, Clark TD, et al. Immunohistochemical demonstration of blood group antigens in neoplastic and normal human urothelium: A comparison with standard red cell adherence. J Urol 130:449–503, 1983.

Foot NC, Papanicolaou GN. Early renal carcinoma in situ detected by means of smears of fixed urinary sediment. JAMA 139:356–358, 1949.

Foot NC, Papanicolaou GN, Holmquist ND, Seybolt JF. Exfoliative cytology of urinary sediments; review of 2,829 cases. Cancer 11:127–137, 1958.

Forni A, Ghetti G, Armell G. Urinary cytology in workers exposed to carcinogenic aromatic amines: A six-year study. Acta Cytol 16:142–145, 1972.

Foså SD. Feulgen-DNA-values in transitional cell carcinoma of the human urinary bladder. Beitr Pathol 155:44–55, 1975.

Foså SD, Kaalhus O. Nuclear size and chromatin concentration in transitional cell carcinoma of the human urinary bladder. Beitr Pathol 157:109–125, 1976.

Fox AJ, White GC. Bladder cancer in rubber workers. Do screening and doctors' awareness distort the statistics? Lancet 1:1009–1011, 1976.

Fradet Y, Cordon-Cardo C, Thomson T, et al. Cell monoclonal antibodies. Proc Natl Acad Sci USA 81:224–228, 1984.

Fradet Y, Cordon-Cardo C, Whitmore WF, et al. Cell surface antigens of human bladder tumors: Definition of tumor subsets by monoclonal antibodies and correlation with growth characteristics. Cancer Res 46:5183–5188, 1986.

Fradet Y, Lockhart C, et al. Performance characteristics of a new monoclonal antibody test for bladder cancer: ImmunoCyt. Can J Urol 4:400–405, 1997.

Framowitz FB, Bard RH, Koss LG. The epithelial origin of a malignant mesodermal mixed tumor of the bladder: Report of case with long-term survival. J Urol 132:2385–2389, 1984.

Framowitz FB, Steinbook ML, Lautin EM, et al. Inverted papilloma of the ureter. J Urol 126:113–116, 1981.

Ganem EJ, Batal JT. Secondary malignant tumors of the urinary bladder metastatic from primary foci in distant organs. J Urol 75:965–972, 1956.

Garner JW, Goldstein AMB, Cosgrove MD. Histologic appearance of the intestinal urinary conduit. J Urol 114:854–857, 1975.

Gelmini S, Crisci A, Salvadori B, et al. Comparison of telomerase activity in bladder carcinoma and exfoliated cells collected in urine and bladder washings, using a quantitative assay. Clin Cancer Res 6:2771–2776, 2000.

Genega EM, Hutchinson B, Reuter VE, Gaudin PB. Immunophenotype of high-grade prostatic adenocarcinoma and urothelial carcinoma. Mod Pathol 13:1186–1191, 2000.

Giacomini G, Bianchi G, Moretti D. Detection of sexually transmitted diseases by urethral cytology, the ignored male counterpart of cervical cytology. Acta Cytol 33:11–15, 1989.

Gill WB, Lu CT, Thomsen D. Retrograde brushing: A new technique for obtaining histologic and cytologic material from ureteral, renal pelvic, and renal calyceal lesions. J Urol 109:573–578, 1973.

Gillenwater JY, Burros HM. Unusual tumors of the female urethra. Obstet Gynecol 31:617–620, 1968.

Gissman L, Diehl V. Molecular cloning and characterization of human papillomavirus DNA derived from a laryngeal papilloma. T Virol 44:393–400, 1982.

Goebbels R, Amberger L, Wernert N, Dhom G. Urothelial carcinoma of the prostate. Appl Pathol 3:242–254, 1985.

Goldstein ML, Whitman T, Renshaw AA. Significance of cell groups in voided urine. Acta Cytol 42:290–294, 1998.

Gowing NF. Urethral carcinoma associated with cancer of the bladder. Br J Urol 32:428–438, 1960.

Grabstald H. Tumors of the urethra in men and women. Cancer 32:1235–1236, 1973.

Grabstald H. Carcinoma of ileal bladder stoma. J Urol 112:332–334, 1974.

Grabstald H, Hilaris B, Henschke U, Whitmore WF Jr. Cancer of the female urethra. JAMA 197:835–842, 1966.

Grabstald H, Whitmore WF, Melamed MR. Renal pelvic tumors. JAMA 218:845–854, 1971.

Granberg-Ohman I, Tribukait B, Wijkstrom H. Cytogentic analysis of 62 transitional cell bladder carcinomas. Cancer Genet Cytogenet 11:69–85, 1984.

Granter SR, Perez-Atayde AR, Renshaw AA. Cytologic analysis of papillary renal cell carcinoma. Cancer 84:303–308, 1998.

Greenlee RT, Hill-Harmon MB, Murray T, Thun M. Cancer statistics 2001. CA Cancer J Clin 51:15–36, 2001.

Grignon DJ, Ro JY, Ayala AG, et al. Primary adenocarcinoma of the urinary bladder. A clinicopathologic analysis of 72 cases. Cancer 67:2165–2172, 1991.

Grignon DJ, Ro JY, Ayala AG, et al. Small cell carcinoma of the urinary bladder. A clinicopathologic analysis of 22 cases. Cancer 69:527–536, 1992.

Grogono JL, Shepheard BGF. Carcinoma of the urachus. Br J Urol 41:222–227, 1969.

Grussendorf-Conen E-I, Deutz FJ, de Villers EM. Detection of human papillomavirus-6 in primary carcinoma of the urethra in men. Cancer 60:1832–1835, 1987.

Guinan P, Vogelzang NJ, Randazzo R. Renal pelvic cancer: a review of 611 patients treated in Illinois 1975–1985. Urology 40:393–399, 1992.

Hajdu SI. Exfoliative cytology or primary and metastatic Wilms' tumors. Acta Cytol 15:339–342, 1971.

Hajdu SI, Savino A, Hajdu EO, Koss LG. Cytologic diagnosis of renal cell carcinoma with the aid of fat stain. Acta Cytol 15:31–33, 1971.

Halling KC, King W, Sokolova IA, et al. A comparison of cytology and fluorescence in situ hybridization for the detection of urothelial carcinoma. J Urol 164:1766–1774, 2000.

Harnden P, Allam A, Joyce AD, et al. Cytokeratin 20 expression by non-invasive transitional cell carcinomas: potential for distinguishing recurrent from non-recurrent disease. Histopathol 27:169–174, 1995.

Harris MJ, Schwinn CP, Morrow JW, et al. Exfoliative cytology of the urinary bladder irrigation specimen. Acta Cytol 15:385–399, 1971.

Hartveit F, Thunold S. Koilocytosis in neoplasia of the urinary bladder. Br J Urol 69:46–48, 1992.

Harving N, Wolf H, Melsen F. Positive urinary cytology after tumor resection: An indicator for concomitant carcinoma in situ. J Urol 140:495–497, 1988.

Helpap B, Bodekar J, Pfitzenmaier N. Histologische und zytologische Aspekte der urotherlialen Atypie (Dysplasie). Pathologe 6:292–297, 1985.

Herr HW. Immunobiology of human bladder cancer. J Urol 115:147–149, 1976.

Herr HW, Badalament RA, Amato DA, et al. Superficial bladder cancer treated with bacillus Calmette-Guérin: A multivariate analysis of factors affecting tumor progression. J Urol 141:22–29, 1989.

Herr HW, Cookson MS, Soloway SM. Upper tract tumors in patients with primary bladder cancer followed for 15 years. J Urol 156:1286–1287, 1996.

Herr HW, Fradet Y, Klein J: Summary of effect of intravesical Bacillus Calmette-Guerin (BCG) on carcinoma in situ of the bladder. Semin Urol Oncol 15:80–85, 1997.

Herr HW, Laudone UP, Badalament RA, et al. Bacillus Calmetter-Guerin therapy alters the progression of superficial bladder cancer. J Clin Oncol 6:1450–1455, 1988.

Herr HW, Pinsky CM, Whitmore WF Jr, et al. Long-term effect of intravesical bacillus Calmette-Guérin on flat carcinoma in situ of the bladder. J Urol 135:265–267, 1986.

Herz F, Barlebo H, Koss LG. Modulation of alkaline phosphatase activity in cell cultures derived from human urinary bladder carcinoma. Cancer 34:1934–1943, 1974.

Hida CA, Gupta PK. Cercariform cells. Are they specific for transitional cell carcinoma? Cancer (Cancer CytoPathol) 87:69–74, 1999.

Hirono I, Shibuya C, Shimizu M, Fushimi K. Carcinogenic activity of processed bracken used as human food. J Natl Cancer Inst 48:1245–1250, 1972.

Hisazumi H, Miyoshi N, Naito K, Misaki T. Whole bladder wall photoradiation therapy for carcinoma in situ of the bladder: A preliminary report. J Urol 131:884–887, 1984.

Hoda RS, Tahir-Kheli N, Decker D, Koss LG. Urine screening on Papnet: Study of 50 cases. Abstract. Acta Cytol 39:201, 1995.

Holmquist ND. Detection of urinary tract cancer in urinalysis specimens in an outpatient population. Am J Clin Pathol 89:499–504, 1988.

Holtz F, Fox JE, Abell MR. Carcinosarcoma of the urinary bladder. Cancer 29:294–304, 1972.

Hom JD, King EB, Fraenkel R, et al. Adenocarcinoma with a neuroendocrine component arising in the urachus. A case report. Acta Cytol 34:269–274, 1990.

Hopenhayn-Rich C, Biggs ML, Fuchs A, et al. Bladder cancer mortality associated with arsenic in drinking water in Argentina. Epidemiology 7:117–124, 1996.

Hopkins SC, Ford KS, Soloway MS. Invasive bladder cancer: support for screening. J Urol 130:61–64, 1983.

Hopman AH, Ramaekeers FC, Raap AK, et al. In situ hybridization as a tool to study numerical chromosome aberrations in solid bladder tumors. Histochem 89:307–316, 1988.

Houston W, Koss LG, Melamed MR. Bladder cancer and schistosomiasis: A preliminary cytological study. Trans R Soc Trop Med Hyg 60:89–91, 1966.

Hruban RH, van der Riet P, Erozan YS, Sidransky D. Brief report: Molecular biology and the early detection of carcinoma of the bladder: The case of Hubert H. Humphrey. N Engl J Med 330:1276–1278, 1994.

Huben RP, Mounzer AM, Murphy GP. Tumor grade and stae as prognostic variables in upper tract urothelial tumors. Cancer 62:2016–2020, 1988.

Hueper WC. Occupational and Environmental Cancers of the Urinary System. New Haven, Yale University Press, 1969.

Ishikawa J, Xu H-J, Hu S-X, et al. Inactivation of the retinoblastoma gene in human bladder and renal cell carcinomas. Cancer Res 51:5736–5743, 1991.

Jacobs JB, Arai M, Cohen SM, Friedell GH. Early lesions in experimental bladder cancer: Scanning electron microscopy of cell surface markers. Cancer Res 36:2512–2517, 1976.

Jao W, Soto JM, Gould VE. Squamous carcinoma of bladder with pseudosarcomatous stroma. Arch Pathol 100:461–466, 1975.

Jewett HJ, Lowell RK, Shelley WM. A study of 364 cases of infiltrating bladder cancer: Relation of certain pathological characteristics to prognosis after extirpation. J Urol 92:668–678, 1964.

Jewett HJ, Strong GH. Infiltrating carcinoma of bladder: Relation of depth of penetration of bladder wall to incidence of local extension and metastases. J Urol 55:366–372, 1946.

Johansson S, Angervall L, Bengston U, Wahlquist L. Uroepithelial tumors of the renal pelvis associated with abuse of phenacetin-containing analgesics. Cancer 33:743–753, 1974.

Johnson TL, Kini SR. Cytologic features of metastatic transitional cell carcinoma. Diagn Cytopathol 9:270–278, 1993.

Kakizoe T, Fujita J, Murase T, et al. Transitional cell carcinoma of the bladder in patients with renal pelvic and ureteral cancer. J Urol 124:17–19, 1980.

Kallioniemi A, Kallioniemi O, Citro G, et al. Identification of gains and losses of DNA sequences in primary bladder cancer by comparative genomic hybridization. Genes Chromosomes Cancer 12:213–219, 1995.

Kalnins ZA, Rhyne AL, Morehead RP, Carter BJ. Comparison of cytologic findings in patients with transitional cell carcinoma and benign urologic diseases. Acta Cytol 14:743–749, 1970.

Kannan V, Bose S. Low grade transitional cell carcinoma and instrument artifact. A challenge in urinary cytology. Acta Cytol 37:899–902, 1993.

Kannan V, Gupta D. Calculus artifact. A challenge in urinary cytology. Acta Cytol 43: 794–800, 1999.

Katz JI, Grabstald H. Primary malignant melanoma of the female urethra. J Urol 116:454–457, 1976.

Kaufman JM, Fam B, Jacobs SC, et al. Bladder cancer and squamous metaplasia in spinal cord injury patients. J Urol 118:967–970, 1977.

Kaye KW, Lange PH. Mode of presentation of invasive bladder cancer: Reassessment of the problem. J Urol 128:31–33, 1982.

Keesee SK, Briggman JV, Thill G, Wu Y-J. Utilization of nuclear matrix proteins for cancer diagnosis. Crit Rev Eukaryot Gene Expr 6:189–214, 1996.

Kennedy SM, Merino MJ, Linehan WM, et al. Collecting duct carcinoma of the kidney. Hum Pathol 21:449–456, 1990.

Kenny GM, Hutchinson WB. Transrectal ultrasound study of prostate. Urology 32:401–402, 1988.

Kern WH. The cytology of transitional cell carcinoma of the urinary bladder. Acta Cytol 19:420–428, 1975.

Kern WH, Bales CE, Webster WW. Cytologic evaluation of transitional cell carcinoma of the bladder. J Urol 100:616–622, 1968.

Khan AU, Farrow GM, Zincke H, et al. Primary carcinoma in situ of the ureter and renal pelvis. J Urol 121:681, 1979.

Kim TS, Seong DH, Ro JY. Small cell carcinoma of the ureter with squamous cell and transitional cell carcinoma components: Report of a case. J Korean Med Sci 16(6):796–800, 2001.

Klein FA, Herr HW, Whitmore WF, et al. An evaluation of automated flow cytometry (FCM) in detection of carcinoma in situ of the urinary bladder. Cancer 50:1003–1008, 1982.

Knappenberger ST, Uson AC, Melicow MM. Primary neoplasms occurring in vesical diverticula: A report of 18 cases. J Urol 83:153–159, 1960.

Kobayashi S, Ohmori M, Miki H, et al. Exfoliative cytology of a primary carcinoma of the renal pelvis. A case report. Acta Cytol 29:1021–1025, 1985.

Konety BR, Nguyen, T-ST, Dhir R, et al. Detection of bladder cancer using a novel nuclear matrix protein, BLCA-4. Clin Cancer Res 6:2618–262, 2000.

Korkolopoulou P, Christodoulou P, Konstantinidou, A-E, et al. Cell cycle regulators in bladder cancer: A multivariate survival study with emphasis on p27Kip1. Hum Pathol 31:751–760, 2000.

Korman HJ, Peabody JO, Cerny JC, et al. Autocrine motility factor receptor as a possible urine marker for transitional cell carcinoma of the bladder. J Urol 155:347–349, 1996.

Koss LG. Tumors of the Urinary Bladder. Atlas of Tumor Pathology. 2nd series, Fascicle 11. Washington DC, Armed Forces Institute of Pathology, 1975.

Koss LG. Some ultrastructural aspects of experimental and human carcinoma of the bladder. Cancer Res 37:2824–2835, 1977.

Koss LG. Mapping of the urinary bladder: Its impact on the concepts of bladder cancer. Hum Pathol 10:533–548, 1979.

Koss LG. Environmental carcinogenesis and cytology [Editorial]. Acta Cytol 24:281–282, 1980.

Koss LG. Urinary tract cytology. In Connolly JC (ed). Carcinoma of the Bladder. New York, Raven Press, 1981, pp 159–163.

Koss LG. Evaluation of patients with carcinoma in situ of the bladder. *In* Sommers CC, Rosen PP (eds). Pathol Annual 17 (Part 2):353–359, 1982.

Koss LG. Tumors of the Urinary Bladder. Atlas of Tumor Pathology. 2nd series, Fascicle 11. Washington DC, Armed Forces Institute of Pathology. Supplement, 1985.

Koss LG. The role of cytology in the diagnosis, detection and follow-up bladder cancer. *In* Denis L, et al (eds). Developments in Bladder Cancer. New York, Alan R. Liss, 1986, pp 97–108.

Koss LG. Precursor lesions of invasive bladder cancer. Eur Urol 14 (Suppl 1): 4–6, 1988.

Koss LG. Cytologic techniques as a diagnostic and prognostic tool in urologic cancer. *In* O'Reilly PH, George NJR, Weiss RM (eds). Diagnostic Techniques in Urology. Philadelphia, WB Saunders, 1990.

Koss LG. Diagnostic Cytology of the Urinary Tract with Histopathologic and Clinical Correlations. Philadelphia, Lippincott-Raven, 1995.

Koss LG, Bartels PH, Bibbo M, et al. Computer discrimination between benign and malignant urothelial cells. Acta Cytol 19:378–391, 1975.

Koss LG, Bartels PH, Bibbo M, et al. Computer analysis of atypical urothelial cells. I. Classification by supervised learning algorithms. Acta Cytol 21: 247–260, 1977.

Koss LG, Bartels PH, Sychra JJ, Wied GL. Computer analysis of atypical urothelial cells. II. Classification by unsupervised learning algorithms. Acta Cytol 21:261–265, 1977.

Koss LG, Bartels PH, Wied GL. Computer-based diagnostic analysis of cells in the urinary sediment. J Urol 123:846–849, 1980.

Koss LG, Czerniak B. Image analysis and flow cytometry of tumors of prostate and bladder; with a comment on molecular biology of urothelial tumors. *In* Pathology and Pathobiology of the Urinary Bladder and Prostate. Chapter 5, Baltimore, Williams & Wilkins, 1992, pp 112–128.

Koss LG, Deitch D, Ramanathan R, Sherman AB. Diagnostic value of cytology of voided urine. Acta Cytol 29:810–816, 1985.

Koss LG, Lavin P. Studies of experimental bladder carcinoma in Fischer 344 female rats. I. Induction of tumors with diet low in vitamin B_6 containing N-2-fluorenylacetamide after single dose of cyclophosphamide. J Natl Cancer Inst 46:585–595, 1971.

Koss LG, Melamed MR, Kelly RE. Further cytologic and histologic studies of bladder lesions in workers exposed to *para*-aminodiphenyl: Progress report. J Natl Cancer Inst 43:233–243, 1969.

Koss LG, Melamed MR, Ricci A, Melick WF, Kelly RE. Carcinogenesis in the human urinary bladder. Observations after exposure to *para*-aminodiphenyl. N Engl J Med 272:767–770, 1965.

Koss LG, Nakanishi I, Freed S. Nonpapillary carcinoma in situ and atypical hyperplasia in cancerous bladders. Further studies of surgically removed bladders by mapping. Urology 9:442–455, 1977.

Koss LG, Tiamson EM, Robbins MA. Mapping cancerous and precancerous bladder changes. A study of the urothelium in ten surgically removed bladders. JAMA 227:281–286, 1974.

Koss LG, Wersto RP, Simmons DA, et al. Predictive value of DNA measurements in bladder washings. Comparison of flow cytometry, image cytophotometry, and cytology in patients with a past history of urothelial tumors. Cancer 64:916–924, 1989.

Kovarik S, Davidsohn I, Stejkal R. ABO antigen in cancer: Detection with the mixed cell agglutination reaction. Arch Pathol 86:12–21, 1968.

Kriegmair M, Baumgartner R, Knuechel R, et al. Fluorescence photodetection of neoplastic urothelial lesions following intravesical instillation of 5-aminolevulinic acid. Urology 44:836–841, 1994.

Krumerman MS, Katatikaru V. Rhabdomyosarcoma of the urinary bladder with intraepithelial spread in an adult Arch Pathol Lab Med 100:395–397, 1976.

Kyo S, Kunimi K, Uchibayashi T, et al. Telomerase activity in human urothelial tumors. Am J Clin Pathol 107:555, 1997.

Lamm DL. BCG immunotherapy for transitional-cell carcinoma in situ of the bladder. Oncology 9:947–952, 1995.

Lamm DL, Blumensten BA, Crawford ED, et al. A randomized trial of intravesical doxorubicin and immunotherapy with Bacille Calmette-Guerin for transitional cell carcinoma of the bladder. N Engl J Med 325:1205–1209, 1991.

Landman J, Chang Y, Kavaler E, et al. Sensitivity and specificity of NMP-22, telomerase, and BTA in the detection of human bladder cancer. Urology 52: 398–402, 1998.

Lange PH, Limas C. Molecular markers in the diagnosis and prognosis of bladder cancer. J Urol 23S:46, 1984.

Larson DM, Gilstad CW, Manson GW, Henry MR. Renal medullary carcinoma: report of a case with positive urinary cytology. Diagn Cytopathol 18: 276–279, 1998.

Laursen B. Cancer of the bladder in patients treated with chlornaphazine. Br Med J 3:684–685, 1970.

Lederer B, Mikuz G, Gäutter W, zur Neiden G. Zytophotometrische Untersuchungen an Tumoren des Ubergangsepithels der Harnblase. Vergleich zytophotometrischer Untersuchungsergebnisse mit dem histologischen Grading. Beitr Pathol 147:379–389, 1972.

Levi PE, Cooper EH, Anderson CK, Williams RE. Analysis of DNA content, nuclear size and cell proliferation of transitional cell carcinoma in man. Cancer 23:1074–1085, 1069.

Leyh H, Hall R, Mazeman E, Blumenstein BA. Comparison of the Bard BTA test with voided urine and bladder wash cytology in the diagnosis and management of cancer of the bladder. Urol 50:49, 1997.

Limas C, Lange P. A, B, H antigen detectability in normal and neoplastic urothelium. Influence of methodologic factors. Cancer 49:2476–2484, 1982.

Limas C, Lange P. T-antigen in normal and neoplastic urothelium. Cancer 58: 1236–1245, 1986.

Lin Y, Miyamoto H, Fujinami K, et al. Telomerase activity in human bladder cancer. Clin Cancer Res 2:929, 1996.

Linker DG, Whitmore WF. Ureteral carcinoma in situ. J Urol 113:777–780, 1975.

Liwnicz BH, Lepow H, Schutte H, et al. Mucinous adenocarcinoma of the renal pelvis: Discussion of possible pathogenesis. J Urol 114:306–310, 1975.

Lomax-Smith JD, Seymour AE. Neoplasia in analgesic nephropathy. A urothelial field change. Am J Surg Pathol 4:565–572, 1980.

Lund F. Mucosal denudation (stripping) for bladder papillomatosis. Scand. J Urol Nephrol 3:204–207, 1969.

MacKenzie AR, Whitmore WF Jr, Melamed MR. Myosarcomas of the bladder and prostate. Cancer 22:833–843, 1968.

Mahadevia PS, Alexander JE, Rojas-Corona R, Koss LG. Pseudosarcomatous stromal reaction in primary and metastatic urothelial carcinoma. A source of diagnostic difficulty. Am J Surg Pathol 13:782–790, 1989.

Mahadevia PS, Karwa GL, Koss LG. Mapping of urothelium in carcinomas of the renal pelvis and ureter. A report of nine cases. Cancer 51:890–897, 1983.

Mahadevia PS, Koss LG, Tar IJ. Prostatic involvement in bladder cancer: Prostate mapping in 20 cystoprostatectomy specimens. Cancer 58:2096–2102, 1986.

Malek RS, Goellner JR, Smith TF, et al. Human papillomavirus infection and intraepithelial, in situ, and invasive carcinoma of the penis. J Urol 42: 159–170, 1993.

Malmgren RA, Soloway MS, Chu EW, et al. Cytology of ileal conduit urine. Acta Cytol 15:506–509, 1971.

Mauri MF, Bonzanini M, Luciani L, Dalla Palma P. Renal collecting duct carcinoma. Report of a case with urinary cytologic findings. Acta Cytol 38: 755–758, 1994.

McKenney JK, Amin MB, Young RH. Urothelial (transitional cell) papilloma of the urinary bladder: A clinicopathologic study of 26 cases. Mod Pathol 16:623–629, 2003.

Meisels A. Cytology of carcinoma of kidney. Acta Cytol 7:239–244, 1963.

Melamed MR, Grabstald H, Whitmore WF Jr. Carcinoma in situ of bladder: Clinico-pathologic study of case with suggested approach to detection. J Urol 96:466–471, 1966.

Melamed MR, Klein FA. Flow cytometry of urinary bladder irrigation specimens. Hum Pathol 15:302–395, 1984.

Melamed MR, Koss LG. Developments in cytological diagnosis of cancer. Med Clin North Am 50:651–666, 1966.

Melamed MR, Koss LG, Ricci A, Whitmore WF Jr. Cytohistological observations on developing carcinoma of urinary bladder in man. Cancer 13:67–74, 1960.

Melamed MR, Voutsa NG, Grabstald H. Natural history and clinical behavior of in situ carcinoma of the human urinary bladder. Cancer 17:1533–1545, 1964.

Melder KK, Koss LG. Automated image analysis in the diagnosis of bladder cancer. Appl Opt 26:3367–3372, 1987.

Melick WF, Escue HM, Naryka JJ, et al. First reported cases of human bladder tumors due to new carcinogen xenylamine. J Urol 74:760–766, 1955.

Melicow MM. Histological study of vesical urothelium intervening between gross neoplasms in total cystectomy. J Urol 68:261–278, 1952.

Melicow MM. Tumors of the bladder: A multifaceted problem. J Urol 112: 467–478, 1974.

Melicow MM. Carcinoma in situ: An historical perspective. Urol Clin North Am 3:5–11, 1976.

Melicow MM, Hollowell JW. Intraurothelial cancer: Carcinoma in situ, Bowen's disease of the urinary system: Discussion of thirty cases. J Urol 68:763–772, 1952.

Melicow MM, Tannenbaum M. Endometrial carcinoma of uterus masculinus (prostate utricle). Report of 6 cases. J Urol 106:892–902, 1971.

Messing EM, Catalona W. Urothelial tumors of the urinary tract. *In* Walsh PC, Retich AB, Vaughan ED Jr et al (eds). Campbells Urology, vol 3, chapter 77. Philadelphia, WB Saunders, 1998, pp 2327–2410.

Mian C, Pycha A, Wiener H, et al. Immunocyt: A new tool for detecting transitional cell cancer of the urinary tract. J Urol 161:1486–1489, 1999.

Michaud DS, Spiegelman D, Clinton SK, et al. Fluid intake and the risk of bladder cancer in men. N Engl J Med 340:1390–1397, 1999.

Mills SE, Wolfe JT III, Weiss MA, et al. Small cell undifferentiated carcinoma of the urinary bladder. A light-microscopic, immunocytochemical, and ultrastructural study of 12 cases. Am J Surg Pathol 11:606–617, 1987.

Mihatsch MJ, Torhorst J, Steinmann E, et al. The morphologic diagnosis of analgesic (phenacetin) abuse. Pathol Res Pract 164:68–79, 1979.

Moll R, Wu X-R, Sun T-T. Uroplakins as biological markers of metastatic transitional cell carcinomas. Am J Pathol 147:1383, 1995.

Morse N, Melamed MR. Differential counts of cell populations in urinary sediment smears from patients with primary epidermoid carcinoma of bladder. Acta Cytol 18:312–315, 1974.

Mostofi FK. Pathology and spread of carcinoma of the urinary bladder. In: Johnston EE, Samuels ML, eds. Cancer of the Genitourinary Tract. New York: Raven Press, 1979:303.

Mostofi FK, Thomson RV, Dean AL Jr. Mucous adenocarcinoma of urinary bladder. Cancer 8:741–758, 1955.

Mount BM, Curtis M, Marshall K, Husk M. Cytologic diagnosis of renal cell carcinoma. Urology 2:421–425, 1973.

Murphy WM. Urinary Cytopathology. Chicago, IL, Am Soc Clin Pathol, 2000.

Murphy WM. Current statues of urinary cytology in the evaluation of bladder neoplasms. Hum Pathol 21:886–896, 1990.

Murphy WM, Deana DG. The nested variant of transitional cell carcinoma: a neoplasm resembling proliferation of Brunn's nests. Mod Pathol 5: 240–243, 1992.

Murphy WM, Rivera-Ramirez I, Medina CA, et al. The bladder tumor antigen (BTA) test compared to voided urine cytology in the detection of bladder neoplasms. J Urol 158:2102, 1997.

Murphy WM, Soloway MS. Developing carcinoma (dysplasia) of the urinary bladder. Pathol Annu 17 (Pt.1):197–217, 1982.

Murphy WM, Soloway MS. Urothelial dysplasia. Urol 127:849–854, 1982.

Murphy WM, von Buedinger RP, Poley RW. Primary carcinoma in situ of the renal pelvis and urethra. Cancer 34:1126–1130, 1974.

Naib ZM. Exfoliative cytology of renal pelvic lesions. Cancer 14:1085–1087, 1961.

Nasuti JF, Fleisher SR, Gupta PK. Significance of tissue fragments in voided urine specimens. Acta Cytol 45:147–152, 2001.

Nazeer T, Ro JY, Tornos C, et al. Endocervical-type glands in the urinary bladder: A clinicopathologic study of six cases. Hum Pathol 27:816–820, 1996.

Nickel JC, Ardern D, Downey J. Cytologic evaluation of urine is important in evaluation of chronic prostatitis. Urology 60:225–227, 2002.

Nortier JL, Martinez M-CM, Schmeiser HH, et al. Urothelial carcinoma associated with the use of a chinese herb (aristolochia fangchi). N Engl J Med 342:1686–1692, 2000.

Oates RD, Stilmant MM, Freedlund MC, Siroky MB. Granulomatous prostatitis following bacillus Calmette-Guérin immunotherapy of bladder cancer. J Urol 140:751–754, 1988.

Obe JA, Rosen N, Koss LG. Primary choriocarcinoma of the urinary bladder. Report of a case with probable epithelial origin. Cancer 52:1405–1409, 1983.

Oliva E, Amin MB, Jimenez R, Young RH. Clear cell carcinoma of the urinary bladder. A report and comparison of four tumors of Mullerian origin and nine of probable urothelial origin with discussion of histogenesis and diagnostic problems. Am J Surg Pathol 26:190–197, 2002.

Omeroglu A, Paner GP, Wojcik EM, Siziopikou K. A carcinosarcoma/sarcomatoid carcinoma arising in a urinary bladder diverticulum. Arch Pathol Lab Med 126:853–855, 2002.

Pamukcu AM, Gorsoy SK, Price JM. Urinary bladder neoplasms induced by feeding bracken fern (*Pteris aquilina*) to cows. Cancer Res 27:917–924, 1964.

Pang S-C. Bony and cartilaginous tumours of the urinary bladder. J Pathol Bacteriol 76:357–377, 1958.

Papanicolaou GN, Marshall VF. Urine sediment smears as diagnostic procedure in cancers of urinary tract. Science 101:519–520, 1945.

Partanen S, Asikainen U. Oat cell carcinoma of the urinary bladder with ectopic adrenocorticotropic hormone production. Hum Pathol 16:313–315, 1985.

Parton I. Primary lymphosarcoma of the bladder. Br J Urol 34:221–223, 1962.

Pedersen-Bjergaard J, Ersboli J, Hansen VL, et al. Carcinoma of the urinary bladder after treatment with cyclophosphamide for non-Hodgkin's lymphoma. N Engl J Med 318:1028–1032, 1988.

Petterson S, Hansson G, Blohme I. Condyloma acuminatum of the bladder. J Urol 115:535–536, 1976.

Peven DR, Hidvegi DF. Clear-cell adenocarcinoma of the female urethra. Acta Cytol 29:142–146, 1985.

Pich A, Chiusa L, Formiconi A, et al. Biologic differences between noninvasive papillary urothelial neoplasms of low malignant potential and low-grade (grade 1) papillary carcinomas of the bladder. Am J Surg Pathol 25: 1528–1533, 2001.

Piper JM, Tonascia J, Matanoski GM. Heavy phenacetin use and bladder cancer in women aged 20 to 49 years. N Engl J Med 313:292–295, 1985.

Piscioli F, Detassis C, Polla E, et al. Cytologic presentation of renal adenocarcinoma in urinary sediment. Acta Cytol 27:383–390, 1983.

Piva A, Koss LG. Cytologic diagnosis of metastatic malignant melanoma in urinary sediment. Acta Cytol 8:398–402, 1964.

Potts IF, Hirst E. Inverted papilloma of the bladder. J Urol 90:175–179, 1963.

Powers CN, Elbadawi A. "Cercariform" cells: a clue to the cytodiagnosis of transitional cell origin of metastatic neoplasm? Diagn Cytopathol 13:15–21, 1995.

Pringle JP, Graham RC, Bernier GM. Detection of myeloma cells in the urine sediment. Blood 43:137–143, 1974.

Prout GR, Griffin PP, Daly JJ. The outcome of conservative treatment of carcinoma in situ of the bladder. J Urol 138:766–770, 1987.

Prout GR, Griffin PP, Daly JJ, Heney NM. Carcinoma in situ of the urinary bladder with and without associated neoplasms. Cancer 52:524–532, 1983.

Prout GR, Lin C-W, Benson R Jr, et. al. Photodynamic therapy with hematoporphyrin derivative in the treatment of superficial transitional-cell carcinoma of the bladder. N Engl J Med 317:1251–1255, 1987.

Pugh RCB. The pathology of cancer of the bladder. An editorial overview. Cancer 32:1267–1274, 1973.

Raab SS, Lenel JC, Cohen MB. Low grade transitional cell carcinoma of the bladder. Cytologic diagnosis by key features as identified by logistic regression analysis. Cancer 74:1621–1626, 1994.

Ramaekers FC, Beck HL, Feitz WF, et al. Application of antibodies to intermediate filament proteins as tissue-specific probes in the flow cytometric analysis of complex tumors. Anal Quant Cytol Histol 8:271–280, 1986.

Ramaekers FC, Beck H, Vooijis GP, Herman CJ. Flow-cytometric analysis of mixed cell populations using intermediate filament antibodies. Exp Cell Res 153:249–253, 1984.

Ramakumar S, Bhuiyan J, Besse JA, et al. Comparison of screening methods in the detection of bladder cancer. J Urol 161:388–394, 1999.

Rehn L. Blasengeschwuelste bei Anilinarbeitern. Arch Klin Chir 50:588–600, 1895.

Rehn L. Blasengeschwuelste bei Fuchsinarbeitern. Arch Klin Chir 53:383–392, 1896.

Reichborn-Kjennerud S, Hoeg K. The value of urine cytology in the diagnosis of recurrent bladder tumors. A preliminary report. Acta Cytol 16:269–272, 1972.

Remick DG, Kumar NB. Benign polyps with prostatic-type epithelium of the urethra and the urinary bladder: A suggestion of histogenesis based on histologic and immunohistochemical studies. Am J Surg Pathol 8:833–839, 1984.

Renshaw AA, Madge R. Cercariform cells for helping distinguish transitional cell carcinoma from non-small cell lung carcinoma in fine needle aspirates. Acta Cytol 41:999–1007, 1997.

Renshaw AA, Nappi D, Weinberg DS. Cytology of grade 1 papillary transitional cell carcinoma. A comparison of cytologic, architectural and morphometric criteria in cystoscopically obtained urine. Acta Cytol 40:676–682, 1996.

Richie JP, Skinner DG. Carcinoma in situ of the urethra associated with bladder carcinoma: The role of urethrectomy. J Urol 119:80–81, 1978.

Richter J, Jiang F, Gorog JP, et al. Marked genetic differences between stage pTa and stage pT1 papillary bladder cancer detected by comparative genomic hybridization. Cancer Res 57:2860–2864, 1997.

Riede CR, Daniltchenko D, Koenig F, et al. Fluorescence endoscopy with 5-aminolevulinic acid reduces early recurrence rate in superficial bladder cancer. J Urol 165:1121–1123, 2001.

Rieger-Christ KM, Cain JW, Braasch JW, et al. Expression of classic cadherins type I in urothelial neoplastic progression. Hum Pathol 32:18–23, 2001.

Rosenkilde OP, Wolf H, Schroeder T, et al. Urothelial atypia and survival rate of 500 unselected patients with primary transitional-cell tumor of the urinary bladder. Scand J Urol Nephrol 22:257–263, 1988.

Rudrick B, Nguyen GK, Lakey WH. Carcinoid tumor of the renal pelvis: report of a case with positive urine cytology. Diagn Cytopathol 12:360–363, 1995.

Rumpelt HJ, Störkel S, Moll R, et al. Bellini duct carcinoma. Further evidence for this rare variant of renal cell carcinoma. Histopathology 18:115–122, 1991.

Sack MJ, Artymyshyn RL, Tomaszewskim JE, Gupta PK. Diagnostic value of bladder wash cytology, with special reference to low grade urothelial neoplasms. Acta Cytol 39:187–194, 1995.

Sacks SA, Waisman J, Apfelbaum HB, et al. Urethral adenocarcinoma (possibly originating in the glands of the Littré). J Urol 113:50–55, 1975.

Sahin AA, Myhre M, Ro JY, et al. Plasmacytoid transitional cell carcinoma. Report of a case with initial presentation mimicking multiple myeloma. Acta Cytol 35:277–280, 1991.

Sandberg AA, Berger CS. Review of chromosome studies in urological tumors. II. Cytogenetics and molecular genetics of bladder cancer. J Urol 151: 545–560, 1994.

Sano ME, Koprowska I. Primary cytologic diagnosis of a malignant renal lymphoma. Acta Cytol 9:194–196, 1965.

Santino AM, Shumaker EJ, Garces J. Primary malignant lymphoma of the bladder. J Urol 103:310–313, 1970.

Sarkis AS, Dalbagni G, Cordon-Cardo C, et al. Association of p53 nuclear overexpression and tumor progression in carcinoma in situ of the bladder. J Urol 152:388–392, 1994.

Sarosdy MF, deVere White RW, Soloway MS, et al. Results of a multicenter trial using the BTA test to monitor for and diagnose recurrent bladder cancer. J Urol 154:379–383, 1995.

Schade ROK, Serck-Hanssen A, Swinney J. Morphological changes in the ureter in cases of bladder carcinoma. Cancer 27:1267–1272, 1971.

Schade ROK, Swinney J. Precancerous changes in bladder epithelium. Lancet 2:943–946, 1968.

Schade ROK, Swinney J. The association of urothelial atypism with neoplasia: Its importance in treatment and prognosis. J Urol 109:619–622, 1973.

Schellhammer PF, Ladaga LE, Fillion MB. Bacillus Calmette-Guérin for superficial transitional cell carcinoma of the bladder. J Urol 135:261–264, 1986.

Schellhammer PF, Whitmore WF Jr. Transitional cell carcinoma of the urethra in men having cystectomy for bladder cancer. J Urol 115:56–60, 1976.

Schellhammer PF, Whitmore WF Jr. Urethral meatal carcinoma following cystourethrectomy for bladder carcinoma. J Urol 115:61–64, 1976.

Schindler S, DeFrias DV, Yu GH. Primary angiosarcoma of the bladder: Cytomorphology and differential diagnosis. Cytopathology 10:137–144, 1999.

Schnadig VJ, Adesokan A, Neal R, Gatalica Z. Urinary cytologic findings in patients with benign and malignant adenomatous polyps of the prostatic urethra. Arch Pathol Lab Med 124:1047–1052, 2000.

Schneider V, Smith MJV, Frable WJ. Urinary cytology in endometriosis of the bladder. Acta Cytol 24:30–33, 1980.

Schujman E, Mukamel E, Slutzker D, et al. Prostatic transitional cell carcinoma: concept of its pathogenesis and classification. Isr J Med Sci 19:794–800, 1983.

Schulte PA, Ringen K, Hemstreet GP, et al. Risk factors of bladder cancer in a cohort exposed to aromatic amines. Cancer 58:2156–2162, 1986.

Schulte PA, Ringen KN, Hemstreet GP, et al. Risk assessment of a cohort exposed to aromatic amines. Initial results. J Occup Med 27:115–121, 1985.

Sedlacek TV, Cunnane M, Carpiniello V. Colposcopy in the diagnosis of penile condyloma. Am J Obstet Gynecol 154:494–496, 1986.

Seemayer TA, Knaack J, Thelmo WL, et al. Further observations on carcinoma in situ of the urinary bladder: Silent but extensive intraprostatic involvement. Cancer 36:514–520, 1975.

Seibel JL, Prasad S, Weiss RE, et al. Villous adenoma of the urinary tract: A lesion frequently associated with malignancy. Hum Pathol 33:236–241, 2002.

Shah N, Saunders MI. A pilot study of postoperative CHART and CHARTWELL in head and neck cancer. Clin Oncol (R Coll Radool) 12:392–396, 2000.

Shenoy UA, Colby TV, Schumann GB. Reliability of urinary cytodiagnosis in urothelial neoplasms. Cancer 56:2041–2045, 1985.

Sharma S, Zippe CD, Pandrangi L, et al. Exclusion criteria enhance the specificity and positive predictive value of NMP22 and BTA stat. J Urol 162:53–57, 1999.

Sharma TC, Melamed MR, Whitmore WF. Carcinoma in situ of the ureter in patients with bladder carcinoma treated by cystectomy. Cancer 26:583–587, 1970.

Sherman AB, Koss LG, Adams SE. Interobserver and intraobserver differences in the diagnosis of urothelial cells. Comparison with classification by computer. Anal Quant Cytol 6:112–120, 1984.

Sherman AB, Koss LG, Adams S, et al. Bladder cancer diagnosis by image analysis of cells in voided urine using a small computer. Anal Quant Cytol 3:239–249, 1981.

Sherman AB, Koss LG, Wyschogrod D, et al. Bladder cancer diagnosis by computer image analysis of cells in the sediment of voided urine using a video scanning system. Anal Quant Cytol Histol 8:177–186, 1986.

Sherwood T. Upper urinary tract tumours following bladder carcinoma: Natural history of urothelial neoplastic disease. Br J Radiol 44:137–141, 1971.

Siddiqui A, Melamed MR, Abbi R, Ahmed T. Mucinous (colloid) carcinoma of urinary bladder following long-term cyclophosphamide therapy for Waldenstrom's macroglobulinemia. Am J Surg Pathol 20:500–504, 1996.

Sidransky D, Frost P, von Eschenbach A, et al. Clonal origin of bladder cancer. N Engl J Med 326:737–740, 1992.

Sidransky D, von Eschenbach A, Tsai YC, et al. Identification of p53 gene mutations in bladder cancers and urine samples. Science 252:706–709, 1991.

Signal SH, Tomaszewski JE, Brooks JJ, et al. Carcinosarcoma of the urinary bladder following long-term cyclophosphamide therapy. Arch Path Lab Med 115:1049–1051, 1991.

Silverman DT, Hartge P, Morrison AS, Devesa SS. Epidemiology of bladder cancer. Hematol Oncol Clin North AM 6:1–30, 1992.

Simeonova PP, Luster MI. Mechanisms of arsenic carcinogenicity: Genetic or epigenetic mechanisms? J Environ Pathol Toxicol Oncol 19:281–286, 2000.

Simon R, Eltze E, Schäfer, et al. Cytogenetic analysis of multifocal bladder cancer supports a monoclonal origin and intraepithelial spread of tumor cells. Cancer Res 61:355–362, 2001.

Simon W, Cordonnier JJ, Snordgrass WT. The pathogenesis of bladder carcinoma. J Urol 88:797–802, 1962.

Skinner DG, Richie JP, Cooper PH, et al. The clinical significance of carcinoma in situ of the bladder and its association with overt carcinoma. J Urol 112:68–71, 1974.

Smart JG. Renal and ureteric tumours in association with bladder tumours. Br J Urol 36:380–390, 1964.

Smith AF. An ultrastructural and morphometric study of bladder tumours. Virchows Arch. [A] 406:7–16, 1985.

Smith AH, Goycolea M, Haque R, Biggs ML. Marked increase in bladder and lung cancer mortality in a region of Northern Chile due to arsenic in drinking water. Am J Epidemiol 147:660–669, 1998.

Sokolova IA, Halling KC, Jenkins RB, et al. The development of a multitarget, multicolor fluorescence in situ hybridization assay for the detection of urothelial carcinoma in urine. J Mol Diag 2:116–123, 2000.

Soloway MS. Surgery and intravesical chemotherapy in the management of superficial bladder cancer. Semin Urol 1:23, 1983.

Soloway MS. Treatment of superficial bladder cancer with intravesical mitomycin C. Analysis of immediate and longterm response in 70 patients. J Urol 134:1107–1109, 1985.

Soloway MS, Briggman V, Carpinito GA, et al. Use of a new tumor marker, urinary NMP22, in the detection of occult or rapidly recurring transitional cell carcinoma of the urinary tract following surgical treatment. J Urol 156:363–367,1996.

Spooner ME, Cooper EH. Chromosome constitution of transitional cell carcinoma of the urinary bladder. Cancer 29:1401–1412, 1972.

Stagier M, Desmet R, Denys H et al. Primary carcinoma in situ of renal pelvis and ureter. Brit J Urol 52:401, 1980.

Stampfer DS, Carpinito GA, Rodriguez-Villanueva J, et al. Evaluation of NMP22 in the detection of transitional cell carcinoma of the bladder. J Urol 159:394–398, 1998.

Starklint H, Kjaergaard J, Jensen NK. Types of metaplasia in forty urothelial bladder carcinomas. A systematic histological investigation. Acta Pathol Microbiol Scand 84:137–142, 1976.

Stein JP, Ginsberg DA, Grossfeld GD, et al. Effect of p21$^{WAPI/CIPI}$ expression on tumor progression in bladder cancer. J Natl Cancer Inst 90:1072–1079, 1998.

Stein JP, Grossfeld GD, Ginsberg DA, et al. Prognostic markers in bladder cancer: A contemporary review of the literature. J Urol 160:645–659, 1998.

Steiner G, Schoenberg MP, Lin JF. et al. Detection of bladder cancer recurrence by microsatellite analysis of urine. Nat Med 3:621–624, 1997.

Steinmaus C, Moore L, Hopenhayn-Rich C, et al. Arsenic in drinking water and bladder cancer. Cancer Invest 18:174–182, 2000.

Sternheimer R. A supravital cytodiagnostic stain for urinary sediments. JAMA 231:636–832, 1975.

Stilmant M, Murphy JL, Merriam JL. Cytology of nephrogenic adenoma of the urinary bladder. Acta Cytol 30:35–40, 1986.

Stitt RB, Colapinto V. Multiple simultaneous bladder malignancies: primary lymphosarcoma and adenocarcinoma. J Urol 96:733–736, 1966.

Su C, Prince CL. Melanoma of the bladder. J Urol 87:365–367, 1962.

Sun TT, Liang F-X, Wu X-R. Uroplakins as markers of urothelial differentiation. In Baskin and Hayward (eds). Advances in Bladder Research, New York, Kluver Academic/Plenum Publ, 1999.

Suprun H, Bitterman W. A correlative cytohistologic study on the interrelationship between exfoliated urinary bladder carcinoma cell types and the staging and grading of these tumors. Acta Cytol 19:265–273, 1975.

Sylora HO, Diamond HM, Kaufman M, et al. Primary carcinoid tumor of the urethra. J Urol 114:150–153, 1975.

Talbert ML, Young RH. Carcinomas of the urinary bladder with deceptively benign-appearing foci: A report of three cases. Am J Surg Pathol 13:374, 1989.

Tanaka T, Yoshimi N, Sawada K, et al. Ki-1-positive large cell anaplastic lymphoma diagnosed by urinary cytology. A case report. Acta Cytol 37:520–524, 1993.

Tawfiek E, Bibbo M, Bagley DH. Ureteroscopic biopsy: Technique and specimen preparation. Urology 50:117–119, 1997.

Taylor DC, Bahagavan BS, Larsen MP, et al. Papillary urothelial hyperplasia. A precursor to papillary neoplasms. Am J Surg Pathol 20:1481–1488, 1996.

Temkin IS. Industrial Bladder Carcinogenesis. New York, Pergamon Press, 1963.

Tenti P, Zappatore R, Romagnoli S, et al. p53 overexpression and human papillomavirus infection in transitional cell carcinoma of the urinary bladder: correlation with histological parameters. J Pathol 178:65–70, 1996.

Thelmo WL, Seemayer TA, Madarnas P, et al. Carcinoma in situ of the bladder with associated prostatic involvement. J Urol 111:491–494, 1974.

Torenbeek R, Blomjous CEM, de Bruin PC, et al. Sarcomatoid carcinoma of the urinary bladder: Clinicopathologic analysis of 18 cases with immunohistochemical and electron microscopic findings. Am J Surg Pathol 18:241–249, 1994.

Travis LB, Curtis RE, Boice JD Jr, Fraumeni JF Jr. Bladder cancer after chemotherapy for non-Hodgkin's lymphoma. N Engl J Med 321:544–545, 1989.

Tribukait B. Flow cytometry in surgical pathology and cytology of tumors of the genito-urinary tract. In Koss LG, Coleman DV (eds). Advances in Clinical Cytology, vol. 2. New York, Masson Publishing, 1984, pp 163–189.

Tribukait B. Flow cytometry in assessing the clinical aggressiveness of genito-urinary neoplasms. World J Urol 5:108–122, 1987.

Tribukait B, Gustafson H, Esposti MD. Ploidy and proliferation of human bladder tumors as measured by flow-cytofluorometric DNA-analysis and its relations to histopathology and cytology. Cancer 43:1742–1751, 1979.

Trillo AA, Kuchler LL, Wood AC, Prater T. Adenocarcinoma of the urinary bladder: histologic, cytologic, and ultrastructural features in a case. Acta Cytol 25:285–290, 1981.

Troster M, Wyatt JK, Alen-Halagah J. Nephrogenic adenoma of the urinary bladder. Histologic and cytologic observations in a case. Acta Cytol 30:41–44, 1986.

Umiker W. Accuracy of cytologic diagnosis of cancer of the urinary tract. Acta Cytol 8:186–193, 1964.

Utz DC, Hanash KA, Farrow GM. The plight of the patient with carcinoma in situ of the bladder. J Urol 103:160–164, 1970.

Utz DC, Zincke H. The masquerade of bladder cancer in situ as interstitial cystitis. Trans Am Assoc Genitourin Surg 75:64–65, 1973.

Valente PT, Atkinson BF, Guerry D. Melanuria. Acta Cytol 29:1026–1028, 1985.

Vallejos H, Del Mistro A, Kleinhaus S, et al. Characterization of human papillomavirus types in condylomata acuminate in children by in situ hybridization. Lab Invest 56:611–615, 1987.

Van Hoeven KH, Artymyshyn RL. Cytology of small cell carcinoma of the urinary bladder. Diagn Cytopathol 14:292–297, 1996.

Van Rhijn BWG, van der Kast TH, Vis AN, et al. FGFR3 and p53 characterize alternative genetic pathways in the pathogenesis of urothelial cell carcinoma. Cancer Res 64:1911–1914, 2004.

Vandersteen DP, Wiemerslage SJ, Cohen MB. Prostatic duct adenocarcinoma: A cytologic and histologic case report with review of the literature. Diagn Cytopathol 17:480–483, 1997.

Videbaek A. Chlornaphazin (Erysan) may induce cancer of the urinary bladder. Acta Med Scand 176:45–50, 1964.

Vlahou A, Schellhammer FF, Mendrinos S, et al. Development of novel proteomic approach for the detection of transitional cell carcinoma of the bladder in urine. Am J Pathol 58:1491–1502, 2001.

Volmar KE, Chan TY, De Marzo AM, et al. Florid von Brunn nests mimicking urothelial carcinoma. A morphologic and immunohistochemical comparison to the nested variant of urothelial carcinoma. Am J Surg Pathol 27:1243–1252, 2003.

Voutsa NG, Melamed MR. Cytology of in situ carcinoma of the human urinary bladder. Cancer 16:1307–1316, 1963.

Wachtel MS, James KE, Miller MA, et al. Bladder washing cytology. Comparison of two analytic methods and two proposed quantitative criteria for carcinoma in situ. Acta Cytol 40:921–928, 1996.

Wagle DG, Moore RH, Murphy GP. Primary carcinoma of the renal pelvis. Cancer 33:1642–1648, 1974.

Wallace D. Cancer of the bladder. Am J Roentgenol Radium Ther Nucl Med 102:581–586, 1968.

Walther M, O'Brien DPD, Birch HW. Condylomata acuminata and verrucous carcinoma of the bladder: Case report and literature review. J Urol 35:362–365, 1986.

Wang CC, Scully RE, Leadbetter WF. Primary malignant lymphoma of the urinary bladder. Cancer 24:772–776, 1969.

Ward E, Halperin W, Thun M, et al. Bladder tumors in two young males occupationally exposed to MBOCA. Am J Ind Med 14:267–272, 1988.

Weaver EJ, McCue PA, Bagley DH, et al. Expression of cytokeratin 20 and CD44 protein in upper urinary tract transitional cell carcinoma. Cytologic-histologic correlation. Anal Quant Cytol Histol 23:339–344, 2001.

Weinberg T. Primary chorionepithelioma of the urinary bladder in a male. Report of a case. Am J Pathol 15:783–795 1939.

Weinstein RS. Changes in plasma membrane structure associated with malignant transformation in human urinary bladder epithelium. Cancer Res 36: 2518–2524, 1976.

Weinstein RS, Coon J, Alroy J, Davidsohn I. Tissue-associated blood group antigens in human tumors. In DeLellis RA (ed). Diagnostic Immunohistochemistry. New York, Masson Publishing, 1981, pp. 239–261.

Weinstein RS, Coon JS, Schwartz D, et al. Pathology of superficial bladder cancer with emphasis on carcinoma in situ. Urology 26(Suppl.):2–10, 1985.

Wheeler JD, Hill WT. Adenocarcinoma involving urinary bladder. Cancer 7: 119–135, 1954.

Whitmore WF Jr. Bladder cancer: An overview. CA Cancer J Clin 38:213–223, 1988.

Whitmore WF, Whitmore WF, Jr, Grabstald H, Mackenzie AR. Preoperative irradiation with cystectomy in the management of bladder cancer. Am J Roentgenol Radium Ther Nucl Med 102:570–576, 1968.

Widran J, Sanchez R, Gruhn J. Squamous metaplasia of the bladder: A study of 450 patients. J Urol 112:479–482, 1974.

Wied GL, Bartels PH, Bahr GF, Oldfield DG. Taxonomic intracellular analytic system (TICAS) for cell identification. Acta Cytol 12:180–204, 1968.

Wijkstrom H, Granberg-Ohman I, Tribukait B. Chromosomal and DNA patterns in transitional cell bladder carcinoma. A comparative cytogenetic and flow-cytofluorometric DNA study. Cancer 53:1718–1723, 1984.

Wojcik EM, Brownlie RJ, Bassler TJ, Miller MC. Superficial urothelial (umbrella) cells. A potential cause of abnormal DNA ploidy results in urine specimens. Anal Quant Cytol Histol 22:411–415, 2000.

Wojcik EM, Saraga SA, Jin JK, Hendricks JB. Application of laser scanning cytometry for evaluation of DNA ploidy in routine cytologic specimens. Diagn Cytopathol 24:200–205, 2001.

Wolf H, Hjøgaard K. Urothelial dysplasia concomitant with bladder tumours as a determinant factor for future new occurrences. Lancet 2:134–136, 1983.

Wolinska WH, Melamed MR. Urinary conduit cytology. Cancer 32:1000–1006, 1973.

Wolinska WH, Melamed MR, Klein FA. Cytology of bladder papilloma. Acta Cytol 29:817, 1985.

Wolinska WH, Melamed MR, Schellhammer PF, Whitmore JWF. Urethral cytology following cystectomy for bladder carcinoma. Am J Surg Pathol 1: 225–234, 1977.

Wu R-L, Osman I, Wu X-R, et al. Uroplakin II gene is expressed in transitional cell carcinoma but not in bilharzial bladder squamous cell carcinoma: Alternative pathways of bladder epithelial differentiation and tumor formation. Cancer Res 58:1291–1297, 1998.

Wu X-R, Lin J-H, Waltz T, et al. Mammalian uroplakins. A group of highly conserved urothelial differentiation-related membrane proteins. J Biol Chem 269:13716–13724, 1994.

Wynder EL, Goldsmith R. The epidemiology of bladder cancer. A second look. Cancer 40:1246–1268, 1977.

Xin W, Raab SS, Michael CW. Low-grade urothelial carcinoma: Reappraisal of the cytologic criteria on ThinPrep. Diagn Cytopathol 29:125–129,2003.

Yamada T, Masawa N, Honma K, et al. Nonpapillary intraepithelial and/or early invasive cancer arisen in the urinary bladder—their developmental and advancing courses. Dokkyo J Med Sci 11:51–69, 1984.

Yamada T, Yokogawa M, Mitani G, et al. Two different types of cancer development in the urothelium of the human urinary bladder with different prognosis. Jpn J Clin Oncol 5:77–90, 1975.

Yamase HT, Powell GT, Koss LG. A simplified method of preparing permanent tissue sections for the erythrocyte adherence test. Am J Clin Pathol 75: 178–181, 1981.

Yates-Bell AJ. Carcinoma in situ of the bladder. Br J Surg 58:359–364, 1971.

Yokoyama S, Hayashida Y, Nagahama J, et al. Primary and metaplastic choriocarcinoma of the bladder. A report of two cases. Acta Cytol 36:176–182, 1992.

Yonekawa M, Hoshida Y, Hanai J, et al. Catheterized urine cytology of mucinous carcinoma arising in the renal pelvis. A case report. Acta Cytol 44: 442–444, 2000.

Young RH. Carcinosarcoma of the urinary bladder. Cancer 59:1333–1339, 1987.

Young RH, Oliva E. Transitional cell carcinomas of the urinary bladder that may be underdiagnosed. A report of four invasive cases exemplifying the homology between neoplastic and non-neoplastic transitional cell lesions. Am J Surg Pathol 20:1448–1454, 1996.

Young RH, Oliva E, Garcia JAS, et al. Urethral caruncle with atypical stromal cells simulating lymphomas or sarcoma: A distinctive pseudoneoplastic lesion of females. A report of six cases. Am J Surg Pathol 20:1190–1195, 1996.

Zaman SS, Sack MJ, Ramchandani P, et al. Cytopathology of retrograde renal pelvis brush specimens: An analysis of 40 cases with emphasis on collecting duct carcinoma and low-intermediate grade transitional cell carcinoma. Diagn Cytopathol 15:312–321, 1996.

Zhang X-M, Elhosseiny A, Melamed MR. Plasmacytoid urothelial carcinoma of bladder: A case report and first description of urinary cytology. Acta Cytol 46:412–416, 2002.

Zhang Z-T, Pak J, Huang H-Y, et al. Role of Ha-ras activation in superficial papillary pathway of urothelial tumor formation. Oncogene 20:1973–1980, 2001.

Zhang ZT, Pak J, Shapiro E, et al. Urothelium-specific expression of an oncogene in transgenic mice induced the formation of carcinoma in situ and invasive transitional cell carcinoma. Cancer Res 59:3512–3517, 1999.

Zincke H, Utz DC, Farrow GM. Review of Mayo Clinic experience with carcinoma in situ. Urology 26(Suppl 4):39–46, 1985.

Zippe C, Pandrangi L, Agarwal A. NMP22 is a sensitive, cost-effective test in patients at risk for bladder cancer. J Urol 161:62–65, 1999.

Zogno C, Schiaffino E, Boeri R, Schmid C. Cytologic detection of metastatic malignant melanoma in urine. A report of three cases. Acta Cytol 41: 1332–1336, 1997.

The Gastrointestinal Tract

The parts of the gastrointestinal tract that are accessible to cytologic investigation are the **esophagus, stomach, duodenum, colon, and the biliary and pancreatic ducts** (Fig. 24-1). The methods of sampling are similar for all the organs, except colon.

METHODS OF SAMPLING

The introduction of **flexible fiberglass optics instruments** has not only revolutionized the endoscopy of the entire gastrointestinal tract but also allowed **direct sampling of any visible lesion by cytology or tissue biopsy.** A variety of instruments specially adapted to the inspection of the esoph-

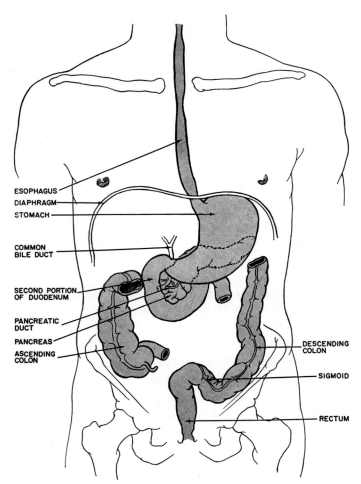

ESOPHAGUS
DIAPHRAGM
STOMACH

COMMON
BILE DUCT

SECOND PORTION
OF DUODENUM

PANCREATIC
DUCT
PANCREAS
ASCENDING
COLON

DESCENDING
COLON

SIGMOID

RECTUM

Figure 24-1   Schematic representation of portions of the gastrointestinal tract accessible to cytologic investigation. The transverse colon is omitted, to demonstrate the pancreas and the duodenum.

agus, stomach, duodenum, and colon are available. Ultra-thin endoscopes with a diameter smaller than 6 mm, provided with a video camera, are now available (Van Damm and Brugge, 1999). These procedures can be performed on any patients with radiographic abnormalities or clinical symptoms, or as a part of **cancer prevention programs** in asymptomatic patients at risk for stomach (in Japan) or colon carcinomas. The instruments may also be used for laser treatment of superficial lesions.

The principles of collection of material for diagnostic sampling are the same for all organs. The instruments are provided with an accessory channel through which a brush, a plastic tube, or a small biopsy forceps may be passed. Thus, **brushing, lavage, or a biopsy** of any area in the gastrointestinal tract may be performed under direct visual control. **Cytologic sampling must be performed prior to biopsy.**

Washings of the esophagus or stomach without endoscopic control are nowadays very rarely used, although this simple technique led to the monumental contributions by Schade (1956, 1959, and 1960A,B) to the diagnosis of early gastric cancer. **An equal volume of 95% alcohol must be added to the fluid immediately after aspiration to preserve the cells.**

Endoscopically directed needle aspiration biopsy for the diagnosis of esophageal and gastric lesions was described

by Layfield et al (1992) in a small number of patients with moderate success. A transbronchial aspiration needle was used in the procedures. There is no evidence that this technique achieved widespread acceptance.

Endoscopic ultrasound-guided needle aspiration biopsy has been proven effective in sampling small lesions of various organs of the gastrointestinal tract (Kosch et al, 1992; Chang et al, 1994; Mallery and Van Damm, 1999; Jhala et al, 2003). Perhaps the most important application of this technique is in sampling of **intramural lesions** and in assessing small lesions of the pancreas (Gress et al, 2001; Afify et al, 2003). For comments on the application of this technique to lesions of the biliary tree, see below.

"Salvage cytology" is a technique proposed by Graham et al (1979) consisting of washing the channel of the endoscopic instrument with saline and collecting the fluid for cytologic analysis into a suction trap. Initially, the technique was intended for use after biopsies (Graham and Spjut, 1979) but Caos et al (1986) reported its successful application without biopsies.

The application of **esophageal and gastro-esophageal balloons and similar techniques** for purposes of cancer detection are described below.

Special methods of cytologic investigation of the colon and rectum and the biliary tract are described further on in this chapter.

PREPARATION OF SMEARS

Preparation of smears from material obtained by endoscopic instruments is an important part of diagnostic evaluation of patients. Special skills are required for handling of **brushes** and **direct needle aspirates.** Brushing is usually performed to sample a visible lesion. Upon completion of brushing, the brush must be carefully, yet rapidly, withdrawn from the instrument and the **smears prepared without delay,** either by the physician or a trained assistant. Usually a brush yields two to four smears. Alternately, the entire brush may be forwarded to the laboratory for further processing (see Chap. 44). Preparation of smears from aspirates is best performed by a trained cytopathologist or technologist by methods described in Chapter 28.

THE ESOPHAGUS

ANATOMY AND HISTOLOGY

The esophagus is a tubular structure with muscular walls which extends from the pharynx across the diaphragm to the cardia of the stomach. The esophageal lumen is slightly narrowed at the level of thyroid cartilage, the bifurcation of the trachea, and the diaphragm. These are the sites wherein esophageal carcinoma tends to occur (see below). The esophagus is **in close proximity to many vital structures.** In the neck, the larynx and the trachea are immediately anterior; the recurrent nerves run along lateral walls of the esophagus, and the vagus nerves descend along its anterior and posterior walls. In the upper thorax, the esophagus is in contact with the trachea and the arch of the aorta. At the level of the heart, the left auricle is in close proximity. Thus, **cancers of esophagus not only may obstruct its lumen, but also may invade and damage several vital organs.**

The esophagus is **lined by nonhornifying squamous epithelium** (Fig. 24-2A). **Islands of gastric epithelium may be found in the areas immediately adjacent to the cardia and, rarely, elsewhere within the esophagus.** Small, **mucus-producing glands** are found in the submucosa. The epithelium rests on a connective tissue layer, the submucosa or the **lamina propria,** which separates the epithelium from the **muscle layers** or the **muscularis propria.**

NORMAL CYTOLOGY

The cytology of the esophageal aspirates, brushings, and washings in the absence of disease is **extremely simple.** The smears are composed essentially of **superficial squamous cells with vesicular nuclei, identical to those observed in sputum samples** (Fig. 24-2B). Less frequent are **smaller squamous cells derived from the deeper layers of the epithelium and provided with nuclei of similar sizes and configuration to the superficial cells. Occasionally, be-**

nign squamous "pearls," may be noted. It is not unusual to find **swallowed cells of respiratory origin, such as dust-containing macrophages and ciliated bronchial cells** (see Chap. 19). Also, **gastric epithelial cells,** singly or in clusters, may occur (see Fig. 24-16). **Foreign material,** especially plant (vegetable) cells, may be present if there is an obstruction of the esophageal lumen. For description of these contaminants, see Chapter 19.

BENIGN DISORDERS

Acute and Chronic Erosive Esophagitis

This group of diseases of varying etiology is very important in diagnostic cytology, because it produces **cells that may be confused with cancer.** Esophagitis may have different causes such as **trauma, acid reflux from the stomach, a reaction to swallowed corrosive liquids, cardiospasm** of long standing, **Plummer-Vinson syndrome** (also known as **sideropenic dysphagia,** a syndrome of atrophy of the esophageal epithelium and iron deficiency anemia), some forms of **avitaminosis, scleroderma** (or **systemic sclerosis of connective tissue,** affecting primarily the skin), **and hiatus hernia.** It is of interest that, in older women, **systemic sclerosis** may be associated with the presence of persisting **fetal DNA,** suggesting that this disease may be an immune response to remote past pregnancies (Artlett et al, 1998). It is not known whether **chronic erosive esophagitis,** a rare, sometimes fatal disease, is related to any of these disorders. A **drug, alendronate,** an inhibitor of bone resorption (osteoporosis) has been shown to cause a **chemical esophagitis** in some patients with erosions and ulcerations of esophageal mucosa and thickening of the esophageal wall. In some cases, the disease is severe and disabling (De Groen et al, 1996).

Histology

The histologic lesion in esophagitis is **mucosal erosions or ulcerations** varying in number, depth, and configuration. There is moderate infiltration of the stroma with inflammatory cells. The surface of the lesion may be covered with granulation tissue or fibrin. **Chronic erosive esophagitis** is characterized by **loss of superficial epithelial layers (mucosal erosions)** (Fig. 24-2C). Squamous metaplasia of the submucosal glands may occur in this disorder.

Cytology

Cells desquamating from the eroded esophageal epithelium are derived from the deep layers and are of the same size as **parabasal squamous cells, occurring singly and in small clusters.** The cytoplasm is evenly distributed and the cells do not vary much in size. In clusters, there is good adherence of the cells to each other. The most outstanding features of the **relatively large, somewhat hyperchromatic nuclei of these cells, sometimes show isolated clumps of chromatin and, occasionally, large nucleoli that may lead to an erroneous diagnosis of cancer** (Fig. 24-2D). Careful attention to cellular detail helps in the correct interpretation of the cytologic findings. The cells seen in erosive esophagi-

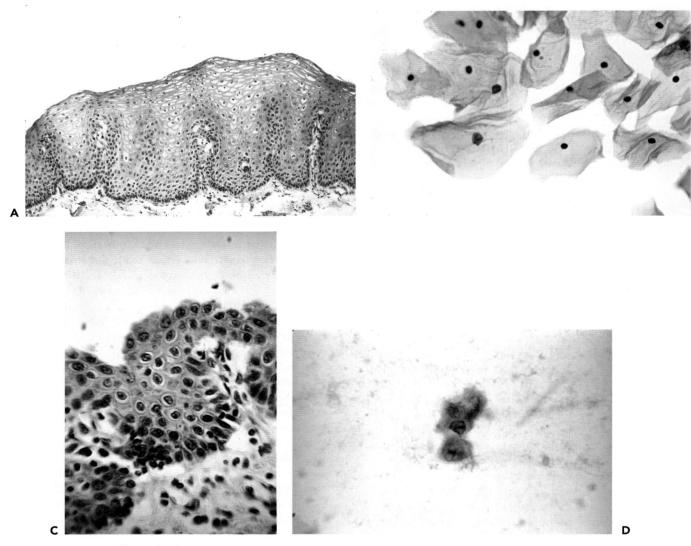

Figure 24-2 Normal esophagus and esophageal erosion. *A.* Normal squamous epithelium lining the esophagus. *B.* Normal squamous cells in an esophagus brush. *C.* Erosive esophagitis. The superficial layers of the squamous epithelium are missing, thus exposing deeper parabasal cells. *D.* Esophageal washing in a case of erosive esophagitis. Small squamous cells with prominent nuclei and nucleoli are shown. (Oil immersion.)

tis may be similar to those observed in **"repair"** of squamous epithelium or in **pemphigus** (see Fig. 21-10).

A recently recognized entity, **eosinophilic esophagitis,** has been observed mainly in children but also in adults (Liacouras, 2003; Dahms, 2004). Clinically, the disease causes painful reflux esophagitis that **mimics gastroesophageal reflux disease (GERD)** but does not respond to antiacid treatment. Dense eosinophilic infiltrate of the esophageal wall has been observed in biopsies (Straumann et al, 2004). There are no reported cases of this entity diagnosed on cytologic sampling.

Herpetic Esophagitis

Clinical Findings and Histology

Many years ago, Berg (1955) emphasized the occurrence of this disease in cancer patients who, in the course of treatment, sustained a **surgical or radiation injury** to the esophagus. **Immunosuppressive therapy, cytotoxic anticancer drugs, and acquired immunodeficiency syndrome (AIDS)** have contributed to an increased frequency of this disease (Lightdale et al, 1977). Most patients have vague complaints referable to the esophagus, such as retrosternal pain or mild dysphagia. Herpetic esophagitis produces **extensive, although superficial, ulcerations** of the esophageal mucosa. In biopsies, **intranuclear eosinophilic inclusions** are observed within the epithelial cells. The use of cytology resulted in primary diagnosis in several cases. Surprisingly, **in some patients, there was no past history of immune deficiency or immunosuppression.** It is, therefore, possible that the disease is more common than hitherto anticipated. We have observed apparent **simultaneous involvement of the esophagus and the bronchial tree.**

Cytology

The disease may be diagnosed in material obtained from the esophagus by washings, or brushing. The cytologic find-

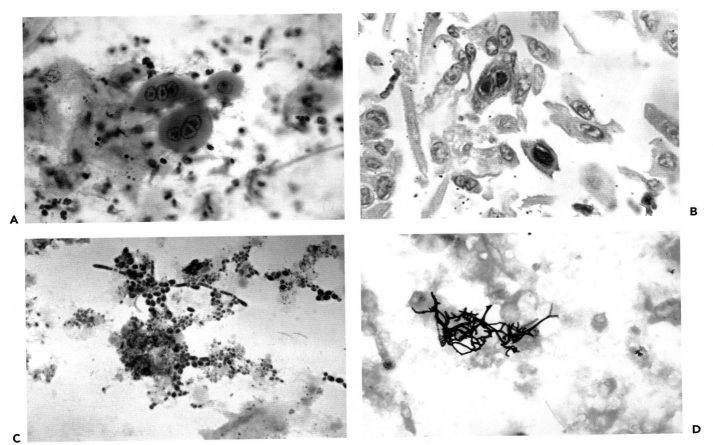

Figure 24-3   Infectious disorders of the esophagus. *A.* Typical cell changes of herpesvirus infection showing large multinucleated squamous cells with eosinophilic intranuclear inclusions. *B.* Another example of cells in herpetic esophagitis with large eosinophilic intranuclear inclusions. *C.* Pseudohyphae and yeast form of *Candida albicans* (moniliasis) in a patient with AIDS. *D.* Nocardia in esophagus. The GMS silver stain shows complex filaments of this bacterium. (*B:* Oil immersion.)

ings are identical with those observed in the material from the female genital tract (see Fig. 10-29), and the respiratory tract (see Chap. 19 and Fig. 19-36). **Multinucleated cells with molded "ground-glass," opaque nuclei and cells with intranuclear eosinophilic inclusions are observed** (Fig. 24-3A,B).

Esophageal Infections in AIDS

Esophagitis is a common early manifestation of AIDS. *Candidiasis* (moniliasis) (Fig. 24-3C), **herpetic esophagitis** (see above), **cytomegalovirus infection** (see Fig. 24-17B), and other infectious agents such as *Nocardia* may be identified in cytologic samples obtained during esophagoscopy (Fig. 24-3D). Geisinger (1995) stressed that **cytologic techniques are much superior to biopsies in the diagnosis of Candida esophagitis.** Teot et al (1993) reported a case with **simultaneous herpetic and cytomegalovirus esophagitis in AIDS.** Borczuk et al (1998) described a case of esophagitis caused by *Trichomonas,* diagnosed in esophageal brushings, in a male patient with AIDS.

Tuberculous esophagitis has been described in India where this disease is prevalent (Jain et al, 1999). The finding of clusters of **elongated epithelioid cells** and occasional

Langhans' type giant cells, in a background of inflammatory exudate, is suggestive of this rare event. Because of a marked increase of tuberculosis in AIDS patients, it may be anticipated that such cases will soon occur in the Western world as well.

Esophageal Diverticula

Esophageal diverticulum is an **outpouching of the esophageal epithelium** through the muscular wall of the organ. A diverticulum distended by accumulated food particles may produce **symptoms of esophageal obstruction** similar to those of cancer. There are no cytologic abnormalities known to occur in the presence of a diverticulum. However, rare **cancers originating within the diverticula** may be diagnosed by cytology (see below).

BARRETT'S ESOPHAGUS (COLUMNAR-LINED ESOPHAGEAL EPITHELIUM)

Clinical and Histologic Data

The syndrome, first described by Barrett in 1950, consists of a **replacement of the distal esophageal squamous epithelium by columnar epithelium of gastric or intestinal** type, associated mainly with chronic gastroesophageal reflux disease **(GERD),** and sometimes with hiatus hernia and esophageal stricture (Mossberg, 1966; Burgess et al, 1971; Spechler and Goyal, 1986; Chandrasoma et al, 2001; Shaheen and Ransohoff, 2002). The segment of the replaced esophageal mucosa may be **short or long** (recent summaries in Glickman et al, 2001 and Spechler, 2002). The symptoms associated with Barrett's syndrome are **dysphagia, regurgitation, heartburn, and pain.** Episodes of **acute obstruction** may occur, sometimes caused by **peptic ulcers, similar to gastric ulcers** (Fig. 24-4). In such cases, the radiologic examination may reveal a stricture that may mimic to perfection the appearance of an esophageal carcinoma (see Fig. 24-4A), although there is usually a preservation of esophageal peristalsis above and below. After treatment, the stricture may regress significantly (Fig. 24-4D). **Barrett's syndrome is, per se, a benign disorder, but has now been recognized as a risk factor for adenocarcinoma of the esophagus and, to a lesser extent, of gastric cardia** (Lagergren et al, 1999). **Cytologic techniques may be used to monitor patients with Barrett's esophagus to identify malignant transformation and precancerous states,** as described below.

Histologic findings show an abrupt transition from the normal squamous epithelium to **mucus-producing columnar epithelium of gastric type or of intestinal type with goblet cells** (see Fig. 24-4C). The epithelium may form **cysts** wherein Rubio et al (1989, 1992) observed occasional presence of **ciliated columnar cells,** although this finding was much more common in papillary carcinomas (see below).

Cytology

Although the diagnosis of uncomplicated Barrett's esophagus is usually established by esophagoscopy and biopsies, **cytologic examination of esophageal brush specimens, aspirates or washings,** may be valuable in establishing baseline data for comparison with future abnormalities occurring during the follow-up of these patients. The **smears, containing mucus-producing benign columnar cells and goblet cells, usually in clusters, characteristic of mucus-producing intestinal epithelium,** are diagnostic of Barrett's esophagus (see Fig. 24-4B). The glandular cells have **small, spherical, nuclei of even sizes.** The peripheral nuclei of the goblet cells may appear a bit darker. We have not

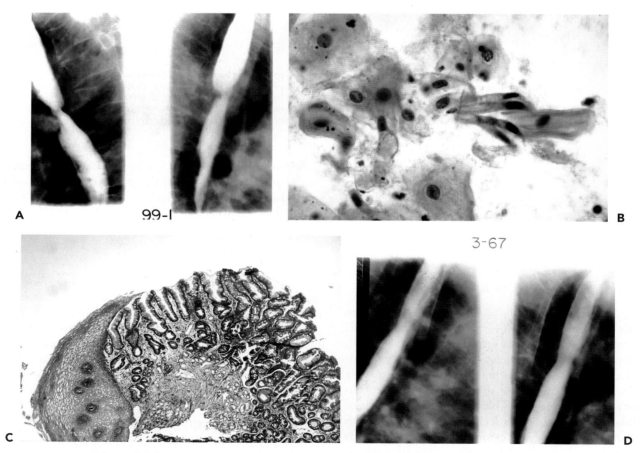

Figure 24-4 **Barrett's esophagus with ulcer formation.** *A.* Narrowing and obstruction of the esophagus in a barium swallow in a 56 year old man. *B.* Brushing of the obstructed area revealed benign columnar cells of intestinal type and normal squamous cells. *C.* Biopsy of the affected area shows a transition between normal squamous epithelium on left and gastric type epithelium on right, characteristic of Barrett's esophagus. *D.* Barium swallow after conservative treatment. The narrowing and the esophageal occlusion seen in A have nearly disappeared and the patient became asymptomatic.

observed the **ciliated columnar cells** described by Rubio (1989), except for **swallowed cells of bronchial origin.** Fennerty et al (1995) attempted to diagnose this disorder by esophageal balloon technique (described below) without success. Malignant changes in Barrett's esophagus are described below.

BENIGN TUMORS

Focal Hyperplasia and Papillomas (Condylomas) of Squamous Epithelium

In 1982, Syrjänen et al described a rare **papilloma-like lesion of the squamous epithelium** of the esophagus, akin to a **condyloma acuminatum,** and postulated that human papillomavirus (HPV) may be a factor in the genesis of this tumor. Winkler et al (1985) confirmed this hypothesis by documenting the presence of HPV antigen in two such lesions and in 11 of 73 **"focal hyperplasias," some of which resembled "flat condylomas" with significant koilocytosis and nuclear abnormalities.** Further evidence that HPV is present in papillomas was provided in case reports (Yamada et al, 1995; Politoske, 1992) and by Lavergne and de Villiers (1999) who confirmed the presence of the virus in 4 of 11 papillomas of the esophagus by molecular analysis. Apparently, none of these lesions progressed to cancer. It is of note, though, that Syrjänen (1982) observed "flat condylomas" at the periphery of invasive esophageal cancers. There is no known cytologic presentation of these lesions but it is likely that koilocytes should be observed in smears.

Granular Cell Tumor or Myoblastoma

A case of **granular cell myoblastoma** of esophagus diagnosed on esophageal brushings was described by Cordoba et al (1998). The lesion is very unusual in this location. The cytologic presentation of this tumor has been described in reference to the lung (see Chap. 20) and the breast (see Chap. 29).

Leiomyoma

We had the opportunity to study esophageal lavage and brush specimens from several cases of leiomyomas of the wall of the esophagus. The tumors could not be recognized in cytologic samples.

SQUAMOUS CARCINOMA AND ITS PRECURSORS

Epidemiology and Clinical Aspects

Squamous carcinoma is, by far, the most common type of esophageal cancer. The disease may affect any part of the esophagus, but occurs preferentially in **segments of slight narrowing:** at the level of the thyroid cartilage, bifurcation of the trachea, and the diaphragm. As a general rule, fully developed esophageal cancers cause **obstruction of the esophagus, resulting in difficulties of swallowing and dysphagia.**

Squamous cancer of the esophagus is a quasi-endemic disorder in northeastern Iran, in parts of China, among the Chinese in Singapore, among Africans in southern Africa, and among men in Brittany (France) (Enzinger and Mayer, 2003). In the United States, the disease is relatively uncommon; African American men appear to be more prone to it than other ethnic groups. In general, the disease is more common in males than in females. Epidemiologic data suggest that intake of hot beverages, cigarette smoking, and alcohol consumption are possible risk factors (Tavani et al, 1994; Enzinger and Mayer, 2003). Recent studies in China failed to reveal any consistent risk factors except, perhaps, diet (Li et al, 1989; Yu et al, 1993). Auerback et al (1965) demonstrated a high frequency of squamous carcinoma in situ of the esophagus among smokers.

The **prognosis of esophageal squamous carcinoma** is stage related. The overall survival is about 20% (Lerut et al, 1992; Goldminc et al, 1993). Izbicki et al (1997) pointed out that the prognosis of patients with clinical stage I disease, confined to the wall of the esophagus, may be modified by finding **occult micrometastasis** in regional lymph nodes stained with an epithelial antibody. Stockeld et al (2002) described the use of **fine needle aspiration (FNA) biopsy technique** for prognosis of esophageal squamous cancer. Aspirates of the esophageal wall, obtained at 2 cm intervals, led to the discovery of microscopic tumor spread in one-third of the 52 investigated patients. The results were more accurate than synchronous esophageal brushing or multiple biopsies. The ratio of benign to malignant cells in the aspirated samples appeared to be of prognostic significance.

Kwong et al (2004) studied chromosomal aberrations in esophageal squamous cancer by comparative genomic hybridization. Numerous gains and losses were observed but **gain in the short arm of chromosome 12** (+12p) predicted poor prognosis after surgery, at least among the Chinese.

Adenocarcinoma occurring in Barrett's esophagus is discussed below.

Human Papillomavirus in Squamous Cancer of the Esophagus

Invariably, as with all squamous cancers, the question of **human papillomavirus (HPV) as a factor in the genesis of this tumor** was raised (Syrjänen, 1987). HPV DNA presence in five invasive esophageal cancers was first reported by Kulski et al (1986). Subsequently, Chang et al (1992) reported the presence of HPV in 25 of 51 (49%) **biopsies** from Chinese patients with invasive esophageal carcinoma. In 16 of these 25 specimens, HPV types 16 and 18 were documented by in situ hybridization. Other types of HPV were observed in the remaining 7 patients. In the same study, 53 of 80 **cytologic preparations,** also from asymptomatic Chinese patients from a high-risk area, were positive for HPV by filter in situ hybridization. HPV was also detected in cells of 2 of 9 patients without cytologic abnormalities, in 3 of 6 patients with "mild dysplasia," in 25 of 31 patients with "moderate dysplasia," in 19 of 28 patients with "severe dysplasia," and in 4 of 6 patients with invasive carcinoma. In an update of this study, Chang et al (2000) reported that 16.9% of 700 Chinese patients with esophageal carcinoma were HPV positive, with 27% of the positive samples containing the "high risk" HPV types 16 and 18.

These data were either confirmed or contested in several papers. Thus, Cooper (1994) and He (1997) observed HPV in about 15% of esophageal cancers. De Villiers et al (1999), known for impeccable laboratory technique, confirmed the presence of HPV of various types in 17% of samples from Chinese patients. Takahashi et al (1998) and Kawaguchi et al (2000) **observed that the presence of HPV was associated with mutations of the p53 gene.**

On the other hand, Smits et al (1995) from the Netherlands, Benamouzig et al (1995) from France, and Mizobuchi et al (1997) from Japan, were unable to identify HPV in their many samples. In a study of 51 patients with squamous carcinoma from three North American cities, only **one** patient's tumor contained HPV type 16 (Turner et al, 1997).

It is quite evident that the issue of the role of HPV in esophageal carcinoma has not been definitely settled but there appears to be little doubt that in tumors from some patients, mainly Chinese and Japanese, the virus is present (Galloway and Daling, 1996). **Since a person-to-person transmission of HPV is unlikely in these patients, an activation of the latent viral infection is a more likely explanation of these findings.**

It is of note that Wang et al (1999) detected **Epstein-Barr virus (EBV)** in squamous cancer in Taiwan.

Histology

Histologic appearance of squamous cancer may vary in the degree of differention from **well differentiated, highly keratinized (verrucous) types** (Fig. 24-5B) **to poorly differentiated squamous cancer** (Fig. 24-5D) **and, rarely, small-cell** (oat cell) type of carcinoma (Rosen et al, 1975; Bogomoletz et al, 1989). **A basaloid variant,** resembling a basal cell carcinoma but with a highly malignant behavior, was described (see Fig. 24-6D) (Abe et al, 1996). **Focal**

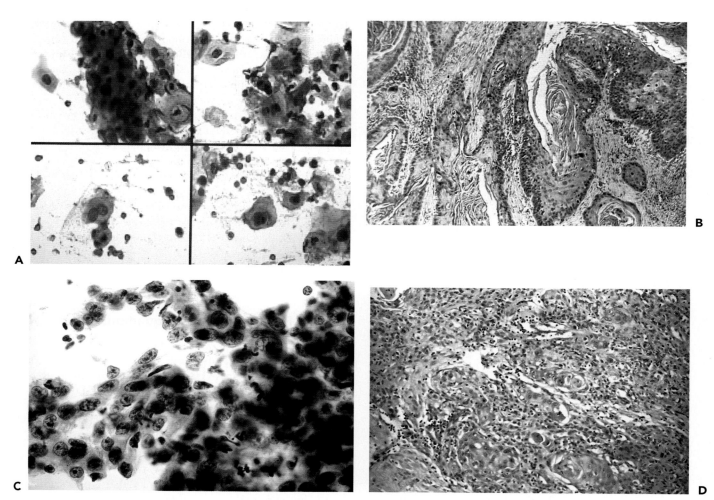

Figure 24-5   Squamous cancer of the esophagus. *A.* Composite image of well differentiated squamous cancer cells observed in typical squamous carcinoma of the esophagus. The cancer cells are markedly keratinized and have obvious enlarged hyperchromatic nuclei. *B.* Invasive squamous carcinoma of the esophagus corresponding to *A. C.* Poorly differentiated squamous carcinoma of the esophagus. The tumor cells are smaller and show marked nuclear abnormalities. *D.* Tissue lesion corresponding to *C. (A:* Images obtained by PAPNET apparatus. With permission of TriPath Imaging, Burlington, NC.)

glandular features may be observed in a substantial proportion of epidermoid carcinomas (Kuwano et al, 1988). Some of the poorly differentiated carcinomas may show **endocrine granules** in electron microscopy (Reyes et al, 1980).

Cytology

As discussed above, these tumors may occur in a variety of grades and degrees of differentiation. The cytologic findings in esophageal washings or brushings closely reflect these structural variants and are similar to those described for bronchogenic carcinomas of similar histologic types (see Chap. 20).

The **well-differentiated squamous carcinoma** produces **heavily keratinized abnormal squamous cells, singly or in clusters, with either completely pyknotic, hyperchromatic nuclei, or with nuclear shadows,** much in the manner described for similar cancers of the bronchus (Fig. 24-5A; see Chap. 20). **Koilocyte-like cells** with large, hyperchromatic nuclei and perinuclear clear zones or halos

are sometimes observed in such tumors. There is no good correlation between these cells and the presence of HPV.

Less well-differentiated squamous cancers of large cell type (epidermoid carcinomas) are characterized by smaller cancer cells with very **scanty basophilic cytoplasm, often forming clusters,** particularly in brush specimens (Figs. 24-5C and 24-6A). The **nuclear abnormalities in the form of enlargement, hyperchromasia and large nucleoli** are usually quite evident. The diagnosis of tumor type depends largely on the finding of squamous cancer cells with eosinophilic cytoplasm, which may be very scarce.

Small cell carcinomas, the most **anaplastic varieties of squamous cancer,** produce **cancer cells that often are very small, with abnormally large, hyperchromatic nuclei and very scanty cytoplasm** (Fig. 24-6C). The corresponding tissue sections may sometimes show the "basaloid" tumor pattern (Fig. 24-6D). Horai et al (1978), Reid et al (1980), and Imai et al (1978) described several examples of such carcinomas. Hoda and Hajdu (1992) pointed out that, **contrary to oat cell carcinoma of the bronchus, cell molding**

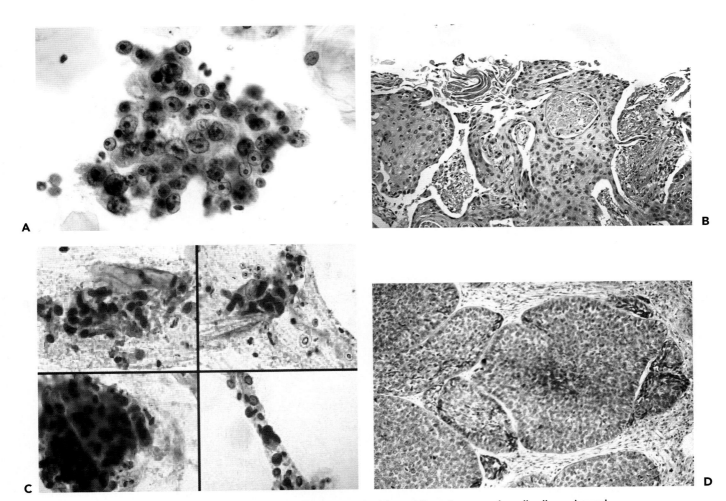

Figure 24-6   **Poorly differentiated squamous (epidermoid) carcinoma and small cell esophageal cancer.** *A.* Esophageal balloon sample shows a cluster of cancer cells from an occult epidermoid carcinoma of the esophagus shown in *B. C.* Composite images of a small-cell (oat cell) carcinoma of the esophagus. Note the very small cancer cells forming clusters and sheets. *D.* Basaloid carcinoma of the esophagus composed of small cells. In spite of its orderly appearance, this tumor is highly malignant. (*C:* Images obtained with the PAPNET apparatus. With permission of TriPath Imaging, Burlington, NC.)

was uncommon in the esophageal tumors and that the evidence of endocrine activity in these tumors was insecure.

Squamous or epidermoid carcinomas of the distal end of the esophagus may extend into the gastric cardia and fail to produce radiographic abnormalities of cancer on cursory examination. Cytologic examination, either by esophageal or gastric brushings, may be of critical diagnostic importance (Fig. 24-7).

The use of fine needle aspiration of the esophageal wall, for diagnosis and prognosis of squamous cancer, proposed by Stockeld et al (2002) was described above.

Precursor Lesions of Squamous Carcinoma and Their Detection: Lessons From China

In the 1961 and 1968 editions of this book, it was anticipated that carcinoma of the esophagus must be preceded by precancerous epithelial changes, such as carcinoma in situ and related abnormalities. In the Western world, the knowledge of precancerous squamous lesions of the esophagus is scarce. There are several cases on record in which squamous carcinoma in situ and related lesions had been observed as incidental findings (previous editions of this book; Imbriglia and Lopusniak, 1949; Auerback et al,

1965; Ushigome et al, 1967; Koss et al, 1998) or as a lesion accompanying invasive carcinoma (Suckow et al, 1962; Kuwano et al, 1988). However, the hypothesis could be confirmed only by the extensive cytologic and histologic studies of esophageal cancer conducted by Chinese investigators.

The stimulus for the Chinese studies was the very high prevalence rate of esophageal cancer in certain areas of central and northern China (Yang, 1980; Shu 1984, 1985). It is of incidental interest that, in the same areas of China, chickens are susceptible to cancer-like tumors of the gullet. The relationship of these tumors to human cancer is not understood. Except for its possible association with diet and human papillomavirus, the causes of human esophageal cancer in China and its relationship to the tumors in poultry, remain unknown at the time of this writing (2004).

The Chinese investigators proposed that prevention of esophageal cancer could be based on the same principles as detection of precursor stages of cancer of the uterine cervix. If cytologic samples, obtained in asymptomatic, high-risk populations, could lead to the discovery of precancerous lesions, then early surgical intervention or photodynamic therapy could prevent invasive esophageal cancer with its very high mortality rate (Yang et al, 2002). The instruments used in the cytologic investigations were small,

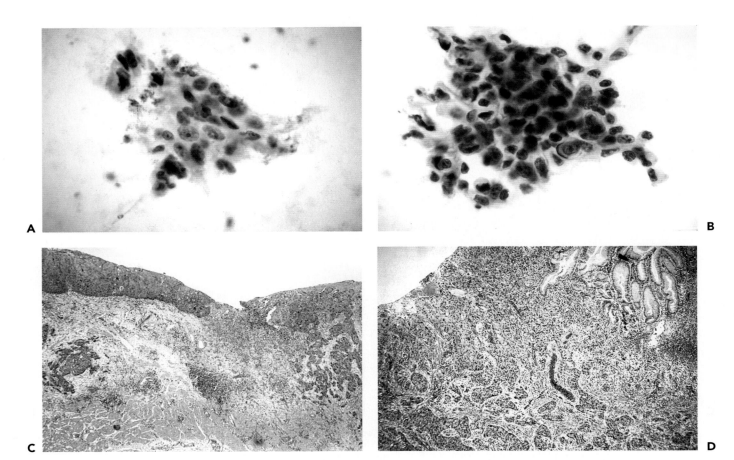

Figure 24-7 Poorly differentiated squamous carcinoma involving distal esophagus and adjacent gastric cardia. The tumor was roentgenologically occult. *A,B.* Clusters of small malignant squamous cells in esophageal lavage. *C.* Squamous carcinoma in situ involving lower esophagus with transition to invasive carcinoma, shown in *D.*

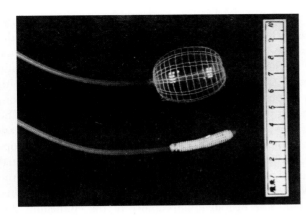

Figure 24-8 Esophageal balloon, collapsed (*bottom*) and distended with air (*top*). Note the rugosity of the surface that serves to obtain cell samples from the esophagus. The balloon is connected to a plastic tube with markers to indicate the position of the balloon in the esophagus. (Courtesy of Dr. Yi-Jing Shu, St. Gallen, Switzerland.)

inflatable **plastic balloons with abrasive surface** (Fig. 24-8), modifications of a gastric balloon that was described in 1950 by Panico et al. The balloon was attached to a narrow-caliber tube with color markers to indicate the position of the balloon in the esophagus. The balloon could be easily swallowed in deflated state, moved by peristalsis to the cardia, inflated, and slowly withdrawn to the level of the cricoid cartilage. At this point, the balloon is deflated and withdrawn. The abrasive surfaces of the balloon contained cells scraped from the surface epithelium that could be examined in smears. The method, which was tested in our institution, caused trivial discomfort to the patients and was well accepted (Greenebaum, 1984).

The **accuracy of balloon sampling** was tested in China on 1,861 patients with overt esophageal cancer, documented by biopsy. The accuracy varied from 87.2% to 99.0%, averaging 94.9% (summary in Shu 1984, 1985). As reported by Shu in 1984, the **cytologic sampling by balloon proved to be much superior to either endoscopy or radiologic examination for the diagnosis of precursor lesions and early invasive squamous carcinoma.** In an elaborate statistical analysis, Dawsey et al (1994A,B) compared the **results of cytologic sampling with the incidence rates of esophageal squamous carcinoma** in the Linxian province of China and concluded that the **esophageal balloon cytology successfully identified persons at increased risk for esophageal cancer.** This was confirmed for the Anyang County of China by Yang et al (2002). It is not known how the balloon method would compare with contemporary endoscopy, which because of cost and limited availability could not be used on a very large scale for purposes of esophageal cancer detection.

Several **other methods** to study esophageal cytology were developed. Jaskiewicz et al (1987) used a **small sponge, attached to a string and packaged in an easy-to-swallow gelatin capsule** to study patients in South Africa. A similar system was described by Sepehr et al (2000) as better acceptable to patients. Qin and Zhou (1992) described an **elastic plastic tube** for esophageal sampling and reported an accuracy of 96% in the diagnosis of cancer.

Results of Screening

The first results of the population survey were presented in the Fourth International Cancer Congress in Florence, Italy in 1974 by an anonymous group representing the Chinese Academy of Medical Sciences. A cytologic survey of 17,471 persons over 30 years of age was conducted in the Henan Province in northern China. **"Dysplasia"** of the esophageal epithelium was observed in 276 patients, mostly below the age of 40, whereas invasive carcinoma in this population usually occurred in patients older than 40. **Follow-up study of the patients with "dysplasia,"** some over a period of 7 to 10 years, disclosed that 30.3% of them developed esophageal carcinoma, in 27.3% the original lesion persisted unchanged, and in 42.4% the changes either regressed to mild dysplasia or reverted to normal. In histologic studies of 67 patients, **the progression of dysplasia of various types to carcinoma in situ could be observed in many specimens.** It was the conclusion of this study that **"marked dysplasia" must be considered a precancerous lesion.** During the intervening years and changing political conditions in China, the names of the investigators became known (summary in Shu 1984, 1985), and the results of several surveys became available.

As related by Shu in 1984, there is no doubt that mass screening for esophageal carcinoma in high-risk areas of China had a major beneficial effect. Before screening was instituted, the diagnosis of carcinoma in situ or early invasive carcinoma was 2 per 1,000 in low-risk areas and 10 per 1,000 in high-risk areas. Screening of 81,187 asymptomatic people over the age of 30 in the high-risk Henan Province resulted in the discovery of 880 esophageal cancers (*a huge prevalence rate of 1%!*), of which 649 (73.7%) were early and treatable by surgery (Shu, 1984). Less is known about survival of these patients, but Dr. Shu assured me that most of the treated patients survived 5 years or longer with a good quality of life. This information must be compared with a survival of about 10% to 25% of patients with invasive squamous cancer of the esophagus commonly observed in the Western world (Ide et al, 1994; Lieberman et al, 1995). Kwong et al (2004) reported that, among Chinese patients with esophagus cancer, those showing a **gain of the short arm of chromosome 12** (+ p12) in the tumor had poor outcome after surgical treatment, regardless of stage of disease.

Screening for Esophageal Squamous Cancer in Countries Other Than China

The accomplishments of the Chinese scholars found several imitators. Thus, Berry et al (1981) attempted a similar project in South Africa (where the rate of esophageal cancer is very high among some black populations), resulting in the discovery of 15 occult invasive carcinomas and carcinomas in situ in 500 patients studied. Dysplasia was illustrated, but the clinical significance of the lesion was not discussed. Similar results were reported by Jaskiewicz et al (1987) from a high-risk rural population in Transkei (South Africa); in five patients, dysplastic changes progressed to invasive cancer.

To our knowledge, the Chinese experience has not been duplicated in the Western countries, except for the work in this laboratory. Greenebaum et al (1984) studied 96 high-risk Montefiore Hospital patients in New York City by the balloon technique. The selected patients had prior cancers of the larynx or pharynx, or were alcoholics and heavy cigarette smokers. Greenebaum unexpectedly found **three occult recurrent oropharyngeal cancers and one carcinoma in situ of the esophagus, observed in a man with prior history of squamous carcinoma of the larynx.** The biopsy of the esophagus disclosed fragments of squamous cancer in the absence of radiologic abnormalities.

Classification of Precancerous Lesions in China

Based on cytologic and histologic criteria, the Chinese investigators divided the precancerous lesions into two groups: **dysplasia and carcinoma in situ. The criteria were derived from the classification of precancerous lesions of the uterine cervix** (see Chap. 11). **Lesions with more orderly epithelial growth, surface differentiation, and relatively minor nuclear abnormalities were classified as** *dysplasia* **and lesions with more significant atypia were classed as** *carcinoma in situ.*

The **dysplasias were further subdivided into mild, moderate, and severe, based mainly on cytologic criteria** (see below). The true significance of dysplasia is not clear. Although, in some patients, the lesions either failed to progress or regress, there is no doubt that, **in a substantial number of untreated patients, invasive cancer of the esophagus was subsequently observed** (Shu 1984, 1985). The same conclusion was reached by Sugimachi et al (1995), who considered "dysplasia" as an early carcinoma of the esophagus. In any event, **the insecure behavior of the precancerous lesions of the esophagus is remarkably similar to lesions of the uterine cervix** (see Chap. 11).

Cytology

Much of the current knowledge of cytology of precursor lesions comes from Chinese sources (summaries in Shu, 1984, 1985; Shen, 1984). There is a remarkable similarity between the cytologic presentation of carcinoma in situ and related lesions of the esophagus and those of the uterine cervix (see Chap. 11). **As in the uterine cervix, the lesions may be conveniently divided into high grade and low grade.**

High-Grade Lesions

The squamous cancer cells derived from high grade lesions **(high grade dysplasia, carcinoma in situ) are of the parabasal variety. The nuclear abnormalities consist of enlargement and hyperchromasia; the cytoplasm is scanty,** resulting in a high nucleocytoplasmic ratio (Fig. 24-9). Cell clustering is common. Shu (1984, 1985) **illustrated several examples of progression of dysplasias to carcinoma in situ and, in some cases, to invasive carcinomas over a period of 2 to 4 years.**

There are very few cases of **carcinoma in situ diagnosed by cytology** in the Western world. Besides the case reported by Imbriglia and Lopusniak (1949), one case of a lesion approaching carcinoma in situ was personally observed in esophageal washings in a 59-year-old man with an esophageal diverticulum and symptoms of obstruction, leading to the clinical diagnosis of esophageal cancer. The lesion was characterized by **typical dyskaryotic (dysplastic) superficial and parabasal squamous cells.** The biopsies, which, unfortunately, were obtained after an initial short course of radiotherapy, localized the lesion to the diverticulum, which was subsequently successfully resected. The histologic appearance of the epithelium disclosed nuclear abnormalities and some degree of disarrangement of the component cells. One **carcinoma in situ** was recognized during balloon screening of a high risk population by Greenebaum et al (1984), and another during analysis of esophageal cytologic abnormalities by a neural net-based scanning system (Koss et al, 1998). In both cases, the **smears contained squamous cancer cells, singly and in clusters, that could not be differentiated from an invasive squamous cancer** (Fig. 24-10). The last patient who had a history of esophageal stricture and necrotizing esophagitis, was alive without evidence of esophageal cancer 3 years after the diagnosis. These anecdotal cases confirm the insecure prognosis of precursor lesions of esophageal squamous carcinoma.

Low-Grade Lesions

Low-grade lesions of the esophagus (mild or moderate dysplasia; Fig. 24-11) are characterized by **well-differentiated superficial and intermediate squamous cells with marked nuclear enlargement and hyperchromasia.** In some patients, **koilocytes** may be observed. The resemblance of these cell abnormalities to dyskaryosis (dysplasia) of cervical squamous cells is remarkable (see Chap. 11).

ADENOCARCINOMA AND ITS PRECURSORS

Clinical Data and Natural History

Although only about 3% of esophageal cancers are adenocarcinomas, this disease has generated an enormous amount of attention because of its **association with "columnar-lined epithelium" or Barrett's esophagus** (Haggitt et al, 1978; recent reviews in Shaheen and Ransohoff, 2002; Enzinger and Mayer, 2003). It is estimated that the presence of this abnormality increases the chances of adenocarcinoma about 50-fold and that **the risk factor** is in proportion to the size of the lesion (Menke-Pluymers et al, 1993; Lagergren et al, 1999). The association of Barrett's esophagus with carcinoma is sometimes referred to as Dawson's syndrome. However, **adenocarcinomas of the esophagus may also occur in the absence of Barrett's syndrome.** The prognosis of esophageal adenocarcinoma is poor with 1-year survival

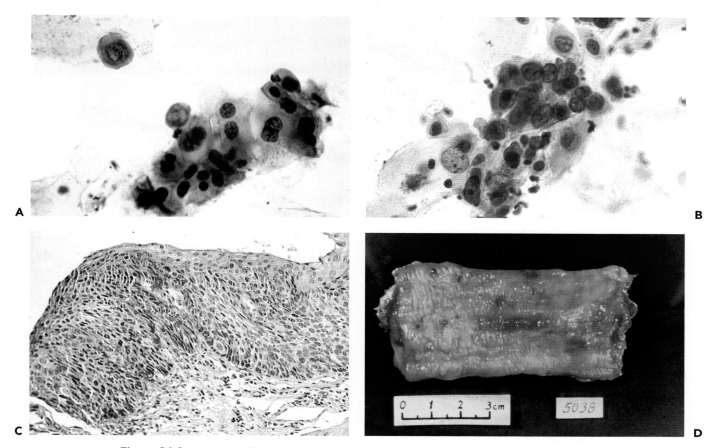

Figure 24-9   Examples of squamous carcinoma in situ from China. *A,B.* Moderately well-differentiated squamous cancer cells. *C.* Squamous carcinoma in situ in biopsy material. *D.* The site of carcinoma in situ as a reddening of mucosa in the resected segment of the esophagus. (*A,B:* High power.) (Photographs courtesy of Dr. Yi-Jing Shu, St. Gallen, Switzerland.)

estimated at 44% but 5-year survival at only 13% (Eloubeidi et al, 2003D).

Histology

Most adenocarcinomas of the esophagus occur in the area of the cardia and originate in islands of gastrointestinal mucosa, less often in the submucosal glands, and usually are histologically similar to gastric adenocarcinoma and its various histologic patterns, described below. **Most tumors are well differentiated and signet ring type of carcinoma is very rare.** Occasionally, **papillary adenocarcinomas, composed of large columnar cancer cells, may be observed** (Fig. 24-12), also possibly related to Barrett's esophagus wherein precancerous lesions of a similarhistologic and cytologic type have been observed (Belladonna et al, 1974). Rubio et al (1989, 1992) observed ciliated glandular cells in dilated glands of papillary adenocarcinomas in patients with Barrett's esophagus.

As frequently happens in areas of the body where two different types of mucosa meet, tumors that have the properties of both **glandular and squamous epithelium** may occur in the lower esophagus. These cancers may be best classified as **mucoepidermoid.** There is no evidence that their behavior is in any way different from the behavior

of pure epidermoid or pure mucus-producing varieties of cancer.

Precursor Lesions

The **sequence of morphologic events in the genesis of adenocarcinoma** became the subject of numerous scientific communications. Briefly summarized, **morphologic precancerous abnormalities in columnar epithelium** (named *dysplasia,* rather than carcinoma in situ) precede invasive carcinoma (Smith et al, 1984; Lee, 1985). These lesions **have been subdivided into "low grade" and "high grade."** The criteria of this classification have been published by Reid et al (1980) and tested as reproducible among expert pathologists by Montgomery et al (2001A).

"High-grade dysplasia" (that we would prefer to classify as **adenocarcinoma in situ**) **consist of nuclear enlargement and hyperchromasia in the columnar epithelial cells, occasionally with branching or distortion of the affected glands and a marked increase in abnormal mitoses** (Reid et al, 1988; Rubio and Riddell, 1989). The lesions are very **similar to precancerous abnormalities and carcinoma in situ of the gastric epithelium** (see Fig. 24-26). The problem with **high-grade esophageal dysplasia is its separation from frank adenocarcinoma, which is not**

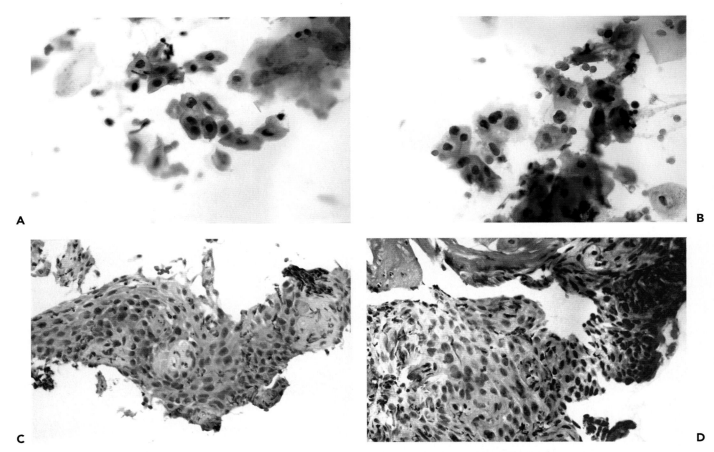

Figure 24-10 Personal case of carcinoma in situ of esophagus. an incidental finding in esophageal brushings. *A,B.* Well-differentiated small squamous cancer cells in esophageal brushings for esophagitis. *C,D.* Low and high power view of a fragment of markedly atypical squamous epithelium of the esophagus, interpreted as carcinoma in situ. The patient was asymptomatic 3 years after the biopsy.

easy either in biopsies or in cytologic samples. Prospective studies of patients with severe dysplasia indicate a high level of **progression to adenocarcinomas of the gastrointestinal type** (Smith et al, 1984; Lee, 1985; Spechler and Goyal, 1986; Rusch et al, 1994; Montgomery et al, 2001B).

Elaborate molecular studies suggested that high grade dysplasia and early adenocarcinoma show similar genetic alterations, regardless whether the Barrett lesion involved short or long segments of the esophagus (Nobukawa et al, 2001). Also, mutation of p53 gene was shown to be frequent in high grade dysplasia and adenocarcinoma than in low-grade dysplasia (Bian et al, 2001). Surgical resection of "severe dysplasia" is curative of the disease but it is not without major complications (Rush et al, 1994). Currently, such lesions may also be treated by endoscopic ablation, using photodynamic therapy or laser surgery (Van Dam and Brugge, 1999).

Much less secure is the identification of low grade or **"mild dysplasia"** which is described as **slight atypia of the columnar epithelial cells** (Robey et al, 1988). According to Montgomery et al (2001A, 2001B), the diagnosis of low-grade dysplasia is fairly reproducible among expert pathologists and shows a **15% to 20% progression rate to invasive cancer.** Patients with Barrett's syndrome are monitored by endoscopic biopsies and by cytologic studies of brush specimens (Spechler, 2002).

Cytology

Invasive Adenocarcinomas and Mucoepidermoid Carcinomas

In brush specimens, the cancer cells derived from adenocarcinomas are usually **well-differentiated columnar cells with conspicuous nuclear abnormalities in the form of enlarged, sometimes hyperchromatic nuclei with large single or multiple nucleoli** (Fig. 24-12A,C). In advanced carcinomas, **these cells occur singly and in small clusters, usually accompanied by evidence of necrosis. Smaller, more spherical cancer cells may also occur in less well-differentiated tumors.** Shurbaji and Erozan (1991) noted that the **findings were not consistent and that nuclear hyperchromasia and large nucleoli were not observed in all the cases.**

In **mucoepidermoid carcinomas,** the cells of glandular derivation **are mixed with occasional squamous cancer cells.** In many such cases, it is not clear **whether the tumor is primarily squamous or glandular,** although the malignant nature of the process is evident.

Precursor Lesions

Cytologic definition of "dysplasia" of columnar epithelium is insecure. Wang et al (1992) described **small clusters**

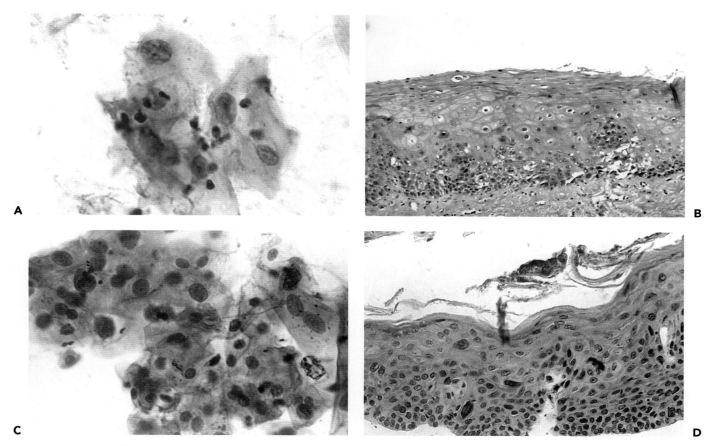

Figure 24-11   Precursor lesions of squamous cancer of the esophagus. *A,B.* Precancerous lesion of the esophagus classified as "mild dysplasia." *A.* Superficial dyskaryotic (dysplastic) squamous cells corresponding to the tissue lesion shown in *B,* which shows only mild focal abnormalities of the squamous epithelium. *C,D.* Precancerous lesion of the esophagus classified as "moderate dysplasia." The balloon smear shown in *C* shows well-differentiated parabasal squamous cancer cells. *D.* The biopsy of the same lesion shows moderate to marked nuclear abnormalities within the squamous epithelium. The lesion shown in *C* and *D* could be classified as high rather than low-grade. (Photographs courtesy of Dr. Yi-Jing Shu, St. Gallen, Switzerland.)

of mildly pleomorphic cells with enlarged nuclei with occasional multiple nucleoli. In a more recent thoughtful review of this topic by Hughes and Cohen (1998), the definition of cytologic abnormalities in dysplasia was not particularly helpful. These authors reviewed the literature and pointed out that the accumulated experience with comparative cytology-histology of these lesions is very small.

Personal experience suggests that the **morphologic distinction of "high-grade or severe dysplasia" from adenocarcinoma is highly subjective.** In cases with **clusters** of mildly or moderately atypical columnar cells with **somewhat enlarged, somewhat hyperchromatic nuclei and the presence of multiple small or single large nucleoli,** the diagnosis of **"atypia" of columnar cells** is justified (Fig. 12-13A,B). **If the atypical cells form clusters, the possibility of an adenocarcinoma cannot be ruled out** (Fig. 12-13C,D). **In all such cases,** the tentative cytologic diagnosis **must be confirmed by biopsies.** The situation is reminiscent of the problems with recognition of early neoplastic abnormalities in endocervical epithelium, discussed at length in Chapter 12.

There is virtually no cytologic experience with the identification of **"mild dysplasia."** Hughes and Cohen (1998)

point out that the separation of the possible neoplastic from reactive changes in the columnar cells is virtually impossible.

Monitoring of precursors of adenocarcinoma by balloon cytology was attempted with diverse results. Fennerty et al (1995) failed to obtain informative samples in a small number of patients. Falk et al (1997), in a much larger series of patients, **compared the inexpensive balloon cytology with brushings.** Brush cytology recognized all of 11 patients with high-grade dysplasia and carcinoma whereas balloon samples failed to recognize two of these patients. For **low-grade dysplasia, both brushings and balloon cytology failed in a substantial proportion of cases.** In two of the patients without disease, atypical cells were observed. This study documented the problem with cytologic diagnosis of low-grade abnormalities.

The monitoring of **epithelial DNA content by flow cytometry** disclosed abnormal, aneuploid DNA histograms in dysplasias and in carcinomas (Haggitt et al, 1988). However, securing adequate cell samples for this procedure by esophageal brushings is difficult. Another approach to progression of dysplasia to adenocarcinoma in tissue samples was discussed by Polkowski et al (1995). These authors reported an

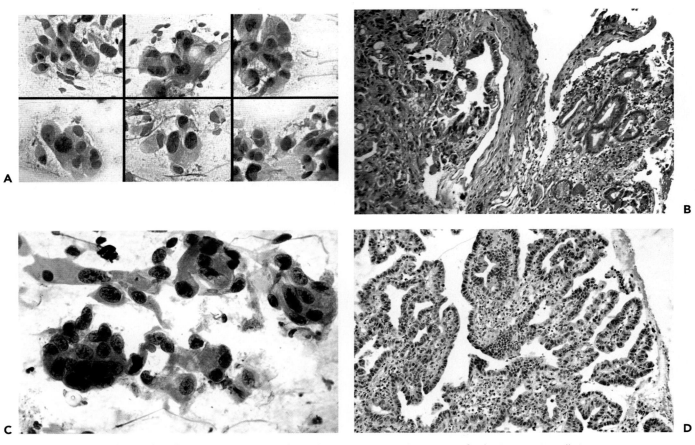

Figure 24-12 **Adenocarcinoma of esophagus.** *A.* Composite picture of columnar cancer cells in a case of esophageal adenocarcinoma shown in *B. C.* Very large columnar cancer cells in another case of esophageal adenocarcinoma in a 43-year-old man without evidence of Barrett's syndrome. The tissue lesion corresponding to *C* is shown in *D.*

increase in the expression of mutated p53 gene and an increase in the proliferative fraction of cells as measured by expression of Ki67 antigen with progression of esophageal dysplasia to adenocarcinoma. To our knowledge, this approach has not been tested in cytologic samples.

CYTOLOGIC FOLLOW-UP OF PATIENTS WITH TREATED ESOPHAGEAL CARCINOMA

The customary treatment of invasive carcinoma of the esophagus is either by surgery, radiotherapy alone or by radiotherapy followed by an attempt at surgical removal of the lesion. Extensive surgical resection for esophageal adenocarcinoma did not improve the survival rate (Hulscher et al, 2002). Combining chemotherapy with cisplatin and radiotherapy **(chemoradiotherapy)** did not improve overall survival of patients (Bosset et al, 1997). In several cases so treated, the observation has been made that, **in spite of the remarkable clinical improvement following radiotherapy, the smears remained positive.** In several of the surgically removed esophagi, there was **disappearance of much of the invasive tumor, but areas of carcinoma in situ**

were not affected by therapy. This situation is reminiscent of the results of radiation treatment of carcinoma of the bladder, discussed in Chapter 23. Undoubtedly, the persisting carcinomas in situ are at the origin of treatment failure in many cases. Stockeld et al (2002) used **serial needle aspiration biopsies** of various parts of the esophagus to rule out the presence of **occult foci of cancer.** The presence of cancer cells in areas of the esophagus grossly free of tumor correlated with poor prognosis.

Brien et al (2001) described **gastric dysplasia-like** epithelial atypia associated with chemoradiotherapy of esophageal cancer. For further discussion of gastric dysplasia, see below.

Radiation changes observed in esophageal cytologic material are closely similar to those described for the uterine cervix (see Chapter 18) and the respiratory tract (see Chap. 19) (Fig. 24-14). The changes may affect both benign and malignant cells (Cabré-Fiol, 1970). **The diagnosis of persisting or residual carcinoma should be made only on cancer cells showing no effect of radiation.**

Radiomimetic changes in esophageal epithelium were described by O'Morchoe et al (1983) in patients receiving **cytotoxic drug therapy** for tumors other than esophageal cancer. Some of these patients also had **herpetic esophagitis** and infections with fungi of the *Candida* species.

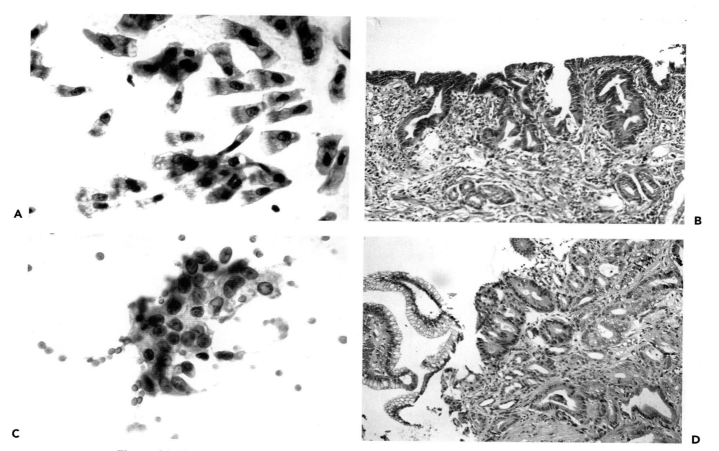

Figure 24-13 Adenocarcinoma in situ of esophagus (severe dysplasia). *A.* Columnar cells with markedly enlarged hyperchromatic nuclei corresponding to the superficial lesion shown in *B. C,D.* Invasive adenocarcinoma of esophagus in a Barrett's patient. *C.* Clusters of cancer cells, some of which are of columnar configuration. *D.* shows a superficially invasive adenocarcinoma.

EFFECTIVENESS OF CYTOLOGY IN THE DIAGNOSIS OF ESOPHAGEAL CANCER

The effectiveness of balloon cytology in the detection of precancerous lesions of the esophagus has been documented in the studies from the People's Republic of China, cited above.

The contributions of cytology in symptomatic patients before widespread use of fiberoptic instruments are best assessed by comparison with other diagnostic techniques: a few **cases of esophageal carcinoma with negative radiographic findings were observed in this laboratory.** The results, of historical interest only, were reported from our laboratory and Papanicolaou's laboratory by Johnson et al in 1955. The cytologic results in 148 cases of esophageal cancer and 135 controls are summarized in Tables 24-1 and 24-2. **In a significant percentage of cases (12%), cytology yielded positive results, whereas the biopsy was either negative or impossible to obtain.** We also reported **three false-positive cases,** based on the presence of atypical squamous cells in cases of erosive esophagitis (see above).

Other older studies (Raskin et al, 1959; Prolla and Kirsner, 1972; Cabré-Fiol, 1970; Drake, 1985) also show a very high rate of accuracy in the diagnosis of esophageal carcinoma, ranging from 90% to 95%. It is of interest that the introduction of fiberoptics and of direct brushing re-

sulted in only slight improvement in the accuracy of cytologic diagnoses of esophageal cancer, when compared with the simpler methods of washings and aspirations. Geisinger (1995) compared the results of cytologic **brushings** with **endoscopic biopsies** in specimens from a broad spectrum of esophageal diseases. There were 18 carcinomas, of which 9 were squamous and 6 adenocarcinomas. In 3 of the 18 carcinomas the diagnosis was established by cytology with negative initial biopsies. One squamous cancer was missed by cytology. Geisinger provided a summary of findings from several papers on this topic. The superiority of brush cytology over biopsies in the diagnosis of esophageal cancer was repeatedly confirmed, thus documenting the clinical value of cytologic techniques.

RARE MALIGNANT TUMORS OF THE ESOPHAGUS

Adenoid Cystic Carcinoma

We have seen one example of this lesion which is most unusual in the esophagus. The tumor has been described in reference to salivary glands and the bronchus (see Chaps. 20 and 32). As is the case in other organs where the tumor is more common, the brush smear disclosed **clusters of small, mo-**

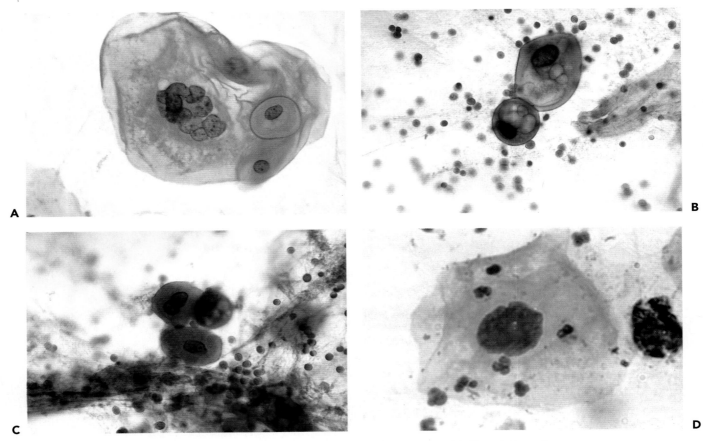

Figure 24-14 Effects of radiotherapy on esophageal squamous epithelium. *A.* Several squamous cells, one being huge in size and provided with multiple nuclei. *B,C.* Cellular enlargement, cytoplasmic vacuole formation, and enlarged hyperchromatic nuclei in an esophagus brush from a 21-year-old woman with mediastinal Hodgkin's disease. *D.* Marked cellular and nuclear enlargement from an esophageal diverticulum resected after a brief course of radiotherapy.

notonous cancer cells with fragments of homogeneous, hyaline material, corresponding to the basement membrane material contained within the cystic spaces in the tumor.

Carcinoma with Pagetoid Changes

An exceptional event is the presence of **pagetoid change** that has been observed in the esophageal epithelium adja-

cent to areas of carcinoma, reported by Yates and Koss (1968). The invasion of the squamous epithelium by large, clear cells of adjacent carcinoma resulted in this readily identifiable histologic pattern, similar to that occurring in the epithelium of the nipple or vulva in Paget's disease (see Chaps. 15 and 29). In the case illustrated here, the **cancer cells shed from the pagetoid area were approximately spherical, had a clear cytoplasm, and were occasionally**

TABLE 24-1

RESULTS OF CYTOLOGIC EXAMINATION OF THE ESOPHAGUS

		Cytology		
	Total Cases	**Positive**	**Suspicious**	**Negative or Insufficient**
Malignant tumors primary in esophagus	148 (100%)	103 (70%)	18	27
No malignant tumor	135	3*	7	125

* Three cases of esophagitis.
(Johnson WD, et al. Cytology of esophageal washings: evaluation of 364 cases. Cancer 8:951–957, 1955.)

TABLE 24-2

COMPARISON OF RESULTS OF CYTOLOGIC EXAMINATION WITH RESULTS OF BIOPSY IN 148 PRIMARY CANCERS OF ESOPHAGUS

		Cytology		
	Total Cases	**Positive**	**Suspicious**	**Negative**
Biopsy				
Positive	117	85	14	18
Negative	18	11	2	5
Impossible to obtain	13	7	2	4
Total	148	102	18	27

(Johnson WD, et al. Cytology of esophageal washings: evaluation of 364 cases. Cancer 8:951–957, 1955.)

arranged in the cell-in-cell pattern, whereas the cells from the main bulk of the tumor were poorly differentiated (Fig. 24-15).

Polypoid Carcinoma (Carcinosarcoma)

Histology

Uncommonly, squamous carcinomas of the esophagus (but also of the larynx, pharynx, and rarely in the vagina) develop into polypoid bulky tumors, the surface of which is formed by a well-differentiated epidermoid carcinoma, sometimes in situ. The bulk of the tumor is composed of elongated spindly cells, occasionally accompanied by bizarre giant cells (Enrile et al, 1973). Experience with these lesions suggests that the spindle and giant cell components represent a peculiar metaplasia of squamous carcinoma and not a benign "pseudosarcoma," as was originally suggested by Stout and Lattes (1957). Still, the latter term is often used to describe this lesion. It must be stressed that, in spite of its ominous appearance, the polypoid carcinoma appears to offer a much better prognosis than ordinary esophageal carcinoma.

Cytology

The cytologic findings in brushings from one of the rare polypoid carcinomas of the esophagus were described by Selvaggi (1992). The smears contained cells of squamous carcinoma and spindly cancer cells, and a few multinucleated giant cells, corresponding exactly to the histologic make-up of the tumor. We observed a similar tumor in the vagina. The smears were composed of malignant squamous cells only (see Chap. 17).

Malignant Melanoma

Several case reports of the very rare primary esophageal melanoma were published (Bullock et al, 1952; Boyd et al, 1954; Broderick et al, 1972; Chaput et al, 1974; Ludwig et al, 1981), occasionally associated with melanosis (De la Pava et al, 1963; Piccone et al, 1970). Summaries of the subject were presented by Mills and Cooper (1983) and by Kanavaros et al (1989). Broderick et al (1972) reported a case of esophageal melanoma with cytologic diagnosis. The malignant cells were clearly pigmented and, accordingly, the accurate diagnosis could be readily established. A similar case was reported by Aldovini et al (1983). One of these very infrequent tumors of the esophagus was diagnosed cytologically by us as cancer but, in the absence of pigment, it was thought to be an epidermoid carcinoma. De la Pava et al (1963) described pigmentation of normal esophageal epithelium as melanosis. This extremely rare condition could be a source of diagnostic error. However, Piccone et al (1970) and Kanavaros et al (1989) described a malignant melanoma developing in melanosis, thus complicating the issue still further.

Sarcomas

Sapi et al (1992) described the cytologic findings in a polypoid tumor of the esophagus, classified as malignant fibrous histiocytoma on the strength of immunocytologic and ultrastructural findings. The smears were characterized by the presence of bizarre tumor giant cells. Clearly, the differential diagnosis in such cases must include polypoid carcinomas, discussed above.

A rare case of rhabdomyosarcoma of the esophagus was described by Shah et al (1995). A case of embryonal rhabdomyosarcoma was described by Willen et al (1989). The cytologic presentation of similar tumors in other organs was described in Chapters 23 and 26.

Choriocarcinoma

A case of an exceedingly rare primary choriocarcinoma of the esophagus was described by Trillo et al (1979). The cytologic features of this tumor are described below in the section on rare gastric tumors, in Chapter 17, discussing rare tumors of the female genital tract, and in Chapter 23, discussing rare tumors of the urinary bladder.

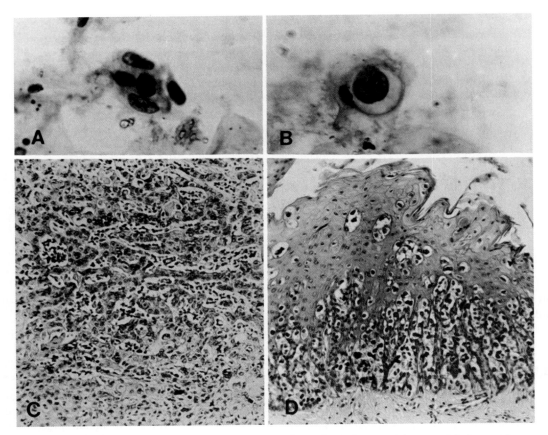

Figure 24-15 Carcinoma at the junction of cardia and esophagus with pagetoid changes in the adjacent esophageal epithelium. *A.* Cluster of poorly differentiated cancer cells (esophageal washings). *B.* Elsewhere in the smear isolated, large cancer cells with clear cytoplasm were noted. *C.* The surgical specimen disclosed a carcinoma of the cardia extending into the esophagus. *D.* The squamous epithelium of esophagus at the edge of the tumor disclosed a typical pagetoid change with large cells with clear cytoplasm.

THE STOMACH

ANATOMY

The stomach is a pouch situated between the esophagus and the duodenum, immediately below the diaphragm; it forms a reservoir of variable capacity within which the preliminary stages of digestion take place. The stomach is divided anatomically into several regions, starting at the esophageal end: the **cardia** (the orifice between the stomach and the esophagus and the adjacent portion of the stomach), a lateral bulge or the **fundus,** the more distal portion of the stomach or **the body,** and the most distal **pyloric area (antrum),** which is separated from the duodenum by a powerful ring of smooth muscle, the **pylorus.** Obstruction of the gastric lumen may occur at either end of the stomach—the cardia or the pylorus (see Fig. 24-1).

From inside out, the stomach is lined by an **epithelium (mucosa),** described in detail below, a **lamina propria,** composed of connective tissue and a thin layer of smooth muscle **(muscularis mucosae),** a powerful layer of smooth muscle or the **muscularis propria,** and the outer layer or the **serosa,** lined by the peritoneum.

HISTOLOGY OF GASTRIC EPITHELIUM (MUCOSA)

Gastric epithelium is by far the most important component of cytologic preparations. The gastric mucosa is composed of **simple tubular glands.** The **lining of the glands of the fundus and the body** of the stomach is complex: the **surface and the necks of the glands are lined by mucus-producing cells.** The deeper portions of the glands contain pepsin-producing chief cells and the eosinophilic parietal cells** that produce hydrochloric acid. The hydrochloric acid is excreted through microscopic canaliculi passing between the chief cells. The **gastric glands of the pyloric area** are fairly uniformly lined by **mucus-producing cells** (Fig. 24-16A).

Electron microscopic studies revealed distinct differences between the cells lining the gastric surface and those lining the neck of the glands. Both cells are mucus-producing but they differ in the type of secretory granules, thus probably performing somewhat different functions. The ultrastructure of the parietal cell fails to reveal any secretory activity. The pepsin-producing chief cells resemble somewhat the exocrine pancreatic and salivary gland cells inasmuch as they contain cytoplasmic secretory granules and

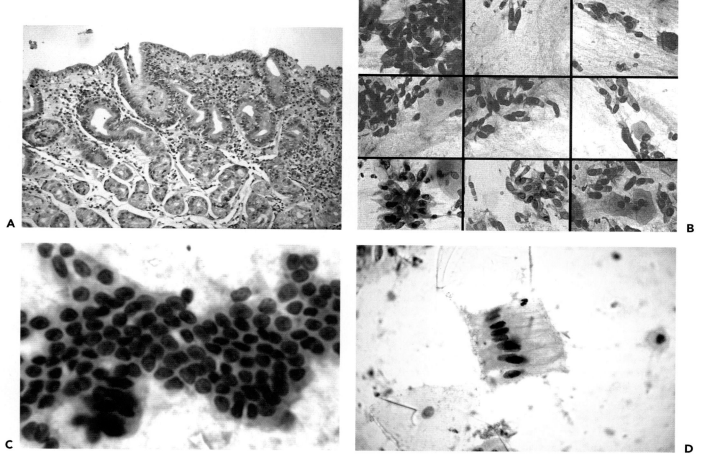

Figure 24-16 **Normal stomach.** *A.* Configuration of normal gastric epithelium (see text). *B.* Benign columnar gastric cells in gastric brushes. *C.* Sheet of benign gastric cells showing the "honeycomb" configuration. *D.* Tall mucus-producing cells from a case of intestinal metaplasia. (*B:* Composite photograph obtained with the PAPNET apparatus. With the permission of TriPath Imaging, Burlington, NC.)

an abundant rough-surfaced reticulum. Argentaffin cells containing dense cytoplasmic granules may be observed in some of the crypts.

CYTOLOGY OF NORMAL STOMACH

The make-up of the specimens varies **according to the method used** to collect the material. **Gastric lavage,** extensively used by Schade and his co-workers (1956A,B, 1959, 1960A,B), yields few normal gastric cells. The **gastric balloon with a rough surface,** devised by Panico et al (1950, 1952) to improve the collection of gastric epithelial cells, yields a richer harvest of cells. The optimal samples of gastric epithelium are obtained by **gastric brushings** during fiberoptic gastroscopy.

In the absence of disease, normal gastric epithelium in brush specimens is represented by columnar cells, occurring singly or forming **cohesive fragments of cells with opaque or clear cytoplasm.** The columnar configuration of the component cells is seen at the edge of such clusters, whereas the center of the cluster shows the "honeycomb" pattern

(Fig. 24-16B,C). The **relatively uncommon, mucus-producing columnar cells** display an abundant, **clear cytoplasm** and have one **flattened surface,** corresponding to the gastric lumen, whereas the **opposite end usually tapers off in the form of a tail** (Fig. 24-16D). Raskin et al (1961) pointed out that such **cells originate from the area of the pyloric antrum.** Such cells are common in **intestinal metaplasia** of the gastric mucosa (see below).

A "**wheel-spokes**" **arrangement of single cells,** with their "tails" directed toward the center may be observed. **Tubular structures** representing entire glands removed by vigorous brushing may also be encountered.

The nuclei of normal gastric cells are located in the approximate **center of the cells.** They are usually spherical, of equal sizes, clear or somewhat opaque, and contain a few granules of chromatin and occasionally a noticeable but very small pink nucleolus. In mucus-producing columnar cells, **the nuclei may be displaced toward the distal end of the cell, a position also observed in goblet cells that play an important role in intestinal metaplasia** (see below). Occasionally, **dense nuclear protrusions,** similar to those observed in endocervical cells, can be observed (see

Chap. 8). When the cytoplasm of the gastric cells is destroyed during processing of the specimens, **"naked" nuclei or nuclei surrounded by cytoplasmic shreds** may be numerous. In **cell blocks,** small fragments of gastric epithelium may occasionally be identified.

Using rapidly fixed material and Papanicolaou stain, **we have not been able to identify with certainty the parietal and the zymogenic (chief) cells** in the smears of gastric specimens. However, Henning and Witte (1957), using air-dried specimens and Pappenheim stain, described the **chief cells** as **plump cells, containing numerous coarse basophilic granules in the cytoplasm; the parietal cells** were described as **small cylindrical cells with a very marked vacuolization of the cytoplasm.** Nieburgs and Glass (1963) identified the chief cells as "darkly stained cells of intermediate size" in brush specimens. Granules were not demonstrated in Papanicolaou stain. The parietal cells were identified by the same authors as "large, pale, round or triangular cells," and, thus, their description is at variance with that given by Henning and Witte, but more in keeping with the histologic appearance of these cells. Takeda (1983) also described the **parietal cells as triangular cells with granular cytoplasm.**

In gastric specimens obtained by **aspiration or washings, swallowed cells of the respiratory and the upper alimentary tract are sometimes present. Ciliated respiratory cells, dust-containing macrophages, and squamous cells of buccal and esophageal origin** may be observed. Also, in the presence of gastric obstruction, **food particles** and, in particular, plant (vegetable) cells, may contaminate the specimen, occasionally rendering it totally useless (see Chap. 19 for detailed description of plant cells).

Other cells present in normal gastric specimens include **sparse polymorphonuclear leukocytes and lymphocytes.** Recognizable **macrophages** may be noted.

BENIGN GASTRIC DISORDERS

Parasites

The flagellated parasite **Giardia lamblia** has been recognized as a common cause of infection of the small intestine and may sometimes be seen in gastric cytology specimens. Symptoms vary from mild to severe gastrointestinal disturbances. *Giardia lamblia* has two stages: cysts and protozoa. The cysts, transmitted in drinking water or by person-to-person contact, are the source of infection. The protozoa, which are released from the cysts, can be recognized in gastric smears as a **flat, pear-shaped small organism, with four pairs of flagella and two nuclei that mimic the appearance of eyeglasses** (Fig. 24-17A). Bloch et al (1987) observed the parasite in the **peritoneal fluid** of a patient with severe infestation.

Trophozoites of the **Acanthamoeba species,** probably a contaminant, were observed by Hoffler and Rubel (1974).

Fungi and Viruses

In patients with AIDS, gastric samples may contain evidence of fungal infection, such as *moniliasis,* which is usually also present in the esophagus. **Cytomegalovirus** infection of gastric epithelium is the most common viral infection and may be associated with **gastric ulcers** (Fig. 24-17B). Other organisms, such as **Helicobacter pylori** are discussed below.

Gastritis and Gastric Ulcer (Type B Gastritis)

Inflammation of the gastric mucosa is a common disorder that may lead to gastric ulceration and may be related to gastric cancer. In 1947, Schindler proposed a subdivision of gastritis into **acute** and **chronic.** In 1990, an attempt was made to standardize the nomenclature of gastritis at a meeting of experts in Sydney, Australia (Price, 1991). The purpose of the **Sydney classification** was to integrate histologic, microbiologic, and endoscopic data to render the classification of gastritis more reproducible.

The reproducibility of histologic classification of gastritis in biopsies is still not optimal (Guarner et al, 1999). These problems cannot be solved by **cytology of the gastric epithelium** which serves mainly to differentiate an inflammatory process from cancer.

Pathogenesis

Until the 1980s, the causes of acute gastritis and of gastric or duodenal ulcer were not clearly understood. Some drugs, such as **lithium,** were shown to be occasionally associated with gastritis. In 1983, an anonymous observation was reported in the journal *Lancet,* suggesting that a not-further-identified bacterium may be associated with gastritis. The observation was confirmed by Marshall and Warren in 1984. The infection with this bacterium, now known as **Helicobacter pylori** (previously known as **Campylobacter pylori**), is very common. The source of the bacterium is drinking water, soil, flies etc. (Sasaki et al, 1999; Suerbaum and Michetti, 2002). Two strains of the bacterium have been sequenced. It is believed that the **bacterial genes can affect human genes encoding cell membrane adhesion molecules** (Ge and Taylor, 1999). Amieva et al (2003) have shown that the bacterium is capable of disrupting the apical tight junctions binding gastric cells. **H. pylori** has now been recognized as the main cause of acute gastritis (also known as pyloric or type B gastritis), ulcer disease, and colitis (Goodwin et al, 1986; Blaser, 1987; Dooley et al, 1989; Cover and Blaser, 1996; Bodger and Crabtree, 1998). There appears to be a relationship between *H. Pylori,* **gastric cancer and malignant lymphomas of the mucosa-associated lymphoid tissue (MALT lymphomas)** (see below).

A related organism *Gastrospirillum hominis* (previously known as *Helicobacter heilmannii*) has been recognized as a less frequent cause of a milder form of chronic gastritis. The two organisms share many pathologic features but have some morphologic differences. *H. pylori* forms **gram-negative curved rods** about 3 μm in length and 0.5 μm in width (Fig. 24-17C,D). *G. hominis* is somewhat longer (3.5 to 7.5 μm), tightly coiled, and can be recognized as straight, spirochete-like structures (summary in Rotterdam et al, 1993).

Both organisms can be identified **in Papanicolaou-**

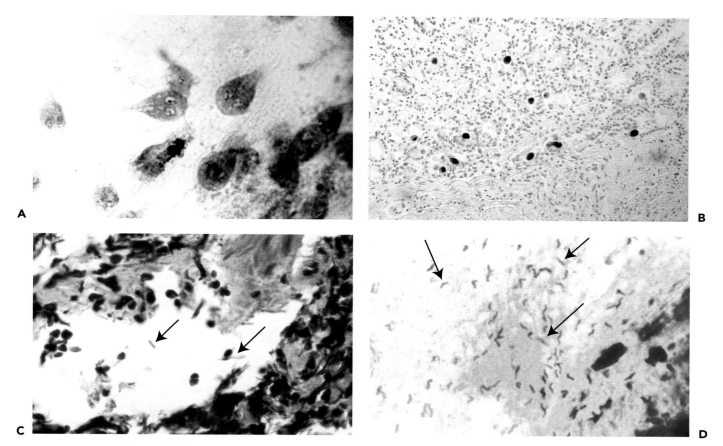

Figure 24-17   Inflammatory gastric disorders. *A. Giardia lamblia* in gastric lavage. Note the triangular configuration of the parasites with the characteristic two-nuclei mimicking eyeglasses. *B.* Cytomegalovirus in a gastric ulcer. The presence of the virus was documented by a specific antibody. *C,D. Helicobacter pylori.* Minuscule corkscrew organisms are seen in the background of the gastric biopsy in *C* and in a gastric brushing in *D* (*arrows*). (*C:* High power; *D:* oil immersion.)

stained cytologic samples but are much easier to demonstrate in **Warthin-Starry silver impregnation or by Giemsa stain and its modifications** (Taylor et al, 1987; Davenport, 1990; Pinto et al, 1991; Mendoza et al, 1993, Ghoussoub and Lachman, 1997). Several observers suggested that the organism may be easier to identify in smears prepared from gastric biopsies than in tissues sections (Faverly et al, 1990).

Chronic Gastric Peptic Ulcer

Clinical Data

Gastric ulcer is a common disease, occurring in patients of all ages, but usually in adults. Most patients have an increased gastric acidity and *Helicobacter pylori* infection. Feared **complications of gastric ulcer include massive gastric hemorrhage and perforation of the gastric wall.** Quite often, particularly when these lesions are small and superficial, the **clinical and radiographic or endoscopic differential diagnosis between a gastric carcinoma and a chronic peptic ulcer may be extremely difficult.** Therefore, these lesions are the **prime target of endoscopic and cytologic studies** (Cantrell, 1971; Prolla et al, 1971; Prolla and Kirsner, 1972).

Histology

Chronic peptic ulcer is an **inflammatory defect in the gastric epithelium** extending for a variable depth into the submucosa and even the muscularis and beyond. The ulcer often undermines one edge of the adjacent epithelium. Depending on the chronicity of the disease, the tissues surrounding the ulcer bed may show **varying degrees of chronic inflammation and fibrosis.** Occasionally, large aggregates of lymphocytes and plasma cells may be noted. **The epithelium surrounding the ulcer shows various degrees of hyperplasia and regeneration.** In the latter case, marked mitotic activity and atypia may be present (Fig. 24-18A,B). There is considerable debate whether gastric carcinoma may develop in peptic ulcer epithelium. Cases do occur wherein this possibility is strongly suggested by histologic findings.

Cytology

Gastric cytology and endoscopic biopsies are the prime methods of differential diagnosis between benign ulcer and carcinoma. Regardless of the technique used to sample the gastric epithelium, the cytologic specimens usually contain **many clusters of gastric epithelial cells.** Necrotic material, fibrin, and inflammatory cells, such as neutrophils or lymphocytes, are usually present in the background. **Cell debris and isolated ("naked") nuclei may be abundant.**

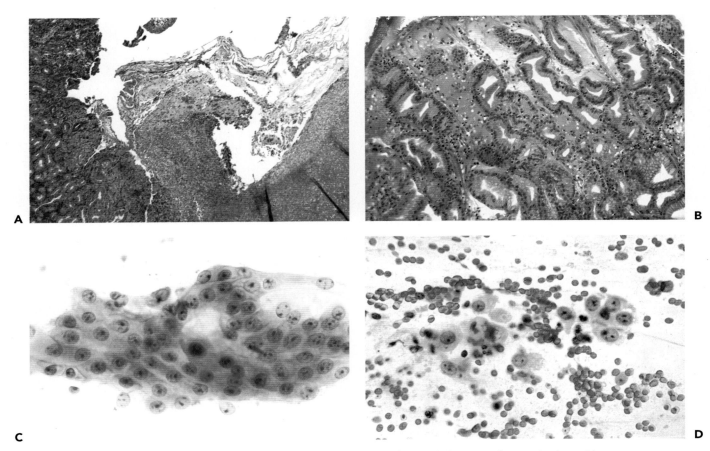

Figure 24-18 Gastric ulcer and gastric repair. *A.* A characteristic crater of a gastric ulcer with its fundus occupied by a fibrin clot. *B.* Gastric biopsy showing atypical proliferation of glands with mitotic activity at the edge of a gastric ulcer. *C,D.* Cells from gastric repair forming a sheet in *C* and appearing singly in *D.* The cells are characterized by the presence of clearly visible nucleoli.

As is the case in other "repair" reactions, the changes in the gastric epithelial cells in peptic ulcers may be difficult to interpret. Flat clusters of cells, arranged side-by-side, are the dominant feature, whereas single cells are relatively few in number (Fig. 24-18C,D). In brush specimens, this important relationship of cells to each other cannot always be fully appreciated because the cell clusters may be thick and unfit for detailed visual analysis. However, the cells at the periphery of such clusters usually are suitable for inspection.

The morphologic features of gastric epithelial cells in ulcer disease are best appreciated in small clusters or in single cells. The cells are **polyhedral rather than columnar** and their **cytoplasm is often opaque.** The principal difficulty in the interpretation of this material is with the **nuclei which are usually enlarged, clear or opaque, and dark, and may contain one or more nucleoli of various sizes** (Fig. 24-18C,D). Drake (1985) stressed nuclear enlargement as a common feature of cells in chronic gastric ulcer and we can confirm his observation.

When conspicuous nuclear and nucleolar enlargement is present in epithelial cells, the differential diagnosis among chronic inflammatory disease, gastric carcinoma, and precancerous abnormalities (both discussed below) **becomes exceedingly difficult. The presence of flat cohesive clusters and few single epithelial cells, the**

absence of significant variability in nuclear sizes, and regular and smooth nuclear membrane are in favor of an inflammatory process, but these criteria are not always helpful. The problem is compounded because occasional gastric carcinomas shed cancer cells with only modest nuclear abnormalities. In such fortunately uncommon cases, the degree of histologic abnormality in a biopsy may also present a diagnostic dilemma that is best solved by additional sampling.

Diagnostic misinterpretation of cytologic findings as cancer in extreme cases of gastric atypia occurs even among observers who combine vast clinical and laboratory experience and thus are best qualified to avoid such mistakes. Prolla and Kirsner (1972) cite five such false positive mistakes among 2,196 patients with benign gastric disease (0.05%).

"Aspirin" Gastritis

Difficult to interpret cytologic abnormalities, similar to those observed in chronic gastric ulcers, may occur in users of **aspirin** and **newer analgesic drugs** who are prone to **erosions of gastric mucosa with episodes of hematemesis. Patients with rheumatoid arthritis** appear to be at significant risk, presumably because of long-term use of large doses of these drugs. In biopsies of the hemorrhagic areas, there is often superficial erosion of the surface epithelium. In more chronic cases, the superficial ulceration may be accompanied by a marked disruption of the mucosal architecture. The glands vary in size and shape and are arranged in a disorderly pattern. The cells lining the **glands, particularly in the deeper portion of the gastric epithelium, show marked abnormalities, such as nuclear enlargement, hyperchromasia, and mitotic activity** (Fig. 24-19A).

Cytology

Cell samples obtained by brushing may show conspicuous abnormalities (Fig. 24-19B–D). The gastric epithelial cells may form **clusters or strips wherein there is variability of nuclear sizes and hyperchromasia of individual nuclei.** Some cells containing **large nucleoli may suggest a gastric carcinoma.** Similar nuclear abnormalities may be observed in columnar or cuboidal **dispersed single cells.** Perhaps the **most disturbing cytologic finding is the presence of clusters of dark nuclei, stripped of cytoplasm.** In the third edition of this book (1979), it was felt that the differential diagnosis of aspirin gastritis from carcinoma was not possible in the absence of clinical history. This view may be somewhat modified today. Although cell clusters may strongly suggest a malignant tumor, the **abnormalities in the single cells, essential to confirm the diagnosis, do not quite measure up to cancer:** the degree of nuclear changes and the size and variability of the nucleoli are less conspicuous than in cancer, but, admittedly, these may be personal perceptions, not easily duplicated.

An accurate **clinical history of analgesic intake may prevent the erroneous diagnosis of gastric carcinoma.** This is particularly important because, within a few weeks after **discontinuation of analgesics, the gastric epithelium recovers** and returns to normal.

Chronic Atrophic Gastritis (Type A Gastritis) and Intestinalization of the Gastric Mucosa

Pathogenesis

Atrophy of gastric epithelia and the replacement of normal gastric epithelium by cells akin to those of mucus-producing epithelium lining the large intestine (**intestinal metaplasia or intestinalization**) usually occur together in the **distal portion of the stomach.** Loss of gastric folds and an **inflammatory infiltrate consisting of lymphocytes and plasma cells in the mucosa and submucosa** are common findings in this disorder which may be observed in a variety of chronic inflammatory conditions and in pernicious anemia.

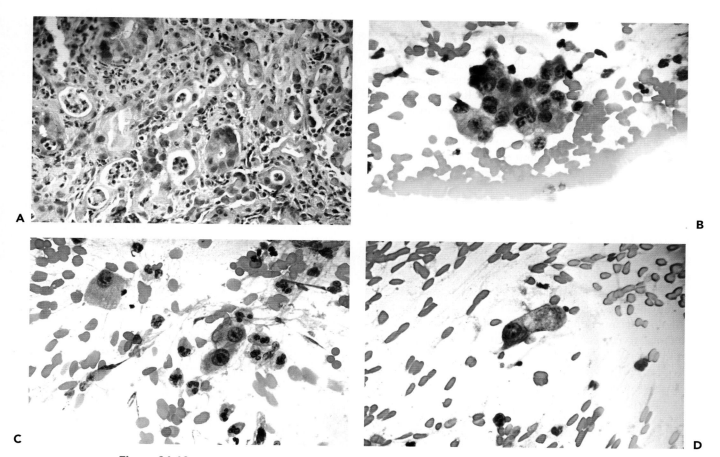

Figure 24-19 **Aspirin gastritis** in a 74-year-old woman with rheumatoid arthritis. *A.* Gastric biopsy showing disorderly arrangement of gastric glands. *B–D.* Gastric brush smears with atypical gastric cells, occurring singly and in clusters. The nuclei of these cells are somewhat enlarged and contain large nucleoli, thus mimicking carcinoma. Six weeks after stopping the medication, the gastric epithelium was normal on biopsy.

Contrary to gastritis type B, described above, **H. pylori is absent** and does not appear to play a role in the genesis of atrophic gastritis which is now considered to be an **autoimmune disease** (Toh et al, 1997).

The significance of intestinal metaplasia as a precancerous event has been studied morphologically (Morson, 1955) and by epidemiologic analysis of gastric cancer-prone populations (Correa, 1982; Rubio et al, 1987; Correa and Chen, 1994). The consensus has developed that, **in populations with a high rate of intestinal metaplasia, there is also a high rate of gastric carcinoma of intestinal type** (see below).

Histology

Intestinal metaplasia consists of large, tall, mucus-producing cells, replacing normal gastric epithelium. The mucus-producing cells are often referred to as goblet cells but are morphologically somewhat different. The metaplastic epithelium also contains **Paneth cells with granular and eosinophilic cytoplasm,** which cannot be identified with reliability in cytologic material. Rubio and Antonioli (1988) reported rare cases of **intestinal metaplasia with ciliated cells.**

Cytology

The condition may be recognized occasionally in cytologic material, which may contain **mucus-producing columnar epithelial cells larger than the normal gastric cells and provided with an abundant, clear cytoplasm** (see Fig. 24-16D). These cells are **more slender than goblet cells** and closely **resemble normal columnar cells desquamating from the colonic mucosa** (see below). **The nuclei are round and even, but are sometimes somewhat larger and darker than normal.** The recognition of intestinal metaplasia in cytologic material is of limited diagnostic significance, except as a warning that the patient may be at risk for gastric carcinoma.

Gastric Tuberculosis

Gastric tuberculosis is on the increase, particularly in patients with AIDS (Brody et al, 1986; Dao et al, 1991). Tuberculosis **may mimic almost any gastric disorder** and cannot be recognized as such either on endoscopy or on radiologic examination. Jain et al (2000) described cytologic findings in gastric brush smears from seven adult patients from India with gastric tuberculosis, confirmed by biopsies. **Slender epithelioid cells were observed in all patients and granulomas, composed of epithelioid and Langhans' type giant cells, were observed in three patients.** Acid fast bacilli could be demonstrated in gastric smears in four of these patients but not in the biopsies. The findings are of note because gastric tuberculosis, previously a very rare disorder, has now been observed in AIDS patients (Brody et al, 1986; Das et al, 1998). For illustrations of cytologic presentation of tuberculosis, see Figures 10-22 and 19-33 (cervix and lung).

Gastric Syphilis

Ulcerative gastric lesions may occur in secondary and tertiary syphilis. Prolla et al (1970) described the cytologic findings in two such cases. Atypical cells, **presumably atypical macrophages or epithelioid cells with large nuclei and prominent nucleoli,** were observed. **Langhans' type giant cells** were also noted.

Other Granulomatous Inflammatory Lesions of the Stomach

The cytologic findings in **granulomatous disorders, regardless of etiology, are similar to those described above for tuberculosis and syphilis** and additional clinical and bacteriologic work-up may be required to determine the nature of the disorder. Thus, markedly atypical giant cells were observed by Bennington et al (1968) in a case of **gastric sarcoidosis.** Drake (1985) described **epithelioid cells and multinucleated giant cells in gastric brushings of a patient with Crohn's disease.**

Malacoplakia

Malacoplakia of the stomach has been described (summary in Flint and Murad, 1984). Cytologic presentation of this rare disorder is discussed in Chapters 19 and 22.

Gastric Amyloidosis

Yang (1995) described a case of gastric amyloidosis observed in a gastric brush specimen. Fragments of eosinophilic material, representing amyloid, were observed in company of normal gastric cells. The diagnosis was confirmed by special stains and electron microscopy.

Ménétrier's Disease

Ménétrier's disease is a disorder of gastric epithelium in which **gastric rugae are markedly thickened** ("hypertophic gastritis"). This disorder **may be associated with gastric polyps and carcinoma** (Appelman, 1984; Wood et al, 1983). There is no known cytologic counterpart of this condition.

Gas Cysts of the Intestine

Gas cysts of the stomach are rare, usually occuring in **disseminated intestinal gas cysts or pneumatosis cystoides intestinorum,** a bizarre disorder of unknown etiology (summary in Koss, 1952). The **cysts are often lined by flattened, multinucleated giant cells of foreign body type.** Such cells were observed in smears in association with gastric carcinoma in a case reported by Bhatal et al (1985).

Pernicious Anemia

Pernicious anemia is a chronic hematologic disorder associated with vitamin B_{12} or folic acid deficiency and atrophic gastritis and, therefore, is a risk factor for gastric cancer (Toh et al, 1997). The issue of specific cytologic abnormalities in pernicious anemia and other states of vitamin B_{12} deficiencies were previously discussed in reference to the uterine cervix and the oral cavity (see Chaps. 17 and 21). Graham and Rheault (1954) and Massey and Rubin (1954) reported in patients with pernicious anemia **gastric and squamous cells with abnormally enlarged nuclei, similar to dyskaryotic (dysplastic) cells.** On the other hand, Schade (1959, 1960B) denied the existence of any specific cytologic or histologic alterations of the gastric mucosa in pernicious anemia. Intestinalization of gastric mucosa (or atrophic gastritis), described above, is, in Schade's experience, a common background of cancers developing in the presence or absence of the hematologic disorder. Personal experience indicates that slightly atypical squamous cells with enlarged nuclei occur quite often in gastric washings of patients with other cancers. A hematologic investigation of several such patients **failed to reveal a relationship between these cell changes and pernicious anemia.** It is entirely possible that the mechanical effects of intubation of the esophagus or, for that matter, a number of dietary deficiencies—such as vitamin B_{12} or folic acid deficiency—may account for these abnormalities. Takeda (1983) illustrated three clusters of enlarged, bland, empty-looking nuclei in gastric cells in pernicious anemia. Drake (1985) also speaks of **"active" gastric cells, with visible nucleoli,** in pernicious anemia. The specificity or, for that matter, diagnostic value, of such changes is in doubt.

Gastric Atypias Caused by Treatment

Chemotherapy by **hepatic artery infusion** for metastatic tumors in the liver **affects gastric epithelium,** causing a radiomimetic effect. **Cell enlargement, with preservation of the normal nucleocytoplasmic ratio, binucleation, and multinucleation of gastric epithelial cells** in gastric brushing material and biopsies, were reported in six patients with secondary gastric ulceration by Becker et al, 1986.

Chemoradiotherapy for esophageal cancer may also lead to significant abnormalities of gastric epithelium that closely **resemble naturally-occurring precancerous lesions (dysplasia)** (Brien et al, 2001). The differential diagnosis between the chemoradiotherapy-induced and naturally occurring precancerous lesions is discussed below.

BENIGN GASTRIC TUMORS

Gastric Polyps

Benign gastric polyps cannot be recognized cytologically **unless fragments of such tumors are present in the exfoliated material processed as a minibiopsy or cell block.** In this case, the interpretation is that of a biopsy specimen. Occasionally, **atypical (adenomatous) polyps may cause the same diagnostic problems as described for gastric ulcer.** Polypoid carcinomas, on the other hand, can be readily distinguished from benign polyps because of their characteristic cytologic presentation, described below.

Benign GIST tumors are discussed below.

MALIGNANT GASTRIC TUMORS

Carcinoma of Stomach

Epidemiology

Gastric carcinoma is exceedingly common in Japan, Korea, certain other areas in Asia, South America, and Eastern Europe. Its **incidence has been declining sharply in the Western world,** even among people of Japanese ancestry living in Hawaii and the continental United States (Haenszel et al, 1976; Craanen et al, 1992; Fuchs and Mayer, 1995). A similar drop has been observed in Europe (Fuchs and Mayer, 1995). Current evidence suggests that the **frequency of tumors in the distal portion of the stomach is decreasing, whereas that of cancers of the proximal stomach (cardia) may be on the rise,** perhaps because of the increased occurrence of Barrett's esophagus, discussed earlier in this chapter (Craanen et al, 1992; Correa and Chen, 1994; Fuchs and Mayer, 1995). It is generally assumed that dietary factors are responsible, although the exact cause-effect relationship between nutrients and gastric cancer has not been established. **Pernicious anemia is a known risk factor** for gastric cancer (Toh et al, 1997). There is also evidence that *H. pylori* may play a role in the genesis of this group of tumors, although the mechanisms are still speculative (Uemura et al, 2001). It is generally assumed that, in cancer, the bacterium interacts with gastric epithelium in a different manner than in gastritis or gastric ulcer (Parsonnet et al, 1991; Forman et al, 1991; Sipponen et al, 1998; Chen et al, 1999; Ge and Taylor, 1999; Suerbaum and Mitchetti, 2002; Amieva et al, 2003).

It has also been shown that diffuse gastric cancer occurs with very **high frequency in families showing mutation of the adhesion gene E cadherin.** In young members of such families, asymptomatic early gastric cancer may be observed (Huntsman et al, 2001).

Clinical Presentation

The clinical symptoms of gastric carcinoma are not specific. In early stages, the disease is often asymptomatic whereas in advanced stages "indigestion," vomiting, hematemesis and melena and, ultimately, pain develop. Severe anemia is often observed.

On endoscopic inspection, gastric carcinomas may appear as a defect of gastric mucosa with raised edges, and thus **may mimic benign gastric ulcers. More often, the tumors are polypoid or present as flat, raised plaques.** A form of gastric cancer with **diffuse infiltration of gastric wall (leather bottle stomach or linitis plastica)** is well known.

Classification and Histology

In 1965, Lauren classified gastric carcinomas into two groups: the **intestinal type** and the **diffuse type.** Lauren documented that the behavior, hence the prognosis, of the two types of tumor were different.

- **The intestinal type of carcinoma is usually associated with intestinal metaplasia, which undergoes transformation to an intramucosal carcinoma (carcinoma in** situ), whence generally **bulky, readily visible tumors are derived.** Intestinal carcinomas are usually **well-differentiated adenocarcinomas,** composed of **large, mucus-producing cells,** are usually located in the distal part of the stomach, and generally have a better prognosis than the diffuse type (Correa, 1992).

■ The less common **diffuse type of gastric carcinoma** (sometimes also called the *gastric type*) is derived from glandular crypts and is usually not accompanied by either intestinal metaplasia or intramucosal carcinoma. The diffuse type of gastric carcinoma is composed of small cancer cells (including the signet ring cell types) and tends to infiltrate the gastric wall early and deeply; hence, it usually appears as a flat or ulcerated lesion, with poor prognosis. A diagram in Figure 24-20 summarizes these events. There are also cases of gastric cancer wherein both types of disease occur in the same stomach.

The confirmatory evidence of this classification scheme was provided by Japanese investigators who studied small, early gastric cancers discovered as a part of the cancer detection effort. **The genesis of the two types of cancer could be confirmed by these studies** (summary in Takeda 1983, 1984). There is other supporting evidence for this concept. In a study of distribution of H-*ras* oncogene product, protein p21, it was documented by Czerniak et al (1989) that, in the intestinal type of gastric cancer, p21 was expressed in areas of intestinal metaplasia and adjacent carcinoma in situ. In the diffuse type, p21 expression was evident in morphologically normal mucosa, apparently the source of cancer. Werner et al (2001) reviewed the molecular bases of the genesis of the two types of gastric carcinoma.

Cytology of Advanced Gastric Carcinoma

The concept of the two types of gastric cancer is not only of theoretical, but also of practical diagnostic and prognostic value and is reflected in histology and cytology of gastric carcinoma. **Carcinomas of the intestinal type shed large, readily recognizable cancer cells, whereas carcinomas of the diffuse type are characterized by smaller, sometimes inconspicuous cancer cells.** Pilotti et al (1977) successfully tested this type of classification of gastric carcinoma by gastric cytology in 78 patients. Takeda et al (1981) applied this classification to cytologic samples in 119 cases of early gastric carcinoma with excellent results. Incidentally, there are no differences in abnormal DNA ploidy values between these two tumor types (Czerniak et al, 1987B).

In **gastric lavage specimens,** the **background of smears** often contains evidence of **inflammation and necrosis** that may obscure the cytologic features. **Direct brush specimens,** particularly if obtained from the surface of the lesion, may also contain a great deal of necrotic material. Perhaps the **easiest to interpret are lavage specimens obtained by means of a jet of fluid under direct gastroscopic control.**

In all types of gastric cancer, the presence of single cancer cells with identifiable malignant features is an important diagnostic prerequisite.

Cytology of Gastric Adenocarcinoma of Intestinal Type

The intestinal-type tumors usually shed **large cancer cells of cuboidal or columnar configuration.** The **size** of the

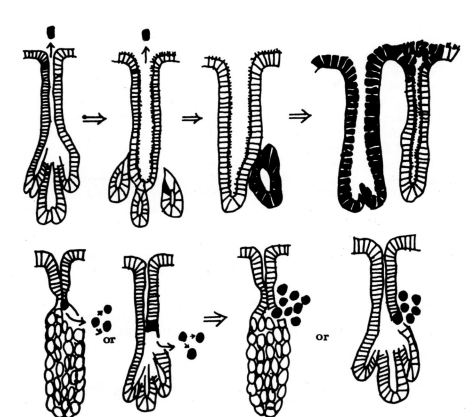

Figure 24-20 Diagrammatic representation of the events in the two types of gastric carcinoma, as suggested by Hattori and Fujita (cited by Takeda, 1984). *Top row:* Events in carcinoma of the intestinal type starting with a single cell transformation (*black cell*), the process involves gastric glands leading to an intramucosal carcinoma (carcinoma in situ), whence bulky, generally well-differentiated gastric cancers are derived. *Bottom row:* Events in carcinoma of diffuse type: the cancer cells, usually small and poorly differentiated (*black*) originate in glandular crypts and infiltrate the adjacent gastric wall without forming a carcinoma in situ. [Modified from Takeda M. Gastric cytology—recent developments. *In* Koss LG, Colman OV (eds). Advances in Clinical Cytology, Vol 2. New York, Masson, 1984, pp 49–65, with permission.]

cancer cells may be variable, but **extreme size differences are rare.** The cancer cells are **dispersed** or form **loosely structured, tri-dimensional clusters, sometimes of papillary configuration,** which differ from tightly knit, honeycomb-type flat clusters of benign gastric cells, often observed in the same smears (Fig. 24-21). Cell clusters are more common in brush specimens than in lavage specimens. Multinucleated giant cancer cells are seen from time to time.

The fragile cytoplasm of the cancer cells may be stripped or damaged, leaving behind **characteristic enlarged, pale or translucent nuclei with a prominent nuclear membrane that is often jagged or indented. Within the nuclei, there are large, single or multiple, spherical or irregular, comma-shaped nucleoli** (Fig. 24-21B). **Nuclear hyperchromasia,** or at least **coarse granularity of the chromatin and opaque appearance of the nuclei, may be observed,** but this feature is not always dominant. Truly **hyperchromatic cancer cells** may be occasionally observed in gastric washings (Fig. 24-21C), most likely representing dead cells removed from the surface of the tumor.

The **differential diagnosis of gastric adenocarcinoma** of intestinal type is mainly with **chronic peptic ulcer** (see above) and **regenerating gastric epithelium, as observed in aspirin gastritis** and chemoradiotherapy-induced changes (Brien et al, 2001). In most instances, the abundance of the characteristic cancer cells in the cytologic specimen is sufficiently persuasive for the diagnosis of cancer to be made. If the evidence is scanty and limited to a few atypical cells, however, the clinical history and roentgenologic findings are of significant assistance in avoiding errors.

Cytology of Gastric Adenocarcinoma of Diffuse ("Gastric") Type

In tumors of this type, the cancer cells are small, often inconspicuous, and approximately spherical in configuration. The nuclei are relatively large, somewhat hyperchromatic, and often contain conspicuous nucleoli (Fig. 24-22A,C). The cytoplasm is scanty, basophilic, often poorly preserved. In direct brush specimens, the recognition of the malignant nature of the small cells is relatively easy (Fig. 24-22A,B). In gastric lavage specimens, the cells are sometimes difficult to identify, particularly if the material contains many contaminating squamous cells and the tumor is very poorly differentiated (Fig. 24-22C,D). In some cases, molding of

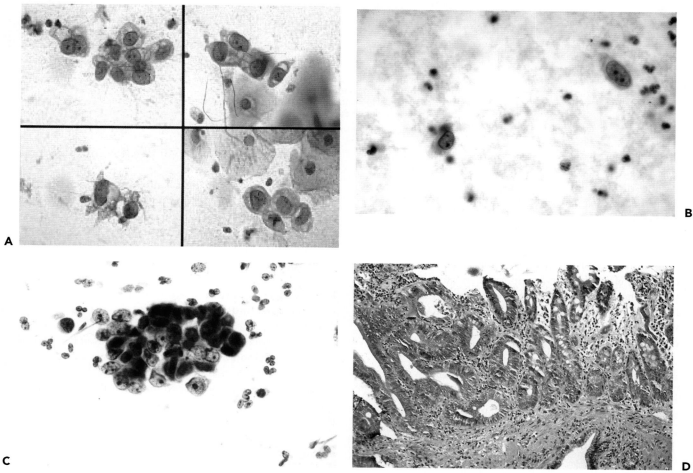

Figure 24-21   Gastric adenocarcinomas (intestinal type). *A.* Composite photograph of columnar and spherical cells of gastric adenocarcinoma with large, prominent nucleoli. *B.* Single gastric cancer cells showing enlarged nuclei and prominent nucleoli. *C.* Cluster of gastric cancer cells with nuclear hyperchromasia and prominent nucleoli. *D.* Gastric carcinoma of intestinal type. (*A:* Composite photograph obtained by PAPNET. With the permission of TriPath Imaging, Burlington, NC.)

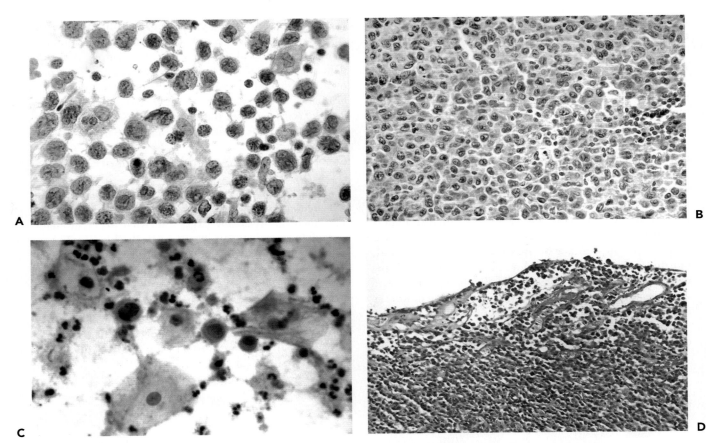

Figure 24-22 **Diffuse gastric type carcinomas.** *A.* Dispersed relatively small cancer cells with nuclear irregularities, some hyperchromasia and prominent nucleoli, corresponding to the tissue pattern shown in *B.* The tumor is composed of sheets of small cells. *C.* Scattered small cancer cells with prominent nucleoli in gastric lavage, also containing squamous cells. *D.* Corresponding tissue lesion with a very poorly differentiated small cell carcinoma.

the small cells may be observed. Rarely, bi- or multinucleated cells may occur.

The **differential diagnosis** of anaplastic carcinomas comprises metastatic (or swallowed) cells of **bronchogenic oat cell carcinoma** and **malignant lymphoma** (see below).

Signet ring-type cells are recognized by their usually large size and **large cytoplasmic vacuoles,** pushing the nucleus to the periphery. Because similarly structured benign cells may also occur, it is important to ascertain that the signet ring cell has the **nuclear characteristics of cancer,** namely large, **clear nuclei with irregularly shaped nuclear membrane and large, irregular nucleoli or large, hyperchromatic nuclei** (Fig. 24-23A,B).

Mixed Types of Gastric Carcinomas

Rarely, **the intestinal and diffuse type of gastric carcinoma may occur simultaneously.** Pilotti et al (1977) identified only 2 such cases in 78 patients with gastric cancer. The cytologic presentation combined the features of both tumor types.

Rare Types of Gastric Carcinoma

The rare **colloid carcinomas** may shed compact clusters of large cancer cells, with large nucleoli, containing cyto-

plasmic mucus that can be visualized with mucicarmine (Fig. 24-23C,D).

Squamous carcinomas or a mixture of squamous and adenocarcinoma **(adenosquamous carcinomas)** may occur in the **area of the cardia** and are similar to esophageal carcinomas of the same type (Fig. 24-24). Usually, the squamous carcinomas are poorly differentiated (epidermoid carcinomas). Keratin-forming squamous cancers are rare. In the presence of a squamous component, **swallowed cancer cells from a tumor of the respiratory tract or esophagus must be considered in the differential diagnosis.**

Rare malignant epithelial tumors combining **features of an adenocarcinoma and a carcinoid have been recognized in cytologic material** (Wheeler et al, 1984). **Large, columnar cells of an adenocarcinoma and small, monotonous cells of a carcinoid** were observed side by side in the same gastric brush smear.

Gastric carcinomas have been observed in **Ménétrier's disease** (Wood et al, 1983; also see above). An unusual association of **gas cysts of the stomach with gastric cancer** was reported by Bhatal et al (1985). **Multinucleated giant cells of foreign body type,** which are characteristic of these cysts were observed in smears **next to malignant cells.**

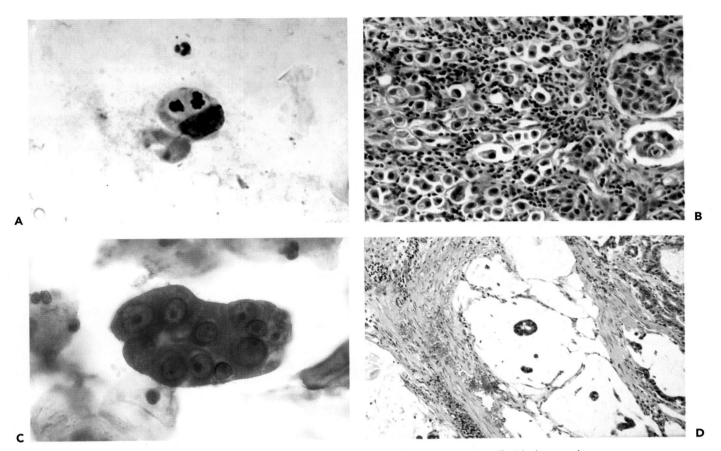

Figure 24-23   **Various features of gastric cancers.** *A.* Signet ring cancer cell with the cytoplasm infiltrated by polymorphonuclear leukocytes, corresponding to the metastatic gastric carcinoma shown in *B. C.* High-power view of mucicermin-stained sharply demarcated cluster of mucus-producing large cancer cells, corresponding to colloid carcinoma, shown in *D.*

PRECURSOR LESIONS OF GASTRIC CARCINOMA: EARLY SUPERFICIAL CARCINOMA AND "DYSPLASIA"

Although it is clear that invasive gastric cancer has to be preceded by a precancerous abnormality of gastric epithelium, the documentation of this sequence of events is rela-

tively recent. The pioneering work in the **recognition of gastric carcinoma in situ and related abnormalities** was performed by Dr. R. O. K. Schade, during his tenure at Newcastle-on-Tyne, UK (Schade 1956A,B, 1959, 1960A,B, 1963). He studied patients who either had vague clinical complaints referable to the gastrointestinal tract or had pernicious anemia and, therefore, were at risk for the

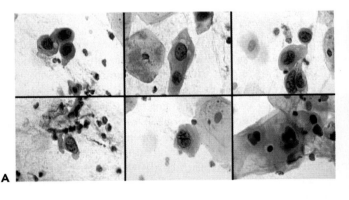

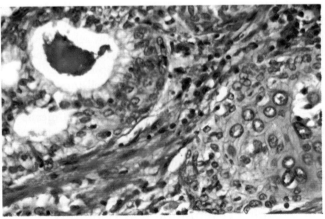

Figure 24-24   **Adenoacanthoma of stomach.** *A.* Composite photograph of cancer cells from the tumor shown in *B.* The tumor has a glandular and squamous component. (*A:* Images obtained with PAPNET apparatus. With permission of TriPath Imaging, Burlington, NC.)

development of gastric cancer. The **cytologic specimens were obtained by washing the stomach with saline through a simple gastric tube on 3 consecutive days** and examining smears obtained from the centrifuged sediment. Within 5 years (1954–1959), Schade was able to diagnose by cytology 41 cases of **very superficially invasive or preinvasive cancer of the stomach, of which 16 were in entirely asymptomatic patients.**

The work of Schade found a following primarily in Japan, where gastric carcinoma is a national scourge, with the hope that early detection of gastric cancer can modify the dismal mortality statistics. There, the **gastric lavage was supplemented by fiberoptic gastroscopy which was initially developed by the Japanese bioindustry specifically for the purpose of gastric cancer detection.** The Japanese health services provided mobile health stations as fully equipped and staffed buses in order to make gastric cancer detection available to all citizens, even those living in small, remote villages. Incidentally, the role of the mobile health stations was subsequently extended to offer cervicovaginal smears and chest x-rays, thus including cervix and lung cancers in the cancer prevention scheme.

The accomplishments of the Japanese scientists have radically altered the outlook on the diagnosis and prognosis of gastric carcinoma (for summaries see Inokuchi, 1966; Kasugai, 1968; Kasugai and Kobayashi, 1974). A large number of papers have documented that the survival of patients treated for superficial carcinoma is vastly superior to survival of treated patients with more advanced gastric cancer. As early as 1966, Inokuchi et al reported a 5-year cure rate of over 90%. Yamazaki et al (1989) reported 5-year survival of 509 treated patients with **early gastric cancer** as close to 100%. By contrast, about one-half of 18 patients with this disorder, who were not treated for various reasons, died of gastric cancer within 5 years. The comparative survival of 350 patients with **occult, but advanced gastric cancer,** treated by curative surgical resection, was 72% after 5 years and 65% after 10 years. On the other hand, all 127 patients with advanced cancer who, for various reasons, were not treated for cure, died within 3 years.

As a consequence of these efforts, the **discovery of gastric cancer in the asymptomatic early stage, notably as superficial carcinoma or carcinoma in situ, has become the rule, rather than the exception in Japan.** The techniques of gastric cancer diagnosis have now achieved worldwide dissemination, particularly fiberoptic gastroscopy combined with gastric cytology and biopsies.

In spite of this progress, the **older, well-tolerated and inexpensive technique of gastric lavage still has its place, particularly in the developing countries, as a means of gastric cancer detection and diagnosis in high-risk patients,** for example, **in patients with pernicious anemia or those with minimal symptoms referable to the upper gastrointestinal tract.**

Endoscopic Presentation and Histology

The extensive Japanese experience in the detection of early gastric cancer has led to the formulation of new concepts of this disease. Although the Japanese investigators recognized that **carcinoma confined to the gastric epithelium (true carcinoma in situ) does exist,** it was also noted that **even a very superficial invasion of the submucosa may occasionally be associated with metastases to the regional lymph nodes.** Hence, it is considered prudent to replace the term *carcinoma in situ* with *superficial or surface gastric carcinoma.*

The **endoscopic appearance** of early (superficial) gastric carcinoma could be separated into three principal types (Fig. 24-25).

■ **Type I is a polypoid lesion,** elevated above the normal level of the epithelium, **usually a carcinoma of intestinal type.**
■ **Type II is a flat lesion,** either slightly elevated above the level of the epithelium or slightly depressed, **usually a carcinoma of intestinal type.**
■ **Type III is a superficially ulcerated lesion,** usually a **carcinoma of diffuse (gastric) type that may be invasive at the time of discovery.**

Type I, II abnormalities are by far more common than type III. A combination of the three types is sometimes observed. It is still not clear how much time is required for the progression of untreated superficial carcinoma of gastric mucosa to fully invasive carcinoma. The progression is likely to be much slower in the intestinal than in the diffuse type of lesions. The evidence at hand strongly suggests, however, that superficial gastric cancers, particularly of the diffuse type, are potentially highly dangerous and must be treated.

Superficial Carcinoma

The histologic appearance of the early lesions is illustrated in Figure 24-25. The early stages of **intestinal type of gastric carcinoma** are characterized by **disorderly glands of variable sizes, lined by cells with hyperchromatic nuclei, often with prominent nucleoli. The diffuse type of lesions** is characterized by an **accumulation of small, often signet-ring type of cancer cells within the epithelium,** infiltrating and often replacing the normal glands.

"Dysplasia" of Gastric Epithelium

Regardless of the diagnostic sophistication of the observer, gastric histology (and cytology) occasionally poses major diagnostic dilemmas. In incidental endoscopic biopsies, there occur epithelial abnormalities that are clearly on the border of cancerous changes in the form of **atrophic gastritis with good preservation of the glandular pattern, but significant nuclear abnormalities within the glands.** Similar lesions were classified as **"dysplasia"** of gastric epithelium (Morson et al, 1980; Jass, 1983). The parallel may be drawn with "dysplasia" occurring in Barrett's esophagus although, to my knowledge, the follow-up of such gastric lesions is limited. Rotterdam et al (1993) cite several follow-up studies that strongly suggest that "severe dysplasia" is a precursor of gastric cancer. The exact clinical significance of such changes is not fully

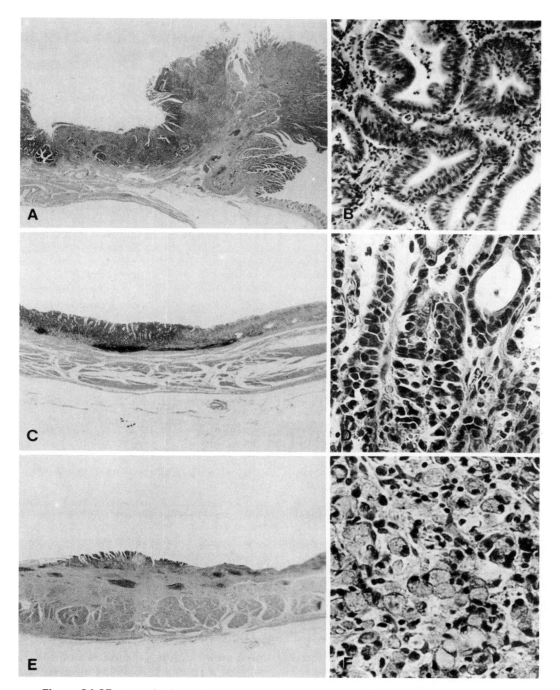

Figure 24-25 Superficial gastric carcinomas. *A,B.* Type I, polypoid lesion; well-differentiated intestinal type of adenocarcinoma. *C,D.* Type II, flat lesion; moderately well-differentiated adenocarcinoma of intestinal type. *E,F.* Type III, ulcerated lesion; signet-ring carcinoma of diffuse type. (Cases courtesy of Prof. S. Shida, Dokkyo University, Mibu, Japan.)

understood, and the therapeutic dilemma is often resolved by surgical intervention that is dictated by prudence, rather than by biologic facts. The **difficulties in the differential diagnosis of gastric "dysplasia" with epithelial abnormalities occurring in chronic gastric ulcers and "aspirin" gastritis have been discussed above and must be considered in the differential diagnosis of such lesions.** The differential diagnosis must also include **gastric epithelial abnormalities** observed in patients

undergoing **chemoradiotherapy for esophageal cancer** (see below).

Cytology

Superficial Carcinoma (Carcinoma In Situ), Intestinal Type

In gastric lavage smears from cases of gastric carcinoma in situ (superficial carcinoma) reported by Schade (1963), abundant cancer cells were present (Fig. 24-26). There was no evidence of necrosis that so often complicates the problem of cytologic diagnosis of advanced and ulcerated gastric cancers. The lesions observed by Schade were mainly of the **intestinal type.** The **cancer cells were large, cuboidal, and contained large, somewhat hyperchromatic nuclei of variable sizes, with prominent multiple nucleoli.** The cytologic findings reflected the tissue abnormality wherein cancer cells lined gastric glands of irregular shape and variable sizes. In superficial carcinoma, cancer cells tend to form more **compact clusters** than in more advanced cancers. The nuclear and nucleolar abnormalities, particularly the latter, become of paramount diagnostic significance.

Schade's observations that **cytologic preparations from superficial carcinomas are easier to interpret than material from advanced gastric cancers** have received ample confirmation from Japanese sources and are also in keeping with personal experience. The specimens are usually free of extensive necrosis and debris and the cancer cells are well preserved (Fig. 24-27).

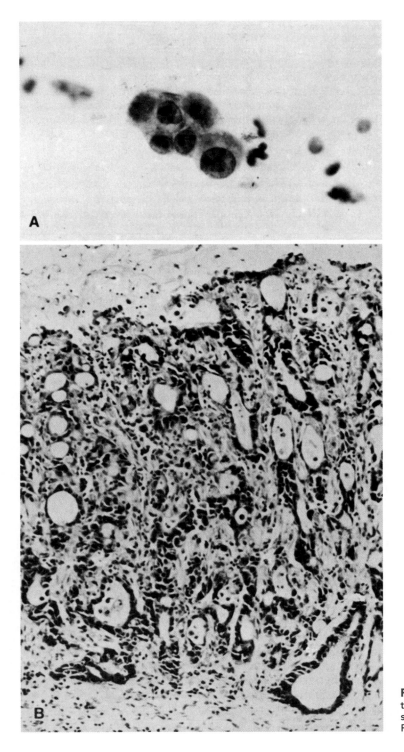

Figure 24-26 Cluster of cancer cells (*A*) and tissue section (*B*) from a case asymptomatic carcinoma in situ of the stomach diagnosed by gastric washings. (Courtesy of Dr. R. O. K. Shade, Newcastle-upon-Tyne, England.)

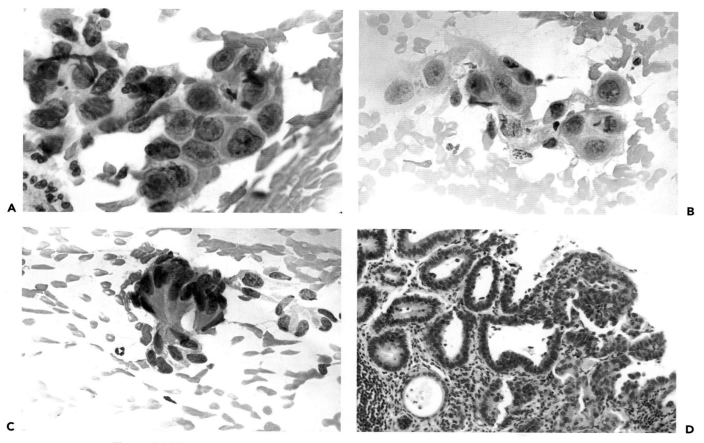

Figure 24-27 Gastric carcinoma in situ. Superficial gastric carcinoma of intestinal type. *A.* High-power view of cohesive cluster of large cancer cells with prominent nucleoli. *B.* Dispersed cancer cells with similar characteristics. *C.* Another cohesive cluster of columnar gastric cells with markedly atypical nuclei. *D.* Tissue lesion showing gastric carcinoma in situ. (Case courtesy of Professor S. Shida, Dokkyo University, Mibu, Japan.)

Superficial Carcinoma, Diffuse Type

The **rare superficial diffuse carcinomas of signet ring type** also shed better preserved cancer cells in which the presence of mucus-containing vacuoles and the morphologic abnormalities of the eccentric nucleus are evident. An example of such cells is shown in Figure 24-23A.

"Dysplasia" of Gastric Epithelium

Our experience with cytology of gastric dysplasia is limited. The lesion may pose major diagnostic dilemmas in the **correlation of cytologic and histologic findings,** as shown in the example illustrated in Figure 24-28. The 54-year-old man had vague abdominal complaints, but no radiographic lesion of note. Cytologic examination of a gastric wash specimen revealed numerous **clusters of highly abnormal large cells with hyperchromatic nuclei and abnormal chromatin patterns** that were diagnosed as gastric carcinoma. The histologic examination of the resected sleeve of the stomach revealed an atrophic gastritis with good preservation of the glandular pattern but significant nuclear abnormalities within the glands. The difficulties of **differential diagnosis between gastric dysplasia and cytologic abnormalities in chronic gastric ulcers and aspirin gastritis** have been discussed above. A careful review of history and knowledge of endoscopic findings is necessary before the diagnosis of gastric "dysplasia" is established. Another potential source of

error is the "dysplasia-like" changes in gastric epithelium caused by **chemoradiotherapy for esophageal cancer** (Brien et al, 2001). These authors suggested that two immunochemical tests, performed on gastric biopsies, may assist in the differential diagnosis between benign gastric epithelial abnormalities and true dysplasia. With the use of **antibody MiB-1,** the proliferation of noncancerous gastric epithelium was **limited** to the depth of gastric glandular crypts whereas, in true dysplasia, the reaction was generalized and involved surface epithelium. Nuclear staining with **antibody to p53** was generally negative in benign lesions and strongly positive in dysplasia.

CYTOLOGY IN THE DIAGNOSIS OF RECURRENT GASTRIC CARCINOMA

After partial gastrectomy for gastric cancer, it may occasionally be possible to diagnose recurring tumor by means of gastric washings. The matter is more often than not of theoretic value only, since in most such cases metastases are present. Offerhaus et al (1984) observed that **"dysplasia" of the residual gastric stump** after resection for gastric carcinoma was a precursor lesion of recurrent gastric cancer. Unfortunately, the study did not include a cytologic component.

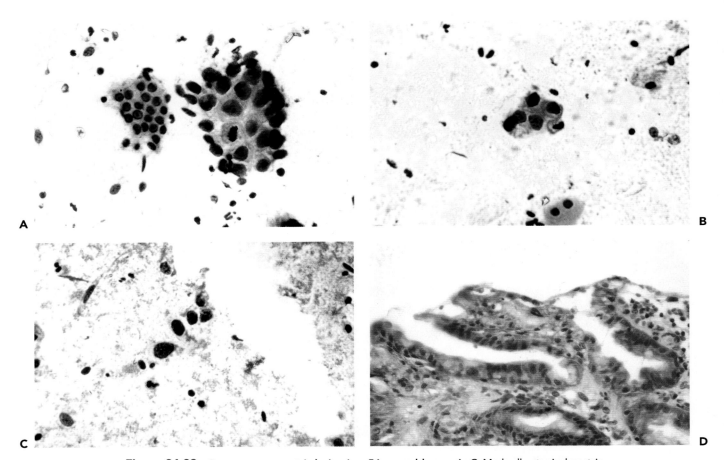

Figure 24-28   Precancerous gastric lesion in a 54-year-old man. *A–C.* Markedly atypical gastric cells with nuclear hyperchromasia. In *C,* the cells are columnar (gastric washings). *D.* Biopsy of gastric epithelium showing moderate atypia of the lining of the glands, interpreted as a precancerous lesion.

RESULTS OF CYTOLOGIC DIAGNOSIS OF GASTRIC CARCINOMA

It may be of some interest that even before the introduction of fiberoptic instruments, specialized laboratories, often directed by gastroenterologists, reported a very high rate of accuracy for gastric cancers diagnosed by cytology **in lavage specimens.** Errors in the diagnosis of gastric cancer in the published series varied from 0% to 4.3%. The results of early personal work in gastric cytology were summarized by McNeer (1967).

Since the introduction of fiberoptic instruments in the 1960s, significant progress has been mainly in the **discovery of early gastric carcinomas** that offer significantly better therapeutic options than more advanced gastric cancer. A dramatic illustration of the change that occurred with the introduction of fiberoptic instruments was provided by Kasugai and Kobayashi (1974), comparing the results of the lavage method and cell samples obtained under direct vision (Table 24-3). In competent hands, combining brush cytology with multiple gastric biopsies, the **diagnosis of *early* gastric cancer** may be achieved in nearly 100% of such lesions.

Still, there is some controversy in reference to the value of brush cytology when compared with direct biopsy of gastric lesion. Thus, Cook et al (1988) suggested that the brushings add very little to biopsies and are a source of

"false-positive" errors. In the hands of Qizilbash et al (1980), the brush specimens were positive in about 89% of the cases of gastric cancer, the biopsy in 93%, and the combination of the two methods in over 95% of the cases. A more optimistic evaluation was offered by Gupta and Rogers (1983), who diagnosed, by brush cytology 21 carcinomas that initially could not be documented by other means. However, these authors also recorded nine unproved, presumably false-positive diagnoses. Hughes et al (1998) studied, by logistic linear regression analysis, the results of gastric brush cytology from 100 patients from several institutions, 50 with documented benign lesions and 50 with gastric cancer. The conclusions of this study, listing the presence of **intact cancer cells, eccentric position of nuclei** and **atypical nuclei** as the three most important features of gastric cancer added little to existing knowledge. Unfortunately, the gastric cancer cases were not subclassified into the intestinal and diffuse types.

In reviewing the accumulated data, it appears that **the most important aspect of gastric cytology is the false-positive rate, the principal sources of error being regenerating gastric epithelium, as in chronic peptic ulcer or aspirin gastritis** (see above). The accuracy of diagnoses obviously depends on quality of the specimens, their technical handling, and the competence and experience of the observer.

TABLE 24-3

COMPARISON OF CYTOLOGIC RESULTS IN THE DIAGNOSIS OF GASTRIC CANCER

	Number of Cases of Gastric Carcinoma	Cytology Positive	Diagnostic Accuracy
Routine lavage	136	110	80.9%
Direct vision lavage			
Early carcinoma	128	122	95.3%
Advanced carcinoma	384	372	96.9%
Direct vision brushing	21	20	95.5%

(Modified from Kasugai T, Kobayashi S. Evaluation of biopsy and cytology in the diagnosis of gastric cancer. Am J Gastroenterol 62:199–203, 1974.)

GASTRIC LYMPHOMAS

Gastric lymphomas account for about 5% of gastric malignant tumors and about one half of malignant lymphomas occurring in the gastro-intestinal tract. Although the general classification of malignant lymphomas is discussed in Chapter 31, gastric lymphomas have specific features that warrant a separate discussion. Of particular interest are the so-called **MALT** lymphomas or malignant lymphomas occurring in the **mucosa-associated lymphoid tissue,** discussed below. The clinical presentation of primary gastric malignant lymphomas is often indolent, mimicking gastric ulcer or gastritis. The tumors have a high curability rate, particularly if diagnosed early (Case Record 13–1995, Massachusetts General Hospital). Therefore, an accurate diagnosis of gastric lymphoma is of great benefit to the patient and cytologic examination of gastric brush specimens may contribute to it. It should be noted, however, that malignant lymphomas develop **beneath** the gastric epithelium, which must be invaded by tumor or ulcerated for the malignant cells to reach the gastric lumen and thus be accessible to cytologic diagnosis.

Large Cell Lymphomas

Nearly all gastric lymphomas are of non-Hodgkin's B cell type. **Large-cell malignant lymphoma of various subtypes is the most frequent form of gastric lymphoma** (Weingrad et al, 1982). The disease is intramural, but may be diagnosed cytologically if the mucosa is involved or if there is an ulcerative lesion. Because of the presence of necrotic material and debris, particularly in the presence of an ulcerated lesion, the diagnosis of lymphoma is difficult in gastric lavage. **Brush specimens,** however, usually show a **nearly pure population of malignant cells** with little debris. In the example shown in Figure 24-29A,B, **medium-sized malignant cells with very scanty cytoplasm were observed in gastric brushings.** The cells formed **loosely structured clusters** and occurred **singly,** a characteristic feature of malignant lymphomas, also emphasized by Lozowski and Hajdu (1984). The **size of the nuclei** was esti-

mated by Lozowski and Hajdu to be twice or three times the size of normal lymphocytes. **Large, prominent, often multiple, nucleoli were noted within the granular nuclei.** Other cytologic features of large-cell gastric malignant lymphoma are similar to those seen in effusions (see Chap. 26). Thus, **nuclear protrusions, nuclear cleavage, and apoptosis (karyorrhexis) may be observed. Large-cell lymphoma** must be differentiated from **small-cell anaplastic carcinoma.** In the latter, **tight cell clusters and cell molding** are evident, features that are **not seen in malignant lymphomas.**

Small-Cell Malignant Lymphomas and MALT Lymphomas

Within recent years, the entity of small cell lymphoma of the stomach has been enriched by the recognition of malignant lymphomas occurring in the **mucosa-associated lymphoid tissue** (**MALT** lymphomas) (Isaacson and Wright, 1984; Isaacson, 1995). These tumors have several unusual features, including an indolent course, an association with *H. pylori,* and a high cure rate. It is speculated that the infection with *H. pylori* leads to a chronic inflammation with accumulation of lymphoid tissue in the gastric wall that becomes transformed into lymphoma (Zucca et al, 1998). **Most, if not all, gastric lesions, previously classified as pseudolymphomas, belong to the category of MALT lymphomas** (Sweeney et al, 1992). Occasionally, MALT lymphomas may progress to a large cell lymphoma (Chan et al, 1990).

The **cytologic diagnosis of small-cell, well-differentiated lymphocytic lymphoma is exceedingly difficult** in suboptimal material obtained by gastric lavage. The principal problem is the presence of lymphocytes in chronic gastritis or gastric ulcer. Also, the cellular and nuclear characteristics of the very small malignant lymphocytes may be insufficient to establish this diagnosis in lavage specimens.

In gastric brush specimens, the characteristic features of small cell lymphomas may be better evident. Immunocytologic stains should be of value in this diagnosis (see Chap. 31). As an example and through the courtesy of Dr. Misao Takeda (formerly of Jefferson Medical College

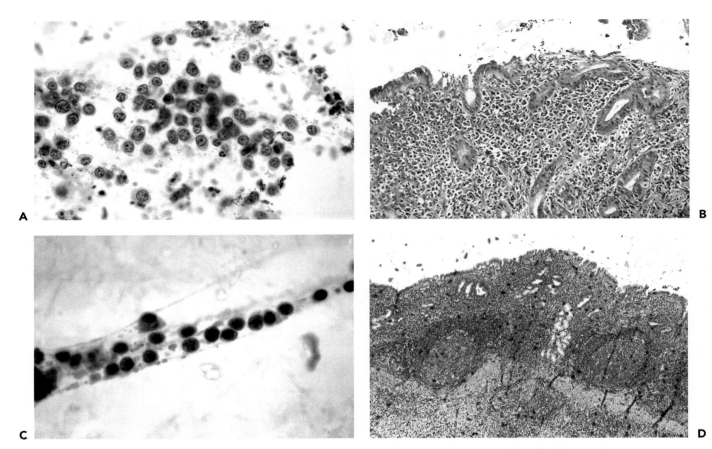

Figure 24-29 **Gastric lymphomas.** *A,B.* Large cell lymphoma. *A.* A cluster of markedly atypical cells of lymphocytic lineage. The cells are characterized by irregular nuclei, prominent nucleoli and very scanty cytoplasm. *B.* The corresponding large cell lymphoma infiltrating gastric wall. *C,D.* Gastric brushing and biopsy in a lesion initially classified as *pseudolymphoma* and now reclassified as *MALT lymphoma.* The smaller cells in the gastric brush are morphologically similar to those shown in a large cell lymphoma in *A.* *D.* The gastric lesion corresponding to *C* with formation of lymphoid follicles. (*C,* higher magnifications). (*C,D* courtesy of Dr. Misao Takeda, Philadelphia.)

in Philadelphia), we had the opportunity to study the gastric smears in a case originally classified as a "pseudolymphoma" but in retrospect is an excellent example of MALT lymphoma (Fig. 24-29C,D). The smears were characterized by **very loosely structured sheets of somewhat enlarged lymphocytic cells, many containing visible nucleoli.** In retrospect, the smaller tumor cells were very similar to cells of a large cell lymphoma (compare Fig. 24-30A with Fig. 24-30C). Scattered plasma cells were also evident. The diagnosis of a malignant lymphoma could be established with confidence in this case.

In the presence of lymphoma, gastric epithelial cells may disclose considerable atypia, similar to that seen in peptic ulcers and probably caused by nonspecific ulcerative or inflammatory changes in the mucosa.

Hodgkin's Disease

Primary gastric Hodgkin's disease is exceedingly rare. However, Hodgkin's disease of adjacent lymph nodes **may sometimes involve the gastric wall.** In such uncommon cases, cancer cells may be observed in exfoliated material but the specific diagnosis cannot be made in the absence of clinical

data. The few clearly malignant and polyhedral cells with hyperchromatic and occasionally double nuclei mimic an epithelial tumor. Raskin et al (1958) and Rubin (1974) reported seeing Reed-Sternberg cells in gastric cytologic material but this has not been our experience.

Performance of Cytology in the Diagnosis of Gastric Lymphoma

As gastric cytology came into widespread use, the early experience with the cytologic diagnosis of malignant lymphomas was variable. Katz et al (1973) reported a relatively poor experience with cytologic diagnosis of these lesions. On the other hand, Kline and Goldstein (1973) reported successful cytologic identification in 9 of 10 patients with this group of diseases. Prolla et al (1970) identified 30 such lesions in 46 patients. Lozowski and Hajdu (1984) studied 29 cases of malignant lymphomas of the gastrointestinal tract, including 24 primary gastric lymphomas. These authors could establish a definite cytologic diagnosis in 5 of 24 gastric lymphomas, 1 of 2 lymphomas of small bowel, and all 3 colonic lymphomas. Sherman et al (1994) studied 27 patients and could establish the cytologic diagnosis in 10 of

18 patients with primary large cell type gastric malignant lymphomas and in 2 of 7 patients with metastatic lymphomas. In 2 of 4 cases with negative biopsies, cytology was suspicious. Suspicious diagnoses were also rendered in two cases of gastritis. **Thus, the role of cytology in the diagnosis of gastric malignant lymphoma is that of an ancillary technique that may occasionally contribute to the diagnosis in cases of biopsy failure or timid interpretation of histologic evidence.**

GASTROINTESTINAL STROMAL TUMORS

A variety of relatively uncommon mesenchymal tumors of gastric and intestinal walls, **previously classified as leiomyomas, leiomyosarcomas, leiomyoblastomas, neurilemomas, gastrointestinal autonomic nerve tumor (GANT), tumors of vascular origin, etc.** are now classified **as gastrointestinal stromal tumors (GISTs)** (Hurlimann and Gardiol, 1991; Franquemont and Frierson, 1992). These tumors have in common certain clinical, molecular, and immunocytochemical features that set them apart from morphologically similar tumors of other organs. These tumors, which may occur in families, are thought to be derived from the interstitial intestinal cells first described many years ago by Ramón

y Cajal that have a growth factor receptor named **c-kit** that can be demonstrated by immunostaining with the **antibody CD117** and, in a somewhat less specific fashion, with the **antibody CD34** (Sarlomo-Rikala et al, 1998; Miettinen et al, 1999). Positive staining with the antibody CD117 has now been declared essential for the diagnosis of GIST (Fletcher et al, 2002). A family with a germline mutation of c-kit was described by Maeyama et al (2001).

About 60% of GISTs are of **spindle cell type,** corresponding to the make-up of smooth muscle or nerve tumors. About 30% of these tumors are composed of large, epithelium-like cells, corresponding to epithelioid leiomyosarcomas, previously also known as leiomyoblastomas. Suster et al (1996) described three patients with **signet ring** type cells. Most of these tumors are **benign** but about one quarter are **malignant** and capable of metastases (Miettinen et al, 1999; Trupiano et al, 2002). Tumor size greater than 5 cm in diameter is an important criterion in poor prognosis (Fletcher et al, 2000). **Stomach** is the most common site of origin of these tumors, followed by **small intestine.** These tumors are **rare** in the **large intestine.** Some of the malignant GISTs appear to respond to a drug known as **imatinib mesylate** (Gleevec, Novartis Pharmaceuticals Corporation, East Hanover, NJ) that is effective in the treatment of chronic myelogenous leukemia (summary in Joensuu et al, 2001; Savage and Antman, 2002;

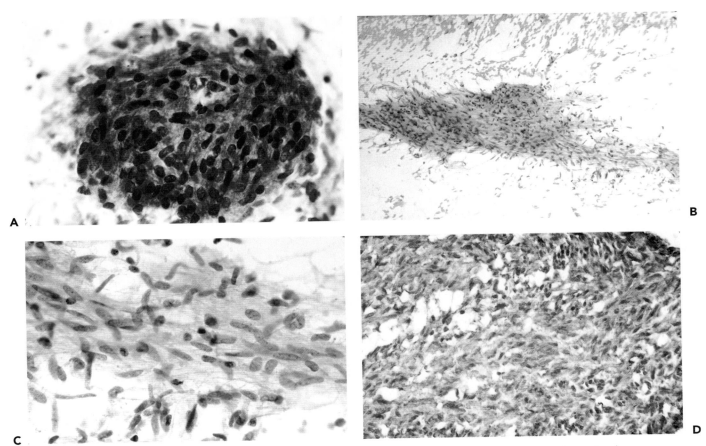

Figure 24-30 Benign gastrointestinal stromal tumor (GIST) in aspirated material. *A.* A sheet of spindly cells forming a whorl. *B.* A sheet of cells, shown in *C* under higher magnification. The cells are spindly in configuration and have virtually no nuclear abnormalities. *D.* Gastric tumor corresponding to *B* and *C,* immunostaining positively for CD34. (Courtesy of Dr. Jacek Sygut, Kielce, Poland.)

Demetri et al, 2002). It must be noted that GISTs, like lymphosarcomas, develop in the gastric wall beneath the gastric epithelium, which must become ulcerated before tumor cells can reach the gastric lumen. In such cases, the **tumor cells may be identified in gastric lavage or brushings.** However, small, nonulcerated tumors may now be aspirated under **endoscopic ultrasound guidance,** a technique described in detail below in reference to bile ducts (Stelow et al, 2003).

Cytology

Benign GISTs

Benign GISTs correspond to leiomyomas or nerve-derived tumors composed of bundles of spindly cells with few, if any, nuclear abnormalities and low mitotic count (< 5 per 50 high power fields). **These tumors can be recognized only in aspiration biopsies.** In a limited number of cases seen by us, the tumor cells in aspirates formed **distinct, loosely structured fragments, sheets or bundles of spindly cells with monotonous elongated nuclei** (Fig. 24-30). A loosely structured matrix was enveloping the cells. Single cells were very rare. The smears had a clean background and were remarkably free of debris or inflammatory cells. Tissue biopsies in such cases were negative for S-100, desmin and myoglobin antibodies but positive for CD117 and CD34. Similar findings have been reported by others (King et al, 1996; Isimbaldi et al, 1998; Li et al, 2001). The differential diagnosis includes an exceedingly rare **solitary fibrous tumor of the gastric serosa** which has a similar cytologic presentation in aspiration biopsy (Shidham et al, 1998).

Malignant GISTs

Before the concept of GIST was formulated, most of these tumors were classified as **leiomyosarcomas,** composed of bundles of **elongated, malignant spindly smooth muscle cells.** Thus, Cabré-Fiol et al (1975) observed three cases of leiomyosarcoma in gastric brush specimens. They reported the presence of characteristic **elongated, spindle-shaped, malignant cells with large, abnormal nuclei** and large nucleoli. Similar cases were described by Qizilbash et al (1980) and by Drake (1985). Prolla and Kirsner (1972) observed elongated malignant cells in bundles *after* gastric biopsies of leiomyosarcomas. In our experience, some **GIST tumors previously classified as leiomyosarcomas may be composed of spindly cells without significant nuclear abnormalities and yet be fully capable of metastases** (Fig. 24-31A,B), an observation confirmed by Li et al (2001). In yet

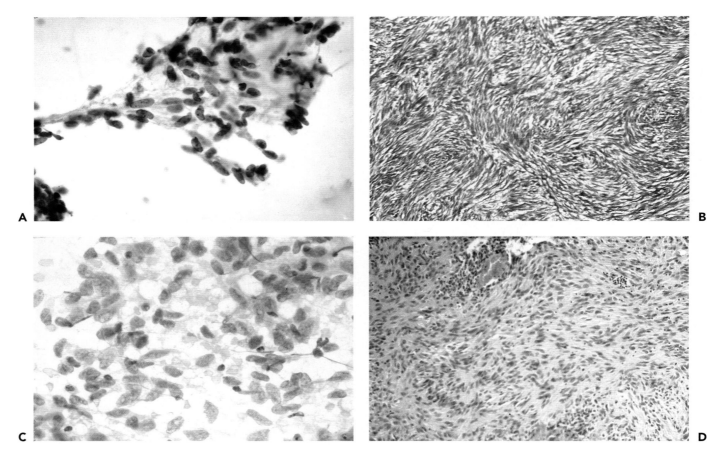

Figure 24-31 Gastric GISTs in aspirated material. *A,B.* Aspiration biopsy of a gastric tumor composed of rather well differentiated spindly cells with only slight nuclear abnormalities. The tumor, which was originally classified as a low grade leiomyosarcoma, produced metastasis. *C,D.* Another example of GIST with relatively slight nuclear abnormalities. The tumor cells shown in *C* are, for the most part, spindly and have rather bland nuclei. The tissue biopsy shows another example of GIST with moderate nuclear abnormalities. (*C,D* courtesy of Dr. Jacek Sygut, Kielce, Poland.)

another case, the spindly cells showed only slight nuclear abnormalities (Fig. 24-31C,D). Thus, the **mere presence of spindly cells in gastric specimens** should be noted as a **warning sign** that a malignant tumor may be present in the gastric wall.

The **epithelioid variant of leiomyosarcomas (leiomyoblastoma) is composed of polygonal cells that mimic an epithelial tumor.** In our experience with aspiration cytology of **malignant GIST tumors** of this type, the smears were composed of epithelioid-type cells with **clearly malignant nuclear features.** The malignant cells were arranged in **loosely structured tissue fragments** (Fig. 24-32A,B). Park et al (1997) reported a case of metastatic **epithelioid leiomyosarcoma** to the liver and emphasized the polygonal configuration and abundant cytoplasm of cancer cells. We also observed a case of malignant GIST tumor wherein the cells formed gland-like structures mimicking an adenocarcinoma (Fig. 24-32C,D). It is evident that only the well differentiated GISTs can be recognized as such in aspiration smears. Tumors composed of clearly malignant cells require clinical data for further classification.

Li et al (2001) described cytologic findings in aspirates of 19 GIST tumors from several institutions. These authors also stressed the tremendous variability of the cytologic presentation of these neoplasms and the absence of features predictive of their metastatic behavior.

OTHER RARE MALIGNANT TUMORS INVOLVING THE STOMACH

A case of **primary gastric melanoma,** with a contributory diagnosis by cytology, was reported by Reed et al (1962). Pigmented malignant cells were observed.

Gorczyca and Woyke (1992) reported a case of **primary gastric choriocarcinoma,** diagnosed in a brush specimen. Bizarre tumor cells, some forming syncytial clusters, were observed. The tumor cells stained for **cytokeratins and human chorionic gonadotropin.** These authors emphasized, however, that **these immunostains may also be positive in pure gastric carcinomas** and, therefore, the morphologic apperance of the tumor cells was of diagnostic importance. **Carcinoids** and other endocrine gastric tumors are discussed below in the colon section.

Metastatic tumors to the stomach may occasionally be diagnosed by gastric washings. Such was the case in a few instances of **mammary carcinoma** observed by us. It should be noted that **patients with mammary carcinoma treated**

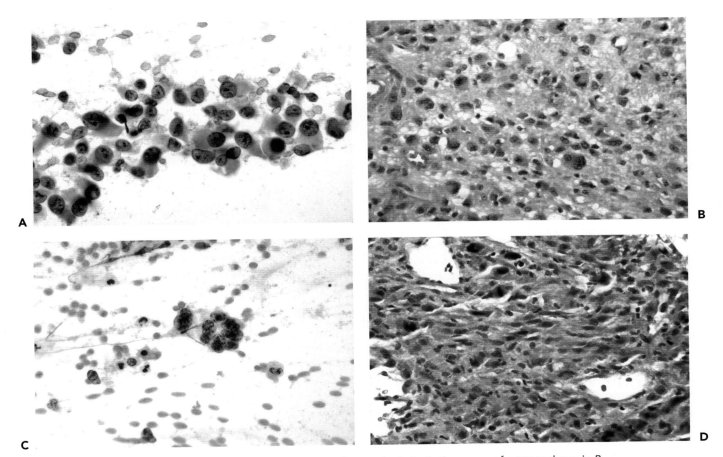

Figure 24-32 **High-grade GIST tumors of stomach.** *A.* Aspiration smear of a tumor shown in *B.* The smear shows clearly malignant cells with nuclear abnormalities. The tissue biopsy in *B* shows a lesion classified initially as an epithelioid leiomyosarcoma. *C,D.* Another example of high-grade GIST tumor. In *C,* The cancer cells show a pseudoglandular arrangement mimicking a gastric carcinoma. *D.* The tissue lesion in the same case, initially diagnosed as leiomyosarcoma.

with steroids are prone to gastric metastases. Somewhat more frequently, **swallowed cancer cells** of **esophageal, laryngeal, and pulmonary origin may be observed in gastric specimens.** This is an **important potential source of diagnostic error** that may result in an unnecessary laparotomy or even gastric resection.

THE COLON AND THE RECTUM

Carcinoma of colon and rectum is the second most lethal cancer in the United States. Because the results of treatment of advanced colonic cancer are unsatisfactory with mortality rate depending on stage of the disease, a major effort is afoot to prevent the disease by recognizing and removing precancerous lesions, or at least to diagnose the disease in early stages.

There are three main approaches to screening for colon cancer: double contrast barium enema, colonoscopy, and detection of occult blood in the stool (summaries in Lieberman, 1998; Winawer, 1999; Bond, 1999).

- **Double contrast barium enema.** This radiologic technique allows the visualization of small space-occupying lesions of the colon. There is considerable debate whether the technique, which is time-consuming and not comfortable for patients, but less expensive than colonoscopy, can assume the role of an effective tool of early cancer detection (Dodd, 1992).
- **Colonoscopy.** Colonoscopy, or inspection of the entire large bowel by fiberoptic instruments, is an expensive and time-consuming technique, requiring the services of a skilled gastroenterologist. There is reasonable consensus that this is, by far, the most effective colon cancer prevention technique, with a relatively small margin of error in the recognition of precursor lesions (reviews in Shinya, 1982; Rex et al, 1997; Inger, 1999).
- **Detection of occult blood in stools.** This is by far the least expensive technique of colon cancer detection that is applicable on a large scale. Slide-like commercial devices are used to detect blood in tiny samples of stool. The slides can be used by the patients in the privacy of their homes or in the physicians' offices. The presence of blood is indicated by a change in color of the slide. Unfortunately, the test is of low specificity, and the presence of blood in stool must be further clarified by additional procedures (Gnauck, 1977). In mass surveys, the test has been shown to be useful in identifying patients at risk (Mandel et al, 1993; Thomas et al, 1995; Scotiniotis et al, 1999).

CYTOLOGIC TECHNIQUES IN THE DIAGNOSIS OF CARCINOMA OF COLON AND ITS PRECURSOR LESIONS

Cytologic techniques have not entered into the mainstream of clinical approaches to colon cancer prevention or diagnosis. Still, there is strong evidence that in skilled hands cytology may be helpful in the diagnosis of colon cancer and its precursor lesions.

Historical Overview

Before the onset of the era of sophisticated radiologic approaches and colonoscopy, the colon has been the target of cytologic investigations for detection or early diagnosis of colonic cancer. Bader and Papanicolaou (1952) used a **rectal-washing apparatus** devised by Loeb (Loeb and Scapier, 1951) to obtain samples from the rectum and lower sigmoid for the diagnosis of cancer located in the descending colon.

The concept of **colonic lavage** for the diagnosis of occult colonic carcinomas was subsequently advocated by Raskin and Pleticka (1964, 1971), who achieved remarkable diagnostic results in selected symptomatic patients without radiologic abnormalities on barium enema.*

Several other lavage techniques were advocated (DeLuca et al, 1974; Katz et al, 1974, 1977). In ulcerative colitis, Katz et al (1977) advocated **segmental lavage of areas of colon** showing strictures, grossly distorted mucosa, or endoscopically inaccessible areas.†

Casts of colon obtained by injecting a soft plastic (Spjut et al, 1963), and even **sponges packed in soluble capsules** (Cromarty, 1977), were used to secure cellular samples from the colon.

Isotonic colon lavage solutions, taken by mouth and used for bowel cleansing before colonoscopy, may also serve as a cell-collecting fluid with satisfactory diagnostic results (Rozen et al, 1990; Rosman et al, 1994). A similar experiment was conducted on 12 patients before colonoscopy by Greenebaum and Brandt (1998; unpublished data) at Montefiore Medical Center but failed to be of value.

For **rectal cancer within the reach of the examiner's finger,** Linehan et al (1983) advocated the preparation of a **smear from the surface of the glove.** The method was successful in the diagnosis of several adenocarcinomas and squamous cancers, as confirmed by Soni and Dhamne (1991) and by Wilson et al (1993).

Current Status

With the widespread use of colonoscopy, **direct brushing techniques** have become the preferred method of collection of cytology specimens. Colorectal cytology is primarily useful in the **identification of cancer or precancerous states**

---

* The method of colonic lavage used by Raskin and Pleticka was as follows: The preparation of a patient was the same as that for a barium enema. A cathartic by mouth, taken 12 hours prior to collection of the material, was necessary. On the morning of the procedure, cleansing enemas were administered until the returns were clear. Actual collection of the cytologic material took place 1 to 2 hours later. From 500 to 1,000 ml of warm Ringer's solution was instilled with the patient in the left decubitus position. Massage of the colon and rotation of the patient were very helpful in obtaining better cytologic material. The fluid was collected after 3 to 5 minutes. Alcohol fixation of the sample was optional. If none was used, immediate centrifugation was advised and smears were prepared from the sediment.
† Katz et al advocated the use of a pulsating saline lavage (500 to 1,000 ml) with the help of a dental irrigation unit attached either to a rigid or flexible colonoscopic instrument. The saline solution was collected in equal volume of 95% ethyl alcohol and the sediment processed after centrifugation as smears or cell blocks.

in high-risk patients (patients with familial polyposis of colon, ulcerative colitis, or patients previously treated for colon cancer) and for the clarification of obscure radiographic or colonoscopic findings. Several observers reported that brushing cytology of colon increases the yield of precancerous lesions and early carcinoma when compared with biopsies (Winawer et al, 1978; Melville et al, 1988; Ehya and O'Hara, 1990).

NORMAL COLON

Histology

The mucosa of the large bowel is composed of a **single or a double layer of columnar cells, arranged in simple tubular glands** (see Fig. 5-6). There are **numerous mucus-producing goblet cells** within the mucosa. The intervening columnar cells have an opaque cytoplasm. Electron microscopic studies have shown that the surface-lining cells are columnar with striated border; **on the surface, there are numerous microvilli with electro-opaque rootlets,** a feature that **may assist in the recognition of colonic cancer cells in metastases** (see Chap. 26). The cytoplasm of the mucus-producing goblet cells is filled with mucus-containing vacuoles that are discharged after reaching the surface of the cell.

Cytology

One of the most difficult tasks in obtaining cytologic specimens from this area is to limit the amount of debris to ensure a clean smear. The **cytologic features of rectal and sigmoid washings or brushings** in the absence of disease are rarely obtained but are simple to interpet. **The epithelial cells are easily recognized as slender columnar cells with pale spherical nuclei located in the approximate center of the cells. They are similar to normal gastric cells** (see Fig. 24-16B). **Depending on the method of securing the specimen, these cells occur singly** and in **loosely structured clusters** (in colonic washings) **or** as **tightly knit clusters or**

bundles of parallel cells (in brush specimens). **Also present are mucus-producing, goblet cells** (described in detail in Chap. 19), macrophages, leukocytes, some **squamous cells of anal origin** and, almost invariably, some debris.

ACUTE INFLAMMATORY DISEASES

Acute Colitis

Disorders such as **amebic colitis** or **acute diverticulitis** result in smears rich in debris and inflammatory exudate containing few, if any, intact epithelial cells (Fig. 24-33). Unless specific **causative agents** (such as *Amoeba histolytica* or ova of *Schistosoma*) are identified, the cytologic diagnosis of colitis must remain nonspecific.

Histoplasmosis

Mullick et al (1996) reported two patients (one with HIV infection) with *Histoplasma capsulatum* infection, causing formation of a colonic and a rectal mass, mimicking cancer. Direct smears disclosed the presence of the fungus, described in detail in Chapter 19.

Cryptosporidiosis

The intracellular parasite *Cryptosporidium,* when ingested, infects the intestinal tract causing a diarrhea that is self-limiting in normal people but may be life-threatening in immuno-compromised patients, particularly those with AIDS (Chen et al, 2002). The diagnosis is usually established on biopsies of the intestine showing small spherical excrescences, measuring about 3 to 5 μm in diameter on the surface of the epithelial cells. There are no recorded cases of cytologic identification of the parasite.

Cytomegalovirus

In AIDS patients, involvement of the colon by this virus is not unusual. For further comments on the recognition of this virus, see above (Fig. 24-17B).

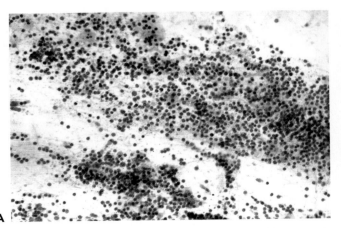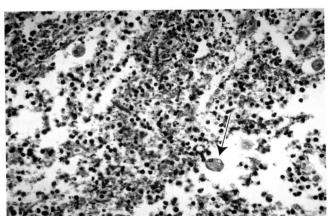

Figure 24-33 *A.* Acute nonspecific colitis in brush smear. The smear is composed mainly of inflammatory cells and some necrotic epithelium. *B.* Amebiasis. The spherical organisms (*arrow*) may be seen in the midst of the inflammatory exudate.

CHRONIC INFLAMMATORY DISEASES

Chronic inflammatory diseases of the bowel are caused by a number of factors, some of which are genetic, as shown with human and animal studies (summary in Podolsky, 2002). Based on clinical and pathological features, two principal forms of inflammatory bowel disease are recognized: **ulcerative colitis** and **Crohn's disease.** Both diseases may lead to a variety of serious complications, including colon cancer. Cytologic techniques have been extensively used in an attempt to identify early cancers in these patients.

Chronic Ulcerative Colitis

The disease usually begins in **young adults** with episodes of bloody diarrhea. The disease may be mild, limited to occasional episodes, moderate, with repeated episodes of diarrhea of longer duration, or severe in which the patients experience continuous diarrhea with numerous bloody bowel movements a day. The fully developed disease is characterized by formation of **confluent mucosal ulcers limited to** various segments of the colon. **Polypoid masses or nodules** may occur at the edge of the ulcers or in the intervening mucosa (Torres et al, 1998).

Patients with ulcerative colitis are **prone to the development of colonic adenocarcinoma,** as had been recognized many years ago (Cook and Goligher, 1975) and repeatedly confirmed (Mellemkjaer et al, 1995). It is generally assumed that colonic cancer in these patients is preceded by epithelial abnormalities which have been named **"dysplasia," rather than "carcinoma in situ"** (summary in Goldman, 1996). Molecular biologic investigation of lesions associated with ulcerative colitis suggested that the mechanism of cancer formation may differ from spontaneously occurring carcinomas (Greenwald et al, 1992; Odze et al, 2000). **Prevention of colonic carcinomas is the goal of treatment of chronic ulcerative colitis.** In patients with "severe dysplasia," colectomy is performed as a precautionary measure. In such specimens, occult invasive carcinomas are sometimes found. The **recognition of "dysplasia" and its differentiation from inflammatory changes, either on colonoscopy or biopsy, often presents a major diagnostic challenge** that may benefit from cytologic examination.

Crohn's Disease

Crohn's disease is the principal disorder in **the differential diagnosis of ulcerative colitis.** Crohn's disease is an **inflammatory disorder of unknown etiology,** but with a strong genetic component, observed mainly in **young adults but also occurring in children** (Podolsky, 2002). The disease is **not limited to the large bowel** as it may also involve **the small intestine** but may be observed in **distal organs** such as the **vulva** and even the **eye.** Contrary to ulcerative colitis which is limited to the mucosa and is diffuse, Crohn's disease is **segmental** and involves the entire thickness of the intestinal wall. **Ulcerations of the mucosa** are accompanied by a **chronic inflammatory reaction in the wall of the intestine,** with frequent formation of **granu-**lomas, and may lead to **fistulous tracts. The role of Crohn's disease as a precancerous condition is still being debated.** However, in the absence of clinical information, **the cytologic presentation of Crohn's disease involving colon may be identical to that of ulcerative colitis.**

Cytology of Chronic Inflmmatory Disease of the Large Bowel

Ulcerative colitis was a natural target of investigations from the very onset of colonic cytology in the 1950s. The principal **purpose of this examination is to separate the precancerous abnormalities ("dysplasia") from inflammatory changes on one hand and fully developed cancer on the other.** Chronic inflammatory changes cause a **"repair reaction"** in the surrounding colonic epithelium and cause **problems of interpretation** that are very similar for all glandular epithelia, such as the **endocervix, Barrett's esophagus, and gastric ulcer** (see Chap. 12; and previous discussion in this chapter).

In colonic smears, there is evidence of an **inflammatory reaction** in the form of leukocytes, fibrin and debris. **The epithelial glandular cells** are usually trapped in the exudate and may appear singly or in loosely structured clusters. **They may be distorted or damaged but usually retain their columnar shape, although they may be somewhat enlarged. Their nuclei are usually pale-staining and may contain visible nucleoli.** As a rule, there is **no nuclear hyperchromasia.** In **Crohn's disease,** the finding of **granulomas,** similar to tuberculous granulomas, may sometimes lead to a specific diagnosis.

Identification of Colonic "Dysplasia"

In ulcerative colitis, the task is **similar to the identification of "dysplasia" in Barrett's esophagus or stomach,** discussed in the first parts of this chapter, and is rendered more difficult by the presence of marked inflammation. Early observers (Galambos et al, 1956; Boddington and Truelove, 1956), using samples obtained by **colonic washings,** emphasized some of the diagnostic problems. In colonic washings, Galambos et al (1955, 1956) described **two types of epithelial cells: the *bland* cells and the *active* cells.** The **bland cells** were larger than normal colonic cells and had **large, clear, pale nuclei,** corresponding to findings in uncomplicated chronic ulcerative colitis. The **active cells** were also larger than normal and their **nuclei were characterized by the presence of large, sometimes irregularly shaped nucleoli.** In the presence of the active cells, **particularly if they displayed variability in size,** the **differential diagnosis between active chronic ulcerative colitis and incipient colonic carcinoma ("dysplasia" in current terminology) was impossible.** Similar difficulties were emphasized by Raskin and Pleticka (1964) and by Prolla and Kirsner (1972). The latter authors also reported the **presence of atypical lymphocytic cells,** which may complicate the cytologic picture still further. Festa et al (1985) compared multiple cytologic samples obtained by colonic lavage and brushings from 41 patients with ulcerative colitis and observed a **wide spectrum of cytologic abnormalities, rang-**

ing from mild to severe atypia, to carcinoma. These observers found that the **morphologic differences between "severe atypia" ("dysplasia") and carcinoma were difficult to ascertain.** The same problem of interpretation occurred with corresponding biopsies. Six carcinomas of the colon (including two **in situ carcinomas, or "severe dysplasia,"** using current nomenclature) were accurately diagnosed. Melville et al (1988) suggested that colonic "dysplasia" could be identified in brush smears because of lesser abnormalities in nuclear configuration when compared with cells of colonic carcinoma. The illustrative evidence in support of this view was not persuasive. In my judgment, all the lesions illustrated had the appearance of cancer cells (see below).

If there is a consensus in this difficult area of cytologic diagnosis, it may be summarized as follows: **the presence of colonic epithelial cells with moderately enlarged, either hyperchromatic or clear nuclei and the presence of distinct, enlarged nucleoli may correspond to "dysplasia" or carcinoma of the epithelium of the diseased colon and should lead to a confirmatory biopsy** (Fig. 24-34). The level of suspicion becomes greater if the nucleoli are not spherical but have a distorted contour.

TUMORS OF THE COLON

Adenomatous Polyps

Clinical and Pathologic Data

Adenomatous polyps are very common **benign colonic neoplasms** that may either cause rectal **bleeding or be completely asymptomatic** and are an incidental finding on endoscopic examination. The polyps may vary in size from tiny, nearly microscopic structures, to substantial tumors that may measure several centimeters in diameter. They consist of a **central connective tissue stalk** surmounted by a **crown of folded colonic epithelium** that may be either normal (see Fig. 7-1) or show varying degrees of **epithelial abnormality, such as "dysplasia" or even foci of carcinoma.** If the glands are tubular, the lesions are referred to as **tubular adenomas.** Another type of polyp, **villous adenoma,** is characterized by **long, delicate stalks and**

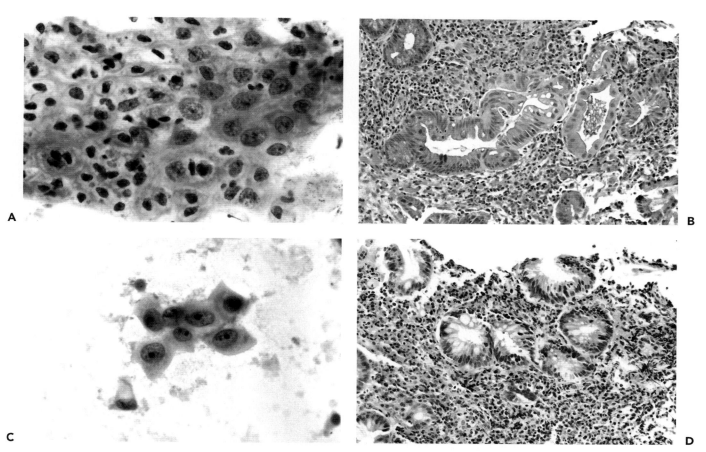

Figure 24-34   Atypias in chronic ulcerative colitis. *A.* Brush smear of a polypoid colonic abnormality in a 50-year-old man with ulcerative colitis. The cells, although forming an adhesive sheet, show significant nuclear abnormalities in the form of enlargement and small nucleoli. *B.* Biopsy of the corresponding colonic lesion showing the pseudopolypoid arrangement of the inflamed epithelium. *C.* Another example of cell abnormalities in chronic ulcerative colitis. The cells shown in *C* under a higher power have a markedly enlarged nuclei and prominent nucleoli and could not be differentiated from cancer cells. *D.* Corresponding area of colonic abnormality in a 49-year-old woman with a 20-year history of ulcerative colitis. Although the glands are atypical, they cannot be classified as malignant. (Courtesy of Dr. June Koizumi, New York Hospital/Cornell Medical Center, New York.)

may become malignant in a high proportion of cases (Takolander, 1975). Mixed patterns of polyps occur.

Polyps are considered to be a stage in the development of colonic carcinoma (see Chap. 7 and Fig. 7-4). Prophylactic removal of polyps reduced the rate of colon cancer and was claimed to be an effective prevention measure (Winawer et al, 1996). Lane (1976) emphasized that most polypoid lesions of colon are benign. For further discussion of colonic carcinoma, see below.

Cytology

In my experience, **benign polyps of the colonic mucosa cannot be identified as such** in brush smears because the cytology is that of benign colon. Thabet and Macfarlane (1962) emphasize the presence of **slender, elongated "needle" cells and of columnar, fan-shaped cells** as characteristic of benign colonic polyps. We were unable to confirm this observation. Occasionally, colonic washings contain thick fragments of tissues that can be embedded in paraffin and identified as polyps in cell blocks.

However, **brush cytology of adenomatous polyps during sigmoidoscopy or colonoscopy, prior to biopsy or removal, may contribute to the discovery of polyps with various degrees of premalignant changes (dysplasia) or foci of carcinoma** (Halpern et al, 1997). The features of colonic "dysplasia" have been discussed above and the features of colonic carcinoma are discussed below.

Adenocarcinoma

Epidemiology and Natural History

The importance of this devastating disease has been mentioned at the beginning of this segment. It is the belief of many epidemiologists, so far unproven, that **dietary factors** are responsible for the frequency of carcinoma of colon. Other **risk factors** for colon cancer include the presence of adenomatous polyps, particularly in familial polyposis of colon, ulcerative colitis, and family history of colon cancer (Winawer et al, 1996; Lynch and de la Chapelle, 2003). Brekkan et al (1972) observed colonic carcinomas developing at **the site of ureterosigmoidostomy.** The sequence of molecular biologic events in the genesis of cancer of the colon, as proposed by Vogelstein and Kinzer, is discussed in Chapter 7. It has been shown that regular intake of **aspirin** or the related drug **sulindac** lowers the risk of colonic cancer (Thun et al, 1991; Heath, 1993; Ladenheim et al, 1995; Wu, 2000; Sandler et al, 2003; Baron et al, 2003).

It is generally accepted that **carcinoma of the colon is preceded by precancerous lesions, such as villous adenomas, adenomatous or tubular benign polyps or epithelial lesions, classified as "dysplasia."** It is the personal view of this writer that the significance of **flat lesions of the colonic epithelium, "aberrant crypts" or flat carcinomas in situ,** which are very difficult to recognize in colonoscopy, has been **severely underestimated** as precursor lesions of colonic cancer, a view also expressed by Pretlow et al (1991). The frequency of **"aberrant crypts," lesions most likely representing early stages of formation of flat carcinomas in situ,** has been emphasized by Japanese observers performing a detailed examination of colonic epithelium, with magnifying colonoscopy and methylene blue staining (Takayama et al, 1998). The crypts usually show mutations of the K-*ras* oncogene (Pretlow et al, 1993). Incidentally, the frequency of "aberrant crypts" may be reduced after treatment with sulindac (Takayama et al, 1998).

Histology

Carcinomas of colon appear to the endoscopist as elevated or ulcerated areas of the colon. Colonic carcinomas are **mucus-producing adenocarcinomas of varying levels of differentiation,** ranging from **well-defined glandular structures to solidly growing, anaplastic cancers, which include signet ring adenocarcinoma. Squamous and mucoepidermoid carcinomas** are occasionally observed (Lundquest et al, 1988), as are very rare carcinomas of other types.

Staging, Grading, and Prognosis

Duke's staging and grading, proposed in the 1930s and 1940s, shown in Tables 24-4 and 24-5, is still widely used with only minor modifications in the assessment and prognosis of colon cancer. Grading indicates a deviation from normal structure of the colonic epithelium and the degree of abnormality of cancer cells. Thus, colonic cancers closely resembling normal gland structure, lined by cells with only slight abnormalities, are tumors grade I. Solidly growing

---

TABLE 24-4

DUKE'S GRADING OF COLONIC CARCINOMAS

Grade	Probability of Metastases
I	18%
II	44%
III	78%

Based on study of 1,726 colonic cancers.
From Dukes CE. J Clin Pathol 2:95–98, 1949.

TABLE 24-5

DUKE'S STAGING OF COLONIC CARCINOMAS

Stage	Definition	Prognosis (5-year Survival)
A	Tumor confined to mucosa or submucosa	95%
B	Invasion of muscularis	50%–60%
C	Metastasis to regional lymph nodes	25%–30%
D	Distant metastasis	0

Based on study of 1,726 colonic cancers.
Dukes CE. J Clin Pathol 2:95–98, 1949.

tumors composed of bizarre or small cancer cells are grade III. The most common gland-forming tumors with intermediate abnormalities are grade II. It has been recently proposed that Duke's staging be replaced by the TNM system (Greene et al, 2002).

Several studies have documented that measuring DNA ploidy in colonic carcinoma may have prognostic significance: diploid tumors with low S-phase appear to have a better prognosis than aneuploid tumors or tumors with high S-phase (Wolley et al, 1982; Wersto et al, 1991; Hixon et al, 1995; Takanishi et al, 1996; Cohn et al, 1997). For further comments on DNA ploidy, see Chapter 47.

Cytology

Today, most colonic carcinomas are diagnosed by colonoscopic biopsies. In the years before fiberoptic colonoscopy, Raskin and Pleticka (1964) reported that up to 20% of malignant lesions of the colon that **could not be definitely identified on the initial radiologic examination (barium enema) could be diagnosed by colonic lavage.** This skilled team diagnosed over 80% of all colonic carcinomas by cytology. Excellent results were also reported by Katz et al (1974, 1977) who used a different lavage method (see above).

With extensive use of colonoscopy, **the role of colonic cytology has been directed toward evaluating high-risk patients, such as those with colonic polyposis, ulcerative colitis, or patients at risk of recurrence at the site of prior colectomy for carcinoma** (DeLuca et al, 1974).

The **cells obtained from well-differentiated adenocarcinomas of the colon** are large, **often columnar or cuboidal in configuration, with large, sometimes irregular, hyperchromatic nuclei with prominent nucleoli, occurring singly and in clusters** (Figs. 24-35 and 24-36). Adenocarcinomas of the **rectum** are identical to colonic cancer (Fig. 24-37C,D). The cytoplasm varies in amount and is often poorly preserved. The diagnosis is based on nuclear abnormalities. Koizumi and Schron (1997) emphasized that in **metastatic colon cancer, the classical hyperchromatic nuclei may be replaced by clear nuclei with large nucleoli** (see Chap. 26 for further comments on this topic). In cell blocks of effluents, fragments of colonic cancer may be observed. It is of note that cells of colonic carcinoma may express the p21 product of the oncogene Ha-*ras,* which may facilitate their recognition in difficult diagnostic situations (Czerniak et al, 1987A).

In **signet ring cell carcinomas, large mucus vacuoles push the large, hyperchromatic nuclei to the periphery of large cells. Poorly differentiated carcinomas** may be represented in smears by **cancer cells of variable sizes, that are often approximately spherical and have large, hyperchromatic nuclei** (Fig. 24-37A,B). In the very rare **small cell carcinomas,** the tumor cells may resemble **similar tumors of lung,** discussed in Chapter 20. Silverman et al (1996) emphasized that **it may be difficult to identify small cell carcinomas in aspiration biopsies as being of colonic origin** because of their similarity to other small cell neoplasms.

Results

Today, the value of colonic cytology is primarily in the evaluation of lesions without clear-cut endoscopic or radio-graphic findings, and in monitoring high-risk patients. However, we have also observed several patients in whom the cytology was consistent with cancer and the initial biopsy or biopsies were nondiagnostic. Thus, cytology may serve as added insurance that a cancer of colon will not be missed. This point was emphasized by Bardawil et al (1990) who reviewed their large experience with colonoscopic brush cytology. These authors stressed the **value of a positive or suspicious cytologic diagnosis, even in the absence of initial histologic evidence of carcinoma.** The diagnoses were ultimately confirmed in all but one patient with a definitive cytologic diagnosis of cancer and in 29 of 34 patients with "suspicious" cytologic findings and initially negative biopsies. Similar results were reported by Halpern et al (1997).

Endocrine Tumors

Tumors with endocrine features, such as benign and malignant **carcinoids** and **endocrine carcinomas,** occur mainly in the small and large intestine but may also be observed in the stomach and the duodenum (Gould and Chejfec, 1978; Gaffey et al, 1990; Caplin et al, 1998). The tumors are derived from argentaffin cells dispersed in the mucosa. Most of these tumors are occult and are an incidental finding but some may have endocrine activity. We observed an example of proliferation of endocrine cells in the wall of the stomach and duodenum of a 12-year-old boy with the classical **Zollinger-Ellison syndrome** of gastric hyperacidity and ulcer formation, caused by secretion of **gastrin.** Most of such cases are associated with **gastrinomas** of the pancreas. In this case, the cells of gastrinoma formed mucosal and submucosal islets of cells or "tumorlets" (Fig. 24-38A,B). Because of their location, the "tumorlets" could not be identified on endoscopic or cytologic examination (Bhagavan et al, 1974). On the other hand, we observed a patient with a **malignant carcinoid** of the duodenum, metastatic to the lung that could be securely diagnosed on a bronchoscopic sample. Small tumor cells with small nuclei of even sizes in the smears and the cell block of the material were characteristic of the disease (Fig. 24-38C,D).

Maligant Lymphoma

The MALT lymphomas, some previously classified as **pseudolymphomas,** discussed above in reference to the stomach, also occur in the the small intestine and the colon. A thickening of the intestinal wall is often seen in these disorders. A point in the differential diagnosis of such lesions is **Whipple's disease,** which may be difficult to distinguish on clinical and radiologic grounds (Whipple, 1907). Whipple's disease, which may affect many other organs besides the intestine, is characterized by large **macrophages, containing a bacterium,** *Tropherima whippelii* (Relman et al, 1992). To our knowledge, there is no record of such a lesion diagnosed by cytologic techniques.

A **large cell B-cell lymphoma of cecum** diagnosed by aspiration biopsy (FNA) was reported by Chen et al (1992).

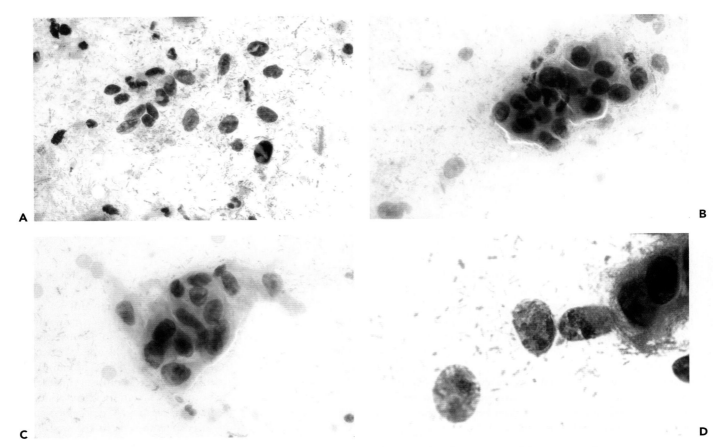

Figure 24-35   Colonic carcinoma in ulcerative colitis. *A.* A brush smear containing cancer cells with enlarged nuclei adjacent to a few normal colonic epithelial cells. *B,C.* Large clusters of colonic cancer cells with large prominent hyperchromatic nuclei. *D.* Oil immersion view of the nuclei of colonic cancer cells to show the coarse configuration of chromatin and prominent large nucleoli.

THE DUODENUM, EXTRAHEPATIC BILE DUCTS, PANCREATIC DUCTS, AND GALLBLADDER*

ANATOMY

The duodenum is the first segment of small bowel, extending for about 25 cm from the pylorus of the stomach around the head of the pancreas in a C-shaped loop to the duodenal-jejunal flexure at the ligament of Treitz. It is divided into four segments, of which the second or descending segment is of special interest in cytology. It is here that the main bile and pancreatic ducts open into the duodenum through a small papilla located on the medial aspect of the duodenum.

The right and left hepatic ducts emerge from the liver and unite in the hilum approximately 1cm from the liver to form the common hepatic duct. **The common hepatic duct** varies in length from about 1 to 5 cm (average 2.0

cm), and is 0.2 to 0.8 cm in diameter, increasing in diameter with age (Thung and Garber, 1991). **The cystic duct** of the gallbladder joins the common hepatic duct to form **the common bile duct** which is about 5 cm in length and 1 mm in diameter, and extends from above the duodenum, behind it and through the head of the pancreas into the papilla in the duodenum. In two-thirds to three-fourths of cases, the main pancreatic duct (duct of Wirsung) joins with the common bile duct as it enters the wall of the duodenum and the papilla to form a dilated common channel or ampulla **(ampulla of Vater)** with a common opening into the duodenum (DiMagno et al, 1982).

The pancreas lies in the retroperitoneum with the head of the pancreas embraced in the curve of the duodenum, the body lying behind the stomach and transverse colon and the tail extending to the hilum of the spleen (Fig. 24-39). The main pancreatic duct (duct of Wirsung) traverses the gland near its posterior surface, receiving branches from all sides, and joining with the common bile duct, or independent of it, enters the duodenal papilla. An accessory pancreatic duct (of Santorini) drains the upper part of the head of the pancreas and may join the main duct or enter the duodenum through a separate orifice.

The gallbladder is a pear-shaped sac that lies under the right lower lobe of the liver, at its inferior edge. It measures

---

* Contributed by Dr. Myron R. Melamed.

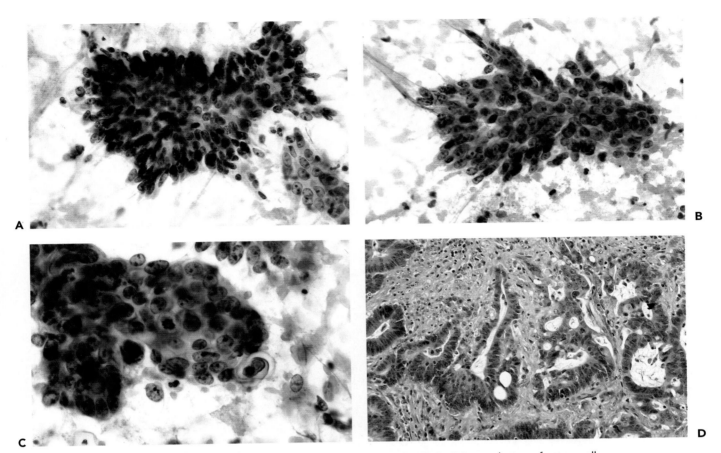

Figure 24-36 **Colonic adenocarcinoma in colonic brushings.** *A–C.* Large clusters of cancer cells with prominent hyperchromatic nuclei and nucleoli, corresponding to the colonic biopsy shown in *D.* In *A* and *B,* the cancer cells have a columnar configuration, whereas in *C,* they are cuboidal in shape. (Photographs courtesy of Dr. June Koizumi, New York Hospital/Cornell Medical Center, New York.)

about 10 cm in length, varies from 3 to 4 cm in width and has a 1 to 2 mm thick wall. The distal end of the gallbladder tapers to an S-shaped neck that connects with the cystic duct. The cystic duct joins the common hepatic duct to form the common bile duct. As much as a liter of bile flows each day from the liver into the gallbladder where water is absorbed, concentrating the bile into a much smaller volume that can be stored within the 50 to 70 ml capacity of the gallbladder. When a fatty meal enters the duodenum, the gallbladder contracts, emptying bile into the duodenum. Figure 24-39 shows a diagrammatic representation of extrahepatic biliary ducts and their relationship with the duodenum and the pancreas.

HISTOLOGY

Duodenum

The villous mucosa of the duodenum undergoes gradual transition from pyloric antral epithelium to tall columnar absorptive epithelium of intestinal type with basal or suprabasal round or oval nuclei, eosinophilic cytoplasm and a deeply eosinophilic brush border at the free surface. There

are interspersed goblet cells and occasional endocrine cells and Paneth cells.

Extrahepatic Bile Ducts

The extrahepatic bile ducts are lined by a single layer of mucin-secreting columnar epithelium with uniform, basally located oval nuclei. Nucleoli are inconspicuous or absent (Fig. 24-40A). In the absence of inflammation, there are few or no goblet cells. A few mucus-secreting glands may be present in the wall of the duct. With inflammation or irritation, the mucosa may undergo hyperplasia with epithelial atypia, increased mitotic activity, gastric or intestinal metaplasia, or sometimes mucinous or squamous metaplasia. Within the terminal portion of the common bile duct, the epithelium forms slender, branching papillary fronds that yield richly cellular brush cytology specimens.

Main Pancreatic Duct

The epithelium of the main pancreatic duct is identical to that of the common bile duct, composed of a single layer of columnar epithelial cells with lightly eosinophilic cyto-

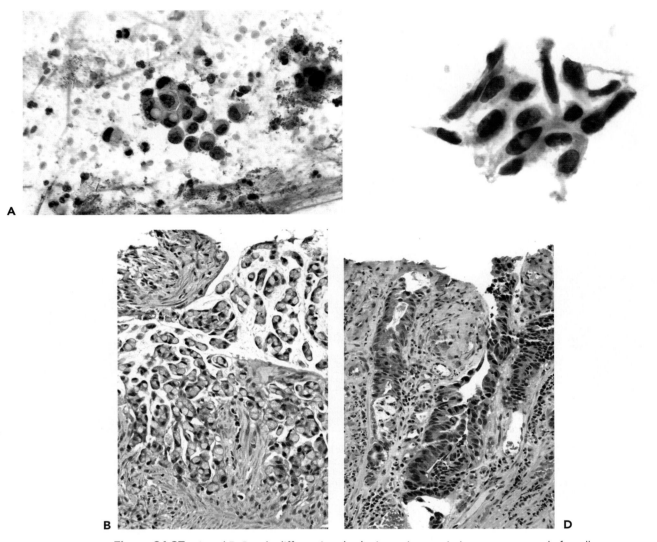

Figure 24-37   A and B: Poorly differentiated colonic carcinoma. *A.* A smear composed of small cancer cells with prominent nuclei and nucleoli and vacuolated cytoplasm corresponding to colloid carcinoma shown in *B.* **C and D: An example of rectal adenocarcinoma.** *C.* Very large columnar cancer cells corresponding to the biopsy shown in *D.* (*C,D:* Photographs courtesy of Dr. June Koizumi, New York Hospital/Cornell Medical Center, New York.)

plasm, basal nuclei and occasional interspersed goblet cells. There may be reactive mucous cell metaplasia or hyperplasia, and occasionally squamous metaplasia (Fig. 24-40B).

Gallbladder

The mucosa of the gallbladder is in branching folds lined by a single layer of tall columnar epithelium with pale eosinophilic cytoplasm and basal or suprabasal smoothly contoured oval nuclei with finely textured chromatin and inconspicuous nucleoli.

INDICATIONS FOR CYTOLOGY

In skilled hands, cytology may contribute significantly to the diagnosis of cancer of the extrahepatic biliary tract, the pancreas or the ampulla of Vater. Although there are pub-

lished examples of presumed precancerous lesions and early invasive carcinomas diagnosed by cytology in symptomatic patients, there is no evidence that this technique is effective in cancer detection.

Obstructive jaundice or **subclinical evidence of bile duct obstruction** (e.g., elevated serum bilirubin, alkaline phosphatase) is the single most important indication for endoscopic bile duct/pancreatic duct cytology. Intraoperative needle aspiration cytology of the gallbladder or imprint/aspiration cytology of the surgically resected gallbladder may have a role in detecting grossly inapparant carcinoma in patients known to be at risk (e.g., cholelithiasis; see below).

METHODS OF INVESTIGATION

Older Sampling Techniques

Cytologic examinations were first carried out on **specimens of duodenal contents,** and on direct collections of bile and

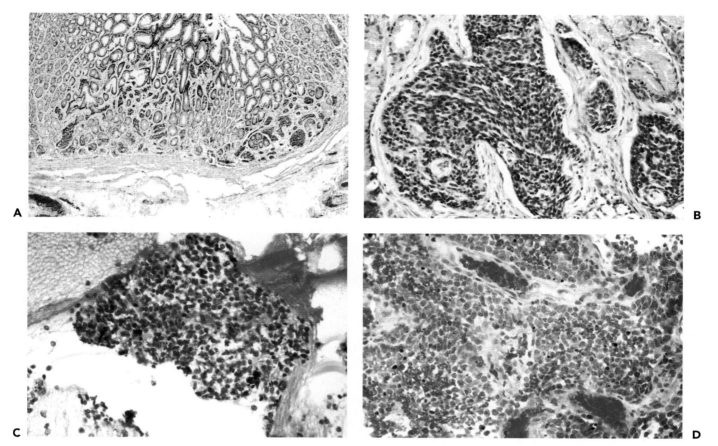

Figure 24-38   Endocrine tumors of the intestine. *A,B.* Low- and high-power view of endocrine tumorlets in a 12-year-old boy with Zollinger-Ellison syndrome. The tumorlets were present within the epithelium and thus could not be identified by cytology (see text). *C,D.* Malignant carcinoid of duodenum identified in brush smear shown in C and corresponding to the tissue biopsy shown in *D.* The lesion metastasized to the liver.

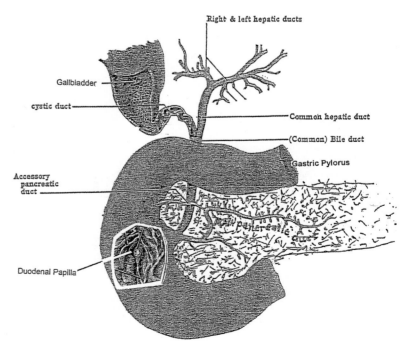

Figure 24-39   Diagrammatic representation of the relationship of extrahepatic biliary and pancreatic ducts, the duodenum, and the pancreas.

pancreatic juice. We must recognize particularly the pioneering efforts of Raskin et al (1958, 1961) in urging the diagnosis of pancreatic and bile duct carcinomas by examination of exfoliated epithelial cells in aspirates of duodenal fluid. Elaborate methods of collecting duodenal contents were devised subsequently to improve specimen quality and diagnostic accuracy (Yamada et al, 1984). Except for carcinomas of the duodenal papilla or ampulla of Vater, however, these specimens usually contained very few poorly preserved tumor cells within a background of necrotic and inflammatory cellular debris. Although Dreiling et al (1960) and Goldstein and Ventzke (1968) claimed diagnostic successes in up to 75% of tumors, the duodenal aspirates generally have been disappointing. Even with improved sampling achieved by **secretin stimulation of the pancreas** (Asnaes and Johansen, 1970; Bourke et al, 1972; Yamada et al, 1984), they failed to gain wide acceptance.

Wertlake and Del Guercio (1976) were, perhaps, the first to demonstrate the feasibility of cancer diagnosis on specimens of bile. Later studies by Cobb and Floyd (1985) and Ishikawa et al (1988) confirmed the diagnostic value of bile cytology. Cell preservation in bile obtained during surgical exploration of the biliary tree has been surprisingly good.

Current Sampling Techniques

Endoscopic Bile and Retrograde Brush Cytology

This technique was made possible by recent advances in endoscopy and is now the most widely used and most effective method of cytologic sampling. With the introduction of endoscopic retrograde cannulation of the common bile duct (**ERCB**) through the ampulla of Vater, it became possible to obtain bile and brush specimens for cytologic examination prior to the introduction of contrast media for radiologic visualization of the duct system. Osnes et al (1975) are credited with introducing this important technique. **Under direct endoscopic visualization, a specially designed brush is threaded into the orifice of the common bile duct (or pancreatic duct) at the ampulla of Vater, and**

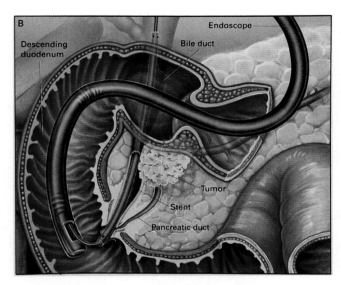

Figure 24-41 Diagrammatic representation of endoscopic retrograde cannulation of the common bile duct (CBD) through the ampulla of Vater. Illustrated here is a tumor of the head of the pancreas that has impinged on and obstructed the CBD as it passes through the pancreas. Brush specimens obtained during the process of opening and stenting the bile duct can provide definitive evidence of carcinoma and exclude inflammatory stricture as a cause of obstruction. (Reprinted from Van Dam J, Brugge WR. Endoscopy of the upper gastrointestinal tract. N Engl J Med 341: 1738–1748, 1999; with permission of publishers of the *New England Journal of Medicine.*)

then into the hepatic ducts and/or main pancreatic duct (Fig 24-41). When the brush is withdrawn, the **adherent cellular material is quickly and evenly spread on one or more glass slides** that are immersed immediately into a 50% alcohol fixative and sent to the laboratory. Alternatively, and preferred by us, **the brush may be placed immediately in normal saline and delivered promptly to the laboratory** for further processing (see Chap. 44). In skilled hands, the endoscopic brushing procedure can be completed within 5 minutes. **Bile** obtained by endoscopic cannulation

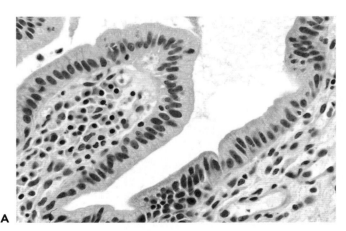

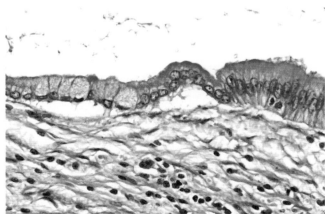

Figure 24-40 Benign epithelia lining the biliary and pancreatic ducts. *A.* Simple columnar epithelium of the extrahepatic biliary and pancreatic ducts. The cells are mucin-secreting with pale staining cytoplasm. They may have cilia. The ovoid nuclei lying in the basal third or half of the cell have delicate chromatin and usually inconspicuous nucleoli. *B.* With inflammation or irritation, the epithelium undergoes hyperplasia with crowding of cells, goblet cell metaplasia (seen here) and increased mucin secretion.

as well as retrograde brush cytology can provide good sampling of well preserved cellular material from selected ducts or areas of interest. We found the brush specimens preferable to bile and consider brush samples the method of choice for cytologic evaluation of patients suspected of harboring carcinoma of the extrahepatic biliary or major pancreatic duct system.

Percutaneous Transhepatic Cytology

When endoscopic retrograde cannulation is unsuccessful or not available, the duct system may be visualized radiographically by percutaneous injection of contrast material into dilated intrahepatic ducts, i.e., by percutaneous transhepatic cholangiography (PTC). Cytologic examinations can be carried out on bile obtained when this procedure is performed, or on subsequent bile drainage specimens. The sensitivity of this method is generally low, but Nilsson et al (1995) reported positive PTC samples in 4 of 8 patients with bile duct cancer. **Cytologic examinations should be included routinely with percutaneous transhepatic cholangiography** and may be diagnostic in some cases.

T-Tube Bile Drainage

Bile can also be a source of cytologic samples. Cressman (1977) reported the cytologic diagnosis of a common duct carcinoma on such a specimen and Muro et al (1983) reported positive cytologic diagnoses of carcinoma in 34 of 100 cases. Simsir et al (1997) found cancer cells present in the saline rinse of biliary stents from 6 of 8 patients with bile duct stenosis caused by cancer.

In an interesting technical modification, Walker et al (1982) used the percutaneous transhepatic cholangiogram and the tip of a decompressing drainage catheter to locate the site of bile duct obstruction as a **guide for percutaneous transhepatic fine needle aspiration.**

Endoscopic Ultrasound-Guided Transmural Needle Aspiration Cytology

The use of this technique is on the increase and we found it to be valuable in some cases (Brugge and Van Dam, 1999; Shin et al, 2002; Stanley, 2003) (Fig. 24-42). The cytologic sample is obtained via a special retractable needle introduced with **ultrasound guidance** during endoscopic retrograde cannulation of the common duct (Howell et al, 1992), and samples are processed according to the preference of the laboratory. Criteria for cytologic diagnosis are the same as brush cytology. **The procedure is advocated in cases of sclerosing tumors, tumors or enlarged lymph nodes extrinsic to the ducts, and tumors beyond reach of the endoscopic brush.** In expert hands, it has had good success without significant complications. Howell et al (1992) obtained positive endoscopic needle aspiration cytology with 100% specificity in 16 of 26 patients, including 10 of 19 with pancreatic carcinoma. Bentz et al (1998) reported 90% sensitivity and 100% specificity in 54 cases of periluminal lymph node aspirates, pancreatic tumors and hepatobiliary lesions. Eloubeidi et al (2003A) reported an accuracy of over 80% of small pancreatic carcinomas with only minor complications. The technique was successful in the diagno-

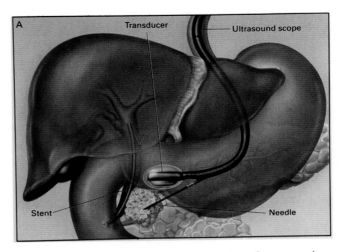

Figure 24-42 Diagrammatic representation of transmural endoscopic fine needle aspiration of pancreatic tumor. If endoscopic brush sampling of the pancreatic duct is unsuccessful or if the tumor is beyond reach of the endoscopic brush, this provides an alternative means of sampling. (Reprinted from Van Dam J, Brugge WR. Endoscopy of the upper gastrointestinal tract. N Engl J Med 341: 1738–1748, 1999; with permission of publishers of the *New England Journal of Medicine.*)

sis of a metastatic carcinoid tumor to celiac lymph nodes (Eloubeidi et al, 2003B).

Percutaneous fine needle aspiration (FNA) of liver and pancreas is described in Chapters 38 and 39.

CYTOLOGY OF DUODENAL ASPIRATES OR WASHINGS

Normal Duodenum

In the absence of disease, there are usually few epithelial cells in the duodenal aspirate. **Cells arising from the duodenal mucosa cannot be clearly differentiated from those of pancreatic or bile duct origin,** which are described and illustrated below. All occur singly or in clusters and have a **columnar configuration with a striated or occasionally ciliated flat luminal surface.** The cells are large and measure 20 to 30 μm in length. Nuclei are round, usually basally placed, and have delicate vesicular chromatin. They often have a small nucleolus. When seen on end in flat clusters, the cells are arranged in a **honeycomb pattern** with the nucleus centrally located within the cytoplasm. In single cells or cells in groups seen from the side, the cytoplasm is generally opaque or sometimes finely vacuolated and may be eosinophilic or cyanophilic. **Goblet cells** may be present singly or in clusters among the columnar cells. They are of approximately the same size as the columnar cells and have a basally placed nucleus with characteristic finely vacuolated supranuclear cytoplasm. In the absence of active disease, the epithelial cells are usually well preserved. The smears contain few macrophages or leukocytes.

Inflammatory Processes

In the presence of active inflammation, most commonly **peptic ulcer, duodenitis** or **pancreatitis,** there is a marked increase in the cellularity of the aspirate. Exfoliated epithelial cells are not well preserved. Most are small and rounded with granular or vacuolated cytoplasm and degenerated nuclei undergoing karyorrhexis or karyolysis and may resemble macrophages (Fig. 24-43). There are numerous stripped or "naked" nuclei, and often a large number of leukocytes and phagocytic macrophages. Orell and Ohlsen (1972) considered **large numbers of stripped nuclei to be characteristic of chronic pancreatitis.** Cheli et al (1974) described an increase in goblet cells in chronic duodenitis.

Parasites and Other Microorganisms

A number of microorganisms have been detected in the duodenal aspirate, including most commonly, the parasite *Giardia lamblia* (see Fig. 24-17A). Joste et al (1999) reported finding *microsporidia* spores in bile from a young man with AIDS and symptoms of cholangitis. The spores are tiny and would be extremely difficult to detect in an inflammatory specimen, even with the help of a silver stain. Papillo et al (1989) identified ova of the liver fluke *clonorchis sinensis* in bile from a patient with cholangiocarcinoma. Wee et al (1995) identified **acid fast bacilli** in T-tube drainage of bile from a patient with hepatobiliary tuberculous pseudotumor, and Kimura et al (1997) detected the fungus, *trichosporon* in bile.

Malignant Tumors

Duodenal aspirates or washings are a poor medium for diagnosis of tumors of the pancreaticobiliary region, particularly when compared with direct brushings, described below. The yield of tumor cells is small and their preservation is generally poor. Only in the rare carcinomas of the **papilla of the ampulla of Vater** is the yield of cancer cells better. The features of the cancer cells are the same as described below for direct brushings of the ducts.

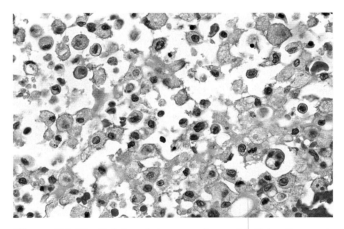

Figure 24-43   **Exfoliated degenerating epithelial cells associated with duodenal ulceration and inflammation.** The cells are rounded with finely vacuolated cytoplasm and pyknotic or lysed nuclei, some resembling macrophages. Leukocytes and red blood cells are few here but are typically present and numerous.

BRUSH CYTOLOGY OF EXTRAHEPATIC BILE AND PANCREATIC DUCTS

Normal Ducts

In the absence of disease, a technically satisfactory **brush** cytology specimen yields abundant benign ductal epithelium, much of which is in irregularly configured flat sheets of cells (Fig. 24-44A) that may be accompanied by granular crystals of yellow or green **bilirubinate** (Fig. 24-44B), **cholesterol crystals** or **crystalline calcium carbonate.** The epithelial cells are in coherent **plaques or strips;** seen on end, the cells comprising such plaques form a **"honeycomb" pattern,** not unlike the pattern of endocervical or gastric cells. A strip of epithelium seen from the side has much the same appearance as the columnar epithelium of bile duct in a histologic section (Fig. 24-44A). Single cells and loose clusters of a few cells are almost always present as well. Some crowding of benign cells caused by inadequate spread of the sample may occur. **"Feathering" of cells** is a brush-induced artifact (Fig. 24-44C) that should not be mistaken for cancer.

The epithelial cells are **columnar** or **cuboidal** with generally pale-staining cytoplasm and a suprabasal **spherical or ovoid nucleus** with delicate chromatin and one or two tiny nucleoli. There may be occasional cytoplasmic vacuoles. There are also tissue fragments containing groups of small, spindly cells with darkly-stained elongated nuclei which are most likely stromal cells (Fig. 24-44D). In the absence of active inflammation, there are few inflammatory cells.

In specimens of **bile,** there are fewer intact plaques of cells and, though sometimes cell preservation is suboptimal, it is adequate for diagnosis in most cases. Cellularity and cell preservation may be improved by saline irrigation of the duct at the time bile is collected (Nishimura et al, 1973).

Atypical Ductal Epithelium

Under a variety of circumstances, some known, such as stones or inflammation, and some unknown, **clusters** of ductal cells may show **nuclear atypia** in the form of isolated enlarged and hyperchromatic nuclei, some showing conspicuous but small nucleoli (Fig. 24-45). The clusters are generally orderly and flat, sometimes infiltrated by polymorphonuclear leukocytes (Fig. 24-45D) and **are not accompanied by single clearly malignant cells.** The interpretation of such atypical clusters may be very difficult, particularly in the presence of obstructive jaundice, as they may reflect changes at the periphery of a carcinoma.

A careful review of the clinical and roentgenologic data is indicated in such cases to rule out **bile stones, an inflammatory process,** or sometimes **extrinsic pressure** on the biliary tree. It has been our policy to report such findings in a conservative fashion, admitting the limitations of cytology in such cases and suggesting a careful follow-up of patients, with additional sampling.

BILE DUCT CARCINOMA

Carcinomas of the extrahepatic bile ducts are relatively uncommon. Edmondson (1967) found 53 cases in a series of

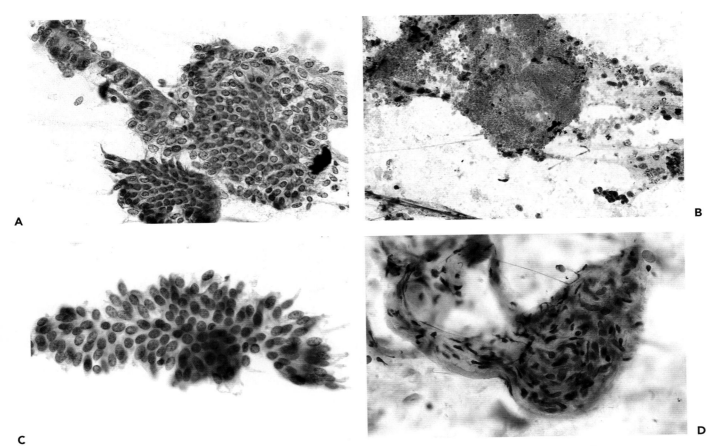

Figure 24-44   Brush cytology of normal biliary or pancreatic ductal epithelium. *A.* The cells obtained by brushing an essentially normal biliary or pancreatic duct are in coherent, flat plaques seen "on end" or from the side. Nuclei are round if the cell is viewed on end and oval if seen from the side. Chromatin is finely textured. Nucleoli may be evident but, in the absence of inflammation, they are inconspicuous. *B.* Inspissated bile in a brushing from a partially obstructed common bile duct. The color may vary from golden-yellow to green. *C.* "Feathering" of ductal cells is a brush-induced artifact. *D.* Spindle stromal cells.

56,000 autopsies (0.1%); 1,380 cases were recorded by the Surveillance, Epidemiology and End Results (SEER) program of the National Cancer Institute over a recent 10-year period in the United States, an estimated incidence of 0.54 cases per 100,000-population (Albores-Saavedra et al, 2000). Most carcinomas are no longer surgically resectable when diagnosed and survival is short. Yet these are potentially curable tumors if confined to the organ of origin and they are amenable to cytologic diagnosis by endoscopic brushing. In fact, short of surgical exploration, endoscopic brush cytology is the only effective means of early diagnosis and is, therefore, of particular interest to the gastroenterologist and cytopathologist.

Extrahepatic bile duct carcinomas occur in patients in their 60s and 70s, are very rare before 40 years of age, and are somewhat more common in men than women. More than 90% of patients present with **symptoms of biliary obstruction,** e.g., jaundice and pruritus. However, tumors narrowing, but not obstructing, the common hepatic or bile duct (see below) or located in the hilum of the liver proximal to the common hepatic duct (**Klatskin's tumor**), may not cause jaundice. About one-third of the patients have a history of cholelithiasis and a surprising number have a history

of prior biliary tract surgery. While there are many conditions that may cause biliary obstruction and jaundice, the most important differential diagnosis of bile duct carcinoma is inflammatory or traumatic **stricture** of bile ducts and **primary sclerosing cholangitis** (see below).

Histology

Carcinomas of extrahepatic bile ducts may grow as polypoid intraluminal tumors but more commonly are nodular or constrictive and diffusely infiltrating the wall of the duct. Three quarters of all extrahepatic bile duct carcinomas are well to moderately differentiated **adenocarcinomas** (Fig. 24-46) and another 4% to 5% each are **adenosquamous, papillary** or **undifferentiated carcinomas** (see below). **Small cell, mucinous** and **signet ring carcinomas** each constitute less than 2% of the bile duct carcinomas.

Brush Cytology

Most carcinomas of the extrahepatic bile ducts are moderately well differentiated and cytologic features are similar to those of other ductal carcinomas. The most abundant

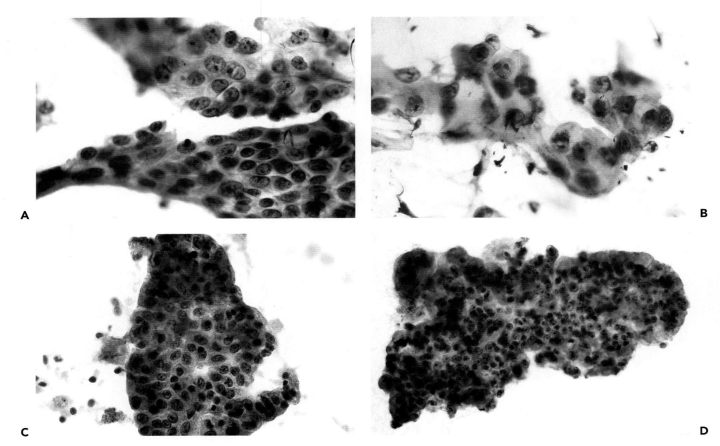

Figure 24-45   Inflammatory atypia in brushings of common bile duct. *A.* Brushing from Ampulla of Vater showing atypia in a patient with gallstones. Though nuclei are enlarged, the epithelial cells form coherent, flat sheets and clearly benign. Nuclear chromatin is delicate and nucleoli are visible but not prominent. *B.* Atypia is more marked in these cells from the same patient. The cells are swollen, with enlarged vesicular nuclei and abundant pale-staining mucinous cytoplasm, and could be considered suspicious. However, nuclear chromatin is delicate and nucleoli, though evident, are not conspicuous. *C.* Reactive epithelial changes in an 82-year-old man with obstructive jaundice. Note the presence of bile pigment. *D.* ThinPrep, same case. There is crowding of cells, mild nuclear hyperchromasia and occasional nuclei with nucleoli. Leukocytes infiltrate the epithelium which retains coherence including well-oriented columnar epithelium at the periphery.

cell samples are obtained from the polypoid tumors. The **tumor cells may be single but also form loosely structured groups that are piled up in three dimensional clusters or disordered flat sheets exhibiting architectural atypia** (Fig. 24-47). **They may also form small papillary clusters, cell-in-cell groups, or occasionally acinar structures** (Fig. 24-47D). Cytologic atypia varies depending upon tumor grade. It is most marked in high-grade carcinomas (Fig. 24-48), and best demonstrated in the few single tumor cells that accompany the cell clusters. Whereas in well-differentiated carcinomas the tumor cells are either somewhat smaller or somewhat larger than normal, in high-grade tumors the tumor cells are three or four times larger than normal may be huge and include mono- or multinucleated giant cells. The cell size and nuclear pallor may increase still further if fixation is delayed even briefly (Fig. 24-48D).

Occasional tumor cells may exhibit cytoplasmic vacuolization and focal mucin secretion, but **mucinous and signet cell carcinomas** are uncommon and yield cells similar to those from other tumors of similar histology observed in other organs.

The most important and most difficult diagnostic task is in the **differential diagnosis of orderly, low-grade adenocarcinoma versus inflammatory or reactive epithelial atypia,** discussed above. The columnar epithelial cells in these two conditions may be similar and nuclear abnormalities of well differentiated carcinomas may not be obvious. However, the tumor cells usually exhibit slight nuclear enlargement, often with irregular nuclear configuration and molding, increased nuclear/cytoplasmic ratio, coarse chromatin clumping and hyperchromasia with visible or even prominent nucleoli. One other important feature in our experience is the **3-dimensional loose aggregation and single cells of carcinoma compared with the flat plaques and fewer single cells of benign reactive atypias.** Benign ductal epithelium is almost always present in the brushings and is useful for comparison with suspect cells. Admittedly, in some cases the distinction cannot be securely made and may require additional sampling.

Bile

Specimens of bile were studied by Nakajima et al (1994) who selected key criteria for diagnosis of carcinoma that

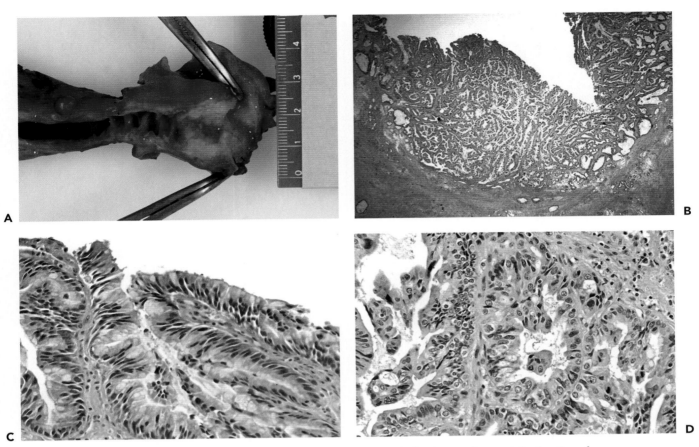

Figure 24-46 Cholangiocarcinoma. *A*. Gross photograph showing carcinoma at the junction of the cystic duct with the common bile duct in a 54-year-old woman with obstructive jaundice. The cystic duct wall is thickened and mucosal folds obliterated. *B*. At low magnification, the ductal epithelium is replaced and the lumen narrowed by the tumor. *C,D*. At higher magnification, the carcinoma is moderately well differentiated, papillary and mucin-secreting.

were similar to cell features described above, and included **loss of honeycomb arrangement, enlarged nuclei, loss of polarity, bloody background and cell-in-cell grouping.** In bile cytology obtained by **transhepatic needle aspiration,** the presence of mucicarmine positive droplets in the tumor cells strongly favors cholangiocarcinoma or metastatic adenocarcinoma over hepatoma. While immunocytochemistry may eventually prove of value, in our experience to date and that of others (Stewart and Burke, 2000), these markers are still of limited value (see below).

RARE TUMORS OF BILE DUCTS

Granular cell tumors of the biliary ducts have been described (Coggins, 1952; Eisen et al, 1991; Butler and Brown, 1998; te Boekhorst et al, 2000; Martin and Stulc, 2000). The cytology of these tumors is discussed in Chapters 20 and 29. A **carcinoid tumor** forming metastases was described by Eloubeidi et al (2003B). A similar case is illustrated in Figure 24-38.

On rare occasions, **squamous carcinoma** or **mixed adenosquamous carcinoma** may arise in the bile duct and cytology samples then contain single or small groups of **keratin-**

ized squamous cancer cells with coarsely textured, irregular, hyperchromatic nuclei and opaque eosinophilic or orangeophilic cytoplasm. Hughes and Niemann (1996) reported two cases of adenosquamous carcinoma diagnosed on brush cytology specimens. When unusual cytologic findings are encountered, one must always consider the possibility of **metastatic carcinoma** to the liver or adjacent hilar lymph nodes causing obstructive jaundice. Dusenberry (1997) reported a case of **hepatoma causing bile duct stricture** in which brushing cytology revealed endothelial cells surrounding clusters of malignant cells, a cytologic feature characteristic of well differentiated hepatoma (see Chap. 38). **Other rare malignant tumors** of the pancreaticobiliary system that deserve brief mention include malignant melanoma and sarcomas (embryonal rhabdomyosarcoma). They are very rare at this site and the cytology of these tumors at other sites is described elsewhere in this text.

PANCREATIC DUCT CARCINOMAS

Brush cytology of pancreatic duct carcinoma is the same as that of extrahepatic bile duct carcinoma (compare Figs. 24-47 and 24-48). In patients whose main pancreatic duct

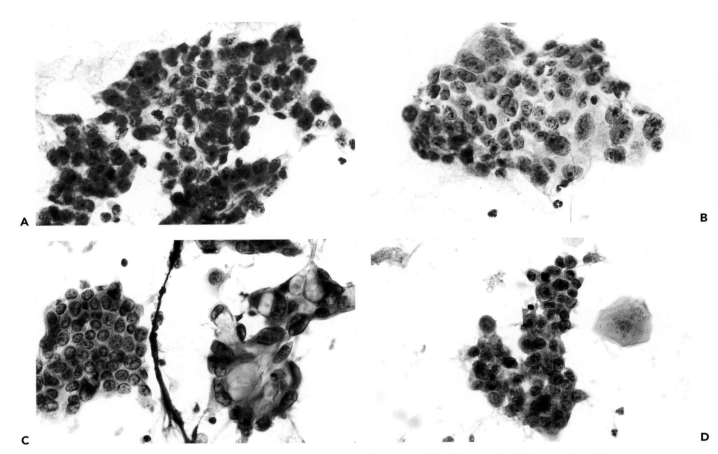

Figure 24-47 Adenocarcinoma in brushing of common bile duct. *A–C.* Cells are enlarged, crowded, overlapping and disarranged with relatively large, coarsely textured, hyperchromatic nuclei. Nucleoli are visible, and may be prominent. Note the gland-like formation in *C. D.* ThinPrep from another case showing cells of adenocarcinoma.

is blocked by carcinoma of the head of the pancreas, it may be possible to cannulate the duct for brushings. If not, a good specimen can be obtained from the dilated distal duct by ultrasound-guided endoscopic transmural needle aspirate (Fig. 24-49). Occasionally, pancreatic duct brushings may result in an unusual diagnosis. Figure 24-50 shows an example of a rare **clear cell carcinoma of pancreas** identified in a brush specimen.

Excellent diagnostic results have been reported with the use of **endoscopic ultrasound devices guided by thin needle aspiration biopsies** (Shin et al, 2002; Eloubeidi et al, 2003A; Stanley, 2003).

PRECANCEROUS LESIONS

Single or multiple areas of **carcinoma in situ ("high-grade dysplasia")** and lesser degrees of epithelial abnormality **("moderate or mild dysplasia")** are commonly present in the extrahepatic bile duct and pancreatic ducts adjacent to or distant from carcinoma.** Albores-Saavedra and Henson (1986) found carcinoma in situ or dysplasia in mucosa adjacent to the invasive carcinoma in 6 of 61 cases. In small series of cases reported by others, precancerous changes accompanying carcinoma ranged from one-third

(Davis et al, 1988) to 45% (Laitio, 1983). Suzuki et al (1989) found carcinoma in situ in 5 of 12 cases. These precursor lesions may be responsible for the high rate of local recurrences following resection of localized tumor. They are characterized in histologic sections by cellular and nuclear abnormalities, hyperplasia and loss of the normal orderly arrangement of the epithelium in an otherwise intact mucosa (Fig. 24-51A,D).

Brush Cytology

Criteria for identification of borderline or precancerous lesions of the main pancreatic and bile ducts are still speculative. They are presumed to be the source of suspicious, though not frankly malignant, cells that commonly accompany the cancer cells in a brush specimen. In several cases seen by us, there were fairly **orderly strips or plaques of columnar or cuboidal epithelium with interspersed large, hyperchromatic nuclei** (Fig. 24-51B,C). In other cytology specimens, dislodged sheets of cells presumed to be from sites of carcinoma in situ have had **overlapping, slightly enlarged but smoothly contoured nuclei** with **granular chromatin, minimal or no hyperchromasia and visible nucleoli.** Distinguishing low level dysplasia from marked inflammatory atypia is difficult in the absence of

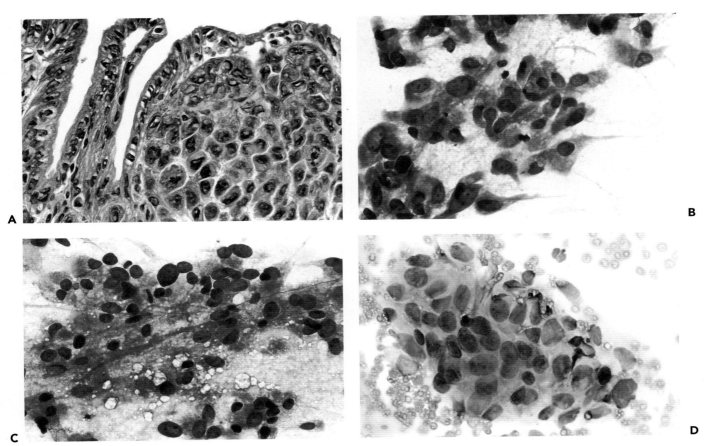

Figure 24-48 Carcinoma of common bile duct in a 77-year-old man. *A.* An area of the tumor showing a focus of anaplastic adenocarcinoma next to a well-differentiated tumor. *B.* A cluster of disarranged, overlapping, predominantly columnar malignant cells with enlarged, hyperchromatic nuclei. *C.* Loosely dissociated cells of adenocarcinoma. *D.* Drying artifact in a brushing of common bile duct carcinoma. Cells are increased in size and pale staining with smudging of chromatin and loss of nuclear detail. (*B,C:* Diff-Quik, Dade Behring Inc., Deerfield, IL.)

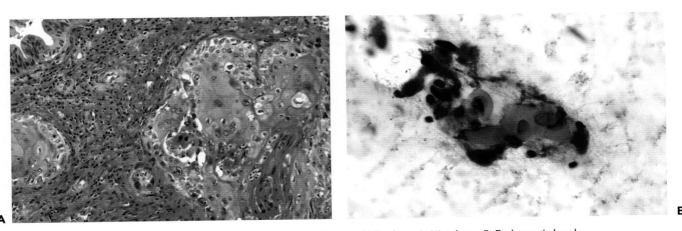

Figure 24-49 Keratinizing squamous carcinoma of bile duct. *A.* Histology. *B.* Endoscopic brush cytology. The cancer cells have densely eosinophilic cytoplasm and hyperchromatic nuclei, resembling squamous cancer cells of other sites. The presence of a few such cells among less differentiated malignant cells is sufficient for diagnosis and classification.

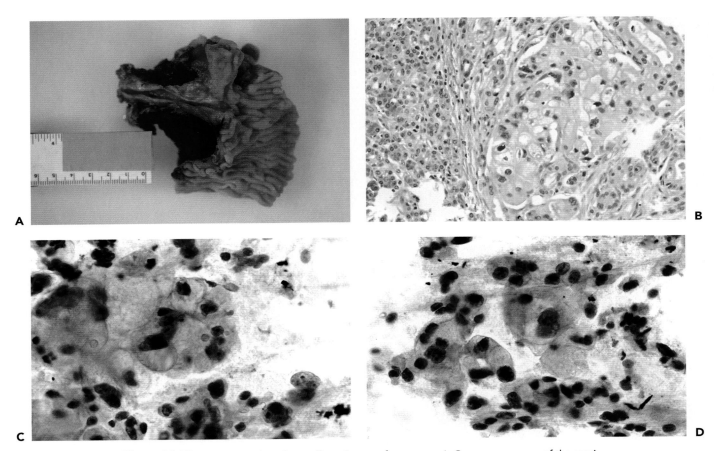

Figure 24-50 **An uncommon clear cell carcinoma of pancreas.** *A.* Gross appearance of the carcinoma arising in the head of the pancreas at the point of junction of the obstructed and dilated common bile with the main pancreatic duct. *B.* Histology of the clear cell carcinoma compared with normal pancreatic parenchyma. The tumor cells are large with abundant, pale-staining "clear" cytoplasm. *C,D.* Tumor cells with abundant pale and delicate cytoplasm and large, irregular hyperchromatic nuclei in a brush cytology specimen form primarily gland-like clusters.

clearly malignant cells. This level of cytologic abnormality warrants repeat examination, which has a high probability of yielding diagnostic cancer cells (see above and Fig. 24-45 for further comments on atypia of bile duct epithelium).

CYTOLOGY OF BILE OBTAINED BY PERCUTANEOUS TRANSHEPATIC ASPIRATES

Bile obtained by percutaneous aspirations contains exfoliated and abraided clusters and single cells of bile duct and hepatic epithelium. Rupp et al (1990), using a device described by Portner and Koolpe (1982), successfully identified 31 of 38 carcinomas, including 21 of pancreatic, 6 of bile duct, 1 of ampullary, 1 of gallbladder origin, and 2 metastatic carcinomas. The specimens varied in cellularity and cellular composition, in degree of cellular preservation and in the presence of blood and inflammatory cells. Bile provides a harsh environment and cellular preservation of epithelium that is not freshly exfoliated may be suboptimal. The reader should be cautioned that, in the presence of chronic obstructive jaundice, the ductal epithelium of bile-filled, distended hepatic ducts and the surrounding hepatocytes may undergo reactive and proliferative changes that mimic carcinoma. However,

nuclear hyperchromasia and structural abnormalities of chromatin seldom approach the level of bile duct carcinoma as described above for brush specimens.

ENDOSCOPIC TRANSMURAL NEEDLE ASPIRATION CYTOLOGY

Cytologic criteria for diagnosis are the same as for percutaneous fine needle aspirates of adenocarcinoma (see Chaps. 38 and 39). The presence of cancer cells in a background of mucin is highly suggestive of an intraductal mucinous adenocarcinoma.

VATERIAN TUMORS

Tumors of the **ampulla of Vater** and/or the **duodenal papilla** are uncommon. They generally present with intermittent jaundice and fever, presumably due to tumor necrosis, and they **mimic the symptoms of biliary calculus.** Obstruction of bile and pancreatic ducts occurs early and duct dilatation often is evident before there is tumor mass. The tumors may be benign (ampullary adenomas) or malignant (ampullary carcinomas).

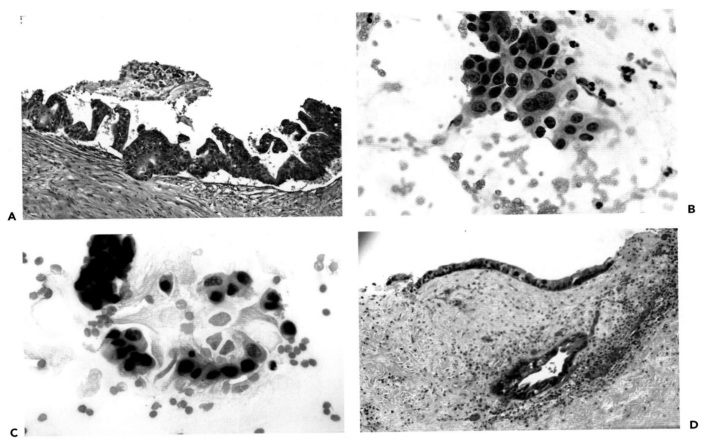

Figure 24-51   Carcinoma in situ of extrahepatic biliary duct. *A.* Histology of carcinoma in situ which may be encountered adjacent to a villous adenoma (see text) or in association with invasive carcinoma. The brush cytology pattern in such cases cannot be differentiated from invasive carcinoma. *B.* Karyomegaly in cells with prominent chromocenters or small nucleoli in a plaque of otherwise benign, unremarkable epithelium. This may reflect focal neoplastic (dysplastic) cellular transformation and, in this case, was seen in the brushing from a patient with carcinoma. The observation is of unknown clinical significance. *C.* Another example of carcinoma in situ. Note the palisade-like arrangement of columnar cancer cells. *D.* Tissue lesion corresponding to *C.* Elsewhere the tumor was invasive.

While **villous adenomas of the ampulla are benign** (Fig. 24-52A), they are considered to be **precursors of adenocarcinoma** (Rosenberg et al, 1986). Foci of carcinoma may be found within the larger adenomas (>12 mm), and co-existing adenoma is frequently found in conjunction with, or at the margins of, adenocarcinoma (Kozuka, 1982; Yamaguchi, 1987; Qizilbash, 1990). **Brush cytology findings of villous adenomas** of the ampulla of Vater were described in four cases by Veronezi-Gurwell et al (1996). The distinguishing feature was the presence of **elongated, slender columnar cells** with elongated, basally placed nuclei, finely granular chromatin and one or more small nucleoli that were either single or formed small groups or sheets (Fig. 24-52B). There may be accompanying bile pigment. In our own experience, the exfoliated epithelial cells closely match normal ductal epithelial cells and we found no reliable cytologic criteria for diagnosis of villous adenoma. The epithelial cells in such cases appeared more rounded and somewhat less uniform than normal, though still columnar or cuboidal. The most useful diagnostic feature was **a grouping of tumor cells into loose three dimensional aggregates** rather than flat clusters.

Ampullary carcinomas yield cells in brushing specimens similar to colonic carcinoma, though usually with less necrosis (see Figs. 24-36 and 24-37). An uncommon tumor that has been observed in the ampulla is a variant of islet cell tumor, a **somatostatinoma,** diagnosed by endoscopic fine needle aspiration cytology by Guo et al (2001).

NONNEOPLASTIC OBSTRUCTIVE PROCESSES

The most common nonneoplastic conditions obstructing the extrahepatic bile ducts are **biliary calculi, bacterial cholangitis, late effects of a stent,** and **primary sclerosing cholangitis** (PSC). Of these, PSC presents the cytopathologist with the **most difficult and most important differential diagnosis** for bile or pancreatic duct carcinoma.

PRIMARY SCLEROSING CHOLANGITIS

Primary sclerosing cholangitis is a chronic, progressive, cholestatic inflammatory disease of the biliary duct system, occurring mainly in men up to the age of 40. The clinical presentation with symptoms and signs of progressing obstructive

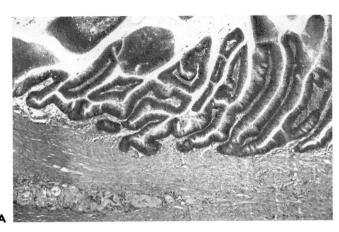

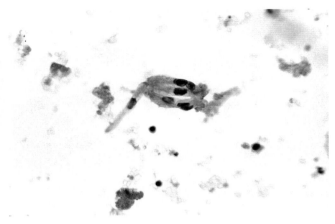

Figure 24-52 **Villous adenoma of duodenum.** *A.* Histology. *B.* Cytology brushings showing elongated epithelial cells (see text). We have not encountered such cells in brushings from a villous adenoma but have seen them in brushing from villous mucosa accompanying carcinoma, as shown here. Note the bile pigment.

jaundice strongly suggest bile duct or pancreatic duct cancer, particularly in the absence of stones. Early in the disease, patients may be asymptomatic or have mild nonspecific symptoms and present with slight elevations of bilirubin or alkaline phosphatase, indicating bile duct obstruction.

The etiology of PSC is unknown but is probably an autoimmune disease. ANCA (antineutrophil cytoplasmic antibodies) are found in most of these patients. PSC is frequently **associated with idiopathic chronic inflammatory bowel disease, most commonly ulcerative colitis.** Intrahepatic bile ducts are involved as well as the extrahepatic duct system and, in some cases, the gallbladder and pancreatic ducts are also involved. The most important complications of PSC are complete obstruction of the common bile duct, bile duct carcinoma which develops in 5% to 10% of these patients, and liver failure late in the course of the disease. In a case seen by us, there was obstruction of the pancreatic duct leading to total atrophy of the exocrine pancreas, sparing the endocrine pancreas. Enns et al (2003) reported that endoscopic retrograde cholangiopancreatography (ERCP) may result in a clinical improvement and that bilirubin levels are an important variable in assessing the status of the patient.

Histologically, the extrahepatic bile ducts exhibit chronic inflammation, fibrosis and stenosis, often with mucosal ulceration.

The experience with **cytologic sampling** of bile ducts in PSC is limited. **Brush cytology** specimens from PSC show **epithelial atypia** with some **crowding and overlapping of nuclei in sheets of cells,** moderate nuclear enlargement and hyperchromasia, and small nucleoli (see Fig. 24-45). In some cases, these cytologic abnormalities may raise suspicion of carcinoma. **Immunocytochemical stains** for p53 and carcinoembryonic antigen (CEA) that are positive in carcinoma and negative or weak in PSC, have been proposed for differential diagnosis. We found them to be of limited value. The differential diagnosis is complicated even more because some of the patients with abnormal cytology were found to have flat or papillary **"dyplasia," or carcinoma in situ** of the mucosa of the bile duct on careful histologic study (Ludwig et al,

1992). At autopsy of patients with PSC, the prevalence of carcinoma reaches 42% (Rosen, et al, 1991).

DIAGNOSTIC ACCURACY OF ERBC

The sensitivity and specificity of cytologic diagnosis by **endoscopic retrograde brush cytology** (ERBC) is highly dependent on the location of the tumor (common bile duct or pancreatic duct), sampling and quality of specimen obtained by the endoscopist and, to a lesser extent, by tumor grade. Brush cytology or ultrasound-guided specimens, obtained by a skilled and experienced endoscopist, properly smeared, fixed and stained, can generally be diagnosed with a high degree of accuracy.

In an early prospective study comparing bile cytology vs. bile duct brushing, Kurzawinski et al (1993) reported positive diagnoses of carcinoma in 69% of 46 patients by brushing and, in 26% of the same group, by bile cytology. There were no false-positive diagnoses and none of those with positive bile cytology had negative brushing cytology.

In a more recent evaluation of bile duct brushing specimens from 131 patients who had biopsy documentation of carcinoma, Kocjan and Smith (1997) achieved sensitivity of 78% with 100% specificity. They reviewed an earlier series to which we have added reports summarizing sensitivity shown in Table 24-6.

In an unpublished series from our own laboratory, Khalbuss and Hussain reviewed 276 bile duct cytology specimens from 187 patients with biliary stricture, of whom 19 had unequivocal evidence of a malignant tumor and 20 were suspicious. All positive cases were confirmed by surgery and pathology (9) or clinical course (10). Of the 20 suspicious cases, 13 had malignant tumors (10 primary in the cholangiopancreatic system) and 2 patients had ampullary villous adenomas. Twelve of 148 patients (8%) with negative brushing cytology proved to have a malignant tumor in the cholangiopancreatic tree (6 bile duct carcinomas; 3 pancreatic carcinomas; 3 ampullary carcinomas).

TABLE 24-6
BILE DUCT BRUSHING SPECIMEN SENSITIVITY FROM PUBLISHED STUDIES*

Year	Authors	No.	Cases Carcinoma	Cytologic Specimen	Sensitivity
Sensitivity Less Than 50%					
1985	Cobb & Floyd	18	Bile duct	Bile	48%
1990	Rabinovitz et al	37	Bile duct	Brushing	
				1st brush	40%
				3rd brush	82%
1991	Foutch et al	17	Bile duct	Brushing	33%
				Bile	6%
1991	Desa et al	24	Bile duct	Brushing	40%
		80	Bile duct	Bile	30%
1994	Ryan and Baldauf	48	Pancreaticobiliary	Brushing	42%
1995	Layfield et al	36	Pancreatic and bile ducts	Brushing	44%
Sensitivity Greater Than 50%					
1977	Harada et al	66	Bile duct	Endoscopic aspirate	83%
			Ampulla	Endoscopic aspirate	100%
1989	Sawada et al	72	Pancreatic	Brushing	85%
1990	Rupp et al	35	Pancreatic and bile duct	Brushing	80%
1990	Scudera et al	20	Pancreatic and bile duct	Brushing	60%
1990	Venu et al	53	Pancreatic and bile duct	Brushing	70%
1991	Witte and Langer	211	Pancreatic and bile duct; and papilla	Brushing	59%
1993	Kurzawinski et al	42	Bile duct	Bile only	33%
		39	Bile duct	Bile & brushing	69%
1996	de Peralta-Venturina et al	55	Pancreaticobiliary	Brushing (68 cases) and bile (8 cases)	100%
1997	Kocjan and Smith	131	Bile duct	Brushing	78%
1999	Trent et al	31	Bile duct	Brushing	80%

* Specificity was 98%–100% in most series.

Kocjan and Smith (1997) **attributed false-negative results to four factors:**

- **Poor sampling on brushing or endoscopic needle aspiration.** These authors suggested that pushing rather than pulling the brush gave better diagnostic results.
- **Overlooking single malignant cells** hidden in a background of inflammatory and necrotic cellular debris
- **Poor recognition of precancerous lesions**
- **Cytologically bland low grade papillary and mucinous tumors**

GALLBLADDER

Indications for Cytology

The purpose of cytologic sampling of the gallbladder is to rule out a primary malignant tumor. The prerequisite for sampling is an enlarged gallbladder, preferably palpable through the abdominal wall. Gallbladder enlargement may have many causes, such as acute or chronic cholecystitis or cholelithiasis, which usually cause clinical symptoms. Painless enlargement may be caused by a cancer of the head of the pancreas obstructing the common bile duct and causing retrograde bile stasis **(Courvoisier's gallbladder).** Primary gallbladder cancer causes symptoms only if associated with stones or in late stages of spread to adjacent organs.

Techniques

Cytologic examination of bile collected in the duodenum or from the common bile duct is of limited value in reference to the gallbladder (Akosa et al, 1995). The gallbladder is out of reach of retrograde endoscopic brushing. The most useful cytologic samples are obtained in thin **needle aspirates of bile from the gallbladder,** either under direct vision at laparotomy or laparascopy, or by ultrasound-guided percutaneous needle aspiration (Zagar et al, 1991). Ishikawa et al (1988) reported that cytologic sampling could be further improved by saline-irrigation at the time of collection. The experience with these techniques in the US is minimal. **Imprint cytology of the gallbladder** was recommended by Vallilengua et al (1995) for detection of dysplasia and occult carcinomas in cholecystectomy specimens of patients at risk.

Inflammatory Lesions

The most common pathologic process involving the gallbladder is chronic cholecystitis, with or without lithiasis (gallstones). **Microcrystalline material and cholesterol crystals** may be present in the bile, usually in association with calculi (Sandmeier and Mihaescu, 2001). Most cases of acute and chronic cholecystitis are nonbacterial and an aspirate of the gallbladder contents reveals a suspension of calcium carbonate and/or cholesterol.

A type of chronic cholecystitis described as **xanthogranulomatous cholecystitis (XGC)** is characterized by a chronically inflamed, thickened gallbladder wall with the presence of many lipid-laden macrophages.

The **association of XGC with carcinoma** of the gallbladder has been repeatedly noted (Goodman and Ishak, 1981; Benbow and Taylor, 1988; Lopez et al, 1991; Krishnani et al, 2000).

Cytology of Xanthogranulomatous Cholecystitis

The cytologic diagnosis of XGC should be considered if a needle aspirate of bile from the gallbladder contains **large foam macrophages with multinucleated giant cells.** Hales and Miller (1987) first reported making this diagnosis by intraoperative fine needle aspirate in a case suspected grossly of carcinoma. Krishnani et al (2000) reported a series of 31 cases of xanthogranulomatous cholecystitis, 11 associated with gallbladder adenocarcinoma.

Krishnani et al described the presence of benign **epithelial cells resembling mesothelial cells** in cohesive clusters as an important morphologic feature of XGC. Other findings, besides the foam cells and **multinucleated giant cells,** were **pink granular background** on May-Grunwald-Giemsa-stained smears. These authors also emphasized the problem with identification of coexisting carcinoma in some cases in the presence of epithelial atypia caused by XGC.

Carcinoma

Carcinoma of the gallbladder is a rare disease of older patients, accounting for fewer than 0.5% of all cancers in women and less than 0.2% of all cancers in men. The incidence is higher in native Americans and Hispanic Americans and there is a **strong association with gallstones,** which are found in more than 80% of cases. Carcinoma is a clinically unsuspected finding in about 2% of cholecystectomy specimens and is most frequent in patients with cholesterol gallstones. The tumors are mainly **adenocarcinomas** of varying degrees of differentiation, though **mucoepidermoid** and **squamous carcinomas** may occur.

Das et al (1998) reported positive cytology in 48 of 82 cases of gallbladder carcinomas with a variety of clinical diagnoses. Sensitivity as high as 88% has been reported by others in a small series of cases (Akosa et al, 1995; Dodd et al, 1996) while 90% sensitivity was reported in a series of 36 cases by Krishnani et al (2000). In a study of 250 patients in whom cholecystectomy was performed for cholelithiasis or cholecystitis, Alonso de Ruiz et al (1982) found **good correlation between histology and the cytology of aspirated bile from the resected gallbladder** in 4 of 6 cases with carcinoma in situ and 7 of 7 cases with invasive carcinoma. There was **poor correlation** with **epithelial hyperplasia and dysplasia.**

The features of adenocarcinoma of gallbladder in needle aspiration biopsy have been described by several observers. In the larger series of cases reported by Akosa et al (1995), Das et al (1998), and Krishnani et al (2000), the cytologic features were those of a **classical adenocarcinoma** with loosely structured clusters of cancer cells with irregular large nuclei and very **prominent nucleoli.** Das et al (1998) reported one case of **mucoepidermoid carcinoma,** five cases of **squamous carcinoma** and two cases of **small cell carcinoma,** all with classical features of these cancers as described elsewhere in this book (see Chap. 20).

Benign Tumors

Papillomas, adenomas, adenomyomas and granular cell tumors have been described in the gallbladder, but are very uncommon. In a series of 1605 cholecystectomies, Kozuka et al (1982) reported 79 invasive carcinomas compared with 18 adenomas, of which 7 had carcinoma in situ. To our knowledge, there are no reports of the cytologic diagnosis of gallbladder adenomas.

BIBLIOGRAPHY

Abe K, Sasano H, Itakura Y, et al. Basaloid-squamous carcinoma of the esophagus. A clinicopathologic, DNA ploidy, and immunohistochemical study of seven cases. Am J Surg Pathol 20:453–461, 1996.

Adler RH. The lower esophagus lined by columnar epithelium: its association with hiatal hernia, ulcer, stricture, and tumor. J Thorac Cardiovasc Surg 45:13–34, 1963.

Afify AM, Al-Khafaji BM, Kim B, Scheiman JM. Endoscopic ultrasound-guided fine needle aspiration of the pancreas. Diagnostic utility and accuracy. Acta Cytol 47:341–348, 2003.

Ahsan N, Berman JJ. Papillary carcinoma of the common bile duct: Diagnosis by bile drainage cytology. Acta Cytol 32:471–474, 1988.

Aka E, Garret M. Diagnosis of the pancreatic carcinoma by cytologic examination of pancreatic duct aspiration fluid during surgery. Ann Surg 167:427–432, 1968.

Akosa AB, Barker F, Desa L, et al. Cytologic diagnosis in the management of gallbladder carcinoma. Acta Cytol 39:494–498, 1995.

Albores-Saavedra J, Henson DE. Tumors of the gall bladder and extrahepatic ducts. Fascicle 22 vol, 2nd series ed. Washington DC, Armed Forces Institute of Pathology, 1986.

Albores-Saavedra J, Henson DE, Klimstra DS. Tumors of the Gall Bladder, Extrahepatic Bile Ducts and Ampulla of Vater. Fascicle 27 vol, 3rd series ed. Washington, DC, Armed Forces Institute of Pathology, 2000.

Aldovini D, Detassis DC, Piscioli D. Primary malignant melanoma of the esophagus. Brush cytology and histogenesis. Acta Cytol 27:65–68, 1983.

Alonso de Ruiz P, Albores-Saavedra J, Henson DE, Monroy MN. Cytopathology of precursor lesions of invasive carcinoma of the gallbladder: A study of bile aspirated from surgically excised gallbladders. Acta Cytol 26:144–152, 1982.

Amieva MR, Vogelmann R, Covacci A, et al. Disruption of the epithelial apical-junctional complex by Helicobacter pylori CagA. Science 300:1430–1434, 2003.

Andersen HA, McDonald JR, Olsen AM. Cytologic diagnosis of carcinoma of esophagus and cardia of stomach. Proc Mayo Clin 24:245–253, 1949.

Anonymous. Unidentified curved bacilli on gastric epithelium in active chronic gastritis [Editorial]. Lancet 1:1273–1275, 1983.

Appelman HD. Pathology of the Esophagus, Stomach, and Duodenum. New York, Churchill Livingstone, 1984, pp 70–119.

Argyres MI, Porter J, Rizeq MN. Diagnosis of clinically unsuspected gall bladder rupture by peritoneal fluid cytology. A case report. Acta Cytol 42:973–977, 1998.

Arnold WT, Hampton J, Olin W, et al. Gastric lesions, including exfoliative cytology. A diagnostic approach. JAMA 173:1117–1120, 1960.

Artlett CM, Smith JB, Jimenez SA. Identification of fetal DNA, cells in skin lesions from women with systemic sclerosis. N Engl J Med 338:1186–1191, 1998.

Asnaes S, Johansen A. Duodenal exfoliative cytology. Duodenal drainage smears after stimulation with secretin. Acta Pathol Microbiol Scand Suppl 212:211–214, 1970.

Auerback O, Stout AP, Hammond EC, et al. Histologic changes in esophagus in relation to smoking habits. Arch Environ Health 14:4–15, 1965.

Ayre JE, Oren BG. New rapid method for stomach-cancer diagnosis; gastric brush. Cancer 6:1177–1181, 1953.

Bader GM, Papanicolaou GN. Application of cytology in diagnosis of cancer of rectum, sigmoid, and descending colon. Cancer 5:307–314, 1952.

Ban-Hock T, van Driel IR, Gleeson PA. Pernicious anemia. N Engl J Med 337:1441–1448, 1997.

Banner B, Beauchamp ML, Liepman M, Woda BA. Interdigitating reticulum-cell sarcoma of the intestine: a case report and review of the literature. Diagn Cytopathol 17:216–222, 1997.

Bardawil RG, D'Ambrosio FG, Hajdu SI. Colonic cytology. A retrospective study with histopathologic correlation. Acta Cytol 34:620–626, 1990.

Barge J, Molas G, Maillard JN, et al. Superficial oesophageal carcinoma: an oesophageal counterpart of early gastric cancer. Histopathology 5:499–510, 1981.

Baron JA, Cole BF, Sandler RS, et al. A randomized trial of aspirin to prevent colorectal adenomas. N Engl J Med 348:891–899, 2003.

Barrett NR. Chronic peptic ulcer of the esophagus and esophagitis. Br J Surg 38:175–182, 1950.

Basque GJ, Boline JE, Holyoke JB. Malignant melanoma of the esophagus; first reported case in a child. Am J Clin Pathol 53:609–611, 1970.

Becker SN, Sass MA, Petras RE, Hart WR. Bizarre atypia in gastric brushings associated with hepatic artery infusion chemotherapy. Acta Cytol 30:347–350, 1986.

Belladonna JA, Hajdu SI, Bains MS, Winawer SJ. Adenocarcinoma in situ of Barrett's esophagus diagnosed by endoscopic cytology. N Engl J Med 291:895–896, 1974.

Bemvenuti GA, Prolla JC, Kirsner JB, Reilly RW. Direct vision brushing cytology in the diagnosis of colorectal malignancy. Acta Cytol 18:477–481, 1974.

Benamouzig R, Jullian E, Chang F, et al. Absence of human papillomavirus DNA detected by polymerase chain reaction in French patients with esophageal carcinoma. Gastroenterology 109:1876–1881, 1995.

Benbow EW, Taylor PM. Simultaneous xanthogranulomatous cholecystitis and primary adenocarcinoma of gall bladder. Histopathol 12:672–682, 1988.

Bennington JL, Porus R, Ferguson B, Hannon G. Cytology of gastric sarcoid. Report of a case. Acta Cytol 12:30–36, 1968.

Bentz JS, Kochman ML, Faigel DO, et al. Endoscopic ultrasound-guided real-time fine-needle aspiration: Clinicopathologic features of 60 patients. Diagn Cytopathol 18:98–109, 1998.

Berg JW. Esophageal herpes; complication of cancer therapy. Cancer 8:731–740, 1955.

Berry AV, Baskind AF, Hamilton DG. Cytologic screening for esophageal cancer. Acta Cytol 25:135–141, 1981.

Bertario L, Russo A, Sala P, et al. Risk of colorectal cancer following colonoscopic polypectomy. Tumori 85:157–162, 1999.

Bhagavan BS, Hofkin GA, Woel GM, Koss LG. Zollinger-Ellison syndrome. Arch Pathol 98:217–222, 1974.

Bhatal PS, Brown RW, Doyle TC, Gray SJ. Pneumatisis cystoides gastrica associated with adenocarcinoma of stomach. Acta Cytol 29:147–150, 1985.

Bian Y-S, Osterheld M-C, Bosman FT, et al. p53 gene mutation and protein accumulation during neoplastic progression in Barrett's esophagus. Mod Pathol 14:397–403, 2001.

Blaser MJ. Gastric campylobacter-like organisms, gastritis and peptic ulcer disease. Gastroenterology 93:371–383, 1987.

Bloch T, Davis TE Jr, Schwenk GR Jr. *Giardia lamblia* in peritoneal fluid. Acta Cytol 31:783–784, 1987.

Boddington MM, Spriggs AI. The epithelial cells in megaloblastic anemias. J Clin Pathol 12:228–234, 1959.

Boddington MM, Truelove SC. Abnormal epithelial cells in ulcerative colitis. Br Med J 1:1318–1328, 1956.

Bodger K, Crabtree JE. *Helicobacter pylori* and gastric inflammation. Br Med Bull 54:139–150, 1998.

Boen ST. Changes in nuclei of squamous epithelial cells in pernicious anemia. Acta Med Scand 159:425–431, 1957.

Bogomoletz WV, Molas G, Gayet B, Potet F. Superficial squamous cell carcinoma of the esophagus. A report of 76 cases and review of the literature. Am J Surg Pathol 13:535–546, 1989.

Bond JH. Screening guidelines for colorectal cancer. Am J Med 106:7S–10S, 1999.

Boon TH, Schade ROK, Middleton GD, Reece MF. An attempt at presymptomatic diagnosis of gastric carcinoma in pernicious anaemia. Gut 5:269–270, 1964.

Borczuk AC, Hagan R, Chipty F, Brandt LJ. Cytologic detection of *Trichomonas* esophagitis in a patient with acquired immunodeficiency syndrome. Diagn Cytopathol 19:313–316, 1998.

Bosset JF, Gignoux M, Triboulet JP, et al. Chemoradiotherapy followed by surgery compared with surgery alone in squamous-cell cancer of the esophagus. N Engl J Med 337:161–167, 1997.

Bourke JB, Swann JC, Brown CL, Ritchie HD. Exocrine pancreatic function studies, duodenal cytology, and hypotonic duodenography in the diagnosis of surgical jaundice. Lancet 1:605–608, 1972.

Boyd DP, Meissner WA, Velkoff CL, Gladding TC. Primary melanocarcinoma of esophagus: report of a case. Cancer 7:266–270, 1954.

Brandborg LL, Taniguchi L, Rubin CE. Exfoliative cytology of nonmalignant conditions of the upper intestinal tract. Acta Cytol 5:187–190, 1961A.

Brandborg LL, Taniguchi L, Rubin CE. Is exfoliative cytology practical for more general use in the diagnosis of gastric cancer? A simplified chymotrypsin technique. Cancer 14:1074–1080, 1961B.

Brandborg LL, Tankersley CB, Uyeda F. "Low" versus "high" concentration chymotrypsin in gastric exfoliative cytology. Gastroenterology 57:500–505, 1960.

Brandt-Rauf PW, Pincus M, Adelson S. Cancer of the gallbladder: a review of forty-three cases. Hum Pathol 13:48–53, 1982.

Brekkan E, Colleen S, Myrvold B, et al. Colonic neoplasia: a late complication of ureterosigmoidostomy. Scand J Urol Nephrol 6:197–202, 1972.

Brenner AJ, Kornstein A, Bandler M, Matzner MJ. Present status of gastric cytology: Study of 60 cases by chymotrypsin method. Am J Gastroenterol 30:415–424, 1958.

Brien TP, Farraye FA, Odze RD. Gastric dysplasia-like epithelial atypia associated with chemoradiotherapy for esophageal cancer: A clinicopathologic and immunohistochemical study of 15 cases. Mod Pathol 14:389–396, 2001.

Broderick PA, Allegra SR, Corvese N. Primary malignant melanoma of the esophagus: a case report. Acta Cytol 16:159–164, 1972.

Brody JM, Miller DK, Zeman RK, et al. Gastric tuberculosis. A manifestation of acquired immunodeficiency syndrome. Radiology 159:347–348, 1986.

Brugge WR, Van Dam J. Pancreatic and biliary endoscopy. N Engl J Med 341:1808–1816, 1999.

Bullock WK, Snyder EN. Carcinoma in situ occurring in pharyngeal diverticulum. Cancer 5:737–739, 1952.

Bultz WC. Giant hypertrophic gastritis: a report of fourteen cases. Gastroenterology 39:183–190, 1960.

Burgess JN, Payne WS, Andersen HA, et al. Barrett esophagus: The column thelial-lined lower esophagus. Mayo Clin Proc 46:728–734, 1971.

Butler JD Jr, Brown KM. Granular cell tumor of the extrahepatic biliary tract. Am Surg 64:1033–1036, 1998.

Cabré-Fiol V. Cytologic diagnosis of esophageal and gastric cancer. *In* Advances in Gastrointestinal Endosopy. Proceedings of the 2nd World Congress of Gastrointestinal Endoscopy. July 1–11, 1970, pp 219–225.

Cabré-Fiol V. Cytology of the digestive system. *In* Marcozzi G, Crespi M (eds). Advances in Gastrointestinal Endoscopy, Padua, Piccin Medical Books, 1972, pp 219–225.

Cabre-Fiol V, Vilardell F. Diagnostic cytologique du cancer du pancreas. Med Chir Dig 4:277–282, 1975.

Cabré-Fiol V, Vilardell F, Sala-Cladera E, Mota AP. Preoperative cytological diagnosis of gastric leiomyosarcoma. A report of three cases. Gastroenterology 68:563–566, 1975.

Cameron AB, Thabet RJ. Recovery of malignant cells from enema returns in carcinoma of colon. Surg Forum 10:30–33, 1959.

Cameron AJ, Ott BJ, Payne WS. The incidence of adenocarcinoma in columnar-lined (Barrett's) esophagus. N Engl J Med 313:857–859, 1985.

Cantrell EG. The benefits of using cytology in addition to gastric radiology. QJ Med 40:239–248, 1971.

Caos A, Olson N, Willman C, Gogel HK. Endoscopic "salvage" cytology in neoplasms metastatic to the upper gastrointestinal tract. Acta Cytol 30:32–34, 1986.

Caplin ME, Buscombe JR, Hilson AJ, et al. Carcinoid tumour. Lancet 352:799–805, 1998.

Carlson SJ, Yokoo H, Vanagunas A. Progression of gastritis to monoclonal B-cell lymphoma with resolution and recurrence following eradication of *Helicobacter pylori*. JAMA 275:937–939, 1996.

Carrie A. Adenocarcinoma of the upper end of the esophagus arising from ectopic gastric epithelium. Br J Surg 37:474, 1950.

Case Record of the Massachusetts General Hospital #13-1995. N Engl J Med 323:1153–1159, 1995.

Chan AO, Luk JM, Hui WM, Lam SK. Molecular biology of gastric carcinoma: from laboratory to bedside. J Gastroenterol Hepatol 14:1150–1160, 1999.

Chan JKC, Ng CS, Isaacson PG. Relationship between high-grade lymphoma and low-grade B-cell mucosa-associated lymphoid tissue lymphoma (MAL-Toma) of the stomach. Am J Pathol 136:1153–1164, 1990.

Chandrasoma PT, Der R, Dalton P, et al. Distribution and significance of epithelial types in columnar-lined esophagus. Am J Surg Pathol 25:1188–1193, 2001.

Chang F, Syrjanen S, Shen Q, Cintorino M, et al. Human papillomavirus involvement in esophageal carcinogenesis in the high-incidence area of China. A study of 700 cases by screening and type-specific in situ hybridization. Scand J Gastroenterol 35:123–130, 2000.

Chang F, Syrjanen S, Wang L, et al. Infectious agents in the etiology of esophageal cancer. Gastroenterology 103:1336–1348, 1992.

Chang KJ, Katz KD, Durbin TE, et al. Endoscopic ultrasound-guided fine-needle aspiration. Gastrointest Endosc 40:694–699, 1994.

Chang KJ, Soetikno RM, Bastas D, et al. Impact of endoscopic ultrasound combined with fine-needle aspiration biopsy in the management of esophageal cancer. Endoscopy 35:962–966, 2003.

Chapman DLS, Klopp CT, Platt LI. Application of balloon technique in detection of cancer. Cancer 6:1174–1176, 1953.

Chaput JD, Gourdier S, Martin E, Larriev H, Etienne J-P. Naevocarcinome primitif de l'oesophage. Sem Hop Paris 50:151–157, 1974.

Cheli R, Astet H, Nicolo G, Ciancomerla G. Cytological findings in chronic non-specific duodenitis. Endoscopy 6:110–115, 1974.

Chen B, Yin H, Dhurandar N. Detection of human papillomavirus in esophageal squamous cell carcinoma by polymerase chain reaction using general consensus primers. Hum Pathol 25:920–923, 1994.

Chen LM, Chao TY, Sheu LF, Hwang WS. Primary cecal lymphoma. Report of a case with preoperative diagnosis by fine needle aspiration and immunocytochemistry. Acta Cytol 36:533–536, 1992.

Chen W, Shu D, Chadwick VS. Helicobacter pylori infection in interleukin-4-deficient and transgenic mice. Scand J Gastroenterol 34:987–992, 1999.

Chen X-M, Keithly JS, Paya CV, LaRusso NF. Cryptosporidiosis. N Engl J Med 346:1723–1731, 2002.

Chinese Academy of Sciences and Honan Province: Coordinating group for research on esophageal carcinoma. Studies on the relationship of dysplasia to carcinoma of the esophagus. Abstract. Proceedings of the 4th International Cancer Congress 4:472, 1974.

Cobb CJ, Floyd WN Jr. Usefulness of bile cytology in the diagnostic management of patients with biliary tract obstruction. Acta Cytol 29:93–100, 1985.

Coggins RP. Granular cell myoblastoma of the common bile duct. Arch Pathol 54:398–402, 1952.

Cohn KH, Ornstein DL, Wang F, et al. The significance of allelic deletions and aneuploidy in colorectal carcinoma: results of a 5-year follow-up study. Cancer 79:223–244, 1997.

Cook IJ, de Carle DJ, Haneman B, et al. The role of brushing cytology in the diagnosis of gastric malignancy. Acta Cytol 32:461–464, 1988.

Cook MG, Goligher JC. Carcinoma and epithelial dysplasia complicating ulcerative colitis. Gastroenterology 68:1127–1136, 1975.

Cooper K. Human papillomavirus DNA sequences in esophagus squamous cell carcinoma. Gastroenterology 107:128–136, 1994.

Cooper WA, Papanicolaou GN. Balloon technique in cytological diagnosis of gastric cancer. JAMA 151:10–14, 1953.

Cordoba A, Manrique M, Zozaya E, et al. Granular-cell tumor of the esophagus: report of a case with a cytologic diagnosis based on esophageal brushing. Diagn Cytopathol 19:455–457, 1998.

Correa P. Precursors of gastric and esophageal cancer. Cancer 50:2554–2565, 1982.

Correa P. Human gastric carcinogenesis: a multistep and multifactorial process—First American Cancer Society Award Lecture on Cancer Epidemiology and Prevention. Cancer Res 52:6735–6740, 1992.

Correa P, Chen VW. Gastric cancer. Cancer Surv 20:55–76, 1994.

Cover TL, Blaser MJ. *Helicobacter pylori* infection, a paradigm for chronic mucosal inflammation: pathogenesis and implications for eradication and prevention. Adv Intern Med 41:85–117, 1996.

Craanen ME, Dekker W, Blok P, et al. Time trends in gastric carcinoma: changing patterns of type and location. Am J Gastroenterol 87:572–579, 1992.

Crespi M, DiMatteo S. The diagnosis of the carcinoma of the stomach in its early phase. Arch Fr Mal Appar Dig 61:285–292, 1972.

Cressman FK. Carcinoma of the common bile duct diagnosis by cytologic examination of T-tube drainage contents. Acta Cytol 21:496–497, 1977.

Cromarty R. Colon cytology simplified using enteric coated encapsulated polyurethane form as a cellular collecting agent. A preliminary report. Acta Cytol 21:158–161, 1977.

Cubilla AL, Fitzgerald PJ. Morphological lesions associated with human primary invasive nonendocrine pancreas cancer. Cancer Res 36:2690–2698, 1976.

Cubilla AL, Fitzgerald PJ. Cancer of the exocrine pancreas. The pathologic aspects. Cancer 35:2–18, 1985.

Czerniak B, Herz F, Koss LG. DNA distribution patterns in early gastric carcinomas: A Feulgen cytometric study of gastric brush smears. Cancer 59:113–117, 1987B.

Czerniak B, Herz F, Koss LG, Schlom J. Oncogene p21 as a tumor marker in the cytodiagnosis of gastric and colonic carcinomas. Cancer 60:2432–2436, 1987A.

Czerniak B, Herz F, Gorczyca W, Koss LG. Expression of ras oncogene p21 protein in early gastric carcinoma and adjacent gastric epithelia. Cancer 64:1467–1473, 1989.

Dag S, Henrik I-S, Lars G, et al. Serial fine needle cytology in the diagnosis of esophageal cancer. Acta Cytol 46:527–534, 2002.

Dahms BBN. Reflux esophagitis: sequelae and differential diagnosis in infants and children including eosinophilic esphagitis. Pediatr Dev Pathol 7:5–16, 2004.

Dao T, Lecointe I, Alix M, et al. Gastric tuberculosis and immunodepression. Gastroenterol Clin Biol 15:864–865, 1991.

Das DK, Tripathi RP, Bhambhani S, et al. Ultrasound-guided fine-needle aspiration cytology diagnosis of gallbladder lesions: a study of 82 cases. Diagn Cytopathol 18:258–264, 1998.

Davenport RD. Cytologic diagnosis of *Campylobacter pylori*-associated gastritis. Acta Cytol 34:211–213, 1990.

Davidson B, Varsamidakis N, Dooley J, et al. Value of exfoliative cytology for investigating bile duct strictures. Gut 33:1408–1411, 1992.

Davis RI, Sloan JM, Hood JM, Maxwell P. Carcinoma of the extrahepatic biliary tract: a clinicopathological and immunohistochemical study. Histopathology 12:623–631, 1988.

Dawsey SM, Lewin KJ, Wang GQ, et al. Squamous esophageal histology and subsequent risk of squamous cell carcinoma of the esophagus: a prospective follow-up study from Linxian, China. Cancer 74:1686–1692, 1994A.

Dawsey SM, Yu Y, Taylor PR, et al. Esophageal cytology and subsequent risk of esophageal cancer. A prospective follow-up study from Linxian, China. Acta Cytol 38: 183–192, 1994B.

Dawson JL. Adenocarcinoma of the middle oesophagus arising in an oesophagus lined by gastric (parietal) epithelium. Br J Surg 51:940–942, 1964.

De Groen PC, Lubbe DF, Hirsch LJ, et al. Esophagitis associated with the use of alendronate. N Engl J Med 335:1016–1021, 1996.

De la Pava S, Nigogsyan G, Pickeren JW, Cabrera A. Melanosis of the esophagus. Cancer 16:48–50, 1963.

De Peralta-Venturina MN, Wong DK, Purslow MJ, Kini SR. Biliary tract cytology in specimens obtained by direct cholangiographic procedures: a study of 74 cases. Diagn Cytopathol 14:334–348, 1996.

De Villiers EM, Lavergne D, Chang F, et al. An interlaboratory study to determine the presence of human papillomavirus DNA in esophageal carcinoma from China. Int J Cancer 81:225–228, 1999.

DeGaetani CF, Sannicola BC, Rigo GP. Primary gastric lymphoplasmacytoid malignant lymphoma (gastric plasmacytoma): an endoscopic cytologic diagnosis. Acta Cytol 21:465–468, 1977.

DeLuca VA Jr, Eisenman L, Moritz M, et al. A new technique for colonic cytology. Acta Cytol 18:421–424, 1974.

Demetri GD, von Mehren M, Blanke CD, et al. Efficacy and safety of imatinib mesylate in advanced gastrointestinal stromal tumors. N Engl J Med 347: 472–480, 2002.

Desa LA, Akosa AB, Lazzara S, et al. Cytodiagnosis in the management of extrahepatic biliary stricture. Gut 32:1188–1191, 1991.

Deschner EE, Long FC, Katz S. Autoradiographic method for an expanded assessment of colonic cytology. Acta Cytol 17:435–438, 1973.

Deyhle P. Coloscopy in the management of bowel disease. Hosp Pract 9: 121–128, 1974.

Dickinson RJ, Dixon MF, Axon ATR. Colonoscopy and the detection of dysplasia in patients with longstanding ulcerative colitis. Lancet 2:620–622, 1980.

DiMagno EP, Shorter RG, Taylor WF, Go VL. Relationships between pancreaticobiliary ductal anatomy and pancreatic ductal and parenchymal histology. Cancer 49:361–368, 1982.

Dodd GD. The role of the barium enema in the detection of colonic neoplasms. Cancer 70:1272–1275, 1992.

Dodd LG, Moffatt EJ, Hudson ER, Layfield LJ. Fine-needle aspiration of primary gallbladder carcinoma. Diagn Cytopathol 15:151–156, 1996.

Dooley CP, Cohen H, Fitzgibbons PL, et al. Prevalance of *Helicobacter pylori* infection and histologic gastritis in asymptomatic persons. N Engl J Med 321:1562–1566, 1989.

Drake M. Gastro-Esophageal Cytology. Basel, S Karger, 1985.

Dreiling DA, Nieburgs HE, Janowitz HD. The combined secretion and cytology test in the diagnosis of pancreatic and biliary tract cancer. Med Clin North Am 44:801–815, 1960.

Dukes CE. The classification of cancer of the rectum. J Pathol 35:323–332, 1932.

Dusenbery D. Biliary stricture due to hepatocellular carcinoma: diagnosis by bile duct brushing cytology. Diagn Cytopathol 16:55–56, 1997.

Dziura BR, Otis R, Hukill P, et al. Gastric brushing cytology: an analysis of cells from benign and malignant ulcers. Acta Cytol 21:187–190, 1977.

Edmondson HA. Tumors of the Gall Bladder and Extrahepatic Bile Ducts. Fascicle 26 vol. Washington, DC, Armed Forces Institute of Pathology, 1967.

Ehya A, O'Hara BJ. Brush cytology in the diagnosis of colonic neoplasms. Cancer 66: 1563–1567, 1990.

Eisen RN, Kirby WM, O'Quinn JL. Granular cell tumor of the biliary tree. A report of two cases and a review of the literature. Am J Surg Pathol 15: 460–465, 1991.

Eloubeidi MA, Chen VK, Eltoum IA, et al. Endoscopic ultrasound-guided fine needle aspiration biopsy of patients with suspected pancreatic cancer: diagnostic accuracy and acute and 30-day complications. Am J Gastroenterol 98:2663–2668, 2003A.

Eloubeidi MA, Chen VK, Volk AL, et al. Recurrent metastatic Klatskin's carcinoid tumor to celiac lymph nodes in a teenager: diagnosis by endoscopic ultrasound-guided fine needle aspiration biopsy with immunocytochemical correlation. Dig Dis Sci 48:2301–2305, 2003B.

Eloubeidi MA, Jhala D, Chhieng DC, et al. Yield of endoscopic ultrasound-guided fine-needle aspiration biopsy in patients with suspected pancreatic carcinoma. Cancer 99:285–292, 2003C.

Eloubeidi MA, Mason AC, Desmond RA, El-Serag HB. Temporal trends (1973–1997) in survival of patients with esophageal adenocarcinoma in the United States: a glimmer of hope? Am J Gastroenterol 98:1627–1633, 2003D.

Enns R, Eloubeidi MA, Mergener K, et al. Predictors of successful clinical and laboratory outcomes in patients with primary sclerosing cholangitis undergoing endoscopic retrograde cholangiopancreatography. Can J Gastroenterol 17:243–248, 2003.

Enrile FT, DeJesus PO, Bakst AA, Baluyot R. Pseudosarcoma of the esophagus (polypoid carcinoma of esophagus with pseudosarcomatous features). Cancer 31:1197–1202, 1973.

Enzinger PC, Mayer RJ. Esophageal cancer. N Engl J Med 349:2241–2252, 2003.

Falk GW, Chittajallu R, Goldblum JR, et al. Surveillance of patients with Barrett's esophagus for dysplasia and cancer with balloon cytology. Gastroenterology 112:1787–1797, 1997.

Faverly D, Fameree D, Lamy V, et al. Identification of *Campylobacter pylori* in gastric biopsy smears. Acta Cytol 34:205–210, 1990.

Feinberg SN. A simple method for the cytologic examination of diarrheal stools. Am J Clin Pathol 57:387–390, 1972.

Fennerty MB, DiTomasso J, Morales TG, et al. Screening for Barrett's esophagus by balloon cytology. Am J Gastroenterol 90:1230–1232, 1995.

Festa VI, Hajdu SI, Winawer SJ. Colorectal cytology in chronic ulcerative colitis. Acta Cytol 29:262–268, 1985.

Filippa DA, Lieberman PH, Weingrad DM. Primary lymphomas of the gastrointestinal tract. Am J Surg Pathol 7:363–373, 1983.

Fletcher CDM, Berman JJ, Corless C, et al. Dignosis of gastrointestinal stromal tumors: A consensus approach. Hum Pathol 33:459–465, 2002; Int J Surg Pathol 10:81–89, 2002.

Flint A, Murad TM. Malakoplakia and malakoplakialike lesions of the upper gastrointestinal tract. Ultrastruct Pathol 7:167–176, 1984.

Fontolliet C, Hurlimann J, Monnier P, et al. Is papilloma of the esophagus a preneoplastic lesion? Schweiz Med Wochenschr 121:754–757, 1991.

Forman D, Newell DG, Fullerton F, et al. Association between infection with *Helicobacter pylori* and risk of gastric cancer: evidence from a prospective investigation. BMJ 302:1302–1305, 1991.

Foutch PG, Kerr DM, Harlan JR, Kummet TD. A prospective, controlled analysis of endoscopic cytotechniques for diagnosis of malignant biliary strictures. Am J Gastroenterol 86:577–580, 1991.

Franquemont DW, Frierson HF Jr. Muscle differentiation and clinicopathologic features of gastrointestinal stromal tumors. Am J Surg Pathol 16:947–954, 1992.

Fraser GM, Kinley CE. Pseudosarcoma with carcinoma of the esophagus. A report of 2 cases. Arch Pathol 85:325–330, 1968.

Fuchs CS, Giovannucci EL, Colditz GA, et al. A prospective study of family history and the risk of colorectal cancer. N Engl J Med 331:1669–1674, 1994.

Fuchs CS, Mayer RJ. Gastric carcinoma. N Engl J Med 333:32–41, 1995.

Fujita S, Hattori T. Cell proliferation, differentiation, and migration in the gastric mucosa: a study on the background of carcinogenesis. Proceedings of the 7th International Symposium, Princess Takamatsu Cancer Research Fund, 1977, pp 21–36.

Fukuda T, Shida S, Takita T, Sawada Y. Cytologic diagnosis of early gastric cancer by the endoscope method with gastrofiberscope. Acta Cytol 11:456–459, 1967.

Gaffey MJ, Mills SE, Lack EE. Neuroendocrine carcinoma of the colon and rectum. A clinicopathologic, ultrastructural, and immunohistochemical study of 24 cases. Am J Surg Pathol 14:1010–1023, 1990.

Galambos JT, Klayman MI. The clinical value of colonic and exfoliative cytology in the diagnosis of cancer beyond the reach of the proctoscope. Surg Gynecol Obstet 101:673–679, 1955.

Galambos JT, Massey BW, Klayman MI, Kirsner JB. Exfoliative cytology in chronic ulcerative colitis. Cancer 9:152–159, 1956.

Galloway DA, Daling JR. Is the evidence implicating human papillomavirus type 16 in esophageal cancer hard to swallow? J Natl Cancer Inst 88:1421–1423, 1996.

Garfinkle JM, Cahan WG. Primary melanocarcinoma of esophagus; first histologically proved case. Cancer 5:921–926, 1952.

Garrett M, Rath H, Pareyman C. Comparison of balloon and lavage techniques in gastric cancer detection and illustration of cytological patterns of gastric cancer. Cancer 13:192–199, 1960.

Ge Z, Taylor DE. Contributions of genome sequencing to understanding the biology of *Helicobacter pylori*. Annu Rev Microbiol 53:353–387, 1999.

Geisinger KR. Endoscopic biopsies and cytologic brushings of the esophagus are diagnostically complementary. Am J Clin Pathol 103:295–299, 1995.

Geisinger KR, Teot LA, Richter JE. A comparative cytopathologic and histologic study of atypia, dysplasia, and adenocarcinoma in Barrett's esophagus. Cancer 69:8–16, 1992.

Ghoussoub RA, Lachman MF. A triple stain for the detection of *Helicobacter pylori* in gastric brushing cytology. Acta Cytol 41:1178–1182, 1997.

Gibbs DD. Exfoliative cytology of the stomach. New York, Appleton-Century-Crofts, 1972.

Giovannucci E, Willett WC. Dietary factors and risk of colon cancer. Ann Med 26: 443–452, 1994.

Glickman JN, Wang H, Das KM, et al. Phenotype of Barrett's esophagus and intestinal metaplasia of the distal esophagus and gastroesophageal junction. Am J Surg Pathol 25:87–94, 2001.

Gnauck R. Screening for colorectal cancer with Haemoccult. Leber Magen Darm 7:32–35, 1977.

Goldman H. Significance and detection of dysplasia in chronic colitis. Cancer 78:2261–2263, 1996.

Goldminc M, Maddern G, Le Prise E, et al. Oesophagectomy by a transhiatal approach or thoracotomy: a prospective randomized trial. Br J Surg 80:367–370, 1993.

Goldstein H, Ventzke LE. Value of exfoliative cytology in pancreatic carcinoma. Gut 9:316–318, 1968.

Goodwin CS, Armstrong JA, Marshall BJ. *Campylobacter pyloridis*, gastritis, and peptic ulceration. J Clin Pathol 39:353–365, 1986.

Gorczyca W, Woyke S. Endoscopic brushing cytology of primary gastric choriocarcinoma. A case report. Acta Cytol 36:551–554, 1992.

Gould VE, Chejfec G. Neuroendocrine carcinomas of the colon. Ultrastructural and biochemical evidence of their secretory function. Am J Surg Pathol 2:1–38, 1978.

Graham DY, Spjut HJ. Salvage cytology: a new alternative fiberoptic technique. Gastrointest Endosc 25:137–139, 1979.

Graham RI, Schade ROK. The distribution of intestinal metaplasia in macroscopic specimen, demonstrated by a histochemical method. Acta Pathol Microbiol Scand 65:53–59, 1965.

Graham RM, Rheault MH. Characteristic cellular changes in epithelial cells in pernicious anemia. J Lab Clin Med 43:235–254, 1954.

Grassi A, Casale V, Fracasso P, et al. Medium-large polyps of the colon: a contribution for their clinical profile and a proper surveillance. J Exp Clin Cancer Res 16:313–319, 1997.

Greene FL, Balch CM, Fleming ID, et al. AJCC Cancer Staging Handbook, 6th ed. New York: Springer, 2002.

Greenebaum E, Brandt LJ. Cytologic study of lavage effluent (GoLYTELY) in colonic adenocarinoma. (1998; unpublished.)

Greenebaum E, Schreiber K, Shu Y-J, Koss LG. Use of esophageal balloon in the diagnosis of carcinomas of the head, neck, and upper gastrointestinal tract. Acta Cytol 28:9–15, 1984.

Greenwald BD, Harpaz N, Yin J, et al. Loss of heterozygosity affecting the p53, Rb and mcc/apc tumor suppressor gene loci in dysplastic and cancerous ulcerative colitis. Cancer Res 52:741–745, 1992.

Gress F, Gottlieb K, Sherman S, Lehman G. Endoscopic ultrasonography-guided fine-needle aspiration biopsy of suspected pancreatic cancer. Ann Intern Med 134:459–464, 2001.

Gretillat PA. Depistage cytologique de quelques cas de carcinome dit "in situ" de l'estomac. Med Wochenschr Schweiz 99:582–583, 1969.

Guarner J, Herrera-Goepfert R, Mohar A, et al. Interobserver variability in application of the revised Sydney classification for gastritis. Hum Pathol 30:1431–1434, 1999.

Guo M, Lemos LB, Bigler S, Baliga M. Duodenal somatostatinoma of the ampulla of vater diagnosed by endoscopic fine needle aspiration biopsy: a case report. Acta Cytol 45:622–626, 2001.

Gupta RK, Rogers KE. Endoscopic cytology and biopsy in the diagnosis of gastroesophageal malignancy. Acta Cytol 27:17–22, 1983.

Haenszel W, Correa P, Cuebllo C, et al. Gastric cancer in Columbia. II. Case-control epidemiologic study of precursor lesions. J Natl Cancer Inst 57:1021–1026, 1976.

Haggitt RC. Adenocarcinoma in Barrett's esophagus: A new epidemic? Hum Pathol 23:475–476, 1992.

Haggitt RC, Reid BJ, Rabinovitch PS, Rubin CE. Barrett's esophagus. Correlation between mucin histochemistry, flow cytometry, and histologic diagnosis for predicting increased cancer risk. Am J Pathol 131:53–61, 1988.

Haggitt RC, Tryzelaar J, Ellis FH, Colcher H. Adenocarcinoma complicating columnar epithelium-lined (Barrett's) esophagus. Am J Clin Pathol 70:1–5, 1978.

Hales MS, Miller TR. Diagnosis of xanthogranulomatous cholecystitis by fine needle aspiration biopsy. A case report. Acta Cytol 31:493–496, 1987.

Halpern M, Gal R, Rath-Wolfson L, et al. Brush cytology and biopsy in the diagnosis of colorectal cancer. A comparison. Acta Cytol 41:628–632, 1997.

Hampton JM, Bacon HE, Myers J. A simplified method for the diagnosis of cancer of the colon by exfoliative cytology. Dis Colon Rectum 5:145–147, 1962.

Hanson J, Thoreson C, Morrissay JF. Brush cytology in the diagnosis of upper gastrointestinal lesions. Gastrointest Endosc 26:33–35, 1980.

Harada H, Sasaki T, Yamamoto N, et al. Assessment of endoscopic aspiration cytology and endoscopic retrograde cholangio-pancreatography in patients with cancer of the hepato-biliary tract. Part II. Gastroenterol Jpn 12:59–64, 1977.

Hatfield ARW, Whittaker R, Gibbs DD. The collection of pancreatic fluid for cytodiagnosis using a duodenoscope. Gut 15:305–307, 1974.

Hawe A, Payne WS, Weiland LH, et al. Adenocarcinoma in the columnar epithelial lined lower (Barrett oesophagus). Thorax 28:511–514, 1973.

Hayashida T, Kidokoro T. End results in early gastric cancer collected from 22 institutions. Stomach Intestine (Japan) [cited by Kobayashi et al, 1970] 4:1077–1085, 1969.

He D, Zhang DK, Lam KY, et al. Prevalence of HPV infection in esophageal squamous cell carcinoma in Chinese patients and its relationship to the p53 gene mutation. Int J Cancer 72:959–964, 1997.

Heath CW Jr. Rheumatoid arthritis, aspirin, and gastrointestinal cancer. J Natl Cancer Inst 85:258–259, 1993.

Henning N, Witte S. Atlas der Gastroenterologischen Cytodiagnostik. Stuttgart, Georg Thieme, 1957.

Henning N, Witte S, Bressel D. The cytologic diagnosis of tumors of the upper gastrointestinal tract (esophagus, stomach, duodenum). Acta Cytol 8:121–130, 1964.

Henson DE, Albores-Saavedra J, Corle D. Carcinoma of the gallbladder. Histologic types, stage of disease, grade, and survival rates. Cancer 70:1493–1497, 1992.

Hishon S, Lovell D, Gummer JWP, et al. Cytology in the diagnosis of oesophageal cancer. Lancet 1:296–297, 1976.

Hixon C, Furlong J, Silbergleit A. Flow cytometry in colon cancer: does flow cytometric cell cycle analysis help predict for short-term recurrence in patients with colorectal carcinoma? J Natl Med Assoc 87:803–806, 1995.

Hoda SA, Hajdu SI. Small cell carcinoma of the esophagus. Cytology and immunohistology in four cases. Acta Cytol 36:113–120, 1992.

Hoffler AS, Rubel LR. Free-living amoebae identified by cytologic examination of gastrointestinal washings. Acta Cytol 18:59–61, 1974.

Horai T, Kobayashi A, Takeishi R, Wada A, Taniguchi H, Taniguchi K, Sano M, Tamura H. A cytologic study on small cell carcinoma of the esophagus. Cancer 41:1890–1878, 1978.

Horn RC. Malignant potential of polypoid lesions colon and rectum. Cancer 28:146–152, 1971.

Howell DA, Beveridge RP, Bosco J, Jones M. Endoscopic needle aspiration biopsy at ERCP in the diagnosis of biliary strictures. Gastrointest Endosc 38:531–535, 1992.

Howell LP, Chow HC, Russell LA. Cytodiagnosis of extrahepatic biliary duct tumors from specimens obtained during cholangiography. Diagn Cytopathol 4:328–334, 1988.

Hsing AW, Hansson, L-E, McLaughlin JK, et al. Pernicious anemia and subsequent cancer: A population-based cohort study. Cancer 71:745–750, 1993.

Huang GJ, K'ai WY. Carcinoma of the Esophagus and Gastric Cardia. New York, Springer-Verlag, 1984, pp 156–190.

Hughes JH, Cohen MB. Is the cytologic diagnosis of esophageal glandular dysplasia feasible? Diagn Cytopathol 18:312–316, 1998.

Hughes JH, Cruickshank AH. Pseudosarcoma of the oesophagus. Br J Surg 56:72–76, 1969.

Hughes JH, Leigh CJ, Raab SS, et al. Cytologic criteria for the brush diagnosis of gastric adenocarcinoma. Cancer 84:289–294, 1998.

Hughes JH, Niemann TH. Adenosquamous carcinoma of the bile duct: cytologic features of brush specimens from two cases. Diagn Cytopathol 15:322–324, 1996.

Hulscher JBF, van Sandick JW, de Boer AGEM, et al. Extended transthoracic resection compared with limited transhiatal resection for adenocarcinoma of the esophagus. N Engl J Med 347:1662–1669, 2002.

Huntsman DG, Carneiro F, Lewis FR, et al. Early gastric cancer in young, asymptomatic carriers of germ-line E-cadherin mutations. N Engl J Med 344:1904–1909, 2001.

Hurlimann J, Gardiol D. Gastrointestinal stromal tumors: an immunohistochemical study of 165 cases. Histopathology 19:311–320, 1991.

Ide H, Nakamura T, Hayashi K, et al. Esophageal squamous cell carcinoma: pathology and prognosis. World J Surg 18:321–330, 1994.

Imai T, Sannohe Y, Okano H. Oat cell carcinoma (apudoma) of the esophagus. Cancer 41:358–364, 1978.

Imbriglia JE, Lopusniak MS. Cytologic examination of sediment from esophagus in case of intra-epidermal carcinoma of esophagus. Gastroenterology 13:457–463, 1949.

Inger DB. Colorectal cancer screening. Prim Care 26:179–187, 1999.

Inokuchi K, Inutsuka S, Furusawa M, et al. Development of superficial carcinoma of the stomach: report of late recurrence. Ann Surg 164:145–151, 1966.

Isaacson PG. The MALT lymphoma concept updated. Ann Oncol 6:319–320, 1995.

Isaacson PG, Jones DB, Sworn MJ, Wright DH. Malignant histiocytosis of the intestine: report of three cases with immunological and cytochemical analysis. J Clin Pathol 35:510–516, 1982.

Isaacson PG, Norton AJ. Malignant lymphoma of the gastrointestinal tract. In Isaacson PG, Norton AJ (eds). Extranodal lymphomas. Edinburgh, Scotland, Churchill Livingstone, 1994, pp 15–65,

Isaacson PG, Wright DH. Extranodal malignant lymphoma arising from mucosa-associated lymphoid tissue. Cancer 53:2515–2524, 1984.

Ishikawa O, Ohhigashi H, Sasaki Y, et al. The usefulness of saline-irrigated bile for the intraoperative cytologic diagnosis of tumors and tumorlike lesions of the gallbladder. Acta Cytol 32:475–481, 1988.

Isimbaldi G, Santangelo M, Cenacchi G, et al. Gastrointestinal autonomic nerve tumor (plexosarcoma): report of a case with fine needle aspiration and histologic, immunologic and ultrastructural study. Acta Cytol 42:1189–1194, 1998.

Iwabuchi M, Sasano H, Hiwatashi N, et al. Serrated adenoma: a clinicopathological DNA ploidy and immunohistochemical study. Anticancer Res 20:1141–1147, 2000.

Izbicki JR, Hosch SB, Pichlmeier U, et al. Prognostic value of immunohistochemically identifiable tumor cells in lymph nodes of patients with completely resected esophageal cancer. N Engl J Med 337:1188–1194, 1997.

Jackson BR. Adenomas of the colon and rectum: histopathology and management. Dis Colon Rectum 17:656–666, 1974.

Jain S, Kumar N, Das DK, Jain SK. Esophageal tuberculosis: Endoscopic cytology as a diagnostic tool. Acta Cytol 43:1085–1090, 1999.

Jain S, Kumar N, Jain SK. Gastric tuberculosis. Endoscopic cytology as a diagnostic tool. Acta Cytol 44:987–992, 2000.

Jaskiewicz K, Venter FS, Marasas WF. Cytopathology of the esophagus in Transkei. J Natl Cancer Inst 79:961–967, 1987.

Jass JR. A classification of gastric dysplasia. Histopathology 7:181–193, 1983.

Jensen O, Schade ROK. The value of a chymotrypsin for a diagnostic gastric lavage. Acta Cytol 6:475–477, 1962.

Jernstrom P, Brewer LA. III. Primary adenocarcinoma of the mid-esophagus arising in ectopic gastric mucous with associated hiatal hernia and reflux esophagitis (Dawson's syndrome). Cancer 26:1343–1348, 1970.

Jhala NC, Jhala DN, Chhieng DC, et al. Endoscopic ultrasound-guided fine-needle aspiration. A cytopathologist's perspective. Am J Clin Pathol 120:351–367, 2003.

Joensuu H, Roberts PJ, Sarlomo-Rikala M, et al. Effect of the tyrosine kinase inhibitor STI571 in a patient with a metastatic gastrointestinal stromal tumor. N Engl J Med 344:1052–1056, 2001.

Johnson WD, Koss LG, Papanicolaou GN, Seybolt JF. Cytology of esophageal washings; evaluation of 364 cases. Cancer 8:951–957, 1955.

Joste NE, Sax PE, Pieciak WS. Cytologic detection of microsporidia spores in bile. A comparison of stains. Acta Cytol 43:98–103, 1999.

Kalnins ZA, Rhyne AL, Dixon FR, Girsh S. Analysis of cytologic findings in patients with gastric carcinoma. Acta Cytol 11:312–318, 1967.

Kanavaros P, Galian A, Periac P, et al. Melanome malin primitif de l'oesophage developpe sur une melanose. Ann Pathol 1:57–61, 1989.

Kasugai T. Evaluation of gastric lavage cytology under direct vision by the fibergastroscope employing Hanks' solution as a washing solution. Acta Cytol 12:345–351, 1968.

Kasugai T, Kobayashi S. Evaluation of biopsy and cytology in the diagnosis of gastric cancer. Am J Gastroenterol 62:199–203, 1974.

Katz S, Katzka I, Platt N, et al. Cancer in chronic ulcerative colitis. Diagnostic role of segmental colonic lavage. Am J Dig Dis 22:355–364, 1977.

Katz S, Klein MS, Winawer SJ, Sherlock P. Disseminated lymphoma involving the stomach. Correlation of endoscopy with directed cytology and biopsy. Am J Dig Dis 18:370–374, 1973.

Katz S, Sherlock P, Winawer SJ. Rectocolonic exfoliative cytology. A new approach. Am J Dig Dis 17:1109–1116, 1972.

Katz S. Newer diagnostic techniques: rectocolonic exfoliative cytology—a new approach. Dis Colon Rectum 17:3–5 1974.

Kaul V, Wani NA, Paljor YD. Primary carcinoma of gall bladder: A review of thirty-six cases. Indian J Pathol Microbiol 32:146–151, 1989.

Kawachi T, Kurisu M, Numanyu N, et al. Precancerous changes in the stomach Cancer Res 36:2673–2677, 1976.

Kawaguchi H, Ohno S, Araki K, et al. p53 polymorphism in human papillomavirus-associated esophageal cancer. Cancer Res 60:2753–2755, 2000.

Kill J, Andersen D, Jensen OM. Biopsy and brush cytology in the diagnosis of gastric cancer. Scand J Gastroenterol 14:189–191, 1979.

Kimura M, Maekura S, Otsuka M, Satou T. Trichosporon detected on bile cytology. Acta Cytol 41:1869–1870, 1997.

King R, Quinonez GE, Gough JC. Fine needle aspiration biopsy diagnosis of a gastrointestinal stromal tumor utilizing transmission electron microscopy. Acta Cytol 40:581–584, 1996.

Kjeldsberg CR, Altshuler HJ. Carcinoma in situ of the colon. Dis Colon Rectum 13:376–381, 1970.

Kline TS, Goldstein F. Malignant lymphoma involving the stomach. Cancer 32:961–968, 1973.

Kline TS, Goldstein F. The role of cytology in the diagnosis of gastric lymphoma. Am J Gastroenterol 62:193–198, 1974.

Kline TS, Yum KK. Fiberoptic coloscopy and cytology. Cancer 37:2553–2556, 1976.

Kobayashi S, Prolla JC, Kirsner JB. Brushing cytology of the esophagus and stomach under direct vision by fiberscopes. Acta Cytol 14:219–223, 1970.

Kobayashi S, Sugiura H, Kasugai T. Reliability of endoscopic observation in diagnosis of early carcinoma of stomach. Endoscopy 4:61–65, 1972.

Kocjan G, Smith AN. Bile duct brushings cytology: potential pitfalls in diagnosis. Diagn Cytopathol 16:358–363, 1997.

Koizumi JH, Schron DS. Cytologic features of colonic carcinoma. Differences between primary and metastatic neoplasms. Acta Cytol 41: 419–426, 1997.

Kosch T, Lorenz R, Zenker K. Local staging and assessment of resectability in carcinoma of the esophagus, stomach and duodenum by endoscopic ultrasonography. Gastrointest Endosc 38:460–467, 1992.

Koss LG. Abdominal gas cysts (pneumatosis cystoides intestinorum hominis): an analysis with report of a case and a critical review of the literature. Arch Pathol 53:523–549, 1952.

Koss LG, Morgenstern N, Tahir-Kheli N, et al. Evaluation of esophageal cytology using a neural net-based interactive scanning system (the PAPNET System). Its possible role in screening for esophageal and gastric carcinoma. Am J Clin Pathol 109:549–557, 1998.

Kozuka S, Tsubone N, Yasui A, Hachisuka K. Relation of adenoma to carcinoma in the gallbladder. Cancer 50:2226–2234, 1982.

Krishnani N, Shukla S, Jain M, et al. Fine needle aspiration cytology in xanthogranulomatous cholecystitis, gallbladder adenocarcinoma and coexistent lesions. Acta Cytol 44:508–514, 2000.

Kurokawa T, Kajitani T, Oota K. Carcinoma of Stomach in Early Phase. Tokyo, Nakayama-Shoten, 1967.

Kurokawa T, Saito T, Yonemura H, et al. Cytological diagnosis of gastric cancer. Exp Med Tuhoku 71:209–224, 1960.

Kurzawinski TR, Deery A, Dooley JS, et al. A prospective study of biliary cytology in 100 patients with bile duct strictures. Hepatology 18:1399–1403, 1993.

Kuwano H, Nagamatsu M, Ohno S, et al. Coexistence of intraepithelial carcinoma and glandular differentiation in esophageal squamous cell carcinoma. Cancer 62:1568–1572, 1988.

Kwong D, Lam A, Guan X, et al. Chromosomal aberrations in esophageal squamous cell carcinoma among Chinese: Gain of 12p predicts poor prognosis after surgery. Hum Pathol 35:309–316, 2004.

Ladenheim J, Garcia G, Titzer D, et al. Effect of sulindac on sporadic colonic polyps. Gastroenterology 108:1083–1087, 1995.

Lagergren J, Bergstrom R, Lindgren A, Nyren O. Symptomatic gastroesophageal reflux as a risk factor for esophageal adenocarcinoma. N Engl J Med 340:825–831, 1999.

Laitio M. Carcinoma of extrahepatic bile ducts: A histopathologic study. Pathol Res Pract 178:67–72, 1983.

Lane N. The precursor tissue of ordinary large bowel cancer. Cancer Res 36:2669–2672, 1976.

Lauren P. The two histological main types of gastric carcinoma: Diffuse and so-called intestinal type carcinoma. An attempt at a histo-clinical classification. Acta Pathol Microbiol Scand 64:31–49, 1965.

Lavergne D, de Villiers EM. Papillomavirus in esophageal papillomas and carcinomas. Int J Cancer 80:681–684, 1999.

Layfield LJ, Reichman A, Weinstein WM. Endoscopically directed fine needle aspiration biopsy of gastric and esophageal lesions. Acta Cytol 36:69–74, 1992.

Layfield LJ, Wax TD, Lee JG, Cotton PB. Accuracy and morphologic aspects of pancreatic and biliary duct brushings. Acta Cytol 39:11–18, 1995.

Lederer B, Schwamberger K, Falser N, et al. Die zytodiagnostik der Magenspülflüssigkeit, eine brauchbare Hilfe bei der Karzinomsuche. Wien Klin Wochenschr 86:464–466, 1974.

Lee A. The Helicobacter pylori genome: New insights into pathogenesis and therapeutics. N Engl J Med 338:832–833, 1998.

Lee JR, Joshi V, Griffin JW Jr, et al. Gastrointestinal nerve tumor. Immunohistochemical and molecular identity with gastrointestinal stromal tumor. Am J Surg Pathol 25:979–987, 2001.

Lee RG. Dysplasia in Barrett's esophagus. Am J Pathol 9:845–852, 1985.

Leong AS, Sormunen RT, Tsui WM, Liew CT. Hep Par 1 and selected antibodies in the immunohistological distinction of hepatocellular carcinoma from cholangiocarcinoma, combined tumours and metastatic carcinoma. Histopathology 33:318–324, 1998.

Lerut T, De Leyn P, Coosemans W, et al. Surgical strategies in esophageal carcinoma with emphasis on radical lymphadenectomy. Ann Surg 216:583–590, 1992.

Lewin KJ, Ranchod M, Dorfman RF. Lymphomas of the gastrointestinal tract: a study of 117 cases presenting with gastrointestinal disease. Cancer 42:693–707, 1978.

Li J-Y, Ershow AG, Chen Z-J, et al. A case-control study of cancer of the esophagus and gastric cardia in Linxian. Int J Cancer 43:755–761, 1989.

Li SQ, O'Leary TJ, Buchner, S-B, et al. Fine needle aspiration of gastrointestinal stromal tumors. Acta Cytol 45:9–17, 2001.

Liacouras CA. Eosinophilic esophagitis in children and adults. J Pediatr Gastroenterol Nutr 37:23–28, 2003.

Lieberman D. How to screen for colon cancer. Annu Rev Med 49:163–172, 1998.

Lieberman MD, Shriver CD, Bleckner S, et al. Carcinoma of the esophagus: prognostic significance of histologic types. J Thorac Cardiovasc Surg 109:130–139, 1995.

Lightdale CJ, Wolf DJ, Marcucci BA, Salyer WR. Herpetic esophagitis in patients with cancer: antemortem diagnosis by brush cytology. Cancer 39:223–226, 1977.

Linehan JJ, Melcher DH, Strachan CJL. Rapid out-patient detection of rectal cancer by gloved digital scrape cytology. Acta Cytol 27:146–151, 1983.

Lipkin M. Proliferative changes in the colon. Am J Dig Dis 19:1029–1032, 1974.

Loeb RA, Scapier J. Rectal washings, technic for cytologic study of recto-sigmoid; preliminary report. Am J Surg 81:298–302, 1951.

Lopez JI, Elizalde JM, Calvo MA. Xanthogranulomatous cholecystitis associated with gall bladder adenocarcinoma. A clinicopathological study of 5 cases. Tumori 77:358–360, 1991.

Lozowski W, Hajdu SI. Preoperative cytologic diagnosis of primary gastrointestinal lymphoma. Acta Cytol 28:563–570, 1984.

Ludwig J, Wahlstrom HE, Batts KP, Wiesner RH. Papillary bile duct dysplasia in primary sclerosing cholangitis. Gastroenterology 102:2134–2138, 1992.

Ludwig ME, Shaw R, de Suto-Nagy G. Primary malignant melanoma of the esophagus. Cancer 48:2528–2534, 1981.

Lundquest DE, Marcus JN, Thorson AG, Massop D. Primary squamous cell carcinoma of the colon arising in a villous adenoma. Hum Pathol 19:362–364, 1988.

Lynch HT, de la Chapelle A. Hereditary colorectal cancer. N Engl J Med 348:919–932, 2003.

MacGregor IL. Carcinoma of the colon and the stomach. A review with comment on epidemiologic associations. JAMA 227:911–915, 1974.

MacMahon B. Risk factors for cancer of the pancreas. Cancer 50:2676–2680, 1982.

Maeyama H, Hidaka E, Ota H, et al. Familial gastrointestinal stromal tumor with hyperpigmentation: association with a germline mutation of the c-kit gene. Gastroenterology 120:210–215, 2001.

Magnus GA. Reassessment of gastric lesion in pernicious anemia. J Clin Pathol 11:289–295, 1958.

Maimon HN, Dreskin RB, Cocco AE. Positive esophageal cytology without detectable neoplasm. Gastrointest Endosc 20:156–159, 1974.

Makhlouf HR, Burke AP, Sobin LH. Carcinoid tumors of the ampulla of Vater: a comparison with duodenal carcinoid tumors. Cancer 85:1241–1249, 1999.

Mallery S, Van Dam J. Interventional endoscopic ultrasonography. J Clin Gastroenterol 29:297, 1999.

Mandel JS, Bond JH, Church TR, et al. Reducing mortality from colorectal cancer by screening for fecal occult blood. N Engl J Med 328:1365–1371, 1993.

Marshall BJ, Warren JR. Unidentified curved bacilli in the stomach of patients with gastritis and peptic ulceration. Lancet 1:1311–1315, 1984.

Martin RCG, Stulc JP. Multifocal granular cell tumor of the biliary tree: case report and review. Gastrointest Endosc 51:238–240, 2000.

Massey BE, Rubin CE. Stomach in pernicious anemia; cytologic study. Am J Med Sci 227:481–492, 1954.

McNeer G. Cytologic interpretation of the gastric aspirate. In McNeer GP, Pack G (eds). Neoplasms of the Stomach. Philadelphia, JB Lippincott, 1967.

McNeer G, Ewing JH. Exfoliated pancreatic cancer cells in duodenal drainage; case report. Cancer 2:643–645, 1949.

Mellemkjaer L, Olsen JH, Frisch M, et al. Cancer in patients with ulcerative colitis. Int J Cancer 60:330–333, 1995.

Melville DM, Richman PI, Shepherd NA, et al. Brush cytology of the colon and rectum in ulcerative colitis: an aid to cancer diagnosis. J Clin Pathol 41:1180–1186, 1988.

Mendoza ML, Martin-Rabadan P, Carrion I, et al. *Helicobacter pylori* infection. Rapid diagnosis with brush cytology. Acta Cytol 37:181–185, 1993.

Menke-Pluymers MB, Hop WC, Dees J, et al. Risk factors for the development of adenocarcinoma in columnar lined (Barrett's) esophagus: the Rotterdam Esophageal Tumor Study Group. Cancer 72:1155–1158, 1993.

Messelt OT. Cytological diagnosis of esophagus cancer. Acta Chir Scand 103:440–444, 1952.

Miettinen M, Sarlomo-Rikala M, Lasota J. Gastrointestinal stromal tumors: recent advances in understanding of their biology. Hum Pathol 30:1213–1220, 1999.

Miettinen M, Sobin LH, Sarlomo-Rikala M. Immunohistochemical spectrum of GISTs at different sites and their differential diagnosis with a reference to CD 117 (KIT). Mod Pathol 13:1134–1142, 2000.

Miller DF, Sikorski JJ, Moritz MM, DeLuca VA. An evaluation of a simplified technique for colonic exfoliative cytology. Acta Cytol 13:53–56, 1969.

Miller MG. The diagnosis of the carcinoma of the stomach its early phase. Arch Fr Mal Dig 61:279–284, 1972.

Mills SE, Cooper PH. Malignant melanoma of digestive system. Pathol Annu 18:1–26, 1983.

Milstoc M. Squamous cell carcinoma of stomach with liver metastasis. NY State J Med 69:2913–2914, 1969.

Minwalla SP, Parry WR. A case of primary malignant melanoma of the esophagus. Br J Surg 48:461–462, 1961.

Misra SP, Misra V, Dwivedi M, Singh M. Fine-needle aspiration biopsy of colonic masses. Diagn Cytopathol 19:330–332, 1998.

Mizobuchi S, Sakamoto H, Tachimori Y, et al. Absence of human papillomavirus-16 and -18 DNA, Epstein-Barr virus DNA in esophageal squamous cell carcinoma. Jpn J Clin Oncol 27:1–5, 1997.

Montgomery E, Bronner MP, Goldblum JR, et al. Reproducibility of the diagnosis of dysplasia in Barrett esophagus: A reaffirmation. Hum Pathol 32:368–378, 2001A.

Montgomery E, Goldblum JR, Greenson JK, et al. Dysplasia as a predictive marker for invasive carcinoma in Barrett esophagus: A follow-up study based on 138 cases from a diagnostic variability study. Hum Pathol 32:379–388, 2001B.

Mori M, Matsukuma A, Adachi Y, et al. Small cell carcinoma of the esophagus. Cancer 63:564–573, 1989.

Morson BC. Carcinoma arising from areas of intestinal metaplasia in the gastric mucosa. Br J Cancer 9:377–385, 1955.

Morson BC, Belcher JR. Adenocarcinoma of oesophagus and ectopic gastric mucosa. Br J Cancer 6:127–130, 1952.

Morson BC, Sobin LH, Grundmann E, et al. Precancerous conditions and epithelial dysplasia in the stomach. J Clin Pathol 33:711–721, 1980.

Mossberg SM. The columnar-lined esophagus Barrett's syndrome—an acquired condition? Gastroenterology 50:671–676, 1966.

Mullick SS, Mody DR, Schwartz MR. Cytology of gastrointestinal histoplasmosis. A report of two cases with differential diagnosis and diagnostic pitfalls. Acta Cytol 40:989–994, 1996.

Muro A, Mueller PR, Ferrucci JT Jr, Taft PD. Bile cytology: A routine addition to percutaneous biliary drainage. Radiology 149:846–847, 1983.

Nakajima T, Tajima Y, Sugano I, et al. Multivariate statistical analysis of bile cytology. Acta Cytol 38:51–55, 1994.

Nieburgs HE, Dreiling MD, Rubio C, Reisman H. The morphology of cells in duodenal-drainage smears: histologic origin and pathologic significance. Am J Dig Dis 7:489–505, 1967.

Nieburgs HE, Glass GBJ. Gastric-cell maturation disorders in atrophic gastritis, pernicious anemia, and carcinoma. Histologic site of origin and diagnostic significance of abnormal cells. Am J Dig Dis 8:135–159, 1963.

Nilsson B, Wee A, Yap I. Bile cytology: Diagnostic role in the management of biliary obstruction. Acta Cytol 39:746–752, 1995.

Nishimura A, Den N, Sato H, Takeda B. Exfoliative cytology of the biliary tract with the use of saline irrigation under choledochoscopic control. Ann Surg 178:594–599, 1973.

Nobukawa B, Abraham SC, Gill J, et al. Clinicopathologic and molecular analysis of high-grade dysplasia and early adenocarcinoma in short- versus long-segment Barrett esophagus. Hum Pathol 32:447–454, 2001.

O'Morchoe PJ, Lee DC, Kozak CA. Esophageal cytology in patients receiving cytotoxic drug therapy. Acta Cytol 27:630–634, 1983.

Odze RD, Brown CA, Hartmann CJ, et al. Genetic alterations in chronic ulcerative colitis-associated adenoma-like DALMs are similar to non-colitic sporadic adenomas. Am J Surg Pathol 24:1209–1216, 2000.

Offerhaus GJA, Stadt J, Huibregtse K, Tytgat GJ. Endoscopic screening for malignancy in the gastric remnant: the clinical significance of dyplasia in gastric mucosa. J Clin Pathol 37:748–754, 1984.

Ojeda VJ, Shilkin KB, Walters MN. Premalignant epithelial lesions of the gall bladder: A prospective study of 120 cholecystectomy specimens. Pathology 17:451–454, 1985.

Okamura T, Korenaga D, Saito A, et al. Reactive changes in the esophageal epithelium a predictability of survival for patients with adenocarcinoma of the upper third of the stomach. Cancer 63:769–773, 1989.

Orell SR, Ohlsen P. Normal and post-pancreatic cytologic patterns of the duodenal juice. Acta Cytol 16:165–171, 1972.

Osnes M, Serck-Hanssen A, Myren J. Endoscopic retrograde brush cytology (ERBC) of the biliary and pancreatic ducts. Scand J Gastroenterol 10:829–831, 1975.

Palmer ED. The Esophagus and Its Diseases. New York, Paul B. Hoeber, 1952.

Panico FG. Cytologic patterns in benign and malignant gastric and esophageal lesions. Surg Gynecol Obstet 94:733–742, 1952.

Panico FG, Papanicolaou GN, Cooper WA. Abrasive balloon for exfoliation of gastric cells. JAMA 143:1308–1311, 1950.

Papillo JL, Leslie KO, Dean RA. Cytologic diagnosis of liver fluke infestation in a patient with subsequently documented cholangiocarcinoma. Acta Cytol 33:865–869, 1989.

Park IA, Kim JS, Ham EK. Fine needle aspiration cytology of gastric epithelioid leiomyosarcoma metastasized to the liver: A case report. Acta Cytol 41:1801–1806, 1997.

Parsonnet J, Friedman GD, Vandersteen DP, et al. *Helicobacter pylori* infection and risk of gastric carcinoma. N Engl J Med 325:1127–1131, 1991.

Parsonnet J, Hansen S, Rodriguez L, et al. *Helicobacter pylori* infection and gastric lymphoma. N Engl J Med 330:1267–1271, 1994.

Petrelli M, Tetangco E, Reid JD. Carcinoma of the colon with undifferentiated, carcinoid, and squamous cell features. Am J Clin Pathol 75:581–584, 1981.

Piccone VA, Klopstock R, LeVeen NH, Sika JP. Primary malignant melanoma of the esophagus associated with melanosis of the entire esophagus. J Thorac Cardiovasc Surg 59:864–870, 1970.

Pilotti S, Rilke F, Clemente C, et al. The cytologic diagnosis of gastric carcinoma related to the histologic type. Acta Cytol 21:48–59, 1977.

Pinto MM, Meriano FV, Afridi S, Taubin HL. Cytodiagnosis of Campylobacter pylori in Papanicolaou-stained imprints of gastric biopsy specimens. Acta Cytol 35:204–206, 1991.

Podolsky DK. Inflammatory bowel disease. N Engl J Med 347:417–429, 2002.

Politoske EJ. Squamous papilloma of the esophagus associated with the human papillomavirus. Gastroenterology 102:668–673, 1992.

Polkowski W, van Lanschot JJ, Ten Kate FJ, et al. The value of p53 and Ki67 as markers for tumour progression in the Barrett's dysplasia-carcinoma sequence. Surg Oncol 4:163–171, 1995.

Pomeranz AA, Garlock JH. Postoperative recurrences of cancer of the colon due to desquamated malignant cells. JAMA 158:1434–1436, 1955.

Porter JM, Kalloo AN, Abernathy EC, Yeo CJ. Carcinoid tumor of the gallbladder: laparoscopic resection and review of the literature. Surgery 112:100–105, 1992.

Portner WJ, Koolpe HA. New devices for biliary drainage and biopsy. AJR Am J Roentgenol 138:1191–1195, 1982.

Pour P, Ghadirian P. Familial cancer of the esophagus in Iran. Cancer 33:1649–1652, 1974.

Pretlow TP, Barrow BJ, Ashton WS, et al. Aberrant crypts: putative preneoplastic foci in human colonic mucosa. Cancer Res 51:564–567, 1991.

Pretlow TP, Brasitus TA, Fulton NC, et al. K-ras mutations in putative preneoplastic lesions in human colon. J Natl Cancer Inst 85:2004–2007, 1993.

Price AB. The Sydney System: Histological division. J Gastroenterol Hepatol 6:209–222, 1991.

Prolla JC, Kirsner JB. Handbook and Atlas of Gastrointestinal Exfoliative Cytology. Chicago, University of Chicago Press, 1972.

Prolla JC, Kobayashi S, Kirsner JB. Gastric cancer, some recent improvements in diagnosis based upon the Japanese experience. Arch Intern Med 124:238–246, 1969.

Prolla JC, Kobayashi S, Kirsner JB. Cytology of malignant lymphomas of the stomach. Acta Cytol 14:291–296, 1970.

Prolla JC, Kobayashi S, Yoshi Y, et al. Diagnostic cytology of the stomach in gastric syphilis. Report of two cases. Acta Cytol 14:333–337, 1970.

Prolla JC, Reilly RW, Kirsner JB, Cockerham L. Direct-vision endoscopic cytology and biopsy in the diagnosis of esophageal and gastric tumors: current experience. Acta Cytol 21:399–402, 1977.

Prolla JC, Xavier RG, Kirsner JB. Morphology of exfoliated cells in benign gastric ulcer. Acta Cytol 15:128–132, 1971.

Prolla JC, Xavier RG, Kirsner JB. Exfoliative cytology in gastric ulcer. Its role in differentiation of benign and malignant ulcers. Gastroenterology 63:33–37, 1972.

Prolla JC, Yoshi Y, Xavier RG, Kirsner JB. Further experience with direct vision brushing cytology of malignant tumors of upper gastrointestinal tract: Histopathologic correlation with biopsy. Acta Cytol 15:375–378, 1971.

Qin D, Zhou B. Elastic plastic tube for detecting exfoliative cancer cells in the esophagus. Acta Cytol 36:82–86, 1992.

Qizilbash AH. Duodenal and peri-ampullary adenomas. Curr Top Pathol 81:77–90, 1990.

Qizilbash AJ, Castelli M, Kowalski MA, Churly A. Endoscopic brush cytology and biopsy in the diagnosis cancer of the upper gastrointestinal tract. Acta Cytol 24:313–318, 1980.

Rabinovitz M, Zajko AB, Hassanein T, et al. Diagnostic value of brush cytology in the diagnosis of bile duct carcinoma: a study in 65 patients with bile duct strictures. Hepatology 12:747–752, 1990.

Raskin HF, Kirsner JB, Palmer WL. Role of exfoliative cytology in the diagnosis of cancer of the digestive JAMA 169:789–791, 1959.

Raskin HF, Kirsner JB, Palmer WL, et al. Gastrointestinal cancer; definitive diagnosis by exfoliative cytology. Arch Surg 76:507–516, 1958.

Raskin HF, Moseley RD Jr, Palmer WL. Carcinoma of the pancreas, biliary tract and liver. CA Cancer J Clin 11:137–148, 166–181, 1961.

Raskin HF, Palmer WL, Kirsner JB. Exfoliative cytology in diagnosis of cancer of the colon. Dis Colon Rectum 2:46–57, 1959.

Raskin HF, Palmer WL, Kirsner JB. Benign and malignant exfoliated gastrointestinal mucosal cells. Arch Intern Med 107:872–884, 1961.

Raskin HF, Pleticka S. Exfoliative cytology of the colon: Fifteen years of lost opportunity. Cancer 28:127–130, 1971.

Raskin HF, Pleticka S. The cytologic diagnosis cancer of the colon. Acta Cytol 8:131–140, 1964.

Raskin HF, Wenger J, Sklar M, et al. Diagnosis of cancer of pancreas, biliary tract, and duodenum by combined cytologic and secretory methods. I. Exfoliative cytology and description of rapid method of duodenal intubation. Gastroenterology 34:996–1008, 1958.

Reece MF, Boon TH, Schade ROK. Exfoliative gastric cytology. Its evaluation in the diagnosis of carcinoma of the stomach. Lancet 2:1163–1164, 1961.

Reed PI, Raskin HF, Graff PW. Malignant melanoma of the stomach. JAMA 182:298–299, 1962.

Reid HAS, Richardson WW, Corrin B. Oat cell carcinoma of the esophagus. Cancer 45:2342–2347, 1980.

Relman DA, Schmidt TM, MacDermott RP, Falkow S. Identification of the uncultured bacillus of Whipple's disease. N Engl J Med 327:293–301, 1992.

Rex DK, Rahmani EY, Haseman JH, et al. Relative sensitivity of colonoscopy and barium enema for detection of colorectal cancer in clinical practice. Gastroenterology 112:17–23, 1997.

Reyes CV, Jao W, Gould VE. Neuroendocrine carcinomas of the esophagus. Ultrastruct Pathol 1:367–376, 1980.

Riberi A, Battersby JS, Vellios F. Epidermoid carcinoma occurring in pharyngoesophageal diverticulum. Cancer 8:727–730, 1955.

Richardson HL, Queen FB, Bishop FH. Cytohistologic diagnosis of material aspirated from stomach; accuracy of diagnosis of cancer, ulcer and gastritis from paraffin-embedded washings. Am J Clin Pathol 19:328–340, 1949.

Robey SS, Hamilton SR, Gupta PK, Erozan YS. Diagnostic value of cytopathology in Barrett esophagus associated carcinoma. Am J Clin Pathol 89:493, 1988.

Rosen CB, Nagorney DM, Wiesner RH, et al. Cholangiocarcinoma complicating primary sclerosing cholangitis. Ann Surg 213:21–25, 1991.

Rosen RG, Garret M, Aka E. Cytologic diagnosis of pancreatic cancer by ductal aspiration. Ann Surg 167:427–432, 1968.

Rosen Y, Moon S, Kim B. Small cell epidermoid carcinoma of the esophagus. An oat-cell-like carcinoma. Cancer 36:1042–1049, 1975.

Rosenberg J, Welch JP, Pyrtek LJ, et al. Benign villous adenomas of the ampulla of Vater. Cancer 58:1563–1568, 1986.

Rosman AS, Federman Q, Feinman L. Diagnosis of colon cancer by lavage cytology with an orally administered balanced electrolyte solution. Am J Gastroenterol 89:51–56, 1994.

Rotterdam H, Sheahan DG, Sommers SC. Biopsy Diagnosis of the Digestive Tract. Raven Press, New York, 1993.

Rozen P, Tobi M, Darmon E, Kaufman L. Exfoliative colonic cytology: A simplified method of collection and initial results. Acta Cytol 34:627–631, 1990.

Rubin CE, Bendit EP. Simplified technique using chymotrypsin lavage for cytological diagnosis of gastric cancer. Cancer 8:1137–1141, 1955.

Rubin CE, Massey BW. Preoperative diagnosis of gastric and duodenal lymphoma by exfoliative cytology. Cancer 7:271–288, 1954.

Rubin CE, Massey BE, Kirsner JB, et al. Clinical value of gastric cytologic diagnosis. Gastroenterology 25:119–138, 1953.

Rubin CE, Nelson JF. Exfoliative cytology as aid in differential diagnosis of gastric lesions discovered roentgenologically. Am J Roentgenol Radium Ther Nucl Med 77:9–24, 1957.

Rubin P. Cancer of the gastrointestinal tract. D. Gastric cancer. JAMA 228:1283–1294, 1974.

Rubin P, Wynder E, Mabuchi K, et al. Cancer of the gastrointestinal tract. I. Esophagus: detection and diagnosis. JAMA 226:1544–1588, 1973.

Rubio CA, Aberg B. Ciliated tumor cells in an adenocarcinoma arising in Barrett's esophagus. A case report. APMIS 97:661–663, 1989.

Rubio CA, Aberg B, Stemmermann G. Ciliated cells in papillary adenocarcinomas of Barrett's esophagus. Acta Cytol 36:65–68, 1992.

Rubio CA, Antonioli D. Ciliated metaplasia in the gastric mucosa in an American patient. Am J Surg Pathol 12:786–789, 1988.

Rubio CA, Auer GU, Kato Y, Liu FS. DNA profiles in dysplasia and carcinoma of the human esophagus. Anal Quant Cytol Histol 3:207–210, 1988.

Rubio CA, Hirota T, Itabashi T. Atypical mitoses in elevated dysplasias of the stomach. Pathol Res Pract 180:372–376, 1985.

Rubio CA, Kato Y, Sugano H, Kitagawa T. Intestinal metaplasia of the stomach in Swedish and Japanese patients without ulcers or carcinoma. Jpn J Cancer Res 78:467–472, 1987.

Rubio CA, Riddell R. Musculo-fibrous anomaly in Barrett's mucosa with dysplasia. Am J Surg Pathol 12:889, 1988.

Rubio CA, Riddell RH. Atypical mitoses in dysplasias of the Barrett's mucosa. Pathol Res Pract 184:1–5, 1989.

Rupp M, Hawthorne CM, Ehya H. Brushing cytology in biliary tract obstruction. Acta Cytol 34:221–226, 1990.

Rusch VW, Levine DS, Haggitt R, et al. The management of high grade dysplasia and early cancer in Barrett's esophagus: a multidisciplinary problem. Cancer 74:1225–1229, 1994.

Ryan ME, Baldauf MC. Comparison of flow cytometry for DNA content and brush cytology for detection of malignancy in pancreaticobiliary strictures. Gastrointest Endosc 40:133–139, 1994.

Saburi R, Ando T, Kakihana M, Tabayashi A, Yamada T. Selective proteolytic lavage method for cytodiagnosis of early gastric cancer. Acta Cytol 11:473–476, 1967.

Sandler RS, Halabi S, Baron JA, et al. A randomized trial of aspirin to prevent colorectal adenomas in patients with previous colorectal cancer. N Engl J Med 348:883–890, 2003.

Sandmeier D, Mihaescu A. Cytodiagnosis of bile microspheroliths: A case report. Diagn Cytopathol 24:247–248, 2001.

Sapi Z, Papp I, Bodo M. Malignant fibrous histiocytoma of the esophagus. Report of a case with cytologic, immunohistologic and ultrastructural studies. Acta Cytol 36:121–125, 1992.

Sarlomo-Rikala M, Kovatich AJ, Barusevicius A, Miettinen M. CD117: a sensitive marker for gastrointestinal stromal tumors that is more specific than CD34. Mod Pathol 11:728–734, 1998.

Sasaki K, Tajiri Y, Sata M, et al. Helicobacter pylori in the natural environment. Scand J Infect Dis 31:275–279, 1999.

Savage DG, Antman KH. Imatinib mesylate—a new oral targeted therapy. N Engl J Med 346:683–693, 2002.

Sawada Y, Gonda H, Hayashida Y. Combined use of brushing cytology and endoscopic retrograde pancreatography for the early detection of pancreatic cancer. Acta Cytol 33:870–874, 1989.

Schade ROK. Cytological diagnosis of gastric carcinoma. Gastroenterologia 85:190–194, 1956A.

Schade ROK. Zytologische Diagnose des Magenkarzinomas. Mit 2 Abbildungen. Ver Dtsch Ges Pathol 39:292–294, 1956B.

Schade ROK. Critical review of gastric cytology. Acta Cytol 3:7–14, 1959.

Schade ROK. Chronic gastritis: A precancerous condition. Acta Unio Int Contra Cancrum 16:1402–1406, 1960A.

Schade ROK. Gastric Cytology: Principles, Methods, and Results. London, Edward Arnold, 1960B.

Schade ROK. Neuere Untersuchungen uber das Magenkarzinom. Dtsch Med Wochenschr 88:1125–1128, 1963.

Scharschmidt BF. The natural history of hypertrophic gastropathy (Ménétrier's disease): report of a case with 16-year follow-up and review of 120 cases from the literature. Am J Med 63:644–652, 1977.

Schindler R. Gastritis. London, UK, Heinemann, 1947.

Scotiniotis I, Lewis JD, Strom BL. Screening for colorectal cancer and other GI cancers. Curr Opin Oncol 11:305–311, 1999.

Scudera PL, Koizumi J, Jacobson IM. Brush cytology evaluation of lesions encountered during ERCP. Gastrointest Endosc 36:281–284, 1990.

Scully RE, Mark EJ, McNelly WF, McNeely BU. Weekly clinicopathological exercises. N Engl J Med 323:100–109, 1988.

Scully RE, Mark EJ, McNeely WF, McNeely BU. Case Records of the Massachusetts General Hospital. Case 13–1995. N Engl J Med 332:1153–1159, 1995.

Selvaggi SM. Polypoid carcinoma of the esophagus on brush cytology (Letter). Acta Cytol 36: 650–651, 1992.

Sepehr A, Razavi P, Saidi F, et al. Esophageal exfoliative cytology samplers. A comparison of three types. Acta Cytol 44:797–804, 2000.

Seybolt JF, Papanicolaou GN. Balloon technique in detection of gastric carcinoma. In Proceedings of the Second National Cancer Conference, New York, American Cancer Society, 1954, pp 1205–1210.

Seybolt JF, Papanicolaou GN. Value of cytology in diagnosis of gastric cancer. Gastroenterology 33:369–377, 1957.

Shah R, Sabanathan S, Okereke CD, Majid MR. Rhabdomyosarcoma of the oesophagus. A case report. J Cardiovasc Surg (Torino) 36:99–100, 1995.

Shaheen N, Ransohoff DF. Gastroesophageal reflux, Barrett esophagus, and esophageal cancer. Scientific review. JAMA 287:1972–1986, 2002.

Sharkey FE, Clark RL, Gray GF. Perianal Paget's disease: report of 2 cases. Dis Colon Rectum 18:245–248, 1975.

Sherman ME, Anderson C, Herman LM, et al. Utility of gastric brushing in the diagnosis of malignant lymphoma. Acta Cytol 38:169–174, 1994.

Shida S. Biopsy smear cytology with the fibergastroscope for direct observation. In Early Gastric Cancer. Gann Monograph 11, Tokyo, University of Tokyo Press, 1971.

Shida S, Koike I, Kotaka H. The differential diagnosis of gastric tumors by roentgenological, gastroendoscopical, and cytological examinations. In Proceeding, First Congress International Society Endoscopy, Tokyo, Hitachi, 1966, pp 577–585.

Shidham VB, Weiss JP, Quinn TJ, Grotkowski CE. Fine needle aspiration cytology of gastric solitary fibrous tumor: a case report. Acta Cytol 42:1159–1166, 1998.

Shin HJ, Lahoti S, Sneige N. Endoscopic ultrasound-guided fine-needle aspiration in 179 cases: the MD Anderson Cancer Center experience. Cancer 96: 174–180, 2002.

Shinya H. Colonoscopy: Diagnosis and Treatment of Colonic Diseases. New York, Igaku-Shoin, 1982.

Shu Y-J. Cytopathology of the esophagus. An overview of esophageal cytopathology in China. Acta Cytol 27:7–16, 1983.

Shu Y-J. Detection of esophageal carcinoma by the balloon technique in the People's Republic of China. In Koss LG, Coleman DV (eds). Advances in Clinical Cytology, Vol. 2. New York, Masson Publishing, 1984, pp 67–102.

Shu Y-J. Cytopathology of Esophageal Cancer. New York, Masson Publishing, 1985.

Shukla S, Krishnani N, Jain M, Pandey R, Gupta RK. Xanthogranulomatous cholecystitis. Fine needle aspiration cytology in 17 cases. Acta Cytol 41: 413–418, 1997.

Shurbaji MS, Erozan YS. The cytopathologic diagnosis of esophageal adenocarcinoma. Acta Cytol 35:189–194, 1991.

Silverman JF, Baird DB, Teot LA, et al. Fine-needle aspiration cytology of metastatic small cell carcinoma of the colon: a report of three cases. Diagn Cytopathol 15:54–59, 1996.

Simsir A, Greenebaum E, Stevens PD, Abedi M. Biliary stent replacement cytology. Diagn Cytopathol 16:233–237, 1997.

Singh PN, Fraser GE. Dietary risk factors for colon cancer in a low-risk population. Am J Epidemiol 148:761–774, 1998.

Sipponen P, Hyvarinen H, Seppala K, Blaser MJ. Review article: Pathogenesis of the transformation from gastritis to malignancy. Aliment Pharmacol Ther 12:61–71, 1998.

Skinner DB, Walther BC, Riddell RH, et al. Barrett's esophagus: Comparison of benign and malignant cases. Ann Surg 198:554–565, 1983.

Smith RRL, Hamilton SR, Boitnott JK, Rogers EL. The spectrum of carcinoma arising in Barrett's esophagus. Am J Surg Pathol 8:563–573, 1984.

Smith-Fourshee JH, Kalnins ZA, Dixon FR, et al. Gastric cytology: evaluation of methods and results in 1,670 cases. Acta Cytol 13:399–406, 1969.

Smithies A, Hatfield AR, Brown BE. The cytodiagnostic aspects of pure pancreatic juice obtained at the time of endoscopic retrograde cholangio-pancreatography (E.R.C.P.). Acta Cytol 21:191–195, 1977.

Smits HL, Tjong-A-Hung SP, ter Schegget J, et al. Absence of human papillomavirus DNA from esophageal carcinoma as determined by multiple broad spectrum polymerase chain reactions. J Med Virol 46:213–215, 1995.

Soni RR, Dhamne BK. Rapid detection of rectal cancer by gloved digital-scrape cytology. Acta Cytol 35:210–214, 1991.

Souquet JC, Berger F, Bonvoisin S, et al. Esophageal squamous cell carcinoma associated with gastric adenocarcinoma. Cancer 63:786–790, 1989.

Spechler SJ. Barrett's esophagus. N Engl J Med 346:836–842, 2002.

Spechler SJ, Goyal RK. Barrett's Esophagus: Pathophysiology, Diagnosis, and Management. New York, Elsevier, 1985.

Spechler SJ, Goyal RK. Barrett's esophagus. N Engl J Med 315:362–371, 1986.

Spjut HJ, Margulis AR, Cook GB. The silicone-foam enema: a source for exfoliative cytological specimens. Acta Cytol 7:79–84, 1963.

Stanley MW. Endoscopic ultrasound-guided fine-needle aspiration. Am J Clin Pathol 120:309–310, 2003.

Steiner PE. Etiology and histogenesis of carcinoma of esophagus. Cancer 9: 436–452, 1956.

Stelow EB, Stanley MW, Mallery S, et al. Endoscopic ultrasound-guided fine needle aspiration of gastrointestinal leiomyomas and gastrointestinal stromal tumors. Am J Clin Pathol 119:703–708, 2003.

Stemmermann GN, Hayashi T. Intestinal metaplasia of the gastric mucosa: A gross and microscopic study of its distribution in various disease states. J Natl Cancer Inst 41:627–634, 1968.

Stewart CJ, Burke GM. Value of p53 immunostaining in pancreatico-biliary brush cytology specimens. Diagn Cytopathol 23:308–313, 2000.

Stockeld D, Ingelman-Sundberg H, Granstrom L, et al. Serial fine needle cytology in the diagnosis of esophageal cancer. Acta Cytol 46:527–534, 2002.

Stout AP. Tumors of the Stomach. Atlas of Tumor Pathology, Sect 6, Fascicle 21. Washington DC, Armed Forces Institute of Pathology, 1953.

Stout AP, Lattes R. Tumors of the Esophagus. Atlas of Tumor Pathology, Sect 5, Fascicle 20. Washington DC, Armed Forces Institute of Pathology, 1957.

Strack PR, Newman HK, Lerner AC, et al. Integrated procedure for the rapid diagnosis of biliary obstruction, portal hypertension and liver disease of uncertain etiology. N Engl J Med 285:1225–1231, 1971.

Strauman A, Sichtin HP, Bucher KA, et al. Eosinophilic esophagitis: red on microscopy, white on endoscopy. Digestion 70:109–116, 2004.

Suckow EE, Yokoo H, Brock DR. Intraepithelial carcinoma concomitant with esophageal carcinoma. Cancer 15:733–740, 1962.

Suerbaum S, Michetti P. Helicobacter pylori infection. N Engl J Med 347: 1175–1186, 2002.

Sugimachi K, Sumiyoshi K, Nozoe T, et al. Carcinogenesis and histogenesis of esophageal carcinoma. Cancer 75:1440–1445, 1995.

Suster S, Fletcher CDM. Gastrointestinal stromal tumors with prominent signet-ring cell features. Mod Pathol 9:609–613, 1996.

Suzuki M, Takahashi T, Ouchi K, Matsuno S. The development and extension of hepatohilar bile duct carcinoma. A three-dimensional tumor mapping in the intrahepatic biliary tree visualized with the aid of a graphics computer system. Cancer 64:658–666, 1989.

Sweeney JF, Muus C, McKeown PP, Rosemurgy AS. Gastric pseudolymphoma: not necessarily a benign lesion. Dig Dis Sci 37:939–945, 1992.

Syrjanen KJ. Human papillomavirus (HPV) infections and their associations with squamous cell neoplasia. Arch Geschwulstforsch 57:417–444, 1987.

Syrjanen KJ, Pyrhonen S, Aukee S, Koskela E. Squamous cell papilloma of the esophagus: a tumour probably caused by human papilloma virus (HPV). Diagn Histopathol 5:291–296, 1982.

Takahashi A, Ogoshi S, Ono H, et al. High-risk human papillomavirus infection and overexpression of p53 protein in squamous cell carcinoma of the esophagus from Japan. Dis Esophagus 11:162–167, 1998.

Takanishi DM, Hart J, Covareli P, et al. Ploidy as a prognostic feature in colonic adenocarcinoma. Arch Surg 131:587–592, 1996.

Takayama T, Katsuki S, Takahashi Y, et al. Aberrrant crypt foci of the colon as precursors of adenoma and cancer. N Engl J Med 339:1277–1284, 1998.

Takeda M. Atlas of Diagnostic Gastrointestinal Cytology. New York, Igaku-Shoin, 1983.

Takeda M. Gastric cytology: Recent developments. In Koss LG, Coleman DV (eds). Advances in Clinical Cytology, Vol 2. New York, Masson Publishing, 1984, pp 49–65.

Takeda M, Gomi K, Lewis PL, et al. Two histologic types of early gastric carcinoma and their cytologic presentation. Acta Cytol 25:229–236, 1981.

Takeda T, Takaso K, Isono S, et al. Cytologic studies on so-called atypical epithelium of the protuberant lesions in the stomach. Acta Cytol 19: 345–350, 1975.

Takolander RJ. Villous papilloma of the colon and rectum. Part I. A clinical study of 213 patients. Ann Chir Gynaecol 64:257–264, 1975.

Tavani A, Negri E, Franceschi S, et al. Risk factors for esophageal cancer in Linxian, People's Republic of China. Cancer Causes Control 3:387–392, 1994.

Taylor DE, Hargreaves JA, Ng L-K, et al. Isolation and characterization of Campylobacter pyloridis from gastric biopsies. Am J Clin Pathol 87:49–54, 1987.

te Boekhorst DS, Gerhards MF, van Gulik TM, Gouma DJ. Granular cell tumor at the hepatic duct confluence mimicking Klatskin tumor. A report of two cases and a review of the literature. Dig Surg 17:299–303, 2000.

Teot LA, Ducatman BS, Geisinger KR. Cytologic diagnosis of cytomegaloviral esophagitis. A report of three acquired immunodeficiency syndrome-related cases. Acta Cytol 37:93–96, 1993.

Thabet RJ, Knoernschild HE, Hausner JL. Millipore filtration technique for colon washings. Cytol Newsletter 2:2–3, 1960.

Thabet RJ, Macfarlane EWE. Cytological field patterns and nuclear morphology in the diagnosis of colon pathology. Acta Cytol 6:325–331, 1962.

Thomas W, White CM, Mah J, et al. Longitudinal compliance with annual screening for fecal occult blood. Minnesota Colon Cancer Control Study. Am J Epidemiol 142:176–182, 1995.

Thorbjarnarson B, Beal JM, Pearce JM. Primary malignant lymphoid tumors of stomach. Cancer 9:712–717, 1956.

Thun MJ, Namboodiri MN, Health CW Jr. Aspirin use and reduced risk of fatal colon cancer. N Engl J Med 325:1593–1596, 1991.

Thung SN, Garber MA. Liver. *In* Sternberg S (ed). Histology for Pathologists. New York, Raven Press, 1991.

Togawa K, Rustagi AK. Human papillomavirus 16 and 18 replication in esophagus squamous cancer cell lines does not require heterologous E1 and E2 proteins. J Med Virol 45:435–438, 1995.

Toh BH, van Driel IR, Gleeson PA. Pernicious anemia. N Engl J Med 337:1411–1488, 1997.

Torres C, Antonioli D, Odze RD. Polypoid dysplasia and adenomas in inflammatory bowel disease: a clinical, pathologic, and follow-up study of 89 polyps from 59 patients. Am J Surg Pathol 22:275–284, 1998.

Traverso G, Shuber A, Levin B, et al. Detection of APC mutations in fecal DNA from patients with colorectal tumors. N Engl J Med 346:311–320, 2002.

Trent V, Khurana KK, Pisharodi LR. Diagnostic accuracy and clinical utility of endoscopic bile duct brushing in the evaluation of biliary strictures. Arch Pathol Lab. Med 123:712–715, 1999.

Trillo AA, Accettullo LM, Yeiter TL. Choriocarcinoma of the esophagus. Histologic and cytologic findings: A case report. Acta Cytol 23:69–74, 1979.

Trupiano JK, Stewart RE, Misick C, et al. Gastric stromal tumors. A clinicopathologic study of 77 cases with correlation of features with nonaggressive and aggressive clinical behaviors. Am J Surg Pathol 26:705–714, 2002.

Turnbull ADM, Goodner JT. Primary adenocarcinoma of the esophagus. Cancer 22:915–918, 1968.

Turner JR, Shen LH, Crum CP, et al. Low prevalence of human papillomavirus infection in esophageal squamous cell carcinomas from North America: analysis by a highly sensitive and specific polymerase chain reaction-based approach. Hum Pathol 28:174–178, 1997.

Uehara H, Nakaizumi A, Iishi H et al. Cytologic examination of pancreatic juice for differential diagnosis of benign and malignant mucin-producing tumors of the pancreas. Cancer 74:826–833, 1994.

Uei Y, Koketsu H, Konda C, Kimura K. Cytodiagnosis of hCG-secreting choriocarcinoma of the stomach. Report of a case. Acta Cytol 17:431–434, 1973.

Uemura N, Okamoto S, Yamamoto S, et al. *Helicobacter pylori* infection and the development of gastric cancer. N Engl J Med 345:784–789, 2001.

Umiker WO, Bolt RJ, Hoekzema AD, Pollard HM. Cytology in diagnosis of gastric cancer, significance of location and pathologic type. Gastroenterology 34:859–866, 1958.

Uras C, Altinkaya E, Yardimci H, et al. Peritoneal cytology in the determination of free tumour cells within the abdomen in colon cancer. Surg Oncol 5:259–263, 1996.

Ushigome S, Spjut HJ, Noon GP. Extensive dysplasia and carcinoma in situ of esophageal epithelium. Cancer 20:1023–1029, 1967.

Vadmal MS, Byrne-Semmelmeier S, et al. Biliary tract brush cytology. Acta Cytol 44:533–538, 2000.

Vallilengua C, Rodriguez Otero JC, et al. Imprint cytology of the gallbladder mucosa. Its use in diagnosing macroscopically inapparent carcinoma. Acta Cytol 39:19–22, 1995.

Van Dam J, Brugge WR. Endoscopy of the upper gastrointestincal tract. N Engl J Med 341:1738–1748, 1999.

van der Heide H, Lantink JA, Wiltink E, Tytgat GNJ. Comparison of whole-gut irrigation with (GoLYTELY) and with a balanced electrolyte solution (BES) as a preparation for colonoscopy. Endoscopy 18:182–184, 1986.

Veen VDAH, Dees J, Blankenstein JD, Blankenstein VM. Adenocarcinoma in Barrett's oesophagus: an overrated risk. Gut 30:14–18, 1989.

Venu RP, Geenen JE, Kini M et al. Endoscopic retrograde brush cytology. A new technique. Gastroenterology 99:1475–1479, 1990.

Veronezi-Gurwell A, Wittchow RJ, Bottles K, Cohen MB. Cytologic features of villous adenoma of the ampullary region. Diagn Cytopathol 14:145–149, 1996.

Waken JK, Bullock WK. Primary melanocarcinoma of the esophagus. Am J Clin Pathol 38:415–421, 1962.

Walker AN, Feldman PS, Covell JL, Tegtmeyer C. Fine needle aspiration under percutaneous transhepatic cholangiographic guidance. Acta Cytol 26:767–771, 1982.

Wang HH, Doria MI Jr, Purohit-Buch S, et al. Barrett's esophagus. The cytology of dysplasia in comparison to benign and malignant lesions. Acta Cytol 36:60–64, 1992.

Wang LS, Chow KC, Wu YC, et al. Detection of Epstein-Barr virus in esophageal squamous cell carcinoma in Taiwan. Am J Gastroenterol 94:2834–2839, 1999.

Warshaw AL, Fernandez-del Castillo C. Pancreatic carcinoma. N Engl J Med 326: 455–465, 1992.

Wasastjerna C, Ekelung P. The amino acid napthylamidase reaction of the bile canaliculi in liver smears. Acta Cytol 18:23–29, 1974.

Wasastjerna C, Ekelung P, Haltia K. The bile canaliculi in cytological aspiration biopsy from patients with liver disorders. Scand J Gastroenterol 5:327–331, 1970.

Wasastjerna C, Thoden CJ, Ekelund P, Haltia K. The bile canaliculi in cytological aspiration biopsies from patients with liver disorders. Scand J Gastroenterol 5:327–331, 1970.

Wee A, Nilsson B, Wang TL, Yap I, Siew PY. Tuberculous pseudotumor causing biliary obstruction. Report of a case with diagnosis by fine needle aspiration biopsy and bile cytology. Acta Cytol 39:559–562, 1995.

Weiden PL, Schuffler MD. Herpes esophagitis complicating Hodgkin's disease. Cancer 33:1100–1102, 1974.

Weingrad DN, DeCosse JJ, Sherlock P, et al. Primary gastrointestinal lymphoma. A 30-year review. Cancer 49:1258–1265, 1982.

Wenger J, Raskin HF. Diagnosis of cancer of pancreas, biliary tract, and duodenum by combined cytologic and secretory methods. II. Secretion test. Gastroenterology 34:1009–1017, 1958.

Werner M, Becker KF, Keller G, Hofler H. Gastric adenocarcinoma: pathomorphology and molecular pathology. J Cancer Res Clin Oncol 127:207–216, 2001.

Wersto RP, Liblit RL, Deitch D, Koss LG. Variability in DNA measurements in multiple tumor samples of human colonic carcinoma. Cancer 67:106–115, 1991.

Wertlake PT, Del Guercio LR. Cytopathology of intra-hepatic bile as component of integrated procedure ("minilap") for hepatobiliary disorders. Acta Cytol 20:42–45, 1976.

Wheeler DA, Chandrasoma P, Carriere CA, Schwinn CP. Cytologic diagnosis of gastric composite adenocarcinoma-carcinoid. Acta Cytol 28:706–708, 1984.

Whipple GH. A hitherto undescribed disease characterized anatomically by deposits of fat and fatty acids in the intestinal mesenteric lymphatic tissues. Bull Johns Hopkins Hosp 18:382–391, 1907.

Willen R, Lillo-Gil R, Willen H, et al. Embryonal rhabdomyosarcoma of the oesophagus. Acta Chir Scand 155:59–64, 1989.

Williams SL, Rogers LW, Quan HQ. Perianal Paget's disease: report of seven cases. Dis Colon Rectum 19:30–40, 1976.

Wilson MS, el Teraifi H, Schofield P. The value of exfoliative cytology in the diagnosis of rectal malignancy. Int. J Colorectal Dis 8:78–80, 1993.

Winawer SJ. Colorectal cancer screening comes of age. N Engl J Med 328:1416–1417, 1993.

Winawer SJ. Natural history of colorectal cancer. Am J Med 106:3S–6S, 1999.

Winawer SJ, Leidner SD, Hajdu SI, Sherlock P. Colonoscopic biopsy and cytology in the diagnosis of colon cancer. Cancer 42:2849–2853, 1978.

Winawer SJ, Sherlock P, Belladona JA, et al. Endoscopic brush cytology in esophageal cancer. JAMA 232:1358, 1975.

Winawer SJ, Zauber AG, Gerdes H, et al. Risk of colorectal cancer in the families of patients with adenomatous polyps. National Polyp Study Workgroup. N Engl J Med 334:82–87, 1996.

Winawer SJ, Zauber AG, Ho MN, et al. Prevention of colorectal cancer by colonoscopic polypectomy. N Engl J Med 329:1977–1981, 1993.

Winkler B, Capo V, Reumann W, et al. Human papillomavirus infection of the esophagus. A clinicopathologic study with demonstration of papillomavirus antigen by the immunoperoxidase technique. Cancer 55:149–155, 1985.

Wisseman CL Jr, Lemon HM, Lawrence KB. Cytologic diagnosis of cancer of descending colon and rectum. Surg Gynecol Obstet 89:24–30, 1949.

Witte S. Intravital fluorescent staining with acridine derivatives in cytodiagnosis of the upper gastrointestinal tract. Acta Cytol 12:15–17, 1968.

Witte S, Langer J. [Endoscopic cytodiagnosis of the pancreas and bile ducts]. Med Klin 86:449–453, 1991.

Wolff WI, Shinya H. Earlier diagnosis of cancer of the colon through colonic endoscopy (colonoscopy). Cancer 34(suppl):912–931, 1974.

Wolley RC, Schreiber K, Koss LG, et al. DNA distribution in human colonic carcinomas and its relationship to clinical behavior. J Natl Cancer Inst 69:15–22, 1982.

Wood GM, Bates C, Brown RC, Losowsky MS. Intramucosal carcinoma of the gastric antrum complicating Ménétrier's disease. J Clin Pathol 6:1071–1075, 1983.

Wu GD. A nuclear receptor to prevent colon cancer. N Engl J Med 342:651–653, 2000.

Yamada T, Murohisa B, Muto Y, et al. Cytologic detection of small pancreatico-duodenal and biliary cancers in the early developmental stage. Acta Cytol 28:435–442, 1984.

Yamada Y, Ninomiya M, Kato T, et al. Human papillomavirus type 16-positive esophageal papilloma at an endoscopic injection sclerotherapy site. Gastroenterology 108:550–553, 1995.

Yamaguchi K, Enjoji M. Carcinoma of the ampulla of Vater: A clinicopathologic study and pathologic staging of 109 cases of carcinoma and 5 cases of adenoma. Cancer 59:506–515, 1987.

Yamazaki H, Oshima A, Murakami R, et al. A long-term follow-up study of patients with gastric cancer detected by mass screening. Cancer 63:613–617, 1989.

Yang CS. Research on esophageal cancer in China: a review. Cancer Res 40:2633–2644, 1980.

Yang H, Berner A, Mei Q, et al. Cytologic screening for esophageal cancer in a high-risk population in Anyang County, China. Acta Cytol 46:445–452, 2002.

Yang M. Detection of amyloid in gastric brushing material. A case report. Acta Cytol 39:255–257, 1995.

Yao T, Kouzuki T, Kajiwara M, et al. "Serrated" adenoma of the colorectum with reference to its gastric differentiation and its malignant potential. J Pathol 187:511–517, 1999.

Yates DR, Koss LG. Paget's disease of the esophageal epithelium. Report of first case. Arch Pathol 86:447–452, 1968.

Yu Y, Taylor PR, Li JY, et al. Retrospective cohort study of risk factors for esophageal cancer in Linxian, People's Republic of China. Cancer Causes Control 4:195–202, 1993.

Zucca E, Bertoni F, Roggero E, et al. Molecular analysis of the progression from *Helicobacter pylori*-associated chronic gastritis to mucosa-associated lymphoid-tissue lymphoma of the stomach. N Engl J Med 338:804–810, 1998.

Index

Pages including f and t denote pages that include figure(s) and table(s).